The Royal Marsden Hospital
Manual of Clinical
Nursing Procedures

The Royal Marsden Hospital Manual of Clinical Nursing Procedures

Eighth Edition

Edited by

Lisa Dougherty
OBE, RN, MSc, DClinP
Nurse Consultant Intravenous Therapy
The Royal Marsden Hospital NHS Foundation Trust

and

Sara Lister
RN, PGDAE, BSc (Hons), MSc, MBACP
Assistant Chief Nurse/Head of School
The Royal Marsden School of
Cancer Nursing & Rehabilitation
The Royal Marsden Hospital NHS Foundation Trust

WILEY-BLACKWELL

A John Wiley & Sons, Ltd., Publication

This edition first published 2011
© 1992, 1996, 2000, 2004, 2008, 2011 The Royal Marsden Hospital

Blackwell Publishing was acquired by John Wiley & Sons in February 2007. Blackwell's publishing programme has been merged with Wiley's global Scientific, Technical, and Medical business to form Wiley-Blackwell.

Registered office
John Wiley & Sons Ltd, The Atrium, Southern Gate, Chichester, West Sussex, PO19 8SQ, UK

Editorial offices
9600 Garsington Road, Oxford, OX4 2DQ, UK
The Atrium, Southern Gate, Chichester, West Sussex, PO19 8SQ, UK
2121 State Avenue, Ames, Iowa 50014-8300, USA

For details of our global editorial offices, for customer services and for information about how to apply for permission to reuse the copyright material in this book please see our website at www.wiley.com/wiley-blackwell.

Library of Congress Cataloging-in-Publication Data

The Royal Marsden Hospital manual of clinical nursing procedures. — 8th ed. / edited by Lisa Dougherty and Sara Lister.
    p. ; cm.
    Manual of clinical nursing procedures
    Includes bibliographical references and index.
    ISBN 978-1-4443-3509-5 (pbk. : alk. paper)
  1. Nursing—Handbooks, manuals, etc. I. Dougherty, Lisa. II. Lister, Sara E. III. Title: Manual of clinical nursing procedures.
    [DNLM: 1. Nursing Care—methods. 2. Nursing Process. 3. Nursing Theory. 4. Patient Care Planning. WY 100.1]
    RT42.R68 2011
    610.73—dc22

                                                                        2010044585

A catalogue record for this book is available from the British Library.

Set in 9.5/11.5 Sabon by Aptara, Inc., New Delhi, India

Printed and bound in Singapore by Ho Printing Singapore Pte Ltd

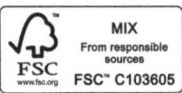

1   2011

Brief table of contents

Detailed table of contents

Chapter 4   Risk management | 129

Part Two   Supporting the patient with human functioning | 153

Chapter 5   Communication | 155

Chapter 6   Elimination   195

Chapter 7   Moving and positioning   279

Chapter 8   Nutrition, fluid balance and blood transfusion   333

Chapter 9   Patient comfort   417

Chapter 10   Respiratory care   533

Part Three   Supporting the patient through the diagnostic process   615

Chapter 11   Interpreting diagnostic tests   617

Chapter 14   Radionuclide investigations and therapy   829

Part Four   Supporting the patient through treatment   867

Chapter 15   Cytotoxic therapy   869

Chapter 16   Medicines management — 933

Chapter 17   Perioperative care   1041

Chapter 18   Vascular access devices: insertion and management   1079

Chapter 19   Wound management   1165

Appendices   1203

List of contributors

Lynn Ansell MPharm, PG Dip Clinical Pharmacy
Formerly Pharmacy Clinical Services Manager
(Chapter 16: Medicines management)

Amanda Baxter RN, RMN, ONC, BSc (Hons), PG Dip
Clinical Nurse Specialist Urology
(Chapter 6: Elimination)

Hannah Brown RN, MN, Dip HE
Formerly Sister
(Chapter 6: Elimination)

Louise Causer RN, ONC, MBA
Clinical Nurse Specialist Nuclear Medicine
(Chapter 14: Radioactive investigations and therapy)

Suzanne Chapman RN, BSc, MSc
Clinical Nurse Specialist Pain Management
(Chapter 9: Patient comfort)

Rebecca Clarke RN, BSc (Hons), MSc
Ward Sister
(Chapter 17: Perioperative care)

Kirsty Cooke CSP, BSc (Hons)
Macmillan Specialist Lymphoedema Therapist
(Chapter 9: Patient comfort)

Jill Cooper Dip COT, MBE, PG Dip, MSc
Lead Occupational Therapist
(Chapter 7: Moving and positioning)

Maria Crisford RN, BSc (Hons), Dip HE
Specialist Sister Colorectal
(Chapter 6: Elimination)

Alison Diffley RN, Advanced Dip, Dip
Clinical Nurse Specialist Counsellor
(Chapter 5: Communication)

Andrew J. Dimech RN, BN, Dip HE, PG Dip, MSc
Intensive Care
Clinical Nurse Specialist Cancer, Critical Care,
    Resuscitation and Outreach
(Chapter 11: Interpreting diagnostic tests)

Shelley Dolan RN, BA (Hons), MSc, PhD
Chief Nurse
(Chapter 4: Risk management)

Pauline Doran-Williams RN, BSc, Dip HE
Specialist Sister Plastic Surgery
(Chapter 19: Wound management)

Lisa Dougherty OBE, RN, MSc, DClinP
Nurse Consultant Intravenous Therapy
(Chapter 11: Interpreting diagnostic tests; Chapter 15:
    Cytotoxic therapy; Chapter 16: Medicines manage-
    ment; Chapter 18: Vascular access devices: insertion and
    management)

Natalie Doyle RN, MSc
Nurse Consultant Rehabilitation
(Chapter 9: Patient comfort)

Steven Edmunds RN, BSc (Hons), Dip HE
Senior Staff Nurse
(Chapter 13: Observations)

Ann Farley RN, BA (Hons)
Specialist Sister Palliative Care
(Chapter 9: Patient comfort)

Andreia Fernandes RN, BSc, PG Dip
Clinical Nurse Specialist Gynaecology-Oncology
(Chapter 6: Elimination; Chapter 9: Patient
    comfort; Chapter 11: Interpreting diagnostic
    tests)

Catherine Forsythe RN, Dip HE, BSc (Hons)
Senior Staff Nurse
(Chapter 11: Interpreting diagnostic tests)

Charlotte Graham RN, BSc
Senior Staff Nurse
(Chapter 13: Observations)

Dimity Grant-Frost RN, BSc
Specialist Sister Palliative Care
(Chapter 2: Assessment, discharge and end of life care)

Jagdesh K. Grewal RN, BA (Hons), PG Dip NE, DMS
Matron
(Chapter 17: Perioperative care)

Oonagh Griffin RD, BSc (Hons)
Dietetic Team Leader
(Chapter 8: Nutrition, fluid balance and blood transfusion)

Diz Hackman Dip Physiotherapy, MCSP, PG Dip, MSc
Clinical Specialist Physiotherapist
(Chapter 7: Moving and positioning)

Kate Hall RN, Dip HE, BSc
Matron
(Chapter 15: Cytotoxic therapy)

Sharlene Haywood RN, BSc (Hons)
Formerly Specialist Sister Rehabilitation Outreach Team
(Chapter 9: Patient comfort)

Beverley Henderson RN, PG Dip Counselling
    Psychotherapy, BSc (Hons)
Clinical Nurse Specialist Counsellor
(Chapter 5: Communication)

Geraldine Heneghan RN, BSc
Sister
(Chapter 11: Interpreting diagnostic tests)

Diana Higgins RN, Dip HE, BA (Hons), MA
PALS and Patient Information Officer
(Chapter 5: Communication)

Claire Hine MCSP, BSc (Hons)
Senior Physiotherapist
(Chapter 7: Moving and positioning)

Justine Hofland RN, BSc (Hons), Dip HE, MSc
Clinical Nurse Director
(Chapter 2: Assessment, discharge and end of
    life care)

Victoria Hollis RN, BN (Hons) MSc
Matron/Nurse Practitioner
(Chapter 13: Observations)

Sonja Hoy RN, PG Dip, PG Cert, BSc (Hons), Dip
Clinical Nurse Specialist Thyroid, Head & Neck, and
    Radiation Protection
(Chapter 14: Radioactive investigations and therapy)

Lorraine Hyde RN, ONC, BSc (Hons)
Matron
(Chapter 15: Cytotoxic therapy)

Beth Jackson RN, Dip HE, BSc (Hons)
Senior Clinical Nurse Specialist Breast Care
(Chapter 19: Wound management)

Kate Jones MCSP, Dip Physiotherapy, MSc
Clinical Specialist Physiotherapist
(Chapter 7: Moving and positioning)

Joanna Lamb RN, BSc (Hons), BA
Ward Sister
(Chapter 13: Observations; Chapter 17: Perioperative care)

Carol Lane RD, BSc (Hons), PG Dip
Dietitian
(Chapter 8: Nutrition, fluid balance and blood transfusion)

Sara Lister RN, BSc (Hons), PGDAE, MSc
Assistant Chief Nurse/Head of School
(Chapter 1: The context of nursing;
    Chapter 2: Assessment, discharge and end of life care;
    Chapter 5: Communication)

Perrie Luke RN, RM, RMN
Sister
(Chapter 10: Respiratory care)

Kate Macfarlane MRCSLT, BSc (Hons), MSc
Speech and Language Therapist/Clinical Lead
(Chapter 5: Communication; Chapter 8: Nutrition, fluid
    balance and blood transfusion)

Jennifer Mackenzie RN, BN
Sister
(Chapter 11: Interpreting diagnostic tests)

Kath Malhotra MCSP, BSc (Hons), PGCE
Lecturer/Practitioner
(Chapter 7: Moving and positioning)

Rebecca Martirani RN, BA
Specialist Sister Infection Prevention
(Chapter 3: Infection prevention and control)

Stacey Magill RN, BN
Senior Staff Nurse
(Chapter 2: Assessment, discharge and end of life care)

Kelly McGovern RN, Dip HE, Dip Cancer
Senior Staff Nurse
(Chapter 2: Assessment, discharge and end of life care)

Hayley McHugh RN, CPPD, BSc (Hons)
Practice Educator
(Chapter 8: Nutrition, fluid balance and blood transfusion)

Chris McNamara RN, BSc (Hons), MSc
Lecturer Practitioner
(Chapter 6: Elimination)

Louise McNamara RN, BN, MSc
Matron
(Chapter 12: Haematological procedures)

Dee Mears DCR, DMS
Superintendent Radiographer
(Chapter 11: Interpreting diagnostic tests)

Helen Mills RN, BSc (Hons), MSc
Head of Quality Assurance
(Chapter 1: The context of nursing)

Carolyn Moore MCSP, SRP
Superintendent Physiotherapist
(Chapter 7: Moving and positioning)

Sarah Newton RD, BSc (Hons)
Dietitian
(Chapter 8: Nutrition, fluid balance and blood
   transfusion)

Gillian M. Parker RN, BSc, ONC
Specialist Sister Urology
(Chapter 6: Elimination)

Natalie Pattison BSc (Hons), MSc, PhD, Dip HE
Clinical Nursing Research Fellow
(Chapter 1: The context of nursing; Chapter 2: Assessment,
   discharge and end of life care)

Karon Payne RN
Transfusion Practitioner
(Chapter 8: Nutrition, fluid balance and blood transfusion)

Abby Peacock Smith RN, BN, CPPD
Sister
(Chapter 10: Respiratory care)

Hannah Perry RN, BSc (Hons)
Specialist Sister Gastrointestinal
(Chapter 6: Elimination)

Scott Pollock Dip SW, BA (Hons), SW, MSc
Complex Discharge Co-ordinator
(Chapter 1: The context of nursing; Chapter 2: Assessment,
   discharge and end of life care)

Stephen Pollock RN, BSc, Dip HE
Charge Nurse
(Chapter 10: Respiratory care)

Jorn Rixen-Osterbro RN, BSc (Hons), Dip HE
Charge Nurse
(Chapter 2: Assessment, discharge and end of life care)

Lara Roskelly RN, Dip N, Dip HE
Sister
(Chapter 10: Respiratory care; Chapter 11: Interpreting
   diagnostic tests)

Steve Scholtes RN, BSc, MSc
Matron
(Chapter 17: Perioperative care)

Richard Schorstein RN, BSc (Hons), PG Dip
Matron
(Chapter 15: Cytotoxic therapy)

Erica Scurr DCR(R), MSc
Lead MRI Superintendent Radiographer
(Chapter 11: Interpreting diagnostic tests)

Clare Shaw RD, BSc (Hons), PG Dip, PhD
Consultant Dietitian
(**Chapter 8: Nutrition, fluid balance and blood transfusion**)

Sian Shepherd RD, BSc (Hons), Advanced Dip
Dietitian
(**Chapter 8**: Nutrition, fluid balance and blood
   transfusion)

Victoria Sinnett DCR(R), MSc
Superintendent Radiographer
(Chapter 11: Interpreting diagnostic tests)

Jenny Smith RN
Senior PALS and Patient Information Officer
(Chapter 5: Communication)

Anna-Marie Stevens RN, RM, ONC, BSc (Hons), MSc
Macmillan Nurse Consultant Palliative Care
(Chapter 6: Elimination; Chapter 9: Patient comfort)

Nicola Tinne RN, BSc, Dip HE
Specialist Sister Head & Neck
(Chapter 19: Wound management)

Joanna Todd RN, BN (Hons), Dip HE
Senior Staff Nurse
(Chapter 13: Observations)

Richard Towers RN, Dip Onc, BSc (Hons), MSc
Lecturer Practitioner/Lead Nurse Counsellor
(Chapter 5: Communication)

Joanna Waller RN, Dip Onc, BN (Hons)
Ward Sister
(Chapter 17: Perioperative care)

Jen Watson RN, BSc, PG Dip
Matron
(Chapter 18: Vascular access devices: insertion and
   management)

Ashworth Paul Weaving RN, BSc, Cert, Advanced Dip
Lead Nurse Infection Prevention and Control
(Chapter 3: Infection prevention and control)

Jennifer Webster BSc (Hons), MSc
Senior Occupational Therapist
(Chapter 7: Moving and positioning)

Linda Wedlake RD, MSc, MMed Sci
Research Dietitian
(Chapter 8: Nutrition, fluid balance and blood
  transfusion)

Helen White MRCSLT, BSc (Hons)
Speech and Language Therapist/Team Leader
(Chapter 5: Communication; Chapter 8: Nutrition, fluid
  balance and blood transfusion)

Barbara Witt RN
Nurse Phlebotomist
(Chapter 11: Interpreting diagnostic tests)

Mary Woods RN, OncCert, BSc (Hons), MSc
Clinical Nurse Specialist/Head of Lymphoedema Services
(Chapter 9: Patient comfort)

Foreword to the eighth edition

As the Chief Nurse of the Royal Marsden Hospital NHS Foundation Trust and a contributor and clinical user for many years, it is a special pleasure and honour to be asked to introduce the eighth edition of *The Royal Marsden Hospital Manual of Clinical Nursing Procedures*. The manual is internationally renowned and used by nurses across the world to ensure their practice is evidence based and effective. As information becomes ever more available to the consumers of healthcare it is essential that the manual is updated frequently so that it reflects the most current evidence to inform our clinical practice.

More than ever in 2011, nurses need to be able to assure the public, patients and their families that care is based on the best available evidence. As nurses seeking to improve our care it is essential that we are able to critically analyse our judgements in the light of current knowledge. For all of us working with patients and their families there is an imperative to question and renew our practice using the many sources of knowledge available to us. In the busy world of clinical practice in a ward, unit or in the community it can be challenging to find time to search for the evidence and this is where *The Royal Marsden Hospital Manual of Clinical Nursing Procedures* is a real practical help.

As in the seventh edition, reviewing the evidence or sources of knowledge has been made more explicit with each level of evidence graded. This grading provides the reader with an understanding of whether the reference comes from a randomized controlled trial, national or international guidance or from expert opinion. At its best, clinical nursing care is an amalgam of a sensitive therapeutic relationship coupled with effective care based on the best evidence that exists. Some areas of practice have attracted international research such as cardiopulmonary resuscitation and infection prevention and control; other areas of practice have not attracted such robust research and therefore it is more of a challenge to ensure evidence-based care. Each time the next edition of the manual is prepared we reflect on the gaps in research and knowledge; this provides the impetus to start developing new concept analyses and develop further research studies. This year there are new areas covered including a chapter on risk management and a section on preparing the patient for diagnostic investigations such as endoscopy or CT scans.

As you look at the list of contributors to the manual you will see that this edition has continued to ask clinically active nurses to share their practice in their chapters. This has the double advantage of ensuring that this manual reflects the reality of practice but also ensures that nurses at the Royal Marsden Hospital NHS Foundation Trust are frequently reviewing the evidence and reflecting upon their care.

A textbook devoted to improving and enhancing clinical practice needs to be alive to the clinical practitioner. You will see that this edition has a new overall format designed to make the manual more effective in clinical care.

As I commend this eighth edition of *The Royal Marsden Hospital Manual of Clinical Nursing Procedures* to you I am aware that it will be used in many different countries and settings. Having had the privilege of visiting and meeting nurses across the world I know that there are more commonalities than differences between us. The common theme is, of course, the need to ensure that we as nurses provide care that is individually and sensitively planned and that it is based on the best available evidence. *The Royal Marsden Hospital Manual of Clinical Nursing Procedures* is a wonderful resource for such evidence and I hope it will be widely used in all clinical settings across the world.

Finally, I would like to pay a warm tribute to the amazing amount of work undertaken by the two editors, Lisa Dougherty and Sara Lister, and to all the nurses and allied health professionals at the Royal Marsden Hospital who have worked so hard on this eighth edition.

Shelley Dolan
Chief Nurse
The Royal Marsden Hospital NHS
Foundation Trust

Introduction and guidelines for use

The first edition of *The Royal Marsden Hospital Manual of Clinical Nursing Procedures* was produced in the early 1980s as a core procedure manual for safe practice within The Royal Marsden Hospital, the first cancer hospital in the world. Thirty years and eight editions later the staff of the hospital are still working together to keep it updated, ensuring that only current evidence-based practice is recommended.

The type of evidence that underpins procedures is made explicit by using a system to categorize the evidence, which is broader than that generally used. It has been developed from the types of evidence described by Rycroft-Malone *et al.* (2004) in an attempt to acknowledge that 'in reality practitioners draw on multiple sources of knowledge in the course of their practice and interaction with patients' (Rycroft-Malone *et al.* 2004, p. 88).

The sources of evidence, along with examples, are identified as follows:

1 *Clinical experience (E):*
   - Encompasses expert practical know-how, gained through working with others and reflecting on best practice.
   - If there is no written evidence to support clinical experience as a justification for undertaking a procedure the text will be referenced as an E but will not be preceded by an author's name.
   - Example: (Dougherty 2008: E). This is drawn from the following article that gives expert clinical opinion: Dougherty, L. (2008) Obtaining peripheral vascular access. In: *Intravenous Therapy in Nursing Practice* (eds L. Dougherty & J. Lamb), 2nd edn. Blackwell Publishing, Oxford.

2 *Patient (P):*
   - Gained through expert patient feedback and extensive experience of working with patients.
   - Example: (Diamond 1999: P). This has been gained from a personal account of care written by a patient, Diamond, J. (1999) *C: Because Cowards Get Cancer Too*. Vermilion, London.

3 *Context (C):*
   - May include Audit and Performance data, Social and Professional Networks, Local and National Policy, guidelines from Professional Bodies (e.g. Royal College of Nursing; RCN) and manufacturer's recommendations.
   - Example: (DH 2001: C). This document gives guidelines for good practice: DH (2001) *Reference Guide to Consent for Examination or Treatment*. Department of Health, London.

4 *Research (R):*
   - Evidence gained through research.
   - Example: (Fellowes *et al.* 2004: R1a). This has been drawn from the following evidence: Fellowes, D., Wilkinson, S. & Moore, P. (2004) Communication skills training for healthcare professionals working with cancer patients, their families and/or carers. *Cochrane Database Syst Rev*, 2, CD003751. DOI: 10.10002/14651858.CD003571.pub2.

The levels that have been chosen are adapted from Sackett, Strauss and Richardson (2000) as follows:

1 (a) Systematic reviews of randomized controlled trials (RCTs).
   (b) Individual RCTs with narrow confidence limits.
2 (a) Systematic reviews of cohort studies.
   (b) Individual cohort studies and low quality RCTs.
3 (a) Systematic reviews of case-controlled studies.
   (b) Case-controlled studies.
4 Case series and poor quality cohort and case-controlled studies.
5 Expert opinion.

The rationale for the system and further explanation is discussed in more detail in Chapter 1.

The Manual is informed by the day-to-day practice in The Royal Marsden NHS Foundation Trust and conversely is the corporate policy and procedure document of the organization. It therefore does not cover all aspects of acute nursing practice or those relating to children's or community nursing. However, it does contain the procedures and changes in practice that reflect modern acute nursing practice.

Core to nursing, wherever it takes place, is the commitment to care for individuals and to keep them safe. Increasing use is being made of the internet to record and access information essential in maintaining this safe environment. This edition of *The Royal Marsden Hospital Manual of Clinical Nursing Procedures* has been significantly revised to reflect the move in professional life to utilize electronic records and web-based information in the process of providing patient care.

A more detailed uniform structure has been introduced for all chapters so that there is a balance to the information included. The number of chapters has been reduced, grouping together similar procedures related to an aspect of human functioning. This is to avoid the need to duplicate material and to make it easier for the reader to find.

The chapters have been organized into four broad sections that represent as far as possible the needs of a patient along their care pathway. The first section, *Managing the patient journey*, presents the generic information that the nurse needs for every patient who enters the acute care environment. The second section, *Supporting the patient with human functioning*, relates to the support a patient may require with normal human functions such as elimination, nutrition, respiration. The third section, *Supporting the patient through the diagnostic process*, includes procedures that relate to any aspects of supporting a patient through the diagnostic process from the simple procedures such as taking a temperature, to preparing a patient for complex procedures such as a liver biopsy. The final section, *Supporting the patient through treatment*, includes the procedures related to specific types of treatment or therapies related to the disease or illness of the patient.

Structure of chapters

The structure of each chapter is consistent throughout the book:

- *Overview*: As the chapters are larger and have considerably more content, each one begins with an overview to guide the reader, informing them of the scope and the sections included in the chapter.
- *Definition*: Each section begins with a definition of the terms and explanation of the aspect of care, with any technical or difficult concepts explained.
- *Anatomy and physiology*: Each section includes a discussion of the anatomy and physiology that relates to the aspect of nursing care in the chapter. If appropriate, this is illustrated with diagrams so the context of the procedure can be fully understood by the reader.
- *Related theory*: If an understanding of theoretical principles is more appropriate background information to help carry out a procedure, this has been included.
- *Evidence-based approaches*: This provides background and presents the research and expert opinion in this area.

If appropriate the indications and contraindications are included as well as any principles of care.

- *Legal and professional issues:* This outlines any professional guidance, law or other national policies that may need to be known about in respect to the procedures. If necessary this includes any professional competences or qualifications that are required in order to perform the procedures.
- *Preprocedural considerations:* When carrying out any procedure there are certain actions that may need to be completed, equipment prepared or medication given beforehand. These are made explicit under this heading.
- *Procedure:* Each chapter includes the current procedures that are used in the acute hospital setting. They have been drawn from the daily nursing practice at The Royal Marsden NHS Foundation Trust. Only procedures where the authors have the knowledge and expertise have been included.

   Each procedure gives detailed step-by-step actions, supported by rationale, and, where available, the known evidence underpinning this rationale has been indicated. Within procedure guidelines, any action steps of the procedure that are a nursing responsibility are highlighted with colour shading, using the same colour as for the headings in that chapter. The manual also includes a few procedures where the primary role of the nurse is to assist another health care practitioner. Within those procedure guidelines, where action steps are carried out by either a doctor or other expert practitioner, rather than being a nursing responsibility, the action steps are highlighted with grey shading, for example, Procedure guideline 10.4: Chest drain: insertion.
- *Problem solving and resolution*: If relevant, each procedure will be followed by a table of potential problems that may be encountered while carrying out the procedure and suggestions as to the cause, prevention and any action that may help resolve the problem.
- *Postprocedural considerations*: Care for the patient doesn't end with the procedure. This new section details any documentation the nurse may need to complete, education/ information that needs to be given to the patient, ongoing observations or referrals to other members of the multiprofessional team.
- *Complications:* Any ongoing problems or potential complications are discussed in a final section and includes evidence-based suggestions for resolution.
- *Illustrations:* The number of colour illustrations has been increased and where relevant they have been used to illustrate the steps of some procedures. This will enable the nurse carrying out the procedures to see in greater detail, for example, the correct position of hands or the angle of a needle.
- *Reference list*: The chapter finishes with a reference list. Only recent texts from the last 10 years have been included unless they are seminal texts. For the first time a list of websites has also been included.

This book is intended as a reference and a resource, not as a replacement for practice-based education. None of the procedures in this book should be undertaken without prior instruction and subsequent supervision from an appropriately qualified and experienced professional. We hope that *The Royal Marsden Hospital Manual of Clinical Nursing Procedures* will continue to be a resource and a contribution to 'continually improving the overall standard of clinical care' (NHSE 1999, p. 3).

References

NHSE (1999) *Clinical Governance: Quality in the New NHS*. Department of Health, London.
NICE (2005) *Violence. The Short-Term Management of Disturbed/Violent Behaviour in Psychiatric In-Patient Settings and Emergency Departments*. National Institute for Health and Clinical Excellence, London.
NICE (2007) *Venous thromboembolism: reducing the risk of venous thromboembolism (deep vein thrombosis and pulmonary embolism) in in-patients undergoing surgery*. National Collaborating Centre for Acute Care.
Pratt, R.J. *et al.* (2007) Epic 2: National evidence-based guidelines for preventing health-care associated infections in NHS hospitals in England. *J Hosp Infect*, 65(1)(Suppl), S1–S12.
Royal College of Surgeons for England, London. www.guidance-nice.org.uk/CG/published/CG46. Accessed 30/4/07.
Rycroft-Malone, J. *et al.* (2004) What counts as evidence in evidence based practice? *J Adv Nurs*, 47(1), 81–90.
Sackett, D.L., Strauss, S.E. and Richardson, W.S. (2000) *Evidence Based Medicine: How to practice and Teach EBM*, 2nd edn. Churchill Livingstone, Edinburgh.

Lisa Dougherty
Sara Lister

Quick reference to the procedure guidelines

Acknowledgements

A book is a team effort and never more so than with this edition of *The Royal Marsden Hospital Manual of Clinical Nursing Procedures*.

Since the first edition was published in 1984, the range of procedures within the manual has grown in complexity and the depth of the theoretical content underpinning them has increased considerably, more so in this edition as the structure has been totally revised. This has demanded more from every author, as they have had to research and write new material as well as revising the evidence base of the existing content. This has been a collaborative task carried out by knowledgeable, expert nurses in partnership with members of the multidisciplinary team including pharmacists, physiotherapists, occupational therapists, dietitians, speech therapists, radiographers and psychological care.

So, we must thank every member of the 'team' who have helped to produce this edition, for their time, effort and perseverance. An additional challenge has been to co-ordinate the increased number of contributors to each chapter. This responsibility has fallen to the lead chapter authors, so, for this, they deserve a special acknowledgement and thanks for their ability to integrate all the contributions and create comprehensive chapters.

We would also like to thank some other key people:

Dale Russell and the library team of the David Adams Library at The Royal Marsden School of Cancer Nursing and Rehabilitation for their help and support in providing the references required by the authors and setting up the end note system.

Stephen Millward and the medical photography team for all the new photographs.

Our families and friends who have encouraged us, stood by us and tolerated our distracted state at times during the last eighteen months.

Finally, our thanks go to Beth Knight, Rachel Coombs, Catriona Dixon and Helen Harvey at Wiley-Blackwell for their advice and support in all aspects of the publishing process.

Lisa Dougherty
Sara Lister

List of abbreviations

5-FU	5-fluorouracil	CAD	coronary artery disease
AAC	augmentive or alternative communication	CARES	Cancer Rehabilitation Evaluation System
A&E	Accident and Emergency	CAUTI	catheter-associated urinary tract infections
ABG	arterial blood gas	CCU	coronary care unit/critical care unit
ABPI	Ankle to Brachial Pressure Index	CD	controlled drug
ADH	antidiuretic hormone	cfu	colony-forming units
ADL	activities of daily living	CJD	Creutzfeldt–Jakob disease
ADR	adverse drug reaction	CML	chronic myeloid leukaemia
AED	automated external defibrillator	CMV	cytomegalovirus
AFO	ankle foot orthosis	CNS	central nervous system
AHP	allied health professional	CO	cardiac output
AIDS	acquired immune deficiency syndrome	COAD	chronic obstructive airways disease
ALARP	as low as reasonably practicable	COMA	Committee on Medical Aspects of Food Policy
ALS	advanced life support		
ALT	alanine aminotransferase	COPD	chronic obstructive pulmonary disease
ANH	acute normovolaemic haemodilution	COSHH	Control of Substances Hazardous to Health
ANP	atrial natriuretic peptide	CPAP	continuous positive airway pressure
ANS	autonomic nervous system	CPET	cardiopulmonary exercise testing
ANTT	aseptic non-touch technique	CPR	cardiopulmonary resuscitation
AORN	Association of Perioperative Registered Nurses	CRP	C-reactive protein
		CSAS	Chemotherapy Symptom Assessment Scale
AP	anteroposterior	CSF	cerebrospinal fluid/colony-stimulating factor
APTR	activated partial thromboplastin ratio	CSS	Central Sterile Services
ARDS	acute/adult respiratory distress syndrome	CSU	catheter specimen of urine
ARSAC	Administration of Radioactive Substances Advisory Committee	CT	computed tomography
		CVAD	central venous access device
AST	aspartate aminotransferase	CVC	central venous catheter
AT	anaerobic threshold	CVP	central venous pressure
ATC	around the clock	CXR	chest X-ray
AV	atrioventricular	DBE	deep breathing exercises
BAL	bronchoalveolar lavage	DF	dorsiflexion
BCG	bacille Calmette-Guérin	DH	Department of Health
BCSH	British Committee for Standards in Haematology	DIC	disseminated intravascular coagulation
		DM	diabetes mellitus
BIA	bio-electrical impedance analysis	DMSO	dimethyl sulphoxide
BLS	basic life support	DNA	deoxyribonucleic acid
BMA	British Medical Association	DNAR	do not attempt resuscitation
BME	black and minority ethnic	DPI	dry powder inhaler
BMI	Body Mass Index	DRE	digital rectal examination
BNF	British National Formulary	DVLA	Driver and Vehicle Licensing Agency
BOC	British Oxygen Company	DVT	deep vein thrombosis
BPI	Brief Pain Inventory	EAPC	European Association of Palliative Care
BSE	bovine spongiform encephalopathy	EBM	evidence-based medicine

EBN	evidence-based nursing	IBCT	incorrect blood component transfused
EBP	evidence-based practice	IC	inspiratory capacity
EBRT	external beam radiotherapy	ICD	implantable cardioverter defibrillator
EBV	Epstein–Barr virus	ICF	intracellular fluid
ECF	extracellular fluid	ICP	intracranial pressure
ECG	electrocardiogram	ICRP	International Commission on Radiological
ECM	extracellular matrix		Protection
EDTA	ethylenediaminetetra-acetic acid	ICS	intraoperative cell salvage
EGFR	epidermal growth factor receptor	ICSI	intracytoplasmic sperm injection
EIA	Equality Impact Assessment	ICU	intensive care unit
ELISA	enzyme-linked immunosorbent assay	IgM	immunoglobulin M
EMLA	eutectic mixture of local anaesthetics	IJV	internal jugular vein
ENT	ears, nose and throat	ILCOR	International Liaison Committee on
EPO	erythropoietin		Resuscitation
ERV	expiratory reserve volume	IMV	intermittent mandatory ventilation
ETT	endotracheal tube	INR	international normalized ratio
EUPAP	European Pressure Ulcer Advisory Panel	IPCT	infection prevention and control team
F(Fr)	French (gauge)	IPEM	Institute of Physics and Engineering in
FBC	full blood count		Medicine
FEES	fibreoptic endoscopic evaluation of	IRMER	Ionizing Radiation (Medical Exposure)
	swallowing		Regulations
FFI	fatal familial insomnia	IRR	infra-red radiation
FFP	fresh frozen plasma	IRV	inspiratory reserve volume
FRC	functional residual capacity	ISC	intermittent self-catheterization
FTSG	full-thickness skin graft	IV	intravenous
FVC	forced vital capacity	IVC	inferior vena cava
GCS	Glasgow Coma Scale	IVF	in vitro fertilization
G-CSF	granulocyte-colony stimulating factor	IUI	intrauterine insemination
GFR	glomerular filtration rate	JPAC	Joint UKBTS/NIBSC Professional Advisory
GGT	gamma-glutamyl transferase		Committee
GI	gastrointestinal	KGF	keratinocyte growth factor
GMC	General Medical Council	KVO	keep vein open
GM-CSF	granulocyte macrophage-colony stimulating	LANSS	Leeds Assessment of Neuropathic Symptoms
	factor		and Signs
GP	general practitioner	LBC	liquid-based cytology
GSL	general sales list	LCT	long-chain triglyceride
GTN	glyceryl trinitrate	LDR	low dose rate
HBsAg	hepatitis B surface antigen	LMA	laryngeal mask airway
HBV	hepatitis B virus	LMN	lower motor neurone
HCA	healthcare assistant	LMWH	low molecular weight heparin
HCAI	healthcare-acquired/associated infection	LPA	Lasting Power of Attorney
HCV	hepatitis C virus	MAC	*Mycobacterium avium intracellulare*
HDN	haemolytic disease of the newborn	MAOI	monoamine oxidase inhibitor
HDR	high dose rate	MAP	mean arterial pressure
HDU	high-dependency unit	MBP	mean blood pressure
HEPA	high-efficiency particulate air	MC&S	microscopy, culture and sensitivity
HIV	human immunodeficiency virus	MCT	medium-chain triglyceride
HLA	human leucocyte antigen	MDA	Medical Devices Agency
HME	heat and moisture exchange(r)	MDI	metered dose inhaler
HOOF	home oxygen ordering form	MDT	multidisciplinary team
HPA	Health Protection Agency	ME	medical examiner
HR	heart rate	MET	medical emergency team
HSC	Health Service Circular/Health and Safety	MEWS	Modified Early Warning System
	Commission	MHRA	Medicines and Healthcare Products
HSE	Health and Safety Executive		Regulatory Agency
IASP	International Association for the Study of	MI	myocardial infarction
	Pain	MIC	minimum inhibitory concentration

MLD	manual lymphatic drainage	PGSGA	patient-generated subjective global assessment
MPQ	McGill Pain Questionnaire	PHCT	primary healthcare team
MRI	magnetic resonance imaging	PICC	peripherally inserted central catheter
MRSA	meticillin-resistant *Staphylococcus aureus*	PN	parenteral nutrition
MSAS	Memorial Symptom Assessment Scale	PNS	peripheral nervous system
MSCC	metastatic spinal cord compression	POA	preoperative assessment
MSU	midstream specimen of urine	POCT	point-of-care testing
NANDA	North American Nursing Diagnosis Association	POM	prescription-only medicine
NBTC	National Blood Transfusion Committee	PPE	personal protective equipment
NCEPOD	National Confidential Enquiry into Patient Outcome and Death	PrP	prion protein
		PSAR	Pain and Assessment Records
NG	nasogastric	PSCC	primary/benign spinal cord compression
NHS	National Health Service	PSD	patient-specific direction
NHSCSP	NHS Cervical Screening Programme	psi	pounds per square inch
NHSE	National Health Service Executive	PT	physiotherapist
NICE	National Institute for (Health and) Clinical Excellence	PTFE	polytetrafluoroethylene
		PTHrp	parathormone-related polypeptide
NIV	non-invasive ventilation	PUO	pyrexia of unknown origin
NMC	Nursing and Midwifery Council	PVC	polyvinylchloride
NMDA	N-methyl-D-aspartate	PVD	peripheral vascular disease
NPSA	National Patient Safety Agency	PWO	partial withdrawal occlusion
NPWT	negative pressure wound therapy	RA	right atrium
NRS	numerical rating scales	RAP	right atrial pressure
NRT	nicotine replacement therapy	RAS	reticular activating system
NSAID	non-steroidal anti-inflammatory drug	RBC	red blood cell
NSF	National Service Framework	RCA	root cause analysis
ODP	operating department practitioner	RCN	Royal College of Nursing
OGD	oesophagogastroduodenoscopy	RCS	Royal College of Surgeons of England
ONS	Oncology Nursing Society	RCUK	Resuscitation Council UK
OSCE	objective structured clinical examination	RIG	radiologically inserted gastrostomy
OT	occupational therapist	RNI	reference nutrient intake
OTC	over the counter	RSV	respiratory syncytial virus
OTFC	oral transmucosal fentanyl citrate	RTO	Resuscitation Training Officer
P	pharmacy medicines	RTOG	Radiation Therapy Oncology Group
PA	posterior anterior	RV	residual volume
PaCO$_2$	partial pressure of carbon dioxide	SA	sinoatrial
PACU	peri-anaesthesia care unit	SABRE	Serious Adverse Blood Reactions and Events
PAD	preoperative autologous donation	SARS	severe acute respiratory syndrome
PART	patient-at-risk team	SBAR	Situation-Background-Assessment-Recommendations
PC	*Pneumocystis carinii*		
PCA	patient-controlled analgesia	SBO	small bowel obstruction
PCEA	patient-controlled epidural analgesia	SCC	spinal cord compression
PCS	postoperative cell salvage	SCI	spinal cord injury
PDPH	postdural puncture headache	SCNS	Supportive Care Needs Survey
PDT	percutaneous dilatational tracheostomy	SDF	stromal cell-derived factor
PE	pulmonary embolism/pulmonary embolus	SGA	subjective global assessment
		SHOT	Serious Hazards of Transfusion
PEA	pulseless electrical activity	SI	Système International
PEEP	positive end-expiratory pressure	SIMV	simulated intermittent mandatory ventilation
PEF(R)	peak expiratory flow (rate)		
PEG	percutaneous endoscopically placed gastrostomy	SIRS	systemic inflammatory response syndrome
		SL	semi-lunar
PEP	postexposure prophylaxis	SLD	simple lymphatic drainage
PET	positron emission tomography	SLE	systemic lupus erythematosus
PF	plantar flexion	SLT	speech and language therapist
PGD	patient group direction	SNRI	serotonin-norepinephrine reuptake inhibitor

SOP	standard operating procedure	TSS	toxic shock syndrome
SPI	Social Problems Inventory	TTO	to take out
SPN	Safer Practice Notice	TURP	transurethral resection of prostate
SRHH	Self Report Health History	TV	tidal volume
SSG	split-thickness or split skin graft	UH	unfractionated heparin
SSI	surgical site infection	UMN	upper motor neurone
SSRI	selective serotonin reuptake inhibitor	UTI	urinary tract infection
SUI	serious untoward incident	V/Q	ventilation/perfusion
SV	stroke volume	VAD	vascular access device
SVC	superior vena cava	VAP	ventilator-associated pneumonia
swg	standard wire gauge	VAT	venous assessment tool
TACO	transfusion-associated circulatory overload	VC	vital capacity
TA-GVHD	transfusion-associated graft-versus-host disease	vCJD	variant Creutzfeldt–Jakob disease
TB	tuberculosis	VDRL	Venereal Disease Research Laboratory
TCA	tricyclic antidepressant	VDS	verbal descriptor scales
TCI	target-controlled infusion	VEGF	vascular endothelial growth factor
TED	thromboembolic deterrent	VF	ventricular fibrillation
TENS	transcutaneous electrical nerve stimulation	VPF	vascular permeability factor
TIVA	total intravenous anaesthesia	VT	ventricular tachycardia
TLC	total lung capacity	VTE	venous thromboembolism
TLD	thermoluminescent	VTM	viral transport medium
TPI	*Treponema pallidum* immobilization	WBC	white blood cell
TPN	total parenteral nutrition	WBP	wound bed preparation
TRALI	transfusion-related acute lung injury	WHO	World Health Organization
TRSC	Therapy Related Symptom Checklist	WOB	work of breathing
TSE	transmissible spongiform encephalopathy	WR	Wassermann reaction

Managing the patient journey

Part one

The context of nursing

The Royal Marsden Hospital Manual of Clinical Nursing Procedures, Eighth Edition. Edited by Lisa Dougherty and Sara Lister.
© 2011 The Royal Marsden Hospital. Published 2011 by Blackwell Publishing Ltd.

4 | # Introduction

Nursing encompasses autonomous and collaborative care of individuals of all ages, families, groups and communities, sick or well and in all settings. Nursing includes the promotion of health, prevention of illness, and the care of ill, disabled and dying people. Advocacy, promotion of a safe environment, research, participation in shaping health policy and in patient and health systems management, and education are also key nursing roles.

(International Council of Nursing 2010)

Factors that shape and direct the nature of healthcare provision

Nursing today is at the heart of healthcare provision in the United Kingdom, and nurses are the largest group of clinical employees (www.nhs.uk) in the NHS. Many factors, from political to economic, from social to technological, shape and direct the nature of healthcare provision and so also affect nursing and the context in which it takes place. These factors are continually changing and evolving and therefore affecting the quality of care for patients.

This chapter will set out the factors that nurses working in hospital settings need to be aware of as they plan, deliver and develop patient care. The factors are discussed under four headings: Political, Economic, Social and Technological, or PEST, a popular model used to structure decision making (Barr and Dowding 2008). The headings are nominal as many factors are complex and overlap with each other. This chapter will also include an explanation of the structure of the rest of the manual, the order of the chapters and the grading system for the evidence of the rationale accompanying the steps in the procedures.

Political factors
High Quality Care for All

Political factors include strategies of the government that impact directly on the current context of health and therefore nursing care. Current national provision has been influenced by *High Quality Care for All* (Darzi 2008), the final report of the NHS Next Stage Review, co-produced by Lord Darzi with the NHS during a year-long process involving more than 2000 clinicians and 60,000 NHS staff, patients, stakeholders and members of the public. The core purpose of this strategy is to increase the quality of all aspects of the health service. Lord Darzi defines quality of care as 'clinically effective, personal and safe' (Darzi 2008, pp.8–9). It is about effectiveness of care, from the clinical procedure the patient receives to their quality of life after treatment. It is also about the patient's entire experience of the NHS and ensuring they are treated with compassion, dignity and respect in a clean, safe and well-managed environment.

In practice, this strategy has meant that resources have been invested in standardizing treatment across the UK and in time may extend to standardizing the practices, procedures and equipment used in treatment. A key strategic aim is to *get the basics right first time* (Darzi 2008, p.5), that is, protecting patient safety by eradicating healthcare-acquired infections and avoidable accidents.

With the change of government in May 2010, the political emphasis shifted to focusing specifically on 'continuously improving those things that really matter to patients – the outcome of their healthcare' (DH 2010b, p.1). This means that the end-result of procedures is going to be more important than the process of achieving them.

'The NHS will be held to account against clinically credible and evidence-based outcome measures, not process targets. We will remove targets with no clinical justification' (DH 2010b, p.4).

For example, in nursing, this may mean an increased analysis of the outcome of the use of certain types of wound care products, the length of time catheters are *in situ* and the effectiveness of pain management processes. However, this approach will be accompanied by a commitment to 'empower and liberate clinicians to innovate, with the freedom to focus on improving healthcare services' (DH 2010b, p.1).

Care Quality Commission

The Care Quality Commission (www.cqc.org.uk), the independent regulator of all health and adult social care in England, is charged with monitoring all healthcare providers across England against the new standards of quality.

Its aim is to make sure better care is provided for everyone, whether that's in hospital, in care homes, in people's own homes or elsewhere. It has a vision of high-quality care, meaning care that:

- is safe
- has the right outcomes, including clinical outcomes (for example, do people get the right treatment and are they well cared for?)
- is a good experience for the people who use it, their carers and their families
- helps to prevent illness, and promotes healthy, independent living
- is available to those who need it when they need it
- provides good value for money.

(www.cqc.org.uk/aboutcqc/whoweare.cfm)

To make this happen the Care Quality Commission has been given statutory powers to enforce standards through prosecution of those statutorily accountable for quality in any healthcare organizations (not just the NHS). These regulatory duties are carried out in the acute care setting through the following pathways.

Registration and enforcement

The Health and Social Care Act, 2008 introduced a new, single registration system that applies to both health and adult social care. From April 2010, all care providers who provide regulated activities (see Box 1.1) will be required by law to be registered with the Care Quality Commission (www.cqc.org.uk/guidanceforprofessionals/introduction toregistration/whoneedstoregister.cfm). To register, all healthcare providers must show they are meeting new essential standards of quality and safety across all the regulated activities they provide (see Box 1.1).

The new system will make sure that people can expect services to meet essential standards of quality and safety that respect their dignity and protect their rights. The new system is focused on outcomes, rather than systems and processes, and places the views and experience of people who use services at the centre. The Care Quality Commission currently publishes results so they are in the public domain. Information is expected to be available more regularly and speedily so that 'Patients will have access to the information they want, to make choices about their care' (DH 2010a, p.3).

Box 1.1 Healthcare activities that need to be registered with the Care Quality Commission

---

Regulated activities that require registration are described in the Health and Social Care Act 2008 (Regulated Activities) Regulations 2009. They include:

- personal care
- accommodation with nursing or personal care
- accommodation for persons who require treatment for substance misuse
- accommodation and nursing or personal care in the further education sector
- treatment of disease, disorder or injury
- assessment or medical treatment for persons detained under the Mental Health Act 1983
- surgical procedures
- diagnostic and screening procedures
- management of supply of blood and blood-derived products
- transport services, triage and medical advice provided remotely
- maternity and midwifery services
- termination of pregnancies
- services in slimming clinics
- nursing care
- family planning services.

The list of regulated activities included in the regulations is based on the level of risk to people who use services. (www.cqc.org.uk/guidanceforprofessionals/ introductiontoregistration/whoneedstoregister.cfm#3)

Assessments of quality

To register, the CQC expects organizations to meet essential standards in quality and safety. Organizations are expected to produce evidence to demonstrate they have met outcomes relating to important aspects of care in respect of:

- involvement and information
- personalized care, treatment and support
- safeguarding and safety
- suitability of staffing
- quality and management
- suitability of management.

Publishing information

This information will then be made available to people so they can make informed decisions about where they have their care. This impacts on nursing as there is an expectation that procedures that define care given are explicit and of course followed.

Patient safety

A key patient safety issue that remains a priority for the NHS has been tackling healthcare-acquired infections. A variety of measures have been put into place following the catastrophic occurrence of deaths from *Clostridium difficile* and MRSA bacteraemias in 2004–5 (Healthcare Commission 2006, 2007).

- *Mandatory surveillance of C. difficile* was introduced in 2004 (because it is a significant cause of morbidity and can be difficult to treat because of its multiple antibiotic resistance).
- *Agreed maximum numbers of MRSA bloodstream infections.* NHS trusts are now required to ensure that their agreed 'ceilings' of the number of MRSA bloodstream infections are not exceeded so that, collectively, the level of infections nationally is maintained at less than half the number in 2003–4. Zero tolerance to infections is encouraged. From July 2010 levels of these infections are published weekly (DH 2010d).
- *Annual Hygiene Code inspections* (for more information, see Chapter 3).

Nurses obviously play a significant role in meeting these measures. A charter for the 'new' role of the matron (DH 2004a) set out ten commitments in respect of a cleaner safer hospital (Box 1.2), building on the principles set down by Florence Nightingale in the 1800s.

> Let whoever is in charge keep this simple question in her head (not, how can I always do this right thing myself, but) how can I provide for this right thing to be always done?
>
> (Nightingale 1859, p.24)

Box 1.2 Commitments of a matron

1 Keeping the NHS clean is everybody's responsibility.
2 The patient environment will be well maintained, clean and safe.
3 Matrons will establish a cleanliness culture across their units.
4 Cleaning staff will be recognized for the important work they do. Matrons will make sure they feel part of the ward team.
5 Specific roles and responsibilities for cleaning will be clear.
6 Cleaning routines will be clear, agreed and well publicized.
7 Patients will have a part to play in monitoring and reporting on standards of cleanliness.
8 All staff working in healthcare will receive education in infection control.
9 Nurses and infection control teams will be involved in drawing up cleaning contracts and matrons have authority and power to withhold payment.
10 Sufficient resources will be dedicated to keeping hospitals clean.

(DH 2004a)

The High Impact Actions for Nursing and Midwifery

A current political initiative in the nursing profession to drive up standards of care is *The High Impact Actions for Nursing and Midwifery* (NHS Institute for Innovation and Improvement 2009). Eight high-impact actions (see Table 1.1) have been selected, from over 600 postings to the High-Impact website, by a group of senior nurses in the NHS. They have been selected as areas where significant improvement to quality can be achieved for patients and have been made available with relevant research evidence developed by academic experts to support day-to-day nursing practice.

The NHS Constitution

The new NHS Constitution aims to make explicit what a person can expect from the NHS so they can feel more empowered as a participant in their own care.

The Constitution was developed in consultation with patients, the public and NHS staff as part of the NHS Next Stage Review led by Lord Darzi. The NHS Constitution was first published on 21 January 2009 and applies to NHS services in England. The Health Act 2009 includes provisions related to the NHS Constitution. These came into force on 19 January 2010 and place a statutory duty on NHS bodies, primary care services, and independent and third sector organizations providing NHS care in England to have regard to the NHS Constitution.

The Constitution:

- outlines the purpose of the NHS and the principles of the NHS, which are the enduring high-level 'rules' that govern the way that the NHS operates and define how it seeks to achieve its purpose
- details NHS values that inspire passion in the NHS and should guide it in the 21st century
- makes explicit rights and pledges. One of the primary aims of the Constitution is to set out clearly what patients, the public and staff can expect from the NHS and what the NHS expects from them in return
- makes explicit rights and pledges for staff, as well as their responsibilities.

Explanations of these are found in Box 1.3.

Table 1.1 High-Impact Actions for Nursing and Midwifery

Category of action	Action	Relevant chapters
Your skin matters	No avoidable pressure sores in the NHS	4, 9
Staying safe, preventing falls	Demonstrate a year-on-year reduction in the number of falls sustained by older people in NHS-provided care	7
Keeping nourished, getting better	Stop inappropriate weight loss and dehydration in NHS-provided care	8
Promoting normal birth	Increase the normal birth rate and eliminate unnecessary caesarean sections through midwives taking the lead role in the care of normal pregnancy and labour, focusing on informing, educating and providing skilled support to first-time mothers and women who have had one previous caesarean section	Not applicable
Important choices – where to die when the time comes	Avoid inappropriate admission to hospital and increase the numbers of people who are able to die in the place of their choice	2
Fit and well to care	Reduce sickness absence in the nursing and midwifery workforce to no more than 3%	Not applicable
Ready to go – no delays	Increase the number of patients in NHS-provided care who have their discharge managed and led by a nurse or midwife where appropriate	2
Protection from infection	Demonstrate a dramatic reduction in the rate of UTIs for patients in NHS-provided care	3, 6

Economic factors

Globally financial resources to pay for healthcare are under considerable constraint. In England for the year 2010–11, 'The Department of Health and the NHS announced that it will deliver £4.35 billion of savings, as their departmental contribution towards £11 billion of savings that are being made across government' (Budget statement, March 23rd 2010).

NHS healthcare providers are responding to this in a variety of ways. These include refining processes of care, ensuring that delays and unnecessary bed days for patients are at a minimum. The distribution of care activities has also been scrutinized across the workforce.

Cost-effectiveness

With increasing emphasis on cost-effectiveness, the necessity of a Registered Nurse to carry out all procedures is constantly questioned. A study entitled *Improving the Effectiveness of the Nursing Workforce* (Centre for Health Economics 2003) has highlighted the shift in roles at the other end of the novice-to-expert continuum, with healthcare assistants taking responsibility for an increasing number of procedures that historically have been the professional domain of nursing (O'Dowd 2003).

Currently in the acute NHS there is no national standard preparation for these roles, nor any regulations governing what healthcare assistants can or cannot do. The Nursing and Midwifery Council is currently looking into options for regulating them (Santry 2010). Whatever happens, nurses continue to be accountable for the patients in their care.

Accountability

Accountability means that if a nurse is delegating care to another professional, healthcare support staff, carer or relative,

Table 1.2 Procedures that could be carried out by a healthcare assistant after relevant training and competency assessment supervised by a Registered Nurse (this is not an exhaustive list)

Procedure	Chapter
Penile sheath application	6
Urinary catheter bag: emptying	6
Stoma care	6
Fluid input: measurement	8
Measuring the weight and height of the patient	8
Blood components: collection and delivery to the clinical area	8
Mouthcare	9
Venepuncture	11
Swab sampling: ear, eye, nose, penile, rectal, throat	11
Urine sampling: midstream specimen of urine: male/female	11
Faecal sampling	11
Pulse measurement	13
Electrocardiogram	13
Blood pressure measurement (manual)	13
Respiratory assessment and pulse oximetry	13
Peak flow reading using a manual peak flow meter	13
Temperature measurement	13
Urinalysis: reagent strip procedure	13
Blood glucose monitoring	13
Antiembolic stockings: assessment, fitting and wearing	17

they must delegate effectively and are accountable for the appropriateness of that delegation. This means that they must:

- establish that anyone they delegate to is able to carry out their instructions
- confirm that the outcome of any delegated task meets required standards
- make sure that everyone they are responsible for is supervised and supported.

(NMC 2008a)

Some of the procedures included in this edition could be carried out by a healthcare assistant (HCA) (Table 1.2). However, it will always be the nurse responsible for those patients on a shift who must ensure that the HCA is competent in carrying out the procedures and knows what to report to the nurse on completing the activity. There is continual debate about the boundaries between the role of the Registered Nurse and the healthcare support worker (Hopwood 2010). This is currently decided locally.

Vigilance

Aiken *et al.* (2002) further emphasized the essential role of the Registered Nurse, describing them as 'the surveillance

> **Box 1.4** Five components of vigilance and how this manual can help the nurse to develop them
>
> 1 *Attaching meaning to what is:* this is described as the ability to differentiate 'adverse signals' indicating danger from the ordinary 'noise' – the normal signs and symptoms. Developing theoretical and professional knowledge is an important part of learning to identify these signals. The reference material in the introductory chapters is essential to developing an understanding of the underlying physiological function or psychological response of the individual so the nurse understands what is normal.
> 2 *Anticipating what might be:* observe, as the normal procedures and responses are described so the abnormal becomes more apparent.
> 3 *Calculating risks:* understanding that there is an inherent risk in every situation. Problem-solving sections help to increase risk awareness and knowledge of the implications of untoward situations associated with procedures.
> 4 *Readiness to act:* developed from a knowledge base, this allows the nurse to know what might be required in a situation and to make sure interventions can be carried out quickly when necessary. The manual has been written by experts who are sharing years of experience of carrying out the procedures. Therefore they know what equipment is needed, have knowledge of the potential problems that might occur and, over time, they have built up solutions to address them.
> 5 *Monitoring the results of interventions:* experts writing chapters have made explicit the source of the rationale for steps in the intervention process, that is, professional knowledge.

system'. It is not just the actions of taking the vital signs, dressing the wound or starting the intravenous drip, it is also 'the watchfulness' that is always part of the nurse's thinking process while activities such as these are completed (Meyer and Lavin 2005). This has been described as vigilance. Vigilance is the search for signals (Lancaster 1998), which are events that the individual determines to be indicators of something significant. Vigilance is not seen; it is only an action that occurs as the result of watching out for and responding to the signals that will suggest to others that vigilance has been happening. Meyer and Lavin (2005) propose that vigilance has five components (Box 1.4).

Benefit of registered nurses delivering care

If qualified nurses deliver care there is also an increased opportunity for patients to benefit from therapeutic nursing. Evidence demonstrates that this does contribute positively to the patient's experience of care (Spilsbury and Meyer 2001). As well as this often hidden aspect of nursing being essential to organizations, it is also essential for patients as they want to feel secure with the nurses caring for them (Williams and Irurita 2004). They want to be assured that the nurses have the ability to assess their needs as individuals as well as recognizing their personal limitations and potential risks.

Advanced practice nursing and other role developments

The other group of nurses whose roles are changing in respect of creating a safer, more efficient health service are those in advanced practice roles. 'Advanced practice' is an umbrella term relating to the skills, knowledge, expertise and attitudes that are firmly grounded in clinical practice, and encompasses aspects of education, research, consultation and case management (Hawkins and Holcombe 1995, NMC 1999, Royal Marsden NHS Trust 2003).

Initially, the *New Deal* for junior doctors (NHSME 1991) began the debate about the areas of medical practice that could be carried out by nurses, with bold statements being made about the potential cost savings (Richardson and Maynard 1995). With the publication of *The Scope of Professional Practice* (UKCC 1992), procedures previously carried out by doctors became the responsibility of nurses and new advanced practice roles evolved. The new advanced practice senior clinical roles such as clinical nurse specialists, nurse consultants and nurse practitioners ensure that experienced and highly skilled nurses stay close to patient care (DH 2006a). The Chief Nursing Officer's 'ten key roles' for nurses in England (DH 2000) provided the legitimacy and authority needed to assume new responsibilities, such as the freedom to admit and discharge patients or order diagnostic investigations. In practice, this means that nurses are undertaking numerous procedures that are more invasive and complex than 30 years ago when the first edition of this manual was published. Specific advanced practice procedures have been made explicit in the manual (Table 1.3).

One of the challenges of advanced practice roles has been assessing competence at this higher level of practice (Lillyman 1998). Benner's (1984) model of skill acquisition offers a framework to define the development from novice through to clinical expert. This and her subsequent work (Benner *et al.* 1996) have been used extensively to articulate the qualities that distinguish an expert nurse and to define expert nursing care. This framework has been used to develop role development profiles, tools that:

> Support competence acquisition in relation to role developments, enabling individuals to take responsibility for planning, managing and evaluating learning and to provide the opportunity for the individual to maintain a record of their own developing competence.
> (Royal Marsden Hospital 2004)

Those activities that have not previously fallen within the scope of nursing practice and for which the nurse has not received education and training may be considered to be role developments. Procedure guidelines are integral to role development and are part of the process of ensuring clinical effectiveness in 'doing the right thing the right way'. Within the UK, there are constant challenges for employers to define and manage these roles because currently there is no national legislative statement of what constitutes an advanced practitioner. This also has implications for the

Table 1.3 Examples of a advanced practice procedures included in the manual

Procedure	Chapter
Urinary catheterization: male	6
Continent urinary diversion stoma drainage tubes: flushing	6
Digital rectal examination	6
Manual evacuation of faeces	6
Log rolling for suspected/confirmed cervical spine instability	7
Blood product request	8
Compression bandaging (standard multilayer)	9
Continuous positive airway pressure	10
Insertion of chest drain	10
Tracheostomy tube change	10
Arterial puncture: radial artery	11
Cervical uterine smear	11
Nasopharyngeal wash: syringe method	11
Nasopharyngeal wash: vacuum-assisted aspirate method	11
Bone marrow aspiration and trephine biopsy	12
Bone marrow harvest	12
Apheresis	12
Extravasation: performing flush-out following an extravasation	15
Cytotoxic therapy: intravesical instillation of cytotoxic drugs	15
Peripheral cannula insertion	18
PICC	18
Implanted ports: insertion and removal of non-coring needles	18
Suturing a simple wound	19

general public as any nurse can call themselves an advanced practitioner.

The NMC initiated national consultation on this aspect of nursing practice in 2005, with the intention of establishing a specific part of the Register for nurses who were functioning as advanced practitioners. In February 2007, a White Paper was published, *Trust, Assurance and Safety – the Regulation of Health Professionals in the Twenty-First Century* (DH 2007a), stating that 'where appropriate, common standards and systems should be developed across professional groups where this would benefit patient safety'. In response to this and the later review by the Council of Regulatory Excellence (2009), the Department of Health published *Advanced Level Nursing: A position statement* (DH 2010e) to assist employers in developing new advanced practice roles and posts and to provide a national benchmark for expected standards of advanced practice.

The benchmark developed by expert practitioners and drawing on previous international work in this area (Australian Nursing and Midwifery Council 2009; Canadian Nurses Association 2008; International Council of Nurses 2008; Scottish Government 2010) has four themes:

- clinical/direct care practice
- leadership and collaborative practice
- improving quality and developing practice
- developing self and others.

All the 28 elements of practice defined under these headings would be an expected part of the role of any nurse working explicitly at an advanced level.

Social factors

This section specifically looks at the current characteristics of society and how they affect the provision of nursing care. The most dominant characteristic currently affecting healthcare is the structure of the 60 million population of the United Kingdom (Office for National Statistics 2008); 16% are over 65 years of age and 2% of those are over 80 years. The NHS spends over 40% of its budget on people over 65 years of age (DH 2007b) so over 65% of those who use inpatient acute hospital services on any given day are older people. This has considerable implications for nursing. The *National Service Framework for Older People* (DH 2001) explicitly sets out standards of care for older people in the care environment.

The aim of Standard 4 of the National Service Framework is to 'ensure that older people receive the specialist help they need in hospital and that they receive the maximum benefit from having been in hospital'. It states explicitly that:

> Older people's care in hospital is to be delivered through appropriate specialist care and by hospital staff who have the right set of skills to meet their needs.
> (www.dh.gov.uk/dr_consum_dh/groups/
> dh_digitalassets/@dh/@en/documents/
> digitalasset/dh_4067211.pdf)

Where relevant, specific care for older people has been included in the manual. However, the principles listed in Box 1.5 are relevant to whatever procedure is being carried out with an older person.

With an increase in the percentage of the population who are older, there is an increase in adults who are vulnerable.

Safeguarding of vulnerable adults

Working with vulnerable people, nurses are likely to identify patients who have been or may be being abused. Many patients who report abuse are fearful as they do not know if they will be taken seriously or what the consequences will be. It may be more difficult to assess if abuse has occurred in a patient with impaired capacity but it should be acknowledged that their lack of capacity makes them more vulnerable. Since 2000 and the launch of *No Secrets* (DH 2000), all staff working with vulnerable patients have a duty to report any suspicions of abuse to the patient's local authority. *No Secrets* required local authorities to develop a multi-agency safeguarding policy as well as each organization having their own local arrangements. It is important to know what the local arrangements are and who to report any safeguarding concerns to within the organization.

Box 1.5 NMC guidelines for the care of the older person

Think People

Nurses capable of delivering safe and effective care for older people are:

- competent, with the right knowledge, skills, attitude and desire to care for older people
- assertive, prepared to challenge poor practice, attitudes and behaviour
- reliable, consistent and dependable
- empathic, compassionate and kind.

Think Process

Delivering quality care that promotes dignity by nurturing and supporting the older person's self-respect and self-worth.

- Communicating with the person, talking with them and listening to what they have to say.
- Assessing need in order to provide individualized care.
- Respecting the person's privacy and dignity.
- Working in partnership with the person, their family, carers and, of course, your colleagues.

Think Place

Diverse settings wherever care is provided for older people.

- Appropriate and safe environments in which to practise dignified care.
- Committed to equality and diversity, providing care in a non-discriminatory, non-judgemental and respectful way.
- With the resources, staff and equipment needed to do the job well.
- Leadership from managers capable of setting and maintaining standards of care and supporting their teams through training, development, supervision and reflection.

(NMC 2009)

No Secrets (DH 2000) is currently under review but it defines a vulnerable adult as a person over the age of 18 years 'who is or may be in need of community care services by reason of mental or other disability, age or illness; and who is or may be unable to take care of him or herself, or unable to protect him or herself against significant harm or exploitation' (DH 2000, p.8). Abuse is described as 'a violation of an individual's human and civil rights by any other person or persons' (DH 2000, p.8). Abuse occurs not only when harm is caused as a result of wilful intent and therefore we need to consider that issues such as neglect and poor practice can also constitute abuse and should be reported in the same way.

If abuse is identified or suspected, it is important to escalate it to the most appropriate person. As abuse in many cases is a criminal act, any evidence must also be kept safe.

Dignity

One of the principles of the NMC Code is: 'Make the care of people your first concern, treating them as individuals and respecting their dignity'. This involves:

- not discriminating in any way against those in your care
- treating people kindly and considerately
- acting as an advocate for those in your care, helping them to access relevant health and social care, information and support.

(NMC 2008b)

An aspect of care that is relevant to everybody but has been raised specifically in respect of the older person is that of dignity. When Milburn (Milburn *et al.* 1995, p.1094) asked patients what care they would like from a nurse, one of the responses was 'being acknowledged and treated as an individual'. Patients described this as being treated with respect, which meant kind, prompt care and regular contact from the nurses. Patients felt care was dignified not only when they were appropriately dressed or covered but also when there was adequate allocation of time, acknowledgement of their views and feelings and the demonstration of discretion and consideration of their feelings (Walsh and Kowanko 2002).

There has been much philosophical debate about the concept of dignity, particularly in the provision of care to a diverse population and the challenges of respecting the values, beliefs and practices of different cultures (Willis 1999), age groups and individuals (Coventry 2006). What does this mean in day-to-day nursing practice?

> The most powerful tool a nurse possesses to maintain and promote dignity is herself, to work with feelings, use them constructively to understand patients and to treat them as valid, worthy and important at a time when they are vulnerable. In order to promote the dignity of another, feelings need to be clarified and understood, to ensure interactions and interventions are patient focused.
>
> (Haddock 1996, p.931)

When performing a physical procedure for a patient, nurses can uphold the dignity of the patient by discussing with them:

- if they would like the procedure to take place
- when is the best time for the procedure to take place
- where they would like it to take place
- who they would like to be there
- if they need any medication before it begins
- if they have any questions
- how much information they would like about the procedure.

(Adapted from Price 2004)

Patients need to feel that they have an equal and influential role in their own healthcare. One of the drivers for nursing practice today is the expectations of patients: 'They are more knowledgeable and expect to be treated as partners and equals and to have choices and options available to them' (DH 2006a, p.6).

We know that patients want more than just a person who can carry out a series of procedures and interventions dictated by their medical condition. Recent research has explored what patients want from their nurse (Milburn *et al.* 1995, Williams and Iruita 2004). In these two studies, the interpersonal aspect of the nurse's role was emphasized as being high on the priority list for patients. From one perspective, the time to listen and talk, that is performing a social function, helps patients to feel respected and valued as human beings. The social interaction while intimate or difficult procedures are being carried out also provides a valuable distraction. As a patient recently commented, 'Having my chemo was so much better when it was given by a friendly chatty nurse, we talked and gossiped about all sorts'.

Specific therapeutic communication is also highly valued by patients:

> … I want them to listen to me when I need them. When I get bad news (about this cancer) I need somebody to sit and listen and to know they don't leave you when you get bad news. They take their time … when you are low, they are there.
>
> (Milburn *et al.* 1995, p.1096)

Frequently even this therapeutic conversation takes place while the nurse is involved in another procedure or care activity with the patient.

Patients also talk about the importance of the nurse in the 'little things'. Reflecting on an episode of hospital care for the treatment of cancer, K.B. Schwartz wrote in *The Boston Globe* that: 'It is quiet acts of humanity that have felt more healing than the high dose radiation and chemotherapy' (Schwartz 1995). These 'little things', such as changing soiled linen or cleaning up the leaking stoma bag, have been described by Darbyshire (1999) as having profound meaning for recovery and, indeed, for cure. He describes this as the essence of nursing, a caring praxis that includes the ability to be with another, sensitively minimizing embarrassing and humiliating experiences.

Practices such as these little, yet very complex, procedures are what helps a patient towards recovery. Giving baths and getting patients to the bathroom are often considered to be the basics of nursing, so are often taken for granted and their complexity and importance are often overlooked. It is when they are carried out by an experienced nurse purposefully and with a patient-centred approach that they make a difference to patients because of the nursing knowledge and skill that are drawn upon (Macleod 1994). The depth of knowledge of the patient and possibilities for recovery influences the timing, pacing and sustainability of action (Benner 1991). Knowledge of the patient is a key component of excellent nursing practice and must be drawn upon when any care activity or procedure is carried out.

Research by Williams and Irurita (2004) found that attention to these interpersonal therapeutic aspects of care provides emotional comfort for patients, which in turn helped patients to feel control over what was happening to them.

Therefore dignity exists when an individual is capable of exerting control over their own behaviour, surroundings and the way in which they are treated by others. They should be capable of understanding information and making decisions. They should feel comfortable with their physical and psychological status quo (Mairis 1994).

Consent

One of the principles in the NHS Constitution is:

> NHS services must reflect the needs and preferences of patients, their families and carers. Patients, their families and carers where appropriate will be involved and consulted on all decisions about their care and treatment.
>
> (DH 2010c, p.3)

The NHS Constitution (DH 2010c) also states that a patient has the right to accept or refuse treatment that is offered and not be given any physical examination or treatment unless they have given valid consent.

The Code (NMC 2008b) states that the nurses have a responsibility to ensure they gain consent and that they must:

- gain consent before treatment or care starts
- respect and support people's rights to accept or decline treatment or care
- uphold people's rights to be fully involved in decisions about their care
- be aware of the legislation regarding mental capacity
- be able to demonstrate that they have acted in someone's best interest if emergency care has been provided.

For consent to be valid, it must be given voluntarily by a competent person who has been appropriately informed and who has the capacity to consent to the intervention in question (NMC 2008c). This will be the patient or someone authorized to do so under a Lasting Power of Attorney (LPA) or someone who has the authority to make treatment decisions as a court-appointed deputy (DH 2009).

The validity of consent does not depend on a signature on a form. Written consent merely serves as evidence of consent. Although completion of a consent form is in most cases not a legal requirement, the use of such forms is good practice where an intervention such as surgery is to be undertaken (DH 2009).

If there is any doubt about the person's capacity to make a decision about consent, the nurse should determine whether or not the person has the capacity to consent to the intervention and that they have sufficient information to be able to make an informed decision (DH 2009). This should be done before the person is asked to sign the form. Documentation is necessary and the nurse should record all discussions relating to consent, details of the assessment of capacity, and the conclusion reached, in the patient's notes (NMC 2008c).

Obtaining consent is a process and not a one-off event (NMC 2008c). Usually the person undertaking the procedure should be the person seeking to obtain consent. There may be situations when a nurse has been asked to seek consent on behalf of other staff. Providing the nurse has had training for that specific area, they may seek to obtain consent (NMC 2008c).

As part of the nursing assessment, the nurse needs to establish if the person is able to read or write. If they are unable, they may be able to make their mark on the form to indicate consent. In this instance, it would be good practice for the mark to be witnessed by a person other than the clinician seeking consent, and for the fact that the person has chosen to make their mark in this way to be recorded in the case notes (DH 2009). The person can direct someone to sign the form on their behalf, but there is no legal requirement for them to do so. If consent has been given validly, the lack of a completed form is no bar to treatment, but a form can be important evidence of such consent (DH 2009).

Consent may be expressed by a person verbally, in writing or by implying (NMC 2008c); an example of implied consent would be where a person, after receiving appropriate information, holds out an arm for their blood pressure to be taken. The nurse should ensure that the person has understood what examination or treatment is intended, and why, for such consent to be valid (DH 2009). It is good practice to obtain written consent for any significant procedure, such as a surgical operation or when the person participates in a research project or a video recording (NMC 2008c).

A competent adult may refuse to consent to treatment or care and nurses must respect that refusal (NMC 2008c).

Mental capacity

The Mental Capacity Act (2005) defines a person who lacks capacity as one who is unable to make a decision for themselves because of an impairment or disturbance in the functioning of their mind or brain. This can be temporary or permanent (DH 2009). Every adult must be presumed to have the mental capacity to consent or refuse treatment (NMC 2008c).

An assessment of a person's capacity must be based on their ability to make a specific decision at the time it needs to be made and not their ability to make decisions in general (DH 2009). A person is unable to make a decision if they cannot do one or more of the following things:

- understand the information given to them that is relevant to the decision
- retain that information long enough to be able to make the decision
- use or weigh up the information as part of the decision-making process
- communicate their decision – this could be by talking or using sign language and includes simple muscle movements such as blinking an eye or squeezing a hand.

(DH 2009)

Where a person lacks the capacity to make a decision for themselves, any decision must be made in that person's best interests (DH 2009).

Patients may have capacity to consent to some interventions but not to others, or may have capacity at some times but not others. Under the Mental Capacity Act, a person must be assumed to have capacity unless it is established that they lack capacity (DH 2009). If there is any doubt, then the healthcare professional should assess the capacity of the patient to take the decision in question (NMC 2010). This assessment and the conclusions drawn from it should be recorded in the patient's notes. Guidance on assessing capacity is given in Chapter 4 of the Mental Capacity Act Code of Practice (2005).

Capacity should not be confused with a healthcare professional's assessment of the reasonableness of the person's decision (DH 2009). A person is entitled to make a decision which may be perceived by others to be unwise or irrational, as long as they have the capacity to do so (NMC 2010). All practical and reasonable measures should be taken to assist the person in making the decision.

Working with patients with learning disabilities

Two significant reports produced in the last few years have an important message for all providers of care to people with learning disabilities: in particular, *Death by Indifference* (Mencap 2007) and the Local Government and Parliamentary Health Service Ombudsmen's response to this report, *Six Lives: The Provision of Public Services for People With Learning Disabilities* (House of Commons 2009). These identified many deficits in health and social care provision to six patients with learning disabilities. As a result of these reports, hospitals and other care providers are being asked to look at how they meet the needs of patients with learning disabilities and ensure there are clear and robust systems for identifying and addressing the needs of this patient group.

It is important to recognize that people with learning disabilities may have additional needs when attending or coming into hospital. We need to work with the patient, their family and carers to identify what additional care and support the patient requires. In doing so, we need to consider the implication of the Mental Capacity Act principles, in particular the presumption of capacity. The information then needs to be shared with all staff who provide care to the patient. This will enable continuity of care and prevent the patient or their carers from having to continually repeat the information to new care providers.

Hospitals need to work with their community partners to facilitate good communication between them both before and after admission and through any ongoing care for people with learning disabilities. For instance, if a patient with learning disabilities is to be admitted to hospital and the Community Learning Disability Nurse has a care plan on how to manage the patient's epilepsy or what their likes and dislikes are, then sharing that information and using the community nurse specialist's professional knowledge and expertise can only help to improve the care provided to the patient. It is therefore beneficial to nurses to know what their local organization arrangements are as well as what community services are available for people with learning disabilities.

Equality and diversity

Another characteristic of the UK population is the diversity of colour, nationality, ethnic origin, religious beliefs and faith, sexual orientations and marital and partnership status. In April 2010, the Equality Act received Royal Assent, providing streamlined law that can be used more effectively to tackle inequalities and discrimination. This law is particularly applicable to all public bodies, including the NHS. There is an expectation that there will be an explicit commitment to equality, diversity and human rights throughout the health and social care system. At strategic level, this means moving towards a single equality scheme; that is, a patient-centred and multifaceted approach is taken to the provision of all services, processes and policy development rather than an approach that puts people into boxes, which can have the effect of ignoring other differences. A generic approach to tackling health inequalities provides the opportunity to review all functions and policies, and to begin embedding equality into the commissioning and provision of services (DH 2010b). In practical terms as nurses, this may mean:

- co-operating with each other and social care organizations to ensure that patients' individual needs are properly managed
- having systems in place to ensure that you are treating patients, their relatives and carers with dignity and respect
- the views of patients, their carers and others are sought and taken into account in designing, planning, delivering and improving healthcare services
- all patients can equally access and have choice in access to services and treatment equitably.

(Adapted from DH 2005)

The competencies expected of every nurses associated with equality and diversity are articulated explicitly in the *NHS Knowledge and Skills Framework* (DH 2004b) (Table 1.4).

Equality Impact Assessment

As part of the commitment to treating all patients equally, all public organizations are legally required to perform an Equality Impact Assessment (EIA). In its simplest form, the EIA process can be seen as a foundation tool for measuring the effect of policy and practice on people and should encourage greater openness about policy making and service development.

An EIA is a means of ensuring that any policy introduced does not affect one or more groups of people, including staff, patients, carers and other users of the organization's services, in an adverse way. EIAs help to identify discrimination by requiring policy and service developers to think about how their policy or service will affect service users and staff and what actions or improvements to it may be required to ensure fairer access to services and employment (Box 1.6).

The outcome of the EIA for this manual will be available on the website of both the Royal Marsden NHS Foundation Trust and the Royal Marsden Manual (www.royalmarsden-manual.com).

Technical factors

The impact of rapid advances in technology on the roles and process of nursing will be considered here. Most obviously, this means that more effective treatments as well as the ability to provide care in different settings are now available (DH 2006a).

Competence

For the nurse, the competencies required in the technical area are increasing. Milburn (Milburn *et al.* 1995), probably not unsurprisingly, found that patients considered that a good nurse is one who knows what she is doing.

The NMC states that:

- you must have the knowledge and skills for safe and effective practice without supervision
- you must keep your knowledge and skills up to date throughout your working life
- you must recognize and work within the limits of your competence.

(NMC 2008a)

Table 1.4 The NHS Knowledge and Skills Framework dimension: equality, diversity and rights

Dimension	Level descriptions			
Core (will relate to all NHS posts)	1	2	3	4
Equality, diversity and rights	Ensure own actions support equality, diversity and rights	Support people's equality, diversity and rights	Promote people's equality, diversity and rights	Enable people to exercise their rights and promote their equality and diversity

Adapted from the *NHS Knowledge and Skills Framework and Development Review Guidance,* Working Draft, version 6, (2003), p.9.
© Crown copyright. Reproduced under the terms of the Click-use Licence.

Box 1.6 Equality impact assessment tool used to assess the procedures in the manual

Section 1

Full title of chapter being screened	
Chapter owner	
Date	
Name and title of people completing Equality Checklist	

Could the Chapter have an impact on staff, patients, carers or other members of the public?

Yes Please complete the rest of the Equality Checklist.
No Please return the Equality Checklist as above

Section 2

What are the purpose and the aims of the Chapter?
Who is intended to benefit from the Chapter and how?

Section 3

Is there any potential or evidence that the Chapter will or could:

Affect people from any social group differently to others?	Yes	No
Discriminate unlawfully against any social group?	Yes	No
Affect the relations between any social groups?	Yes	No
Prevent the Trust from achieving the aims of its Equality and Diversity policy?	Yes	No

If Yes, please identify which potential social groups could be affected.

There is an expectation that on qualifying, the nurse will have the competence to carry out fundamental procedures.

Competence is defined in the dictionary as having 'The ability to do something successfully or efficiently' (Pearsall 1998, p.374). There is considerable debate as to what is needed to achieve this, whether it is just technical ability to perform a skill or whether associated knowledge and the appropriate attitude are also important (Arthur *et al*. 2001, Darbyshire 1999, Musk 2004, Ray 1987). However, the NMC states that a registered nurse 'must have the knowledge and skills for safe and effective practice when working without direct supervision' (NMC 2008a).

This manual has been structured to enable nurses to develop competence, recognizing that competence is not just about knowing how to do something but also about understanding the rationale for doing it and the impact it may have on the patient.

Developing skills

Competence develops over time. Benner's (1984) model of skill acquisition offers a framework to define the development from novice through to clinical expert. Based on the Dreyfus model (1982), which distinguishes between the level of skilled performance that can be achieved through principles and theory based in the classroom and context-dependent judgements and skill that can only be acquired in real situations, the manual is relevant to competence development at all levels.

- *Stage 1: Novice*. As a novice, the related *anatomy and physiology*, *related theory and preprocedural considerations* will provide 'objective attributes' (Benner 1984), that is, knowledge of features of the task that can be gained away from the situation, for example understanding of venous anatomy of the arm. The procedures will give 'context-free rules' (Benner 1984) to guide actions that are not determined by the patient as an indivdual. This is the first step to technical competence (Ray 1987).
- *Stage 2: Advanced beginner*. The advanced beginner is one who has got some clinical experience and can use the *evidence-based approaches* to understand what they have seen in practice and the procedures as a reminder of the steps to follow to undertake a procedure. Chapters 2 and 5 will also be important at this stage to introduce the nurse to professional aspects of care that are essential in carrying out any procedure holistically as they progress to becoming a competent practitioner.
- *Stage 3: Competent*. At this stage, the nurse should be familiar with carrying out core procedures, but they may need to develop problem-solving skills in respect of specific procedures. The *problem-solving tables* and *complications sections* will help them to develop these skills.
- *Stage 4: Proficient*. Proficient nurses perceive situations as a whole. They will have integrated knowledge, skills and attitudes (Benner 1984). The manual will provide a useful reference to alert them to changes in practice and using the *evidence-based approaches* sections will heighten their awareness of the new evidence underpinning practice.
- *Stage 5: Expert*. The manual will be useful to the expert to highlight areas where further research needs to be done to establish the evidence underpinning practice. It will also be a useful reference to guide them as they learn those procedures that are new to their role.

Developing new roles has obvious risks attached to it and although every individual nurse is accountable for their own actions, every healthcare organization has to take vicarious liability for the care, treatment and procedures that take place. An organization will have expectations of all its nurses in respect of keeping patients, themselves and the environment safe. There are the obvious ethical and moral reasons for this: 'Nurses have a moral obligation to protect those we serve and to provide the best care we have available' (Wilson 2005, p.118). So there is an increasing requirement to demonstrate competencies in specific areas. This has become part of the risk management process of an NHS organization.

Evidence-based practice

The moral obligation described above extends to the evidence upon which we base our practice. Nursing now exists in a healthcare arena that routinely uses evidence to support decisions and practice and nurses must justify their rationales for practice. Where historically, nursing and specifically clinical procedures were based on rituals rather than research (Ford and Walsh 1994, Walsh and Ford 1989), evidence-based practice (EBP) now forms an integral part of practice, education, management, strategy and policy. Best Research for Best Health (DH 2006b) outlines a health research strategy to ensure practice is underpinned by world-class research. Building research evidence that ranges from prevention of ill health, promotion of health, disease management, patient care, delivery of healthcare and its organization to public health and social care is essential in striving to improving health (DH 2006b). Critical appraisal of research and evidence is also essential for healthcare staff to understand and appropriately carry out evidence-based practice.

Nursing care must be appropriate, timely and based on the best available evidence. NHS staff now have open access to these resources to facilitate EBP, which increases the likelihood of the care that is delivered to patients being based upon evidence of what works (Rycroft-Malone *et al.* 2004a). Defining and exploring the concept of EBP should help to further clarify the expectations that nurses now have to meet.

What is evidence-based practice?

This has been described by Sackett, a pioneer in introducing EBP in UK healthcare, as:

> ... the conscientious, explicit and judicious use of current best evidence in making decisions about the care of the individual patients. The practice of evidence-based medicine means integrating individual clinical expertise with the best available external clinical evidence from systematic research.
>
> (Sackett *et al.* 1996, p.72)

Despite the emphasis on research in EBP, it is important to note that where research evidence is lacking, other forms of evidence can be equally informative when making decisions about practice. Evidence-based practice goes much wider than research-based practice and encompasses clinical expertise as well as other forms of knowing, such as those outlined in Carper's seminal work (1978) on nursing. These include:

- empirical evidence
- aesthetic evidence
- ethical evidence
- personal evidence.

This issue is evident throughout this manual where clinical expertise and guidelines inform the actions and rationale of the procedures. Indeed, these other types of evidence are highly important as long as we can still apply scrutiny to their use. Porter (2010) describes a wider empirical base upon which nurses make decisions and argues for nurses to take into account and be transparent about other forms of knowledge such as ethical, personal and aesthetic knowing, echoing Carper (1978). By doing this, and through acknowledging limitations to these less empirical forms of knowledge, nurses can justify their use of them to some extent. Furthermore, in response to Paley's (2006) critique of EBP as a failure to holistically assess a situation, nursing needs to guard against cherry-picking, ensure EBP is not brandished ubiquitously and indiscriminately and know when judicious use of, for example, experiential knowledge (as a form of personal knowing) might be more appropriate.

Greenhalgh (2002), another EBP pioneer, describes later developments in the evidence-based medicine (EBM) and EBP movement and how intuitional and clinical knowledge was allowed its place.

Medicine and nursing have undoubtedly been shaped in recent years by the move toward EBP and the pressure to revisit and review practice regularly. Traynor (2009) discussed how nursing, as well as lower status groups in medicine, embraced the shift to EBP as an exercise in the 1990s and suggested that this may be in part due to nurses' status as a profession and the subsequent desire to acquire technical knowledge. Regardless of what the impetus has been for nursing to adopt EBP as integral to its practice, the use of evidence is now widespread, expected and accepted practice.

Evidence-based nursing (EBN) and EBP are differentiated by Scott and McSherry (2009) in that EBN involves additional elements in its implementation. Evidence-based nursing is regarded as an ongoing process by which evidence is integrated into practice and clinical expertise is critically evaluated against patient involvement and optimal care (Scott and McSherry 2009). For nurses to implement EBN, four key requirements are outlined:

- to be aware of what EBN means
- to know what constitutes evidence
- to understand how EBN differs from EBM and EBP
- to know how to engage with and apply the evidence.
  (Scott and McSherry 2009)

We contextualize our information and decisions to reach best practice for patients and the ability to use research evidence and clinical expertise together with the preferences and circumstances of the patient to arrive at the best possible decision for that patient is recognized (Guyatt *et al.* 2004).

Leaders of EBP such as Greenhalgh and Sackett have changed their focus away from solely the evidence of effectiveness through research to consider other areas of evidence (Greenhalgh 2002, Paley 2006, Traynor 2009). Thus the evidence required today to support all of these principles needs to come from a range of sources, as proposed by Higgs and Jones, who consider that evidence should be: 'Knowledge derived from a variety of sources that has been subjected to testing and has been found to be credible' (Higgs and Jones 2008, p.311). Credibility, as raised above, is a key issue (McKenna *et al.* 2000, Scott and McSherry 2009). As such, the emphasis and value of expert opinion highlighted here should in no way allow nurses to disregard research evidence (McKenna *et al.* 2000). Moreover, nurses' and midwives' professional code now insists on use of best available evidence (NMC 2008b).

Knowledge can be gained that is both propositional, that is from research and generalizable, and non-propositional, that is implicit knowledge derived from practice (Rycroft-Malone *et al.* 2004b). In more tangible, practical terms, evidence bases can be drawn from a number of different sources, and this pluralistic approach needs to be set in the context of the complex clinical environment in which nurses work in today's NHS (Pearson *et al.* 2007, Rycroft-Malone *et al.* 2004b). The evidence bases can be summarized under four main areas.

1 Research.
2 Clinical experience/expertise/tradition.
3 Patient, clients and carers.
4 The local context and environment.
   (Pearson *et al.* 2007, Rycroft-Malone *et al.* 2004b)

These four areas can also be regarded as corresponding to the empirical, personal, ethical and aesthetic categories of evidence which Carper (1978) espoused. What can be regarded as evidence to facilitate clinical decision making needs further consideration. When making clinical decisions, clinicians use evidence that relates to the four principal interests of:

■ *feasibility*: practical and possible
■ *appropriateness*: fits or is suitable for a situation
■ *meaningfulness*: personal experience, opinions, values of the patient
■ *effectiveness*: achieves the intended outcome.
   (Pearson *et al.* 2007)

In the clinical environment, practitioners will draw upon and integrate these forms of evidence in order to deliver person-centred care, which underpins EBN. Of the sources of evidence available, research has been regarded as the best form. However, in some areas of nursing practice there is a lack of evidence available to support decisions made in practice (Pearson *et al.* 2007). In addition, there is also debate about the types of evidence available to support practice. Within nursing, qualitative research is the prevalent design used, whilst within the field of evidence-based practice there is the perception that quantitative evidence is superior to that which is qualitative (Rolfe and Gardner 2006), although this has been debated (Hewitt-Taylor 2003). Narrative, intuitional and clinical practices still have their place

with EBP, especially where evidence is lacking (Greenhalgh 1999, 2002). Indeed, there are different opinions on the value of different types of research for EBP and it is important to consider, as Mulhall suggests, that: 'No single design has precedence over another, rather the design chosen must fit the particular research question' (Mulhall 1998, p.5). In practice, this can be a challenge and there will continue to be debate and discussion on the relative merits of different research designs in evidence-based practice. This will be discussed further when considering the grading of evidence.

Clinical experience and expertise play a fundamental role in terms of evidence-based nursing and practice. However, there remains some contention in relation to the terminology, role and status within the literature (Rolfe and Gardner 2006, Pearson *et al.* 2007). A clear distinction is apparent between experience, as a source of knowledge or evidence, and expertise, which is the application of evidence to practice, but these terms are often used interchangeably. A nurse may have many years of experience, been qualified for 20 years, but may not have developed knowledge as a result of this and thus is not able to apply this to develop expertise when making decisions related to her clinical practice. On the other hand, a nurse may have both experience and expertise but these are difficult to capture, make explicit and ensure they are verified for a wider audience (Rycroft-Malone *et al.* 2004b). Expert opinion does have a role both within hierarchies of evidence and within the definitions of evidence-based practice, although it is often regarded as poorer evidence compared to research (Rolfe and Gardner 2006). Guidelines and consensus practices may be informed by expert opinion. What is perhaps most important is the blending of this knowledge with research and the sharing of this with others to contribute to evidence-based decision making in practice (Rycroft-Malone *et al.* 2004b).

The involvement of patients in decision making about their own care and wider consultation in relation to the development of services within the NHS is a principle that has been developed and supported by the Department of Health in relation to healthcare generally and cancer care more specifically (DH 1995, 2000, 2010a). Individual experiences and preferences should be central to the practice of evidence-based healthcare and recent policy has tried to address this with a specific strategy to ensure inclusion through cancer care (DH 2010a). However, the inclusion of the patient's values, experiences and preferences into evidence-based practice can be complicated and difficult to achieve (Rycroft-Malone *et al.* 2004b). For example, a patient may request a new treatment but the research evidence may not be there to support it. This is particularly contentious, with the role of the National Institute for Health and Clinical Excellence (NICE) being to appraise treatments upon which subsequent funding decisions are based. Equally, the patient may decline a treatment for which there is research evidence because in their experience, it has unwelcome side-effects. We now have a policy driver (DH 2010a) to encourage us to work towards the patient and carer having a greater role in the decision and care they receive. We must also be mindful that without patient participation, the research we use as evidence to underpin our practice would not be possible (Staley 2009).

The context within which healthcare is delivered, whilst not traditionally recognized as a base for evidence, has been suggested to contain sources of evidence that would impact upon evidence-based patient care (Rycroft-Malone *et al.* 2004b). This is clinical knowledge from clinical experience and professional practice. Practitioners will draw upon both local and national sources to underpin their practice and these would include, for example, policies, patient stories, cultural context and professional networks. For some, it may include the use of some of the procedures contained in this edition. Moreover, in today's NHS in cancer and other specialties, it is evident that NICE guidance, the NHS Cancer Plan, published patient stories, patient satisfaction surveys and other sources will influence the delivery of patient care. What we have yet to determine is how to appraise and integrate this systematically into the evidence-based agenda in which we work.

Systems and challenges of grading evidence

Within the arena of evidence-based practice today, we must assess the quality of the evidence before it is used to inform practice. Hierarchies of evidence have been developed by a range of individuals and organizations in an attempt to identify the 'best' evidence to inform a particular decision that needs to be made in relation to a particular treatment, procedure or area of practice (Sackett *et al.* 2000). A key underlying assumption of using such a system is that not all evidence is equivalent (Rycroft-Malone 2006) and the quality of the evidence base therefore needs to be judged in some way. Making such judgements about evidence is complex and difficult to achieve. However, an explicit approach, as will be found in this manual, may help to facilitate critical appraisal of these judgements, provide confidence when applying evidence in practice and improve communication of this information (Grade Working Group 2004).

As Mantzoukas' (2009) review of nursing research within the hierarchies of evidence recently outlined, one of the challenges for nursing is that many of the hierarchies of evidence do not consider some of the evidence bases discussed in this chapter and put a lower value on research evidence that is not a meta-analysis or cluster randomized controlled trial (CRCT). To address this problem, some writers such as Rolfe and Gardner (2006) have sought to challenge this and move from an 'exclusive' hierarchy to an 'inclusive' hierarchy that does not only consider evidence from research programmes but considers all sources of evidence together. How this is achieved is under discussion in the literature, so in the interim we have established, after much debate, a process to grade the procedures in this edition which captures all the evidence bases, not only the research.

Grading evidence in The Royal Marsden Hospital Manual of Clinical Nursing Procedures

The evidence underpinning all the procedures has been reviewed and updated. To reflect the current trends in EBP, the evidence presented to support the procedures within this edition of *The Royal Marsden Hospital Manual of Clinical Nursing Procedures* has been graded, with this grading made explicit to the reader. The rationale for the system adopted will now be outlined.

As we have seen, there are many sources of evidence and ways of grading evidence and this has led us to a decision to consider both of these factors when referencing the procedures. You will therefore see that references will identify if the source of the evidence was from:

- clinical experience (Dougherty and Lamb 2008, E)
- patient (Diamond 1998, P)
- context and guidelines (DH 2010a, C)
- research (Fellowes *et al.* 2004, R).

If there is no written evidence to support a clinical experience or guidelines as a justification for undertaking a procedure, the text will be referenced as an 'E' but will not be preceded by an author's name.

For the evidence that comes from research, this referencing system will be taken one step further and the research will be graded using a hierarchy of evidence. The levels that have been chosen are adapted from Sackett *et al.* (2000) and can be found in Box 1.7.

Taking the example above of Fellowes *et al.* (2004), this is a systematic review of RCTs from the Cochrane Centre and so would be identified in the references as: Fellowes *et al.* (2004, R1a).

Through this process we hope that the reader will be able to more clearly identify the nature of the evidence upon which the care of patients is based and that this will assist when using these procedures in practice. You may also like to consider the evidence base for other procedures and policies in use in your own organization.

Box 1.7 Levels of evidence

1a Systematic reviews of RCTs.
1b Individual RCTs with narrow confidence limits.
2a Systematic reviews of cohort studies.
2b Individual cohort studies and low-quality RCTs.
3a Systematic reviews of case–control studies.
3b Case–control studies.
4 Case series and poor-quality cohort and case–control studies.
5 Expert opinion.

RCTs, randomized controlled trials.
(Adapted from Sackett *et al.* 2000).

Implementing evidence in practice

The implementation of evidence in practice in an organization, be that at a local level in a ward, throughout a hospital or in the community, can be demanding and requires planning, determination and time and the participation of individuals, teams and the organization to effect this change. It is beyond the scope of this chapter to cover the process in detail but some key factors to consider in the successful implementation of EBP are the evidence which has been explored in detail in this chapter, the context and facilitation (Rycroft-Malone *et al.* 2002, Scott and McSherry 2009). It can be useful to consider questions such as: how appropriate is the research to your group of patients/families/staff? Will the proposed research answer the issues you have? Is it transferable and is it justified to implement it? Did the design meet the stated research question and was the design appropriate? Was it methodologically rigorous?

Implementation of evidence in practice is most likely to occur when evidence is robust and inclusive, the context is receptive to change and the process is facilitated by someone who has the skills to effect change. Practice development teams in organizations are well placed to assist with the implementation of evidence in practice but the onus is also in the individual nurse who has a professional, moral and ethical duty to ensure that their practice is up to date, and who needs to willingly engage and apply evidence to practice.

Conclusion

This chapter has discussed the current context of healthcare, identifying the issues that influence the use and development of nursing procedures in the delivery of patient-centred care. The procedures in this book affect the whole person. They range from those that are observational and physically non-invasive to those involving intrusion into both the physical body and the psychological persona. The intent also varies; some are diagnostic, others therapeutic and some are supportive with the aim of increasing well-being. This chapter seeks to remind you of the importance of seeing procedures not just as tasks but as part of the whole for the patient.

It is important to remember that even if a procedure is very familiar to us and we are very confident in carrying it out, it may be new to the patient, so time must be taken to explain it and gain consent, even if this is only verbal consent. The diverse range of technical procedures that patients may be subjected to should act as a reminder not to lose sight of the unique person undergoing such procedures and the importance of individualized patient assessment in achieving this.

Website

www.nhs.uk/choiceintheNHS/Rightsandpledges/
NHSConstitution/Documents/COI_NHSConstitution
WEB2010.pdf.

When a nurse
Encounters another
What occurs is never a neutral event
A pulse taken
Words exchanged
A touch
A healing moment
Two persons
Are never the same.

(Anon in Dossey *et al.* 2005)

Nurses have a central role to play in helping patients to manage the demands of the procedures described in this manual. It must not be forgotten that for the patient, the clinical procedure is part of a larger picture, which encompasses an appreciation of the unique experience of illness. Alongside this we need to be mindful of the evidence upon which we are basing the care we deliver. We hope that through increasing the clarity with which the evidence for the procedures in this edition is presented, you will be better able to underpin the care you deliver to your patients in your day-to-day practice.

References

Aiken, L.H., Clarke, S.P., Sloane, D.M., Sochalski, J. and Silber, J.H. (2002) Hospital nurse staffing and patient mortality, nurse burnout and job dissatisfaction. *JAMA*, 288 (16), 1987–1993.

Arthur, D., Pang, S. and Wong, T. (2001) The effect of technology on the caring attributes of an international sample of nurses. *International Journal of Nursing Studies*, 38 (1), 37–43.

Australian Nursing and Midwifery Council (2009) *Nurse Practitioners: Standards and Criteria for the Accreditation of Nursing and Midwifery Courses Leading to Registration, Enrolment, Endorsement and Authorisation in Australia—with Evidence Guide.* www.anmc.org.au/userfiles/ANMC_Nurse_Practitioner(1).pdf

Barr, J. and Dowding, L. (2008) *Leadership in Healthcare.* Sage, Thousand Oaks, CA.

Benner, P.E. (1991) The role of experience, narrative, and community in skilled ethical comportment. *Advanced Nursing Science*, 14 (2), 1–21.

Benner, P.E. (1984) *From Novice to Expert : Excellence and Power in Clinical Nursing Practice.* Addison-Wesley, Menlo Park, CA.

Benner, P.E., Tanner, C.A. and Chesla, C.A. (1996) *Expertise in Nursing Practice: Care, Clinical Judgment and Ethics.* Springer, New York.

Canadian Nurses Association (2008) *Advanced Practice: A National Framework.* www.cna-aiic.ca/CNA?documents/pdf/publications/ANP_National_Framework_e.pdf

Carper, B. (1978) Fundamental patterns of knowing in nursing. *ANS Advances in Nursing Science*, 1 (1), 13–23.

Centre for Health Economics (2003) *Improving the Effectiveness of the Nursing Workforce: Short Report of Analysis of NISCM Data Set.* University of York, Centre for Health Economics, York.

Council for Regulatory Excellence (2009) *Advanced Practice: Report to the four UK Health Departments.* Unique ID 17/2008. www.chre.org.uk

Coventry, M.L. (2006) Care with dignity: a concept analysis. *Journal of Gerontological Nursing*, 32 (5), 42–48.

Darbyshire, P. (1999) Nursing, art and science: revisiting the two cultures. *International Journal of Nursing Practice*, 5 (3), 123–131.

Darzi, Lord (2008) *High Quality Care for All: NHS Next Stage Review Final Report.* Department of Health, London.

DH (1995) *Improving the Quality of Cancer Services*. Department of Health, London.

DH (2000) *No Secrets: Guidance on Developing and Implementing Multi-Agency Policies and Procedures to Protect Vulnerable Adults from Abuse*. Department of Health, London.

DH (2001) *National Service Framework for Older People*. Department of Health, London.

DH (2004a) *A Matron's Charter: An Action Plan for Cleaner Hospitals*. Department of Health, London.

DH (2004b) *NHS Knowledge and Skills Framework*. Department of Health, London.

DH (2005) *Promoting Equality and Human Rights in the NHS – A Guide for Non-Executive Directors of NHS Boards*. Department of Health, London.

DH (2006a) *Modernising Nursing Careers*. Department of Health, London.

DH (2006b) *Best Research for Best Health*. Department of Health, London.

DH (2007a) *Trust, Assurance and Safety – the Regulation of Health Professionals in the Twenty-First Century*. Department of Health, London.

DH (2007b) *A Recipe for Care – Not a Single Ingredient*. Department of Health, London.

DH (2009) *Reference Guide to Consent for Examination of Treatment*, 2nd edn. Department of Health, London.

DH (2010a) *The Handbook to the NHS Constitution*. Department of Health, London.

DH (2010b) White Paper. *Equity and Excellence: Liberating the NHS*. Department of Health, London.

DH (2010c) *The NHS Constitution: The NHS Belongs to Us All*. Department of Health, London.

DH (2010d) *Revision to the Operating Framework for the NHS in England 2010/11*. Department of Health, London.

DH (2010e) *Advanced Level Nursing: A Position Statement*. Department of Health, London.

Diamond, J. (1998) *C: Because Cowards Get Cancer Too*. Vermilion, London.

Dossey, B.M., Keegan, L. and Guzzetta, C.E. (2005) *Holistic Nursing: A Handbook for Practice*, 4th edn. Jones and Bartlett, Sudbury, MA.

Dougherty, L. and Lamb, J. (2008) *Intravenous Therapy in Nursing Practice*, 2nd edn. Blackwell Publishing, Oxford.

Dreyfus, S.E. (1982) Formal models vs human situational understanding: inherent limitations on modelling of business expertise, in *From Novice to Expert: Excellence and Power in Clinical Nursing Practice* (ed. P.E. Benner). Addison-Wesley, Menlo Park, CA, pp.133–155.

Fellowes, D., Wilkinson, S. and Moore, P. (2004) Communication skills training for health care professionals working with cancer patients, their families and/or carers. *Cochrane Database of Systematic Reviews*, 2, CD003751.

Ford, P. and Walsh, M. (1994) *New Rituals for Old: Nursing Through the Looking Glass*. Butterworth-Heinemann, Oxford.

Grade Working Group (2004) Grading quality of evidence and strength of recommendations. *BMJ*, 328, 1490–1498.

Greenhalgh, T. (1999) Narrative based medicine: narrative based medicine in an evidence based world. *BMJ*, **318** (7179), 323–325.

Greenhalgh, T. (2002) Intuition and evidence – uneasy bedfellows? *British Journal of General Practice*, **52** (478), 395–400.

Guyatt, G., Cook, D. and Haynes, B. (2004) Evidence based medicine has come a long way. *BMJ*, **329** (7473), 990–991.

Haddock, J. (1996) Towards further clarification of the concept 'dignity'. *Journal of Advanced Nursing*, **24** (5), 924–931.

Hawkins, J.W. and Holcombe, J.K. (1995) Titling for advanced practice nurses. *Oncology Nursing Forum*, **22** (8 Suppl), 5–9.

Healthcare Commission (2006) Investigation into outbreaks of *Clostridium difficile* at Stoke Mandeville Hospital. Healthcare Commission, London.

Healthcare Commision (2007) Investigation into outbreaks of *Clostridium difficile* at Maidstone and Tunbridge Wells NHS Trust. Healthcare Commission, London.

Hewitt-Taylor, J. (2003) Reviewing evidence. *Intensive and Critical Care Nursing*, **19** (1), 43–49.

Higgs, J. and Jones, M. A. (2008) *Clinical Reasoning in the Health Professions*, 3rd edn. Butterworth-Heinemann, Edinburgh.

Hopwood, L. (2010) A study to explore the contribution to patient care made by Registered Nurses and non-registered healthcare staff and their ability to understand their own and each other's roles (unpublished). Available from Greenwich School of Management. www.greenwich-college.ac.uk/.

House of Commons (2009) *Six Lives: The Provision of Public Services for People With Learning Disabilities*. Stationery Office, London.

International Council of Nursing (2010) The ICN definition of nursing. http://www.icn.ch/definition.htm.

Lillyman, S. (1998) Assessing competence, in *Advanced and Specialist Nursing Practice* (eds P. McGee and G. Castledine), Blackwell Science, Oxford, pp.119–129.

MacLeod, M. (1994) 'It's the little things that count': the hidden complexity of everyday clinical nursing practice. *Journal of Clinical Nursing*, 3 (6), 361–368.

Mairis, E.D. (1994) Concept clarification in professional practice – dignity. *Journal of Advanced Nursing*, **19** (5), 947–953.

McKenna, H., Cutcliffe, J. and McKenna, P. (2000) Evidence-based practice: demolishing some myths. *Nursing Standard*, **14** (16), 39–42.

Mantzoukas, S. (2009) The research evidence published in high impact nursing journals between 2000 and 2006: a quantitative content analysis. *International Journal of Nursing Studies*, 46 (4), 479–489.

Mencap (2007) *Death by Indifference*. MENCAP, London. www.mencap.org.uk/displaypagedoc.asp?id=284.

Mental Capacity Act (2005) Code of Practice. Stationery Office, London.

Meyer, G. and Lavin, M.A. (2005) Vigilance: the essence of nursing. *Online Journal of Issues in Nursing*, **10** (3), 8.

Milburn, M., Baker, M., Gardner, P., Hornsby, R. and Rogers, L. (1995) Nursing care that patients value. *British Journal of Nursing*, **4** (18), 1094–1099.

Musk, A. (2004) Proficiency with technology and the expression of caring: can we reconcile these polarized views? *International Journal for Human Caring*, 8 (2), 13–21.

NHS Institute of Innovation and Improvement (2009) *High Impact Actions for Nursing and Midwifery*. NHS Institute of Innovation and Improvement, London.

NHSME (1991) *Junior Doctors: The New Deal*. NHS Management Executive, London.

Nightingale, F. (1859) *Notes on Nursing*. JB Lippincott, Philadelphia.

NMC (1999) *Scope of Practice: A Higher Level of Practice*. Nursing and Midwifery Council, London.

NMC (2008a) *Accountability*. Nursing and Midwifery Council, London.

NMC (2008b) *The Code: Standards of Conduct, Performance and Ethics for Nurses And Midwives*. Nursing and Midwifery Council, London.

NMC (2008c) *Consent*. Nursing and Midwifery Council, London. www.nmc-uk.org/Nurses-and-midwives/Advice-by-topic/A/Advice/Consent.

NMC (2009) *Guidelines for Care of the Older Person.* Nursing and Midwifery Council, London.

NMC (2010) *Advice Sheet: Mental Capacity Act 2005.* Nursing and Midwifery Council, London.

O'Dowd, A. (2003) Who should perform the caring role? *Nursing Times,* 99 (10), 10–11.

Office for National Statistics (2008) News release: population grows to 61.4 million. www.statistic.gov.uk.

Paley, J. (2006) Evidence and expertise. *Nursing Inquiry,* 13 (2), 82–93.

Pearsall, J. (1998) *The New Oxford Dictionary of English.* Oxford University Press, Oxford, p. 374.

Pearson, A., Field, J. and Jordan, Z. (2007) *Evidence-Based Clinical Practice in Nursing and Health Care: Assimilating Research, Experience, and Expertise.* Blackwell Publishing, Oxford.

Porter, S. (2010) Fundamental patterns of knowing in nursing: the challenge of evidence-based practice. *ANS Advances in Nursing Science,* 33 (1), 3–14.

Price, B. (2004) Demonstrating respect for patient dignity. *Nursing Standard,* 19 (12), 45–51; quiz 52.

Ray, M.A. (1987) Technological caring: a new model in critical care. *Dimensions in Critical Care Nursing,* 6 (3), 166–173.

Richardson, G. and Maynard, A. (1995) *Fewer Doctors? More Nurses? A Review of the Knowledge Base of Doctor–Nurse Substitution.* Centre for Health Economics, University of Leeds, Leeds.

Rolfe, G. and Gardner, L. (2006) Towards a geology of evidence-based practice – a discussion paper. *International Journal of Nursing Studies,* 43 (7), 903–913.

Royal Marsden Hospital (2004) *Developing Your Role: A Guide for Nurses.* Royal Marsden NHS Foundation Trust, London.

Royal Marsden NHS Trust (2003) *Advanced Nursing Practice at the Royal Marsden NHS Trust 1999–2002.* Royal Marsden NHS Trust, London.

Rycroft-Malone, J. (2006) The politics of the evidence-based practice movements: legacies and current challenges. *Journal of Research in Nursing,* 11 (2), 95–109.

Rycroft-Malone, J., Harvey, G., Kitson, A. *et al.* (2002) Getting evidence into practice: ingredients for change. *Nursing Standard,* 16 (37), 38–43.

Rycroft-Malone, J., Harvey, G., Seers, K., Kitson, A., McCormack, B. and Titchen, A. (2004a) An exploration of the factors that influence the implementation of evidence into practice. *Journal of Clinical Nursing,* 13 (8), 913–924.

Rycroft-Malone, J., Seers, K., Titchen, A., Harvey, G., Kitson, A. and McCormack, B. (2004b) What counts as evidence in evidence-based practice? *Journal of Advanced Nursing,* 47 (1), 81–90.

Sackett, D.L., Strauss, S.E. and Richardson, W.S. (2000) *Evidence-Based Medicine: How to Practice and Teach EBM,* 2nd edn. Churchill Livingstone, Edinburgh.

Sackett, D.L., Rosenberg, W.M., Gray, J.A., Haynes, R.B. and Richardson, W.S. (1996) Evidence based medicine: what it is and what it isn't. *BMJ,* 312 (7023), 71–72.

Santry, C. (2010) We need to be clear about our primary responsibility. *Nursing Times,* 106 (4), 4–5.

Schwartz, K.B. (1995) A patient's story. *Boston Globe Magazine,* 16th July. www.theschwartzcenter.org/story/index.html.

Scott, K. and McSherry, R. (2009) Evidence-based nursing: clarifying the concepts for nurses in practice. *Journal of Clinical Nursing,* 18 (8), 1085–1095.

Scottish Government (2010) *Advanced Nursing Practice Roles: Guidance for NHS Boards.* www.knowledge.scot.nhs.uk/media/clt/ResourceUploads/188860/Advanced%20%Practice%20Guidance%20-%20Final_.pdf

Spilsbury, K. and Meyer, J. (2001) Defining the nursing contribution to patient outcome: lessons from a review of the literature examining nursing outcomes, skill mix and changing roles. *Journal of Clinical Nursing,* 10 (1), 3–14.

Staley, K. (2009) *Exploring Impact: Public Involvement in NHS, Public Health and Social Care Research.* INVOLVE, Eastleigh. www.invo.org.uk/pdfs/Involve_Exploring_Impactfinal28.10.09.pdf.

Traynor, M. (2009) Indeterminacy and technicality revisited: how medicine and nursing have responded to the evidence based movement. *Sociology of Health and Illness,* 31 (4), 494–507.

UKCC (1992) *The Scope of Professional Practice: A UKCC Position Statement.* United Kingdom Central Council for Nursing, Midwifery and Health Visiting, London.

Walsh, K. and Kowanko, I. (2002) Nurses' and patients' perceptions of dignity. *International Journal of Nursing Practice,* 8 (3), 143–151.

Walsh, M. and Ford, P. (1989) *Nursing Rituals, Research and Rational Actions.* Heinemann Nursing, Oxford.

Williams, A.M. and Irurita, V.F. (2004) Therapeutic and non-therapeutic interpersonal interactions: the patient's perspective. *Journal of Clinical Nursing,* 13 (7), 806–815.

Willis, W.O. (1999) Culturally competent nursing care during the perinatal period. *Journal of Perinatal and Neonatal Nursing,* 13 (3), 45–59.

Wilson, C. (2005) Said another way. My definition of nursing. *Nursing Forum,* 40 (3), 116–118.

Assessment, discharge and end of life care

The Royal Marsden Hospital Manual of Clinical Nursing Procedures, Eighth Edition. Edited by Lisa Dougherty and Sara Lister.
© 2011 The Royal Marsden Hospital. Published 2011 by Blackwell Publishing Ltd.

Overview

This chapter will give an overview of a patient's care from assessment through to discharge and will include care of the dying and procedures after death.

Assessment is considered to be the first step in the process of individualized nursing care. It provides information that is critical to the development of a plan of action that enhances personal health status. It also decreases the potential for, or the severity of, chronic conditions and helps the individual to gain control over their health through self-care (RCN 2004). Assessment forms an integral part of patient care and should be viewed as a continuous process.

Inpatient assessment and the process of care

Definition

Assessment is a systematic, deliberate and interactive process that underpins every aspect of nursing care (Heaven and Maguire 1996). It is the process by which the nurse and patient together identify needs and concerns. It is seen as the cornerstone of individualized care, a way in which the uniqueness of each patient can be recognized and considered in the care process (Holt 1995).

Related theory

Principles of assessment

The process of assessment requires nurses to make accurate and relevant observations, to gather, validate and organize data and to make judgements to determine care and treatment needs. A nursing assessment should have physical, psychological, emotional, spiritual, social and cultural dimensions, and it is vital that these are explored with the person being assessed. The patient's perspective of their level of daily activity functioning (Horton 2002) and their educational needs are essential to help maximize their understanding and self-care abilities (Alfaro-Lefevre 2002). It is only after making observations of the person and involving them in the process that the nurse can validate their perceptions and make appropriate clinical judgements.

Effective patient assessment is integral to the safety, continuity and quality of patient care and fulfils nurses' legal and professional obligations in practice. The main principles of assessment are outlined in Box 2.1.

Structure of assessment

Structuring patient assessment is vital to monitor the success of care and to detect the emergence of new problems. Different conceptual or nursing models, such as that of Roper *et al.* (2000), provide frameworks for a systematic approach

---

Box 2.1 Principles of assessment

1 Patient assessment is patient focused, being governed by the notion of an individual's actual, potential and perceived needs.
2 It provides baseline information on which to plan the interventions and outcomes of care to be achieved.
3 It facilitates evaluation of the care given and is a dimension of care that influences a patient's outcome and potential survival.
4 It is a dynamic process that starts when problems or symptoms develop, which continues throughout the care process, accommodating continual changes in the patient's condition and circumstances.
5 It is essentially an interactive process in which the patient actively participates.
6 Optimal functioning, quality of life and the promotion of independence should be primary concerns.
7 The process includes observation, data collection, clinical judgement and validation of perceptions.
8 Data used for the assessment process are collected from several sources by a variety of methods, depending on the healthcare setting.
9 To be effective, the process must be structured and clearly documented.

(Alfaro-Lefevre 2002, NMC 2008, Teytelman 2000, White 2003)

---

to assessment (such as Roper's Activities of Daily Living), implying that there is a perceived value in the co-existence of a variety of perspectives. There remains, however, much debate about the effectiveness of such models for assessment in practice, some arguing that individualized care can be compromised by fitting patients into a rigid or complex structure (Kearney 2001, Tierney 1998). Nurses therefore need to take a pragmatic approach and utilize assessment frameworks that are appropriate to their particular area of practice. This is particularly relevant in today's rapidly changing healthcare climate where nurses are taking on increasingly advanced roles, working across boundaries and setting up new services to meet patients' needs (DH 2006a).

Nursing models represent a set of concepts and statements integrated into a meaningful conceptual framework (Kozier *et al.* 2003) representing different theoretical approaches to nursing care.

Nursing models can serve as a guide to the overall approach to care within a given healthcare environment and therefore provide a focus for the clinical judgements and decision-making processes that result from the process of assessment. It has been argued that whilst nursing models have not been widely implemented in clinical practice, nurses do use them as a way to consider the process of nursing (Wimpenny 2001). During any patient assessment, nurses engage in a series of cognitive, behavioural and practical steps but do not always recognize them as discrete decision-making entities (Ford and McCormack 1999). Nursing models give novice practitioners a structure with which to identify these processes and to reflect on their practice in order to develop analytical, problem-solving and judgement skills needed to provide an effective patient assessment.

Nursing models have been developed according to different ways of perceiving the main focus of nursing. These include adaptation models (e.g. Roy 1984), self-care models (e.g. Orem *et al.* 2001) and activities of daily living models (e.g. Roper *et al.* 2000). Each model represents a different view of the relationship between four key elements of nursing: health, person, environment and nursing. It is important that the appropriate model is used to ensure the focus of assessment data collected is effective for particular areas of practice (Alfaro-Lefevre 2002, Murphy *et al.* 2000). Nurses must also be aware of the rationale for implementing a particular model since the choice will determine the nature of patient care in their day-to-day work. The approach should be sensitive enough to discriminate between different clinical needs and flexible enough to be updated on a regular basis (Allen 1998, Smith and Richardson 1996).

In the context of cancer care, the Cancer Action Team (2007) has published guidance for a holistic common assessment of the supportive and palliative care needs of adults with cancer. The content of the assessment is divided into five domains including background information and assessment preferences, physical needs, social and occupational needs, psychological well-being and spiritual well-being. The guidance recommends that a structured assessment should be undertaken at key points throughout the person's cancer illness trajectory, recognizing the importance of assessment as an ongoing process (Cancer Action Team 2007, NICE 2004).

Incorporating these key dimensions, the framework of choice at the Royal Marsden Hospital is based on Gordon's Functional Health Patterns (Gordon 1994; see Box 2.2). The framework facilitates an assessment that focuses on patients' and families' problems and functional status and applies clinical cues to interpret deviations from the patient's usual patterns (Johnson 2000). The model is applicable to all levels of care, allowing all problem areas to be identified. The information derived from the patient's initial functional

health patterns is crucial for interpreting both the patient's and their family's pattern of response to the disease and treatment. It is therefore considered particularly applicable for the cancer and palliative care settings where patients' needs and responses vary enormously along their illness trajectory.

Evidence-based approaches
Methods of assessment

Assessment information is collected in many different formats and consists of both objective and subjective data. Nurses working in different settings rely on different observational and physical data that may include assessment of vital signs, physical systems, symptoms and laboratory results. Subjective data are based on what the patient perceives and may include descriptions of their concerns, support network, their awareness and knowledge of their abilities/disabilities, their understanding of their illness and their attitude to and readiness for learning (Coyne *et al.* 2002, White 2003). A variety of methods have been developed to facilitate nurses in eliciting both objective and subjective assessment data on the assumption that if assessment is not accurate, all other nursing activity will also be inaccurate.

Studies of patient assessment by nurses are few but they indicate that discrepancies between nurses' perceptions and those of their patients are common (Brown *et al.* 2001, Lauri *et al.* 1997, McDonald *et al.* 1999, Parsaie *et al.* 2000). Communication is therefore key for, as Suhonen *et al.* (2000) suggest, 'there are two actors in individual care, the patient and the nurse' (p.1254). Gaining insight into patients' preferences and individualized needs is facilitated by meaningful interaction and depends both on patients' willingness and capability in participating in the process and nurses' interviewing skills. The initial assessment interview not only allows the nurse to obtain baseline information about the patient, but also facilitates the establishment of a therapeutic relationship (Crumbie 2006). Patients may find it difficult to disclose some problems and these may only be identified once the nurse–patient relationship develops and the patient trusts that the nurse's assessment reflects concern for their well-being.

Assessment interviews

An assessment interview needs structure to progress logically in order to facilitate the nurse's thinking (an example of such a structure can be found in Box 2.3) and to make the patient feel comfortable in telling their story. It can be perceived as being in three phases: the introductory, working and end phases (Crumbie 2006). It is important at the beginning to emphasize the confidential nature of the discussion and to take steps to reduce anxiety and ensure privacy since patients may modify their words and behaviour depending on the environment (Neighbour 1987).

In the middle working phase, various techniques can be employed to assist with the flow of information. Open questions are useful to identify broad information that can then be

---

Box 2.2 Gordon's functional health patterns

- Health perception–health management.
- Nutrition–metabolic.
- Elimination.
- Activity–exercise.
- Sleep–rest.
- Cognitive–perceptual.
- Self-perception–self-concept.
- Coping–stress tolerance.
- Role–relationship.
- Sexuality–reproductivity.
- Value–belief.

(Gordon 1994)

Box 2.3 Carrying out a patient assessment using functional health patterns

Pattern	Assessment and data collection are focused on
Health perception–management	■ The person's perceived level of health and well-being, and on practices for maintaining health. ■ Habits that may be detrimental to health are also evaluated. ■ Actual or potential problems related to safety and health management may be identified as well as needs for modifications in the home or for continued care in the home.
Nutrition and metabolism	■ The pattern of food and fluid consumption relative to metabolic need. ■ Actual or potential problems related to fluid balance, tissue integrity. ■ Problems with the gastrointestinal system.
Elimination	■ Excretory patterns (bowel, bladder, skin). ■ Excretory problems such as incontinence, constipation, diarrhoea and urinary retention may be identified.
Activity and exercise	■ The activities of daily living requiring energy expenditure, including self-care activities, exercise and leisure activities. ■ The status of major body systems involved with activity and exercise is evaluated, including the respiratory, cardiovascular and musculoskeletal systems.
Sleep and rest	■ The person's sleep, rest and relaxation practices. ■ Dysfunctional sleep patterns, fatigue, and responses to sleep deprivation may be identified.
Cognitive and perceptual ability	■ The ability to comprehend and use information. ■ The sensory functions, neurological functions.
Perception/concept of self	■ The person's attitudes toward self, including identity, body image and sense of self-worth. ■ The person's level of self-esteem and response to threats to their self-concept may be identified.
Stress and coping	■ The person's perception of stress and its effects on their coping strategies. ■ Support systems are evaluated, and symptoms of stress are noted. ■ The effectiveness of a person's coping strategies in terms of stress tolerance may be further evaluated.
Roles and relationships	■ The person's roles in the world and relationships with others. ■ Satisfaction with roles, role strain or dysfunctional relationships may be further evaluated.
Sexuality and reproduction	■ The person's satisfaction or dissatisfaction with sexuality patterns and reproductive functions. ■ Concerns with sexuality may be identified.
Values and belief	■ The person's values, beliefs (including spiritual beliefs) and goals that guide their choices or decisions.

(Adapted from Gordon 1994)

---

explored more specifically with focused questions to determine the nature and extent of the problem. Other helpful techniques include restating what has been said to clarify certain issues, verbalizing the implied meaning, using silence and summarizing (Morton 1993). It is important to recognize that there may be times when it is not possible to obtain vital information directly from the patient; they may be too distressed, unconscious or unable to speak clearly, if at all. In such situations, appropriate details should be taken from relatives or friends and recorded as such. Effort should equally be made to overcome language or cultural barriers by the use of interpreters.

The end phase involves a further summary of the important points and an explanation of any referrals made. In order to gain the patient's perspective on the priorities of care and to emphasize the continuing interest in their needs, a final question asking about their concerns can be used (Alfaro-Lefevre 2002). Examples include: 'Tell me the most important things I can help you with', 'Is there anything else you would like to tell me?', 'Is there anything that we haven't covered that still concerns you?' or 'If there are any changes or you have any questions, do let me know'.

Box 2.4 is a summary of the types of assessment.

Preprocedural considerations
Assessment tools

The use of assessment tools enables a standardized approach to be used to obtain specific patient data. This can facilitate the documentation of change over time and the evaluation of clinical interventions and nursing care (Conner and Eggert 1994). Perhaps more importantly, assessment tools encourage patients to engage in their care and provide a vehicle for communication to allow nurses to follow patients' experiences more effectively. An example of this comes from the European-wide cancer nursing WISECARE project (Kearney 2001). Nurses developed systematic measurements

Box 2.4 Types of patient assessment

- **Mini assessment**
  A snapshot view of the patient based on a quick visual and physical assessment. Consider patient's ABC (airway, breathing and circulation), then assess mental status, overall appearance, level of consciousness and vital signs before focusing on the patient's main problem.

- **Comprehensive assessment**
  An in-depth assessment of the patient's health status, physical examination, risk factors, psychological and social aspects of the patient's health that usually takes place on admission or transfer to a hospital or healthcare agency. It will take into account the patient's previous health status prior to admission.

- **Focused assessment**
  An assessment of a specific condition, problem, identified risks or assessment of care; for example, continence assessment, nutritional assessment, neurological assessment following a head injury, assessment for day care, outpatient consultation for a specific condition.

- **Ongoing assessment**
  Continuous assessment of the patient's health status accompanied by monitoring and observation of specific problems identified in a mini, comprehensive or focused assessment.

(Ahern and Philpot 2002, Holmes 2003, White 2003)

Box 2.5 Examples of assessment tools used in cancer care

Generic assessment tools

Cancer Rehabilitation Evaluation System (CARES) (Ganz *et al.* 1992).

Problems checklist (Osse *et al.* 2004).

Supportive Care Needs Survey (SCNS) (Bonevski *et al.* 2000).

Specific assessment tools

Piper Fatigue Scale (Piper 1997).

Oral assessment (Eilers *et al.* 1988).

Chemotherapy Symptom Assessment Scale (C-SAS) (Brown *et al.* 2001).

Pain and Assessment Records (PSAR) (Bouvette *et al.* 2002).

for four chemotherapy treatment-related symptoms and this enhanced care by directly linking nursing interventions to patients' reports of their experience. Improvements in outcomes were demonstrated and patients perceived their feelings and experience had been better considered in their treatment plan (Kearney 2001).

Assessment tools in clinical practice can be used to assess patients' general needs, for example the supportive care needs survey (Bonevski *et al.* 2000), or to assess a specific problem, for example the oral assessment guide (Eilers *et al.* 1988). The choice of tool depends on the clinical setting although in general, the aim of using an assessment tool is to link the assessment of clinical variables with measurement of clinical interventions (Frank-Stromborg and Olsen 2004). To be useful in clinical practice, an assessment tool must be simple, acceptable to patients, have a clear and interpretable scoring system and demonstrate reliability and validity (Brown *et al.* 2001).

Nurse researchers and clinicians have developed a broad spectrum of tools to assess the problems frequently encountered by patients (Box 2.5). More tools are used in practice to assess treatment-related symptoms than other aspects of care, possibly because these symptoms are predictable and of a physical nature and are therefore easier to measure. The most visible symptoms are not always those that cause most distress, however (Holmes and Eburn 1989), an acknowledgement of the patient's subjective experience is therefore an important element in the development of assessment tools (McClement *et al.* 1997, Rhodes *et al.* 2000).

The use of patient self-assessment tools appears to facilitate the process of assessment in a number of ways. It enables patients to indicate their subjective experience more easily, gives them an increased sense of participation (Kearney *et al.* 2000) and prevents them from being distanced from the process by nurses rating their symptoms and concerns (Brown *et al.* 2001). Many authors have demonstrated the advantages of increasing patient participation in assessment by the use of patient self-assessment questionnaires (Rhodes *et al.* 2000). A number of patient self-report tools have been developed for cancer patients as a result, and whilst many have been established for research purposes, an increasing number are being used very effectively in everyday clinical practice (Box 2.6).

The methods used to facilitate patient assessment are important adjuncts to assessing patients in clinical practice. There is a danger that too much focus can be placed on the framework, system or tool that prevents nurses thinking about the significance of the information that they are gathering from the patient (Harris *et al.* 1998). Rather than following assessment structures and prompts rigidly, it is essential that nurses utilize their critical thinking and clinical judgement throughout the process in order to continually develop their skills in eliciting information about patients' concerns and using this to inform care planning (Edwards and Miller 2001).

Box 2.6 Examples of specific patient self-assessment tools used in cancer care

- Self Report Health History (SRHH) (Skinn and Stacey 1994).
- Memorial Symptom Assessment Scale (MSAS) (Portenoy *et al.* 1994).
- Concerns Checklist in Oncology Outpatient Setting (Dennison and Shute 2000).
- Therapy Related Symptom Checklist (TRSC) (Williams *et al.* 2001).
- Social Problems Inventory (SPI) (Wright *et al.* 2001).
- Symptoms and Concerns Checklist (Lidstone *et al.* 2003).

Principles of an effective nursing assessment

The admitting nurse is responsible for ensuring that an initial assessment is completed when the patient is admitted. The patient's needs identified following this process then need to be documented in their care plan.

The following box (Box 2.7) discusses each area of assessment indicating points for consideration and suggesting questions that may be helpful to ask the patient as part of the assessment process.

Box 2.7 Points for consideration and suggested questions for use during the assessment process

1 Cognitive and perceptual ability

Communication

The nurse needs to assess the level of sensory functioning with or without aids/support such as hearing aid(s), speech aid(s), glasses/contact lenses, and the patient's capacity to use and maintain aids/support correctly. Furthermore, it is important to assess whether there are or might be any potential language or cultural barriers during this part of the assessment. Knowing what the norm within the culture will facilitate understanding and lessen miscommunication problems (Galanti 2000).

- *How good are the patient's hearing and eyesight?*
- *Is the patient able to express their views and wishes using appropriate verbal and non-verbal methods of communication in a manner that is understandable by most people?*
- *Are there any potential language or cultural barriers to communicating with the patient?*

Information

During this part of the assessment the nurse will assess the patient's ability to comprehend the present environment without showing levels of distress. This will help to establish whether there are any barriers to the patient understanding their condition and treatment. It may help them to be in a position to give informed consent.

- *Is the patient able and ready to understand any information about their forthcoming treatment and care? Are there any barriers to learning?*
- *Is the patient able to communicate an understanding of their condition, plan of care and potential outcomes/responses?*
- *Will he or she be able to give informed consent?*

Neurological

It important to assess the patient's ability to reason logically and decisively, and determine that he or she is able to communicate in a contextually, coherent manner.

- *Is the patient alert and orientated to time, place and person?*

Pain

To provide optimal patient care, the assessor needs to have appropriate knowledge of the patient's pain (Wilson 2007) and an ability to identify the pain type and location. Assessment of a patient's experience of pain is a crucial component in providing effective pain management. Dimond (2002) asserts that it is unacceptable for patients to experience unmanaged pain or for nurses to have inadequate knowledge about pain. Pain should be measured using an assessment tool that identifies the quantity and/or quality of one or more of the dimensions of the patient's experience of pain.

Assessment should also observe for signs of neuropathic pain including descriptions such as shooting, burning, stabbing, allodynia (pain associated with gentle touch) (Australian and New Zealand College of Anaesthetists 2005, Jensen *et al.* 2003, Rowbotham and Macintyre 2002).

- *Is the patient pain free at rest and/or on movement?*
- *Is the pain a primary complaint or a secondary complaint associated with another condition?*
- *What is the location of the pain and does it radiate?*
- *When did it begin and what circumstances are associated with it?*
- *How intense is the pain, at rest and on movement?*
- *What makes the pain worse and what helps to relieve it?*
- *How long does the pain last, for example, continuous, intermittent?*
- *Ask the patient to describe the character of pain using quality/sensory descriptors, for example, sharp, throbbing, burning.*

For further details regarding pain assessment, see Chapter 9.

2 Activity and exercise

Respiratory

Respiratory pattern monitoring addresses the patient's breathing pattern, rate and depth.

In this section it is also important to assess and monitor smoking habits. It is helpful to document the smoking habit in the format of pack-years. A *pack-year* is a term used to describe the number of cigarettes a person has smoked over time. One pack-year is defined as 20 manufactured cigarettes (one pack) smoked per day for 1 year. At this point in the assessment, it would be a good opportunity, if appropriate, to discuss smoking cessation. A recent meta-analysis indicates that if interventions are given by nurses to their patients with regard to smoking cessation the benefits are greater (Rice and Stead 2008).

- *Does the patient have any difficulty breathing?*
- *Is there any noise when they are breathing such as wheezing?*
- *Does breathing cause them pain?*
- *How deep or shallow is their breathing?*
- *Is their breathing symmetrical?*
- *Does the patient have any underlying respiratory problems such as COPD, emphysema, tuberculosis, bronchitis, asthma or any other airway disease?*

For further details, see Chapter 10.

Cardiovascular

A basic assessment is carried out and vital signs such as pulse (rhythm, rate and intensity) and blood pressure should be noted. Details of cardiac history should be taken for this part of the assessment. Medical conditions and previous surgery should be noted.

- *Does the patient take any cardiac medication?*
- *Does he/she have a pacemaker?*

For further information, see Chapter 13.

Physical abilities – personal hygiene/mobility/toileting – independence with the activities of daily living

The aim during this part of the nursing assessment is to establish the level of assistance required by the person to tackle activities of daily living such as walking and steps/stairs. An awareness of obstacles to safe mobility and dangers to personal safety is an important factor and part of the assessment.

The nurse should also evaluate the patient's ability to meet personal hygiene, including oral hygiene, needs. This should include the patient's ability to make arrangements to preserve standards of hygiene and the ability to dress appropriately for climate, environment and their own standards of self-identity.

- *Is the patient able to stand, walk and go to the toilet?*
- *Is the patient able to move up and down, roll and turn in bed?*
- *Does the patient need any equipment to mobilize?*
- *Has the patient good motor power in their arms and legs?*
- *Does the patient have any history of falling?*
- *Can the patient take care of their own personal hygiene needs independently or do they need assistance?*
- *What type of assistance do they need: help with mobility or fine motor movements such as doing up buttons or shaving?*

It might be necessary to complete a separate manual handling risk assessment – see Chapter 4.

For further information, see Chapters 7 and 9.

3 Elimination

Gastrointestinal

During this part of the assessment it is important to determine a baseline with regard to independence.

- *Is the patient able to attend to their elimination needs independently and is he/she continent? Are bowel movements within the patient's own normal pattern and consistency?*
- *What are the patient's normal bowel habits?*
- *Does the patient have any underlying medical conditions such as Crohn's disease or irritable bowel syndrome?*
- *Does the patient have diarrhoea or is he/she prone to or have constipation?*
- *How does this affect the patient?*

Genitourinary

The assessment is focused on the patient's baseline observations with regard to continence/incontinence. It is also important to note whether there is any penile or vaginal discharge or bleeding.

Does the patient have a urinary catheter *in situ*? If so, list the type and size. Furthermore, note the date the catheter was inserted and/or removed. Urinalysis results should also be noted here.

- *How often does the patient need to urinate? (Frequency)*
- *How immediate is the need to urinate? (Urgency)*
- *Do they wake in the night to urinate? (Nocturia)*
- *Are they able to maintain control over their bladder at all times? (Incontinence – inability to hold urine)*

See Chapter 6 for further information.

4 Nutrition

Oral care

As part of the inpatient admission assessment, the nurse should obtain an oral health history that includes oral hygiene beliefs, practices and current state of oral health. During this assessment it is important to be aware of treatments and medications that affect the oral health of the patient.

If deemed appropriate, use an oral assessment tool to perform the initial and ongoing oral assessment.

(Continued)

Box 2.7 (*Continued*)

During the admission it is important to note the condition of the patient's mouth.

- Lips – pink, moist, intact
- Gums – pink, no signs of infection or bleeding
- Teeth – dentures, bridge, crowns, caps

For full oral assessment, see Chapter 9.

Hydration

An in-depth assessment of hydration and nutritional status will provide the information needed for nursing interventions aimed at maximizing wellness and identifying problems for treatment. The assessment should ascertain whether the patient has any difficulty eating or drinking. During the assessment the nurse should observe signs of dehydration, for example dry mouth, dry skin, thirst or whether the patient shows any signs of altered mental state.

- *Is the patient able to drink adequately? If not, please explain why not.*
- *How much and what does the patient drink?*
- *Note the patient's alcohol intake in the format of units per week and the caffeine intake measured in the amount of cups per day.*

Nutrition

A detailed diet history provides insight into a patient's baseline nutritional status. Assessment includes questions regarding chewing or swallowing problems, avoidance of eating related to abdominal pain, changes in appetite, taste or intake, as well as use of a special diet or nutritional supplements. A review of past medical history should identify any conditions and highlight increased metabolic needs, altered gastrointestinal function and the patient's capacity to absorb nutrients.

- *What is the patient's usual daily food intake?*
- *Do they have a good appetite?*
- *Are they able to swallow/chew the food – any dysphagia?*
- *Is there anything they don't or can't eat?*
- *Have they experienced any recent weight changes or taste changes?*
- *Are they able to eat independently?*

(Arrowsmith 1999, DH 2005, Malnutrition Advisory Group 2000)

For further information, see Chapter 8

Nausea and vomiting

During this part of the assessment you want to ascertain whether the patient has any history of nausea and/or vomiting. Nausea and vomiting can cause dehydration, electrolyte imbalance and nutritional deficiencies (Marek 2003), and it can also affect a patient's psychosocial well-being. They may become withdrawn, isolated and unable to perform their usual activities of daily living.

Assessment should address questions such as:

- *Does the patient feel nauseous?*
- *Is the patient vomiting? If so, what is the frequency, volume, content and timing?*
- *Does nausea precede vomiting?*
- *Does vomiting relieve nausea?*
- *When did the symptoms start? Did they coincide with changes in therapy or medication?*
- *Does anything make the symptoms better?*
- *Does anything make the symptoms worse?*
- *What is the effect of any current or past antiemetic therapy including dose, frequency, duration, effect, route of administration?*
- *What is the condition of the patient's oral cavity?*

(Perdue 2005)

5 Skin

A detailed assessment of a patient's skin may provide clues to diagnosis, management and nursing care of the existing problem. A careful skin assessment can alert the nurse to cutaneous problems as well as systemic diseases. In addition, a great deal can be observed in a person's face, which may give insight to his or her state of mind.

- *Does the patient have any wounds or sore places on their skin?*
- *Does the patient have any dry or red areas?*

Furthermore, it is necessary to assess whether the patient has any wounds and/or pressure sores. If so, you would need to complete a further wound assessment. For further information about wound care, see Chapter 19.

6 Controlling body temperature

This assessment is carried out to establish baseline temperature and determine if the temperature is within normal range, and whether there might be intrinsic or extrinsic factors for altered body temperature. It is important to note whether any changes in temperature are in response to specific therapies (e.g. antipyretic medication, immunosuppressive therapies, invasive procedures or infection (Bickley 2007)). White blood count should be recorded to determine whether it is within normal limits. See Chapters 11 and 13 for further information.

- *Is the patient feeling excessively hot or cold?*
- *Have they been shivering or sweating excessively?*

7   Sleep and rest

This part of the assessment is carried out to obtain sleep and rest patterns and reasons for variation. Description of sleep patterns, routines and interventions applied to achieve a comfortable sleep should be documented. The nurse should also include the presence of emotional and/or physical problems that may interfere with sleep.

- *Does the patient have enough energy for desired daily activities?*
- *Does the patient tire easily?*
- *Has he/she any difficulty falling asleep or staying asleep?*
- *Does he/she feel rested after sleep?*
- *Does he/she sleep during the day?*
- *Does he/she take any aids to help them sleep?*
- *What are the patient's normal hours for going to bed and waking?*

8   Stress and coping

Assessment is focused on the patient's perception of stress and on his or her coping strategies. Support systems should be evaluated and symptoms of stress should be noted. It includes the individual's reserve or capacity to resist challenge to self-integrity, modes of handling stress. The effectiveness of a person's coping strategies in terms of stress tolerances may be further evaluated (adapted from Gordon 1994).

- *What are the things in the patient's life that are stressful?*
- *What do they do when they are stressed?*
- *How do they know they are stressed?*
- *Is there anything they do to help them cope when life gets stressful?*
- *Is there anybody who they go to for support?*

9   Roles and relationships

The aim is to establish the patient's own perception of the roles and responsibilities in their current life situation The patient's role in the world and their relationships with others are important to understand. Assessment in this area includes finding out about the patient's perception of the major roles and responsibilities they have in life, satisfaction or disturbances in family, work or social relationships. An assessment of home life should be undertaken which should include how they will cope at home post discharge from hospital and how home will cope while they are in hospital, for example dependants, animals or children and if there are any financial worries.

- *Who is at home?*
- *Are there any dependants (include children, pets, anybody else they care for)?*
- *What responsibilities does the patient have for the day-to-day running of the home?*
- *What will happen if they are not there?*
- *Do they have any concerns about home while they are in hospital?*
- *Are there any financial issues related to their hospital stay?*
- *Will there be any issues related to employment or study while they are in hospital?*

10   Perception/concept of self

Body image/self-esteem

Body image is highly personal, abstract and difficult to describe. The rationale for this section is to assess the patient's level of understanding and general perception of self. This includes their attitudes about self, perception of abilities (cognitive, affective or physical), body image, identity, general sense of worth and general emotional pattern. An assessment of body posture and movement, eye contact, voice and speech patterns should also be included.

- *How do you describe yourself?*
- *How do you feel about yourself most of the time?*
- *Has it changed since your diagnosis?*
- *Have there been changes in the way you feel about yourself or body?*

11   Sexuality and reproduction

Understanding sexuality as the patient's perceptions of their own body image, family roles and functions, relationships and sexual function can help the assessor to improve assessment and diagnosis of actual or potential alterations in sexual behaviour and activity.

Assessment in this area is vital and should include relevant feelings about the patient's own body, their need for touch, interest in sexual activity, how they communicate their sexual needs to a partner, if they have one, and the ability to engage in satisfying sexual activities.

(Continued)

30

Box 2.7 (*Continued*)

This may also be an opportunity to explore with the patient issues related to future reproduction if this is relevant to the admission. Below are a few examples of questions that can be used.

- *Are you currently in a relationship?*
- *Has your condition had an impact on the way you and your partner feel about each other?*
- *Has your condition had an impact on the physical expression of your feelings?*
- *Has your treatment or current problem had any effect on your interest in being intimate with your partner?*

12 Values and beliefs

Religious, spiritual and cultural beliefs

The aim is to assess the patient's spiritual, religious and cultural needs to provide culturally and spiritually specific care while concurrently providing a forum to explore spiritual strengths that might be used to prevent problems or cope with difficulties. Assessment is focused on the patient's values and beliefs, including spiritual beliefs or on the goals that guide his or her choices or decisions. A patient's stay in hospital may be influenced by their religious beliefs or other strongly held principles, cultural background, ethnic origin. It is important for nurses to have knowledge and understanding of the diverse cultures of their patients and take their different practices into account.

- *Are there any spiritual/cultural beliefs that are important to you?*
- *Do you have any specific dietary needs related to your religious, spiritual or cultural beliefs?*
- *Do you have any specific personal care needs related to your religious, spiritual or cultural beliefs (i.e. washing rituals, dress)?*

13 Health perception and management

Relevant medical conditions, side-effects/complications of treatment

Assessment of the patient's perceived pattern of health and well-being and how health is managed should be documented here. Any relevant history of previous health problems, including side-effects of medication, experienced previously should be noted. Examples of other useful information that should be documented are compliance with medication regimen, use of health promotion activities such as regular exercise and if the patient has annual check-ups.

- *What does the patient know about their condition and planned treatment?*
- *How would they describe their own current overall level of fitness?*
- *What do they do to keep well: exercise, diet, annual check-ups or screening?*

Postprocedural considerations
Decision making and nursing diagnosis

The purpose of collecting information through the process of assessment is to enable the nurse to make a series of clinical judgements, otherwise known as nursing diagnoses, and subsequently decisions about the nursing care each individual needs. The decision-making process is based upon the clues observed, analysed and interpreted and it has been suggested that expert nurses assess the situation as a whole and make judgements and decisions intuitively (King and Clark 2002, Hedburg and Satterlund Larsson 2003, Peden-McAlpine and Clark 2002), reflecting Benner's (1984) renowned novice-to-expert theory. However, others argue that all nurses use a logical process of clinical reasoning in order to identify patients' needs for nursing care and that, while this becomes more automatic with experience and perhaps more subconscious, it should always be possible for a nurse to explain how they arrive at a decision about an individual within their care (Gordon 1994, Putzier and Padrick 1984, Rolfe 1999). A further notion is that of a continuum, where our ability to make clinical judgements about our patients lies on a spectrum, with intuition at one end and linear, logical decisions (based on clinical trials, for example) at the other (Cader *et al.* 2005, Thompson 1999). Factors that may influence the process of decision making include time, complexity of the judgement or decision to be made, as well as the knowledge, experience and attitude of the individual nurse.

Nursing diagnosis is a term which describes both a clinical judgement that is made about an individual's response to health or illness, and the process of decision making that leads to that judgement; Box 2.8 illustrates the process of making a nursing diagnosis. The importance of thorough assessment within this process cannot be overestimated. The gathering of comprehensive and appropriate data from patients, including the meanings attributed to events by the patient, is associated with greater diagnostic accuracy and

---

Box 2.8 The process of nursing diagnosis

- Collect information using an appropriate assessment framework.
- Identify clusters of information and consider possible nursing judgements (nursing diagnoses).
- Collect further information to verify these judgements.
- Arrive at an accurate nursing judgement (nursing diagnosis).

(Gordon 1994, Tanner *et al.* 1987)

Box 2.9 Characteristics of conditions labelled as nursing diagnoses

1 Nurses can identify the condition through a process of diagnostic reasoning (assessment, problem identification).
2 The condition can be resolved primarily by nursing interventions.
3 Nurses assume accountability for patient/outcomes.
4 Nurses assume responsibility for research on the condition and its treatment.

(Gordon 1994)

---

thus more timely and effective intervention (Alfaro-Lefevre 2002, Gordon 1994, Hunter 1998).

The concept of a 'nursing diagnosis' has historically generated much debate within the nursing literature, and it is therefore important to clarify the difference between a nursing diagnosis and a patient problem or care need. 'Patient problems' or 'needs' are common terms used within nursing to facilitate communication about nursing care (Hogston 1997). As patient problems/needs may involve solutions or treatments from disciplines other than nursing, the concept of a 'patient problem' is similar to but broader than a nursing diagnosis. Nursing diagnoses describe problems that may be dealt with by nursing expertise (Leih and Salentijn 1994) (Box 2.9).

The term 'nursing diagnosis' also refers to a standardized nursing language, to describe patients' needs for nursing care, that originated in America over 30 years ago and has now been developed, adapted and translated for use in numerous other countries. The language of nursing diagnosis provides a classification of over 200 terms (NANDA-I 2009), representing judgements that are commonly made with patients/clients about phenomena of concern to nurses, enabling more consistent communication and documentation of nursing care (see Box 2.10 for an example of a nursing diagnosis).

Most significantly, the use of common language enables nurses to clearly and consistently express what they do for patients and why, making the contribution of different nursing roles clearly visible within the multidisciplinary care pathway (Delaney 2001, Elfrink *et al.* 2001, Grobe 1996, Moen *et al.* 1999). Secondly, an increasingly important reason for trying to structure nursing terms in a systematic way has been the need to create and analyse nursing information in a meaningful way for electronic care records (Clark 1999, Westbrook 2000). The term 'nursing diagnosis' is not commonly used within the UK as no definitive classifications or common languages are in general use; however, for the aforementioned reasons, the adaptation and implementation of standard nursing languages within clinical practice in the UK are being explored (Chambers 1998, Lyte and Jones 2001, Westbrook 2000).

Planning and implementing care

Nursing diagnoses provide a focus for planning and implementing effective and evidence-based care. This process consists of identifying nursing-sensitive patient outcomes and determining appropriate interventions that will enable the individual to reach their desired outcome. However, while nurses may gather valuable information through the assessment process, it is often the case that very little of this is translated into the documentation (Ford and Walsh 1994), resulting in the standard of care bearing little relationship to

---

Box 2.10 Example of a nursing diagnosis

Label

Definition
Provides a clear meaning of the diagnosis.

Acute pain: an unpleasant sensory and emotional experience associated with actual or potential tissue damage or described in terms of such damage (IASP 2007). Sudden or slow onset of any intensity from mild to severe with an anticipated or predictable end and a duration of <3 months.

Defining characteristics
Cues to determine if the condition or response described by the diagnosis is present for the patient/client.

For example:
- The patient states they have pain.
- Pain assessment: numerical rating scale (0–10) pain score >2.
- Evidence of noxious stimuli, e.g. surgery, trauma.
- Guarding of injury.
- Reduction in patient's normal mobility.

Refer to NANDA-I (2009) for a complete list of defining characteristics.

Related factors
Factors that contribute to the diagnosis being present. Individualized to each patient or client.

Injury agents (biological, chemical, physical, psychological).

(Adapted from NANDA-I 2009)

Box 2.11 Examples of measurable and non-measurable verbs for use in outcome statements

Measurable verbs (use these to be specific)

- State; verbalize; communicate; list; describe; identify.
- Demonstrate; perform.
- Will lose; will gain; has an absence of.
- Walk; stand; sit.

Non-measurable verbs (do not use)

- Know.
- Understand.
- Think.
- Feel.

(Alfaro-Lefevre 2002, pp.134–135)

the written documentation (Ballard 2006, Ford and Walsh 1994). Therefore, when planning care, it is vital:

- to determine the immediate priorities and recognize whether patient problems require nursing care or whether a referral should be made to someone else
- to identify the anticipated outcome for the patient, noting what the patient will be able to do and in what time frame. The use of 'measurable' verbs that describe patient behaviour or what the patient says facilitates the evaluation of patient outcomes (see Box 2.11)
- to determine the nursing interventions, that is, what nursing actions will prevent or manage the patient's problems so that the patient's outcomes may be achieved
- to record the care plan for the patient which may be written or individualized from a standardized/core care plan or a computerized care plan.

(Alfaro-Lefevre 2002, Shaw 1998, White 2003)

Outcomes should be patient focused and realistic, stating how the outcomes or goals are to be achieved and when the outcomes should be evaluated. Patient-focused outcomes centre on the desired results of nursing care, that is, the impact of care on the patient, rather than on what the nurse does. Outcomes may be short, intermediate or long term, enabling the nurse to identify the patient's health status and progress (stability, improvement or deterioration) over time. Setting realistic outcomes and interventions requires the nurse to distinguish between nursing diagnoses that are life-threatening or an immediate risk to the patient's safety and those that may be dealt with at a later stage. Identifying which nursing diagnoses/problems contribute to other problems (for example, difficulty breathing will contribute to the patient's ability to mobilize) will make the problem a higher priority. By dealing with the breathing difficulties, the patient's ability to mobilize will be improved.

The formulation of nursing interventions is dependent on adequate information collection and accurate clinical judgement during patient assessment. As a result, specific patient outcomes may be derived and appropriate nursing interven-

tions undertaken to assist the patient to achieve those outcomes (Hardwick 1998). Nursing interventions should be specific to help the patient achieve the outcome and should be evidence based. When determining what interventions may be appropriate in relation to a patient's problem, it may be helpful to clarify the potential benefit to the patient after an intervention has been performed, as this will help to ensure its appropriateness.

It is important to continue to assess the patient on an ongoing basis whilst implementing the care planned. Assessing the patient's current status prior to implementing care will enable the nurse to check whether the patient has developed any new problems that require immediate action. During and after providing any nursing action, the nurse should assess and reassess the patient's response to care. The nurse will then be able to determine whether changes to the patient's care plan should be made immediately or at a later stage. If there are any patient care needs that require immediate action, for example consultation or referral to a doctor, recording the actions taken is essential. Involving the patient and their family or friends will promote the patient's well-being and self-care abilities. The use of clinical documentation in nurse handover will help to ensure that the care plans are up to date and relevant (Alfaro-Lefevre 2002, White 2003).

Evaluating care

Effective evaluation of care requires the nurse to critically analyse the patient's health status to determine whether the patient's condition is stable, has deteriorated or improved. Seeking the patient's and family's views in the evaluation process will facilitate decision making. By evaluating the patient's outcomes, the nurse is able to decide whether changes need to be made to the care planned. Evaluation of care should take place in a structured manner and on a regular basis by a Registered Nurse. The frequency of evaluation depends on the clinical environment within which the individual is being cared for as well as the nature of the nursing diagnosis (problem) to which the care relates. Questions such as:

- What are the patient's self-care abilities?
- Is the patient able to do what you expected?
- If not, why not?
- Has something changed?
- Are you missing something?
- Are there new care priorities?

will help to clarify the patient's progress (Alfaro-Lefevre 2002, White 2003). It is helpful to consider what is observed and measurable to indicate that the patient has achieved the outcome.

Documenting

Nurses have a professional responsibility to ensure that healthcare records provide an accurate account of treatment, care planning and delivery, and are viewed as a tool of communication within the team. There should be 'clear evidence of the care planned, the decisions made, the care delivered and the information shared' (NMC 2009, p.8) (Box 2.12).

Box 2.12 The Royal Marsden Hospital guidelines for nursing documentation

General principles

1   Records should be written legibly in black ink in such a way that they cannot be erased and are readable when photocopied.
2   Entries should be factual, consistent, accurate and not contain jargon, abbreviations or meaningless phrases (e.g. 'observations fine').
3   Each entry must include the date and time (using the 24-hour clock).
4   Each entry must be followed by a signature and the name printed as well as:
    ■   the job role (e.g. staff nurse or clinical nurse specialist)
    ■   if a nurse is a temporary employee (i.e. an agency nurse), the name of the agency must be included under the signature.
5   If an error is made, this should be scored out with a single line and the correction written alongside with date, time and initials. Correction fluid should not be used at any time.
6   All assessments and entries made by student nurses must be countersigned by a Registered Nurse.
7   Healthcare assistants:
    ■   can write on fluid balance and food intake charts
    ■   who have demonstrated achievement of the learning outcomes for observing and monitoring the patient's condition as defined in *The Royal Marsden Hospital Health Care Assistant Role Assessment and Development Profile* (2001) can write on observation charts
    ■   must not write on prescription charts, assessment sheets, care plans or progress notes.

Assessment and care planning

1   The first written assessment and the identification of the patient's immediate needs must begin within 4 hours of admission. This must include any allergies or infection risks of the patient and the contact details of the next of kin.
2   The following must be completed within 24 hours of admission and updated as appropriate:
    ■   completion of nutritional, oral, pressure sore and manual handling risk assessments
    ■   other relevant assessment tools, for example pain and wound assessment.
3   All sections of the nursing admission assessment must be completed at some point during the patient's hospital stay with the identification of the patient's care needs. If it is not relevant or if it is inappropriate to assess certain functional health patterns, for example the patient is unconscious, then indicate the reasons accordingly.

   The ongoing nursing assessment should identify whether the patient's condition is stable, has deteriorated or improved.
4   Care plans should be written wherever possible with the involvement of the patient, in terms that they can understand, and include:
    ■   patient-focused, measurable, realistic and achievable goals
    ■   nursing interventions reflecting best practice
    ■   relevant core care plans that are individualized, signed, dated and timed.
5   Update the care plan with altered or additional interventions as appropriate.
6   The nursing documentation must be referred to at shift handover so it needs to be kept up to date.

Principles of assessment

■   Assessment should be a systematic, deliberate and interactive process that underpins every aspect of nursing care (Heaven and Maguire 1996).
■   Assessment should be seen as a continuous process (Cancer Action Team 2007).

Structure of assessment

■   The structure of a patient assessment should take into consideration the specialty and care setting and also the purpose of the assessment.
■   When caring for individuals with cancer, assessment should be carried out at key points during the cancer pathway and dimensions of assessment should include background information and assessment preferences, physical needs, social and occupational needs, psychological well-being and spiritual well-being (Cancer Action Team 2007).
■   Functional health patterns provide a comprehensive framework for assessment, which can be adapted for use within a variety of clinical specialties and care settings (Gordon 1994).

Methods of assessment

■   Methods of assessment should elicit both subjective and objective assessment data.
■   An assessment interview must be well structured and progress logically in order to facilitate the nurse's thinking and to make the patient feel comfortable in telling their story.
■   Specific assessment tools should be used, where appropriate, to enable nurses to monitor particular aspects of care, such as symptom management (e.g. pain, fatigue), over time. This will help to evaluate the effectiveness of nursing interventions whilst often providing an opportunity for patients to become more involved in their care (Conner and Eggert 1994).

(Continued)

34

Box 2.12 (*Continued*)

Decision making and nursing diagnosis

■ Nurses should be encouraged to provide a rationale for their clinical judgements and decision making within their clinical practice (NMC 2009).

■ The language of nursing diagnosis is a tool that can be used to make clinical judgements more explicit and enable more consistent communication and documentation of nursing care (Clark 1999, Westbrook 2000).

Planning and implementing care

■ When planning care, it is vital that nurses recognize whether patient problems require nursing care or whether a referral should be made to someone else.

■ When a nursing diagnosis has been made, the anticipated outcome for the patient must be identified in a manner which is specific, achievable and measurable (NMC 2009).

■ Nursing interventions should be determined in order to address the nursing diagnosis and achieve the desired outcomes (Gordon 1994).

Evaluating care

■ Nursing care should be evaluated using measurable outcomes on a regular basis and interventions adjusted accordingly (Box 2.10).

■ Progress towards achieving outcomes should be recorded in a concise and precise manner. Using a method such as charting by exception can facilitate this (Murphy 2003).

Documenting and communicating care

■ The content and quality of record keeping are a measure of standards of practice relating to the skills and judgement of the nurse (NMC 2009).

■ In addition to the written record of care, the important role that the nursing shift report, or 'handover', plays in the communication and continuation of patient care should be considered, particularly when considering the role of electronic records (Ballard 2006).

(Reproduced with kind permission of the Royal Marsden Hospital NHS Foundation Trust 2005)

The content and quality of record keeping are a measure of standards of practice relating to the skills and judgement of the nurse (NMC 2009).

Preoperative assessment

Definition

Preoperative assessment (also known as surgical preassessment, anaesthetic assessment, preoperative evaluation and preoperative screening) is defined as 'the clinical investigation that precedes anaesthesia for surgical or non-surgical procedures' (Garcia-Miguel *et al.* 2003). It is a process that is completed prior to surgery to help evaluate the risks to the patient attached to their upcoming surgery. It ideally allows time prior to the surgery to properly manage and optimize any co-morbidities that may affect the perioperative care of the patient. Because general anaesthesia is considered a risk to the patient, it is necessary to 'consider the patient's health and quality of life and to question whether the proposed benefits of surgery outweigh the attendant risks' (Avidan *et al.* 2003, p.4).

Related theory

Traditionally patients were admitted to hospital 1–2 days preoperatively to allow for the appropriate assessment, tests and investigations to be completed prior to their surgery. Once they were admitted, it was frequently found that patients were presenting with complicated, newly identified or inappropriately managed co-morbidities so surgery was often delayed or cancelled. It was also found that a large number of cancelled operations occurred because patients did not arrive for their scheduled operation fasted. Some did not arrive because the date provided was inconvenient (due to childcare or work-related concerns) or the surgery was no longer wanted or needed.

Preoperative assessment clinics were established to address these issues. It has been found that providing patients with a time and place to explore their concerns and gain the information they need has increased the attendance of patients and therefore made more effective use of operating theatre time and other associated resources (NICE 2003, p.32).

According to the *National Good Practice Guidance on Preoperative Assessment for Inpatient Surgery* (Modernisation Agency 2003), preoperative assessment clinics were created with several objectives in mind.

■ Provide the opportunity to further explain and discuss any information provided by the surgeon to the patient. This process should aid in minimizing any patient fears or anxieties, through ensuring that the patient understands the upcoming surgery, as well as what the recovery following the surgery will entail.

- Assist in the assessment of the patient's fitness for the surgery, as well as anaesthesia and postoperative recovery. This will provide information for a comprehensive assessment of the risks and benefits of the required surgery and anaesthesia. This comprehensive assessment allows the patient to make an informed decision with regard to the risks and benefits of the desired surgery.
- Identify any co-morbidities that may require intervention prior to admission and surgery. This should allow enough time to take appropriate action before admission to make changes to the patient's treatment regimen, such as discontinuation of anticoagulants or implementation of antihypertensive medications.
- Assist in ensuring that the patient is in optimum health prior to surgery, through further referrals to secondary care specialists as necessary, for example cardiologists.
- Perform necessary investigations prior to surgery and ensure that the results of these investigations are actioned (for example, haematological investigations).
- Identify the need for and arrange supply of any specialist equipment and special requirements for the postoperative period (for example, critical care beds, bariatric equipment).
- Provide information to the patient about any specific preoperative preparation that may be required (for example, fasting, bowel preparation). This may also include involving members of the multidisciplinary team such as clinical nurse specialists, physiotherapists or dietitians.
- Give the patient a point of contact for further questions or concerns, or if they want to postpone or cancel the surgery.
- Provide information to the patient on what they should anticipate in the postoperative period. This may include leaflets and videos to help the patient understand the planned procedure. This would also include discussion with the anaesthetist about pain control, intubation and potential critical care admission.
- Provide any assistance with health promotion activities such as smoking cessation, weight loss and alcohol use that will help to improve the outcome in the perioperative and postoperative periods. This may include further referrals to primary care services such as stop smoking services or dietetic advice.
- Identify any cultural, religious or communication needs for the patient.
- Identify any discharge planning needs prior to the date of admission. This will allow for the appropriate services to be contacted before admission, and facilitate a prompt discharge date.
- Provide the appropriate preoperative documentation for the multidisciplinary team.

Evidence-based approaches

The preoperative assessment (POA) should include a comprehensive medical history, physical examination and the ordering of appropriate investigations.

Principles of care

Principles table 2.1 provides an overview of issues to be considered. More detailed information can be found in the related references.

Principles table 2.1 Preoperative history taking

Principle	Rationale
Medical history Medical history should start with the history of the presenting illness. For the preoperative assessment, this starts with the reason why the patient is having the planned procedure. It is important to include how the patient first presented with the symptoms of the condition, and any treatments provided. Details of treatments such as previous chemotherapy or radiotherapy are important to obtain within the health history. A full history of current and previous medical problems should be taken. This would include any history of disorders such as diabetes mellitus, hypertension, asthma, epilepsy, strokes or cardiac symptoms such as chest pains or shortness of breath. It is valuable to obtain information such as dates of diagnosis, severity, treatments required and any history of hospitalizations for the disorders.	This information enables the assessor to document the scope of the disease, how well it is controlled and how it affects the patient's everyday life. It is through obtaining a comprehensive history of 'the patient's medical problems, previous surgeries, and responses to questions [that] set the framework for further enquiry to establish a complete history' (Sweitzer 2008, p.23).
Family history This includes assessment for common familial illnesses, such as hypertension, coronary artery disease, stroke, diabetes and hypercholesterolaemia.	This alerts the anaesthetist to potential medical problems.

(Continued)

Principles table 2.1 (*Continued*)

Principle	Rationale

Body system review
It is essential to assess each of the following body systems in more detail.
■ *Cardiovascular system*
   – Cardiac function.
   – History of cardiovascular disease such as ischaemia, anaemias and clotting disorders.
   – Blood pressure.
   – Patient's risk of thrombosis, excessive bleeding.
■ *Respiratory system*
   – History of respiratory disease such as asthma, chronic obstructive pulmonary disease.
   – Respiratory infections.
■ – *Gastrointestinal*
   – Digestive history.
   – Nutritional and BMI status.
   – Hepatic functioning.
   – Renal function including urination patterns.
■ *Central nervous system*
   – History of neurological disease such as epilepsy, transient ischaemic attacks.
   – Pain profile.
■ *Endocrine system*
   – Thyroid function.
   – Blood glucose levels measured with HbA_{1c} test.
   – History of any other endocrine disorder.
■ *Musculoskeletal system*
   – This should include a review of the range of movement and any musculoskeletal disease that may either give the patient pain or restrict their movement.
	It is important to assess each body system as this contributes to the information about the patient's overall health status.

Surgical and anaesthetic history Assessors must gather history of previous surgery. It is also important to find out about previous anaesthetic problems such as postoperative nausea and vomiting, as well as a history of malignant hyperthermia. The anaesthetic assessment also includes any cardiovascular, hepatic or pulmonary impairment, bleeding disorders, significant history of reflux or a hiatus hernia, breathing difficulties such as sleep apnoea, paroxysmal nocturnal dyspnoea or orthopnoea.	History of previous major surgeries or recent anaesthetics gives the assessor a good idea of the fitness of patient for the planned surgery. Identifying these factors is important in assessing the potential risk in performing the designated procedure on the patient. The American Society of Anesthesiologists (ASA) developed a scale with which to classify patients on the basis of their existing co-morbidities (see Table 2.1). The ASA status was developed to help identify potential risks, as it was shown that 'patient co-morbidity appears to be the most important factor in assessing the likelihood of an adverse outcome' (Tung 2008, p.4).
Medications and allergies A full list of the patient's current medications, including over-the-counter medications and vitamin and herbal supplements, is essential. If a patient is taking steroids or opiates, these require careful titration peri or postoperatively. Specific medications may need to be discontinued days or weeks prior to surgery (Figure 2.1). The patient's allergy status should be determined and specific details of reactions recorded. Medication 'intolerance' should also be documented to avoid severe side-effects such as nausea and vomiting.	Many medications interact with anaesthetic agents or will negatively affect the patient in the peri- or postoperative period. These include anticoagulants, diabetic medications, calcium channel antagonists, beta-blockers and some antidepressants.

Principle	Rationale
History of previous anaphylactic reactions should be thoroughly documented to avoid potential incidents. Patients who are allergic to latex will need to be first on the theatre list, and theatre staff will need to be alerted to avoid complications.	

Social history

Social history encompasses social situations such as home life and occupation.	Within the social history, the assessor develops a general idea about the social practices of the patient that may affect their fitness for surgery but also influence their recovery.
It is important to know about the patient's past and current *occupational* picture.	The patient's occupation will give the assessor a picture of not only the patient's home and financial situation, but also potential occupational disorders such as respiratory or musculoskeletal disorders.
Understanding the patient's *support systems* such as family or wider community is important. It is also necessary to explore smoking, drug and alcohol use.	This will allow the assessor to pick up on potential 'road blocks' for a timely discharge. If the patient is found to have little or no available support in the community, the assessor has the opportunity to initiate any discharge planning or Social Services referrals prior to admission. This allows for the patient to avoid any potential delays in their discharge.
Alcohol: it is imperative to communicate to the patient the importance of honesty with regard to alcohol or drug intake. Many patients will often admit to usage, but may deny they have excessive intake or a problem. It is important to assess the amount consumed on a daily or weekly basis. The maximum recommended consumption of alcohol for males is 28 units per week, and for females 21 units per week.	Long-term abuse of alcohol, tobacco products or drugs can lead to organ damage, related medical complications, and therefore a higher incidence of perioperative morbidity and mortality. Perioperative events such as delirium tremens are considered medical emergencies.
Smoking behaviour is important to assess. The length of time an individual has smoked, the number smoked a week, the pattern of their smoking, i.e. times of day, smoking with specific activities such as waking up, going to sleep or managing stress. Preoperative smoking cessation is important and help with this should be offered during the assessment. 'At least 8 weeks of abstinence is required for maximal benefit' (Fernandez Perez *et al.* 2008, p.137), but the beneficial effects of smoking cessation can be seen within as little as 12 hours (Fernandez Perez *et al.* 2008).	Smoking-related lung disease is prevalent in the UK with at least 26% of the population as known smokers. The extent of smoking-related effects is dependent upon the amount, and the length of time, of smoking. Smokers have hyper-reactive airways that lead them to become more susceptible to incidents of laryngospasm or bronchospasm. They have an increased chance of developing postoperative lung infections due to a compromised ability to clear secretions. Smoking also affects the liver, which may mean that the patient will require higher dosages of medications. Postoperative healing is also affected by smoking as nicotine is a vasoconstrictor. Long-term smoking leads to chronic obstructive pulmonary disease (COPD), peripheral vascular disease (PVD) and coronary artery disease (CAD) (Haddock and Burrows 1997).

Table 2.1 American Society of Anesthesiologists (ASA) physical status classification

Classification	Remarks
ASA 1	Healthy patient without organic, biochemical, or psychiatric disease
ASA 2	A patient with mild systemic disease (e.g. mild asthma, well-controlled hypertension). No significant impact on daily activity. Unlikely impact on anaesthesia and surgery
ASA 3	Significant or severe systemic disease that limits normal activity (e.g. renal failure on dialysis or class 2 congestive heart failure). Significant impact on daily activity. Likely impact on anaesthesia and surgery
ASA 4	Severe disease that is a constant threat to life or requires intensive therapy (e.g. acute MI, respiratory failure requiring mechanical ventilation). Serious limitation of daily activity. Major impact on anaesthesia and surgery
ASA 5	Moribund patient who is equally likely to die in the next 24 hours with or without surgery
ASA 6	Brain-dead organ donor

The Royal Marsden Foundation NHS Trust
Peri-operative Guidelines for Drug Therapy

■ Medication to Omit
□ Medication to Omit unless specifically asked to give by Doctor (see comments below)
▨ Medication to continue can be given up to 2 hours before surgery, with a sip of water

BNF Category	Drug Name / Group	Comments
Gastro-intestinal System	H₂ antagonists, e.g. ranitidine	
	Proton pump inhibitors, e.g. lansoprazole	
Cardiovascular System	Alpha antagonists, e.g. doxazosin	
	Anti-arrythmics, e.g. digoxin, amiodarone	
	Beta-blockers, e.g. atenolol	Avoid stopping suddenly. Continue iv if prolonged NBM
	Calcium antagonists, e.g. amlodipine	
	Loop & thiazide diuretics, e.g. furosemide, bendroflumethiazide	
	Nitrates, e.g. isosorbide mononitrate	
	ACE inhibitors, e.g. lisinopril	Consult Anaesthetist. May cause hypotension on induction of anaesthesia
	Angiostensin receptor II antagonists, e.g. losartan	Consult Anaesthetist. May cause hypotension on induction of anaesthesia
	Aspirin	If to be withheld, stop 7-10 days pre-op
	Clopidogrel	Stop 7 days pre-op unless Cardiologist states continue
	Dipyridamole	If procedure high risk, omit on day of surgery
	Low molecular weight heparin, e.g. tinzaparin, enoxaparin	Omit 12 hrs pre-op
	Potassium sparing diuretics, e.g. spironolactone, amiloride	Omit on day of surgery. May contribute to hyperkalaemia post-op
	Warfarin	Stop 3 days pre-op. If appropriate admit 3 days pre-op and start a heparin infusion until 4 hrs before surgery. Aim for APPT ratio < 1.5
Respiratory System	Aminophylline / Theophylline	
	Inhalers, e.g. salbutamol, beclometasone	
Central Nervous System	Anti-epileptics, e.g. phenytoin	
	Antipsychotics, e.g. haloperidol, risperidone	
	Benzodiazepines, e.g. diazepam	
	Opioid analgesics, e.g. morphine, methadone, codeine	Consult Anaesthetist to plan post-op analgesia
	Paracetamol	
	Parkinson's treatment, e.g. co-careldopa, co-beneldopa	
	Selective serotonin re-uptake inhibitors (SSRIs), e.g. paroxetine, fluoxetine	
	Anti-dementia drugs, e.g. donepezil, rivastigmine, galantamine (acetylcholinesterase inhibitors)	May prolong neuromuscular blockade and exaggerate muscle relaxation with succinylcholine-type muscle relaxants. Alert anaesthetist to the potential for prolonged neuromuscular blockade. Omit rivastigmine and glantamine 24-48 hours prior to surgery. It is recommended to stop donepezil 2-3 weeks prior to surgery; however these patients may not return to their baseline mental function, therefore may be unethical to stop
	Lithium	Check levels pre-op. Continue for minor surgery. Discuss with Anaesthetist plan for major surgery. Restart ASAP post-op
	Non-steroidal anti-inflammatory (NSAIDs), e.g. diclofenac, COX II inhibitors	Increased risk of bleeding. Can stop 1-3 days pre-op depending on half-life. Stop Piroxicam 7 days pre-op
	Tricyclic antidepressants, e.g. amitriptyline	Increased risk of arrhythmias. Consult Anaesthetist
	Clozapine	Stop 12 hrs pre-op. Restart ASAP. Contact pharmacy for advice
	Monoamine-oxidase inhibitors (non-reversible), e.g. phenelzine	Stop 14 days pre-op (discuss with Psychiatrist). If not withdrawn inform Anaesthetist
	Reversible MAOIs, e.g. moclobemide	Omit on day of surgery
Infections	Antibiotics	
	Anti-virals, e.g. HIV antiretroviral drugs, aciclovir	

Figure 2.1 Guide to preoperative medication. Reproduced with permission from Dr. David Chisholm, Anaesthetist, The Royal Marsden Hospital NHS Foundation Trust, 2010.

BNF Category	Drug Name / Group	Comments
Endocrine System	Corticosteroids, e.g. prednisolone (Current or stopped within last 3 months)	May need additional hydrocortisone bolus intra/post operation:- **Minor surgery**: 25mg hydrocortisone at induction (or usual oral dose) **Moderate surgery**: 25mg hydrocortisone at induction (or usual oral dose) then 25mg hydrocortisone TDS for 24 hours and then restart usual steroid dose **Major surgery**: 25mg hydrocortisone at induction (or usual oral dose) then 50mg TDS hydrocortisone for 48-72 hours and then restart usual steroid dose
	Desmopressin (DDAVP)	
	Hormone antagonists, e.g. tamoxifen, anastrozole	Thromboprophylaxis and TEDS
	Hormone replacement therapy (HRT)	Thromboprophylaxis and TEDS
	Levothyroxine	
	Progesterone only oral contraceptives	Thromboprophylaxis and TEDS
	Combined oral contraceptives (i.e. containing oestrogen)	Omit 4 weeks prior to major sugery institute thromboprophylaxis and TEDS. Advise on alternative family planning
	Glibenclamide, Glipizide, Gliclazide, Tolbutamide & Glitazones (e.g. pioglitazone)	Refer to Anaesthetist. Omit all oral hypoglycaemics on morning of surgery
	Insulin	Continue until morning of surgery. Omit morning dose & breakfast. **Minor surgery:** Re-start s/c insulin post-op with first meal. **Major surgery:** Omit breakfast and S/C insulin and start intravenous sliding scale insulin
	Metformin	Refer to Anaesthetist. Omit 48-72 hrs pre-op in patients with renal impairment
Malignant Disease & Immunosuppression	Drugs to prevent adverse effects, e.g. allopurinol	Seek advice from Oncologist/Haematologists
	DMARDS, e.g. methotrexate for Rheumatoid Arthritis	Continue unless at risk of renal complications. Discuss with specialist
	Immunosuppressants, e.g. azathioprine, ciclosporin	Seek advice from Oncologist/Haematologists
	Cytotoxics, e.g. alkylating agents, antimetabolites	Seek advice from Oncologist/Haematologists
Complementary Alternative Medicines	Echinacea (activates cell-mediated immunity allergic reactions, poor wound healing, increased risk of infection, reduced action of immunosuppressive medicines).	Discontinue as far in advance as possible before surgery
	Ephedra (causes dose-dependent increases in blood pressure and heart rate. Risk of MI and stroke from tachycardia and hypertension. Long-term use depletes endogenous catecholamines & may cause intraoperative haemodynamic instability. Interacts with MAOIs).	Discontinue 24 hrs before surgery
	Garlic (inhibits platelet aggregation (may be irreversible) so may increase risk of bleeding, especially when combined with other platelet inhibitors).	Discontinue at least 7 days before surgery
	Ginkgo (inhibits platelet activating factor so may increase risk of bleeding, especially when combined with other platelet inhibitors).	Discontinue at least 36 hrs before surgery
	Ginseng (lowers blood glucose & inhibits platelet aggregation so can lead to hypoglycaemia risk of bleeding. Platelet inhibition may be irreversible and increased).	Discontinue at least 7 days before surgery
	Kava (sedates and reduces anxiety so could increase sedative effect of anaesthetics. Has potential for tolerance).	Sedates & reduces anxiety Discontinue at least 24 hrs before surgery
	St John's Wort (inhibits neurotransmitter serotonin, norepinephrine and dopamine reuptake by neurons. Induces cytochrome P450 therefore concentrations of alfentanil, midazolam, and lidocaine may be reduced. Also reduces concentrations of digoxin, warfarin and ciclosporin).	Discontinue at least 5 days before surgery
	Valerian (sedates via modulation of GABA transmission and receptor function so increases the sedative effect of anaesthetics, especially those via GABA receptor e.g. midazolam. Long-term use could increase amount of anaesthetic required).	Reduce dose gradually over several weeks before surgery: risk of benzodiazepine-like withdrawal. If a patient is dependent on valerian, can be taken up until day of sugery. Benzodiazepines can be used to treat withdrawal in the post-operative period
Nutrition & Blood	Drugs for nutrition, e.g. iron, folic acid, calcium, magnesium	Continue unless specifically asked not to
This information applies to all types of surgery (minor or major). Please contact local pharmacy for administration advice if the patient requires a prolonged NBM period.		

Figure 2.1 (Continued)

Physical examination

Within the POA, baseline vital signs and a physical examination are essential and should be completed by a trained assessor. The physical examination should include specific attention to the respiratory and cardiac systems, as they are 'most obviously affected by anaesthetics and which themselves exert an influence on the course of anaesthesia and the postoperative period' (Cashman 2001, p.9). Examination of further organ systems, such as abdominal or neurological systems, should also be completed if indicated by the patient's history. For example, patients with known alcohol or drug abuse should be further examined for hepatic and neurological impairments. Principles table 2.2 lists elements of a physical examination.

Principles table 2.2 Preoperative: physical examination

Principle	Rationale
Airway assessment Within the preoperative assessment it is vital to perform an airway assessment. This includes: ■ range of motion of the neck and jaw ■ mouth opening ■ dentition ■ history of temporomandibular joint dysfunction and other airway abnormalities. The airway assessment should include neck and jaw flexion, condition of the teeth and the ability to protrude the lower incisors in front of the upper incisors.	If there are any problems with the airway the anaesthetist needs to be told so that appropriate equipment can be ordered for the day of surgery. Patients with prominent incisors, receding jaw, a thick or short neck, obesity and a poor mouth opening (less than three finger widths between upper and lower teeth) may indicate a difficult intubation (Behar *et al.* 2007).
Cardiac assessment Patients should be assessed for the presence of hypertension, peripheral oedema, exertional dyspnoea, persistent cough, raised jugular venous pressure, inspection of pulses for irregularities and also for poor circulation to extremities. Auscultation of the heart should assess for signs of heart murmurs. The bases of the lungs should be auscultated for crackles.	Patients with a history of unstable angina, congestive heart failure, symptomatic arrhythmias and severe valvular heart disease are deemed a higher risk for complications in the perioperative or postoperative period (Avidan *et al.* 2003). The type of murmur plays an important part in the assessment of the patient's surgical risk, as severe valvular dysfunction can indicate a high surgical risk. This may indicate signs of fluid overload.
Respiratory assessment The respiratory examination should include: ■ observation for signs of cyanosis or clubbing of the finger nails ■ signs of tachynopea, use of accessory muscles, abnormal chest expansion or barrel chest ■ lung fields should also be percussed to assess for signs of hyper-resonance or dullness ■ auscultation should be performed for abnormal breath sounds such as wheezes or crackles, and for reduced breath sounds ■ peak flow testing should also be performed to test for lung function.	This may indicate signs of respiratory disease, such as carcinoma. (Thomas and Monaghan 2008). This may indicate signs of lung disease, anxiety or respiratory distress. (Thomas and Monaghan 2008). This may indicate pulmonary complications such as COPD, consolidation, pleural effusion, or neoplasm (Thomas and Monaghan 2008). Reduced breath sounds may indicate pleural effusion, pneumothorax, neoplasm or infection such as pneumonia. Crackles may indicate signs of infection or fluid. Wheeze may indicate COPD, asthma or neoplasm (Bickley 2007, Thomas and Monaghan 2008). The value will depend on the patient's age, sex and height. Lower values may indicate a degree of airway obstruction and help to provide the assessor with an indicator of possible obstructive airway disease.

Legal and professional issues

Who should perform the preoperative assessment?

The POA should only be performed by assessors trained and deemed competent in the process. Assessors can include not only doctors or anaesthetists but also nurses or operating department practitioners (ODPs). The role of the assessor is broad (Box 2.13), but they should be competent in the following procedures:

- take a comprehensive health history
- perform a physical examination
- order appropriate investigations.

Box 2.13 Role of the assessor in the preoperative assessment clinic

---

- Work to guidelines and competencies agreed by the anaesthetists, surgeons and other allied health professionals to ensure a consistent approach.
- Take a targeted history and conduct a relevant physical examination of the patient, including airway assessment.
- Refer patients who fall outside the agreed criteria to the anaesthetist, who may then make further referrals.
- Arrange and perform investigations in accordance with NICE guidelines.
- Ensure that the results of tests are evaluated and refer abnormal investigation results to the available anaesthetist, surgeon and/or primary care, according to local guidelines.
- Refer a patient back to primary care or another healthcare professional to optimize the patient's medical condition, according to local guidelines.
- Take responsibility for following up referrals to ensure the patient remains in the preoperative system.
- Liaise actively with the anaesthetic department.
- Arrange and co-ordinate any assessment and/or investigations needed near time of surgery.
- Take responsibility for all communication with the patient throughout their preoperative journey.
- Commence necessary planning for the perioperative stay and to ensure a timely discharge.
- Identify factors that may influence the dates of surgery offered, for example school holidays.
- Collate all information prior to surgery and ensure that the multidisciplinary documentation is available for anaesthetists to see at least 48 hours prior to admission.
- Communicate approximate length of operation, any special requirements and essential resources to the waiting list office, bed management, operating theatre department and/or theatre scheduler.
- Contact all patients failing to attend preoperative assessment to identify the reason. Act on the reason, following local protocols for the management of DNAs in preoperative assessment.

(Modernisation Agency 2003, p.14)

The Association of Anaesthetists of Great Britain and Ireland (2001, p.6) states that trained staff 'play an essential role when, by working to agreed protocols, they screen patients for fitness for anaesthesia and surgery' although they are not qualified to make the final decision about a patient's fitness for surgery, but play an important role in 'identifying problem patients'. Non-complicated patients often do not require further assessment by an anaesthetist until the day of admission. Patients considered complicated by the trained assessor are further reviewed by an anaesthetist. According to the American Society of Anesthesiologists, although 'Non-anaesthetic personnel may gather and correlate information, the final responsibility for determining the medical status of the patient, developing and discussing with them a plan of anaesthetic care rests with the anaesthetists' (Cashman 2001).

While the POA can be performed by non-anaesthetic personnel such as nurses, it is vital that the anaesthetist in charge of the patient's case is aware of the patient's co-morbidities. According to Cashman (2001), anaesthetic involvement 'enhances the anaesthetist's awareness of the patient's medical condition and facilitates planning of perioperative care... in preventing anaesthetic morbidity and mortality and ensuring a smooth course of anaesthetic administration' (pp.8–9).

Preprocedural considerations

Preoperative investigations

Another aspect of the preoperative assessment is the ordering and interpreting of preoperative investigations. Investigations are often ordered to establish baseline values, support or refute differential diagnoses, and support or monitor the management of existing disease processes. The results of the physical examination and history taking direct the practitioner to the types of preoperative investigations necessary. Research shows that investigations are often ordered based on routine rather than on patient health indicators or for aiding in perioperative management. *Preoperative Tests: The Use of Routine Preoperative Tests for Elective Surgery* (NICE 2003) is an evidence-based guide for the ordering and use of routine preoperative testing in elective surgeries. The investigations are based on ASA status (see Table 2.1), the age of the patient and their co-morbidities. Principles table 2.3 lists various laboratory tests.

Electrocardiograms

A standard 12-lead electrocardiogram is frequently performed if indicated by the age of the patient, risk factors, co-morbidities and findings of the physical examination. The patient's ASA grading and the surgical grading of the planned surgery may also indicate an ECG. The ECG will indicate if there is ischaemia, infarction, conduction abnormalities and dysrhythmias (Mangano 1990). The proportion of patients with an abnormal ECG increases with age and presence of co-morbidities. An ECG can also be completed

Principles table 2.3 Preoperative: laboratory tests

Test	Rationale
Haematology	
Full blood count (FBC), including haemoglobin, haematocrit	Patients with a history of smoking, malignancy, respiratory and cardiac disease may be at increased risk for anaemia and polycythaemia.
White blood count	Patients with a history of recent chemotherapy and radiotherapy treatment, malignancy or recent infection.
Platelet count	Patients with a history of bleeding tendencies, renal or hepatic disease, or recent treatment with chemotherapy should have platelet count assessed.
Coagulation screening, including prothrombin and activated partial thromboplastin time	This is not recommended unless the patient: ■ is taking anticoagulants ■ has a history of bleeding disorders ■ has a history of postsurgical bleeding ■ has a bleeding history (such as liver disease or malignancy) (Chee *et al.* 2008).
Group and save or cross-match	Having the blood tested prior to the date of surgery gives the blood bank more time to find the appropriate blood required for the specific patient. Patients with unusual blood typing or rare antibodies may need to have special blood obtained from an outside blood bank, and having the sample collected in advance will decrease the chance of errors and of the patient having their surgery postponed.
Serum biochemistry	
Glycosylated haemoglobin (HbA$_{1c}$) level	Patients presenting with a history of steroid use, obesity, cardiovascular disease. Patients who have symptoms suggestive of diabetes. The HbA$_{1c}$ is a more accurate measurement of the patient's long-term glucose control and compliance.
Baseline serum creatinine and blood urea nitrogen level	Patients with history of renal dysfunction, diabetes, cardiovascular disease or obesity, or use of medications such as steroids or diuretics.
Liver function tests, such as albumin	Patients presenting with liver disease or malignancy, alcohol abuse, malnutrition and jaundice. Because the liver and kidneys aid the metabolism and elimination of many anaesthetics and medications, it is vital to ensure adequate organ function.
Electrolyte levels	Patients presenting with a history of renal dysfunction, diabetes, malignancy, malnutrition, vomiting or diarrhoea, or use of medications such as diuretics or chemotherapy, should have electrolyte levels taken preoperatively. The patient may require preoperative prescribing of supplements, such as potassium, to optimize electrolyte levels prior to surgery. Electrolyte imbalances such as hypokalaemia or hyponatraemia can be potentially life-threatening in the perioperative period.

Test	Rationale
Other	
Thyroid function testing	Patients with a history of hypo- or hyperthyroidism. Patients with untreated or severe thyroid disease are at increased risk of developing thyroid storm related to the stress of surgery or illness (Weinberg *et al.* 1983).
Urinalysis	Patients who are presenting with symptoms of a urinary tract infection or those presenting for procedures of the urinary tract such as cystoscopy. Evidence has shown that 'the major source of organisms causing bacteraemia is pre-existing urinary infection' and if there is any doubt regarding possible infection of the urinary tract then 'antibiotics should be given to prevent systemic spread' (Bavetta *et al.* 1990, p.735).
Pregnancy testing	Pregnancy testing should be completed based on findings of the medical history, and date of last menstrual cycle, ideally on the day of admission, unless the patient suspects she may be pregnant, as it provides a more up-to-date and accurate assessment of the patient's pregnancy status.

to establish a baseline prior to surgery for postoperative comparison.

Imaging: chest X-ray (CXR)

A CXR can give the practitioner valuable information to support or refute potential diagnoses or further assess the severity of a specific disease. Patients presenting with history of cardiovascular or respiratory symptoms or disease processes should have a CXR completed preoperatively. If the patient has had a CXR within the last 6 months, it does not need to be repeated unless new problems have arisen or the existing problems have worsened.

Cardiopulmonary exercise testing

Dr Paul Older (Older and Smith 1988) introduced the concept of cardiopulmonary exercise testing (CPET) (Figure 2.2). CPET is a dynamic, non-invasive test, involving the use of an exercise bicycle (cycle ergometer) where the work rate is gradually and imperceptibly increased in a stepped or ramped manner until the patient is unable to continue. This enables examination of the ability of the patient's cardiorespiratory system to adapt to a 'stress' situation of increased oxygen demand, in effect mimicking the conditions of surgery.

Cardiopulmonary exercise testing relies upon accurate breath-by-breath measurements of pulmonary gas exchange through a mouthpiece measuring respiratory gas exchange. In addition, electrocardiography, blood pressure, pulse oximetry and heart rate are monitored during exercise (American Thoracic Society (ATS)/American College of Chest Physicians (ACCP) 2003, Wasserman *et al.* 2005). From the CPET, two

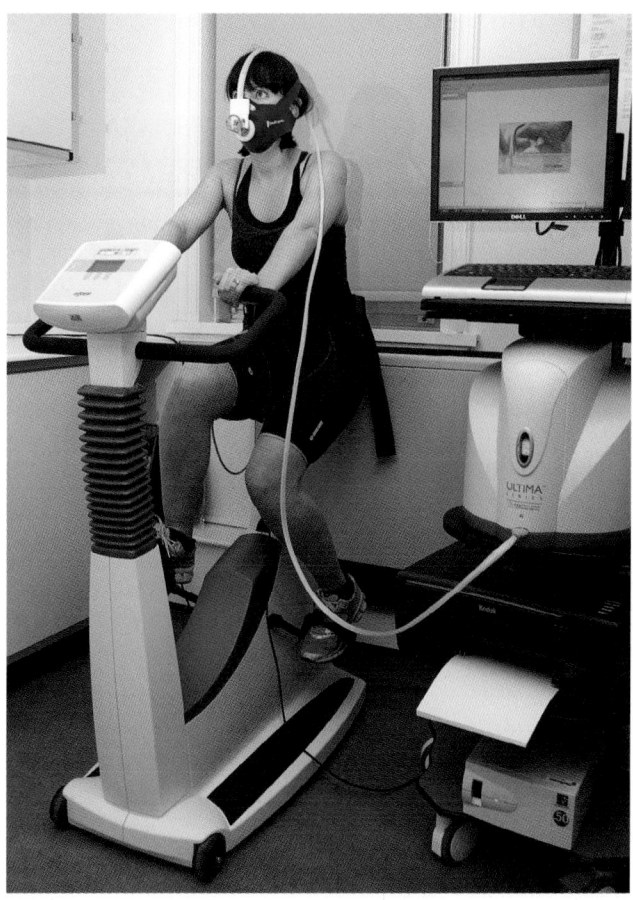

Figure 2.2 Cardiopulmonary exercise testing (CPET).

key indicators are derived: the body's maximum oxygen uptake (VO_{2max}) and the point at which anaerobic metabolism exceeds aerobic metabolism (anaerobic threshold, AT). Together these broadly indicate the ability of the cardiovascular system to deliver oxygen to the peripheral tissues and the ability of the tissues to utilize that oxygen. In addition, the AT has been shown to be a useful predictor of postoperative cardiac complications in abdominal surgery (Older et al. 1999).

Exercise testing is commonly used to reproduce common symptoms such as impaired exercise capacity, fatigue and exertional breathlessness. This enables accurate physiological measurements to be obtained, assisting with the overall assessment of suitability for surgery, and can predict postoperative mortality and morbidity (Cooper and Storer 2008). This assessment will reveal to both the healthcare professional and the patient what needs to be considered if optimum results are to be achieved from surgery (Bassett 2002).

Cardiopulmonary exercise testing is often referred to as 'the gold standard for measuring exercise tolerance'. It enables clinicians to triage patients to the appropriate level of care after surgery, allowing the efficient use of intensive care facilities (Davies and Wilson 2007, MacGregor et al. 2009). It is also useful to assist surgeons in assessing treatment options more easily (Older et al. 1993). The patient is then in a better position to evaluate their own risk/benefit ratio for surgery and thus make a more informed decision on consent for an operation (ATS/ACCP 2003, Lee et al. 2006).

Further referrals

During the patient's preoperative assessment, it is often deemed necessary to refer for further expert assessment or advice. This is helpful in providing valuable information regarding the patient's condition and creating an appropriate plan of action for the patient in the perioperative or postoperative period. Patients are seen by a specialist to further assess whether they are in the optimum condition for the desired surgery and/or if their health can be 'optimized' prior to surgery to improve their postoperative outcomes. According to Cherian and Tomlinson (2001), perioperative 'optimization' involves identifying whether a patient's health status can be improved.

Discharge planning

Definition

Discharge planning is defined by Rorden and Taft (1990) as 'a process made up of several steps or phases whose immediate goal is to anticipate changes in patient care needs and whose long-term goal is to ensure continuity of health care'.

Related theory

Discharge planning should involve the development and implementation of a plan to facilitate the transfer of an individual from hospital to an appropriate setting and include the multidisciplinary team, the patient and their family and carers. Furthermore, it involves building on, or adding to, any assessments undertaken prior to admission (DH 2003a). It is acknowledged that the activities required to achieve a safe and timely discharge of patients back into the community are complex (DH 2010).

The nurses' ability in this task is central to a good discharge and requires them to have a clear understanding of how to assess the patient's and carer's needs (Atwal 2002, Reilly et al. 1996). Determining the discharge needs of a patient returning to the community is, as suggested by Foust (2007, p.73), 'a first and complex step' in the discharge planning process.

One of the key elements of the Clinical Governance agenda is improved quality and effectiveness (DH 1998a). Good-quality discharge should reduce delayed discharges (Tarling and Jauffur 2006) and facilitate meeting the targets set by various Department of Health publications (DH 2000a, 2002, 2004a). It is evident from the literature that there is growing pressure to ensure patients have a better discharge experience and that hospitals work to improve the discharge planning processes (Maramba et al. 2004, Mistiaen et al. 2007, Salter 1996).

Therefore all hospitals should have a discharge policy which is developed, agreed and ideally jointly published with all the relevant local health and social service agencies. The Department of Health (2003b) states in its guidance on discharge policy development that this 'will need to be understood by staff' and highlights the importance of training through induction and ongoing education programmes. Standards should be applicable to the planning and delivery of care at all stages: preadmission and admission; the period as an inpatient; predischarge; the discharge process and postdischarge (Health Services Accreditation 1996). Patient preadmission clinics are an ideal opportunity to assess care required on discharge (DH 2003a). It is worth ensuring that the information gathered at preadmission is shared with community staff, as they may be able to commence their assessments prior to admission, and with the ward staff responsible for planning the patient's discharge.

Poor discharge planning is considered detrimental to a patient's physical and psychological well-being (Smith 1996). Patients may return home with insufficient support, resulting in unnecessary readmissions to hospital or struggling at home with inadequate care (Rosswurm and Lanham 1998). Poor discharge planning can result in patients remaining in hospital for longer periods of time than is necessary (Wells et al. 2002). A lack of proactive planning for discharge on or even before admission leads to a longer length of stay (DH 2004a). Therefore it is essential that discharge planning is an ongoing process from preassessment through to the day the patient returns to the community. Given the potential benefits of good discharge planning to patients and their carers and the evidence identifying the impact of poor discharge planning, it is clearly in the best interests of all concerned to ensure that discharge planning is given priority and is seen as a core activity in patient care (Foust 2007, Maramba *et al.* 2007).

Your Guide to the National Health Service (NHSE 2001) states that from the moment a patient arrives:

> Arrangements for discharging you from hospital will begin, and your discharge plan will be agreed with you, taking account of your needs. When you are ready to leave hospital, the nurses and doctors will talk to you about what will happen to you during your recovery and you will be told who to contact in an emergency.
>
> If you need ongoing care at home, your GP, midwife, health visitor, community nurse or Social Services department will be there to help you.
>
> If you need any medical equipment for your return home, the NHS and your Social Services department will aim to provide it promptly. If you need your home to be adapted in any way, your Social Services department will assess your needs.
>
> (NHSE 2001, p.30)

All patients, whether short- or long-stay, those with few or simple needs or those with complex needs, should receive comprehensive discharge planning commenced at the earliest opportunity (DH 2010).

Evidence-based approaches
Principles of discharge planning

The key principles for effective discharge planning are as follows.

- Unnecessary admissions are avoided and discharge is facilitated by a whole-system approach to care planning.
- Patients and carers should be actively involved in the process (DH 1995, DH 2004b).
- Discharge planning should commence on the initial contact with patients.
- Complex discharge should be co-ordinated by a named person.
- Discharge is a core nursing task (Atwal 2002).
- Discharge planning should be a multidisciplinary process by which resources to meet the needs of patients and carers are put in place (Salter 1996).
- Effective use is made of transitional, intermediate and enablement care services, so that patients achieve their optimal outcome and acute hospital beds are used appropriately.
- Patients and carers understand the discharge planning process and their rights, and receive appropriate information to enable them to make informed decisions about their future care.

(Adapted from DH 2003a)

The discharge planning process and the primary/secondary care interface

The discharge planning process can be initiated by any member of the primary healthcare team (PHCT) or Social Services staff in the patient's home, prior to admission, in preadmission clinics or on hospital admission (Huber and McClelland 2003). Importance is attached to developing a primary care-led NHS, reinforced by the government's White Paper *The New NHS: Modern, Dependable* (DH 1998b). The focus on quality, patient-centred care and services closer to where people live will be dependent on primary, secondary and tertiary professionals working together (Davis 1998).

However, it is important to note that the Community Care (Delayed Discharges) Act (DH 2003b) introduced a system of reimbursement to NHS bodies from Social Services departments for delays caused by the failure of Social Services departments to provide timely assessment and/or services for a patient being discharged from an acute hospital bed. An awareness of the process and required timescales is essential to ensure that a patient's discharge is not delayed because Social Services have had insufficient time to respond to a request for an assessment.

The discharge planning process takes into account a patient's physical, psychological, social, cultural, economic and environmental needs. It involves not only patients but also families, friends, informal carers, the hospital multidisciplinary team and the community health/social services teams (Maramba *et al.* 2004, Salentera *et al.* 2003), with the emphasis on health and social services departments working jointly. However, a new emphasis is being placed on personalized care in the community, with patients purchasing and managing their own care package (Darzi 2008). Giving patients greater control and choice over the services they need requires the professionals to ensure that they have provided information regarding all the possible alternatives for care open to the patient and their carers (Darzi 2008).

As well as patient experience, discharge planning is considered a factor in reducing the length of stay in hospital, which has a financial impact for the NHS (DH 2004a, Bull and Roberts 2001, Mardis and Brownson 2003, Nazarko 1998). Given the huge cost of inpatient care, it is financially sensible to ensure that procedures are in place, and complied with, to facilitate patients being discharged at the earliest opportunity. However, the notion of a seamless service may be idealistic because of increasing time constraints and the complex care needs of high-dependency patients (Smith 1996).

Occasionally the discharge process may not proceed as planned; a discharge may be delayed for a number of reasons and a system should be in place to record this (for example, see Figure 2.3). Patients may take their own discharge against medical advice and this should be documented accordingly (see Box 2.14). When patients are assessed as requiring care or equipment but decline these, this does not negate the nurse's duty to ensure a discharge is safe. A discussion

DISCHARGE DELAY MONITORING FORM
Please refer to accompanying guidelines

Ward
Week commencing

Were there any delayed discharges this week (please tick) YES ☐ NO ☐

If yes please complete form fully.

Please complete this form for patients who no longer need clinical care in a comprehensive cancer centre, but who stay in the hospital because of 'delayed or lack of appropriate Community/Social Services or internal failures to plan the discharge properly'

Patient's Details: (Give full address inc. postcode) **Hospital No:** _____

Name: _____ **Consultant:** _____

Address: _____

_____

_____ **Postcode:** _____

Expected Date of Discharge: _____ | **Actual Date of Discharge:** _____

Reason for Delay in Discharge: (Please tick the appropriate boxes)

Royal Marsden NHS Trust Failure	☐	Other Hospital Failure	☐
Hospice Failure	☐	Transport Failure	☐
		Internal Social Services Failure	☐
Community Health Service Failure e.g. D/N, Macmillan	☐	External Social Services Failure	☐
Identify Health Authority _____		*Identify Social Services Dept.* _____	
Patient/Relative choice	☐	Other	☐
(Don't count if 24 hours' notice given to relatives)		Please specify _____	

Full details of delay: Please complete

_____

_____

_____

_____

Signature: _____ **Print Name:** _____

Please send completed forms to Complex Discharge Co–Ordinator / Tracking Officer

Figure 2.3 Discharge delay monitoring form. Reproduced with kind permission of the Royal Marsden Hospital NHS Foundation Trust (2006).

Box 2.14 Patients taking discharge against medical advice

Nursing staff responsibility
If a patient wishes to take their own discharge, the ward sister/co-ordinator should contact:

- a member of the medical team
- the manager on call
- the complex discharge co-ordinator.

The complex discharge co-ordinator will inform Social Services if appropriate. Out of hours, following a risk assessment, the manager on call will contact the local Social Services department, if appropriate, and inform the hospital Social Services department the following day.

Medical staff responsibility
The doctor, following consultation with the patient, should complete the appropriate form prior to the patient leaving the hospital. The form must be signed by the patient and the doctor and filed in the medical notes. The doctor must immediately contact the patient's GP.

should take place with the patient and carer to assess how they intend to manage without the required care/equipment in place. It is crucial that the community services are aware of assessed needs that are not being met through patient choice or lack of resources. It is critical that the community team who will be supporting the patient when they return home are notified and where possible this should be in writing, such as sending them a copy of the patient refusal of equipment form. Some patients receiving news of a poor prognosis may prefer to go home to die and plans would need to be set up at short notice (Figure 2.4).

The role of informal carers

Engaging and involving patients and informal carers as equal partners is central to successful discharge planning (DH 2003a, Holzhausen 2001). The Picker Report (Garrett and Boyd 2008), an independent patient survey, identified that 16% of patients questioned reported that they did not feel involved in their discharge. The hospital discharge process is also a critical time for informal carers (Higginson and Costantini 2008) yet Holzhausen (2001) suggests they do not feel involved in the discharge process. It may

| Name: | | Hospital No: | |

Checklist for Discharge

This form should be used to assist with planning an urgent discharge home for a patient with terminal care needs. It should be used in conjunction with the discharge policy.

Sign and date to confirm when arranged and equipment given. Document relevant information in the discharge planning section of the nursing documentation. Document if item or care is not applicable.

Appoint a designated ward based discharge lead:

Name:.. Designation:.. Contact No:...........

	Date & Time	Signature, Print Name & Job Title
Patient / Family issues		
Meeting with patient/family to discuss: patient's condition and prognosis		
Plan agreed and discussed with patient and carers. Explain the level of care that will be provided in the community. Ensure an understanding that there will not be 24-hour nursing presence.		
Communication with District Nurse and Community Palliative Care Team		
Discuss • Patient and family needs • The role of each service and the timing and frequency of visits • Community Service cover at night (to support family) e.g. Marie Curie or other local services • The need to complete the Continuing Care Application Form, if necessary		
Agreed planned date and time of district nurse's first visit..		
Agreed planned date and time of community palliative care team first visit...		
Night nursing service Start date.....................................		
Communication with GP and Community Palliative Care Medical Team–Medical Responsibilities **(Hospital medical team to organize – the nurse to confirm when arranged)**		
Registrar to discuss with GP the patient needs and their prognosis, medication and the need to review the patient in the community for death certification purposes.		
Oxygen cylinder/ concentrator (delete as appropriate) ordered through GP and delivery date organized for.................................		
Medical summary faxed to GP ☐ **copy with patient** ☐		
Registrar to discuss with the Palliative Care Medical Team the patient's needs and proposed plan of care		
Adequate supply of drugs prescribed for discharge (TTOs) including crisis drugs, i.e. Midazolam and morphine sulphate		
Medical letter or authorization for drugs to be administered by community nurses.		
'Do Not Attempt Resuscitation' letter for Community Staff		
'Do Not Attempt Resuscitation' letter for Ambulance Crew		

Figure 2.4   Checklist for patients being discharged home for urgent palliative care.

be the first time they are confronted with the reality of their role, the effect it may have on their relationship with the person needing care, their family and their employment (Hill and Macgregor 2001). Research suggests that if carers are unsupported, this can result in early readmission of the patient (Holzhausen 2001).

The Carers Act 1995 was implemented to support carers in a practical way by providing information, helping carers to remain at work and to care for themselves. Under the Act, carers are entitled to their own assessment and many support services can be provided, including respite, at no charge.

Throughout discharge planning, carers' needs should be acknowledged. Carers may have different needs from patients and there may be conflicting opinions about how the patient's care needs can be met. It is not uncommon for patients to report that their informal carer is willing to provide all care but the carer is not in agreement with this. Healthcare professionals should allow carers sufficient time, provide appropriate information to enable them to make decisions, provide written information on the discharge plan and ensure adequate support is in place before discharge (Hill and Macgregor 2001). This will promote a successful and seamless transfer from hospital to home.

Communication and discharge planning

Effective, safe discharge planning needs to be patient and carer focused. Therefore it is dependent on a multidisciplinary approach and the sharing of good practice (Ashby and Mendelson 2009, Martin 2001). There is consistent evidence to suggest that best practice in hospital discharge involves multidisciplinary teamwork throughout the process (Borill *et al.* 2001). The multidisciplinary approach, where all staff have a clear understanding of their roles and responsibilities, will also help to prevent inappropriate readmissions and delayed discharges (Stewart 2000). This approach also promotes the highest possible level of independence for the patient, their partner and family by encouraging appropriate self-care activities.

Ineffective discharge planning has been shown to have detrimental effects on a patient's psychological and physical well-being and their illness experience (Cook 2001, Kissane 2004). Planning care, providing adequate information and involving patients, families and healthcare professionals will keep disruption to a minimum. Poor discharge planning can also result in patients remaining in hospital for longer than is necessary (Wells *et al.* 2002).

To achieve the best quality of life for patients and carers, there needs to be good co-ordination in terms of care planning and delivery of that care over time (Speck 1992). Discharge co-ordinators are generally health or social care professionals who have both hospital and community experience. Their role is to advise on and help with planning the care patients may need when leaving hospital, particularly when the nursing and care needs are complex. McKenna *et al.* (2000) cite poor communication between hospital and community. Discharge processes (DH 2004a) endorse the value of co-ordination in a climate of shorter hospital stays and timely patient discharge.

For complex discharges, it is helpful if a key worker, for example the discharge co-ordinator, is appointed to manage the discharge and, where appropriate, for family meetings/case conferences to take place and include the patient/carer, multidisciplinary team and PHCT and representatives (Health Services Accreditation 1996, Salter 1996). Additionally, a guide to planning a complex discharge (Box 2.15) can highlight the communication required by the multidisciplinary team.

Box 2.15 Guide to arranging a complex discharge home

NB: This is not an exhaustive list and MUST BE DISCUSSED with the complex discharge co-ordinator/specialist sister, discharge planning, palliative care.

Complex discharge definition

- A large package of care involving different agencies.
- The patient's needs have changed since admission, with different services requiring co-ordination.
- The family/carer requires intensive input into discharge planning considerations (e.g. psychological interventions):
  - patients who are entitled to Continuing NHS Funded Care and who require a package of care on discharge
  - patients for repatriation.

1 **Comprehensive assessment by nurse on admission and document care accordingly**

   (a) Provisional discharge date set.

- This will only be an approximate date, depending on care needs, equipment, and so on.
- It should be reviewed regularly with multidisciplinary team.
- Discharge should **not** be arranged for a Friday or weekend.

(b) Referrals to relevant members of multidisciplinary team.

For example, occupational therapist, physiotherapist, Social Services.

(c) Referral to community health services (in liaison with multidisciplinary team).

For example, District Nurse (who may be able to arrange for night sitters), Community Palliative Care Team.

(d) Request equipment from District Nurse and discuss with family.

For example, hoist, hospital bed, pressure-relieving mattress/cushion, commode, nebulizer.
- **If oxygen is required,** medical team to complete Home Oxygen Ordering Form (HOOF) and Home Oxygen Consent Form (HOCF) for oxygen cylinders and concentrators at home. Fax to relevant oxygen supplier.

2 **Discuss at ward multidisciplinary meeting, arrange family meeting/case conference as required, and invite all appropriate healthcare professionals, including community staff**

(a) Appoint discharge co-ordinator at the multidisciplinary meeting.
- To act as co-ordinator for referrals and point of contact for any discharge concerns.
- To plan and prepare the family meeting/case conference and to arrange a chairperson and minute-taker for the meeting.
- Primary team nurse to liaise with discharge co-ordinator.

(b) Formulate a discharge plan at meeting.
- At the meeting, formulate a discharge plan in conjunction with patient, carers, and all hospital and community personnel involved and agree a discharge date; an occupational therapist home visit may be required.

(c) Ascertain discharge address.
- Liaise with services accordingly.
- It is important to agree who will care for patient/where the patient will be cared for, for example ground/first floor.
- Ascertain type of accommodation patient lives in so that the equipment ordered will fit in appropriately.
- **NB: If not returning to own home, a GP will be required to take patient on as a temporary resident.**

(d) Confirm PROVISIONAL discharge date.
- This will depend on when community services and equipment can be arranged.
- This must be agreed with the patient and family/informal carer/s.

3 **Ascertain whether District Nurse is able to undertake any necessary clinical procedures in accordance with their primary care trust policy, for example care of skin-tunnelled catheters. Consider alternative arrangements if necessary**

(a) Confirm equipment agreed and delivery date.
- **NB: Family must be informed of delivery date and also requested to contact ward to inform that this has been received.**

(b) Confirm start date for care.
- For example, Social Services/District Nurse/community palliative care.

(c) Confirm with patient/family agreed discharge date.
- Liaise with complex discharge co-ordinator for Community Services Arrangements Form.
- Check community services are able to enter patient's home as necessary.

4 **Forty-eight hours prior to discharge, fax and telephone District Nurse with Community Care Referral Form and discuss any special needs of patient, for example syringe driver, oxygen, wound care, intravenous therapy, MRSA or other infection status. Give written information and instructions**

(a) Arrange transport and assess need for escort/oxygen during transport.
- Should be in place for any change in patient's condition/treatment plan.

(b) Ongoing review.
- **If there is a change**, notify/liaise with multidisciplinary team and community services.

(c) If NO change within 24 hours of discharge, confirm that:
  - patient is medically fit for discharge
  - all community services are in place as agreed
  - patient has drugs to take out (TTO) and next appointment
  - access to home, heating and food are checked.
- Ensure patient has drugs TTO with written and verbal instructions.
- Next in/outpatient appointment as required.
- Check arrangements for patient to get into home (front door key), heating, food and someone there to welcome them home, as appropriate.

5 **Hospital equipment: for example syringe drivers: ensure clearly marked and arrangements made for return**

6 **After discharge, follow-up phone call to patient by ward nurse/complex discharge co-ordinator as agreed to ensure all is well**

Discharge at end of life

The *End of Life Care Strategy* (DH 2008) requires that assessment is made of the patient's preferred place of care and where they wish to be cared for at the end of life. There may be occasions when a patient is reaching the end of life and the decision is made that their preferred place of care/death is home. Then every effort must be made to ensure that all practicable steps are taken to allow that to happen (Vaartio *et al.* 2006). It is important to contact the District Nurses, the community palliative care team and (where available) the community matron at the earliest opportunity. A fast-track NHS Continuing Care Funding application may need to be submitted to access funding for the care provision. The patient may also require essential equipment to enable them to return home, such as bed, commode or hoist; again, these should be ordered at the first opportunity. Once care and equipment are in place and discharge is proceeding, ensure that a medical review takes place and that the GP, District Nurses and community palliative care team are provided with a copy of the discharge summary. Telephone contact with the GP prior to discharge is essential to ensure they visit the patient at home.

Anticipated patient outcomes

- To ensure patients have a safe and timely discharge from hospital to the community.
- To ensure patients and carers are involved throughout the discharge planning process.
- To provide patients and carers with written and verbal information to meet their needs on discharge.
- To provide continuity of care between the hospital and the agreed environment by facilitating effective communication.

(Adapted from DH 2004a)

Preprocedural considerations

It is essential that nurses are aware of their trust's discharge procedures and protocols.

Single assessment process

Referred to in *The NHS Plan* (DH 2000a) and reinforced in *The National Service Framework for Older People* (DH 2001a), the Single Assessment Process is designed to replace fragmented assessments carried out by different agencies with one seamless procedure (Hunter 2001). The aim is to produce a single, centrally held, electronic summary/tool containing all the information needed to assess and provide for an older person's health and social care needs. The end result will be a comprehensive 'individual care plan' that will lay out their full needs and entitlements (Hunter 2001). Although there has been a high level of commitment to the Single Assessment Process from both health and social care professionals, implementation has occurred at different rates. It appears that more progress has been made in the community rather than hospitals and general practitioner practices (NHS Connecting for Health 2005). Work continues on the development of a data-sharing system that will allow previous assessments, carried out before a hospital admission, to be shared across the NHS, preventing the need for patients to go through the assessment process more than once.

Intermediate care

The National Bed Enquiry (DH 2000b), *The NHS Plan* (DH 2000a) and *The National Service Framework for Older People* (DH 2001a) signalled the development of intermediate care as one of the major initiatives for services in the future. It is recognized that older people are best cared for at home if at all possible. To aid the transition period from hospital to home, intermediate care teams may provide a period of intensive care/rehabilitation following a hospital stay, which may take place in a care home or in the individual's own home. It is likely to be limited to a maximum of 6 weeks but there are local variations in practice. Intermediate care needs to have a person-centred approach involving patients and carers in all aspects of assessment, goal setting and discharge planning. Its success depends on local knowledge of the service and interagency collaboration (Hancock 2003). There is growing evidence suggesting that intermediate care initiatives reduce admissions to acute hospitals and residential/nursing home placements (DH 2002).

Discharge to a care home

Discharge to a care home (whether a residential or nursing home) requires careful thought as giving up their own home is one of the most traumatic events that a person has to consider. A thorough multidisciplinary assessment is essential, taking into account the individual needs of the patient and carer and exploring all the options before agreeing on a care home. Placements can be delayed while waiting for a vacancy and it may be necessary to consider an interim placement (DH 2003a).

In 2001 there were important changes in the funding arrangements for adults requiring registered nursing care in nursing homes in England (DH 2001b). All adults needing the skills and knowledge of a Registered Nurse to meet all or certain elements of their care needs have that care paid for by the NHS. The amount of funding, paid directly to the nursing home, is dependent on a comprehensive assessment of the patient's care needs by a Registered Nurse, who will usually be employed by the local primary care trust. NHS-funded nursing care was originally provided via payment 'bands', which relate to the level of nursing care required. However, the *National Framework* (DH 2006b), which came into effect in October 2007, replaced the banding system with a weekly rate for NHS-funded nursing care.

NHS continuing healthcare

NHS Continuing Healthcare is a general term that describes the care that people need over an extended period of time as the result of disability, accident or illness, to address both physical and mental health needs. It may require services from the NHS and/or social care. It can be provided in a range of settings, for example, from a care home to care in people's own homes. NHS Continuing Healthcare is a package of care arranged and funded solely by the NHS. It should be awarded when it is established (through multidisciplinary comprehensive assessment) that an individual's primary care need is a health need. There has been inconsistency in applying the criteria nationally (House of Commons Health Committee 2005), resulting in the Department of Health producing a *National Framework for NHS Continuing Healthcare* (DH 2006b).

In October 2009 the new national tools for NHS Continuing Care were launched. These replace any previous tools, including the fast-track assessment for those patients who have a rapidly deteriorating condition. There is a legal obligation to inform patients of their right to be assessed for NHS Continuing Care funding. There is a booklet informing patients of their rights and outlining the process (DH 2007). Patients who may be entitled to funding through this process could be paying unnecessarily for their care through Social Services as they will have been financially assessed.

Procedure guideline 2.1 Discharge planning

Preprocedure

Action	Rationale
This is the initial assessment (at the preadmission clinic or within the first 24–48 hours of admission).	
1 The admitting nurse is responsible for ensuring that an initial assessment is completed when the patient is admitted and is documented in the patient's care plan. Assessment should be ongoing and regularly reviewed with the multidisciplinary team.	To enable the physical, psychological and social care needs of the patient and carers to be identified at an early stage (Biddington 2000, C; DH 2000c, C).
2 An expected date of discharge must be established and the patient should be aware of this.	To ensure planning for discharge commences (Biddington 2000, C).
3 Clarify whether the patient has dependants, for example elderly relatives, children or a disabled partner, who require care/support. If so, establish who is looking after them and whether they receive any services.	Arrangements may need to be made for alternative carers or an increase in services. Notification may need to be made, for example to school nurse/teacher if patient has children at school. E
4 Establish who else is involved in giving care/support and the type of help given, for example local support group, voluntary agency, church.	To assess the support that the patient and carers may require at home so that appropriate services can be mobilized. To establish social network in order to co-ordinate care between voluntary and statutory agencies. E
5 Ascertain the type of accommodation the patient is living in, for example house, bungalow (council or privately owned), residential or nursing home, sheltered housing.	To identify any potential accommodation needs which may entail social work intervention, adaptations or housing advice re unsuitable accommodation or homelessness. E
6 Ensure that the home address and telephone number of the patient are documented accurately in the care plan. Establish where the patient will be going on discharge and document the discharge address if different from the permanent address.	Personal information may not have been updated on previous nursing or medical records. It is crucial that this information is accurate when making referrals to community services, to ensure appropriate service provision. E
7 Ensure that the patient is registered permanently with a GP, and with a GP on a temporary basis if going to a different address on discharge. Check the names, addresses and telephone numbers with the patient.	Community nursing services are unable to accept the patient without medical support. Accurate information is required to establish which District Nurse will have responsibility for patient care. It is important for the patient that medical care can be provided at home. E

(Continued)

Procedure guideline 2.1 (*Continued*)

8 Establish whether any statutory community health or Social Services have been involved before the patient's admission. Include the health visitor when the patient has children under the age of 5 years.	To enable contact for exchange of information. Valuable information can be obtained from community services to assist in assessing potential needs on discharge (DH 2003a, C).

Procedure

9 Assess the patient's ability to carry out activities of daily living at home prior to admission, for example were they able to climb stairs? Consider patient's current level of functioning and whether this will change as a result of treatment and/or rehabilitation.	To establish at an early stage whether an occupational therapy/physiotherapist assessment is required. Home assessment by occupational therapy may be required prior to discharge, which may involve complex planning and preparation (DH, 2001c, C; Kumar 2000).
10 Refer to other hospital personnel as soon as potential needs are recognized, for example occupational therapist, physiotherapists, dietitian, speech and language therapist. Referral as soon as possible after admission is essential: do not wait until treatment is completed and discharge is imminent.	To ensure multidisciplinary planning and co-ordination. Considerable time may be needed to arrange community services and early referral helps to prevent discharge delays. E
11 Patients identified as requiring local authority Social Services support are referred to the Social Services department. Some hospitals use a 'trigger' form as an aid to assessment, an example of which can be found in Box 2.16.	To ensure early and appropriate referral to the Social Services department for assessment. E
12 A discharge planning care plan should be commenced. All members of the multidisciplinary team should document in the care plan their assessment, plans and action taken.	To facilitate multidisciplinary planning, co-ordination and communication. E
13 Where there is a designated discharge co-ordinator, they can act as a resource offering support and education to the ward team in the preparation of discharge plans, especially for those patients requiring a complex package of care.	To facilitate effective discharge planning and utilize expertise appropriately. E
14 Formulate a discharge plan in conjunction with patient and carers and all involved hospital and community personnel and agree a discharge date.	To collate information and co-ordinate planning (DH 2004a, C).
15 For complex discharges, a discharge planning meeting should be held.	To co-ordinate continuity of care planning. E
16 The ward-based nurse is responsible for arranging and co-ordinating community nursing services (including the Community Palliative Care Team) in consultation with the discharge co-ordinator, if applicable.	To facilitate continuity of care between hospital and community. E
17 Refer to the community nursing services with a minimum of 48 hours' notice. If a complex package of care is being organized, more notice will be required. Invite community nurses to visit the ward where appropriate.	Community nurses may wish to assess the patient's nursing care needs and ensure preparation of the home prior to discharge. They need time to liaise with other agencies to co-ordinate care and to obtain any equipment required. E
18 Ascertain whether community nurses are able to carry out necessary clinical procedures in accordance with their trust policy, for example care of skin-tunnelled catheters. Consider alternative arrangements if necessary. Give written information and instructions.	District Nurses may not have been trained in certain procedures or may be unfamiliar with particular equipment. E

19	Details of patient's MRSA status (or other infections) must be given to community personnel and written in requirements.	To reduce risk of cross-infection. Community staff require full knowledge of the patient's history and nursing referral details (Halm *et al.* 2003, E; Smith 2003, E, C).
20	Complete the community care referral form or update letter. The form/letter should be completed and signed and a copy provided for all community services.	Provide information for community staff to ensure that they have accurate information (Halm *et al.* 2003, E).
21	Ensure any essential medical/nursing aids or equipment have been obtained before discharge by community services, for example oxygen, nebulizers, commode, pressure-relieving mattress, hoist.	Some equipment may not be available or may take some time to obtain. Equipment may be loaned from the community and appropriate legislation procedures must be followed for safety reasons (DH 2001c, C).
22	Home assessment by occupational therapy may be required prior to discharge.	
23	Patients requiring community nursing, physiotherapy, occupational therapy, stoma care, speech therapy and/or dietetic support on discharge will be referred by the appropriate hospital-based healthcare professional to their equivalent in the community.	To ensure continuity of specialist care. E

Leaving the hospital on discharge

24	Medical staff are responsible for assessing the patient's medical fitness for discharge and for liaising with other members of the multidisciplinary team regarding arrangements for meeting the patient's care needs in the community.	To ensure that both health and social care needs are taken into consideration when formulating discharge plans (DH 2003a, C).
25	Ensure that patient and, with their agreement, carers have full information regarding the patient's medical condition and care required.	To prepare carers and to enable patient/carer support. E
26	Teach the patient and carers any necessary skills, allowing sufficient time to practise before discharge. This should include information on the safe use of equipment, for example a hoist, and identify if there are any trust protocols regarding assessing competency to use equipment.	To enable the patient to be as independent as possible and promote an understanding of self-care techniques. E
27	Ensure that the patient has a door key and can gain entrance to their residence. Wherever possible, ensure that someone is at home to receive the patient.	The patient may have left their key with a neighbour. It is helpful for someone to be available to welcome the patient and attend to any immediate needs. E
28	Book transport if required with 48 hours' notice, using relevant form. Specify if patient needs a stretcher or chair, or requires escort. Ensure that transport is also booked for return clinic appointment if necessary.	The patient may not have private transport facilities and may be too weak to use public transport. E
29	Cancel transport if discharge date or outpatients department appointment is altered.	To prevent a waste of resources. E
30	Patients should be given an appropriate supply of medication and, where necessary, a supply of wound dressings or medical equipment. The community nurses should be informed about exactly what the patient is being discharged with; they may require a signed prescription.	To ensure the safe and continuous administration of medication and use of equipment at home. Time is needed to obtain supplies in the community. E

(Continued)

Procedure guideline 2.1 *(Continued)*

31 Discharge plans should not be altered without consultation with all the hospital personnel who have been involved in the planning, for example occupational therapist, social worker, discharge co-ordinator, and also patient/family/carers.	If there is no consultation this causes considerable confusion and stress for the patient/carers, and all involved services. It may result in the patient being unsupported at home. E
32 If discharge is cancelled or postponed, or if the patient dies, ensure that all relevant community services are informed.	To avoid distress to relatives. To avoid wasted visits and promote good community relations. E
33 Weekend discharge: patients who require a high level of health and Social Services support should generally not be discharged home on a Friday or Saturday or a public holiday. This applies particularly to patients who were previously unknown to community services. (NB: it may be appropriate, under the Community Care (Delayed Discharges) Act, 2003, to discharge patients if agreement has been obtained with local authority Social Services or if a patient has a poor prognosis and wishes to return home.)	All community services will be operating at a reduced level and emergency medical back-up may be difficult to obtain. E
Note: assessment and planning for weekend leave are as important as for final discharge.	
34 Inform the patient and carers of potential side-effects of treatment and management.	To alleviate anxiety and to promote patient comfort, knowledge and safety. E
35 Ensure that patient and carers have information on local support groups or national specialist organizations as appropriate.	Some patients may benefit from the kind of support offered by the organizations. E
36 Reinforce any special instructions with written information or by giving an approved patient education booklet.	To promote an understanding of disease and treatment. To confirm arrangements made. To enable the patient to contact the appropriate services. E
37 Information on community services arranged, including names and telephone numbers and expected date of first visit, should be given to the patient and carers prior to discharge. This information should also be documented in the patient's care plan.	To confirm arrangements made. To enable the patient to contact the appropriate services. E
38 Ensure that arrangements have been made to provide patient with food at home on discharge and that there will be adequate heating.	To supply immediate needs. E
39 Ensure that the patient and carers are given verbal and written information on the dosage, route, frequency and side-effects of any medication and how to obtain further supplies.	Lack of information makes it difficult for the GP to provide the medical care required (DH 2003a, C).

Postprocedure

40 A follow-up phone call should be made to establish how the patient is managing.	To ensure services are in place. E

Box 2.16 Patients with particular care needs on discharge

- Live alone.
- Are frail and/or elderly.
- Have care needs which place a high demand on carers.
- Have a limited prognosis.
- Have serious illnesses and will be returning to hospital for further treatments.
- Have continuing disability.
- Have learning difficulties.
- Have mental illness or dementia.
- Have dependants.
- Have limited financial resources.
- Are homeless or live in poor housing.
- Do not have English as their first language.
- Have been in hospital for an 'extended stay'.
- Require aids/equipment at home.

(DH 1989, 2004a)

Postprocedural considerations

Discharge delays

A discharge delay is when a patient remains in hospital beyond the date agreed by the multidisciplinary team and beyond the time when they are medically fit to leave (DH 2003a). For every patient who is 'delayed', the trust is required to inform the Strategic Health Authority through the SITREP reporting mechanism which is normally captured at a point in time each week. It is the responsibility of health authorities, in collaboration with Social Services departments, to monitor the way in which discharges from hospitals are being undertaken and, if problems occur, to establish the reasons, so that any necessary changes are made to address the local needs (DH 1989). Each hospital should have at least a basic system of audit and quality control of discharge practice and procedures.

Care of the dying patient

Definitions

Terminal illness

Describes any disease which is at an advanced stage or has no known cure.

Palliative care

The term used for care, wherever and by whomever provided, which seeks to improve quality of life through the prevention and relief of suffering in the time leading up to death (Higgins 2010). Palliative care is applicable from early in the course of an illness, in conjunction with other therapies which aim to prolong life (WHO 2002; www.who.int/cancer/palliative/en).

Terminal phase

'The ill-defined period of irreversible decline that heralds imminent death. This is usually a period of several days, but may be as short as a few hours, or as long as a couple of weeks' (Back 1992). The expression 'terminal care' applies to care given during this period of time.

Anatomy and physiology

In the days and hours leading up to an expected death, the following are common.

- A weaker pulse (but regular unless previously arrhythmic).
- A gradual drop in blood pressure (though at this stage it should not be routinely taken).
- Shallower, slower breathing which varies in depth, often in a Cheyne–Stokes pattern.
- A decreasing level of consciousness leading eventually to coma, except in those few patients who remain awake until a few minutes before they die.
- Cooling and clamminess of the skin from the periphery inwards.
- Cyanosis of the skin on the extremities and around the mouth.
- Eventual loss of all signs of cardiorespiratory function and the corneal reflex – death is said to occur at this point (Fürst 2004).

Related theory

Care of the person who has reached the final stage of their life is a key aspect of maintaining human dignity and is enormously important for relatives and friends who will remember this period perhaps better than any other during the cancer journey. Unrelieved suffering of patients at the end of life is associated with increased relative distress and can unnecessarily complicate the already difficult period of bereavement. Nursing care during this period does not simply represent a continuation of previously given care, nor necessarily the complete cessation of all 'active treatment' measures which may previously have been undertaken. As with all aspects of nursing care, assessment of the individual patient and their relatives, exceptional communication and good multiprofessional working will help to determine the appropriate next steps for each individual.

Cancer has a well-defined trajectory (Figure 2.5) and it is usual for physical deterioration to take place over several weeks, with a terminal phase lasting hours to days at the end of life. However, sometimes patients can experience sudden death, either as a result of treatment and its side-effects or from complications of the disease itself, including bleeding, infection, pulmonary embolism or a cardiac event. Those deaths which follow the former pattern will be discussed here.

Care of the dying patient starts with a recognition from the multiprofessional team that the terminal phase has begun. It is perhaps the single most important factor in enabling the achievement of all the factors associated with

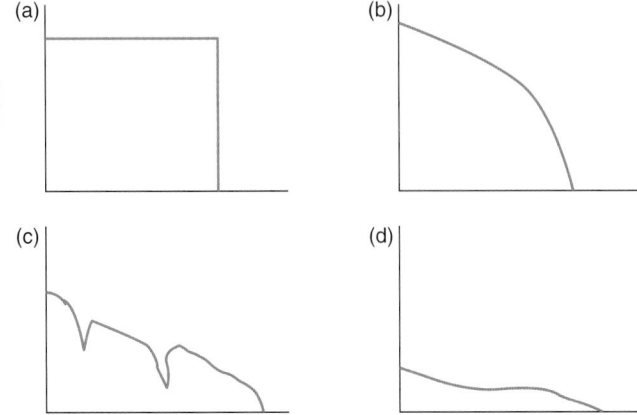

Figure 2.5 Different death trajectories: y axis = health status, x axis = time. (a) Sudden death. (b) Typical cancer death. (c) Typical death from end-organ failure. (d) Typical death from dementia. From Glare and Christakis 2004.

a 'good death' (Faull and Nyatanga 2005). The terminal phase can be difficult to identify, and often there are barriers from healthcare professionals reluctant to make a diagnosis of dying. In an attempt to overcome some of these barriers, four basic criteria for recognizing the terminal phase are widely acknowledged (and are associated with the Liverpool Care Pathway, to be discussed later in this chapter) (Kinder and Ellershaw 2003). The presence of two or more of the following, commonly preceded by a progressive period of decline, and where no other reversible cause is present, is said to denote the terminal phase of life:

- the patient is bedbound
- the patient is semi-comatose or comatose
- the patient is only able to take sips of fluid
- the patient is no longer able to take tablets.

Evidence-based approaches

Palliative care is relatively new as a specialty in nursing and medicine and its evidence base is therefore comparatively small, though growing. Nursing care of the dying patient should have as its main priority meeting personal needs which will allow the patient to have a 'good' death. It has been suggested that the following characteristics are central to a 'good' death from medical, nursing and patient perspectives: (1) control, (2) comfort, (3) closure, (4) trust in healthcare providers, (5) recognition of impending death, and (6) an honouring of personal beliefs and values (Kehl 2006).

The WHO (2002) suggests that palliative care:

- provides relief from pain and other distressing symptoms
- affirms life and regards dying as a normal process
- intends neither to hasten nor postpone death
- integrates the psychological and spiritual aspects of patient care

- offers a support system to help patients live as actively as possible until death
- offers a support system to help the family cope during the patient's illness and in their own bereavement
- uses a team approach to address the needs of patients and their families, including bereavement counselling if indicated
- enhances quality of life and may also positively influence the course of an illness
- is applicable early in the course of illness, in conjunction with other therapies that are intended to prolong life, such as chemotherapy and radiation therapy, and includes those investigations needed to better understand and manage distressing clinical complications.

Legal and professional issues
Advance directives

Advance directives, formerly known as 'living wills', allow people to make a legal decision to refuse, in advance, a proposed treatment, or the continuation of that treatment, if at the necessary time the person lacks the capacity to consent to it. Advance directives can only be made by those who are deemed to have the mental capacity to do so, and allow only for the refusal of treatments – they cannot enforce the provision of specified treatments in the same circumstances (Mental Capacity Act 2005, sections 24–26).

Decisions to refuse life-sustaining treatments must be made in writing, be signed and witnessed, and must expressly state that the decision stands even if the person's life is at risk. Advance directives can be withdrawn verbally or in writing and are not considered valid if the person has conferred lasting power of attorney on another person. Furthermore, advance directives are invalidated if the person has done anything which is clearly inconsistent with the original advance decision made, for example, any change in religious faith.

The Mental Health Capacity Act 2005 (sections 24–26) forms the legal basis for advance directives.

Assisted suicide and euthanasia

Euthanasia is the intentional killing, by act or omission, of a person whose life is thought not to be worth living. Assisted suicide is similar in intentionality but differs in that it involves one person (whether a healthcare professional or not) providing the means for another to end his or her own life, whilst not participating in the act itself (Wyatt 2009). At present, both are illegal in the United Kingdom, despite current campaigns to change the law, and it is, therefore, unlawful for any registered nurse to participate in this process.

It must be remembered, however, that those who approach healthcare professionals with a request for assisted suicide or euthanasia will be doing so from a position of significant vulnerability and deserve compassion and respect. Commonly, requests for assisted suicide or euthanasia stem from a fear of pain, indignity and dependence (Wyatt 2009) and it is imperative to ensure that patients are offered adequate opportunities to express these fears, and the specialist physical, psychosocial and spiritual support necessary to minimize their distress.

Artificial hydration

One of the most contentious issues in day-to-day palliative care practice is that of hydration at the end of life, and clear, compassionate communication with patients and their relatives about this aspect of care is therefore essential, as many will be concerned about the impact of poor oral hydration on themselves or their loved one. There is currently no conclusive research in favour of either giving or withholding artificial hydration in end-of-life care, especially in terms of its impact on the length of remaining life. However, studies of the experiences of hospice nurses suggest that artificial hydration has no benefit and, at worst, may contribute to increased respiratory secretions (see Table 2.2) and oedema elsewhere in the body (Watson *et al.* 2009) and so most palliative care practitioners usually favour stopping artificial hydration on the grounds of preventing increased symptomatology. It is important that the distress of (most often) the relatives is acknowledged in these situations, and their concerns explored. Once the rationale for discontinuing artificial hydration is offered and the patient and/or relatives have been reassured, it is important to support a decision which serves the best interests of the patient first, and their relatives as well. It may be necessary to negotiate a contract whereby a small amount of artificial hydration is given for an agreed period, on the understanding that this will be discontinued if it is causing distress to the patient. As ever, complex situations require skilled and experienced communication (see Chapter 5).

Preprocedural considerations
Communication

Excellent communication is paramount in all areas of nursing practice, but perhaps most emphatically so in dealing with dying patients and their relatives. Skilful, truthful communication at the end of life affords people the dignity of making educated decisions about the management of their condition and how and where they want to spend their remaining time. Whilst each individual's information needs will be different and require careful assessment, healthcare professionals tend to underestimate patients' desire for information and preferences about decision making (Fallowfield 2005). A large UK study showed that the vast majority of cancer patients want all possible information, though the timing of such information and the depth of detail desired were variable (Jenkins *et al.* 2001). Cultural and spiritual influences must be taken into account when assessing the information needs of patients in the terminal phase of life.

It is critical that nurses have the necessary training and skills for effective therapeutic communication with terminally ill patients and their relatives. For more detailed information about communication, see Chapter 5.

Prognosis

Prognostication simply means predicting an outcome (Glare and Christakis 2004) – and in the care of those who are dying, patients and their families may want information about the likely time remaining before death occurs. This can be difficult to know with much certainty but is generally easier to gauge the closer death is to occurring. Whilst studies show that patients and their relatives tend to have different information needs regarding prognosis (relatives generally wanting more detailed information than patients) (Clayton and Tattersall 2006), it is important that these are carefully assessed to ensure that the needs of all those involved with the patient can be met. Discussions surrounding prognosis should be undertaken by professionals confident in advanced communication skills and with the appropriate experience to offer an approximation on the grounds of their clinical knowledge and experience. The principles of breaking bad news (see Chapter 5) should be adhered to in undertaking discussions about prognosis.

Procedure

The importance of individually tailored care for those in the terminal phase of their lives and their relatives cannot be overemphasized. No framework, pathway or care plan is a substitute for careful assessment, information giving, listening, referral and skilled intervention. Each person will require slightly different care in one way or another and, as with all areas of nursing care, assumptions should never be made solely on the basis of previous preferences, sociocultural or religious stereotypes.

Nonetheless, some principles and interventions, whilst not to be applied without bearing in mind the individual's needs, are important and should be routinely considered, even if not undertaken for each patient.

The Liverpool Care Pathway (LCP) provides guidance on many different aspects of terminal care including comfort measures, the anticipatory prescription of medicines, the discontinuation of inappropriate interventions (including resuscitation) and care of the relatives (both before and after the death of the patient). The pathway was developed in the late 1990s by the specialist palliative care teams at the Royal Liverpool University Hospital and the Marie Curie Centre in Liverpool in response to an obvious disparity in the quality of end-of-life care in the general setting as opposed to a specialist palliative care setting (such as a hospice). The LCP was seen as a means of enabling professionals of all specialties to provide the best possible multidisciplinary care for their patients as they enter the terminal phase of life (Kinder and Ellershaw 2003). The pathway is adaptable by individual institutions according to local practices, but in essence comprises three sections: (1) initial assessment and care of the dying patient, (2) ongoing care of the dying patient, and

Table 2.2 Common symptoms observed in the terminal phase of life

Symptom	Management changes
Pain	Levels of pain may increase, decrease or remain stable. Analgesics may need to be rationalized and/or administered via a different route (e.g. via a subcutaneous syringe pump) as the patient may no longer be able to swallow (for further information, see Chapter 9)
	Levels of consciousness, lucidity and respiratory rate will all be commonly altered during the terminal phase. It is important to bear this in mind when assessing the effect and side-effects of analgesic medications
	Some discomfort can be caused by immobility and pressure on the skin. If appropriate (i.e. if it will not cause patient or relative distress), the patient should be moved to a pressure-relieving mattress. Otherwise regular skin care should be carried out as tolerated (see Chapter 9 for further information)
Nausea/vomiting	Nausea and vomiting may increase, decrease or remain stable. Antiemetics may need to be rationalized and/or administered via a different route (e.g. via a subcutaneous syringe pump) as the patient may no longer be able to swallow
	Because the insertion of a nasogastric tube is considered a fairly invasive and uncomfortable procedure, it is unlikely to be appropriate for the management of nausea and vomiting in the terminal care setting. Those nasogastric tubes already *in situ* should remain unless causing distress to the patient
	Injectable hyoscine hydrobromide (Buscopan) or octreotide should be considered to dry gastric secretions in those patients with mechanical vomiting secondary to bowel obstruction
Respiratory secretions	'Noisy', 'bubbly' breathing or 'death rattle' in the terminal phase of life affects approximately 50% of dying patients (O'Donnell 1998) and is the result of fluid pooling in the hypopharynx
	Changing the position of the patient in the bed may reduce the noisiness of breathing. It is important to reassure the family that the patient is not drowning or choking, and is unlikely to be distressed by the symptom themselves
	Antimuscarinic (hyoscine butylbromide) or anticholinergic drugs (glycopyrronium or hyoscine hydrobromide) are often used in this setting and can be administered subcutaneously via a syringe pump
Agitation/restlessness	Confusion, delirium, agitation and restlessness are all terms used to describe patient distress in the last 48 hours of life. The symptom is fairly common, with up to 88% of patients experiencing symptoms in the last days or hours of life (Lawlor *et al.* 2000). Careful assessment should include consideration of any precipitating factors including: medications, reversible metabolic causes, constipation, urinary retention, hypoxia, withdrawal from drugs or alcohol, uncontrolled symptoms and existential distress
	Clear, concise communication, continuity of carers if possible, the presence of familiar objects and people and a safe immediate environment can all be helpful nursing interventions
	Where the cause of the symptoms cannot be established or cannot be reversed, anxiolytics, antipsychotics or sedation may need to be considered. This may need to be discussed with relatives instead of the patient. It is important that the nurse is present for these conversations in order to facilitate reassurance of the relatives throughout
Breathlessness	Breathlessness may be a new symptom in the terminal phase or may worsen from its pre-existing state. Careful assessment is important as this symptom will usually involve physiological, psychological and environmental factors
	Low-dose opioids and anxiolytics can be of use for breathlessness, though as with other medications, the route of administration may need to be altered. Nebulized bronchodilators and oxygen may also be of benefit. Where the symptom is causing severe distress and is intractable, sedation may need to be considered in discussion with the patient and relatives
	Relaxation exercises, open windows or electric fans and massage may also be of benefit if the patient can tolerate these
Constipation	The focus of care with regard to constipation should remain on patient comfort. Oral laxatives are inappropriate if the patient cannot swallow and rectal interventions should only be undertaken if the patient is clearly distressed by this symptom

Table 2.3 The Liverpool Care Pathway (LCP) – key stages and patient goals

Stage	Focus/stage specifics	Assessment/patient goals
Initial assessment	Medical assessment, including the cessation of inappropriate therapy and medication, forward planning for treatment symptoms and an assessment of appropriate nursing care needs	■ Physical assessment ■ Assessment of comfort ■ Psychological assessment ■ Assessment of psychological needs/insight into condition ■ Assessment of religious/spiritual needs ■ Assessment of communication needs
Ongoing assessment	Four-hourly nursing assessment of symptom control	■ Pain ■ Agitation ■ Respiratory tract secretions ■ Nausea and emesis ■ Other symptoms such as dyspnoea ■ Oral hygiene ■ Elimination needs ■ Safe delivery of medication ■ Mobility/pressure area care ■ Psychological support ■ Religious/spiritual support ■ Needs of family/significant other
Care after death	Discussion with family Correct documentation	■ Last Offices ■ Property/valuables ■ Family information ■ Bereavement booklet ■ Informing GP/appropriate organizations

Reproduced from Jevon (2010).

(3) care of family and carers after death of the patient. The key stages and patient goals of the LCP are demonstrated in Table 2.3. *Care of the Dying: A Pathway to Excellence* (Ellershaw and Wilkinson 2003) is a key reference book in understanding the development, implementation and evaluation of the LCP.

The LCP is a useful tool in prompting the multiprofessional team to consider different aspects of caring for the dying patient and their relatives. It makes provision for regular assessment of the patient and relatives, and acts as a central source of multidisciplinary documentation about care given in the last days of life. The Department of Health's *End-of-Life Care Strategy* (DH 2008), which seeks to ensure equitable access to excellent palliative care nationwide, recommends the use of the LCP across all healthcare settings as a means of providing a high standard of care in the last days and hours of life.

The LCP, and indeed all good palliative care, always integrates physical, psychological, social and spiritual aspects of care, at no time more important than in the terminal phase of life. Some principles of care are outlined for each of these areas below.

Physical care

Table 2.2 lists the most common physical symptoms present during the terminal phase of life and any management changes specific to care of the patient who is dying. The first four symptoms are the most common.

Psychosocial care

Ongoing psychosocial assessment, support and care of the patient and their relatives are extremely important as death approaches. However, provision may need to be adjusted according to the changing needs of the patient – many will experience increasing anxiety and distress, increased feelings of social isolation and, alongside this, a decrease in physical energy available to them for dealing with these concerns. Relatives will naturally be distressed by the increasing illness of the patient and may exhibit signs of grief even before death occurs. Nurses should ensure that, wherever possible, the physical environment is conducive to patients and relatives being able to express their thoughts and emotions, and that appropriately trained staff are available to listen and support them.

Preferred priorities of care

An important aspect of meeting the psychosocial needs of patients and their relatives in the last days of life is to ensure that, wherever possible, preferred priorities of care are discussed and met. These include preferred place of care and death and other difficult issues which have traditionally

60

not been discussed, to the detriment of the patient. A formal document, developed as part of the Department of Health's *End-of-Life Care Strategy* (DH 2008), is available to support these discussions (www.endoflifecareforadults. nhs.uk).

Spiritual and religious care

As death approaches, many people will be seeking answers to life's big questions: its nature, meaning and purpose and what, if any, form it takes after death. Some may find these answers in religion, others in their own philosophy or that of others. Many nurses acknowledge the struggle to provide spiritual or religious support because they feel inadequately skilled or knowledgeable (Kissane and Yates 2003). However, assessment, even if simple, communication and onward referral will ensure that appropriate care can be given without compromising the integrity of the healthcare professional, nor denying the patient the opportunity to explore these central life issues.

Those with specific religious beliefs may have certain religious practices which need to be undertaken before or after death. It is important to try to discuss these with the patient, as even where relatives share a common faith, there may be differences in the way each person practises. It is, as always, vital that assumptions are not made on the basis of a previously disclosed religious preference – for example, not all Catholic believers will want to be given the sacrament of the sick. Each patient and their relatives should have the opportunity to express their needs and nurses should ensure that, wherever possible, these are met. Further information about religious/cultural perspectives and practices is given in Table 2.4.

Postprocedural considerations

Nursing care does not end when the death of the patient occurs. Last Offices should be performed with as much attention to detail and respect for the individual as any other procedure.

Last Offices

Definitions

The term 'Last Offices' is historically related to the Latin *officium*, meaning service or duty. It is used to refer to the final act performed on a person's body. Last Offices, sometimes referred to as 'laying out', is the term for the nursing care given to a deceased patient which demonstrates continued respect for the patient as an individual (NMC 2008). Nursing care continues even after death. Last Offices includes health, safety and legal requirements, making the person's body safe to handle, respecting religious, cultural and spiritual requirements, and making the person who has died as pleasant as possible for others to see.

Patients, even though they have died, are still referred to as patients or people throughout this section.

Related theory

After-death care is the final act a nurse will carry out for the patient and remains associated with ritual (Pattison 2008b). Nursing care for a patient who has died has historical roots dating back to the 19th century (Wolf 1988). However, contemporary nursing has moved away from the ritualistic practices of cleansing, plugging, packing and tying the patient's orifices to prevent the leakage of body fluids to encompass much more than simply dealing with a dead body (Pattison 2008b, Pearce 1963). Consideration now has to be given to legal issues surrounding death, the removal (or non-removal) of equipment, washing and grooming, and ensuring correct identification of the patient (Costello 2004). The *End-of-Life Care Strategy* (DH 2008) emphasizes care after a patient has died, and in particular it points to the value of integrated care pathways in managing administrative and psychosocial care. This corresponds to 'good death' theory where being treated with dignity is an underlying premise (Kehl 2006, Smith 2000), and good death encompasses all stages of dying and death (Pattison 2008b). This principle, therefore, continues after death.

Carrying out such an intimate act, that in many cultures would be carried out only by certain family or community members, requires careful consideration by nurses and adequate preparation of procedures that include family members where possible. Since 60.6% of all men and women who die in England and Wales will die in an institution (hospice, hospital, care home) (ONS 2009), it is predominantly nurses who will have to carry out after-death care, prior to patients being moved to mortuaries or funeral homes. Quested and Rudge (2001) suggested that this aspect of care is largely invisible to other healthcare workers.

Death threatens the orderly continuation of social life, according to Seale (1998). Last Offices can mark the social transition of the person as well as the biological death of the patient, and begins the process of handing over care to the family and funeral director. Last Offices can be considered as an important act in the rite of passage in moving the deceased person into the world of the dead (Van Gennep 1972) and is a procedure that people in all cultures recognize.

Evidence-based approaches
Rationale

Last Offices has its foundation in traditional cultures and is a nursing routine which does not have a large amount of research-based evidence (Cooke 2000). The administration of Last Offices can have symbolic meaning for nurses, often providing a sense of closure. It can be a fulfilling experience as it is the final demonstration of respectful, sensitive care given to a patient (Nearney 1998) and also the family (Speck 1992).

Table 2.4 Cultural and religious factors to be considered at Last Offices

	Beliefs about death	Cultural or religious routines	Preparing the body	Postmortem/ transplantation	Specific 'burial' requirements	For further information contact
Buddhism	Death is viewed as very important as it is a time of transition before rebirth as they move towards Nirvana – the freedom from suffering death and rebirth	There is no one specific ritual but a state of calm is necessary. An example may be: ■ a monk called to recite prayers/lead meditation ■ the family wanting the body to remain in one place for up to 7 days for the rebirth to take place. However, it is recognized this is not possible in a healthcare setting	At all times the body should be treated with greatest care and respect When washing has taken place, the body should be wrapped in a plain white sheet	No objections	Prefer cremation as symbol of impermanence of the body	The Buddhist Hospice Trust 01983 526945 www.buddhisthospice.org.uk
Christianity Anglican/ Church of England	God's forgiveness is available to all who ask because of the selfless/sinless death of Jesus Christ on the cross. As Christ was resurrected, death has been overcome and eternal life is a gift from God, available to all who believe and seek forgiveness	Priest or minister may attend to say prayers. Primarily to support relatives and friends	No specific requests	No objections	No preference	Hospital Chaplaincies Council 020 7898 1894 www.nhs-chaplaincy-spiritualcare.org.uk
Non-conformist/ Free Church		Prayers may be offered but these will be informal in most situations	No specific requests	No objections	No preference	
Roman Catholicism		Priest requested to recite prayers for the dying and then prayers for the dead	A religious icon such as a crucifix or rosary may accompany the patient's body	No objections	Burial has in the past been preferred	
Church of Jesus Christ of Latter Day Saints Mormon Church	Earthly life is viewed as a test to see if individuals are fit to return to God on death. Death is viewed as a temporary separation from loved ones		The body should be washed and dressed in a shroud. Some may wear a religious undergarment which must remain in place after the patient has died	No religious objection	Burial preferred	The Church of Jesus Christ of Latter Day Saints 0121 712 1200 www.ldschurch.org
Christian Scientist	There are no specific rituals associated with death		Females only to touch female body	This is generally not supported unless there is a legal requirement for it	Prefer cremation	For details of local Christian Science Church www.christianscience.org.uk

Table 2.4 (*Continued*)

	Beliefs about death	Cultural or religious routines	Preparing the body	Postmortem/transplantation	Specific 'burial' requirements	For further information Contact
Hinduism	Hindus believe that all human beings have a soul that passes through successive cycles of birth and re-birth. It is believed that eventually the soul will be purified and join the cosmic consciousness	Last rites include: tying a thread around the neck or wrist to bless the dying person, sprinkling holy water from the River Ganges on them, placing a sacred Tulsi leaf in their mouth if possible, placing the person on a sheet or mat on the floor to symbolize close-ness to Mother Earth, freedom from physical constraints and the easing of the soul's departure	Close family members usu-ally wash the body led by the eldest son. They may be dis-tressed if a non-Hindu touches the body so gloves should be worn. A female must only be touched by a female and a male by a male The body should be covered by a plain white sheet All religious objects should remain in place	Only if absolutely necessary. If a postmortem does take place, the organs must be returned to the body	Cremation within 24 hours of death arranged by the eldest son	National Council of Hindu Temples (UK), www.hinducounciluk.org
Islam	Death is a mark of transition from one state of being to another. Muslims are encouraged to accept death as part of the will of Allah	The time before death is im-portant for extending forgive-ness to family and friends The Koran is recited until the point of death	The body should be turned to the right (Quibla (Mecca)) if this hasn't happened before the patient dies The relatives will close the eyes and bandage the lower jaw so the mouth doesn't gape Flex the joints of the arms and legs to stop them becoming rigid A complete cleansing (Ghusal) will then take place performed by the relatives (this may take place after the body has been removed from the ward) The body will be wrapped in a Caffan. If there isn't one avail-able, a sheet will do A female must be handled by female nursing staff and a male by male staff Maintaining modesty and dignity is essential	This is not acceptable, primarily because it will delay burial but also because the person may still be able to perceive pain	Burial will take place as quickly as possible	Muslim Council of Great Britain http://www.mcb.org.uk/downloads/Death-Bereavement.pdf
Jehovah's Witness	When a person dies their existence stops for ever	There are no special rituals or practices to perform	No special requirements are to be observed		Funeral must be modest and dignified	his@wtbts.org.uk www.watchtower.org

Religion	Belief about death	Care of the dying/body	Cremation/burial	Contact
Judaism	Death is the end of life but eternal life is offered if they have the right relationship with God	Orthodox Jews don't permit the touching or moving of a dying person. Following death, the rabbi will be requested to perform Last Rites. It is important that somebody stays with the body until a member of Jewish Burial Society or family member arrives. The family may want to keep watch with the body to pray even if it is in the mortuary. The body will receive the ritual washing (Taharah) performed by either trained members of the synagogue or the Jewish Burial Society. If the rabbi cannot be contacted, essential procedures can be performed by healthcare staff: ■ close eyes and mouth ■ all catheters and drains and the fluid in them must be left as they are considered part of the body ■ open wounds must be covered ■ the body must be laid flat with hands open and arms parallel to the body ■ DON'T wash the body ■ Traditionally the body is covered by a plain white sheet with the feet facing the door	This is not permitted by Orthodox Jews except where the law requires it. Reform Jews permit it on the grounds of the furthering of medical knowledge. Cremation is permitted for non-Orthodox Jews	The Burial Society of the United Synagogue 020 8343 3456. The Office of the Chief Rabbi (Orthodox), 735 High Road, North Finchley, London WC1N 9HN. 020 8343 6301. Union of Liberal and Progressive Synagogues, Montagu Centre, 21 Maple Street, London W1T 4BE
Sikhism	Life after death is a continuous cycle of rebirth; the person's soul is their essence	Prior to the death, comfort may be derived from reciting verses from the holy book (Guru Granth Sahib). The relatives may wish to prepare the body but this shouldn't be assumed. The five Ks should be left on the body. 1 Kesh – uncut hair symbolic of sanctity and a love of nature 2 Kangha – a wooden comb symbolizing cleanliness 3 Kara – a steel band worn on the right wrist symbolic of strength and restraint 4 Kirpan – a sword or dagger symbolizing the readiness to fight against injustice 5 Kaccha – unisex undershorts symbolizing morality. The body must be touched only by staff of the same sex. The eyes and mouth closed. The face straight and clean	Cremation. No objections	Sikh Educational and Cultural Association (UK) 01474 332356

64

Many parts of this nursing procedure are based on general principles of infection prevention and control, and safe working. Furthermore, there is a cultural requirement to continue with the practice of Last Offices, as 'rituals serve to express symbolic meanings important to groups of people functioning within a subculture' (Wolf 1988, p.59). This is particularly important with something as profound as death. Rituals have a role in providing comfort and structure at a traumatic time, which Neuberger (2004) suggests can be valuable for families. Nurses approaching this act of care with compassion might enable families to see that their family member was respected and cared for, even after death. Nurses demonstrate the respect they have for a person who has died and the family, who may now 'own' the body, through rituals associated with Last Offices (Pattison 2008b).

Contemporary nursing practice and education increasingly shy away from ritualistic practices as they are considered irrational and unscientific (Philpin 2002) but Last Offices remains a notable exception. However, this is not to say that nurses carrying out Last Offices do it 'without thinking about it in a problem-solving way' (Walsh and Ford 1989, p.9) or in a way that does not recognize the individual needs of deceased patients and their carers. Instead, they are carried out with insight into the meanings attached to the accomplishment of this aspect of nursing care (Philpin 2002).

This aspect of care is usually carried out on the ward. In institutions without mortuary technicians, nurses may also rarely be called on to aid a family to view a patient who has died in the hours after death in the mortuary (Figure 2.6) or in a 'chapel of rest' (Figure 2.7).

There is no national guidance for how to prepare patients who have died for the mortuary or funeral home. *Patients Who Die in Hospital* (DH 1997) and *What to Do After a Death* (DWP 2006) deal with death in hospital and focus on procedures around the legalities of organizing funerals.

Figure 2.6   Mortuary.

Figure 2.7   Chapel of rest.

Specific guidance might potentially disallow individual variation and personalization of after-death care in respect to patient wishes, cultures and religions. There is, however, national guidance on infection prevention and control in relation to people who have died. Care of the patient who has died must take into account health and safety guidelines to ensure families, healthcare workers, mortuary staff and undertakers are not put at risk (HSAC 2003). This chapter incorporates this guidance into broader national guidance where appropriate. It aims to ensure that patients who have died are treated with respect and dignity even after death, that legalities are adhered to, and that appropriate infection prevention and control measures are taken.

Indications

- When a patient's death has been verified and documented.
- For adult patients who have died in hospital or in a hospice.

Contraindications

When to consult for further guidance before undertaking procedure:

- if a patient who has died is indicated for a postmortem
- if a patient who has died is a candidate for organ donation.

Legal and professional issues

In administering Last Offices, nurses need to know the legal requirements for care of patients after death and it is essential that correct procedures are followed. Every effort should be made to accommodate the wishes of the patient's relatives (Neuberger 2004). The UK is an increasingly multicultural and multifaith society which presents a challenge to nurses who need to be aware of the different religious and cultural rituals that may accompany the death of a patient. There are notable cultural variations within and between people of different faiths, ethnic backgrounds and national origins. This can affect approaches to death and dying (Neuberger 2004) and needs to remembered when administering Last Offices in order to avoid presumptions. While those who have settled in a society where there is a dominant faith or culture other than their own might appear to increasingly adopt that dominant culture, they may choose to retain their different practices at times of birth, marriage or death (Neuberger 1999). Approaches to death and dying also reveal as much of the attitude of society as a whole as they do about individuals within that society (Field *et al.* 1997).

Practices relating to Last Offices will vary depending on the patient's cultural background and religious practices (Nearney 1998). The following sections provide a guide to cultural and religious variations in attitudes to death and how individuals may wish to be treated. The information that follows is not designed to be a 'factfile' (Gilliat-Ray 2001, Gunaratnam 1997, Smaje and Field 1997) of information on culture and religion that seeks to give concrete information. Such a 'factfile' would not be appropriate as we need to be aware that whilst death and death-related beliefs, rituals and traditions can vary widely between specific cultural groups, within any given religious or cultural group there may be varying degrees of observance of these issues (Green and Green 2006), from orthodox to agnostic and atheist. Categorizing individuals into groups with clearly defined norms can lead to a lack of understanding of the complexities of religious and cultural practice and can depersonalize care for individuals and their families (Neuberger 1999, Smaje and Field 1997).

Last Offices for an expected death may be very different to those given to a patient who has died suddenly or unexpectedly (Docherty 2000) or in a critical care setting, so these issues will be dealt with later in this chapter. In certain cases the patient's death may need to be referred to the coroner or medical examiner for further investigation and possible postmortem (DH 2003c). If those caring for the deceased are unsure about this then the person in charge of the patient's care should be consulted before Last Offices are commenced.

Prior to the patient's death, whenever possible it is good practice to ascertain if the patient wishes to donate organs or tissue following their death. For further information on this, visit www.nhsorgandonor.net.

Preprocedural considerations

Before undertaking Last Offices several other events must take place.

Confirmation of death

Death should be confirmed or verified by appropriate healthcare staff. At present, confirmation of death is usually done by a medical doctor but can be undertaken by nurses in certain healthcare settings, if death is *expected* and local policy permits this (RCN 1996). Unexpected deaths must be confirmed by a medical doctor (and usually a senior medical doctor). Confirmation of death must be recorded in the medical and nursing notes (and care pathway documentation if necessary).

A registered medical doctor who has attended the deceased person during their last illness is required to give a medical certificate of the cause of death (Home Office 1971). The certificate requires the doctor to state on which date they last saw the deceased alive and whether or not they have seen the body after death (this may mean that the certificate is completed by a different doctor from the one who confirmed death). Out-of-hours medical examiners can now certify death where there is a cultural/religious requirement to bury, cremate or repatriate patients quickly (DH 2008). Medical examiners can also certify for reportable deaths where a postmortem is not deemed necessary (DH 2008). The medical examiner (ME) is a primary care trust-appointed but independent health professional who determines the need for coroner referral. For those who need a quick burial within 24 hours, this remains at the discretion of the local births and deaths registrar in each council and depends on the individual opening hours and on-call facilities. Local hospital policy should outline procedures for out-of-hours death registration and certification, and burial is usually easier to accommodate than cremation within 24 hours.

Repatriation to another country needs further documentation, alongside the death certification and registration documents, and this varies according to which country repatriation is to. Only a coroner or medical examiner is authorized to permit the body to be moved out of England or Wales. A 'Form of Notice to a Coroner of Intention to Remove a Body Out of England' (Form 104) is required which can be obtained from coroners or registrars. This form needs to be given to the coroner along with any certificate for burial or cremation already issued. The coroner's office will acknowledge receipt of notice and inform when repatriation can occur. Coroner authorization normally takes up to 4 working days so that necessary enquiries can be made. In urgent situations, this can sometimes be expedited. The coroner's office and relevant High Commission will have further information. In terms of infection control, packing may be required by different countries and those involved with repatriation must be informed if there is a danger of infection (HSAC 2003). Funeral directors would assist with transportation issues.

Referral to a coroner

If the patient's death is to be referred to a coroner or ME, this will affect how their body is prepared. The need for referral to a coroner or ME needs to be ascertained with the person verifying the death (DH 2008). Preparation in this situation differs according to how the patient died. Broadly, two types of death are referred to the coroner.

- Those from a list of cases where the coroner must be informed (which includes deaths within 24 hours of an operation, for example).

■ Cases where the treating doctor is unable to certify the cause of death (Home Office 2002, HTA 2006).

The Department of Health website at www.dh.gov.uk gives more information about when to refer to the coroner or ME and when postmortems are indicated.

Requirement for a postmortem

Postmortems can affect preparation after death, depending on whether this is a coroner's postmortem (sometimes referred to as a legal postmortem because it cannot be refused) or a postmortem requested by the consultant doctor-in-charge to answer a specific query on the cause of death (also referred to as a hospital or non-legal postmortem). A coroner's post-mortem might require specific preparation but the coroner or ME will advise on this and should be contacted as soon as possible after death to ascertain any specific issues. Individual hospitals, institutions and NHS trusts should provide further guidance on these issues. If the patient is to be referred to the coroner, cap off catheters and ensure there is no possibility of leakage. Do not remove any invasive devices until this has been discussed with the coroner (HTA 2006).

If the patient is *not* to be referred to the coroner, invasive and non-invasive attachments, such as central venous access catheters, peripheral venous access cannulas, Swan–Ganz catheters, tracheal tubes (tracheostomy/endotracheal) and drains, can be removed prior to Last Offices.

Organ donation

Consider whether the patient is a candidate for organ or tissue donation. Patients who previously expressed a wish to be a donor (or carry a donor card), or whose family has expressed such a wish, might need specific preparation (see further resources at the end of the chapter and contact local or regional transplant co-ordinators).

Organ donation is an important consideration at the end of life. Current law is an opt-in system for donation, there-fore express wishes must be made by families (next of kin) or patients.

Infectious patient

If the patient was infectious, it needs to be established whether it is a notifiable infection, for example, hepatitis B, C or tuberculosis, or non-notifiable (Healing *et al.* 1995, HPA 2010, HSAC 2003). There are additional requirements for patients with bloodborne infections, so the senior nurse on duty should be consulted and local infection control policy adhered to. In the UK, notifiable infections must be reported via a local authority 'proper officer' which is the attending doctor's duty. Infection prevention and control contacts in local trusts or services can provide more help and guidance around notification. Placing the patient who has died in a body bag is advised for all notifiable diseases and a number of non-notifiable infectious diseases (i.e. HIV, transmissible

spongiform encephalopathies, e.g. Creutzfeldt–Jakob disease). A label identifying the infection must also be attached to the patient's body. Specific guidance is outlined in Procedure guideline 2.2.

Certain extra precautions are required when handling a patient who has died from an infectious disease. However, the deceased will pose no greater threat of an infectious risk than when they were alive. It is assumed that staff will have practised universal precautions when caring for all patients, and this practice must be continued when caring for the deceased patient (HSAC 2003).

Porters, mortuary staff, undertakers and those involved with Last Offices must also be informed if there is a danger of infection (HSAC 2003) or radiation (see Chapters 3 and 14).

Informing the next of kin

Inform and offer support to relatives and/or next of kin to ensure that the relevant individuals are aware of the patient's death and any specific care or practices can be carried out (Wilkinson and Mula 2003). The support of a hospital chaplain or other religious leader or other appropriate person should be offered. If the relative(s) or next of kin are not contactable by telephone or by the GP, it may be necessary to inform the police of the death.

Some families and carers may wish to assist with Last Offices, and within certain cultures it may be unacceptable for anyone but a family member or religious leader to wash the patient (Green and Green 2006). It may also be required for somebody of the same sex as the patient to undertake Last Offices (Neuberger 2004). Families and carers should be sup-ported and encouraged to participate if possible as this may help to facilitate the grieving process (Berry and Griffie 2001).

Families and carers should also be supported in adhering to infection prevention and control procedures.

There are a few, very rare, exceptions where it is not pos-sible for families to participate in Last Offices.

■ If the patient has had any of the following infections pri-or to death: typhus, severe acute respiratory syndrome, yellow fever, anthrax, plague, rabies and smallpox. As-sistance with Last Offices or viewing is not permitted be-cause of the high risk of transmission of these infections (Healing *et al.* 1995).

■ The patient who has died was exposed to radiation. Pa-tients may have been treated with radioactive material as therapy or may have been exposed to it in accidental circumstances. Always seek expert radiation protection advice before beginning Last Offices in such cases.

Patient considerations

Ascertain any social, cultural, spiritual and/or religious con-siderations that should be observed during the procedure. Spiritual needs involved in preparation of the patient who has died can be diverse but the final sections in this chapter give up-to-date guidance about religious considerations in

Procedure guideline 2.2 Last Offices

Essential equipment

- Disposable plastic apron
- Disposable plastic gloves
- Bowl of warm water, soap, patient's own toilet articles. Disposable wash cloths and two towels
- Disposable razor or patient's own electric razor, comb and equipment for nail care
- Equipment for mouth care including equipment for cleaning dentures
- Identification labels × 2
- Documents required by law and by organization/insitution policy, for example Notification of Death cards
- Shroud or patient's personal clothing: night-dress, pyjamas, clothes previously requested by patient, or clothes which comply with deceased patient/family/cultural wishes

- Body bag if required (if there is actual or potential leakage of bodily fluids and/or if there is infectious disease). Labels for the patient's body defining the nature of the infection/disease (HSAC 2003)
- Gauze, tape, dressings and bandages if wounds, puncture sites or intravenous/arterial devices
- Valuables/property book
- Plastic bags for clinical and domestic (household) waste
- Laundry skip and appropriate bags for soiled linen
- Clean bedlinen
- Record books for property and valuables
- Bags for the patient's personal possessions
- Disposable or washable receptacle for collecting urine, if appropriate
- Sharps bin, if appropriate

Optional equipment

- Caps/spigots for urinary catheters (if catheters are to be left *in situ*)
- Goggles
- Full gowns
- 3M masks (if highly infectious) (HSAC 2003)

- Petroleum jelly
- Suction equipment and absorbent pads (where there is the potential for leakage)
- Card or envelope to offer lock of hair, as appropriate

Preprocedure

Action	Rationale
1 Apply gloves and apron, gowns/masks/goggles if the patient is infectious.	Personal protective equipment (PPE) must be worn when performing Last Offices, and is used to protect yourself and all your patients from the risks of cross-infection (Fraise and Bradley 2009, E, HSAC 2003, C; Pratt *et al.* 2007, C, R2b; RCN 2005, C).
2 If the patient is on a pressure-relieving mattress or device, consult the manufacturer's instructions before switching off.	If the mattress deflates too quickly, it may cause a manual handling challenge to the nurses carrying out Last Offices.

Procedure

3 Lay the patient on their back with the assistance of additional nurses and straighten any limbs as far as possible (adhering to your own organization's manual handling policy).	To maintain the patient's privacy and dignity (NMC 2008, C) and for future nursing care of the body. Stiff, flexed limbs can be difficult to fit easily into a mortuary trolley, mortuary fridge or coffin and can cause additional distress to any carers who wish to view the body. However, if the patient's body cannot be straightened, force should not be used as this can be corrected by the funeral director (Green and Green 2006, E).
4 Remove all but one pillow. Close the mouth and support the jaw by placing a pillow or rolled-up towel on the chest or underneath the jaw. Do not bind the patient's jaw with bandages.	To avoid leaving pressure marks on the face which can be difficult to remove.
5 Remove any mechanical aids such as syringe drivers, heel pads, and so on. Apply gauze and tape to syringe driver/IV sites and document disposal of medication (adhering to your own organization's disposal of medication policy). Consider leaving prosthetics *in situ* as appropriate (e.g. limb, dental or breast prosthetics).	To prepare the body for burial or cremation. E

(Continued)

Procedure guideline 2.2 (*Continued*)

6 Close the patient's eyes by applying light pressure to the eyelids for 30 seconds. If this is unsuccessful then a little sticky tape such as Micropore can be used, and leaves no mark. Alternatively, moistened cotton wool may be used to hold the eyelids in place.	To maintain the patient's dignity (NMC 2008, C) and for aesthetic reasons. Closure of the eyelids will also provide tissue protection in case of corneal donation (Green and Green 2006, E).
7 Drain the bladder by applying firm pressure over the lower abdomen. Have a disposable or washable receptacle at the ready to collect urine.	Because the patient's body can continue to excrete fluids after death (Green and Green 2006, E).
8 Leakages from the oral cavity, vagina and bowel can be contained by the use of suctioning, drainage and incontinence pads respectively. Patients who do continue to have leakages from their orifices after death should be placed in a body bag following Last Offices. The packing of orifices can cause damage to the patient's body and should only be done by professionals who have received specialist training. It might be helpful to manage self-limiting leakages with absorbent pads and gently rolling the patient who has died to aid drainage of potential leakages.	Leaking orifices pose a health hazard to staff coming into contact with the patient's body(Green and Green 2006, E; HSAC 2003, C). Ensuring that the patient's body is clean will demonstrate continued respect for the patient's dignity (NMC 2008, C). The packing of orifices is considered unnecessary, as it increases the rate of bacterial growth that can occur when these areas of the patient's body are not allowed to drain naturally (Berry and Griffie 2001, E). However, there are certain situations where it is necessary (in severe leakage or where repatriation is required). A body bag is also necessary in these cases.
9 Exuding wounds or unhealed surgical scars should be covered with a clean absorbent dressing and secured with an occlusive dressing (e.g. Tegaderm). Stitches and clips should be left intact. Consider leaving intact recent surgical dressings for wounds that could potentially leak, for example large amputation wounds. Reinforcement of the dressing should be sufficient.	The dressing will absorb any leakage from the wound site. (Naylor *et al.* 2001, R2b). Open wounds and stomas pose a health hazard to staff coming into contact with the body (RCN 2005, C). Disturbing recent large surgical dressings may encourage seepage and leakage (Travis 2002, E).
10 Stomas should be covered with a clean bag.	
11 Remove drainage tubes, unless otherwise stated. Record the tubes and devices that have been removed and those that have been left *in situ*. Open drainage sites need to be sealed with an occlusive dressing (e.g. Tegaderm).	Open drainage sites pose a health hazard to staff coming into contact with the patient's body (RCN 2005, C). When a death is being referred to the coroner or ME or for postmortem, all lines, devices and tubes should be left in place (Green and Green 2006, C).
12 Wash the patient, unless requested not to do so for religious/cultural reasons or carer's preference. Male patients should be shaved unless they chose to wear a beard in life.	For hygienic and aesthetic reasons. As a mark of respect and point of closure in the relationship between nurse and patient (Cooke 2000, C).
If shaving a man, apply water-based emollient cream to the face.	To prevent brown streaks on the skin.
13 It may be important to family and carers to assist with washing, thereby continuing to provide the care given in the period before death.	It is an expression of respect and affection, part of the process of adjusting to loss and expressing grief (Berry and Griffie 2001, E).
14 Mouth and teeth should be cleaned with foam sticks or a toothbrush. Insert clean dentures if the patient normally used them. Apply petroleum jelly to the lips and perioral area.	Teeth and mouth are cleaned for hygienic and aesthetic reasons (Cooke 2000, C) and to remove debris. Petroleum jelly can prevent skin excoriation or corrosion if stomach contents aspirate.

15 Remove all jewellery (in the presence of another nurse) unless requested by the patient's family to do otherwise. Jewellery remaining on the patient should be documented on the 'Notification of Death' form. Record the jewellery and other valuables in the patient's property book and store the items according to local policy. Avoid the use of the names of precious metals or gems when describing jewellery to prevent potential later confusion. Instead, use terms such as 'yellow metal' or 'red stone'. Rings left on the patient's body should be secured with tape, if loose.	To meet with legal requirements, cultural practices and relatives' wishes (Green and Green 2006, C).
16 Dress the patient in personal clothing or white garment, traditionally called a shroud (depending on organizational policy or the family's wishes).	For aesthetic reasons for family and carers viewing the patient's body or religious or cultural reasons and to meet the family's or carers' wishes (Green and Green 2006, C).
17 Ensure the correct hospital or organizational irremovable patient identification label is attached to the patient's wrist and attach a further identification label to one ankle. Complete any documents such as Notification of Death cards. Copies of such cards are usually required (refer to hospital policy for details). Tape one securely to clothing or shroud.	To ensure correct and easy identification of the patient's body in the mortuary (Green and Green 2006, C).
18 Wrap the patient's body in a sheet, ensuring that the face and feet are covered and that all limbs are held securely in position.	To avoid possible damage to the patient's body during transfer and to prevent distress to colleagues, for example portering staff (Green and Green 2006, E).
19 Secure the sheet with tape.	Pins must not be used as they are a health and safety hazard to staff. E
20 Place the patient's body in a body bag as leakage of body fluids may be anticipated. The patient may also have a known infectious disease.	To avoid actual or potential leakage of fluid, whether infection is present or not, as this poses a health hazard to all those who come into contact with the deceased patient. The sheet will absorb excess fluid (HSAC 2003, C).

Postprocedure

21 Tape the second Notification of Death card to the outside of the sheet (or body bag).	For ease of identification of the patient's body in the mortuary (Green and Green 2006, E).
22 Request the portering staff to remove the patient's body from the ward and transport to the mortuary.	To avoid decomposition which occurs rapidly, particularly in hot weather and in overheated rooms. Many pathogenic organisms survive for some time after death and so decomposition of the patient's body may pose a health and safety hazard for those handling it (Cooke 2000, E). Autolysis and growth of bacteria are delayed if the patient's body is cooled.
23 Screen off the beds/area that will be passed as the patient's body is removed.	To avoid causing unnecessary distress to other patients, relatives and staff.
24 Remove gloves and apron. Dispose of equipment according to local policy and wash hands.	To minimize risk of cross-infection and contamination (Fraise and Bradley 2009, E).
25 Record all details and actions within the nursing documentation.	To record the time of death, names of those present, and names of those informed (NMC 2009, C).
26 Transfer property and patient records to the appropriate administrative department.	The administrative department cannot begin to process the formalities such as the death certificate or the collection of property by the next of kin until the required documents are in its possession (Green and Green 2006, C).

Problem-solving table 2.1 Prevention and resolution (Procedure guideline 2.2)

Problem	Cause	Prevention	Action
Relatives not present at the time of the patient's death	Possible unexpected death; non-contactable family	Preparation of family for event of death where appropriate	Inform the relatives as soon as possible of the death Consider also that they may want to view the patient's body before Last Offices are completed
Relatives or next of kin not contactable by telephone or by the general practitioner	Out-of-date or missing contact information	Ensure next of kin contact information is documented and up to date	If within the UK, local police will go to next of kin's house. If abroad, the British Embassy will assist
Death occurring within 24 hours of an operation	n/a	In relation to documentation, ensure information around circumstance of death is documented and handed over to relevant healthcare staff	All tubes and/or drains must be left in position. Spigot or cap off any cannulas or catheters. Treat stomas as open wounds. Leave any endotracheal or tracheostomy tubes in place. Machinery can be disconnected (discuss with coroner) but settings must be left alone Postmortem examination will be required to establish the cause of death. Any tubes, drains, and so on may have been a major contributing factor to the death
Unexpected death	n/a	As above	As above. Postmortem examination of the patient's body will be required to establish the cause of death
Unknown cause of death	n/a	As above	As above
Patient brought into hospital who is already deceased	n/a	Not preventable but where possible, ensure patients' families are prepared for all eventualities, particularly if palliative care patients whose death is expected, and that family know who to call and what to do in the event of death	As above, unless patient seen by a medical practitioner within 14 days before death. In this instance, the attending medical officer may complete the death certificate if they are clear as to the cause of death
Patient who dies after receiving systemic radioactive iodine	There is a potential risk of exposure to radiation (IPEM 2002)	Radiation protection should be undertaken (see Chapter 14)	Ensure those in contact with the patient's body are aware and pregnant nurses should not carry out Last Offices for these patients. For further information see Chapter 14
Patient who dies after insertion of gold grains, colloidal radioactive solution, caesium needles, caesium applicators, iridium wires or iridium hair pins	There is a potential risk of exposure to radiation (IPEM 2002)	Radiation protection should be undertaken (see Chapter 14) when removing wires. Physicist may remove radioactive wires/needles, and so on, themselves, depending on source	Inform the physics department as well as appropriate medical staff. Once a doctor has verified death, the sources are removed and placed in a lead container. A Geiger counter is used to check that all sources have been removed. This reduces the radiation risk when completing the Last Offices procedures. Record the time and date of removal of the sources. Ensure those in contact with the patient's body are aware and pregnant nurses should not carry out Last Offices for these patients. For further information see Chapter 14

Problem	Cause	Prevention	Action
Patient and/or relative wishes to donate organs/tissues for transplantation	n/a	Discussion around transplantation should occur with families/next of kin wherever appropriate (as deemed by clincial team). Exceptions apply	As stated in the Human Tissue Act 1961, patients with malignancies can only donate corneas and heart valves (and more recently, tracheas). Contact local transplant co-ordinator as soon as decision is made to donate organs/tissue and before Last Offices is attempted. Obtain verbal and written consent from the next of kin, as per local policy. Prepare patient who has died as per transplant co-ordinator's instructions. For further guidance see: www.uktransplant.org.uk
Patient to be moved straight from ward to undertakers	n/a	n/a	Contact senior nurse for hospital. Contact local Register Office as Certificate for Burial or Cremation ('green' document) needs to be obtained. Liaise with chosen funeral directors and the deceased's family. Perform Last Offices as per religious/cultural/family wishes. Obtain written authority for removal of person by the funeral directors, from the next of kin. Document all actions and proceedings (Travis 2002)
Relatives want to see the person who has died after removal from the ward	n/a	n/a	Inform the mortuary staff in order to allow time for them to prepare the body. Occasionally nurses might be required to undertake this in institutions where there are no mortuary staff. The patient's body will normally be placed in the hospital viewing room. Ask relatives if they wish for a chaplain or other religious leader or appropriate person to accompany them. As required, religious artefacts should be removed from or added to the viewing room. The nurse should check that the patient's body and environment are presentable before accompanying the relatives into the viewing room. The relatives may want to be alone with the deceased but the nurse should wait outside the viewing room in order that support may be provided should the relatives become distressed. After the relatives have left, the nurse should contact the portering service who will return the deceased patient to the mortuary
Patient has an implantable cardioverter defibrillator (ICD) which could potentially delay death certification (Goldstein *et al.* 2004). There are risks (potential explosion) associated around cremation with both pacemakers (Dimond 2004) and ICDs (MHRA 2002)	n/a	Knowledge of device *in situ* prior to death	Nurses must inform funeral directors and mortuary staff about patients with cardiac pacemakers *in situ* and ensure it is clearly documented (Dimond 2004; Royal Marsden NHS Foundation Trust 2006,). For patients with ICDs, the implants should be disabled once death has been confirmed (Goldstein *et al.* 2004) since these can delay pronunciation of death. This will prevent the chance of shocks being delivered to a patient who has already died or who is dying. The MHRA (2002) highlights that taping a small magnet over the skin does not always disable ICDs. However, cardiac technicians can reprogramme ICDs to non-shock mode (MHRA 2002). Nurses should consult local protocols and guidance for clear information on what should be done in specific areas

Last Offices. It should be noted that this is guidance only and the patient's previous wishes should be established where possible and should always take precedence (Pattison 2008a). If not documented, try to determine the patient's previous wishes from family or carers. The patient's last will and testament might have instruction on this, or an Advance Directive might have information. Families, carers or members of the patient's community or faith may wish to participate in Last Offices (with consent of the next of kin or as expressed in the patient's wishes when they were alive). If this is the case, they must be adequately prepared for this with careful and sensitive explanation of the procedure to be undertaken.

Families may request other items to accompany the patient who has died to the mortuary and funeral home. This might be an item of sentimental value, for instance, and in this case it should be at the discretion of those caring for the patient and the nurse-in-charge (local policy might also specify). Certain religious artefacts must never be removed from the patient, even after death, for example, the five Ks in Sikhism (Kesh – uncut hair, Kangha – the wooden comb which fixes uncut hair into a bun, Kara – an iron, steel or gold bracelet worn on the right wrist, Kirpan – a symbolic sword worn under clothing in a cloth sheath or as a brooch or pendant, and Kach – undergarments) (Neuberger 2004).

Table 2.4 lists the cultural and religious factors to be considered at Last Offices but these are only guidelines: individual requirements may vary even amongst members of the same faith. Families may require all, part or none of these actions to be carried out. They are adapted from Green and Green (2006), Neuberger (2004), Pattison (2008a, b) and Speck (1992).

Varying degrees of adherence and orthodoxy exist within all the world's faiths. The given religion of a patient may occasionally be offered to indicate an association with particular cultural and national roots, rather than to indicate a significant degree of adherence to the tenets of a particular faith. If in doubt, consult the family members concerned.

Regardless of the faith that the patient's record states they hold, wishes for Last Offices may differ from the conventions of their stated faith. Sensitive discussion is needed by nurses to establish what is wanted at this time. If patients are of a faith not listed in Table 2.4 or hold no religious beliefs, ask the relatives to outline the patient's previously expressed wishes, if any, or establish the family's wishes. Furthermore, the patient may be non-denominational and/or the family members may be multi-denominational so all possibilities must be taken into account.

Additional considerations

It is important to inform other patients, particularly if the person has died in an area where other people are present (such as a bay or open ward) and might know the patient. Senior staff should offer guidance in the event of uncertainty about how to deal with the situation.

Finally, Last Offices should be carried out within 2–4 hours of death. This is because rigor mortis can occur relatively soon after death, and this time is shortened in warmer environments (Berry and Griffie 2001).

Postprocedural considerations
Immediate care
Relatives' time with patient after death

Since there is a time limit to how long a patient should remain in the heat of a ward (there could potentially be early onset of rigor mortis), the senior nurse will have to exercise discretion over when to send the patient to the mortuary. This will vary according to family circumstances (there could be a short delay in a relative travelling to the ward/area) and the ward situation (side rooms are obviously easier for the family/other patients). As a general rule, 1–2 hours would be considered the upper limits for a patient to remain in the ward area, after Last Offices have been carried out.

Viewing the patient in the chapel of rest

Families may wish to view the patient in the chapel of rest again (Figure 2.7). It is important to ensure that the patient is in a presentable state before taking the family to see them.

Spiritual, emotional and bereavement support

The bereaved family may find it difficult to comprehend the death of their family member and it can take great sensitivity and skill to support them at this time. Explaining all procedures as fully as possible can help understanding of the practices at the end of life. Offering bereavement care services may be useful to families for that difficult period immediately after death and in the future. National services such as CRUSE (www.cruse.org.uk) can be useful if local services are not available.

Relatives may express extreme distress; this is a difficult situation to handle and other family members are likely to be of most comfort and support at this point. The family member may wish for their GP to be contacted.

Maintain a high degree of sensitivity when outlining the process after a patient has died since families frequently have to attend the hospital in the very near future in order to collect the documentation for registering the death.

Education of patient and relevant others

Helping the family to understand procedures after death is the role of many people in hospital but primarily this will fall upon those who first meet with the family after their relative has died. The Home Office leaflet *What to Do After a Death* (DWP 2006) can help families.

If the family states that they feel the death was unnatural or even that it was interfered with, we have a responsibility to explore these feelings and even outline their legal entitlement to a postmortem.

- Prepare the family for what they might see.
- Invite the family into the bed space/room.

- Accompany family but respect their need for privacy should they require it.
- Anticipate questions.
- Offer the family the opportunity to discuss care (at that time or in the future).
- Offer to contact other relatives on behalf of the family.
- Advise about the bereavement support services that can be accessed. Arrange an appointment if requested.
- Provide them with a point of contact with the hospital.

Some families may wish for a memento of the patient, such as a lock of hair. Try to anticipate and accommodate these wishes as much as possible.

Websites and useful addresses

For further information about organ donation contact the following website or your local transplant co-ordinator:
www.uktransplant.org.uk

For further information about bereavement and bereavement advice: Cruse Bereavement Care,
www.crusebereavementcare.org.uk

For advice following a death: Citizens Advice Bureau,
www.citizensadvice.org.uk

Hospital Chaplaincies Council:
www.nhs-chaplaincy-spiritualcare.org.uk

For specific guidance on religious practices

National Spiritual Assembly of the Bahais of the United Kingdom
Email: nsa@bahai.org.uk
Website: www.bahai.org.uk

Buddhist Hospice Trust
Website: www.buddhisthospice.org.uk

Hindu Council UK
Website: www.hinducounciluk.org

Jainism
Website: www.jainism.org

Jehovah's Witnesses
Email: his@wtbts.org.uk
Website: www.watchtower.org

Rastafarianism
Website: www.rastafarian.net

Zoroastrian Trust Funds of Europe
Email: secretary@ztfe.com
Website: www.ztfe.com

The BBC Religion and Ethics websites also provide useful information.
www.bbc.co.uk/religion/religions/judaism
www.bbc.co.uk/religion/religions/sikhism
www.bbc.co.uk/religion/religions/zoroastrian

References

Ahern, J. and Philpot, P. (2002) Assessing acutely ill patients on general wards. *Nursing Standard*, 16 (47), 47–54.

Alfaro-Lefevre, R. (2002) *Applying Nursing Process: Promoting Collaborative Care*. Lippincott, Williams and Wilkins, Philadelphia.

Allen, D. (1998) Record-keeping and routine practice: the view from the wards. *Journal of Advanced Nursing*, 27 (6), 1223–1230.

Arrowsmith, H. (1999) A critical evaluation of the use of nutritional screening tools by nurses. *British Journal of Nursing*, 8 (22), 1483–1490.

Ashby, M and Mendelson, D. (2009) Family carers: ethical and legal issues, in *Family carers in palliative care: A guide for health and social care professionals* (eds Hudson, P and Payne, S.). Oxford University Press, Oxford .

Association of Anaesthetists of Great Britain and Ireland (2001) Preoperative Assessment: the role of the Anaesthetist. www. nhshealthquality.org/nhsqis/files/Anaesthesia.pdf.

American Thoracic Society/American College of Chest Physicians (2003) ATS/ACCP statement on cardiolpulmonary exercise testing. *American Journal of Respiratory and Critical Care Medicine*, 67, 211–277.

Atwal, A. (2002) Nurses' perceptions of discharge planning in acute health care: a case study in one British teaching hospital. *Journal of Advanced Nursing, 39* (5), 450–458.

Australian and New Zealand College of Anaesthetists (ANZCA) (2005) Acute pain management: scientific evidence. www.anzca. edu.au/resources/books-and-publications/acutepain.pdf.

Avidan, M., Harvey, A.M.R., Ponte, J. *et al.* (2003) *Perioperative Care, Anaesthesia, Pain Management and Intensive Care*. Churchill Livingstone, Edinburgh.

Back, I.N. (1992) Terminal restlessness in patients with advanced malignant disease. *Palliative Medicine*, 6, 293–298.

Ballard, E.C. (2006) Improving information management in ward nurses' practice. *Nursing Standard*, 20 (50), 43–48.

Bassett, A. (2002) Patient assessment, in *Sabiston Textbook of Surgery: The Biological Basis of Modern Surgical Practice*, 18th edn (eds C.M. Townsend, Beauchamp, R.D., Evers, B.M. and Mattox, K.). Elsevier Inc, Toronto.

Bavetta, S., Olsha, O. and Fenely, J. (1990) Spreading sepsis by cystoscopy. *Postgraduate Medical Journal*, 66 (779), 734–735.

Behar, J., Gogalniceanu, P. and Bromley, L. (2007) Anaesthesia: introduction and preoperative assessment. *Student BMJ*, 15, 12–14.

Benner, P.E. (1984) *From Novice to Expert: Excellence and Power in Clinical Nursing Practice*. Addison–Wesley, Menlo Park, CA.

Berry, P. and Griffie, J. (2001) Planning for the actual death, in *Textbook of Palliative Nursing* (eds B. Ferrell and N. Coyle). Oxford University Press, Oxford. pp.382–394.

Bickley, L. (2007) *Bates' Guide to Physical Examination and History Taking*, 9th edn. Lippincott, Williams and Wilkins, Philadelphia.

Biddington, W. (2000) Reviewing discharge planning processes and promoting good practice. *Journal of Clinical Nursing*, 14 (5), 4–6.

Bonevski, B, Sanson-Fisher, R., Girgis, A. *et al.* (2000) Evaluation of an instrument to assess the needs of patients with cancer. *Cancer*, 88, 215–217.

Borill, C, West, M., Dawson, J. *et al.* (2001) *Team Working and Effectiveness in Health Care*. Aston Centre for Health Service Organisation Research, Aston, Yorkshire. www.itslifejimbutnotasweknowit. org.uk/files/Team_effectiveness.pdf

Bouvette, M., Fothergill-Bourbonnais, F. and Perreault, A. (2002) Implementation of the pain and symptom assessment record (PSAR). *Journal of Advanced Nursing*, 40 (6), 685–700.

74

Brown, V, Sitzia, J., Richardson, A. *et al.* (2001) The development of the Chemotherapy Symptom Assessment Scale (C–SAS): a scale for the routine clinical assessment of the symptom experiences of patients receiving cytotoxic chemotherapy. *International Journal of Nursing Studies*, **38** (5), 497–510.

Bull, M.J. and Roberts, J. (2001) Components of a proper hospital discharge for elders. *Journal of Advanced Nursing*, 35(4), 571–581.

Cader, R., Campbell, S. and Watson, D. (2005) Cognitive continuum theory in nursing decision-making. *Journal of Advanced Nursing*, 49 (4), 397–405.

Cancer Action Team (2007) *Holistic Common Assessment of Supportive and Palliative Care Needs for Adults with Cancer: Assessment Guidance*. Cancer Action Team, London.

Cashman, J.N. (2001) The preoperative visit, in *Preoperative Assessment* (ed. J. Cashman). BMJ Books, London, pp.3–20.

Chambers, S. (1998) Nursing diagnosis in learning disabilities nursing. *British Journal of Nursing*, 7 (19), 1177–1181.

Chee, Y.L., Crawford, J.C., Watson, H.G. and Greaves, M. (2008) Guidelines on the assessment of bleeding risk prior to surgery or invasive procedures. *British Journal of Haematology*, 140, 496–504.

Cherian, V.T. and Tomlinson, A.A. (2001) Preoperative optimisation, in *Preoperative Assessment* (ed. J. Cashman). BMJ Books, London, pp.93–132.

Clark, J. (1999) A language for nursing. *Nursing Standard*, **13** (31), 42–47.

Clayton, J.M. and Tattersall, M.H.N. (2006) Communication in Palliative Care, in *Textbook of Palliative Medicine* (eds E. Bruera, I. Higginson, C. Ripamonti and C. von Guten). Hodder Arnold, London.

Conner, F.W. and Eggert, L.L. (1994) Psychosocial assessment for treatment planning and evaluation. *Journal of Psychosocial Nursing and Mental Health Services*, 32 (5), 31–42.

Cook, D. (2001) *Patient autonomy versus paternalism. Critical Care Medicine*, 20(2), N24–25.

Cooke, H. (2000) *A Practical Guide to Holistic Care at the End of Life*. Butterworth Heinemann, Oxford.

Cooper, C. and Storer, T. (2008) *Exercise Testing And Interpretation: A Practical Approach*. Cambridge University Press, Cambridge.

Costello, J. (2004) *Nursing the Dying Patient: Caring in Different Contexts*. Palgrave Macmillan, Basingstoke.

Coyne, P.J., Lyne, M.E. and Watson, A.C. (2002) Symptom management in people with AIDS. *American Journal of Nursing*, **102** (9), 48–57.

Crumbie, A. (2006) Taking a history, in *Nurse Practitioners: Clinical Skills and Professional Issues* (ed. M. Walsh). Butterworth Heinemann, Edinburgh, pp.14–26.

Darzi, Lord (2008) *Our NHS, Our Future: Next Stage Review*. Department of Health, London.

Davies, S. and Wilson, R. (2007) Cardiopulmonary exercising testing for the surgical patient. *Care of the Critically Ill*, 23(4), 110–118.

Davis, S. (1998) Primary–Secondary Care Interface. Proceedings of conference, 25 March. NHS Executive, June, Issue 2.

Delaney, C. (2001) Health informatics and oncology nursing. *Seminars in Oncology Nursing*, 17 (1), 2–6.

Dennison, S. and Shute, T. (2000) Identifying patient concerns: improving the quality of patient visits to the oncology outpatient department – a pilot audit. *European Journal of Oncology Nursing*, 4 (2), 91–98.

DH (1989) *Discharge of Patients from Hospital. Health Circular (89) 5*. HMSO, London.

DH (1997) *Patients Who Die in Hospital: HSG(97)43*. Department of Health, London. http://webarchive.national-archives.gov.uk/+/www.dh.gov.uk/en/Publicationsandstatistics/Lettersandcirculars/Healthserviceguidelines/DH_4018378.

DH (1998a) *A First Class Service: Quality in the New NHS*. NHSE, London.

DH (1998b) *The New NHS: Modern, Dependable*. HMSO, London.

DH (2000a) *The NHS Plan. A Plan for Investment, A Plan for Reform*. HMSO, London.

DH (2000b) *Shaping the Future NHS: Long Term Planning for Hospitals and Related Services. Consultation Document on the Findings of the National Bed Enquiry*. HMSO, London.

DH (2000c) *Patient and Public Involvement in the NHS*. HMSO, London.

DH (2001a) *The National Service Framework for Older People*. HMSO, London.

DH (2001b) *NHS Funded Nursing Care in Nursing Homes: What It Means for You*. HMSO, London.

DH (2001c) *Guide to Integrating Community Equipment Services*. HMSO, London.

DH (2002) *National Service Framework for Older People – Intermediate Care: Moving Forward*. HMSO, London.

DH (2003a) *Discharge from Hospital: Pathway, Process and Practice*. HMSO, London.

DH (2003b) *Delayed Transfers of Care: Planning for Implementation of Reimbursement and Improving Hospital Discharge Practice*. HMSO, London.

DH (2003c) *A Guide to the Post-mortem Examination Procedure*. Department of Health, London.

DH (2004a) *Achieving Timely 'Simple' Discharge from Hospital – a Toolkit for the Multi-disciplinary Team*. HMSO, London.

DH (2004b) *Carers and Disabled Children Act 2000 and Carers (Equal Opportunities) Act 2004. Combined Policy Guidance*. HMSO, London.

DH (2005) *Choosing a Better Diet: A Food and Health Action Plan*. Department of Health, London.

DH (2006a) *Modernising Nursing Careers: Setting the Direction*. Department of Health, London.

DH (2006b) *National Framework for NHS Continuing Healthcare and NHS-funded Nursing Care in England. Consultation Document*. HMSO, London.

DH (2007) *NHS Continuing Healthcare and NHS-Funded Nursing Care: Public Information Leaflet*. Department of Health, London. http://webarchive.nationalarchives.gov.uk/+/www.dh.gov.uk/prod_consum_dh/groups/dh_digitalassets/@dh/@en/documents/digitalasset/dh_079516.pdf.

DH (2008) *End-of-Life Care Strategy*. Department of Health, London.

DH (2010) *'Ready to Go'. Planning the discharge and the transfer of patients from hospital and intermediate care*. Department of Health, London.

DWP (2006) *What to Do After a Death*. Department of Work and Pensions, London.

Dimond, B. (2002) *Legal Aspects of Pain Management*. Quay Books, Salisbury.

Dimond, B. (2004) Health and safety considerations following the death of a patient. *British Journal of Nursing*, **13** (11), 675–676.

Docherty, B. (2000) Care of the dying patient. *Professional Nurse*, **15** (12), 752.

Edwards, M. and Miller, C. (2001) Improving psychosocial assessment in oncology. *Professional Nurse*, 16 (7), 1223–1226.

Eilers, J., Berger, A.M. and Peterson, M.C. (1988) Development, testing and application of the oral assessment guide. *Oncology Nursing Forum*, 15 (3), 325–330.

Elfrink, V., Bakken, S., Coenen, A., McNeil, B. and Bickford, C. (2001) Standardized nursing vocabularies: a foundation for quality care. *Seminars in Oncology Nursing*, 17 (1), 18–23.

Ellershaw, J. and Wilkinson, S. (2003) *Care of the Dying: A Pathway to Excellence.* Oxford University Press, Oxford.

Fallowfield, L. (2005) Communication with the patient and family, in *Oxford Textbook of Palliative Medicine* (eds D. Doyle, G. Hanks, N. Cherny and K. Calman). Oxford University Press, Oxford.

Faull, C. and Nyatanga, B (2005) Terminal care and dying, in *Handbook of Palliative Care* (eds C. Faull, Y. Carter and L. Daniels). Wiley-Blackwell, Oxford.

Fernandez Perez, E.R., Gajic, O., Sprung, J. and Warnder, D.O. (2008) Pulmonary diseases, in *Preoperative Assessment and Management*, 2nd edn (ed. B.J. Sweitzer). Lippincott Williams and Wilkins, Philadelphia, pp.124–147.

Field, D., Hockley, J. and Small, N. (1997) *Death, Gender and Ethnicity.* Routledge, London.

Ford, P. and McCormack, B. (1999) Determining older people's need for registered nursing in continuing health care: the contribution of the Royal College of Nursing's Older People's Assessment Tool. *Journal of Clinical Nursing*, 8 (6), 731–742.

Ford, P. and Walsh, M. (1994) *New Rituals for Old: Nursing Through The Looking Glass.* Butterworth-Heinemann, Oxford.

Foust, J.B. (2007) Discharge planning as part of daily nursing practice. *Applied Nursing Research*, 20 (2), 72–77.

Fraise, A.P. and Bradley, T. (eds) (2009) *Ayliffe's Control of Healthcare-associated Infection: A Practical Handbook,* 5th edn. Hodder Arnold, London.

Frank-Stromborg, M. and Olsen, S.J. (eds) (2004) *Instruments for Clinical Health-Care Research,* 3rd edn. Jones and Bartlett, Sudbury, MA.

Fürst, C.J. (2004) The terminal phase, in *Oxford Textbook of Palliative Medicine* (eds D. Doyle, G. Hanks, N. Cherny and K. Calman). Oxford University Press, Oxford.

Galanti, G. (2000) An introduction to cultural differences. *Western Journal of Medicine*, 172 (5), 335–336.

Ganz, P.A., Schag, C.A., Lee, J.J. and Sim, M.S. (1992) The CARES: a generic measure of health-related quality of life for patients with cancer. *Quality of Life Research*, 1 (1), 19–29.

Garcia-Miguel, F.J., Serrano-Aguilar, P.G. and Lopez-Bastida, J. (2003) Preoperative assessment. *Lancet*, 362, 1749–1757.

Garrett, E. and Boyd, J. (2008) *Key Findings Report: Adult Inpatient Survey Results 2007.* Picker Institute Europe, Oxford. www.nhssurveys.org/survey/613.

Glare, P. and Christakis, N. (2004) Predicting survival in patients with advanced disease, in *Oxford Textbook of Palliative Medicine* (eds D. Doyle, G. Hanks, N. Cherny and K. Calman). Oxford University Press, Oxford.

Goldstein, N.E., Lampert, R., Bradley, E. *et al.* (2004) Management of implantable cardioverter defibrillators in end-of-life care. *Annals of Internal Medicine*, 141 (11), 835–838

Gordon, M. (1994) *Nursing Diagnosis, Process and Application.* Mosby, St Louis.

Green, J. and Green, M. (2006) *Dealing with Death: A Handbook of Practices, Procedures and Law,* 2nd edn. Jessica Kingsley Publishers, London.

Grobe, S.J. (1996) The nursing intervention lexicon and taxonomy: implications for representing nursing care data in automated patient records. *Holistic Nursing Practice*, 11 (1), 48–63.

Gunaratnam, Y. (1997) Culture is not enough: a critique of multiculturalism in palliative care, in *Death, Gender and Ethnicity* (eds D. Field, J. Hockley and N. Small). Routledge, London, pp.166–186.

Haddock, J. and Burrows, C. (1997) The role of the nurse in health promotion: an evaluation of a smoking cessation programme in surgical pre-admission clinics, *Journal of Advanced Nursing*, 26, 1098–1110.

Halm, J., Gagner, S, Goering, M. *et al.* (2003) Interdisciplinary rounds: impact on patients, family and staff. *Clinical Nurse Specialist*, 17 (3), 133–142.

Hancock, S. (2003) Intermediate care and older people. *Nursing Standard*, 17 (48), 45–51.

Hardwick, S. (1998) Clarification of nursing diagnosis from a British perspective. *Assignment*, 4 (2), 3–9.

Harris, R, Wilson-Barnett, J., Griffiths, P. and Evans, A. (1998) Patient assessment: validation of a nursing instrument. *International Journal of Nursing Studies*, 35, 303–313.

Healing, T.D., Hoffman, P.N. and Young, S.E.J. (1995) The infection hazards of human cadavers. *Communicable Disease Report*, 5 (5), R61–R68

Health Services Accreditation (1996) *Service Standards for Discharge Care.* NHS, East Sussex.

Heaven, C.M. and Maguire, P. (1996) Training hospice nurses to elicit patient concerns. *Journal of Advanced Nursing*, 23, 280–286.

Hedberg, B. and Satterlund Larsson, U. (2003) Observations, confirmations and strategies – useful tools in decision-making process for nurses in practice? *Journal of Clinical Nursing*, 12 (2), 215–222.

Higgins, D. (2010) Care of the dying patient: a guide for nurses, in *Care of the Dying and Deceased Patient* (ed. P. Jevon). Wiley-Blackwell, Oxford.

Higginson, I.J. and Costantini, M (2008) Dying with cancer, living well with cancer. *European Journal of Cancer*, 44, 1414–1424.

Hill, M. and Macgregor, G. (2001) *Health's Forgotten Partners? How Carers are Supported Through Hospital Discharge.* Carers UK, London. www.carershealthmatters.org.uk.

Hogston, R. (1997) Nursing diagnosis and classification systems: a position paper. *Journal of Advanced Nursing*, 26 (3), 496–500.

Hollins, S. (2006) Religions, Culture and Healthcare. Radcliffe, Oxford.

Holmes, H.N. (ed.) (2003) *Three-Minute Assessment.* Lippincott, Philadelphia.

Holmes, S. and Eburn, E. (1989) Patients' and nurses' perceptions of symptom distress in cancer. *Journal of Advanced Nursing*, 14 (7), 575–581.

Holt, P. (1995) Role of questioning in patient assessment. *British Journal of Nursing*, 4, 1145–1146.

Holzhausen, F. (2001) *'You Can Take Him Home Now'. Carers' Experiences of Hospital Discharge.* Carers National Association, London.

Home Office (1971) *Report of the Committee on Death Certification and Coroners.* CMND 4810. HMSO, London.

Home Office (2002) When Sudden Death Occurs: Coroners and Inquests. www.nnuh.nhs.uk/docs%5Cleaflets%5C90.pdf.

Horton, R. (2002) Differences in assessment of symptoms and quality of life between patients with advanced cancer and their specialist palliative care nurses in a home care setting. *Palliative Medicine*, 16 (6), 488–494.

House of Commons Health Committee (2005) *NHS Continuing Care, Sixth Report of Session 2004–2005*, Vol. 1. House of Commons Publications, Norwich, pp.399–391.

HPA (2010) The Infection Hazards of Human Cadavers: Guidelines on Precautions to Be Taken With Cadavers of Those Who Have Died With a Known or Suspected Infection. www.vfda.net/CadaverPolicyUK.pdf.

HSAC (2003) *Safe Working and the Prevention of Infection in the Mortuary and Postmortem Room.* Health and Safety Advisory Committee /HSE, London.

HTA (2006) *Human Tissue Authority. Code of Practice – consent.* www.hta.gov.uk/_db/_documents/2006-07-04_Approved_by_Parliament_-_Code_of_Practice_1_-_Consent.pdf.

Huber, D.L. and McClelland, E. (2003) Patient preferences and discharge planning transitions. *Journal of Professional Nursing*, 19 (4), 204–210.

Hunter, M. (1998) Rehabilitation in cancer care: a patient-focused approach. *European Journal of Cancer Care*, 7 (2), 85–87.

Hunter, M. (2001) Will social services suffer in new regime? *Community Care*, 13 (87), 10–11.

IASP (2007) *IASP Pain Terminology*. International Association for the Study of Pain, Seattle. www.iasp-pain.org/AM/Template.cfm?Section=General_Resource_Links&Template=/CM/HTMLDisplay.cfm&ContentID=3058.

IPEM (2002) *Medical and Dental Guidance Notes. A Good Practice Guide on All Aspects of Ionising Radiation Protection in the Clinical Environment*. Institute of Physics and Engineering in Medicine, York.

Jenkins, V., Fallowfield, L. and Saul, J. (2001) Information needs of patients with cancer: results from a large study in UK cancer centres. *British Journal of Cancer*, 84 (1), 48–51.

Jensen, T.S, Wilson, P. and Rice, A. (2003) *Clinical Pain Management: Chronic Pain*. Arnold, London.

Jevon, P. (ed) (2010) *Care of the Dying Patient: A Guide for Nurses*. Wiley-Blackwell, Oxford.

Johnson, T. (2000) Functional health pattern assessment on-line: lessons learned. *Computers in Nursing*, 18 (5), 248–254.

Kearney, N. (2001) Classifying nursing care to improve patient outcomes: the example of WISECARE. *NT Research*, 6 (4), 747–756.

Kearney, N., Miller, M., Sermeus, W. *et al.* (2000) Collaboration in cancer nursing practice. *Journal of Clinical Nursing*, 9, 429–435.

Kehl, K.A. (2006) Moving toward peace: an analysis of the concept of a good death. *American Journal of Hospice Palliative Care*, 23 (4), 277–286.

Kinder, C. and Ellershaw, J. (2003) How to use the Liverpool Care Pathway for the Dying Patient, in *Care of the Dying: A Pathway to Excellence* (eds J. Ellershaw and S. Wilkinson S). Oxford Univerity Press, Oxford.

King, L. and Clark, J.M. (2002) Intuition and the development of expertise in surgical ward and intensive care nurses. *Journal of Advanced Nursing*, 37 (4), 322–329.

Kissane, D. (2004) Bereavement, in *Oxford Textbook of Palliative Medicine*, 3rd edn (eds D. Doyle, G. Hanks, N. Cherny and K. Calman). Oxford University Press, Oxford.

Kissane, D. and Yates, P. (2003) Psychological and existential distress, in *Palliative Nursing: A Guide to Practice* (eds M. O'Connor and S. Aranda). Radcliffe Medical Press, Oxford.

Kozier, B., Erb, G., Berman, A. *et al.* (2003) *Fundamentals of Nursing: Concepts, Process and Practice*, 7th edn. Addison Wesley, Menlo Park, CA.

Kumar, S. (2000) *Multidisciplinary Approach to Rehabilitation*. Butterworth Heinemann, London.

Lauri, S., Lepisto, M. and Kappeli, S. (1997) Patients' needs in hospital: nurses' and patients' views. *Journal of Advanced Nursing*, 25, 339–346.

Lawlor, P.G., Gagnon, B., Mancini, I.L. *et al.* (2000) Occurrence, causes, and outcome of delirium in patients with advanced cancer: a prospective study. *Archives of Internal Medicine*, 160 (6), 786–794.

Lee, J., Chaloner, E. and Hollingsworth, S. (2006) The role of cardiopulmonary fitness and its genetic influences on surgical outcomes. *British Journal of Surgery*, 93, 147–157.

Leih, P. and Salentijn, C. (1994) Nursing diagnoses: a Dutch perspective. *Journal of Clinical Nursing*, 3 (5), 313–320.

Lidstone, V., Butters, E., Seed, P. T., Sinnott, C., Beynon, T. and Richards, M. (2003) Symptoms and concerns amongst cancer outpatients: identifying the need for specialist palliative care. *Palliative Medicine*, 17 (7), 588–595.

Lyte, G. and Jones, K. (2001) Developing a unified language for children's nurses, children and their families in the United Kingdom. *Journal of Clinical Nursing*, **10** (1), 79–85.

MacGregor, T., Patel, N., Blick, C., Arya, M. and Muneer, A. (2009) Is there a role for cardiopulmonary exercise testing before major urological surgery? *BJU International*, 104 (5), 579–580.

Malnutrition Advisory Group (2000) *Explanatory Notes for the Screening Tool for Adults at Risk of Malnutrition*. Malnutrition Advisory Group, Maidenhead.

Mangano, D.T. (1990) Preoperative assessment of the patient with ischemic heart disease, in *Preoperative Cardiac Assessment* (ed. D.T. Mangano). J.B.Lippincott Company, Philadelphia, pp.1–55.

Maramba, P.J., Richards, S., Myers, A.L. and Larrabee, J.H. (2004) Discharge planning process: applying a model for evidence-based practice. *Journal of Nursing Care Quality*, 19 (2),123–129.

Mardis, R. and Brownson, K. (2003) Length of stay at an all-time low. *Health Care Manager*, 22 (2), 122–127.

Marek, C. (2003) Anti-emetic therapy in patients receiving cancer chemotherapy. *Oncology Nursing Forum*, 30, 259–269.

Martin, J. (2001) Benchmarking – how do you do it? *Nursing Times*, 97 (42), 30–31.

McClement, S.E., Woodgate, R.L. and Degner, L. (1997) Symptom distress in adults with cancer. *Cancer Nursing*, 20 (4), 236–243.

McDonald, M.V., Passik, S., Dugan, W. *et al.* (1999) Nurses' recognition of depression in their patients with cancer. *Oncology Nursing Forum*, **26** (3), 593–599.

McKenna, H., Keeney, S., Glenn, A. *et al.* (2000) Discharge planning: an exploratory study. *Journal of Advanced Nursing*, 9, 594–601.

Mental Capacity Act (2005) Stationery Office, London.

MHRA (2002) *Removal of Implantable Cardioverter Defibrillators*. MHRA, London.

Mistiaen, W., van Cauwelaert, P., Muylaert, P. and de Worm, E. (2007) Thousand Carpentier-Edwards pericardial valves in the aortic position: what has changed in the last 20 years and what are the effects on hospital complications? *Journal of Heart Valve Disease*, 16, 1–6.

Modernisation Agency (2003) *National Good Practice Guidance on Preoperative Assessment for Inpatient Surgery*. Department of Health, London.

Moen, A., Henry, S.B. and Warren, J.J. (1999) Representing nursing judgements in the electronic health record. *Journal of Advanced Nursing*, **30** (4), 990–997.

Morton, P.G. (1993) *Health Assessment in Nursing*, 2nd edn. Springhouse, Philadelphia.

Murphy, E.K. (2003) Charting by exception. *AORN Journal*, **78** (5), 821–823.

Murphy, K., Cooney, A., Casey, D. *et al.* (2000) The Roper, Logan and Tierney (1996) model: perceptions and operationalization of the model in psychiatric nursing within a Health Board in Ireland. *Journal of Advanced Nursing*, 31 (6), 1333–1341.

NANDA-I (2009) *Nursing Diagnoses: Definitions and Classifications 2009–2011*. North American Nursing Diagnosis Association–International, Philadelphia.

Naylor, W., Laverty, D. and Mallett, J. (2001) *The Royal Marsden Hospital Handbook of Wound Management in Cancer Care*, Blackwell Science, Oxford.

Nazarko, L. (1998) Improving discharge: the role of the discharge co-ordinator. *Nursing Standard*, **12** (49), 35–37.

Nearney, L. (1998) Last offices, part 1. *Nursing Times*, **94** (26), Insert.

Neighbour, R. (1987) *The Inner Consultation*. MTP Press, Lancaster.

Neuberger, J. (1999) Cultural issues in palliative care, in *Oxford Textbook of Palliative Medicine* (eds D. Doyle, G. Hanks and N. MacDonald). Oxford University Press, Oxford, pp.777–780.

Neuberger, J. (2004) *Caring for People of Different Faiths*. Radcliffe Medical Press, Abingdon.

NHS Connecting for Health (2005) *CRDB SAP Action Team Output V1.0*. Crown Copyright.

NHSE (2001) *Your Guide to the National Health Service*. HMSO, London.

NICE (2003) *Preoperative Tests: The Use of Routine Preoperative Tests for Elective Surgery [CG3]*. National Institute for Health and Clinical Excellence, London.

NICE (2004) *Guidance on Cancer Services: Improving Supportive and Palliative Care for Adults with Cancer*. National Institute for Health and Clinical Excellence, London.

NMC (2008) *The Code: Standards of Conduct, Performance and Ethics for Nurses and Midwives*. Nursing and Midwifery Council, London.

NMC (2009) *Record Keeping: Guidance for Nurses and Midwives*. Nursing and Midwifery Council, London.

O'Donnell, V. (1998) The pharmacological management of respiratory secretions. *Journal of Palliative Nursing*, 4, 199–203.

Older, P. and Smith, R. (1988) Experience with the preoperative invasion measurement of haemodynamic, respiratory and renal function in 100 elderly patients scheduled for major abdominal surgery, *Anaesthesia Intensive Care*, 16, 389–395.

Older, P., Smith, R., Courtney, P. and Hone, R. (1993) Preoperative evaluation of cardiac failure and ischaemia in elderly patients by cardiopulmonary exercise testing. *Chest*, 104, 701–704.

Older, P., Hall, A. and Hader, R. (1999) Cardiopulmonary exercise testing as a screening test for perioperative management of major surgery in the elderly. *Chest*, 116, 355–362.

ONS (2009) *Mortality Statistics Deaths Registered in 2008*. OPSI, Kew.

Orem, D.E., Taylor, S.G. and Renpenning, K. (2001) *Nursing: Concepts of Practice*, 6th edn. Mosby, St Louis, MO.

Osse, B.H., Vernooij, M.J., Schade, E. and Grol, R.P. (2004) Towards a new clinical tool for needs assessment in the palliative care of cancer patients: the PNPC instrument. *Journal of Pain and Symptom Management*, 28 (4), 329–341.

Parsaie, F.A., Golchin, M. and Asvadi, I. (2000) A comparison of nurse and patient perceptions of chemotherapy treatment stressors. *Cancer Nursing*, 23 (5), 371–374.

Pattison, N. (2008a) Care of patients who have died. *Nursing Standard*, 22 (28), 42–48.

Pattison, N. (2008b) Caring for patients after death. *Nursing Standard*, 22 (51), 48–56.

Pearce, E. (1963) *A General Textbook of Nursing*. Faber and Faber, London.

Peden-McAlpine, C. and Clark, N. (2002) Early recognition of client status changes: the importance of time. *Dimensions of Critical Care Nursing*, 21 (4), 144–150.

Perdue, C. (2005) Understanding nausea and vomiting in advanced cancer. *Nursing Times*, 101 (4), 32.

Philpin, S. (2002) Rituals and nursing: a critical commentary. *Journal of Advanced Nursing*, 38 (2), 144–151.

Piper, B.F. (2004) Measuring fatigue, in *Instruments for Clinical Health-Care Research*, 3rd edn (eds M. Frank-Stromborg and S.J. Olsen). Jones and Bartlett, Sudbury, MA, pp.538–569.

Portenoy, R.K., Thaler, H.T., Kornblith, A.B. et al. (1994) The Memorial Symptom Assessment Scale: an instrument for the evaluation of symptom prevalence, characteristics and distress. *European Journal of Cancer*, 30A (9), 1326–1336.

Pratt, R.J., Pellowe, C.M., Wilson, J.A. et al. (2007) epic2: National evidence-based guidelines for preventing healthcare-associated infections in NHS hospitals in England. *Journal of Hospital Infection*, 65S, S1–S64.

Putzier, D.J. and Padrick, K.P. (1984) Nursing diagnosis: a component of nursing process and decision making. *Topics in Clinical Nursing*, 5 (4), 21–29.

Quested, B. and Rudge, T. (2001) Procedure manuals and textually mediated death. *Nursing Inquiry*, 8 (4), 264–272.

RCN (1996) *Verification of Death by Registered Nurses*. Issues in Nursing and Health, 38. Royal College of Nursing, London.

RCN (2004) *Nursing Assessment and Older People. A Royal College of Nursing Toolkit*. Royal College of Nursing, London.

RCN (2005) *Good Practice in Infection Prevention and Control. Guidance for Nursing Staff*. Royal College of Nursing, London.

Reilly, D., McNeely, M., Doerner, D. et al. (1999) Self-reported exercise tolerance and the risk of serious perioperative complications. *Archives of Internal Medicine*, 159, 2185–2192.

Rhodes, V.A., McDaniel, R., Homan, S. et al. (2000) An instrument to measure symptom experience: symptom occurrence and symptom distress. *Cancer Nursing*, 23 (1), 49–54.

Rice, V.H. and Stead, L.F. (2008) Nursing interventions for smoking cessation. *Cochrane Database of Systematic Reviews*, 1, CD001188.

Rolfe, G. (1999) Insufficient evidence: the problems of evidence-based nursing. *Nurse Education Today*, 19 (6), 433–442.

Roper, N., Logan, W. and Tierney, A.J. (2000) *The Roper Logan Tierney Model of Nursing: Based on Activities of Living*. Churchill Livingstone, Edinburgh.

Rorden, J.W. and Taft, E. (1990) *Discharge Planning Guide for Nurses*. W.B. Saunders, Philadelphia.

Rosswurm, M.A. and Lanham, D.M. (1998) Discharge planning for elderly patients. *Journal of Gerontological Nursing*, 24 (5), 14–21.

Rowbotham, D.J. and Macintyre, P.E. (2002) *Clinical Pain Management: Acute Pain*. Arnold, London.

Roy, C. (1984) *Introduction to Nursing: an Adaptation Model*, 2nd edn. Prentice-Hall, New Jersey.

Royal Marsden NHS Foundation Trust (2006) After death care, in *Critical Care Unit Guidelines*. Internal Document, Royal Marsden NHS Foundation Trust, London.

Royal Marsden NHS Trust (2005) *Guidelines for Nursing Documentation*. Royal Marsden NHS Trust, London.

Salentera, S., Eriksson, E., Junnola, T. et al. (2003) Clinical judgement and information seeking by nurses and physicians working with cancer patients. *Psycho-Oncology*, 12, 280–290.

Salter, M. (1996) Nursing the patient in the community, in *Nursing the Patient with Cancer* (ed. V. Tschudin). Prentice-Hall, Hemel Hempstead, pp.438–451.

Seale, C. (1998) *Constructing Death. The Sociology of Dying and Bereavement*. Cambridge University Press, Cambridge.

Shaw, M. (1998) *Charting Made Incredibly Easy*. Lippincott, Williams and Wilkins, Philadelphia.

Skinn, B. and Stacey, D. (1994) Establishing an integrated framework for documentation: use of a self-reporting health history and outpatient oncology record. *Oncology Nursing Forum*, 21 (9), 1557–1566.

Smaje, C. and Field, D. (1997) Absent minorities? Ethnicity and the use of palliative care services, in *Death, Gender and Ethnicity* (eds D. Field, J. Hockley and N. Small). Routledge, London, pp.142–165.

Smith, A. (2003) Antibiotic resistance, in *Infection Control in the Community* (eds J. Lawrence and D. May). Churchill Livingstone, London, pp.319–332.

Smith, G. and Richardson, A. (1996) Development of nursing documentation for use in the outpatient oncology setting. *European Journal of Cancer Care*, 5, 225–232.

Smith, R. (2000) A good death. An important aim for health services and for us all. *BMJ*, 320, 129–130.

Smith, S. (1996) Discharge planning: the need for effective communication. *Nursing Standard*, 10 (38), 39–41.

Speck, P. (1992) Care after death. *Nursing Times*, 88 (6), 20.

Stewart, W. (2000) Development of discharge skills: a project report. *Nursing Times*, 96 (41), 37.

Suhonen, R., Valimaki, M. and Katajisto, J. (2000) Developing and testing an instrument for the measurement of individual care. *Journal of Advanced Nursing*, 32 (5), 1253–1263.

Sweitzer, B.J. (2008) Overview of preoperative evaluation and testing, in *Preoperative Assessment and Management*, 2nd edn (ed. B.J. Sweitzer). Lippincott Williams and Wilkins, Philadelphia, pp.14–50.

Tanner, C.A., Padrick, K.P., Westfall, U.E. and Putzier, D.J. (1987) Diagnostic reasoning strategies of nurses and nursing students. *Nursing Research*, 36 (6), 358–363.

Tarling, M. and Jauffur, H. (2006) Improving team meetings to support discharge planning. *Nursing Times, 102 (26), 32–35.*

Teytelman, Y. (2000) Effective nursing documentation and communication. *Seminars in Oncology Nursing*, 18 (2), 121–127.

Thomas, J. and Monaghan, T. (2008). *Oxford Handbook of Clinical Examination and Practical Skills*. Oxford University Press, Oxford.

Thompson, C. (1999) A conceptual treadmill: the need for 'middle ground' in clinical decision making theory in nursing. *Journal of Advanced Nursing*, 30 (5), 1222–1229.

Tierney, A.J. (1998) Nursing models; extant or extinct? *Journal of Advanced Nursing*, 28 (1), 77–85.

Travis, S. (2002) *Procedure for the Care of Patients Who Die in Hospital*. Royal Marsden NHS Trust, London.

Tung, A. (2008) Risk reduction and risk assessment, in *Preoperative Assessment and Management*, 2nd edn (ed. B.J. Sweitzer). Lippincott Williams and Wilkins, Philadelphia, pp.1–13.

Vaartio, H., Leino-Kilpi, H., Salentera, S. and Suominen, T. (2006). Nursing advocacy: how is it defined by patients and nurses, what does it involve and how is it experienced? *Scandinavian Journal of Caring Sciences*, 20 (3), 282–292.

Van Gennep A. (1972) *The Rites of Passage*. Chicago University Press, Chicago.

Walsh, M. and Ford, P. (1989) *Nursing Rituals, Research and Rational Action*. Butterworth Heinemann, Oxford.

Wasserman, K., Hansen, J., Sue, D. *et al.* (2005) *Principles of Exercise Testing and Interpretation Including Pathophysiology and Clinical Applications*, 4th edn. Lippincott, Williams and Wilkins, London.

Watson, M., Lucas, C., Hoy, A. and Wells, J. (eds) (2009) Ethical Issues, in *Oxford Handbook of Palliative Care* (eds M. Watson, C. Lucas, A. Hoy and I. Back). Oxford University Press, Oxford.

Weinberg, A.D., Brennan, M.D., Gorman, C.A. *et al.* (1983) Outcome of anesthesia and surgery in hypothyroid patients. *Archives of Internal Medicine* 143 (5), 893–897.

Wells, D.L., LeClerc, C.M., Craig, D., Martin, D.K. and Marshall, V.W. (2002) Evaluation of an integrated model of discharge planning: achieving quality discharges in an efficient and ethical way. *Canadian Journal of Nursing Research*, 34 (3), 103–122.

Westbrook, A. (2000) Nursing language. *Nursing Times*, 96 (14), 41.

White, L. (2003) *Documentation and the Nursing Process*. Delmar Learning, Clifton Park, NY.

WHO (2002) Guidance on Palliative Care. www.who.int/cancer/palliative/en.

Wilkinson, S. and Mula, C. (2003) Communication in care of the dying, in *Care of the Dying: A Pathway to Excellence* (eds J. Ellershaw and S. Wilkinson). Oxford University Press, Oxford, pp.74–89.

Williams, P.D., Ducey, K.A., Sears, A.M., Williams, A.R., Tobin-Rumelhart, S.E. and Bunde, P. (2001) Treatment type and symptom severity among oncology patients by self-report. *International Journal of Nursing Studies*, 38 (3), 359–367.

Wilson, B. (2007) Nurses' knowledge of pain. *Journal of Clinical Nursing*, 16 (6), 1012–1020.

Wimpenny, P. (2001) The meaning of models of nursing to practising nurses. *Journal of Advanced Nursing*, 40 (3), 346–354.

Wolf, Z. (1988) *Nurses' Work: The Sacred and the Profane*. University of Pennsylvania Press, Philadelphia.

Wright, E.P., Selby, P.J., Crawford, M. *et al.* (2003) Feasibility and compliance of automated measurement of quality of life in oncology practice. *Journal of Clinical Oncology*, 21 (2), 374–382.

Wyatt, J. (2009) *Matters of Life and Death*. Inter-Varsity Press, Nottingham.

Chapter 3

Infection prevention and control

Procedure guidelines

The Royal Marsden Hospital Manual of Clinical Nursing Procedures, Eighth Edition. Edited by Lisa Dougherty and Sara Lister.
© 2011 The Royal Marsden Hospital. Published 2011 by Blackwell Publishing Ltd.

Overview

This chapter describes the steps to be taken to minimize the risk of individuals acquiring infections during the course of care or treatment. Patients are most at risk but healthcare staff are also legally obliged to take reasonable and practicable precautions to protect themselves, other staff and anyone else who may be at risk in their workplace (Health and Safety at Work, etc. Act 1974). The chapter describes the **standard precautions** that must be taken with all patients at all times regardless of their known infection status, and the additional precautions that need to be taken with some patients. Additional precautions can be required either because the patient is colonized or infected with micro-organisms that may pose a particular risk to others, or because they are particularly vulnerable to infection themselves. The chapter also describes the specific precautions that must be taken during invasive procedures, in particular aseptic technique. Related issues such as the safe management of healthcare waste are also considered briefly.

Infection prevention and control

Definitions

'Infection prevention and control' has been defined as the clinical application of microbiology in practice (RCN 2010). More simply, it is a collective term for those activities intended to protect people from infections. Such activities are carried out as part of daily life by most individuals; for example, people wash their hands before eating to protect themselves from infection. The term is most often used in relation to healthcare, in particular with reference to preventing patients acquiring those infections most often associated with healthcare (such as wound infection) and preventing the transmission of micro-organisms from one patient to another (sometimes referred to as cross-infection).

Defined in Box 3.1 are some other terms used when discussing infection prevention and control. Confusion may sometimes arise because some of these terms are synonymous or have meanings which overlap, or are used in different ways by different people or organizations and this has been highlighted wherever possible.

Related theory

People who are in hospital or receiving healthcare elsewhere have an increased vulnerability to infection. There are many reasons for this, including reduced immunity and the use of invasive devices and procedures that bypass the body's normal defences. In addition, being in hospital puts them in closer proximity to other people with infectious conditions. However, many infections acquired by patients receiving healthcare are preventable, as has been amply demonstrated by the 50% reduction in MRSA bacteraemia (bloodstream

infections caused by meticillin-resistant *Staphylococcus aureus*) in English NHS hospitals between 2005 and 2008 (Health Protection Agency 2010a) and recent dramatic falls in the number of cases of *Clostridium difficile* infection in England (Health Protection Agency 2010b). These reductions have been achieved by the systematic application and monitoring of established practices for the prevention and control of infection, including diligent hand hygiene and correct aseptic technique.

Common healthcare-associated infections

The 2006 national prevalence survey of patients in hospital in England with infections identified a prevalence rate of around 8%; that is, eight out of every 100 patients in hospital at the time of the survey had an infection. The most common types of infection were gastrointestinal infections (22%), urinary tract infections (20%), pneumonia (14%) and surgical site infections (13.8%) (Hospital Infection Society/Infection Control Nurses Association 2007). Less common types of infection, for example bacteraemia (bacteria infecting the bloodstream), may be more severe, so *all* procedures must be carried out in such a way as to minimize the risk of any infection.

Causes of infection

Infections are normally caused by micro-organisms. These are life forms too small to see with the naked eye. In some cases, for example prion diseases such as Creutzfeldt–Jakob disease (CJD), it can be unclear if the causative agent is actually living or not, while at the other extreme, infection control precautions will be applied to prevent the transmission of visible parasites such as scabies mites or enteric worms that may be metres in length (although their eggs are microscopic). The term 'infectious agent' is therefore often used to describe anything that may be transmitted from one person to another, or from the environment to a person, and subsequently cause an infection or parasitic infestation.

The major groups of micro-organisms are described below. Which group an infectious agent belongs to will have significant implications for the treatment of an infected individual – for example, antibiotics target bacteria but have no effect on viral infections – but for infection prevention and control it is more important to understand the *route of transmission* as this will dictate if any additional, transmission-based, precautions need to be in place.

Types and classification of micro-organisms

Historically, the classification of micro-organisms was based on physical characteristics such as their size, shape or ability to retain a particular stain to make them visible under the microscope. Some of these distinctions are still useful, but classification is increasingly based on genetic characteristics, as analysis reveals the actual relationships between organisms. This can lead to confusion as new discoveries

Box 3.1 Terms used when discussing infection prevention and control

Infectious agent

Anything that may be transmitted from one person to another, or from the environment to a person, and subsequently cause an infection or parasitic infestation. Infectious agents are most often micro-organisms such as bacteria or viruses.

Pathogen

A micro-organism that is capable of causing infection. Many micro-organisms are opportunistic pathogens; that is, they will cause infection in vulnerable individuals but not, normally, in healthy adults.

Colonization

When micro-organisms are present on or in a person but not currently causing any harm, that person is said to be colonized with those organisms. For example, human beings are normally colonized with huge numbers of several different species of bacteria.

Healthcare-associated infection (HCAI)

Any infection acquired as a result of a healthcare-related intervention or an infection acquired during the course of healthcare that the patient may reasonably expect to be protected from. For example, a person may acquire viral gastroenteritis in many circumstances but if they acquire it in hospital from another patient, it should be regarded as healthcare associated. This has replaced the term 'hospital-acquired infection'.

Cross-infection

Cross-infection is one term given to the transmission of infectious agents between patients within the healthcare setting. It may be direct transmission from one person to another, or indirect, for example via an incorrectly cleaned piece of equipment.

Universal precautions

Correctly called universal blood and body fluid precautions, these are the precautions that are taken with all blood and 'high-risk' body fluids. They are based on the principle that any individual may be infected with a bloodborne virus, such as HIV or hepatitis B, and so pose a risk of infection; no individual can be regarded as completely 'risk free'. They are incorporated within standard precautions.

Standard precautions

The phrase 'standard precautions' is sometimes used interchangeably with 'universal precautions' (see above) but is used in this chapter and elsewhere (e.g. Health Protection Scotland 2009, Siegel *et al.* 2007) to describe the actions that should be taken in every care situation to protect patients and others from infection, regardless of what is known of the patient's status with respect to infection. Standard precautions include:

- hand hygiene at the '5 moments' described by the WHO (2009), including before and after each patient contact
- care in the use and disposal of sharps
- the correct use of personal protective equipment for contact with all blood, body fluids, secretions and excretions (except sweat)
- providing care in a suitably clean environment with adequately decontaminated equipment
- the safe disposal of waste
- the safe management of used linen.

Transmission-based precautions

Additional infection control precautions taken with patients known or strongly suspected to be infected or colonized with organisms that pose a significant risk to other patients. The precautions will vary depending on the route by which the organism travels from one individual to another, but there will be common elements. Transmission-based precautions can be divided into:

- contact
- enteric
- droplet
- airborne.

Contact precautions

Additional infection control precautions to be taken with patients known or strongly suspected to be infected or colonized with pathogenic micro-organisms that are mainly transmitted through touch or physical contact. Contact precautions normally consist of isolation of the patient in a single room, where possible, and use of gloves and apron for any procedure involving contact with the patient or their immediate environment (Siegel *et al.* 2007).

(Continued)

> **Box 3.1** (*Continued*)
>
> *Enteric precautions*
>
> Additional infection control precautions to be taken with patients suffering symptoms of infectious gastroenteritis, that is diarrhoea or vomiting that does not have an obvious mechanical or non-infectious cause. Enteric precautions should be taken from the first instance of diarrhoea or vomiting, regardless of whether a causative organism has been identified, until there is a definitive diagnosis that the symptoms do not have an infectious cause. Enteric precautions consist of prompt isolation of the patient in a single room with the door closed and use of gloves and apron for any procedure involving contact with the patient or their immediate environment (Chadwick *et al.* 2000, DH/HPA 2008).
>
> *Droplet precautions*
>
> Additional infection control precautions taken with patients known or strongly suspected to be infected or colonized with pathogenic micro-organisms that are mainly transmitted via droplets of body fluid expelled by an infected person. These are most often respiratory secretions expelled during coughing and sneezing but can include droplets from other sources such as projectile vomiting or explosive diarrhoea. The droplets are relatively large (>5 micrometres diameter) and do not remain suspended in the air for long so special ventilation is not normally required. Droplet precautions consist of isolation of the patient in a single room with the door closed and use of gloves and apron for any procedure involving contact with the patient or their immediate environment. Staff entering the room should wear a mask (Siegel *et al.* 2007).
>
> *Airborne precautions*
>
> Additional infection control precautions taken with patients known or strongly suspected to be infected or colonized with pathogenic micro-organisms that are mainly transmitted through the airborne route. These organisms are present in smaller droplets expelled by an infected person and so remain suspended in the air. Droplet precautions consist of prompt isolation of the patient in a single room, if possible with negative pressure ventilation or a positive pressure lobby, with the door closed, and use of gloves and apron for any procedure involving contact with the patient or their immediate environment. Staff entering the room should wear a fitted respirator (Siegel *et al.* 2007).
>
> Some guidelines merge droplet and airborne precautions in order to provide a single set of instructions for staff caring for patients with any respiratory or airborne infection.
>
> Isolation
>
> Isolation is the practice of nursing a patient in a single-occupancy room to reduce the risk of spread of pathogens and to reinforce and facilitate additional infection control precautions.
>
> *Source isolation*
>
> The practice of isolating a patient for the main purpose of preventing the spread of organisms from that patient.
>
> *Protective isolation*
>
> The practice of isolating a patient for the main purpose of preventing the spread of organisms to that patient, normally used for patients with impaired immune systems.
>
> Cohorting
>
> When the number of patients with a particular infection or carrying a particular organism exceeds the single room capacity of a healthcare provider, they may be nursed together in a cohort. This is most often done for highly infectious conditions such as norovirus. Patients who require isolation but have different infections cannot be cohort nursed together because of the risk of cross-infection between them.
>
> Barrier nursing
>
> The practice of nursing a patient who is carrying an infectious agent that may be a risk to others in such a way as to minimize the risk of transmission of that agent to others.
>
> Reverse barrier nursing
>
> The practice of nursing an individual who is regarded as being particularly vulnerable to infection in such a way as to minimize the transmission of potential pathogens to that person.

lead to species being reclassified and renamed. It should be noted that there can also be a wide variety of characteristics within each species, leading to significant variations in the severity of infection caused by different strains of the same organism. A good example of this is *Escherichia coli*. Every human being carries millions of these bacteria with no ill effects but infection with the toxin-producing O157 strain can cause serious illness.

This section describes the different types of organisms that may be encountered in a healthcare environment as well as the differences between and within the different types (Goering *et al.* 2007, Wilson 2000).

Bacteria

Bacteria are probably the most important group of micro-organisms in terms of infection prevention and control because they are responsible for many opportunistic infections in healthcare. A healthy human being will typically be host to one *quadrillion* (1000 trillion, or 10^{15}) bacteria – around ten times as many organisms as there are cells in the human body. In normal circumstances the relationship between these bacteria and their host is commensal (i.e. their presence does not cause the host any problems) and may be mutually beneficial. For example, *E. coli* present in the gut can be an aid to digestion. However, when circumstances change, these commensal organisms can cause infections. If the *E. coli* in the example above are transferred from the gut to the urinary tract, a urinary tract infection can result.

Whether or not any particular situation will result in an infection depends on a wide range of factors and is not always predictable. What is certain is that bacterial infections cannot occur when bacteria are not present, hence the importance of measures designed to minimize the risk of transmission. However, the presence of bacteria does not necessarily indicate an infection – as noted above, many millions of bacteria live on and in the human body without causing harm – so the diagnosis of a bacterial infection and any decision about treatment must be made by considering a combination of the patient's symptoms and laboratory results that may indicate the presence of any particular bacteria (Wilson 2000).

Bacteria are what are known as *prokaryotes*, as opposed to *eukaryotes*, the term used for more complex organisms such as humans. This means that bacterial cells are much smaller and simpler than human cells, typically about the size of some of the structures such as mitochondria that exist within a mammalian cell. This small size means that bacteria do not have separate structures (such as a nucleus) within their cells. What bacteria do have and mammalian cells do not is a cell wall that contains the rest of the cell and gives it a distinctive shape (Goering *et al.* 2007). Some of these shapes are illustrated in Table 3.1. In terms of healthcare-associated infections, the most important bacteria are generally rod shaped or spherical.

The structure of the cell wall determines another important distinction in medically significant bacteria: whether they are Gram positive or Gram negative. The 'Gram' in these terms refers to Gram staining, named after its Dutch inventor, Hans Christian Gram (1853–1938), who devised

Table 3.1 Bacterial shapes and arrangements

	Shape/arrangement	Notes/example
	Coccus (sphere)	Different species divide in one plane to make pairs and chains or in multiple planes to make clusters
	Chain	Streptococcus
	Pair (diplococci)	Neisseria
	Cluster	Staphylococcus
	Straight rod	Escherichia coli
	Spore-forming rod	Clostridium difficile
	Comma-shaped	Vibrio cholerae
	Spiral-shaped	Treponema pallidum, which causes syphilis

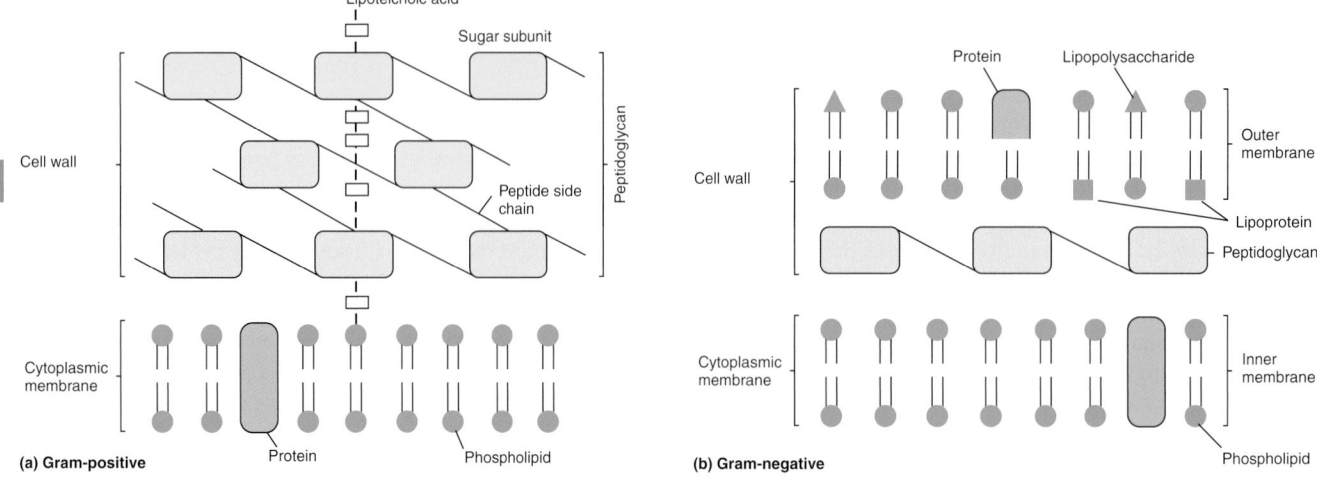

Figure 3.1   Gram-positive (a) and Gram-negative (b) bacterial cell walls. Used with permission from Elliot (2007).

the stain in 1884. Put simply, the structure of the cell wall determines whether or not the bacteria are able to retain a particular stain in the presence of an organic solvent such as acetone. The structure of the cell wall determines other characteristics of the bacteria, including their susceptibility to particular antibiotics, so knowing whether the cause of a bacterial infection is Gram positive or negative can help to determine appropriate treatment (Goering *et al.* 2007). The structure of the two different types of cell wall is shown in Figure 3.1.

Other structures visible outside the cell wall may include pili, which are rigid tubes that help the bacteria attach to host cells (or, in some cases, other bacteria for the exchange of genetic material), flagellae, which are longer, mobile projections that can help bacteria to move around, and capsules, that can provide protection or help the bacteria to adhere to surfaces. These are illustrated in Figure 3.2. The presence or absence of different structures will play a part in determining an organism's pathogenicity – its ability to cause an infection and the severity of that infection (Goering *et al.* 2007).

A final bacterial structure to consider is the spore. Bacteria normally reproduce by a process called binary fission – they create a copy of their genetic material and split themselves in two, with each 'daughter' cell being an almost-exact copy of the parent (there are mechanisms by which bacteria can transfer genetic material between cells and so acquire characteristics such as antibiotic resistance, but they are beyond the scope of this chapter). However, some bacteria, notably *Clostridium difficile*, have the capacity, in adverse conditions, to surround a copy of their genetic material with a tough coat. Because this structure is created within the bacterial cell, it is sometimes referred to as an endospore, but is more often simply called a *spore*. The parent cell then dies and disintegrates, leaving the spore to survive until conditions are suitable for it to germinate into a normal, 'vegetative' bacterial cell that can then reproduce (Goering

et al. 2007). Spores are extremely tough and durable. They are not destroyed by boiling (hence the need for high-temperature steam under pressure in sterilizing autoclaves) or by the alcohol handrubs widely used for hand hygiene – hence the need to physically remove them from the hands by washing with soap and water when caring for a patient with *Clostridium difficile* infection (DH/HPA 2008).

Some medically significant bacteria are listed in Table 3.2.

A few bacteria do not easily fit into the Gram-positive/negative dichotomy. The most medically significant of these are the *Mycobacteria*, which are responsible for diseases including tuberculosis and leprosy (Goering *et al.* 2007).

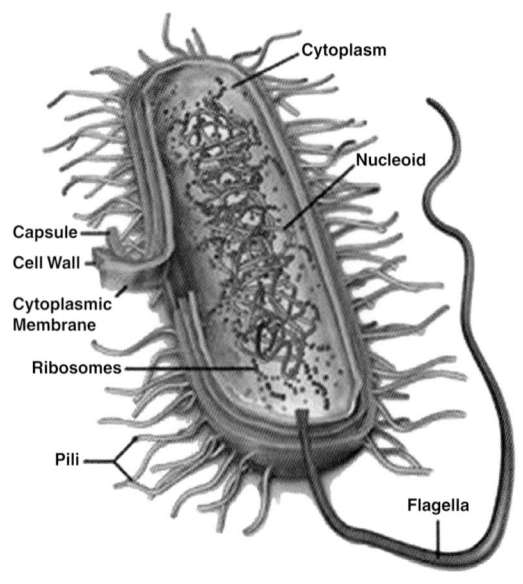

Figure 3.2   Bacterial structures.

Table 3.2 Medically significant bacteria

	Spherical	Rod-shaped
Gram positive	Staphylococcus aureus	Clostridium difficile
	Streptococcus spp	Clostridium tetanii
		Bacillus spp
Gram negative	Neisseria meningitides	Pseudomonas aeruginosa
	Neisseria gonorrhoeae	Escherichia coli
		Legionella pneumophila
		Acinetobacter baumanii
		Salmonella

Viruses

Viruses are much smaller, and even simpler, than bacteria. They are often little more than a protein capsule containing some genetic material. They do not have cells, and some people do not even consider them to be alive. They have genes and will evolve through natural selection, but have no metabolism of their own. The most significant characteristic of viruses is that they can only reproduce within a host cell, by using the cell's own mechanisms to reproduce the viral genetic material and to manufacture the other elements required to produce more virus particles. This often causes the death of the cell concerned (Goering *et al.* 2007).

The small size of viruses (poliovirus, for example, is only 30 nanometres (nm) across) means that most are smaller than the wavelengths of visible light. They can only be 'seen' with a specialist instrument such as an electron microscope, which will only be available in a very few hospital microbiology laboratories. Diagnosis of viral infections is normally by the patient's symptoms, with confirmation by laboratory tests designed to detect either the virus itself or antibodies produced by the patient's immune system as a response to infection (Wilson 2000).

There are viruses that specifically infect humans, or other animals, or plants, or even bacteria. This is one characteristic that can be used in classifying them. However, the main basis for classification is by the type of genetic material they contain. This can be DNA or RNA, and may be in a double strand, as seen in other organisms' DNA, or in a single strand. Other characteristics include the shape of the viral particle and the sort of disease caused by infection.

The life cycle of all viruses is similar and can be summarized as follows (Goering *et al.* 2007).

1 *Attachment*: a virus particle attaches to the outside of a host cell. Viruses are generally very limited in the types of cell that they can attach to, and normally infect only a single species or a limited range of related host organisms. Even a wide-ranging virus such as rabies is restricted to infecting mammals.

2 *Penetration*: the virus particle enters the host cell. The exact mechanism of this depends on the virus and the type of host.

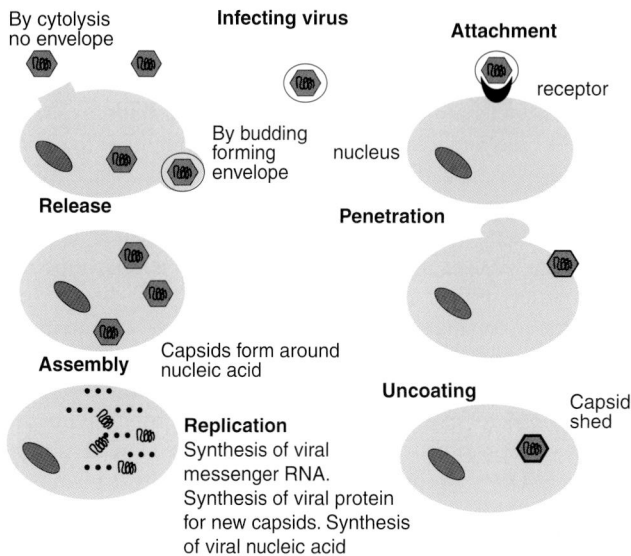

Figure 3.3   The viral life cycle. Used with permission from Perry (2007).

3 *Uncoating*: the virus particle breaks down and exposes the viral genetic material.

4 *Replication*: the instructions contained in the viral genes cause the host cell mechanisms to create more viral particles.

5 *Release*: the new viral particles are released from the cell. Some viruses may 'bud' from the surface of the cell, acquiring their enclosing membranes in the process, but often release occurs due to cell rupture and destruction.

This process is illustrated in Figure 3.3.

A final point to consider in relation to viral structure and infection prevention and control is the presence or absence of a lipid envelope enclosing the viral particle. Those viruses that have a lipid envelope, such as herpes zoster virus (responsible for chicken pox and shingles), are much more susceptible to destruction by alcohol than those without, for example norovirus, which is a common cause of viral gastroenteritis.

Fungi

Like bacteria, fungi exist in many environments on Earth, including, in some cases, as commensal organisms on human beings. Unlike bacteria, they are eukaryotic, so their cells share some characteristics with other eukaryotes such as humans, but they are distinct from both animals and plants. Fungi are familiar to us as mushrooms and toadstools and the yeast that is used in brewing and baking. They also have many uses in the pharmaceutical industry, particularly in the production of antibiotics. Fungi produce spores, both for survival in adverse conditions, as bacteria do, and to provide a mechanism for dispersal in the same way as plants (Goering *et al.* 2007).

A few varieties of fungi are able to cause opportunistic infections in humans. These are usually found in one of two forms: either as single-celled yeast-like forms that reproduce in a similar fashion to bacteria, by dividing or budding, or as plant-like filaments called *hyphae*. A mass of hyphae together forms a *mycelium*. Some fungi may appear in either form, depending on environmental conditions. Fungal infections are referred to as *mycoses*. Superficial mycoses such as ringworm and thrush usually involve only the skin or mucous membranes and are normally mild, if unpleasant, but deeper mycoses involving major organs can be life threatening. These most frequently occur in patients who have severely impaired immune systems and may be an indicator of such impairment; for example, pneumonia caused by *Pneumocystis jiroveci* (previously *carinii*) is considered a clinical indication of AIDS. Superficial infections are generally transmitted by physical contact, whereas deeper infections can result, for example, from spores being inhaled. This is why it is important to ensure that patients with impaired immunity are protected from situations where the spores of potentially pathogenic fungi are likely to be released, for example during building work (Goering *et al.* 2007).

Protozoa

Protozoa are single-celled animals, some species of which are medically important parasites of human beings, particularly in tropical and subtropical parts of the world where diseases such as malaria are a major public health issue. Unlike bacteria, their relationship with humans is almost always parasitic – that is, their presence has an adverse effect on the host. The life cycles of protozoa can be complex, and may involve stages in different hosts.

Medically important protozoa include *Plasmodium*, the cause of malaria, *Giardia* and *Cryptosporidium*, which can cause gastroenteritis, and *Trichomonas*, which is a sexually transmitted cause of vaginitis.

The most common routes of infection with protozoa are by consuming them in food or water or via an insect vector such as a mosquito (Goering *et al.* 2007). Cross-infection in the course of healthcare is uncommon but not unknown.

Helminths

'Helminth' is a generic term for parasitic worms. A number of worms from three different groups affect humans: tapeworms, roundworms (nematodes) and flukes. Transmission is generally by ingestion of eggs or larvae, or of infected animals or fish, but some are transmitted via an insect vector and some, notably the nematode *Strongyloides*, have a larval stage that is capable of penetrating the skin.

Helminth infections can affect almost every part of the body, and the effects can be severe. For example, the *Ascaris* worm can cause bowel obstruction if there are large numbers present; *Brugia* and *Wuchereria* obstruct the lymphatic system and eventually cause elephantiasis as a result; and infection with *Toxocara* (often after contact with dog faeces)

can result in epilepsy or blindness. However, cross-infection in healthcare is not normally considered a significant risk.

Arthropods

Arthropods (insects) are most significant in infectious disease in terms of their function as vectors of many viral, bacterial, protozoan and helminth-caused diseases. Some flies lay eggs in the skin of mammals, including humans, and the larvae feed and develop in the skin before pupating into the adult form, and some, such as lice and mites, are associated with humans for the whole of their life cycle. Such arthropod infestations can be uncomfortable, and there is often significant social stigma attached to them, possibly because the creatures are often visible to the naked eye. The activity of the insects and the presence of their saliva and faeces can result in quite severe skin conditions that are then vulnerable to secondary fungal or bacterial infection (Goering *et al.* 2007).

Lice

Species of *Pediculus* infest the hair and body of humans, feeding by sucking blood from their host. The adult animal is around 3 mm long and wingless, moving by means of claws. It cannot jump or fly, and dies within 24 hours if away from its host, so cross-infection is normally by direct contact or transfer of eggs or adults through sharing personal items.

Scabies

Scabies is caused by the mite *Sarcoptes scabiei*, an insect less than 1 mm long, which burrows into the top layers of skin. Infestation usually starts around the wrists and in between the fingers because acquisition is normally by close contact with an infected individual. The female mites lay eggs in these burrows and the offspring can spread to other areas of skin elsewhere on the body. The burrows are visible as a characteristic rash in the areas affected. In immunocompromised hosts or in those unable to practise normal levels of personal hygiene, very high levels of infestation can occur, often with thickening of the skin and the formation of thick crusts. This is known as 'Norwegian scabies' and is associated with a much higher risk of cross-infection than the normal presentation. Scabies is most often associated with long-stay care settings, but there have been reported outbreaks associated with more acute healthcare facilities.

Prions

Prions are thought to be the causative agents of a group of diseases called transmissible spongiform encephalopathies (TSEs), the most well known of which are Creutzfeldt–Jakob disease (CJD) and its variant (vCJD), which has been associated with the bovine spongiform encephalopathy (BSE) outbreak in Great Britain in the late 1980s and early 1990s. TSEs cause serious, irreversible damage to the central nervous system and are fatal. They are characterized by 'plaques' in the brain that are surrounded by holes that give the appearance of a sponge, hence the name. It used to be thought that this group of diseases was caused by so-called 'slow' viruses but they are now widely thought to be caused by prions, although this theory is not universally accepted. The theory is described below (Weaving 2007).

The prion protein (PrP) is a normally occurring protein found on the surface of some cells (PrPC). The disease-causing form of the protein (PrPCJD) appears to have an identical amino acid sequence but has a different three-dimensional shape. When the normal protein PrPC is exposed to the disease-causing form PrPCJD, it changes its conformation to that of PrPCJD. PrPCJD appears to progressively accumulate and be deposited in the brain, resulting in the characteristic 'plaques'. This process is slow compared to the replication of most micro-organisms and 'classic' CJD normally appears in older people.

One of the characteristics of vCJD is that it affects a much younger age group, although the incubation period still appears to be a number of years. There are currently no reliable tests to identify infection before the onset of symptoms, which has led to the worry that there could be a large pool of asymptomatic carriers of the vCJD infectious agent who may act as a reservoir for onward transmission via healthcare procedures. Routes of transmission already confirmed for CJD and vCJD include dura mater and corneal grafts, treatment with human-derived growth hormone, blood transfusion and surgical instruments. The infectious agent does not appear to be affected by decontamination processes such as autoclaving and chemical disinfectants to the same extent as more familiar micro-organisms such as bacteria or viruses. This has led to extensive reviews of decontamination procedures in the UK and has resulted in an increased emphasis on effective washing to remove any residual organic material that may harbour the infectious agent, and on the tracking of instruments to individual patients to facilitate any look-back exercise should any patient be identified as suffering from CJD or vCJD at a later date.

Creutzfeldt–Jakob disease is a sporadic illness that affects around one person in every million and probably arises from a spontaneous genetic mutation. It should also be noted that only a very small number of people have developed vCJD. It appears that a combination of exposure to the infectious agent and genetic susceptibility is necessary for progression to the disease (related TSE have a very strong genetic component), and there are numerous measures in place to prevent both the infectious agent entering the food chain and onward transmission through healthcare interventions. These appear to be the only routes of infection – there is no evidence of transmission via any other route. However, there is much that is unclear about the disease and the causative agent.

Mechanisms of infection

Whether or not a particular infectious agent will cause an infection in any given circumstance is dependent on

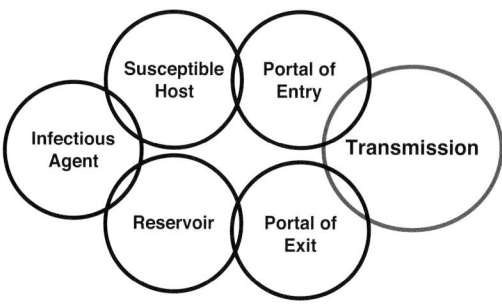

Figure 3.4 The chain of infection. A useful tool for seeing how to prevent transmission. How would you break each of the links in the chain?

many different factors, including how easily that agent can be transmitted and its *pathogenicity* or *virulence* – its ability to cause disease and the severity of the infection produced. However, it is generally accepted that for infection to occur, certain linked requirements need to be met. These links are often referred to as the *chain of infection* (Damani 2003). While the chain of infection will not be strictly accurate in every case – some 'links' may be missing or will overlap – it is an extremely useful model to consider how infection can be prevented, by breaking the 'links' in this chain. Some links are easier to break than others – for example, it is often easier to prevent an infectious agent entering a susceptible person than it is to prevent it leaving an infected one.

The chain of infection is illustrated in Figure 3.4 and the links are listed, with examples of how infection can be prevented at each link, in Table 3.3.

Modes of transmission

The mode of transmission is the method by which an infectious agent passes from one person or place to another. Considering the mode of transmission allows you to implement the measures required to prevent it.

Direct contact

This is person-to-person spread of infectious agents through physical contact between people. It occurs through normal nursing activities and can happen during aseptic procedures if technique is poor. It can be prevented through good hand hygiene and the use of barriers such as aprons and gloves.

Indirect contact

This occurs when someone comes into contact with a contaminated object. Many items in the healthcare environment can become contaminated, but the most likely routes of spread are inadequately decontaminated items of equipment used for diagnosis or treatment. Transmission is prevented by effective cleaning and decontamination and good hand hygiene.

Table 3.3 Links in the chain of infection

Link	Definition	Example	Examples of breaking the chain
Infectious agent	A potentially pathogenic micro-organism or other agent	Any potential pathogen	Removal of infectious agents through cleaning; destruction of micro-organisms through sterilization of equipment; treatment of patient with bacterial infection with antibiotics
Reservoir	Any location where micro-organisms or other agents may exist or reproduce	Human beings; the healthcare environment; stagnant water	Cleaning equipment and the environment; removing stagnant water by flushing low-use taps and showers and changing flower water regularly; minimizing the number of people present in high-risk situations such as surgery
Portal of exit	The route by which the infectious agent leaves the reservoir	Diarrhoea or vomit may carry norovirus; droplets expelled during coughing or sneezing may contain respiratory pathogens	Asking a patient with active tuberculosis infection to wear a mask in communal areas of the hospital
Mode of transmission	See Modes of transmission		
Portal of entry	The route by which the infectious agent enters a new host	Organisms introduced into a normally sterile part of the body through use of an invasive device, for example urinary catheter; inhalation of airborne pathogens	Avoiding unnecessary invasive devices; using strict aseptic technique; staff members wearing masks when dealing with infectious agents that may be inhaled
Susceptible host	The person that the infectious agent enters has to be susceptible to infection	The very old and very young are more susceptible, as are people with underlying chronic illnesses	Ensuring adequate nutrition and personal hygiene; providing vaccination to healthcare workers

Droplet transmission

When people cough, sneeze or even talk, they expel droplets of respiratory secretions and saliva. These droplets will travel about a metre from the person expelling them, and may contain the agents responsible for respiratory infections such as influenza or tuberculosis. Transmission is prevented through isolating the affected patient and using masks, aprons and gloves to provide a barrier, and also through good hand hygiene as there will almost always also be transmission by indirect contact.

Airborne transmission

Airborne transmission also involves droplets or particles containing infectious agents, but on a small enough scale that the particles can remain suspended in the air for long periods of time. Infections spread via this route include measles and chicken pox. Prevention is as for droplet transmission.

Parenteral transmission

This is a form of contact transmission, where blood or body fluids containing infectious agents come into contact with mucous membranes or exposed tissue. In healthcare, this can occur through transplantation or infusion, which is why blood and organs for transplantation are screened for bloodborne viruses such as HIV, or through an inoculation injury where blood splashes into the eyes or a used item of sharp equipment penetrates the skin (often called a 'needlestick' injury). Transmission is prevented by good practice in handling and disposing of sharps and the appropriate use of protective equipment, including eye protection.

Faecal–oral transmission

This occurs when an infectious agent present in the faeces from the gastrointestinal tract of an infected person is subsequently ingested by someone else and enters their gastrointestinal tract. It is the route of much gastrointestinal illness and water- and foodborne disease. There are often several steps involved; for example, someone with infectious diarrhoea whose hand hygiene is insufficiently effective is likely to contaminate any food they prepare, which will then expose anyone who eats it to infection. Transmission is prevented through isolating any patient with symptoms of gastroenteritis, effective hand hygiene (with soap and water as many of these organisms may be less susceptible to alcohol) by both staff and patients, appropriate use of gloves and aprons, and good food hygiene.

Vector transmission

Many diseases are spread through the action of a vector, most often an insect that travels from one person to another to feed. This route is not currently a concern in healthcare in England, but in parts of the world where malaria is endemic, for example, protecting patients from vectors such as mosquitoes will be an important element of nursing care.

These definitions are useful for considering the different routes by which infectious agents can spread but there is overlap between the different categories: droplet and airborne spread, for example, or indirect contact and faecal–oral. Many agents will be spread by more than one route, or there may be a combination of routes involved. In norovirus infection, for example, the overall mode of spread is faecal–oral but if someone is infected with norovirus, they may vomit and create an aerosol of droplets that contain the virus. Those droplets may be ingested directly from the atmosphere or they may settle on food, surfaces or equipment in the immediate vicinity. Anyone touching those surfaces will pick up the virus on their hands (indirect contact) and transmit it to their mouth either directly or via food.

Sources of infection

An individual may become infected with organisms already present on their body (endogenous infection) or introduced from elsewhere (exogenous infection). The majority of HCAIs are endogenous, hence the importance of procedures such as effective skin decontamination prior to invasive procedures.

Indicators and effects of infection

Generally, infection is said to have occurred when infectious agents enter a normally sterile area of the body and cause symptoms as a result. There are obvious exceptions to this – for example, the digestive tract is not sterile, being home to trillions of micro-organisms, but many types of infectious gastroenteritis are caused by particular organisms entering this area – but it is a useful working definition. The symptoms of infection are listed below. Not all symptoms will be present in all cases, and it should be noted that many symptoms are due to the body's response to infection and so may not be present in severely immunocompromised patients.

Symptoms of infection

- *Heat*: the site of the infection may feel warm to the touch, and the patient may have a raised temperature.
- *Pain*: at the site of the infection.
- *Swelling*: at the site of the infection.
- *Redness*: at the site of the infection.
- Pus.

- Feeling of general malaise.
- *In gastrointestinal infection*: abdominal pain and tenderness; nausea; diarrhoea and/or vomiting.
- *In urinary tract infection*: frequency of micturition; often confusion in the elderly; loin pain and/or abdominal discomfort.

Evidence-based approaches

Rationale

The principle of all infection prevention and control is preventing the transmission of infectious agents. However, the measures taken to reduce the risk of transmission must be reasonable, practicable and proportionate to the risk of transmission and the effects of infection with any particular agent. For example, while *Staphylococcus aureus* can cause severe infections, it is carried by around a third of the population and so isolating every patient carrying it would not be practicable. Meticillin-resistant *Staphylococcus aureus* (MRSA) can cause equally serious infections, is resistant to many of the antibiotics that would normally be used to treat these infections and is carried by far fewer people, so it is both reasonable and practicable to take additional precautions to prevent its spread in healthcare. These may include isolation in an acute hospital but it would not be reasonable to segregate a colonized individual in a mental health unit where social interaction may form part of their care and the risk to other individuals is less.

The management of any individual who is infected or colonized with an organism that may pose a risk to other individuals must be based on a risk assessment that takes into account how easily the infectious agent can be passed to other people; the susceptibility to infection of other people being cared for in the same area and the likely consequences of their becoming infected; the practicality of implementing particular infection prevention and control precautions within that area or institution (the number of single rooms available, for example); and the individual's other nursing needs. The infection prevention and control policies of health and social care providers are based on generic risk assessments of their usual client or patient group and should be adhered to unless there are strong reasons to alter procedures for a particular individual's care. In such circumstances, the advice of the infection prevention and control team (IPCT) should be sought first. Nurses working in independent and social care settings should seek advice from the IPCT of the local primary care organization or local health protection unit of the Health Protection Agency.

Indications

Infection prevention and control precautions must be taken with all patients, regardless of whether or not they are known to be carrying any particular infectious agent that may cause a hazard to others. This is because it is impossible to guarantee whether or not any given individual is free of any particular infectious agent and because many common micro-organisms may cause infections in some circumstances. The indications for additional infection control precautions are that an individual is particularly vulnerable to infection because of some deficiency in their normal defence mechanisms or that they are known to be infected or colonized with an infectious agent that may pose a particular risk to others.

Contraindications

As mentioned previously, precautions to prevent the spread of infection must be based on a risk assessment that takes in all the relevant factors. In some cases precautions will need to be modified because of a patient's physical or psychological needs. Isolation, for example, has been demonstrated to have an adverse psychological effect on some individuals (Morgan *et al.* 2009).

Anticipated patient outcomes

The anticipated outcome is that no patient will acquire micro-organisms from any other individual during the course of healthcare or suffer an avoidable infection.

Legal and professional issues

In England, the Health and Safety at Work, etc. Act 1974 is the primary piece of legislation relating to the safety of people in the workplace. It applies to all employees and employ-

ers, and requires them to do everything that is reasonable and practicable to prevent harm coming to anyone in the workplace. It requires employers to provide training and appropriate protective equipment and employees to follow the training that they have received, use the protective equipment provided, and report any situations where they believe inadequate precautions are putting anyone's health and safety at serious risk. This dovetails with the requirements of the Nursing and Midwifery Council (NMC 2008a) for nurses to promote and protect the well-being of those in their care and to report their concerns in writing if problems in the environment of care are putting people at risk.

The requirement to protect individuals from healthcare-associated infections is further emphasized in England by the Health and Social Care Act 2008. This legislation is monitored and enforced by the Care Quality Commission, which assesses care providers against the requirements of the Code of Practice for health and adult social care on the prevention and control of infections and related guidance (DH 2010a). Often referred to as the Hygiene Code, this has been applied to NHS hospitals in England, in one form or another, for some years but from October 2010 applies to all providers of health or adult social care. Each provider must be registered with the Care Quality Commission and declare compliance with the ten criteria of the Hygiene Code. These criteria are summarized in Table 3.4.

Nurses need to be aware of the measures that are in place in their workplace to ensure compliance with the Code of Practice. For example, many hospital trusts have a programme

Table 3.4 Criteria of the 2010 Hygiene Code of Practice

Compliance criterion	What the registered provider will need to demonstrate
1	Systems to manage and monitor the prevention and control of infection. These systems use risk assessments and consider how susceptible service users are and any risks that their environment and other users may pose to them.
2	Provide and maintain a clean and appropriate environment in managed premises that facilitates the prevention and control of infections
3	Provide suitable accurate information on infections to service users and their visitors
4	Provide suitable accurate information on infections to any person concerned with providing further support or nursing/medical care in a timely fashion
5	Ensure that people who have or develop an infection are identified promptly and receive the appropriate treatment and care to reduce the risk of passing on the infection to other people
6	Ensure that all staff and those employed to provide care in all settings are fully involved in the process of preventing and controlling infection
7	Provide or secure adequate isolation facilities
8	Secure adequate access to laboratory support as appropriate
9	Have and adhere to policies designed for the individual's care and provider organizations that will help to prevent and control infections
10	Ensure, so far as is reasonably practicable, that care workers are free of and are protected from exposure to infections that can be caught at work and that all staff are suitably educated in the prevention and control of infection associated with the provision of health and social care

From DH (2010a). © Crown copyright. Reproduced under the terms of the Click-use Licence.

of regular visits to clinical areas by senior staff who will carry out an inspection against the criteria of the Code as if they were an external assessor. This programme ensures that senior staff are familiar with the Code and that everyone is familiar with the inspection process. In addition, nurses may need to carry out activities to promote compliance and provide evidence of assurance, such as audits of hand hygiene performance or compliance with aseptic technique. One such set of audits in place in many hospitals in England is the package produced by the Department of Health (2007a) and known collectively as *Saving Lives*. These are discussed in more detail later.

In addition to healthcare-specific requirements, items of legislation and regulation have also been devised with the objective of reducing the risk of infection in any situation that apply to healthcare as much as they do to any other business or workplace. These include legislation and regulation relating to food hygiene (Food Safety Act 1990), water quality (Health and Safety Commission 2001), waste management (Hazardous Waste Regulations 2005) and other issues that are peripheral to healthcare but must be taken into account when developing policies and procedures for an NHS trust or other healthcare provider.

Competencies

The NMC Code (NMC 2008a) states that all nurses must work within the limits of their competence. This means not carrying out aseptic procedures, for example, without being competent and confident that they can be carried out without increasing the risk of introducing infection through lack of knowledge or technique. However, there are some procedures for infection prevention and control that must be carried out as part of every care activity, and so all nurses must be competent in these if they are to provide any level of physical care at all. These include:

- hand hygiene
- use of personal protective equipment such as gloves and aprons
- appropriate segregation and disposal of waste, in particular used sharps items and other equipment designated as single use
- appropriate decontamination of reusable equipment after use.

Preprocedural considerations

Equipment

All infection prevention and control measures have the objective of preventing the transmission of infectious agents, whether by removing them from items that may be contaminated (hand hygiene and cleaning) or establishing a barrier (personal protective equipment and isolation). There are therefore some items that should be available for effective infection prevention and control in any situation where healthcare is provided.

Equipment for hand hygiene

It is essential that wherever care is provided, there are facilities for hand hygiene. Hand wash basins in clinical areas should have taps that can be turned on and off without using the hands; that is, they should be non-touch or lever operated (DH 2006b). Basins used solely by clinical staff for hand hygiene should not have plugs (to encourage hand washing under running water) or overflows (because they are difficult to clean effectively and can be a reservoir for organisms such as *Pseudomonas* that may cause infection in vulnerable individuals (NHS Estates 2001). Basins that are also used by patients may require plugs, which will require careful management with some client groups to reduce the risk of flooding. In all cases, the taps should be positioned so that water does not fall directly into the outflow as this may lead to splashes containing organisms from within the drain. Taps should be of a mixer type that allows the temperature to be set before handwashing starts. Access to basins must be unobstructed by any furniture or equipment to ensure that they can easily be used whenever required.

Liquid soap dispensers should be positioned close to hand wash basins and care should be taken to ensure that soap cannot drip onto the floor from the dispenser and cause a slip hazard. Soap should be simple and unscented to minimize the risk of adverse reactions from frequent use. There is no advantage to using soap or detergents combined with or containing antimicrobial agents for routine handwashing. These preparations carry a higher risk of adverse reactions and should not be used routinely. Bar soap should not be used. A paper towel dispenser should be fixed to the wall close to the hand wash basin. Hand towels should be of adequate quality to ensure that hands are completely dried by the proper use of one or two towels. To conveniently dispose of these towels, a suitable bin with a pedal-operated lid should be positioned close to the basin, but not so that it obstructs access to the basin.

Alcohol-based handrub should be available at the point of care in every clinical area for use immediately before care and between different care activities on the same patient (NPSA 2008). Dispensers may be attached to the patient's bed or bedside locker, and free-standing pump-top bottles can be used where appropriate, such as on the desk in a room used for outpatient clinics. Dispensers should not be sited close to sinks unless this is unavoidable because of the risk of confusion with soap, particularly if the dispensers are similar. Smaller sized personal-issue bottles are appropriate where there is a risk that handrub may be accidentally or deliberately drunk, such as in paediatric areas or when caring for a patient with alcohol dependency (NPSA 2008). *Note*: Antiseptic handrubs based on non-alcoholic antiseptics are available but evidence suggests that alcohol is the most useful agent in terms of range and speed of antimicrobial activity (WHO 2009).

Equipment for waste disposal

Also available should be disposal bags for domestic and clinical waste and a sharps bin if the procedure is to involve the use of any sharp single-use items (DH 2006a). The sharps bin should always be taken to the point of use (Pratt *et al.* 2007); do not transport used sharps in any other way or in any other container. Bags and containers used for hazardous waste should be coloured according to their final disposal method (DH 2006a).

Personal protective equipment (PPE)

Other equipment required for infection prevention and control will depend on the activity being carried out, but basic PPE to provide a barrier to body fluids and micro-organisms – non-latex disposable gloves, disposable aprons and eye protection as a minimum – should be readily available in the clinical area (Pratt *et al.* 2007), and particularly where regular use is anticipated. For example, it is appropriate to have dispensers for gloves and aprons situated outside isolation rooms. All PPE sold in the UK must comply with the relevant regulations and standards, including being 'CE' marked to demonstrate that they meet these standards (Department of Trade and Industry 2002).

Disposable gloves

Gloves will be necessary in some circumstances but should be worn only when required (Infection Control Nurses Association 2002). Non-sterile disposable gloves are most usefully available packaged in boxes of 100 ambidextrous gloves, in small, medium and large sizes. These boxes should be located close to the point of use, ideally in a fixed dispenser to make removing the gloves from the box as easy as possible. In the past, natural rubber latex was a commonly used material for these gloves but concerns about latex sensitivity mean that many healthcare organizations have adopted gloves made of alternative materials such as vinyl. There is some evidence that vinyl may be a less effective barrier than latex, but all gloves carry a risk of failure, often not visible to the naked eye (Korniewicz *et al.* 2002), hence the need for hand hygiene regardless of whether or not gloves are worn. Whatever the material, these gloves are single use – they should be used for the task for which they are required and then removed and disposed of. They cannot be cleaned and reused for another task (MHRA 2006, Pratt *et al.* 2007).

Disposable aprons

Single-use disposable aprons may be obtained either in a box or linked together on a roll. Presentation is not important as long as it is compatible with the dispensers in use and the product meets the requisite standards (i.e. is 'CE' marked). Aprons are normally made of thin polythene and are available in a range of colours. Different coloured aprons can be used to designate staff doing different tasks or working in different areas to give a visible reminder of the risk of cross-infection. As with disposable gloves, disposable aprons should be used for the task for which they are required and then removed and disposed of (MHRA 2006, Pratt *et al.* 2007).

Sterile gloves

Single-use sterile gloves, both latex and latex free, should be available in any area where their use is anticipated. Sterile gloves are packed as a left-and-right pair and are manufactured in a wide range of full and half sizes (similar to shoe sizes) so as to fit closely and provide the best possible compromise between acting as a barrier and allowing the wearer to work normally. Natural rubber latex is still one of the best materials for this, so sterile gloves are more often made of this than of alternative materials. Care must be taken to ensure alternatives are available for patients with sensitivity to latex.

Sterile gowns

To provide 'maximal barrier precautions' during surgery or other invasive procedures carrying a high risk of infection, or where infection would have serious consequences such as insertion of a central venous catheter, a sterile gown will be required in addition to sterile gloves. Modern sterile gowns are most often single-use disposable products made of water-repellent material as multiple-use fabric gowns may, over time, lose their effectiveness as a barrier.

Eye protection

Eye protection will be required in any situation where the mucous membranes of the eyes may be exposed to body fluid droplets generated during aerosol-generating procedures or surgery with power tools. Both single-use and multiple-use options are available. Goggles are normally sufficient as long as they are worn in conjunction with a fluid-repellent mask. If greater protection is required, or a mask is not worn for any reason, a face shield should be used. Face shields may also be more appropriate for people who wear glasses; prescription glasses will often not provide sufficient protection and should not be relied upon.

Masks and respirators

If dealing with organisms spread by the airborne or droplet route, a facemask or respirator will be required. When using a respirator (usually used to prevent the transmission of respiratory viruses), a good fit is essential to ensure that there is no leakage around the sides. Staff who are likely to need to use respirators should be 'fit tested' using a taste test to ensure that they have the correct size. A taste test consists of wearing the respirator while being exposed to a strong-tasting vapour (normally inside a hood to contain the vapour); if the subject can taste the vapour then the respirator is not properly fitted. Fit testing is normally carried out by the infection prevention and control team or occupational health department. Note that facial hair under the edge of the respirator will prevent a proper seal; staff with beards may therefore be unable to work safely if a respirator is required.

Single-use masks and respirators are normally the best option (and should be strictly single use). In the past, some materials used in mask manufacture would become wet from exhaled moisture and lose their barrier properties; modern products contain fluid-resistant materials and will last for the full duration of an episode of use. Multiple-use respirators are sometimes required, often for people whose face shape does not allow a good seal with disposable products (DH 2010b).

Assessment and recording tools

Assessment for infection prevention and control should take place at every level in an organization providing healthcare, from completing an assessment of infection risks (both to and from the patient) as part of the care planning process to the audit of compliance in a team, unit or hospital (DH 2010a). As mentioned previously, the Care Quality Commission assesses care providers in England against the requirements of the Hygiene Code. Other external assessors may also require evidence that procedures are in place to reduce the risk of healthcare-associated infection. Such evidence may include audits of compliance with hand hygiene against the WHO '5 moments' when hand hygiene should be performed at the point of care (WHO 2009) or audits to demonstrate that all the elements of a procedure that carries a particular risk of infection have been carried out. Such procedures are sometimes referred to as 'high-impact interventions' because the risk of infection is such that improving adherence to good practice when they are carried out can have a significant impact on an organization's infection rates. The English Department of Health's *Saving Lives* toolkit (DH 2007a) is a collection of guidelines for high-impact interventions in the form of care bundles, and audits of those care bundles that can be used both for practice improvement and as evidence of good practice for internal and external assessment. All nurses should know which of these tools are being used in their workplace and actively participate in their completion.

At the level of individual patients, all additional precautions for infection prevention should be documented within the patient's individual plan of care, which should include regular reassessment and changes as necessary as the patient's condition alters. For example, a patient given antibiotics for a chest infection may be at risk of developing *Clostridium difficile* infection; if they develop diarrhoea, they will need to be isolated immediately but if the diarrhoea settles following treatment, they will no longer require isolation once they have been free of symptoms for 48 hours (DH/HPA 2008). When a procedure is carried out that requires additional precautions, for example aseptic technique, it should be documented in the record of that procedure that those precautions were adhered to or, if not, the reasons why they could not be implemented.

Specific patient preparations
Education

All patients should be informed about the risks of healthcare-associated infection and the measures that are known to reduce the risk of infection. In particular, patient education programmes that encourage the patient to ask healthcare workers 'Did you wash your hands?' have been demonstrated to increase compliance with hand hygiene (McGuckin *et al.* 2001). In addition, patients who are infected or colonized with infectious agents that require additional precautions to be implemented to reduce the risk of infection to other patients must be clearly told the nature of the infectious agent and its mode of spread, the risk to others, the details of the precautions required and the rationale behind them. Patients are likely to suffer anxiety if they are infected or colonized by such agents and this can be alleviated through being provided with clear information. Similarly, there are adverse psychological effects of isolation and other precautions (Gammon 1998) and these are more likely to be mitigated if the patient has a clear understanding of why they are being implemented (Ward 2000).

Procedure guideline 3.1 Handwashing

Essential equipment

- Hand wash basin
- Liquid soap
- Paper towels
- Domestic waste bin

Preprocedure

Action	Rationale
1 Remove any rings, bracelets and wristwatch still worn and roll up sleeves. (Note: It is good practice to remove all hand and wrist jewellery and roll up sleeves before entering any clinical area and the English Department of Health has instructed NHS trusts to implement a 'bare below the elbows' dress code.)	Jewellery inhibits good handwashing. Dirt and bacteria can remain beneath jewellery after handwashing. Long sleeves prevent washing of wrists and will easily become contaminated and a route of transmission of micro-organisms (DH 2010c, C).
2 Cover cuts and abrasions on hands with waterproof dressing.	Cuts and abrasions can become contaminated with bacteria and cannot be easily cleaned. Repeated handwashing can worsen an injury (WHO 2009, C). Breaks in the skin will allow the entry of potential pathogens.

(Continued)

93

Procedure guideline 3.1 (Continued)

3 Remove nail varnish and artificial nails (most uniform policies and dress codes prohibit these). Nails must also be short and clean.	Long and false nails and imperfections in nail polish harbour dirt and bacteria that are not effectively removed by hand-washing (WHO 2009, C).

Procedure

4 Turn on the taps and where possible direct the water flow away from the plughole. Run the water at a flow rate that prevents splashing.	Plugholes are often contaminated with micro-organisms that could be transferred to the environment or the user if splashing occurs (NHS Estates 2001, C).
5 Run the water until hand hot.	Warm water is more pleasant to wash with than cold so handwashing is more likely to be carried out effectively. E Water that is too hot could cause scalding. Soap is more effective in breaking down dirt and organic matter when used with hand-hot water (DH 2001, C).
6 Wet the surface of hands and wrists.	Soap applied directly onto dry hands may damage the skin. E The water will also quickly mix with the soap to speed up handwashing.
7 Apply liquid soap and water to all surfaces of the hands.	Liquid soap is very effective in removing dirt, organic material and any loosely adherent transient flora. Tablets of soap can become contaminated, potentially transferring micro-organisms from one user to another, but may be used if liquid soap is unavailable (DH 2001, C). To ensure all surfaces of the hands are cleaned. E
8 Rub hands together for a minimum of 10–15 seconds, with particular attention to between the fingers and the tips of fingers and thumbs (see Action Figure 8a). The areas that are most frequently missed through poor hand hygiene technique are shown in Action Figure 8b.	To ensure all surfaces of the hands are cleaned. Areas that are missed can be a source of cross-infection (Fraise and Bradley 2009, E).
9 Rinse soap thoroughly off hands.	Soap residue can lead to irritation and damage to the skin. Damaged skin does not provide a barrier to infection for the healthcare worker and can become colonized with potentially pathogenic bacteria, leading to cross-infection (DH 2001, C).
10 Turn off the taps using your wrist or elbow. If the taps are not lever-type, turn them off using a paper hand towel to prevent contact.	To avoid re-contaminating the hands. E

Postprocedure

11 Dry hands thoroughly with a disposable paper towel from a towel dispenser.	Damp hands encourage the multiplication of bacteria and can potentially become sore (DH 2001, C).
12 Dispose of used paper towels in a black bag in a foot-operated waste bin.	Paper towels used to dry the hands are normally non-hazardous and can be disposed of via the domestic waste stream (DH 2006a, C). Using a foot-operated waste bin prevents contamination of the hands. E

Action Figure 8a   1. Rub hands palm to palm. 2. Rub back of each hand with palm of other hand with fingers interlaced. 3. Rub palm to palm with fingers interlaced. Rub with back of fingers to opposing palms with fingers interlocked. Rub tips of fingers. Rub tips of fingers in opposite palm in a circular motion. 4. Rub each thumb clasped in opposite hand using a rotational movement. 5. Rub each wrist with opposite hand. 6. Rinse hands with water.

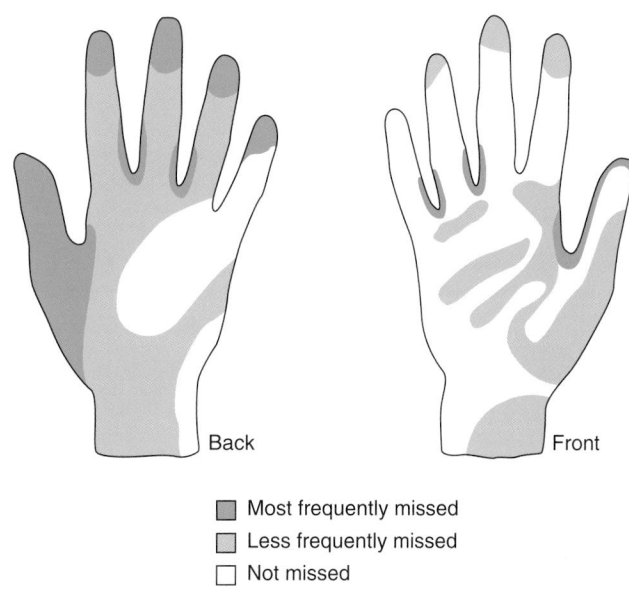

Back   Front

■ Most frequently missed
□ Less frequently missed
□ Not missed

Action Figure 8b   Areas most commonly missed following handwashing. Reproduced by kind permission of the *Nursing Times* where this first appeared in 1978.

Procedure guideline 3.2 Hand decontamination using alcohol handrub

Essential equipment

- Alcohol-based handrub

Procedure

Action	Rationale
1 Dispense the amount of handrub indicated in the manufacturer's instructions into the palm of one hand.	Too much handrub will take longer to dry and may consequently cause delays; too little will not decontaminate hands adequately. E
2 Rub the alcohol handrub into all areas of the hands, until the hands are dry, using the illustrated actions in Action Figure 2.	To ensure all areas of the hands are cleaned. Alcohol is a rapid-acting disinfectant, with the added advantage that it evaporates, leaving the hands dry. This prevents contamination of equipment, whilst facilitating the application of gloves (WHO 2009, C, E).

1 Apply a small amount (about 3 ml) of the product in a cupped hand

2 Rub hands together palm to palm, spreading the handrub over the hands

3 Rub back of each hand with palm of other hand with fingers interlaced

4 Rub palm to palm with fingers interlaced

5 Rub back of fingers to opposing palms with fingers interlocked

6 Rub each thumb clasped in opposite hand using a rotational movement

7 Rub tips of fingers in opposite palm in a circular motion

8 Rub each wrist with opposite hand

9 Wait until product has evaporated and hands are dry (do not use paper towels)

10 The process should take 15–30 seconds

cleanyourhands® campaign

NHS
National Patient Safety Agency

Action Figure 2   Alcohol handrub hand hygiene technique – for visibly clean hands. Adapted from WHO (2009). © Crown copyright. Reproduced under the terms of the Click-use Licence.

Procedure guideline 3.3 Putting on and removing non-sterile gloves

Essential equipment

- Non-sterile gloves

Preprocedure

Action	Rationale
1 Clean hands before putting on gloves.	Hands must be cleansed before and after every patient contact or contact with patient's equipment (Pratt *et al.* 2007, C).

Procedure

2 Remove gloves from the box singly (see Action Figure 2), to prevent contamination of the gloves lower down. If it is likely that more than two gloves will be required (i.e. if the procedure requires gloves to be changed part-way through), consider removing all the gloves needed before starting the procedure.	To prevent cross-contamination. E
3 Holding the cuff of the glove, pull it into position, taking care not to contaminate the glove from the wearer's skin (see Action Figure 3). This is particularly important when the second glove is being put on, as the gloved hand of the first glove can touch the skin of the ungloved second hand if care is not taken.	To prevent cross-contamination. E
4 During the procedure or when undertaking two procedures with the same patient, it may be necessary to change gloves. Gloves are single-use items and must not be cleansed and reused.	Disposable gloves are single-use items. They cannot be cleaned and reused for the same or another patient (MHRA 2006, C).
5 If gloves become damaged during use they must be replaced.	Damaged gloves are not an effective barrier. E
6 Remove the gloves when the procedure is completed, taking care not to contaminate the hands or the environment from the outside of the gloves.	The outside of the glove may be contaminated. E
7 Remove the first glove by firmly holding the outside of the glove wrist and pulling off the glove in such a way as to turn it inside out (see Action Figure 7).	Whilst removing the first glove, the second gloved hand continues to be protected. By turning the glove inside out during removal, any contamination is contained inside the glove. E
8 Remove the second glove by slipping the fingers of the ungloved hand inside the wrist of the glove and pulling it off whilst at the same time turning it inside out (see Action Figure 8).	By putting the fingers inside the glove, they will not be in contact with the potentially contaminated outer surface of the glove. E

Postprocedure

9 Dispose of used gloves as 'hazardous infectious waste' (see Action Figure 9), that is, into an orange waste bag, unless instructed otherwise by the infection prevention and control team.	All waste contaminated with blood, body fluids, excretions, secretions and infectious agents thought to pose a particular risk should be disposed of as hazardous infectious waste. Orange is the recognized colour for hazardous infectious waste that does not require incineration and may be made safe by alternative treatment (DH 2006a, C).
10 After removing the gloves, decontaminate your hands.	Hands may have become contaminated (Pratt *et al.* 2007, C).

(Continued)

Procedure guideline 3.3 *(Continued)*

Action Figure 2   Remove gloves from the box.

Action Figure 3   Holding the cuff of the glove, pull it into position.

Action Figure 7   Remove the first glove by firmly holding the outside of the glove wrist, then pull off the glove in such a way as to turn it inside out.

Action Figure 8   Remove the second glove by slipping the thumb of the ungloved hand inside the wrist of the glove and pulling it off while turning it inside out.

Action Figure 9   Dispose of used gloves.

Procedure guideline 3.4 Putting on and removing a disposable apron

Essential equipment

- Disposable apron

Preprocedure

Action	Rationale
1 Remove an apron from the dispenser or roll using clean hands and open it out.	To make it easy to put on. E

Procedure

Action	Rationale
2 Place the neck loop over your head and tie the ties together behind your back, positioning the apron so that as much of the front of your body is protected as possible (see Action Figures 2a,2b).	To minimize the risk of contamination being transferred between your clothing and the patient, in either direction. E
3 If gloves are required, don them as described in Procedure guideline 3.3. At the end of the procedure, remove gloves first.	The gloves are more likely to be contaminated than the apron and therefore should be removed first to prevent cross-contamination (DH 2010b, C).
4 Remove the apron by breaking the ties and neck loop; grasp the inside of the apron and dispose of it (see Action Figure 4).	The inside of the apron should be clean. E

Postprocedure

Action	Rationale
5 Dispose of used aprons as 'hazardous infectious waste', that is, into an orange waste bag, unless instructed otherwise by the infection prevention and control team.	All waste contaminated with blood, body fluids, excretions, secretions and infectious agents thought to pose a particular risk should be disposed of as hazardous infectious waste. Orange is the recognized colour for hazardous infectious waste that does not require incineration and may be made safe by alternative treatment (DH 2006a, C).
6 After removing the apron, decontaminate your hands.	Hands may have become contaminated (Pratt et al. 2007, C).

Action Figure 2a Place the neck loop of the apron over your head.

Action Figure 2b Tie the ties together behind your back, positioning the apron so that as much of the front of your body is protected as possible.

Action Figure 4 Remove the apron by breaking the neck loop and ties.

Procedure guideline 3.5 Putting on and removing a disposable mask or respirator

Essential equipment

- Disposable surgical mask or respirator

Preprocedure

Action	Rationale
1 Remove surgical-type masks singly from the box, or remove individually wrapped items from their packaging, with clean hands.	To prevent contamination of the item or others in the box or dispenser. E
2 Remove glasses, if worn.	Glasses will obstruct the correct positioning of the mask or respirator and may be dislodged and damaged. E

Procedure

3 Place the mask/respirator over nose, mouth and chin (see Action Figure 3).	To ensure correct positioning. E
4 Fit the flexible nose piece over the bridge of your nose if wearing a respirator.	To ensure the best fit. E
5 Secure the mask or respirator at the back of the head with ties or fitted elastic straps and adjust to fit (see Action Figure 5).	To ensure the mask/respirator is comfortable to wear and remains in the correct position throughout the procedure. E
6 If wearing a respirator, perform a fit check. First, breathe in – respirator should collapse or be 'sucked in' to the face. Then breathe out – respirator should not leak around the edges.	To ensure that there is a good seal around the edge of the respirator so that there is no route for non-filtered air to pass in either direction. Note that this check should be carried out whenever a respirator is worn and is not a substitute for prior fit testing (DH 2010b, C, E).
7 Replace glasses, if worn.	To restore normal vision. E
8 At the end of the procedure, or after leaving the room in which the respirator is required, remove by grasping the ties or straps at the back of the head and either break them or pull them forward over the top of the head. Do not touch the front of the mask/respirator (see Action Figures 8a, 8b).	To avoid contaminating the hands with material from the outside of the mask/respirator (DH 2010b, C, E).
9 Dispose of used disposable items as 'hazardous infectious waste', that is, into an orange waste bag, unless instructed otherwise by the infection prevention and control team.	All waste contaminated with blood, body fluids, excretions, secretions and infectious agents thought to pose a particular risk should be disposed of as hazardous infectious waste. Orange is the recognized colour for hazardous infectious waste that does not require incineration and may be made safe by alternative treatment (DH 2006a, C).

Postprocedure

10 Clean reusable items according to the manufacturer's instructions, usually with detergent and water or a detergent wipe.	To avoid cross-contamination and ensure the item is suitable for further use (DH 2010b, C, E).

Procedure guideline 3.5 (*Continued*)

Action Figure 3 Place the mask over your nose, mouth and chin.

Action Figure 5 Secure the mask at the back of the head with ties.

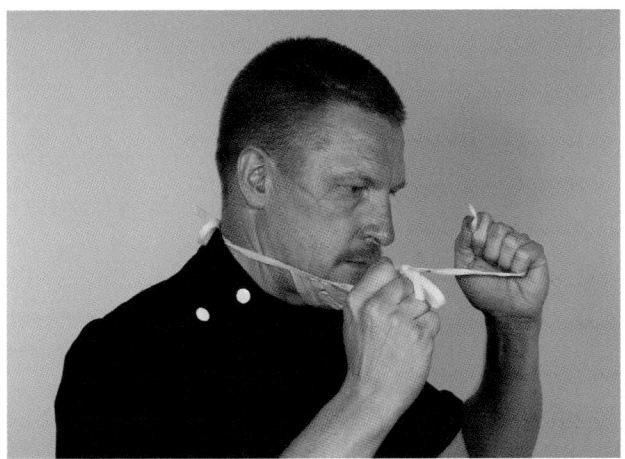

Action Figure 8a After use, remove the mask by untying or breaking the ties and pulling them forward.

Action Figure 8b Do not touch the front of the mask.

Procedure guideline 3.6 Putting on or removing goggles or a face shield

Purpose: To protect the mucous membranes of the eyes, nose and mouth from body fluid droplets generated during aerosol-generating procedures or surgery with power tools.

Essential equipment

■ Reusable or disposable goggles or face shield

Preprocedure

Action	Rationale
1 Remove eye protection from any packaging with clean hands.	To prevent cross-contamination. E

(*Continued*)

Procedure guideline 3.6 *(Continued)*

Procedure

2 Apply demister solution according to manufacturer's instructions, if required.	To ensure good visibility throughout the procedure. E
3 Position item over eyes/face and secure using ear pieces or headband; adjust to fit.	To ensure the item is comfortable to wear and remains in the correct position throughout the procedure. E
4 At the end of the procedure, remove by grasping the ear pieces or headband at the back or side of the head and lifting forward, away from the face. Do not touch the front of the goggles or face shield (see Action Figure 4).	To avoid contaminating the hands with material from the outside of the eye protection (DH 2010b, C, E).

Postprocedure

5 Dispose of used disposable items as 'hazardous infectious waste', that is, into an orange waste bag, unless instructed otherwise by the infection prevention and control team.	All waste contaminated with blood, body fluids, excretions, secretions and infectious agents thought to pose a particular risk should be disposed of as hazardous infectious waste. Orange is the recognized colour for hazardous infectious waste that does not require incineration and may be made safe by alternative treatment (DH 2006a, C).
6 Clean reusable items according to the manufacturer's instructions, usually with detergent and water or a detergent wipe.	To avoid cross-contamination and ensure the item is suitable for further use. E

Action Figure 4 Don and remove eye protection by grasping the earpieces; do not touch the front.

Procedure guideline 3.7 Donning sterile gloves: open technique

Purpose: To have a barrier between the nurse's hands and the patient to prevent the transmission of infectious agents in either direction, and to prevent contamination of a vulnerable area or invasive device through contact with non-sterile gloves.

Note that in steps 4 and 5, below, either glove can be put on first. Simply exchange 'left' and 'right' in the description if you wish to put on the right-hand glove first.

Essential equipment

- Sterile disposable gloves
- All other equipment required for the procedure for which the gloves are required

Preprocedure

Action	Rationale
1 Clean hands using soap and water or alcohol-based handrub.	Hands must be cleansed before and after every patient contact or contact with patient's equipment (Pratt *et al.* 2007, C).
2 Prepare all the equipment required for the procedure, including setting up the sterile field and tipping sterile items on to it from packets if you do not have an assistant, but do not touch any sterile item before putting on gloves.	To avoid contaminating gloves with non-sterile packets. E

Procedure

3 Open the packet containing the gloves and open out the inside packaging on a clean surface so that the fingers of the gloves are pointed away from you, taking care not to touch the gloves or allow them to come into contact with anything that is non-sterile (see Action Figure 3).	To prevent contamination of the gloves and to put them in the best position for putting them on. E
4 Hold the cuff of the left-hand glove with your right fingertips, at the uppermost edge where the cuff folds back on itself. Lift this edge away from the opposite edge to create an opening. Keeping them together, slide the fingers of the left hand into the glove, taking care not to contaminate the outside of the glove, while keeping hold of the folded edge in the other hand and pulling the glove onto the hand. Spread the fingers of the left hand slightly to help them enter the fingers of the glove (see Action Figure 4a, 4b, 4c).	To prevent contamination of the outside of the glove. E
5 Open up the right-hand glove with your left hand fingertips by sliding them beneath the folded-back cuff. Taking care not to touch the left-hand glove or the outside of the right-hand glove, and keeping the fingers together, slide the fingers of the right hand into the right-hand glove. Again, spread your fingers slightly once inside the body of the glove to help them into the glove fingers (see Action Figures 5a, 5b).	To prevent contamination of the outside of the glove. E
6 When both gloves are on, adjust the fit by pulling on the body of the glove to get your fingers to the end of the glove fingers (see Action Figures 6a, 6b).	To ensure the gloves are comfortable to wear and do not interfere with the procedure. E

(Continued)

Procedure guideline 3.7 (*Continued*)

Postprocedure

7 Remove the gloves when the procedure is completed, taking care not to contaminate the hands or the environment from the outside of the gloves.	The outside of the glove is likely to be contaminated. E
8 First, remove the first glove by firmly holding the outside of the glove wrist and pulling off the glove in such a way as to turn it inside out.	Whilst removing the first glove, the second gloved hand continues to be protected. By turning the glove inside out during removal, any contamination is contained inside the glove. E
9 Then remove the second glove by slipping the fingers of the ungloved hand inside the wrist of the glove and pulling it off whilst at the same time turning it inside out.	By putting the fingers inside the glove, the fingers will not be in contact with the potentially contaminated outer surface of the glove. E
10 Dispose of used gloves as 'hazardous infectious waste', that is, into an orange waste bag, unless instructed otherwise by the infection prevention and control team.	All waste contaminated with blood, body fluids, excretions, secretions and infectious agents thought to pose a particular risk should be disposed of as hazardous infectious waste. Orange is the recognized colour for hazardous infectious waste that does not require incineration and may be made safe by alternative treatment (DH 2006a, C).
11 After removing the gloves, decontaminate your hands.	Hands may have become contaminated (Pratt *et al.* 2007, C).

Action Figure 3 Open the packet containing the gloves onto a clean surface and open out the inside packaging so that the fingers of the gloves point away from you.

Action Figure 4a Hold the cuff of the first glove with the opposite hand and slide the fingertips of the other hand (that the glove is to go on) into the opening.

Action Figure 4b Keep hold of the folded edge and pull the glove onto your hand.

Action Figure 4c Spread your fingers slightly to help them enter the fingers of the glove.

Action Figure 5a Slide the fingertips of your gloved hand beneath the folded cuff of the second glove.

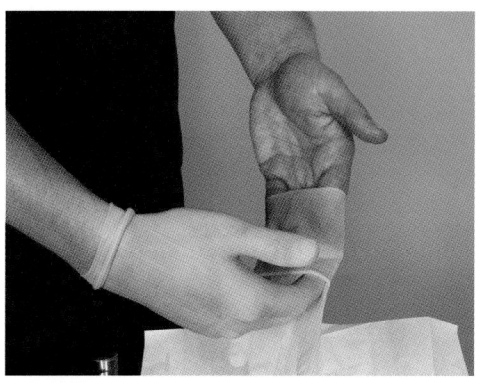

Action Figure 5b Slide the fingertips of your ungloved hand into the opening of the second glove.

Action Figure 6a Pull the glove onto your hand, again spreading your fingers slightly to help them enter the fingers of the glove.

Action Figure 6b When both gloves are on, adjust the fit.

Procedure guideline 3.8 Donning a sterile gown and gloves: closed technique

Note 1: These procedures will normally require participants to also wear a mask and eye protection.

Note 2: An assistant is required to open sterile gloves and tie the back of the gown.

Essential equipment

- Sterile disposable gloves
- Sterile disposable or reusable gown

Preprocedure

Action	Rationale
1 Prepare the area where gowning and gloving will take place. Open the gown pack with clean hands. Do not touch the inside of the package.	To ensure that there is adequate room to don gown and gloves and to avoid contaminating either. E

(Continued)

Procedure guideline 3.8 (*Continued*)

2 Wash your hands using a surgical scrub technique with either antiseptic hand wash solution or soap. Dry using a separate sterile paper towel for each hand and forearm. If hands have been washed with soap, apply an antiseptic handrub to the hands and forearms.	To both disinfect and physically remove matter and micro-organisms from the hands (WHO 2009, C).

Procedure

3 Open the inner layer of the gown pack, if present (see Action Figures 3a, 3b).	To allow the gown to be removed. E
4 Grasp the gown on its inside surface just below the neck opening (this should be uppermost if the gown pack has been opened correctly) and lift it up, holding it away from the body and any walls or furniture. The gown should fall open with the inside facing towards you (see Action Figure 4).	To open out the gown while keeping its outer surface sterile. E
5 Insert the free hand into the corresponding sleeve of the gown, pulling the gown towards you, until your fingers reach, but do not go beyond, the cuff of the sleeve (see Action Figure 5).	To pull on the gown while keeping its outer surface sterile. E
6 Release the inside surface of the gown and insert that hand into the corresponding sleeve, again until your fingers reach, but do not go beyond, the cuff of the sleeve. The assistant should help by pulling on the ties of the gown (see Action Figure 6.)	To pull on the gown while keeping its outer surface sterile. E
7 The assistant opens a pair of sterile gloves and presents the inner packaging for you to take. Place this on the sterile area of the open gown package so that the fingers of the gloves point towards you (see Action Figure 7).	To prepare the gloves for donning while keeping them and the gown sterile. E
8 Open the inner packaging of the gloves. The fingers should be towards you, the thumbs uppermost and the cuffs folded over. Keeping your hands within the sleeves of the gown, slide the thumb of your right hand (still inside the sleeve) between the folded-over cuff and the body of the right glove. Pick up that glove. Grasp the cuff of that glove on the opposite side with the other hand (still inside its sleeve) and unfold it, pulling it over the cuff of the sleeve and the hand inside. Then push your right hand through the cuff of the sleeve into the glove. Repeat the process with the left hand. Once both hands are inside their respective gloves, there is no risk of contaminating the outside of the gloves or gown with your bare hands (see Action Figures 8a, 8b, 8c, 8d, 8e, 8f, 8g).	To don the gloves while keeping their outer surface sterile and ensuring that there is no risk of contaminating the outside of the gown. E
9 If you need to change a glove because it is damaged or contaminated, pull the sleeve cuff down over your hand as you do so and don the replacement glove using the technique above.	To minimize the risk of contaminating the gown or the sterile field. E
10 Dispose of used gloves and disposable gowns as 'hazardous infectious waste', that is, into an orange waste bag, unless instructed otherwise by the infection prevention and control team.	All waste contaminated with blood, body fluids, excretions, secretions and infectious agents thought to pose a particular risk should be disposed of as hazardous infectious waste. Orange is the recognized colour for hazardous infectious waste that does not require incineration and may be made safe by alternative treatment (DH 2006a, C).

Postprocedure

11 At the end of the procedure, remove gown and gloves as a single unit by pulling the gown away from you so as to turn it and the gloves inside out (see Action Figures 11a, 11b).

12 Consign reusable gowns as infected linen according to local arrangements.

To minimize any risk to laundry workers from contaminated items (NHS Executive 1995, C).

13 After removing the gloves and gown, decontaminate your hands.

Hands may have become contaminated (Pratt *et al.* 2007, C).

Action Figure 3a   Open the gown pack with clean hands onto a clean surface. Do not touch the inner packet until after the surgical scrub.

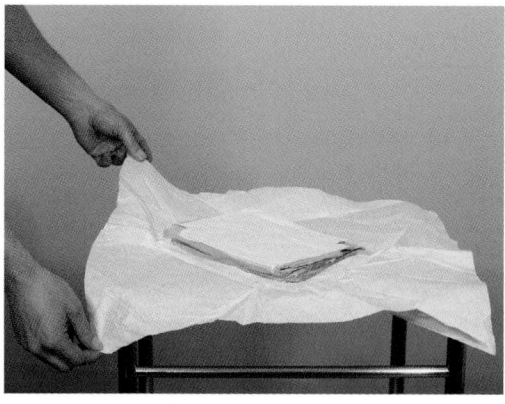

Action Figure 3b   Open the inner layer of the pack; use sterile towels to dry hands and forearms if required.

Action Figure 4   Lift up the gown by its inner surface and hold it away from the body.

Action Figure 5   Put one hand into the corresponding sleeve and use the other hand to pull the gown towards you. Your hand should not go beyond the cuff.

(Continued)

Procedure guideline 3.8 (*Continued*)

Action Figure 6   Put the other hand into the other sleeve. Again, your hand should not go beyond the cuff.

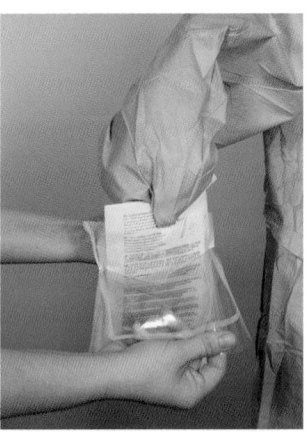

Action Figure 7   The assistant opens a pair of sterile gloves and presents the inner packaging for you to take.

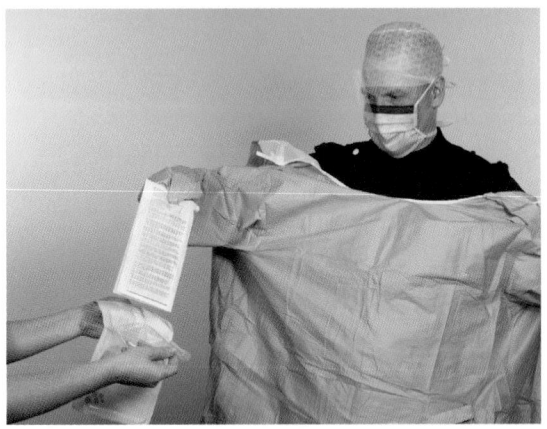

Action Figure 8a   Take the gloves, keeping your hands inside your sleeves.

Action Figure 8b   Open the inner glove packet on the sterile open gown package so that the glove fingers point towards you.

Action Figure 8c   Slide the thumb of one hand (still inside the sleeve) under the folded-over cuff of the corresponding glove.

Action Figure 8d Push your hand through the cuff and into the glove.

Action Figure 8e Pull the glove into position using the other hand (still inside its sleeve).

Action Figure 8f Repeat the process with the other glove.

Action Figure 8g Adjust the fit when both gloves are on.

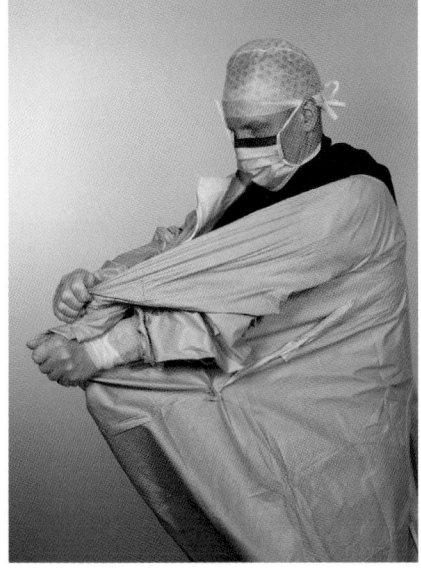

Action Figure 11a At the end of the procedure, remove gown and gloves as a single unit by pulling the gown away from you.

Action Figure 11b Turn it and the gloves inside out.

Aseptic technique

Evidence-based approaches
Rationale

Aseptic technique is the practice of carrying out a procedure in such a way that you minimize the risk of introducing contamination into a vulnerable area or contaminating an invasive device. Aseptic technique is required whenever you are carrying out a procedure that involves contact with a part of the body or an invasive device where introducing micro-organisms may increase the risk of infection. Note that the area or device on which you are working will not necessarily be sterile – wounds, for example, will be colonized with micro-organisms – but your aim must be to avoid introducing additional contamination.

Aseptic non-touch technique (ANTT®) is the practice of avoiding contamination by not touching key elements such as the tip of a needle, the seal of an intravenous connector after it has been decontaminated, or the inside surface of a sterile dressing where it will be in contact with the wound. An example of non-touch technique is illustrated in Figure 3.5. Gloves are normally worn for ANTT but they are mainly for the practitioner's, rather than the patient's, protection. Non-sterile gloves are therefore perfectly acceptable.

As with other infection prevention and control measures, the actions taken to reduce the risk of contamination will

Figure 3.5 Avoiding contamination by avoiding contact with the key elements. With permission from ICU Medical Europe S.R.L.

depend on the procedure being undertaken and the potential consequences of contamination. Examples of different aseptic techniques and the measures required for them are given in Table 3.5. It is therefore difficult to provide a procedure guideline that will apply to the whole range of aseptic procedures. To provide a context, the following procedure contains steps for changing a wound dressing but is presented as a guide to aseptic technique in general. Local guidance and training should be sought before carrying out specific procedures. Some specific procedures are described in other chapters of this manual.

Table 3.5 Examples of aseptic procedures

Procedure	Precautions required
Surgical joint replacement	Must be carried out in an operating theatre with specialist ventilation by a team who will wear sterile gowns and gloves, or even full body suits with individual exhaust systems to eliminate airborne contamination
Urinary catheterization	Can be carried out in an open ward by a practitioner wearing an apron and sterile gloves
Peripheral intravenous cannulation	Can be performed wearing non-sterile gloves and using an appropriate non-touch technique

Procedure guideline 3.9 Aseptic technique, for example, changing a wound dressing

Essential equipment (will vary depending on procedure)

- Sterile dressing pack containing gallipots or an indented plastic tray, low-linting swabs and/or medical foam, disposable forceps, gloves, sterile field, disposal bag. Please note that there may be different packs specifically for particular procedures, for example IV packs. Usage and availability of these will vary locally so reference is generally made to 'sterile dressing pack'
- Fluids for cleaning and/or irrigation. Normal saline is normally appropriate
- Hypo-allergenic tape (if required)
- Appropriate dressing (if required)
- Alcohol handrub (handwashing is an acceptable alternative but will take more time and may entail leaving the patient; alcohol handrub is most appropriate for hand hygiene during a procedure as long as hands are physically clean)
- Any other material as determined by the procedure being carried out
- Any extra equipment that may be needed during procedure, for example sterile scissors

- Traceability system for any reusable surgical instruments and patient record form
- Detergent wipe for cleaning trolley

Preprocedure

Action	Rationale
1 Check that all the equipment required for the procedure is available and, where applicable, is sterile (i.e. that packaging is undamaged, intact and dry; that sterility indicators are present on any sterilized items and have changed colour where applicable).	To ensure that only sterile products are used (MHRA 2010, C); to ensure that the patient is not disturbed unnecessarily if items are not available and to avoid unnecessary delays during the procedure. E
2 Explain and discuss the procedure with the patient.	To ensure that the patient understands the procedure and gives their valid consent (NMC 2008b, C).

Procedure

3 Clean hands with alcohol handrub or wash with soap and water and dry with paper towels.	Hands must be cleaned before and after every patient contact and before commencing the preparations for aseptic technique, to prevent cross-infection (Pratt *et al.* 2007, C).
4 Clean trolley with detergent and water or detergent wipes and dry with a paper towel. If disinfection is also required (e.g. by local policy), use disposable wipes saturated with 70% isopropyl alcohol and leave to dry.	To provide a clean working surface (Fraise and Bradley 2009, E); alcohol is an effective and fast-acting disinfectant that will dry quickly (Fraise and Bradley 2009, E).
5 Place all the equipment required for the procedure on the bottom shelf of the clean dressing trolley.	To maintain the top shelf as a clean working surface. E
6 Take the patient to the treatment room or screen the bed. Ensure that any fans in the area are turned off and windows closed. Position the patient comfortably and so that the area to be dealt with is easily accessible without exposing the patient unduly.	To allow any airborne organisms to settle before the sterile field (and in this case, the wound) is exposed. Maintain the patient's dignity and comfort. E
7 Put on a disposable plastic apron.	To reduce the risk of contaminating clothing or contaminating the wound or any sterile items from clothing. E
8 Take the trolley to the treatment room or patient's bedside, disturbing the curtains as little as possible.	To minimize airborne contamination. E
9 Loosen the adhesive or tape on the existing dressing.	To make it easier to remove the dressing. E
10 Clean hands with alcohol handrub.	Hands should be cleaned before any aseptic procedure (WHO 2009). Using alcohol handrub avoids having to leave the patient to go to a sink. E
11 Open the outer cover of the sterile pack and, once you have verified that the pack is the correct way up, slide the contents, without touching them, onto the top shelf of the trolley.	To minimize contamination of the contents. E
12 Open the sterile field using only the corners of the paper.	So that areas of potential contamination are kept to a minimum. E
13 Open any other packs, tipping their contents gently onto the centre of the sterile field.	To prepare the equipment and, in the case of a wound dressing, reduce the amount of time that the wound is uncovered. E
14 Where appropriate, loosen the old dressing.	To minimize trauma when removing the old dressing. E

(Continued)

Procedure guideline 3.9 *(Continued)*

15 Clean hands with alcohol handrub.	Hands may have become contaminated by handling outer packets or the old dressing (Pratt *et al.* 2007, C).
16 Carefully lift the plastic disposal bag from the sterile field by its open end and, holding it by one edge of the open end, place your other hand in the bag. Using it as a sterile 'glove', arrange the contents of the dressing pack and any other sterile items on the sterile field.	To maintain the sterility of the items required for the procedure while arranging them so as to perform the procedure quickly and efficiently. E
17 With your hand still enclosed within the disposal bag, remove the old dressing from the wound. Invert the bag so that the dressing is contained within it and stick it to the trolley below the top shelf. This is now the disposal bag for the remainder of the procedure for any waste other than sharps.	To minimize risk of contamination, by containing dressing in bag. E To ensure that any waste can be disposed of without contaminating the sterile field. E
18 Pour any solutions into gallipots or onto indented plastic tray.	To minimize risk of contamination of lotion. E
19 Put on gloves, as described in Procedure guideline 3.3 or 3.7. The procedure will dictate whether gloves should be sterile or non-sterile.	Gloves should be worn whenever any contact with body fluids is anticipated (Pratt *et al.* 2007). Sterile gloves provide greater sensitivity than forceps for procedures that cannot be carried out with a non-touch technique and are less likely to cause trauma to the patient. E
20 Carry out the relevant procedure according to the guidelines.	

Postprocedure

21 Make sure the patient is comfortable.	To minimize the risk of causing the patient distress or discomfort. E
22 Dispose of waste in orange plastic waste bags. Remove apron and gloves and discard into orange waste bag.	To prevent environmental contamination. Orange is the recognized colour for hazardous infectious waste (DH 2006a, C).
23 Draw back curtains or help the patient back to the bed area and ensure that they are comfortable.	To minimize the risk of causing the patient distress or discomfort. E
24 Check that the trolley remains dry and physically clean. If necessary, wash with liquid detergent and water or detergent wipe and dry thoroughly with a paper towel.	To remove any contamination on the trolley and so minimize the risk of transferring any contamination elsewhere in the ward (Pratt *et al.* 2007, C).
25 Clean hands with alcohol handrub or soap and water.	Hands should be cleaned after any contact with the patient or body fluids (WHO 2009, C).
26 Document the procedure clearly, including details of who carried it out, any devices or dressings used, particularly any left *in situ*, and any deviation from prescribed procedure. Fix any record labels from the outside packaging of any items used during the procedure on the patient record form and add this to the patient's notes.	Provides a record of the procedure and evidence that any items used have undergone an appropriate sterilization process (DH 2007b, C; NMC 2009, C).

Source isolation

Evidence-based approaches

Rationale

Source isolation is used for patients who are infected with, or are colonized by, infectious agents that require additional precautions over and above the standard precautions used with every patient in order to minimize the risk of transmission of that agent to other vulnerable persons, whether patients or staff. Common reasons for source isolation include infections that cause diarrhoea and vomiting, entailing the use of enteric precautions; infections that are spread through the air, entailing the use of airborne or droplet precautions; and infection or colonization with antibiotic-resistant bacteria, requiring contact precautions. Note that the patient's other nursing and medical needs must always be taken into account and infection control precautions may need to be modified accordingly.

Patients requiring source isolation are normally cared for in a single room, although outbreaks of infection may require affected patients to be nursed in a cohort, that is, isolated as a group. A single-occupancy room will physically separate patients who present a risk from others who may be at risk, and will act as a reminder to any staff dealing with that patient of the need for additional infection control precautions. Single-occupancy rooms used for source isolation should have en-suite toilet and bathroom facilities wherever possible, and contain all items required to meet the patient's nursing needs during the period of isolation (e.g. instruments to assess vital signs), which should remain inside the room throughout the period of isolation. If this is not possible because insufficient equipment is available on the ward, any items taken from the room must be thoroughly cleaned and disinfected (normally with a chlorine solution) before being used with any other patient.

The air pressure in the room should be negative or neutral in relation to the air pressure in the rest of the ward (note that some airborne infections will require a negative pressure room). A lobby will provide an additional degree of security and space for donning and removing personal protective equipment and performing hand hygiene. Some facilities have lobbies that are ventilated so as to have positive pressure with respect to both the rest of the ward and the single-occupancy room; this allows the room to be used for both source and protective isolation. Where insufficient single rooms are available for source isolation, they should be allocated to those patients who pose the greatest risk to others, using a tool such as the Lewisham Isolation Prioritization System (LIPS) to prioritize patients (Breathnach *et al.* 2010) (Figure 3.6). As a general rule, patients with enteric symptoms, that is diarrhoea and vomiting, or serious airborne infections, such as tuberculosis, will have the highest priority for single-occupancy rooms. If this situation arises, it will mean that additional precautions will be required for some patients on the open ward, for example gloves and aprons will still be required while caring for someone colonized with MRSA even if they are not isolated.

Principles of care

Attending to the patient in isolation

Meals

Meals should be served on normal crockery and the patient provided with normal cutlery. Cutlery and crockery should be washed in a dishwasher able to thermally disinfect items, that is, with a final rinse of 80°C for 1 minute or 71°C for 3 minutes. Disposable cutlery and crockery should only be used if specifically instructed by the infection prevention and control team. Disposables and uneaten food should be discarded in the appropriate bag.

Contaminated crockery is a potential vector for infectious agents, particularly those causing enteric disease, but thermal disinfection will minimize this risk (Fraise and Bradley 2009).

Urine and faeces

Wherever possible, a toilet should be kept solely for the patient's use. If this is not available, a commode should be left in the patient's room. Gloves must be worn by staff when dealing with body fluids. Bedpans and urinals should be bagged in the isolation room and taken directly to the sluice for disposal. They should not be emptied before being placed in the bedpan washer or macerator unless the contents volume needs to be measured for a fluid balance or stool chart. Gloves and apron worn in the room should be kept on until the body waste is disposed of and then removed (gloves first) and discarded as infected waste.

This will minimize the risk of infection being spread from excreta, for example via a toilet seat or a bedpan (Pratt *et al.* 2007) and the risk of hands or clothing being contaminated by body waste.

Spillages

As elsewhere, any spillage must be mopped up immediately, using the appropriate method for the fluid spilt, and the area dried. This removes the risk of anyone slipping and removes and disinfects any contaminated fluid that may carry a risk of infection.

Bathing

If an en-suite bathroom is not available, the patient must be bathed elsewhere on the ward. The patient does not need to use the bathroom last but the bathroom must be thoroughly cleaned after use so bathing them last will minimize any delays to other patients that this may cause. However, if the patient requires an early bath, for example because they are leaving the ward for an examination elsewhere, this must be catered for.

Thorough cleaning and disinfection of the bathroom will minimize the risk of cross-infection to other patients.

Step 1	Identify infection or condition
Step 2	Use score card to record: • ACDP hazard group • Mode of transmission • Evidence for transmission • Assess prevalence of infection in the hospital • Determine antibiotic resistance • Assess susceptibility of other patients • Assess dispersal characteristics of patient
Step 3	Add all scores and compare total to chart to determine priority for isolation

Score card *(Document score in patient's notes)*

Patient name	Date		Name and designation of person scoring
Significant details	e.g. micro-organism/s		

Criteria	Classification	Score	Comments
ACDP	2	5	
	3	10	
	4	40	
Route	Air-borne	15	
	Droplet	10	
	Contact/faeco-oral	5	
	Blood-borne	0	
Evidence of transmission	Strong (published)	10	
	Moderate (consensus)	5	
	Poor	0	
	Nil	-10	
Significant resistance	Yes	5	Such as MRSA, VRE, ESBL, Gent resistance
	No	0	
High susceptibility of other patients with serious consequences	Yes	10	Specific for various infections and patient populations
	No	0	
Prevalence in the hospital	Sporadic	0	
	Endemic	-5	This reflects the burden of infection in the hospital and cohort measures may be more applicable
	Epidemic	-5	See above
Dispersal	High risk	10	This includes diarrhoea, projectile vomiting, coughing, confused wandering infected patients, etc.
	Medium risk	5	
	Low risk	0	
TOTAL SCORE			

Using the score to determine the priority for isolation:

Score	Priority for isolation
0 - 20	Low
25 - 35	Medium
35+	High

INFECTION/CONDITION IDENTIFIED	ACDP category	Evidence for transmission in healthcare	Mode of transmission	Score and priority for isolation	Specific guidance
Adenovirus	2	Moderate	Contact / droplet / faeco-oral	20	Not usually problem in immune competent adults. **A problem in newborns, children and immunodeficient individuals**
Antibiotic resistant organisms including GRE, ESBL, acinetobacter and VRE (MRSA is below)	2	Strong	Contact	35	Dependant on site of body and where patient is sited in the hospital High risk is : External site, e.g. catheter Patient in intensive care or high dependency unit
Atypical mycobacteria	3	Weak	Air borne	(25)	**Rarely requires isolation**
Campylobacter	2	Poor	Faeco-oral	10	
Chickenpox (varicella)	2	Strong	Air borne	30-40	More infectious than shingles. Usually infectious for up to five days following first crop of vesicles - longer in immunodeficient individuals
CJD (TSE)	3	Nil	Blood / tissue	10	
Clostridium difficile	2	Strong	Faeco-oral/ possibly droplet	35-45	Isolate in the presence of diarrhoea and until there has been no diarrhoea for at least 48 hours
Cryptococcus	2	Nil	Nil	5	Problem in pregnant women and babies
Cytomegalovirus	2	Nil	Contact	10	
Diarrhoea with or without vomiting (assume potential gastroenteritis or C. difficile until negative specimen result and definitive alternative diagnosis available)	2	Strong	Faecal-oral	>45	Isolate until symptom-free for 48 hours or until negative specimen result and definitive alternative diagnosis available
Diphtheria/pharyngeal	2	Strong	Droplet	>35	
Hepatitis A & E	2	Poor	Faecal-oral	25	Isolate for 14 days after onset of jaundice
Hepatitis B & C	2	Poor	Blood	10	
Impetigo	2	Strong	Contact	20	May be a problem in children and immunodeficient
Influenza (clinical diagnosis)	2	Strong	Droplet	25-35	Immunodeficient individuals are particularly susceptible and should avoid contact with influenza cases. Cohort in outbreaks or pandemics
Legionnaires disease (legionellosis)	2	Nil	Air borne	20	
Lice	2	Strong- body lice Poor- head/ pubic lice	Contact	10-20	Head and pubic lice are less transmissible than body lice in hospital environment
Measles	2	Strong	Droplet	>35	
Meningitis undiagnosed (viral or bacterial)	2 or 3	Moderate	**Droplet** / faeco-oral	30-40	All meningitis cases should be isolated until cause is established. Meningococcal meningitis requires isolation until patient has received 48 hours of treatment
MRSA	2	Strong	Contact	>35	Risk assess for isolation: High risk includes: • Major dispersers, i.e. dry or flaky skin, expectorating infected sputum • Surgical especially in orthopaedic, cardiac or neurosurgery areas • Patients with multiple devices and interventions, e.g. ITU, NICU & SCBU • PVL, MRSA Medium risk includes: • Positive screening swab but otherwise well and not in areas identified above. These patients may be cohorted
Mumps	2	Moderate	Droplet	30-40	
Palliative care	N/a	N/a	N/a		Cannot be scored in the same way as infectious agents but must be taken into account when prioritising use of single rooms. Need to consider condition and all nursing needs vs risk to other patients if a potentially infected individual is not isolated
RSV	2	Strong	Droplet	25	**A problem in newborn, children and immunodeficiency**
Rotavirus	2	Strong	**Droplet/ faeco-oral**	25	**A problem in newborn, children and immunodeficiency**
Rubella	2	Moderate	Droplet		Susceptibility of non immune may be an issue. Medium risk paediatrics and women's health
Salmonella or Shigella	2	Strong	Faeco-oral	>30	Dependant on potential for dispersal
Scabies (confirmed)	2	Strong	Contact	20	Medium risk for patients who are incontinent or have diarrhoea
Scarlet fever	2	Moderate	Droplet	30	
Shingles (herpes zoster)	2	Moderate	Contact	30	No isolation needed if lesions are covered or dried Medium risk is : weeping lesions, non-immune women of child bearing age, babies and children and immunodeficient
Streptococcus pyogenes (Group A strep)	2	Strong	**Droplet / contact**	25	Remain isolated for 24 hours following treatment
TB-non-pulmonary	3	Nil	Contact	15	Dependant on site and stage of disease
TB-open pulmonary or exuding lesion	3	Strong	Contact / air-borne	35	Isolated for period of 10-14 days following commencement of treatment **MDRTB patients should remain in isolation throughout hospital stay** High risk: Patients who have a cough. MDRTB
Typhoid fever	3	Weak	Faeco-oral	25	Dependant on potential for dispersal
Verotoxin producing strains of Escherichia coli (e.g. E.coli O157)	3	Poor	Faeco-oral	25	Medium risk for patients who are incontinent or have diarrhoea
VHF- Lassa / Ebola / Marburg	4	Blood/contact/ droplet	**Droplet/ blood/ contact**	>70	Blood and body fluids are highly infectious — **transfer to regional Infectious diseases facility**
Wound oozing/infected	2	Blood/contact	**Contact**		

Figure 3.6 Lewisham Isolation Prioritization System (LIPS). Used with permission of Lewisham Healthcare NHS Trust. For more information and updates contact Lewisham Healthcare NHS Trust. ACDP, Advisory Committee on Dangerous Pathogens; CJD, Creutzfeldt-Jakob disease; ESBL, extended–spectrum beta lactamase producers; Gent, gentamicin; GRE, glycopeptide–resistant enterococci; ITU, intensive care unit; MDRTB, multi-drug resistant tuberculosis; MRSA, meticillin resistant Staphylococcus aureus; NICU, neonatal intensive care unit; PVL, Panton–Valentine leukocidin; RSV, respiratory syncytial virus; SCBU, special care baby unit; TB, tuberculosis; TSE, transmissible spongiform encephalopathy; VHF, viral haemorrhagic fever; VRE, vancomycin–resistant enterococci.

Linen

Place infected linen in a red water-soluble alginate polythene bag, which must be secured tightly before it leaves the room. Just outside the room, place this bag into a red linen bag which must be secured tightly and not used for other patients. These bags should await the laundry collection in the area designated for this.

Placing infected linen in a red alginate polythene bag confines the organisms and allows laundry staff to recognize the potential hazard and avoid handling the linen (NHSE 1995, C).

Waste

Orange waste bags should be kept in the isolation room for disposal of all waste generated in the room. The top of the bag should be sealed and labelled with the name of the ward or department before it is removed from the room.

Cleaning the isolation room

1 Domestic staff must be instructed on the correct procedure to use when cleaning an isolation room, including an explanation as to why isolation is essential to reduce the risk of cross-infection, the materials and solutions used, and the correct colour coding for these materials. This will reduce the risk of mistakes and ensure that appropriate precautions are maintained (DH 2001, R1b).

2 Isolation rooms must be cleaned last, to reduce the risk of the transmission of contamination to 'clean' areas (NPSA 2009, E).

3 Separate cleaning equipment must be used for isolation rooms. Cross-infection may result from shared cleaning equipment (Wilson 2006, E).

4 Cleaners must wear gloves and plastic aprons while cleaning isolation rooms to minimize the risk of contaminating hands or clothing. Some PPE may also be required for the safe use of some cleaning solutions.

5 Floor (hard surface: carpeted rooms should not be used as isolation rooms). This must be washed daily with a disinfectant as appropriate. All excess water must be removed. Daily cleaning will keep the bacterial count reduced. Organisms, especially Gram-negative bacteria, multiply quickly in the presence of moisture and on equipment (Wilson 2006, E).

6 Cleaning solutions must be freshly made up each day and the container emptied and cleaned daily. Disinfectants may lose activity over time; cleaning solutions can easily become contaminated (Dharan et al. 1999).

7 After use, the bucket must be cleaned and dried. Contaminated cleaning equipment and solutions will spread bacteria over surfaces being cleaned (Dharan et al. 1999).

8 Mop heads should be laundered in a hot wash daily as they become contaminated easily (Wilson 2006, E).

9 Furniture and fittings should be damp-dusted daily using a disposable cloth and a detergent or disinfectant solution by nursing or cleaning staff as dictated by local protocol, in order to remove dirt and a proportion of any organisms contaminating the environment (Wilson 2006, E).

10 The toilet, shower and bathroom area must be cleaned at least once a day and if they become contaminated, using a non-abrasive hypochlorite powder, cream or solution. Non-abrasive powders or creams preserve the integrity of the surfaces. E

Cleaning the room after a patient has been discharged

1 The room should be stripped. All bedlinen and other textiles must be changed and curtains changed (reusable curtains must be laundered and disposable curtains discarded as infectious waste). Dispose of any unused disposable items. Curtains and other fabrics readily become colonized with bacteria (Patel 2005, E); paper packets cannot be easily cleaned. E

2 Impervious surfaces, for example locker, bedframe, mattress cover, chairs, floor, blinds, soap dispenser, should be washed with soap and water, or a combined detergent/chlorine disinfectant if sporicidal activity is required, and dried. Relatively inaccessible places, for example ceilings, may be omitted. Wiping of surfaces is the most effective way of removing contaminants; spores from, for example, Clostridium difficile will persist indefinitely in the environment unless destroyed by an effective disinfectant; bacteria will thrive more readily in damp conditions; inaccessible areas are not generally relevant to any infection risk (Wilson 2006, E).

3 The room can be reused as soon as it has been thoroughly cleaned and restocked. Effective cleaning will have removed infectious agents that may pose a risk to the next patient.

Discharging the patient from isolation

If the patient no longer requires isolation but is still to be a patient on the ward, inform them of this and the reasons why isolation is no longer required before moving them out of the room. Also inform them if there is any reason why they may need to be returned to isolation, for example if enteric symptoms return.

If the patient is to be discharged home or to another health or social care setting, ensure that the discharge documentation includes details of their condition, the infection control precautions taken while in hospital and any precautions or other actions that will need to be taken following discharge. Suitable accurate information on infections must be supplied to any person concerned with providing further support or nursing/medical care in a timely fashion (DH 2010a).

Procedure guideline 3.10 Source isolation: preparing an isolation room

Essential equipment

- Single-occupancy room
- Patient equipment
- Personal protective equipment
- Hand hygiene facilities
- Patient information material

Preprocedure

Action	Rationale
1 Identify the most suitable room available for source isolation, taking into account the risk to other patients and staff and the patient's other nursing needs.	To ensure the best balance between minimizing the risk of cross-infection and maintaining the safety and comfort of the isolated patient. E

Procedure

Action	Rationale
2 Remove all non-essential furniture and equipment from the room. The remaining furniture should be easy to clean. Ensure that the room is stocked with any equipment required for patient care and sufficient but not excessive numbers of any disposable items that will be required.	To ensure the availability of everything required for patient care while minimizing the number of items that will require cleaning or disposal at the end of the isolation period and the amount of traffic of people and equipment into and out of the room. E
3 Ensure that a bin for clinical waste with an orange bag is present in the room. This will be used for all waste generated in the room. The bag must be sealed before it is removed from the room.	For containing contaminated rubbish within the room and minimizing further spread of infection. E
4 Place a container for sharps in the room.	To contain contaminated sharps within the infected area (DH 2006a, C).
5 Keep the patient's personal property to a minimum. All belongings taken into the room should be washable, cleanable or disposable. Contact the infection prevention and control team for advice as to how best to clean or wash specific items.	The patient's belongings may become contaminated and cannot be taken home unless they are washable or cleanable. E
6 Ensure that all PPE required is available outside the room. Wall-mounted dispensers offer the best use of space and ease of use but if necessary, set up a trolley outside the door for PPE and alcohol handrub. Ensure that this does not cause an obstruction or other hazard.	To have PPE readily available when required. E
7 Explain the reason for isolation and the precise precautions required to the patient, their family and other visitors, providing relevant patient information material where available. Allow the patient to ask questions and ask for a member of the infection prevention and control team to visit the patient if ward staff cannot answer all questions to the patient's satisfaction.	Compliance is more likely if patients and their visitors understand the reasons for isolation; the patient's anxiety will be reduced if they have as much information as possible about their condition. E
8 Fix a suitable notice outside the room where it will be seen by anyone attempting to enter the room. This should indicate the special precautions required while preserving the patient's confidentiality.	To ensure all staff and visitors are aware of the need for additional infection control precautions. E
9 Move the patient into the single-occupancy room.	
10 Arrange for terminal cleaning of the bed space that the patient has been occupying.	To remove any infectious agents that may pose a risk to the next patient to occupy that bed (NPSA 2009, C).

Postprocedure

11 Assess the patient daily to determine if source isolation is still required; for example, if enteric precautions have been required, has the patient been without symptoms for 48 hours?	There is often limited availability of isolation rooms (Wigglesworth and Wilcox 2006, R) so they must be used as effectively as possible. E

Procedure guideline 3.11 Source isolation: entering the isolation room

Essential equipment

- Personal protective equipment as dictated by the precautions required. Gloves and apron are the usual minimum; a respirator will be required for droplet precautions; eye protection if an aerosol-generating procedure is planned
- Any equipment required for any procedure you intend to carry out in the room

Preprocedure

Action	Rationale
1 Collect all equipment needed.	To avoid entering and leaving the infected area unnecessarily. E

Procedure

Action	Rationale
2 Ensure you are 'bare below the elbow' (see Procedure guideline 3.1).	To facilitate hand hygiene and avoid any contamination of long sleeves or cuffs that could be transferred to other patients. E
3 Put on a disposable plastic apron.	To protect the front of the uniform or clothing, which is the most likely area to come in contact with the patient. E
4 Put on a disposable well-fitting mask or respirator of the appropriate standard if droplet or airborne precautions are required, for example: (a) Meningococcal meningitis before completion of 24 hours of treatment (b) Pandemic influenza (c) Tuberculosis, if carrying out aerosol-generating procedure or the TB may be multiresistant.	To reduce the risk of inhaling organisms (DH 2010b, NICE 2006, C).
5 Don eye protection if instructed by infection prevention and control team (e.g. for pandemic influenza) or if conducting an aerosol-generating procedure (e.g. bronchoscopy or intubation) in a patient requiring airborne/droplet precautions.	To prevent infection via the conjunctiva (DH 2010b, C).
6 Clean hands with soap and water or alcohol handrub.	Hands must be cleaned before patient contact (WHO 2009, C).
7 Don disposable gloves if you are intending to deal with blood, excreta or contaminated material, or if providing close personal care where contact precautions are required.	To reduce the risk of hand contamination (Pratt et al. 2007, C).
8 Enter the room, shutting the door behind you.	To reduce the risk of airborne organisms leaving the room (Kao and Yang 2006, R1a) and to preserve the patient's privacy and dignity.

Procedure guideline 3.12 Source isolation: leaving the isolation room

Essential equipment

- Orange waste bag
- Hand hygiene facilities

Action	Rationale
Procedure	
1 If wearing gloves, remove and discard them in the orange waste bag.	To avoid transferring any contamination on the gloves to other areas or items (Pratt *et al.* 2007, C).
2 Remove apron by holding the inside of the apron and breaking the ties at neck and waste. Discard it into the orange waste bag.	To avoid transferring any contamination on the apron to other areas or items (Pratt *et al.* 2007, C).
3 Clean hands with soap and water or alcohol handrub. Do not use alcohol handrub when patients require enteric precautions: wash with soap and water.	Hands must be cleaned after contact with the patient or their immediate environment (WHO 2009); alcohol is less effective against *Clostridium difficile* spores and some enteric viruses and in the presence of organic material such as faeces (Fraise and Bradley 2009, E).
4 Leave the room, shutting the door behind you.	To reduce the risk of airborne spread of infection (Kao and Yang 2006, R1a).
5 Clean hands with soap and water or alcohol handrub. If the patient requires enteric precautions, hands should be cleaned with soap and water.	Hands must be cleaned after contact with the patient or their immediate environment (WHO 2009, C). Alcohol is not effective on all organisms that cause enteric infections (Fraise and Bradley 2009, E).

Procedure guideline 3.13 Source isolation: transporting infected patients outside the source isolation area

Action	Rationale
Procedure	
1 Inform the department concerned about the procedure required, the patient's diagnosis and the infection control precautions required at the earliest opportunity.	To allow the department time to make appropriate arrangements. E
2 If possible and appropriate, arrange for the patient to have the last appointment of the day.	The department concerned and any intervening areas will be less busy, so reducing the risk of contact with other vulnerable individuals, and additional cleaning required following any procedure will not disrupt subsequent appointments. E
3 Inform the portering service of the patient's diagnosis and the infection control precautions required; ensure that this information has been passed to any porters involved in transfer and reinforce the precautions required.	Explanation and reinforcement will minimize the risk of cross-infection through failure to comply with infection control precautions (Fraise and Bradley 2009, E).
4 Escort the patient if necessary.	To attend to the patient's nursing needs and to remind others of infection control precautions if required. E

5	If the patient has an infection requiring droplet or airborne precautions that may present a risk to people encountered in the other department or in transit, they will need to wear a mask or respirator of the appropriate standard. Provide the patient with the mask and explain why it is required and how and when it is to be worn (i.e. while outside their single-occupancy room) and assist them to don it if necessary.	To prevent airborne cross-infection. E Providing the patient with relevant information will reduce anxiety.

Protective isolation

Evidence-based approaches
Rationale

Protective isolation is used to minimize the exposure to infectious agents of patients who are particularly at risk of infection. Although the evidence that protective isolation successfully reduces the incidence of infection is limited (Wigglesworth 2003), probably because many infections are endogenous (i.e. caused by the patient's own bacterial flora), it is used to reduce the risk of exogenous infection (cross-infection from other people or the environment) in groups who have greatly impaired immune systems (Fraise and Bradley 2009), such as autologous and allogenic bone marrow transplant patients. Patients who have compromised immune systems often have greatly reduced numbers of a type of white blood cell called a neutrophil; this condition is known as neutropenia and those people suffering from it are described as neutropenic. Neutropenia is graded from mild to severe according to how few neutrophils are in the circulation and hence how much the risk of infection is raised.

Single-occupancy rooms used for protective isolation should have neutral or positive air pressure with respect to the surrounding area. High-efficiency particulate air (HEPA) filtration of the air in the room may reduce exposure to airborne pathogens, particularly fungal spores. A room with positive pressure ventilation must not be used for any patient infected or colonized with an organism that may be spread through an airborne route; in this circumstance if an immunocompromised patient has such an organism, they should be nursed in a room with neutral air pressure or with a positive pressure lobby.

Principles of care
Diet for the immunocompromised patient

- Educate the patient in the importance of good food hygiene in reducing their exposure to potential pathogens; they should choose only cooked food from the hospital menu and avoid raw fruit, salads and uncooked vegetables. Stress the importance of good hand hygiene before eating or drinking. Uncooked foods are often heavily colonized by micro-organisms, particularly Gram-negative bacteria (Moody et al. 2006); potential pathogens on the hands may be inadvertently consumed while eating or drinking.
- Educate the patient's family in the importance of good food hygiene, particularly good hand hygiene, and advise that any food brought in for the patient should be in undamaged, sealed tins and packets obtained from well-known, reliable firms and within the expiry date. Correctly processed and packaged foods are more likely to be of an acceptable food hygiene standard.
- Provide the patient with filtered water or sealed cartons of fruit juice (not fresh) to drink (Vonberg et al. 2005). Do not supply bottled water. Tap water may occasionally be contaminated with potential pathogens; long-life fruit juice has been pasteurized to remove micro-organisms; bottled water very often contains more micro-organisms than tap water.

Discharging the neutropenic patient

- Crowded areas, for example shops, cinemas, pubs and discos, should be avoided. Although the patient's white cell count is usually high enough for discharge, the patient remains immunocompromised for some time (Calandra 2000, E).
- Pets should not be allowed to lick the patient, and new pets should not be obtained. Pets are known carriers of infection (Lefebvre et al. 2006).
- Certain foods, for example take-away meals, soft cheese and pâté, should continue to be avoided. These foodstuffs are more likely to be contaminated with potential pathogens (Gillespie et al. 2005).
- Salads and fruit should be washed carefully, dried and, if possible, peeled, to remove as many pathogens as possible (Moody et al. 2006).
- Any signs or symptoms of infection should be reported immediately to the patient's general practitioner or to the discharging hospital. Any infection may have serious consequences if left untreated.

Procedure guideline 3.14 Protective isolation: preparing the room

Essential equipment

- Single-occupancy room
- Patient equipment
- Personal protective equipment
- Hand hygiene facilities inside and outside the room
- Patient information material detailing the other infection prevention precautions required
- Cleaning materials for the room

Preprocedure

Action	Rationale
1 Identify the most suitable room available for protective isolation, taking into account the risk to the patient, the patient's other nursing needs and other demands on the available single rooms.	To ensure the best balance between minimizing the risk of infection, maintaining the safety and comfort of the isolated patient and the availability of single rooms for other purposes. E

Procedure

2 Remove all non-essential furniture and equipment from the room. The remaining furniture should be easy to clean. Ensure that the room is stocked with any equipment required for patient care and sufficient numbers of any disposable items that will be required.	To ensure the availability of everything required for patient care while minimizing the amount of cleaning required and the amount of traffic of people and equipment into and out of the room. E
3 Ensure that all PPE required is available outside the room. Wall-mounted dispensers offer the best use of space and ease of use but if necessary, set up a trolley outside the door for PPE and alcohol handrub. Ensure that this does not cause an obstruction or other hazard.	To have PPE readily available when required. E
4 Ensure that the room is thoroughly cleaned before the patient is admitted.	Effective cleaning will remove infectious agents that may pose a risk to the patient (NPSA 2009, C).
5 Explain the reason for isolation and the precise precautions required to the patient, their family and other visitors, providing relevant patient information material where available. Allow the patient to ask questions and ask for a member of the infection prevention and control team to visit the patient if ward staff cannot answer all questions to the patient's satisfaction.	Compliance is more likely if patients and their visitors understand the reasons for isolation; the patient's anxiety will be reduced if they have as much information as possible about their condition. E
6 Fix a suitable notice outside the room where it will be seen by anyone attempting to enter the room. This should indicate the special precautions required while preserving the patient's confidentiality.	To ensure all staff and visitors are aware of the need for additional infection control precautions. E
7 Move the patient into the single-occupancy room.	
8 Ensure that surfaces and furniture are damp-dusted daily using disposable cleaning cloths and detergent solution, and the floor is mopped daily using soap and water.	Damp-dusting and mopping remove micro-organisms without distributing them into the air. E

Procedure guideline 3.15 Protective isolation: entering the isolation room

Essential equipment

- Hand hygiene facilities
- Disposable plastic apron
- Additional equipment, including PPE, for any procedure to be undertaken

Preprocedure

Action	Rationale
1 Collect all equipment needed.	To avoid entering and leaving the room unnecessarily.

Procedure

Action	Rationale
2 Ensure you are 'bare below the elbow' (see Procedure guideline 3.1).	To facilitate hand hygiene and to avoid transferring any contamination to the patient from long sleeves or cuffs. E
3 Put on a disposable plastic apron.	To provide a barrier between the front of the uniform or clothing, which is the most likely area to come in contact with the patient. E
4 Clean hands with soap and water or alcohol handrub.	To remove any contamination from the hands which could be transferred to the patient (WHO 2009, C).
5 Close the room door after entering.	To reduce the risk of airborne transmission of infection from other areas of the ward and ensure that air conditioning and filtration work as efficiently as possible. E

Visitors

Action	Rationale
1 Ask the patient to nominate close relatives and friends who may then, after instruction (see steps 1–5, above), visit freely. The patient or their representative should ask other acquaintances and non-essential visitors to avoid visiting during the period of vulnerability.	The incidence of infection increases in proportion to the number of people visiting but unlimited visiting by close relatives and friends diminishes the sense of isolation that the patient may experience; large numbers of visitors are difficult to screen and educate. E
2 Exclude any visitor who has had symptoms of infection or been in contact with a communicable disease in the previous 48 hours.	Individuals may be infectious both before and after developing symptoms of infection (Chadwick *et al.* 2000, C).
3 Educate all visitors to decontaminate their hands before entering the isolation room.	Hands carry large numbers of potentially pathogenic microorganisms that can be easily removed (WHO 2009, C).
4 Visiting by children, other than very close relatives, should be discouraged.	Children are more likely to have been in contact with infectious diseases but are less likely to be aware of this, and are more likely to develop infections because they have less acquired immunity. E

Prevention and management of inoculation injury

Related theory

Healthcare workers are at risk of acquiring bloodborne infections such as human immunodeficiency virus (HIV), the virus that causes acquired immune deficiency syndrome (AIDS), hepatitis B and hepatitis C. While the risk is small, five episodes of occupationally acquired HIV infection had nonetheless been documented in the UK up to 2002 (Health Protection Agency 2005). In 2006–7, 914 incidents of occupational exposure to bloodborne viruses were reported, of which between one-fifth and one-third could have been prevented through proper adherence to universal precautions and the safe disposal of hazardous waste (Health Protection Agency 2008). An understanding of the risk of infection and the preventive measures to be taken is essential in promoting a safer work environment (UK Health Departments 1998).

Bloodborne viruses are present in both the blood and other high-risk fluids that should be handled with the same precautions as blood. High-risk fluids include:

- cerebrospinal fluid
- peritoneal fluid
- pleural fluid
- pericardial fluid
- synovial fluid
- amniotic fluid
- semen
- vaginal secretions
- breast milk
- any other body fluid or unfixed tissue or organ containing visible blood (including saliva in dentistry).

Body fluids that do not need to be regarded as high risk, unless they are bloodstained, are:

- urine
- faeces
- saliva
- sweat
- vomit.

The most likely route of infection for healthcare workers is through the percutaneous inoculation of infected blood via a sharps injury (often called a needlestick injury) or by blood or other high-risk fluid splashing onto broken skin or a mucous membrane in the mouth, nose or eyes. These incidents are collectively known as inoculation injuries. Blood or another high-risk fluid coming into contact with intact skin is not regarded as an inoculation injury. It carries little or no risk due to the impervious nature of intact skin.

Evidence-based approaches

If the guidance in Box 3.2 is followed, it has been shown to reduce the risk of sharps injuries.

Complications

In the event of an inoculation injury occurring, prompt and appropriate action will reduce the risk of subsequent infection. These actions are described in Box 3.3 and should be taken regardless of what is thought to be known about the status of the patient whose blood has been inoculated. HIV, for example, has a 3-month 'window' following infection during which the patient has sufficient virus in their blood to be infectious but before their immune system is producing sufficient antibodies to be detected by the normal tests for HIV status.

Box 3.2 Actions to reduce the risk of inoculation injury

- Do not re-sheath used needles.
- Ensure that you are familiar with the local protocols for the use and disposal of sharps (e.g. location of sharps bins) and any other equipment before undertaking any procedure involving the use of a sharp item.
- Do not bend or break needles or disassemble them after use: discard needles and syringes into a sharps bin immediately after use.
- Handle sharps as little as possible.
- Do not pass sharps directly from hand to hand; use a receiver or similar receptacle.
- Discard all used sharps into a sharps container at the point of use: take a sharps container with you to the point of use if necessary. Do not dispose of sharps into anything other than a designated sharps container.
- Do not fill sharps bins above the mark that indicates that it is full.
- Sharps bins that are not full or in current (i.e. immediate) use should be kept out of reach of children and with any temporary closure in place.
- Sharps bins in use should be positioned at a height that enables safe disposal by all members of staff and secured to avoid spillage.
- Wear gloves in any situation where contact with blood is anticipated.
- Avoid wearing open footwear in any situation where blood may be spilt or where sharps are used.
- Always cover any cuts or abrasions, particularly on the hands, with a waterproof dressing while at work. Wear gloves if hands are particularly affected.
- Wear facial protection consisting of a mask and goggles or a face shield in any situation that may lead to a splash of blood or other high-risk fluid to the face. Do not rely on prescription glasses – they may not provide sufficient protection.
- Clear up any blood spillage promptly and disinfect the area. Use any materials or spillage management packs specifically provided for this purpose in accordance with the manufacturer's instructions.

(UK Health Departments 1998)

Management of waste in the healthcare environment

Definition

Waste is defined as 'any substance or object the holder discards, intends to discard or is required to discard' (European Parliament 2008).

Evidence-based approaches
Rationale

Waste material produced in the healthcare environment may carry a risk of infection to people who are not directly

---

Box 3.3 Actions to take in the event of inoculation injury

- Encourage any wound to bleed to wash out any foreign material that has been introduced. Do not squeeze the wound, as this may force any virus present into the tissues.
- Wash any wound with soap and water. Wash out splashes to mucous membranes (eyes or mouth) with large amounts of clean water.
- Cover any wound with a waterproof dressing to prevent entry of any other foreign material.
- Ensure the patient is safe then report the injury as quickly as possible to your immediate line manager and occupational health department. This is because postexposure prophylaxis (PEP), which is medication given after any incident thought to carry a high risk of HIV transmission, is more effective the sooner after the incident it is commenced (DH 2008).
- Follow any instructions given by the occupational health department.
- Co-operate with any action to test yourself or the patient for infection with a bloodborne virus but do not obtain blood or consent for testing from the patient yourself; this should be done by someone not involved in the incident.
- Complete a report of the incident according to local protocols.

(UK Health Departments 1998)

---

involved in providing healthcare but who are involved in the transport or disposal of that waste. All waste disposal is subject to regulation and hazardous waste is subject to further controls, depending on the nature of the hazard (DH 2006a). To ensure that everyone involved in waste management is aware of, and protected from, any hazard presented by the waste with which they are dealing, and that the waste is disposed of appropriately, a colour coding system is used. The colours in general use are shown in Table 3.6.

Waste receptacles are plastic bags or rigid plastic containers of the appropriate colour (see Table 3.7).

Legal and professional issues

The producer of hazardous waste is legally responsible for that waste, and remains responsible for it until its final disposal by incineration, alternative treatment or landfill (DH 2006a). In order to track waste to its point of origin, for example if it is necessary to identify where waste has been disposed of into the wrong waste stream, healthcare organizations should have a system of identifying waste according to the ward or department where it is produced. This may be through the use of labelling or dedicated waste carts for particular areas. When assembling sharps bins, always complete the label on the outside of the bin, including the date and the initials of the assembler. When sharps bins are closed and disposed of, they should be dated and initialled at each stage.

Table 3.6 Waste colours code

Colour	Description
	Waste which requires disposal by incineration Indicative treatment/disposal required is incineration in a suitably permitted or licensed facility.
	Waste which may be "treated" Indicative treatment/disposal required is to be "rendered safe" in a suitably permitted or licensed facility, **usually alternative treatment plants (ATPs). However this waste may also be disposed of by incineration.**
	Cytotoxic and cytostatic waste Indicative treatment/disposal required is **incineration** in a suitably permitted or licensed facility.
	Offensive/hygiene waste* Indicative treatment/disposal required is **landfill** in a suitably permitted or licensed site. This waste should not be compacted in unlicensed/permitted facilities.
	Domestic (municipal) waste Minimum treatment/disposal required is **landfill** in a suitably permitted or licensed site. Recyclable components should be removed through segregation. Clear/opaque receptacles may also be used for domestic waste.
White	**Amalgam waste** For **recovery**

*The use of yellow/black for offensive/hygiene waste was chosen as these colours have historically been universally used for the sanitary/offensive/hygiene waste stream.
From DH (2006a). © Crown copyright. Reproduced under the terms of the Click-use Licence.

Table 3.7 Waste containers

Waste receptacle	Waste types	Example contents	Indicative treatment/disposal
"Over-stickers" with the radioactive waste symbol may be used on yellow packaging.	Healthcare waste contaminated with radioactive material	Dressings, tubing etc. from treatment involving low level radioactive isotopes	Appropriately licensed incineration facility
	Infectious waste contaminated with cytotoxic and/or cytostatic medicinal products	Dressings/tubing from cytotoxic and/or cytostatic treatment	Incineration
SHARPS	Sharps contaminated with cytotoxic and cytostatic medicinal products[1]	Sharps used to administer cyto-toxic products	Incineration
	Infectious and other waste requiring incineration including anatomical waste, diagnostic specimens, reagent or test vials, and kits containing chemicals	Anatomical waste from theatres	Incineration
SHARPS	Partially discharged sharps not contaminated with cytoproducts[1]	Syringe body with residue medicinal product	Incineration
Solid / Liquid	Medicines in original packaging	Waste in original packaging with original closures	Incineration
Solid / Liquid	Medicines NOT in original packaging	Waste tablets not in foil pack or bottle	Hazardous waste incineration
	Infectious waste, potentially infectious waste and autoclaved laboratory waste	Soiled dressings	Licensed/permitted treatment facility
SHARPS	(i) Sharps not contaminated with medicinal products[2] Or (ii) Fully discharged sharps contaminated with medicinal products other than cytotoxic and cytostatic medicines	Sharps from phlebotomy	Suitably authorized incineration or alternative treatment facility[1]
	Offensive/hygiene waste	Human hygiene waste and non-infectious disposable equipment, bedding and plaster casts	Deep landfill

(Continued)

Table 3.7 (*Continued*)

Waste receptacle	Waste types	Example contents	Indicative treatment/disposal
Black bag or clear bag is acceptable.	Domestic waste	General refuse,[3] including confectionery products, flowers, etc.	Landfill
WHITE CONTAINER	Amalgam waste	Dental amalgam waste	Recovery

(From DH (2006a). © Crown copyright. Reproduced under the terms of the Click-use Licence.

[1]The authorisation type and content for alternative treatments in Northern Ireland Scotland England and Wales may differ. Not all facilities are authorised to process all types of waste. **Important: It is not acceptable practice to intentionally discharge syringes, etc., containing residual medicines in order to dispose of them in the fully discharged sharps receptacle. Partially discharged syringes contaminated with residual medicines should be disposed of in the yellow- or purple-lidded sharps receptacle shown above.**

[2]The requirements for packaging are significantly affected by the presence of medicinal waste and the quantity of liquid present in the container.

[3]General refuse is that waste remaining once recyclates (that is, paper, cardboard) have been removed.

Management of soiled linen in the healthcare environment

As with waste, soiled linen must be managed so as to minimize any risk to any person coming into contact with it. This is done by clearly identifying any soiled linen that may present a risk through the use of colour coding and limiting any contact with such linen through the use of water-soluble bags to contain the linen so that laundry staff do not have to handle it before it goes into the washer (NHS Executive 1995).

Linen that may present a risk may be described as foul, infected or infested. The management of all hazardous linen is similar, so the following procedure applies to any linen that is wet with blood or another high-risk body fluids (see Prevention and management of inoculation injury) or faeces, or has come from a patient in source isolation for any reason, that is where enteric, contact or droplet/airborne precautions are in place, or from a patient who is infested with lice, fleas, scabies or any other ectoparasite. Note that this procedure can be much more easily carried out by two people working together.

Procedure guideline 3.16 Safe disposal of foul, infected or infested linen

Essential equipment

- Disposable gloves and apron
- Water-soluble laundry bag
- Red plastic or linen laundry bag in holder
- Orange waste bin

Preprocedure

Action	Rationale
1 Assemble all the required equipment.	To avoid having to fetch anything else during the procedure and risk spreading contamination to other areas. E
2 Put on disposable gloves and apron.	To minimize contamination of your hands or clothing from the soiled linen. E
3 Separate the edges of the open end of the water-soluble laundry bag.	To make it easier to put the soiled linen in the bag. E

(Continued)

Procedure guideline 3.16 (Continued)

Procedure

4 Gather up the foul, infected or infested linen in such a way that any gross contamination (e.g. blood, faeces) is contained within the linen.	To minimize any contamination of the surrounding area. E
5 If there are two people, one holds the water-soluble laundry bag open while the other puts the soiled linen into it. If one person, hold one edge of the open end of the water-soluble bag in one hand and place the soiled linen in the bag with the other. In either case, take care not to contaminate the outside of the bag.	So as to remove the need for laundry workers to handle foul, infected or infested linen before it is washed (NHS Executive 1995, C).
6 Tie the water-soluble bag closed using the tie provided or by knotting together the edges of the open end.	To keep the soiled laundry inside the bag. E
7 Place the full water-soluble bag of soiled linen into the red outer laundry bag. Do not touch this bag.	To identify the linen as requiring special treatment. E
8 Remove gloves and apron and dispose of them into an orange waste bag.	To avoid transferring contamination to other areas (DH 2006a, C).
9 Wash hands and forearms with soap and water.	To avoid transferring contamination to other areas (WHO 2009, C).
10 Close the red outer laundry bag and transfer it to the designated collection area.	To ensure it does not cause an obstruction and is transferred to the laundry at the earliest opportunity. E

References

Breathnach, A., Zinna, S., Riley, P. and Planche, T. (2010) Guidelines for prioritisation of single-room use: a pragmatic approach. *Journal of Hospital Infection*, 74 (1), 89–91.

Calandra, T. (2000) Practical guide to host defence mechanisms and the predominant infections encountered in immunocompromised patients, in *Management of Infections in Immunocompromised Patients, Part I, Chapter 1* (eds M.P. Glauser and P.A. Pizzo). W.B. Saunders, London, pp.3–16.

Chadwick, P.R., Beards, G., Brown, B. *et al.* (2000) Management of hospital outbreaks due to small round structured viruses. *Journal of Hospital Infection*, 45 (1), 1–10. www.hpa.org.uk/web/HPAwebFile/HPAweb_C/1194947408355.

Damani, N.N. (2003) Principles of infection control, in *Manual of Infection Control Procedures*, 2nd edn. Cambridge University Press, Cambridge.

Department of Trade and Industry (2002) *Product Standards: Personal Protective Equipment: Guidance Notes on the UK Personal Protective Equipment Regulations 2002 (S.I. 2002 No. 1144)*. Department of Trade and Industry, London. www.bis.gov.uk/files/file11263.pdf.

DH (2001) Standard principles for preventing hospital-acquired infection. *Journal of Hospital Infection*, 47 (Supplement), S21–S37.

DH (2006a) *Health Technical Memorandum 07-01: Safe Management of Healthcare Waste*. Department of Health, London. www.dh.gov.uk/prod_consum_dh/groups/dh_digitalassets/documents/digitalasset/dh_073328.pdf.

DH (2006b) *Health Technical Memorandum 64: Sanitary Assemblies*. Stationery Office, London.

DH (2007a) *Saving Lives: Reducing Infection, Delivering Clean and Safe Care*. Stationary Office, London. www.dh.gov.uk/en/Publicationsandstatistics/Publications/PublicationsPolicyAndGuidance/DH_078134.

DH (2007b) *Health Technical Memorandum 01-01: Decontamination of Reusable Medical Devices, Part A – Management and Environment (English edition)*. Department of Health, London.

DH (2008) *HIV Post-Exposure Prophylaxis: Guidance from the UK Chief Medical Officers' Expert Advisory Group on AIDS*. Department of Health, London. www.dh.gov.uk/prod_consum_dh/groups/dh_digitalassets/@dh/@en/documents/digitalasset/dh_089997.pdf.

DH (2010a) *The Health and Social Care Act 2008: Code of Practice for Health and Adult Social Care on the Prevention and Control of Infections and Related Guidance*. Department of Health, London. www.dh.gov.uk/prod_consum_dh/groups/dh_digitalassets/documents/digitalasset/dh_110435.pdf.

DH (2010b) *Pandemic (H1N1) 2009 Influenza: A Summary of Guidance for Infection Control in Healthcare Settings*. Department of Health, London. www.dh.gov.uk/prod_consum_dh/groups/dh_digitalassets/@dh/@en/@ps/documents/digitalasset/dh_110899.pdf.

DH (2010c) *Uniforms and Workwear: Guidance on Uniform and Workwear Policies for NHS Employers*. Department of Health, London. www.dh.gov.uk/prod_consum_dh/groups/dh_digitalassets/@dh/@en/@ps/documents/digitalasset/dh_114754.pdf.

126

DH/HPA (2008) *Clostridium difficile Infection: How to Deal with the Problem*. Department of Health/Health Protection Agency, London. www.hpa.org.uk/web/HPAwebFile/HPAweb_C/1232006607827.

Dharan, S., Mourouga, P., Copin, P. *et al.* (1999) Routine disinfection of patients' environmental surfaces. Myth or reality? *Journal of Hospital Infection*, **42** (2), 113–117.

Elliott, T., Worthington, A., Osman, H. and Gill, M. (2007) *Lecture Notes: Medical Microbiology and Infection*, 7th edn. Blackwell Publishing, Oxford.

European Parliament (2008) Directive 2008/98/EC of the European Parliament and of the Council of 19 November 2008 on waste and repealing certain Directives. *Official Journal of the European Union* 22.11.2008. eur-lex.europa.eu/LexUriServ/LexUriServ.do?uri=OJ:L:2008:312:0003:0030:EN:PDF.

Food Safety Act 1990. HMSO, London.

Fraise, A.P. and Bradley, T. (eds) (2009) *Ayliffe's Control of Health care-associated Infection: A Practical Handbook*, 5th edn. Hodder Arnold, London.

Gammon, J. (1998) Analysis of the stressful effects of hospitalisation and source isolation on coping and psychological constructs. *International Journal of Nursing Practice*, **4** (2), 84–96.

Gillespie, I.A., O'Brien, S.J., Adak, G.K. *et al.* (2005) Foodborne general outbreaks of *Salmonella enteritidis* phage type 4 infection, England and Wales, 1992–2002: where are the risks? *Epidemiology and Infection*, **133** (5), 795–801.

Goering, R., Dockrell, H., Zuckermann, M. *et al.* (2007) *Mims' Medical Microbiology*, 4th edn. Mosby, London.

Hazardous Waste (England and Wales) Regulations 2005 and the List of Wastes (England) Regulations 2005. HMSO, London.

Health and Safety at Work etc. Act 1974. HMSO, London.

Health and Safety Commission (2001) *Legionnaires' Disease: The Control of Legionella Bacteria in Water Systems. Approved Code of Practice and Guidance*, 3rd edn (L8). Health and Safety Executive, London.

Health Protection Agency (2005) *Occupational Transmission of HIV: Summary of Published Reports March 2005 Edition: Data to December 2002*. Health Protection Agency, London. www.hpa.org.uk/web/HPAwebFile/HPAweb_C/1194947320156.

Health Protection Agency (2008) *Eye of the Needle: United Kingdom Surveillance of Significant Occupational Exposures to Bloodborne Viruses in Healthcare Workers*. Health Protection Agency, London. www.hpa.org.uk/web/HPAwebFile/HPAweb_C/1227688128096.

Health Protection Agency (2010a) *Results from the Mandatory Surveillance of MRSA Bacteraemia*. Health Protection Agency, London. www.hpa.org.uk/web/HPAweb&HPAwebStandard/HPAweb_C/1233906819629.

Health Protection Agency (2010b) *Clostridium difficile Mandatory Surveillance*. Health Protection Agency, London. www.hpa.org.uk/web/HPAweb&HPAwebStandard/HPAweb_C/1179746015058.

Health Protection Scotland (2009) *Standard Infection Control Precautions*. www.hps.scot.nhs.uk/haiic/ic/standardinfectioncontrolprecautions-sicps.aspx.

Hospital Infection Society/Infection Control Nurses Association (2007) *The Third Prevalence Survey of Healthcare-associated Infections in Acute Hospitals in England 2006: Report for Department of Health England*. Department of Health, London. www.dh.gov.uk/prod_consum_dh/groups/dh_digitalassets/documents/digitalasset/dh_078389.pdf.

Infection Control Nurses Association (2002) *A Comprehensive Glove Choice*. Fitwise, Edinburgh.

Kao, P.H. and Yang, R.J. (2006) Virus diffusion in isolation rooms. *Journal of Hospital Infection*, **62** (3), 338–345.

Korniewicz, D.M., El-Masri, M., Broyles, J.M. *et al.* (2002) Performance of latex and nonlatex medical examination gloves during simulated use. *American Journal of Infection Control*, **30** (2), 133–138.

Lefebvre, S., Waltner-Toews, D., Peregrine, A. *et al.* (2006) Prevalence of zoonotic agents in dogs visiting hospitalized people in Ontario: implications for infection control. *Journal of Hospital Infection*, **62** (3), 458–466.

McGuckin, M., Waterman, R., Storr, J. *et al.* (2001) Evaluation of a patient empowering hand hygiene programme. *Journal of Hospital Infection*, **48** (3), 222–227.

MHRA (2006) *DB 2006(04) Single-use Medical Devices: Implications and Consequences of Reuse*. Medicines and Healthcare Products Regulatory Agency, London. www.mhra.gov.uk.

MHRA (2010) Guidance notes on medical devices which require sterilization, in *EC Medical Devices Directives: Guidance for Manufacturers on Clinical Investigations to Be Carried Out In the UK, Updated March 2010*. MHRA, London, pp.40–41. www.mhra.gov.uk.

Moody, K., Finlay, J., Mancuso, C. *et al.* (2006) Feasibility and safety of a pilot randomized trial of infection rate: neutropenic diet versus standard food safety guidelines. *Journal of Pediatric Hematology/Oncology*, **28** (3), 126–133.

Morgan, D.J., Diekema, D.J., Sepkowitz, K. and Perencevich, E.N. (2009) Adverse outcomes associated with contact precautions: a review of the literature. *American Journal of Infection Control*, **37**, 85–93.

NHS Estates (2001) *Infection Control in the Built Environment*. Stationery Office, London.

NHS Executive (1995) *HSG (95) 18 Hospital Laundry Arrangements for Used and Infected Linen*. NHS Executive, London.

NICE (2006) *Clinical Guideline 33: Tuberculosis*. National Institute for Health and Clinical Excellence, London. www.nice.org.uk/nicemedia/live/10980/30018/30018.pdf.

NMC (2008a) *The Code: Standards of Conduct, Performance and Ethics for Nurses and Midwives*. Nursing and Midwifery Council, London. www.nmc-uk.org/aDisplayDocument.aspx?documentID=5982.

NMC (2008b) *Consent*. Nursing and Midwifery Council, London.

NMC (2009) *Record Keeping: Guidance for Nurses and Midwives* Nursing and Midwifery Council, London.

NPSA (2008) *Patient Safety Alert Second Edition 2 September 2008: Clean Hands Save Lives*. National Patient Safety Agency, London. www.nrls.npsa.nhs.uk/resources/type/alerts/?entryid45=59848&q=0%C2%ACclean+hands%C2%AC%20.

NPSA (2009) *Revised Healthcare Cleaning Manual*. National Patient Safety Agency, London. www.nrls.npsa.nhs.uk/EasySiteWeb/getresource.axd?AssetID=61814&type=full&servicetype=Attachment.

Patel, S. (2005) Minimising cross-infection risks associated with beds and mattresses. *Nursing Times*, **101** (8), 52–53.

Perry, C. (2007) *Infection Prevention and Control*. Blackwell Publishing, Oxford.

Pratt, R.J., Pellowe, C.M., Wilson, J.A. *et al.* (2007) epic2: National evidence-based guidelines for preventing healthcare-associated infections in NHS hospitals in England. *Journal of Hospital Infection*, **65S**, S1–S64. www.epic.tvu.ac.uk/PDF%20Files/epic2/epic2-final.pdf.

RCN (2010) *Infection Prevention and Control*. www.rcn.org.uk/development/practice/infection_control.

Siegel, J.D., Rhinehart, E., Jackson, M., Chiarello, L. and the Healthcare Infection Control Practices Advisory Committee (2007) *Guideline for Isolation Precautions: Preventing Transmission of*

Infectious Agents in Healthcare Settings. Centers for Disease Control, Atlanta, GA. www.cdc.gov/ncidod/dhqp/pdf/isolation2007.pdf.

UK Health Departments (1998) *Guidance for Clinical Health Care Workers: Protection Against Infection with Blood-borne Viruses. Recommendations of the Expert Advisory Group on AIDS and the Advisory Group on Hepatitis.* Deaprtment of Health, London. www.dh.gov.uk/en/Publicationsandstatistics/Lettersandcirculars/Healthservicecirculars/DH_4003818.

Vonberg, R.P, Eckmanns, T., Bruderek, J. *et al.* (2005) Use of terminal tap water filter systems for prevention of nosocomial legionellosis. *Journal of Hospital Infection,* **60** (2), 159–162.

Ward, D. (2000) Infection control: reducing the psychological effects of isolation. *British Journal of Nursing,* **9** (3), 162–170.

Weaving, P. (2007) Creutzfeldt Jakob disease. *British Journal of Infection Control,* **8** (5), 26–29.

WHO (2009) *WHO Guidelines on Hand Hygiene in Health Care: First Global Patient Safety Challenge. Clean Care is Safer Care.* World Health Organization, Geneva. whqlibdoc.who.int/publications/2009/9789241597906_eng.pdf.

Wigglesworth, N. (2003) The use of protective isolation. *Nursing Times,* **99** (07), 26.

Wigglesworth, N. and Wilcox, M.H. (2006) Prospective evaluation of hospital isolation room capacity. *Journal of Hospital Infection,* **63** (2), 156–161.

Wilson, J. (2000) *Clinical Microbiology: An Introduction for Healthcare Professionals,* 8th edn. Baillière Tindall, London.

Wilson, J. (2006) *Infection Control in Clinical Practice,* 3rd edn. Baillière Tindall, London.

Risk management

The Royal Marsden Hospital Manual of Clinical Nursing Procedures, Eighth Edition. Edited by Lisa Dougherty and Sara Lister.
© 2011 The Royal Marsden Hospital. Published 2011 by Blackwell Publishing Ltd.

Overview

The fundamental goal for every healthcare professional is to ensure that their patients are treated in a safe environment and protected wherever possible from harm. This manual is devoted to ensuring that the care nurses give to patients is consistently of a high quality and based on sound evidence of good practice. Whilst nurses are obliged to keep updated in their practice and only undertake roles and activities for which they feel they have the knowledge, skills and experience (NMC 2008), keeping patients safe involves a deeper understanding of the hazards which may exist along a patient's pathway of care.

This chapter will look at the ways in which risks to patients and staff can be identified at an early stage and managed appropriately. The management of risk is everybody's business and as the main caregivers in the NHS, it is essential that nurses understand the key principles of risk management and ensure that they know how to keep their patients, colleagues and indeed themselves safe.

Risk management

Definitions

Risk management can be defined as the culture, processes and structures that are directed towards the effective management of potential opportunities and adverse effects (Standards Australia and Standards New Zealand 2009) or, in relation to nursing, the way in which individuals and teams make sure their patients and staff are kept safe by having appropriate systems to identify and manage hazards and risks.

The language of risk is often confusing to healthcare professionals so before looking further into risk management, it is important to understand the basic definitions.

- *Hazard:* a situation, object, property, substance, phenomenon or activity with the potential to cause harm (HSE 2010).
- *Adverse event:* any event or circumstances leading to unintentional harm or suffering relating to treatment. Adverse events may be preventable or non-preventable (WHO 2005).
- *Risk:* the likelihood that something will occur that will have an impact on the achievement of aims and objectives (Standards Australia and Standards New Zealand 2009) or the probability that a specific adverse event (or patient safety incident) will occur in a specific time period or as the result of a specific situation (NPSA 2007).
- *Clinical risk:* the chance of an adverse outcome resulting from clinical investigation, treatment or patient care (NPSA 2007).
- *Inherent clinical risk:* the permanent or currently unavoidable clinical risk that is associated with a particular clinical investigation or treatment (NPSA 2007).

- *Clinical risk management:* the use of techniques to minimize the occurrence of near misses, errors and incidents in the processes of clinical activity and thereby reducing unwanted outcomes (NPSA 2009, Standards Australia and Standards New Zealand 2009).
- *Patient safety incident:* any unintended or unexpected incident which could have or did lead to harm for one or more patients receiving healthcare.

A patient safety incident is an umbrella term used to describe a single incident or a series of incidents that occur over time. Terms such as adverse, error or mistake suggest individual causality and blame and can often prevent the development of full understanding and learning from the incident.

The main categories of patient safety incidents as defined by the National Patient Safety Agency in 2009 were:

- medication incident
- consent incident
- surgical incident
- anaesthetic incident
- medical device incident
- medical records/clinical information, breaches in confidentiality
- radiotherapy and systemic isotope incidents
- diagnostic radiology
- pathology.

(NPSA 2009)

Patient safety incidents may include:

- incidents that staff are involved in
- incidents that staff may have witnessed
- incidents that caused no harm or minimal harm
- incidents with more serious outcomes
- prevented patient safety incidents (also known as near misses).

A medicine could be described as a *hazard* if it has the potential to cause harm. However, the *risk* of that harm may be very small provided effective controls/measures are in place. If the patient could suffer harm as a result of taking the medication, the *adverse event* may be described as a *clinical risk*, and a *patient safety incident* if the harm occurred unexpectedly or unintentionally.

If the *hazard* is considered as selecting the wrong drug because of look-alike packaging, there is a *clinical risk* to the patient, a *risk* to the members of staff involved and a *risk* to the organization. If the organization identified the hazard and changed the packaging, this could be defined as successful *clinical risk management*. If a healthcare professional still administered the wrong drug following the mitigating action, this would be described as a *patient safety incident* (NPSA 2009).

Accident

An unplanned, undesired non-clinical event that could have or did lead to the injury or death of any person affected by the organization's activities. This definition therefore includes injuries to staff, visitors and contractors. It also applies to any incident involving a patient that is not directly related to their clinical care; for example, a patient fall would be included as an accident.

Non-clinical incident

An incident which is not related to the clinical area of patients but which could have or did lead to harm to an individual or to the organization. Examples of non-clinical incidents include:

- accident to member of staff, patient, visitor or other person
- security incident
- violence, aggression
- ionizing radiation incident (non-clinical)
- equipment (non-medical) incident
- environmental incident, for example chemical spillage, flood, fire, waste disposal
- food safety incident (NPSA 2009).

Non-clinical prevented incident

A situation in which an event or omission, or a sequence of events or omissions, fails to develop further, whether or not as the result of compensating action, thus preventing harm/injury.

Serious untoward incident

A serious untoward incident (SUI) is an accident or incident involving a patient, member of staff, visitor on NHS property, contractor or other person to whom the organization owes a duty of care, that causes actual serious injury or unexpected death.

SUIs may include:

- permanent harm to one or more patients, staff, visitors or members of the public or where the outcome requires life-saving intervention or major surgical/medical intervention or will shorten life expectancy
- unexpected death of a baby, child or young person
- a scenario that prevents or threatens to prevent a provider organization's ability to continue to deliver healthcare services, for example, actual or potential loss or damage to property, reputation or the environment
- serious abuse or physical attack of a person on NHS property
- an incident likely to attract adverse media coverage or public concern for the organization or the wider NHS (NPSA 2009).

Never events

Serious, largely preventable patient safety incidents that should not occur. The core sets of 'never events' are updated by the NPSA on an annual basis and currently include (NPSA 2009):

- wrong site surgery
- retained instrument post operation

- wrong route administration of chemotherapy
- misplaced nasogastric or orogastric tube not detected prior to use
- inpatient suicide using non-collapsible rails (mental health)
- escape from medium- or high-security mental health services
- in-hospital maternal death from postpartum haemorrhage after elective caesarean section
- intravenous administration of mis-selected concentrated potassium chloride.

Never events are immediately reportable to the NPSA and may affect healthcare organizations' registration with the Care Quality Commission. Healthcare providers may also be subject to financial penalties if never events occur within their organization.

Evidence-based approaches

Raising the profile of risk management in the UK

Risk management and risk prevention have come to dominate the healthcare agenda in the UK (Southgate and Dauphinee 1998, Vincent 2006).

Across the world, several notable incidents involving one or more deaths have led to a refocusing of the safety culture (Alaszewski 2002, Flynn 2002). In the UK, the events that occurred at the Bristol Royal Infirmary were instrumental in the regulation of healthcare. Events such as those that happened at Bristol and more recently at the Mid-Staffordshire NHS Foundation Trust (Francis 2010) have highlighted key issues such as culture, leadership, lack of critical analysis, inward looking and in some cases lack of clinical ownership (Francis 2010, Heyman et al. 2010, Weick and Sutcliffe 2003). The Department of Health has drawn upon Bristol, Mid-Staffordshire and other evidence from major global incidents in medications and screening to support the urgency of improving risk management and the safety and consistency of healthcare treatments and outcomes (Heyman et al. 2010).

The Bristol Inquiry findings provided supporting arguments for reforms designed to develop a more systematic approach to setting, delivering and monitoring standards in healthcare (DH 1998).

- Clear national standards for services and treatments, through National Service Frameworks (NSFs) and a new National Institute for Clinical Excellence (NICE).
- Local delivery of high-quality healthcare, through clinical governance underpinned by modernized professional self-regulation and extended life-long learning.
- Effective monitoring of progress through a new Commission of Health Improvement, a framework for assessing performance in the NHS and a new national survey of patient and user experience. The Commission for Health Improvement (CHI) was replaced in 2004 by the

Healthcare Commission, which in 2009 became part of the Care Quality Commission (CQC) together with the Commission for Social Care Inspection and the Mental Health Act Commission (CQC 2009).

The reforms in monitoring risk and safety in the NHS at this time involved working in partnership with the public, nurses, doctors and allied healthcare professionals. The government, however, made it clear that the responsibility for managing risk and quality lay with the individual staff and professions within the NHS, and 'failure would not be tolerated' (DH 1998).

The quality agenda

The quality agenda has been a key driving force in the development and funding of health services in the new millennium. Nurses, doctors and allied healthcare professionals (AHPs) need to demonstrate that they are not only managing risk and preventing harm, but that they are also achieving key clinical outcomes for their patients. The increase in regulation of health services, in the form of clinical audit, professional peer review and external regulation, and the sharing of this information with the public have enabled patients to make choices regarding the treatment and care they receive. Nurses now find themselves in the position of explaining to patients how they are ensuring their safety, particularly with issues such as hand hygiene and cleanliness.

As with all public services, regulatory oversight of the NHS has increased notably since the 1980s. It is conducted at arm's length from the government through a number of external bodies (Power 2007).

Hutter (2006) summarized this trend as a move from government to governance. *High Quality Care for All* (DH 2008), the final report of the Next Stage Review, was a landmark document for the future of healthcare in the UK. In the report, Lord Darzi described quality as having three key components in relation to doing the best for patients: patient experience, effectiveness of care and patient safety, or, from a patient's viewpoint:

- be nice to me
- make me better
- do me no harm.

Table 4.1 outlines Darzi's seven steps to quality, all of which relate to staff throughout the NHS, from those in the clinical areas delivering hands-on care to the leaders of organizations at trust board level.

Care Quality Commission (CQC)

The CQC was established by the Health and Social Care Act 2008 to bring together the Healthcare Commission, the Commission for Social Care Inspection and the Mental Health Act Commission, the three former regulatory bodies in the health and adult social care system in England. The creation of a super-agency is intended to overcome barriers between health and social care where the distinctions between their services increasingly blur.

From 1 April 2009, for the first time, healthcare providers were obliged to register with the CQC their compliance with the Hygiene Code and from 1 April 2010, with the CQC's Essential Standards of Quality and Safety. These quality standards are divided into 28 outcomes, which must be consistently achieved, 16 of those outcomes relating directly to care delivered to patients by frontline staff.

The CQC has powers of enforcement and is required to adopt a risk-based approach and efficiently target action where it is needed (DH 2007, DH 2008). In relation to governmental efforts to control healthcare-associated

Table 4.1 Darzi's seven steps to enhancing quality

Step	Enhancing and improving quality	Description
1	Bring clarity to quality	Further development of NICE and evidence portal
2	Measuring quality	The introduction of quality metrics and 'scorecards' to demonstrate quality performance against quality targets
3	Publish quality performance	As from April 2010, all NHS and Foundation trusts are obliged to publish quality accounts. These demonstrate how the above measures of quality have been achieved and the quality objectives for the organization
4	Recognize and reward quality	Commissioning for Quality and Innovation (CQUINS) provide financial incentives in relation to preset quality indicators
5	Raise standards	A National Quality Board and Quality Observatory will ensure quality standards are set and met within the health service
6	Safeguard quality	From 1 April 2009 healthcare organizations were obliged to register with the newly formed CQC regarding compliance with the Hygiene Code and from 1 April 2010 regarding compliance with the Quality Standards for Health
7	Staying ahead	Professionals are encouraged to introduce best practice models from the UK and abroad

infections and quality standards, the CQC is able to fine hospitals, close wards, suspend services and increase inspection visits where hygiene or care quality requirements are not being met. In the wake of the Mid-Staffordshire NHS Trust case (Healthcare Commission 2009) and the subsequent independent enquiry (Francis 2010), risk scrutiny is to be strengthened by the establishment of 'risk summits'. Inspectors, health watchdogs and regional NHS chiefs will vet the safety of every hospital and share information so that patterns in sub-standard care can be identified. Other reforms include faster alert systems to identify trusts with high mortality rates and risk profiling to identify organizations threatened by management changes and high staff turnover or vacancy rates (Francis 2010).

Risk management and organizational change

Making sure patients come to no harm is a key component of ensuring high-quality care for all. The quality agenda described above has a key focus on establishing and measuring targeted outcomes and establishing very clear reporting structures.

Running alongside the quality agenda in the NHS has been an increasing focus on and use of formal risk-based management approaches (Power 2007). This has also been stimulated by a wider strengthening of faith in its importance to the functioning of a well-governed organization, which is internally and externally accountable for how it handles uncertainty and risk (Power 2007). The leaders of healthcare organizations are being held to account for the levels of risk and harm within their organizations, making investment in robust systems for managing risk, from ward to board, a very high priority.

The publication of *An Organization with a Memory* (DH 2000) and *Building a Safer NHS for Patients* (DH 2001) highlighted from international research the need for organizations to learn more when things go wrong. With the publication of patient safety data such as infection rates in hospitals, patients are also lobbying for better, safer care in hospitals. It is estimated that around 10% of patients (900,000 using 2002–3 admission rates) admitted to NHS hospitals have experienced a patient safety incident and that up to half of these could have been prevented. This study also estimated that 72,000 of these incidents might have contributed to a patient's death (Vincent 2006). Whilst the majority of those incidents relate to system failures involving many healthcare professionals, nurses have a key role to play not only in preventing harm but also in the analysis of patient safety incidents which inevitably occur, and the dissemination of lessons learned to prevent reoccurrence of incidents.

The quality agenda has provided the NHS with a much greater focus on managing risk and maintaining patient safety than ever before but with such pressure to achieve excellent clinical outcomes comes the risk of professionals being apprehensive in reporting when adverse incidents occur. Quality agendas such as the one outlined above are, however, officially viewed as a method for promoting re-flective cultures in which learning rather than blame and defensiveness predominates (Berta *et al.* 2005).

The vision for the NHS is one where patients and staff will be enabled to report errors and guided by this information, healthcare services will individually and collectively progress through continuous improvement.

Development of a 'No Blame' culture

Organizational culture is difficult to define and assess (Davies *et al.* 2000) but there is wide agreement that one of the key impediments to openness in NHS institutions is fear of professionally harmful consequences such as loss of job and/or reputation and litigation (Meurier 2000). Reason (2006) has argued that the source of such fears lies in the myth that errors are the exception rather than the norm in healthcare and must therefore be the fault of flawed individuals.

Fear of blame can lead professionals to draw back from openness and instead take refuge behind professional lines. For example, an in-depth study by Shaw *et al.* (2007) revealed that frontline nurses felt unfairly targeted when patient incidents occurred. As a result, they became less open to new ideas of treatment and to participating confidently in multidisciplinary practice.

Approaches that refocus attention on wider issues and underlying factors of patient incidents are thought to be more helpful because they avoid prior assumption of personal blame, promote open reporting and stimulate learning from mistakes (Vincent 2006). The Being Open policy (NPSA 2005) requires all NHS organizations to establish an infrastructure which facilitates openness between staff, patients and carers following an incident. Research confirms that patients would welcome prompt disclosure and an apology when incidents occur (Carthey 2005).

Developing a 'no blame' culture within the NHS has been key in recent developments in patient safety, though dilemmas still remain for many nurses when working with staff who have been involved in patient safety incidents. Studies have shown that the best way of reducing error rates and preventing harm is to target failures in systems, and involve staff in reducing risk and participating in learning from near misses rather than taking actions against individual members of staff (Macrea 2008).

The National Reporting and Learning Service of the NPSA provides examples of frequently reported patient safety incidents and then suggests ways to redesign systems, increase learning and reduce risk. Recently published examples include reducing the risk of harm from chest drains and from prescribing and administering controlled drugs (NPSA 2010). Dr Lucian Leape from the Harvard School of Public Health suggests that individuals and organizations confront two myths concerning patient safety.

- *The perfection myth*: if people try hard enough, they will not make any errors.
- *The punishment myth*: if we punish people when they make errors, they will make fewer of them.

The National Patient Safety Agency has a key role both in producing guidance and offering support to professionals, and in the analysis and benchmarking of safety data across healthcare services to identify trends and lessons learned (NPSA 2009). It recognizes that healthcare will always involve risks, but that by adopting a culture of openness and transparency, and tackling the root causes of patient safety incidents, risks can be reduced.

The National Patient Safety Agency (NPSA)

The NPSA was established in 2001. Its two main aims were, firstly, to identify trends and patterns in patient safety problems through its National Reporting and Learning System (NRLS) and secondly, to support staff at the local level to report incidents with a view to ensuring a high national profile for improving patient safety. Subsequently, the agency has undergone several significant changes. In 2005, its remit was expanded to cover safety aspects of hospital design, food and cleanliness, safety issues in research and support for local performance concerns.

The launch of the Never Events Policy for England in March 2009 (NPSA 2009) is the most recent attempt to set patient safety targets. It defines eight core events considered absolutely preventable, including wrong site surgery, inpatient suicide using non-collapsible rails, and wrong route administration of chemotherapy. The never events framework lists highly specific and selected risks but is intended to act as a spur to the risk and patient safety agenda.

The risk management process

Risk management is a central part of any organization's strategic and operational management processes. It is integral to the business planning process in order to ensure that the organization can achieve its core objectives. Risk management, undertaken systematically and robustly, will help ensure a successful trust, one that prospers while delivering an excellent high-quality and safe service to its patients.

Health and safety management is inseparable from risk management. Legally healthcare trusts are required to have a health and safety policy (DH 1999). The term 'risk management' is used as an overarching concept but it explicitly includes the management of health, safety, fire and security, clinical, operational, financial and strategic risks.

Figure 4.1 depicts an organizational model for managing risk, which is based on the Australian/New Zealand risk management standard 4360:2004 (Standards Australia and Standards New Zealand 2009) and is internationally recognized.

The risk management process made easy

As can be seen from Figure 4.1, the risk management process comprises seven key stages (Standards Australia and Standards New Zealand 2009).

1 Establishing the context.
2 Risk identification.
3 Risk analysis.
4 Risk evaluation.
5 Risk treatment.
6 Monitoring and reviewing risks.
7 Communication and consultation.

Stage 1 – establishing the context

A key component of the context of risk management which impacts upon every level of the process is the individual and organizational commitment to maintain an open dialogue with staff and others about risk issues, to listen to staff concerns and to communicate effectively to all relevant parties about risk-related issues. Nurses working within any organization need to ensure that they are familiar with the risk management strategy and how risks are managed and recorded at an organizational level (NPSA 2009).

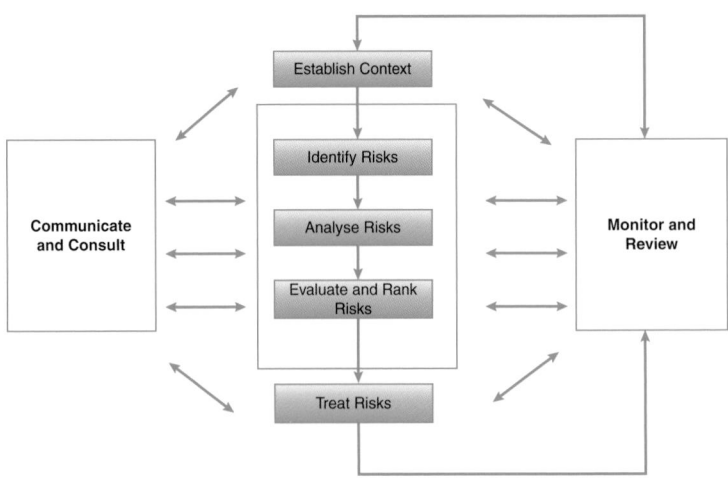

Figure 4.1 The risk management process. Standards Australia and Standards New Zealand (2009) under license 101-c097 SAI Global.

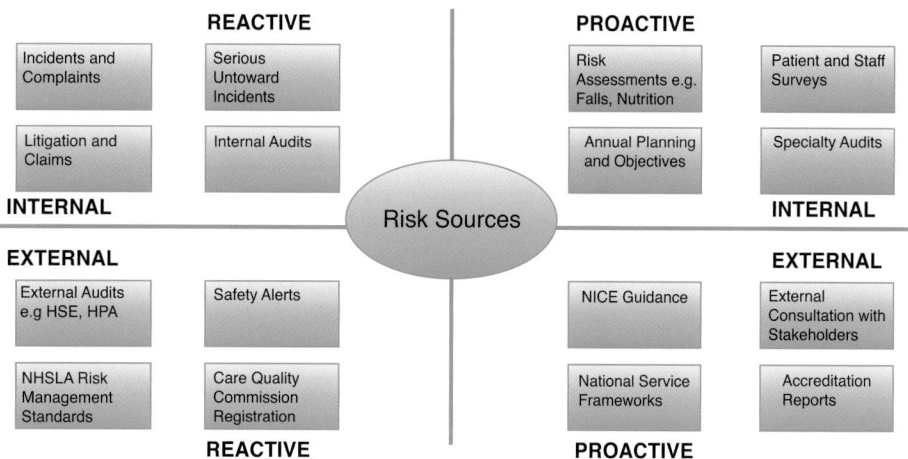

Figure 4.2 Risk sources. Standards Australia and Standards New Zealand (2009) under license 101-c097 SAI Global.

Stage 2 – risk identification and analysis

To prevent harm, it is important to understand not only what is likely to go wrong but also how and why it may go wrong. Hopkinson (2001) states that 'the objective of the risk identification element is to ensure that all significant risks are listed so that they can be analysed and evaluated'. This step requires considering the activity within the context of the physical and emotional environment and the culture of the organization and the staff who perform the activity.

This is a small step but essential to the process, as risks that are not identified will not be managed. Risks are identified from a wide range of sources, as illustrated in Figure 4.2.

As can be seen, risk identification is undertaken in many ways and includes incident reporting forms, use of specific risk assessment forms such as falls, pressure sore, nutrition, complaints, legal claims, adverse events and adverse trend analysis, Health and Safety Executive visits, trust health and safety audit inspections, and NHS Litigation Authority standards. Healthcare organizations are now obliged to assess the key risks for the organization and there is an expectation that wards and departments will meet regularly to discuss and analyse particular risks in their clinical areas. This is known as proactive risk assessment.

Stages 3 and 4 – risk analysis and evaluation

The data collected from the risk identification process have to be analysed to ensure that decisions can be made about prioritizing and treating the risks. This stage involves considering the consequence (how bad?) and the likelihood (how often?).

A widely used system for risk analysis and evaluation in trusts is the three-step 5 × 5 risk-scoring matrix as detailed in Steps A–C.

- Step A involves assessing the severity/consequence score (how bad?).
- Step B involves assessing the likelihood of the consequence occurring (how often?).
- Step C involves assessing the consequence × the likelihood and applying a risk grading score.

Step A: consequence score

The most appropriate domain for the identified risk is chosen from the left-hand side of the table. Then the individual works along the columns in the same row to assess the severity of the risk on the scale of 1 to 5 to determine the consequence score, which is the number given at the top of the column.

Consequence score (severity levels) and examples of descriptors					
	1	2	3	4	5
Domains	**Negligible**	**Minor**	**Moderate**	**Major**	**Catastrophic**
Impact on the safety of patients, staff or public (physical/ psychological harm)	Minimal injury requiring no/ minimal intervention or treatment	Minor injury or illness, requiring minor intervention	Moderate injury requiring professional intervention	Major injury leading to long-term incapacity/disability	Incident leading to death

(Continued)

	Consequence score (severity levels) and examples of descriptors *(Continued)*				
	1	2	3	4	5
Domains	**Negligible**	**Minor**	**Moderate**	**Major**	**Catastrophic**
	No time off work	Requiring time off work for >3 days Increase in length of hospital stay by 1–3 days	Requiring time off work for 4–14 days Increase in length of hospital stay by 4–15 days RIDDOR/agency reportable incident An event which impacts on a small number of patients	Requiring time off work for >14 days Increase in length of hospital stay by >15 days Mismanagement of patient care with long-term effects	Multiple permanent injuries or irreversible health effects An event which impacts on a large number of patients
Quality/complaints/audit	Peripheral element of treatment or service suboptimal Informal complaint/ enquiry	Overall treatment or service suboptimal Formal complaint (stage 1) Local resolution Single failure to meet internal standards Minor implications for patient safety if unresolved Reduced performance rating if unresolved	Treatment or service has significantly reduced effectiveness Formal complaint (stage 2) complaint Local resolution (with potential to go to independent review) Repeated failure to meet internal standards Major patient safety implications if findings are not acted on	Non-compliance with national standards with significant risk to patients if unresolved Multiple complaints/ independent review Low performance rating Critical report	Totally unacceptable level or quality of treatment/service Gross failure of patient safety if findings not acted on Inquest/ombudsman enquiry Gross failure to meet national standards
Human resources/organizational development/staffing/ competence	Short-term low staffing level that temporarily reduces service quality (<1 day)	Low staffing level that reduces the service quality	Late delivery of key objective/service due to lack of staff Unsafe staffing level or competence (>1 day) Low staff morale Poor staff attendance for mandatory/key training	Uncertain delivery of key objective/ service due to lack of staff Unsafe staffing level or competence (>5 days) Loss of key staff Very low staff morale No staff attending mandatory/key training	Non-delivery of key objective/service due to lack of staff Ongoing unsafe staffing levels or competence Loss of several key staff No staff attending mandatory training/ key training on an ongoing basis
Statutory duty/inspections	No or minimal impact or breach of guidance/ statutory duty	Breach of statutory legislation Reduced performance rating if unresolved	Single breach in statutory duty Challenging external recommendations/ improvement notice	Enforcement action Multiple breaches in statutory duty Improvement notices Low performance rating Critical report	Multiple breaches in statutory duty Prosecution Complete systems change required Zero performance rating Severely critical report

Adverse publicity/reputation	Rumours Potential for public concern	Local media coverage Short-term reduction in public confidence Elements of public expectation not being met	Local media coverage Long-term reduction in public confidence	National media coverage with <3 days service well below reasonable public expectation	National media coverage with >3 days service well below reasonable public expectation. MP concerned (questions in the House) Total loss of public confidence
Business objectives/ projects	Insignificant cost increase/schedule slippage	<5% over project budget Schedule slippage	5–10% over project budget Schedule slippage	Non-compliance with national objectives 10–25% over project budget Schedule slippage Key objectives not met	Incident leading >25% over project budget Schedule slippage Key objectives not met
Finance including claims	Small loss Risk of claim remote	Loss of 0.1–0.25% of budget Claim less than £10,000	Loss of 0.25–0.5% of budget Claim(s) between £10,000 and £100,000	Uncertain delivery of key objective/loss of 0.5–1.0% of budget Claim(s) between £100,000 and £1 million Purchasers failing to pay on time	Non-delivery of key objective/loss of >1% of budget Failure to meet specification/ slippage Loss of contract/ payment by results Claim(s) >£1 million
Service/business interruption/Environmental impact	Loss/interruption of >1 hour Minimal or no impact on the environment	Loss/interruption of >8 hours Minor impact on environment	Loss/interruption of >1 day Moderate impact on environment	Loss/interruption of >1 week Major impact on environment	Permanent loss of service or facility Catastrophic impact on environment

Step B: likelihood score (L)

This involves assessing the likelihood of the consequence occurring.

Likelihood score	1	2	3	4	5
Frequency	**Rare**	**Unlikely**	**Possible**	**Likely**	**Almost certain**
How often might it/does it happen?	This will probably never happen/recur	Do not expect it to happen/recur but it is possible it may do so	Might happen or recur occasionally	Will probably happen/recur but it is not a persisting issue	Will undoubtedly happen/recur, possibly frequently

Step C: risk scoring = consequence × likelihood (C × L)
This involves multiplying the consequence score by the likelihood score to come up with a risk level.

	Likelihood				
Likelihood score	**1**	**2**	**3**	**4**	**5**
	Rare	Unlikely	Possible	Likely	Almost certain
5 Catastrophic	5	10	15	20	25
4 Major	4	8	12	16	20
3 Moderate	3	6	9	12	15
2 Minor	2	4	6	8	10
1 Negligible	1	2	3	4	5

The risk scores are not intended to be precise mathematical measures of risk but the system allows healthcare professionals and managers to arrive at a consistent risk evaluation score and subsequent risk level. Risks can then be prioritized and action taken accordingly. Within each range of risk, there is a range of scores that will further help the process of prioritization. These levels can be simplified into the following format.

1–3	Low risk – quick, easy measures implemented immediately and further action planned when resources permit. Can be managed at local level with appropriate procedures.
4–6	Moderate risk – actions implemented as soon as possible but no later than a year. Requires escalation to senior manager.
8–12	High risk – actions implemented as soon as possible and no later than 6 months. Escalation to senior level.
15–25	Extreme risk – requires urgent action. Escalation to trust board/Strategic Health Authority.

In summary, where a risk is adequately addressed by existing controls or can be resolved by some immediate action, it will be the responsibility of all staff to ensure that the control is implemented in their ward or area and that any necessary action is taken. In cases where the risk cannot be immediately resolved, it is the responsibility of the manager to escalate the risk through the trust risk management structures so that the risk may be reviewed by senior management and placed on a document know as the *risk register*.

A risk register is a log of risks which have been evaluated but not yet fully controlled; these are therefore risks that may impact upon patient safety or the trust's objectives.

The risk register includes details of the nature of the risk, the severity, likelihood and overall rating, the service which owns the risk, the controls currently in place, the forum where progress in mitigating the risk is monitored, and progress achieved.

Stage 5 – risk treatment

Where risks have been identified, action must be taken to control these risks by reducing the potential impact or likelihood to an acceptable level. The overall purpose of risk treatment is to determine what will be done to mitigate the risk and who will be responsible for the treatment action(s). Risks are more likely to be acted upon if responsibility is allocated to an individual. Risk treatment options are evaluated in terms of feasibility, cost and benefits with the aim of choosing the most appropriate and practical way of reducing risk to a tolerable level. Risk action plans may seek to reduce the likelihood of occurrence, minimize the consequences, transfer or share the risk, or retain the risk.

The following list of risk reduction approaches can be used.

- *Avoid the risk:* for example, by deciding not to proceed with the activity likely to generate risk (where this is practicable); for example, withdrawing equipment from use or terminating activity.
- *Reduce the likelihood of the risk materializing:* audit and compliance programmes, policies and procedures, preventive maintenance, supervision and training.
- *Reduce the potential impact if the risk does materialize:* for example, through contingency planning, minimizing exposure to the risk.
- *Transfer of risk:* this involves another party bearing or sharing some part of the risk. Mechanisms include the use of contracts, insurance arrangements and organizational structures such as partnership and joint ventures.

Stage 6 – monitoring and reviewing risks

Continuous monitoring and review of risks ensure that new risks are detected and managed, action plans are implemented and managers and stakeholders kept informed. The availability of regular information on risks can assist in identifying trends like trouble spots or other changes that have arisen. It is essential that this information is accurate, complete and based on the most recently available data. Ongoing review is also required to ensure that risk management treatment plans remain relevant. In reality, the factors that affect risk assessments are ever changing and it is therefore important for this process to be ongoing to ensure that the risk management system remains effective.

Stage 7 – communication and consultation

At every stage of the risk management process, it is important that healthcare professionals, ward and departmental teams, managers and the risk management team communicate and consult both which each other and with key stakeholders, which may include the patient and their family. Key decisions regarding risk issues need to be made collaboratively in order for the whole process to remain open and transparent. Essential to nurses being successful and confident in managing risk is their understanding of their own and others' contribution to the risk management process and maintaining effective communication throughout the organization.

The two scenarios below demonstrate the way in which the risk management process can be put into practice in the ward setting. The first scenario demonstrates the 'procedure' for undertaking proactive risk assessment of a situation, and the second outlines the procedure for managing risk following a patient safety incident.

Scenario One

Mrs M is a 75-year-old woman admitted for a course of chemotherapy. She lives with her daughter who is her main carer. On admission she is appears to be a very thin, frail woman who is slightly unsteady on her feet. She walks with the aid of a walking frame but requires supervision. Mrs M's daughter also cares for her mother-in-law so is unable to stay with her mother in hospital.

Risk management stages	Action
1 Establish the context	As part of the induction process to any clinical area, you should ensure that you fully understand the risk management procedures for the organization, including the documentation required to ensure that a full assessment of the patient is undertaken.
	Prior to the patient arriving on the ward, ensure you have the appropriate documentation available, including any risk assessment you may require, for example falls risk assessment.
	Introduce yourself to the patient and her daughter and explain the admission assessment process.
	Show the patient and her daughter around the ward, explain the ward values and routines and introduce her to her 'neighbours', if appropriate.
2 Risk identification	Undertake a full patient admission assessment, including risk assessments such as a falls assessment, pressure ulcer risk assessment (see Chapter 19), venous thrombosis assessment (VTE), nutritional assessment (see Chapter 8). Include the patient's daughter in the risk assessments to gain a full picture of the patient's needs.
3/4 Risk analysis and evaluation	Formulate an action/care plan based on the assessment of risk above and agree the plan with the patient and her daughter, especially concerning discharge planning.
5 Risk treatment	Communicate the results of the risk assessment and implement the actions required to the rest of the multiprofessional ward team and make referrals to other professionals as required.
6 Monitoring and reviewing risk	Ensure the patient's risk treatment/care plans are reviewed regularly throughout her stay. Her risk status may change as she progresses through her treatment pathway and risk assessments may need to be repeated.
7 Communication and consultation	Ensure multidisciplinary meetings, ward handovers and ward rounds include regular discussions regarding the patient's risk treatment/care plan.
1–7	Prior to discharge, meet once again with the patient and her daughter to assess the potential risks on discharge and the actions that the patient and her daughter are able to undertake to mitigate those risks, together with any support they may need to manage them. This may include referral to community services, home care teams, local authority support. Depending on the level of risk identified, a full multiprofessional team risk assessment may need to be undertaken.

Scenario Two

You hear a loud commotion in the ward and on investigation find that Mr S, an 80-year-old patient who is 2 days post abdominal surgery, appears to have fallen out of bed and is lying on the floor next to his bed. He is in considerable pain, though there are no obvious signs of injury or haemorrhage.

Risk management stages	Actions
	Remain calm and breathe deeply. The patient will become more anxious if you are not calm, which may result in further harm.
	Call for immediate help from both the senior nurse and the medical team. The immediate priority is to prevent further harm to the patient.
1/2 Establish the context/Risk identification	Undertake an initial assessment of the patient without moving him and commence any first aid procedures required, for example securing peripheral lines and abdominal wounds, whilst awaiting the medical team.
	Offer the patient reassurance throughout by explaining exactly what is happening. The patient will be confused and alarmed. An understanding of exactly what is happening will reduce this anxiety.
2 Risk identification	Assist the medical team in their initial assessment.
2 Risk identification and 3/4 Risk analysis and evaluation	Once the patient is safe to be lifted back into bed, transfer the patient back to bed whilst following the trust's manual handling procedures. There is the potential for a second incident in relation to manual handling so even during patient safety incidents, it is important to prevent further incidents.
2 Risk identification, 3/4 Risk analysis and evaluation and 5 Risk treatment	Depending on the level of injuries sustained, undertake any further nursing observations or care required and adjust the patient's plan of care to include extra care needs.
2–7	Explain to the patient exactly what has happened and what is going to happen to prevent reoccurrence of the incident. If appropriate, explain the situation to the patient's next of kin. Risk monitoring and communication: communication is essential, ensuring that the patient and their family know the staff are being open and transparent regarding the incident.
3/4 Risk analysis and evaluation If there is serious injury to the patient then a formal root cause analysis is likely to be undertaken, led by the risk co-ordinator. The nurse can do an immediate assessment of obvious causes of the fall	Evaluate the root cause of the fall, for example bed guard not in place, patient confused, restless.
5 Risk treatment The risk plan should mitigate the future risks of reoccurrence of the incident	Undertake a risk assessment regarding the patient's risk of falling again and formulate a risk treatment plan. This may include the use of bed safety sides, or one-to-one nursing care.
3/4 Risk analysis and evaluation This scoring assessment should be undertaken in line with the organization's incident reporting policy and in collaboration with senior staff if appropriate	Complete an incident form, outlining the action which is being taken to mitigate the reoccurrence of such an incident. Include a risk score, for example if the patient fell because his bed guard was not correctly in place but this is now included in the risk treatment plan, together with extra nursing observation. What is the likelihood of the patient falling out of bed again? What are the potential consequences if the patient were to fall out of bed again?
7 Communication and consultation Communicating the action needed to prevent the reoccurrence of incidents and any lessons learned is key in the management of risk within wards, departments and organizations	Discuss the incident and the risk score with the senior nurse/risk co-ordinator and plan how lessons learned from the incident can be shared with the whole team. Consider whether any of the staff require further training on the management of falls prevention.

Box 4.1 Priorities in the event of a patient safety incident

Immediate

- Mitigate harm by taking immediate action within the scope of professional practice and call for help if the patient is at risk of further injury or harm.
- Remain calm and offer an initial explanation to the person or people involved.
- Take action to prevent immediate reoccurrence of the incident.
- Report the incident to a senior member of staff.

Short term

- Complete an incident form (depending on the organization, this may be in electronic format), assessing the likelihood and consequence of the risk reoccurring.

- You may be asked to be involved in a root cause analysis (RCA) event. This is a structured process for analysing how the incident occurred, what the main causes of the incident were and how it can be prevented in the future.
- Discuss the incident one to one with your manager, identifying any areas of specific training or support you may require to prevent reoccurrence of the incident.

Long term

- Ensure that actions resulting from the RCA or incident investigation are followed up and completed.
- Work with the ward/departmental team to audit the lessons learned and actions taken.

Legal and professional issues

However well intentioned healthcare organizations may be, the nature of healthcare means that at times things do not go to plan. Nurses from novice to expert can find patient safety incidents extremely stressful and at times upsetting. It is important that if a nurse is involved in an adverse event, they seek and are given appropriate support and guidance in order to learn from the event and prevent its reoccurrence in the future. The nurse has an obligation to report any incidents which occur, and to act in a transparent and open manner. Box 4.1 highlights the action which should be taken if a nurse believes an incident has occurred. Nurses can test their knowledge of risk management by working through a checklist (Box 4.2).

Box 4.2 Risk management – how do you do?

		Yes	No
1	Have you undergone risk management training within your organization?		
2	Do you understand the organization's risk management and incident reporting policies?		
3	Do you comply at all times with the relevant risk management strategies and policies?		
4	Do you know what the three top risks are in your clinical area and what action has been put in place to mitigate those risks?		
5	Do you report to your line manager if you have any concerns regarding risks or patient safety?		
6	Do you follow up to see if any action has been taken?		
7	Are you familiar with/ have you had training on the specific patient risk assessments in your organization? Manual handling? Pressure area assessments? Nutritional assessments? Infection control assessments? Falls assessments?		
8	Are you competent to use all the equipment you are currently using?		
9	Do you identify with your line manager any areas of your practice in which you require further training?		
10	Do you discuss risk management with your patients and their families where appropriate?		
11	Do you know how to complete an incident form?		
12	Have you had training on how to undertake root cause analysis?		
13	Do you regularly access the National Patient Safety Agency website to keep updated?		

The assessment and mitigation of important clinical risks

In clinical practice there are some risks that have been highlighted nationally and internationally as both largely preventable and, if they occur, causing major morbidity, suffering and high financial costs. Three key examples of these are the prevention of:

- venous thromboembolism (VTE)
- pressure ulcers
- falls.

Venous thromboembolism

Related theory

The prevention of venous thromboembolism

Each year over 25,000 people in England die from VTE contracted in hospital (House of Commons Health Select Committee 2005).

The main danger is from pulmonary embolism (PE). A thrombus forms in the lower limb or pelvic veins and then travels in the blood and lodges in the lungs, leading to acute massive PE, which has a high mortality rate. The initial thrombus is called a deep vein thrombosis (DVT). A DVT is itself a cause of substantial morbidity and may lead to the development of post-thrombotic syndrome (in around 30% of people with DVT), which is associated with chronic swelling and ulceration of the legs. Add this burden of morbidity to the 25,000 deaths and it becomes a massive health problem (NICE 2010). It is possible to greatly reduce the risk of VTE by using four main approaches to prevention, and sometimes a combination.

- The use of antiembolic compression stockings.
- The use of prophylactic anticoagulation.
- Early mobilization after surgery.
- External compression and decompression devices in those who cannot mobilize.

(Dolan and Fitch 2007, House of Commons Health Select Committee 2005, NICE 2007)

On admission or preferably prior to admission, all patients should have a risk assessment to assess both their individual risk for developing VTE and any risk factors for preventive therapies (National Clinical Guidelines Centre 2009).

Risk factors for the development of VTE

- Active cancer or cancer treatment.
- Age over 60 years.
- Critical care admission.
- Dehydration.
- Known thrombophilias.
- Obesity (Body Mass Index >30 kg/m^2).
- One or more significant co-morbidities.
- Individual history or first-degree relative with a history of VTE.
- Use of hormone replacement therapy.
- Use of oestrogen-containing contraceptive therapy.
- Varicose veins with phlebitis.
- Pregnancy and up to 6 weeks following birth (special considerations).

(National Clinical Guidelines Centre 2009)

Antiembolic stockings (graduated elastic compression stockings)

Graduated compression (antiembolic) stockings promote venous flow and reduce venous stasis not only in the legs but also in the pelvic veins and inferior vena cava (National Clinical Guidelines Centre 2009, NICE 2007, Roderick et al. 2005).

Thigh-length graduated compression/antiembolic stockings should be fitted from the time of admission to hospital unless contraindicated, for example peripheral arterial disease or diabetic neuropathy (NICE 2007) and until the patient has returned to their usual level of mobility. For details on measurement and fitting, see Chapter 17.

The use of prophylactic anticoagulation with low molecular weight heparin

Heparin interrupts the clotting cascade and can prevent clots. Different types of heparin affect clotting at varying levels and work in slightly dissimilar ways, depending on whether they are unfractionated heparin (UH) or low molecular weight heparin (LMWH). In addition, factor Xa inhibitors prevent the formation and development of thrombi.

Unfractionated heparin and LMWH are comparable in preventing VTE, but the advantage of LMWH over UH is that it has been shown to have a better side-effect profile with fewer adverse events (Lechler et al. 2006). Patients also rarely need to have regular clotting tests that are recommended for those on UH. The side-effects of LMWH include thrombocytopenia, liver abnormalities, skin rashes and minor bruising and so it should be used cautiously in patients who have renal failure (Dolan and Fitch 2007, National Clinical Guidelines Centre 2009, NICE 2007, Wilson 2007).

Patients who are at risk from VTE and are assessed as being able to receive LMWH should commence prophylactic treatment as soon as they have been assessed as at risk and continue with it as long as the risk remains. Patients will receive an injection which is administered subcutaneously once a day. There are several LMWH preparations available for use in the UK and Europe. Many patients will continue with LMWH on discharge from hospital and will therefore need to be taught how to self-administer or, if unable to undertake this, their family or a professional carer will need to administer the once-daily dose (National Clinical Guidelines Centre 2009, NICE 2007).

Intermittent pneumatic compression devices

Pneumatic compression devices, usually in the form of a calf boot attached to an external pump which constantly inflates and deflates, are used to promote venous return. They are most useful in patients who have been assessed as having high risk factors and are immobile following surgery or critical illness. The device can be used in combination with VTE compression stockings and LMWH.

The device is often applied in theatre or in critical care and is then used until the risk has reduced or the patient is unable to tolerate it. With all external compression devices, it is important that the device is regularly removed and skin integrity is assessed. Only pneumatic compression devices that are CE marked and have been assessed as safe to use as a medical device should be used (National Clinical Guidelines Centre 2009).

Pressure ulcers

Definition

Pressure ulcers are areas of localized tissue damage caused by excess pressure, shearing or friction forces (Benbow 2006). The extent of this damage can range from persistent erythema to necrotic ulceration involving muscle, tendon and bone (RCN 2005).

Related theory

The three major extrinsic factors that are identified as being significant contributors in the development of pressure ulcers are pressure, shearing and friction. These factors should be removed or diminished to reduce injury (RCN 2005).

- *Pressure.* The blood pressure at the arterial end of the capillaries is approximately 35 mmHg, while at the venous end it drops to 16 mmHg (the average mean capillary pressure is about 17 mmHg) (Guyton and Hall 2000, Tortora and Grabowski 2008). External pressures exceeding this will cause capillary obstruction as the capillaries close when the pressure between the bed surface and the bony prominence exceeds 16–32 mmHg (Landis 1930, S. Hampton, personal communication, October 2006). Tissues that are dependent on these capillaries are deprived of their blood supply and will eventually become ischaemic and die (Bridel-Nixon 1999, Tong 1999). The pressure near bony prominences can be up to five times greater and is known as the 'cone of pressure'; thus a surface redness can hide extensive tissue damage nearer the bone. It also explains why a small ulcer can open into a large, undetermined ulcer with overhanging edges and sinus formation (S. Hampton, personal communication, October 2006).
- *Shearing.* This may occur when the patient slips down the bed or is dragged up the bed. As the skeleton moves over the underlying tissue, the microcirculation is destroyed

and the tissue dies of anoxia. In more serious cases, lymphatic vessels and muscle fibres may also become torn, resulting in a deep pressure ulcer (Clay 2000, Collier 1999, Simpson *et al.* 1996).
- *Friction.* A component of shearing, which causes stripping of the stratum corneum, leading to superficial ulceration (Johnson 1989, Waterlow 1988). Poor lifting and moving techniques may be a major contributory factor (NICE 2003).

The most common sites for pressure ulcer development are areas where soft tissue is compressed between a prominence (such as the sacrum) and an external surface (such as a mattress or seat of a chair) (Hess 2005).

Evidence-based approaches

Rationale

Pressure ulcers are a major healthcare issue and are associated with pain, infection, prolonged hospital stay and in extreme cases can be a causative factor in a patient's death (Bennett *et al.* 2004, RCN 2005). Many pressure ulcers are preventable if there is a systematic and multiprofessional approach to their prevention and continuous assessment of skin integrity (Beldon 2006).

A 3-year clinical audit published in 2009 reported overall pressure ulcer prevalence in UK hospitals of 10.2–10.3%. Over half of pressure ulcers are hospital acquired (57–63%) (Phillips and Buttery 2009). Another study, published in 2004, reported that the mean incidence of pressure damage amongst hospital inpatients in the UK was approximately 40 cases per 1000 admissions in the population at risk (Bennett *et al.* 2004). NPSA data from 2009 demonstrate that of the pressure ulcers reported to the NRLS each year, 13% were grade 1, 47% were grade 2, 23% were grade 3 and 17% were grade 4 (NHS Institute for Innovation and Improvement 2010, NPSA 2009). See Box 4.3.

Identifying at-risk patients

The European Pressure Ulcer Advisory Panel (EPUAP 2003) recommends that assessment of at-risk patients should be ongoing and frequency of reassessment should be dependent on changes in the patient's condition or environment.

Many predisposing factors are involved in the development of pressure ulcers. An individual's potential to develop pressure ulcers may be influenced by the following intrinsic factors.

Box 4.3 Grades of pressure ulcers
Grade 1: non-blanchable erythema of intact skin.
Grade 2: presents clinically as an abrasion or blister.
Grade 3: superficial lesions.
Grade 4: deep lesions, extensive destruction, tissue necrosis or damage to muscle, bone or supporting structures.
(EPUAP 2003)

143

- Reduced mobility or immobility.
- Acute illness.
- Level of consciousness.
- Extremes of age.
- Vascular disease.
- Severe, chronic or terminal illness.
- Previous history of pressure damage.
- Malnutrition and dehydration.
- Neurologically compromised.
- Obesity.
- Poor posture.
- Use of equipment such as seating or beds which do not provide appropriate pressure relief (NHS Institute for Innovation and Improvement 2010, RCN 2005).

Older people and pregnant women are also at risk, as are people from black and minority ethnic backgrounds whose skin colour may mean that early signs of pressure ulcers are not as readily identifiable (NHS Institute for Innovation and Improvement 2010).

Grades of pressure ulcers

If a pressure ulcer develops then classification of the wound may assist in determining the most appropriate treatment. These classifications are valuable in describing the state of the ulcer and the most pertinent care required by the patient (see Box 4.3).

Preprocedural considerations

Equipment

A wide variety of devices are available to help relieve pressure over susceptible areas, for example cushions, static/dynamic mattresses and replacement beds. These devices differ in function, complexity and costs and the choice must be based on meeting the patient's individual need, sound criteria for decision making and effective use of available resources (Table 4.2). The data currently available to evaluate the clinical effectiveness of pressure-relieving devices are variable but the following are supported by some data.

- Patients with pressure ulcers should have access to pressure- relieving support surfaces and strategies, for example mattresses and cushions, 24 hours a day and this applies to all support surfaces.
- All individuals assessed as having a grade 1–2 pressure ulcer should, as a minimum provision, be placed on a high-specification foam mattress or cushion with pressure-reducing properties. Observation of skin changes, documentation of positioning and repositioning schemes must be combined in the patient's care.
- If there is any potential or actual deterioration of affected areas or further pressure ulcer development, an alternating pressure (AP) (replacement or overlay) or sophisticated continuous low pressure (CLP) system (e.g. low air loss, air fluidized, air flotation, viscous fluid) should be used.

- Depending on the location of ulcer, individuals assessed as having grade 3–4 pressure ulcers (including intact eschar where depth and therefore grade cannot be assessed) should be, as a minimum provision, placed on an AP mattress or sophisticated CLP system.
- If AP equipment is required, the first choice should be an overlay system. However, circumstances such as patient weight or patient safety indicate the need for a replacement system.

In 2005, NICE in collaboration with the RCN created a clinical guideline in pressure ulcer management (NICE 2005, RCN 2005). This included data looking at evidence-based practice, cost-effectiveness and economic evaluations of the different devices, drugs and procedures, amongst others, in the management of pressure ulcers (see Table 4.2). In 2009 the Nursing Executive Centre in the US also looked at the prevention of pressure ulcers and their approach is linked to ward organization, spot audits of assessment and pressure-relieving devices (Nursing Executive Centre 2009).

Assessment tools

There are several risk assessment tools in pressure ulcer development such as those developed by Norton, Braden and Waterlow (Braden and Bergstrom 1987, Norton *et al.* 1985, Waterlow 1991, 1998). Particular areas of care have also constructed their own hybrid assessment tool as a result of professional discussion and tailoring to specific patient needs (Birtwistle 1994, Chaplin 2000, Lindgren *et al.* 2002). NICE (2003) cautions professionals to use risk assessment tools as an *aide mémoire* and recommends their use in conjunction with clinical judgement (Chaplin 2000, RCN 2005). Some of the most commonly used tools include the following.

Norton scale

Using the Norton scale (Table 4.3) patients with a score of 14 or below are considered to be at greatest risk of pressure ulcer development. A score of 14–18 is not considered at risk but will require reassessment and a score of 18–20 indicates minimal risk. The 'cut-off' point for 'at-risk' patients was later raised to 15 or 16 by Norton (Norton *et al.* 1985, Anthony *et al.* 2008). Norton acknowledged that the scale was not intended as a universal tool and age and nutrition are not included.

Waterlow scale

The Waterlow scale (Figure 4.3) Defines a score of 11–15 as being 'at risk', 16–20 as 'high risk' and over 20 as 'very high risk' (Waterlow 2005). In a study of the Norton and Waterlow scales, 75.7% of patients identified as 'at risk' by the Waterlow scale developed a pressure ulcer, whereas 62% of those with a score of 16 or less on the Norton Scale developed ulcers (Smith *et al.* 1986) This may suggest that the Waterlow Scale gives a more accurate prediction of patient risk.

Table 4.2 A selection of mechanical methods for relieving pressure

Aid	Use	Advantages	Disadvantages
Silicone-filled mattress pad/cushion (e.g. Transoft)	Waterlow 10 or patients on prolonged bedrest, able to move spontaneously	Relieves pressure by distributing it over a greater area. Comfortable. Machine (industrial) washable. Acceptable in community settings as well as in hospital. Can be used for incontinent patients. Relatively cheap purchase price. Plastic protective covers available	If the patient is very incontinent of urine, even if the plastic side is uppermost, there is seepage into the core material. Stitching comes undone after several launderings. Not recommended for routine use in pressure ulcer prevention
Roho air-filled mattress/cushions	High–medium-risk patients, Waterlow 10–15	Interlinked air cells transfer air with movement. Patient can be nursed sitting or recumbent. Non-mechanical. Washable	Can be punctured and is expensive to repair. Often incorrectly inflated due to lack of understanding and education. Can be mechanically cleaned in sterile supply department
Alternating pressure beds	High–medium-risk patients, Waterlow 15	Mechanical alteration of pressure. Reduce the frequency of (but not need for) repositioning. Available on hire at short notice	Must be checked and maintained. May increase pressures in very thin patients. Punctures possible. Patients may complain of nausea due to movement of cells
Pressure redistributing foam mattress	Moderate risk as above	Two-way multi-stretch foam and flexible covers, less expensive than beds	Should be audited 6 monthly for cross-infection risk. Should be placed on meshed mattress board, not solid, and turned monthly
Dynamic air mattress or low air loss bed	Moderate–high-risk patients, Waterlow 15–20	Equalizes pressure and weight and can be programmed to adjust air support to give optimal pressure redistribution. Warm	Expensive to buy, but can be hired. Makes some patients feel 'sea-sick'. Reduces self-motivated movement. Cells can become quite hard
Air fluidized bed	High-risk patients, Waterlow 20, or indicated because of medical condition	As near to levitation as possible! Warm, sterile air produces a beneficial environment for healing wounds. One nurse can manage even a very heavy or debilitated patient on their own. Can be used for incontinent patients or those with heavy wound exudate. May help to alleviate severe pain	Expensive to hire. Need to reinforce floors before it can be installed. Minimizes self-motivation. Can be difficult for the patient to get in and out of bed even with help. Available on hire basis only

It is important to remember the risk of cross-infection with the use of special beds. Most companies provide adequate cleaning/sterilizing of their equipment. Sheepskin is not a pressure-relieving device and can become hard and matted with washing although it has been commended for helping with shearing in the past (Hampton and Collins 2004). See also www.nice.org.uk/page.aspx?o=cg029fullguideline.

Table 4.3 The Norton Scale

Physical condition	Score	Mental condition	Score	Activity	Score	Mobility	Score	Incontinent	Score
Good	4	Alert	4	Ambulant	4	Full	4	Not	4
Fair	3	Apathetic	3	Walk/help	3	Slightly limited	3	Occasionally	3
Poor	2	Confused	2	Chairbound	2	Very limited	2	Usually/urine	2
Very bad	1	Stuporous	1	Bedfast	1	Immobile	1	Doubly	1

Used with permission from Norton *et al.* (1985) and Braden and Bergstrom (1987).

146

	Date (Day/Month/Year)									
	Time									
GENDER	Male	1								
	Female	2								
AGE	14–49	1								
	50–64	2								
	65–74	3								
	75–80	4								
	81+	5								
BUILD	Average	0								
	Above average	1								
	Obese	2								
	Below average	3								
APPETITE (select one option ONLY)	Average	0								
	Poor	1								
	NG Tube/fluids only	2								
	NBM/anorexic	3								
VISUAL ASSESSMENT OF AT RISK SKIN AREA (may select one or more options)	Healthy	0								
	Thin and fragile	1								
	Dry	1								
	Oedematous	1								
	Clammy (Temp↑)	1								
	Previous pressure sore or scarring	2								
	Discoloured	2								
	Broken	3								

Name: _____ Hospital No: _____

Instruction for use:
1. Score on admission and update weekly or if significant change in patient's condition
2. Add scores together and insert total score
3. Document actions taken in the evaluation section
4. If total score is 10+ initiate core care plan At Risk of Pressure Damage/Pressure Ulcer Formation

10+ AT RISK   15+ HIGH RISK   20+ VERY HIGH RISK

Figure 4.3   Waterlow pressure ulcer risk assessment. Adapted from the Waterlow Pressure Sore/Ulcer Risk Assessment Scoring System, available from www.judywaterlow.fsnet.co.uk, with permission and acknowledgement of the copyright holder, J. Waterlow, 1991, revised 1995, 1998 and 2005. (Continued)

MOBILITY (select one option ONLY)	Fully	0							
	Restless/fidgety	1							
	Apathetic	2							
	Restricted	3							
	Inert (due to ↓ consciousness/traction)	4							
	Chairbound	5							
CONTINENCE (select one option ONLY)	Continent/catheterized	0							
	Occasional incontinence	1							
	Incontinent of urine	2							
	Incontinent of faeces	2							
	Doubly incontinent	3							
TISSUE MALNUTRITION (may select one or more options)	Smoking	2							
	Anaemia	2							
	Peripheral vascular disease	5							
	Cardiac failure	5							
	Cachexia	8							
NEUROLOGICAL DEFICIT (score depends on severity)	Diabetes, CVA, MS, motor/sensory paraplegia, epidural	4–6							
MAJOR SURGERY TRAUMA (up to 48 hours post surgery)	Above waist	2							
	Orthopaedic, below waist, spinal, >2 hours on theatre table	5							
MEDICATION	Cytotoxics, high dose steroids, anti-inflammatory	4							
TOTAL SCORE									
NURSE SIGNATURE									

Figure 4.3   (*Continued*)

Braden scale

The Braden scale (Table 4.4) is based on six subscores (sensory perception, activity, moisture, nutrition, mobility, and friction and shearing) which are scored from 1 to 4 depending on the severity of the condition (with the exception of friction and shearing which is scored 1–3). The total score is then added up with a possible range of 6 to 23. The lower the score, the higher the risk of developing a pressure ulcer. Hospital patients are considered to be at risk if their score is 16 or below.

The Braden Scale was originally designed as a pressure ulcer predictor, unlike the Norton and Waterlow Scales which assess risk (Waterlow 2005).

Table 4.4 Braden Scale for predicting pressure sore risk

Sensory perception	1. *Completely limited*	2. *Very limited*	3. *Slightly limited*	4. *No impairment*
Ability to respond meaningfully to pressure related discomfort	Unresponsive (does not moan, flinch or grasp) to painful stimuli, due to diminished level of consciousness or sedation	Responds only to painful stimuli. Cannot communicate discomfort except by moaning or restlessness	Responds to verbal commands, but cannot always communicate discomfort or need to be turned	Responds to verbal commands. Has no sensory deficit that would limit ability to feel or voice pain or discomfort
	or	*or*	*or*	
	limited ability to feel pain over most of body surface	has a sensory impairment that limits the ability to feel pain or discomfort over half of the body	has some sensory impairment that limits ability to feel pain or discomfort in 1 or 2 extremities	
Moisture	1. *Constantly moist*	2. *Very moist*	3. *Occasionally moist*	4. *Rarely moist*
Degree to which skin is exposed to moisture	Skin is kept moist almost constantly by perspiration, urine and so on. Dampness is detected every time patient is moved or turned	Skin is often, but not always moist. Linen must be changed at least once a shift	Skin is occasionally moist, requiring an extra linen change approximately once a day	Skin is usually dry, linen only requires changing at routine intervals
Activity	1. *Bedfast*	2. *Chairfast*	3. *Walks occasionally*	4. *Walks frequently*
Degree of physical activity	Confined to bed	Ability to walk severely limited or non-existent Cannot bear own weight and/or must be assisted into chair or wheelchair	Walks occasionally during day, but for very short distances, with or without assistance. Spends majority of each shift in bed or chair	Walks outside the room at least twice a day and inside room at least once every 2 hours during waking hours
Mobility	1. *Completely immobile*	2. *Very limited*	3. *Slightly limited*	4. *No limitations*
Ability to change and control body position	Does not make even slight changes in body or extremity position without assistance	Makes occasional slight changes in body or extremity position but unable to make frequent or significant changes independently	Makes frequent though slight changes in body or extremity position independently	Makes major and frequent changes in position without assistance
Nutrition	1. *Very poor*	2. *Probably inadequate*	3. *Adequate*	4. *Excellent*
Usual food intake pattern: 1 NBM: nothing by mouth 2 IV: intravenously 3 TPN: total parenteral nutrition	Never eats a complete meal. Rarely eats more than 1/3 of any food offered. Eats 2 servings or less of protein (meat or dairy products) per day. Takes fluids poorly. Does not take a liquid dietary supplement	Rarely eats a complete meal and generally eats only about 1/2 of any food offered. Protein intake includes only 3 servings of meat or dairy products per day. Occasionally will take a dietary supplement	Eats over half of most meals. Eats a total of 4 servings of protein (meats, dairy products) each day. Occasionally will refuse a meal, but will usually take a supplement if offered	Eats most of every meal. Never refuses a meal. Usually eats a total of 4 or more servings of meat and dairy products. Occasionally eats between meals. Does not require supplementation

	or is NBM 1 and/or maintained on clear fluids or IV 2 for more than 5 days	*or* receives less than the optimum amount of liquid diet or tube feeding	*or* is on a tube feeding or TPN 3 regimen that probably meets most of nutritional needs
Friction and shear	**1.** *Problem* Requires moderate to maximum assistance in moving. Complete lifting without sliding against sheets is impossible. Frequently slides down in bed or chair, requiring frequent repositioning with maximum assistance. Spasticity, contractures or agitation lead to almost constant friction	**2.** *Potential problem* Moves feebly or requires minimum assistance. During a move skin probably slides to some extent against sheets, chair, restraints, or other devices. Maintains relatively good position in chair or bed most of the time but occasionally slides down	**3.** *No apparent problem* Moves in bed and in chair independently and has sufficient muscle strength to lift up completely during move. Maintains good position in bed or chair at all times
TOTAL SCORE	Total score of 12 or less represents **high risk**		

Assess	Date	Evaluator/signature/title	Assess	Date	Evaluator/signature/title
1	/ /		3	/ /	
2	/ /		4	/ /	
Name: last, first, middle		Attending physician	ID number		

High risk: total score <12; moderate risk: total score 13–14; low risk: total score 15–16 if under 75 years old or 15–18 if over 75 years old.

Postprocedural considerations

Ongoing care

Treatment of pressure ulcers is the same as for any other wound. The aetiology and underlying or related pathology, as well as the wound itself, must be assessed in order to provide the most appropriate treatment. Care should be aimed at relief of pressure, the minimization of symptoms from predisposing factors and the provision of the ideal microenvironment for wound healing.

When positioning patients, prolonged pressure on bony prominences must be minimized. An awareness of interface pressures, for example creased bedlinen and night clothing, is also important to avoid increased friction and further skin breakdown. Regular repositioning is recommended after assessing other factors such as patient's medical condition, comfort, overall plan of care and the support surface. Where appropriate or possible, patients and their families should be familiarized with the importance of pressure ulcer prevention.

For management see Chapter 19.

Prevention of falls

Related theory

In the UK the average rate of falls in acute hospitals in 2008 was 5.4 incidents per 1000 bed-days (NPSA 2009). This equates to 30 falls per week in an 800-bed acute trust. The physical and psychological costs to the patient and financial costs for the health economy are high. Falls may result in a loss of confidence or independence which, in turn, may lead to a need for increased or extended support from the NHS (Ward *et al.* 2010). Preventing falls in the older person has been well described in national guidance and all prevention programmes should include particular reference to the care of the older person (Age UK 2008, Becker *et al.* 2003, Oliver *et al.* 2007, Ward *et al.* 2010).

The prevention of falls is complex and as with many other types of risk assessment and prevention, a systematic multiprofessional approach is recommended. Individual needs and the different environmental factors associated with different settings – for example, home, care home or hospital – will need to be assessed regularly.

There are many techniques which have been demonstrated to reduce the incidence of falls, including exercise programmes, identification bracelets, alarm systems and risk assessments (Ward *et al.* 2010). Part of the Chief Nursing Officer for England's programme of 'High Impact Actions for Care' includes 'Staying Safe – Preventing Falls' (Ward *et al.* 2010), the aim of which is to demonstrate a year-on-year reduction in the number of falls sustained by older people in NHS-provided care. However, patient safety must always be carefully balanced with patient independence and their right to make informed choices (NHS Institute for Innovation and Improvement 2010). Following on from this, Ipswich Hospital Trust developed a checklist for nurses to use on the wards regularly throughout the day (NHS Institute for Innovation and Improvement 2009).

- Hydration: making sure patients have something to drink.
- Checking toilet needs.
- Ensuring patients have the right footwear.
- Decluttering the area.
- Making sure patients can reach what they need, such as the call bell.
- Making sure bedrails are correctly fitted.
- Ensuring patients have an appropriate walking aid, if applicable.

Key principles of risk management

Related theory

Good risk management awareness and practice at all levels is a critical success factor for any organization. In healthcare it can mean the difference between success and failure, not only in terms of an individual patient clinical outcome but also of the organization as a whole (Roberts 2002).

Nurses have a pivotal role to play in risk management and promoting safety and, indeed, a moral obligation to protect those we serve and to provide the best possible care (Wilson 2005).

Nurses are not only the main caregivers in wards and departments but also have a surveillance role, ensuring that they remain vigilant and able to identify risks which may adversely affect the patient experience. When discussing the vigilant nurse, Meyer and Lavin (2005) suggest five components, which are key in the role of the nurse.

- *Attaching meaning to what is*: this is described as the ability to differentiate 'adverse signals', which indicate that there are dangers, from the ordinary 'noise', the normal signs and symptoms.
- *Anticipating what might be*: observe, as the normal procedures and response are described so the abnormal becomes more apparent.

- *Calculating risks*: understanding that there is an inherent risk in every situation.
- *Readiness to act*: developed from a knowledge base, this allows the nurse to know what might be required in a situation and to make sure interventions can be carried out quickly when necessary.
- *Monitoring* the results of interventions.

Patients want to be assured that nurses have the ability to assess their needs as well as recognize their limitations and potential risks. With this comes the need for the nurse to have knowledge of risk and how it works within the organization. Understanding the policies, processes and procedures for managing risk is then a key component of ongoing learning for all nurses and healthcare professionals.

References

Age UK (2008) *Ways to Make Tasks Easier Around the Home.* England.

Alaszewski, A. (2002) The Impact of the Bristol Royal Infirmary disaster and inquiry on public services in the UK. *Journal of Interprofessional Care,* 16, 371–378.

Anthony, D., Parbooteeah, S., Saleh, M. and Papanikolou, P. (2008) Norton Waterlow and Braden Score: a review of the literature and a comparison between scores and clinical judgement. *Journal of Clinical Nursing,* 17 (5), 646–653.

Becker, C., Kron, M., Lindemann, U. *et al.* (2003) Effectiveness of a multifaceted intervention on falls in nursing home residents. *Journal of the American Geriatrics Society,* 51 (3), 306–313.

Beldon, P. (2006) Topical negative pressure dressings and vacuum-assisted closure. *Wound Essentials,* 1, 110–114.

Benbow, M. (2006) An update on VAC therapy. *Journal of Community Nursing,* 20 (4), 28–32.

Bennett, G., Dealey, C. and Posnett, J. (2004) The cost of pressure ulcers in the UK. *Age and Aging,* 33 (3), 230–235.

Berta, W., Teare, G., Gilbart, E. *et al.* (2005) The contingencies of organizational learning in long-term care: factors that affect innovation adoption. *Health Care Management Review,* 30, 282–292.

Birtwistle, J. (1994) Pressure sore formation and risk assessment in intensive care. *Care of the Critically Ill,* 10 (4), 154–155, 157–159.

Braden, B.J. and Bergstrom, N. (1987) A conceptual schema for the study of aetiology of pressure sores. *Rehabilitation Nursing,* 12 (1), 8–12.

Bridel-Nixon, J. (1999) Pressure sores, in *Nursing Management of Chronic Wounds,* 2nd edn (eds M. Morison, C. Moffatt, J. Bridel-Nixon and S. Bale). Mosby, London.

Carthey, J. (2005) Being Open With Patients and Their Carers Following Patient Safety Incidents. Clinical Governance Bulletin, 5.5. National Patient Safety Agency, London.

Chaplin, J. (2000) Pressure sore risk assessment in palliative care. *Journal of Tissue Viability,* 10 (1), 27–31.

Clay, M. (2000) Pressure sore prevention in nursing homes. *Nursing Standard,* 14 (44), 45–50.

Collier, M. (1999) Pressure ulcer development and principles for prevention, in *Wound Management: Theory and Practice* (eds M. Miller and D. Glover). Nursing Times Books, London.

CQC (2009) *Mental Health Act Commission 13th Biannual Report 2007–2009: Coercion and Consent.* Care Quality Commission, London.

Davies, H., Nutley, S. and Mannion, R. (2000) Organisational culture and quality of health care. *Quality in Health Care*, **9**, 111–119.

DH (1998) *A First Class Service. Quality in the New NHS.* Department of Health, London.

DH (1999) HSC 1999/123. Governance in the new NHS. Controls Assurance Statements 1999/2000. Risk Management and Organizational Controls. Department of Health, London.

DH (2000) *An Organization with a Memory.* Department of Health, London.

DH (2001) *Building a Safer NHS for Patients.* Department of Health, London.

DH (2007) *The Future Regulation of Health and Adult Social Care in England. Response to Consultation.* Department of Health, London.

DH (2008) *High Quality Care For All: NHS Next Stage Review Final Report.* Department of Health, London.

Dolan, S. and Fitch, M. (2007) The management of venous thromboembolism in cancer patients. *British Journal of Nursing*, **16** (21), 1308–1312.

EPUAP (2003) Pressure Ulcer Prevention Guidelines. www.epuap.org.uk.

Flynn, R. (2002) Clinical governance and governmentality. *Health, Risk and Society*, **4**, 155–173.

Francis, R. (2010) Mid-Staffordshire NHS Foundation Trust Inquiry (2005–2009). Independent Inquiry into Care Provided by Mid Staffordshire NHS Foundation Trust. HC375-1 2009/10. Department of Health, London.

Guyton, A.C. and Hall, J.E. (2000) *Textbook of Medical Physiology*, 10th edn. W.B. Saunders, Philadelphia.

Hampton, S. and Collins, F. (2004) *Tissue Viability: The Prevention, Treatment and Management of Wounds.* Whurr, London.

Health and Safety Executive (2010) Guidance on risk management. www.hse.gov.uk/risk/theory/alarpglance.htm.

Healthcare Commission (2009) Investigation into Mid Staffordshire Foundation Trust. Healthcare Commission, London.

Hess, C.T. (2005) Pressure ulcers, in *Wound Care Clinical Guide*, 5th edn. Lippincott, Williams and Wilkins, Philadelphia, pp.79–93.

Heyman, B, Shaw, M., Alaszewski, A. and Titterton, M. (2010) *Risk, Safety, and Clinical Practice. Health Care Through the Lens of Risk.* Oxford University Press, Oxford.

Hopkinson, M. and Hopkinson, J.B. (2001) Risk management in the NHS: adapting risk management techniques for the commercial world. *Healthcare Risk Report*, **7** (2), 19–20.

House of Commons Health Select Committee (2005) Health Committee Report on the Prevention of Venous Thromboembolism in Hospitalised Patients. www.publications.parliament.uk/pa/cm200405/cmselect/cmhealth/99/9902.html.

Hutter, B.M. (2006) Risk, regulation, and management, in *Risk In Social Science* (eds P. Taylor-Gooby and J. Zinn). Oxford University Press, Oxford.

Johnson, A. (1989) Granuflex wafers as a prophylactic pressure sore dressing. *Care: Science and Practice*, **7** (2), 55–58.

Landis, E.M. (1930) Micro-injection studies of capillary blood pressure in human skin. *Heart*, **15**, 209–228.

Lechler, E., Schramm, W. and Flobach, W. (2006) The venous thrombotic risk in non-surgical patients: epidemiological data and efficacy/safety profile of a low molecular weight heparin (enoxaparin). *Haemostasis*, 26, 49–56.

Lindgren, M., Unosson, M., Krantz, A.N. *et al.* (2002) A risk assessment scale for the prediction of pressure sore development, reliability and validity. *Journal of Advanced Nursing*, 38 (2), 190–199.

Macrea, C. (2008) Learning from patient safety incidents: creating participative risk regulation in healthcare. *Health, Risk and Society*, **10** (1) 53–67.

Meurier, C. (2000) Understanding the nature of errors in nursing: using a model to analyse critical incident reports of errors, which had resulted in an adverse or potentially adverse event. *Journal of Advanced Nursing*, **32**, 202–207.

Meyer, G. and Lavin, M.A. (2005) Vigilance: the essence of nursing. www.nursingworld.org/ojin/topic22/tpc22.6htm.

National Clinical Guidelines Centre (2009) *Venous Thromboembolism: Reducing the Risk of Venous Thromboembolism (Deep Vein Thrombosis and Pulmonary Embolism) in Patients Admitted to Hospital.* National Clinical Guidelines Centre, London.

NHS Institute for Innovation and Improvement (2009) *Staying Safe – Preventing Falls.* www.institute.nhs.uk/building_capability/hia_supporting_info/staying_safe_preventing_falls.html.

NHS Institute for Innovation and Improvement (2010) Your Skin Matters. Extract from literature review – High Impact Actions for Nurses and Midwives. NHS Institute for Innovation and Improvement, London.

NICE (2003) Pressure Ulcer Risk Assessment and Prevention. National Institute for Health and Clinical Excellence, London. www.nice.org.uk.

NICE (2005) *Pressure Ulcer Management.* CG 29. National Institute for Health and Clinical Excellence, London.

NICE (2007) *Venous Thromboembolism: Reducing the Risk of Thromboembolism (Deep Vein Thrombosis and Pulmonary Embolism) with Inpatients Undergoing Surgery.* CG46. National Institute for Health and Clinical Excellence, London.

NICE (2010) *Quality Standards Programme: Quality Standard for Venous Thromboembolism (VTE) Prevention.* National Institute for Health and Clinical Excellence, London.

NMC (2008) *The Code: Standards of Conduct, Performance and Ethics for Nurses and Midwives.* Nursing and Midwifery Council, London.

Norton, D., McLaren, R. and Exton-Smith, A. (1985) *An Investigation of Geriatric Nursing Problems in Hospital.* Churchill Livingstone, Edinburgh.

NPSA (2005) Being Open When Patients Are Harmed. National Patient Safety Agency, London.

NPSA (2007) *Healthcare Risk Assessment Made Easy.* National Patient Safety Agency, London.

NPSA (2009) Never Events Framework 2009/10. National Patient Safety Agency, London.

NPSA (2009) The Organization Patient Safety Incident Reports. National Patient Safety Agency, London.

NPSA (2010) *National Reporting and Learning Service: Learning from Patient Safety Incidents* National Patient Safety Agency, London.

Nursing Executive Centre (2009) *Pressure ulcer prevention best practice: bedside report.* Advisory Board Company, Washington DC.

Oliver, D., Connelly, J., Victor, C. *et al.* (2007) Strategies to prevent falls and fractures in hospitals and care homes and effect of cognitive impairment: systematic review and meta-analyses. *BMJ*, **324**, 82.

Philips, L. and Buttery, J. (2009) Exploring pressure ulcer prevention and preventative care. *Nursing Times,* 105 (16), 34–36.

Power, M. (2007) *Organized Uncertainty: Designing a World of Risk Management.* Oxford University Press, Oxford.

RCN (2005) The Management of Pressure Ulcers in Primary and Secondary Care: A Clinical Practice Guideline. www.nice.org.uk/page.aspx?o=cg029fullguideline.

Reason, J. (2006) Resisting cultural change, in *Clinical Governance in a Changing NHS* (eds M. Lugon and J. Secker-Walker). Royal Society of Medicine Press, London.

Roberts, G. (2002) *Risk Management in Healthcare.* Witherby and Co, London.

Roderick, P., Ferris, G., Wilson, K. et al. (2005) Towards evidence-based guidelines for the prevention of venous thromboembolism: systematic reviews of mechanical methods, oral anticoagulation, dextran and regional anaesthesia as thromboprophylaxis. Health Technology Assessment, 9 (49), 1–78.

Shaw, M., Heyman, B., Reynolds, L. *et al.* (2007) Multi-disciplinary teamwork in a UK regional secure mental health unit: a matter for negotiation? *Social Theory and Health,* 5, 356–375.

Simpson, A., Bowers, K. and Weir-Hughes, D. (1996) *Clinical Care: Pressure Sore Prevention.* Whurr, London.

Smith, K.P., Zardiackas, L.D. and Didlake, R.H. (1986) Cortisone, vitamin A and wound healing: the importance of measuring wound surface area. *Journal of Surgical Research*, 40 (2), 49–52.

Southgate, L. and Dauphinee, D. (1998) Maintaining standards in British and Canadian medicine: the developing role of the regulatory body. *BMJ,* **316,** 697–700.

Standards Australia and Standards New Zealand (2009). *Risk management principles and guidelines. ISO 31000.* International Organization for Standardization. www.iso.org

Tong, A. (1999) Back to basics wound care. *Nursing Times,* **1** (1), 20–23.

Tortora, G.J. and Grabowski, S.R. (2008) *Principles of Anatomy and Physiology,* 12th edn. John Wiley, Chichester.

Vincent, C. (2006) *Patient Safety.* Elsevier, London.

Ward, L., Fenton, K. and Maher, D. (2010) The high impact actions for nursing and midwifery 3: staying safe, preventing falls. *Nursing Times,* **106** (29), 12–13.

Waterlow, J. (1988) Prevention is cheaper than cure. *Nursing Times,* 84 (25), 69–70.

Waterlow, J. (1991) A policy that protects. *Professional Nurse,* **6** (5), 258–264.

Waterlow, J. (1998) The treatment and use of the Waterlow card. *Nursing Times,* **94** (7), 63–67.

Waterlow, J. (2005) From costly treatment to cost-effective prevention: using Waterlow. *Wound Care,* **10** (9 Suppl), S25–S30.

Weick, K. and Sutcliffe, K. (2003) Hospitals as cultures of entrapment: a re-analysis of the Bristol Royal Infirmary. *California Management Review,* **45,** 73–84.

Wilson, C. (2005) Said another way: my definition of nursing. *Nurse Forum,* **40** (3), 116–118.

Wilson, E. (2007) Preventing deaths from VTE in hospital 2: thromboprophylaxis. *Nursing Times* 103 (38), 26.

WHO (2005) World Alliance for Patient Safety: WHO draft guidance for adverse event reporting and learning systems. WHO Production Services, Geneva, Switzerland.

152

Supporting the patient with human functioning

Part two

Communication

The Royal Marsden Hospital Manual of Clinical Nursing Procedures, Eighth Edition. Edited by Lisa Dougherty and Sara Lister.
© 2011 The Royal Marsden Hospital. Published 2011 by Blackwell Publishing Ltd.

Overview

The aim of this chapter is to define and describe effective communication.

It will consider the process of offering psychological support to patients and focus upon the management of factors that contribute to or compromise this process. The medium of communication can take many forms; this chapter is mostly concerned with interpersonal communication using language comprising verbal (including tone) and non-verbal expression.

There are specific sections on denial and collusion, anxiety, depression, anger management, delirium and finally, assisting those with sensory impairment to communicate, including a section on surgical voice restoration.

Communication

Definition

Communication is a universal word with many definitions, many of which describe it as a transfer of information between a source and a receiver (Kennedy Sheldon 2009). In nursing, this communication is primarily interpersonal: the process by which information, meanings and feelings are shared through the exchange of verbal and non-verbal messages between two or more people (Brooks and Heath 1993, Wilkinson 1991).

Anatomy and physiology

Physiologically being able to produce speech and to hear are the two dominant physical processes in respect of communication.

The human voice is produced by exhaled air vibrating the vocal cords in the larynx to set up sound waves in the column of air in the pharynx, nose and mouth. Pitch is controlled by the tension on the vocal cords: the tighter they are, the more they vibrate and the higher the pitch. The sounds produced are amplified by the physical spaces of the pharynx and nose and modified by the lips, tongue and jaw into recognizable speech. The muscles of the face, tongue and lips help us to enunciate words (Tortora and Derrickson 2009) (Figure 5.1).

The ear contains receptors for sound waves and the external or outer ear is designed to collect them and direct them inward. As the waves strike the tympanic membrane, it vibrates due to the alternate compression and decompression of the air. This vibration is passed on through the malleus, incus and stapes of the middle ear. As the stapes vibrates, it pushes the oval window. The movement of the oval window sets up waves in the perilymph of the cochlea that ultimately lead to the generation of nerve impulses that travel to the auditory area of the cerebral cortex (Tortora and Derrickson 2009) (Figure 5.2).

The physiological process of communication is, however, much greater than just speech and hearing. The central nervous system is central to both verbal and non-verbal communication. Not only does it continually receive information but it also selects that which is important to respond to, so that overstimulation is avoided. Communication issues may arise if any of these processes are altered.

Related theory

There are many theories about interpersonal communication and nurses are encouraged to consider Heron's (2001) Six Category Intervention Analysis (Box 5.1) to reflect upon their own and other health professionals' communication. The main aim is to support and maintain the patient's optimum level of communication while remaining aware of the impact of their disease and its management on the patient's ability and/or motivation to speak. We need to be aware of different coping styles and attitudes of the patient and key people in their lives, other co-morbidities, disease progression, fluctuating cognitive abilities and treatment side-effects. All these factors demand a flexible approach when supporting communication throughout the length of the patient pathway (White 2004).

Non-verbally, people communicate via gestures, body language, posture, facial expression, clothing, furniture, touch, music and art. Communication can be heavily

---

Box 5.1 Heron's six category intervention analysis (2001)

Authoritative

1 *Prescriptive.* A prescriptive intervention seeks to direct the behaviour of the client, usually behaviour that is outside the practitioner–client relationship.
2 *Informative.* An informative intervention seeks to impart knowledge, information and meaning to the client.
3 *Confronting.* A confronting intervention seeks to raise the consciousness of the client about some limiting attitude or behaviour of which he is relatively unaware.

Facilitative

4 *Cathartic.* A cathartic intervention seeks to enable the client to discharge or abreact painful emotion, primarily grief, fear and anger.
5 *Catalytic.* A catalytic intervention seeks to encourage self-discovery, self- directed learning, living and problem solving in the client.
6 *Supportive.* A supportive intervention seeks to affirm the worth and value of the client's person, qualities, attitudes or actions.

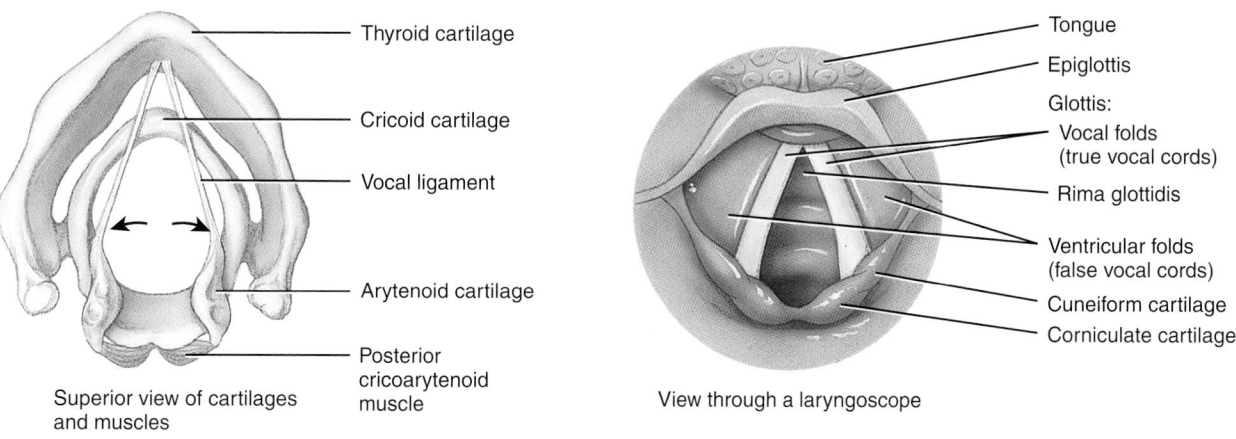

Superior view of cartilages and muscles

View through a laryngoscope

(a) Movement of vocal folds apart (abduction)

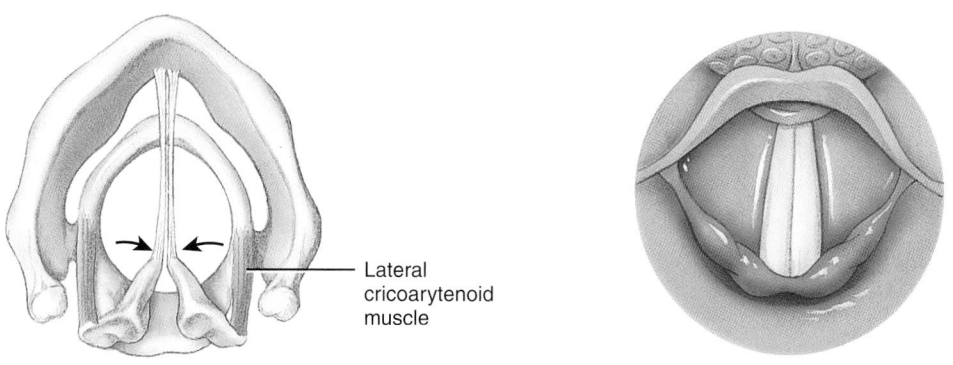

(b) Movement of vocal folds together (adduction)

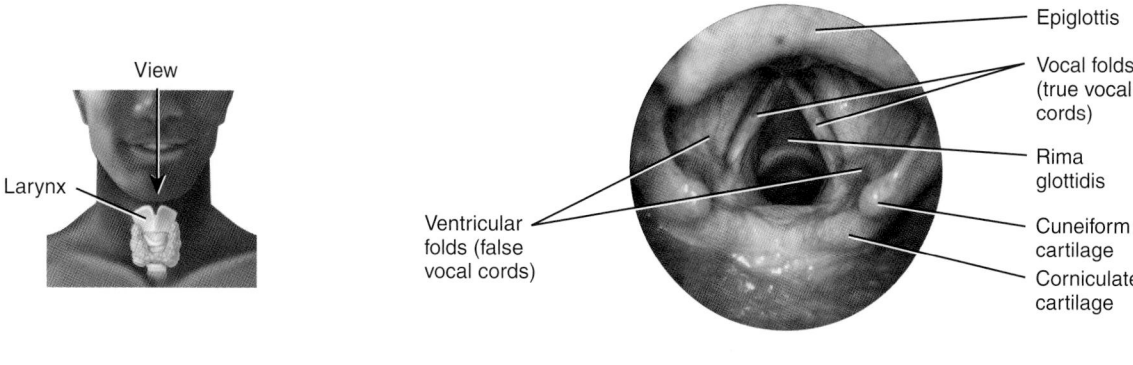

(c) Superior view

Figure 5.1 Movement of the vocal cords. Reproduced from Tortora and Derrickson (2009).

influenced by a multitude of external and internal factors, for example illness, culture, class, self-esteem, immediate environment, gender, status, mood, depression, and the influence of these factors needs to be carefully considered in each circumstance. All patients and relatives should be assessed for their psychological needs and tailored support offered to meet individual needs.

Evidence-based approaches

'Effective communication is widely regarded to be a key determinant of patient satisfaction, compliance and recovery' (Chant *et al.* 2002, p.13), yet poor communication is one of the most common causes of complaints in healthcare (Cambell 2006). Supportive communication is

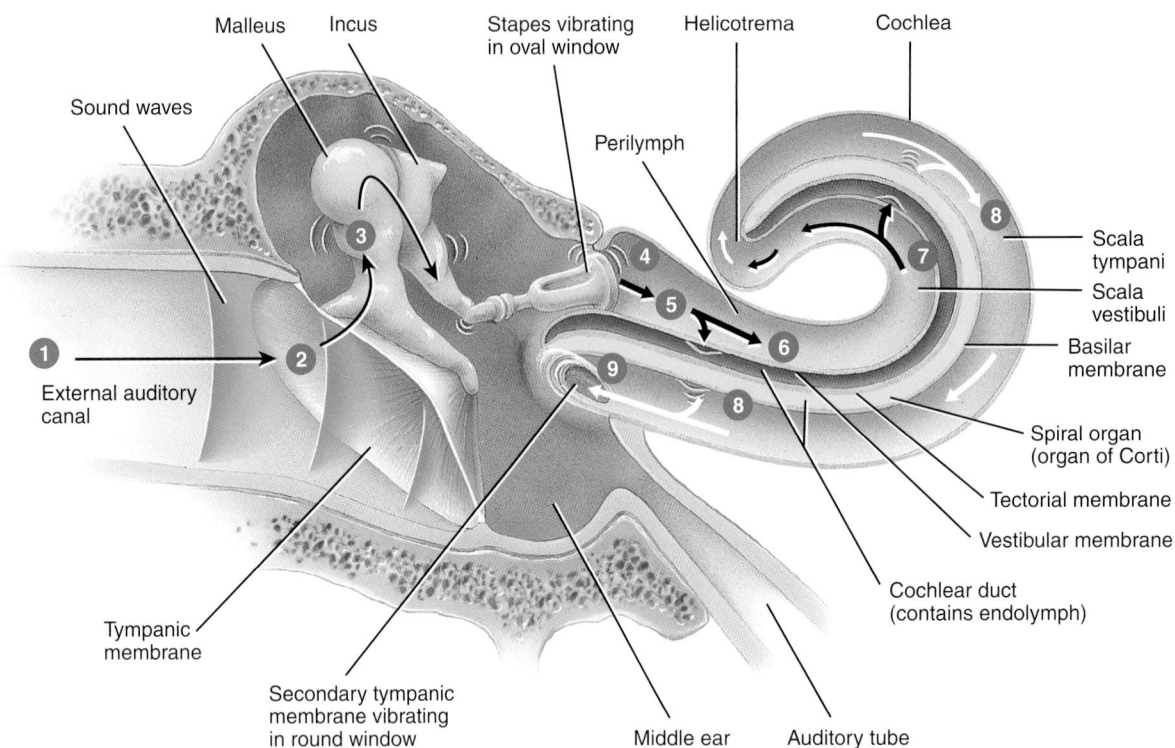

Figure 5.2 Events in the stimulation of auditory receptors in the right ear. Reproduced from Tortora and Derrickson (2009).

important to create an environment where the individual patient feels heard and understood and can be helped appropriately. Communication needs to be highly flexible – dependent upon cultural, social and environmental factors. Nurses need to communicate effectively with patients in order to deliver individualized safe care and treatment and to manage psychosocial concerns appropriately. People with illness want to be approached with a 'caring and humane attitude' that respects their privacy and dignity (Maben and Griffiths 2008). Patients want their personal values to be respected and to be treated as equals by health professionals. This can be achieved by taking the time to communicate, not controlling dialogue, listening and offering emotional support (Smith *et al.* 2005) and by striving for open, clear and honest communication (Baile *et al.* 2000, Heyland *et al.* 2006, Jenkins *et al.* 2001, Smith *et al.* 2005). The patient's dignity can be promoted by enabling the expression of concerns in a safe environment.

Patients want to be able to experience a meaningful connection and a sense of 'being known' by the staff they encounter (Thorne *et al.* 2005). Nurses need to be able to accurately assess how much patients want to share their thoughts and feelings without assuming that they either do or do not wish to. Communication occurs in a time-pressured environment. Practical and technical tasks demand the nurse's time and tend to be prioritized above psychological support. The resulting

communication may be limited and prevent effective exploration of psychological care issues. Without effective exploration, patients are not sufficiently encouraged to engage with and manage their own care. Nurses need to be aware of and consider what other features of the environment contribute to the nature of the dialogue that takes place, for example the wearing of uniform (Edwards 2005, Hargie and Dickson 2004). Patients may not expect to discuss psychosocial issues with nurses because of the communication bias toward physical and medical issues. The task-orientated short communication encounters that emerge do not encourage the disclosure of psychosocial concerns (Silverman *et al.* 2005).

Patient satisfaction is not necessarily related to the acquisition of specific communication skills (Thorne *et al.* 2005) but staff still need to be able to enquire about the nature and manner of support that patients wish for (so that satisfaction can be achieved wherever possible).

Listening and appropriate verbal responses that demonstrate empathy remain the key skills; if nothing else is achieved, adopting these qualities will be beneficial to patients and be a valuable use of time.

Listening

Listening is a skill often assumed to be natural. Rarely would we consider that we were physically unable to listen

> **Box 5.2** How to let someone know you are listening to them
>
> - Non-verbal encouragement.
> - Verbal characteristics.
> - Questioning.
> - Paraphrasing.
> - Clarifying.
> - Summarizing.
> - Empathy.

and perhaps this makes us pay little attention to this crucial skill area (Box 5.2).

The physical act of hearing is distinct from that of 'listening'. Hearing can be considered to be passive, but listening requires active processing and the attachment of meaning.

It might be difficult for us to answer the question 'How do we listen?' and perhaps a procedure of 'how to listen' would not do justice to the sophistication and success of good listeners. However, there are ways of describing the constituent parts of listening that, if followed, would make the person speaking appreciate that they were being listened to.

Problems can emerge as two people may interpret the meaning of the same dialogue differently. For example, if you have asked the question, 'How are you?' and the patient replies 'Getting by', do you assume they are doing well and coping or that this means they are struggling and 'putting on a brave face'?

Hopefully, you will be attending to numerous non-verbal cues to decipher what the patient actually means. If there is a suggestion of 'incongruence', where the patient says 'Getting by' in a low and sad-sounding voice, coupled with a simultaneous lowering of the head, we might consider the latter assumption. Alternatively, if the patient sounds upbeat and looks you in the face with a smile you might be reassured they mean the former.

There are strategies to promote successful listening, for example 'summarizing' and 'clarifying' (at suitable moments) what the patient is saying.

Non-verbal responses

Non-verbal communication generally indicates information transmitted without speaking. Included in this would be the way you sit or stand, facial expression, gestures and posture, whether you nod or smile and the clothes worn: all will have an impact on the total communication taking place (Hargie and Dickson 2004).

Egan (2002) usefully describes the acronym SOLER to summarize the constituent elements of non-verbal communication: facing the patient **Squarely**; maintaining an **Open** posture; **Leaning** slightly towards the patient to convey interest; having appropriate **Eye** contact, not staring nor

avoiding (cultural dimension needs to be considered with this); and being **Relaxed**. By learning an awareness of these factors and making this behaviour part of your normal demeanour, patients will be encouraged to talk more openly, facilitating emotional disclosure.

Saying nothing says something, so there is always communication however reluctant you or the patient are.

It can be argued that non-verbal information is more powerful than verbal information, for example in the case of 'incongruence' where the verbal message indicates one thing and the non-verbal suggests another. There is a tendency to believe the non-verbal message over the verbal in these instances.

This highlights the need to communicate with genuine compassion. Without this, supportive communication can be severely reduced in its effectiveness.

Non-verbal communication becomes even more important in the case of people whose verbal communication is impaired, for example by stroke, trauma or surgery. Patients need to be supported, ensuring, for example, that they have constant access to pen and paper; communication boards can be used to good effect and it is worth considering the use of information technology and communication software, if available. The experience of losing the ability to speak can be very isolating and frustrating and preparation of the patient and practice with communication aids is important to maximize the success of communication. It is essential that people with a speech deficit are given more time to communicate their needs, and we must be patient and persist with interaction until a satisfactory level of understanding is gained.

We can use non-verbal behaviour to encourage patients to talk by nodding/making affirming noises, for example 'Hmmm'. This 'affirming' is mostly done naturally, for example at points of eye contact, as specific points are made and during slight pauses in dialogue. It can be especially important to affirm when the patient is talking about psychological or emotional issues as they will need you to validate that this is an acceptable topic of conversation.

Verbal responses

The way things are said makes a big difference, so attention needs to be paid to the tone, rate and depth of speech. This means sounding alert, interested and caring, but not patronizing. Speech should be delivered at an even rate: not too fast or too slow (unless presenting difficult or complex information).

Questioning

One skill that needs to be used in close collaboration with listening is that of questioning. When specific information is required, for example in a crisis, closed questions are indicated. Closed questions narrow the potential answer (Silverman *et al.* 2005) and allow the gathering of specific information for a purpose. Closed questions therefore are ones which are likely to generate a short 'yes or no' answer, for example 'Are you all right?'.

In care situations with significant life-changing implications, however, a broader assessment of the patient's perspective is required and there is a need to show compassion and support psychosocial issues. Open questions and listening are therefore required. Open questions do the opposite of closed questions; they broaden the potential answer (Silverman *et al.* 2005) and hand the initiative and agenda over to the patient. So instead of asking 'Are you all right?', ask 'How are you today?' or 'What has your experience of treatment been like?'.

It is good to include a psychological focus to make it clear that this is part of what you are interested in; for example, 'How did that make you feel?' or 'What are your main concerns?'.

Open questions cannot be used in isolation as the opportunity for open discussion can easily be blocked by failing to ensure that the rest of the fundamental communication elements are in place. Attention must therefore be paid to protecting sufficient time, verbal space (not interrupting) and encouragement (in the form of nonverbal cues, paraphrasing, clarifying and summarizing), so that the patient and/or relative can express their feelings and concerns.

Open questions may not be appropriate with people who have a communication problem, perhaps following head and neck surgery or where complex communication is going to be difficult, as for those whose first language is not English.

Try to use one question at a time: it is easy to ask more than one question in a sentence and this can make it unclear where your focus is and lead the patient to answer only one part of your question.

Open questions can also be helpful to respond to cues that the patient may give as to their underlying psychological state. Cues can be varied, numerous and difficult to define, but essentially these are either verbal or non-verbal hints of underlying unease or worry. Concerns may be easier to recognize where they are expressed verbally and unambiguously (del Piccolo *et al.* 2006).

Reflecting back

You can repeat the same words back to the patient: this signals that their focus is a legitimate topic for discussion (Perry and Burgess 2002), but if this technique is overused it can sound unnatural (Silverman *et al.* 2005).

When it is used, it needs to be done with thought and include 'something of you in your response' (Egan 2002, p.97), meaning that you remain alert and caring.

Paraphrasing

This technique involves telling the patient what they have told you but using different words that retain the same meaning; for example:

Patient: I need to talk to them but whenever they start to talk to me about the future, I just start to get wound up and shut down.

Nurse: So when your family try to talk, you get tense and you stop talking ….

Clarifying

The aim of this technique is to reduce ambiguity and help the patient define and explore the central or pivotal aspect of issues raised. Many of us may be reluctant to explore emotional or psychological issues too much, just in case the issues raised are too emotional and hard to deal with (Perry and Burgess 2002). However, if the principles of good communication are applied and a focus on the patient's agenda is maintained, distressing and difficult situations can be moved forward positively.

The use of open questions is likely to raise certain issues that would benefit from further exploration. Clarification encourages the expression of detail and context to situations, helping to draw out pertinent matters, perhaps not previously considered by either patient or health professional. A mixture of open or closed questions can be used in clarification (Box 5.3).

It might be necessary for you to clarify your own position too, perhaps acknowledge that you don't know something and cannot answer certain questions, for example 'Will the treatment work?'.

Sometimes not knowing can be a valuable position, enabling you to seek out the patient's experience and not just assume it. Our experience might be relevant, but each patient and relative will require the opportunity to tell it in their words and to feel 'heard'.

Summarizing

This intervention can be used as a way of opening or closing dialogue. An opening can be facilitated by recapping a previous discussion or outlining your understanding of the patient's position. Summarizing can be used to punctuate a longer conversation and highlight specific issues raised.

Box 5.3 Open and closed questions

- Are you feeling like that now? (closed)
- You seem to be down today, am I right? (closed)
- Can you describe how the experience made you feel? (closed)
- You say that you've not had enough information: can you tell me what you do know? (open)
- You mention that you are struggling: what kinds of things do you struggle with? (open)
- You say it's been hard getting this far: what has been the hardest thing to cope with? (open)

This serves several purposes.

- It informs your patient that you have listened and understood their position.
- It allows the patient to correct any mistakes or misconceptions generated.
- It brings the conversation from the specific to the general (which can help to contextualize issues).
- It gives an opportunity for agreement to be reached about what may need to happen.

Examples of summarizing:

> It sounds like you are tired and are struggling to manage the treatment schedule. It also sounds like you don't have enough information and we could support you more with that …

Summarizing can be a useful opportunity to plan and agree what actions are necessary. Avoid getting caught up with planning, though: the important issue is that you have listened and understood. In our nursing role, we are familiar with 'doing' and correcting problematic situations and although interventions can be helpful in psychosocial issues, sometimes it is necessary not to act and to just 'be' with the patient, accepting their experience as it is, however emotionally painful.

Recognizing when to act and when to sit with distress can be difficult. However, it is important for us to develop this awareness and to accept that sometimes there are no solutions to difficult situations. The temptation to always correct problems might only serve to negate the patient's experience of being listened to.

Empathy

Sharing time and physical space with other people demands the development of a relationship. In nursing, the relationship with patients is defined by many factors, for example physical and medical care. In clinical roles it might be possible to be emotionally detached and to exist behind a 'professional mask' (Taylor 1998, p.74) but when working in a supportive role, a shared experience and bond are generated, inclusive of feelings.

Recognizing our own feelings is important to allow us to understand and to 'tolerate another person's pain' (McKenzie 2002, p.34). Nurses demonstrate empathy when there is a 'desire to understand the client (patient) as fully as possible and to communicate this understanding' (Egan 2002, p.97).

This means attempting to understand what the patient might be going through, taking into consideration their physical, social and psychological environment. This inferred information can be used to 'connect' with the patient, all the time checking that our interpretation of their experience is accurate (we can be wrong even if we have experienced similar things).

Rogers (1975, p.2) seminally described the skill of empathy as: 'The ability to experience another person's world as if it were one's own, without losing the "as if" quality'. That means allowing ourselves to get into the patient's shoes and experience some of what they might be experiencing, without allowing ourselves to enter the experience wholly (it isn't our experience). Empathy allows for an opportunity to 'taste' and therefore attempt to understand the patient's perspective. Understanding emotions and behaviours in this way encourages an acceptance and positive negotiation of them. Maintaining the 'as if' quality protects us from adopting too great an emotional load. Having too much of a sense of loss or sorrow may prevent us from offering effective support, as we are drawn to focus on our own feelings more than is necessary or helpful (for ourselves or the patient).

Empathy may not always come easily, especially if a patient is angry. What can be very useful in the development and use of empathy is the ability to step back from the situation and reflect upon what it is that you, as the nurse, feel and how this relates to what is happening for the patient.

Barriers to effective communication

Poor communication with patients can negatively affect decision making and quality of life (Fallowfield *et al.* 2001, Thorne *et al.* 2005).

The environmental conditions in which nurses work, with competing professional demands and time pressures, can reduce the capacity to form effective relationships with patients (Henderson *et al.* 2007).

There is a personal, emotional impact when providing a supportive role for patients with psychological and emotional issues (Botti *et al.* 2006, Dunne 2003, Turner *et al.* 2007) and it is therefore likely that blocking or avoidance of patients' emotional concerns relates to emotional self-preservation for the nurse.

When communicating and assessing patient's needs, nurses may be anxious about eliciting distress and managing expressed concerns. They may lack confidence in their ability to clarify patients' feelings without 'causing harm to the patient or getting into difficulty themselves' (Booth *et al.* 1996, p.526). As a consequence, nurses can make assumptions, rather than assessing concerns properly (Booth *et al.* 1996, Kelsey 2005, Roberts and Snowball 1999, Schofield *et al.* 2008). To illustrate this point, Kruijver *et al.* (2001) demonstrated how nurses verbally focus upon physical issues, which accounted for 60% of communication with patients. Nurses often recognize this bias and suggest that they feel greater competence discussing physical rather than psychological issues and seek better skills to help them to manage challenging situations (McCaughan and Parahoo 2000). Being supported practically and emotionally by supervisors and/or senior staff can be seen to decrease blocking behaviours (Booth *et al.* 1996). Clinical supervision can aid the transfer of communication skills into practice (Heaven *et al.* 2006).

Institutions, work environments and the nature of the senior staff within them can influence the nature of communication (Booth *et al.* 1996, Chant *et al.* 2002, McCabe 2004, Menzies-Lyth 1988, Wilkinson 1991). Nurses may improve their own practice by identifying where environmental barriers lie and attempting to mitigate the features of the clinical environment that inhibit psychological care.

Despite the difficulties outlined, it has been argued that nurses can communicate well when they are facilitated to provide individual patient-focused care (McCabe 2004).

Legal and professional issues

Effective communication is central to a number of explicit standards of *The Code* (NMC 2008a) (see Appendix 1).

Make the care of people your first concern, treating them as individuals and respecting their dignity.

- You must listen to the people in your care and respond to their concerns and preferences.
- You must make arrangements to meet people's language and communication needs.
- You must share with people, in a way they can understand, the information they want or need to know about their health.
- You must uphold people's rights to be fully involved in their care.

There are four essential features of maintaining dignity in communication.

1 *Attitude*. Being aware of the other person's experience, our attitudes towards them and how this affects the care provided.
2 *Behaviour*. Being respectful and kind, asking permission, giving your full attention and using understandable language.
3 *Compassion*. Being aware of and in touch with our own feelings and 'acknowledging the person beyond their illness' (Chochinov 2007, p.186).
4 *Dialogue*. Being able to demonstrate an appropriate knowledge of the patient's history, experience and family context. You might usefully make educated guesses about the likely experiences of the patient, for example 'It must have been difficult to have received the news at that point in your life'.

The Code also makes explicit the responsibility to be aware of the legislation regarding mental capacity, a factor that can have a significant impact on communication. The Mental Capacity Act (2005) sets out guidance. Firstly, always presume people have mental capacity unless they:

- are unable to understand information given to them to make choices
- can understand but are unable to retain the information
- are unable to weigh up and relate the information accurately to their situation

- are unable to communicate their wishes or choices (by any means).

(BMA 2007)

If any of these factors are in question, the Mental Capacity Act (2005) recommends that determining an individual's decision-making capacity is best achieved through multi-disciplinary assessment. A separate assessment of capacity must take place for every decision involving the individual. Brady Wagner (2003) specifies four key areas that need to be fulfilled in order to have the capacity to make a decision.

1 Understanding the diagnosis and other information given regarding treatment and non-treatment options.
2 Manipulating those options and consequences in relation to one's personal values and goals.
3 Reasoning through a decision.
4 Communicating the preference/decision.

The mental capacity of an individual needs to be considered in any communication but particularly if it involves the patient making a decision about treatment or care options and in respect of consent. At any time before making any referral for further support, it is important that the patient fully understands and consents.

The Equality Act (2010) reinforces the duty to ensure that everybody, irrespective of their disability, sex, gender, race, ethnic origin, age, relationship status, religion or faith, has equal access to information and is communicated with equitably. This means, for example, that provision is necessary to meet the information needs of blind and partially sighted people (Section 21 of the Disability Discrimination Act, October 1999).

People from black and minority ethnic (BME) groups constitute 6% of the population in the United Kingdom (Dein 2006). Originating primarily from the Caribbean, Africa, South Asia and China, the majority of people falling into this group continue to maintain strong cultural links with their countries of origin even after being resident in the United Kingdom for several generations.

Communication needs are individual and information requirements are also culturally sensitive. People may hold different beliefs about why they have developed an illness, for instance thinking that they are being punished for something that they may or may not have done (Dein 2006).

Medical language is full of technical vocabulary and jargon which is often difficult to comprehend even for native English speakers. Macdonald (2004) suggests that people from BME groups may often come from communities where the opportunity for education is limited, thus making it increasingly difficult for them to comprehend the information that has been provided, particularly when their first language might not be English. Macdonald states that 'sentences should be short, clear and precise' (2004, p.131).

Patients from different ethnic backgrounds will often take a family member to health-related appointments. The family member is there to assist in the dialogue between the patient and the medical/nursing practitioner. Macdonald (2004) discusses the fact that communication is a two-way process and suggests that for it to be effective, the information provided needs to be patient focused. The process of translation and interpretation is never without potential problems, however, and it is important to try to find more effective ways of ensuring that the information provided is not misunderstood or misinterpreted.

In addition to the written word, there are also a number of reputable telephone helplines that can facilitate the translation from one language to another. It is good practice that these services be utilized rather than relying on family or friends of the patient (MacDonald 2004). The reason for this is because the latter may not fully understand what they are being asked to translate, or might misconstrue or misrepresent what is being said (Macmillan Cancer Relief 2004).

Competencies

Communication is such an essential aspect of the role of anybody in healthcare that the Knowledge and Skills Framework specifies the competencies in communication expected at different levels (Table 5.1). Nurses are expected to be competent as a minimum to level 3. This is a baseline and much work has been done in developing programmes to advance communication skills further.

The consistency of the success of training interventions has been widely discussed (Chant *et al.* 2002, Heaven *et al.* 2006, Schofield *et al.* 2008). The NHS 'Connected' programme (www.connected.nhs.uk) has been developed initially to develop further the skills of key members of multidisciplinary teams in cancer care (Fellowes *et al.* 2003).

Ongoing development of communication skills should include learning how to negotiate barriers to good communication in the clinical environment, tailoring and individualizing communication approaches for different patients, conflict resolution and negotiation skills (Gysels *et al.* 2005, Roberts and Snowball 1999, Schofield *et al.* 2008, Wilkinson 1991).

Courses with a behavioural component of communication training, that is, role playing situations in the classroom, are preferable as this is indicated to influence effectiveness (Gysels *et al.* 2005).

If an issue appears to be beyond the scope of practice of the nurse, it is essential that further advice and help are sought to manage a patient's psychosocial needs.

Supporting yourself and using supervision are key factors in being able to support other people. This means having a balanced lifestyle, knowing when you are under pressure and putting structures in place to support yourself. Make use of colleagues and friends who understand the burdens of the type of work you do. Sharing support issues and developing a good team spirit are good practices. Try to establish for yourself where and who you can go to for debriefing after distressing experiences. Do not ignore your own needs.

163

Preprocedural considerations

Time

In an acute hospital environment time is always pressured. For effective, supportive communication to take place, the patient needs to know that they have the nurse's attention for a set period of time. It is therefore essential to be realistic and proactive with the patient to negotiate a specific conversation for a prescribed length of time at a prearranged point in the day. It is important to be realistic but also to keep to the arrangement, otherwise there is the potential for the patient to consider that their psychological needs are not important (Towers 2007).

Environment

Conversations in a hospital environment can be very difficult, especially if privacy is sought. However, there are still actions that can be taken to make the environment as conducive as possible to enable supportive communication to take place (Towers 2007) (Box 5.4). This preliminary work might seem insignificant and time consuming but it underlines the importance of your communication to the patient and illustrates your interest in them.

Assessment

Nurses need to make careful assessments of the patient's psychological care needs. Every patient needs to be assessed for their coping style and their perception of support should be discussed at key stages in the journey of their illness. Patients' needs are diverse and hence individual discussion is necessary

Table 5.1 Knowledge and Skills Framework: four dimensions of communication competence

1	2	3	4
Establish and maintain communication with other people on routine and operational matters	Establish and maintain communication with people about routine and daily activities, overcoming any differences in communication between the people involved	Establish and maintain communication with individuals and groups about difficult or complex matters, overcoming any problems in communication	Establish and maintain communication with various individuals and groups on complex potentially stressful topics in a range of situations

Adapted from *NHS Knowledge and Skills Framework and Development Review Guidance*. Working draft, version 6 (2003).

Box 5.4 Making the environment conducive to supportive communication

- Can the patient safely and comfortably move to a more suitable area to talk with more privacy?
- Do they wish to move?
- Do they wish other people/members of the family to be there?
- Clear a space if necessary, respecting the patient's privacy and property.
- Check whether sitting on one side or another is preferable to them.
- Remove distractions, for example switch off a television, with the patient's permission.
- Is the patient able to sit comfortably?
- Will the patient be too hot or cold?
- As far as possible, choose a seat for yourself that is comfortable, and on the same level as the patient.
- Position your seat so you can have eye contact with each other easily without having to turn significantly.
- If you are in an open area on a ward, draw the curtains (with the patient's permission), to give you some privacy. Obviously, this does not prevent sound transfer and it is worth acknowledging the limitations of privacy.

Figure 5.3 Distress thermometer.

to enable professionals to understand and negotiate the desire for hope and control in care and treatment (Hack *et al.* 2005). Assessment and recording tools may support this discussion.

Recording tools

The Distress Thermometer is a validated instrument for measuring distress (Gessler *et al.* 2008, Mitchell 2007, Ransom *et al.* 2006). It is similar to a pain analogue scale (0 = no distress, 10 = extreme distress) and is thus simple to use and understand (Mitchell *et al.* 2009) (Figure 5.3). The tool helps to establish which of the broad range of

challenges that may face any unwell person is dominant at any given time. It provides a language to help patients talk about what is concerning them (Mitchell 2007). The patient marks where they feel they are at that moment or for an agreed period preceding the assessment. Trigger questions included with the Distress Thermometer can then be used to explore the nature of the distress, for example exploring family difficulties, financial worries, emotional or physical problems. A score of over 5 would warrant some supportive discussion and exploration of whether other support is necessary or desired. It may be that no further referral is necessary and the structured discussion this tool provides is sufficient in lowering the level of distress (NCCN 2010).

Principles of supportive communication

The process in Principles table 5.1 is not a rigidly prescribed sequence as skills and strategies may be used differently depending upon the situation.

Principles table 5.1 Supportive communication

Principle	Rationale
Consider whether the patient is comfortable and doesn't need pain relief or to use the toilet before you begin.	Pain and the medication used to treat it and other distractions and discomforts may limit a patient's ability to reason and concentrate. E
Protect the time for psychosocial focus of conversation. This involves telling other staff that you don't wish to be disturbed for a prescribed period.	Patients may observe how busy nurses are and withhold worries and concerns unless given explicit permission to talk (McCabe 2004, R3b).
Set a realistic time boundary for your conversation at the beginning.	You may only have 10 minutes and therefore you need to articulate the scope of your available time; this will help you to avoid distraction and give your full attention during the time available. E
Introduce yourself and your role and check what the patient wishes to be called.	This helps to establish initial rapport (Silverman *et al.* 2005, R5).

Spend a short time developing a rapport and indicating your interest in the patient, for example comment on a picture by the bedside.	Patients want to feel known. P
Be ready to move the conversation on to issues that may be concerning the patient.	Be aware that some patients may stay with neutral topics as the central focus of the conversation and withhold disclosure of psychosocial concerns until later in a conversation (Silverman *et al.* 2005, R5).
Suggest the focus of conversation, for example 'I would like to talk about how you have been feeling' or 'I wondered how you have been coping with everything'.	This indicates to the patient that you are interested in their psychological issues. E
Respond to and refer to cues.	Patients frequently offer cues – either verbal or non-verbal hints about underlying emotional concerns – and these need to be explored and clarified (Oguchi *et al.* 2010, R3b).
Responding to cues: 'I noticed you seemed upset earlier. I have 10 minutes to spare in which we can talk about it if you wish' or 'You have seemed a little frustrated. Is now a good time to talk about how I can help you with this?'.	
If the patient does not wish to talk, respect this (it is still important that you have offered to talk and the patient may well wish to talk at another time).	The patient may not wish to talk at that moment or may prefer to talk to someone else. E
Ask open questions: prefix your question with 'what', 'how' or 'why'.	Open questions encourage patients to talk (Hargie and Dickson 2004, R5).
Use closed questions sparingly.	If patients have a complicated issue to discuss, closed questions can help them be specific and can be used for clarification as well as when closing dialogue (Hargie and Dickson 2004, R5).
Add a psychological focus where you can, for example 'how have you felt about that?'.	This will help elicit information about psychological and emotional issues (Ryan *et al.* 2005, R3a).
Listen carefully and feed back your understanding of what is being said at opportune moments.	Listening is a key skill – it is an active process requiring concentration, verbal and non-verbal affirmations (Silverman *et al.* 2005, Wosket 2006, R5).
Be empathic (try to appreciate what the other person may be experiencing and recognize how difficult that is for them).	Empathy is about creating a human connection with your patient (Egan 2002, R5).
Allow for silences.	This can give rise to further expression and useful thinking time for yourself and the patient (Silverman *et al.* 2005, R5).
Initially avoid trying to 'fix' people's concerns and the problems that they express. It might be more powerful and important to simply sit, listen and show your understanding.	As an individual is listened to, they may feel comfort, relief and a sense of human connection essential for support (Egan 2002, R5).
Ask the patient how they think you may be able to help them.	The patient will know what they need better than we do. E
Avoid blocking (see Box 5.5).	Blocking results in failing to elicit the full range of concerns a patient may have (Back *et al.* 2005, R3a).
When you are nearing the end of the time you have agreed to be with the patient, let the patient know, that is, suggest that soon you will need to stop your discussion.	The patient can find this easier to accept if you have clearly expressed the time you had available in the first place (Towers 2007, R5).

(Continued)

Principles table 5.1 (*Continued*)

Acknowledge that you may not have been able to cover all concerns and summarize what has been discussed, checking with the patient how accurate your understanding is.	The patient can correct any misinterpretations and this can lead to satisfactory agreement about the meeting. It also signifies closure of a meeting (Hargie and Dickson 2004, R5).
If further concerns are raised at this point, you will need to make it clear that you cannot support them at the current time. Let the patient know when you or other staff may be available to talk again, or where else they may get further support.	Clarity and honesty are important, as is working within boundaries. Knowing the limits of your time and expertise will help to prevent confusion about where the patient can receive types of support. E
Agree any action points and follow up as necessary. If needs remain unmet, offer support from a clinical nurse specialist or a counselling service, if available. You must discuss what this means and be realistic with regard to waiting times. Consent from the patient for any further referral is essential (unless you consider the patient to be at risk).	Having made a suitable assessment, you can involve further support if appropriate. E
Document your conversation, having agreed with the patient what is appropriate to share with the rest of the team.	It is essential to document your conversation so other members of the team are informed and to meet your professional requirements (NMC 2008a, C; NMC 2009, C).
Reflect upon your own practice.	You may have unintentionally controlled the communication or blocked expression of emotion. Reflection will increase your self-awareness and help develop your skills. E
Consider your own support needs. If you are affected by any discussions you have had, seek discussion with supportive senior members of staff or consider debriefing and/or supervision.	Clinical supervision supports practice, enabling registered nurses to maintain and improve standards of care (NMC 2008b, C).

Box 5.5 Characteristics of blocking behaviours

Blocking can be defined as:

- failing to pick up on cues (ignoring emotional content)
- selectively focusing on the physical/medical aspects of care
- premature or false reassurance, for example telling people not to worry
- inappropriate encouragement or trivializing, for example telling someone they look fine when they have expressed altered body image
- passing the buck, for example suggesting it is another professional's responsibility to answer questions or sort out the problem (doctors or counsellors, for example)
- changing the subject, for example asking about something mundane or about other family members to deflect the conversation away from issues that may make the nurse feel uncomfortable
- jollying along, for example 'You'll feel better when you get home'
- using closed questions (any question that can be answered with a yes or a no is a closed question).

(Faulkner and Maguire 1994)

Informing patients

Definition

Principles of providing information to patients and discussing procedures to be carried out.

Related theory

Research conducted by the Picker Institute (Ellins and Coulter 2005) shows that 80% of people actively seek information about how to cope with health problems. Information is of prime importance in helping to support people in the decision-making process, particularly when they are vulnerable and feeling anxious. It is important that high-quality, reliable and evidence-based information should be accessible to patients, their relatives and carers at the right time, making it an integral part of their care (DH 2008). This is reiterated in the White Paper *Our Health, Our Care, Our Say* (DH 2006), which states that 'people with a long-term condition and/or long-term need for support – and their carers – should routinely receive information about their condition' and the services available to them. Information prescriptions represent good practice for supporting the information needs of individuals (DH 2009).

Evidence-based approaches

With any procedure, it is essential that the patient (assuming consciousness and ability to make rational decisions) is psychologically prepared and consented. This requires careful explanation and discussion before a procedure is carried out.

As nurses, we can become so familiar with procedures that we expect them to be considered 'routine' by our patients. This can prevent us from providing thorough and necessary information and gaining acceptance and co-operation from our patients. We therefore need to avoid assuming that repetitive or frequent procedures do not require consent, explanation and potential discussion, for example taking a temperature.

It is important to consider giving information in small amounts and checking whether the patient understands what has been said after each part has been explained. Keep language simple and clarify common and complex medical terms, for example 'cannula', 'catheter'.

Check frequently whether the patient wishes you to continue to provide them with the same level of information. If confusion is arising, consider whether you are providing too much detail or using too many medical terms. Be aware whether the patient is paying attention or appears anxious (e.g. fidgety/non-attentive behaviour). Do not ignore these cues: name them. For example: 'I notice you seem a little anxious while I am describing this …' or 'You seem concerned about the procedure, what can I do to help?'. This recognition of behaviour will help to fully explore and support the patient's concerns.

Prior to starting, establish how the patient can communicate with you during the procedure, for example confirm that they can ask questions, request more analgesia or ask for the procedure to stop (if this is realistic).

Information must be presented accurately and calmly and without 'false reassurance', for example do not say something 'will not hurt' or it 'will not go wrong', when it might. It is better to explain the risk and likely outcome. Explain that working with the nurse and co-operating with instructions are likely to improve the outcome and that every effort will be made to reduce risk and manage any problems efficiently.

Respect any refusal unconditionally; however, you may wish to explore the reasons for refusal and explain the potential (realistic) consequences. Document carefully and discuss with the multidisciplinary team. If a patient has had a procedure before, do not assume that they are fully aware of the potential experience or risk involved, which may well have changed.

Attention to good communication, honesty, confidence and calmness will help to reassure the patient, thus gaining their compliance and improving the potential outcome (Maguire and Pitceathly 2002).

Giving the right amount of information is important; for example, it has been shown that getting the level of information wrong (too much or too little) at diagnosis can sig-nificantly affect the subsequent level of coping (Fallowfield *et al.* 2002). Getting the level right can be achieved by simply asking how much people want to know and frequently checking if the level of information is satisfactory for the individual.

Preprocedural considerations
Patient information

Patient information in this context refers to information about disease, its treatment, effects and side-effects, and the help and support available to people living with a chronic condition, their relatives and carers.

When writing information for patients and carers, consideration should be given to information already available on the chosen topic. The purpose of the information may be to:

- address frequently asked questions
- inform about a treatment or service
- reduce anxiety
- give reference material.

Ideas should be shared with other members of the team or clinical unit, and patients and carers involved, from the outset. The content of the material should be accurate and evidence based and meet the current Department of Health and NHS Litigation Authority requirements.

When writing the information, everyday language should be used as if speaking face to face and avoiding the use of jargon; 16% of adults in England do not have the literacy levels expected of an 11-year-old (DfES 2003). However, there is no need to be patronizing or use childish language. The Plain English campaign (www.plainenglish.co.uk) offers a downloadable guide entitled *How to write plain English*.

Information should be dated and carry a planned review date. Sources of information should be acknowledged. This gives the reader confidence in the material.

The provision and production of information must take into account diversity in ethnicity, culture, religion, language, gender, age, disability, socio-economic status and literacy levels, as stated in the Department of Health publication *Better Information, Better Choice, Better Health* (2004). See Principles table 5.2 for the provision of information.

Information should be ratified according to local trust policy. Where a trust does not produce patient information materials to meet specific patient needs, suitable alternative sources of information should be sought.

Other sources of information

Patients and their families may benefit from information and support available in the wider community, away from

Principles table 5.2 Provision of information

Principle	Rationale
Review the changing context of the patient's situation.	What may have been relevant before may now not be the same. People's circumstances and needs change. E
Prepare for discussion, ensuring you are familiar with the procedure, disease process, medication or other aspect of care to be discussed.	Accurate information giving is an essential part of nursing care. E
If possible, discuss the procedure some time before it is to be carried out for the first time. Provide the patient with leaflets, DVDs or video if available so the patient has time to review the information at their own pace.	Give patients the opportunity to digest information in their own time (Lowry 1995, E). In certain groups it can be demonstrated to improve clinical outcomes, satisfaction, chances of meeting the targeted discharge date and return to prior functional status sooner (Lookinland and Pool 1998, R2b).
Introduce yourself.	Ensure the patient understands who you are and your role and specific aim. Promote patient satisfaction (Delvaux et al. 2004, R1b).
Maintain a warm and approachable demeanour. Do not rush.	Promote patient satisfaction (Delvaux et al. 2004, R1b).
Explain that you have a procedure to carry out, considering privacy in giving information.	Promote dignity/preserve confidentiality (NMC 2008a, C).
Name the procedure. Elicit, clarify and check the information received by the patient.	Promote understanding and patient satisfaction. E
Explain the procedure, avoiding the use of medical jargon. Be prepared to repeat information or rephrase until the patient understands. (If the patient doesn't understand, they haven't consented.)	Establish mutual understanding. Gain compliance with procedure: minimize risk (NMC 2008a, C). Improve outcome (Fellowes et al. 2004, R1a). Help patients manage side-effects and adhere to care and treatment (Chelf et al. 2001, R3a).
Confirm consent: ensure that the patient is happy for you to proceed. Allow the patient an opportunity to ask further questions or say no to the procedure. (If the patient fully understands what is involved, they may decide that they are not ready to proceed.)	Respecting the rights of the individual (NMC 2008a, C). Obtaining consent correctly (NMC 2008c, C; see also Appendix 1).
Start the procedure, reiterating the main issues as you go along and keeping the patient updated on progress.	To maintain open dialogue and address issues and questions, as they arise. E
Make it clear when the procedure has finished and what has been achieved. Offer opportunity for discussion of implications, disclosing as much information as the patient wishes.	So that the patient is aware and has the information they need and want (Jenkins et al. 2001, R2b).

the environment of statutory health services. Sources of additional information include:

- *disease-specific national charities*, for example the Multiple Sclerosis Society or the British Heart Foundation: these organizations produce written material in booklet and fact sheet format, as well as having websites
- *the 'illness memoir' and internet blogs*: personal accounts are easily accessible online and through bookstores. It may help patients to hear other people's stories as this can reduce the sense of isolation and powerlessness and promote hope (Chelf et al. 2001). It must be borne in mind that not everyone will benefit from these sources of information
- *peer support*: the therapeutic benefits of groups are extensively documented (NICE 2004) and most of the support charities will have a directory of local and national groups available.

Managing challenging issues with communication

Denial and collusion

Definitions

Denial is a complex phenomenon but most commonly can be defined as a strategy offering 'psychological protection against the perception and processing of subjectively painful or distressing information' (Goldbeck 1997, p.586).

Collusion is when two or more parties develop a 'secret' understanding, that is, withholding information from another person. It is important that health professionals resist invitations to collude with information that the patient has inaccurately understood (Macdonald 2004).

Related theory

A diagnosis of any potentially life-threatening illness can be experienced in many different ways and elicit strong emotional responses. Patients are likely to be distressed and experience a wide range of emotions which may arguably be lessened if 'healthcare professionals (HCPs) were truthful and open with patients about their diagnosis and prognosis' (Wilkinson *et al.* 2005, p.124).

Numerous coping strategies, including denial, may be used when someone is given a potentially life-threatening diagnosis such as cancer. Denial is not an uncommon reaction to a threatening diagnosis and is a well-recognized phenomenon in clinical practice (Vos and Haes 2007). Ten percent of patients deny the gravity of their diagnosis but usually still ask about potential treatments (Maguire 2000). As healthcare professionals, the more we understand about denial, the better equipped we are likely to feel to cope with it.

Literature on denial tends to be limited to the cancer field and prevalence rates are difficult to assess. Vos (2008) found that most lung cancer patients displayed some level of denial, which increased over the course of the illness. This outcome warrants the conclusion that in clinical practice, 'denial in this group of patients has to be considered as a normal phenomenon and not as a sign of disturbed coping' (Vos 2008, p.1170).

Healthcare professionals may view denial as a normal and acceptable response to a potentially life-threatening diagnosis or they may consider it problematic, especially as it can be seen to generate discomfort and uncertainty for them and the patient's family.

Family members and healthcare professionals can collude with patient denial, perhaps as a means of protecting the patient or themselves from facing the full impact and pain of the situation. Healthcare professionals need to be aware of the pitfalls of colluding with patient or family denial and consider how they may contribute to it.

The concept of denial has been considered from different theoretical perspectives over time. Historically, in early psychoanalytic teaching denial was felt to be a maladaptive, immature defence which needed to be confronted. The emphasis was on the pathological nature of denial. More recently, this view is being challenged.

As human beings, we live our lives in our own individual, unique way and also deal with a life-threatening diagnosis in our own way. For some people, focusing on hope and cure is the priority, whilst for others it is first necessary to prepare themselves and their family for the possibility that their illness may be incurable. Denial is a complex, fluid process, as is living with a life-threatening diagnosis. Patients' understanding of what is happening to them can fluctuate from minute to minute.

> Denial is not an 'all or none' phenomenon. A patient may accept his illness in the morning, but by evening deny that he has it.
>
> (Dein 2005, p.251)

Medical and nursing staff, family members and patients may all 'be in denial' at some point – to protect either themselves or those they care about.

Evidence-based approaches
Assessment of denial

In order to try to understand as fully as possible the emotions that patients are experiencing and the resources they have for coping, a careful assessment of each patient's circumstances is important.

Healthcare professionals need to establish what information the patient has been given, before assuming that the patient is experiencing denial. We need to be sure that patients have been given adequate, digestible information, if necessary on several occasions.

It is helpful to view denial as a process and to see its expression along a continuum. This needs to be acknowledged in the assessment process.

Repeated assessments of denial may help us to understand how various factors might influence denial and to better understand its dynamic nature.

Denial can generate discomfort and uncertainty in staff. Recognizing and understanding it can help healthcare professionals cope with the challenge of caring for a patient who is using denial as a coping mechanism.

Complications

Balancing the reality of the illness with reasonable hope is often difficult for all concerned. When working with patients whom we think are in denial, the challenge for healthcare professionals is not so much the confrontation of denial but rather the avoidance of collusion with it (Houldin 2000).

Principles table 5.3 Supporting a patient in denial

Principle	Rationale
Healthcare professionals should aim to provide honest information to patients with the use of good communication skills, to the depth and detail the patient requests.	This enables patients to have control over the rate at which they absorb and integrate news and information that may have life-threatening implications for them (Maguire 2000, R5).
Useful skills are those of listening, reflecting and summarizing.	This will establish a supportive relationship which in the future may provide the patient with the security to acknowledge the gravity of the information they have been given. E
If denial is affecting a treatment regime or decisions for the future, it may need to be gently challenged. This can be done by either questioning any inconsistencies in the patient's story or asking if at any point they have thought that their illness may be more serious.	These questions may help the patient get closer to knowledge they may already have about the seriousness of their illness. With the right support, they might be able to face their fears and be more fully involved in decisions about future care and treatment. E
If the patient remains in denial it shouldn't be challenged any further (Dein 2005).	'Confrontation, if pursued in an insensitive or dismissive way or in the absence of adequate trust and support mechanisms, may increase denial, may reduce treatment compliance, or may even precipitate a complete breakdown in the health care professional–patient relationship' (Goldbeck 1997, p.586; Maguire 2000, R5).
The delivery of bad news and information giving needs to be recorded clearly. The degree to which the patient accepts the information is variable and needs to be respected and carefully documented.	Good communication can help prevent patients receiving mixed messages. E

Collusion can leave healthcare professionals, patients and relatives feeling confused. Recognizing collusion, challenging it and discussing our concerns with colleagues is important. Working with our multiprofessional team helps to improve communication and to ensure a collaborative approach to care. Drawing on the richness of experience of others can help.

Clinical supervision can provide a safe reflective space for healthcare professionals to explore their practice. It is an ideal place to explore the complex phenomenon of denial and collusion, as well as find support and if necessary challenge.

See Principles table 5.3.

Anxiety

Definition

Anxiety is a feeling of fear and apprehension about a real or perceived threat. The source of the feeling may or may not be known (Kennedy Sheldon 2009).

Anatomy and physiology

Anxious feelings can result in physical symptoms related to the flight or fight response as physically the body responds to the threat, real or otherwise. The sympathetic nervous system releases adrenaline that is responsible for an increase in heart rate and therefore palpitations and raised blood pressure, faster, shallower breathing (hyperventilation), dizziness, dry mouth and difficulty swallowing, relaxation of sphincters leading to an increase in urinary and faecal elimination, reduction in blood supply to the intestines leading to feelings of 'butterflies', knotted stomach and nausea, increase in perspiration as the body seeks to cool down the tense muscles, and musculoskeletal pains (particularly in the back and neck) (Powell and Enright 1990). These are all unpleasant physical symptoms for the patient and can escalate further if not managed at an early stage.

Related theory

There are a number of theories about anxiety, its causes and therefore how to manage it (Powell and Enright 1990). To be effective in supporting and communicating with a patient with anxiety, it is necessary to know that there are three aspects of feeling anxious.

- *Bodily sensations.*
- *Behaviour:* how the individual behaves when faced with the fear, especially if the behaviour involves avoiding it.
- *Thinking:* this is the ideas, beliefs and mental pictures about what might happen in the situation feared (Powell 2009).

Principles table 5.4 Supporting an anxious individual

Principle	Rationale
Be alert to the signs and symptoms of anxiety.	Early recognition and intervention may help to prevent worsening of symptoms. E
Encourage the patient to talk about the source of their anxiety if they can.	Patients may find some benefit from expressing their concerns and being heard. E
Listen and only when the patient has expressed all their fears offer information or gently challenge misinformation about treatment, processes or outcomes if this is the source of the anxiety.	Information about a procedure, particularly an operation, can reduce anxiety and improve outcomes (Scott 2004, R3a; Nordahl *et al.* 2003, R2b).
If the patient doesn't know why they are feeling anxious, encourage them to describe what is happening in their body, when it started, what makes it worse, what makes it better.	Patient feels listened to and less alone, which may increase their sense of security and therefore reduce anxiety. E
Ask the patient if they have had the feelings before. What has helped previously (coping mechanisms) and what do they think may help this time?	The patient is encouraged to take control and apply their own coping mechanisms. E

Anxiety is a normal response to threatening events but can become a problem when it is frequent, exaggerated, experienced out of context or interfering with an individual's life (Blake and Ledger 2007). As levels of anxiety increase, awareness and interaction with the environment decrease, and recall and general function are also impaired (Kennedy Sheldon 2009). At the extreme, anxiety may become a panic attack.

Evidence-based approaches

Research has recently demonstrated that the most effective way of helping an individual with the more acute levels of anxiety is through a cognitive behavioural approach (Donohoe and Ricketts 2006, NICE 2007). Some of these principles are applicable to communicating with a patient with general anxiety associated with their illness and treatment. One of the key interventions is educating the patient, normalizing their response to their situation but also giving information about the situations and circumstances that may be triggering the anxiety (Donohoe and Ricketts 2006). Referring the patient for relaxation therapy can also help them physiologically, as they will learn how to release the muscular tension that may lead to headaches, backaches and other aches and pains (Blake and Leger 2007, Powell 2009).

See Principles table 5.4.

Panic attacks (acute anxiety)

Related theory

A panic attack is a discrete period of intense fear or discomfort that is accompanied by a range of somatic or cognitive symptoms (Donohoe and Ricketts 2006) (Box 5.6).

Panic attacks occur in up to 5% of the population with a sudden onset of symptoms such as dizziness, difficulty in breathing and thoughts of losing control or dying. The more these thoughts intrude, the more extreme the physiological response becomes (Powell 2009). The immediate response for many individuals is to try and leave the situation as soon as possible. This brings immediate relief but increases the likelihood of further apprehension and repeated attack at a later date (Powell 2009).

Box 5.6 Criteria for a panic attack

A discrete period of intense fear or discomfort in which four (or more) of the following symptoms develop abruptly and reach a peak within 10 minutes.

- Palpitations, pounding heart or accelerated heart rate.
- Sweating.
- Trembling or shaking.
- Sensations of shortness of breath or smothering.
- Feeling of choking.
- Chest pain or discomfort.
- Nausea or abdominal distress.
- Feeling dizzy, unsteady, light-headed or faint.
- De-realization or depersonalization.
- Fear of losing control or going crazy.
- Fear of dying.
- Pins and needles in extremities.
- Chills or hot flushes.

(Donohoe and Ricketts 2006)

An indication for many individuals that a panic attack is beginning is a feeling of tightness in the chest or being aware that their breathing is fast. If not managed, this progresses to hyperventilation (Powell 2009).

Evidence-based approaches

Managing acute anxiety (including panic attacks) can help to avoid the development of panic disorder and generalized anxiety disorder. Nurses can support patients to avoid anxiety attacks by taking time to talk issues through. If the anxiety has progressed further and the patient is experiencing the warning signs that they are on the verge of hyperventilation, it is helpful to:

- remind them that the symptoms they are feeling are not harmful
- help them to actively release tension in the upper body by encouraging them to sit up and drop their shoulders in a sideways widening direction. This makes hyperventilation more difficult since the chest and diaphragm muscles are stretched outwards
- breathe slowly … in to a count of 4 and out to a count of 4. Slowing your own breathing down can help the patient
- encourage them to concentrate on breathing out and trying to breathe through their nose.

(Adapted from Powell 2009)

A panic or anxiety attack does not necessarily mean that the patient has a pathological disorder. Prompt treatment and management are important to prevent transient anxiety turning into a disorder (NICE 2007).

Preprocedural considerations

Pharmacological support
Panic disorder

Benzodiazepines, antipsychotics and sedating antihistamines are associated with a worse long-term outcome and pharmacological interventions should be either tricyclic or selective serotonin reuptake inhibitor (SSRI) antidepressant medication (see Depression, Pharmacological support).

Generalized anxiety disorder

Again, antidepressant medication should be considered and this should be an SSRI unless otherwise indicated. Other medication has also been shown to be effective: serotonin-norepinephrine reuptake inhibitors (SNRIs) (venlafaxine) and antihistamines/benzodiazepines in short-term use (NICE 2004).

Box 5.7 Rebreathing technique instructions for a patient

- Make a mask of your hands and put them over your nose and mouth and keep them there (Figure 5.4).
- Breathe in and out through your nose once.
- Breathe in your own exhaled air through your nose.
- Breathe out hard through your mouth.

This should be done slowly without holding your breath. Repeat this four or five times but no more. Remain calm and relaxed while doing it.

(Adapted from Powell 2009)

Non-pharmacological support
The rebreathing technique

This involves the patient rebreathing the air they have just breathed out (Box 5.7). This air is high in carbon dioxide so has less oxygen. This means that there will be a lower amount of oxygen in the blood, thus activating the parasympathetic nervous system and promoting relaxation (Blake and Ledger 2007).

After the panic attack, it is important to reflect with the patient about what happened and try to identify any triggers. Explanation and education about physiological responses can help to show the patient the importance of slowing their breathing which will in turn give them a sense of control.

If these panic attacks continue or if the patient has a history of anxiety then the management of this will include a referral for psychological support (with consent). Medication may be indicated after assessment (NICE 2007).

See Principles table 5.5.

Figure 5.4 Hand position for rebreathing technique.

Principles table 5.5 Supporting an individual having a panic attack

Principle	Rationale
Firstly, exclude any physical reasons for the patient's distress such as an acute angina episode or asthma attack.	If the panic attack has a physical cause management needs to be instigated as soon as possible. E
Remain calm and stay with the patient.	The patient will not be reassured by others reacting with tension or anxiety about the situation. E
Maintain eye contact with the patient. Consider holding the patient's hand.	This helps the patient to be connected to reality and engage with your attempts to support them. Some patients may be reassured by physical touch (but assess each individual) for appropriateness. E
Guide the patient to breathe deeply and slowly, demonstrating where necessary.	This gives the patient an activity to concentrate on and may help normalize any carbon dioxide and oxygen blood imbalance. E

Depression

Definition

Currently, depression can be defined as:

> ... a range of mental health disorders characterised by the absence of a positive affect (a loss of interest and enjoyment in ordinary things and experiences), low mood and a range of associated emotional, cognitive, physical and behavioural symptoms. It is often accompanied by anxiety, and can be chronic even in milder presentations.
>
> (NICE 2009a)

Depression describes a group of related disorders whose definition has changed over time.

Related theory

Depression is a common psychological response in patients with a chronic physical illness such as heart disease, diabetes and cancer. When this occurs, it is referred to as a 'co-morbid' depression. Co-morbid depression is difficult to detect as symptoms can be similar to the expected side-effects of the illness or treatment. For example, undetected depression rates in adult patients with cancer can be as high as 50% (Brown *et al.* 2009, Trask 2004). Depression can be found in 20% of patients with a chronic physical illness (NICE 2009a), which is 2–3 times higher than individuals in good health. It is therefore essential that patients with a long-term physical illness are regularly assessed for anxiety and depression.

Box 5.8 sets out some of the symptoms of depression (NICE 2009a).

Box 5.8 Symptoms that indicate a diagnosis of clinical depression

Behavioural

- Tearfulness.
- Irritability.
- Socially withdrawn.
- Changes to sleep patterns.
- Lowered appetite.
- Lack of libido.
- Fatigue.
- Diminished activity.
- Attempts at self-harm or suicide.

Physical

- Exacerbation of pre-existing pains.
- Pains secondary to increased muscle tension.
- Agitation and restlessness.
- Changes in weight.

Cognitive

- Poor concentration.
- Reduced attention.
- Pessimistic thoughts.
- Recurring negative thoughts about oneself, past and future.
- Mental slowing.
- Rumination.

Emotional

- Feelings of guilt.
- Worthlessness.
- Deserving of punishment.
- Lowered self-esteem.
- Loss of confidence.
- Feelings of helplessness.
- Suicidal ideation.

Depression can be accompanied by anxiety and can be diagnosed as either depression or mixed depression and anxiety. The incidence of depression in the UK has been quoted as 2.6% (2.3% male, 2.8% female). However, the figure for mixed anxiety and depression rises to 11.4% (9.1% male, 13.6% female) (NICE 2009a, p.18).

A normal low mood is differentiated from what is medically diagnosed as a depressive episode by the length of time the low mood is experienced. Low mood that persists for 2 weeks or more or rapid-onset/severe low mood are reasons for concern. The presence of other depressive symptoms contributes to a diagnosis as well as a consideration of how this low mood affects the individual's ability to interact socially. Generally, depression is a time-limited disorder with the potential for full recovery within 6–8 months (NICE 2008a). However, if a chronic physical illness is present, this may be different. Severe depression may be accompanied by psychotic symptoms, that is, hallucinations or delusional thoughts.

Evidence-based approaches

Approaches to treatment of depression are influenced by the severity of the condition. Diagnosing depression has improved following the introduction of ICD-10 which lists 10 depressive symptoms, dividing them into:

- sub-threshold   <4 symptoms
- mild   4 symptoms
- moderately depressed   5–6 symptoms
- severe   7 or more symptoms with or without psychosis.

Symptoms need to be present for greater than 2 weeks.
Core management skills include risk assessment plus the following.

- Good communication skills are required to enable the nurse to elicit information from the patient (Brown et al. 2009, Strong et al. 2004) and show understanding of the problem. See Principles table 5.6.
- A sufficient understanding of the signs and symptoms of anxiety and depression and ability to make a preliminary assessment.
- A sufficient understanding of antidepressant medication to enable an explanation of its actions to the patient.
- An ability to 'refer on' when it is recognized that the issues are beyond the scope of experience. This must be done with the patient's consent.
- Awareness of the stigma attached to a diagnosis of depression, and protection of the patient's privacy and dignity.
- Sensitivity to diverse cultural ethnic and religious backgrounds considering variations in presentations of low mood.

- Awareness of any cognitive impairments or learning disabilities to ensure that specialist therapists are involved (where needed).

Use of hospital psychological care departments can assist with the care and treatment of patients as well as providing a supervisory and support framework for staff. Working with psychological care departments can help nurses develop their assessment skills of anxiety and depression helping them to identify the appropriate time for a referral to a specialist service if required (Towers 2007).

Preprocedural considerations
Pharmacological support

There are four main types of antidepressant (RCPsych Depression leaflet 2010). When prescribing antidepressants, the two main considerations are the presence of other physical health problems and the side-effects of the drugs which may affect the underlying physical disease.

There is minimal difference between the effectiveness of each type of antidepressant; however, there are clear differences in the side-effects of the different classes and types of antidepressants.

The therapeutic effect of antidepressants may take months to appear and treatment should continue for at least 6 months after a response to the treatment.

Selective serotonin reuptake inhibitors are safer in overdose than tricyclic antidepressants (TCAs), which can be dangerous. There is, however, an increased risk of gastrointestinal bleeding with SSRIs so they should be avoided in patients taking non-steroidal anti-inflammatory drugs.

Monoamine oxidase inhibitors can affect blood pressure, particularly when certain food types are eaten.

Serotonin-norepinephrine reuptake inhibitors are not appropriate for patients with heart conditions as they too increase blood pressure.

Table 5.2 lists the most commonly prescribed antidepressants (RCP, BSRM, NCPCS 2008).

Nurses have an important role in exploring with the patient any concerns they may have regarding taking an antidepressant. The patient should be equipped with all the necessary information regarding the optimum time to take the medication and the expected length of time before any therapeutic effect becomes apparent. Medication should be taken for at least 6 months following remission.

Discontinuation of treatment usually requires titration of doses. Therefore treatment must not be stopped abruptly and should be monitored by the prescribing doctor or nurse. Concerns regarding addiction require further information and reassurance confirming that this is unlikely to happen with the more modern antidepressant treatments. Further information on pharmacological intervention can be found in the NICE guidelines on depression (NICE 2009a).

Table 5.2 Most commonly prescribed antidepressants

Medication	Trade name	Group
Amitriptyline	Tryptizol	Tricyclic
Clomipramine	Anafranil	Tricyclic
Citalopram	Cipramil	SSRI
Dosulepin	Prothiaden	Tricyclic
Doxepin	Sinequan	Tricyclic
Fluoxetine	Prozac	SSRI
Imipramine	Tofranil	Tricyclic
Lofepramine	Gamanil	Tricyclic
Mirtazapine	Zispin	NaSSA
Moclobemide	Manerix	MAOI
Nortriptyline	Allegron	Tricyclic
Paroxetine	Seroxat	SSRI
Phenelzine	Nardil	MAOI
Reboxetine	Edronax	SNRI
Sertraline	Lustral	SSRI
Tranylcypromine	Parnate	MAOI
Trazodone	Molipaxin	Tricyclic related
Venlafaxine	Efexor	SNRI

SSRI, selective serotonin reuptake inhibitor; SNRI, serotonin and noradrenaline reuptake inhibitor; MAOI, monoamine oxidase inhibitor; NaSSA, noradrenergic and specific serotonergic antidepressant.

Non-pharmacological support

Nurses can be involved in assessing depression in patients with physical illness. NICE guidance sets out a four-step model for managing a patient with depression. The first

Principles table 5.6 Communicating with a depressed patient

Principle	Rationale
Initiate the conversation, develop rapport.	Good assessment is not possible without good communication. E
Show understanding, caring and acceptance of behaviours, including tears or anger.	Accepting the patient as they are without attempting to block or contain their emotions helps them to express their feelings accurately. E
Encourage patient to identify their own abilities or strategies for coping with the situation.	Promote self-efficacy. E

Box 5.9 Managing the patient with depression: NICE guidance, step 1

Key questions:
1 During the last month, have you often been bothered by:
   - feeling down, depressed or hopeless?
   - having little interest or pleasure in doing things?
2 How long have you felt like this for? (NICE 2009a, p.4)

If the patient answers 'yes' to question 1 and the time scale is longer than 2 weeks, it is important that a referral is made for further assessment by a healthcare professional with clinical competence in managing depression, such as a clinical psychologist or a registered mental health nurse, so they can determine if the patient has been bothered by 'feelings of worthlessness, poor concentration or thoughts of death' (NICE 2009a, p.4).

Other questions should assess for the following.
- Other physical health problems that may be significantly affecting their mood such as uncontrolled pain, sleep disruption, excessive nausea and vomiting, physical limitations on their independence or body image disturbance.
- A history of psychological illness such as depression.
- A consideration of the medication the patient is taking, specifically medication for mental health problems. Have they been able to take it and absorb it or have they had any digestive issues?
- Social support for the patient: who else is around to support the person, are they isolated?

(Adapted from NICE 2009a)

step (Box 5.9) could be managed by a nurse in an acute environment.

Assessment of how the patient's low mood has affected their usual daily activities such as eating, dressing and sleeping is important. The nurse can also encourage the patient to engage with activities that would be the normal for them.

Suicidal ideation

Definition

This is where someone has thoughts about suicide – it does not necessarily mean they are intending to act upon them.

Related theory

National statistics for UK suicide indicate that there are approximately 11 suicides per 100,000 population per year. Males outnumber females by approximately 3:1 (Office for National Statistics: www.statistics.gov.uk/cci/nugget.asp?id=1092).

See Principles table 5.7.

Principles table 5.7 Communicating with a patient who is expressing suicidal ideation

Principle	Rationale
Explore low mood, anxiety and agitation with patients.	These factors indicate increased risk (Hermes *et al.* 2009, R3a).
Assess for risk: this can be as simple as making a statement remarking upon the person's low mood and asking them if they have ever thought of hurting themselves.	Most people will answer truthfully (Sobczak 2009, R3a).
Explore any expressions of suicidal ideas for intention to act. This can be achieved by asking if the patient has a plan.	Suicidal thoughts do not mean that people are at risk but you do need to establish what the risk is.
Crucially you will also need to explore what stops people from acting and what changes might cause them to act. If you consider the patient is at risk, explain to them that you need to refer them for further support.	Assessing suicidal risk needs to be simple (Billings 2004, R5).
Inform and involve the consultant and psychological support services.	

Anger, aggression and violence management

Definition

Anger is 'an emotional state that may range in intensity from mild irritation to intense fury and rage. Anger has physical effects including raising the heart rate and blood pressure and the levels of adrenaline and noradrenaline' (Mednet 2010).

Related theory

Nurses may be exposed to anger and aggression. Poor communication is frequently a precursor to aggressive behaviour (Duxbury and Whittington 2005). Aggression and abuse tend to be discussed synonymously in the literature and are reported to occur with some frequency in nursing (McLaughlin *et al.* 2009). Anger is felt or displayed when someone's annoyance or irritation has increased to a point where they feel or display extreme displeasure. Verbal aggression is the expression of anger via hostile language; this language causes offence and may result in physical assault. Verbal abuse may actually be experienced as worse than a minor physical assault (Adams and Whittington 1995). Whatever the cause of anger or conflict, people can behave in a number of challenging ways and with varying degrees of resistance to social and hospital rules. People may simply refuse to comply with a request or may behave more aggressively, for example by pushing someone aside (without intent to harm) or by deliberately striking out at others. Mental capacity issues should be considered when assessing the causes of aggressive behaviours.

When patients do feel anger, they may feel too depleted by experiences of disease and treatment to express it (Bowes *et al.* 2002).

For some people, anger may be the least distressing emotion to display. Sometimes helplessness, sadness and loss are far harder to explore and show to others. Anger therefore can be a way of controlling intimacy and disclosure, but it can escalate to threatening, abusive or violent behaviour.

Evidence-based approaches

Prevention is the most effective method of managing anger; that is, diffusing stressful or difficult interactions before they become a crisis. There are situations encountered within practice where challenging or difficult behaviour can be seen to be related to underlying stress and difficulty in a person's situation. Anger, aggression and violence may have 'biological, psychological, social and environmental roots' (Krug 2002, p.25). People frequently get angry when they feel they are not being heard or when their control of a situation and self-esteem are compromised. Many health professionals are unfortunately renowned for failing to acknowledge patients as people and this can stimulate an angry and arguably legitimate behavioural response. Institutional pressures can influence healthcare professionals to act in controlling ways and may contribute to patients' angry responses (Gudjonsson *et al.* 2004). Patients are often undergoing procedures that threaten them and they may consequently feel vulnerable and react aggressively as a result. Another source of anger can be when personal beliefs in the form of rules are broken by others. We therefore need to strive to be aware of individual and cultural values and work with them to avoid frustration and upset.

People also can become angry when they feel that they have not been communicated with honestly or are misled about treatments and their outcomes. To prevent people's frustration escalating into anger or worse, health professionals need to ensure that they are communicating with people openly, honestly and frequently.

Some patients may appear or sound aggressive when they are not intending to be and the nurse must therefore use good judgement to clarify their behaviour in these instances. Nurses need to be aware of their own boundaries and capabilities when dealing with challenging or abusive situations.

Threats, uncertainty and disempowerment may predispose people to anger and living with and being treated for any serious condition can be sufficiently threatening and disempowering, for example those affected by cancer (Faulkner and Maguire 1994).

It is frequently possible to engage with and manage some of the underlying features without endangering anyone. People who are behaving aggressively probably do not normally act that way and may apologize when helped.

Box 5.10 Warning signs that a patient is angry

- Tense angry facial signs, restlessness and increased volume of speech.
- Prolonged eye contact and a refusal to communicate.
- Unclear thought process, delusions or hallucinations.
- Verbal threats and reporting angry feelings.

Talking down or de-escalation of situations where someone is being non-compliant can be achieved with careful assessment of the situation and skilful communication. NICE (2005) clinical guidelines on managing disturbed and violent behaviour recommend remaining calm when approaching someone and offering them choices. It is acknowledged, however, that there is little research indicating the correct procedure to follow.

Box 5.10 lists signs indicating that people may be angry. It is necessary to engage people sensitively and carefully to attempt to help them whilst maintaining a safe environment for all.

Principles table 5.8 Communicating with a patient who is angry

Principle	Rationale
Remain calm.	
Verbally acknowledge the person's distress/anger and suggest you wish to help.	The person may respond positively and accept help. E
Acknowledge issues that may be contributing, for example being kept waiting.	This helps the person feel that their concerns are understood. E
Consider what causes there may be, for example medication or disease (consider diabetes – hypo/hyperglycaemia), medical, circumstantial and so on.	Several factors might be influencing the behaviour. E
Consider safety – try to move to another area (ideally where you can sit down). If others might be intimidated or in danger, be clear about moving one of the parties away where practical, but do not endanger yourself in the process.	Maintain safety for all. E
If a person's behaviour is hostile and intimidating, tell them you are finding their behaviour threatening and state clearly you wish them to stop/desist (see Box 5.11 for suggested phrases).	Some people may not be aware of the impact of their behaviour and will change it when it is pointed out that it is unacceptable. E
Assess individual situations and make use of relatives or friends if they are present and can be of assistance in diffusing the situation.	Sometimes people will listen more to a person who is close to them. E
Create some physical distance or summon assistance if the patient does not concur and continues to be threatening, abusive or passively non-compliant (e.g. refuses to move).	Maintaining safety for all. E

(Continued)

Principles table 5.8 (*Continued*)

Warn the person that you will contact security staff/police if necessary – avoid threatening language. If possible, make a personal or practical appeal.	People need clear information about the consequences of their actions. E
Attempt to talk the individual down, that is, calm them down by remaining calm and professional yourself, keeping your voice at a steady pace and a moderate volume. Try to engage the person in conversation.	Your behaviour will have an impact on theirs. E
Avoid personalizing the anger but do not accept unwarranted personal criticism.	If we personalize then we are likely to react in a way that exacerbates the situation but neither should you accept abuse. E
You may suggest walking with the patient to discuss issues but ensure you remain in a public/safe environment.	Changing the environment may help to recontextualize behaviour and movement channels agitation. E
The key communication skills discussed in the skills section will be helpful here but fundamentally you need to listen to what the grievance is, treat the person as an individual, preserve their dignity and attempt to help where you realistically can. Avoid passing the buck or blocking in another way.	People need to be heard and understood. E
If a patient is no longer abusive or threatening but is struggling to reduce their anger, they may benefit from some further psychological support or medication to help them feel calmer.	The short-term use of some medication may be beneficial. C
In rare and extreme circumstances where patients are violent and do not respond to de-escalation attempts and where the safety of other people is compromised, you must take immediate action by involving security and the police. If an ambulant outpatient, you need to ask them to leave if their behaviour is not acceptable.	Maintaining safety for all. E
Restraint and sedation may be required in some cases. Follow individual hospital security/emergency procedures in these instances.	

The ideal outcome for an encounter with an angry, aggressive or threatening person is that safety is not compromised and the healthcare professional is able to talk the person down, helping them to express the reason why they are angry. Follow-up support should be offered to help stop the person repeating the same behaviour. However, people should also be made aware of potential sanctions if they are unable to comply, for example withdrawal of treatment, involvement of the police and so on.

See Principles table 5.8.

Legal and professional issues

Nurses may be inclined to accept aggressive behaviour as part of the job (Mclaughlin *et al.* 2009) due to being encouraged to be caring, compassionate and accepting of others. Despite this, nurses have the right to work without feeling intimidated or threatened and should not tolerate verbal or physical abuse, threats or assault. Personal comments, sarcasm and innuendo are all unacceptable.

Employers have a responsibility to adhere to Management of Health and Safety at Work Regulations (HM Government 2000). This involves providing a safe environment for people to work in and one that is free from threats and abuse. With any physical assault, the police should be involved.

Preprocedural considerations
Pharmacological support

Short-term use of a benzodiazepine, for example diazepam or lorazepam, may be indicated. Assess this carefully, that is, do not assume that it is necessary. Once a situation is more under control, you can ask if the person feels less angry and whether they feel that they need further support. Suggesting this at the wrong time or insensitively may inflame the situation.

Box 5.11 Phrases that might help when talking with an angry person

- I can see that you are angry about this…
- I would like to help you try to sort this out, how can I do that?
- In order for me to help you, I need you to stop shouting.
- You are shouting at me and I can't help you until you stop.
- Please stop (unacceptable behaviour), you are making me and these other people quite frightened.
- Can you tell me what is making you so angry so that I might be able to help you sort it out?

Try to agree with the patient where possible (this can be a good way to diffuse tensions):

- I can see how that would annoy you … let's see what we can do about it.
- What might I/we do, for you to … (comply with the rules/ request)?

Box 5.12 Signs and symptoms of delirium

- Difficulty maintaining attention on features of the environment.
- Easily distractible.
- Unable to have a coherent conversation.
- Unable to recall recent events.

Other observable features include:

- disorientation
- rambling speech
- disinhibition
- slow responses
- disturbance of sleep patterns
- rapid mood changes or a significant change of attitude
- distress
- hallucinations and being irrationally frightened of objects.

(Irving and Foreman 2006)

A psychiatrist may prescribe an antipsychotic medication for short-term use, for example Risperidone.

See also Box 5.11 for phrases that might help when talking with an angry person.

It can be distressing to be exposed to threatening or abusive people and it is good practice to seek a debriefing interview. This can help you and the institution reflect upon the experience and procedures in place to manage such situations. Check with your occupational health or human resources department to establish where you can access support facilities.

Delirium

Definition

Delirium is an altered state of consciousness or acute confusion caused by a severe medical illness (Sendelbach *et al.* 2009).

Related theory

In most cases, delirium is caused by a general medical condition, intoxication or withdrawal of medication/substances which act upon the neurochemical balance of the brain (Ross 1991). Causative factors like infection, post anaesthesia and medication (especially analgesics) need to be considered, particularly for sudden onset of delirium in the hospital environment.

Figures for the incidence of delirium vary, but up to 25% may experience a delirium whilst hospitalized. Up to 50% of postoperative patients may develop delirium (NICE 2008b). There is an increased prevalence for inpatients over the age of 65 years. Age, the severity of illness, pre-existing cognitive decline, immobility and malnutrition all increase risk (Irving *et al.* 2006).

The disturbance can develop quickly and fluctuate during the course of a 24-hour period (DSM IV 1994). Environmental cues during the daytime act as stabilizing factors and this makes symptoms typically worse at night. The disturbance can resolve within hours/days or can last longer if co-existing with other problems like dementia. A patient's behaviour may change to indicate potential delirium before a full set of diagnostic symptoms is observable (Duppils and Wikblad 2004) (Box 5.12). There is considerable morbidity and mortality associated with delirium, delaying recovery and rehabilitation (Irving *et al.* 2006, NICE 2008b). Recognizing and addressing delirium is important because of the distress it causes patients, families and staff (Lawlor *et al.* 2000). A marked feature of delirium is the variety and fluctuating nature of symptoms.

Evidence-based approaches

Nurses play a critical role in the prevention, early detection (Milisen *et al.* 2005) and management of delirium. Delirium is frequently iatrogenic (i.e. caused by medical intervention) and hence can often be corrected once the causative factor has been identified.

Addressing the causative factors as part of good nursing and medical care will help prevent the development of delirium. This means ensuring hydration and nutritional requirements are met and any electrolyte imbalances are monitored and corrected.

Nurses need to be aware that patients over the age of 65 (especially those having anaesthesia) will be highly prone to developing delirium so need to be monitored carefully over a period of time to pick up any early signs. The effect of analgesia (especially opiates) also needs to be considered.

The emergence of delirium can also be significant at the end of life and significantly complicate care (Delgado-Guay *et al.* 2008). Terminal restlessness is a term often used to describe this agitated delirium in end-of-life care, where the causes may require specific management different from that of other types of delirium (Travis *et al.* 2001). A progressive shutdown of body organs in the last 2–3 days of life (Lawlor *et al.* 2000) leads to irresolvable systemic imbalances. The management of delirium in end-of-life care therefore shift from a focus on reversing the cause to alleviating the symptoms. Nurses should avoid medicating symptoms unless this is in the patient's best interests.

Principles of care

Initial screening for any cognitive issues on admission is important to identify predictive factors and establish a baseline of cognitive functioning. Involving the family can be crucial to an accurate assessment where there are existing changes.

Once identified, delirium should be managed by attempting to establish the potential reversible causes. This will include:

- newly started medications
- changes in dosage
- opioid toxicity, withdrawal from opioids or alcohol
- use of corticosteroids
- metabolic imbalances or organ failure affecting the processing and excretion of drugs
- infections
- hypercalcaemia
- constipation.

Legal and professional issues

In the case of medium to longer term delirium, another person may make decisions upon the patient's behalf – this person will have 'lasting power of attorney' and may have been nominated by the patient. It could be a professional, friend or a member of the family. This person will need to be registered with the public guardian and is bound to act in the patient's best interests.

The Mental Capacity Act sets out protection for liability when caring for someone with reduced capacity. This is reliant upon accurate and suitable assessment of capacity and best interests.

Restraint

Restraint is a difficult ethical issue requiring careful consideration. Restraint takes many forms and must be meticulously judged for the potential to benefit or harm an individual. As a general rule, restraint should be a last resort to protect the individual and/or others from harm.

Wherever possible, nurses must attempt to create an environment where restraint is not going to be necessary. It is a rare requirement and all feasible steps to avoid the use of restraint must be explored.

Any action taken must be the 'least harmful' intervention in the circumstance. The aim is to balance the patient's right to independence with their and others' safety. If restraint is required, nurses must explain to the patient why they are doing what they are doing (regardless of the patient's perceived capacity) and reduce the negative impact upon the patient's dignity as much as possible.

An example of justified restraint would be use of mittens in a patient recovering from sedation or anaesthesia who is attempting to remove cannula, drains or catheters (behaviour likely to cause them harm). Regular review and documentation are necessary and the mittens should be removed as soon as the potential harm has passed (RCN 2008).

Documentation

Delirium is under-reported in nursing and medical note taking (Irving *et al.* 2006). Documentation outlining the onset of behaviours and symptoms is instrumental in assisting the medical team to identify the cause and likely solution to the problem. The documentation of the assessment and subsequent care must be detailed and accurate.

Preprocedural considerations
Pharmacological support

Once diagnosed, symptoms that do not respond to non-pharmacological interventions can be treated with prescribed medication: antipsychotics, for example olanzapine, and/or sedatives, for example haloperidol (NICE 2009b). As far as possible, benzodiazepines are avoided as these are associated with delirium (BNF 2011). However, they may be used if delirium is caused by alcohol withdrawal.

Use of medication for sedation in the end stages of life needs individual consideration and the family must be involved and communicated with regularly.

It is worth noting that health professionals and family members can mistake the agitation of delirium for symptoms of pain. If opioids are increased as a result, there will be a potential worsening of the delirium (Delgado-Guay *et al.* 2008).

Non-pharmacological support

Creating an environment conducive to orientation is important wherever possible, for example a quiet well-lit environment, where normal routines take place. Nurses must help patients to maximize their independence through activity as mobilization is seen to assist with orientation (Neville 2006). Nursing interventions include creating a well-lit room with familiar objects, limited staff changes (possibly

Principles table 5.9 Communicating with an individual with delirium

Principle	Rationale
It is essential to ensure that aids for visual and hearing impairments are functional and are being used.	To maximize ability to communicate normally. E, C
Adjust environment to promote the patient's orientation, for example visible clock or calendar, photographs of family.	Maintain/promote orientation. E, C
Background noise should be kept to a minimum.	This can be very distracting for the patient. E, C
The healthcare professional should introduce themselves to the patient (do not assume they remember you). If possible, limit the number of individuals involved in care.	Promote consistency and reduce potential for confusion. E
Give simple information in short statements. Use closed questions.	Closed questions are less taxing and only require a yes or no answer. E, R5
It is important to give explicit explanation of any procedures or activities carried out with the individual.	Maintain respect and dignity. E, C

requiring one-to-one nursing care), reduced noise stimulation and the presence of family or familiar friends.

Liaison with the patient's family is important so that they understand what is happening and what they can do to help. It must be recognized how distressing it can be to witness or spend time with a delirious member of the family. The family should therefore be given the opportunity to talk about their concerns and be updated with information about the cause and management.

Safety is a priority and patients must be observed carefully to prevent any injury occurring to themselves or others.

See Principles table 5.9.

Acquired communication disorders

Definitions

Aphasia/dysphasia (terms can be used interchangeably) is an acquired communication disorder that impairs a person's ability to process language. It does not affect intelligence but does affect how someone uses language. Any injury to the brain has the potential to change a person's ability to speak, read, write and understand others.

Aphasia may be temporary or permanent. Aphasia does *not* include speech impairments caused by damage to the muscles involved with speech, that is, dysarthria.

Dysarthria is a motor speech disorder. Neurological and muscular changes may cause difficulty in producing or sustaining the range, force, speed and co-ordination of the movements needed to achieve appropriate breathing, phonation, resonance and articulation for speech (Royal College of Speech and Language Therapists 2006). Speech may sound flat, slurred, nasal or have a jerky rhythm; pitch, loudness and breath control can also be affected.

Dyspraxia of speech is different from dysarthria as it is not caused by muscle weakness or sensory loss but is a disorder of initiating and sequencing purposeful/voluntary movement. Verbal expression may be hesitant with sound substitutions, for example saying 'tup of tea' for 'cup of tea'.

Dysphonia is a voice disorder and may be related to disordered laryngeal, respiratory and vocal tract function and reflect structural, neurological, psychological and behavioural problems as well as systemic conditions (Mathieson 2001).

Anatomy and physiology

Language

It is now recognized that many areas of the brain are involved with language processing and the complex relationship between structure and function is not fully understood. Distortion and/or compression can occur at some distance from a problem (like a primary or secondary tumour). This means that any consequent cognitive and language impairments may have no direct relationship with the location of brain tumours (Gaziano and Kumar 1999, Gehring *et al.* 2008, Meyer and Levin 1996, Murdoch 1990, Scheibal *et al.* 1996).

Speech

Speech (dysarthria), voice (dysphonia) and swallowing (dysphagia) can be impaired by any brain tumour or head and neck cancers involving the ventricular system, brainstem, cerebellum and cranial nerves (V, VII, IX, X, XI, XII). The management of swallowing difficulties is covered in Chapter 8.

Related theory

The brain is the organ of the body that is, above all others, linked with our sense of self. The importance of effective communication is considered at the beginning of this chapter and this need becomes more apparent with any communication disorder. Speech and language shape our thoughts, and language is necessary to make sense of or give meaning to our world. It is the currency of friendship (Parr *et al.* 1997) and is intrinsic and essential to our well-being. Its value and complexity may not become apparent until it is disrupted.

One of the key issues for patients with aphasia (disruption of language processing) is when we expect them to make sense of their disease, its treatment and management options. To do this, they need to use the very medium that is damaged – language. This may have an obvious or more subtle impact upon how the patient's psychological, emotional and social needs are met.

When patients have difficulty communicating, their sense of identity can become fragile and may be further undermined when they are in a hospital. Understandably, in this environment, the focus is on their medical diagnosis, prognosis, treatments and side-effects. Facilitating their communication strengths allows us to help them understand, as well as supporting, acknowledging and respecting their individual needs.

Barriers to communication

- *Poor memory*: delayed language processing can further compromise short-term memory problems.
- *Reduced concentration and short attention span*: acute post surgical; during and after radiotherapy treatment to the brain.
- *Distractibility*: increased sensitivity to background noise or visual distractions.
- *Generalized fatigue*: already using extra energy to process language, it becomes too effortful to chat.
- Previous communication style and communication needs.

Evidence-based approaches

Communication is a neurological function and the speech and language therapist has a key role in the specialist assessment and management of disorders/disruptions to this vital function (Giordana and Clara 2006). Patients with diseases affecting their central nervous system require input from a well-co-ordinated multiprofessional team (NICE 2006), to support their complex changing care needs throughout the patient pathway (NICE 2004, NICE 2006, NSF 2005, RCP, BSRM, NCPCS 2008).

Box 5.13 Suggestions to facilitate realistic expectations and successful use of AAC

- An early referral to the speech and language therapist to assess the appropriateness of the use of AAC.
- With the addition of any aid (no matter how simple or sophisticated), communication becomes more complex and difficult as it involves another step in the process, that is, changes from a two-way to a three-way process.
- Patients need to be motivated to use aids.
- The use of aids requires planning, extra concentration and time, listening, watching and interpretation by both patient and conversation partner.

Preprocedural considerations

Equipment

Communication aids

Communication aids or equipment are referred to as augmentive or alternative communication (AAC). AAC may range from basic picture charts or books to electronic aids and computer programs and may support communication when the patient presents with a severe dysarthria or a severe expressive and/or receptive aphasia. Box 5.13 provides suggestions to facilitate realistic expectations and successful use of AAC.

Patients with various forms of communication difficulty

The person with aphasia

See Principles table 5.10.

The person with impaired speech (dysarthria)

See Principles table 5.11.

The person with impaired voice (dysphonia)

See Principles table 5.12.

The person who is blind or partially sighted

See Principles table 5.13.

The person who is deaf or hard of hearing

See Principles table 5.14.

Communication for an individual with a laryngectomy

Definition

Laryngectomy involves removal of the larynx, resulting in loss of voice and a permanent tracheostoma on the neck.

Principles table 5.10 Supporting communication for the person with aphasia

Principle	Rationale
Be aware of where the aphasic patient is within their disease trajectory.	
Be aware if the patient has impaired attention, concentration and/or memory.	This will affect what you say and how you check for understanding. E
Minimize distractions – both visual and auditory.	Make it easier for both parties to concentrate. E
Allow enough time, with a calm, friendly, encouraging approach.	Develop and maintain rapport. E
Use a notebook to record key information.	This minimizes miscommunication particularly if the information is new or complex, the patient is anxious or their memory function is impaired. E
Frequent signposting and checking understanding.	To make sure the patient understands the purpose of the conversation. E
Talk directly to the patient and ask them what is/isn't helpful.	
Have a pen and paper for both people to use during the conversation.	Writing or drawing can support what is being said. E
Speech should be clear, slightly slower and of normal volume.	
Use straight-forward language, avoiding jargon.	Medical terminology is inevitably long and complex but can be clearly written in the notebook for future reference. E
Say one thing at a time and pause between 'chunks' of information.	Allow time for understanding and for questions. E
Structure questions carefully and make use of closed questions.	Limit the need for complex expression. E
Regularly check the patient's understanding.	
Declare a change of topic clearly.	It can be harder for some patients to recognize when the topic has changed. E
Be prepared for their and your frustration. You might have to come back to a topic at another time.	Abilities may fluctuate, so what helps one moment might not work another time. E

Principles table 5.11 Supporting communication for the person with dysarthria

The dysarthria may range from mild, slightly slurred or imprecise speech to being unintelligible (this is different from aphasia where language is not affected).

Principle	Rationale
Be encouraging but honest and open if you are having difficulty understanding.	This allows the patient to repeat things or express things in another way that may be more understandable. E
Ask if they use any strategies to help their speech.	Patients may well know what helps most. E
Encourage a slower rate of speech and regular pauses.	Ensure adequate breathing between words and phrases. E
Find a quiet environment to speak.	Reduce distractions and make it easier to concentrate. E
Allow more time than usual.	
Have pen and paper to hand, and encourage writing when necessary.	Provide another medium of communication. E

Principles table 5.12 Supporting communication for the person with dysphonia

The dysphonia may fluctuate from a mild hoarseness to not being able to voice at all. Early referral to a speech and language therapist for assessment and advice on vocal hygiene may be required.

Principle	Rationale
Have pen and paper to hand, encourage writing when necessary.	Provide another medium of communication. E
Encourage the patient to talk gently and avoid either shouting or whispering.	This can strain the voice. E
Avoid having to talk where there is background noise.	The individual would then need to strain unnecessarily. E
Face-to-face communication is preferable. Keep telephone calls to a minimum.	The patient will then be able to use non-verbal communication to transmit their message. E
Encourage regular sips of water.	To maintain hydration and keep the throat area moist. E
Use closed questions so the individual doesn't need to make lengthy replies.	Discourage lengthy responses to questions. E
Discourage frequent throat clearing. Instead, encourage a firm swallow if possible or gentle throat clearing.	
Be aware if the room atmosphere is dry (placing a bowl of water beside the radiator will help humidify/moisten the air).	A humid atmosphere is preferable to reduce local irritation. E

Principles table 5.13 Communication with someone who is blind or partially sighted

Sight loss may vary from mild to complete. Any sight loss is a significant issue when caring for patients. They will rely more on other senses, especially their hearing. Good communication practice is essential and you may need to be the eyes for the patient and relay information they are not aware of, for example the patient's visitor has arrived and is waiting. It is important to be open about the visual impairment and identify the preferred method(s) for each person. No single method will suit all. Even the same person might use different methods at different times and under different circumstances.

Blind and partially sighted people have the same information needs as everyone else and need accessible information in a suitable format such as large-print documents, Braille or audio information. Access to information facilitates informed decisions and promotes independence.

Principle	Rationale
Always say who you are when you arrive.	Normal cues are not available to the blind or partially sighted. E
In situations where there might be confusion as to who is being spoken to, use the patient's name or a light touch when you are addressing them.	As above.
Explain precisely where you are.	So people can orientate towards you. E
Ensure glasses are clean and within reach.	
Clear and careful explanations and checking understanding verbally are essential.	We communicate a substantial essence of meaning non-verbally. Blind people therefore do not receive this information so it is harder to gain full understanding. E
Indicate to a patient when you are leaving.	Normal cues are not available to the blind or partially sighted. E

Principles table 5.14 Communicating with someone who is deaf or hard of hearing

As with blindness, the severity of the impairment will vary. If a hearing aid is used, make sure it is fitted and working. Remember that hearing aids amplify everything, even background noise. More severe hearing loss will not benefit from an aid and these patients might rely on lip reading and/or signing or writing.

Principle	Rationale
Find a suitable place to talk: somewhere quiet with no noise or distractions, with good lighting. Make sure that the light is not behind you.	So the person can clearly see your face, and lip reading and expression can contribute to understanding. E, C
Be patient and allow extra time to for the consultation/conversation.	It is likely to take longer than normal. E
Depending on the purpose of the consultation, writing down a summary of the key points made might be helpful.	This will ensure the person has a record of what is said in case they have misunderstood or misheard what is said. E
If the person is wearing a hearing aid, do not assume they can hear you. Ask if it is on and if they still need to lip read.	
If an interpreter is required always remember to talk directly to the person you are communicating with, not the interpreter.	This is respectful and confirms that it is them you are addressing. E
Make sure you have the listener's attention before you start to speak.	Otherwise they may miss crucial information. E
Contextualize the discussion by giving the topic of conversation first.	Signposting helps people understand. R5, E
Talk clearly but not too slowly, and do not exaggerate your lip movements.	Lip reading is easier for people when you talk fairly normally. E
Use natural facial expressions and gestures and try to keep your hands away from your face.	Blocking your face will make understanding more difficult. E
Use plain language; avoid waffling, jargon and unfamiliar abbreviations.	Plain language will be more easily understood. E
Check that the person understands you. Be prepared to repeat yourself as many times as necessary.	Many people need to have information repeated to understand it. E

Anatomy and physiology

The larynx is found in the neck at the level of the third and sixth cervical vertebrae. It lies anterior to the oesophagus, situated at the top of the trachea (Mathieson 2001). The larynx is made of bone and cartilage held together by muscles and membranes. As the upper airway is shared with the food passage, the main function of the larynx is to protect the airway from saliva, and food and drink from entering the trachea and lungs. The larynx allows production of a cough to clear unwanted materials from the airway (Corbridge 1998) and is used for voicing. Within the larynx, held between the thyroid cartilage and the arytenoids lie the vocal folds; as air from the trachea passes up towards the vocal folds, they vibrate to make sound. This is then directed up towards the resonating cavities, pharynx and nasal cavities to the mouth where the lips and tongue articulate to produce voice.

Related theory

Once the vocal cords have been removed, another vibrating source needs to be created. There are a variety of communication options post laryngectomy, including oesophageal speech, artificial larynx and surgical voice restoration.

Box 5.14 lists the variety of ways in which communication is restored post laryngectomy.

Box 5.14 Ways in which communication is restored after laryngectomy

- *Oesophageal voice* involves getting air into the oesophagus (Searl and Reeves 2007) either by inhaling or injecting air into the back of the mouth. Instead of the vocal cords vibrating, the walls of the pharynx vibrate. Sound then moves up into mouth where recognizable speech is produced.
- An *artificial larynx* involves using a battery-powered device which is placed against the neck cheek or intraorally (Searl and Reeves 2007). When the button is pushed, a vibration occurs in the head of the device and it is this vibration through the tissues that creates sound as the patient mouths the words.
- *Surgical voice restoration* (SVR) (Figure 5.5) allows communication to be restored by use of a voice prosthesis which may also be referred to as a valve.

Surgical voice restoration has become the most popular, with success rates of up to 90% reported (Op de Coul *et al.* 2000). SVR entails creating a fistula between the posterior wall of the trachea and the anterior wall of the oesophagus, into which a one-way voice prosthesis is placed. By closing off the tracheostoma, pulmonary air is diverted through the prosthesis into the oesophagus where the walls vibrate to make sound (van As-Brooks and Fuller 2007).

The prosthesis is a silicone device, which fits into the tracheo-oesophageal puncture (TEP) and acts as a one-way valve, preventing food and drink from entering the trachea from the oesophagus (Figure 5.6). A puncture created at the time of the laryngectomy is known as a primary puncture whilst a secondary puncture is created some time after the laryngectomy operation. Postoperatively, patients with a primary puncture are fed via a stoma gastric tube, which enables the puncture to remain patent, avoids food contamination around the healing pharynx and decreases the risk of fistula formation (Karlen and Maisel 2001, Rhys-Evans *et al.* 2003).

Preprocedural considerations

Equipment

Voice prostheses

Voice prostheses have been available in Britain for over 25 years (Singer 2004) and there are a number of devices on the market, mainly Blom-Singer and Provox products. All work according to the same principle with a one-way valve, two flanges, one anterior and one posterior, to secure the prosthesis *in situ* in the TEP and a strap to attach to the neck (Figure 5.7). The prostheses come in a variety of diameters and lengths and it is the role of the

Figure 5.5 Surgical voice restoration. Image courtesy of InHealth Technologies.

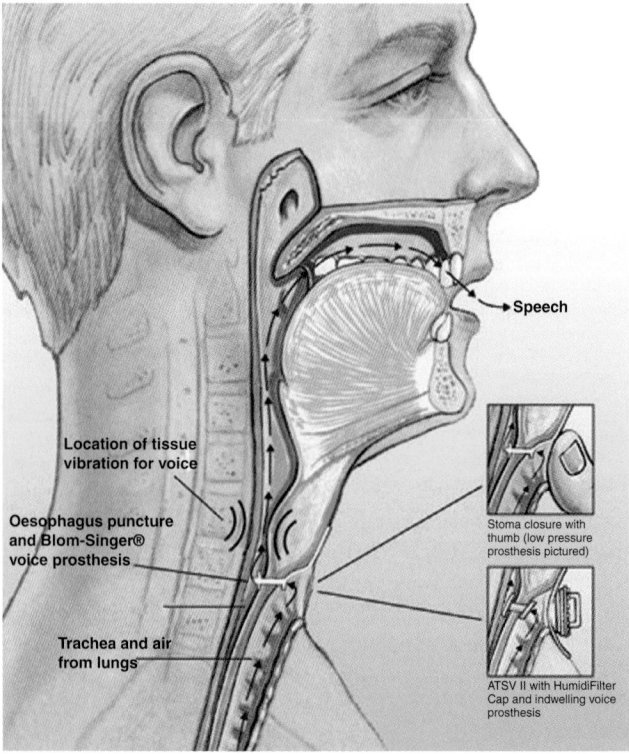

Figure 5.6 Voice prosthetics. Image courtesy of InHealth Technologies.

(a)

Flange

Hole where air enters

Retention collar (in pharynx)

Duckbill tip (in pharynx)

Slit shows where it opens

(b)

Flange

Hole where air enters

Retention collar
(in pharynx)

Low-pressure tip
(in pharynx)

Flap valve inside

(c)

Flange

Hole where air enters

Low-pressure tip

Flap valve (inside)

Retention collar (in pharynx)

(d)

Flange (cut off after insertion)

Retention collar
with radiopaque
edge (in pharynx)

Hole where air enters

Low-pressure valve, inside

Figure 5.7 Laryngectomy voice rehabilitation. (a) Duckbill valve. (b) Low-pressure valve, 16 Fr gauge. (c) Low-pressure valve, 20 Fr gauge. (d) Indwelling valve, 20 Fr gauge.

Table 5.3 Competencies for cleaning a voice prosthesis in a laryngectomy patient

Knowledge and understanding	Skills
Altered anatomy following a laryngectomy	An ability to recognize a laryngectomee versus a patient with a tracheostomy
The function of a voice prosthesis	An ability to recognize a voice prosthesis *in situ*
The importance of keeping the prosthesis clean	An ability to provide the patient/carer with relevant physical preparation for cleaning the prosthesis
Principles of brush selection	An ability to perform a safe cleaning technique with the appropriate equipment
Complications which may arise during or after cleaning, their cause and preventive measures	An ability to evaluate your cleaning technique with regard to demonstrating knowledge, recognizing difficulties, their cause and future preventive measures

Figure 5.8 Prosthesis brush.

187

Procedure guideline 5.1 Voice prosthesis: cleaning *in situ*

Essential equipment

- Non-sterile gloves and eye protection
- Light source
- Nebulizer
- Gauze pads
- Sterile water
- Tape
- Prosthesis brush (Figure 5.8)
- Tweezers
- Long cotton buds
- Clinically clean tray

Preprocedure

Action	Rationale
1 Explain and discuss the procedure with the patient.	To ensure that the patient understands the procedures and gives their valid consent (NMC 2008c, E).

Procedure

2 Settle the patient in a chair or upright in bed and arrange lighting to illuminate the stoma.	To ensure the patient is comfortable and well supported. E
3 Ask the patient to use the nebulizer.	To loosen secretions in trachea.
4 Wet the gauze and wipe around the stoma, wiping away from stoma.	To ensure clean stomal area and prevent water entering trachea. E
5 Remove the tape and clean behind the strap, replace with new tape.	To ensure stomal area is fully cleaned and prosthesis is secured. E
6 Using tweezers, carefully remove any dry crusts from around the prosthesis and trachea.	To ensure breathing is not impeded. E
7 Wet the cotton buds and carefully clean the outside of the prosthesis.	To ensure air can enter the prosthesis. E
8 Wet the prosthesis brush and carefully insert into barrel of prosthesis, turning one way only, and remove. Hold the strap of prosthesis during the procedure.	To ensure barrel of prosthesis is clean to allow air flow. To ensure the prosthesis does not become dislodged. E

Postprocedure

9 Record the procedure.	To maintain accurate records (NMC 2009).

Problem-solving table 5.1 Prevention and resolution (Procedure guideline 5.1)

Problem	Cause	Prevention	Action
Loss of the prosthesis or stoma gastric catheter	Accidental dislodgement or excessive coughing	Teach patients how to insert stent or catheter whilst on the ward	Immediately insert either stent or catheter. Check the patient has not inhaled the prosthesis; if they have, call for urgent ENT
Peripheral leak	Voice prosthesis too long		Specialized SLT or other trained clinician to downsize as appropriate

Central leakage	Food debris preventing closure of prosthesis	Thickener added to all drinks	Clean with a brush
Loss of voice	Debris blocking barrel of prosthesis		Clean with a brush
	Due to incorrectly sized prosthesis		Specialized SLT or other trained clinician to change device
	Due to oedema in the TEP or voicing technique		Specialized SLT to advise

189

Procedure guideline 5.2 Voice prosthesis: changing a Blom-Singer exdwelling duckbill voice prosthesis

The patient should be fully informed about the procedure. The specialist clinician must have identified the rationale for changing the prosthesis, usually due to a centrally leaking voice prosthesis. This is an advanced practice procedure and should only be undertaken if the appropriate theoretical and practical knowledge and skills have been gained through attendance at either a recognized workshop or inhouse training.

Essential equipment

- Non-sterile gloves and eye protection
- Light source
- Stent
- Catheter
- Appropriate size voice prosthesis with introducer stick
- Lubricating jelly
- Tape
- Cup of coloured water
- Clinically clean tray
- Tissues

Preprocedure

Action	Rationale
1 Explain and discuss the procedure with the patient.	To ensure that the patient understands the procedures and gives his/her valid consent (NMC 2008c, E).

Procedure

2 Settle the patient in a chair or upright in bed and arrange lighting to illuminate the stoma.	To ensure the patient is comfortable and well supported. E
3 Place a little lubricating jelly on the stent.	To ease insertion. E
4 Ask the patient to swallow and then open their mouth as the prosthesis is pulled out via the strap.	To minimize amount of saliva entering the fistula and reduce the risk of coughing. E
5 Immediately insert the stent fully and tape to the patient's neck.	To keep the fistula patent and prevent saliva from entering the fistula, resulting in coughing. E
6 Place the new prosthesis on the inserter stick, securing with flange.	To prevent prosthesis from dislodging from introducer during insertion. E
7 Remove stent, ensuring patient's mouth is open, and replace with prosthesis. A slight click may be felt as the posterior retention collar on the prosthesis passes into the pharynx.	To insert prosthesis. E
8 Gently pull the prosthesis forward.	To ensure it is fully through into the pharynx. E

(Continued)

Procedure guideline 5.2 *(Continued)*

9 If prosthesis comes out, reinsert stent.	To keep the fistula patent and prevent saliva from entering the fistula, resulting in coughing. Repeat steps 5–12. E
10 Place tape on the strap of the prosthesis onto the patient's neck.	To keep strap out of the way and further secure voice prosthesis. E
11 Give the patient some coloured water to drink and check for leakage from the prosthesis.	To ensure prosthesis is not leaking. If it is, clean with a brush or remove and repeat steps 4–12. E
12 Ask patient to voice by occluding the stoma.	To ensure voice prosthesis is fully through. If no voice, clean with a brush or remove and repeat steps 4–12. E
13 If unable to insert the voice prosthesis, prevent leak or achieve voice, insert a catheter and tape firmly to the chest. Call the Speech and Language Therapist.	To ensure patient can eat and drink safely as TEP blocked by catheter. Provide pen and paper for communication. E

Postprocedure

9 Record the procedure.	To maintain accurate records (NMC 2009).

specialist speech and language therapist to choose the most appropriate model for the patient, taking into account the patient's requirements. Prostheses can be either exdwelling, meaning the patient can be taught to self change, or indwelling, requiring the input of a specialist clinician, including a specialist speech and language therapist, ENT doctor or a nurse experienced in fitting and managing voice prostheses.

One of the care requirements is cleaning a voice prosthesis. This is an advanced practice role of a specialist nurse who has met the required competencies (see Table 5.3).

Websites and useful addresses

Action for Blind People
Helpline: 0800 915 4666
Website: www.actionforblindpeople.org.uk

Depression Alliance
Telephone: 0845 123 23 20
Website: www.depressionalliance.org

Depression UK
Email: info@depressionuk.org
Website: www.depressionuk.org

NHS patient information toolkit, version 2.0 (2003)
Website: www.nhsidentity.nhs.uk/
patientinformationtoolkit/patientinfotoolkit.pdf

Plain English Campaign
Telephone: 01663 744409
Website: www.plainenglish.co.uk

RNIB See It Right
Telephone: 020 7388 1266
Helpline: 0303 123 9999
Website: www.rnib.org.uk

RNID
Telephone: 020 7296 8000
Textphone: 020 7296 8001
Information Line (freephone):
Telephone: 0808 808 0123
Textphone: 0808 808 9000
Website: www.rnid.org.uk

Royal College of Psychiatrists
Leaflet on delirium:
www.rcpsych.ac.uk/mentalhealthinfo/problems/
physicalillness/delirium.aspx

Royal College of Speech and Language Therapists
Telephone: 020 7378 1200
Website: www.rcslt.org

Speakability
Helpline: 0808 808 9572
Website: www.speakability.org.uk

Stroke Association
Helpline: 0845 3033 100
Website: www.stroke.org.uk

References

Adams, J. and Whittington, R. (1995) Verbal aggression to psychiatric staff: traumatic stressor or part of the job? *Psychiatric Care*, 2 (5), 171–174.

Back, A.L., Arnold, R.M., Baile, W.F. *et al.* (2005). Approaching difficult communication tasks in oncology. *CA*, 55 (3), 164.

Baile, W.F., Buckman, R., Lenzi, R. *et al.* (2000) SPIKES – a six-step protocol for delivering bad news: application to the patient with cancer. *Oncologist*, 5 (4), 302–311.

Billings, C.V. (2004) Psychiatric inpatient suicide: focus on intervention. *Journal of the American Psychiatric Nurses Association*, 10, 190–192.

Blake, C. and Ledger, C. (2007) *Insight into Anxiety*. Waverley Abbey Insight Series. CWR, Farnham.

Booth, K., Maguire, P., Butterworth, T. and Hillier, V. (1996) Perceived professional support and the use of blocking behaviours by hospice nurses. *Journal of Advanced Nursing*, 24, 522–527.

Botti, M., Endacott, R., Watts, R. *et al.* (2006) Barriers in providing psychosocial support for patients with cancer. *Cancer Nursing*, 29 (4), 309–316.

Bowes, D.E., Tamlyn, D. and Butler, L.J. (2002) Women living with ovarian cancer: dealing with an early death. *Health Care for Women International*, 23 (2), 135–148.

Brady Wagner, L. (2003) Clinical ethics in the context of language and cognitive impairment: rights and protections. *Seminars in Speech and Language*, 24 (4), 275–284.

British Medical Association (2007) *Mental Capacity Act. Guidance for Health Professionals*. BMA, London.

BNF (2011) *British National Formulary*. BMT Group and RPS Publishing, London.

Brooks, W.D. and Heath, R.W. (1993) *Speech Communication*. WC Brown, Dubuque, IA.

Brown, R.F., Byland, C.L., Kline, N. *et al.* (2009) Identifying and responding to depression in adult cancer patients. *Cancer Nursing*, 32 (3), E1–E7.

Cambell, S. (2006) A project to promote better communication with patients. *Nursing Times*, 102 (19), 28–30

Chant, S. Jenkinson, T., Randle, J. and Russell, G. (2002) Communication skills: some problems in nurse education and practice. *J Clin Nurs*, 11, 12–21.

Chelf, J.H., Agre, P., Axelrod, A. *et al.* (2001) Cancer-related patient education: an overview of the last decade of evaluation and research. *Oncology Nursing Forum*, 28 (7), 1139–1147.

Chochinov, H.M. (2007) Dignity and the essence of medicine: the A, B, C, and D of dignity conserving care. *BMJ (Clinical Research Ed)*, 335 (7612), 184–187.

Corbridge, R. J. (1998) *Essential ENT Practice*. Arnold, London.

Deakin, K., Lee, K., Robinson, S. and Hermes, B. (2009) Suicide risk assessment: 6 steps to a better instrument. *Journal of Psychosocial Nursing and Mental Health Services*, 47 (6), 44–49.

Dein, S. (2005) Working with the patient who is in denial. *European Journal of Palliative Care*, 12 (6), 251–253.

Dein, S. (2006) *Culture and Cancer Care: Anthropological Insights in Oncology*. Open University Press, Maidenhead.

Delgado-Guay, M.O., Yennurajalingam, S. and Bruera, E. (2008) Delirium with severe symptom expression related to hypercalcemia in a patient with advanced cancer: an interdisciplinary approach to treatment. *Journal of Pain and Symptom Management*, 36 (4), 442.

Del Piccolo, L., Goss, C. and Bergvik, S. (2006) The fourth meeting of the Verona Network on Sequence Analysis. 'Consensus finding on the appropriateness of provider responses to patient cues and concerns'. *Patient Education and Counseling*, 61, 473–475.

Delvaux, N., Razavi, D., Marchal, S. *et al.* (2004) Effects of a 105 hours psychological training program on attitudes, communication skills and occupational stress in oncology: a randomised study. *British Journal of Cancer*, 90, 106–114.

DH (2004) *Better Information, Better Choice, Better Health*. Department of Health, London.

DH (2006) *Our Health, Our Care, Our Say: A New Direction for Community Services*. Department of Health, London.

DH (2008) *Information Accreditation Scheme*. Department of Health, London. www.dh.gov.uk/en/Healthcare/PatientChoice/BetterInformationChoicesHealth/Informationaccreditation/index.htm.

DH (2009) *Information Prescriptions*. Department of Health, London. www.dh.gov.uk/en/Healthcare/PatientChoice/Better InformationChoicesHealth/Informationprescriptions/index.htm.

DfES (2003) *The Skills for Life Survey*. Department for Education and Skills, Norwich. www.dfes.gov.uk/research/data/uploadfiles/RB490.pdf.

Donohoe, G. and Ricketts, T. (2006) Anxiety and panic. In: Feltham, C. and Horton, I. (eds) *The Sage Handbook of Counselling and Psychotherapy*. Sage, London.

DSM-IV (1994) *Diagnostic and Statistical Manual of Mental Disorders*, 4th edn. American Psychiatric Association, Washington, DC.

Dunne, K. (2003) The personal cost of caring. Guest editorial. *International Journal of Palliative Nursing*, 9 (6). 232.

Duppils, G.S. and Wikblad, K. (2004) Delirium: behavioural changes before and during the prodromal phase. *Journal of Clinical Nursing*, 13 (5), 609–616.

Duxbury, J. and Whittington, R. (2005) Causes and management of patient aggression and violence: staff and patient perspectives. *Journal of Advanced Nursing*, 50 (5), 469–478.

Edwards, P. (2005) An overview of the end-of-life discussion. *International Journal of Palliative Nursing*, 11 (1), 21–27.

Egan, G. (2002) *The Skilled Helper. A Problem–Management and Opportunity–Development Approach to Helping*, 7th edn. Brooks/Cole, Pacific Grove, CA.

Ellins, J. and Coulter, A. (2005) *How Engaged are People in their Healthcare? Findings of a National Telephone Survey*. Picker Institute, Oxford.

Equality Act (2010). www.equalities.gov.uk/equality_act_2010.aspx

Fallowfield, L., Ratcliffe, D., Jenkins, V. and Saul, J. (2001) Psychiatric morbidity and its recognition by doctors in patients with cancer. *British Journal of Cancer*, 84, 1011–1015.

Fallowfield, L., Jenkins, V.A. and Beveridge, H.A. (2002) Truth may hurt but deceit hurts more: communication in palliative care. *Palliative Medicine*, 16, 297–303.

Faulkner, A. and Maguire, P. (1994) *Talking to Cancer Patients and their Relatives*. Oxford University Press, Oxford.

Fellowes, D., Wilkinson, S.M., Leliopoulou, C. and Moore, P. (2003) Communication Skills Training for Health Care Professionals Working with Cancer Patients, Their Families and/or Carers: A Systematic Review. Cochrane Collaboration. www.cochrane.org/reviews/en/ab003751.html.

Fellowes, D., Wilkinson, S. and Moore, P. (2004) Communication skills for health care professionals working with cancer patients, their families and/or carers. *Cochrane Database of Systematic Reviews*, 2, CD003751.

Gaziano, J.E. and Kumar, R. (1999) Primary brain tumours. In: Sullivan, P. and Guilford, A.M. (eds) *Swallowing Intervention in Oncology*. Singular Publishing Group, San Diego, pp. 65–76.

Gehring, K., Sitskoorn, M.M., Aaronson, N.K. and Taphoorn, J.B. (2008) Interventions for cognitive deficits in adults with brain tumours. *Lancet Neurology*, 7, 548–560.

Gessler, S., Low, J., Daniells, E. *et al.* (2008) Screening for distress in cancer patients: is the distress thermometer a valid measure in the UK and does it measure change over time? A prospective validation study. *Psycho-Oncology*, **17** (6), 538.

Giordana, M.T. and Clara, E. (2006) Functional rehabilitation and brain tumours patients. A review of outcome. *Journal of Neurological Sciences*, **27**, 240–244.

Goldbeck, R. (1997) Denial in physical illness. *Journal of Psychosomatic Research*, **43** (6), 575–593.

Gudjonsson, G.H., Rabe-Hesketh, S. and Szmukler, G. (2004) Management of psychiatric in-patient violence: patient ethnicity and use of medication, restraint and seclusion. *British Journal of Psychiatry*, **184**, 258–262.

Gysels, M. Richardson, R. and Higginson, I.J. (2005) Communication training for health professionals who care for patients with cancer: a systematic review of effectiveness. *Journal of Supportive Care in Cancer*, **13** (6), 356–366.

Hack, T.F., Degner, L.F. and Parker, P.A. (2005). The communication goals and needs of cancer patients: a review. *Psycho-Oncology*, **14** (10), 831.

Hargie, O. and Dickson, D. (2004) *Skilled Interpersonal Communication: Research Theory and Practice*, 4th edn. Routledge, London.

Heaven, C., Clegg, J. and Maguire, P. (2006) Transfer of communication skills training from workshop to workplace: the impact of clinical supervision. *Patient Education and Counseling*, **60**, 313–325.

Henderson, A., van Eps, M.A., Pearson, K. *et al.* (2007) 'Caring for' behaviours that indicate to patients that nurses 'care about' them. *Journal of Advanced Nursing*, **60** (2), 146.

Hermes, B., Deakin, K., Lee, K. and Robinson, S. (2009) Suicide risk assessment: 6 steps to a better instrument. *Journal of Psychosocial Nursing and Mental Health Services*, **47** (6), 44–49.

Heron, J. (2001) *Helping the Client: A Creative Practical Guide*. Sage Publications, London.

Heyland, D.K., Dodek, P., Rocker, G. *et al.* (2006) What matters most in end-of-life care: perceptions of seriously ill patients and their family members. *Canadian Medical Association Journal*, **174** (5), 627–633.

HM Government (2000) *Management of Health and Safety at Work: Management of Health and Safety at Work Regulations 1999 Approved Code of Practice & Guidance*, HSE, Sudbury.

Houldin, A. (2000) *Patients with Cancer. Understanding the Psychological Pain*. Lippincott, Philadelphia.

Irving, K. and Foreman, M. (2006) Practice development – delirium. Delirium, nursing practice and the future. *International Journal of Older People Nursing*, **1** (2), 121–127.

Irving, K., Fick, D. and Foreman, M. (2006) Practice development – delirium. Delirium: a new appraisal of an old problem. *International Journal of Older People Nursing*, **1** (2), 106–112.

Jacobsen P., Donovan, K., Trask, P. *et al.* (2005) Screening for psychologic distress in ambulatory cancer patients. *Cancer*, **103** (7), 1494–1502.

Jenkins, V., Fallowfield, L. and Saul, J. (2001) Information needs of patients with cancer: results from a large study in UK cancer centres. *British Journal of Cancer*, **84**, 48–51.

Karlen, R.G., and Maisel, R.H. (2001) Does primary tracheoesophageal puncture reduce complications after laryngectomy and improve patient communication? *American Journal of Otolaryngology*, **22** (5), 324–328.

Kelsey, S. (2005) Improving nurse communication skills with cancer patient. *Cancer Nursing Practice*, **4** (2), 27–31.

Kennedy Sheldon, L. (2009) *Communication for Nurses*. Jones and Bartlett, Sudbury, MA.

Krug, E.G. (2002) *World Report on Violence and Health*. World Health Organization, Geneva.

Kruijver, I.P.M., Kerkstra, A., Bensing, J.M. and van de Weil, H.B.M. (2001) Communication skills of nurses during interactions with simulated cancer patients. *Journal of Advanced Nursing*, **34** (6), 772–779.

Lawlor, P.G., Gagnon, B., Mancini, I.L. *et al.* (2000) Occurrence, causes, and outcome of delirium in patients with advanced cancer: a prospective study. *Archives of Internal Medicine*, **160** (6), 786–794.

Lookinland, S. and Pool, M. (1998) Study on effect of methods of pre-operative education in women. *AORN Journal*, **67** (1), 203–213.

Lowry, M. (1995) Knowledge that reduces anxiety: creating patient information leaflets. *Professional Nurse*, **10** (5), 318–320.

Maben, J. and Griffiths, P. (2008) *Nurses in Society: Starting the Debate*. King's College, London.

Macdonald, E. (2004) *Difficult Conversations in Medicine*. Oxford University Press, Oxford.

Macmillan Cancer Relief (2004) *Macmillan Black and Minority Ethnic Toolkit – Effective Communication with African-Caribbean and African Men Affected by Prostrate Cancer*. Macmillan Cancer Relief, London.

Maguire, P. (2000) *Communication Skills for Doctors*. Arnold, London.

Maguire, P. and Pitceathly, C. (2002) Key communication skills and how to acquire them. *British Medical Journal*, **325**, 697–700.

Mathieson, L. (2001) *The Voice and Its Disorders*, 6th edn. Whurr, London.

McCabe, C. (2004) Nurse–patient communication: an exploration of patients' experiences. *Journal of Clinical Nursing*, **13**, 41–49.

McCaughan, E. and Parahoo, K. (2000) Medical and surgical nurses' perceptions of their level of competence and educational needs in caring for patients with cancer. *Journal of Clinical Nursing*, **9**, 420–428.

McKenzie, R. (2002) The importance of philosophical congruence for therapeutic use of self in practice. In: Freshwater, D. (ed) *Therapeutic Nursing. Improving Patient Care through Self-awareness and Reflection*. Sage Publications, London, pp. 22–38.

McLaughlin, S., Gorley, L. and Moseley, L. (2009) The prevalence of verbal aggression against nurses. *British Journal of Nursing*, **18** (12), 25.

Mednet (2010) www.medterms.com/script/main/art.asp?articlekey= 33843

Mental Capacity Act (2005) www.opsi.gov.uk/acts/acts2005/ ukpga_ 20050009_en_1

Menzies-Lyth, I. (1988) *Containing Anxiety in Institutions: Selected Essays*. Free Association Books, London.

Milisen, K., Lemiengre, J., Braes, T. and Foreman, M.D. (2005) Multicomponent intervention strategies for managing delirium in hospitalized older people: systematic review. *Journal of Advanced Nursing*, **52** (1), 79–90.

Mitchell, A.J. (2007) Pooled results from analysis of the accuracy of distress thermometer and other ultra short methods of detecting cancer related mood disorders. *Journal of Clinical Oncology*, **25**, 4670–4681.

Mitchell, A.J., Baker-Glenn, E.A., Park, B. *et al.* (2010) Can the Distress Thermometer be improved by additional mood domains? Part II. What is the optimal combination of Emotion Thermometers? *Psycho-Oncology*, **19** (2), 134–140.

Murdoch, B.E. (1990) *Acquired Speech and Language Disorders. A Neuro-Anatomical and Functional Neurological Approach*. Chapman and Hall, London.

NCCN (2010) Distress Management. Clinical Practice Guidelines in Oncology. www.nccn.org.

192

Neville, S. (2006) Practice development – delirium. Delirium and older people: repositioning nursing care. *International Journal of Older People Nursing*, **1** (2), 113–120.

NICE (2004) *Clinical Guidelines for the Management of Anxiety (Panic Disorder, With or Without Agoraphobia, and Generalised Anxiety Disorder) in Adults in Primary, Secondary and Community Care (CG 22)*. National Institute for Health and Clinical Excellence, London.

NICE (2005) *CG25 The Short-Term Management of Disturbed/Violent Behaviour in In-Patient Psychiatric Settings and Emergency Departments Violence*. National Institute for Health and Clinical Excellence, London.

NICE (2006) *Guidance on Cancer Services: Improving Outcomes for People with Tumours of the Brain and Central Nervous System*. National Institute for Health and Clinical Excellence, London.

NICE (2007) *Depression: Management of Depression in Primary and Secondary Care*. National Institute for Health and Clinical Excellence, London.

NICE (2008a) *Depression in Adults* (Update): *Final Scope*. National Institute for Health and Clinical Excellence. www.nice.org.uk/guidance/index.jsp?action=download&o=42260.

NICE (2008b) *Delirium: Final Scope*. National Institute for Health and Clinical Excellence. www.nice.org.uk/guidance/index.jsp?action=download&o=41170.

NICE (2009a) *Depression in Adults with a Chronic Physical Health Problem. Quick Reference Guide for Healthcare Professionals in General Hospital Settings*. National Institute for Health and Clinical Excellence, London.

NICE (2009b) *Delirium Draft Guideline*. National Institute for Health and Clinical Excellence. www.nice.org.uk/nicemedia/pdf/DeliriumDraftFullGuideline061109.pdf.

NMC (2008a) *The Code: Standards of Conduct, Performance and Ethics for Nurses and Midwives*. Nursing and Midwifery Council, London.

NMC (2008b) *Clinical Supervision for Registered Nurses*. Nursing and Midwifery Council, London www.nmc-uk.org/Nurses-and-midwives/Advice-by-topic/A/Advice/Clinical-supervision-for-registered-nurses/.

NMC (2008c) *Consent*. Nursing and Midwifery Council, London www.nmc-uk.org/Nurses-and-midwives/Advice-by-topic/A/Advice/Consent.

NMC (2009) *Record Keeping: Guidance for Nurses and Midwives*. Nursing and Midwifery Council, London.

Nordahl, G., Olofsson, N., Asplund, K. and Sjoling, M. (2003) The impact of preoperative information on state anxiety, postoperative pain and satisfaction with pain management. *Patient Education and Counseling*, **51** (2), 169.

NSF (2005) *The National Service Framework for Long-Term Conditions*. Department of Health, London.

Oguchi, M., Jansen, J., Butow, P. et al. (2010) Measuring the impact of nurse cue-response behaviour on cancer patients emotional cues. *Patient Education and Counseling*, April 27, epub ahead of print.

Op de Coul, B.M., Hilgers, F.J., Balm, A.J. et al. (2000) A decade of postlaryngectomy vocal rehabilitation in 318 patients: a single Institution's experience with consistent application of provox indwelling voice prostheses. *Archives of Otolaryngology, Head and Neck Surgery*, **126** (11), 1320–1328.

Parr, S., Byng, S., Gilpin, S. and Ireland, C. (1997) *Talking About Aphasia*. Open University Press, Buckingham.

Perry, K.N. and Burgess, M. (2002) *Communication in Cancer Care*. Blackwell Publishing, Oxford.

Powell, T. (2009) *The Mental Health Handbook*, 3rd edn. Speechmark, Milton Keynes.

Powell, T. and Enright, S. (1990) *Anxiety and Stress Management*. Routledge, London.

Ransom, S., Jacobsen, P.B. and Booth-Jones, M. (2006) Validation of the Distress Thermometer with bone marrow transplant patients. *Psycho-Oncology*, **15** (7), 604.

RCN (2008) *Let's Talk About Restraint. Rights, Risks and Responsibility*. Royal College of Nursing, London. www.rcn.org.uk/__data/assets/pdf_file/0007/157723/003208.pdf.

RCP, BSRM, NCPCS (2008) *Long-term Neurological Conditions: Management at the Interface Between Neurology, Rehabilitation and Palliative Care: Concise Guidance to Good Practice No 10*. Royal College of Physicians, British Society of Rehabilitation Medicine, National Council for Palliative Care Services, London.

RCPsych Depression leaflet (2010) Royal College of Psychiatrists Public Education Editorial Board. www.rcpscy.ac.uk.

Rhys-Evans, P.H., Montgomery, P.Q., Gullane, P.J. (eds) (2003) *Principles and Practice of Head and Neck Oncology*. Taylor and Francis, London.

Roberts, D. and Snowball, J. (1999) Psychosocial care in oncology nursing: a study of social knowledge. *Journal of Clinical Nursing*, **8**, 39–47.

Rogers, C.R. (1975) Empathic: an unappreciated way of being. *Counselling Psychologist*, **5**, 2–10.

Ross, C.A. (1991) CNS arousal systems: possible role in delirium. *International Psychogeriatrics*, **3** (2), 353–371.

Royal College of Speech and Language Therapists (2006) Therapists guidance on best practice in service organisation and provision. *Communicating Quality*, (3).

Ryan, H., Schofield, P., Cockburn, J. et al. (2005) Original article: How to recognize and manage psychological distress in cancer patients. *European Journal of Cancer Care*, **14** (1), 7–15.

Scheibal, R.S., Meyer, C.A. and Levin, V.A. (1996) Cognitive dysfunction following surgery for intra-cerebral glioma. Influence of histopathology, lesion, location and treatment. *Journal of Neuro-oncology*, **30**, 61–69.

Schofield, P., Carey, M., Bonevski, B. and Sanson-Fisher, R. (2006) Barriers to the provision of evidence-based psychosocial care in oncology. *Psycho-Oncology*, **15** (10), 863.

Schofield, P.E., Butow, P.N., Thompson, J.F. and Tattersall, M.H.N. (2008) Physician communication. *Journal of Clinical Oncology*, **26** (2), 297–302.

Scott, A. (2004) Managing anxiety in ICU patients: the role of pre-operative information provision. *Nursing in Critical Care*, **9** (2), 72–79.

Searl, J.P. and Reeves, S. (2007) Nonsurgical voice restoration following total laryngectomy. In: Ward, E.C. and van As-Brooks C.J. (eds) *Head and Neck Cancer – Treatment, Rehabilitation and Outcomes*. Plural Publishing, San Diego.

Sendelbach, S., Guthrie, P. and Schoenfelder, D. (2009) Acute confusion/delirium: identification, assessment, treatment, and prevention. *Journal of Gerontological Nursing*, **35** (11), 11–18.

Silverman, J., Kurtz, S. and Draper, J. (2005) *Skills for Communicating with Patients*, 2nd edn. Radcliffe Publishing, Oxford.

Singer, M.I. (2004) The development of successful tracheoesophageal voice restoration. *Otolaryngology Clinics of North America*, **37** (3), 507–517.

Smith, C., Dickens, C. and Edwards, S. (2005) Provision of information for cancer patients: an appraisal and review. *European Journal of Cancer Care*, **14**, 282–288.

Sobczak, J.A. (2009) Managing high-acuity-depressed adults in primary care. *Journal of the American Academy of Nurse Practitioners*, **21** (7), 362–370.

Strong, V., Sharpe, S., Cull, A. et al. (2004) Can oncology nurses treat depression? A pilot project. *Journal of Advanced Nursing*, **46** (5), 542–548.

193

Taylor, B. (1998) Ordinariness in nursing as therapy. In: McMahon, R. and Pearson, A. (eds) *Nursing as Therapy*. Stanley Thornes, Cheltenham, pp. 64–75.

Thomas, S.P., Groer, M., Davis, M. *et al.* (2000) Anger and cancer: an analysis of the linkages. *Cancer Nursing*, **23**, 344–349.

Thorne, S.E., Kuo, M., Armstrong, E.-A. *et al.* (2005) 'Being known': patients' perspectives of the dynamics of human connection in cancer care. *Psycho-Oncology*, **14** (10), 887.

Tortora, G.J. and Derrickson, B.H. (2009) *Principles of Anatomy and Physiology*, 12th edn. John Wiley, Hoboken, NJ.

Towers, R. (2007) Providing psychological support for patients with cancer. *Nursing Standard*, **28** (12), 50–58.

Trask, P.C. (2004) Assessment of depression in cancer patients. *Journal of the National Cancer Institute Monographs*, **32**, 80–92.

Travis, S., Conway, J., Daly, M. and Larsen, P. (2001) Terminal restlessness in the nursing facility: assessment, palliation, and symptom management. *Geriatric Nursing*, **22** (6), 308–312.

Turner, J., Clavarino, A., Yates, P. *et al.* (2007) Oncology nurses' perceptions of their supportive care for patients with advanced cancer: challenges and educational needs. *Psycho-Oncology*, **16**, 149–157.

Van As-Brooks, C.J. and Fuller, D.P. (2007) Prosthetic tracheoesophageal voice restoration following total laryngectomy. In: Ward, E.C. and van As-Brooks C.J. (eds) *Head and Neck Cancer – Treatment, Rehabilitation and Outcomes*. Plural Publishing, San Diego.

Vos, M. (2008) Denial in lung cancer patients: a longitudinal study. *Psycho-Oncology*, **17**, 1163–1171.

Vos, M.S. and Haes, J. (2007) Denial in cancer patients, an explorative review. *Psycho-Oncology*, **16** (1), 12.

White, H. (2004) Acquired communication and swallowing difficulties in patients with primary brain tumours. In: Booth, S. and Bruera, E. (eds) *Palliative Care Consultations Primary and Metastatic Brain Tumours*. Oxford University Press, Oxford, pp. 117–134.

Wilkinson, S. (1991) Factors which influence how nurses communicate with cancer patients. *Journal of Advanced Nursing*, **16**, 677–688.

Wosket, V. (2006) *Egan's Skilled Helper Model: Developments and Applications in Counselling*. Routledge, London.

Zabora, J., Brintzenhofeszoc, K., Curbow, B. *et al.* (2001) The prevalence of psychological distress by cancer site. *Psycho-oncology*, **10**, 19–28.

194

Elimination

The Royal Marsden Hospital Manual of Clinical Nursing Procedures, Eighth Edition. Edited by Lisa Dougherty and Sara Lister.

Overview

This chapter will provide an overview of elimination and is divided into three main sections. The first reviews urinary elimination, examining penile sheaths, urinary catheterization, urinary diversions and bladder irrigation. The second section reviews faecal elimination, examining diarrhoea, constipation, enemas, suppositories, digital rectal examination and manual evacuations. The final section examines stoma care, intestinal bowel obstruction and ileus.

Normal elimination

Assisting the patient with normal elimination

Evidence-based approaches

Principles of care

Elimination is a sensitive issue and providing effective care and management for problems associated with it can be prob-

lematic. The difficulties associated with this can be minimized if the nurse seeks to respect the patient's dignity when carrying out procedures such as assisting them with using a bedpan or a commode.

Preprocedural considerations

It is essential that the procedure is explained clearly to the patient to ensure consent is obtained and patient co-operation is agreed. A manual handling assessment is vital in order to establish if additional equipment such as a hoist is required.

Pharmacological support

Skin breakdown as a result of incontinence is a common problem with either faecal and/or urinary incontinence (Gray *et al.* 2007). Current nursing practice includes the use of a wide range of skin moisturizers and barrier creams but there is little known about their efficacy or effectiveness (Gray *et al.* 2007). A recent review suggests that the use of barrier creams with a pH near to that of normal skin can be useful in prevention of skin problems but more research is required (Beeckman *et al.* 2009).

Procedure guideline 6.1 **Slipper bedpan use: assisting a patient**

Essential equipment

- Disposable apron and gloves
- Slipper bedpan and paper cover
- Toilet paper

- Manual handling equipment as appropriate
- Additional nurse if required
- Wash bowl, warm water, disposable wipes and a towel

Preprocedure

Action	Rationale
1 Take the equipment to the bedside and explain the procedure to the patient.	To ensure that the patient understands the procedure and gives their valid consent (NMC 2008a, C).
2 Carry out appropriate manual handling assessment prior to commencing procedure and establish whether an additional nurse or equipment such as a hoist is necessary.	To maintain a safe environment. E

Procedure

3 Take the equipment to the bedside and explain the procedure to the patient.	To ensure that the patient understands the procedure and gives their valid consent (NMC 2008a, C).
4 Wash hands, put on gloves and apron.	To ensure procedure is as clean as possible (Fraise and Bradley 2009, E).
5 Close door/draw curtains around the patient's bed area.	To maintain privacy and dignity and avoid any unnecessary embarrassment for the patient (NMC 2008b, C).
6 Remove the bedclothes and, providing there are no contraindications (e.g. if patient is on flat bed rest), assist the patient into an upright sitting position.	An upright, 'crouch-like' posture is considered anatomically correct for defaecation. Poor posture adopted while using a bedpan has been shown to cause extreme straining during defaecation. Patients should therefore be supported with pillows in order to achieve an upright position on the bedpan (Taylor 1997, E).

7 Ask the patient to raise their hips/buttocks and insert the bedpan beneath the patient's pelvis, ensuring that the wide end of the bedpan is between the legs, and the narrow end is beneath the buttocks.	A slipper bedpan provides more comfort for a patient who is unable to sit upright on a conventional bedpan (Nicol 2008, E).
8 Offer patients the use of pillows and encourage them to lean forward slightly.	To provide support and optimize positioning for defaecation (Taylor 1997, E).
9 If the patient is unable to adopt a sitting/upright position, then roll them onto one side, using appropriate manual handling equipment, and insert a slipper bedpan with the narrow/flat end underneath their buttocks and wide end between their legs. Then roll the patient onto their back and so onto the bedpan.	To ensure that the patients is in optimum position for eliminating. E
10 Once the patient is on the bedpan, encourage them to move their legs slightly apart and check to ensure that their positioning is correct.	To avoid any spillage onto the bedclothes and reduce risk of contamination and cross-infection. E
11 Cover the patient's legs with a sheet.	To maintain privacy and dignity (NMC 2008b, C).
12 Ensure that toilet paper and call bell are within patient's reach and leave the patient, but remain nearby.	To maintain privacy and dignity (NMC 2008b, C).
13 When the patient has finished using the bedpan, bring washing equipment to the bedside, remove the bedpan, and replace paper cover. Assist patient with cleaning perianal area using warm water and soap. Apply a small amount of barrier cream to the perineal/buttock area if appropriate.	Talcum powder should not be used and barrier creams should be applied sparingly, gently layered on in the direction of the hair growth rather than rubbed into the skin (Le Lievre 2002, E).
14 Offer a bowl of water for the patient to wash their hands.	For infection prevention and control and patient's comfort (Fraise and Bradley 2009, E).
15 Ensure bedclothes are clean, straighten sheets and rearrange pillows, assisting patient to a comfortable position. Ensure call bell is within reach of the patient.	For patient comfort. P
16 Take bedpan to the dirty utility (sluice) room and, where necessary, measure urine output and note characteristics (see Figure 6.1, The Bristol Stool Chart) and amount of faeces.	To monitor and evaluate patient's elimination patterns. E

Postprocedure

17 Dispose of contents safely and place bedpan in the washer/disposal unit.	For infection prevention and control (Fraise and Bradley 2009, E).
18 Remove disposable apron and gloves. Wash hands using soap and water.	For infection prevention and control (Fraise and Bradley 2009, E).
19 Record any urine output/bowel action in patient's documentation.	To maintain accurate documentation (NMC 2009, C).

Procedure guideline 6.2 Commode use: assisting a patient

Essential equipment

- Disposable apron and gloves
- Commode with conventional bedpan inserted below seat
- Toilet paper

- Manual handling equipment as appropriate
- Additional nurse if required
- Wash bowl, warm water, disposable wipes and a towel

Preprocedure

Action	Rationale
1 Carry out appropriate manual handling assessment prior to commencing procedure and ensure that patient's weight does not exceed the maximum recommended for commode (see manufacturer's guidelines).	To maintain a safe environment. E
2 Wash hands, put on gloves and apron.	For infection prevention and control (Fraise and Bradley 2009, E).
3 Take the equipment to the bedside and explain the procedure to the patient.	To ensure that the patient understands the procedure and gives their valid consent (NMC 2008a, C).

Procedure

4 Close door/draw curtains around the patient's bed area.	To maintain privacy and dignity and avoid any unnecessary embarrassment for the patient (NMC 2008b, C).
5 Remove the commode cover. Assist the patient out of the bed/chair and onto the commode.	
6 Ensure the patient's feet are positioned directly below their knees and flat on the floor. The use of a small footstool and/or pillows may help to achieve a comfortable position.	An upright, crouching posture is considered anatomically correct for defaecation. Pillows and a footstool can provide support and optimize positioning for defaecation (Taylor 1997, E).
7 Once the patient is on the commode, encourage them to move their legs slightly apart and check to ensure that their positioning is correct.	To avoid any spillage and reduce risk of contamination and cross-infection. P
8 Cover the patient's knees with a towel or sheet.	To maintain privacy and dignity (NMC 2008b, C).
9 Ensure that toilet paper and call bell are within patient's reach and leave the patient, but remain nearby.	To maintain privacy and dignity (NMC 2008b, C).
10 When the patient has finished using the commode, bring washing equipment to the bedside. Assist patient with cleaning perianal area using toilet paper and, where necessary, warm water and soap. Apply a small amount of barrier cream to the perineal/buttock area if appropriate.	Talcum powder should not be used and barrier creams should be applied sparingly, gently layered on in the direction of the hair growth rather than rubbed into the skin (Le Lievre 2002, E).
11 Offer a bowl of water for the patient to wash their hands.	For infection control and patient dignity (Fraise and Bradley 2009, E).
12 Assist the patient to stand and walk to bed/chair, ensuring that they are comfortably positioned. Ensure call bell is within reach of the patient.	For patient comfort. P

Postprocedure

13 Replace cover on the commode and return to the dirty utility (sluice) room.	To reduce any risk of contamination or cross-infection (Fraise and Bradley 2009, E) and to avoid patient embarrassment (NMC 2008b, C).

14 Remove pan from underneath the commode and where necessary, measure urine output, and note characteristics (see Figure 6.1) and amount of faeces.	To monitor and evaluate patient's elimination patterns. E
15 Dispose of contents safely and place pan in the washer/disposal unit.	For infection prevention and control (Pratt *et al.* 2007, C).
16 Clean commode using Actichlor plus solution.	
17 Remove disposable apron and gloves. Wash hands.	For infection control purposes (Fraise and Bradley 2009, E).
18 Record any urine output/bowel action in patient's documentation.	To maintain accurate documentation (NMC 2009, C).

Urinary elimination

Definition

Urinary elimination is the excretion of urine from the body (Thibodeau and Patton 2007).

Anatomy and physiology

The urinary tract (Figure 6.2) consists of the two kidneys, two ureters, the bladder and urethra. The urinary system produces, stores and eliminates urine. The kidneys are responsible for excreting wastes such as urea and ammonium and for the reabsorption of glucose and amino acids. They are involved with the production of hormones including calcitrol, renin and erythropoietin. The kidneys also have homoeostatic functions including the regulation of electrolytes, acid/base balance and blood pressure (Tortora and Derrickson 2009).

Each kidney excretes urine into a ureter, which arises from the renal pelvis on the medial aspect of each kidney. In adults the ureters are approximately 25–30 cm long and 2–4 mm in diameter (Tortora and Derrickson 2009). The ureters are muscular tubes, which propel urine from the kidneys to the urinary bladder. They enter the bladder through the back of the bladder, running within the wall of the bladder for a few centimetres. Ureterovesical valves prevent the backflow of urine from the bladder to the kidneys.

The bladder sits on the pelvic floor and is a hollow, muscular, distensible organ which stores urine until it is convenient to expel it. Urine enters the bladder via the ureters and exits via the urethra. As the bladder fills, stretch receptors in the muscular wall signal the parasympathetic nervous system to contract the bladder, initiating the conscious desire to expel urine. In order for urine to be expelled, both the automatically controlled internal sphincter and the voluntary controlled external sphincter must be opened.

Urine leaves the bladder via the urethra. In females this lies in front of the anterior wall of the vagina and is approximately 3.8 cm long. In males it passes through the prostate and penis and is approximately 20 cm long (Tortora and Derrickson 2009).

Penile sheaths

Definition

Penile sheaths are external devices made from a soft and flexible latex or silicone tubing which are applied over the penis to direct urine into a urinary drainage bag from where it can be conveniently emptied. They are used by men to manage urinary incontinence.

Evidence-based approaches
Rationale

Penile sheaths (also known as conveens) are only to be considered once other methods of promoting continence have failed, as the promotion and treatment of incontinence should be the primary concern of the nurse (Pomfret 2003). They should be considered as a preferable alternative to other methods of continence control, such as pads which quickly can become sodden (Pomfret 2003) and cause skin problems, and catheters, which have several potential complications (Fader *et al.* 2001).

Indications

Penile sheaths may be used to relieve incontinence when no other means is practicable or when all other methods have failed. Penile sheaths are associated with many common problems which are identified by Woodward (2007); these include difficulty in fitting, leaking, kinking, falling off, allergies and urinary tract infections.

Contraindications

Penile sheaths are contraindicated for men with very small or retracted penises (Booth 2009).

Preprocedural considerations
Equipment

Silicone types are now preferred due to concerns about latex allergies (Booth and Lee 2005) (Figure 6.3).

THE BRISTOL STOOL FORM SCALE

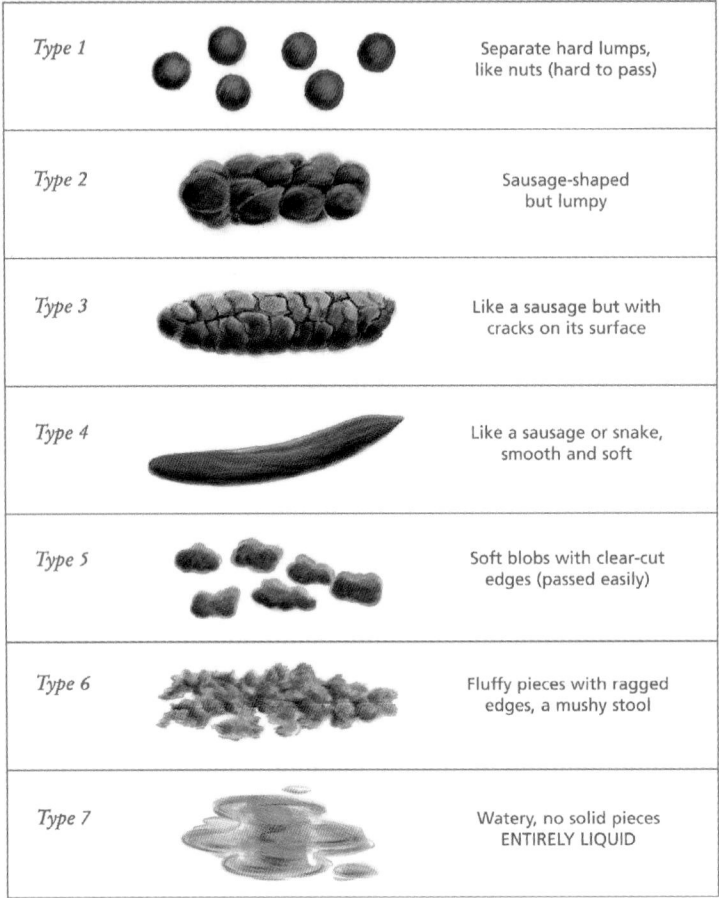

Type 1	Separate hard lumps, like nuts (hard to pass)
Type 2	Sausage-shaped but lumpy
Type 3	Like a sausage but with cracks on its surface
Type 4	Like a sausage or snake, smooth and soft
Type 5	Soft blobs with clear-cut edges (passed easily)
Type 6	Fluffy pieces with ragged edges, a mushy stool
Type 7	Watery, no solid pieces ENTIRELY LIQUID

Figure 6.1 Bristol Stool Form Chart. Reproduced by kind permission of Dr K.W. Heaton, Reader in Medicine at the University of Bristol. © 2000 Norgine Ltd.

Sizing and fitting

As modern sheaths come in a variety of sizes and the correct size can be determined by measuring the girth of the penile shaft, one of the most important considerations is to move away from the mentality that one size fits all. The penis should be measured in the flaccid state (Potter 2007). Most devices come with a manufacturer's sheath sizing guide with different diameters cut into it, so that the correct size can be easily determined. Sheaths are available in a variety of different sizes, which generally increase in increments of 5–10 mm, and in either standard or short lengths (Robinson 2006). Silicone sheaths are advantageous as they are transparent, allowing the patient's skin to be observed and to breathe by allowing the transmission of water vapour and oxygen (Booth and Lee 2005).

Fixation

The main methods in current use follow two different approaches. First, the sheaths can be self-adhesive, so that the sheath itself has a section along its length with adhesive on the internal aspect that sticks to the penile shaft as it is applied. The second method is a double-sided strip of hypoallergenic or foam material applied in a spiral around the penis (which increases the surface area of the conveen adhered to the penis) and then the sheath is applied over the top. Newer devices have been developed which move away from the condom catheter-based system and employ a unique hydrocolloid 'petal' design which adheres only to a small area of the glans penis around the meatus, ensuring a comfortable and secure fit and are ideal for men with a retracted penis (Wells 2008).

Figure 6.2   Anatomy of the female genitourinary tract.

Figure 6.3   Penile sheath.

Procedure guideline 6.3 Penile sheath application

Essential equipment

- Bowl of warm water and soap
- Non-sterile gloves
- Selection of appropriate penile sheaths
- Bactericidal alcohol handrub

- Disposable plastic apron
- Drainage bag and stand or holder
- Hypoallergenic tape or leg strap
- Catheter leg bag

Preprocedure

Action	Rationale
1 Explain and discuss the procedure with the patient.	To ensure that the patient understands the procedure and gives his valid consent (NMC 2008a, C).
2 Screen the bed.	To ensure patient's privacy. To allow dust and airborne organisms to settle before the field is exposed (NMC 2008b, C).
3 Assist the patient to get into the supine position with the legs extended.	To ensure the appropriate area is easily accessible. E
4 Do not expose the patient at this stage of the procedure.	To maintain patient's dignity and comfort (NMC 2008b, C).
5 Wash hands using bactericidal soap and water or bactericidal alcohol handrub.	To reduce risk of infection (Fraise and Bradley 2009, E).
6 Put on a disposable plastic apron.	To reduce risk of cross-infection from micro-organisms on uniform (Fraise and Bradley 2009, E).
7 Prepare the trolley, placing all equipment required on the bottom shelf.	The top shelf acts as a clean working surface. E
8 Take the trolley to the patient's bedside, disturbing screens as little as possible.	To minimize airborne contamination (Fraise and Bradley 2009, E).

(Continued)

Procedure guideline 6.3 (*Continued*)

Procedure

Procedure	Rationale
9 Remove cover, maintaining the patient's privacy, and position a disposable pad under the patient's buttocks and thighs.	To ensure urine does not leak onto bedclothes. E
10 Clean hands with a bactericidal alcohol handrub.	Hands may have become contaminated by handling the outer packs (Fraise and Bradley 2009, E).
11 Put on non-sterile gloves.	To reduce risk of cross-infection (Fraise and Bradley 2009, E).
12 Retract the foreskin, if necessary, and clean the penis with soap and water. Dry completely and reduce or reposition the foreskin.	To remove old adhesive and ensure sheath sticks to the skin and to prevent retraction and constriction of the foreskin behind the glans penis (paraphimosis) which may occur if this is not performed. E
13 Trim any excess pubic hair from around the base of the penis.	To prevent sheath from painfully pulling pubic hair when applied. E
14 Apply sheath following manufacturer's guidelines, ensuring that there is a space between the glans penis and the sheath. Squeeze the sheath gently around the penile shaft.	To prevent the sheath from rubbing the glans penis and causing discomfort and potential skin irritation and to ensure sheath has adhered to penis (Pomfret 2003, C).
15 Connect catheter bag and ensure tubing is not kinked.	To facilitate drainage of urine into catheter bag. E
16 Dispose of equipment in a orange plastic clinical waste bag and seal the bag before moving the trolley.	To prevent environmental contamination. Orange is the recognized colour for clinical waste (DH 2005a, C).
17 Draw back the curtains once the patient has been covered.	To maintain the patient's dignity (NMC 2008b, C).
18 Record information in relevant documents; this should include: ■ reasons for applying penile sheath ■ date and time of application, sheath type ■ length and size ■ manufacturer ■ any problems negotiated during the procedure ■ a review date to assess the need for reapplication.	To provide a point of reference or comparison in the event of later queries (NMC 2009, C).

Problem-solving table 6.1 **Prevention and resolution (Procedure guideline 6.3)**

Problem	Cause	Action	Prevention
Leaking or back flow of urine under the sheath	Penile sheath is the wrong size	Remeasure penile shaft and select the correct size	Measure penile shaft using the sizing tool
Twisting or kinking of sheath	Lack of care taken when applying / drainage tube unsecured	Secure drainage bag to leg or stand	Assess patients mobility before application and select suitable type and method of securing the drainage bag
Difficulty fitting sheath to patient with retracted penis	Anatomy of the patient	Observe the penile length when the patient is sitting. If the length of the penis is less than 5 cm when sitting use a hydro-colloid petal design sheath	—

Urinary catheterization

Definition

Urinary catheterization is the insertion of a specially designed tube into the bladder using aseptic technique, for the purposes of draining urine, the removal of clots/debris and the instillation of medication.

Related theory

Urinary catheterization is an invasive procedure and should not be undertaken without full consideration of the benefits and risks. The presence of a catheter can be a traumatic experience for patients and have huge implications for body image, mobility, pain and discomfort (Clifford 2000, RCN 2008).

Evidence-based approaches

Rationale

Indications

Urinary catheterization may be carried out for the following reasons.

- To empty the contents of the bladder, for example before or after abdominal, pelvic or rectal surgery, before certain investigations and before childbirth, if thought necessary.
- To determine residual urine.
- To allow irrigation of the bladder.
- To bypass an obstruction.
- To relieve retention of urine.
- To introduce cytotoxic drugs in the treatment of papillary bladder carcinomas.
- To enable bladder function tests to be performed.
- To measure urinary output accurately, for example when a patient is in shock, undergoing bone marrow transplantation or receiving high-dose chemotherapy.
- To relieve incontinence when no other means is practicable.
- To avoid complications during the insertion of radioactive material (e.g. caesium into the cervix/womb, brachytherapy for the prostate).

Legal and professional issues

Competencies

The Nursing and Midwifery Council (NMC 2008b) states that nurses performing urinary catheterization should have:

- a good knowledge of the urinary tract anatomy and physiology
- a sound knowledge of the principles of aseptic technique
- a knowledge of equipment and devices available
- awareness of infection control practice and legislation

- practice within the limits of competence and be able to recognize when they need to seek help from more experienced staff
- understanding of the issues of informed consent and a knowledge of the Mental Capacity Act
- the ability to deliver care based on the best available evidence or best practice.

Preprocedural considerations

Patients should be assessed individually as to the ideal time to change their catheters. The use of a catheter diary will help to ascertain a pattern of catheter blockages so changes can be planned accordingly.

Equipment

'A catheter is a hollow tube that is used to remove fluid from, or instil fluid into, a body cavity or viscus' (Pomfret 1996, p.245).

Catheter selection

A wide range of urinary catheters are available, made from a variety of materials and with different design features. Careful assessment of the most appropriate material, size and balloon capacity will ensure that the catheter selected is as effective as possible, that complications are minimized and that patient comfort and quality of life are promoted (Pomfret 1996, Robinson 2001). Types of catheter are listed in Table 6.1 and illustrated in Figure 6.4, together with their suggested use. Catheters should be used in line with the manufacturer's recommendations, in order to avoid product liability (Fraise and Bradley 2009, NHS Supply Chain 2008, RCN 1994).

Balloon size

In the 1920s, Fredrick Foley designed a catheter with an inflatable balloon to keep it positioned inside the bladder. Balloon sizes vary from 2.5 mL for children to 30 mL. The

Figure 6.4 Catheter types.

Table 6.1 Types of catheter

Catheter type	Material	Uses
Balloon (Foley) two-way catheter: two channels, one for urine drainage and second, smaller channel for balloon inflation	Latex, PTFE-coated latex, silicone elastomer coated, 100% silicone, hydrogel coated	Most commonly used for patients who require bladder drainage (short, medium or long term)
Balloon (Foley) three-way irrigation catheter: three channels, one for urine, one for irrigation fluid; one for balloon inflation	Latex, PTFE-coated latex, silicone, plastic	To provide continuous irrigation (e.g. after prostatectomy). Potential for infection is reduced by minimizing need to break the closed drainage system (Mulhall *et al.* 1993)
Non-balloon (Nelaton) or Scotts, or intermittent catheter (one channel only)	PVC and other plastics	To empty bladder or continent urinary reservoir intermittently; to instil solutions into bladder

PTFE, polytetrafluoroethylene; PVC, polyvinylchloride.

latter is used to aid haemostasis after prostatic surgery. Large balloon catheters (30 mL) weigh approximately 48 g, causing pressure on the bladder neck and pelvic floor and potential damage to these structures (Kristiansen *et al.* 1983, Pomfret 2000, Robinson 2001). These catheters are associated with leakage of urine, pain and bladder spasm as they can cause irritation to the bladder mucosa and trigone (Robinson 2001, Stewart 1998). Large balloons are inclined to sit higher in the bladder, allowing a residual pool of urine to collect below the balloon and thus providing a reservoir for infection (Getliffe 1996a, Pomfret 2000).

Consequently, a 5–10 mL balloon is recommended for adults and a 3–5 mL balloon for children.

Care should be taken to use the correct amount of water to fill the balloon because too much or too little may cause distortion of the catheter tip. This may result in irritation and trauma to the bladder wall, consequently causing pain, spasm, bypassing and haematuria. If underinflated, one or more of the drainage eyes may become occluded or the catheter may become dislodged. Overinflation risks rupturing the balloon and leaving fragments of it inside the bladder (Pomfret 2000, Robinson 2001).Catheter balloons should only be inflated once; deflation/reinflation or topping up are not recommended by the manufacturers as distortion of the balloon may occur (Nazarko 2009, Robinson 2004a).

Catheter balloons ought to be filled only with sterile water (Hart 2008). Tap water and 0.9% sodium chloride should not be used as salt crystals and debris may block the inflation channel, causing difficulties with deflation (Head 2006). Any micro-organisms which may be present in tap water can pass through the balloon into the bladder (Falkiner 1993, Stewart 1998).

Catheter size

Urethral catheters are measured in charrières (ch). The charrière is the outer circumference of the catheter in millimetres and is equivalent to three times the diameter. Thus a 12 ch catheter has a diameter of 4 mm.

Potential side-effects of large-gauge catheters include:

- pain and discomfort
- pressure ulcers, which may lead to stricture formation
- blockage of paraurethral ducts
- abscess formation (Blandy and Moors 1989, Crow *et al.* 1986, Edwards *et al.* 1983, Roe and Brocklehurst 1987, Winn 1998)
- bypassing – urethral leakage.

The most important guiding principle is to choose the smallest size of catheter necessary to maintain adequate drainage (McGill 1982, Robinson 2006). If the urine to be drained is likely to be clear, a 12 ch catheter should be considered. Larger gauge catheters may be necessary if debris or clots are present in the urine (Pomfret 1996, Winn 1998).

Length of catheter

There are three lengths of catheter currently available:

- female length: 23–26 cm
- paediatric: 30 cm
- standard length: 40–44 cm.

The shorter female length catheter is often more discreet and less likely to cause trauma or infections because movement in and out of the urethra is reduced. Infection may also be caused by the longer catheter looping or kinking (Pomfret 2000, Robinson 2001). In obese women or those in wheelchairs, however, the inflation valve of the shorter catheter may cause soreness by rubbing against the inside of the thigh, and the catheter is more likely to pull on the bladder neck; therefore, the standard length catheter should be used (Evans *et al.* 2001, Godfrey and Evans 2000, Pomfret 2000).

Tip design

Several different types of catheter tip are available in addition to the standard round tip (Figure 6.5). Each tip is designed to overcome a particular problem.

Tiemann tip   Whistle-tipped   Roberts catheter   Standard tip
catheter

Figure 6.5 Catheter tips.

- The *Tieman-tipped catheter* has a curved tip with one to three drainage eyes to allow greater drainage. This catheter has been designed to negotiate the membranous and prostatic urethra in patients with prostatic hypertrophy.
- The *whistle-tipped catheter* has a lateral eye in the tip and eyes above the balloon to provide a large drainage area. This design is intended to facilitate drainage of debris, for example blood clots.
- The *Roberts catheter* has an eye above and below the balloon to facilitate the drainage of residual urine.

Catheter material

A wide variety of materials are used to make catheters. The key criterion in selecting the appropriate material is the length of time the catheter is expected to remain in place. Three broad timescales have been identified.

- Short term (1–7 days): e.g. PVC and intermittent catheters.
- Short to medium term (up to 28 days): e.g. PTFE.
- Medium to long term (6 weeks–12 weeks): e.g. hydrogel and silicone coated.

The principal catheter materials are as follows.

Polyvinyl chloride (PVC)

Catheters made from PVC or plastic are quite rigid. They have a wide lumen, which allows a rapid flow rate, but their rigidity may cause some patients discomfort. They are mainly used for intermittent catheterization or postoperatively. They are recommended for short-term use only (Pomfret 1996).

Latex

Latex is a purified form of rubber and is the softest of the catheter materials. It has a smooth surface, with a tendency to allow crust formation. Latex absorbs water and consequently the catheter may swell, reducing the diameter of the internal lumen and increasing its external diameter (Pomfret 2000, Robinson 2001). It has been shown to cause urethral irritation (Wilksch *et al.* 1983) and therefore should only be considered when catheterization is likely to be short term.

Hypersensitivity to latex has been increasing in recent years (Woodward 1997) and latex catheters have been the cause of some cases of anaphylaxis (Young *et al.* 1994).

Woodward (1997) suggests that patients should be asked whether they have ever had an adverse reaction to rubber products before catheters containing latex are utilized.

Teflon (polytetrafluoroethylene [PTFE]) or silicone elastomer coatings

A Teflon or silicone elastomer coating is applied to a latex catheter to render the latex inert and reduce urethral irritation (Slade and Gillespie 1985). Teflon is recommended for short-term use and silicone elastomer-coated catheters are used for long-term catheterization.

All silicone

Silicone is an inert material which is less likely to cause urethral irritation. Silicone catheters are not coated and therefore have a wider lumen. The lumen of these catheters, in cross-section, is crescent or D-shaped, which may induce formation of encrustation (Pomfret 1996). Because silicone permits gas diffusion, balloons may deflate and allow the catheter to fall out prematurely (Barnes and Malone-Lee 1986, Studer *et al.* 1983). These catheters may be more uncomfortable as they are more rigid than the latex-cored types (Pomfret 2000). All-silicone catheters are suitable for patients with latex allergies. Silicone catheters are recommended for long-term use.

Hydrogel coatings

Catheters made of an inner core of latex encapsulated in a hydrophilic polymer coating are commonly used for long-term catheterization. The polymer coating is well tolerated by the urethral mucosa, causing little irritation. Hydrogel-coated catheters become smoother when rehydrated, reducing friction with the urethra. They are also inert (Nacey and Delahunt 1991), and are reported to be resistant to bacterial colonization and encrustation (Roberts *et al.* 1990, Woollons 1996). Hydrogel-coated catheters are recommended for long-term use.

Conformable catheter

Conformable catheters are designed to conform to the shape of the female urethra, and allow partial filling of the bladder. The natural movement of the urethra on the catheter, which is collapsible, is intended to prevent obstructions (Brocklehurst *et al.* 1988). They are made of latex and have a silicone elastomer coating. Conformable catheters are approximately 3 cm longer than conventional catheters for women.

Other materials

Research into new types of catheter materials is ongoing, particularly examining materials that resist the formation of biofilms (bacterial colonies that develop and adhere to the catheter surface and drainage bag) and consequently reduce the instances of urinary tract infections (Pratt *et al.* 2007).

Catheters coated with a silver alloy have been shown to prevent urinary tract infections (Saint *et al.* 1998). However, the studies that demonstrated this benefit were all small scale and a number of questions about the long-term effects of using such catheters, such as silver toxicity, need to be addressed. Argyria is a condition caused by the deposition of silver locally or systemically in the body, and can give rise to nausea, constipation and loss of night vision (Bardsley 2009, Cymet 2001, Pratt *et al.* 2007). There is some suggestion in the research that the use of silver alloy-coated catheters does reduce the onset of bacteriuria and may be beneficial when catheterization is in high-risk situations, for example diabetic and intensive care patients (Saint *et al.* 2000). However, research trials analysed by the Cochrane Collaboration (Schumm and Lam 2008) indicate that this asymptomatic bacteraemia was only seen in the first 5–7 days; after this, the catheter type made little difference (Plowman *et al.* 2001, Pratt *et al.* 2007).

Catheters coated with antibiotics such as gentamicin, rifampicin, nitrofurazone and nitrouroxone have been investigated in the search to find a product that will reduce instances of catheter-associated urinary tract infections (CAUTI). They may have a role to play in the management of trauma patients; nitrofurazone-impregnated catheters were shown to reduce urinary infections when compared with standard catheters in a trial by Stensballe *et al.* (2007). Whether this effect would be present in non-trauma patients and in the management of patients with long-term catheters is unknown. However, issues such as antibiotic sensitivity or resistance have not been fully investigated or assessed (Schumm and Lam 2008).

The cost implications for routine use of these impregnated catheters would be huge for the NHS (Johnson *et al.* 2006). However, a recent review of impregnated catheters found that silver alloy (antiseptic)-coated or nitrofurazone-impregnated (antibiotic) urinary catheters do reduce infections in hospitalized adults, and siliconized catheters may reduce adverse effects in men, but the evidence is weak (Schumm and Lam 2008). Trials with a specific catheter may be appropriate on an individual patient basis when other types of catheter management of recurrent infections have failed (Brosnahan *et al.* 2006).

Drainage bags

A wide variety of drainage systems are available. Selecting a system involves consideration of the reasons for catheterization, the intended duration, the wishes of the patient, and infection control issues (Wilson and Coates 1996).

Urine drainage bags should only be changed according to clinical need, that is when that catheter is changed or if the bag is leaking, or at times dictated by the manufacturer's instructions, for example every 5–7 days (Pratt *et al.* 2007, Wilson 1998). Urine drainage bags positioned above the level of the bladder and full bags cause urine to reflux, which is associated with infection. Therefore bags should always be positioned below the level of the bladder to maintain an unobstructed flow and emptied appropriately. Urine drainage bags should be hung on suitable stands to avoid contact with the floor. In situations when dependent drainage is not possible, the system should be clamped until dependent drainage can be resumed (Kunin 1997). When emptying drainage bags, clean separate containers should be used for each

patient and care should be taken to avoid contact between the drainage tap and the container (Pratt *et al.* 2007).

Urine drainage bags are available in a wide selection of sizes ranging from the large 2 litre bag, which is used more commonly in non-ambulatory patients and overnight, to 350–750 mL leg bags (Figure 6.6, Figure 6.7). There are also large drainage bags that incorporate urine-measuring devices, which are used when very close monitoring of urine output is required (Figure 6.8).

There are a number of different styles of drainage bags, from the new body-worn 'belly bags' (Pomfret 2007) to the standard leg-worn bags. They allow patients greater mobility and can be worn under the patient's own clothes and therefore are much more discreet, helping to preserve the patient's privacy and dignity. Shapes vary from oblong to oval and some have cloth backing for greater comfort in contact with the skin. Others are ridged to encourage an even distribution of urine through the bag, resulting in better conformity to the leg. The length of the inlet tube also varies (direct, short, long and adjustable length) and the intended position on the leg, that is thigh, knee or lower leg, determines which length is used (Robinson, 2006, 2008). The patient should be asked to

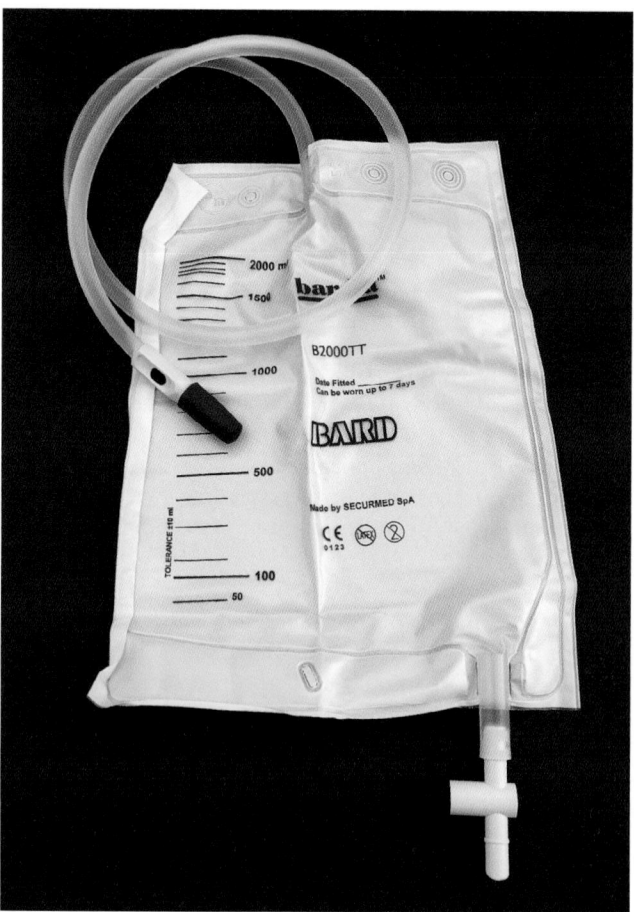

Figure 6.6 Urinary catheter bag, standard.

Figure 6.7   Urinary catheter leg bag.

Figure 6.8   Urinary catheter with urometer.

identify the most comfortable position for the bag (Pomfret 2007). The majority of drainage bags, even the new belly bag, are fitted with an antireflux valve to prevent the backflow of urine into the bladder (Madeo and Roadhouse 2009). Several different tap designs exist and patients must have the manual dexterity to operate the mechanism (Robinson 2008). Most leg bags allow for larger 1–2 litre bags to be connected via the outlet tap, to increase capacity for night-time use.

Leg drainage bag supports

A variety of supports are available for use with these bags, including sporran waist belts, leg holsters, knickers/pants and leg straps (Doherty 2006, Roe 1992).

Leg straps

The use of thigh straps (e.g. Simpla G-Strap) and other fixation devices (e.g. Bard StatLock, Comfasure, Clinimed CliniFix) helps to immobilize the catheter and thus reduce the trauma potential to the bladder neck and urethra (Eastwood 2009). It is particularly appropriate for men, due to the longer length and weight of the tube being used; however, some women may also find the extra support more comfortable. Guidance from the Royal College of Nurses (RCN 2008) and NHS Scotland (NHSQIS 2004) reiterates the importance of catheter tetherage to promote patient comfort and to limit the potential complications of catheter migration and subsequent need for recatheterization. The application of these devices is not without potential complications; for example, restriction of the circulation to the limb may give rise to deep vein thrombosis while tension and traction to the urethra can cause trauma and necrosis, especially in men (Bierman and Carigan 2003).

Catheter valves

Catheter valves, which eliminate the need for drainage bags, are also available. The valve allows the bladder to be emptied intermittently and is particularly appropriate for patients who require long-term catheterization, as they do not require a drainage bag.

Catheter valves are only suitable for patients who have good cognitive function, sufficient manual dexterity to manipulate the valve and an adequate bladder capacity. It is important that catheter valves are released at regular intervals to ensure that the bladder does not become overdistended. (These valves must not be used on patients following certain operations to the prostate or bladder, as pressure caused by the distending bladder may cause perforation or rupture; in most of these instances the urethral catheter is only required for a short period of time and free drainage is the preferred method.) As catheter valves preclude free drainage, they are unlikely to be appropriate for patients with uncontrolled detrusor overactivity, ureteric reflux or renal impairment (Fader et al. 1997). Catheter valves are designed to fit with linked systems so it is possible for patients to connect to a drainage bag. This may be necessary when access to toilets may be limited, for example overnight or on long journeys.

Catheter valves are licensed by the Department of Health to remain *in situ* for 5–7 days, and this corresponds with most manufacturers' recommendations (Pomfret 1996). Little research into the advantages and disadvantages of catheter valves has been completed.

Pharmacological support
Anaesthetic lubricating gel

The use of anaesthetic lubricating gels is well recognized for male catheterization, but there is some controversy over their use for female catheterization. In male patients the gel is instilled directly into the urethra and then external massage is used to move the gel down its length, unless a conforming gel such as Instillagel is used and then this is not necessary. In female patients the anaesthetic lubricating gel or plain lubricating gel is applied to the tip of the catheter only, if it is used at all. It has been suggested that most of the lubricant is wiped off the catheter at the urethral introitus so therefore it fails to reach the urethral tissue (Muctar 1991).

These differences in practice imply that catheterization is a painful procedure for men but is not so for women. This assumption is not based on any empirical or biological evidence. Other than the differences in length and route, the male and female urethra are very similar except for the presence of lubricating glands in the male urethra (Tortora and Derrickson 2009). The absence of these lubricating glands in the female urethra suggests that there is perhaps a greater need for the introduction of a lubricant (Wilson 2008). Women have complained of pain and discomfort during catheterization procedures (Mackenzie and Webb 1995), suggesting that the use of anaesthetic lubricating gels must be reconsidered (BAUN 2000, 2009, Woodward 2005). The literature does highlight a couple of issues on the use of lidocaine gel. If it is not instilled far enough in advance, that is, more than 4 minutes, it will have only a lubricating effect (Association for Continence Advice 2003/2008, Tanabe *et al.* 2004) and if the gel is not instilled up the urethra, it will not dilate or anaesthetize it (Bardsley 2005, NICE 2003). There is a need for caution with the use of lidocaine in the elderly, those with cardiac dysrhythmias and those with sensitivity to the drug, as there is a danger of injury to the urothelial lining of the urethra during the procedure, allowing systemic absorption of the drug (BNF 2011).

Trauma can occur during catheterization, which in turn can increase the risk of infection. Using single-use lubrication gels with antiseptic properties can reduce these risks (BNF 2011, Pratt *et al.* 2007). Since there is a lack of research to clarify the efficacy of lubricating gels, practice must be based on the research evidence that is available and the physiology and anatomy of the urethra.

Procedure guideline 6.4 Urinary catheterization: male

Essential equipment

- Sterile catheterization pack containing gallipots, receiver, low-linting swabs, disposable towels
- Disposable pad
- Sterile gloves
- Selection of appropriate catheters
- Sterile anaesthetic lubricating jelly
- Universal specimen container

- 0.9% sodium chloride
- Bactericidal alcohol handrub
- Hypoallergenic tape or leg strap for tethering
- Sterile water
- Syringe and needle
- Disposable plastic apron
- Drainage bag and stand or holder

Preprocedure

Action	Rationale
1 Explain and discuss the procedure with the patient.	To ensure that the patient understands the procedure and gives his valid consent (NMC 2008a, C).
2 Screen the bed.	To ensure patient's privacy (Fraise and Bradley 2009, E).
3 Assist the patient to get into the supine position with the legs extended.	To ensure the appropriate area is easily accessible. E
4 Do not expose the patient at this stage of the procedure.	To maintain patient's dignity and comfort (NMC 2008b, C).
5 Wash hands using bactericidal soap and water or bactericidal alcohol handrub.	To reduce risk of infection (Fraise and Bradley 2009, E).
6 Put on a disposable plastic apron and two pairs of sterile gloves.	To reduce risk of cross-infection from micro-organisms on uniform (Fraise and Bradley 2009, E).

7 Prepare the trolley, placing all equipment required on the bottom shelf.	The top shelf acts as a clean working surface. E
8 Take the trolley to the patient's bedside, disturbing screens as little as possible.	To minimize airborne contamination (Fraise and Bradley 2009, E).

Procedure

9 Open the outer cover of the catheterization pack and slide the pack onto the top shelf of the trolley.	To prepare equipment. E
10 Using an aseptic technique, open the supplementary packs.	To reduce the risk of introducing infection into the bladder (NICE 2003, C).
11 Remove cover, maintaining the patient's privacy, and position a disposable pad under the patient's buttocks and thighs.	To ensure urine does not leak onto bedclothes. E
12 Remove top pair of gloves and dispose.	Gloves may have become contaminated by handling outer packs (Bardsley and Kyle 2008, E).
13 Place sterile towels across the patient's thighs and under buttocks.	To create a sterile field. E
14 Wrap a sterile topical swab around the penis. Retract the foreskin, if necessary, and clean the glans penis with 0.9% sodium chloride or sterile water.	To reduce the risk of introducing infection to the urinary tract during catheterization. E
15 Insert the nozzle of the lubricating jelly into the urethra. Squeeze the gel into the urethra, remove the nozzle and discard the tube. Massage the gel along the urethra.	Adequate lubrication helps to prevent urethral trauma. Use of a local anaesthetic minimizes the discomfort experienced by the patient (Bardsley 2005, P).
16 Squeeze the penis and wait approximately 5 minutes.	To prevent anaesthetic gel from escaping. To allow the anaesthetic gel to take effect. E
17 Grasp the penis behind the glans, raising it until it is almost totally extended. Maintain grasp of penis until the procedure is finished.	This manoeuvre straightens the penile urethra and facilitates catheterization (Stoller 2004, P). Maintaining a grasp of the penis prevents contamination and retraction of the penis.
18 Place the receiver containing the catheter between the patient's legs. Insert the catheter for 15–25 cm until urine flows.	The male urethra is approximately 18 cm long (Bardsley 2005, P).
19 If resistance is felt at the external sphincter, increase the traction on the penis slightly and apply steady, gentle pressure on the catheter. Ask the patient to strain gently as if passing urine.	Some resistance may be due to spasm of the external sphincter. Straining gently helps to relax the external sphincter. E
20 When urine begins to flow, advance the catheter almost to its bifurcation.	Advancing the catheter ensures that it is correctly positioned in the bladder. E
21 Gently inflate the balloon according to the manufacturer's direction, having ensured that the catheter is draining properly beforehand.	Inadvertent inflation of the balloon in the urethra causes pain and urethral trauma (Getliffe and Dolman 2003, E).
22 Withdraw the catheter slightly and attach it to the drainage system.	To ensure that the balloon is inflated and the catheter is secure. E

(Continued)

Procedure guideline 6.4 *(Continued)*

23 Support the catheter, if the patient desires, either by using a specially designed support, for example Simpla G-Strap, or by taping the catheter to the patient's leg. Ensure that the catheter does not become taut when patient is mobilizing or when the penis becomes erect. Ensure that the catheter lumen is not occluded by the fixation device or tape.	To maintain patient comfort and to reduce the risk of urethral and bladder neck trauma. Care must be taken in using adhesive tapes as they may interact with the catheter material (Fillingham and Douglas 2004, E; Pomfret 1996, P).
24 Ensure that the glans penis is clean and then reduce or reposition the foreskin.	Retraction and constriction of the foreskin behind the glans penis (paraphimosis) may occur if this is not done (Pomfret 2003, E).

Postprocedure

25 Make the patient comfortable. Ensure that the area is dry.	If the area is left wet or moist, secondary infection and skin irritation may occur (Pomfret 2003, E).
26 Measure the amount of urine.	To be aware of bladder capacity for patients who have presented with urinary retention. To monitor renal function and fluid balance. It is not necessary to measure the amount of urine if the patient is having the urinary catheter routinely changed (Pomfret 2003, E).
27 Take a urine specimen for laboratory examination, if required (see Chapter 11).	For further information, see Procedure guideline 11.1
28 Dispose of equipment in an orange plastic clinical waste bag and seal the bag before moving the trolley.	To prevent environmental contamination. Orange is the recognized colour for clinical waste (DH 2005a, C).
29 Draw back the curtains.	
30 Record information in relevant documents; this should include: ■ reasons for catheterization ■ date and time of catheterization ■ catheter type, length and size ■ amount of water instilled into the balloon ■ batch number ■ manufacturer ■ any problems negotiated during the procedure ■ a review date to assess the need for continued catheterization or date of change of catheter.	To provide a point of reference or comparison in the event of later queries (NMC 2009, C).

Procedure guideline 6.5 Urinary catheterization: female

Essential equipment

- Sterile catheterization pack containing gallipots, receiver, low-linting swabs, disposable towels
- Disposable pad
- Sterile gloves
- Selection of appropriate catheters
- Sterile anaesthetic lubricating jelly
- Universal specimen container

- 0.9% sodium chloride or antiseptic solution
- Bactericidal alcohol handrub
- Hypoallergenic tape or leg strap for tethering
- Sterile water
- Syringe and needle
- Disposable plastic apron
- Syringe and needle
- Drainage bag and stand or holder

Preprocedure

Action	Rationale
1 Explain and discuss the procedure with the patient.	To ensure that the patient understands the procedure and gives her valid consent (NMC 2008a, C).
2 Screen the bed.	To ensure patient's privacy. To allow dust and airborne organisms to settle before the sterile field is exposed (Fraise and Bradley 2009, E).
3 Assist the patient to get into the supine position with knees bent, hips flexed and feet resting about 60 cm apart.	To enable genital area to be seen. E
4 Do not expose the patient at this stage of the procedure.	To maintain the patient's dignity and comfort (NMC 2008b, C).
5 Ensure that a good light source is available.	To enable genital area to be seen clearly. E
6 Wash hands using bactericidal soap and water or bactericidal alcohol handrub.	To reduce risk of cross-infection (Fraise and Bradley 2009, E).
7 Put on a disposable apron and two pairs of sterile gloves.	To reduce risk of cross-infection from micro-organisms on uniform (Bardsley and Kyle 2008, E; Fraise and Bradley 2009, E).

Procedure

8 Prepare the trolley, placing all equipment required on the bottom shelf. (Also see Catheter selection.)	To reserve top shelf for clean working surface. E
9 Take the trolley to the patient's bedside, disturbing screens as little as possible.	To minimize airborne contamination (Fraise and Bradley 2009, C).
10 Open the outer cover of the catheterization pack and slide the pack on the top shelf of the trolley.	To prepare equipment. E
11 Using an aseptic technique, open supplementary packs.	To reduce risk of introducing infection into the urinary tract. E
12 Remove cover, maintaining the patient's privacy, and position a disposable pad under the patient's buttocks.	To ensure urine does not leak onto bedclothes. E
13 Remove top pair of gloves and dispose.	Gloves may have become contaminated by handling outer packs (Bardsley and Kyle 2008, E).
14 Place sterile towels across the patient's thighs.	To create a sterile field. E
15 Using low-linting swabs, separate the labia minora so that the urethral meatus is seen. One hand should be used to maintain labial separation until catheterization is completed.	This manoeuvre provides better access to the urethral orifice and helps to prevent labial contamination of the catheter. E
16 Clean around the urethral orifice with 0.9% sodium chloride or an antiseptic solution, using single downward strokes.	Inadequate preparation of the urethral orifice is a major cause of infection following catheterization. To reduce the risk of cross-infection (Fraise and Bradley 2009, E).
17 Insert the nozzle of the lubricating jelly into the urethra. Squeeze the gel into the urethra, remove the nozzle and discard the tube. Allow 5 minutes for the gel's antiseptic and anaesthetic effects to occur.	Adequate lubrication helps to prevent urethral trauma. Use of a local anaesthetic minimizes the patient's discomfort (Woodward 2005, P).
18 Place the catheter, in the receiver, between the patient's legs.	To provide a temporary container for urine as it drains. E

(Continued)

Procedure guideline 6.5 (*Continued*)

19 Introduce the tip of the catheter into the urethral orifice in an upward and backward direction. Advance the catheter until 5–6 cm has been inserted.	The direction of insertion and the length of catheter inserted should relate to the anatomical structure of the area. E
20 Either remove the catheter gently when urinary flow ceases or advance the catheter 6–8 cm.	This prevents the balloon from becoming trapped in the urethra.
21 Inflate the balloon according to the manufacturer's directions, having ensured that the catheter is draining adequately.	Inadvertent inflation of the balloon within the urethra is painful and causes urethral trauma (Getliffe and Dolman 2003, P).
22 Withdraw the catheter slightly and connect it to the drainage system.	To ensure that the balloon is inflated and the catheter is secure. E
23 Support the catheter, if the patient desires, either by using a specially designed support, for example Simpla G-Strap, or by taping the catheter to the patient's leg. Ensure that the catheter does not become taut when patient is mobilizing. Ensure that the catheter lumen is not occluded by the fixation device or tape.	To maintain patient comfort and to reduce the risk of urethral and bladder neck trauma. Care must be taken in using adhesive tapes as they may interact with the catheter material (Pomfret 1996, P).

Postprocedure

24 Make the patient comfortable and ensure that the area is dry.	If the area is left wet or moist, secondary infection and skin irritation may occur. E
25 Measure the amount of urine.	To be aware of bladder capacity for patients who have presented with urinary retention. To monitor renal function and fluid balance. It is not necessary to measure the amount of urine if the patient is having the urinary catheter routinely changed (Fillingham and Douglas 2004, E).
26 Take a urine specimen for laboratory examination if required (see Chapter 11).	For further information, see Procedure guideline 11.1.
27 Dispose of equipment in an orange plastic clinical waste bag and seal the bag before moving the trolley.	To prevent environmental contamination. Orange is the recognized colour for clinical waste (DH 2005a, C).
28 Draw back the curtains.	
29 Record information in relevant documents; this should include: ■ reasons for catheterization ■ date and time of catheterization ■ catheter type, length and size ■ amount of water instilled into the balloon ■ batch number and manufacturer ■ any problems negotiated during the procedure ■ a review date to assess the need for continued catheterization or date of change of catheter.	To provide a point of reference or comparison in the event of later queries (NMC 2009, C).

Postprocedural considerations

Documentation

To ensure adequate documentation of the process of urinary catheterization, the following information should be recorded in the patient's notes.

■ Note patient's consent and understanding of the procedure, plus allergy status.
■ Reason for catheterization.
■ Type of catheter inserted, gauge and length.
■ Manufacturer and batch number plus expiry date.
■ Date and time of insertion.

- Size of balloon and volume of sterile water used to inflate it.
- Cleansing procedure and type of lubricant used.
- Any difficulties experienced or clinical observations noted.
- Plan of action, i.e. duration of catheterization/predicted date for change of long-term catheter.
- Signed and printed by person performing the procedure.

(NMC 2008b, NMC 2009, RCN 2008)

Suprapubic catheterization

Definition

Suprapubic catheterization is the insertion of a catheter through the anterior abdominal wall into the dome of the bladder. The procedure is performed under general or local anaesthesia, using a percutaneous system (Kirkwood 1999, Robinson 2008).

Evidence-based approaches

Rationale

The National Patient Safety Agency (NPSA 2009) has recently published a rapid response report stating that the insertion of a suprapubic catheter should be undertaken by experienced urology staff using ultrasound imaging and that the first catheter change should also be performed by them.

Indications

Suprapubic catheterization does offer some advantages over urethral catheterization (Rigby 2009). The risk of patients developing urinary tract infection is reduced, as the bacterial count on the abdominal skin is less than around the perineal and perianal areas, although bacteriuria and encrustation still occur in susceptible patients (Simpson 2001, Winn 1998). Urethral integrity is retained and it allows for the resumption of normal voiding after surgery. Clamping the suprapubic catheter allows urethral voiding to occur, and the clamp can be released if voiding is incomplete. Pain and catheter-associated discomfort are reduced. Patient satisfaction is increased as, for some, their level of independence is increased and sexual intercourse can occur with fewer impediments (Barnes *et al*. 1993, Fillingham and Douglas 2004, Hammarsten and Lindquist 1992, Wilson 1998).

There are a number of risks and disadvantages associated with suprapubic catheterization.

- Bowel perforation and haemorrhage at the time of insertion.
- Infection, swelling, encrustation and granulation at insertion site.
- Pain, discomfort or irritation for some patients.
- Bladder stone formation and possible long-term risk of squamous cell carcinoma.
- Urethral leakage.

(Addison and Mould 2000)

Preprocedural considerations

Equipment

A number of different suprapubic catheters are available. A trocar is used with all types of catheters in order to make the tract through which the catheter is threaded. Specifically designed catheters incorporate a fixing plate, which requires sutures to secure the catheter to the skin of the abdomen. For long-term use, a Foley catheter is adequate. Large charrière size (18–22 ch) hydrogel-coated or 100% silicone catheters are recommended (Winder 1994).

Postprocedural considerations

Care of a suprapubic catheter is the same as for a urethral catheter. Immediately following insertion of a suprapubic catheter, aseptic technique should be employed to clean the insertion site (Robinson 2008). Dressings may be required if secretions soil clothing, but they are not essential. Once the insertion site has healed (7–10 days), the site and catheter can be cleaned during bathing using soap, water and a clean cloth (Fillingham and Douglas 2004).

Intermittent catheterization

Some patients need a catheter long term to empty their bladder. This is often managed by teaching them intermittent self-catheterization.

Evidence-based approaches

Indications

Patients suitable for intermittent self-catheterization include those:

- with a bladder capable of storing urine without leakage between catheterizations
- who can comprehend the technique
- with a reasonable degree of dexterity and mobility to position themselves for the procedure and manipulate the catheter
- who are highly motivated and committed to carrying out the procedure (Colley 1998).

This procedure may be required by patients who have undergone continent reconstruction to manage initial postoperative incontinence. Patients with a Mitrofanoff reconstruction will need to perform this procedure for life.

Intermittent self-catheterization (ISC) is not a new technique, although it has become noticeably more popular in recent years. The procedure involves the episodic introduction of a catheter into the bladder to remove urine. After this the catheter is removed, leaving the patient catheter free between catheterizations. In hospital, this should be a sterile procedure because of the risks of hospital-acquired infection. However, in the patient's home a clean technique may be used (Lapides *et al*. 2002, Wilson 1998). Catheterization should be carried

213

out as often as necessary to stop the bladder becoming over-distended and to prevent incontinence (Bennett 2002). How frequent this is depends on the individual but may vary from once a week, to once a day, to 4–6 times a day.

The advantages of intermittent catheterization over indwelling urethral catheterizations include improved quality of life, as patients are free from bulky pads or indwelling catheters and drainage bags, greater patient satisfaction and greater freedom to express sexuality. In addition, urinary tract complications are minimized and normal bladder function is maintained (Bakke and Malt 1993, Bakke *et al.* 1997, Chai *et al.* 1995, Webb *et al.* 1990, Wright 2009).

Preprocedural considerations
Equipment

Nelaton catheters are generally used to carry out intermittent self-catheterizations. These catheters are available in standard, female and paediatric lengths and in charrière sizes 6–24; as they are not left in the bladder, they do not have a balloon (Winder 1995). They are normally manufactured from plastic but there is also a non-PVC, chlorine-free catheter available. Some Nelaton catheters are coated with a lubricant which is activated by soaking the catheter in water for a short while; others are packaged with a lubricant gel which coats the catheter as it slides out of the packaging (these catheters are for single use only). Lubricated Nelaton catheters are also available with an integral drainage bag, useful when toilet facilities are unavailable or the environment is not conducive to performing a clean procedure safely or comfortably.

Uncoated catheters, which require separate lubrication, may be reused by a single patient for up to a week, but the catheter must be rinsed in running water and properly dried after use; between uses, it should be kept in a clean bag or container (Barton 2000, Lapides *et al.* 2002).

Procedure guideline 6.6 Urinary catheterization: intermittent self-catheterization: male

Essential equipment

- Lubricating gel
- Appropriately sized catheter. If carrying out this procedure in hospital, a new catheter must be used every time

Preprocedure

Action	Rationale
1 Wash hands using bactericidal soap and water or bactericidal alcohol handrub.	To prevent infection (Fraise and Bradley 2009, E).
2 Stand in front of a toilet or a low bench with a suitable container if it is easier.	To catch urine. E
Standing in front of a mirror is helpful for patients with a large abdomen.	For ease of observation.

Procedure

3 Clean glans penis with water. If the foreskin covers the penis, it will need to be held back during the procedure.	To reduce risk of infection (Fraise and Bradley 2009, E).
4 Open catheter packaging or container. If using an uncoated catheter, a water-soluble lubricating gel may be applied to the surface of the catheter. If using a coated catheter, pre-soak it in water to activate the slippery coating.	To prepare catheter and to ease insertion. E
5 Hold penis, with the non-dominant hand, upwards towards your stomach.	To prevent trauma to the penoscrotal junction. E
6 Hold the catheter with the dominant hand, being careful not to touch the part of the catheter entering the body, and gently insert it into the opening of the urethra. Advance the catheter into the bladder.	To reduce the risk of introducing an infection (Fraise and Bradley 2009, E).
There will be a change of feeling as the catheter passes through the prostate gland and into the bladder. It may be a little sore on the first few occasions only. If there is any resistance, do not continue. Withdraw the catheter and contact a nurse or doctor.	The prostate gland surrounds the urethra just below the neck of the bladder and consists of much firmer tissue. This can enlarge and cause an obstruction, especially in older men. E

214

7	Drain the urine into the toilet or suitable container. When the urine stops flowing slowly remove the catheter, halting if more urine starts to flow.	To ensure that the bladder is completely emptied.
8	Before removing the catheter from the urethra, put a finger over the funnel end of the catheter and then remove the catheter from the urethra.	To trap urine in the catheter and prevent spillage on to clothing or the floor. E
9	Hold the catheter over the toilet or suitable container and remove finger from the funnel end to release the trapped urine.	
10	If using a coated catheter, dispose of the catheter in a suitable receptacle.	To prevent environmental contamination.
	If the catheter is uncoated and is to be reused, wash through with tap water.	To remove urine.
	Allow to drain then dry the outside of the catheter.	To reduce risk of infection.
	Store in a dry container (as per manufacturer's instructions). These catheters may be used for 5–7 days.	
11	Wash hands with soap and water.	To reduce the risk of infection.

Procedure guideline 6.7 Urinary catheterization: intermittent self-catheterization: female

Essential equipment

- Mirror
- Appropriately sized catheter. If carrying out this procedure in hospital, a new catheter must be used every time
- Lubricating gel

Preprocedure

Action	Rationale
1 Wash hands using bactericidal soap and water or bactericidal alcohol handrub.	To reduce risk of cross-infection (Fraise and Bradley 2009, E).
2 Take up a comfortable position, depending on mobility (e.g. sitting on toilet; standing with one foot placed on toilet seat).	To facilitate insertion of intermittent catheter. E

Procedure

3 Spread the labia (the lips at the entrance to the vagina) and wash genitalia, from front to back, with soap and water, then dry.	To reduce the risk of introducing infection (Fraise and Bradley 2009, E).
4 Open catheter packaging or container. If using an uncoated catheter, a water-soluble lubricating gel may be applied to the surface of the catheter. If using a coated catheter, presoak it in water to activate the slippery coating (Barton 2000).	To prepare catheter and to ease insertion. E
5 Find the urethral opening above the vagina. A mirror can be used to help identify it. Gently insert the catheter into the urethra, taking care not to touch the part of the catheter entering the body.	To reduce risk of introducing an infection.

(Continued)

Procedure guideline 6.7 (*Continued*)

6 Drain the urine into the toilet or suitable container. When the urine stops flowing, slowly remove catheter, halting if more urine starts to flow.	To ensure that the bladder is completely emptied.
7 Before removing the catheter from the urethra, put a finger over the funnel end of the catheter and then remove the catheter from the urethra.	To trap urine in the catheter and prevent spillage on to clothing or the floor. E
8 Hold the catheter over the toilet or suitable container and remove finger from the funnel end to release the trapped urine.	To prevent spillage on to clothing or the floor.

Postprocedure

9 If using a coated catheter, dispose of it in a suitable receptacle.	To prevent environmental contamination.
If the catheter is uncoated and is to be reused, wash through with tap water.	To remove urine.
Allow to drain then dry the outside of the catheter.	To reduce risk of infection.
Store in a dry container (as per manufacturer's instructions). These catheters may be used for 5–7 days.	
10 Wash hands with soap and water.	To reduce the risk of infection.

Problem-solving table 6.2 **Prevention and resolution (Procedure guidelines 6.4, 6.5, 6.6 and 6.7)**

Problem	Cause	Prevention	Action
Urethral mucosal trauma	Incorrect size of catheter		Recatheterize the patient using the correct size of catheter. Check the catheter support and apply or reapply as necessary
	Procedure not carried out correctly or skilfully. Movement of the catheter in the urethra		
	Creation of false passage as a result of too rapid insertion of catheter		Nurse may need to remove the catheter and wait for the urethral mucosa to heal
Patient has a vasovagal attack	This is caused by the vagal nerve being stimulated so that the heart slows down, leading to a syncope faint		Lie the patient down in the recovery position. Inform doctors
Male Paraphimosis	Failure to retract foreskin after catheterization or catheter toilet		Always retract the foreskin
Female No drainage of urine	Incorrect identification of external urinary meatus	Ensure sufficient light to observe the area. Revise the female anatomy prior to the procedure	Check that catheter has been sited correctly. If catheter has been wrongly inserted in the vagina, leave it in position to act as a guide, reidentify the urethra and catheterize the patient. Remove the inappropriately sited catheter

| Difficulty in visualizing the urethral orifice | This can be due to vaginal atrophy and retraction of the urethral orifice | The index finger of the 'dirty' hand may be inserted in the vagina, and the urethral orifice can be palpated on the anterior wall of the vagina. The index finger is then positioned just behind the urethral orifice. This then acts as a guide, so the catheter can be correctly positioned (Jenkins 1998) |

Procedure guideline 6.8 Urinary catheter bag: emptying

Essential equipment

- Swabs saturated with 70% isopropyl alcohol
- Sterile jug
- Disposable gloves

Preprocedure

Action	Rationale
1 Explain and discuss the procedure with the patient.	To ensure that the patient understands the procedure and gives their valid consent (NMC 2008a, C).
2 Wash hands using bactericidal soap and water or bactericidal alcohol handrub, and put on disposable gloves.	To reduce risk of cross-infection (Fraise and Bradley 2009, E).

Procedure

3 Clean the outlet valve with a swab saturated with 70% isopropyl alcohol.	To reduce risk of infection (Fraise and Bradley 2009, E).
4 Allow the urine to drain into the jug.	To empty drainage bag and accurately measure volume of contents. E
5 Close the outlet valve and clean it again with a new alcohol-saturated swab.	To reduce risk of cross-infection (Fraise and Bradley 2009, E).
6 Cover the jug and dispose of contents in the sluice, having noted the amount of urine if this is requested for fluid balance records.	To reduce risk of environmental contamination (DH 2005a, C).
7 Wash hands with bactericidal soap and water.	To reduce risk of infection (Fraise and Bradley 2009, E).

Procedure guideline 6.9 Urinary catheter removal

Essential equipment

- Dressing pack containing sterile towel, gallipot, foam swab or non-linting gauze
- Disposable gloves
- Needle and syringe for urine specimen, specimen container
- Syringe for deflating balloon

(Continued)

Procedure guideline 6.9 (*Continued*)

Preprocedure

Action	Rationale
1 Catheters are usually removed early in the morning.	So that any retention problems can be dealt with during the day. E
2 Explain procedure to patient and inform them of potential postcatheter symptoms, such as urgency, frequency and discomfort, which are often caused by irritation of the urethra by the catheter.	So that patient knows what to expect, and can plan daily activity.

Procedure

Action	Rationale
3 Clamp below the sampling port until sufficient urine collects. Take a catheter specimen of urine using the sampling port.	To obtain an adequate urine sample and to assess whether postcatheter antibiotic therapy is needed (Fraise and Bradley 2009, E).
4 Wearing gloves, use saline to clean the meatus and catheter, always swabbing away from the urethral opening. *Note*: in women, never clean from the perineum/vagina towards the urethra.	To reduce risk of infection (Fraise and Bradley 2009, E). To help reduce the risk of bacteria from the vagina and perineum contaminating the urethra. E
5 Release leg support.	For easier removal of catheter. E
6 Having checked volume of water in balloon (see patient documentation), use syringe to deflate balloon.	To confirm how much water is in the balloon. To ensure balloon is completely deflated before removing catheter. E
7 Ask patient to breathe in and then out; as patient exhales, gently (but firmly with continuous traction) remove catheter.	To relax pelvic floor muscles. E
Male patients should be warned of discomfort as the deflated balloon passes through the prostate gland.	It is advisable to extend the penis as per the process for insertion to aid removal. E

Postprocedure

Action	Rationale
8 Clean meatus and make the patient comfortable.	To maintain patient comfort and dignity. E
9 Encourage patient to exercise and to drink 2–3 litres of fluid per day.	To prevent urinary tract infections. E

Complications

Infections

Catheterization carries an infection risk. Catheter-associated infections are the most common hospital-acquired infection, possibly accounting for up to 35–40% of all hospital infection (Roadhouse and Wellstead 2004).

Key areas have been identified as having a direct link with the development of urinary tract infection.

- Assessing the need for catheterization and the length of time the catheter is *in situ* (Nazarko 2007).
- Selection of the most appropriate type of catheter and drainage system to be used.
- The aseptic conditions and process by which the catheter is inserted and maintained as a closed drainage system.

- Training and competence of the person performing the procedure and those undertaking the aftercare, that is, patients, relatives and health professionals.

The maintenance of a closed drainage system is central in reducing the risk of catheter-associated infection. It is thought that micro-organisms reach the bladder by two possible routes: from the urine in the drainage bag or via the space between the catheter and the urethral mucosa (Getliffe 1995, Gould 1994). To reduce the risk of infection, it is important to keep manipulation of the closed system to a minimum; this includes unnecessary emptying, changing the drainage bags or taking samples. There is now an intregal catheter and drainage bag available to reduce the number of potential disconnection sites and infection risk. Before handling catheter drainage systems, hands must be decontaminated and a pair of clean non-sterile gloves should be worn (Pratt *et al.* 2007). All urine samples should only be obtained via the specially designed sampling ports using an aseptic technique.

Urinary tract infections (male): meatal cleaning

Cleaning the urethral meatus, where the catheter enters the body, is a nursing procedure intended to minimize infection of the urinary tract for men (DH and CMO 2003, Mangnall and Watterson 2006). Studies examining the use of a variety of antiseptic, antimicrobial agents or soap and water found that there was no reduction in bacteriuria when using any of these preparations for meatal cleaning compared to routine bathing or showering (Pratt *et al.* 2007). Further studies support the view that vigorous meatal cleaning is unnecessary and may compromise the integrity of the skin, thus increasing the risk of infection (Leaver 2007, Saint and Lipsky 1999). Therefore it is recommended that routine daily personal hygiene with soap and water (NICE 2003) is all that is needed to maintain meatal hygiene (Pomfret and Tew 2004, Pratt *et al.* 2007). Nursing intervention is necessary if there is a poor standard of hygiene or a risk of contamination (Gilbert 2006); removal of a smegma ring, where the catheter meets the meatus, is important to prevent ascending infections and meatal trauma (Wilson 2005).

A urinary tract infection (UTI) may be introduced during catheterization because of faulty aseptic technique, inadequate urethral cleaning or contamination of catheter tip. UTI may be introduced via the drainage system because of faulty handling of equipment, breaking the closed system or raising the drainage bag above bladder level causing urine reflux.

If a UTI is suspected a catheter specimen of urine must be sent for analysis. The patient should be encouraged to have a fluid intake of 2–3 litres a day. Medical staff should be informed if the problem persists so antibiotics can be prescribed.

Table 6.2 details other complications that may arise if a patient is catheterized.

Urinary diversions

Definition

A urinary diversion is a surgically created system for removing urine from the body when either the bladder or urethra is either non-existent or no longer viable.

Evidence-based approaches

Rationale

Invasive bladder cancer is the most common condition for which urinary diversions are performed. Other conditions that may lead to urinary diversion include:

- pelvic cancers, for example gynaecological cancers, sarcoma
- congenital abnormalities, for example bladder extrophy

- neuropathic bladder, a condition where the nerve impulses do not reach the bladder as the result of an underlying disease or injury, for example myelomeningocoele
- trauma
- irreparable fistula
- interstitial cystitis
- radiation fibrosis
- intractable incontinence (Black 1994, Taylor 2005).

There are two main types: a urostomy, which is an incontinent diversion where the urine is stored in a body-worn pouch, and continent urinary diversions. Continent urinary diversions differ in that a system is created to collect and store urine before it is removed from the body.

The main aim in selection of urinary diversion is to provide patients with a diversion which gives the lowest potential for complications and the best quality of life and, for those patients with cancer, the best cancer control (Parekh *et al.* 2006).

Indications

A urinary diversion is formed to:

- eliminate urine from the body if the lower urinary tract is defective or absent
- preserve the upper urinary tract
- avoid metabolic disturbance
- store the urine either internally or externally until convenient to empty.

Continent diversions:

- store an adequate volume of urine at low pressure
- offer patients a choice of urinary diversion
- improve or maintain the individual's body image, psychological and social well-being by removing the necessity of wearing external devices, for example urostomy pouch or incontinence pads (Leaver 2002, Randles 1990).

Principles of care

Patients are selected carefully for urinary diversion, particularly for the continent types of diversions. Patients' general levels of health, co-morbidities, renal and hepatic function are all taken into consideration when deciding on the type of urinary diversion. Intestinal disease such as Crohn's disease, urinary stress incontinence, bladder cancer involving the bladder neck or prostatic urethra and previous pelvic radiotherapy are contraindications for continent diversion and will dictate the types of diversions offered to patients (Hautmann *et al.* 2006, Meyer *et al.* 2005).

Patients undergoing continent diversions must be motivated towards self-care, those needing to self-catheterize must be dextrous enough to manipulate Nelaton catheters and good anal sphincter control is a must for those undergoing a rectal bladder.

Table 6.2 Complications of catheterizaction

Problem	Cause	Suggested action
Inability to tolerate indwelling catheter	Urethral mucosal irritation	Nurse may need to remove the catheter and seek an alternative means of urine drainage
	Psychological trauma	Explain the need for and the functioning of the catheter
	Unstable bladder	
	Radiation cystitis	
Inadequate drainage of urine	Incorrect placement of a catheter	Resite the catheter
	Kinked drainage tubing	Inspect the system and straighten any kinks
	Blocked tubing, for example pus, urates, phosphates, blood clots	If a three-way catheter, such as a Foley, is in place, irrigate it. If an ordinary catheter is in use, milk the tubing in an attempt to dislodge the debris, then attempt a gentle bladder washout. Failing this, the catheter will need to be replaced; a three-way catheter should be used if the obstruction is being caused by clots and associated haematuria
Fistula formation	Pressure on the penoscrotal angle	Ensure that correct strapping is used
Penile pain on erection	Not allowing enough length of catheter to accommodate penile erection	Ensure that an adequate length is available to accommodate penile erection
Formation of crusts around the urethral meatus	Increased urethral secretions collect at the meatus and form crusts, due to irritation of urothelium by the catheter (Fillingham and Douglas, 2004)	Correct catheter toilet
Leakage of urine around catheter	Incorrect size of catheter	Replace with the correct size, usually 2 ch smaller
	Incorrect balloon size	Select catheter with 10 mL balloon
	Bladder hyperirritability	Use Roberts tipped catheter
		As a last resort, bladder hyperirritability can be reduced by giving diazepam or anticholinergic drugs (Nazarko 2009)
Unable to deflate balloon	Valve expansion or displacement	Check the non-return valve on the inflation/deflation channel. If jammed, use a syringe and needle to aspirate by means of the inflation arm above the valve
	Channel obstruction	Obstruction by a foreign body can sometimes be relieved by the introduction of a guidewire through the inflation channel
		Inject 3.5 mL of dilute ether solution (diluted 50/50 with sterile water or 0.9% sodium chloride) into the inflation arm
		Alternatively, the balloon can be punctured suprapubically using a needle under ultrasound visualization
		Following catheter removal, the balloon should be inspected to ensure it has not disintegrated, leaving fragments in the bladder
		Note: steps above should be attempted by or under the directions of a urologist. The patient may require cystoscopy following balloon deflation to remove any balloon fragments and to wash the bladder out
Dysuria	Inflammation of the urethral mucosa	Ensure a fluid intake of 2–3 litres per day. Advise the patient that dysuria is common but will usually be resolved once micturition has occurred at least three times. Inform medical staff if the problem persists
Retention of urine	May be psychological	Encourage the patient to increase fluid intake. Offer the patient a warm bath. Inform medical staff if the problem persists

Encouraging patients' independence in living with a urinary diversion is a key aim of care. Practical help, advice and support are employed in encouraging patients to continue with all necessary activities of daily living.

Methods of urinary diversion

Urinary diversions may be divided into two main types.

- Incontinent diversions, whereby urine is stored in an external body-worn appliance, for example ileal conduit, colonic conduit, cutaneous ureterostomy.
- Continent diversions where urine is stored in an internal pouch, for example Mitrofanoff, Mainz, orthotopic neobladder.

Incontinent diversions

An ileal conduit is the most common form of urostomy; the colon (colonic conduit) may also be used. Urostomy comes from the Greek words *uros* meaning urine and *stoma* meaning mouth or opening (Nazarko 2008). Approximately 1500 urostomies were formed in the UK in 2006 (Burch 2008).

A section of bowel is isolated, along with its mesentery vessels, and the remaining ends of the bowel are anastomosed to restore continuity. The isolated section is mobilized, the proximal end is closed and the ureters, once resected from the bladder, are implanted at this end. The distal end is brought out onto the surface of the abdominal wall and everted to form a spout (Figure 6.9), as in an ileostomy (Fillingham and Fell 2004). Urine from a urostomy will contain mucus from the bowel used in its construction (Taylor 2005).

A cutaneous ureterostomy is another form of incontinent diversion, whereby the ureters are brought out onto the abdominal wall together (one stoma) or separately (two stomas). This may be a permanent or temporary procedure,

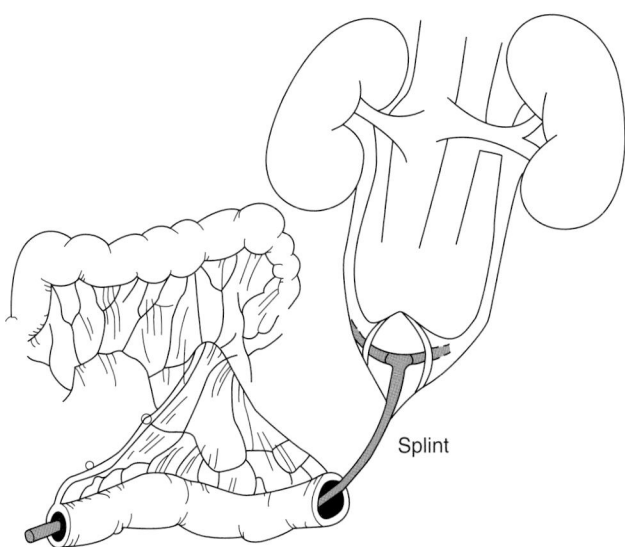

Figure 6.9 Urostomy.

Splint

221

Box 6.1 Types of continent cutaneous diversion with catheterizable stomas

1 Mitrofanoff pouch.
2 Kock pouch.
3 Benchekroun pouch.
4 Mainz pouch.
5 Indiana pouch.
6 Le bag.
7 Miami.

and may be used for patients with poor renal function and when less extensive abdominal surgery is indicated. Stomas formed in this way are often small and flush to the abdomen. They are prone to stenosis and it is often difficult to maintain a leak-proof appliance (Fillingham and Fell 2004).

Continent diversions

All continent diversions consist of three components.

- A reservoir to store urine, which may be the bladder itself, an augmented bladder or one made completely out of ileum or colon.
- A continence mechanism to retain urine in the reservoir, which may be an existing valve or sphincter, such as the ileocaecal valve, urethral sphincter or anal sphincter. A valve may also be constructed using the same tissue used to construct the reservoir, such as a flutter valve created by the intussusception of a segment of bowel or a flap valve created by tunnelling a narrow tube between muscle and mucosal layers of the reservoir (Leaver 2002).
- A channel or tunnel to let the urine out, which may be formed by utilizing other tube/tunnel-like structures such as the appendix, ureter, urethra or fallopian tube. Alternatively, a segment of ileum or colon can be used (Leaver 2002).

There are three main types of continent diversion: continent cutaneous diversion, rectal bladder and orthotopic neobladder.

Continent cutaneous diversion

There are a number of different types of continent cutaneous diversions (Box 6.1), which differ in construction, use different structures to form the reservoir and the tunnel and different techniques to create the continence mechanism. The outcomes for patients and the nursing care involved are essentially similar in most cases. The most commonly performed procedure of this type in the UK is arguably the Mitrofanoff (Leaver 1996) (Figure 6.10).

In this type of diversion, urine drains into the urinary reservoir constructed from bowel or bladder through the ureters. One end of the tissue used to construct the channel is buried in a submuscular tunnel in the bladder, forming an obstructing flap valve. The other end is brought to the surface of the abdominal wall to form a continent stoma.

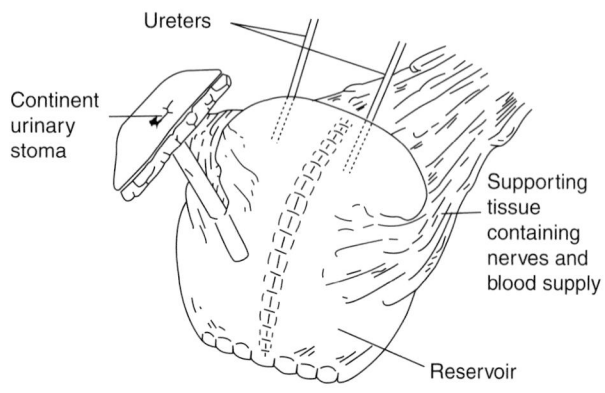

Figure 6.10 Continent urinary diversion.

As the bladder fills with urine, more pressure is put on the valve, causing it to become even more obstructed. A catheter is passed into the stoma along the channel, through the valve and into the bladder when the patient wants to empty their bladder (Leaver 1996). Patients can self-catheterize into the continent urinary stoma every 4–6 hours to empty the urine reservoir (Figure 6.11).

Rectal bladder

A type of rectal bladder, the ureterosigmoidostomy, is the oldest known continent urinary diversion (Fisch and Hohenfellner 1992). In this procedure the ureters are directly implanted into the sigmoid colon, where the urine and faeces mix and are evacuated via the anus. This procedure became unpopular because of continual complications of infection, electrolyte imbalance, loss of renal function, renal calculi, the high rate of incontinence, especially at night, and its poor reputation for morbidity and mortality (Leaver 2002).

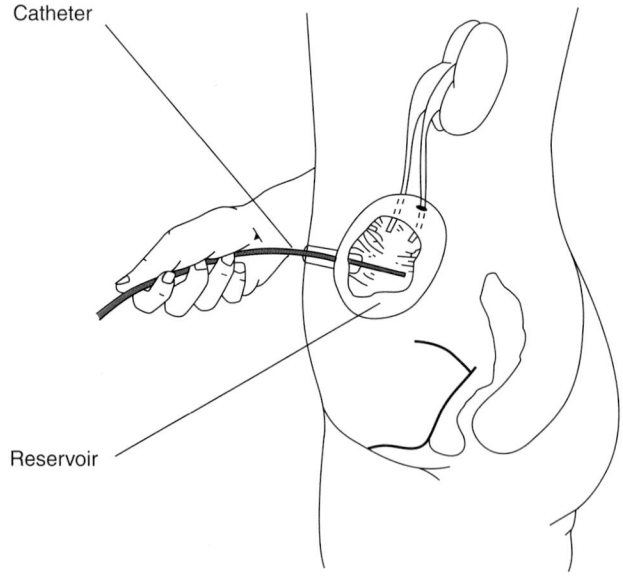

Figure 6.11 Self-catheterization into the continent urinary stoma.

Improved understanding of how some complications arise, development in surgical techniques and greater ability to manage electrolyte imbalances have all led to renewed interest in the rectal bladder (D'Elia *et al.* 2004, Leaver 2002). High-pressure peristalsis in the bowel has been shown to cause the reflux of faeces into the kidneys If the bowel is detubularized, this high pressure can be overcome. To detubularize the rectum, it is opened longitudinally and closed transversely to form a pouch, which remains continuous with the sigmoid colon (Figure 6.12a). The ureters are implanted in a serous lined extramural tunnel into this pouch which is called the sigma-rectum pouch or Mainz Sigma II (D'Elia *et al.* 2004). This modified pouch acts as a reservoir for urine until the patient is ready to void. The patient can, in time, distinguish between needing to void urine and opening their bowels even though both events take place via the rectum (Leaver 2002).

Orthotopic neobladder

In this type of diversion the neobladder is constructed by using the ileum or a section of the large colon and then it is anastomosed to the urethra to allow voiding in the conventional way (Parekh *et al.* 2006) (Figure 6.12b). Therefore this procedure is only suitable for patients in whom the urethra is left intact. This procedure was initially contraindicated in females as the urethra was routinely removed during cystectomy and it was thought that females would be unable to maintain continence. Better understanding of the anatomy of female continence mechanism and anatomical dissection has led to more women being offered this type of diversion (Meyer *et al.* 2005).

The ability to pass urine naturally via the urethra and maintaining a normal anatomical appearance are the major advantages of this procedure. Patients need to use the Valsalva manoeuvre to empty the neobladder but some patients find this difficult and may need to perform clean intermittent self-catheterization. Pelvic floor exercises should be taught preoperatively and performed on a daily basis. Continence can be problematic; most patients (83–96%) achieve continence during the day, and nocturnal continence rates are 74–83% (Meyer *et al.* 2005).

Preoperative preparation, assessment and care

Preoperative care can be divided into two sections:

- physical
- psychological.

Physical

It is important to ensure that patients undergoing the formation of a rectal bladder have good anal sphincter

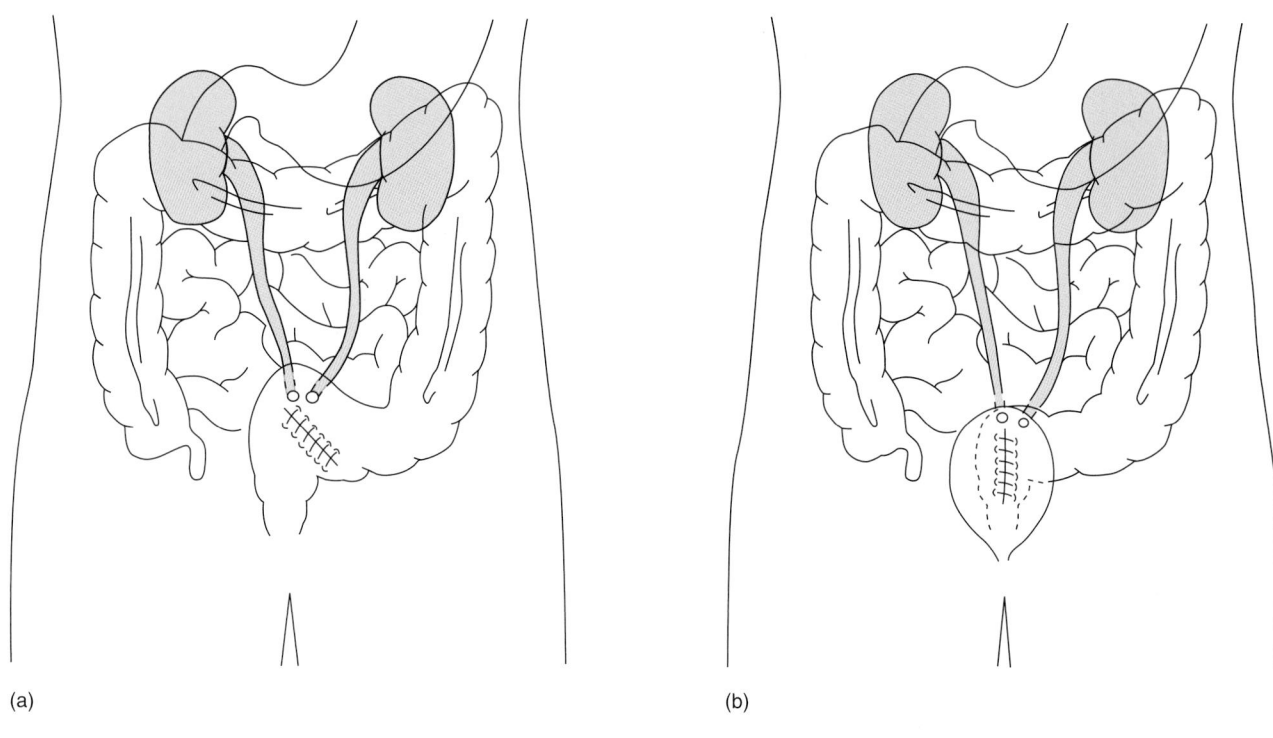

(a)   (b)

Figure 6.12   (a) Mainz Sigma II or rectal bladder. (b) Orthotopic neobladder.

control. This can be established with the porridge test. A sloppy porridge enema is instilled into the patient's rectum and the patient needs to hold 300–350 mL for 3–4 hours without leaking. It is important that during this time the patient performs as many usual activities as possible, such as walking, climbing stairs, and so on. The porridge imitates the contents of the rectum postoperatively (Leaver 2002).

Patients having an orthotopic neobladder need to be taught intermittent self-catheterization (see Procedure guidelines 6.6 and 6.7) and pelvic floor exercises (Kegel exercises) (Perimenis and Koliopanou 2004, Varol and Studer 2004).

Bowel preparation is often undertaken as it is thought to improve surgical visibility and prevent contamination of the surgical field. The regimen used depends on the surgeon's preference. Patients undergoing this procedure are at risk of developing hypovolaemia and electrolyte imbalance. Therefore, it is important that the fluid loss is replaced orally or intravenously (Woodhouse *et al.* 1989). The need for bowel preparation is currently being questioned and it is not used by centres following an enhanced recovery programme. These programmes improve patient recovery and reduce hospital stay.

Patients undergoing an incontinent diversion will need to have the site for their stoma marked; often patients who are having a continent diversion will also have a stoma sited in case the planned surgery cannot be performed. For information on stoma siting, see the section on Stoma care.

Psychological

Once patients have been selected as suitable candidates, psychological preparation should begin as soon as possible. Boore (1978), Hayward (1978) and Varol and Studer (2004) have illustrated the importance of preoperative information and explanation in reducing postoperative physical and psychological stress to the individual following the formation of a stoma. Their research is also applicable to patients receiving continent urinary diversion stomas.

Patients should receive a full explanation of their operation and the type or types of urinary diversion which are available for them, including all the advantages and disadvantages of each diversion. The amount and type of information should be adapted to the individual's requirements. The specialist urology nurse is valuable in the preoperative stage (Varol and Studer 2004). Many patients focus on the lack of appliance wearing in these types of surgery and are blind to the complications of the surgery itself (Leaver 2002). They should be shown pictures of the appropriate urinary diversion and encouraged to familiarize themselves with the equipment: pouches, wafers, catheters and bladder syringes. The specialist nurse should also discuss issues such as body image, sexuality, fears and concerns.

It is important to provide written information, diagrams, DVDs, internet websites and equipment for the patient to take home. This helps clarify and reinforce the verbal information given during the consultation.

Procedure guideline 6.10 Continent urinary diversion stoma: self-catheterization

Essential equipment

- Catheter for catheterization depending upon the size of the stoma
- Tissues
- Clean jug or bowl
- Gauze

Preprocedure

Action	Rationale
1 Explain and discuss the procedure with the patient.	To ensure that the patient understands the procedure and gives their valid consent. (NMC 2008a, C).
2 Collect all equipment necessary for the procedure.	To ensure all the equipment required is easily available. E
3 Take the equipment to the toilet, bathroom or screened bed area. Ensure there is a good light and a full-length mirror.	To ensure the patient's privacy. To ensure patient can see the stoma clearly. E
4 The equipment should be arranged on a clean surface and within easy reach for the procedure.	To reduce the risk of contamination by surface bacteria. So the equipment is easily available. E
5 The patient needs to remove any inhibiting clothing.	To ensure the patient can examine the stoma. E
6 The patient should wash their hands with soap and water, then dry them.	To ensure the hands are clean (Fraise and Bradley 2009, E).

Procedure

Action	Rationale
7 The patient should look at the stoma, if necessary with the aid of a hand or full-length mirror.	To look for mucus and swelling around the stoma. E
8 The patient should wipe away any mucus with a tissue soaked in warm water and gently pat dry.	To ensure the opening of the stoma is clear and mucus does not block the catheter during insertion into the stoma. E
9 If a lubricated catheter is to be used, follow manufacturers' guidelines. If not, lubricate tip of catheter with water-soluble lubricant.	To act as a lubricant to allow the catheter to enter the urinary reservoir without causing internal trauma. E
10 Ensure the untipped end of the catheter is in a receiver, such as a jug, bowl or toilet.	To ensure the urine goes into a bowl and not onto the patient. E
11 The patient can either use a mirror to guide the tube into the opening of the stoma or feel the opening with two fingers slightly apart with the stoma between.	To act as a guide to pass the catheter into the continent urinary stoma. E
12 Insert the catheter gently into the stoma, following the pathway inside (usually towards the middle of the abdomen) until urine starts to flow, then insert tube a further 4–6 cm to reduce risk of contamination.	The direction of insertion and the diameter of catheter inserted depend on the type, size and shape of continent urinary stoma. E To negotiate continence device. E
13 When all the urine has stopped flowing, advance the catheter to ensure the bladder is completely empty. Slowly remove the catheter using a rotating action. If urine starts flowing again wait until it stops before removing the catheter any further.	To ensure complete emptying of the urinary reservoir. The rotating action reduces the suction effect and pain due to friction (Leaver 1996, C). It may dislodge any debris or mucus blocking the tube and allow the urine to flow (Leaver 1996).
14 Remove the tube. Cover the end of the catheter with a finger just before it is removed from the tunnel. Hold the catheter over the receptacle before removing the finger.	To trap urine in catheter and stop it leaking on to the patient (Colley 1998). To allow complete drainage of the tube.

Postprocedure

15 Dispose of catheter in orange bin disposal bag.	To ensure safe disposal (DH 2005a, C).
16 Cover the stoma with a non-adherent dressing and secure with skin-protective tape.	To prevent mucus staining the patient's clothing. E
17 The patient should wash their hands with soap and water, and then dry them.	To remove any urine on the hands.
18 The patient can then dress, collect equipment and dispose of any soiled dressings.	To prevent cross-infection (Fraise and Bradley 2009, E).

Procedure guideline 6.11 Continent urinary diversion stoma drainage tubes: flushing

Essential equipment

- Syringe with appropriate tip to engage tube
- Sterile 0.9% sodium chloride or water sufficient to perform procedure: 20–100 mL
- Gloves
- Antiseptic solution

Preprocedure

Action	Procedure
1 Explain and discuss the procedure with patient.	To ensure that the patient understands the procedure and gives their valid consent (NMC 2008a, C).
2 Screen the bed. Ensure that the patient is in a comfortable position allowing access to the drainage tube.	For the patient's privacy and to reduce the risk of cross-infection. (Fraise and Bradley 2009, E).
3 Perform the procedure using aseptic technique.	To minimize the risk of cross-infection.
4 Move trolley to the bedside, disturbing the curtains as little as possible.	To minimize airborne contamination.
5 Open the outer wrappings of the packs and put them on the top shelf of the trolley. Prepare fluid to carry out the flush by decanting it into a sterile receiver ready to be drawn into a syringe.	To commence preparation of equipment for procedure (Fraise and Bradley 2009, E).
6 Prepare the sterile field.	To minimize airborne contamination.
7 Wash hands with bactericidal alcohol handrub.	To commence preparation of equipment for procedure (Fraise and Bradley 2009, E).

Procedure

8 If possible, clamp drainage tube.	To prevent leakage, if possible, when the drainage tube is disconnected. E
9 Place a sterile towel under the junction of the drainage tube and drainage bag and disconnect.	To create a sterile field and reduce the risk of cross-infection.
10 Clean hands with a bactericidal alcohol handrub and put on gloves.	To remove organisms from the surface of the hands and so reduce the risk of introducing infection into the drainage tube (Fraise and Bradley 2009, E).

(Continued)

Procedure guideline 6.11 *(Continued)*

11 Draw up correct volume of irrigation fluid. Introduce catheter tip into drainage tube, release clamp if applied previously, and gently inject the sterile water into the drainage tube.	To flush the possible blockage from the tube. E
12 Remove syringe. Allow drainage tube to drain into sterile receptacle.	To assess the presence of a blockage in the drainage tube. E
13 Connect new drainage bag.	To prevent introduction of bacteria into the drainage tube via the original bag.
14 Measure fluid collected from drainage tube, subtracting the volume of fluid used to flush tube.	To accurately record drainage from the tube. Observe for further blockages. E

Postprocedure

15 Make the patient comfortable, remove equipment, clean trolley and wash hands.	To reduce the risk of cross-infection.
Repeat steps 11 and 12 as often as necessary to remove debris.	

Problem-solving table 6.3 Prevention and resolution (Procedure guidelines 6.10 and 6.11)

Problem	Cause	Prevention	Suggested action
Unable to flush drainage tube using moderate force	Severe blockage Displaced tube		Inform medical staff of situation, suggest investigation to determine the position of the tube
No fluid draining from tube after flushing	Dehydration Displaced tube Re-blocked tube	Encourage the patient to maintain good fluid intake	Assess the patient's nutritional state, skin turgor, fluid balance chart, mucous membranes. Review patient with medical team. If good fluid intake has been established and the tube is in position, repeat process
Cannot insert the catheter into the stoma	Using too large a catheter. Unable to locate opening. Opening occluded, for example due to swelling	Use an appropriate size catheter, not too large	Advise the patient to try a smaller sized catheter, and to use a magnifying mirror to find the opening. Advise the patient to rest for 10 minutes to let the stoma relax and then to insert catheter. A warm bath may help to dilate the opening. If still unable to catheterize, then patient should contact the hospital
			Doctor may give subcutaneous injection of steroid to reduce swelling. A needle and syringe may be used to draw off a quantity of urine to take pressure off the valve and thus allow the catheter to be inserted. If the catheter remains occluded, a suprapubic catheter may be inserted to allow the swelling to subside and drain urine from the reservoir. The stoma may need to be dilated by a doctor

Problem	Cause	Prevention	Suggested action
Partial insertion only of catheter is possible	Tubing kinked. Stricture in the stoma		Remove tubing and try with fresh tubing of the same size. Or try with a size smaller tubing. If unable to catheterize, contact the hospital
Patient has not catheterized for 4 hours and feels distended; is easily catheterized but no urine is passed	Tubing not reaching the reservoir. Tubing kinked. Tube is doubling back on itself. Tube blocked with mucus		Insert tubing further. Do not use force. If there is resistance then stop. Contact the hospital Try coughing. The increased intra-abdominal pressure may dislodge the plug of mucus. While the tube is inserted, flush it with tap water Remove tubing, examine for mucus and reinsert once it is clear. Flush the urinary reservoir
Stoma leaks urine between catheterizations	Reservoir not emptied regularly. Plug blocking tubing, preventing complete drainage. Stoma failure		Must catheterize every 3–4 hours. If the patient has drunk large amounts of alcohol (a diuretic) or is taking diuretic medication, it may be necessary to catheterize more frequently. Flush reservoir at least twice a day. If still leaking, inform the hospital. Surgical fashioning of the stoma may be necessary
Staining of blood during catheterization	Trauma due to rough technique		Lubricate the tube well and insert gently into stoma. If blood staining continues or increases in amount, inform the hospital

227

Postoperative considerations

Postoperative stage 1

Incontinent diversions

Urine will dribble from the stoma every 20–30 seconds and it starts draining immediately. Normal output is 1500 mL/ 24 hours (Cottam 1999), but may be less after periods of reduced fluid intake, for example at night. Urinary stents (fine-bore catheters) may be in place from the ureters past the anastomosis and out of the stoma. They are placed to maintain patency and protect the suturing until primary healing is completed (Black 2000). Stents are left *in situ* for 7–10 days.

See section on Stoma care for further information.

Continent diversions

Extensive experience has shown that to allow healing of the continent diversion and to reduce the risk of urine leaking into the peritoneum, it is important that the reservoir is kept empty for at least 7 days and possibly for several weeks. The length of time required will vary depending on the type of diversion and the surgeon's preference. Patients will have a number of drainage tubes in place and special attention to urinary output and the patency and support of these tubes is required (Figure 6.13). The drains and catheters used are unique to the type of diversion and determined by the

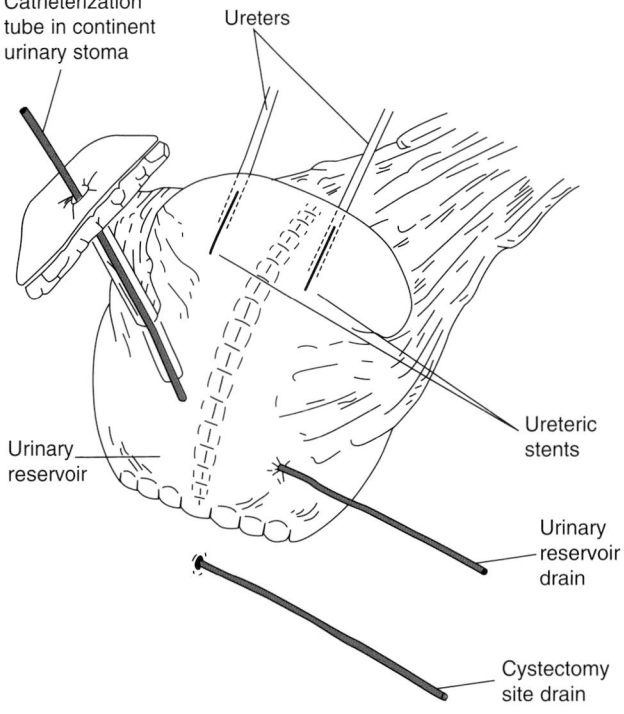

Figure 6.13 Siting of wound drains to reduce risk of haematoma and abscess formation.

228

surgeon's preference. It is important that each drainage tube is identified and labelled appropriately.

There will often be one or two fine-bore catheters placed in the ureters (ureteric stents), which will initially drain most of the urine. One or two catheters may be present in the new reservoir to keep it drained; these can become blocked with debris or mucus (which is produced by the bowel) so they should be flushed with 20 mL of sterile 0.9% sodium chloride four times daily starting from day 1 postoperatively. If the catheters do block there is a high risk that the new reservoir will become distended and anastomotic leaks may occur (Perimenis and Koliopanou 2004). Any difficulties in flushing these catheters should be reported to the specialist nurse and medical staff.

After 5 days the emphasis of the procedure changes from maintaining the patency of the catheters to removal of all mucus present in the reservoir. Fifty millilitres of sterile 0.9% sodium chloride should be gently instilled and drawn back. The solution and mucus removed are then discarded, and the process is repeated until no further mucus is obtained. This may require a total of 400–600 mL of sterile 0.9% sodium chloride. It is important that no force is used to draw back the flush solution; if resistance is felt, the bladder syringe should be removed and the solution allowed to drain. It is important that mucus is removed as it is implicated in the formation of stones (Hensle *et al.* 2004).

Ureteric stents may be removed 7 days after the operation although this does vary from patient to patient and with surgeon preference. The removal of the other catheters is dependent on the type of diversion and surgeon preference.

Postoperative stage 2
Incontinent diversions

See section on Stoma care for further information.

Continent cutaneous diversion

In this type of diversion the catheter via the cutaneous stoma and the pouch catheter remain in place for up to 6 weeks from the date of surgery. Therefore patients will be discharged home for a few weeks with these catheters although only one needs to be on free drainage. Patients need to be taught how to care for these catheters before discharge.

Patients are readmitted for activation of their diversion. Both catheters are clamped to allow the reservoir to fill up with urine which helps the patient to establish the sensations experienced as this happens. If no sensations are felt then a voiding programme needs to be established to avoid overfilling. A catheter is released after 2–3 hours, depending on how the patient tolerates the sensation. This process is repeated 1–2 times to continue to expand the pouch. The pouch capacity at this stage is 250–300 mL; generally pouches are constructed to hold 500 mL and it may

take several weeks to reach this target. Patients continue to expand their pouch at their own pace once they are discharged.

Once the pouch has been initially stretched, the catheter is removed and the catheterization procedure is explained and demonstrated (see Procedure guideline 6.10). Patients should be supervised during the catheterization process until they are competent and confident with the procedure. Generally, patients remain in hospital for 1–2 days.

Ongoing care
Rectal bladder

Ureteric stents are usually removed 10 days postoperatively and the rectal catheter 12 days later. Patients often experience frequency and incontinence and need support, encouragement and reassurance. Patients need to stretch their new bladder by attempting to resist the urge to empty it for increasingly longer periods of time. Voiding will eventually be every 2–4 hours, often emptying once at night (Leaver 2002).

Orthotopic neobladder

Patients with a neobladder will have a urethral catheter in place and may also have a suprapubic catheter, depending on surgeon preference. The urethral catheter may be removed before they are discharged or they may go home with catheter(s) in place and return to hospital 1–2 weeks later to have their catheter removed. If the patient is discharged home with catheter(s) in place they will need to be taught how to care for their catheter(s). Those patients who go home with catheters in place will need to be admitted for activation of their neobladder.

When the urethral catheter is removed patients should be advised to expect some urinary incontinence in the first few days or weeks; it usually happens just before the next void and at night time, so patients are advised to get up to void 1–2 times a night. If the patient has a suprapubic catheter in place, this may be released after each void to check any residual volume of urine that may be present. When the residual volume is less than 100 mL, the catheter may be removed.

The neobladder needs to be stretched by patients resisting the urge to empty it for increasingly longer periods of time. Neobladders are constructed to hold approximately 500 mL of urine and it will take many weeks to build up to this volume. As the neobladder capacity expands, continence will improve (Varol and Studer 2004). Patients should be taught voiding techniques and advised to continue performing pelvic floor (Kegel) exercises. They should also be given equipment and advised on how to manage their incontinence whilst their bladder compliance improves.

Specific discharge plans

All patients who have undergone any type of urinary diversion have similar discharge needs. They are taught how to recognize a urinary tract infection and advised to drink at least 2–3 litres of fluid daily to reduce the risk of this happening. All patients undergoing continent diversion are advised to wear a medical alert bracelet, so that if they are found unconscious at any time a doctor or nurse will be aware of the surgery that has been performed.

Patients should be discharged with adequate supplies to last until a prescription is obtained from the general practitioner. Written information should include how to care for their diversion, how to obtain supplies of any equipment needed and details of healthcare professionals they should contact in the event of any difficulties. Arrangements should be made for a home visit from the community nurse and/or stoma nurse and/or continence nurse.

Education of patient and relevant others

Before patients are discharged they should be informed about the following.

■ To empty the pouch every 4–6 hours to prevent overdistension and to always empty the pouch before participating in strenuous activities to minimize the pressure put on the pouch. If the pouch becomes too full there is a risk of trauma to, or rupture of, the pouch, leakage of urine via the tunnel or, because of increased pressure on the valve, it may make catheterization difficult or impossible (Busuttil-Leaver 2004).
■ To ensure an undisturbed sleep by reducing the amount of fluid the patient drinks 3 hours before going to sleep. The patient should catheterize or void before going to sleep and on waking.
■ To keep a catheter available at all times (in suit, car, handbag, at work and at home), in case the patient needs to empty the urine.
■ A small amount of mucus may leak from the continent urinary stoma and a piece of gauze can be worn to protect clothing.

Patients should be informed that it will take time to become accustomed to and gain confidence in their new continent urinary diversion.

Teaching intermittent self-catheterization of a continent urinary diversion stoma

Intermittent self-catheterization is when patients insert a self-catheterization (Nelaton type) catheter into the urinary reservoir via the continent urinary stoma using a clean technique (see Chapter 3). It is performed to evacuate or instil fluids, after which the tube is removed.

Intermittent self-catheterization may be carried out for the following reasons.

■ To empty the contents of the urinary reservoir every 4–6 hours. If the reservoir is left too long between emptying, it can become overstretched and lose its elasticity.

■ To allow irrigation of the urinary reservoir for the removal of mucus which may occlude the continent urinary stoma and potentially lead to stone formation.

Intermittent self-catheterization should be taught in a place that offers privacy, with a good clear light and a mirror (bathroom, toilet or at the patient's bedside). It is a clean and not a sterile procedure. Patients can learn self-catheterization with the aid of a mirror or by touch, and are observed and assisted by a nurse until they are proficient (see Procedure guideline 6.10).

This procedure should always be performed aseptically in hospital. At home it is performed as a clean technique.

Complications

A number of complications have been identified; these may be short-term 'teething' problems while the pouch settles down and the patient becomes familiar with it. However, some patients require further surgery or treatment to rectify problems to ensure their pouch function is acceptable. The most common complications are:

■ infection
■ stenosis of the stoma
■ leakage via the stoma
■ inability to empty pouch
■ loss of tunnel
■ high-pressure bladder system
■ stone formation. A number of factors have been implicated in this process; these include urinary stasis, increased mucus production from the intestinal segment and colonization with urea-splitting bacteria
■ metabolic acidosis
■ renal damage
■ pouch rupture
■ incontinence
■ skin irritation with Mainz II if anal sphincter leaks
■ secondary malignancy following Mainz II due to the high risk posed by the mixture of urine and faeces in the bowel. Neoplasms usually are seen 20–30 years after surgery (Stewart 1986). Yearly endoscopic follow-up should be carried out from the 12th postoperative year in order to detect any tumours early (McCahill et al. 1992, Wagstaff et al. 1991, Woodhouse 1994, Woodhouse and Christofides 1998).

Bladder irrigation

Definition

Bladder irrigation is the continuous washing out of the bladder with sterile fluid, usually 0.9% normal saline (Ng 2001).

Evidence-based approaches
Rationale
Indications

Bladder irrigation is performed to prevent the formation and retention of blood clots, for example following prostatic surgery. However, there is evidence emerging that postoperative bladder irrigation can be safely eliminated by modifying the surgical technique used for suprapubic prostatectomy (Okorie *et al.* 2010). On rare occasions bladder irrigation is performed to remove heavily contaminated material from a diseased urinary bladder (Cutts 2005, Fillingham and Douglas 2004, Scholtes 2002).

Principles of care

There are a number of risks associated with bladder irrigation (including introducing infection) and the procedure should not be undertaken lightly (McCarthy and Hunter 2001, NICE 2003). Prior to taking a decision to use bladder maintenance solutions, patients should be assessed (Rew 1999). The guiding principle for effective catheter management always involves addressing the individual needs of the patient (Godfrey and Evans 2000). Assessment of all aspects of catheter care and irrigation should be undertaken, including:

- patient activity and mobility (catheter positioning, catheter kinking)
- diet and fluid intake
- standards of patient hygiene
- patient's and/or carer's ability to care for the catheter (Getliffe 1996a, Ng 2001, Rew 1999, Rew 2005).

An important aspect of management for patients in whom a clear pattern of catheter history can be established is the scheduling of catheter changes prior to likely blockages (Getliffe 1996b, Yates 2004). In patients in whom no clear pattern emerges, or for whom frequent catheter changes are traumatic, acidic bladder washouts can be beneficial in reducing catheter encrustations (Getliffe 1996a, McCarthy and Hunter 2001, Rew 1999, Yates 2004). The administration of catheter maintenance solutions to eliminate catheter encrustation can also be timed to coincide with catheter bag changes (every 5–7 days) so that the catheter system is not opened more than necessary (Yates 2004).

Preprocedural considerations
Equipment
Catheters used for irrigation

A three-way urinary catheter must be used for irrigation in order that fluid may simultaneously be run into, and drained out from, the bladder (Cutts 2005, Getliffe 1996a, Ng 2001). A large-gauge catheter (16–24) is often used to accommodate any clot and debris which may be present. This catheter is commonly passed in theatre when irrigation is required, for example after prostatectomy (Forristal and Maxfield 2004). Occasionally, if a patient is admitted with a heavily contaminated bladder, for example blood clots, bladder irrigation may be started on the ward. If the patient has a two-way catheter, this must be replaced with a three-way type (Scholtes 2002).

It is recommended that a three-way catheter is passed if frequent intravesical instillations of drugs or antiseptic solutions are prescribed and the risk of catheter obstruction is not considered to be very great. In such cases, the most important factor is minimizing the risk of introducing infection and maintaining a closed urinary drainage system, for which the three-way catheter allows (Figure 6.14).

Occasionally blood clots can cause a catheter blockage which requires the catheter and drainage tube to be 'milked' using rubber-tipped 'milking' tongs in order to prevent damaging the catheter. This encourages the removal of clots from within the drainage system and ensures the catheter remains free flowing (Lowthian 1991).

Pharmacological support

The agent most commonly recommended for irrigation is 0.9% sodium chloride which should be used in every case unless an alternative solution is prescribed. 0.9% sodium chloride is isotonic; consequently it does not affect the body's fluid or electrolyte levels, enabling large volumes of the solution to be used as necessary (Cutts 2005). In particular, 3-litre bags of 0.9% sodium chloride are available for irrigation purposes. It has been proposed that sterile water should never be used to irrigate the bladder as it can be readily absorbed by osmosis (Addison 2000a). However, a recent study has demonstrated that sterile water is a safe irrigating fluid for transurethral resection of prostate (TURP) (Moharari *et al.* 2008).

Although not a common complication, absorption of irrigation fluid can occur during bladder irrigation. This can produce a potentially critical situation, as absorption leads to electrolyte imbalance and circulatory overload (Getliffe 1996a). Absorption is most likely to occur in theatre where glycine irrigation fluid, devoid of sodium or potassium, is forced under pressure into the prostatic veins (Forristal and Maxfield 2004). The 0.9% sodium chloride cannot be used during surgery as it contains electrolytes which interfere with diathermy (Forristal and Maxfield 2004). However, the risk of absorption still remains while irrigation continues postoperatively. For this reason it is important that fluid balance is monitored carefully during irrigation (Scholtes 2002).

Figure 6.14 Closed urinary drainage system with provision for intermittent or continuous irrigation.

Procedure guideline 6.12 **Commencing bladder irrigation**

Essential equipment

- Sterile dressing pack
- Antiseptic solution
- Bactericidal alcohol handrub
- Clamp
- Disposable irrigation set
- Infusion stand
- Sterile jug
- Absorbent sheet
- Gloves

Medicinal products

- Sterile irrigation fluid

Preprocedure

Action	Rationale
1 Explain and discuss the procedure with the patient.	To ensure that the patient understands the procedure and gives their valid consent (NMC 2008a, C).

Procedure guideline 6.12 *(Continued)*

2 Screen the bed. Ensure that the patient is in a comfortable position, allowing the nurse access to the catheter.	For the patient's privacy and to reduce the risk of cross-infection (Fraise and Bradley 2009, E).

Procedure

3 Perform the procedure using an aseptic technique.	To minimize the risk of infection (Fraise and Bradley 2009, E).
4 Open the outer wrappings of the pack and put it on the top shelf of the trolley.	To prepare equipment. E
5 Insert the end of the irrigation giving set into the fluid bag and hang the bag on the infusion stand. Allow fluid to run through the tubing so that air is expelled.	To prime the irrigation set so that it is ready for use. Air is expelled in order to prevent discomfort from air in the patient's bladder. E
6 Clamp the catheter and place absorbent sheet under the catheter junction.	To prevent leakage of urine through the irrigation arm when the spigot is removed. E To contain any spillages.
7 Clean hands with a bactericidal alcohol handrub. Put on gloves.	To minimize the risk of cross-infection (Fraise and Bradley 2009, E).
8 Place a sterile paper towel under the irrigation inlet of the catheter and remove the spigot.	To create a sterile field. To prepare catheter for connection to irrigation set (Scholtes 2002, E).
9 Discard the spigot and gloves.	To prevent reuse and reduce risk of cross-infection (Fraise and Bradley 2009, E).
10 Put on sterile gloves. Clean around the end of the irrigation arm with sterile low-linting gauze and an antiseptic solution.	To remove surface organisms from gloves and catheter and to reduce the risk of introducing infection into the catheter (Fraise and Bradley 2009, E).
11 Attach the irrigation giving set to the irrigation arm of the catheter. Keep the clamp of the irrigation giving set closed.	To prevent overdistension of the bladder, which can occur if fluid is run into the bladder before the drainage tube has been unclamped (Scholtes 2002, E).
12 Release the clamp on the catheter tube and allow any accumulated urine to drain into the catheter bag. Empty the urine from the catheter bag into a sterile jug.	Urine drainage should be measured before commencing irrigation so that the fluid balance may be monitored more accurately (Scholtes 2002, E).
13 Discard the gloves.	These will be contaminated, having handled the cathether bag (Fraise and Bradley 2009, E).
14 Set irrigation at the required rate and ensure that fluid is draining into the catheter bag.	To check that the drainage system is patent and to prevent fluid accumulating in the bladder. C

Postprocedure

15 Make the patient comfortable, remove unnecessary equipment and clean the trolley.	To reduce the risk of cross-infection (Fraise and Bradley 2009, E).
16 Wash hands.	To reduce the risk of cross-infection (Fraise and Bradley 2009, E).

Problem-solving table 6.4 Prevention and resolution (Procedure guideline 6.12)

Problem	Possible cause	Prevention	Suggested action
Fluid retained in the bladder when the catheter is in position	Fault in drainage apparatus, for example:		
	blocked catheter		'Milk' the tubing. Wash out the bladder with 0.9% sodium chloride
	kinked tubing		Straighten the tubing
	overfull drainage bag	Empty the drainage bag every 4 hours	Empty the drainage bag
	catheter clamped off		Unclamp the catheter
Distended abdomen related to an overfull bladder during the irrigation procedure	Irrigation fluid is infused at too rapid a rate	Monitor fluid drainage rate every 15 minutes	Slow down the infusion rate
	Fault in drainage apparatus		Check the patency of the drainage apparatus
Leakage of fluid from around the catheter	Catheter slipping out of the bladder		Insert the catheter further in. Decompress balloon fully to assess the amount of water necessary. Refill balloon until it remains *in situ*, taking care not to overfill beyond safe level (see manufacturer's instructions)
	Catheter too large or unsuitable for the patient's anatomy		If leakage is profuse or catheter is uncomfortable for the patient, replace the catheter with one of smaller size
Patient experiences pain during the lavage or irrigation procedure	Volume of fluid in the bladder is too great for comfort		Reduce the fluid volume within the bladder
	Solution is painful to raw areas in the bladder		Inform the doctor. Administer analgesia as prescribed
Retention of fluid with or without distended abdomen, with or without pain	Perforated bladder		Stop irrigation. Maintain in recovery position. Call medical assistance. Monitor vital signs. Monitor patient for pain, tense abdomen

233

Procedure guideline 6.13 Care of the patient during bladder irrigation

Essential equipment

- Sterile dressing pack
- Antiseptic solution
- Bactericidal alcohol handrub
- Clamp
- Disposable irrigation set
- Infusion stand
- Sterile jug
- Absorbent sheet

(Continued)

Procedure guideline 6.13 *(Continued)*

Medicinal products

- Sterile irrigation fluid

Procedure

Action	Rationale
1 Adjust the rate of infusion according to the degree of haematuria. This will be greatest in the first 12 hours following surgery (average fluid input is 6–9 litres during the first 12 hours, falling to 3–6 litres during the next 12 hours). The aim is to obtain a drainage fluid which is rosé in colour.	To remove blood from the bladder before it clots and to minimize the risk of catheter obstruction and clot retention (Scholtes 2002, E).
2 Check the volume in the drainage bag frequently when infusion is in progress, for example half-hourly or hourly, or more frequently as required.	To ensure that fluid is draining from the bladder and to detect blockages as soon as possible, also to prevent overdistension of the bladder and patient discomfort. To empty catheter drainage bags before they reach capacity.
3 Using rubber-tipped 'milking' tongs, 'milk' the catheter and drainage tube, as required.	To remove clots from within the drainage system and to maintain an efficient outlet (Lowthian 1991, E).
4 Annotate the fluid balance chart accurately. The fluid balance of all patients having bladder irrigation must be monitored.	So that urine output is known and any related problems, for example renal dysfunction, may be detected quickly and easily. E

Postprocedural considerations

Documentation

Bladder irrigation recording chart

The bladder irrigation recording chart (Figure 6.15) is designed to provide an accurate record of the patient's urinary output during the period of irrigation. Record the time (column A) and the fluid volume in each bag of irrigating solution (column B) as it is put up.

When the irrigating fluid has all run from the first bag into the bladder, record the original volume in the bag in column C. Record the corresponding time in column A. Do not attempt to estimate the fluid volume run-in while a bag is in progress as this will be inaccurate. If, however, a bag is discontinued, the volume run-in can be calculated by measuring the volume left in the bag and deducting this from the original volume. This should be recorded in column C (Scholtes 2002).

The catheter bag should be emptied as often as is necessary, the volume being recorded in column D and the corresponding time in column A. The catheter bag must also be emptied whenever the bag of irrigating fluid is empty, and the volume recorded in column D.

When each bag of fluid has run through, add up the total volume drained by the catheter in column D, and write this in red. Subtract from this the total volume run-in (column C) to find the urine output (D − C = E). Write this in column E. Draw a line across the page to indicate that this calculation is complete and continue underneath for the next bag.

Faecal elimination

Definition

Faecal elimination is the process of elimination – simply the expulsion of the residues of digestion, faeces, from the digestive tract (Thibodeau and Patton 2007). The act of expelling faeces is called defaecation.

Anatomy and physiology

This section will consider the normal structure and function of the bowel, which includes the small and large intestine (Figure 6.16). The small intestine begins at the pyloric sphincter of the stomach, coils through the abdomen and opens into the large intestine at the ileocaecal junction. It is approximately 6 m in length and is divided into three segments: the duodenum (25 cm), jejunum (2.5 m) and ileum (3.5 m) (Thibodeau and Patton 2007). The mucosal surface of the small intestine is covered with finger-like processes called villi, which increase the surface area available for absorption and digestion. A number of digestive enzymes are also secreted by the small intestine (Tortora and Derrickson 2009).

Movement through the small bowel is divided into two types, namely segmentation and peristalsis, and is controlled by the autonomic nervous system. Segmentation refers to the localized contraction of the intestine, which mixes the intestinal contents and brings particles of food into contact with the mucosa for absorption. Once the majority of a meal

Patient name:			Hospital no:		
(A) Date and time	**(B) Volume put up**	**(C) Volume run in**	**(D) Total volume out**	**(E) Urine**	**(F) Urine running total**
10/7/06					
10.00	2000				
10.30			700		
11.10			850		
11.40		2000	600		
			2150	150	150
11.45	2000				
12.30			500		
13.15			700		
14.20		2000	800		
			2400	400	550
14.25	2000				
15.30			850		
17.00	Irrigation stopped	1200	800		
			1650	450	1000

Figure 6.15 Bladder irrigation recording chart.

has been absorbed through this process, intestinal content is then pushed along the small intestine by repeated peristaltic wave-like actions. Intestinal content usually remains in the small bowel for 3–5 hours (Tortora and Derrickson 2009).

The total volume of fluid, including ingested liquids and gastrointestinal secretions, that enters the small intestine daily is about 9.3 litres. The small intestine is responsible for absorbing around 90% of the nutrients, electrolytes and water within this volume by diffusion, facilitated diffusion, osmosis and active transport (Tortora and Derrickson 2009). Water is able to move across the intestinal mucosa in both directions, but is influenced by the absorption of nutrients

and electrolytes. As various electrolytes and nutrients are actively transported out of the lumen, they create a concentration gradient, promoting water absorption, via osmosis, in order to maintain an osmotic balance between intestinal fluid and blood. This ultimately leads to only about 1 litre of effluent passing through into the colon (Thibodeau and Patton 2007, Tortora and Derrickson 2009, Wood 1996).

From the ileocaecal sphincter to the anus, the colon is approximately 1.5–1.8 m in length. Its main function is to eliminate the waste products of digestion by the propulsion of faeces towards the anus. In addition, it produces mucus to lubricate the faecal mass, thus aiding its expulsion. Other

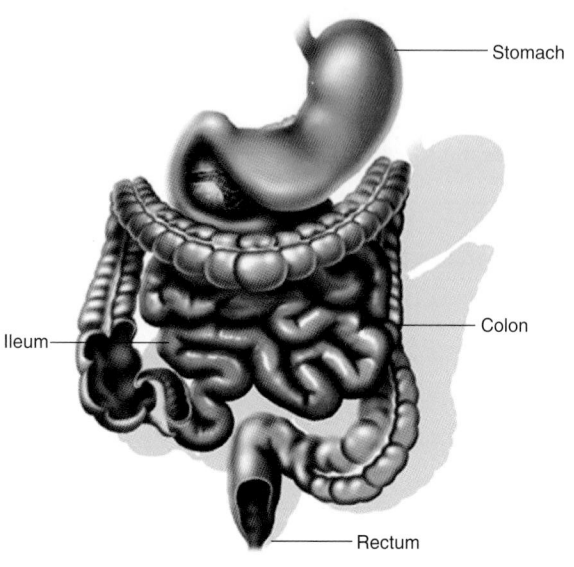

Figure 6.16 The gastrointestinal tract.

functions include the absorption of fluid and electrolytes, including sodium and potassium, the storage of faeces and the synthesis of vitamins B and K by bacterial flora (Thibodeau and Patton 2007, Tortora and Derrickson 2009).

Faeces consist of the unabsorbed end-products of digestion, bile pigments, cellulose, bacteria, epithelial cells, mucus and some inorganic material. They are normally semi-solid in consistency and contain about 70% water (Tortora and Derrickson 2009). The colon absorbs about 2 litres of water in 24 hours, so if faeces are not expelled they will gradually become hard due to dehydration and more difficult to expel. If there is insufficient roughage (fibre) in the faeces, colonic stasis occurs, which leads to continued water absorption and further hardening of the faeces. The movement of faeces through the colon towards the anus is by mass peristalsis, a gastrocolic reflex initiated by the presence of food in the stomach, which begins at the middle of the transverse colon and quickly drives the colonic contents into the rectum. This mass peristaltic movement generally occurs 3–5 times a day (Perdue 2005). In response to this stimulus, faeces move into the rectum (Norton 1996b, Taylor 1997, Tortora and Derrickson 2009).

Diarrhoea

Definition

The term diarrhoea originates from the Greek for 'to flow through' (Bell 2004) and can be characterized according to its onset and duration (acute or chronic) or by type (e.g. secretory, osmotic or malabsorptive). Diarrhoea can also be defined in terms of stool frequency, consistency, volume or weight (Metcalf 2007).

Related theory

Diarrhoea is a serious global public health problem, in particularly in low-income and middle-income countries. The World Health Organization (2003) believes that over 3 million episodes happen each year, with many people dying. The disease pathogens are most commonly transmitted via the faecal–oral route (Ejemot *et al.* 2009).

Acute diarrhoea

Acute diarrhoea is very common, usually self-limiting, lasts less than 2 weeks and often requires no investigation or treatment (Shepherd 2000). Causes of acute diarrhoea include:

- dietary indiscretion (eating too much fruit, alcohol misuse)
- allergy to food constituents
- infective:
  - travel associated
  - viral
  - bacterial (usually associated with food)
  - antibiotic related.

Chronic diarrhoea

Chronic diarrhoea generally lasts longer than 2–4 weeks (Metcalf 2007) and may have more complex origins. Chronic causes can be divided as follows (Thomas *et al.* 2003).

- *Colonic*: colonic neoplasia, ulcerative colitis and Crohn's disease, microscopic colitis.
- *Small bowel*: small bowel bacterial overgrowth, coeliac disease, Crohn's disease, Whipple's disease, bile acid malabsorption, disaccharidase deficiency, mesenteric ischaemia, radiation enteritis, lymphoma, giardiasis.
- *Pancreatic*: chronic pancreatitis, pancreatic carcinoma, cystic fibrosis.
- *Endocrine*: hyperthyroidism, diabetes, hypoparathyroidism, Addison's disease, hormone-secreting tumours.
- *Other causes*: laxative misuse, drugs, alcohol, autonomic neuropathy, small bowel resection or intestinal fistulas, radiation enteritis.

Preprocedural considerations
Assessment

The cause of diarrhoea needs to be identified before effective treatment can be instigated. This may include clinical investigations such as stool cultures for bacterial, fungal and viral pathogens or a more formal medical evaluation of the gastrointestinal tract (Kornblau *et al.* 2000).

Ongoing nursing assessment is essential for ensuring individualized management and care. The lack of a systematic approach to assessment and poor documentation cause problems in effective management of diarrhoea (Cadd *et al.* 2000, Smith 2001). Nurses need to be aware of contributing factors and be sensitive to patients' beliefs and values in order to provide holistic care. A comprehensive assessment is therefore essential and should include the following.

- History of onset, frequency and duration of diarrhoea: patient's perception of diarrhoea is often related to stool consistency (Metcalf 2007).
- Consistency, colour and form of stool, including the presence of blood, fat, mucus. Stools can be graded using a scale such as the Bristol Stool Form Chart (see Figure 6.2), where diarrhoea would be classified as types 6 or 7 (Longstreth *et al.* 2006).
- Associated symptoms: pain, nausea, vomiting, fatigue, weight loss or fever.
- Physical examination: check for gaping anus, rectal prolapse and prolapsed haemorrhoids (Nazarko 2007).
- Recent lifestyle changes, emotional disturbances or travel abroad.
- Fluid intake and dietary history, including any cause-and-effect relationships between food consumption and bowel action.
- Regular medication, including antibiotics, laxatives, oral hypoglycaemics, appetite suppressants, antidepressants, statins, digoxin or chemotherapy (Nazarko 2007).
- Effectiveness of antidiarrhoeal medication (dose and frequency).
- Significant past medical history: bowel resection, pancreatitis, pelvic radiotherapy.
- Hydration status: evaluation of mucous membranes and skin turgor.
- Perianal or peristomal skin integrity: enzymes present in faecal fluid can cause rapid breakdown of the skin (Nazarko 2007).
- Stool cultures for bacterial, fungal and viral pathogens: to check for infective diarrhoea (Pellatt 2007). Treatment may not be commenced until results are available except if the patient has been infected by *Clostridium difficile* in the past.
- Blood tests: full blood count, urea and electrolytes, liver function tests, vitamin B_{12}, folate, calcium, ferritin, ESR (erythrocyte sedimentation rate) and C-reactive protein.
- Patient's preferences and own coping strategies including non-pharmacological interventions and their effectiveness (Cadd *et al.* 2000, Chelvanayagam and Norton 2004, King 2002, Kornblau *et al.* 2000).

All episodes of acute diarrhoea must be considered potentially infectious until proven otherwise. The risk of spreading the infection to others can be reduced by adopting universal precautions such as wearing of gloves, aprons and gowns, disposing of all excreta immediately and, ideally, nursing the patient in a side room with access to their own toilet (King 2002). Advice should always be sought from infection control teams. At this stage nursing care should also include educating patients about careful handwashing.

Diarrhoea can have profound physiological and psychosocial consequences on a patient. Severe or extended episodes of diarrhoea may result in dehydration, electrolyte imbalance and malnutrition. Patients not only have to cope with increased frequency

of bowel movement but may have abdominal pain, cramping, proctitis and anal or perianal skin breakdown. Food aversions may develop or patients may stop eating altogether as they anticipate subsequent diarrhoea following intake. Consequently, this may lead to weight loss and malnutrition. Fatigue, sleep disturbances, feelings of isolation and depression are all common consequences for those experiencing diarrhoea. The impact of severe diarrhoea should not be underestimated; it is highly debilitating and may cause patients on long-term therapy to be non-compliant, resulting in a potentially life-threatening problem (Kornblau *et al.* 2000).

Once the cause of diarrhoea has been established, management should be focused on resolving the cause and providing physical and psychological support for the patient. Most cases of chronic diarrhoea will resolve once the underlying condition is treated, for example drug therapy for Crohn's disease or dietary management for coeliac disease. Episodes of acute diarrhoea, usually caused by bacteria or viruses, generally resolve spontaneously and are managed by symptom control and the prevention of complications (Shepherd 2000).

Pharmacological support

The treatment for diarrhoea depends on the cause.

Antimotility drugs such as loperamide or codeine phosphate may be useful in some cases, for example in blind loop syndrome and radiation enteritis. These drugs reduce gastrointestinal motility to relieve the symptoms of abdominal cramps and reduce the frequency of diarrhoea (Shepherd 2000). It is important to rule out any infective agent as the cause of diarrhoea before using any of these drugs, as they may make the situation worse by slowing the clearance of the infective agent.

In the case of bacterial diarrhoea, treatment with antibiotics is recommended only in patients who are very symptomatic and show signs of systemic involvement (Metcalf 2007). Not uncommonly, *Salmonella* can become resistant to commonly used antimicrobial agents such as amoxicillin (Metcalf 2007). When dealing with antibiotic-associated diarrhoea, most patients will notice a cessation of their symptoms with discontinuation of the antibiotic therapy. If diarrhoea persists, it is important to exclude pseudomembranous colitis by performing a sigmoidoscopy and sending a stool for cytotoxin analysis. However, over the last few years there has been increasing evidence supporting the use of probiotics in cases of diarrhoea associated with antibiotics (McFarland 2007). Researchers believe that probiotics restore the microbial balance in the intestinal tract previously destroyed by inciting antibiotics (Hickson *et al.* 2007). There are a variety of probiotic products available and their effectiveness appears to be related to the strain of bacteria causing the diarrhoea (Hickson *et al.* 2007, McFarland 2007).

Fluid replacement

The prevention and/or correction of dehydration is the first step in managing an episode of diarrhoea. Adults normally require 1.5–2 litres of fluid in 24 hours. The person who has diarrhoea will require an additional 200 mL for each loose stool. Dehydration can be corrected by using intravenous fluids and electrolytes or by oral rehydration solutions. The extent of dehydration dictates whether a patient can be managed at home or will need to be admitted to hospital (Nazarko 2007). Nursing care should also include monitoring signs or symptoms of electrolyte imbalance, such as muscle weakness and cramps, hypokalaemia, tachycardia and hypernatraemia (Metcalf 2007).

Non-pharmacological support

Maintaining dignity

Preserving the patient's privacy and dignity is essential during episodes of diarrhoea. The nurse has an important role in minimizing the patient's distress by adjusting language and using terms that are appropriate to the individual to reduce embarrassment (Smith 2001) and by listening to the patient's preference for care (Cadd *et al.* 2000). Additionally, the use of deodorizers and air fresheners to remove the smell caused by offensive diarrhoea contributes to the person's dignity. Stoma deodorants are thought to be more effective and samples can be obtained from company representatives (Nazarko 2007).

Skin care

It is important that the patient has easy access to clean toilet and washing facilities and that requests for assistance are answered promptly. Skin care is also essential to prevent bacteria present in faecal matter from destroying the skin's cellular defences and causing skin damage. This is particularly important with diarrhoea since it has high levels of faecal enzymes that come into contact with the perianal skin (Le Lievre 2002). The anal area should be gently cleaned with warm water immediately after every episode of diarrhoea. Frequent washing of the skin can alter the pH and remove protective oils from the skin. Products aimed at maintaining healthy peristomal skin have been used to protect perianal skin in patients with diarrhoea (Nazarko 2007). Soap should be avoided, unless it is an emollient, to avoid excessive drying of the skin and gentle patting of the skin is preferred for drying to avoid friction damage. Talcum powder should not be used and barrier creams should be applied sparingly, gently layered on in the direction of the hair growth rather than rubbed into the skin (Le Lievre 2002). The use of incontinence pads should be carefully considered in a person with severe episodes of diarrhoea. This particular material does not adsorb fluid stools, protect the skin from damage or contain smells.

Faecal collection devices can be useful if the person is cared for in bed as undue movement may cause leakage (Nazarko 2007, Wilson 2008). This type of device is fitted over the anus and fluid stools drain into a drainage bag similar to a drainable stoma bag.

Diet

A diet rich in fibre can cause diarrhoea. In this case the person should be advised to reduce the amount and space it out over the day (Nazarko 2007). Chilli and other spices can irritate the bowel and should be avoided. Sorbitol (artificial sweetener), beer, stout and high doses of vitamins and minerals should also be avoided.

Faecal incontinence

Faecal incontinence is a clinical symptom associated with diarrhoea (Nazarko 2007). When it is not possible to treat the cause of the diarrhoea, a care plan should be created to prevent complications and manage incontinence (NICE 2007). Factors that can contribute to the development of faecal incontinence are (Nazarko 2007):

- damage or weakness of the anal sphincter: obstetric damage, haemorrhoidectomy, sphincterotomy or degeneration of the internal anal sphincter muscle
- severe diarrhoea
- faecal loading (impaction): immobility, lack of fluids
- neurological conditions: spinal cord injury, Parkinson's disease
- cognitive deficits.

Diarrhoea can potentially disrupt a person's well-being. Community nurses and hospital-based specialist nurses have an essential role in supporting those affected by this condition. Diagnosis, treatment and management of diarrhoea and potential faecal incontinence can take place at home where individuals are more familiar with the environment.

Constipation

Definition

Constipation results when there is a delayed movement of intestinal content through the bowel (Walsh 1997). It has been defined as persistent, difficult, infrequent or incomplete defaecation, which may or may not be accompanied by hard, dry stools (Norton 2006, Thompson *et al.* 1999). There is a lack of consensus amongst both healthcare professionals and the general public as to what actually constitutes constipation (Norton 2006, Perdue 2005).

Anatomy and physiology

The rectum is very sensitive to rises in pressure, even of 2–3 mmHg, and distension will cause a perineal sensation with a subsequent desire to defaecate. A co-ordinated reflex empties the bowel from mid-transverse colon to the anus. During this phase the diaphragm, abdominal and levator ani muscles contract and the glottis closes. Waves of peristalsis occur in the distal colon and the anal sphincter relaxes, allowing the evacuation of faeces (Tortora and Derrickson 2009). The stimulus to defaecate varies in individuals according to habit, and if a decision is made to delay defaecation, the stimulus disappears and a process of retroperistalsis occurs whereby the faeces move back into the sigmoid colon (Perdue 2005). If these natural reflexes are inhibited on a regular basis, they are eventually suppressed and reflex defaecation is inhibited, resulting in such individuals becoming severely constipated.

Related theory

It has been estimated that up to 27% of a given population experience constipation (Cook *et al.* 1999, Longstreth *et al.* 2006). Constipation is a common symptom in cancer and palliative care. Constipation has been reported in 55% of patients in their last week of life (Conill *et al.* 1997) and 70–100% of patients receiving treatment in hospital (McMillan 1999). It can affect this patient group at any stage of their disease and for a variety of reasons.

Constipation occurs when there is either a failure of colonic propulsion (slow colonic transit) or a failure to evacuate the rectum (rectal outlet delay) or a combination of these problems (Norton 1996a, Norton 2006, Teahon 1999).

The management of constipation depends on the cause and there are numerous possible causes, with many patients being affected by more than one causative factor (Figure 6.17).

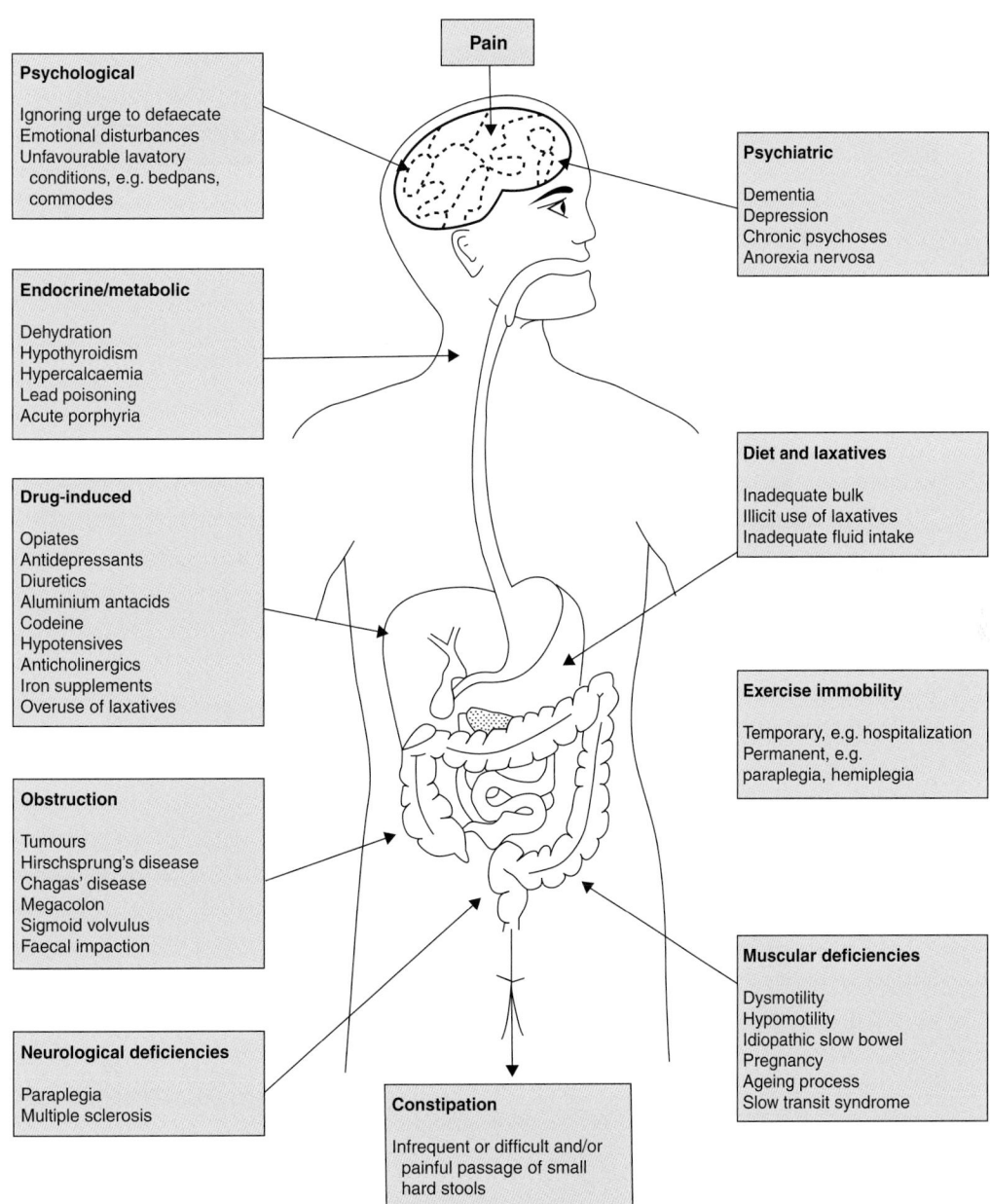

Figure 6.17   Classification of constipation: combined sources.

While constipation is not life-threatening, it does cause a great deal of distress and discomfort. Particularly, constipation can be associated with abdominal pain or cramps, feelings of general malaise or fatigue and feelings of bloatedness. Nausea, anorexia, headaches, confusion, restlessness, retention of urine, faecal incontinence and halitosis may also be present in some cases (Maestri-Banks 1998, Norton 1996b).

The effective treatment of constipation relies on the cause being identified by thorough assessment. Constipation can be categorized as primary, secondary or iatrogenic (Perdue 2005). Factors that lead to the development of primary constipation are extrinsic or lifestyle related and include:

- an inadequate diet (low fibre)
- poor fluid intake
- a lifestyle change
- ignoring the urge to defaecate (see Figure 6.18).

Constipation that is attributed to an intrinsic disease process or conditions such as anal fissures, colonic tumours or hypercalcaemia is classified as secondary constipation,

Correct position for opening your bowels

Step one

Knees higher than hips

Step two

Lean forwards and put elbows on your knees

Step three

Bulge out your abdomen
Straighten your spine

Correct position

Knees higher than hips
Lean forwards and put elbows on your knees
Bulge out yout abdomen
Straighten your spine

Figure 6.18 Correct positioning for opening your bowel. Reproduced by kind permission of Ray Addison and Wendy Ness. © Norgine Ltd.

whereas iatrogenic constipation generally results from treatment or medication (Perdue 2005). Constipation of unknown cause must be investigated in order to ensure that appropriate treatment is instigated (Taylor 1997, Teahon 1999).

Preprocedural considerations

Assessment

Undertaking a detailed history from the patient is pivotal in establishing the appropriate treatment plan. At present, there is no comprehensive assessment tool that has been validated. It is of vital importance that nurses adopt a proactive preventive approach to the assessment and management of constipation. Kyle *et al.* (2005a) have developed the Eton Scale, a constipation risk assessment tool.

There are a variety of factors that may affect normal bowel functioning which should be considered within an assessment, including:

- nutritional intake/recent changes in diet
- fluid intake
- mobility, for example lack of exercise
- medication, for example analgesics, antacids, iron supplements, tricyclic antidepressants
- lack of privacy, for example having to use shared toilet facilities, commodes or bedpans
- medical conditions, including disease process or symptoms, for example cancer, vomiting
- radiological investigations of the bowel involving the use of barium
- change in patient's normal routine/lifestyle/home circumstances
- change in psychological status, for example depression.

In addition to the identification of these risks/contributing factors, it is important to take a careful history of a patient's bowel habits, taking particular note of the following.

- Any changes in the patient's usual bowel activity. How long have these changes been present and have they occurred before?
- Frequency of bowel action.
- Volume, consistency and colour of the stool. Stools can be graded using a scale such as the Bristol Stool Form Chart (see Figure 6.2) where constipation would be classified as types 1 or 2 (Longstreth *et al.* 2006).
- Presence of mucus, blood, undigested food or offensive odour.
- Presence of pain or discomfort on defaecation.
- Use of oral or rectal medication to stimulate defaecation and its effectiveness.

A digital rectal examination (DRE) can also be performed, providing the nurse has received suitable training or instruction, to assess the contents of the rectum and to identify conditions which may cause discomfort such as haemorrhoids or anal fissures (Hinrichs and Huseboe 2001, Peate 2003, RCN 2006, Winney 1998). See the section on Digital rectal examination for further information.

Additional investigations such as an abdominal X-ray may be necessary to exclude bowel obstruction (Christer *et al.* 2003, Edwards *et al.* 2003, Fallon and O'Neill, 1997, Kyle *et al.* 2005a, Maestri-Banks 1998, Thompson *et al.* 2003).

Over recent years, international criteria (the Rome Criteria) have been developed and revised (Longstreth *et al.* 2006) which can help to more accurately and consistently define constipation. According to the new Rome III Criteria, an individual who is diagnosed with constipation should report having at least two of the following symptoms within the last 3 months where those symptoms began at least 6 months prior to diagnosis (Longstreth *et al.* 2006, Norton 2006).

- Straining for at least 25% of the time.
- Lumpy or hard stool for at least 25% of the time.
- A sensation of incomplete evacuation for at least 25% of the time.
- A sensation of anorectal obstruction or blockage for at least 25% of the time.
- Manual manoeuvres used to facilitate defaecation at least 25% of the time (e.g. manual evacuation).
- Less than three bowel movements a week.
- Also, in such patients, loose stools are rarely present without the use of laxatives.

It is important to recognize that although the Rome Criteria are the most used definition of constipation, their application to cancer and palliative care patients has its limitations (Stevens *et al.* 2008). The rationale for this is that many cancer and palliative care patients have constipation which is caused by a physical process or a drug so they do not have functional constipation. Also, many in this group of patients require treatment before 12 weeks.

The myth that daily bowel evacuation is essential to health has persisted through the centuries. It is thought that less than 10% of the population have a bowel evacuation daily (Edwards *et al.* 2003). This myth has resulted in laxative abuse becoming one of the most common types of drug abuse in the Western world. The annual cost to the NHS of prescribing medications to treat constipation is in the region of £45 million (DH 2005b).

An individual's bowel habit is dictated by their diet, lifestyle and environment, and the notion of what is a 'normal' bowel habit varies considerably. Studies have revealed that in the USA and UK, 95–99% of people pass at least three stools per week (Ehrenpreis 1995) and 'normal' bowel movement has been defined as ranging between three times a day and three times a week (Nazarko 1996). Given that there is such a wide normal range, it is important to establish the patient's usual bowel habit and the changes that may have occurred. Many patients are too embarrassed to discuss bowel function and will often delay reporting problems, despite the sometimes severe impact these symptoms have on their quality of life (Cadd *et al.* 2000). Generally complaints will be either that the patient has diarrhoea or is constipated. These should be seen as symptoms of some underlying disease or malfunction and managed accordingly. The nurse's priority is to effectively assess the nature and cause of the problem, to help find appropriate solutions and to inform and support the patient. This requires sensitive communication skills to dispel embarrassment and ensure a shared understanding of the meanings of the terms used by the patient (Smith 2001).

Pharmacological support

Laxatives

Laxatives can be defined simply as substances that cause evacuation of the bowel by a mild action (Mosby 2006). A laxative with a mild or gentle effect is also known as an aperient and one with a strong effect is referred to as a cathartic or a purgative. Purgatives should be used only in exceptional circumstances, that is, where all other interventions have failed, or when they are prescribed for a specific purpose. The aim of laxative treatment is to achieve comfortable rather than frequent defaecation and, wherever possible, the most natural means of bowel evacuation should be employed, with preference given to use of oral laxatives where appropriate (Fallon and O'Neill 1997, Perdue 2005). The many different types of laxatives available may be grouped into types according to the action they have (see Table 6.3).

Bulking agents

Bulking agents are usually the first line of laxative treatment and work by retaining water and promoting microbial growth in the colon, increasing faecal mass and stimulating peristalsis (Peate 2003). Ispaghula husk (Isogel, Regulan) and sterculia (Normacol) both trap water in the intestine by the formation of a highly viscous gel which softens faeces, increases weight and reduces transit time (Butler 1998). These agents need plenty of fluid in order to work (2–3 litres per day), so their appropriateness should be questioned for those with advanced cancer or for the older patient (Hinrichs and Huseboe 2001, Maestri-Banks 1998, Perdue 2005). They also take a few days to exert their effect (Maestri-Banks 1998) and so are not suitable to relieve acute constipation. Also, they are contraindicated in some patients, including those who have bowel obstruction, faecal impaction, acute abdominal pain and reduced muscle tone, or those who have had recent bowel surgery. Increasing the bulk may worsen impaction, lead to increased colonic faecal loading or even intestinal obstruction (Norton 1996a), and in some cases may increase the risk of faecal incontinence. Other potentially harmful effects include malabsorption of minerals, calcium, iron and fat-soluble vitamins, and reduced bio-availability of some drugs (Taylor 1997). Another problem initially is that bulk laxatives tend to distend the abdomen, often making the individual feel full and uncomfortable. Sometimes this leads to temporary anorexia (Taylor 1997).

Stool softeners

Stool-softening preparations, such as docusate sodium and glycerol (glycerine) suppositories, act by lowering the surface tension of faeces which allows water to penetrate and soften the stool (Hinrichs and Huseboe 2001, Peate 2003). They may also have a weak stimulatory effect (Barrett 1992), but drugs of this type are often given in combination with a chemical stimulant (Shepherd 2000). Softening agents usually take 1–3 days to work (Day 2001).

Liquid paraffin acts as a lubricant as well as a stool softener by coating the faeces and allowing easier passage. However, its use should be avoided as there are a number of problems associated with this preparation. It interferes with the absorption of fat-soluble vitamins and can also cause skin irritation and changes to the bowel mucosa, while accidental inhalation of droplets of liquid paraffin may result in lipoid pneumonia (BNF 2011, Maestri-Banks 1998, Peate 2003).

Osmotic agents

These can be divided into two subgroups: lactulose and magnesium preparations.

Lactulose is a synthetic disaccharide which exerts an osmotic effect in the small bowel. Distension of the small bowel induces propulsion which in turn reduces transit time. Colonic bacteria metabolize lactulose into a short-chain organic salt which is then absorbed; therefore the osmotic effect does not continue throughout the colon (Barrett 1992). This process of metabolism also produces gas which

Table 6.3 Types of laxative

Type of laxative	Example	Brand names and sources
Bulk producers	Dietary fibre	Bran, wholemeal bread, Fybogel (ispaghula), Normacol (sterculia)
	Mucilaginous polysaccharides	
	Methylcellulose	
Stool softeners	Synthetic surface active agents, liquid paraffin	Agarol, Dioctyl, Petrolager, Milpar
Osmotic agents	Sodium, potassium and magnesium salts	Magnesium sulphate, milk of magnesia, lactulose
Stimulant laxatives	Sodium picosulphate, glycerine	Senna, Senokot, bisacodyl, Dulcolax, co-danthrusate, Picolax, glycerol

in turn stimulates colonic movements and increases bacterial growth. This results in increased stool weight and thus colonic transit time is shortened (Spiller 1994). However, bowel action may still take up to 3 days to occur following administration (Shepherd 2000) and flatulence, cramps and abdominal discomfort are associated with high dosages.

Magnesium preparations also exert an osmotic effect on the gut and additionally they stimulate the release of cholecystokinin. This encourages intestinal motility and fluid secretion (Nathan 1996). They have a rapid effect, working within 2–6 hours, so fluid intake is important with these preparations as patients may experience diarrhoea and dehydration (Hinrichs and Huseboe 2001). These preparations should be avoided in patients with renal or hepatic impairment (Taylor 1997).

Stimulant laxatives

Laxatives including bisacodyl, danthron and senna stimulate the nerve plexi in the gut wall, increasing peristalsis and promoting the secretion of water and electrolytes in the small and large bowel (Maestri-Banks 1998, Peate 2003, Shepherd 2000). Abdominal cramping may be increased if the stool is hard and a stool softener may be used in combination with this group of drugs (ABPI 1999, Taylor 1997). Long-term use of these laxatives should be avoided, except for patients on long-term opiates, as they may lead to impaired bowel function such as atonic non-functioning (cathartic) colon (ABPI 1999, Hinrichs and Huseboe 2001, Taylor 1997).

Preparations containing danthron are restricted to certain groups of patients, that is, the terminally ill as some studies on rodents have indicated a potential carcinogenic risk (ABPI 1999, Shepherd 2000, Taylor 1997). Danthron preparations should not be used for incontinent patients, especially those with limited mobility, as prolonged skin contact will colour the skin pink or red and superficial sloughing of the discoloured skin will occur (ABPI 1999, Taylor 1997).

Methylnaltrexone

Methylnaltrexone bromide is a parenteral preparation that is a peripherally acting selective antagonist of opioid binding to the mu-receptor, thus reversing peripherally mediated opioid-induced constipation but not centrally mediated analgesic effects (Thomas *et al.* 2008). The indications for use are opioid-induced constipation in patients with advanced illness receiving palliative care and who are unable to take oral laxatives. It is necessary to exclude bowel obstruction prior to its use and it should be used under the advice of a palliative care team.

Non-pharmacological support

Diet

Dietary manipulation may help to resolve mild constipation, although it is much more likely to help prevent constipation from recurring. Increasing dietary fibre increases stool bulk,

which in turn improves peristalsis and stool transit time. This results in a softer stool being delivered to the rectum (Norton 1996b). The government's strategy on food and health aims to increase the UK average daily fibre intake from the current 13.8 to 18.0 g (this recommended amount is based on the Englyst method; British Nutrition Foundation 2004, DH 1998).

There are two types of fibre: insoluble fibre is contained in foods such as wholegrain bread, brown rice, fruit and vegetables and soluble fibre is contained in foods such as oats, pulses, beans and lentils. It is recommended that fibre should be taken from a variety of both soluble and insoluble foods and eaten at times spread throughout the day (British Nutrition Foundation 2004, Edwards *et al.* 2003, Food Standards Agency 2006, Teahon 1999). Care should be taken to increase dietary fibre intake gradually as bloating and abdominal discomfort can result from a sudden increase, particularly in the older person and those with slow-transit constipation (Bush 2000, Cummings 1994, Edwards *et al.* 2003, Norton 1996a). Other sources of dietary laxatives can be encouraged with care; for example, prunes contain diphenylisatin and onions contain indigestible sugars (Norton 1996a).

Dietary changes need to be made in combination with other lifestyle changes. Daily fluid intake should be between 2.0 and 2.5 litres (Day 2001, Taylor 1997, Teahon 1999). Fruit juices such as orange and prune juice can help stimulate bowel activity (Winney 1998) and coffee has been shown to stimulate colonic motor and bowel activity (Addison 1999a, Brown *et al.* 1990). The motor response takes place within minutes of drinking coffee and can last for up to 90 minutes (Addison 2000a).

There is a need for further studies to examine the role of dietary manipulation in the management of constipation, particularly the function of dietary fibre and fluid intake (Addison 2000b).

Positioning

Patients should be advised not to ignore the urge to defaecate and to allow sufficient time for defaecation (Norton 1996a). It is important that the correct posture for defaecation is adopted; crouching or a 'crouch-like' posture is considered anatomically correct (Taylor 1997) and the use of a footstool by the toilet may enable patients to adopt a better defaecation posture (Edwards *et al.* 2003, NICE 2007, Norton 1996a, Taylor 1997) (see Figure 6.18). The use of the bedpan should always be avoided if possible as the poor posture adopted while using a bedpan has been shown to cause extreme straining during defaecation (Taylor 1997). Where possible, patients should be supported to get to a bathroom.

Exercise

Where possible, patients should be encouraged to increase their level of exercise; physical activity has been found to have a positive effect on peristalsis, particularly after eating (Thompson *et al.* 2003). Therapies such as homoeopathy

Table 6.4 Classification of laxatives

Type of laxative	How it works	Name of drug	Special notes for patients
Bulk forming	These drugs act by holding onto water so the stool remains large and soft and encourages the gut to move	Fybogel	If your nurse or doctor is unsure if your bowel has a normal activity or is concerned about the amount of fluid you are taking, this drug may not be considered for you
Stimulant	Will cause water and electrolytes to accumulate in the bowel and will stimulate the bowel to move	Senna tablet/liquid Bisacodyl tablet/suppositories	This group of drugs will be avoided if your bowel is not moving very well as they can cause abdominal cramps
Mixed stimulant and softener	2-in-1 preparations	Co-Danthramer liquid and capsules available	This drug may cause your urine to change colour
		Docusate tablets	Mild stimulant
Softeners	Attract and retain water in the bowel	Milpar (liquid paraffin and magnesium hydroxide) Docuaste Arachis oil enema	If you have an allergy to nuts please tell your nurse or doctor as an arachis oil enema should be avoided
Osmotic	Act in the bowel by increasing stimulation of fluid secretion and movement in the bowel	Lactulose Movicol Phosphate enema Microlax enema	Can cause bloating and excess wind and abdominal discomfort Powdered sachet that needs to be dissolved in about 150 mL fluid

and reflexology can also be utilized (Edwards *et al.* 2003, Emly *et al.* 1997, Rankin-Box 2000).

However, overall, laxatives are the most commonly used treatment for constipation (Table 6.4). In general, they should be used as a short-term measure to help relieve an episode of constipation as long-term use can perpetuate constipation and a dependence on laxatives can develop (Butler 1998). However, in cancer and palliative care patients where drugs such as opioids may need to be maintained then laxative therapy may need to continue for longer periods of time.

Enemas

Definition

An enema is the administration of a substance in liquid form into the rectum, either to aid bowel evacuation or to administer medication (Higgins 2006).

Evidence-based approaches
Rationale
Indications

Enemas may be prescribed for the following reasons.

- To clean the lower bowel before surgery, X-ray examination of the bowel using contrast medium or before endoscopy examination.

- To treat severe constipation when other methods have failed.
- To introduce medication into the system.
- To soothe and treat irritated bowel mucosa.
- To decrease body temperature (due to contact with the proximal vascular system).
- To stop local haemorrhage.
- To reduce hyperkalaemia (calcium resonium).
- To reduce portal systemic encephalopathy (phosphate enema).

Contraindications

Enemas are contraindicated under the following circumstances.

- In paralytic ileus.
- In colonic obstruction.
- Where the administration of tap water or soap and water enemas may cause circulatory overload, water intoxication, mucosal damage and necrosis, hyperkalaemia and cardiac arrhythmias.
- Where the administration of large amounts of fluid high into the colon may cause perforation and haemorrhage.
- Following gastrointestinal or gynaecological surgery, where suture lines may be ruptured (unless medical consent has been given).
- Frailty.
- Proctitis.
- The use of microenemas and hypertonic saline enemas in patients with inflammatory or ulcerative conditions of the large colon.

- Recent radiotherapy to the lower pelvis unless medical consent has been given (Davies 2004).

Evacuant enemas

An evacuant enema is a solution introduced into the rectum or lower colon with the intention of it being expelled, along with faecal matter and flatus, within a few minutes. The osmotic activity increases the water content of the stool so that rectal distension follows and induces defaecation by stimulating rectal motility (Barrett 1992, Roe 1994).

The following solutions are often used.

- Phosphate enemas with standard or long rectal tubes in single-dose disposable packs. Although these are often used for bowel clearance before X-ray examination and surgery, there is little evidence to support their use due to the associated risks and contraindications. Davies (2004) and Bowers (2006) highlight the risk of phosphate absorption resulting from pooling of the enema due to lack of evacuation and also the risk of rectal injury caused by the enema tip. Studies have found that if evacuation does not occur, patients may suffer from hypovolaemic shock, renal failure and oliguria. When using this type of enema, it is vital that good fluid intake is encouraged and maintained.
- Dioctyl sodium sulphosuccinate 0.1% and sorbitol 25% in single-dose disposable packs are used to soften impacted faeces.

- Sodium citrate 450 mg, sodium alkylsulphoacetate 45 mg and ascorbic acid 5 mg in single-dose disposable packs.

Retention enemas

A retention enema is a solution introduced into the rectum or lower colon with the intention of being retained for a specified period of time. Two types of retention enema are in common use.

- Arachis oil (may be obtained in a single-dose disposable pack). This needs to be used cautiously as it is contraindicated in patients with peanut allergies (Day 2001).
- Prednisolone.

Enemas containing arachis oil enhance the lubricating process, as well as softening impacted faeces (Butler 1998). These work by penetrating faeces, increasing the bulk and softness of stools. They work most effectively when warmed to body temperature and retained for as long as possible (Clarke 1988).

All types of enemas need to be prescribed and checked against the prescription before administration. It is essential that the implications and procedure are fully explained to the patient, so as to relieve anxiety and embarrassment.

Legal and professional issues

Administration requires skill and knowledge from the practitioner and adherence to the Nursing and Midwifery Council's (NMC 2008c) *Standards for Medicines Management*.

245

Procedure guideline 6.14 Enema administration

Essential equipment

- Disposable incontinence pad
- Disposable gloves
- Topical swabs
- Lubricating jelly

- Rectal tube and funnel (if not using a commercially prepared pack)
- Solution required or commercially prepared enema

Preprocedure

Action	Rationale
1 Explain and discuss the procedure with the patient.	To ensure that the patient understands the procedure and gives their valid consent (NMC 2008a, C).
2 Wash hands.	For infection prevention and control (Fraise and Bradley 2009, E).
3 Ensure privacy.	To avoid unnecessary embarrassment and to promote dignified care (NMC 2008b, C).
4 Allow patient to empty bladder first if necessary.	A full bladder may cause discomfort during the procedure (Higgins 2006, E).
5 Ensure that a bedpan, commode or toilet is readily available.	In case the patient feels the need to expel the enema before the procedure is completed. P

(Continued)

Procedure guideline 6.14 (*Continued*)

Procedure

6 Warm the enema to room temperature by immersing in a jug of hot water.	Heat is an effective stimulant of the nerve plexi in the intestinal mucosa. An enema at room temperature or just above will not damage the intestinal mucosa. The temperature of the environment, the rate of fluid administration and the length of the tubing will all have an effect on the temperature of the fluid in the rectum (Higgins 2006, E).
7 Assist the patient to lie on the left side, with knees well flexed, the upper higher than the lower one, and with the buttocks near the edge of the bed.	This allows ease of passage into the rectum by following the natural anatomy of the colon. In this position gravity will aid the flow of the solution into the colon. Flexing the knees ensures a more comfortable passage of the enema nozzle or rectal tube (Higgins 2006, E).
8 Place a disposable incontinence pad beneath the patient's hips and buttocks.	To reduce potential infection caused by soiled linen. To avoid embarrassing the patient if the fluid is ejected prematurely following administration. P
9 Wash hands and put on disposable gloves.	For infection prevention and control (Fraise and Bradley 2009, E).
10 Place some lubricating jelly on a topical swab and lubricate the nozzle of the enema or the rectal tube.	This prevents trauma to the anal and rectal mucosa which reduces surface friction (Higgins 2006, E).
11 Expel excessive air from enema and introduce the nozzle or tube slowly into the anal canal while separating the buttocks. (A small amount of air may be introduced if bowel evacuation is desired.)	The introduction of air into the colon causes distension of its walls, resulting in unnecessary discomfort to the patient. The slow introduction of the lubricated tube will minimize spasm of the intestinal wall (evacuation will be more effectively induced due to the increased peristalsis). C
12 Slowly introduce the tube or nozzle to a depth of 10.0–12.5 cm.	This will bypass the anal canal (2.5–4.0 cm in length) and ensure that the tube or nozzle is in the rectum. C
13 If a retention enema is used, introduce the fluid slowly and leave the patient in bed with the foot of the bed elevated by 45° for as long as prescribed.	To avoid increasing peristalsis. The slower the rate at which the fluid is introduced, the less pressure is exerted on the intestinal wall. Elevating the foot of the bed aids in retention of the enema by the force of gravity. C
14 If an evacuant enema is used, introduce the fluid slowly by rolling the pack from the bottom to the top to prevent backflow, until the pack is empty or the solution is completely finished.	The faster the rate of flow of the fluid, the greater the pressure on the rectal walls. Distension and irritation of the bowel wall will produce strong peristalsis which is sufficient to empty the lower bowel (Higgins 2006, E).
15 If using a funnel and rectal tube, adjust the height of the funnel according to the rate of flow desired.	The forces of gravity will cause the solution to flow from the funnel into the rectum. The greater the elevation of the funnel, the faster the flow of fluid. E
16 Clamp the tubing before all the fluid has run in.	To avoid air entering the rectum and causing further discomfort. E
17 Slowly withdraw the tube or nozzle.	To avoid reflex emptying of the rectum. E
18 Dry the patient's perineal area with a gauze swab.	To promote patient comfort and avoid excoriation. P
19 Ask the patient to retain the enema for 10–15 minutes before evacuating the bowel.	To enhance the evacuant effect. C

20	Ensure that the patient has access to the nurse call system, is near to the bedpan, commode or toilet, and has adequate toilet paper.	To enhance patient comfort and safety. To minimize the patient's embarrassment. P

Postprocedure

21	Remove and dispose of equipment.	
22	Wash hands.	For infection prevention and control (Fraise and Bradley 2009, E).
23	Record in the appropriate documents that the enema has been given, its effects on the patient and its results (colour, consistency, content and amount of faeces produced), using the Bristol Stool Form Chart (see Figure 6.2).	To monitor the patient's bowel function (Gill 1999, C).
24	Observe patient for any adverse reactions.	To monitor the patient for complications (Peate 2003, C).

247

Problem-solving table 6.5 Prevention and resolution (Procedure guideline 6.14)

Problem	Cause	Prevention	Action
Unable to insert the nozzle of enema pack or rectal tube into the anal canal	Tube not adequately lubricated. Patient in an incorrect position	Ensure patient is relaxed and in the correct position	Apply more lubricating jelly. Ask the patient to draw knees up further towards the chest. To ensure the patient is relaxed before inserting the nozzle or rectal tube
	Patient apprehensive and embarrassed about the situation. Patient unable to relax anal sphincter		Ensure adequate privacy and give frequent explanations to the patient about the procedure. Ask the patient to take deep breaths and 'bear down' as if defaecating.
Unable to advance the tube or nozzle into the anal canal	Spasm of the canal walls	Ask the patient to take slow deep breaths to help them relax	Wait until spasm has passed before inserting the tube or nozzle more slowly, thus minimizing spasm. Ask patient to take slow deep breaths to help them to relax.
Unable to advance the tube or nozzle into the rectum	Blockage by faeces		Withdraw tubing slightly and allow a little solution to flow and then insert the tube further
	Blockage by tumour		If resistance is still met, stop the procedure and inform a doctor.
Patient complains of cramping or the desire to evacuate the enema before the end of the procedure	Distension and irritation of the intestinal wall produce strong peristalsis sufficient to empty the lower bowel	Encourage the patient to retain the enema	Stop instilling the enema fluid and wait with the patient until the discomfort has subsided.
Patient unable to open bowels after an evacuant enema	Reduced neuromuscular response in the bowel wall		Inform the doctor that the enema was unsuccessful and reassure the patient.

Suppositories

Definition

A suppository is a medicated solid formulation that melts at body temperature when inserted into the rectum (Moppett and Parker 1999).

Evidence-based approaches

Rationale

Indications

The use of suppositories is indicated under the following circumstances.

- To empty the bowel prior to certain types of surgery and investigations.
- To empty the bowel to relieve acute constipation or when other treatments for constipation have failed.
- To empty the bowel before endoscopic examination.
- To introduce medication into the system.
- To soothe and treat haemorrhoids or anal pruritus.

Contraindications

The use of suppositories is contraindicated when one or more of the following pertain.

- Chronic constipation, which would require repetitive use.
- Paralytic ileus.
- Colonic obstruction.
- Malignancy of the perianal region.
- Low platelet count.
- Following gastrointestinal or gynaecological operations, unless on the specific instructions of the doctor.

Methods of administration of suppositories

The use of suppositories dates back to about 460 BC. Hippocrates recommended the use of cylindrical sup-positories of honey smeared with ox gall (Hurst 1970). The torpedo-shaped suppositories commonly used today came into being in 1893, when it was recommended that they were inserted apex (pointed end) first (Moppett 2000).

This practice has been questioned by Abd-el-Maeboud *et al.* (1991) who suggest that suppositories should be inserted blunt end first. This advice is based on anorectal physiology; if a suppository is inserted apex first, the circular base distends the anus and the lower edge of the anal sphincter fails to close tightly. The normal squeezing motion (reverse vermicular contraction) of the anal sphincter therefore fails to drive the suppository into the rectum. These factors can lead to anal irritation and expulsion of the suppository (Moppett 2000). The study by Abd-el-Maeboud *et al.* (1991) remains the only research evidence supporting this practice. Whilst their work demonstrated that patients found insertion and retention of suppositories much easier and more comfortable using the base-first method, the isolated nature of this research means that manufacturers' instructions continue to recommend apex end first. Therefore this area of practice remains somewhat unclear: the Abd-el-Maeboud *et al.* (1991) study, coupled with the anatomical and physiological rationale, would imply that blunt end first is preferable.

Types of suppository

There are several different types of suppository available. Retention suppositories are designed to deliver drug therapy, for example analgesia, antibiotic, non-steroidal anti-inflammatory drug (NSAID). Those designed to stimulate bowel evacuation include glycerine, bisacodyl and sodium bicarbonate. Lubricant suppositories, for example glycerine, should be inserted directly into the faeces and allowed to dissolve. They have a mild irritant action on the rectum and also act as faecal softeners (BNF 2011). However, stimulant types, such as bisacodyl, must come into contact with the mucous membrane of the rectum if they are to be effective as they release carbon dioxide, causing rectal distension and thus evacuation.

Procedure guideline 6.15 **Suppository administration**

Essential equipment

- Disposable incontinence pad
- Disposable gloves
- Topical swabs or tissues

- Lubricating jelly
- Suppository(ies) as required (check prescription before administering a medicinal suppository, e.g. aminophylline)

Preprocedure

Action	Rationale
1 Explain and discuss the procedure with the patient. If you are administering a medicated suppository, it is best to do so after the patient has emptied their bowels.	To ensure that the patient understands the procedure and gives their valid consent (NMC 2008a, C). To ensure that the active ingredients are not prevented from being absorbed by the rectal mucosa and that the suppository is not expelled before its active ingredients have been released (Moppett 2000, E).
2 Wash hands.	To ensure the procedure is as clean as possible and for infection control reasons (Fraise and Bradley 2009, E).
3 Ensure privacy.	To ensure privacy and dignity for the patient (NMC 2008b, C).
4 Ensure that a bedpan, commode or toilet is readily available.	In case of premature ejection of the suppositories or rapid bowel evacuation following their administration. P

Procedure

5 Assist the patient to lie on the left side, with the knees flexed, the upper higher than the lower one, with the buttocks near the edge of the bed.	This allows ease of passage of the suppository into the rectum by following the natural anatomy of the colon. Flexing the knees will reduce discomfort as the suppository is passed through the anal sphincter (Moppett 2000, E).
6 Place a disposable incontinence pad beneath the patient's hips and buttocks.	To avoid unnecessary soiling of linen, leading to potential infection and embarrassment to the patient if the suppositories are ejected prematurely or there is rapid bowel evacuation following their administration. E
7 Wash hands.	For infection prevention and control (Fraise and Bradley 2009, E).
8 Place some lubricating jelly on the topical swab and lubricate the blunt end of the suppository if it is being used to obtain systemic action. Separate the patient's buttocks and insert the suppository blunt end first, advancing it for about 2–4 cm. Repeat this procedure if a second suppository is to be inserted.	Lubricating reduces surface friction and thus eases insertion of the suppository and avoids anal mucosal trauma. Research has shown that the suppository is more readily retained if inserted blunt end first (Abd-el-Maeboud *et al.* 1991, R2b). (For further information, see Suppositories.) The anal canal is approximately 2–4 cm long. Inserting the suppository beyond this ensures that it will be retained (Abd-el-Maeboud *et al.* 1991, R2b).
9 Once the suppository(ies) has been inserted, clean any excess lubricating jelly from the patient's perineal area.	To ensure the patient's comfort and avoid anal excoriation (Moppett 2000, E).
10 Ask the patient to retain the suppository(ies) for 20 minutes, or until they are no longer able to do so. If a medicated suppository is given, remind the patient that its aim is not to stimulate evacuation and to retain the suppository for at least 20 minutes or as long as possible.	This will allow the suppository to melt and release the active ingredients. Inform patient that there may be some discharge as the medication melts in the rectum (Henry 1999, E).

Postprocedure

11 Remove and dispose of equipment. Wash hands.	For infection prevention and control (Fraise and Bradley 2009, E).
12 Record that the suppository(ies) have been given, the effect on the patient and the result (amount, colour, consistency and content, using the Bristol Stool Chart – see Figure 6.2) in the appropriate documents.	To monitor the patient's bowel function (Gill 1999, C).
13 Observe patient for any adverse reactions.	To monitor for any complications (Peate 2003, E).

Digital rectal examination

Definition

A digital rectal examination (DRE) is an invasive procedure that can be carried out, as part of a nursing assessment, by a qualified nurse who has received suitable education and training (RCN 2006). The procedure involves the nurse inserting a lubricated gloved finger into the rectum.

Evidence-based approaches
Rationale
Indications

This examination should only be performed in the following circumstances (RCN 2006).

- To establish whether faecal matter is present in the rectum and if so, to assess the amount and consistency.
- To assess the need for rectal medication and to evaluate its efficacy in certain circumstances, for example in patients who have diminished anal/rectal sensation.
- For digital stimulation to trigger defaecation by stimulating the rectoanal reflex (RCN 2006, Weisner and Bell 2004).
- To assess anal sphincter function and tone.
- To assess anal/rectal sensation.

Legal and professional issues

This examination should not be a primary investigation for constipation but should only be performed after a full assessment. Discussion with medical staff should occur to confirm diagnosis and jointly plan appropriate interventions to treat the constipation (RCN 2006). As nursing roles develop, clinical nurse specialists and nurse practitioners may be increasingly involved in areas of care that neces-

sitate undertaking DRE as part of a physical assessment or procedure. Such instances may include:

- the assessment of prostate size, consistency, mobility and anatomical limits
- during procedures such as the placement of a rectal probe/sensor prior to urodynamic studies or the placement of catheters used in the treatment of constipation or anismus (RCN 2006).

Preprocedural considerations
Specific patient preparations

Before carrying out a DRE, the perineal and perianal area should be checked for signs of rectal prolapse, haemorrhoids, anal skin tags or lesions, foreign bodies or infestations. The condition of the skin should be noted, as should the type and amount of any discharge or leakage. If any of these abnormalities are seen, a DRE should not be carried out until advice is taken from a specialist nurse or medical practitioner (RCN 2006).

Precautions

Special care should be used in performing DRE in patients when disease processes or treatments in particular affect the anus or the bowel mucosa. These conditions include (RCN 2006):

- active inflammation of the bowel, for example ulcerative colitis
- recent radiotherapy to the pelvic area
- rectal/anal pain
- rectal surgery or trauma to the anal/rectal area
- obvious rectal bleeding
- spinal injury patients, because of autonomic dysreflexia
- patients with known allergies, for example latex
- patients with a history of abuse.

Procedure guideline 6.16 Digital rectal examination

Essential equipment

- Disposable incontinence pad
- Disposable gloves (check if patient allergic to latex)
- Lubricating gel
- Tissues or topical swabs

Preprocedure

Action	Rationale
1 Explain and discuss procedure with the patient.	To ensure that the patient understands the procedure and gives their valid consent (NMC 2008a, C).
2 Ensure privacy.	To avoid unnecessary embarrassment to the patient and to promote dignity and privacy (NMC 2008b, C).
3 Ensure that a bedpan, commode or toilet is readily available.	DRE can stimulate the need for bowel movement (Weisner and Bell 2004, E).

Procedure

4 Assist the patient to lie in the left lateral position with knees flexed, the upper knee higher than the lower knee, with the buttocks towards the edge of the bed.	This allows ease of digital examination into the rectum by following the natural anatomy of the colon. Flexing the knees reduces discomfort as the examining finger passes the anal sphincter (Kyle *et al.* 2005b, C).
5 Place a disposable incontinence pad beneath the patient's hips and buttocks.	To reduce potential infection caused by soiled linen. To avoid embarrassing the patient if faecal staining occurs during or after the procedure. E
6 Wash hands with bactericidal soap and water or bactericidal alcohol handrub and put on disposable gloves.	For infection prevention and control (Fraise and Bradley 2009, E).
7 Place some lubricating gel on a swab and gloved index finger. Inform patient you are about to proceed.	To minimize discomfort as lubrication reduces friction and to ease insertion of the finger into the anus/rectum. Lubrication also helps minimize anal mucosal trauma (Kyle *et al.* 2005b, C). Assists with patient co-operation with the procedure (NMC 2008b, C).
8 Observe anal area prior to the insertion of the finger into the anus for evidence of skin soreness, excoriation, swelling, haemorrhoids, rectal prolapse and infestation. Proceed to insert finger into the anus/rectum.	May indicate incontinence or pruritus. Swelling may be indicative of possible mass or abscess. Abnormalities such as bleeding, discharge or prolapse should be reported to medical staff before any examination is undertaken (RCN 2006, C).
9 On insertion of finger, assess anal sphincter control; resistance should be felt.	Digital insertion with resistance indicates good internal sphincter tone, poor resistance may indicate the opposite (Addison 1999b, E).
10 Digital examination may feel faecal matter within the rectum; note consistency of any faecal matter.	May establish loaded rectum and indicate constipation and the need for rectal medication (RCN 2006, C).
11 Clean anal area after the procedure.	To prevent irritation and soreness occurring. Preserves patient dignity and personal hygiene.

Postprocedure

12 Remove gloves and dispose of equipment in appropriate clinical waste bin. Wash hands with bactericidal soap and water.	For infection prevention and control (Fraise and Bradley 2009, E).
13 Assist patient into a comfortable position and offer toilet facilities as appropriate.	To promote comfort. P
14 Document findings and report to medical team.	To ensure continuity of care and ensure appropriate corrective action may be initiated (RCN 2006, C).

Manual evacuation

Definition

Manual evacuation of the rectum is an invasive procedure involving digital removal of faeces, which should only be performed when necessary, generally as a last resort, and after individual assessment (RCN 2006, Rigby 2003).

Related theory

Managing bowel problems such as constipation and prolonged bowel evacuation in patients following spinal cord injury requires a multimodality approach. This includes dietary fibre, digital stimulation, enemas, suppositories, stool softeners and abdominal massage (Addison and White 2002, Amir *et al.* 1998). Digital stimulation is a method of initiating the defaecation reflex by dilating the anus, with either a finger or an anal dilator (Weisner and Bell 2004), but is only useful if the rectum is full.

Autonomic dysreflexia is unique to patients with spinal cord injury. It is an abnormal response from the autonomic nervous system to a painful (noxious) stimulus perceived below the level of spinal cord injury (Harrison 2000, Powell and Rigby 2000). Distended bowel caused by constipation or impaction can lead to autonomic dysreflexia and therefore it is important that an effective programme of bowel management is established and followed (Harrison 2000).

Evidence-based approaches

Rationale

Advances in oral, rectal and surgical treatments have reduced the need for manual evacuations to be performed; however, for certain groups of patients, such as those with spinal injuries, spina bifida or multiple sclerosis, this procedure may be the only suitable bowel-emptying technique forming a long-standing, integral part of their bowel routine (Kyle *et al.* 2005b).

Manual evacuation of faeces can be distressing, it may be painful and it can be a dangerous procedure. In particular, stimulation of the vagus nerve in the rectal wall can slow the patient's heart, in addition to the risk of bowel perforation and bleeding (Kyle *et al.* 2005b, Powell and Rigby 2000).

Indications

Indications for assisted evacuation of bowels (manual evacuation or digital stimulation) include (RCN 2006):

- faecal impaction/loading
- incomplete defaecation
- inability to defaecate
- if other bowel-emptying techniques have failed
- neurogenic bowel dysfunction
- patients with spinal injury.

Patients are at risk of rectal trauma if these procedures are not performed with care or knowledge. The nurse should be aware of any conditions that may contraindicate performance of these procedures (see Precautions, Digital rectal examination).

Legal and professional issues

Nurses who have received appropriate training may perform manual evacuation and, in addition, they should ensure that their employer has defined policies and procedure for undertaking this role (RCN 2006, Withell 2000). If appropriate, the patient and their personal carer may wish for the carer to maintain their established programme of bowel management (Harrison 2000).

Preprocedural considerations

Specific patient preparations

If this procedure is used as an acute intervention, the patient's pulse rate should be recorded before and during the process. Patients with a spinal injury should also have their blood pressure measured before, during and at the end of the procedure. A baseline blood pressure measurement should be available for comparison (RCN 2006). Every time the procedure is performed, the consistency of the stool should be noted before continuing. If the stool is hard and dry, lubricant suppositories should be inserted and left for 30 minutes before commencing. If the stool is too soft to remove effectively, consider delaying the procedure for 24 hours to allow further water reabsorption to occur. During the procedure the nurse should observe the patient for signs of:

- distress, pain or discomfort
- bleeding
- autonomic dysreflexia: hypertension, bradycardia, headache, flushing above the level of the spinal injury, sweating, pallor below the level of spinal injury, nasal congestion (Harrison 2000)
- collapse (RCN 2006).

Procedure guideline 6.17 Manual evacuation of faeces

Essential equipment

- Disposable incontinence pad
- Disposable gloves (check if patient is allergic to latex)
- Lubricating gel
- Receiver and/or yellow bag
- Specimen pot (if required)
- Bedpan or commode (if appropriate)
- Tissues or topical swabs

Preprocedure

Action	Rationale
1 Explain and discuss procedure with the patient.	To ensure that the patient understands the procedure and gives their valid consent (NMC 2008a, C).
2 Ensure privacy.	To avoid unnecessary embarrassment to the patient.

Procedure

3	Take the patient's pulse. In spinal injury patients a blood pressure reading should also be taken (RCN 2006, C).	Provides a baseline measurement. Stimulation of the vagus nerve in the rectal wall can lead to a reduction in pulse rate (Powell and Rigby 2000, E). In spinal cord injury, stimulus below the level of injury may result in symptoms of autonomic dysreflexia including hypertension (Kyle *et al.* 2005b, C).
4	Assist the patient to lie in the left lateral position with knees flexed, the upper knee higher than the lower knee, with the buttocks towards the edge of the bed.	This allows ease of digital insertion into the rectum, by following the natural anatomy of the colon. Flexing the knees reduces discomfort as the finger passes the anal sphincter (Kyle *et al.* 2005b, C).
5	Place a disposable incontinence pad beneath the patient's hips and buttocks.	To reduce potential infection caused by soiled linen. To avoid embarrassing the patient if faecal staining occurs during or after the procedure.
6	Wash hands with bactericidal soap and water or bactericidal alcohol handrub and put on disposable gloves.	For infection prevention and control (Fraise and Bradley 2009, E).
7	Place some lubricating gel on a swab and gloved index finger.	To minimize discomfort as lubrication reduces friction and to ease insertion of the finger into the anus/rectum. Lubrication also helps minimize anal mucosal trauma (Kyle *et al.* 2005b, C).
8	Inform the patient you are about to proceed.	Assists with patient co-operation with the procedure (NMC 2008b, C).
9	Observe anal area prior to the insertion of the finger into the anus for evidence of skin soreness, excoriation, swelling, haemorrhoids or rectal prolapse.	May indicate incontinence or pruritus. Swelling may be indicative of possible mass or abscess. Abnormalities such as bleeding, discharge or prolapse should be reported to medical staff before any examination is undertaken (RCN 2006, C).
10	Proceed to insert finger into the anus/rectum. Proceed with caution in those patients with spinal cord injury.	The majority of spinal cord injury patients will not experience any pain (Kyle *et al.* 2005b, C).
11	If the stool is type 1 (see Figure 6.2), remove one lump at a time until no more faecal matter is felt.	To relieve patient's discomfort (Kyle *et al.* 2005b, C).
12	If a solid faecal mass is felt, split it and remove small pieces with hooked finger until no more faecal matter is felt.	To relieve patient discomfort (Kyle *et al.* 2005b, C).
13	Check the patient's pulse at least once during the procedure. In spinal injury patients a blood pressure reading should also be taken at least once during the procedure or at any sign of distress (RCN 2006, C). If the patient is displaying a reduction in pulse rate or change in rhythm, or in the spinal cord injury patient, a raised blood pressure, STOP the procedure and if possible sit the patient up and administer appropriate medications as prescribed (Kyle et al. 2005b, C).	Stimulation of the vagus nerve in the rectal wall can lead to a reduction in pulse rate (Powell and Rigby 2000). In spinal cord injury, stimulus below the level of injury may result in symptoms of autonomic dysreflexia, including hypertension (Kyle *et al.* 2005b, C).
14	If faecal mass is too hard to break up, or more than 4 cm across, stop the procedure and discuss with the multidisciplinary team.	To avoid unnecessary pain and damage to the anal sphincter. The patient may require the procedure to be carried out under anaesthetic (Kyle *et al.* 2005b, C).
15	As faeces is removed, it should be placed in an appropriate receiver.	To assist in appropriate disposal and reduce contamination or cross-infection risk.

(Continued)

Procedure guideline 6.17 (Continued)

16 Encourage patients who receive this procedure on a regular basis to have a period of rest or, if appropriate, to assist using the Valsalva manoeuvre.	Patient and nurse education is required to use this technique safely and so further guidance should be sought before introducing this manoeuvre as it may lead to complications such as haemorrhoids (Kyle *et al.* 2005b, C).
17 Wash and dry the patient's anal region and buttocks.	To ensure patient feels comfortable and clean. P

Postprocedure

18 Remove gloves and dispose of equipment in appropriate clinical waste bin. Wash hands.	For prevention and control of infection (Fraise and Bradley 2009, E).
19 Assist patient into a comfortable position.	To promote comfort. P
20 Document findings and report to medical team.	To ensure continuity of care and assist in nursing diagnosis so appropriate actions may continue (RCN 2006, C).

254

Stoma care and intestinal (bowel) obstruction and ileus

Stoma care

Definition

Stoma is a word of Greek origin meaning mouth or opening (Taylor 2005).

Anatomy and physiology

The gastrointestinal tract stretches from the mouth to the anus (see Figure 6.16). It is responsible for absorption of carbohydrates, proteins, fats, water, electrolytes, vitamins and bile salts.

The small bowel is divided into three sections: the duodenum, the jejunum and the ileum. Its primary function is digestion and absorption of nutrients, vitamins, minerals, fluids and electrolytes.

The colon (large bowel) consists of the caecum, ascending colon, transverse colon, descending colon, sigmoid colon, rectum and anal canal. It is about 1.5–1.8 metres long and approximately 6 cm in diameter (Thibodeau and Patton 2007). The colon has four main functions (Nazarko 2007).

- *Reabsorption*: around 1 litre of water in 24 hours and bile salts that are secreted from the liver to enable digestion to happen.
- *Creation of vitamins and biotin*: the bacteria in the colon form vitamin K, essential for blood clotting, vitamin B_5, necessary for the manufacture of neurotransmitters and hormones, and biotin, a substance required in glucose metabolism.
- *Elimination*: of indigestible residue of food and excess metabolites.

- *Formation and storage of faeces*: as the end-products of digestion pass through the colon, they become thicker and more formed and are stored in the colon until they can be eliminated.

The rectum and anal canal include internal and external sphincters which are the mechanisms responsible for controlling bowel function. Therefore disturbance of this results in loss of bowel control and incontinence.

An understanding of the relevant anatomy and physiology is key to understanding the functions of different types of stoma formation.

Related theory

Approximately 13,500 people undergo stoma formation surgery every year in the UK (Baxter and Salter 2000). The most common underlying conditions resulting in the need for stoma surgery are colorectal cancer, bladder cancer, ulcerative colitis and Crohn's disease. Other causes of stoma surgery include:

- cancer of the bowel
- cancer of the pelvis, for example gynaecological cancer
- trauma
- neurological damage
- congenital disorders
- ulcerative colitis
- Crohn's disease
- diverticular disease
- familial polyposis coli
- intractable incontinence
- fistula
- radiation enteritis.

Therefore stoma surgery affects many people regardless of gender, age and culture.

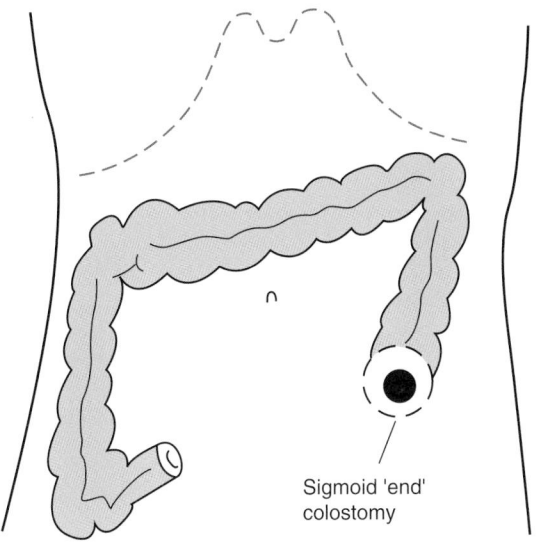

Figure 6.19 Sigmoid 'end' colostomy.

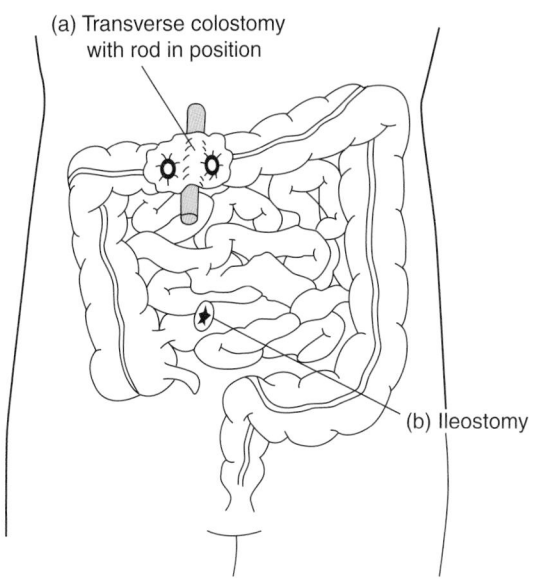

Figure 6.21 (a) Transverse colostomy. (b) Ileostomy.

Types of stoma

Colostomy

A colostomy may be formed from any section of the large bowel. Its position along the colon will dictate the output and consistency of faeces. Therefore an understanding of the anatomy and physiology is essential to fully care for stoma patients.

The most common site for a colostomy is on the sigmoid colon. This will produce a semi-solid or formed stool and is generally positioned in the left iliac fossa and is flush to the skin (Black 2000). Stomas formed higher up along the colon will produce a slightly more liquid stool. A colostomy tends to act on average 2–3 times per day, but this can vary between individuals.

Colostomies can either be permanent (end) (Figures 6.19 and 6.20) or temporary (loop) (Figures 6.21 and 6.22).

Permanent (end) colostomies are often formed following removal of rectal cancers, as in abdominoperineal resections of the rectum, whereas a temporary (loop) colostomy may be formed to divert the faecal output, to allow healing of a surgical join (anastomosis) or repair, or to relieve an obstruction or bowel injury (Taylor 2005). This type of stoma is often referred to as a defunctioning stoma, which indicates that the bowel distal to the stoma is being rested (Black 2000, Taylor 2000).

As is evident from Figures 6.20 and 6.22, end and loop colostomies are very different in appearance. An end colostomy tends to be flush to the skin and sutured to the abdominal wall and consists of an end-section of bowel,

Figure 6.20 End colostomy. With permission from Dansac Ltd.

Figure 6.22 Loop colostomy with bridge *in situ*.

Figure 6.23 End ileostomy. With permission from Dansac Ltd.

whereas a loop colostomy is larger in size. During the perioperative period it is supported by a stoma bridge or rod (Figure 6.22). This is placed under the section of bowel and is generally left in place for 3–10 days following surgery and then removed (Wright and Burch 2008).

Ileostomy

Ileostomies are formed when a section of ileum is brought out onto the abdominal wall. This is generally positioned at the end of the ileum on the right iliac fossa, but can be anywhere along the ileum. Consequently, the output tends to be looser, more liquid stool, as waste is being eliminated before the water is absorbed from the large bowel (colon). Due to the more acidic, abrasive nature of the stool at this stage, a spout is formed with this type of stoma. The ileum is everted to form a spout which allows the effluent to drain into an appliance, without coming into contact with the peristomal skin (Black 2000) (Figure 6.23). This prevents skin breakdown and allows for better management. The average output from an ileostomy is 200–600 mL per day.

Ileostomies can also be either permanent (end) (Figure 6.23) or temporary (loop). Permanent ileostomies are often formed following total colectomies (removal of the entire colon) for diverticular disease. Loop ileostomies are more common and are often formed to allow healing of a surgical join (anastomosis) lower down, to allow healing of an ileo-anal pouch or to aid healing of diseased bowel (Taylor 2005). These are sometimes held in place by a stoma bridge or rod. Refer to Procedure guideline 6.19 for more information on bridge/rod care and removal.

Evidence-based approaches

Stoma care has developed greatly over the years and is mainly based on experiential learning. Although an evidence base for this does exist, it mainly centres around clinical practice and experience.

Stoma care is very individual and requires full holistic patient assessment. The primary aim is to promote patient independence by providing care and advice on managing the stoma, therefore allowing the patient to continue with all the necessary activities of daily living.

Rationale
Indications

Stoma care is essential:

- to collect faeces or urine in an appropriate appliance
- to achieve and maintain patient comfort and security
- to maintain psychological adaptation and independence of the patient.

Legal and professional issues

As already discussed, stoma care is primarily based on experience and therefore the development of skills. It is a basic nursing task that all qualified nurses should be able to carry out. It has recently been recognized that many of the basic nursing skills are being carried out by healthcare assistants and carers. Therefore there is an increasing demand for education in this area. Stoma care often develops due to nurses who have an interest in this area and then further build on their skills. Due to the increasing demand for good effective stoma care, many courses and conferences now exist to improve patient care and enhance interest.

Preprocedural considerations
Equipment

Many of the appliances now available are very similar in style, colour and efficiency and often there is very little to choose between them when the time comes for the ostomate to decide what to wear.

The aim of good stoma care is to return patients to their place in society (Black, 1994). One of the ways in which this can be facilitated is to provide them with a safe, reliable appliance. This means that there should be no fear of leakage or odour and the appliance should be comfortable, unobtrusive, easy to handle and disposable. The ostomate should be allowed a choice from the management systems available. It is also important to identify and manage early on problems with the stoma or peristomal skin. When choosing the appropriate management system for the new ostomate, factors which need to be considered include:

- type of stoma
- type of effluent
- patient's cognitive ability
- manual dexterity
- lifestyle
- condition of peristomal skin
- siting of stoma
- patient preference (Black 2000, Kirkwood 2006).

What is the stoma type?

COLOSTOMY   ILEOSTOMY   NOT KNOWN   UROSTOMY

Is the output
FAECES or URINE?

FAECES   URINE

Is the output
FORMED?

Is the output
LOOSE?

CLOSED APPLIANCE

Transparent (clear) or non-transparent (opaque).

One- or two-piece systems.

Different sizes available.

Single use.

Change when half full.

Flushable pouches available.

UROSTOMY APPLIANCE

Must have a tap.

Can connect to a night drainage bag.

Transparent (clear) or non-transparent (opaque).

One- or two-piece systems.

Empty when about half full.

Change every 1 to 3 days.

DRAINABLE APPLIANCE

Transparent (clear) or non-transparent (opaque).

One- or two-piece systems.

Different sizes available.

Empty when about half full.

Change every 1 to 3 days.

Figure 6.24 Flow chart for choosing appliances. International Ostomy Forum group (2006) Observation Index. Dansac Ltd.

Pouches

Although some people whose stomas were created several years ago are wearing non-disposable rubber bags, most appliances used today are made from an odour-proof plastic film. These pouches usually adhere to the body by a hydrocolloid wafer or flange (Taylor 2000). Pouches may be opaque or clear and often have a soft backing to absorb perspiration. They usually have a built-in integral filter containing charcoal to neutralize any odour. The type of pouch used will depend on the type of stoma and effluent expected. Refer to Figure 6.24 to assist pouch selection.

Choosing the right size

It is important that the flange of the appliance fits snugly around the stoma within 0.3 cm of the stoma edge (Kirkwood 2006). This narrow edge is left exposed so that the appliance does not rub on the stoma. Stoma appliances usually come with measuring guides to allow for choice of size. During the initial weeks following surgery, the oedematous

Figure 6.25 Stoma equipment. (a) Drainable bowel stoma pouch. (b) Urostomy pouch. (c) Closed bag.

stoma will gradually reduce in size and the appliances will be changed accordingly.

Fear of malodour when using pouches

Pouches usually have a built-in integral filter containing charcoal to neutralize any odour when flatus is released; therefore, smell is only noticeable when emptying or changing an appliance (Rudoni and Sica 1999). There are also various deodorizers available. These come in the form of drops or powders that may be put into the pouch or sprays, which can be sprayed into the air just before changing or emptying the pouch (Burch and Sica 2005). The individual should be reassured that any problems with odour or leakage will be investigated and that in most circumstances the problem will be solved with alternative appliances or accessories (Black 1997, Bryant 1993).

Drainable pouches are used when the effluent is fluid or semi-formed, that is, ileostomy or transverse colostomy (Figure 6.25a). These pouches have specially designed filters, which are less likely to become blocked or leak faecal fluid. They need to be emptied regularly and the outlet rinsed carefully and then closed with a clip or 'roll-up' method. They may be left on for up to 3 days.

Urostomy pouches have a drainage tap for urine and should be emptied regularly (Figure 6.25b). They can be attached to a large bag and tubing for night drainage. These pouches can remain on for up to 3 days.

Closed pouches are mainly used when formed stool is expected, for example sigmoid colostomy (Figure 6.25c). They have a flatus filter and need to be changed once or twice a day.

One- or two-piece systems

All types of pouch (closed, drainable or with a tap) fall into one of two broad categories: one-piece or two-piece systems.

- *One-piece*: this comprises a pouch attached to an adhesive wafer that is removed completely when the pouch is changed. This is an easier system for an ostomate with dexterity problems, for example arthritis, peripheral neuropathy, to handle.
- *Two-piece*: this comprises a wafer onto which a pouch is clipped or stuck. It can be used with sore and sensitive skin because when the pouch is removed, the flange is left intact and so the skin is left undisturbed.

Plug system

Patients with colostomies may be able to stop the effluent by inserting a plug into the stoma lumen. This plug swells in the moist environment and behaves as a seal. This system should only be introduced by a stoma nurse specialist (Taylor 2000).

Solutions for skin and stoma cleaning

Mild soap and water, or water only, is sufficient for skin and stoma cleaning. It is important that all soap residues are removed as they may interfere with pouch adhesion. Detergents, disinfectants and antiseptics cause dryness and irritation and should not be used. The stoma is not a wound or a lesion and should be regarded as a resited urethra or anus.

See Table 6.5 for a summary of products used in managing problems associate with stoma.

Deodorants

Aerosols

Use: To absorb or mask odour. *Method*: One or two puffs into the air before emptying or removing appliance. *Examples*: Limone, Naturcare, FreshAire.

Drops and powders

Use: For deodorizing bag contents. *Method*: Before fitting pouch or after emptying and cleaning drainable pouch, squeeze tube two or three times. *Examples*: Ostobon deodorant powder, Nodor S drops, Saltair No-roma.

Preoperative assessment and care

Preoperative care can be divided into two sections: physical and psychological.

Physical

- Firstly, physical care consists of surgical preparation, which can be in the form of bowel preparation where patients are required to take laxatives to cleanse their bowel prior to surgery. This arguably improves surgical visibility and prevents contamination. This depends on the surgeon's preference and needs to be checked with the patient's surgical team on admission.
- Due to the current developments regarding reducing patients' hospital stay, many hospitals are carrying out

Table 6.5 A summary of products used for problems associated with stoma

Accessory	Product example	Use	Precautions
Creams	Chiron barrier cream (ABPI 1999)	Sensitive skin as a protective measure	Grease from creams can prevent adherence of the appliance
Protective films	Cavilon no sting barrier film, LBF	To prevent irritation and give protection	If contains alcohol, avoid on broken skin
Protective wafers	Stomahesive	To cover and protect skin	Allergies (rare)
Seals/washers	Cohesive seals Hollister barrier rings	Provide skin protection around the stoma. Useful to fill gaps and dips in skin	Allergies (rare)
Pastes	Stomahesive adapt paste	Useful to fill gaps and dips in skin and provide a smoother surface for applying the pouch	If contains alcohol, avoid on broken skin Should not be used as a solution to an ill-fitting pouch
Protective paste	Orabase paste	Protect raw, sore areas	
Powders	Ostoseal protective powder	Protect sore, wet areas and aid healing	Can sometimes affect adherence
Adhesive preparations	Saltair solution	To improve adherence of product	Should not be used as a solution to an ill-fitting pouch
Adhesive removers	Appeel Adhesive remover aerosols	Aids removal of pouch if patient experiencing pain when pouch removed	Some contain alcohol and should not be used on broken skin
Stoma baseplate securing tape	Hydroframe	To improve patient security. Useful for patients with parastomal hernias	Should not be used as a solution to an ill-fitting pouch
Thickening agents	Gel-X capsules, Ostosorb gel	To help solidify loose stoma output	If output is loose, cause should be investigated
Convex devices	Adapt ring convex inserts, soft seal	Useful for retracted stomas	Bruising and ulceration if used incorrectly
Aerosols	Limone, FreshAire	To mask and absorb odour	Avoid patient associating aerosol spray with stoma
Drops and powders	Nodor S Drops	Deodorizing bag contents	

259

enhanced recovery programmes for colorectal patients. This involves intensive input preoperatively, where selected patients are required to take nutritional drinks and develop skills in changing a stoma bag. This will improve recovery and management and consequently reduce hospital stay. These enhanced recovery programmes are relatively new and are still being trialled in many centres.

- Finally, stoma siting is one of the most important tasks to be carried out by a doctor, stoma care nurse or ward nurse or anyone with appropriate knowledge and skills. This minimizes future difficulties such as the stoma interfering with clothes or skin problems caused by leakage of the appliance due to a badly sited stoma (Bass *et al.* 1997, Qin and Bao-Min 2001).

Patient assessment is necessary taking into account:

- physical problems
- disabilities
- mental state
- visual impairment
- manual dexterity
- lifestyle
- work
- leisure/sporting activities
- ethnicity.

The following guidelines should be adhered to when siting a stoma.

- Locate the rectus muscle: this reduces the risk of herniation later (Myers 1996). The muscle can be identified by asking the patient to lie flat and raise their head. The muscle may also be palpated and easily felt when the patient coughs.
- Identify a flat area of skin on the abdomen, as this facilitates safe adhesion of the appliance.
- Avoid skin creases, especially in the region of the groin or the umbilicus, to avoid urine or faecal matter tracking along the skin creases.

- Avoid any previous or proposed scars, which may lead to skin creases and difficulty applying a bag.
- Avoid bony prominences and pendulous breasts as this may hinder vision of the stoma.
- Avoid the waistline or belt areas, as the patient's clothing may put pressure on the stoma which may lead to leaks or trauma of the stoma.
- Ideally the patient should be able to see their stoma as this will make postoperative self-care easier.

All these factors need to be carefully considered and discussed with the patient whilst siting the stoma. Patient involvement is important as it allows the patient control and enhances their coping strategies. Make sure that you get the patient to adopt various positions before making a final decision on the stoma site, for example lying flat, sitting, standing, bending, as this sometimes changes the decision based on skin creases and patient comfort. Consideration must be given to any bending or lifting involved with the patient's work and any other activities in which the patient partakes. Account must also be taken of any weight gain or loss in the postoperative period, as this may change the contours of the abdomen and hence the position of the stoma.

Once the site has been chosen, it should be clearly marked with a permanent marker pen, preferably a few days before the surgery. Offering the patient a bag to wear prior to surgery allows them time to adapt to their proposed surgery. This procedure should then be documented in the medical notes, stating any complications or issues discussed.

Psychological

Psychological preparation of the individual facing stoma surgery should begin as soon as surgery is considered, preferably by utilizing the skills of a trained stoma care nurse. It is important that the information and discussions are tailored to the individual's needs, taking into account their level of anxiety and distress (Borwell 1997).

It is important that patients meet all members of the multidisciplinary team who are involved in their care and that they fully understand the need for the stoma surgery. This needs to be explained in order to obtain informed consent. It is beneficial if the patient is met in preassessment or at home prior to surgery to discuss the implications of stoma care and the patient's role in rehabilitation. At this point it is also helpful to provide the patient with written information and access to self-help support groups.

Stoma counselling is often best carried out by the specialist stoma care nurse involved in the patient's care. This provides an ideal opportunity to discuss issues such as:

- body image
- family relationships
- sexual relationships
- depression and anger
- fears and concerns.

It is often beneficial to provide patients with some patient information/literature to take home. This gives them an opportunity to digest the information and write down any questions that they have. There are many different aids available, such as information booklets, samples of various products, diagrams, DVDs and internet websites. These help to reinforce and clarify the verbal information given to the patient.

Specific patient preparation
Patient education

Patients undergoing stoma formation have to make major physical and psychological adjustments following surgery. If surgery is elective, patient education should begin in the preoperative period (O'Connor 2005). Adequate pre- and postoperative support is mandatory to improve quality of life for stoma patients (Bloeman *et al.* 2009). Individual holistic patient assessment is key as it is important to identify appropriate teaching strategies for each patient. One of the most important ways in which a nurse can support the patient is to teach them stoma care, ensuring independence before discharge (Burch and Sica 2005). It is important that the patient is able to independently change their stoma bag, recognize problems and obtain support and supplies once discharged home. Providing patients with adequate information and input helps to promote patient decision making by allowing them control (Henderson 2003).

You will wear gloves when changing an appliance. This practice should be explained to patients so that they do not feel it is just because they have a stoma that gloves are worn. (It is recognized that it could be difficult to attach an appliance with gloves *in situ*, due to adhesive, but once the stoma has been cleaned of excreta and blood, gloves may be removed to apply bag.)

Procedure guideline 6.18 **Stoma care**

Essential equipment

Clean tray holding:

- Tissues, wipes
- New appliance
- Measuring device/template
- Scissors

- Disposal bags for used appliances, tissues and wipes
- Relevant accessories, for example adhesive remover, protective film, seals/washers
- Bowl of warm water
- Soap (if desired)
- Jug for contents of appliance
- Gloves

Preprocedure

Action	Rationale
1 Explain and discuss the procedure with the patient.	To ensure that the patient understands the procedure and gives their valid consent (NMC 2008a, C). To familiarize the patient with the procedure.
2 Ensure that the patient is in a suitable and comfortable position where they will be able to watch the procedure, if well enough. A mirror may be used to aid visualization.	To allow good access to the stoma for cleaning and for secure application of the stoma bag. The patient will become familiar with the stoma and will also learn much about the care of the stoma by observation of the nurse (Bryant 1993, P).
3 Use a small protective pad to protect the patient's clothing from drips if the effluent is fluid and apply gloves for nurse's protection.	Avoids the necessity for renewing clothing or bedclothes and demoralization of the patient as a result of soiling. E

Procedure

4 If the bag is of the drainable type, empty the contents into a jug before removing the bag.	For ease of handling the appliance and prevention of spillage. E
5 Remove the appliance. Peel the adhesive off the skin with one hand while exerting gentle pressure on the skin with the other.	To reduce trauma to the skin. Erythema as a result of removing the appliance is normal and quickly settles (Broadwell 1987, C).
6 Fold appliance in two to ensure no spillage and place in disposal bag.	To ensure safe disposal according to environmental policy (DH 2005a, C).
7 Remove excess faeces or mucus from the stoma with a damp tissue.	So that the stoma and surrounding skin are clearly visible. E
8 Examine the skin and stoma for soreness, ulceration or other unusual phenomena. If the skin is unblemished and the stoma is a healthy red colour, proceed.	For the prevention of complications or the treatment of existing problems. E
9 Wash the skin and stoma gently until they are clean.	To promote cleanliness and prevent skin excoriation. E
10 Dry the skin and stoma gently but thoroughly.	The appliance will attach more securely to dry skin. E, C
11 Measure the stoma and cut appliance leaving 3 mm clearance. Apply a clean appliance.	Appliance should provide skin protection. The aperture should be cut just a little larger than the stoma so that effluent cannot cause skin damage. This should be no more than 3 mm from the stoma (Kirkwood 2006, C).

Postprocedure

12 Dispose of soiled tissues and the used appliance in a disposable bag and place it in an appropriate plastic bin. At home the bag should be placed in a plastic bag, tied and disposed of in a rubbish bag.	To ensure safe disposal. E
13 Wash hands thoroughly using bactericidal soap and water or bactericidal alcohol handrub.	To prevent spread of infection by contaminated hands. (Fraise and Bradley 2009, E)

Procedure guideline 6.19 Stoma bridge or rod removal

Essential equipment

Clean tray holding:

- Tissues
- New appliances
- Disposal bags for used appliances and tissues
- Relevant accessories, for example belt
- Bowl of warm water
- Soap if desired
- Jug for contents of appliance
- Gloves

Preprocedure

Action	Rationale
1 Explain and discuss the procedure with the patient.	To ensure that the patient understands the procedure and gives their valid consent (NMC 2008a, C).
2 Ensure the patient is in a suitable and comfortable position.	To allow good access to the stoma for cleaning and for secure application of stoma bag. E
3 Apply gloves.	To reduce risk of cross-infection (Fraise and Bradley 2009, E).
4 If the bag is of the drainable type, empty the contents into a jug before removing the bag.	For ease of handling the appliance and prevention of spillage. E

Procedure

5 Remove the appliance. Peel the adhesive off the skin with one hand while exerting gentle pressure on the skin with the other.	To reduce trauma to the skin. Erythema as a result of removing the appliance is normal and quickly settles (Broadwell 1987, C).
6 Remove excess faeces or mucus from the stoma with a damp tissue.	So that the stoma and surrounding skin are clearly visible. E
7 Slide the bridge gently to one side to ensure the mobile wing of the bridge is away from the stoma. Turn this wing so that it becomes flush with the bridge. Gently slide the bridge through the stoma loop (see Action Figure 7).	To prepare bridge for removal. E
8 Fold the bridge in half so that the bridge appears in a 'C' shape. Gently slide the bridge through the stoma loop (see Action Figure 7).	
9 Examine the skin and stoma for soreness, ulceration or other unusual phenomena. If the skin is unblemished and the stoma is a healthy red colour, proceed. If the skin is red and/or broken, apply barrier cream. If the stoma is not a healthy red colour inform medical and/or stoma care nurse.	For the prevention of complications or the treatment of existing problems (see Table 6.5). E
10 Wash the skin and stoma gently until they are clean.	To promote cleanliness and prevent skin excoriation. E
11 Dry the skin and stoma gently but thoroughly.	The appliance will attach more securely to dry skin. E
12 Apply a clean appliance.	To contain effluent from the stoma. E

13	Dispose of soiled tissues, the bridge and the used bag.	To prevent environmental contamination. E
14	Wash hands with bactericidal soap and water or bactericidal alcohol handrub.	To reduce risk of cross-infection (Fraise and Bradley 2009, E).

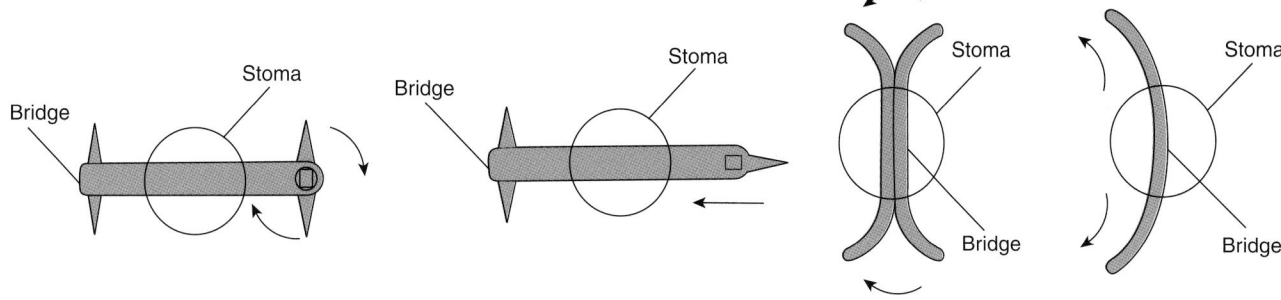

Action Figure 7   Removal of stoma bridge or rod.

Postprocedural considerations

Immediate care

Colostomy function

In the first few days a sigmoid colon stoma will produce hae-moserous fluid and wind. By day 5 there should be some fae-cal fluid and then by day 7–14, semi-formed stool (Cottam 1999). A closed appliance may be used. In the case of a stoma formed in the transverse colon, only a small amount of water will be reabsorbed from the faecal matter, so the faecal matter will be unformed. This means a drainable pouch will need to be used.

Patients with a sigmoid colostomy may find that whole-meal foods assist in producing a formed stool once or twice daily (Black 1998, Myers 1996). Medications that reduce peristaltic action, for example codeine phosphate, may also be used to control diarrhoea. The only means of controlling a sigmoid colostomy, however, is by regular irrigation or by use of a Conseal plug system. Stoma care nurses will need to assess patients before teaching them how to perform the irrigation procedure or to use Conseal plugs.

Ileostomy function

For the first few days the stoma will produce haemoserous fluid and wind. By days 5–10 there will be brown faecal matter (Cottam 1999). The fluid output after surgery can be as much as 1500 mL/24 hours but this will gradually reduce to 500–850 mL/24 hours as the bowel settles down (Black 2000). Sometimes the output from a stoma remains high (>1000 mL/24 hours), which may be due to the amount of small bowel removed at surgery or an underlying bowel condition; these patients require careful management.

It is important that fluid balance recordings are made and serum electrolytes are measured as patients are at risk of so-dium and/or magnesium depletion (Burch 2004). Patients with a high-output stoma may need to be managed by specialist teams which include gastroenterologists, dietitians and stoma care nurses. The effluent takes on a porridge-like consistency when a normal intake of food is established. A drainable appliance is therefore used. The effluent contains enzymes, which will excoriate the skin, so if the pouch leaks, it must be changed promptly to prevent skin breakdown. The effluent cannot be controlled and is often more active after meals (Black 1997, Myers 1996). Sometimes medication, for example codeine or loperamide, which reduces peristaltic action, may be used to control excessive watery output.

Urostomy/ileal conduit function

Urine will dribble from the stoma every 20–30 seconds and it starts draining immediately. Normal output is 1500 mL/24 hours (Cottam 1999), but may be less after periods of reduced fluid intake, for example at night. Urinary stents (fine-bore catheters) may be in place from the ureters past the anastomosis and out of the stoma. They are placed to maintain patency and protect the suturing until primary healing is completed (Black 2000). Stents are left *in situ* for 7–10 days.

Postoperative stages

Stage I

In theatre, an appropriately sized transparent drainable appliance should be applied, which should be left on for approximately 2 days. For the first 48 hours postoperatively, the stoma should be observed for signs of ischaemia or necrosis and the stoma colour (a pink and healthy appearance indicates a good blood supply), size and stoma output should be noted, as should the presence of any devices, such as ureteric stents or bridge with a loop stoma (Kirkwood 2006).

Table 6.6 Decision tool to use when selecting appropriate bag/pouch

Type of stoma	Expected postoperative output	Recommended bag to be used	Expected stoma output on discharge	Recommended bag to be used on discharge
Colostomy	Haemoserous fluid Flatus Liquid/loose stool	Clear drainable bag	Soft formed stool Bowel action 1–3 times a day	Closed opaque bag
Ileostomy	Haemoserous fluid Liquid/loose stool Flatus	Clear drainable bag	Loose stool Approximately >600 mL per day	Opaque drainable bag
Urostomy	Urine Mucus	Clear drainable bag with tap	Urine 0.5 mL/kg/h	Opaque drainable bag with tap

Table 6.6 recommends the most appropriate bag type to use on each type of stoma and the expected output. The drainable appliance should always be emptied frequently, gas should be allowed to escape and the appliance should not be allowed to get more than half full with effluent. If the appliance becomes too full, leaks may occur and the weight from the effluent or the pressure from gas may cause the appliance to fall off (Black 1997). A leak-proof, odour-resistant well-fitted appliance does much to promote patient confidence at this time (Kirkwood 2006). The first time a bowel stoma acts, the type, appearance, quantity and consistency of the matter passed should be recorded; this includes any flatus that may be passed (Kirkwood 2006).

Immediately postoperatively patients would not be expected to perform their own stoma care but would be encouraged to observe the nurse caring for them and discuss it with the nurse. During appliance changes, observations should be made of the following.

- *Stoma*: colour, size and general appearance: oedematous, flush with abdomen, retracted.
- *Peristomal skin*: presence of any erythema, broken areas, rashes.
- *Stoma/skin margin (mucocutaneous margin)*: sutures intact, tension on sutures, separation of stoma edge from skin (mucocutaneous separation).

Any abnormalities should be reported to the stoma care nurse and medical staff (Black 2000, Burch 2004, Kirkwood 2006) (Figure 6.26).

Viewing the stoma may be difficult for the patient, who may be very aware of other people's reaction to it (Price 1990). The patient's reaction to their stoma should be observed and recorded.

Stage II

As the patient's condition improves, they should be encouraged to participate in the care of their stoma. A demonstration change of the appliance should be given with a full explanation of the principles of stoma care. This will be followed by further opportunities to discuss any problems or raise new

queries. Care procedures should be divided into small successive stages and patients should be given support to work through these stages until they are able to take on the care of their stoma. Provided the patient agrees, it is useful to involve the patient's partner or close friends or relatives at this stage. Their acceptance of the stoma may encourage the patient and help to restore the patient's self-esteem (Salter 1995). They may now be ready to discuss appliances and choose the one that they wish to use at home. Preparation for discharge will be discussed (Black 1994, Heywood Jones 1994).

Stage III

Ideally, the patient should now be independent, eating a normal diet, be ready for discharge and should be competent in stoma care. If the family or close friends are closely involved during all stages and are supportive, patients are better able to adapt to the threat of mutilating surgery and altered pattern of elimination (Price 1990). The family or close friends are also likely to require support and information so that they are in a position to help the ostomate. Acceptance of the stoma is a gradual process and, on discharge from hospital, patients may only be beginning to adapt to life with a stoma (Salter/RCN 1997).

Ongoing care
Body image

Stoma formation creates many issues for the patient and many struggle with body image. Studies suggest that this is often overlooked (Opus 2010). The circumstances in which the stoma is formed will influence psychological recovery (Black 2000). Communication is key and it is important to allow the patient and family to discuss their concerns and anxieties. Therefore stoma care nurses play a vital role in supporting the patient and family. It is important to promote patient independence and acceptance.

Diet

All patients should be encouraged to eat a wide variety of foods. Our digestive system reacts in an individual way to

Ostomy Forum - Observation index

Stoma / Status		Skin / Condition		Output / Consistency	
A Normal	above skin level	A Normal	as rest of skin	A Normal	For patient and stomatype
B Flush	mucosa level with the skin	B Erythema	red	B Fluid	
C Retracted	below skin level	C Macerated	excoriated; moist	C Thick	
D Prolapsed	notable increasing length of stoma	D Eroded	excoriated; moist and bleeding	D Solid	
E Hernia	bowel entering parastomal space	E Ulcerated	skin defect reaching in to subcutaneous layer	E Hard	
F Stenosis	tightening of stoma orifice	F Irritated	irritant causing skin to be inflamed, sore, itchy and red	F High output	Uro>2500ml/24 hrs Ileo>1500ml/24 hrs
G Granulomes	nodules/granulation on stoma	G Granuloma	nodules/over granulation tissue on skin	G Too low output	Uro<1200ml/24 hrs Ileo<500ml/24 hrs
H Separation	mucocutaneous separation	H Predisposing factors	underlying diseases, e.g. eczema and psoriasis	H Excessive flatus	
I Recessed	stoma in a skin fold or a crease	I CPD*	greyish, nodules on skin, often caused by urine	I Excessive odour	
J Necrosis	lack of blood supply causing partial or complete tissue death	J Infected	e.g. fungus, folliculitis	J Excessive mucus production	
K Laceration	mucosa that is jagged/torn or ulcerated due to trauma	Z Others	e.g. Pyoderma gangrenosum	K Blood	
L Oedematous	gross swelling of the stoma		* Chronic Papillomatous Dermatitis	L Non functioning stoma	(e.g. sub-ileus)
Z Others				Z Others	

Figure 6.26 Ostomy observational index. (With permission from Dansac Ltd.) (*Continued*)

Psychological

A — Normal for patients based on HTF

B — Low in spirits

C — Worry about diagnosis/disease

D — Worry about stoma management

E — Previous emotional problems (coping strategies, earlier problems/losses/diseases)

F — Body image/self perception

G — Others

Social

A — Resumed normal social activity for patient based on HTF

B — Started working/schooling/education

C — Avoiding working/schooling/education

D — Avoiding social gatherings due stoma related problems and fears (leakage/odour/noise)

E — Financial worries/concerns

F — Social isolation

Z — Others

Sexuality

A — Normal for patient based on the HTF

B — Physical post surgery difficulties:
  1. abdominal, surgical pain
  2. discharge/seepage problems
  3. erectile dysfunction
  4. lubrication
  5. dyspareunia
  6. retrograde ejaculations

C — Psychological post surgery difficulties:
  1. fear of failure
  2. fear of pain
  3. fear of leakage from pouch/rectum
  4. fear of odor/noise
  5. fear of rejection from partner
  6. fear of forming new relationships
  7. loss of sexual desire

Z — Other

www.lindegaard.dk

E01-78.300 06/06 ©2006 Dansac A/S and Salford Royal Hospitals NHS Trust

dansac
Dedicated to Stoma Care

Figure 6.26 (Continued)

different foods and so it is important that patients try a wide range of foods on several occasions and that none should be specifically avoided (Bridgewater 1999). Patients can then make decisions about different foods based on their own experience of their own reaction. Explanations should be given of how the gut functions, how it has been changed since surgery and the effects certain foodstuffs may cause.

Colostomy and ileostomy formation means the loss of the anal sphincter so passage of wind cannot be controlled. High-fibre foods such as beans and pulses produce wind as they are broken down in the gut; hence individuals who eat large quantities of these foodstuffs may be troubled by wind. There are several non-food causes of wind, such as chewing gum, eating irregularly and drinking fizzy drinks, which should be considered before blaming a particular food (Bridgewater 1999). Eating yoghurt or drinking buttermilk may help reduce wind for these patients. Green vegetables, pulses and spicy food are examples of foods that may cause colostomy and ileostomy output to increase or become watery. Boiled rice, smooth peanut butter, apple sauce and bananas are some of the foods that may help thicken stoma output (Black 2000, Bridgewater 1999).

Some foods, for example tomato skin and pips, may be seen unaltered in the output from an ileostomy (Black 1997, Blackley 1998, Hulten and Palselius 1996). Celery, dried fruit, nuts and potato skins are some of the foods which can temporarily block ileostomies (Black 2000, Bridgewater 1999). The blockage is usually related to the amount eaten (Wood 1998). The offending food can be tried at another time in small quantities, ensuring it is chewed well and not eaten in a hurry (Bridgewater 1999).

There are no dietary restrictions with a urostomy. It must be stressed, however, that an adequate fluid intake must be maintained to minimize the risk of urinary tract infection. The recommended fluid intake for all individuals is 1.5–2.0 litres per day (Bridgewater 1999). Fluid intake should be increased in hot weather or at times when there is an increase in sweating, for example exercise, fever. Beetroot, radishes, spinach and some food dye may discolour urine; some drugs may also have this effect, for example metronidazole, nitrofurantoin. Urine may develop a strong odour following consumption of asparagus or fish (Bridgewater 1999).

Fear of malodour

This is a common fear for patients with bowel stomas, often based on hearsay or experience with other ostomists in hospital or the community. Appliances are odour free when fitted correctly. Flatus may be released via charcoal filters and deodorizers are available. The individual must be reassured, however, that any problems that occur postoperatively will be investigated, with a good possibility of their being solved by such means as the use of alternative appliances (Black 2000, Burch 2004).

Sex and the ostomate

The possibility of sexual impairment for both men and women after stoma surgery depends on the nature of the operation, and the ensuing damage to the nerves and tissues involved. The psychological impact of the surgery and its effect on the individual's body image must also be taken into consideration. Surgery that results in physical sexual disability will have psychological repercussions, while some sexual difficulties may be of psychological origin (Black 2004, Borwell 1997, Salter 1996). Impairment may be permanent or temporary. In the latter case, resolution of the difficulty may take anything up to 2 years. Pre- and postoperative counselling should be offered for both patient and partner.

All patients may experience loss of libido and sexual desire. Ejaculatory disturbances occur following cystectomy so men facing this surgery should be offered sperm banking prior to surgery. Erectile dysfunction is a common complication of pelvic surgery and there are a number of treatment options available. These include oral medications (sildenafil, tadalafil, vardenafil), sublingual apomorphine, intraurethral and intracavernosal alprostadil, vacuum devices and penile implants (Ashford 1998, Kirby et al. 1999, Newey 1998).

Female patients may experience dyspareunia; this may be due to narrowing or shortening of the vagina, a reduction in the volume of vaginal secretions or changes in genital sensations (Black 2004, Borwell 1999, Schover 1986). The use of a lubricant, adopting different positions during lovemaking or encouraging greater relaxation by extending foreplay may help resolve painful intercourse (Black 2004, Borwell 1999, Bryant 1993).

Discharge planning

Discharge planning for the patient with a stoma should commence once the patient is admitted. It is important to set a provisional discharge date and set realistic goals with the patient. The patient needs to be discharged home with:

- adequate stoma supplies (approx. 2 weeks' supply)
- contact details of community stoma care nurse
- prescription details of products being used
- information on delivery company, if relevant.

Continuity of care for these patients is crucial. Effective communication and collaboraton between healthcare professionals are key to psychological adaptation and successful rehabilitation (Borwell 2009).

Follow-up support

The patient is discharged with adequate supplies until a prescription is obtained from the general practitioner. Written reminders are provided of how to care for the stoma, how to obtain supplies of appliances, and any other information that may be required. The patient should have details of non-medical stoma clinics, details about the relevant agencies and information about voluntary associations. Arrange-

		Tick Box	Date, Signature & Print Name
1.	Planned date of discharge: _____	Yes ☐ No ☐	
2.	Is the patient independent with stoma care	Yes ☐ No ☐	
3.	Community stoma care nurse informed	Yes ☐ No ☐	
4.	District nurses informed if necessary	Yes ☐ No ☐ N/A ☐	
5.	Date of first home visit by community stoma care nurse	**Date:**	
6.	Patient given contact details of community stoma care nurse Nurses NAME: _____ Contact telephone number: _____	Yes ☐ No ☐	
7.	If patient has chosen to use a delivery company, company informed and first order placed	Yes ☐ No ☐	
8.	Outpatient appointment made: _____	Yes ☐ No ☐	
9.	Patient given two weeks supply of stoma products	Yes ☐ No ☐	

Figure 6.27 Discharge checklist. From The Royal Marsden Hospital NHS Foundation Trust, Stoma Care Pathway.

ments should also have been made for a home visit from the stoma care nurse and/or the community nurse (Blackley 1998, Cronin 2005). Figure 6.27 provides an example of a discharge checklist.

Obtaining supplies

All NHS patients with a permanent stoma are entitled to free prescriptions for their stoma care products, and should complete the relevant forms for exemption from payment. Appliances can then be obtained from the local chemist, free home delivery services or directly from the appropriate manufacturers.

Complications

As a healthcare professional providing support and care to stoma patients, it is important to be able to distinguish normal from abnormal. The observational index (see Figure 6.26) provides a reference guide to use when observing, recording and reporting. If any of the complications are noted, it is important to ensure that the medical team and/or stoma care nurse is informed. Advice on how to manage these problems should be obtained from your specialist stoma care nurse. Recognition of problems and complications early can prevent more serious complications later.

Intestinal (bowel) obstruction and ileus

Definition

Intestinal obstruction occurs when the passage of contents through the bowel lumen is inhibited, either by mechanical (anatomical) or non-mechanical causes.

Table 6.7 Types of bowel obstruction

Type of obstruction	Causes
Mechanical – extrinisic causes	Tumours (benign or malignant), intussusceptions, adhesions (malignant, postoperative or radiation injury), bands (congenital), stenosis, hernias, malrotation/volvulus, aneurysm/embolus/telangiectasia/haematoma, abdominal trauma
Mechanical – intrinsic causes	Tumours, tuberculosis enteritis, Crohn's disease, toxic megacolon, radiation injury, diverticulitis, malrotation/volvulus, mesenteric cysts, congenital defects, Meckel's diverticulum, haematoma
Mechanical – intraluminal causes	Faecal impaction, gallstone ileus, ingested foreign objects, gastric bezoars, meconuim ileus, barium impaction
Neurogenic	Hirschsprung's disease, abdominal trauma, constipation secondary to spinal cord damage or compression, chemotherapy, severe electrolyte imbalance
Pseudo-obstruction (Ogilvie's syndrome)	Abdominal malignancy/carcinomatosis, chest infection, myocardial infarction, cerebrovascular accident, renal failure, puerperium, severe electrolyte imbalance

Adapted from Yamada (2009).

The alternative term 'ileus' is sometimes used to describe the failure of passage of intestinal contents in the absence of any mechanical obstruction (Morton *et al.* 2005).

Related theory

Intestinal obstructions can be divided into those which occur in the large or small bowel, and can be further subdivided into the types of intestinal obstruction detailed in Table 6.7.

Intestinal obstructions are caused by a physical narrowing or internal blockage of the gut lumen, extrinsic compression of the bowel, or a disruption or failure in motility. In cancer patients, malignant bowel obstruction can be either partial or complete, with acute or gradual onset of symptoms (Letizia and Norton 2003).

Obstruction can occur at a single site or, in the case of disseminated intra-abdominal disease, such as intra-abdominal carcinomatosis, in multiple sites (Lynch and Sarazine 2006). Bowel obstruction is a common complication in patients with end-stage cancer, in particular where the primary tumour is abdominal or pelvic in origin. The reported incidence of the condition is between 5% and 42% in advanced ovarian cancer and from 4% to 24% in advanced colorectal cancer (Ripamonti *et al.* 2001).

Intestinal obstruction is a potentially devastating complication for the patient, with a vast number of possible clinical causes, and is a condition which can rapidly progress to cause life-threatening complications (Shih *et al.* 2003). Intestinal obstruction precipitates a cascade of pathophysiological events which lead to complex and unpleasant symptoms. Thoughtful nursing assessment and evaluation, and meticulous symptom control, can make an important contribution to improving the experience of the patient in bowel obstruction.

Small bowel obstruction
Aetiology

The most common cause of small bowel obstruction (SBO) in adults is adhesions, accounting for approximately 65–75%

of cases, and it is estimated that 93–100% of patients who undergo transperitoneal surgery will develop postoperative adhesions (Menzies and Ellis 1990). The second most common cause of SBO is hernias, which are thought to account for around 25% of cases (Turnage and Bergen 2002). SBO by primary small bowel neoplasm is uncommon (3% of cases), but approximately 10% of SBO are caused by luminal compression from gastric, pancreatic, gynaecological or colonic neoplasms.

Pathophysiology

When the small bowel becomes obstructed or static, large volumes of fluid and swallowed air accumulate in the lumen of the intestine, proximal to the obstruction. Oral fluid intake, saliva and gastric, biliary and pancreatic juices contribute to the accumulated fluid. Swallowed air is high in nitrogen and is not well absorbed by the bowel lumen. Initially peristalsis continues but in an unco-ordinated fashion, propelling luminal contents toward the site of obstruction (Ripamonti and Mercadente 2004). These bursts of peristalsis above the level of obstruction cause pain, which is often cramping and intermittent in nature (Morton *et al.* 2005).

Over time, as the obstructive process progresses, the bowel wall and lumen become oedematous and distended. The permeability of capillaries in the bowel wall is increased by the building pressure in the gut lumen, which in turn forces fluid and electrolytes from the capillaries into the abdominal cavity. This extravasation of fluid and electrolytes, coupled with fluid loss from vomiting, can precipitate hypovolaemia, hyponatraemia and hypokalaemia. Furthermore, the distension and hyperactive state of the bowel cause damage to the epithelial cells of the bowel wall, initiating an inflammatory response, activating cyclo-oxygenase pathway and release of prostaglandins (Murphy-Ende 2001).

In proximal SBO, the abdominal pain tends to be more severe, abdominal distension is typically minimal, and emesis is frequent, bilious and tends to relieve pain. It is commonly more frequent early in the course of obstruction. Nausea may be described as building in 'waves' and may be relieved after vomiting (Scott Brown *et al.* 2007). Distal SBO tends to present with moderate abdominal distension and intermittent or constant pain. Vomiting is typically intermittent.

As obstruction progresses further, eventually peristaltic action of the bowel decreases, and this stasis encourages proliferation of bacteria. If the patient continues to eat and drink, bacterial fermentation causes gas production, leading to further abdominal distension. This bacterial overgrowth can cause the bowel contents proximal to the obstruction to become faeculent and malodorous within hours of the obstruction developing (Morton *et al.* 2005).

Large bowel obstruction (colonic obstruction)
Aetiology

By contrast, most obstructions of the large intestine (colon) are caused by malignant neoplasms, sigmoid diverticulitis and volvulus. These three causes account for 90% of cases of large bowel obstruction. In a study in the USA, malignancy was found to be the most common cause of colonic obstruction, contributing to 50% of cases (Turnage and Bergen 2002). Ten percent to 28% of patients with colorectal cancer will go on to develop a malignant obstruction in the course of their disease, and 20–50% of patients with ovarian cancer present with large bowel obstruction (Ripamonti *et al.* 2008).

Pathophysiology

The process of large bowel obstruction mimics that of small bowel obstruction. Normal colonic flora continue to produce methane and ammonia which contribute to distension of the bowel. In the presence of a competent ileocaecal valve, accumulating fluid and gas are unable to decompress into the adjacent small bowel. As a result, the intraluminal pressure builds and when this pressure exceeds that of the capillary pressure, ischaemia can occur. In colonic obstruction, changes in intestinal flora and translocation of bacteria from the mesentery can also cause sepsis.

Figure 6.28 illustrates the 'cascade' process of bowel obstruction.

Evidence-based approaches

The nursing management of the patient in bowel obstruction is multidimensional. Whilst there are essentially two basic approaches to resolving bowel obstruction (surgery or medical management), the nurse should work with the multidisciplinary team to provide care appropriate to the individual. The nurse can play an important role in assessing, evaluating and treating the side-effects of bowel obstruction, and in supporting and educating the patient. This section outlines the risks and benefits of medical and surgical management and provides an evidence-based approach to addressing some of the common symptoms of intestinal obstruction.

Surgical or medical management

Where possible, small bowel obstruction is medically treated with supportive measures (Morton *et al.* 2005). A Norwegian study of 154 patients by Fevang *et al.* (2002) supported this; 91 patients in their study had small bowel obstruction without evidence of strangulation and, following conservative management, 79% of these obstructions were successfully resolved. Where ileus or pseudo-obstruction (e.g. Ogilvie's syndrome) is the cause of symptoms, surgical management is not appropriate.

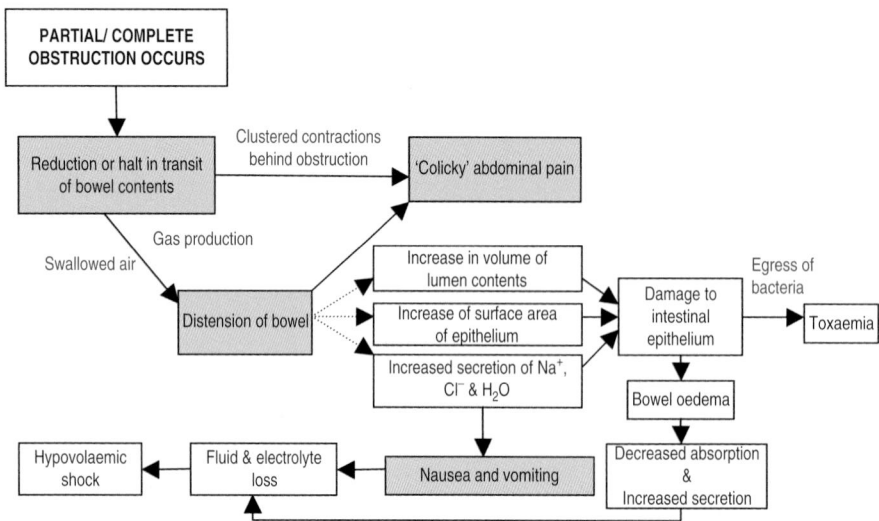

Figure 6.28 Cascade process of bowel obstruction. Reproduced from Ripamonti *et al.* (2008).

By contrast, colonic obstruction more commonly requires relieving by a surgical approach, although in the instance of a volvulus, decompression by colonoscopy may be possible. Endoscopic placement of colonic stent may be used as a palliative relief of obstruction by inoperable tumours of the colon, and studies have shown clinical improvement in symptoms in over 75% of patients (Camunez *et al.* 2000, Mainar *et al.* 1999). If the patient's condition fails to improve following medical management of colonic obstruction, or if the patient has a complete obstruction and competent ileocaecal valve, surgical management is recommended.

The medical/pharmacological approach is particularly favoured in the management of malignant bowel obstruction, where surgery may be contraindicated by complications such as diffuse intra-abdominal spread of disease, massive ascites, poor nutritional status and poor performance status (Lynch and Sarazine 2006). A multidisciplinary steering group for the European Association for Palliative Care (EPAC) concluded that surgery to relieve malignant obstruction should not be routinely undertaken in patients with poor prognostic criteria (Ripamonti *et al.* 2001). Pharmacological management of intestinal obstruction revolves around use of analgesics, antispasmodics and antiemetics to manage symptoms. Corticosteroids have also been used to successfully reverse obstruction in malignant obstruction (Feuer and Broadley 1999). They reduce peritumoural and perineural oedema, thereby helping to relieve obstruction, and have an antiemetic action (Ripamonti *et al.* 2001).

Principles of care

Nursing care of the patient in bowel obstruction is focused on competent assessment and treatment of symptoms and on supporting the patient through what can be a traumatic experience, which may have life-changing consequences. The nurse should work with the whole multidisciplinary team in endeavouring to control the patient's symptoms. The nurse should advocate for the patient, both informing and involving the patient in decisions about their care whenever possible throughout the episode.

Preprocedural considerations
Pharmacological support
Analgesia

Good pain relief is an essential part of the management of bowel obstruction. Where pain can be effectively managed, an episode of bowel obstruction may be less distressing for the patient. Pain should be regularly assessed using an appropriate assessment tool, allowing the patient to describe and rate their pain, to that analgesia can be appropriately titrated.

The pain associated with bowel obstruction is usually described by patients as severe. With reference to the World Health Organization analgesic ladder, such pain should be treated with opioids (Lynch and Sarazine 2006). Opioids can be effectively delivered via the subcutaneous route, allowing

for 24-hour infusion and intermittent bolus breakthrough dose administration. Intravenous administration produces rapid analgesia but of short duration, necessitating 4-hourly administration of doses. In addition, buccal or transdermal opioids may be appropriate, as both avoid the oral route, although the transdermal route should be reserved for when opioid requirements are stable. The opioid dose must always be carefully titrated against the effect and should usually be administered parenterally (Hanks *et al.* 2001).

Antiemesis

The nausea and vomiting associated with bowel obstruction can be very distressing for the patient. The nurse has a role in supporting the patient, providing reassurance, and assessing and managing symptoms appropriately.

Antiemesis in bowel obstruction is focused on decompression of the bowel, management of gastrointestinal secretions, and management of bowel spasm. A wide-bore nasogastric tube, such as a Ryle's tube, may be inserted to decompress the stomach. This can be used to aspirate stomach contents to relieve nausea and distension. Nasogastric tubes should not be used for long-term management of bowel obstruction as they are associated with pain, epistaxis, infection and psychological distress (Ripamonti and Mercadente 2004) and can cause pressure ulcers on the nose if they are in place long term. If long-term gastric decompression is required in the patient with irreversible malignant bowel obstruction, a venting gastrostomy may be placed. Palliative venting gastrostomy reduces episodes of emesis and allows patients with bowel obstruction near the end of life to drink a free fluid diet which they may find comforting, improving their quality of life at a distressing time (Lynch and Sarazine 2006).

Antiemetics should be prescribed with care. Prokinetic antiemetics which promote gastric emptying and peristalsis, such as metoclopramide or domperidone, should be avoided in patients with complete obstruction. The prokinetic action of these drugs stimulates bowel contraction and can cause increased pain as they contribute to the dysrhythmic, spasmodic contraction of bowel. Antiemesis can be better achieved using a dopamine receptor agonist such as prochlorperazine or haloperidol, blocking chemoreceptor trigger zones and preventing transmission to the vomiting centre in the brain. In addition, corticosteroids may be used to reduce inflammation and oedema in the bowel, and have the benefit of both an antiemetic effect and co-analgesic properties (Feur and Broadley 1999). Studies have shown that corticosteroids may play a role in relieving obstruction in the patient with malignant bowel obstruction, by reducing peritumour oedema (Laval *et al.* 2000). The subcutaneous infusion route provides an opportunity to provide constant delivery of antiemesis, avoiding the oral route.

Increased production of secretions can also contribute to nausea, and a somatostatin analogue, such as octreotide, has antivasointestinal properties and may help to reduce bowel secretions (Ripamonti and Mercadente 2004). Octreotide inhibits release and activity of GI hormones, modulates GI function by reducing gastric acid secretion, reduces intestinal motility and decreases bile flow but increases mucus production. It plays an important role in reducing GI contents and increasing absorption of water and electrolytes at intracellular level (Ripamonti *et al.* 2008). Consequentially, secretions throughout the whole GI tract are reduced and patients may suffer from a dry mouth; therefore diligent and regular mouthcare is necessary to alleviate the discomfort associated with dry mouth, and the possible increased risk of oral infections because of reduced saliva production.

Non-pharmacological support

Hydration

Fluid resuscitation should be commenced and essential electrolytes such as potassium should be replaced as indicated by blood results. Patients in bowel obstruction can become profoundly dehydrated from vomiting and as fluid and electrolytes leave the oedematous bowel and enter the abdominal cavity. This causes hypotension, tachycardia and derangement of electrolytes. The nurse should make an assessment of the patient's hydration status (see Chapter 8) and keep an accurate record of fluid input and output, remembering to record nasogastric losses.

In the patient with bowel obstruction receiving end-of-life care, thought should be given to whether it is appropriate to commence intravenous hydration, as artificially hydrating such patients may be contraindicated, and the benefits and burdens of IV hydration should be discussed with the patient and their family (Lynch and Sarazine 2006).

Nutrition

Enteral feeding is usually contraindicated in bowel obstruction so the patient in bowel obstruction is at risk of nutritional deficiency. In order to prevent exacerbation of nausea and vomiting, and abdominal pain and distension, the benefits of total parenteral nutrition (TPN) may be considered. The indication for TPN is to maintain or restore a patient's nutritional status, and the prevention and correction of complications associated with malnutrition. The nutritional benefits of TPN are greater if it is delivered over an extended period, and it is not particularly beneficial for short-term use (Bozzetti *et al.* 2001).

In patients with inoperable bowel obstruction due to malignancy, the use of TPN is controversial as it can lead to complications and can make prolonged hospital stay necessary, which can be a barrier to timely and appropriate discharge at the end of life (Philip and Depczynski 1997).

Food and eating are often of great importance to patients emotionally, socially and culturally, as well as physically. For those patients who are unable to eat or drink due to inoperable and irreversible malignancy, long-term gastric decompression offers effective palliation of distension and vomiting, whilst allowing the patient to drink and eat for comfort, venting the stomach when necessary

to alleviate symptoms. This may allow them to continue an active lifestyle without the discomfort, aesthetic problems and inconvenience of a nasogastric tube (Ripamonti *et al.* 2001).

Psychosocial and emotional care

The nurse can play a crucial role in supporting the obstructed patient with psychosocial, emotional and cultural issues surrounding bowel obstruction. For some patients and their families, it can be a difficult subject to discuss and the nurse can help facilitate good communication about the condition. For the patient who has an operable obstruction, there is the possible challenge of a stoma to contemplate, and the psychosocial, emotional, cultural and psychosexual implications of this.

For many patients, the eating and sharing of food have great emotional, social and cultural significance, and when these activities are curtailed by obstruction, the patient may experience a sense of loss. The nurse can work in conjunction with the patient and their family to try and control symptoms, and help to restore as normal a lifestyle as possible. Patients at the end of life should be given choices about how they would like their condition managed, and where possible should be treated in such a way that their care can be given at home if this is clinically and practically feasible.

Websites

Medic-Alert Foundation: www.medicalert.org.uk

Sexual Dysfunction Association:
www.sexualdysfunctionassociation.com

Urostomy Association: www.uagbi.org

References

Abd-el-Maeboud, K.H., El-Naggar, T. and El-Hawi, E.M.M. (1991) Rectal suppositories. Commonsense mode of insertion. *Lancet*, **338**, 798–800.

ABPI (1999) *ABPI Compendium of Data Sheets and Summaries of Product Characteristics 1999–2000*. Datapharm Publications, Leatherhead, Surrey.

Addison, R. (1999a) Practical procedures for nurses No. 37.1. Fluid intake and continence care. *Nursing Times*, **95**(49), 12.

Addison, R. (1999b) Practical procedures for nurses No. 33.1. Digital rectal examination 1. *Nursing Times*, **95** (40), 1–2.

Addison, R. (2000a) Fluid intake: how coffee and caffeine affect continence. *Nursing Times*, **96** (40) (Suppl), 7–8.

Addison, R. (2000b) Fluids, fibre and constipation. *Nursing Times*, **96** (31) (Suppl), 11–12.

Addison, R. and Mould, C. (2000) Risk assessment in suprapubic catheterisation. *Nursing Standard*, **14** (36), 43–46.

Addison, R. and White, M. (2002) Spinal injury and bowel management. *Nursing Times*, **98** (4), 61.

Amir, I., Sharma, R., Bauman, W. and Korsten, M. (1998) Bowel care for the individual with spinal cord injury. Comparison of four approaches. *J Spinal Cord Med*, **21** (1), 21–24.

Ashford, L. (1998) Erectile dysfunction. *Professional Nurse,* **13** (9), 603–608.

Association for Continence Advice (2003/2008) *Notes on Good Practice.* Association for Continence Advice, London.

Bakke, A. and Malt, U.F. (1993) Social functioning and general well-being in patients treated with clean intermittent catheterization. *Journal of Psychosomatic Research,* **37** (4), 371–380.

Bakke, A., Digranes, A. and Hoisaeter, P.A. (1997) Physical predictors of infection in patients treated with clean intermittent catheterization: a prospective 7-year study. *British Journal of Urology,* **79** (1), 85–90.

Bardsley, A. (2005) Use of lubricant gels in urinary catheterisation. *Nursing Standard,* **20** (8), 41–46.

Bardsley, A. (2009) Coated catheters – reviewing the literature. *Journal of Community Nursing,* **23** (2), 15–17.

Bardsley, A. and Kyle, G. (2008) The use of gloves in uretheral catheterisation. *Continence UK,* **2**(1), 65–68.

Barnes, D.G., Shaw, P.J., Timoney, A.G. and Tsokos, N. (1993) Management of the neuropathic bladder by suprapubic catheterisation. *British Journal of Urology,* **72** (2), 169–172.

Barnes, K.E. and Malone-Lee, J. (1986) Long-term catheter management: minimizing the problem of premature replacement due to balloon deflation. *Journal of Advanced Nursing,* **11** (3), 303–307.

Barrett, J.A. (1992) Faecal incontinence, in *Clinial Nursing Practice. The Promotion and Management of Continence* (ed. B. Roe). Prentice Hall, New York, pp. 196–219.

Barton, R. (2000) Intermittent self-catheterisation. *Nursing Standard,* **15** (9), 47–55.

Basch, A. (1987) Symptom distress changes in elimination. *Seminars in Oncology Nursing,* **3** (4), 287–92.

Bass, E.M., Del Pino, A., Tan, A. *et al.* (1997) Does preoperative stoma marking and education by the enterostomal therapist affect outcome? *Diseases of the Colon and Rectum,* **40** (4) 440–442.

BAUN and Astratech Healthcare (2009) *Clean Intermittent Catheterisation. The Patient's Journey.* British Association of Urological Nurses, Bathgate, Scotland.

BAUN (2000) *Guidelines for Female Urethral Catheterisation using 2% Lignocaine Gel (Instillagel).* British Association of Urological Nurses. Fitwise, Bathgate, Scotland.

Baxter, A. and Salter, M. (2000) Stoma care nursing. *Nursing Standard,* **14,** 59.

Beeckman, D., Schoonhoven, L. Verhaeghe, S. *et al.* (2009) Prevention and treatment of incontinence-associated dermatitis: literature review. *Journal of Advanced Nursing,* **65** (6), 1141–1154.

Bell, S. (2004) Investigations and management of chronic diarrhoea in adults, in *Bowel Continence Nursing* (eds C. Norton and S. Chelvanayagam). Beaconsfield Publishers, Beaconsfield, Bucks, pp. 92–102.

Bennett, E. (2002) Intermittent self-catheterisation and the female patient. *Nursing Standard,* **17** (7), 37–42.

Bierman, S. and Carigan, M. (2003) The prevention of adverse events associated with urinary tract catheterization. *Managing Infection Control,* September, 43–49.

Black, P. (1994) Stoma care: a practical approach. *Nursing Standard,* **8** (34). RCN Nurs Update, Learning Unit 045.

Black, P. (1997) Practical stoma care. *Nursing Standard,* **11** (47), 49–53.

Black, P. (1998) Colostomy. *Professional Nurse,* **13** (12), 851–857.

Black, P. (2000) Practical stoma care. *Nursing Standard,* **14** (41), 47–55.

Black, P. (2004) Psychological, sexual and cultural issues for patients with a stoma. *British Journal of Nursing,* **13** (12), 692–697.

Blackley, P. (1998) *Practical Stoma, Wound and Continence Management.* Research Publications, Australia.

Blandy, J.P. and Moors, J. (1989) *Urology for Nurses.* Blackwell Scientific, Oxford.

Bloemen, J.G., Visschers, R.G., Truin, W., Beets, G.L. and Konsten, J.L. (2009) Long-term quality of life in patients with rectal cancer: association with severe postoperative complications and presence of a stoma. *Diseases of the Colon and Rectum,* **52** (7), 1251–1258.

BNF (2011) *British National Formulary.* BMJ Group and RPS Publishing, London.

Boore, J.R.P. (1978) *A Prescription for Recovery: The Effects of Pre-operative Preparation of Surgical Patients on Post-operative Stress, Recovery and Infection.* Royal College of Nursing, London.

Booth, F. (2009) Ensuring penile sheaths do their job properly. *Nursing and Residential Care,* **11** (11), 550–554.

Booth, F. and Lee, L. (2005) A guide to selecting and using urinary sheaths. *Nursing Times,* **101** (47), 43–46.

Borwell, B. (1997) Psychological considerations of stoma care nursing. *Nursing Standard,* **11** (48) 49–55.

Borwell, B. (1999) Sexuality and stoma care, in *Stoma Care in the Community: A Clinical Resource dor Practitioners* (ed. P. Taylor). Nursing Times Books, London, pp.110–135.

Borwell, B. (2009) Continuity of care for the stoma patient: psychological considerations. *British Journal of Community Nursing,* **14** (8), 330–331.

Bowers, B. (2006) Evaluating the evidence for administering phosphate enemas. *British Journal of Nursing,* **15** (7), 378–381.

Bozzetti, F., Braga, M., Gianotti, L., Gavazzi, C. and Mariani, L. (2001) Postoperative enteral versus parenteral nutrition in malnourished patients with gastrointestinal cancer: a randomised multicentre trial. *Lancet,* **358** (9292), 1487–1492.

Bridgewater, S.E. (1999) Dietary considerations, in *Stoma Care in the Community: A Clinical Resource dor Practitioners* (ed. P. Taylor). Nursing Times Books, London.

British Nutrition Foundation (2004) Dietary fibre. www.nutrition.org.uk.

Broadwell, D.C. (1987) Peristomal skin integrity. *Nursing Clinics of North America,* **22** (2), 321–332.

Brocklehurst, J.C., Hickey, D.S., Davies, I., Kennedy, A.P. and Morris, J.A. (1988) A new urethral catheter. *BMJ,* **296** (6638), 1691–1693.

Brosnahan, J., Jull, A. and Tracy, C. (2006) Types of urethral catheters for management of short-term voiding problems in hospitalised adults (review). The Cochrane Collaboration. *The Cochrane Library,* Issue 2. John Wiley, New York.

Brown, S.R., Cann, P.A. and Read, N. (1990) Effect of coffee on distal colon function. *Gut,* **31,** 450–453.

Bryant, R.A. (1993) Ostomy patient management: care that engenders adaptation. *Cancer Investigations,* **11** (5), 565–577.

Burch, J. (2004) The management and care of people with stoma complications. *British Journal of Nursing,* **13** (6), 307–308, 310, 312, 314–318.

Burch, J. (2008) Nutrition for people with stomas 1: overview of issues. *Nursing Times,* **104** (48) 25–25.

Burch, J. and Sica, J. (2005) Stoma care accessories: an overview of a crowded market. *British Journal of Community Nursing,* **10** (1), 24–31.

Bush, S. (2000) Fluids, fibre and constipation. *Nursing Times,* **96** (31) (Suppl), 11–12.

Busuttil-Leaver, R.B. (2004) Reconstructive surgery for the promotion of continence, in *Urological Nursing,* 3rd edn (eds S. Fillingham and J. Douglas). Baillière Tindall, Edinburgh, pp.135–159.

Butler, M. (1998) Laxatives and rectal preparations. *Nursing Times,* **94** (3), 56–58.

Cadd, A., Keatinge, D., Henssen, M. *et al.* (2000) Assessment and documentation of bowel care management in palliative care: incorporating patient preferences into the care regimen. *Journal of Clinical Nursing,* **9,** 228–235.

273

Campbell, T. and Lunn, D. (1999) Colorectal cancer. Part 3: patient care. *Professional Nurse*, 15 (2), 117–121.

Camunez, F., Echenagusia, A., Simo, G., Turegano, F., Vazquez, J. and Barreiro-Meiro, I. (2000) Malignant colorectal obstruction treated by means of self-expanding metallic stents: effectiveness before surgery and in palliation. *Radiology*, 216 (2), 492–497.

Chai, T., Chung, A.K., Belville, W.D. and Faerber, G.J. (1995) Compliance and complications of clean intermittent catheterization in the spinal cord injured patient. *Paraplegia*, 33 (3), 161–163.

Chelvanayagam, S. and Norton, C. (2004) Nursing assessment of adults with faecal incontinence, in *Bowel Continence Nursing* (eds C. Norton and S. Chelvanayagam). Beaconsfield Publishers, Beaconfield, Bucks, pp. 45–62.

Christer, R., Robinson, L. and Bird, C. (2003) Constipation. Causes and cures. *Nursing Times*, 99 (25), 26–27.

Clarke, B. (1988) Making sense of enemas. *Nursing Times*, 84 (30), 40–44.

Clifford, E. (2000) Urinary catheters: reducing the incidence of problems. *Community Nurse*, 6 (4), 35–36.

Colley, W. (1998) Catheter care – 1. *Nursing Times*, 94 (24), suppl 1–2.

Conill, C., Verger, E., Henriques, I. *et al.* (1997) Symptom prevalence: I the last week of life. *Journal of Pain and Symptom Management*, 14 (6), 328–331.

Cook, T., Frall, S., Gough, A. and Lennard, F. (1999) The conservative management of constipation in adults. *J Assoc Chart Physiother Women's Health*, 85, 24–28.

Cottam, J. (1999) Recovering after stoma surgery (Know How Series). *Community Nurse*, 5 (9), 24–25.

Crawshaw, A. (2004) How to establish a rectal irrigation service. *Gastrointestinal Nursing*, 2 (2), 29–31.

Cronin, E. (2005) Best practice in discharging patients with a stoma. *Nursing Times*, 101 (47), 67–68.

Crow, R.A., Chapman, R.C., Roe, B.H. and Wilson, J.A. (1986) *A Study of Patients with Indwelling Catheters and Related Nursing Practice*. University of Surrey, Guildford.

Cummings, J.H. (1994) Non-starch polysaccharides (dietary fibre) including bulk laxatives in constipation, in *Constipation* (eds M.A. Kamm and J.E. Lennard-Jones). Wrightson Biomedical, Petersfield, Hampshire, pp. 307–314.

Cutts, B. (2005) Developing and implementing a new bladder irrigation chart. *Nursing Standard*, 20 (8), 48–53.

Cymet, T. (2001) Do silver alloy catheters increase the risk of systemic argyria? *Archives of Internal Medicine*, 161 (7), 1014–1015.

Davies, C. (2004) The use of phosphate enemas in the treatment of constipation: use of laxatives. *British Journal of Nursing*, 12 (19), 1130–1136.

Day, A. (2001) The nurse's role in managing constipation. *Nursing Standard*, 16 (8), 41–44.

D'Elia, G., Pahernik, S., Fisch, M. *et al.* (2004) Mainz Pouch II technique: 10 year experience. *BJU International*, 93, 1037–1042.

DH (1998) *Nutritional Aspects of the Development of Cancer. Report on Health and Social Subjects 48*. HMSO, London.

DH (2005a) *Hazardous Waste (England) Regulations*. Department of Health, London.

DH (2005b) *Prescription Cost Analysis, England 2004*. HMSO, London.

DH and Chief Medical Officer (2003) *Winning Ways: Working Together to Reduce Healthcare Associated Infection in England: Report of the Chief Medical Officer*. Department of Health, London.

Doherty, W. (2006) Male urinary catheterisation. *Nursing Standard*, 20 (35), 57–63.

Eastwood, L. (2009) Safe and secure – improving practice in the UK. *Journal of Community Nursing*, 23 (5), 30–32.

Edwards, C., Dolman, M. and Horton, N. (2003) Down, down and away! An overview of adult constipation and faecal incontinence, in *Promoting Continence. A Clinical and Research Resource*, 2nd edn (eds K. Getliffe and E. Dolman). Baillière Tindall, London, pp. 185–226.

Edwards, L.E., Lock, R., Powell, C. and Jones, P. (1983) Post-catheterisation urethral strictures. A clinical and experimental study. *British Journal of Urology*, 55 (1), 53–56.

Ehrenpreis, E.D. (1995) Definitions and epidemiology of constipation, in *Constipation. Etiology, Evaluation and Management* (eds S.D. Wexner and D.C.C. Bartolo). Butterworth Heinemann, Philadelphia, pp. 3–8.

Ejemot, R., Ehir, J., Meremikwu, M. and Critchley, J. (2008) Hand washing for preventing diarrhea. *Cochrane Database of Systematic Reviews*, 1, CD004265.

Emly, M., Wilson, L. and Darby, J. (1997) Abdominal massage for adults with learning disabilities. *Nursing Times*, 97 (30) (Suppl), 61–62.

Evans, A., Painter, D. and Feneley, R. (2001) Blocked urinary catheters: nurses' preventive role. *Nursing Times*, 97 (1), 37–38.

Fader, M., Pettersson, L., Brooks, R. *et al.* (1997) A multicentre comparative evaluation of catheter valves. *British Journal of Nursing*, 6 (7), 359, 362–364, 366–367.

Fader, M., Pettersson, L., Dean, G. *et al.* (2001) Sheaths for urinary incontinence: a randomized trial. *British Journal of Urology*, 87, 367–372.

Falkiner, F.R. (1993) The insertion and management of indwelling urethral catheters – minimizing the risk of infection. *Journal of Hospital Infection*, 25 (2), 79–90.

Fallon, M. and O'Neill, B. (1997) Clinical review. ABC of palliative care. Constipation and diarrhoea. *BMJ*, 315, 1293–1296.

Feuer, D.J. and Broadley, K.E. (1999) Systematic review and meta-analysis of corticosteroids for the resolution of malignant bowel obstruction in advanced gynaecological and gastrointestinal cancers. Systematic Review Steering Committee. *Annals of Oncology*, 10 (9), 1035–1041.

Fevang, B.T., Jensen, D., Svanes, K. and Viste, A. (2002) Early operation or conservative management of patients with small bowel obstruction? *European Journal of Surgery*, 168 (8-9), 475–481.

Fillingham, S. and Douglas, J. (2004) *Urological Nursing*, 3rd edn. Baillière Tindall, Edinburgh.

Fillingham, S. and Fell, S. (2004) Urological stomas, in *Urological Nursing*, 2nd edn (eds S. Fillingham and J. Douglas). Baillière Tindall, London, pp. 207–225.

Fisch, M. and Hohenfellner, R. (1992) The sigma-rectum pouch (Mainz II pouch), in *Continent Urinary Diversion* (eds R. Hohenfellner and R. Wammeck). Churchill Livingstone, Edinburgh.

Food Standards Agency (2006) Starchy foods – fibre. www.eatwell.gov.uk/healthydiet/nutritionessentials/starchfoods/.

Forristal, H. and Maxfield, J. (2004) Prostatic problems, in *Urological Nursing*, 3rd edn (eds S. Fillingham and J. Douglas). Baillière Tindall, London, pp. 161–184.

Fraise A.P. and Bradley C. (eds) (2009) *Ayliffe's Control of Healthcare Associated Infection: A Practical Handbook*, 5th edn. Hodder Arnold, London.

Gardiner, A. (2004) Rectal irrigation for relief of functional bowel disorders. *Nursing Standard*, 19 (9), 39–42.

Getliffe, K. (1995) Care of urinary catheters. *Nursing Standard*, 10 (1), 25–31.

Getliffe, D.A. (1996a) Bladder instillations and bladder washouts in the management of catheterized patients. *Journal of Advanced Nursing*, 23, 548–554.

Getliffe, D.A. (1996b) The use of bladder wash-outs to reduce urinary catheter encrustation. *British Journal of Urology*, 73, 696–700.

274

Getliffe, K. and Dolman, M. (2003) *Promoting Continence: A Clinical and Research Resource*, 2nd edn. Baillière Tindall, London.

Gilbert, R. (2006) Taking a midstream specimen of urine. *Nursing Times*, 102 (18), 22–23.

Gill, D. (1999) Practical procedures for nurses. Stool specimen assessment. Part 1: Assessment. *Nursing Times*, 96, 26.

Godfrey, H. and Evans, H. (2000) Management of long-term urethral catheters: minimizing complications. *British Journal of Nursing*, 9 (2), 74–80.

Gould, D. (1994) Keeping on tract. . . . *Nursing Times*, 90 (40), 58–64.

Gray, M., Bliss, D., Doughty, D. *et al.* (2007) Incontinence-associated dermatitis: a consensus. *Journal of Skin and Wound Care*, 15, 170–175.

Hammarsten, J. and Lindqvist, K. (1992) Suprapubic catheter following transurethral resection of the prostate: a way to decrease the number of urethral strictures and improve the outcome of operations. *Journal of Urology*, 147 (3), 648–651.

Hanks, G., De Conno, F., Cherny, N. *et al.* (2001) Expert working group of the research network of the European Association for Palliative Care. Morphine and alternative opioids in cancer pain: the EAPC recommendations. *British Journal of Cancer*, 84 (5), 587–593.

Harrison, P. (2000) *HDU/ICU Managing Spinal Injury, Critical Care*. Spinal Injuries Association, London.

Hart, S. (2008) Urinary catheterization. *Nursing Standard*, 22 (27), 44–48.

Hautmann, R.E., Volkmer, B.G., Schumacher, M.C. *et al.* (2006) Long-term results of standard procedures in urology: the ileal neobladder. *World Journal of Urology*, 24, 305–314.

Hayward, J. (1978) *Information – A Prescription Against Pain*. Royal College of Nursing, London.

Head, C. (2006) Insertion of a urinary catheter. *Nursing Older People*, 18 (10), 33–36.

Henderson, S. (2003) Power imbalance between nurses and patients: a potential inhibitor of partnership in care. *Journal of Clinical Nursing*, 12 (4), 501–509.

Henry, C. (1999) The advantages of using suppositories. *Nursing Times*, 95 (17), 50–51.

Hensle, T.W., Bingham, J., Lam, J. and Shabsigh, A. (2004) Preventing reservoir calculi after augmentation cystoplasty and continent urinary diversion: the influence of an irrigation protocol. *BJU International*, 93 (4), 585–587.

Heywood Jones, I. (1994) Stoma care. *Community Outlook*, 4 (12), 22–23.

Hickson, M., D'Souza, A.L., Muthu, N. *et al.* (2007) Use of probiotic Lactobacillus preparation to prevent diarrhoea associated with antibiotics: randomised double blind placebo controlled trial. *BMJ*, 335 (7610), 80.

Higgins, D. (2006) How to administer an enema. *Nursing Times*, 102 (20), 24–25.

Hinrichs, M. and Huseboe, J. (2001) Research-based protocol: management of constipation. *Journal of Gerontology Nursing*, 27 (2), 17–28.

Hogan, C.M. (1998) The nurse's role in diarrhoea management. *Oncology Nursing Forum*, 25 (5), 879–886.

Hulten, L. and Palselius, I. (1996) Are dietary restrictions necessary for ileostomy surgery? *Eurostoma*, 13, 20.

Hurst, A. (1970) *Selected Writings of Sir Arthur Hurst (1879–1944)*. Ballantyne, Spottiswode.

Jenkins, S.C. (1998) Digital guidance of female urethral catheterization. *British Journal of Urology*, 82 (4), 589–590.

Johnson, J.R., Kuskowski, M.A. and Wilt, T.J. (2006) Systematic review: antimicrobial urinary catheters to prevent catheter-associated urinary tract infection in hospitalized patients. *Annals of Internal Medicine*, 144 (2), 116–126.

King, D. (2002) Determining the cause of diarrhoea. *Nursing Times*, 98 (23) (Suppl), 47–48.

Kirby, R.S., Carson, C.C. and Goldstein, I. (1999) *Erectile Dysfunction: A Clinical Guide*. Isis Medical Media, Oxford.

Kirkwood, L. (1999) Continence. Taking charge. *Nursing Times*, 95 (6), 63–64.

Kirkwood, L. (2006) Postoperative stoma care and the selection of appliances. *Journal of Community Nursing*, 20 (3), 12–18.

Kornblau, A., Benson, A., Catalono, R. *et al.* (2000) Management of cancer treatment-related diarrhea: issues and therapeutic strategies. *Journal of Pain and Symptom Management*, 19 (2), 118–129. PubMed.

Kristiansen, P., Pompeius, R. and Wadstrom, L.B. (1983) Long-term urethral catheter drainage and bladder capacity. *Neuro-ourology and Urodynamics*, 2 (2), 135–143.

Kunin, C.M. (1997) *Urinary Tract Infections: Detection, Prevention, and Management,* 5th edn. Williams and Wilkins, Baltimore, MD.

Kyle, G., Prynn, P., Oliver, H. and Dunbar, T. (2005a) The Eton Scale: a tool for risk assessment for constipation. *Nursing Times*, 101 (18 Suppl), 50–51.

Kyle, G., Oliver, H. and Prynn, P. (2005b) *The Procedure for the Digital Removal of Faeces. Guidelines 2005*. Norgine, Uxbridge.

Lapides, J., Diokno, A.C., Silber, S.M. and Lowe, B.S. (2002) Clean, intermittent self-catheterization in the treatment of urinary tract disease. *Journal of Urology*, 167 (4), 1584–1586.

Laval, G., Girardier, J., Lassauniere, J.M., Leduc, B., Haond, C. and Schaerer, R. (2000) The use of steroids in the management of inoperable intestinal obstruction in terminal cancer patients: do they remove the obstruction? *Palliative Medicine*, 14 (1), 3–10.

Leaver, R.B. (1996) Continent urinary diversions – the Mitrofanoff principle, in *Stoma Care Nursing – A Patient-Centred Approach* (ed. C. Myers). Edward Arnold, London, pp. 166–179.

Leaver, R.B. (2002) Continent urinary diversions and rectal bladders, in *The Essentials of Pouch Care Nursing* (ed. J. Williams). Whurr Publishing, London, pp. 128–142.

Leaver, R.B (2007) The evidence for urethral meatal cleansing. *Nursing Standard*, 21 (41), 39–42.

Le Lievre, S. (2002) An overview of skin care and faecal incontinence. *Nursing Times*, 98 (4) (Suppl), 58–59.

Letizia, M. and Norton, E. (2003) Successful management of malignant bowel obstruction. *Journal of Hospice and Palliative Nursing*, 5 (3), 152–160.

Longstreth, G.F., Thompson, W., Chey, W. *et al.* (2006) Functional bowel disorders. *Gastroenterology*, 130, 1480–1491.

Lowthian, P. (1991) Using bladder syringes sparingly. *Nursing Times*, 87 (10), 61–64.

Lynch, B. and Sarazine, J. (2006) A guide to understanding malignant bowel obstruction. *International Journal of Palliative Nursing*, 12 (4), 164–171.

Mackenzie, J. and Webb, C. (1995) Gynopia in nursing practice: the case of urethral catheterization. *Journal of Clinical Nursing*, 4 (4), 221–226.

Madeo, M. and Roadhouse, A. (2009) Reducing the risk associated with urinary catheters. *Nursing Standard*, 23 (29), 47–55.

Maestri-Banks, A. (1998) An overview of constipation – causes and treatment. *International Journal of Palliative Nursing*, 4 (6), 271–275.

Mainar, A., De Gregorio Ariza, M.A., Tejero, E. *et al.* (1999) Acute colorectal obstruction: treatment with self-expandable metallic stents before scheduled surgery – results of a multicenter study. *Radiology*, 210 (1), 65–69.

Mangnall, J. and Watterson, L. (2006) Principles of aseptic techniques in urinary catheterisation. *Nursing Standard*, 21 (8), 49–56.

McCahill, P.D., Whittle, D.I. and Jacobs, S.C. (1992) Toxic shock syndrome: a complication of continent urinary diversion. *Journal of Urology*, **147** (3 I), 681–682.

McCarthy, K. and Hunter, I. (2001) Importance of pH monitoring in the care of long term catheters. *British Journal of Nursing*, **10** (19), 1240–1246.

McFarland, L. (2007). Diarrhoea associated with antibiotic use. *BMJ*, **335**, 54–55.

McGill, S. (1982) Catheter management: it's the size that's important. *Nursing Mirror*, **154** (14), 48–49.

McMillan, S.C. (1999) Assessing and managing narcotic induced constipation in adults with cancer. *Cancer Control*, **6** (2), 198–204.

Menzies, D. and Ellis, H. (1990) Intestinal obstruction from adhesions – how big is the problem? *Annals of the Royal College of Surgeons of England*, **72** (1), 60–63.

Metcalf, C. (2007). Chronic diarrhoea: investigation, treatment and nursing care. *Nursing Standard*, **21** (21), 48–56.

Meyer, J.P., Fawcett, D., Gillatt, D. and Persad, R. (2005) Orthotopic neobladder reconstruction – what are the options? *BJU International*, **96**, 439–497.

Moharari, R., Khajavi, M., Khademhosseini, P. *et al.* (2008) Sterile water as an irrigation fluid for transurethral resection of the prostate: anesthetical view of the records of 1600 cases. *Southern Medical Journal*, **101** (4), 373–375.

Moppett, S. (2000) Which way is up for a suppository? *Nursing Times*, **96** (19 Suppl), 12–13.

Moppett, S. and Parker, M. (1999) Insertion of a suppository. (Practical procedures for nurses, part 29). *Nursing Times*, **95** (23), supplement.

Morton, P.G., Fontaine, D.K., Hudak, C.M. and Gallo, B.M. (eds) (2005) *Critical Care Nursing: A Holistic Approach*, 8th edn. Lippincott Williams and Wilkins, New York, pp.962–991.

Mosby (2006) *Mosby's Dictionary of Medicine, Nursing and Health Professions*. Mosby Elsevier, St Louis, MO.

Muctar, S. (1991) The importance of a lubricant in transurethral interventions. *Urologue (B)*, 32, 153–155.

Mulhall, A.B., King, S., Lee, K. and Wiggington, E. (1993) Maintenance of closed urinary drainage systems: are practitioners aware of the dangers? *Journal of Clinical Nursing*, 2, 135–140.

Murphy-Ende, K. (2001) Palliation of gastrointestinal obstructive disorders. *Nursing Clinics of North America*, **36** (4), 761–778.

Myers, C. (1996) *Stoma Care Nursing: A Patient-Centred Approach*. Arnold, London.

Nacey, J.N. and Delahunt, B. (1991) Toxicity study of first and second generation hydrogel-coated latex urinary catheters. *British Journal of Urology*, **67** (3), 314–316.

NANDA-I (2007) *Nursing Diagnoses: Definitions and Classifications 2007–2008*. North American Nursing Diagnosis Association International, Philadelphia.

Nathan, A. (1996) Laxatives. *Pharmaceutical Journal*, **257**, 52–55.

Nazarko, L. (1996) Preventing constipation in older people. *Professional Nurse*, **11** (12), 816–818.

Nazarko, L. (2007) Managing diarrhoea in the home to prevent admission. *British Journal of Community Nursing*, **508** (11), 510–512.

Nazarko, L. (2008) Caring for a patient with a urostomy in a community setting. *British Journal of Community Nursing*, **13** (8), 354–361.

Nazarko, L. (2009) Providing effective evidence-based catheter management. *British Journal of Nursing* (Continence supplement), 18 (7), S4–12.

Newey, J. (1998) Causes and treatment of erectile dysfunction. *Nursing Standard*, **12** (47), 39–40.

Ng, C. (2001) Assessment and intervention knowledge of nurses in managing catheter patency in continuous bladder irrigation following TURP. *Urology Nursing*, **21** (2), 97–108.

NHS Supply Chain (2008) www.supplychain.nhs.uk/portal/page/portal/public/NHS.

NHSQIS (2004) *Urinary Catheterisation and Catheter Care: Best Practice Statement*. NHS Quality Improvement Scotland. www.nhshealthquality.org/nhsqis/files/CATHURIN_BPS_JUN04.pdf.

NICE (2003) *Infection Control, Prevention of Healthcare associated Infection in Primary and Community Care. Clinical Guideline 2*. National Institute for Health and Clinical Excellence, London.

NICE (2007) *The Management of Faecal Incontinence in Adults. Clinical Guideline 49*. National Collaborating Centre for Acute Care, London.

Nicol, M. (2008) *Essential Nursing Skills*, 3rd edn. Mosby Elsevier, Edinburgh.

Nicol, M., Barin, C. and Bedford-Turner, S. (2000) *Essential Nursing Skills*. Mosby International, Edinburgh.

NMC (2008a) *Consent*. Nursing and Midwifery Council, London. www.nmc-uk.org/Nurses-and-midwives/Advice-by-topic/A/Advice/Consent.

NMC (2008b) *The Code: Standards of Conduct, Performance and Ethics for Nurses and Midwives*. Nursing and Midwifery Council, London.

NMC (2008c) *Standards for Medicines Management*. Nursing and Midwifery Council, London.

NMC (2009) *Record Keeping: Guidance for Nurses and Midwives*, Nursing and Midwifery Council, London.

Norton, C. (1996a) The causes and nursing management of constipation. *British Journal of Nursing*, **5** (20), 1252–1258.

Norton, C. (1996b) *Nursing for Continence*, 2nd edn. Beaconsfield Publishers, Beaconsfield, Bucks.

Norton, C. (2006) Constipation in older patients. Effects on quality of life. *British Journal of Nursing*, **15** (4), 188–192.

NPSA (2009) *Minimising Risks Of Suprapubic Catheter Insertion (Adults Only): NPSA/2009/RRR005*. National Patient Safety Agency, London. www.nrls.npsa.nhs.uk/resources/patient-safety-topics/medical-device-equipment/?entryid45=61917andp=2.

O'Connor, G. (2005) Teaching stoma management skills: the importance of self care. *British Journal of Nursing*, **14** (6), 320–325.

Okorie, C., Salia, M., Liu, P. and Plisters, L. (2010) Modified suprapubic prostatectomy without irrigation is safe. *Urology*, **75** (3), 701–705.

Opus (2010) Pre and post op steps to improve body image. *Gastrointestinal Nursing*, **8** (2), 34.

Parekh, D.J., Bochner, B.H. and Dalbagni, G. (2006) Superficial and muscle-invasive bladder cancer: principles of management and outcome assessments. *Journal of Clinical Oncology*, **24** (35), 5519–5527.

Peate, I. (2003) Nursing role in the management of constipation: use of laxatives. *British Journal of Nursing*, **12** (19), 1130–1136.

Pellatt, G. (2007) Clinical skills: bowel elimination and management of complications. *British Journal of Nursing*, **16** (6), 351–355.

Perdue, C. (2005) Managing constipation in advanced cancer care. *Nursing Times*, **101** (21), 36–40.

Perimenis, P. and Koliopanou, E. (2004) Postoperative management and rehabilitation of patients receiving an ileal orthotopic bladder substitution. *Urology Nursing*, **24** (5), 383–386.

Petticrew, W. (1997) Treatment of constipation in older people. *Nursing Times*, **93** (48), 55–56.

Philip, J. and Depczynski, B. (1997) The role of total parenteral nutrition for patients with irreversible bowel obstruction secondary to gynecological malignancy. *Journal of Pain and Symptom Management*, **13** (2), 104–111.

Plowman, R., Graves, N., Esquivel, J. and Roberts, J. (2001) An economic model to assess the cost and benefits of the routine use of silver alloy coated catheters to reduce the risk of urinary tract infections in catheterised patients. *Journal of Hospital Infection*, 48, 33–42.

Pomfret, I.J. (1996) Catheters: design, selection and management. *British Journal of Nursing*, 5 (4), 245–251.

Pomfret, I.J. (2003) Back to basics: an introduction to continence issues. *Journal of Community Nursing*, 16 (7), 36–41.

Pomfret, I. and Tew, L.E. (2004) Urinary catheters and associated UTI's. *Journal of Community Nursing*, 18 (9), 15–19.

Potter, J. (2007) Male urinary incontinence – could penile sheaths be the answer? *Journal of Community Nursing*, 21 (5), 40–42.

Powell, M. and Rigby, D. (2000) Management of bowel dysfunction. Evacuation difficulties. *Nursing Standard*, 14 (47), 47–54.

Pratt, R.J., Pellowe, C., Wilson, J. *et al.* (2007) epic2: National evidence-based guidelines for preventing healthcare-associated infections in NHS hospitals in England. *Journal of Hospital Infection*, 65S, S1–S64.

Price, B. (1990) *Body Image: Nursing Concepts and Care*, Prentice-Hall, New York.

Qin, W. and Bao-Min, Y. (2001) The relationship between site selection and complications in stomas. *World Council on Enterostomal Therapy*, 21 (2), 10–12.

Randles, J. (1990) The Mitrofanoff pouch. *Nursing*, 4 (18), 20–22.

Rankin-Box, D. (2000) An alternative approach to bowel disorders. *Nursing Times*, 96 (19 Suppl), 24–25.

RCN (1994) *Guidelines on Male Catheterisation: The Role of the Nurse*. Royal College of Nursing, London.

RCN (2006) *Digital Rectal Examination and Manual Removal of Faeces: Guidance for Nurses*. Royal College of Nursing, London.

RCN (2008) *Catheter Care – RCN Guidance for Nurses*. Royal College of Nursing, London.

Rew, M. (1999) Use of catheter maintenance solutions for long-term catheters. *British Journal of Nursing*, 8 (11), 708–715.

Rew, M. (2005) Caring for catheterized patients: urinary catheter maintenance. *British Journal of Nursing*, 14 (2), 87–92.

Rigby, D. (2003) Manual evacuation of faeces. *Nursing Times*, 99 (1) (Suppl), 48.

Rigby, D. (2009) An overview of suprapubic catheter care in community practice. *British Journal of Community Nursing*, 14 (7), 278–284.

Ripamonti, C. and Mercadente, S. (2004) Pathophysiology and management of malignant bowel obstruction, in *Oxford Textbook of Palliative Medicine*, 3rd edn (eds D. Doyle, G. Hanks, N. Cherny and K. Calman). Oxford University Press, Oxford, pp.496–507.

Ripamonti, C., Twycross, R., Baines, M. *et al.* (2001) Clinical-practice recommendations for the management of bowel obstruction in patients with end-stage cancer. *Supportive Care in Cancer*, 9 (4), 223–233.

Ripamonti, C., Easson, A. and Gerdes, H. (2008) Management of malignant bowel obstruction. *European Journal of Cancer*, 44, 1106.

Roadhouse, A.J. and Wellstead, A. (2004) The prevention of indwelling catheter related urinary tract infections – the outcome of a performance improvement project. *British Journal of Infection Control*, 5 (5), 22–24.

Roberts, J.A., Fussell, E.N. and Kaack, M.B. (1990) Bacterial adherence to urethral catheters. *Journal of Urology*, 144 (2 I), 264–269.

Robinson, J. (2001) Urethral catheter selection. *Nursing Standard*, 15 (25), 39–42.

Robinson, J. (2004) A practical approach to catheter-associated problems. *Nursing Standard*, 18 (31), 38–42.

Robinson, J. (2006) Continence: sizing and fitting a penile sheath. *British Journal of Community Nursing*, 11 (10), 420–427.

Robinson, J. (2008) Insertion, care and management of suprapubic catheters. *Nursing Standard*, 23 (8), 49–56.

Roe, B.H. (1992) Indwelling catheters, in *Clinical Nursing Practice: The Promotion and Management of Continence* (ed. B.H. Roe). Prentice-Hall, London, pp.177–191.

Roe, B.H. (1994) *Clinical Nursing Practice: The Promotion and Management of Continence*. Prentice-Hall, New York.

Roe, B.H. and Brocklehurst, J.C. (1987) Study of patients with indwelling catheters. *Journal of Advanced Nursing*, 12 (6), 713–718.

Rudoni, C. and Sica, J. (1999) NaturCare from AlphaMed: the non–scented ostomy deodorant. *British Journal of Nursing*, 8 (17), 1168–1170.

Saint, S. and Lipsky, B.A. (1999) Preventing catheter-related bacteriuria. Should we? Can we? How? *Archives of Internal Medicine*, 159 (8), 800–808.

Saint, S., Elmore, J.G., Sullivan, S.D., Emerson, S.S. and Koepsell, T.D. (1998) The efficacy of silver alloy-coated urinary catheters in preventing urinary tract infection: a meta-analysis. *American Journal of Medicine*, 105 (3), 236–241.

Saint, S., Veenstra, D.L., Sullivan, S.D., Chenoweth, C. and Fendrick, A.M. (2000) The potential clinical and economic benefits of silver alloy urinary catheters in preventing urinary tract infection. *Archives of Internal Medicine*, 160 (17), 2670–2675.

Salter, M. (1995) Advances in ileostomy care. *Nursing Standard*, 9 (49), 33–40.

Salter, M. (1996) Sexuality and the stoma patient, in *Stoma Care Nursing: A Patient-Centred Approach* (ed. C. Myers). Arnold, London.

Salter, M. and Royal College of Nursing (1997) *Altered Body Image: The Nurse's Role*, 2nd edn. Baillière Tindall, London.

Scholtes, S. (2002) Management of clot retention following urological surgery. *Nursing Times*, 98 (28), 48–50.

Schover, L.R. (1986) Sexual rehabilitation of the ostomy patient, in *Ostomy Care and The Cancer Patient: Surgical and Clinical Considerations* (eds D.B. Smith and D.E. Johnson). Grune and Stratton, Orlando, FL, pp.103–119.

Schumm, K. and Lam, T. (2008) Types of urethral catheters for management of short-term voiding problems in hospitalised adults. *Cochrane Database of Systematic Reviews*, 2, CD004013.

Scott Brown, M., Spence, R. and Johnston, P. (eds) (2007) *Emergencies in Oncology*. Oxford University Press, Oxford, pp.239–242.

Shepherd, M. (2000) Treating diarrhoea and constipation. *Nursing Times*, 96 (6) (Suppl), 15–16.

Shih, S.C., Jeng, K.S., Lin, S.C. *et al.* (2003) Adhesive small bowel obstruction: how long can patients tolerate conservative treatment? *World Journal of Gastroenterology*, 9 (3), 603–605.

Simpson, L. (2001) Indwelling urethral catheters. *Nursing Standard*, 15 (46), 47–53.

Slade, N. and Gillespie, W.A. (1985) *The Urinary Tract and the Catheter: Infection and Other Problems*. Wiley, Chichester.

Smith, S. (2001) Evidence-based management of constipation in the oncology patient. *European Journal of Oncology Nursing*, 5 (1), 18–25.

Spiller, R.C. (1994) *Diarrhoea and Constipation*. Libra Pharmaceuticals, Petroc Press, Reading, Berks.

Stensballe, J., Tvede, M., Looms, D. *et al.* (2007) Infection risk with nitrofurazone-impregnated urinary catheters in trauma patients. *Annals of Internal Medicine*, 147 (5), 285–294.

Stevens, A., Droney, J. and Riley, J. (2008) Managing and treating opioid induced constipation in patients with cancer. *Gastrointestinal Nursing*, 6 (9), 1–6.

Stewart, E. (1998) Urinary catheters: selection, maintenance and nursing care. *British Journal of Nursing*, 7 (19), 1152–1154, 1156, 1158–1161.

Stewart, M. (1986) Urinary diversion and bowel cancer. *Annals of the Royal College of Surgeons of England*, 68 (2), 98–102.

278

Stoller, M. (2004) Retrograde instrumentation of the urinary tract, in *Smith's General Urology*, 16th edn (eds E.A. Tanagho, J.W. McAninch and D.R. Smith). Lange Medical Books/McGraw-Hill, New York, pp.163–174.

Studer, U.E., Bishop, M.C. and Zingg, E.J. (1983) How to fill a silicone catheter balloon. *Urology*, 22 (3), 300–302.

Tanabe, P., Steinmann, R., Anderson, J., Johnson, D., Metcalf, S. and Ring–Hurn, E. (2004) Factors affecting pain scores during female urethral catheterization. *Academic Emergency Medicine*, 11 (6), 699–702.

Taylor, C. (1997) Constipation and diarrhoea, in *Nursing in Gastroenterology* (eds L. Bruce and T.M.D. Finlay). Churchill Livingstone, Oxford, pp. 27–54.

Taylor, P. (2000) Choosing the right stoma appliance for a colostomy. *Community Nurse*, 6 (9), 35–38.

Taylor, P. (2005) An introduction to stomas: reasons for their formation. *Nursing Times*, 101 (29), 63–64.

Teahon, E. (1999) Constipation, in *Essential Coloproctology for Nurses* (eds T. Porret and N. Daniel). Whurr, London, pp. 206–221.

Thibodeau, G. and Patton, K.T. (2007a) *Anatomy and Physiology*, 6th edn. Mosby Elsevier, St Louis, MO.

Thibodeau, G. and Patton, K. (2007b) Anatomy of the digestive system, in *Anatomy and Physiology*, 6th edn (eds G. Thibodeau and K. Patton). Mosby, St Louis, MO, pp. 925–960.

Thomas, J., Karver, S., Cooney, G.A. *et al.* (2008) Methylnaltrexone for opioid induced constipation in advanced illness. *New England Journal of Medicine*, 22, 1070–1071.

Thomas, P., Forbes, A., Green, J. *et al.* (2003) Guidelines for the investigation of chronic diarrhoea, 2nd edn. *Gut*, 52 (5), v1–15.

Thompson, M.J., Boyd-Carson, W., Trainor, B. *et al.* (2003) Management of constipation. *Nursing Standard*, 18 (14–16), 41–42.

Thompson, W.G., Longstreth, G.F., Drossman, D.A. *et al.* (1999) Functional bowel disorders and functional abdominal pain. *Gut*, 45, 1143–1147.

Tortora, G.J. and Derrickson, B.H. (2009) *Principles of Anatomy and Physiology*, 12th edn. John Wiley, Hoboken, NJ.

Turnage, R.T. and Bergen, P. (2002) Intestinal obstruction and ileus, in *Sleisenger and Fordtran's Gastrointestinal and Liver Disease: Pathophysiology, Diagnosis, Management*, 7th edn (eds M. Feldman, L.S. Friedman and M.H. Sleisenger). Saunders, Philadelphia.

Varol, C. and Studer, U.E. (2004) Managing patients after ileal orthotopic bladder substitution. *BJU International*, 93, 266–270.

Wagstaff, K.E., Woodhouse, C.R.J., Rose, G.A., Duffy, P.G. and Ransley, P.G. (1991) Blood and urine analysis in patients with intestinal bladders. *British Journal of Urology*, 68 (3), 311–316.

Walsh, M. (1997) *Watson's Clinical Nursing and Related Sciences*, 5th edn. Baillière Tindall, London.

Webb, R.J., Lawson, A L. and Neal, D.E. (1990) Clean intermittent self-catheterisation in 172 adults. *British Journal of Urology*, 65 (1), 20–23.

Weisner, P. and Bell, S. (2004) Bowel dysfunction: assessment and management in the neurological patient, in *Bowel Continence Nursing* (eds C. Norton and S. Chelvanayagam). Beaconsfield Publishers, Beaconsfield, Bucks.

Weller, B. (1989) *Encyclopaedic Dictionary of Nursing and Health Care*. Baillière Tindall, Eastbourne.

Wells, M. (2008) Managing urinary incontinence with Bioderm external continence device. *British Journal of Nursing*, 17S (9), 24–29.

Wilksch, J., Vernon-Roberts, B., Garrett, R. and Smith, K. (1983) The role of catheter surface morphology and extractable cytotoxic material in tissue reactions to urethral catheters. *British Journal of Urology*, 55 (1), 48–52.

Wilson, L.A. (2005) Urinalysis. *Nursing Standard*, 19 (35), 51–53.

Wilson, M. (1998) Infection control. *Professional Nurse*, 13 (5), S10–13.

Wilson, M. (2008). Diarrhoea and its possible impact on skin health. *Nursing Times*, 104 (18), 49–52.

Wilson, M. and Coates, D. (1996) Infection control and urine drainage bag design. *Professional Nurse*, 11 (4), 245–246, 248–249, 251–252.

Winder, A. (1994) Suprapubic catheterisation. *Community Outlook*, 4 (12), 25–26.

Winder, A. (1995) Intermittent self catheterisation. *Journal of Community Nursing*, 9 (2), 24–27.

Winn, C. (1998) Complications with urinary catheters. *Professional Nurse*, 13 (5 Suppl), S7–10.

Winney, J. (1998) Constipation. *Nursing Standard*, 13 (11), 49–56.

Withell, B. (2000) A protocol for treating acute constipation in the community setting. *British Journal of Community Nursing*, 5 (3), 110–117.

Wood, S. (1996) Nutrition and the short bowel syndrome, in *Stoma Care Nursing: A Patient-Centred Approach* (ed. C. Myres). Edward Arnold, London, pp. 79–89.

Wood, S. (1998) Nutrition and stoma patients. *Nursing Times*, 94 (48), 65–67.

Woodhouse, C.R.J. (1994) *The Infective Metabolic and Histological Consequences of Enterocystoplasty*. European Board of Urology, European Update Series, Vol 3, Union Européenne Des Médecins Spécialistes, Brussels.

Woodhouse, C.R.J. and Christofides, M. (1998) Modified ureterosigmoidostomy (Mainz II) – technique and early results. *British Journal of Urology*, 81 (2), 247–252.

Woodhouse, C.R.J., Malone, P.R., Cumming, J. and Reilly, T.M. (1989) The Mitrofanoff principle for continent urinary diversion. *British Journal of Urology*, 63 (1), 53–57.

Woodward, S. (1997) Complications of allergies to latex urinary catheters. *British Journal of Nursing*, 6 (14), 786–788, 790, 792–793.

Woodward, S. (2005) Use of lubricant in female urethral catheterization. *British Journal of Nursing*, 14 (19), 1022–1023.

Woodward, S. (2007) The BioDerm external continence device. Evidence and assessment for use. *British Journal of Neuroscience Nursing*, 3 (12), 580–584.

Woollons, S. (1996) Urinary catheters for long-term use. *Professional Nurse*, 11 (12), 825–830.

World Health Organization (WHO) (2003) *Treatment of Diarrhoea: A Manual for Physicians and Other Senior Health Workers*. World Health Organization, Geneva.

Wright, D. (2009) Urinary catheterisation: the infection control aspects. *Journal of Community Nursing*, 23 (3), 11–14.

Wright, S. and Burch, J. (2008) Pre and post operative care, in *Stoma Care* (ed J. Burch). Wiley-Blackwell, Oxford, pp. 119–141.

Xue, Y. (2008) Hand washing for preventing diarrhea. *Journal of Advanced Nursing*, 64 (1), 14–15.

Yamada, T. (ed.) (2009) *Textbook of Gastroenterology*, 5th edn. Wiley-Blackwell, Chichester.

Yates, A. (2004) Crisis management in catheter care. *Journal of Community Nursing*, 18 (5), 28–30.

Young, A.E., Macnaughton, P.D., Gaylard, D.G. and Weatherly, C. (1994) A case of latex anaphylaxis. *British Journal of Hospital Medicine*, 52 (11), 599–600.

Moving and positioning

Overview

The aim of this chapter is to provide guidance on various aspects of moving and positioning patients, acknowledging the need to be clinically effective and, where possible, evidence based. It relates to moving and positioning of adults and does not specifically cover positioning in children or neonates.

The main objectives of the chapter are to:

1 outline the general considerations of moving and positioning
2 provide guidance on the principles of moving and positioning whether the patient is in bed, sitting or preparing to mobilize
3 consider optimal moving and positioning including modifications for patients with different clinical needs.

The principles of moving and positioning will relate to the effect on the patient, but the practitioner needs to ensure that they consider their own position regarding the safety aspects of manual handling. For recommendations and further information on safe manual handling, refer to government (HSE 2004) and local trust policy (HSE 1992), the manual handling advisor, or the physiotherapist (PT).

In this chapter the general principles of moving and positioning will be discussed first followed by considerations of positioning for patients with specific clinical needs, which will require modification or additional considerations of the general principles. The first specific clinical area covered will be moving and positioning of unconscious patients and patients with an artificial airway. Following this, there will be a section looking at additional considerations and modifications for patients with different respiratory requirements. The next section of the chapter will relate to the specific moving and positioning needs of patients with a neurological problem, including the management of patients with spinal cord compression. The final clinical area to be considered will relate to considerations and modifications necessary for upper and lower limb amputees.

All terms marked with an asterisk are explained in the Glossary at the end of the chapter.

Moving and positioning

Definition

The verb 'to position' is defined as 'a way in which someone or something is placed or arranged' (Pearsall 2001). In medical terms, the word 'position' relates to body position or posture. Moving and positioning lie within the broader context of manual handling, which incorporates 'transporting or supporting a load (including lifting, putting down, pushing, pulling, carrying or moving) by hand or bodily force' (HSE 1992).

Anatomy and physiology

The human body is a complex structure relying on the musculoskeletal system to provide support and to assist in movement. The musculoskeletal system is an integrated system consisting of bones, muscles and joints.

Whilst bones provide the structural framework for protecting vital organs and providing stability, skeletal muscles maintain body alignment and help movement (Tortora and Derrickson 2009). In order for skeletal muscles to provide this function, they often cross at least one joint and attach to the articulating bones that help form the joint so that when a muscle contracts, movement of a joint can occur in one direction. Muscles tend to work in synergy with each other (rather than in isolation) not just to create but also to control the movement. The ability of a muscle to either contract or to extend assists their function (Figure 7.1). However, muscles will waste if not used and can also become shortened if not stretched regularly.

Joints are supported not just by the muscles but also by ligaments which are strong connective tissue structures attached either side of the joint, for example the knee (Figure 7.2). Ligaments can also become shortened if they are maintained in one position repeatedly or over a long period of time, which can prevent full joint movement.

Evidence-based approaches
Rationale

Moving and positioning are important aspects of patient care because together they can affect the patient physically, physiologically and psychologically. They can have a major influence on the patient's recuperation and well-being, addressing impairments in order to optimize their function and participation in society.

Positioning is often a good starting point to maximize the benefit of other interventions such as bed exercises, breathing exercises, optimizing rest and mobilizing in order to facilitate recovery and maximize function. However, although it is important, it must not be seen in isolation and is just one aspect of patient management within the context of preventative, rehabilitative, supportive and palliative rehabilitation models (Dietz 1981) where the overall goal is to assist independence.

It is important to frequently evaluate the effect that moving and positioning have on the individual with different pathologies to ensure that the intervention is helping to achieve the desired result or goal. This relates to considering whether the moving and positioning procedure is being clinically effective and, where possible, is evidence based.

There are several points to consider with regard to the clinical effectiveness of moving and positioning.

- Is the timing right for moving the patient? For example, is the pain relief adequate?
- Is it being carried out in the correct way? This relates to manual handling with regard to preventing trauma to

Coracoid process and
supraglenoid tubercle

Shoulder joint

Scapula

Tendons

ORIGINS
from scapula
and humerus

BELLY
of triceps
brachii
muscle

BELLY
of biceps
brachii
muscle

Humerus

Tendon

INSERTION
on ulna

Tendon

INSERTION
on radius

Elbow joint

Ulna

Radius

(a) Origin and insertion of a skeletal muscle

Biceps brachii
muscle

Effort (E) = contraction
of biceps brachii

L

Load (L) = weight of
object plus forearm

F

Fulcrum (F) = elbow joint

(b) Movement of the forearm lifting a weight

Figure 7.1 Relationship of skeletal muscles to bones: origin and insertion of skeletal muscle. Reproduced from Tortora and Derrickson (2009).

Lateral condyle
of femur

Anterior
cruciate
ligament

Lateral
meniscus

Fibular
collateral
ligament

Anterior ligament
of head of fibula

Fibula

Patellar
surface
of femur

Posterior
cruciate
ligament

Medial
condyle
of femur

Medial
meniscus

Transverse
ligament of
the knee

Tibial
tuberosity

Tibial
collateral
ligament

Tibia

Figure 7.2 Anterior view of the right knee (tibiofemoral) joint. Reproduced from Tortora and Derrickson (2009).

both the patient and the practitioner. It is well known that nurses have a high incidence of work-related musculo-skeletal injuries (Nelson *et al.* 2006) so that approved patient handling techniques are essential for safe practice.

- Is the required position taking into account all the pertinent needs of the patient? This emphasizes the need to consider the patient in a holistic manner and take into account any co-morbidities as well as the primary focus that is being addressed.
- Is it achieving the desired or a detrimental result?

Indications

Assistance in moving and positioning is indicated for patients who have difficulty moving or require periods of rest when normal function is impaired.

Contraindications

There are no general contraindications for moving and positioning. The severity of an illness may leave no choice except bed rest, but the rest itself is rarely beneficial.

Patients who are unstable may also need medical attention prior to any moving or change in position.

Principles of care

The principles of positioning are based on patterns of posture which maximize function with the minimal amount of effort (Gardiner 1973) and without causing damage to the body system (Pope 1996). These basic principles of positioning can be applied regardless of a patient's pathology. The aim is to reduce impairment, facilitate function and alleviate symptomatic discomfort and to assist future rehabilitation where appropriate.

The main principles underpinning all interventions regarding patient positioning and mobilization focus on the short- and long-term goals of rehabilitation and management for each specific patient. It is imperative that a thorough assessment is carried out prior to any intervention in order to plan appropriate goals of treatment. It may be necessary to compromise on one principle, depending on the overall goal. For example, for the palliative patient, it may be that the primary aim of any intervention is to facilitate comfort at the cost of reducing function. Regular reassessment is necessary to allow for modification of plans to allow for changes in status.

Effects of bed rest/decreased mobility

Patients with acute medical conditions and decreased mobility are at risk of developing secondary complications of bed rest such as pulmonary embolus (PE) (Reidel 2001), deep vein thrombosis (DVT) or respiratory infection (Convertino *et al.* 1997). Historically patients complaining of pain, dyspnoea, neurological dysfunction and fatigue were advised to rest. However, inactivity can cause a variety of problems (Creditor 1993, Doyle *et al.* 2004) including:

- deconditioning of many of the body's systems (particularly in cardiorespiratory and musculoskeletal systems)
- deterioration of symptoms
- fear of movement
- loss of independence
- social isolation.

Therefore, patients should be encouraged or assisted to mobilize or change position, at frequent intervals. The use of rehabilitation programmes in the patient with critical illness has the potential to decrease time on the critical care unit, shorten overall hospital stay and prevent readmission (Thomas 2009). Early referral to therapy services is advantageous.

If bed rest is unavoidable then the following factors should be taken into account:

- patient comfort and adequate support
- avoidance of the complications of prolonged bed rest
- the optimum frequency of position change.

Active movements, as advised by the physiotherapist, should be practised where possible in order to (Adam and Forrest 1999):

- maintain full joint range
- maintain full muscle length and extensibility
- assist venous return
- maintain sensation of normal movement.

Active ankle movements (Figure 7.3) are to be encouraged to assist the circulation, as failure to exercise the calf muscle for prolonged periods may result in limited or poor blood circulation in the lower leg and increases the risk of DVT (O'Donovan *et al.* 2006).

Risk assessment

There is an absolute requirement to assess the risks arising from moving and handling patients that cannot reasonably be avoided. Once the risk of not moving the patient is deemed to be greater than moving the patient (see previous rationale), consider the following (TILE).

T Task/operation: achieving the desired position or movement.
I Individual: this refers to the handler/s. In patient handling, this relates to the skills, competencies and physical capabilities of the handlers. It is also important to consider health status, gender, pregnancy, age and disability.

(a) (b)

Figure 7.3 (a) Ankle in dorsiflexion (DF). (b) Ankle in plantarflexion (PF).

L   Load: in the case of patient handling, the load is the patient.

E   Environment: before positioning or moving the patient, think about the space, placement of equipment and removal of any hazards.

There have recently been initiatives looking at specific areas to improve patient care following the publication of *High Impact Actions for Nursing and Midwifery* in 2009 (www.institute.nhs.uk). One area identified in this report is falls prevention with the aim of demonstrating a reduction in the number of falls in older people within NHS care. Local initiatives and action plans are currently being formulated to address this issue.

The key points to be considered are summarized in Box 7.1 and discussed further in Chapter 4.

Effective use of therapeutic handling in the context of use of a comprehensive competency-based training tool can benefit patient outcome, enabling balance and motor training in early rehabilitation with minimal risk to staff (Mehan *et al.* 2008). Where there is any doubt about patients with complex needs, seek advice from the PT or the occupational therapist (OT) for assessment.

Consent must be obtained before any intervention is started. Consent is the voluntary and continuing permission of the patient to receive a particular treatment based on an adequate knowledge of the purpose, nature and likely risks of the treatment including the likelihood of its success and any alternatives to it. Permission given under any unfair or undue pressure is not consent (NMC 2008). This is discussed in more detail in Chapter 1.

Legal and professional issues

For recommendations and further information on safe manual handling refer to professional guidance, government, local trust policy (HSE 1992) and the manual handling advisor or the physiotherapist.

Preprocedural considerations

Before positioning or moving the patient consider the following factors.

Assessment

Pressure/skin care

The risk of skin damage when the patient is positioned or moved will be increased by factors including incontinence, profuse perspiration, poor nutrition and obesity (Hickey 2003a). Direct pressure to the skin and friction during movement of patients are two of the most common causes of injury to the skin that can lead to pressure ulcers. Correct moving and handling of the patient will minimize the risk of pressure ulcer formation (see Chapter 4).

Skin integrity should be assessed using the Waterlow Scale (see Chapter 19) prior to positioning and vulnerable areas protected with specialist pressure-relieving equipment or additional use of pillows/towels. Use of special beds or cushions may be required depending on individual assessment.

Minimize contact with other surfaces where possible to ensure optimum skin condition. Care should be taken when lying the patient directly over the greater trochanter as this increases pressure at this interface and the risk of developing pressure sores (Hawkins *et al.* 1999).

Wounds

Consider the location of wounds and injuries when selecting a comfortable position. Ideally positions should avoid pressure on or stretching through any wounds and consideration should be given to the timing of dressing changes, which should be done before positioning to avoid disturbing the patient twice.

Sensation

Take extra care in positioning patients with decreased sensation as numbness and paraesthesia* may result in skin damage as the patient is unaware of pressure/chaffing. These patients may not be able to adjust their position or alert nursing staff in the normal way so it is very important to check the patient's skin regularly for areas of redness or breakdown.

Box 7.1 Risk assessment

1 Assess the patient clinically.
2 Consider realistic clinical goals and functional outcomes in discussion with the patient and ascertain the level at which the patient will be able to participate in the task.
3 Consider whether the proposed intervention involves hazardous manual handling and reduce the hazard by:
   (a) adapting the technique
   (b) introducing equipment. Studies advocate the use of assistive devices to promote safer patient handling for patients with complex needs following assessment (Nelson *et al.* 2006, Rockefeller 2008), with a positive impact on patient outcomes with no detrimental effect on staff handling following assessment (Nelson *et al.* 2008)
   (c) seeking advice/assistance from appropriately skilled colleagues.
4 Risk assessment should be an ongoing process and be constantly updated.
5 After the procedure, document the risk assessment in the communication section of the patient's care plan, being sure to include the date, the number of staff involved and the equipment needed to perform the task. Also document any changes in the patient's condition, such as skin redness. It is important to also document the intended duration of time for which the patient should be maintained in this new position.

(CSP 2008)

Oedema/swelling

Where possible, swollen limbs should not be left dependent but be supported on pillows/footstool as elevation will help to maximize venous return and minimize further swelling. Oedema may result in pain, fragile skin or loss of joint movement.

Pain

Ensure the patient has optimal pain relief before moving. Patients who are pain free at rest may need additional analgesic cover before movement. It is important to allow adequate time for any medication to take effect. See also Chapter 9.

Weakness

Consider the patient's ability to maintain the position. Additional support may be required in the form of pillows or towels to maintain the desired posture.

Limitations of joint and soft tissue range (contractures)

Soft tissue changes and contractures occur through disuse in normal muscle (Jones and Moffatt 2002). As a result, restrictions in joint range may mean that positions need to be modified or become inappropriate.

If there is the potential for any joint or soft tissue restrictions then liaise with the PT or OT regarding any specific exercises or positions necessary for the patient to avoid contractures. This may affect position choice or may involve incorporating appropriate splinting to maintain muscle length.

Communication and involvement with the multidisciplinary team will aid interventions such as physiotherapy as treatment could occur at the same time as positional changes. This potentially allows for more physical assistance in moving the patient without involving other staff, allows collaborative working such as changing sheets, repositioning and assessment of pressure areas, and will minimize unnecessary disturbance of the patient (Hough 2001).

Fracture or suspected fracture

Patients with unstable fractures or suspected fractures should not be moved and the area should be well supported. A change of position could result in pain, fracture displacement and associated complications. Patients with osteoporosis* or metastatic bony disease with unexplained bony pain should be treated as having a suspected fracture. Risk factors for osteoporosis increase with age and include being female, Caucasian and postmenopausal, having a low BMI, a positive family history, a sedentary lifestyle and smoking. Before an osteoporotic lesion becomes apparent radiologically, at least 50% of bone mass must be lost so

that pain may precede radiological changes (McGarvey 1990).

Altered tone

Tone can be altered by positioning with either positive or negative consequences. For further information on patients with neurological impairment and the unconscious patient, see below.

Spinal stability

It is important to establish spinal stability before positioning or moving the patient. The specifics of moving and positioning a patient with spinal cord compression are discussed later in this chapter.

Medical devices associated with treatment

Care should be taken to avoid pulling on lines or causing occlusion if the patient has a catheter, intravenous infusion, venous access device or drain. Pulling on devices may cause pain/injury to the patient and be detrimental to care. Prior to procedure ensure that electrical pumps have been disconnected and sets are untangled and flowing freely. Ensure these are reconnected once the patient is repositioned.

Medical status/cardiovascular instability

The defining parameter for mobilization is that the patient's oxygen transport system is capable of increasing the oxygen supply to meet metabolic demand (Pryor and Prasad 2008). Patients who are medically unstable may become more unstable during movement. Therefore, patients who are acutely unwell should be monitored carefully during any change of position.

Fatigue

Fatigue can be a distressing symptom, so advice and help should be given to the patient to pace their everyday activities. Barsevick et al. (2002) describe energy conservation as 'the deliberate planned management of one's personal energy resources in order to prevent their depletion'. Therefore, prioritizing activities may help to avoid engaging in tasks that are unnecessary or of little value (Cooper 2006).

Cognitive state

It is important to explain to the patient the reasons for moving and positioning appropriate to their level of understanding. Always explain what will happen step by step and give clear instructions to the patient to enable them to participate in the movement.

It is known that impaired cognition* and depression are intrinsic risk factors for falls in older people (DH 2001).

Privacy and dignity

In order to maintain privacy and dignity (CSP 2008) during positioning, ensure the environment is as private as possible by shutting the door and/or the curtains prior to moving the patient. It may be appropriate to ask visitors to wait outside. The process of uncovering the patient may make them feel vulnerable and/or distressed, so keep them covered as much as is practically possible during the procedure. Make sure catheter bags and drains are hung as discreetly as possible under the patient's bed/chair.

Patient explanation/instruction

Explain to the patient the reasons for changing their position and where possible gain their verbal consent. If patients are fully informed of the planned change in position they may be able to participate with the manoeuvre and reduce the need for assistance.

Documentation/liaison with multidisciplinary team (MDT)

It is important to check to see if there are any instructions or indications regarding positioning or moving the patient in their documentation. If unsure then check with the MDT as this may provide guidance on what positions are more appropriate and any special precautions that need to be considered prior to moving and positioning.

Equipment

Sliding sheets are used to assist patients to roll or change position in bed. Due to the slippery surface of the slide sheet fabric, friction is reduced and it is easier to move or relocate the patient with very minimal effort or discomfort.

285

Procedure guideline 7.1 **Positioning the patient: supine**

Essential equipment

- Pillows/towels
- Sliding sheets/manual handling equipment if indicated following risk assessment in accordance with local manual handling policy
- Bed extension for tall patients

Preprocedure

Action	Rationale
1 Explain and discuss the procedure with the patient.	To ensure that the patient understands the procedure and gives their valid consent (NMC 2008, C).
2 Wash hands thoroughly or use an alcohol-based handrub.	To reduce the risk of contamination and cross-infection (Fraise and Bradley 2009, E).
3 Ensure that the bed is at the optimum height for handlers. If two handlers are required try to match handlers' heights as far as possible.	To minimize the risk of injury to the practitioner (Smith 2005, C).

Procedure

4 **Either:** Place one pillow squarely under the patient's head according to patient comfort. For patients with an airway or head and neck surgery, take care not to occlude or displace tubes or increase pressure to vulnerable areas.	To support the head in a neutral position and to compensate for the natural lordosis* of the cervical spine. E To ensure the airway is patent. E To increase patient support and comfort. E
Or: Use two pillows in a 'butterfly' position so that two layers of pillow support the head with one layer of pillow under each shoulder.	This may be necessary for the patient with pain, breathlessness (see Moving and positioning of the patient with respiratory compromise) or an existing kyphosis*. E
Or: Use a folded towel under the patient's head if this provides natural spinal alignment.	To prevent excessive neck flexion. E
5 Ensure the patient lies centrally in the bed.	To ensure spinal and limb alignment. E

(Continued)

Procedure guideline 7.1 *(Continued)*

6 Place pillows and/or towels under individual limbs to provide maximum support for the patient with painful, weak or oedematous limbs.	To ensure patient comfort. E, P
7 Ensure the patient's feet are fully supported by the mattress. For taller patients use a bed extension if required.	To ensure patient comfort. E
8 Place a pillow at the end of the hospital bed to support the ankles at 90° of flexion if the patient has weakness or is immobile around the ankle.	To ensure patient comfort. E To prevent loss of ankle movement. E

Positioning the patient: sitting in bed

Evidence-based approaches

Rationale

Indications

- Patients should be encouraged to sit up in bed periodically if their medical condition prevents them from sitting out in the chair (Figure 7.4). If the patient is unable to participate fully in the procedure, manual handling equipment should be used to help achieve the desired position.

Attention should also be given to sitting posture. Poor posture is one of the most common causes of low back pain which may frequently be brought on by sitting for a long time in a poor position (McKenzie 2006) as it causes an increase in pressure in the disc (Norris 1995).

Contraindications

Post lumbar puncture, patients should lie flat to prevent dural headache in accordance with local policy.

Spinal instability

Refer to Moving and positioning of the patient with actual or suspected spinal cord compression (SCC) or spinal cord injury (SCI).

Figure 7.4 Sitting up in bed.

Procedure guideline 7.2 Positioning the patient: sitting in bed

Essential equipment

- Pillows
- Manual handling equipment may be required, for example sliding sheets or a hoist, depending on local policy

Preprocedure

Action	Rationale
1 Explain and discuss the procedure with the patient.	To ensure that the patient understands the procedure and gives their valid consent (NMC 2008, C).

| 2 | Wash hands thoroughly or use an alcohol-based handrub. | To reduce the risk of contamination and cross-infection (Fraise and Bradley 2009, E). |
| 3 | Ensure that the bed is at the optimum height for handlers. If two handlers are required try to match handlers' heights as far as possible. | To minimize the risk of injury to the practitioner (Smith 2005, C). |

Procedure

4	Ask the patient to sit up in bed. The angle at which the patient sits may be influenced by pain, fatigue, abdominal distension or level of confusion/agitation.	To encourage haemodynamic* stability. E To enable effective breathing patterns, maximizing basal expansion (Pryor and Prasad 2008, R4). To assist in functional activities such as eating and drinking. E
5	Ask the patient to position their hips in line with the hinge of the automatic mattress elevator or backrest of the bed.	To ensure good postural alignment, that is, flexing at the hip when sitting up in bed. E To prevent strain on the spine. E
6	Place a pillow under the patient's knees or use the electrical control of the bed to slightly bend the patient's knees. Extra care should be taken if the patient has a femoral line or is on haemofiltration*.	To reduce strain on the lumbar spine. E To maintain the position. E
7	Place a pillow under individual or both upper limbs for patients with a chest drain, upper limb weakness, trunk weakness, surgery involving shoulder/upper limb/breast/thorax, fungating wounds involving axilla, breast and shoulder, upper limb/truncal lymphoedema or fractures involving ribs or upper limbs.	To provide upper limb support. E To maintain trunk alignment. E To encourage basal expansion (Pryor and Prasad 2008, E).

287

Positioning the patient: side-lying

Evidence-based approaches

Rationale

Indications

This can be a useful position for patients with:

- compromised venous return, for example pelvic/abdominal mass, pregnancy
- global motor weakness
- risk of developing pressure sores
- unilateral pelvic or lower limb pain

- altered tone (see Moving and positioning the patient with neurological impairment)
- fatigue
- chest infection, for gravity-assisted drainage of secretions
- lung pathology (see Moving and positioning the patient with respiratory compromise)
- abdominal distension, for example ascites*, bulky disease, to optimize lung volume (see Moving and positioning the patient with respiratory compromise).

Contraindications

- Suspected or actual spinal fracture or instability.

Procedure guideline 7.3 **Positioning the patient: side-lying**

See Figure 7.5.

Essential equipment

- Pillows
- Manual handling equipment may be required following risk assessment, for example sliding sheets or a hoist, depending on local policy

(Continued)

Figure 7.5 Side-lying.

Procedure guideline 7.3 (*Continued*)

Preprocedure

Action	Rationale
1 Explain and discuss the procedure with the patient.	To ensure that the patient understands the procedure and gives their valid consent (NMC 2008, C).
2 Wash hands thoroughly or use an alcohol-based handrub.	To reduce the risk of contamination and cross-infection (Fraise and Bradley 2009, E).
3 Ensure that the bed is at the optimum height for handlers. If two handlers are required try to match handlers' heights as far as possible.	To minimize the risk of injury to the practitioner (Smith 2005, C).

Procedure

4 Place one or two pillows in a 'butterfly' position under the patient's head, ensuring the airway remains patent. Extra care should be taken for those patients with a tracheostomy, central lines or recent head and neck surgery.	To support the head in mid-position. E To support shoulder contours. E
5 Ask/assist the patient to semi-flex the lowermost leg at the hip and the knee. Extra care should be taken with the degree of flexion for those patients who have hip or knee pain or loss of movement, fracture involving the femur or pelvis, leg oedema, femoral lines or other venous access devices.	To support the patient in a stable position and prevent rolling. E
6 **Either:** Ask/assist the patient to semi-flex the uppermost leg at the hip and knee. Use a pillow to support under the leg placed on the bed. **Or:** Place a pillow between the patient's knees.	To prevent lumbar spine rotation. E To support the pelvic girdle. E To aid pressure care. E
7 Place the underneath arm in front with scapula protracted* (this would not be appropriate for patients with shoulder pathology). Extra care should be taken with patients with low tone in the affected arm, swollen arms or who have access lines in that arm.	To promote patient comfort. E To promote shoulder alignment. E To provide additional support and comfort. E

Procedure guideline 7.4 Positioning the patient: lying down to sitting up

See Figures 7.6, 7.7 and 7.8.

Essential equipment

■ Manual handling equipment may be required dependent on risk assessment, for example sliding sheets or a hoist, depending on local policy

Preprocedure

Action	Rationale
1 Explain and discuss the procedure with the patient.	To ensure that the patient understands the procedure and gives their valid consent (NMC 2008, C).
2 Wash hands thoroughly or use an alcohol-based handrub.	To reduce the risk of contamination and cross-infection (Fraise and Bradley 2009, E).
3 Ensure that the bed is at the optimum height for patients or handlers. If two handlers are required try to match handlers' heights as far as possible.	To minimize the risk of injury to the practitioner (Smith 2005, C).

Procedure

4 Ask the patient to bend both knees and turn their head towards the direction they are moving. Abdominal wounds should be supported by the patient's hands. Extra care should be taken with patients who have joint pathology, oedema, ascites or positional vertigo*.	To assist the patient to roll using their bodyweight. E
5 Ask patient to reach towards the side of the bed with the uppermost arm and roll on to their side.	
6 Ask the patient to bend their knees and lower their feet over the edge of the bed.	
7 Ask the patient to push through the underneath elbow and the upper arm on the bed to push up into sitting. As the patient sits up, monitor changes in pain or dizziness which could indicate postural hypotension or vertigo. Be aware that the patient with neurological symptoms or weakness may not have safe sitting balance.	To help to lever the patient into a sitting position using the weight of their legs. E
8 Achieve upright sitting position with appropriate alignment of body parts.	To ensure safe sitting position achieved. E

289

Figure 7.6 Lying to sitting (stage 1).

Figure 7.7 Lying to sitting (stage 2).

Figure 7.8 Lying to sitting (stage 3).

Positioning the patient: in a chair/wheelchair

Preprocedural considerations
Equipment

Pressure cushion

This is a piece of equipment designed to evenly redistribute the weight of a patient to provide pressure relief for those who are vulnerable to skin breakdown (see Chapter 4). They are an effective aid to increasing patients' sitting tolerance. There are various types available and they are usually provided by the OT dependent on the specific needs of the patient.

Procedure guideline 7.5 **Positioning the patient: in a chair/wheelchair**

Essential equipment

- Upright chair with arms that support elbow to wrist – if using a wheelchair, make certain that the chair has been measured by an occupational therapist (OT) to ensure correct fit and position of the foot rests
- Manual handling equipment may be required following risk assessment, for example a hoist, depending on local policy
- Pillows/rolled-up towel
- Footstool if the patient has lower limb oedema
- Pressure cushion

Procedure	
Action	**Rationale**
1 Place a pressure cushion in the chair and ask the patient to sit well back in the chair. They should have a maximum 90° angle at their hips and knee joints. The patient may not be able to achieve this position if they have pain, abdominal distension or hip/back pain. It may be necessary to refer the patient to the OT for chair raises, a specialized cushion or appropriate seating if a comfortable or safe position cannot be achieved.	Patients with reduced mobility are at greater risk of pressure skin damage. To provide a stable base of support for balance. E To ensure good body alignment. E To achieve a safe sitting position. E
2 Place a pillow or rolled-up towel in the small of the patient's back as is comfortable for the patient.	To allow the patient's back to be supported in a good position. E
3 Ensure the patient's feet are resting on the floor or supported surface. Use pillows or a rolled-up towel to support under the feet if necessary. Make sure the patient's feet are supported on the foot rests if using a wheelchair.	To provide postural alignment and support the lumbar spine. E

4 If the patient has lower leg oedema, use a foot stool, ensuring the whole leg and foot are supported and avoiding hyperextension* at the knees.	To improve venous drainage. E
5 Discourage the patient from crossing their legs.	To reduce risk of developing a DVT (O'Donovan *et al.* 2006, R4).

Moving the patient from sitting to standing

Preprocedural considerations

If the patient stands from the side of a hospital bed, it is helpful to raise the bed slightly to reduce the work of standing for the patient to ensure that the hips are level or higher than the knees with the feet in contact with the floor.

A physiotherapy referral may be appropriate. See Figure 7.9 and Figure 7.10.

Procedure guideline 7.6 Moving from sitting to standing: assisting the patient

See Figures 7.9 and 7.10

Essential equipment

- Walking aid if required (if previously issued by physiotherapist)
- Suitable non-slip, well-fitting, supportive and flat footwear (if not available then bare feet are preferable to socks or stockings which may slip) (Figure 7.11)

Procedure

Action	Rationale
1 Ask the patient to lean forward and 'shuffle' (by transferring their weight from side to side) and bring their bottom closer to the front of the chair or edge of the bed.	To bring the patient's weight over their feet. E

(Continued)

Figure 7.9 Sitting to standing (stage 1).

Figure 7.10 Sitting to standing (stage 2).

(a)

(b)

Figure 7.11 Examples of a supportive shoe.

Procedure guideline 7.6 *(Continued)*

2 Ask the patient to move their feet back so they are slightly tucked under the chair with their feet hip width apart.	To provide a stable base prior to moving. E
3 Instruct the patient to lean forward from their trunk.	To help initiate movement. E To facilitate a normal pattern of movement. E
4 Instruct the patient to push through their hands on the arms of the chair or surface on which they are sitting as they stand. Encourage a forward and upward motion whilst extending their hips and knees.	To minimize energy expenditure. E
5 Once standing, ask the patient to stand still for a moment to ensure balance is achieved before attempting to walk.	To ensure safe static standing. E

Problem-solving table 7.1 **Prevention and resolution (Procedure guidelines 7.1, 7.2, 7.3, 7.4, 7.5 and 7.6)**

Problem	Cause	Prevention	Action
Increase in pain/nausea	Change in posture and position of joints and soft tissues. Patients who are symptom controlled at rest may suffer incidental pain when moving	Preprocedural symptom control Ongoing assessment of symptoms and adjustment of medication	Assist the patient to move slowly and offer support and reassurance where needed

Problem	Cause	Prevention	Action
Change in medical status	Change in position may cause a drop in blood pressure or trigger cardiovascular instability	Monitor carefully	Always have two people present if the patient is at risk of cardiovascular instability Be prepared to return to original position
Bowel/ bladder elimination	Change in position may stimulate bladder and bowels	Put pads and pants on the patient before moving, where appropriate	It may be necessary to stop and clean the patient before continuing to move or position
Increase in loss of fluid, e.g. wound	Change in position may cause breakdown of primary healing or increase in muscular activity which may increase fluid loss	Give support to wounds during movement where possible	Stop and alert medical team for assessment
Loss of consciousness, fainting	Change in position may cause decrease in blood pressure	Allow adequate time for the patient to adjust to a more upright position. Sit patient up in bed and then sit over the edge of the bed and allow time for positional adjustment in blood pressure before attempting to stand	Call for help and follow emergency procedure Refer to local procedure for managing a falling patient
Fall	Multifactoral	Risk assessment and planning	Call for help and follow emergency procedure Refer to local procedure for managing a falling patient
Poor adherence to/ toleration of sitting position	Discomfort Reduced tolerance Cognitive issues	Use pillows/towels to ensure patient is well supported and comfortable A timed goal often helps with patient compliance. Start with a short time, for example 30 minutes, and build up the time slowly. Always tell the patient how long they are aiming to sit out for and make sure the call bell is within reach	Combine sitting out with a meal time as this can help the patient to eat more easily and also help to distract the patient from the length of time they have to sit out
Inability to maintain the position	Patients who are weak and/ or fatigued may be at risk of slipping or falling	Careful positioning of towels and pillows may be needed to maintain a central safe posture in the chair	Observe the patient regularly

293

Moving and positioning the unconscious patient

Definition

Consciousness is a state of awareness of self, environment and one's response to that environment. To be fully conscious means that the individual appropriately responds to the external stimuli. An altered level of consciousness represents a decrease in this full state of awareness and response to environmental stimuli (Boss 1998).

Anatomy and physiology

Physiological changes in the unconscious patient

Unconsciousness is a physiological state in which the patient is unresponsive to sensory stimuli and lacks awareness of self and the environment (Hickey 2003b). There are many central nervous system conditions that can result in the patient being in an unconscious state. The depth and duration of unconsciousness span a broad spectrum of presentations from fainting, with a momentary loss of consciousness, to prolonged coma lasting several weeks, months or even years. The physiological changes that occur in unconscious patients will depend on the cause of unconsciousness, on the length of immobility while unconscious, outcome and quality of care. Also drugs, for example some muscle relaxants such as those used in intensive care, can contribute to muscle weakness, raised intraocular and intracranial pressure, electrolyte imbalances and airway tone (Booij 1996). Unconsciousness can lead to problematic changes for patients which have implications for nursing interventions, including moving and positioning.

Evidence-based approaches
Principles of care

The general principles of care already mentioned earlier in the chapter are all relevant to this section. However, there are some other general principles that also need to be considered for these patients.

Sedation

In the critically ill patient sedation is an essential part of the management. In addition to managing the primary neurological problem, the nurse must also incorporate a rehabilitation framework to maintain intact function, prevent complications and disabilities, and restore lost function to the maximum that is possible.

Communication

There is evidence that unconscious patients are aware of what is happening to them and can hear conversations around them (Jacobson and Winslow 2000, Lawrence 1995). It is therefore important to tell them what is going to happen, that is that they are going to be moved, and explain the procedure just as it would be explained to the conscious patient.

Immobility

The human body is designed for physical activity and movement. Therefore any lack of exercise, regardless of reason, can result in multisystem deconditioning, anatomical and physiological changes. Guidance from a physiotherapist for passive exercises early in the period of unconsciousness may help in the prevention of further complications. There is, however, no evidence to justify the inclusion of regular passive movements within the standard management of a patient's care. Intervention will be specific to the patient's presentation (Harrison 2000, Pryor and Prasad 2008).

The risk of deep vein thrombosis and pulmonary embolism is increased in the unconscious patient. This is due to several factors including blood pooling in the legs, hypercoagulability and prolonged pressure from immobility in bed (Hickey 2003a).

Effects of immobility of muscle

- *Decreased muscle strength:* the degree of loss varies with the particular muscle groups and the degree of immobility. The antigravitational muscles of the legs lose strength twice as quickly as the arm muscles and recovery takes longer.
- *Muscle atrophy:* this means loss of muscle mass. When the muscle is relaxed, it atrophies about twice as rapidly as in a stretched position. Increased muscle tone prevents complete atrophy so patients with upper motor neurone disease lose less muscle mass than those with lower motor neurone disease (Hickey 2003a). For more information see Moving and positioning the patient with neurological impairment.

Respiratory function

Due to the immobility of the unconscious patient, there is an increased threat of developing respiratory complications such as atelectasis, pneumonia, aspiration and airway obstruction. Respiratory assessment should be carried out prior to moving and changing position in order to provide a baseline that can be referred to following the procedure. The assessment should include checking patency of the airway, monitoring the rate, pattern and work of breathing, pulse oximetry* to check oxygen saturations* and blood gases to assess adequacy of gaseous exchange.

Patients may require mechanical ventilation for the following reasons.

- Inability to ventilate adequately, for example post anaesthesia or inspiratory muscle fatigue or weakness.
- Inability to protect own airway or presenting with upper airway obstruction.
- Ability to breathe adequately but inadvisable, for example with an acute head injury.

Mechanical ventilation may be required for days, weeks or even months (MacIntyre and Branson 2009). It is worth remembering that mechanically ventilated patients often cannot express any sort of preference for certain body positions. If the patient is intubated with an endotracheal tube they are at increased risk of developing nosocomial infections (Hickey 2003a) so it is important that lung volumes and respiratory mechanics should be continuously monitored (Hickey 2003a). For more information see Moving and positioning the patient with respiratory compromise.

Cardiovascular function

Immobility can cause changes in cardiovascular function, for example increased cardiac workload, decreased cardiac output and decreased blood pressure. In addition, the positioning of the unconscious patient will cause central fluid shift, from the legs to the thorax and head, so the head of the unconscious patient with raised intracranial pressure may need to be elevated to at least 30° (Hickey 2003a).

Changes in cardiovascular function may be secondary to neurological changes so the patient's neurological function should be monitored. Hypovolaemia*, sepsis or cardiogenic shock* are other factors that should be considered as they will cause cardiovascular instability and should be treated accordingly (Geraghty 2005).

Moving and positioning the patient with an artificial airway

Definition

Some patients, whether unconscious or not, may not be able to maintain a 'safe' airway and therefore may require an artificial airway to support the respiratory system. Patients may have a particular airway depending upon their individual need and presentation. The different airways include:

- nasal
- endotracheal
- tracheostomy.

For more detailed information regarding these and specific care issues and including anatomy and physiology see Chapter 10.

Evidence-based approaches

Principles of care

Maintaining a patent artificial airway

When moving patients with an artificial airway, it is important to maintain neutral head and neck alignment within the movement plane. It is sensible to have one member of staff in sole charge of looking after the patient's artificial airway to avoid risks of trauma, dislodgement and occlusion and, if ventilated, prolonged disconnection from oxygen source. Also changing position will alter the neck musculature and it is important to ensure the tracheostomy tapes are tied securely before and after moving the patient.

With newly formed tracheostomies there is an increased risk of dislodgement 7–10 days following the procedure as the surrounding fascia and muscle need to repair to form

the tract (Hough 2001). During this time it is important to have the following equipment by the patient's bedside:

- tracheal dilators
- two spare tracheostomy tubes, one a size smaller
- tracheostomy tapes
- spare inner cannula
- inner tube cleaners, oxygen supply and tracheostomy mask
- humidification
- suction equipment
- Ambu-bag.

These are essential in case the patient's airway is compromised (for guidance on how to use this equipment see Chapter 10).

Emergency situations

The three most significant life-threatening emergency situations with a tracheostomy tube are blockage, displacement and haemorrhage. These are discussed in more depth in Chapter 10. If any of these occur whilst moving your patient, stop and call for assistance immediately.

Staff should not be moving a patient with a tracheostomy, particularly a new tracheostomy, unless they are experienced in managing these emergency situations or working alongside someone who is.

Legal and professional issues
Consent

If an individual is unconscious an understanding of the Mental Capacity Act is essential. This is discussed in more detail in Chapter 1.

Preprocedural considerations

It is important to ensure regular positional changes as with any patient unable to move themselves (Harrison 2000) to help maintain pressure areas and reduce complications of prolonged bed rest. Ideally the patient should be moved 2 hourly and positions alternated between side-lying and supine.

It is important to consider fitting antiembolic stockings on the patient if appropriate and in line with local trust policy. These help reduce the risk of venous thromboembolism (Geraghty 2005).

Equipment
Artificial airway

If the patient has a tracheostomy, ensure the appropriate equipment is at the bedside (see Principles of care, Maintaining a patent artificial airway) and the tracheostomy tapes are tightly secured.

Procedure guideline 7.7 Positioning the unconscious patient or patient with an airway in supine

Essential equipment

- Manual handling equipment may be required following risk assessment, for example sliding sheets or a hoist, depending on local policy
- Pillows
- Towels
- Splints (Figure 7.13, Figure 7.14)
- Bed extension for tall patients
- At least three members of staff to move patient; refer to local trust policy
- If patient has artificial airway, one extra staff member to be in charge of airway
- Appropriate emergency airway equipment at bedside in line with local trust policy

---

Preprocedure

Action	Rationale
1 Explain the procedure to the patient. If the patient is alert and has an airway, ensure they understand the procedure and give their valid consent.	To inform the patient of the procedure, even if unconscious (NMC 2008, C).
2 Wash hands thoroughly or use an alcohol-based handrub.	To reduce the risk of contamination and cross-infection (Fraise and Bradley 2009, E).
3 Ensure that the bed is at the optimum height for handlers. If two handlers are required try to match handlers' heights as far as possible.	To minimize the risk of injury to the practitioner (Smith 2005, C).
4 It is important to document the patient's vital signs prior to moving.	This will provide a baseline for any changes that may occur during the moving or positioning procedure.

Procedure

5 Head: maintain proper alignment of head and neck; support with pillow or towel roll.	Helps to maintain a patent airway. P
6 Elevate the head of the bed by 30°.	Helps reduce the risk of nosocomial pneumonia (Drakulovic *et al.* 1999: R1b). This facilitates the drainage of secretions from the oropharynx, minimizes the risk of aspiration, assists the maintenance of adequate cerebral perfusion pressure and promotes an effective breathing pattern (Hickey 2003a, E).
7 Body: position in alignment with spine (utilize towels and pillows).	This helps to maintain correct alignment of the body and minimize complications such as contractures. It will also help to maintain musculoskeletal function (Geraghty 2005, E).
8 Limbs: **Upper:** Support arms and wrists on pillows and towels (Figure 7.12) or splints (Figure 7.13); flex the arms at the elbow.	To prevent shoulder drag and wrist drop (Geraghty 2005, E).
Lower: Place a pillow between the knees, use pillows or splints to flex the ankles parallel to the feet, align the hips with the head (Figure 7.14).	To prevent skin breakdown and foot drop (Geraghty 2005, E). To prevent internal rotation of the upper leg (Hickey 2003a, E).

Postprocedure

9 Monitor colour, temperature and pulses of the limbs.	To enhance pulmonary function, prevent atelectasis and hypostatic pneumonia (Geraghty 2005, E) and to help preserve musculoskeletal function and prevent deep vein thrombosis (Hickey 2003a, E).

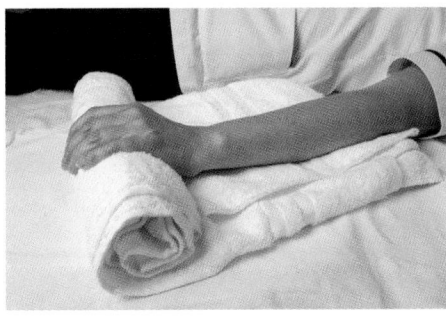

Figure 7.12   Hand resting on towel.

Figure 7.13   Hand resting in splint.

Figure 7.14   Foot resting in splint.

Procedure guideline 7.8 Positioning the unconscious patient or patient with an airway in side-lying

Essential equipment

- Manual handling equipment may be required following risk assessment, for example sliding sheets or a hoist, depending on local policy
- Pillows
- Towels
- Splints
- Bed extension for tall patients
- Minimum of three members of staff to move patient
- If patient has artificial airway, one extra staff member to be in charge of airway, and appropriate emergency equipment at bedside in line with local trust policy

Preprocedure

Action

1 Explain the procedure to the patient. If the patient is alert and has an airway, ensure they understand the procedure and are aware of what is going on.

Rationale

To inform the patient of the procedure, even if unconscious (NMC 2008, C).

Procedure guideline 7.8 (*Continued*)

2 Wash hands thoroughly or use an alcohol-based handrub.	To reduce the risk of contamination and cross-infection (Fraise and Bradley 2009, E).
3 Ensure that the bed is at the optimal height for patients or handlers. If two handlers are required try to match handlers' heights as far as possible.	To minimize the risk of injury to the practitioner (Smith 2005, C).

Procedure

4 Place one or two pillows in 'butterfly' position under the patient's head ensuring the airway remains patent. Extra care should be taken for those patients with a tracheostomy, central lines or recent head and neck surgery.	To support the head in mid-position. E To support shoulder contours. E
5 Ask/assist the patient to semi-flex the lowermost leg at the hip and the knee. Extra care should be taken with the degree of flexion for those patients who have hip or knee pain or loss of movement, fracture involving the femur or pelvis, leg oedema, femoral lines or other venous access devices.	To support the patient in a stable position and prevent rolling. E
6 **Either:** Ask/assist the patient to semi-flex the uppermost leg at the hip and knee. Use a pillow to support under the leg placed on the bed. **Or:** Place a pillow between the patient's knees.	To prevent lumbar spine rotation. E To support the pelvic girdle. E To aid pressure care. E
7 Place the underneath arm in front with scapula protracted (this would not be appropriate for patients with shoulder pathology). Extra care should be taken with patients with low tone in the affected arm, swollen arms or who have access lines in that arm.	To promote patient comfort. E To promote shoulder alignment. E To provide additional support and comfort. E

Problem-solving table 7.2 **Prevention and resolution (Procedure guidelines 7.7 and 7.8)**

Problem	Cause	Prevention	Action
Change in medical status	With any change in position, transient changes in vital signs also occur	It is essential, due to the patient's inability to communicate, that any changes in respiratory and cardiovascular status are closely monitored with any positional change or intervention (Harden 2008, Hough 2001)	If oxygen saturation (SaO_2) drops and does not return to its usual value within 5 minutes, or heart rate (HR) increases or decreases by over 10 bpm and does not settle, the patient should be returned gently to the previous position (Hough 2001)
Joint muscle trauma	Joints and muscles of the unconscious patient are relatively unprotected and prone to trauma (Pryor and Prasad 2008)	Ensure upon changing position that all limbs are in appropriate positions and not overstretched	Once repositioned, ensure limbs are well supported

Problem	Cause	Prevention	Action
Risk of excess pressures on structures	Structures positioned without due care and attention	Also if patient is in side-lying, ensure the ear is not twisted under the head (Hough 2001)	Move patient's head to change position of ear to a more comfortable position
Artificial airway patency blocked	Change of position of neck or of airway	Ensure endotracheal/ tracheostomy tube is secure. This may involve checking the cuff pressure and the endotracheal/tracheostomy ties (see Chapter 10) as movement will alter the soft tissue distribution which will impact on these Monitor vital signs closely to ensure return to normal values within 5 minutes (Hough 2001)	Call for assistance immediately. Refer to Chapter 10 for more specific guidance on emergency management of the airway

Postprocedural considerations

The general principles of care mentioned earlier in the chapter are relevant to this section. However, there are also some other general principles that need to be considered for these patients. It is important to ensure regular positional changes as with any patient unable to move themselves (SIA 2000) to help maintain pressure areas and reduce complications of prolonged bed rest. Ideally, the patient should be moved 2 hourly and positions alternated between side-lying and supine.

Documentation

Alterations in level of consciousness, in cardiovascular and respiratory systems will also need to be recorded.

Moving and positioning the patient with respiratory compromise

Definition

The causes of respiratory compromise may be multifactoral and should be established before undertaking positioning interventions. Compromise may be due to medical intervention (e.g. side-effects of medication), metabolic, surgical or primary respiratory pathologies. The guidelines regarding principles of moving and positioning are applicable to these patients but particular observation is required regarding their response to the intervention.

Anatomy and physiology

Both skeletal and muscular structures that make up the thoracic cage and surround the lungs play a vital role in respiration (see Chapter 10 for more details). Compromise of one or more of these (e.g. abdominal muscle dysfunction due to abdominal surgery, ascites or deconditioning) may lead to an alteration in normal respiratory function and the ability to generate an effective cough (Hodges and Gandevia 2000).

Evidence-based approaches
Principles of care

The main aim of positioning management of the patient with respiratory symptoms is to:

- maximize ventilation/perfusion (V/Q) matching
- minimize the work of breathing (WOB)
- maximize the drainage of secretions.

In many instances positioning, as outlined above, may enhance medical management by the use of the effects of gravity upon the cardiovascular and respiratory systems. This may reduce the need for more invasive intervention (Jones and Moffatt 2002) such as mechanical ventilation. Therefore, the most advantageous positioning should be integrated into the overall 24-hour plan, and positions that may have an adverse effect should be avoided (ACPRC 1996).

The general principles of care mentioned earlier in the chapter are all relevant to this section.

Positioning to maximize ventilation/perfusion matching

Definition

For optimal gaseous exchange to take place, it is necessary that the air and the blood are in the same area of lung at the same time. Matching of these is expressed as a ratio of alveolar ventilation to perfusion (V/Q). A degree of mismatch can occur either due to adequate ventilation to an underperfused area (dead space) or inadequate ventilation to a well-perfused area (shunt).

Anatomy and physiology

The function of the lungs is to exchange oxygen and carbon dioxide between the blood and atmosphere. Oxygen from the atmosphere comes into close contact with blood via the alveolar capillary membrane. Here it diffuses across into the blood and is carried around the body. The amount of oxygen that reaches the blood depends on the rate and depth of the breath, the compliance of the chest and any airway obstruction.

In a self-ventilating individual in the upright position, ventilation will be preferential in the dependent regions as:

- the apex of the lung is more inflated and therefore has less potential to expand
- the bases of the lung are compressed by the weight of the lungs and the blood vessels and therefore have more potential to inflate.

Perfusion to the alveoli is approximately equal to that of the systemic circulation but as the pressure is far less, the distribution is gravity dependent. The variability in the distribution of perfusion throughout the lung is far greater than that of ventilation.

Evidence-based approaches
Principles of care

In a self-ventilating upright position, V/Q is not exactly matched even in a healthy lung but is regarded as optimal in the bases (Figure 7.15) as there is the greatest perfusion and ventilation. Similarly in a side-lying position, the effect of gravity alters the distribution of perfusion and ventilation so that the dependent area of lung, that is, the bottom of the lung, has the best V/Q ratio.

In a patient receiving mechanical ventilation, especially in a mandatory mode (where the ventilator rather than the patient initiates and terminates the breath), the distribution of ventilation and perfusion will alter (Figure 7.16). As ventilation is driven by a positive pressure, rather than the negative pressure when self-ventilating, air will take the path of least resistance. Ventilation will therefore be optimal in the apex of the lungs in the upright position or the non-dependent/uppermost lung in side-lying. This can, however, be altered further in the presence of lung pathology. Perfusion will remain preferentially delivered to the bases (in the upright position) or the dependent/lowermost lung (in side-lying) and have a higher gradient (variability from apex to bases) than in self-ventilating patients as the positive pressure displaces blood from areas of highest ventilation. These two situations mean that the V/Q ratio of those receiving mechanical ventilation can have a higher degree of mismatch. Strategies such as positive end-expiratory pressure (PEEP) and a higher oxygen delivery will help to overcome this.

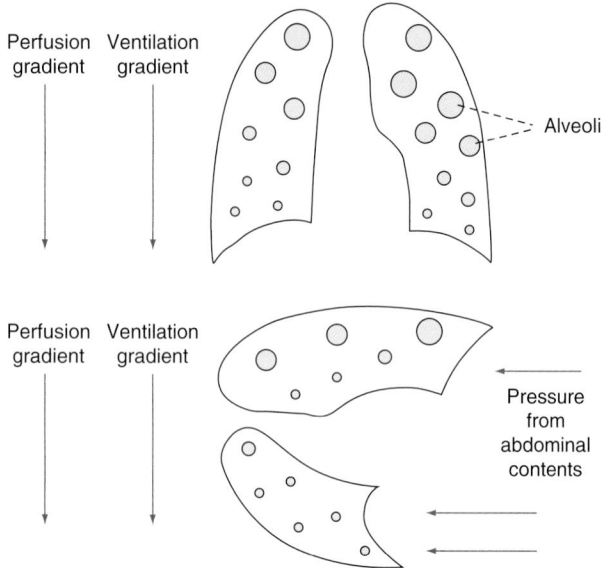

Figure 7.15 Effect of gravity on the distribution of ventilation and perfusion in the lung in the upright and lateral positions. Reproduced with permission from Nelson Thornes Ltd from Hough (2001).

Preprocedural considerations

The general principles of care mentioned earlier in the chapter are all relevant to this section. However, there are also some other general principles that need to be considered for these patients.

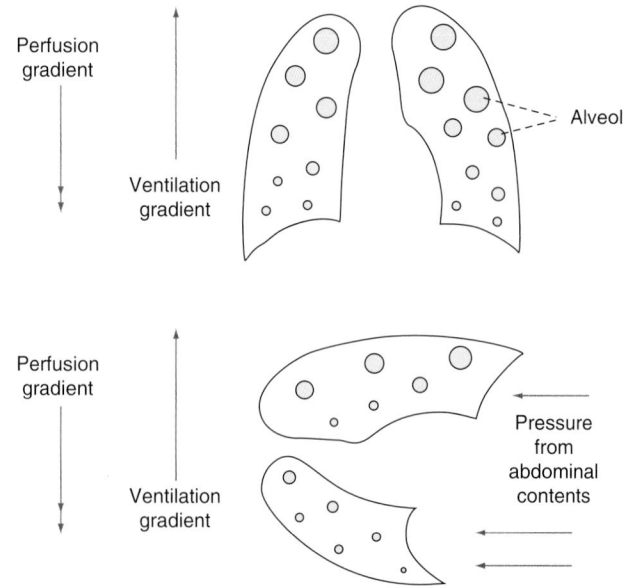

Figure 7.16 Effect of controlled mandatory ventilation on ventilation and perfusion gradients. In contrast to spontaneous respiration, the perfusion gradient increases downwards and the ventilation gradient is reversed. Reproduced with permission from Nelson Thornes Ltd from Hough (2001).

Pharmacological support

Oxygen requirements

Repositioning can cause a temporary fall in oxygen saturation or a raised respiratory rate. If the fall is greater than 4% or recovery time is protracted, supplemental oxygen delivery may be required for several minutes before, during and after moving.

Procedure guideline 7.9 Positioning the patient to maximize V/Q matching with unilateral lung disease in a self-ventilating patient

Equipment

- Pillows/towels
- Sliding sheets/manual handling equipment if indicated following risk assessment in accordance to local manual handling policy
- Bed extension for tall patients

Preprocedure

Action	Rationale
1 Explain and discuss the procedure with the patient.	To ensure that the patient understands the procedure and gives their valid consent (NMC 2008, C).
2 Wash hands thoroughly or use an alcohol-based handrub.	To reduce the risk of contamination and cross-infection (Fraise and Bradley 2009, E).
3 Ensure that the bed is at the optimum height for handlers. If two handlers are required try to match handlers' heights as far as possible.	To minimize the risk of injury to the practitioner (Smith 2005, C).

Procedure

4 Position in side-lying on the unaffected side. Refer to the general principles of moving and positioning the patient in side-lying (see Procedure guideline 7.3).	Ventilation and perfusion are both preferentially distributed to the dependent areas of lung.

Procedure guideline 7.10 Positioning the patient to maximize V/Q matching for widespread pathology in a self-ventilating patient

Equipment

- Pillows/towels
- Sliding sheets/ manual handling equipment if indicated following risk assessment in accordance with local manual handling policy
- Bed extension for tall patients

Preprocedure

Action	Rationale
1 Explain and discuss the procedure with the patient.	To ensure that the patient understands the procedure and gives their valid consent (NMC 2008, C).
2 Wash hands thoroughly or use an alcohol-based handrub.	To reduce the risk of contamination and cross-infection (Fraise and Bradley 2009, E).

(Continued)

Procedure guideline 7.10 (*Continued*)

3 Ensure that the bed is at the optimum height for handlers. If two handlers are required try to match handlers' heights as far as possible.	To minimize the risk of injury to the practitioner (Smith 2005, C).

Procedure

4 Position the patient in high sitting as discussed in the general principles of moving and positioning of the patient in sitting in bed or chair (see Procedure guidelines 7.2 and 7.5).	The effects of shunting mean perfusion will best match ventilation in high supported sitting (Dean 1985, R4, E).

Problem-solving table 7.3 Prevention and resolution (Procedure guidelines 7.9 and 7.10)

Problem	Cause	Prevention	Action
Reduced oxygen saturations. This will be evident by looking at the saturation level on the oximeter* if present or observation of patient colour and work of breathing	Movement causes an increase in oxygen demand from the tissues. If this is not matched by adequate delivery then saturations levels will be lower	Preoxygenate prior to movement if patient is requiring high levels of oxygen or is ventilated	Increase the concentration of oxygen delivered until satisfactory saturations are achieved. Aim to reduce this as much as possible but consider that a higher level of oxygen may be required in the altered position If this is still not tolerated, return the patient to previous position
Raised or tense shoulders/increased effort in breathing	Use of accessory muscles to assist with respiration	Use pillows/towels to support upper limbs in positions where they are not able to actively fix and thereby alter their function	Reassurance to patient Increase oxygen concentration until respiratory rate returns to normal If position remains poorly tolerated, return to the previous position

Positioning to minimize the work of breathing

Anatomy and physiology

At rest, inspiration is an active process whereas expiration is passive. The main muscle involved in inspiration is the diaphragm (Figure 7.17). The diaphragm contracts, thereby increasing the volume of the thoracic cavity. Additionally, the external intercostals work by pulling the sternum and rib cage upwards and outwards, likened to a pump and bucket handle (Figure 7.18). When increased ventilation is required (e.g. with exercise or in disease), the accessory muscles (scalene and sternocleidomastoid) assist with this process.

If this situation is prolonged, as in respiratory disease, the diaphragm activity reduces and the accessory muscles have to do a higher proportion of the work. This can be observed in a patient who adopts a posture of raised shoulders.

Although expiration should be passive in normal conditions, the internal intercostals and muscles of the abdominal wall (transversus abdominis, rectus abdominis and the internal and external obliques) are utilized in times of active expiration to push the diaphragm upwards, reducing the volume of the thoracic cavity and forcefully expelling air. This can be observed clinically when the abdominal wall visibly contracts and pulls in the lower part of the rib cage during expiration.

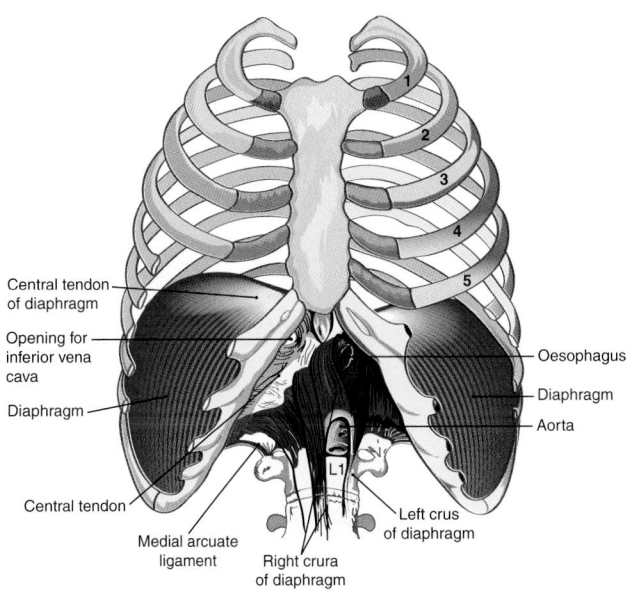

Figure 7.17 The diaphragm as seen from the front. Note the openings in the vertebral portion for the inferior vena cava, oesophagus and aorta.

Evidence-based approaches

Principles of care

Many people suffering with long-term breathlessness adopt positions that will best facilitate their inspiratory muscles. The aim of any position is to restore a normal rate and depth of breathing in order to achieve efficient but adequate ventilation (see Box 7.2).

Preprocedural considerations

The general procedural considerations mentioned earlier in the chapter are all relevant to this section. However, there are also some other general principles that need to be considered for these patients.

Box 7.2 Positioning to minimize the work of breathing

There are certain resting positions that can help reduce the work of breathing, as shown in Figure 7.19.

1 High side-lying (see Figure 7.19a).
2 Forward lean sitting (see Figure 7.19b).
3 Relaxed sitting (see Figure 7.19c).
4 Forward lean standing (see Figure 7.19d).
5 Relaxed standing (see Figure 7.19e).

These positions serve to:

■ support the body, reducing the overall use of postural muscle and oxygen requirements
■ improve lung volumes
■ optimize the functional positions of the respiratory (thoracic and abdominal) muscles (Dean 1985).

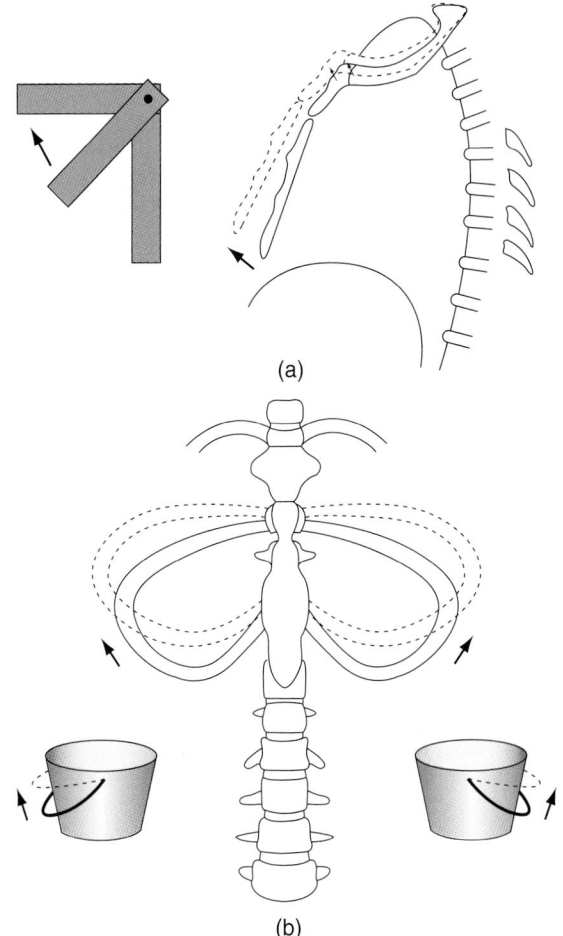

(a)

(b)

Figure 7.18 Movement of chest wall on inspiration. (a) The upper ribs move upwards and forwards, increasing the anteroposterior dimension of the thoracic cavity. As a result, the sternum also rises forwards. (b) The lower ribs move like bucket handles, increasing the lateral dimension of the thorax. Reproduced with kind permission from Aggarwal and Hunter (2007).

Pharmacological support

Administering nebulizers

If prescribed, administering nebulizers approximately 15 minutes prior to moving will help to dilate the airways, making breathing more efficient and ensuring better oxygen delivery to the blood.

Oxygen requirements

Repositioning can cause a temporary fall in oxygen saturation or a raised respiratory rate. If the fall is greater than 4% or recovery time is protracted, supplemental oxygen delivery may be required for several minutes before, during and after moving.

303

(a)

(b)

(c)

(d)

(e)

Figure 7.19 Positions to support breathing.

Non-pharmacological support
Pacing

It may be necessary to allow the patient time to rest during the process of getting into a new position to limit the exertion and therefore increased respiratory demand.

Environment

A breathless patient may be anxious about carrying out a task that could exacerbate their breathlessness. By reducing additional stressors such as noise and a cluttered environment, this can be minimized.

Positioning to maximize the drainage of secretions

Anatomy and physiology

The trachea branches into two bronchi, one to each lung (Figure 7.20). Each main bronchus then divides into lobar and then segmental bronchi (upper, middle and lower on the right, upper and lower on the left), each one branching into two or more segmental bronchi with a smaller and smaller diameter, until they reach the bronchioles and finally alveoli.

The walls of the airways are lined with epithelium which contains cilia. The cilia constantly beat in a co-ordinated movement, propelling the mucus layer towards the pharynx. The mucus layer traps any dust particles/foreign objects which can then be transported along the 'mucociliary escalator', an important part of the lungs' defence mechanism. An increased volume of mucus is produced in response to airway irritation and in some disease states.

A reduced ability to effectively remove this mucus can lead to an increased bacterial load and therefore may compromise respiratory functioning by causing airway obstruction. Consequently leading to segmental atelectasis or lobar collapse, long term this can lead to chronic inflammation and airway destruction.

Preprocedural considerations

The general principles of care mentioned earlier in the chapter and the preprocedural considerations to minimize the

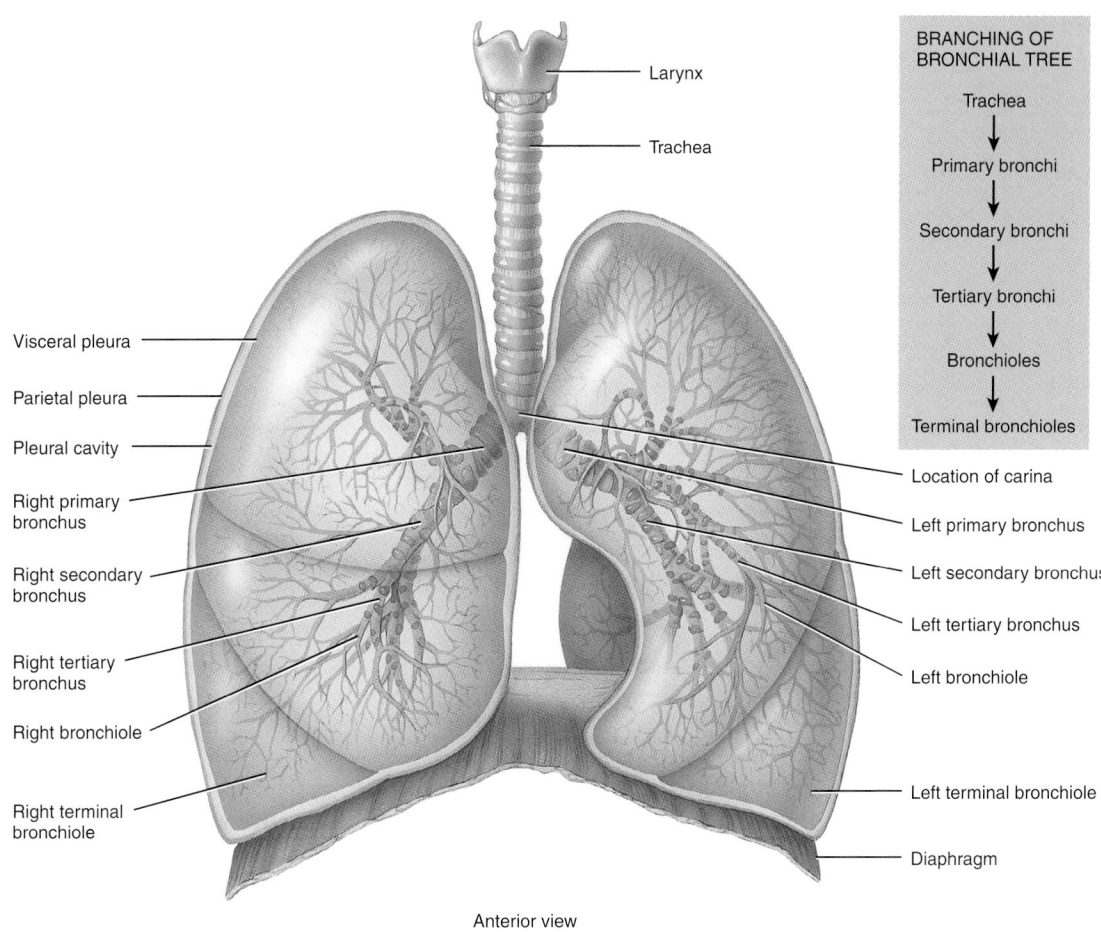

Figure 7.20   The bronchial tree. Reproduced from Tortora and Derrickson (2009).

Procedure guideline 7.11 Positioning to maximize the drainage of secretions

Equipment

- Pillows/towels
- Sliding sheets/manual handling equipment if indicated following risk assessment in accordance with local manual handling policy
- Bed extension for tall patients

Preprocedure

Action	Rationale
1 Explain and discuss the procedure with the patient.	To ensure that the patient understands the procedure and gives their valid consent (NMC 2008, C).
2 Wash hands thoroughly or use an alcohol-based handrub.	To reduce the risk of contamination and cross-infection (Fraise and Bradley 2009, E).
3 Ensure that the bed is at the optimum height for handlers. If two handlers are required try to match handlers' heights as far as possible.	To minimize the risk of injury to the practitioner (Smith 2005, C).

(Continued)

Procedure guideline 7.11 (*Continued*)

Procedure	
4 Auscultate the chest.	To determine most affected area and therefore area to be treated. E
5 Position patient with segment to be drained uppermost.	Use gravity to facilitate drainage of secretions. Bronchopulmonary segment needs to be perpendicular to gravity. E
6 Leave to drain for 10 minutes if tolerated.	Suggested optimal duration (Fink 2002, R).
7 Physiotherapy techniques such as breathing/manual techniques may be carried out whilst in position.	To further assist the removal of secretions. E

Problem-solving table 7.4 **Prevention and resolution (Procedure guideline 7.11)**

Problem	Cause	Prevention	Action
Reduced oxygen saturations. This will be evident by looking at the saturation level on the oximeter* if present or observation of patient colour and work of breathing	Movement causes an increase in oxygen demand from the tissues. If this is not matched by adequate delivery then saturation levels will be lower Positions to drain secretions may not comply with positions to match V/Q	Preoxygenate prior to movement if patient is requiring high levels of oxygen or is ventilated	Increase the concentration of oxygen delivered until satisfactory saturations are achieved. Aim to reduce this as much as possible but consider that a higher level of oxygen may be required in the altered position If this is still not tolerated, return the patient to previous position
Large volume of secretions/ increased audible secretions/ coughing	Drainage of distal secretions into more proximal airway	Clear airway prior to movement Regular airway clearance following movement	Clear airway of any secretions either by coughing or suctioning

work of breathing are all relevant to this section. However, there are also some other preprocedural considerations that need to be taken into account for these patients.

Non-pharmacological support
Humidification

Drainage of secretions will be optimized if the patient and therefore the mucus layer and cilia are well hydrated. This can be ensured by adequate humidification (see Chapter 10).

The problem-solving, postprocedural considerations and complications in general principles of moving and positioning patients and respiratory compromise also apply to these patients. Refer to relevant sections in this chapter.

Moving and positioning the patient with neurological impairment

The general principles of positioning discussed earlier can be applied for this group of patients. However, the complexity of these patients highlights the difficulty of a uniform approach to overall management. Therefore, this section will look at some of the variations in presentation of this patient group and suggest some principles to be considered when positioning these patients.

This will cover recommendations for assisting patients presenting with physical neurological symptoms affecting their central nervous systems (CNS) and peripheral nervous systems (PNS) as a consequence of their disease or treatment itself. These may include:

- hemiparesis or monoparesis*
- hemi-aesthesia*
- peripheral motor/sensory neuropathies*
- spinal cord compression/injury.

Definitions

Neurological insult through disease or illness can cause damage to patients' central, peripheral and autonomic nervous systems, affecting the relay of messages to and from nerves to enable normal motor and sensory function. Sequelae associated with neurological deficit include altered tone, abnormal movement patterns, sensory, cognitive, perceptual* and speech and language problems.

Anatomy and physiology

The nervous system is a complex organ which allows us to automatically and volitionally adjust to internal and external environments. This maintains equilibrium of body systems and enables effective, efficient motor and cognitive function. It can be considered in three main areas: central nervous system, peripheral nervous system and autonomic nervous system (ANS). The CNS consists of two parts: the brain and spinal cord. The brain consists of four lobes (frontal, temporal, parietal and occipital), the midbrain, pons, medulla oblongata and cerebellum. Each has individual and joint roles, and interconnects with the others via a complex system of pathways producing automatic and volitional movement and cognitive function. These connect with every part of the body via the PNS, consisting of cranial and spinal nerves which carry motor and sensory (afferent) fibres. The ANS, made up of sympathetic and parasympathetic components, regulates structures not under conscious control, for example arterial blood pressure, gastrointestinal motility and secretion, urinary bladder emptying, sweating, body temperature, activated mainly by centres in the brainstem, spinal cord and hypothalamus. Illness, disease and/or side-effects of treatment can affect any or all of these systems which will have implications for clinical practice and patient management.

Related theory

Disease or damage to the central or peripheral nervous system can lead to temporary or permanent complex physical, cognitive, psychological and psychosocial problems (Brada 1995, Ellison and Love 1997, Guerrero 1998, Kirshblum *et al.* 2001, Lindsay *et al.* 2004, Tookman *et al.* 2004). These may include:

- weakness: unilateral, bilateral or global
- altered tone
- sensory changes
- balance problems
- perceptual problems
- visual problems
- cognitive problems
- dysphagia*

Box 7.3 The physical benefits of movement

- Sensorimotor appreciation.
- Posture and balance control.
- Maintenance of joint and soft tissue range of movement.
- Maximization of functional independence.
- Minimization of tonal changes such as spasticity (Hawkins *et al.* 1999).
- Cardiorespiratory fitness (Convertino *et al.* 1997).

- dysphasia*
- behavioural changes
- autonomic dysfunction
- dysarthria*.

If a person with a neurological presentation is unable to move, they are deprived of the physical benefits of movement (see Box 7.3).

Effective management of patients with neurological impairment requires holistic assessment including consideration of altered tone, abnormal patterns of movement, abnormal reflex activity and joint protection.

Abnormal reflex activity

For the patient with neurological deficit moving and positioning can help to manage the positional influences of unwanted reflex activity for those with altered tone (Davies 1985, Edwards 2002a, Jackson 1998, Stokes 2004). Positions suggested relate to the desire to avoid the development of abnormal patterns of movement associated with altered tone through minimizing the influence of primitive developmental reflexes (Bobath 1990). The three reflexes whose 'release' can be influenced are: (i) the tonic labyrinthine reflex; (ii) the symmetrical tonic neck reflex; and (iii) the asymmetrical tonic neck reflex (Davies 1985, Davies 2000, Jackson 1998). Davies (2000) describes these primitive reflexes as follows.

The tonic labyrinthine reflex is evoked by changes in the position of the head in space, originating at otolithic organs of the labyrinths and believed to be integrated at brainstem levels. In supine, extensor tone increases throughout the body with resultant extension of head, spine and limb extension and shoulder retraction. In prone, flexor tone* increases throughout the body. This may only be seen as a reduction in extensor tone* in a patient with severe spasticity. The influence of head position relative to the body will also be noticed in sitting or standing and may affect functional movement or position.

The symmetrical tonic neck reflex is a proprioceptive reflex, elicited by stretching of the muscles and joints of the neck. When the head extends, extensor tone in the arms and flexor tone in the legs increase. When the head is flexed, the extensor tone in the lower limbs increases, with more flexor tone in the arms. This position can be seen where the patient sits unsupported or is half lying in bed with their head flexed; their affected leg extends and affected arm

307

flexes more. This can also be seen when a patient is sitting unsupported in a chair or wheelchair.

The asymmetrical tonic neck reflex is elicited as a proprioceptive response from the muscles of the joints and neck. Extensor tone increases in the limbs on the same side to which the head is turned. The limbs on the occipital side show an increase in flexor tone. Patients who have poor mobility dependent on a wheelchair may have an increase in lower limb flexor tone on their weak side as well as affecting their arm. Here, a flexion contracture of the knee may develop, requiring effective management strategies recommended by therapists following individual patient assessment.

Professionals agree that positioning is a key element of rehabilitation and management of patients with neurological deficit (Bobath 1990, Carter and Edwards 2002, Davies 1985, Hawkins *et al.* 1999, Lynch and Grisogono 1991, Raine *et al.* 2009). An optimal position is not always possible due to variables such as the patient's medical condition and presence of contractures (Edwards 1998). There appears to be an overall lack of consensus in clinicians' actual practice regarding the key components of the positions necessary to limit the onset of spasticity and unwanted patterns of movement (Chatterton *et al.* 2001, Jackson 1998, Mee and Bee 2007). Prevention of complications is an important aim (Bobath 1990, Carter and Edwards 2002, Davies 1985, Lynch and Grisogono 1991, Mee and Bee 2007, Raine *et al.* 2009). Davies (1985, 2000) describes positioning for stroke patients and urges the avoidance of flat supine positioning due to its influence on the tonic neck and labyrinthine reflexes potentially resulting in an increase in inappropriate extensor activity throughout the body. Edwards (1998) recommends a variety of postures especially for patients with hypertonus.

A survey of physiotherapists identified that the most common aims of positioning for patients with stroke were modulation of muscle tone (93%), prevention of damage to affected limbs (92%) and supporting and stabilizing body segments (91%) (Chatterton *et al.* 2001). Expert opinion identifies that these factors promote recovery where recovery is likely (Barnes 2001, Edwards 1998, Hawkins *et al.* 1999, Pope 2002).

Altered tone and abnormal patterns of movement

Tone is defined clinically as 'the resistance that is encountered when the joint of a relaxed patient is moved passively' (Britton 1998). Alterations in tone will affect functional recovery in patients with neurological problems and require careful management. This can be through positioning, splinting if required and oral and focal pharmacological intervention (Barnes 2008).

Increased tone and spasticity are disorders of spinal proprioceptive reflexes. Spasticity is defined as:

a motor disorder characterised by a velocity dependent increase in tonic stretch reflexes (muscle tone) with exaggerated tendon jerks, resulting from hyperexcitabil-

ity of the stretch reflex, as one component of the upper motor neurone syndrome.

(Barnes 2001, p.1)

Normal movement is dependent on a neuromuscular system that can receive, integrate and respond appropriately to multiple intrinsic and extrinsic stimuli. Where this is altered through CNS or PNS disease, abnormal movement patterns will exist which will affect patients functionally. Key components include:

- normal postural tone
- reciprocal innervation of muscles
- sensory: motor feedback and feedforward mechanism
- balance reactions (Edwards 2002b)
- biomechanical properties of muscle (Edwards 1998).

The influence of altered tone and abnormal patterns of movement is key to therapeutic theories regarding the recovery of motor control in patients with neurological problems. Patients may attempt to perform functional skills as prerequisites of activities of daily living, but without appropriate background postural tone and normal properties of muscle, these movements will be performed in an abnormal way.

Joint protection

Positioning is suggested as a strategy to prevent hemiplegic shoulder pain and to prevent loss of range of movement (Ada *et al.* 2005, Dean *et al.* 2000, Kaplan 1995). This aims to prevent the patient's functional deterioration (Gloag 1985). Dean *et al.* (2000) identified that these complications often prevent a patient's full participation in rehabilitation, contributing to poor upper limb functional outcome. Several factors were described for this.

- Glenohumeral subluxation due to lack of muscular activity around the shoulder.
- Trauma to the shoulder complex through unsuitable exercise.
- Trauma through inappropriate handling of the patient by staff during transfers.

Dean *et al.* (2000) acknowledged that consistency in education was essential for these common problems. Ada *et al.* (2005) recommended that patients with little upper limb function in the early stages after a stroke undergo a programme of positioning of the affected shoulder. Their study showed statistical significance in maintaining shoulder range when compared with patients who received standard upper limb care of arm support and exercise only. Such specific joint positioning requires assessment by the physiotherapist for each individual patient.

Soft tissue changes and contractures

With increased tone, joint range and subsequent function are at risk. Restriction in the range of movement is not always simply through increased tone of the relevant muscles. The surrounding soft tissues, tendons, ligaments and the joints themselves can develop changes leading to an increased likelihood of them being maintained in a shortened position (Barnes 2008); a secondary biomechanical component of spasticity is often seen in patients with functional mobility problems. Adaptation of the mechanical properties of muscle also contributes to increased tone in patients with hypertonia (O'Dwyer *et al.* 1996). It is possible, but not proven, that maintaining a joint through a full range of movement may prevent the longer term development of soft tissue contractures (Barnes 2008).

Evidence-based approaches

Principles of care

The general principles of care mentioned earlier in the chapter are all relevant to this section. However, there are also some other principles that need to be considered for these patients. For those with acute and long-standing neurological issues, principles of moving and positioning can be applied at any time along their treatment trajectory for those with rehabilitation potential, deteriorating function and those requiring palliative management. Posture and postural control will be affected in these patients. 'Posture' describes the biomechanical alignment and orientation of the body to the environment (Shumway-Cook and Woollacott 2001), 'postural control' provides orientation and balance (Lundy-Ekman 2007). Positional influences in the patient with neurological impairment may affect spinal, pelvic and shoulder girdle alignment with risk of soft tissue shortening due to the following potential problems.

- Flattened lumbar spine.
- Extended thoracic spine.
- Pelvis tilted backwards.
- Retracted hip.
- Elevated shoulder, retracted scapula.
- Feet tend toward plantarflexion (Shumway-Cook and Woollacott 2001).

Therefore, additional considerations should be applied for the neurological patient with severe tonal management issues. These should always be discussed with the physiotherapist.

Preprocedural considerations

The general principles of moving and positioning patients can be applied when assisting those with complex neurological impairment. Patients with neurological impairment may be able to participate in usual transfer techniques but risk assessment will consider several additional factors. This section will identify considerations for staff in their decision making. Where there is any doubt when moving patients with complex needs, guidance should be sought from a physiotherapist/occupational therapist.

Patients with neurological deficits may vary in their presentation on a daily basis. The additional considerations for positioning and moving patients with neurological impairment are listed in Box 7.4.

Box 7.4 Considerations for moving patients with neurological impairment

- Variations in tone, for example flaccidity or spasm.
- Cognitive problems including attention deficit.
- Behavioural problems.
- Communication problems.
- Variable client ability, for example 'on/off' periods for patients with Parkinson's disease and patients with changing presentations, for example multiple sclerosis, degenerative conditions.
- Sensory and proprioceptive problems, including reduced midline awareness.
- Pain/altered sensitivity.
- Decreased balance and co-ordination.
- Visual disturbance.
- Varying ability over 24 hours, for example, fatigue at the end of the day, at night.
- Effects of medication.
- Varying capability of the patient according to the experience and/or skill mix of handler(s).
- Post surgery, presence of tracheotomy, chest and other drains.
- Traumatic and non-traumatic spinal injury – risk of spinal instability.
- Importance of maintaining privacy and dignity.

(CSP 2008, p.26)

Equipment

Splints and orthoses

In advanced spasticity, it is often the soft tissue changes that contribute most to subsequent disability, such as limb deformity leading to poor function and problems with regard to hygiene, positioning, transferring and feeding and making the individual prone to pressure sores (O'Dwyer *et al.* 1996). Therapeutic splinting may maintain and assist function (Edwards 1998, Raine *et al.* 2009, Shumway-Cook and Woollacott 2001).

An orthosis or splint is an external device designed to apply, distribute or remove forces to or from the body in a controlled manner in order to control body motion and prevent alteration in the shape of body tissues (see Figure 7.12 and Figure 7.13). The aim is to compensate for weak or absent muscle function or to resist unopposed action of spastic muscle (Edwards and Charlton 1996). They may help gain alignment for proximal and truncal activity (Raine *et al.* 2009) and enable more balanced and efficient walking (Hesse 2003). As with all therapeutic interventions, they should only be used after detailed assessment and based on sound clinical reasoning.

Seating

Appropriate seating is also advocated as an adjunct to management for effective postural support (Kirkwood and Bardslay 2001, Pope 1996, 2002, Raine *et al.* 2009).

Occupational therapists and physiotherapists will consider this for management of patients with complex needs.

Environment and positioning

Problems of perception* are considered to be one of the main factors limiting functional motor recovery following stroke (Baer and Durward 2004). These can affect patients with disease or illness affecting their CNS. Here, the patient fails to respond appropriately to stimuli presented on their hemiplegic side, the contralateral side to the brain lesion (Baer and Durward 2004, Lindsay *et al.* 2004). Environmental factors such as correct positioning are essential for ensuring optimal level of function for each individual (Edwards 2002a). Clinical management strategies include:

- addressing the patient from the affected side
- deliberate placement of items such as drinks on that side

- advice to carers to position themselves on the patient's affected side whilst talking to them in order to orientate them to their affected side
- positioning the patient on their affected side, enabling function with their sound side.

Limited evidence exists to suggest the benefit of these approaches (Baer and Durward 2004). However, it is recognized as a useful treatment adjunct for these patients, through promotion of sensory awareness/appreciation, including perception and body image and enabling function (Bobath 1990, Davies 1985, Edwards and Carter 2002, Grieve and Gnanasekaran 2008, Lynch and Grisogono 1991, Raine *et al.* 2009).

Rehabilitation opportunity

Patients with neurological illness or disease present with an assortment of clinical symptoms. Positioning can assist in their holistic management and allow future opportunity for rehabilitation where their illness or disease allows.

Procedure guideline 7.12 Positioning the neurological patient with tonal problems

Essential equipment

- Pillows or towels (as guidance or basic positioning)

Optional equipment

- Hand/foot resting splint if required
- Resting splint if required

Medicinal products

- Analgesia as required
- Antispasmodics as required

Preprocedure

Action	Rationale
1 Explain the procedure to the patient.	To ensure that the patient understands the procedure and gives their valid consent (NMC 2008, C).
2 Wash hands thoroughly or use an alcohol-based handrub.	To reduce the risk of contamination and cross-infection (Fraise and Bradley 2009, E).
3 Ensure that the bed is at the optimum height for handlers. If two handlers are required try to match handlers' heights as far as possible.	To minimize the risk of injury to the practitioner (Smith 2005, C).

Procedure

4 Follow basic advice for positioning the patient in supine, side-lying and sitting in bed as described in the above procedure guidelines for positioning patients.	To promote alignment of body segments for patients with high or low tone due to abnormal influences of primitive developmental reflexes resulting in asymmetrical posture (Bobath 1990, E; Davies 1985, E; Edwards and Carter 2002, E; Lynch and Grisogono 1991, R4).
	To ensure patient comfort. E

5a Consider and apply possible modifications as specified below for the supine (see Action Figure 5a1(a)).

- Place pillow under hemiplegic hip for alignment.
- Place additional pillows or wedge under knees and/or head.
- Place pillow to support feet in neutral/plantargrade position:
  - Apply foot resting splint (ankle foot orthosis (AFO) (see Action Figure 5a2 and Figure 7.14) to weak foot and ankle if recommended. NB: Ensure the splint is fitted correctly
  - Place pillow under weak arm.
- Apply resting splint for hand/forearm if required.

To control pelvic and spinal alignment. E

To optimize patient comfort. E

To maintain joint and soft tissue range (ACPIN 1998, C; E; Barnes 2001, R4; Edwards 1998, E).

To maintain soft tissue and joint range (Edwards 1998, E; Shumway-Cook and Woollacott 2001, E).

5b Consider and apply possible modifications as specified below for side-lying (see Action Figure 5a1(b)).

- Place pillow under head and in front of trunk.
- Place pillow in front of trunk.
- Place patient's affected arm on pillow. Apply resting splint for hand/forearm if required.

To support the patient's affected shoulder and upper limb due to a risk of trauma, pain, muscle and soft tissue shortening (Ada *et al.* 2005, R2b, E; Dean *et al.* 2000, R2b).

To reduce the influence of primitive developmental reflexes and asymmetrical posturing of head and trunk in patients with high or low tone. E

May be effective in maintaining opposing trunk muscles. E

To maintain soft tissue and joint range (Barnes 2001, R4; Edwards 1998, E; Shumway-Cook and Woollacott 2001, E).

311

Postprocedure

The general principles of care mentioned earlier in the chapter are all relevant to this section.

6 For patients requiring use of an external splint to maintain joint position and range, skin condition must be closely monitored.

To monitor skin integrity and pressure care. E

Action Figure 5a1   Positioning the patient with neurological weakness. (a) Supine: affected arm supported on pillow. (b) Side-lying: affected arm supported on pillow.

(a)

(b)

Action Figure 5a2   (a) Ankle foot orthosis. (b) Ankle foot orthosis *in situ*.

Problem-solving table 7.5 Prevention and resolution (Procedure guideline 7.12)

Problem	Cause	Prevention	Action
Unable to position patient's legs in bed due to increased tone – legs remain 'stiff'	Abnormal tone (high or low) affecting limbs secondary to CNS involvement (cortical/spinal)	Assess for other noxious stimuli which may increase tone in patients with CNS disease Ensure pain control Ensure bowel management Ensure effective catheter drainage Assess for infection	Use leg flexion position in bed control **And/or** Position small folded pillow/rolled towel under patient's knees Avoid contact of patient's feet against end of bed – this can stimulate increased tone in legs Liaise with physiotherapist (PT)
Unable to achieve comfortable position for patient with CNS involvement Patient's limbs may demonstrate persistent increased tone despite positioning	Possible causes: ■ inadequate pain control ■ inadequate antiepilepsy medication ■ other noxious stimuli	Assess for other noxious stimuli which may increase tone in patients with CNS disease Ensure pain control Ensure bowel management Assess for infection	Reassess patient Ensure adequate analgesia Ensure adequate antiepilepsy medication Possibly a medical review required

Patient's arm remains flexed/unable to position in bed	Abnormal tone (high or low) affecting limbs due to CNS involvement		Position small flat pillow under patient's affected arm to provide support **Or** Position small flat pillow across patient's abdomen to support both upper limbs Use of resting splint if indicated for patient management – liaise with PT and/ or OT
Patent is unaware of affected side	Sensory/motor inattention		Ensure patient's environment is made available to them Ensure affected limbs are supported by pillows/folded/ rolled towel as required (refer to positioning for patients with neurological deficits)

313

Postprocedural considerations

The general principles of care mentioned earlier in the chapter are all relevant to this section. However, there are also some other general principles that need to be considered for these patients.

Ongoing care

Where the patient requires use of an external splint to maintain joint position and joint range, skin integrity must be closely monitored (see Chapter 9), including skin/pressure care, and any adverse effects treated accordingly following assessment.

Documentation

The general principles of care mentioned earlier in the chapter are all relevant to this section. However, in addition, instructions regarding the appropriate use of splints should be clearly documented in the patient's care plan including application, removal and timing of wear.

Education of patient and relevant others

The patient and carer(s) should be given written information regarding use of any splints or orthotics including application, removal and timing of wear according to the therapist's advice. Environmental and clinical management strategies should be explained to the patient and carers for effective holistic management.

Moving and positioning of the patient with actual or suspected spinal cord compression (SCC) or spinal cord injury (SCI)

Definition

Spinal cord compression or injury is when the function of the spinal cord becomes compromised.

Anatomy and physiology

The spinal cord is about 45 cm in length and extends from the base of the brain, surrounded by the vertebrae, to the pelvis. Nerves situated within the spinal cord (upper motor neurones: UMNs) carry the messages between the brain and spinal nerves along the spinal tract. Spinal nerves branch out from the spinal cord to the other parts of the body (lower motor neurones: LMNs). These exit and enter at each vertebral level to communicate with specific areas of the body.

Following damage to the spinal cord through traumatic vertebral displacement or tumour/oedema growth, 'spinal shock'* may occur (see Complications). Within the confines of the vertebral canal, the oedematous cord is compressed against the surrounding bone. A complex series of physiological and biochemical reactions occur due to resulting oedema and vascular damage. Circulation of blood and oxygen is disrupted; ischaemic tissue necrosis follows with an immediate cessation of conductivity within the spinal cord neurones. This can persist for 2–6 weeks (SIA 2000).

Related theory

Spinal cord compression (Figure 7.21) or injury encompasses the following.

- *Traumatic spinal cord injury (SCI).* This is damage or trauma to the spinal cord that results in loss of or impaired function causing reduced mobility or feeling.

Figure 7.21 Spinal cord compression (metastatic).

Common causes include trauma (for example, car accident, gunshot, falls, sports injuries) or disease (for example, transverse myelitis, polio, spina bifida, Friedreich's ataxia). The spinal cord does not have to be severed in order for a loss of functioning to occur. It is estimated that 500–700 people sustain traumatic SCI in the UK each year (SIA 2000).

- *Primary/benign spinal cord compression (PSCC)*
- *Degenerative conditions.* These include osteoporosis and spondylosis (Mann *et al.* 2000).
- *Haematoma* (Kalina *et al.* 1995)
- *Primary tumours.* These include intradural extramedullary tumours (neurofibromas, meningiomas: Lohani and Sharma 2004), intramedullary tumours (ependymomas) and low-grade astrocytomas (Britton and Ng 1998).
- *Metastatic spinal cord compression (MSCC).* This is an oncological emergency defined as compression of the dural sac and its contents (spinal cord and cauda equina) by an extradural mass (Loblaw *et al.* 2003). Causes include:
  - direct soft tissue extension from vertebral bony metastases
  - tumour growth through intravertebral foramina (e.g. from retroperitoneal tumours or paravertebral lymphadenopathy)
  - compression due to bony collapse
  - intramedullary metastases (rare).

  The true incidence of MSCC is unknown due to current restrictions in detection rate and coding systems in the UK (NICE 2008). Postmortem evidence indicates it is present in 5–10% of patients with advanced cancer.

Classification

SCC is classified as either stable or unstable.

- *Stable:* this is where spinal alignment is intact with no further risk of progression of neurological symptoms as the spine is still able to maintain and distribute weight appropriately.
- *Unstable:* this is where spinal fractures/lesions pose a risk of spinal cord injury and potentially irreversible neurological symptoms due to (potential) abnormal movement at the fracture site.

Additionally, it can be further classified as complete or incomplete.

- *Complete spinal cord injury:* refers to when the cord 'loses all descending neuronal control below the level of the lesion' (Lundy-Ekman 2007, p.230).
- *Incomplete spinal cord injury:* refers to when 'the function of some ascending and/or descending fibres is preserved within the spinal cord' (Lundy-Ekman 2007, p.230).

Clinical presentation

Clinical presentation of SCC is dependent on the location of the compression, the duration of its presence and consequently the level of neural function that is spared. The patient presents with loss of all voluntary movement and sensation below the level of the injury/lesion. There is also progressive loss of sympathetic and parasympathetic activity throughout the area (SIA 2000).

In SCC, early diagnosis is crucial in order to at best prevent and otherwise minimize irreversible neurological damage.

Common symptoms include:

- radicular* pain
- limb weakness
- difficulty walking
- sensory loss
- cauda equina signs (saddle anaesthesia, bladder or bowel dysfunction)
- sexual dysfunction (NICE 2008).

Stable spine

The general principles of care mentioned earlier in the chapter are all relevant to this group of patients. However, patients need to be assessed for adequate pain control prior to moving and positioning, and care should be taken to avoid excessive rotation of the spine when turning.

Unstable spine

For patients with an unstable spine or severe mechanical pain suggestive of spinal instability, specific instructions for moving must be followed until bony and neurological stability are radiologically confirmed (NICE 2008, SIA 2000). This is to ensure spinal alignment and reduce the risk of further spinal damage (NICE 2008, SIA 2000).

'Careful handling, positioning and turning can prevent secondary cord damage during transfer and movements for patients with spinal cord injury' (SIA 2000). Procedure guidelines 7.1, 7.3 and 7.12 are relevant to moving patients with metastatic spinal cord compression. However, this patient group will require additional considerations to enable safe practice without compromising their clinical condition. These may include:

- lateral surface transfer, for example bed to trolley using PAT lateral transfer board. Manual support of the patient's head and neck should be applied for any flat surface transfer (SIA 2000). This ensures appropriate spinal alignment and patient comfort
- log rolling for personal/pressure care for patients with unstable SCC.

Evidence-based approaches
Rationale

When moving and turning the patient with confirmed/suspected spinal instability who is being nursed flat, log rolling

must be used. This is a technique to maintain neutral spinal alignment. It is an essential method to enable the patient to use a slipper pan and also to maintain pressure areas through regular turning every 2–3 hours (NICE 2008). Patients should only be moved with adequate numbers of staff who have been fully trained in moving patients with spinal cord compression/injury. Differing methods are recommended dependent on the level of the lesion/injury (SIA 2000).

- Cervical lesions (T4 and above):
  - pelvic twist for pressure care
  - log roll with five people required.
- Thoracolumbar lesions:
  - log roll with four people required (SIA 2000).

Contraindications

The pelvic twist is contraindicated in the presence of thoracolumbar or pelvic injury/damage and pre-existing spinal deformity or rigidity, for example ankylosing spondylitis (SIA 2000).

Principles of care

The general principles of care mentioned earlier in the chapter are all relevant to individuals with SCC. However, there are some other factors that need to be considered for these patients. Early and accurate diagnosis and, if appropriate, treatment is imperative to optimize neurological functioning. Timely referral to rehabilitation services is imperative for assessment, appropriate intervention and thorough discharge planning to enable smooth transition back into the community (CAT 2009, NICE 2008). Active rehabilitation may be postponed until the medical team has confirmed that the patient's spine is stable. However, there is a significant role for members of the rehabilitation team in the management of these patients in terms of:

- assessment of motor recovery
- minimizing further complications such as chest infections which may arise as a result of prolonged bed rest
- effective, co-ordinated discharge planning. The positioning and moving needs of these patients are often complex and so discharge planning may be lengthy and multifaceted, requiring ongoing support and rehabilitation in the community to optimize functional independence (Bray and Cooper 2004).

For patients with complex symptoms, e.g. spinal instability, weakness, sensory impairment, refer to the physiotherapist.

Preprocedural considerations

Patients may be able to assist with moving, positioning and transfers depending on:

- spinal stability
- pain

- level of lesion
- muscle power
- sensory impairment
- exercise tolerance
- patient confidence.

Implications for moving and positioning of early and accurate diagnosis and treatment for MSCC

The neurological status of the patient at the time of diagnosis is a significant prognostic factor for the functional outcome (Maranzano and Latini 1995, NICE 2008). Eighty percent of patients maintain or improve functional mobility if ambulatory compared to 10% if paraplegic* prior to treatment (Pigott *et al.* 1994). Therefore, it is essential that motor function is preserved through good handling prior to treatment; further cord damage may be provoked through inappropriate mobilization before, during and after treatment (NICE 2008). Until spinal stability is confirmed, patients with suspected SCC should be nursed flat to maintain neutral spinal alignment and minimize the risk of further damage (NICE 2008, SIA 2000).

Pain management – pharmacological and non-pharmacological

As already discussed, spinal and radicular pain can be an indicator of SCC in the first instance but in relation to moving and handling, it can also be suggestive of changes in neurology once gradual sitting and mobilization commence (NICE 2008). Implementation of a pain assessment chart can enable continuity of care, allowing accurate assessment and evaluation of all pharmacological (i.e. non-steroidal anti-inflammatory drugs, opiates, bisphosphonates and epidural) and non-pharmacological interventions (i.e. relaxation and therapeutic management).

Equipment
Spinal brace/cervical collar

Where there is confirmed or risk of spinal instability due to vertebral collapse, patients will require external spinal support. This may be in the form of a spinal brace or collar. A properly fitted hard collar (Figure 7.22) must be used when there is suspicion of spinal instability (NICE 2008, SIA 2000). This is available from surgical appliances/

Figure 7.22 Hard collar *in situ.*

orthotic or some physiotherapy departments. Manufacturer's product details and care instructions are provided upon issue. Staff should be guided by medical advice and local policy.

Moving and handling aids

Patients may be able to assist with transfers using transfer boards, standing aids, mobility aids, frames, crutches and sticks. If they are unable to assist, there are a variety of moving and handling aids, for example lateral patient transfer boards, hoists and standing hoists, which maintain the safety of both the patient and the carer (HSE 1992). For lesions affecting cervical and thoracolumbar spine or where injuries make turning difficult, an electric turning bed can be used (SIA 2000).

Assessment and recording tools

The focus of an initial neurological assessment is to establish the level of cord injury and act as a baseline against which future improvements or declines may be compared (SIA 2000). Standard assessments, including pain, motor and sensory charts, should be used as a baseline and updated with any change in a patient's presentation. Assessments will depend on local policy and may include:

- ASIA Spinal Cord Injury Classification (ASIA 2001)
- Spinal Cord Independence Measure (SCIM III) (Catz and Itzkovich 2007, Catz *et al.* 2007, Itzkovich *et al.* 2007)
- Pain assessment chart, for example Visual Analogue Scale (Tiplady *et al.* 1998)
- manual handling risk assessment.

Procedure guideline 7.13 Log rolling for suspected/confirmed cervical spinal instability

See Figure 7.23

Essential equipment

- Pillows
- Collar or spinal brace
- A minimum of five people are needed to move a person with cervical spinal instability

Optional equipment

- Slipper pan
- Clean sheets
- Hygiene equipment
- Continence pads
- Pressure care

Preprocedure

Action	Rationale
1 Explain and discuss the procedure with the patient.	To ensure that the patient understands the procedure and gives their valid consent (NMC 2008, C).
2 Wash hands thoroughly or use an alcohol-based handrub.	To reduce the risk of contamination and cross-infection (Fraise and Bradley 2009, E).
3 Ensure that the bed is at the optimum height for handlers. If two or more handlers are required try to match handlers' heights as far as possible.	To minimize the risk of injury to the practitioner (Smith 2005, C).
4 Ensure there are sufficient personnel available to assist with the procedure (minimum five for patients with cervical spinal instability).	Four staff to maintain spinal alignment and one to perform personal/pressure care check during the procedure (SIA 2000, C).

Procedure

5 Assess patient's motor and sensory function.	To provide a baseline to compare against after the procedure (SIA 2000, C).
6 Lead practitioner stabilizes the patient's neck, supporting the patient's head.	To co-ordinate and lead log roll. E To take responsibility for providing instructions and ensuring all other practitioners are ready before commencing the manoeuvre (SIA 2000, C).
7 Ideally, the lead practitioner's hands should offer support for the entire cervical curve from the base of the skull to C7.	To immobilize patient's head. E To ensure spinal alignment is monitored throughout the procedure (SIA 2000, C).
8 The second practitioner stands at the thorax. Position hands over the patient's lower back and shoulder.	To ensure the lower spine remains aligned (SIA 2000, C).
9 The third practitioner stands at the hip area. Place one hand on the patient's lower back and the other under the patient's upper thigh.	To prevent movement at thoracolumbar site (SIA 2000, C).
10 The fourth practitioner stands at the patient's lower leg. Place hands under knee and ankle.	To ensure the lower spine remains aligned (SIA 2000, C).
11 Ensure there is a fifth person standing on opposite side of bed.	To position the equipment or take care of hygiene needs. E To assess upper back and occiput. This needs to be carried out once a day to check pressure areas (SIA 2000, C).

(Continued)

Procedure guideline 7.13 *(Continued)*

12 The lead practitioner holding the head provides clear instructions to the team; for example, 'We will roll on three: One, two, three'.	To ensure co-ordinated approach to the move. E
13 Each practitioner remains in place whilst the necessary action is performed.	
14 The person holding the head then provides clear instructions to return to supine.	To complete the move. E
15 Additional stages of procedure in order to leave the patient in a lateral position.	
(a) All practitioners must stay in place until the practitioner holding the patient's head confirms neutral spine alignment.	To ensure the lower spine remains aligned (SIA 2000, C). To ensure patient comfort. E
(b) Position patient between 30° and 50° lateral tilt.	To ensure pressure care. E To prevent excessive pressure being exerted on lower trochanter (SIA 2000, C).
(c) The fifth person places pillow lengthwise behind patient from shoulder to hip.	To ensure the lower spine remains aligned (SIA 2000, C). To ensure patient comfort. E
(d) The fifth person places pillow under patient's upper thigh lengthwise from hip to foot.	To ensure the lower spine remains aligned (SIA 2000, C). To ensure patient comfort. E
(e) Fifth person places pillow between foot and end of bed.	To ensure the lower spine remains aligned (SIA 2000, C). To ensure patient comfort. E

Postprocedure

16 Reassess and record neurological symptoms.	To ensure clinical status maintained (SIA 2000, C).

Figure 7.23 Log rolling and positioning of the patient with spinal cord compression or injury. Note, in practice five people are needed for this manoeuvre. Reproduced with kind permission of the Spinal Injuries Association (2000).

Procedure guideline 7.14 Positioning for suspected/confirmed cervical spinal instability: pelvic twist to right

See Figure 7.24. This procedure is for cervical injuries only. It is contraindicated in the presence of thoracolumbar or pelvic trauma.

Essential equipment
- Collar or spinal brace
- Foam wedge or pillows

Optional equipment
- Equipment required for the purpose of the log roll, for example slipper pan, clean sheets, hygiene equipment, pads or pressure care

Preprocedure

Action	Rationale
1 Explain and discuss the procedure with the patient.	To ensure that the patient understands the procedure and gives their valid consent (NMC 2008, C).
2 Wash hands thoroughly or use an alcohol-based handrub.	To reduce the risk of contamination and cross-infection (Fraise and Bradley 2009, E).
3 Ensure that the bed is at the optimum height for handlers. If two handlers are required try to match handlers' heights as far as possible.	To minimize the risk of injury to the practitioner (Smith 2005, C).
4 Ensure there are five people available to assist with the procedure.	

Procedure

5 The lead practitioner stands at the head. Place hands firmly on patient's shoulders.	To take responsibility for providing instructions and ensuring all other practitioners are ready before commencing the manoeuvre. E To prevent movement of unstable cervical spine. E
6 A second practitioner positions themselves on the opposite side of the bed to which the patient will be turned.	
7 The third practitioner assists the second practitioner to lift the patient's leg to allow them to place their left hand under the leg to the right hip and their right hand under the patient's lumbar region.	To prevent an angle of more than 30°. E
8 The patient's left hip is then upwardly rotated by the second practitioner.	The second practitioner's hands provide a barrier against friction during the turn. E
9 Both the lead and second practitioners maintain their position whilst the third practitioner places a folded pillow beneath the patient's left buttock above the sacrum. Place additional pillow under upper buttock if required.	To prevent undue pressure risk to sacral/buttock region (SIA 2000, C).
10 Place two pillows below the patient's left leg.	To support the left leg. E
11 Position a pillow at the foot end of the bed.	Minimize the risk of foot drop (SIA 2000, C).

Postprocedure

12 In the event of a worsening of pain or neurological symptoms, reassessment by medical team.

320

Figure 7.24 Pelvic twist for patient with unstable cervical spine. Note, in practice five people are needed for this manoeuvre. Reproduced with kind permission of the Spinal Injuries Association (2000).

Procedure guideline 7.15 Log rolling for suspected/confirmed thoracolumbar spinal instability

Essential equipment

- Pillows
- Collar or spinal brace

Optional equipment

- Slipper pan
- Clean sheets
- Hygiene equipment
- Pads
- Pressure care

Preprocedure

Action	Rationale
1 Explain and discuss the procedure with the patient.	To ensure that the patient understands the procedure and gives their valid consent (NMC 2008, C).
2 Wash hands thoroughly or use an alcohol-based handrub.	To reduce the risk of contamination and cross-infection (Fraise and Bradley 2009, E).
3 Ensure that the bed is at the optimum height for patients or handlers. If two handlers are required try to match handlers' heights as far as possible.	To minimize the risk of injury to the practitioner (Smith 2005, C).

4 Ensure there are sufficient personnel available to assist with the procedure (minimum four for patients with thoracolumbar spinal instability).	Three staff to maintain spinal alignment and one to perform personal/pressure care check during the procedure (SIA 2000, C).
5 Assess patient's motor power and sensation as per local documentation agreement.	For assessment before and after log roll (SIA 2000, C).

Procedure

6 The lead practitioner stands at the patient's thorax and positions hands over the patient's lower back and shoulder.	To co-ordinate and lead log-roll. E To take responsibility for providing instructions and ensuring all other practitioners are ready before commencing the manoeuvre (SIA 2000, C). To ensure the lower spine remains aligned (SIA 2000, C).
7 The second practitioner stands at the hip area. Place one hand on the patient's lower back and the other under the patient's upper thigh.	To prevent movement at thoracolumbar site (SIA 2000, C).
8 The third practitioner stands at the patient's lower leg. Place hands under knee and ankle.	To ensure the lower spine remains aligned (SIA 2000, C).
9 Ensure there is a fourth person standing on opposite side of bed.	To position the equipment or take care of hygiene needs. E To assess upper back and occiput. E To be carried out once a day to check pressure areas (SIA, 2000 C).
10 The lead practitioner provides clear instructions to the team, for example 'We will roll on three: One, two, three'.	To ensure co-ordinated approach to the move. E
11 Each practitioner remains in place whilst the necessary action is performed.	
12 The person holding the head then provides clear instructions to return to supine.	To complete the move. E
13 Additional stages of procedure in order to leave the patient in a lateral position:	
(a) All practitioners must stay in place until the practitioner holding the patient's head confirms neutral spine alignment.	To ensure the lower spine remains aligned (SIA 2000, C). To ensure patient comfort. E
(b) Position patient between 30° and 50° lateral tilt.	To ensure pressure care. E To prevent excessive pressure being exerted on lower trochanter (SIA, 2000 C).
(c) The fourth person places pillow lengthwise behind patient from shoulder to hip.	To ensure the lower spine remains aligned (SIA 2000, C). To ensure patient comfort. E
(d) The fourth person places pillow under patient's upper thigh lengthwise from hip to foot.	To ensure the lower spine remains aligned (SIA 2000, C). To ensure patient comfort. E
(e) Fourth person places pillow between foot and end of bed.	To ensure the lower spine remains aligned (SIA 2000, C). To ensure patient comfort. E

Postprocedure

14 Reassess and record neurological symptoms. In the event of a worsening of pain or neurological symptoms, reassessment by medical team.	To ensure clinical status maintained (SIA 2000, C).

Procedure guideline 7.16 Early mobilization of the patient in bed

Essential equipment

- Collar/spinal brace for patients with unstable spine

Preprocedure

Action	Rationale
1 Explain and discuss the procedure with the patient.	To ensure that the patient understands the procedure and gives their valid consent (NMC 2008, C).
2 Wash hands thoroughly or use an alcohol-based handrub.	To reduce the risk of contamination and cross-infection (Fraise and Bradley 2009, E).
3 Ensure that the bed is at the optimum height for patients or handlers. If two handlers are required try to match handlers' heights as far as possible.	To minimize the risk of injury to the practitioner (Smith 2005, C).
4 Ensure there are sufficient personnel available to assist with the procedure (minimum four for patients with thoracolumbar spinal instability).	Three staff to maintain spinal alignment and one to perform personal/pressure care check during the procedure (SIA 2000, C).

Procedure

5 Assess stabilization of neurological symptoms.	To assess and evaluate clinical symptoms (NICE 2008, C).
6 Confirm mobilization status with medical staff.	
7 Ensure collar/brace is *in situ* for patients with unstable spine.	To ensure safety and stability (NICE 2008, C; SIA 2000, C).
8 Assist the patient to move from supine to sitting at 60° in bed over 3–4 hours.	
9 Perform regular close monitoring of blood pressure and neurological symptoms.	To assess and evaluate clinical symptoms (NICE 2008, C).
10 On confirmation of stable symptoms, assist patient to sit over edge of bed unsupported (see Procedure guideline 7.4).	To ensure safe handling (CSP 2008, C; HSE 1992, C).
11 Closely monitor any changes in symptoms.	To assess and evaluate clinical symptoms (NICE 2008, C).
12 On confirmation of stable symptoms, proceed to standard principles of mobilization (see Procedure guideline 7.6) and follow risk assessment consideration. Refer to the general principles for moving patients with neurological impairment.	To ensure safe handling (CSP 2008, C; HSE 1992, C).

Postprocedural considerations
Ongoing care

Reassessment by the medical team will be necessary in the event of an increase in pain or neurological symptoms.

Documentation

Any changes in (neurological) presentation and/or function must be documented both prior to and following any procedure.

Problem-solving table 7.6 Prevention and resolution (Procedure guidelines 7.13, 7.14, 7.15 and 7.16)

Problem	Cause	Prevention	Action
1 **Autonomic dysreflexia (mass reflex):** ■ Severe hypertension (abrupt rise in blood pressure) – systolic blood pressure can easily exceed 200 mmHg	Overstretching of bladder or rectum (urinary obstruction being the most common cause) Ingrown toenail or other painful stimuli Fracture (#) below level of lesion	Closely monitor urinary drainage Ensure effective bowel management regime	THIS IS A MEDICAL EMERGENCY: Identify or eliminate the most common (most lethal) cause of autonomic dysreflexia, which is non-drainage of urine
■ Bradycardia ■ 'Pounding' headache ■ Flushed or blotchy appearance of skin above the level of lesion ■ Profuse sweating above the level of lesion ■ Pallor below the level of lesion ■ Nasal congestion ■ Non-drainage of urine	Pressure sore/burn/scald/sunburn UTI/bladder spasm Renal or bladder calculi Visceral pain or trauma Pregnancy/delivery DVT/PE Severe anxiety/emotional distress (Lundy-Ekman 2007, SIA 2000)		If this is not the cause, then proceed to investigate alternative causes according to the causes list Reassure the patient throughout because anxiety increases the problem Remove the noxious stimulus, for example recatheterize immediately in the event of a blocked catheter Do not attempt a bladder washout because there is no guarantee that the fluid will be returned If possible, sit the patient up, or tilt the bed head-up, to induce some element of postural hypotension If symptoms remain unresolved after removal of noxious stimulus, or if the noxious stimulus cannot be identified, administer a proprietary chemical vasodilator, such as sublingual glyceryl trinitrate (GTN) or captopril 25 mg, sublingually. Nifedipine capsules, which were previously recommended for use in treating or preventing autonomic dysreflexia, are being withdrawn as they have been implicated in episodes of severe hypotension Record blood pressure and give further reassurance Monitor patient's condition Refer to local SIU for a specialist opinion/referral (SIA 2000)

323

(Continued)

Problem-solving table 7.6 (*Continued*)

Problem	Cause	Prevention	Action
2 **Orthostatic hypotension**	Loss of sympathetic vaso-constriction Loss of muscle-pumping action for blood return	Antiembolic stockings Careful assessment and monitoring during early mobilization/upright positional changes	Medical review
3 **Pain** Increased pain on movement to the extent that it is perceived by the patient as severe or does not reverse with rest	Potential extension of spinal cord compression	Ensure patients with unstable spine are moved appropriately	Nurse patient flat Reassess spinal stability prior to further movement (NICE 2008)
4 **Respiratory function** Reduced respiratory function in patient with cervical level SCC	Ineffective use of main respiratory muscles for effective ventilation for tetraplegic patients with lesions at C3 and above Most patients with tetraplegia* at C4 and above are able to make sufficient respiratory effort to avoid the need for mechanical ventilation. They will, however, require oxygen therapy (SIA 2000)	Avoid flat lying for long periods Ensure effective GI clearance/management – constipation and impaction of the bowel are a common complication of SCI management. This may place undue pressure on the diaphragm and lessen breathing space for effective respiratory function (SIA 2000) Closely monitor respiratory function, especially for patients undergoing radiotherapy as radiotherapy-induced oedema may cause symptoms to present at a higher cord level, impairing respiratory effort and function	Sit patient as upright as tolerated Ensure appropriate head/neck support as required – collar/cervicothoracic brace for unstable cervical spinal involvement
5 **Cardiac syncope***	A cervical collar applied too tightly may cause cardiac syncope (SIA 2000)	Ensure appropriate fit of cervical collar	Check cervical collar is not too tight Liaise with orthotist/PT
6 **Cardiac syncope:** 2° hypoxia following initial injury 2° turning to left side	Sustained hypoxia increases vagal activity with a high risk of cardiac syncope (SIA 2000) Turning the patient on to their left side for prolonged periods can increase vagal stimulation and may induce cardiac syncope This problem is not usual during routine turning or twisting to the left side for pressure relief	Avoid turning the patient on to their left side for prolonged periods (e.g. during a back wash or sheet change)	Administer high concentrations of oxygen and the use of atropine (SIA 2000) Measure dynamic trend of the patient's observations (SIA 2000) Turning the patient onto their right side does not have the same effect

Complications

There are a number of potential long-term complications that may occur during or after moving and positioning SCC/SCI patients. These are due to initial injury, the subsequent effects of changes in bowel and bladder functions and paralysis* associated with their disease or injury through autonomic and peripheral nervous system dysfunction, and those associated with bed rest.

1 *Spinal shock:* following initial injury/lesion development, spinal shock can occur due to the loss of vasomotor tone throughout the paralysed areas of the body.

This is most pronounced in cases of tetraplegia. Patients present with hypotension, bradycardia and poikilothermia*. This is due to a temporary/permanent loss of reflexes and muscle tone/control potentially leading to a compromised cardiac output. The patient must be closely monitored throughout and following any procedure or transfer, as recommended by medical staff.

2 *Autonomic dysfunction:* following injury/lesion development, secondary effects occur due to autonomic dysfunction, a potential complication for all patients with complete spinal cord lesions above the level of T6 (see Problem-solving table 7.6).

- *Autonomic dysreflexia:* a mass reflex due to excessive activity of the sympathetic nervous system elicited by noxious stimuli below the level of the lesion. **This is a medical emergency;** unresolved, it can cause fatal cerebral haemorrhage. Patients present with severe hypertension (abrupt rise in blood pressure), systolic blood pressure can easily exceed 200 mmHg, bradycardia, 'pounding' headache, flushed or blotchy appearance of skin above the level of lesion, profuse sweating above the level of lesion, pallor below the level of lesion, nasal congestion, non-drainage of urine.
- *Orthostatic hypotension:* extreme fall in blood pressure on assuming an upright position (systolic >20 mmHg, diastolic >10 mmHg). More common in tetraplegia than quadriplegia (Krassioukov *et al.* 2009, Lundy-Ekman 2007).
- *Poor thermoregulation:* compensatory sweating above the level of lesion and loss of ability to shiver below the level of lesion.

Patients should avoid exposure to excessive heat/cold temperatures; peripheral vasodilation means that the patient's core temperature can soon equal the environmental temperature through circulatory conduction – 'poikilothermia*. Ensure that the patient's body temperature is maintained at an appropriate level during all procedures, treatments, investigations and transfers. Active warming should be undertaken cautiously for fear of causing skin damage (SIA 2000, C).

3 *Pressure care:* risk to skin integrity and the development of pressure sores due to a lack of movement, poor circulation and altered sensation.

4 *Circulation:* risk of DVT due to the loss of vasomotor tone throughout the paralysed areas of the body. Application of thigh-length thromboembolic deterrent (TED) stockings can replace some of the lost muscle resistance, as well as reducing the risk of DVT (SIA 2000).

Moving and positioning the patient with an amputation

Definition

Amputation refers to the loss of a part or whole of a limb normally as a result of trauma or vascular disease (Figure 7.25).

Related theory

The level of the amputation and the surgical technique can affect both the cosmetic appearance as well as the potential functional ability for the individual.

There are certain levels of amputation that provide a residual limb suitable for a prosthetic fitting, function and cosmesis. Cosmetic appearance will depend to some extent on the level of the amputation and what prosthetic options this leaves. It is essential that one of these levels is selected rather than the boundary of the dead or diseased tissue with the viable tissue.

(Engstrom and van de Ven 1999)

Evidence-based approaches
Rationale
Indications

Positioning and moving patients both before and after amputation are indicated for all patients undergoing upper or lower limb amputation whatever the level.

This is in order to:

- prevent problems arising as a consequence of reduced mobility
- maintain range of movement and muscle strength in order to rehabilitate the patient early postoperatively and to regain maximum function as soon as possible.

Contraindications (with regard to certain positions)

- Leaving the limb on the amputated side unsupported as this can:
  - exacerbate pain
  - hinder wound healing
  - increase stump oedema.

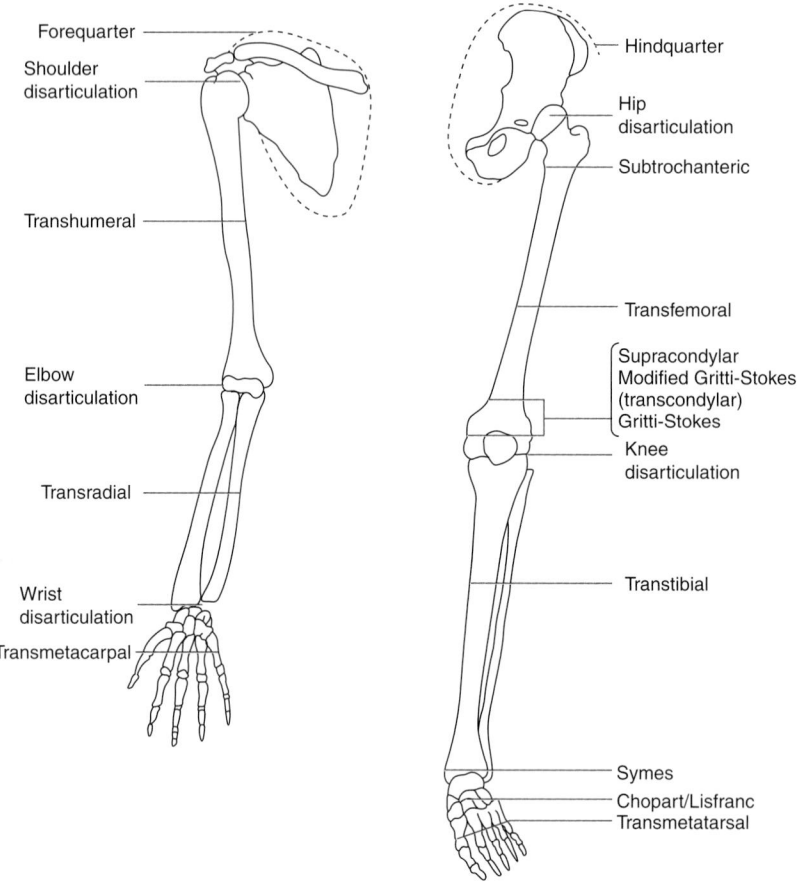

Figure 7.25 Levels of amputation in the upper and lower limb. Reproduced from Engstrom and van de Ven (1999).

Principles of care

The main goals of moving and positioning with regard to amputee management are to:

- maximize function by preventing contractures (particularly if the patient's goal is prosthetic rehabilitation)
- help to control stump oedema in order to assist wound healing
- assist the regaining of functional independence as soon as possible.

There are also two important points to consider when assisting an amputee patient.

- Firstly, any level of amputation, either of an upper or lower limb, will alter the patient's centre of gravity, potentially resulting in decreased balance. This in turn will increase the risk of falls for these patients.
- Secondly, body symmetry and posture will be altered which can also affect balance and may lead to poor postural habits that will hinder recovery and function.

Where possible, the process of positioning starts at the preoperative stage when the affected limb is often painful and the patient is frequently less able to mobilize. As a result, the patient may adopt positions of comfort that can lead to contractures. These positions are often maintained post amputation due to comfort and habit but are also due to changes in muscle balance (Engstrom and van de Ven 1999). For example, above-knee amputees may adopt a flexed and abducted position of their stump due to an alteration in muscle balance and pain but this can lead to contracture over time if not corrected.

Contractures can profoundly affect the potential for prosthetic rehabilitation and overall function so early correct positioning is paramount in this cohort of patients (Munin *et al.* 2001).

Preoperatively, patients should also be encouraged to keep as mobile as possible within pain limits to reduce the effects of deconditioning.

Pain, including phantom limb pain*, can be a major problem with these patients in the early postoperative stages.

In order to ensure that everyone works together towards a common goal, BACPAR (2006) recommends a comprehensive assessment by key professionals to establish rehabilitation goals. This assessment should be carried out as soon as possible following the decision to amputate and will need to undergo regular review.

The general principles of care mentioned earlier in the chapter are all relevant to this section. However, in addition, particular attention should be given to any possible balance issues for both upper limb and lower limb amputations as previously mentioned.

Note: Following lower limb amputation patients should be mobilized with caution, particularly if a prosthetic assessment is planned. This is because standing for long periods or hopping can:

- negatively influence stump oedema and wound healing
- overtire a patient, particularly elderly patients or those who are physically deconditioned prior to the amputation
- encourage the patient to adopt poor gait patterns due to excessive weight bearing on the remaining limb, leading to difficulty with prosthetic rehabilitation.

Preprocedural considerations

Equipment

Stump board

This will be required when sitting out in a wheelchair to ensure that the limb is fully supported and help prevent knee flexion contractures for below-knee (transtibial) amputees (Figure 7.26).

Wheelchair and seating cushion

Occupational therapy will assess and provide a wheelchair and a suitable cushion for lower limb amputees. If a patient has a bilateral lower limb amputation then they will need a specially adapted wheelchair with the wheels set back in order to provide sufficient stability.

(a)

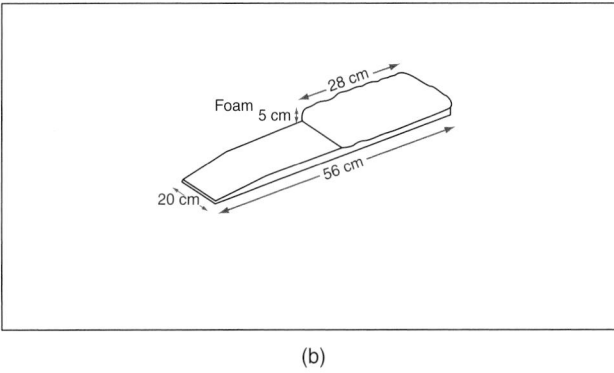

(b)

Figure 7.26 Two designs of stump board. (a) An adjustable stump board: the angle can be varied for comfort. (b) A fixed stump board: this slides underneath the wheelchair cushion. Reproduced from Engstrom and van de Ven (1999).

Procedure guideline 7.17 Positioning the preoperative and postoperative amputation patient

Essential equipment:

- Stump board (for below-knee amputees sitting out in wheelchair)
- Pillows
- Hoists and appropriate amputee and rehabilitation slings or sliding sheets may be required if the patient presents as a manual handling risk

Preprocedure

Action	Rationale
1 Explain and discuss the procedure with the patient.	To ensure that the patient understands the procedure and gives their valid consent (NMC 2008, C).
2 Wash hands thoroughly or use an alcohol-based handrub.	To reduce the risk of contamination and cross-infection (Fraise and Bradley 2009, E).
3 Ensure that the bed is at the optimum height for the patient and handlers. If two handlers are required try to match handlers' heights as far as possible.	To minimize the risk of injury to the practitioner and patient (Smith 2005, C).

(Continued)

Procedure guideline 7.17 (Continued)

Procedure

Upper limb amputee

4 Ensure patient is maintaining full range of motion of all remaining joints of the upper limb.	To prevent contractures in case of possible prosthetic rehabilitation and functional use. E

Below-knee amputee

5 Maintain knee extension.

■ In bed: do not place a towel or pillow under the knee unless it is supporting the whole of the stump; that is, do not encourage the knee to be maintained in a flexed position.	To prevent knee flexion contracture. E To assist stump oedema management. E To promote healing. E
■ In chair: use a stump board on the wheelchair if one has been issued. If the patient is sitting out in the chair then support the amputation with a footstool and pillows.	To support knee joint. E To prevent excessive knee flexion. E To aid stump oedema management (White 1992, R4, E). To protect the residual limb. E

Above-knee amputee

6 Maintain hip in a neutral position.

■ In bed: ensure the patient is periodically lying supine.	To maintain hip extension. E To prevent hip flexion contracture. E
Or:	
■ Consider prone-lying or side-lying with the hip in neutral position.	To avoid shortening of hip flexors and abductors. E
■ In sitting: ensure that the patient does not place a towel or pillow under stump.	To prevent excessive hip flexion. E

Problem-solving table 7.7 Prevention and resolution (Procedure guideline 7.17)

Problem	Cause	Prevention	Action
Painful stump following transfer or change of position	Fear of movement Pressure on distal end of stump over wound Stump dependent leading to increased oedema and reduced blood flow Unsupported stump	Reassure patient Ensure that stump is well supported following change in position Ensure adequate analgesia prior to movement and support stump wherever possible during the procedure	Explain procedure to patient prior to moving position. E Ensure that there is no pressure over the wound site following the procedure. E
Wound breakdown	Unsupported stump during movement Infection	Ensure that stump is well supported during and following change in position	Ensure that there is no pressure over the wound site following the procedure. E Seek medical review

No pillows or one
pillow

Arms positioned wherever
comfortable for patient

Residual limb lying flat
(with knee straight if t/t)
No pillow

Nurse call bell placed within
patient's reach

Head turned to sound side

Patient wearing a watch to
time period prone

Both hips completely flat
on bed

Remaining leg supported
on a pillow to prevent toes
from digging into bed

Footboard and bedclothes
turned right back out of
the way

Points to remember

1. To roll prone, the amputee must turn towards
   the sound side, the nurse ensuring that the
   residual limb is lowered gently.
2. Intially the amputee lies prone for about 10
   minutes.
3. The amputee should then build up to lying
   prone for 30 minutes three times a day.

Figure 7.27   The correct position for prone lying (t/t denotes transtibial). Reproduced from Engstrom and van de Ven (1999).

Complications

1 *Limb contracture* can occur due to:
   - immobility
   - alteration in muscle balance around the joints
   - pain
   - habit.

   In order to help prevent limb contracture, the patient
   will require adequate analgesia to control pain. It is also
   important to remind them if they are tending to adopt
   positions of their stump which could lead to limb contracture. The physiotherapist may recommend that the
   patient adopt certain positions for periods during the
   day to help prevent contractures such as prone-lying for
   above-knee amputees (Figure 7.27).
2 *Ongoing phantom limb pain.* This can be a persistent
   problem and will need referral to the pain team for appropriate management.
3 *Wound infection or delayed healing.* Review by medical
   team for appropriate management.

Websites

http://spinal.co.uk
www.asia-spinalinjury.org
http://guidance.nice.org.uk/CG75

Glossary

Ascites – the intraperitoneal accumulation of a watery fluid.
Cardiac syncope – fainting with unconsciousness of any cardiac cause.

Cardiogenic shock – occurs when there is failure of the pump
action of the heart resulting in reduced cardiac output.

Cognition – the mental processes involved in gaining knowledge and comprehension, including thinking, knowing,
remembering, judging and problem solving. These are higher-
level functions of the brain and encompass language, imagi-
nation, perception and planning.

Dysarthria – a speech disorder resulting from motor weakness, inco-ordination or stiffness of muscles used for speaking.

Dysphagia – an impairment of swallowing that may involve any structures from the lips to the gastric cardia.

Dysphasia/aphasia – an acquired communication disorder that impairs a person's ability to process language. It does not affect intelligence but does affect how someone can use language. Speaking, understanding what is said, reading and writing are all communication skills and may all be changed by injury to the brain. Aphasia may be temporary or permanent. It does not include speech impairments caused by damage to the muscles involved with speech – that is *dysarthria*.

Extensor tone – an increase in the tone of muscles which move the limbs into an extended position.

Flexor tone – an increase in tone in the muscles which flex the joints.

Haemodynamic(s) – the physical factors that govern blood flow. Literally means 'blood movement'.

Haemofiltration – a renal replacement therapy similar to haemodialysis which is almost always used to treat acute renal failure.

Hemi-aesthesia/paraesthesia – sensory loss affecting one half of the body.

Hemiparesis/hemiplegia – weakness or paralysis affecting one half of the body.

Hyperextension – the excessive extension of a limb or joint.

Hypovolaemia – a blood disorder consisting of a decrease in the volume of circulating blood.

Kyphosis – anatomical convexity of the spine (normally thoracic).

Lordosis – anatomical anterior concavity of the cervical and lumbar vertebrae.

Monoparesis – weakness or paralysis affecting one limb.

Osteoporosis – a reduction in the quantity and quality of bone by the loss of both bone mineral and protein content.

Oximeter – an instrument for measuring the proportion of oxygenated haemoglobin in the blood.

Oxygen saturation – the proportion of oxygenated haemaglobin in the blood.

Paraesthesia – abnormal touch sensation, e.g. pins and needles or tingling.

Paralysis – complete loss of motor function.

Paraplegia – paresis or paralysis of both lower limbs and trunk.

Paresis – partial loss of motor function.

Perception – interpretation of sensation into meaningful forms.

Peripheral motor/sensory neuropathies – dysfunction or pathology affecting one or more peripheral nerves.

Phantom limb pain – painful sensation in the part of the extremity that has been amputated.

Poikilothermia – having a body temperature that varies with the temperature of its surroundings.

Protract – extend or push forward part of the body, for example scapula.

Radicular – nerve root symptoms, for example pain or loss of sensation within a dermatome.

Spinal shock – a temporary suppression of spinal cord activity caused by oedema at and below the level of the lesion in spinal cord injury.

Tetraplegia – paresis or paralysis of arms, trunk, lower limbs and pelvic organs from damage to cervical spinal cord.

Vertigo – dizziness or giddiness.

References

ACPIN (1998) *Clinical Practice Guidelines on Splinting Adults with Neurological Dysfunction*. Association of Chartered Physiotherapists Interested in Neurology, Chartered Society of Physiotherapy, London.

ACPRC (1996) *Physiotherapy Management of the Spontaneously Breathing, Acutely Breathless, Adult Patient: A Problem Solving Approach*. Chartered Society of Physiotherapy, London.

Ada, L., Goddard, E., McCully, J. *et al.* (2005) Thirty minutes of positioning reduces the development of shoulder external rotation contracture after stroke: a randomized controlled trial. *Archives of Physical Medicine and Rehabilitation*, 86 (2), 230–234.

Adam, S. and Forrest, S. (1999) ABC of intensive care: other supportive care. *British Medical Journal*, 319 (7203), 175–178.

Aggarwal, R. and Hunter, A. (2007) How exactly does the chest wall work? *Student BMJ*, 15.

ASIA (American Spinal Injury Association) (2002) Impairment Scale. American Spinal Injury Association, Atlanta, GA. www.asia-spinalinjury.org/publications/2006_Classif_worksheet.pdf.

BACPAR (2006) *Clinical Guidelines for the Pre and Post Operative Management of Adults with Lower Limb Amputation*. Chartered Society of Physiotherapy, London.

Baer, M.P. and Durward, B. (2004) Stroke, in *Physical Management in Neurological Rehabilitation*, 2nd edn (ed. M. Stokes). Elsevier Mosby, Edinburgh, pp. 75–101.

Barnes, M.P. (2001) Spasticity: a rehabilitation challenge in the elderly. *Gerontology*, 47 (6), 295–299.

Barnes, M.P. (2008) An overview of the clinical management of spasticity, in Barnes, M.P. and Johnson, G.R. (eds) *Upper Motor Neurone Syndrome and Spasticity: Clinical Management and Neurophysiology*, 2nd edn. Cambridge University Press, Cambridge, pp. 1–9.

Barsevick, A.M., Whitmer, K., Sweeney, C. and Nail, L.M. (2002) A pilot study examining energy conservation for cancer treatment-related fatigue. *Cancer Nursing*, 25 (5), 333–341.

Bobath, B. (1990) *Adult Hemiplegia: Evaluation and Treatment*, 3rd edn. Heinemann Medical, Oxford.

Booij, L.H.D.J. (1996) Fundamentals of anaesthesia and acute medicine, in *Neuromuscular Transmission*. BMJ Books, London, pp. 124–159.

Boss, B.J. (1998) Nursing management of adults with common neurologic problems, in *Adult Health Nursing*, 3rd edn (eds P. Gauntlett Beare and J.L. Myers). Mosby, St Louis, MO, pp. 904–947.

Brada, M. (1995) Central nervous system tumours, in Horwich, A. (ed) *Oncology: A Multidisciplinary Textbook*. Chapman and Hall, London, pp. 395–416.

Bray, J. and Cooper, J. (2004) The contribution of occupational therapy to palliative medicine, in *The Oxford Textbook of Palliative Medicine*, 3rd edn (eds D. Doyle, G. Hanks, N. Cherny and K. Calman). Oxford University Press, Oxford, pp. 1035–1041.

Britton, J. and Ng, V. (1998) Clinical neuro-imaging, in *Neuro-oncology for Nurses* (ed. D. Guerrero). Whurr, London, pp. 81–123.

Britton, T.C. (1998) Abnormalities of muscle tone and movement, in *Neurological Physiotherapy* (ed. M. Stokes). Mosby, London. pp. 57–65.

CAT (2009) *Cancer and Palliative Care Rehabilitation Care Pathways (Draft)*. Cancer Action Team, London.

Catz, A. and Itzkovich, M. (2007) Spinal Cord Independence Measure: comprehensive ability rating scale for the spinal cord lesion patient. *Journal of Rehabilitation and Research Development*, **44** (1), 65–68.

Catz, A., Itzkovich, M., Tesio, L. *et al.* (2007) A multicenter international study on the Spinal Cord Independence Measure, version III: Rasch psychometric validation. *Spinal Cord*, **45** (4), 275–291.

Chatterton, H.J., Pomeroy, V.M. and Gratton, J. (2001) Positioning for stroke patients: a survey of physiotherapists' aims and practices. *Disability and Rehabilitation*, **23** (10), 413–421.

Convertino, V.A., Bloomfield, S.A. and Greenleaf, J.E. (1997) An overview of the issues: physiological effects of bed rest and restricted physical activity. *Medicine and Science in Sports and Exercise*, **29**(2), 187–190.

Cooper, J. (2006) *Occupational Therapy in Oncology and Palliative Care*, 2nd edn. John Wiley, Chichester.

Creditor, M.C. (1993) Hazards of hospitalization of the elderly. *Annals of Internal Medicine*, **118** (3), 219–223.

CSP (2008) *Guidance on Manual Handling in Physiotherapy*, 3rd edn. CSP, London.

Davies, P.M. (1985) *Steps to Follow: A Guide to the Treatment of Adult Hemiplegia, Based on the Concept of K. and B. Bobath*. Springer-Verlag, Berlin.

Davies, P.M. (2000) *Steps to Follow: The Comprehensive Treatment of Adult Hemiplegia*. Springer-Verlag, Berlin.

Dean, C.M., Mackey, F.H. and Katrak, P. (2000) Examination of shoulder positioning after stroke: a randomised controlled pilot trial. *Australian Journal of Physiotherapy*, **46** (1), 35–40.

Dean, E. (1985) Effect of body position on pulmonary function. *Physical Therapy*, **65**(5), 613–618.

DH (2001) *National Service Framework for Older People*. Department of Health, London.

Dietz, J.H. (1981) *Rehabilitation Oncology*. John Wiley, New York.

Doyle, D., Hanks, G., Cherny, N. and Calman, K. (eds) (2004) *Oxford Textbook of Palliative Medicine*, 3rd edn. Oxford University Press, Oxford.

Drakulovic, M.B., Torres, A., Bauer, T. T., Nicolas, J.M., Nogue, S. and Ferrer, M. (1999) Supine body position as a risk factor for nosocomial pneumonia in mechanically ventilated patients: a randomised trial. *Lancet*, **354**(9193), 1851–1858.

Edwards, S. (1998) Physiotherapy management of established spasticity in spasticity rehabilitation, in *Spasticity Management* (ed. G. Shean). Churchill Communications Europe, London, pp. 71–90.

Edwards, S. (2002a) Abnormal tone and movement as a result of neurological impairment, in Edwards, S. (ed) *Neurological Physiotherapy: A Problem Solving Approach*, 2nd edn. Churchill Livingstone, Edinburgh, pp. 63–86.

Edwards, S. (2002b) An analysis of normal movement as the basis for the development of treatment techniques, in Edwards, S. (ed)

Neurological Physiotherapy: A Problem Solving Approach, 2nd edn. Churchill Livingstone, Edinburgh, pp.35–68.

Edwards, S. and Carter, P. (2002) General principles of treatment, in *Neurological Physiotherapy: A Problem Solving Approach*, 2nd edn (ed. S. Edwards). Churchill Livingstone, Edinburgh, pp.121–154.

Edwards, S. and Charlton, P. (1996) Splinting and the use of orthoses in the management of patients with neurological disorders, in *Neurological Physiotherapy: A Problem Solving Approach*. Churchill Livingstone, London, pp. 161–188.

Ellison, D. and Love, S. (1997) Classification and general concepts of CNS neoplasms and astrocytic neoplasms, in *Neuropathology: a Reference Text of CNS Pathology*. Mosby, London.

Engstrom, B. and van de Ven, C. (eds) (1999) *Therapy for Amputees*, 3rd edn. Churchill Livingstone, Edinburgh.

Fink, J. (2002) Positioning versus postural drainage. *Respiratory Care*, **47** (7), 769–777.

Fraise, AP and Bradley, T. (eds) (2009) *Ayliffe's Control of Healthcare Associated Infection: A Practical Handbook*, 5th edn Hodder Arnold, London.

Gardiner, M.D. (1973) *The Principles of Exercise Therapy*, 3rd edn. Bell, London.

Geraghty, M. (2005) Nursing the unconscious patient. *Nursing Standard*, **20** (1), 54–64.

Gloag, D. (1985) Rehabilitation after stroke: 1– What is the potential? *British Medical Journal (Clinical Research Edition)*, **290** (6469), 699–701.

Grieve, J.I. and Gnanasekaran, L. (2008) *Neuropsychology for Occupational Therapists: Cognition in Occupational Performance*, 3rd edn. Blackwell, Oxford.

Guerrero, D. (1998) *Neuro-Oncology for Nurses*. Whurr, London.

Harden, B. (2008) *Respiratory Physiotherapy: An On-Call Survival Guide*, 2nd edn. Elsevier Health Sciences, Edinburgh.

Harrison, P. (2000) *Managing Spinal Injury: Critical Care*. Spinal Injury Association, Milton Keynes.

Hart, S. (2008) Aseptic technique, in *The Royal Marsden Hospital Manual of Clinical Nursing Procedures*, 7th edn. Wiley-Blackwell, Oxford, pp. 51–69.

Hawkins, S., Stone, K. and Plummer, L. (1999) An holistic approach to turning patients. *Nursing Standard*, **14** (3), 51–56.

Hesse, S. (2003) Rehabilitation after stroke: evaluation, principles of therapy, novel treatment approaches and assistive devices. *Topics in Geriatric Medicine*, **19** (2), 109–126.

Hickey, J.V. (2003a) Management of the unconscious neurological patient. in Hickey, J.V. (ed) *The Clinical Practice of Neurological and Neurosurgical Nursing*, 5th edn. Lippincott Williams and Wilkins, Philadelphia, pp. 345–357.

Hickey, J.V. (2003b) Neurological assessment, in Hickey, J.V. (ed) *The Clinical Practice of Neurological and Neurosurgical Nursing*, 5th edn. Lippincott Williams and Wilkins, Philadelphia, pp. 159–184.

Hodges, P.W. and Gandevia, S.C. (2000) Changes in intra-abdominal pressure during postural and respiratory activation of the human diaphragm. *Journal of Applied Physiology*, **89** (3), 967–976.

Hough, A. (2001) *Physiotherapy in Respiratory Care: An Evidence-Based Approach to Respiratory and Cardiac Management*, 3rd edn. Nelson Thornes, Cheltenham.

HSE (1992) *Manual Handling Operations Regulations 1992*. HMSO, London.

HSE (2004) *Getting to Grips with Manual Handling: A Short Guide*. Health and Safety Executive, Sudbury. www.hse.gov.uk/pubns/indg143.pdf.

Itzkovich, M., Gelernter, I., Biering-Sorensen, F. *et al.* (2007) The Spinal Cord Independence Measure (SCIM) version III: reliability and validity in a multi-center international study. *Disability and Rehabilitation*, **29** (24), 1926–1933.

331

Jackson, J. (1998) Specific treatment techniques, in *Neurological Physiotherapy*. Mosby, London, pp. 299–311.

Jacobson, A.F. and Winslow, E.H. (2000) Caring for unconscious patients. *American Journal of Nursing*, **100** (1), 69.

Jones, M. and Moffatt, F. (2002) *Cardiopulmonary Physiotherapy*. BIOS, Oxford.

Kalina, P., Drehobl, K.E., Black, K., Woldenberg, R. and Sapan, M. (1995) Spinal cord compression by spontaneous spinal subdural haematoma in polycythemia vera. *Postgraduate Medical Journal*, **71** (836), 378–379.

Kaplan, M.C. (1995) Hemiplegic shoulder pain – early prevention and rehabilitation. *Western Journal of Medicine*, **162** (2), 151–152.

Kirkwood, C.A. and Bardsley, G.I. (2001) Seating and positioning in spasticity, in *Upper Motor Neurone Syndrome and Spasticity: Clinical Management and Neurophysiology*. Cambridge University Press, Cambridge, pp. 122–141.

Kirshblum, S., O'Dell, M.W., Ho, C. and Barr, K. (2001) Rehabilitation of persons with central nervous system tumors. *Cancer*, **92** (4 Suppl), 1029–1038.

Krassioukov, A., Eng, J.J., Warburton, D.E. and Teasell, R. (2009) A systematic review of the management of orthostatic hypotension after spinal cord injury. *Archives of Physical Medicine and Rehabilitation*, **90**(5), 876–885.

Lawrence, M. (1995) The unconscious experience. *American Journal of Critical Care*, **4** (3), 227–232.

Lindsay, K.W., Bone, I. and Callander, R. (2004) *Neurology and Neurosurgery Illustrated*, 4th edn. Churchill Livingstone, Edinburgh.

Loblaw, D.A., Laperriere, N.J. and Mackillop, W.J. (2003) A population-based study of malignant spinal cord compression in Ontario. *Clinical Oncology*, **15** (4), 211–217.

Lohani, B. and Sharma, M.R. (2004) Patterns of spinal tumours in Nepal: a clinico-radiological study. *Nepal Journal of Neuroscience*, **1**, 113–119.

Lundy-Ekman, L. (2007) Motor neurons, in *Neuroscience: Fundamentals for Rehabilitation*, 3rd edn. Saunders Elsevier, St Louis, MO, pp. 188–242.

Lynch, M. and Grisogono, V. (1991) *Strokes and Head Injuries: A Guide for Patients, Families, Friends, and Carers*. John Murray, London.

MacIntyre, N.R. and Branson, R.D. (2009) *Mechanical Ventilation*, 2nd edn. Saunders Elsevier, St Louis, MO.

Mann, F.A., Kubal, W.S. and Blackmore, C. (2000) Improving the diagnosis of cervical spine injury in the very elderly: implications of epidemiology of injury. *Emergency Radiology*, **7** (1), 35–41.

Maranzano, E. and Latini, P. (1995) Effectiveness of radiation therapy without surgery in metastatic spinal cord compression: final results from a prospective trial. *International Journal of Radiation Oncology Biology Physics*, **32**(4), 959–967.

McGarvey, C.L. (1990) *Physical Therapy for the Cancer Patient*. Churchill Livingstone, New York.

McKenzie, R. (2006) *Treat Your Own Back*. Spinal Publications, New Zealand.

Mee, L.Y. and Bee, W.H. (2007) A comparison study on nurses' and therapists' perception on the positioning of stroke patients in Singapore General Hospital. *International Journal of Nursing Practice*, **13** (4), 209–221.

Mehan, R., Mackenzie, M. and Brock, K. (2008) Skilled transfer training in stroke rehabilitation: a review of use and safety. *International Journal of Therapy and Rehabilitation*, **15** (9), 382–389.

Munin, M.C., Espejo-de Guzman, M.C., Boninger, M.L. *et al.* (2001) Predictive factors for successful early prosthetic ambulation among lower-limb amputees. *Journal of Rehabilitation Research and Development*, **38** (4), 379–384.

Nelson, A., Matz, M., Chen, F. *et al.* (2006) Development and evaluation of a multifaceted ergonomics program to prevent injuries associated with patient handling tasks. *International Journal of Nursing Studies*, **43** (6), 717–33.

Nelson, A., Collins, J., Siddharthan, K., Matz, M. and Waters, T. (2008) Link between safe patient handling and patient outcomes in long-term care. *Rehabilitation Nursing*, **33**(1), 33–43.

NICE (2008) *CG75 Metastatic Spinal Cord Compression: Full Guideline*. National Institute for Clinical Excellence, London. www.nice.org.uk/nicemedia/live/12085/42668/42668.pdf.

NMC (2008) *Consent*. Nursing and Midwifery Council, London. www.nmc-uk.org/Nurses-and-midwives/Advice-by-topic/A/Advice/Consent.

Norris, C.M. (1995) Spinal stabilisation 2. Limiting factors to end stage motion in the lumbar spine. *Physiotherapy*, **81**(2), 64–72.

O'Donovan, K.J., Bajd, T., Grace, P.A. *et al.* (2006) An investigation of recommended lower leg exercises for induced calf muscle activity. Proceedings of the 24th IASTED International Conference on Biomedical Engineering. Innsbruck, Austria, ACTA Press.

O'Dwyer, N.J., Ada, L. and Neilson, P.D. (1996) Spasticity and muscle contracture following stroke. *Brain*, **119** (Pt 5), 1737–1749.

Pearsall, J. (2001) *The Concise Oxford Dictionary*, 10th edn. Oxford University Press, Oxford.

Pigott, K.H., Baddeley, H. and Maher, E.J. (1994) Pattern of disease in spinal cord compression on MRI scan and implications for treatment. *Clinical Oncology*, **6** (1), 7–10.

Pope, P. (1996) Postural management and seating, in *Neurological Physiotherapy* (ed. S. Edwards). Mosby, London, pp. 135–160.

Pope, P. (2002) Postural management and special seating, in Edwards, S. (ed) *Neurological Physiotherapy: A Problem Solving Approach*, 2nd edn. Churchill Livingstone, Edinburgh. pp. 189–218.

Pryor, J.A. and Prasad, S.A. (2008) *Physiotherapy for Respiratory and Cardiac Problems: Adults and Paediatrics*, 4th edn. Churchill Livingstone Elsevier, Edinburgh.

Raine, S., Meadows, L. and Etherington-Lynch, M. (2009) *Bobath Concept. Theory and Clinical Practice in Neurological Rehabilitation*. Wiley-Blackwell, Chichester.

Riedel, M. (2001) Acute pulmonary embolism 1: pathophysiology, clinical presentation, and diagnosis. *Heart*, **85**(2), 229–240.

Rockefeller, K. (2008) Using technology to promote safe patient handling and rehabilitation. *Rehabilitation Nursing*, **33** (1), 3–9.

Shumway-Cook, A. and Woollacott, M.H. (2001) Clinical management of the patient with reach, grasp and manipulation disorders, in *Motor Control: Theory and Practical Applications*, 2nd edn. Lippincott Williams and Wilkins, Philadelphia; London, pp. 545.

SIA (2000) *Managing Spinal Injury: Critical Care*. www.spinal.co.uk/pdf/SIA%20Critical%20care.pdf.

Smith, J. (2005) *The Guide to the Handling of People*, 5th edn. Backcare in collaboration with the Royal College of Nursing and the National Back Exchange, London, p. 234.

Stokes, M. (2004) *Physical Management in Neurological Rehabilitation*, 2nd edn. Elsevier Mosby, Edinburgh.

Thomas, A.J. (2009) Exercise intervention in the critical care unit – what is the evidence? *Physical Therapy Reviews*, **14** (1), 50–59.

Tiplady, B., Jackson, S.H., Maskrey, V.M. and Swift, C.G. (1998) Validity and sensitivity of visual analogue scales in young and older healthy subjects. *Age and Ageing*, **27** (1), 63–66.

Tookman, A.J., Hopkins, K. and Scharpen-von-Heusson, K. (2004) Rehabilitation in palliative medicine, in Doyle, D., Hanks, G., Cherny, N. and Calman, K. (eds) *Oxford Textbook of Palliative Medicine*, 3rd edn. Oxford University Press, Oxford, pp. 1019–1032.

Tortora, G.J. and Derrickson, B. (2009) *Principles of Anatomy and Physiology*, 12th edn. John Wiley, Hoboken, NJ.

White, E.A. (1992) Wheelchair stump boards and their use with lower limb amputees. British *Journal of Occupational Therapy*, **55**(5), 174–178.

332

Chapter 8

Nutrition, fluid balance and blood transfusion

The Royal Marsden Hospital Manual of Clinical Nursing Procedures, Eighth Edition. Edited by Lisa Dougherty and Sara Lister.
© 2011 The Royal Marsden Hospital. Published 2011 by Blackwell Publishing Ltd.

Overview

Good nutrition, the supply of optimal nutrients and fluid to meet requirements, is an essential component of health, with poor nutrition contributing to ill health and prolonged recovery from illness or disease. It is therefore crucial that the nutritional status of all patients is assessed and considered during the whole of the patient's care. This chapter addresses how fluid and nutrition can influence body composition, how to identify patients who are malnourished or at risk of malnutrition and, most importantly, how the patient's nutritional needs can be met.

The provision of food and fluids to patients is an integral part of basic care. In normal circumstances adequate nutritional intake enables the body to maintain homoeostasis of body composition and function but in disease states this balance can be altered. The majority of patients will achieve adequate nutrition through the oral route of diet and fluids but, for some, additional artificial nutritional support or products such as blood will be required to maintain optimal body composition and function. This chapter describes how the patient's needs can be assessed and met through oral, enteral and parenteral routes of nutrition, fluid or blood products.

Fluid balance

Definition

In the human homoeostatic state, the intake of fluids equals fluid excreted from the body, thereby maintaining optimal hydration. In nursing practice, this term refers to the procedure of measuring fluid input and output to determine fluid balance (Marieb and Hoehn 2010, Scales and Pilsworth 2008).

Anatomy and physiology

Body composition

The human body is made up of approximately 60% water (this varies with age, gender and percentage of fatty tissue) (Alexander *et al.* 2000, Scales and Pilsworth 2008, Urden *et al.* 2002). Bodily water/fluid is essential to life and vital for:

- controlling body temperature
- the delivery of nutrients and gases to cells
- the removal of waste
- acid–base balance and
- the maintenance of cellular shape (Baumberger-Henry 2008).

Total body water is distributed between two main compartments: intracellular fluid (ICF, within the cell) and extracelluar fluid (ECF, outside the cell). ECF is further divided into the intravascular space, within the blood vessels (known as plasma), the interstitial space which surrounds the cells and the transcellular space. The transcellular space contains specialized fluids such as cerebrospinal fluid but does not readily exchange fluid with other compartments so is rarely considered in fluid management (Bishop 2008, Haskal 2007).

Bodily fluid is a composition of water and a variety of dissolved solutes which Marieb and Hoehn (2010) classify as electrolytes and non-electrolytes. Non-electrolytes include glucose, lipids, creatine and urea and are molecules that do not dissociate in solution and have no electrical charge. Electrolytes such as potassium, sodium, chloride, magnesium and bicarbonate all dissociate in solution into charged ions that conduct electricity. Concentration of these solutes varies depending on the compartment in which they are contained; for example, ECF has a high sodium content (135–145 mmol/L) and is relatively low in potassium (3.5–4.5 mmol/L) and ICF is the reverse – high in potassium but lower in sodium. The movement and distribution of fluid and solutes between compartments are controlled by the semi-permeable phospholipid cellular membranes that separate them (Baumberger-Henry 2008).

Transport and movement of water and solutes

Water can readily and passively pass across the membrane and does so by osmosis (see Table 8.1) in response to changing solute concentrations. The amount of solute in solution determines the osmolarity – the higher the solute concentration, the higher the osmolarity; this is also referred to as the osmotic pressure (or pull). Electrolytes move across the membrane via the protein channels, some by diffusion (see Table 8.1) and also via a passive mode of transport where solutes move towards an area of low solute concentration. Sodium and potassium are an exception to this rule, as they are required to move against the concentration gradient in order to preserve higher intravascular sodium concentrations. Energy is utilized to pump sodium out of the cell via the protein channels and pump potassium back into the cell, known as the sodium/potassium pump (see Table 8.1).

The movement of water and solutes out of the intravascular space and into the interstitial space is dependent on opposing osmotic and hydrostatic pressures. Hydrostatic pressure is caused by the pumping action of the heart and the diameter (resistance) of the vessels/capillaries forcing water and molecules that are small enough to pass through the membrane out of the vessel and into the interstitial fluid. Within the vascular system, only the capillaries have semi-permeable membranes so it is here this 'filtration' occurs. At the arteriole end of the capillary, the hydrostatic pressure exceeds the osmotic pressure, moving solutes out of the plasma and into the interstitial space. At the venous end, hydrostatic pressure is reduced and the osmotic pressure within the vessel (plasma) is higher so water is

Table 8.1 Molecule transport modes

Transport mode	Description	Diagram
Osmosis	Movement of water from an area of low solute concentration to an area of high solute concentration	
Diffusion	Movement of solutes from an area of high concentration to an area of low concentration	
Facilitated diffusion	Movement of solutes from an area of high concentration to an area of low concentration, facilitated by a carrier molecule (e.g. glucose only enters the cell carried by insulin)	
Active transport	Movement of solutes against the concentration gradient from an area of low concentration to an area of high concentration. This transport requires energy synthesized within the cell (i.e. the sodium/potassium pump)	

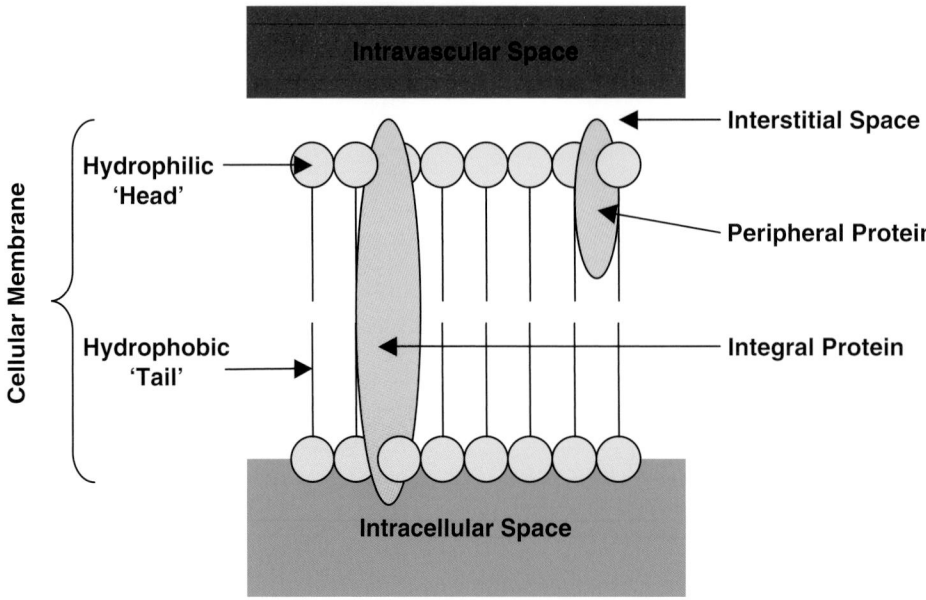

Figure 8.1 Cellular membrane.

pulled back into the vessel and circulating volume (van Wissen and Breton 2004). The osmotic pressure is provided by plasma proteins that are too large to pass through the membrane even under pressure. Oedema can result if the membranes become permeable to protein; osmotic pressure is then reduced, resulting in excess of water moving into the interstitial space. Pulmonary oedema is caused by this mechanism at the site of the lungs. Sepsis or a systemic inflammatory response is an example of a condition where the capillary membranes become more permeable to protein.

Osmolarity and fluid balance

Sodium is the most influential electrolyte in fluid balance and is the primary cation (positively charged ion) of the ECF. The concentration of sodium in the ECF has the most profound effect on its osmolarity and therefore water balance. If ECF osmolarity increases (for example, with increased intake of sodium, reduced fluid intake, increased loss of fluid), osmoreceptors of the hypothalamus detect very slight changes (1–2% increase) in plasma osmolarity (Marieb and Hoehn 2010) and trigger the thirst response which in turn encourages oral fluid intake in an attempt to restore the balance (Figure 8.1).

Hormonal mechanisms and the kidneys are highly influential in fluid and electrolyte balance and again are also triggered in response to changing osmolarity and/or plasma volumes. Antidiuretic hormone (ADH) is released from the posterior pituitary gland (in response to stimulus of the osmoreceptors in the hypothalamus) (van Wissen and Breton 2004) and acts on the tubules and collecting ducts of the kidneys, inhibiting water excretion and encourag-

ing water reabsorption. If plasma osmolarity falls (indicating water excess), these mechanisms are suppressed by a negative feedback loop; the osmoreceptors are no longer stimulated. This in turn inhibits ADH release; renal tubules no long conserve water and thirst is reduced, leading to a reduction of oral intake and restoration of balance. ADH is also released in the renin-angiotensin response to a reduction in blood pressure (detected by baroreceptors in blood vessels); more detailed information on this mechanism can be found in Chapter 13.

Aldosterone is a mineralocorticoid and is secreted by the adrenal cortex in response to increased osmolarity and/ or decreased blood pressure (part of the renin-angiotensin system). It acts on the renal tubules, initiating the active transport of sodium (and hence water) from the tubules and collecting ducts back into the plasma and circulating volume (Baumberger-Henry 2008).

These homoeostatic mechanisms are very effective in maintaining fluid and electrolyte balance in health and act to compensate for fluid imbalances to ensure effective cellular function. However, these compensatory mechanisms are not sustainable and will eventually fail if ill health or imbalance persists. For example, in continued haemorrhage, the body will compensate by conserving water and vasoconstricting vessels in an attempt to increase blood pressure and volume. Continued haemorrhage and failure to replace lost fluids will lead to cellular and organ dysfunction which in turn lead to organ failure and possible death (Adam and Osborne 2005).

Dehydration is a particular concern in ill health as often fluid intake is reduced (poor appetite, nil by mouth, nausea) and often coincides with an increased output (vomiting, diarrhoea, haemorrhage, drains, fever). The elderly are at particular risk of dehydration as the effectiveness of the thirst response diminishes with age (Ainslie *et al.* 2002, Mentes 2006). When the osmolarity of the ECF increases, it encourages water out of the cell into the ECF, which eventually leads to cellular dehydration, impaired metabolism, disturbed cellular shape and impaired cellular function.

If the osmolarity of the ECF falls, water moves into the cell. If this continues, it will lead to water toxicity, causing cells to expand and eventually burst. Care should therefore be taken when administering intravenous fluids, as fluids that are of lower osmolarity than ECF (hypotonic) will cause a shift of water into the cells. Conversely, hypertonic solutions will cause a shift of fluid from the cells, causing dehydration. Maintenance fluids should usually be isotonic (have the same osmolarity as ECF) (Sheppard and Wright 2006).

Evidence-based approaches

Fluid and electrolyte balance monitoring and management are integral and vital to nursing care (Jevon and Ewens 2007). Alexander *et al.* (2000) suggest that nurses must have a good understanding of the concepts involved in fluid balance in order to recognize or anticipate imbalances and implement the correct interventions/care. Understanding of the physiological mechanisms will ensure that tasks such as fluid balance charting are carried out with understanding and thought.

Fluid balance charting allows healthcare professionals to carefully monitor the fluid input and output and calculate the fluid balance. This is usually measured over a 24-hour period (Jevon and Ewens 2007). A positive fluid balance indicates that the input has exceeded the output, and a negative result the reverse. Although fluid balance charts are a good indication of fluid balance, this is not an exact measurement, for several reasons. Some losses are insensible such as those from perspiration, respiratory secretions and immeasurable bowel losses. The calculation of fluid balance also relies heavily on the accurate measuring and charting of input and output, a skill documented in the literature as often being done poorly by nurses (Callum *et al.* 1999, Mooney 2007). For such measurements to be taken accurately may require additional interventions such as the need for catheterization. Current recommendations highlight that the benefits of accurate fluid balance measurements outweigh the risks associated with such procedures (Callum *et al.* 1999, NICE 2007). Table 8.2 shows the possible routes and sources of fluid intake and output.

The National Confidential Enquiry into Perioperative Deaths (Callum *et al.* 1999) highlights how important effective fluid balance management is and states that imbalance can lead to 'serious postoperative morbidity and mortality'. Of the patients reviewed, 20% were found to have poorly kept fluid balance records, emphasizing the need for effective monitoring and record keeping; the report suggests that accurate fluid balance recording should be

Table 8.2 Fluid intake and output

Intake	Output
Oral	**Urine output**
Food and drinks	*Normally approx 1500 mL/per day*
Normally 2000 mL/per day	
Parenteral/intravenous	**Faeces**
Maintenance fluids, IVI, intermittent drugs, flushes	*Normally approx 100 mL/per day*
Additional to or replaces oral intake	
Enteral	**Perspiration**
Nasal gastric/nasal jejostomy, percutaneous gastric jejostomy feed, flushes	*Normally approx 200 mL/day*
Additional to or replaces oral intake	**Gastric secretions**
	Vomit, nasal gastric/gastrostomy drainage
	Additional to normal output
	Wounds and drains
	Additional to normal output
	Insensible losses
	Perspiration, respiratory secretions
	Additional to normal output

From Sheppard and Wright (2006).

as important as the recording of prescriptions and medicine administration. Studies have suggested that nurses may not be aware of the importance of the task (Scales and Pilsworth 2008) and Bryant (2007) identified a knowledge deficit amongst colleagues regarding the assessment of fluid status and subsequent management, which led to an increase in training in this skill. The *National Service Framework for Older People* (DH 2001a) also recognizes the importance of fluid status assessment and subsequent fluid management in the older population.

Although a very useful tool, fluid balance charting should not be used in isolation. When considering fluid and electrolyte balance, additional triggers such as physical assessment and monitoring plasma levels of electrolytes should be integral to the observation and care of a patient with actual or potential fluid and electrolyte imbalances (NICE 2007).

Table 8.3 Assessment of fluid status

Assessment	Usual findings	Indications	
Symptoms		**Fluid deficit**	**Fluid overload**
History To establish any condition, medication or lifestyle that may contribute to or predispose the patient to a fluid imbalance	Differs for each patient	For example, chronic or acute diarrhoea, medication such as diuretics, poor oral fluid intake	Ingestion of too much water/fluid, renal failure/dysfunction
Thirst *Ask the patient*	Occasional; resolved by taking an oral drink	Unusually thirsty	No thirst, normal
Mucosa and conjunctiva *Inspect*	Usually moist and pink	Dry and whitened mucosa, dry conjunctiva and 'sunken' eyeballs	Moist, pink and glistening
Clinical signs			
Heart rate	Usual resting 60–100 bpm	Raised	Normal or raised
Peripheral pulse character	Radial pulse is felt just under the skin at the wrist, light palpation with two or three fingers	Thready, difficult to palpate	Bounding, easy to palpate
Blood pressure	Patient's own normal should be used as a guide	BP will fall if blood volume falls beyond compensatory mechanisms. Patient may experience postural hypotension	Rise in blood pressure, or may remain normal
Central venous pressure	3–10 mmHg	Low	Raised
Respiratory rate	12–20 breaths/min	High, to meet increased oxygen demands of compensatory mechanisms	High, if overload present
Capillary refill	Usually 2–3 seconds	Slower	Faster
Urine output	0.5–1 mL/kg	Low	Increase, if good renal function
Lung sounds, auscultation	Vesicular breath sounds, 'rustling' heard mainly on inspiration	Normal	Additional sounds (crackles) may indicate fluid overload
Skin turgor	Following a gentle pinch, the fold of skin should return to normal	Skin will take much longer to 'bounce' back to normal. Unreliable in elderly who may have lost some elasticity of their skin	May be normal; however, may be oedematous therefore skin remains dented/pinched
Serum electrolyte levels			
Sodium	135–145 mmol/L	Raised	Lowered
Potassium	3.5–5 mmol/L	May be lowered if cause of fluid deficit is GI losses	Normal
Urea	2.5–6.4 mmol/L	Decreased	Normal

Table 8.3 (*Continued*)

Assessment	Usual findings	Indications	
Symptoms		Fluid deficit	Fluid overload
Creatinine	Male: 63–116 µmol/L Female: 54–98 µmol/L	Normal, but eventually rises with prolonged poor renal perfusion	Normal
	This is a basic examination of serum electrolytes in fluid balance. There are several conditions and treatments that may affect these so they should not be used in isolation to assess or treat fluid imbalance.		
Serum osmolarity	275–295 mosmol/kg	Increased	Decreased
Urine osmolarity	50–1400 mosmol/kg	Increased	Decreased
Daily weight	A person's daily weight should be fairly stable; large losses or gain in weight may indicate fluid imbalance	Reduced each day	Increased each day
Temperature	36.5–37.5°C	May be elevated and this may also contribute to the fluid deficit (increased insensible losses)	Normal

From Adam and Osbourne (2006), Epstein *et al.* (2006), Flanagan *et al.* (2007), Levi (2005).

Nursing assessment is discussed in detail in Chapter 2 and the assessment of a patient's fluid status should be an integral part of any admission and subsequent daily assessments, particularly if the patient is critically ill and/or a fluid deficit has been identified. See Table 8.3 for details of what should be included in a fluid status assessment.

Within fluid management, and particularly fluid resuscitation, there is an ongoing debate surrounding the benefits of the use of colloids over crystalloid for fluid replacement. Perel and Roberts (2007) conducted a systematic review of the evidence and concluded that there is no apparent benefit to the patient when using colloid rather than crystalloid. The UK Adult Resuscitation Guidelines (Resuscitation Council 2005) agree that there is no benefit in choosing colloid over crystalloid but they do recommend that dextrose is avoided due to the redistribution of fluid from the intravascular space and because it may cause hyperglycaemia.

Rationale
Indications

Any patient who has shown signs or symptoms of a fluid imbalance or those having undergone surgery or acute illness that has led to critical care admission should have their fluid intake and output monitored and fluid balance calculated on an hourly basis (Mooney 2007). The decision to monitor fluid balance should be a multidisciplinary one; however, it is the responsibility of the bedside nurse to ensure this is done so accurately.

Legal and professional issues

The Code (NMC 2008a) clearly states that clear and accurate records must be kept; this includes fluid balance charts. Nurses should have an understanding of the mechanisms of fluid balance and identify potential imbalances and the problems associated with these imbalances.

Preprocedural considerations

In order to monitor fluid balance, both input and output must be accurately measured. Below are procedural guidelines for measuring input and output. If the patient is awake, able to take oral fluids and is mobile, they must be educated about the fact that their fluid balance is being monitored and each drink must be recorded, as should each episode of passing urine, bowel motion or vomiting and so on. It is helpful to provide a cup with markings showing volume.

It is important to note that patients may have other means of urine output, for example an ileal conduit, ureteric stents, suprapubic catheterization, neo bladder. The same concepts can be utilized to measure the output, by attaching an urometer to the catheter or the urostomy bag.

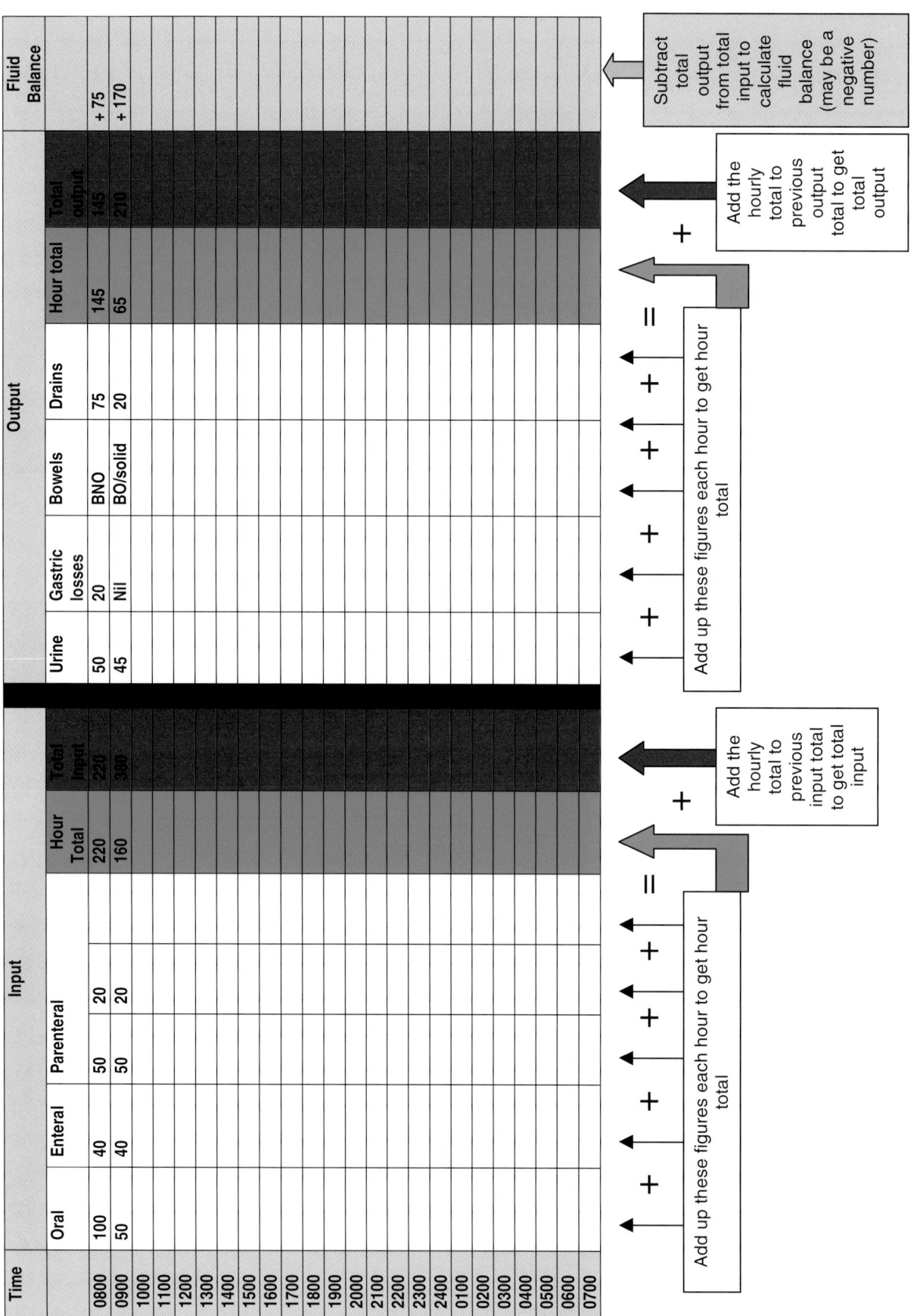

Time	Input					Output							Fluid Balance
	Oral	Enteral	Parenteral		Hour Total	Total Input	Urine	Gastric losses	Bowels	Drains	Hour total	Total output	
0800	100	40	50	20	220	220	50	20	BNO	75	145	145	+ 75
0900	50	40	50	20	160	360	45	Nil	BO/solid	20	65	210	+ 170
1000													
1100													
1200													
1300													
1400													
1500													
1600													
1700													
1800													
1900													
2000													
2100													
2200													
2300													
2400													
0100													
0200													
0300													
0400													
0500													
0600													
0700													

Add up these figures each hour to get hour total

Add the hourly total to previous input total to get total input

Add up these figures each hour to get hour total

Add the hourly total to previous output total to get total output

Subtract total output from total input to calculate fluid balance (may be a negative number)

Figure 8.2 Example of a fluid balance chart.

Procedure guideline 8.1 Fluid input: measurement

Essential equipment

- Fluid balance chart
- Appropriate pumps for fluid or feeding

Preprocedure

Action	Rationale
1 Educate the patient about the fact that their fluid input is being monitored and ask them to alert you to any oral intake.	To ensure the patient is aware of the need to record any oral intake so this can be noted accurately (Baraz *et al.* 2009, R4).
2 Obtain fluid balance chart and document patient's name and the date commenced.	To ensure chart is correctly labelled for the correct patient, allowing accurate documentation (Powell-Tuck *et al.* 2009, C).
3 Ensure pumps available for intravenous fluids, nasogastric/jejunostomy feeds.	To enable accurate hourly record of intake (Reid *et al.* 2004, E)

Procedure

4 Measure oral fluid intake hourly, noting it on the fluid balance chart (see Figure 8.2).	To obtain accurate real-time fluid balance status (Sumnall 2007, E).
5 Note any enteral or parenteral intake.	To obtain accurate real-time fluid balance status and ensure all possible input considered (Alexander *et al.* 2000, E).
6 Add together the values for oral, enteral and parenteral intake for the hour.	To assess hourly fluid intake (Scales and Pilsworth 2008, E).
7 Add this value to the cumulative total for intake (see Figure 8.2).	To assess total intake and enable calculation of the fluid balance (Scales and Pilsworth 2008, E).

Postprocedure

8 Once output totals are calculated (see Procedure guideline 8.6), subtract output from input.	To calculate fluid balance (Powell-Tuck *et al.* 2009, C).
9 Document on chart and in patient's notes.	To ensure accurate documentation (NMC 2009, C).

Procedure guideline 8.2 Fluid output: monitoring/measuring output if the patient is catheterized

Essential equipment

- Urometer
- Measuring jugs (with volume indicators)
- Gloves, apron, goggles
- Bedpan/urinary bottles/commode
- Bile drainage bag/gastrostomy drainage bag
- Scales

Procedure guideline 8.2 (*Continued*)

Preprocedure

Action	Rationale
1 Determine sources of fluid output (see Table 8.2) and note them on the fluid balance chart.	To ensure all possibilities have been considered and to ensure accurate (as possible) output determination (Scales and Pilsworth 2008, E).

Procedure

2 Explain to the patient that it is necessary to monitor their urine output and that you will be doing so every hour.	To ensure the patient is not alarmed by frequent observation and that they are kept informed about current care (Bryant 2007, E).
3 Attach a urometer to the catheter, using an aseptic technique (see Chapter 3, Procedure guideline 3.9).	To allow accurate assessment of hourly urine output, to prevent cross-infection (Fraise and Bradley 2009, E).
4 Each hour, on the hour, note the volume of urine in the urometer, recording this on the fluid balance chart.	To determine urine output and to keep accurate records of this, thus enabling assessment of fluid balance (Scales and Pilsworth 2008, E).
5 Empty the urometer into the collection bag (until the bag is full; this will then need emptying).	To ensure urometer is empty for the next hour's determination. E
6 Add recorded urine output to the other values for output, giving an hourly total.	To allow for fluid balance determination (see Table 8.2). E

Postprocedure

7 Once all output has been determined, noted on chart and total hourly output calculated, subtract total output from total input.	To calculate hourly fluid balance (Levi 2005, E).

Procedure guideline 8.3 Fluid output: monitoring/measuring output if the patient is not catheterized

Essential equipment

- Measuring jugs (with volume indicators)
- Gloves, apron, goggles
- Bedpan/urinary bottles/commode
- Scales

Preprocedure

Action	Rationale
1 Determine sources of fluid output (see Table 8.2) and note on the fluid balance chart.	To ensure all possibilities have been considered to ensure accurate (as possible) output determination (Scales and Pilsworth 2008, E).

Procedure

2 Explain to the patient that it is necessary to measure their urine output.	To ensure that the patient knows that any urine they pass needs to be measured in order to record output and to obtain their co-operation in ensuring accuracy of measurement (Chung *et al.* 2002, R4).

3	Supply the patient with urinary bottles and/or bedpans and ask them to use these even if they are able to mobilize to the toilet; ask them to inform you of each episode.	To ensure the urine is kept for measuring and not disposed of (Chung *et al.* 2002, R4).
4	Use protective equipment for bodily fluids when handling used bottle or bedpan.	To prevent cross-infection (Fraise and Bradley 2009, E).
5	Place bedpan/bottle on to scales, subtracting appropriate value to compensate for weight of item.	To obtain value of urine in millilitres. E
6	If no scales available, use a jug with volume markings; pour urine into jug (using universal precautions), noting level of urine.	To measure urine volume. E
7	Once noted, dispose of urine appropriately.	To prevent contamination and/or cross-infection (Fraise and Bradley 2009, E).
8	Record value on fluid balance chart, adding this to the rest of the output values for the hour.	To determine fluid output for the hour (Sumnall 2007, E).

Postprocedure

9	Once all output has been determined, noted on chart and total hourly output calculated, subtract total output from total input.	To calculate hourly fluid balance (Levi 2005, E).

Procedure guideline 8.4 Fluid output: measuring output from drains

Essential equipment

- Measuring jugs (with volume indicators)
- Gloves, apron, goggles
- Tape and pen

Preprocedure

Action	**Rationale**
1 Determine sources of fluid output (see Table 8.2) and note them on the fluid balance chart.	To ensure all possibilities have been considered to ensure accurate (as possible) output determination (Scales and Pilsworth 2008, E).

Procedure

2	Explain to the patient that the output from the drains will be monitored hourly.	To inform the patient about current care and to ensure they are not alarmed by the frequent observations (Bryant 2007, E).
3	If the drain is drainable, empty contents into jug, noting volume; use universal precautions.	To determine volume of fluid drained and prevent cross-infection (Fraise and Bradley 2009, E).
4	If it is not possible to drain the fluid out of the bag, use a suitable pen and mark the level the fluid reaches each hour. Date and time each marking.	To determine drainage each hour. To ensure consistency in reading and to communicate to other members of the multi-disciplinary team regarding drainage (Sumnall 2007, E).
5	Note volume/drainage on fluid balance chart.	To determine drainage each hour (Sumnall 2007, E).

(Continued)

Procedure guideline 8.4 (*Continued*)

6 Add this figure to the rest of the output values for the hour.	To determine accurate total fluid lost each hour (Sumnall 2007, E).

Postprocedure

7 Once all output has been determined, noted on chart and total hourly output calculated, subtract total output from total input.	To calculate hourly fluid balance (Levi 2005, E).

Procedure guideline 8.5 Fluid output: monitoring output from gastric outlets, nasogastric tubes, gastrostomy

Essential equipment

- Urometer
- Measuring jugs (with volume indicators)
- Gloves, apron, goggles
- Bile drainage bag/gastrostomy drainage bag

Preprocedure

Action	Rationale
1 Determine sources of fluid output (see Table 8.2) and note them on the fluid balance chart.	To ensure all possibilities have been considered to ensure accurate (as possible) output determination (Scales and Pilsworth 2008, E).

Procedure

2 Explain to the patient that it is necessary to monitor drainage every hour.	To inform the patient of current care and interventions (Bryant 2007, E).
3 Ensure gastric outlet device has a drainage bag attached.	To collect any output for measurement. E
4 If instructed, leave the bag open to drain (this may differ depending on condition).	To enable drainage. E
5 Drain contents into marked jug every hour (if quantity allows), using universal precautions.	To determine volume and prevent cross-infection (Fraise and Bradley 2009, E).
6 Attach a urometer if output is high.	To ensure accurate reading and for ease of measuring. E
7 Note volume on fluid balance chart, adding this value to the rest of the output values for that 1 hour.	To enable determination of fluid balance (Sumnall 2007, E).

Postprocedure

8 Once all output has been determined, noted on chart and total hourly output calculated, subtract total output from total input.	To calculate hourly fluid balance (Levi 2005, E).

Procedure guideline 8.6 Fluid output: monitoring output from bowels

Essential equipment

- Measuring jugs (with volume indicators)
- Gloves, apron, goggles
- Bedpan/commode
- Scales
- Rectal tube 'Flexiseal' (if required)

Preprocedure

Action	Rationale
1 Determine sources of fluid output (see Table 8.2) and note them on the fluid balance chart.	To ensure all possibilities have been considered to ensure accurate (as possible) output determination (Scales and Pilsworth 2008, E).

Procedure

2 Explain to the patient that it is necessary to monitor volume of fluid excreted, including that from the bowel, particularly if the stool is loose/watery.	To keep the patient informed about current care and observations, to ensure co-operation in monitoring fluid output (Bryant 2007, E).
3 Provide the patient with bedpans, even if able to mobilize to the bathroom; ask them to place the bedpan over the toilet bowl.	To enable inspection and measurement of fluid lost via the bowel. E
4 If stool is loose enough, this can be transferred into a jug and the volume measured, or use scales.	To quantify fluid output from stool (Scales and Pilsworth 2008, E).
5 If the stool is formed and it is not possible to accurately quantify, still note on fluid balance chart that bowels were opened.	To take into account any insensible losses (Mooney 2007, E).
6 A rectal tube may be suitable in some patients; please refer to local policy regarding use of rectal tube. Note any output on the fluid balance chart.	To ensure correct use of tube and to quantify any fluid losses from the bowel. E
7 Add losses to the previous losses for the hour.	To calculate hourly fluid output (Sumnall 2007, E).

Postprocedure

8 Once all output has been determined, noted on chart and total hourly output calculated, subtract total output from total input.	To calculate hourly fluid balance (Levi 2005, E).

Procedure guideline 8.7 Fluid output: monitoring output from stoma sites

Essential equipment

- Measuring jugs (with volume indicators)
- Gloves, apron, goggles

Preprocedure

Action	Rationale
1 Determine sources of fluid output (see Table 8.2) and note them on the fluid balance chart.	To ensure all possibilities have been considered to ensure accurate (as possible) output determination (Alexander *et al.* 2000, E).

(Continued)

Procedure guideline 8.7 (*Continued*)

Procedure

2 Explain to the patient that you are monitoring hourly output.	To ensure the patient understands why their stoma is being checked hourly. To ensure they are up to date with current care (Bryant 2007, E).
3 Check that the stoma bag is drainable; if not, change (see Chapter 6 for further information and Procedure guidelines on stomas and changing stoma bags).	To ensure ease of draining bag contents and to reduce the number of times the adhesive flange is removed, in order to protect the skin. E
4 Using protective equipment, empty the contents of the stoma bag into the measuring jug, noting volume.	To determine output from stoma for 1 hour and prevent cross-infection (Fraise and Bradley 2009, E).
5 Dispose of contents using protective equipment, adhering to local policy.	To ensure correct disposal of contents and prevent cross-infection (Fraise and Bradley 2009, E).
6 Note volume of stool on chart; add to other losses for the hour.	To ensure correct documentation of output and allow calculation of fluid balance (Association of Surgeons of Great Britain and Ireland 2008, C).
7 Add hourly total (all outputs) to cumulative output (see Figure 8.2).	To enable fluid balance determination (Sumnall 2007, E).

Postprocedure

8 Once all output has been determined, noted on chart and total hourly output calculated, subtract total output from total input.	To calculate hourly fluid balance. E

Problem-solving table 8.1 Prevention and resolution (Procedure guidelines 8.1, 8.2, 8.3, 8.4, 8.5, 8.6 and 8.7)

Problem	Cause	Prevention	Action
Non-compliance/co-operation from patients	Usually misunderstanding or lack of education regarding importance of monitoring fluid balance	Effective patient education and teaching	Determine effective teaching methods, considering individual needs, for example poor hearing, illiteracy. Re-educate the patient, using appropriate means
Inability to record input due to lack of pumps to regulate intravenous fluids or enteral feeds	Not available, unable to use, inappropriate	Request more equipment from appropriate sources, request training	Calculate drip rates on free-flowing fluids to ensure correct hourly input calculated
Insensible losses	Inability to measure some losses	N/A	Note on chart if perspiration is excessive or if bowels opened and immeasurable, to highlight possible inaccuracy in fluid balance

Problem	Cause	Prevention	Action
Leaking drains	Inevitable with some drains	Inevitable with some drains; however, surrounding opening may require further suturing; request surgical review if necessary	Utilize stoma bag/wound drainage bag to collect drainage, to enable measurement
Incorrect fluid balance calculation	Incorrect fluid input determination Incorrect fluid output determination Incorrect calculation	Appropriate teaching and education for nurses performing these procedures, competency checking	Ensure nurses are educated appropriately, access information and education if unsure of procedure or technique

Postprocedural considerations

Every hour the findings of fluid monitoring should be recorded; any deficit or change in fluid balance should be reported. Any imbalance noted will require action and a management plan. The nurse recording the fluid balance should have an appreciation of the importance of fluid imbalance management and should notify the appropriate person.

Complications

Correct fluid balance monitoring is essential in the successful management of actual or potential fluid balance disturbances (Jevon and Ewens 2007). Over- or underestimation of the fluid status could lead to incorrect management, resulting in fluid overload (hypervolaemia), dehydration (hypovolaemia) (Bryant 2007) and/or electrolyte disturbances, all of which will ultimately lead to organ dysfunction.

Cook *et al.* (2004) describe the importance of correct fluid balance monitoring and recording, not only volumes but the type of fluid administered. They explain that the accurate recording of fluid balance should have the same emphasis and importance as prescription charting.

Fluid overload/hypervolaemia

Underestimating the fluid balance may lead to continued or increased administration of IV fluids, which if monitored incorrectly could result in circulatory overload. Excess IV fluid administration is not the only cause of circulatory overload, which can also result from acute renal failure, heart failure and intake of excessive sodium.

In health, homoeostatic mechanisms exist to compensate and redistribute excess fluids but in ill health, these mechanisms are often inadequate, leading to increasing circulatory volumes. As the volume within the circulatory system rises, so does the hydrostatic pressure, which when excessive results in leaking of fluid from the vessels into the surrounding tissues. This is evident as oedema, initially apparent in the ankles and legs or buttocks and sacrum if the patient is in bed. This can progress to generalized oedema,

where even the tissues surrounding the eyes become puffy and swollen.

A bounding pulse and an increased blood pressure are also signs of fluid overload, as is an increased cardiac output and raised central venous pressure (Edwards 2000).

One of the most dangerous symptoms of fluid overload is pulmonary oedema, which occurs when the hydrostatic pressure within the vessels causes congestion within the pulmonary circulation, increasing the hydrostatic pressure there and causing fluid to leak into the lungs and pulmonary tissues (Casey 2004). This presents with respiratory symptoms, including shortness of breath, increased respiratory rate, a cough, often associated with pink frothy sputum and finally reduced oxygen saturations due to inadequate gaseous exchange at the alveolar level (Casey 2004). Left untreated, this can be fatal as the lungs are failing to provide essential cells and organs with oxygen, which would eventually cause organ dysfunction and then failure.

Cardiac ischaemia can also result from fluid overload, not only from the reduced availability of oxygen to the cardiac cells due to the pulmonary oedema, but also from the increase in volume causing the cardiac muscle to stretch, leading to cell damage (Alexander *et al.* 2000).

Treatment of hypovolaemia would involve restricting fluid intake, monitoring electrolytes and using diuretics in an attempt to offload some of the excess fluid. Vasodilators may also be considered to reduce the pressure in the vessels. If these mechanisms fail, it may be necessary to use renal replacement therapy to drive the fluid out of the circulation.

In some cases fluid overload is part of the disease process. However, with effective monitoring and fluid balance recording and assessment, it may be possible to avoid the devastating complications.

Hypovolaemia/dehydration

Dehydration refers to a negative fluid balance, when the fluid output exceeds the fluid intake (Jevon 2010). Overestimation of the fluid balance may lead to inadequate replacement of lost fluids. Dehydration can, however, be caused by

347

a loss of fluids to 'third spaces' such as ascites or lost due to a reduction in colloid osmotic pressure (hypoalbuminaemia) (Casey 2004), losses which are not easy to account for. Fluid balance charts should therefore always be used in association with physical assessment of the patient, weight measurement and laboratory results.

There are three categories of dehydration (Mentes 2006) – isotonic, hypertonic and hypotonic – each related to the type of fluid and solutes lost. Isotonic describes the loss of both water and sodium from the ECF; hypertonic is excessive loss of water only, which leads to a rise in ECF sodium, causing a shift in fluid from the intracellular space to the extracellular. Hypotonic dehydration results from excessive sodium loss, particularly in the overuse of diuretics.

Dehydration can ultimately cause a reduction in circulating volume. As with any change in a homoeostatic state, the body in health has the ability to compensate but in ill health these mechanisms are often inadequate. Untreated dehydration will quickly lead to a drop in blood pressure and a rise in heart rate (to compensate for the fall in blood pressure). A fall in blood pressure will firstly lead to inadequate renal perfusion, causing a rise in metabolites, acidosis, acute renal failure and eventual toxaemia. Untreated, other organs will suffer from underperfusion, possibly resulting in ischaemia, organ dysfunction and eventual organ failure (Sumnall 2007).

Additional signs and symptoms of dehydration are thirst, weight loss, decreased urine output, dry skin and mucous membranes, fatigue and increased body temperature (Goertz 2006).

Treatment of dehydration includes the replacement of lost fluid and electrolytes but caution must be exercised. If the dehydration is mild, slower fluid replacement is advised, in order to prevent further complications in shifts in electrolytes. However, if hypovolaemia exists with the signs and symptoms of circulatory shock, low blood pressure and organ dysfunction, aggressive fluid replacement is advised (Jevon 2010).

Nutritional status

Definitions

Nutritional status refers to the state of a person's health as determined by their dietary intake and body composition. Nutritional support refers to any method of giving nutrients which encourages an optimal nutritional status. It includes modifying the types of foods eaten, dietary supplementation, enteral tube feeding and parenteral nutrition (NCCAC 2006).

Anatomy and physiology

The normal process of ingestion of food or fluids is via the oral cavity to the gastrointestinal tract.

Figure 8.3 Pharyngeal stage of swallowing.

The normal swallow involves a number of stages, starting with the oral preparatory stage which is influenced by the sight and smell of food. Food or liquid is placed in the mouth and the lips are closed. After chewing and mixing with saliva, it forms a cohesive mass (bolus) that is held on the centre of the tongue. Swallowing is a voluntary task that requires intact functioning of the cranial nerves in addition to intact motor and sensory input for lips, jaw, teeth, tongue and palate.

The pharyngeal stage of swallowing, which is involuntary (see Figure 8.3), occurs as the food bolus crosses the mandible/tongue base as the palate closes, sealing entry to the nasal cavity and reducing risk of nasal regurgitation. Movement of the tongue base and posterior pharyngeal wall squeezes the bolus down the pharynx. Involuntary movements of the larynx (voice box), vocal cords and epiglottis protect the airway and open the cricopharyngeus. The bolus travels from the cricopharyngeus to the gastro-oesophageal junction and peristaltic action then transfers the bolus down the oesophagus (Logemann 1998).

The gastrointestinal tract is the site where food is ingested, digested and absorbed, thus enabling nutrients to be used by the body for growth and maintenance of body functions. Food ingested is moved along the gastrointestinal tract by peristaltic waves through the oesophagus, stomach, small intestine and large intestine. The passage of food and fluid through the gastrointestinal tract is dependent on the autonomic nervous system, gut hormones such as gastrin and cholecystokinin, the function of exocrine glands such as the parotid, pancreas and liver and psychological aspects such as anxiety. Sphincters situated between the stomach and duodenum, the ileocaecal valves and the anal sphincter also regulate the rate of passage of food and fluids through the tract.

Before food can be absorbed, it must be digested and broken down into molecules that can be transported across the intestinal epithelium which line the gastrointestinal tract. This process is dependent on digestive enzymes secreted by the pancreas and lining of the intestinal tract which act on specific nutrients. Bile, from the liver, is required to emulsify fat, thus enabling it to be broken down by digestive enzymes. The absorption of nutrients is dependent on an active, or energy-dependent, transport across the intestinal epithelium lining the digestive tract. Villi, finger-like projections, increase the surface area of the small intestine to aid absorption. Most nutrients are absorbed from the small intestine although some require specific sites within the gastrointestinal tract; for example, vitamin B_{12} is absorbed in the terminal ileum. Mucosa shed into the lumen of the intestine is broken down and absorbed along with fluid and electrolytes secreted into the lumen during the process of digestion. The volumes of fluid secreted into the gut are large and may amount to 8–9 L a day when combined with an oral intake of 1.5–2 L daily. The majority of fluid is reabsorbed in the small intestine with the remainder being absorbed in the large intestine. Bacteria in the large intestine metabolize non-starch polysaccharides (dietary fibre), increasing faecal bulk and producing short chain fatty acids which are absorbed and metabolized for energy.

Related theory

Bodyweight is the most widely used measure of nutritional status in clinical practice. However, whilst weight provides a simple, readily obtainable and usually fairly precise measure, it remains a one-dimensional metric and as such has limitations. In contrast, an understanding of anatomy and physiology and in particular the changes that can occur in body composition, in addition to frank weight gain or loss, provides valuable clinical insight (Battezzati *et al.* 2003). In the so-called 'two-compartment' model of body composition, bodyweight is described in terms of, firstly, fat-free mass, that is bones, muscles and organs, which includes the hepatic carbohydrate energy store glycogen, and secondly, fat mass or adipose tissue (van Loan 2003). Water comprises up to 60% of total bodyweight. It is distributed throughout the fat-free and fat compartments with approximately two-thirds present as intracellular and one-third as extracellular fluid. Thus, a healthy 70 kg male comprises 42 kg of water which amounts to 60% of total bodyweight. This is made up of 28 L of intracellular fluid and 14 L of extracellular fluid. The same 'typical' male contains approximately 12 kg of muscle, also referred to as lean body mass, and 12 kg of fat (Geissler and Powers 2005).

Body composition and nutritional status are closely linked and are dependent upon a number of factors including age, sex, metabolic requirements, dietary intake and the presence of disease. Depletion of lean body mass occurs in both acute trauma and chronic inflammatory conditions and negatively affects functional and immune capacity (Roubenoff and Kehayias 1991). Loss of skeletal lean body mass is a natural phenomenon of ageing and similarly compromises functional capacity. Shifts in body water compartments are readily observed in conditions such as ascites and oedema (Bedogni *et al.* 2003). Both of these conditions result from an abnormally increased extracellular water compartment and, despite a gain in total bodyweight, are indicative of worsening outcome.

The physiological characteristics of the different body compartments can be exploited by various assessment tools and techniques to determine changes indicative of nutritional risk (Bedogni *et al.* 2006). Such changes are masked if weight alone is used as the sole measurement.

Evidence-based approaches

Rationale

Nutritional support, to maintain or replete body composition, should be considered for anybody unable to maintain their nutritional status by taking their usual diet (NCCAC 2006). These include the following.

- Patients unable to eat their usual diet (e.g. because of anorexia, mucositis, taste changes or dysphagia) should be given advice on modifying their diet.
- Patients unable to meet their nutritional requirements, despite dietary modifications, should be offered oral nutritional supplements.
- Patients unable to take sufficient food and dietary supplements to meet their nutritional requirements should be considered for an enteral tube feed.
- Patients unable to eat at all should have an enteral tube feed. Reasons for complete inability to eat include carcinoma of the head and neck area or oesophagus, surgery to the head or oesophagus, radiotherapy treatment to the head or neck and fistulae of the oral cavity or oesophagus.
- Parenteral nutrition (PN) may be indicated in patients with a non-functioning or inaccessible gastrointestinal (GI) tract who are likely to be 'nil by mouth' for 5 days or longer. Reasons for a non-functioning or inaccessible GI tract include bowel obstruction, short bowel syndrome, gut toxicity following bone marrow transplantation or chemotherapy, major abdominal surgery, uncontrolled vomiting and enterocutaneous fistulae. Enteral nutrition should always be the first option when considering nutritional support.

Patients in any group may have an increased requirement for nutrients due to an increased metabolic rate, as found in those with burns, major sepsis, trauma or cancer cachexia (Bozzetti 2001, Thomas 2007, Todorovic and Micklewright 2004). Patients should have nutritional requirements estimated prior to the start of nutritional support and should be monitored regularly.

Methods of assessing of nutritional status

Before the initiation of nutritional support, the patient must be assessed. The purpose of assessment is to identify whether a patient is undernourished, the reasons why this may have occurred and to provide baseline data for planning and evaluating nutritional support (NCCAC 2006). It is helpful to use more than one method of assessing nutritional status. For example, a dietary history may be used to assess the adequacy of a person's diet but does not reflect actual nutritional status, whereas percentage weight loss does give an indication of nutritional status. However, percentage weight loss taken in isolation gives no idea of dietary intake and likelihood of improvement or deterioration in nutritional status (NCCAC 2006).

Bodyweight and weight loss

Body Mass Index (BMI) or comparison of a patient's weight with a chart of ideal bodyweight gives a measure of whether the patient has a normal weight, is overweight or underweight, and may be calculated from weight and height using the following equation:

$$\mathrm{BMI} = \frac{\text{Weight (kg)}}{\text{Height (m)}^2}$$

Tables are available to allow the rapid and easy calculation of BMI (BAPEN 2003a). These comparisons, however, are not a good indicator of whether the patient is at risk nutritionally, as an apparently normal weight can mask severe muscle wasting.

Of greater use is the comparison of current weight with the patient's usual weight. Percentage weight loss is a useful measure of the risk of malnutrition:

$$\% \text{ Weight loss} = \frac{\text{Usual Weight} - \text{Actual Weight}}{\text{Usual Weight}} \times 100$$

A patient would be identified as malnourished if they had any of the following:

- BMI less than 18.5 kg/m^2
- unintentional weight loss greater than 10% within the last 3–6 months
- BMI less than 20 kg/m^2 and unintentional weight loss greater than 5% within the last 3–6 months.

(NCCAC 2006)

Sick children should have their weight and height measured frequently. It may be useful to measure on a daily basis (Shaw and Lawson 2007). These measurements must be plotted onto centile charts. A single weight or height cannot be interpreted as there is much variation of growth within each age group. It is a matter of concern if a child's weight begins to fall across the centiles or if the weight plateaus.

Obesity and oedema may make interpretation of bodyweight difficult; both may mask loss of lean body mass and potential malnutrition (Pennington 1997).

Accurate weighing scales are necessary for measurement of bodyweight. Patients who are unable to stand may require sitting scales.

It is often not appropriate to weigh palliative care patients who may experience inevitable weight loss as disease progresses. Psychologically, it may be difficult for patients to see that they are continuing to lose weight. Measures of nutritional status such as clinical examination and current food intake may still be used in addition to measures of bodyweight.

Skinfold thickness and bio-electrical impedance

Skinfold thickness measurements can be used to assess stores of body fat. They are rarely used in routine nutritional assessment due to the insensitivity of the technique and the variation between measurements made by different observers. They are more appropriate for long-term assessments or research purposes and the technique should only be used by practitioners who are practised in using skinfold thickness calipers because of the potential for intra-investigator variation in results (Durnin and Womersley 1974).

Bio-electrical impedance analysis (BIA) is a simple, non-invasive and relatively inexpensive technique for measuring body composition (Janssen *et al.* 2000). This technique works well in healthy individuals but may be of limited use in some hospital patients with abnormal hydration status (for example, severe dehydration or ascites) and is also less reliable at the extremes of BMI ranges (Kyle *et al.* 2004).

Clinical examination

Observation of the patient may reveal signs and symptoms indicative of nutritional depletion.

- *Physical appearance*: emaciated, wasted appearance, loose clothing/jewellery.
- *Oedema*: will affect weight and may mask the appearance of muscle wastage. May indicate plasma protein deficiency and is often a reflection of the patient's overall condition rather than a measure of nutritional status.
- *Mobility*: weakness and impaired movement may result from loss of muscle mass.
- *Mood*: apathy, lethargy and poor concentration can be features of undernutrition.
- *Pressure sores and poor wound healing*: may reflect impaired immune function as a consequence of undernutrition and vitamin deficiencies (Thomas and Bishop 2007).

Specific nutritional deficiencies may be identifiable in some patients. For example, thiamine deficiency characterized by dementia is associated with high alcohol consumption. Rickets is seen in children with vitamin D deficiency.

A more structured approach can be taken by using an assessment tool such as SGA or patient-generated SGA (PG-SGA) (Bauer *et al.* 2002). This involves a systematic evaluation of muscle and fat sites around the body and assessment for oedema in the ankles or sacral area in immobile patients. Such an assessment can be used to determine whether the patient is malnourished and can be repeated to assess changes in nutritional status.

Dietary intake

Nutrient intake can be assessed by a diet history (Thomas and Bishop 2007). A 24-hour recall may be used to assess recent nutrient intake and a food chart may be used to monitor current dietary intake. A diet history may also be used to provide information on food frequency, food habits, preferences, meal pattern, portion sizes, the presence of any eating difficulty and changes in food intake (Reilly 1996). A food chart on which all food and fluid taken is recorded is a useful method for monitoring nutritional intake, especially in the hospital setting or when dietary recall is not reliable (Thomas and Bishop 2007).

Biochemical investigations

Biochemical tests carried out on blood may give information on the patient's nutritional status. The most commonly used are as follows.

- *Plasma proteins.* Changes in plasma albumin may arise due to physical stress, changes in circulating volume, hepatic and renal function, shock conditions and septicaemia. Plasma albumin and changes in plasma albumin are not a direct reflection of nutritional intake and nutritional status as it has been shown that they may remain unchanged despite changes in body composition (NCCAC 2006). In addition, albumin has a long half-life of 21 days, so it cannot reflect recent changes in nutritional intake. It may be useful to review serum albumin concentrations in conjunction with C-reactive protein (CRP), which is an acute-phase protein produced by the body in response to injury or trauma. CRP greater than 10 mg/L and serum albumin less than 30 g/L suggests 'illness'. CRP less than 10 mg/L and serum albumin less than 30 g/L suggests protein depletion (Elia 2001). Prealbumin and retinol binding protein levels are more sensitive measures of nutrition support, reflecting recent changes in dietary intake rather than nutritional status. However, they may be expensive to measure or not measured routinely in hospital.
- *Haemoglobin.* This is often below haematological reference values in malnourished patients (men 13.5–17.5 g/dL, women 11.5–15.5 g/dL). This can be due to a number of reasons, such as loss of blood from circulation, increased destruction of red blood cells or reduced production of erythrocytes and haemoglobin, for example due to dietary deficiency of iron or folate.
- *Serum vitamin and mineral levels.* Clinical examination of the patient may suggest a vitamin or mineral deficiency. For example, gingivitis may be due to a deficiency of vitamin C, vitamin A, niacin or riboflavin. Goitre is associated with iodine deficiency, and tremors, convulsions and behavioural disturbances may be caused by magnesium deficiency (Shenkin 2001). Serum vitamin and mineral levels are rarely measured routinely, as they are expensive and often cannot be performed by hospital laboratories.
- *Immunological competence.* Total lymphocyte count may reflect nutritional status although levels may also be depleted with malignancy, chemotherapy, zinc deficiency, age and non-specific stress (Bodger and Heatley 2001).

If a patient is considered to be malnourished by one or more of the above methods of assessment then referral to a dietitian should be made immediately (Burnham and Barton 2001).

Methods for calculation of nutritional requirements

The body requires protein, energy, fluid and micronutrients such as vitamins, minerals and trace elements to function optimally. Nutritional requirements should be estimated for patients requiring any form of nutritional support to ensure that these needs are met.

Energy requirements may be calculated using equations such as those derived by Schofield (1985), which take into account weight, age, sex, activity level and clinical injury, for example post surgery, sepsis or ventilator dependency. An easier and more appropriate method is to use bodyweight and allowances based on the patient's clinical condition (Table 8.4). Careful adjustments may be necessary in cases of oedema or obesity, in order to avoid overfeeding (Horgan and Stubbs 2003).

Fluid and nitrogen (or protein) requirements can be calculated in a similar way. If additional nitrogen is being given in situations where losses are increased, for example due to trauma, GI losses or major sepsis, then additional energy intake is required to assist in promoting a nitrogen balance. Improvement in nitrogen balance is the single nutritional parameter most consistently associated with improved outcome, and the primary goal of nutrition support should be the attainment of nitrogen balance (Gidden and Shenkin 2000). Additional fluid of 500–750 mL is necessary for every 1°C rise in temperature in pyrexial patients (Thomas 2007).

Table 8.4 Guidelines for estimation of patient's daily energy and protein requirements (per kilogram bodyweight)

	Normal	Pyrexia or extreme sepsis
Energy (kcal)	25	25–35
(kJ)	105	105–146
Nitrogen (g)	0.17 (0.14–0.2)	0.2–0.3
Protein (g)	1 (0.87–1.25)	1.25–1.87
Fluid (mL)	30–35	30–35 plus 2–2.5 mL per °C in temperature above 37°C

Vitamin and mineral requirements calculated as detailed in the Committee on Medical Aspects of Food Policy (COMA) Report 41 on dietary reference values (COMA and DH 1991) apply to groups of healthy people and are not necessarily appropriate for those who are ill. A patient deficient in a vitamin or mineral may benefit from additional supplements to improve a condition. Macronutrient and micronutrient requirements for children are also listed in the COMA Report. Calculations are usually done with the reference nutrient intake (RNI). The child's actual bodyweight, not the expected bodyweight, is used when calculating requirements. This is to avoid excessive feeding. For a very small child, the height age instead of the chronological age is the basis of calculation (Shaw and Lawson 2007).

Methods for measuring height and weight of an adult patient

Taking an accurate height and weight of a patient is an essential part of nutrition screening. Accurate measurements of bodyweight may also be required for estimating body surface area and calculating drug dosages, such as for chemotherapy. All patients should have height and weight measured on admission to hospital and weight should be taken at regular intervals during their hospital stay according to local policy and individual clinical need.

Preprocedural considerations

Check that the patient is able to stand or sit on the appropriate scales. The patient should remove outdoor clothing and shoes before being weighed and having height measured.

When obtaining a height measurement, check that the patient is able to stand upright whilst the measurement is taken. For patients who are unable to stand then height may be determined by measuring ulna length and using conversion tables (BAPEN 2003a).

It may not be possible to weigh patients who cannot be moved or are unable to sit or stand. Alternative methods to obtain weight should be explored, for example bed scales which can be placed under the wheels of the bed, scales as an integral part of a bed or a patient hoist with weighing facility.

Equipment
Scales

Scales (either sitting or standing) must be calibrated and positioned on a level surface. If electronic or battery scales are used then they must be connected to the mains or have appropriate working batteries prior to the patient getting on the scales.

Stadiometer

These are devices for measuring height and may be mounted on weighing scales or wall mounted.

Tape measure

Required if estimating height from ulna length. The tape measure should use centimetres, be disposable or made of plastic that can be cleaned with a detergent wipe between patient uses.

Assessment tools

Identification of patients who are malnourished or at risk of malnutrition is an important first step in nutritional care. There are a number of screening tools available which

---

Procedure guideline 8.8 **Measuring the weight and height of the patient**

Essential equipment

- Scales
- Stadiometer (preferably fixed to the wall)

Optional equipment

- Tape measure

Preprocedure

Action	Rationale
1 Position the scales for easy access and apply the brakes (if appropriate).	To ensure that the patient can get on and off the scales easily and to avoid accidents should the scales move. E
2 Ask the patient to remove shoes and outdoor garments. The patient should be wearing light indoor clothes only (see Action Figure 2).	Outdoor clothes and shoes will add additional weight and make it difficult to obtain an accurate bodyweight. E

352

Procedure

3 Ensure that the scales record zero then ask the patient to stand on scales (or sit if using sitting scales). Ask the patient to remain still and check that the patient is not supporting any weight on any object, for example wall, stick or feet on the floor.	To record an accurate weight (NMC 2009, C).
4 Note the reading on the scale and record immediately, taking care that it is legible. Check with the patient that the weight reflects their expected weight and that the weight is similar to previous weights recorded. This may require conversion of weight from kg to stones and pounds or vice versa.	To check that the weight is correct. If the weight is not as expected then the patient should be re-weighed. E
5 Ensure that the patient has removed their shoes and then ask them to stand straight with heels together. If the stadiometer is wall mounted, the heels should touch the heel plate or the wall. With a freestanding device the person's back should be toward the measuring rod.	Shoes will provide additional height and make the measurement inaccurate. E To ensure that the patient is standing upright. If the person does not have their back against the measuring rod then the measuring arm may not reach the head. E
6 The patient should look straight ahead and with the bottom of the nose and the bottom of the ear in a parallel plane. The patient should be asked to stretch to reach maximal height.	To ensure an accurate height is measured. E
7 Record height to the nearest millimetre.	To record an accurate measurement of the patient's height (NMC 2009, C).
8 To estimate the height of a patient from ulna length, ask the patient to remove long-sleeved jacket, shirt or top.	To be able to access their left arm for measurement purposes. E
9 Measure between the point of the elbow (olecranon process) and the midpoint of the prominent bone of the wrist (styloid process) on the left side if possible.	To obtain measurement of the length of the ulna. E
10 Estimate the patient's height to the nearest centimetre, using a conversion table.	To estimate the patient's height (BAPEN 2003a, C).

Postprocedure

11 Document height and weight in patient's notes.	To record the accurate measurement of patient's height and weight (NMC 2009, C).

Action Figure 2   Weighing a patient.

Problem-solving table 8.2 Prevention and resolution (Procedure guideline 8.8)

Problem	Cause	Prevention	Action
Patient unable to stand on scale	Poorly positioned scales Patient balance not sufficient	Check with patient prior to asking them to stand on scales if they are able to do so. Offer sitting scales if necessary	Ensure both sitting and standing scales are available in the hospital
Weight obtained appears too low	Patient may have put pressure on scales prior to them reaching zero	Ensure zero is visible before patient touches scales	Check weight with patient once obtained Re-weigh patient to check correct weight
Weight obtained appears too high	Patient may be wearing outdoor clothes, shoes or be carrying a bag, drainage bag and so on Patient may have fluid retention, for example oedema or ascites	Ensure that the patient is wearing light indoor clothes before standing on the scales Check whether patient has fluid retention	Check weight with patient once obtained Re-weigh patient to check correct weight
Patient is unable to stand	Patient is unwell or has physical disability	Discuss the procedure with patient before undertaking height measurement	Consider estimating height from ulna measurement

354

consider different aspects of nutritional status. National screening initiatives have demonstrated that 28% of patients admitted to hospital were found to be at risk of malnutrition – high risk (22%) and medium risk (6%) (BAPEN 2009). Particular diagnoses, such as cancer, increase the risk of malnutrition.

All patients who are identified as at risk of malnutrition should undergo a nutritional assessment. Subjective global assessment (SGA) is a comprehensive assessment but necessitates more time and expertise to carry out than most screening tests. Some more simple screening tools, including the malnutrition universal screening tool (MUST) (BAPEN 2003a), based on the patient's Body Mass Index, weight loss and illness score, are less time consuming. Other tools may be specific to the patient's age or diagnosis (Kondrup et al. 2003). The most important feature of using any screening tool is that patients identified as requiring nutritional assessment or intervention have a nutritional care plan initiated and are referred to the dietitian for further advice if appropriate.

Postprocedural considerations

Consideration must be given to the patient's weight and whether this reflects a change in their clinical condition. The weight may be being used as part of a nutritional screening or assessment or for planning of treatment, for example medication. Any significant changes should be interpreted in the light of potential changes in body composition and incorporated into the patient's care plan. For example, a loss of weight may require further questioning about dietary intake and the commencement of a nutritional care plan.

After taking a measurement of height it is useful to check with the patient that the figure obtained is approximately the height that is expected. However, it is important to consider that patients may report a loss in height with increasing years. A cumulative height loss from age 30 to 70 years may be about 3 cm for men and 5 cm for women and by age 80 years it increases to 5 cm for men and 8 cm for women (Sorkin et al. 1999).

Provision of nutritional support: oral

Evidence-based approaches
Rationale

An essential part of providing diet for a patient is to ensure that the patient is able to consume the food and fluid in a safe and pleasant environment. Some patients may require assistance with feeding or drinking and a system should be in place to ensure that these patients receive the required attention at each meal time and beverage service provided.

Box 8.1 Food and nutrition benchmark ('food' includes drinks)

Agreed patient/client-focused outcome: patients/clients are enabled to consume food (orally) which meets their individual needs

Indicators/information that highlight concerns which may trigger the need for benchmarking activity:

- Patient satisfaction surveys
- Complaints figures and analysis
- Audit results: including catering audit, nutritional risk assessments, documentation audit, environmental audit (including dining facilities)
- Contract monitoring, for example wastage of food, food handling and/or food hygiene training records

- Ordering of dietary supplements/special diets
- Audit of available equipment and utensils
- Educational audits/student placement feedback
- Litigation/Clinical Negligence Scheme for Trusts
- Professional concern
- Media reports
- *Sustainable Food and the NHS* (King's Fund 2005), *Food and Nutritional Care in Hospitals* (Council of Europe 2003)

Factor	Benchmark of best practice
1 Screening/assessment to identify patients'/clients' nutritional needs	Nutritional screening progresses to further assessment for all patients/clients identified as 'at risk' using a screening tool that assesses Body Mass Index and weight changes, for example MUST (NCCAC 2006)
2 Planning, implementation and evaluation	Plans of care based on ongoing nutritional assessments are of care for those patients who require advised, implemented and evaluated nutritional assessment
3 A conducive environment (acceptable sights, smells and sounds)	The environment is conducive to enabling the individual patients/clients to eat. Implementation of Protected Mealtimes
4 Assistance to eat and drink	Patients/clients receive the care and assistance they require with eating and drinking. Provision of eating aids where appropriate
5 Obtaining food	Patients/clients/carers, whatever their communication needs, have sufficient information to enable them to obtain their food. Examples include the NHS menu provision and utilizing menu translation services
6 Food provided	Food that is provided by the service meets the needs and preferences of individual patients/clients through audit of patient feedback and equality and diversity co-operatives
7 Food availability	Patients/clients have set mealtimes. Flexibility is also important, ensuring a replacement meal is offered if a meal is missed and patients can access a lighter meal or snacks at any time
8 Food presentation	Food is presented to patients/clients in a way that takes into account portion capacity and what appeals to them as individuals
9 Monitoring	The amount of food patients actually eat is monitored, recorded and leads to action when there is cause for concern
10 Eating to promote health	All opportunities are used to encourage the patients/clients to eat to promote their own health

Other factors which may influence future food intake (e.g. surgery, chemotherapy or radiotherapy) also need to be taken into consideration when planning nutritional support, as clinical experience shows these may exert a deleterious effect on appetite and the ability to maintain an adequate nutritional intake (Newman *et al.* 1998).

DH 2001b. © Crown copyright. Reproduced under the terms of the Click-Use Licence.

It is essential that meals are appetizing and strictly comply with any dietary restriction that is relevant to the patient. For example, those with food allergies, texture modifications, religious or cultural dietary requirements need to be clearly identified with the senior ward nurse, before assistance with feeding commences. Eating and drinking are pleasurable experiences and the psychosocial aspect of this cannot be overestimated. The inability to participate in mealtimes can be socially isolating (Ekberg *et al.* 2002, Gaziano 2002).

Supporting the dignity of the patient throughout the process is also imperative to its success and acceptance.

Provision of food and nutrition in a hospital setting

Many factors, including being in hospital, need to be taken into consideration when planning nutritional support. Within the *Essence of Care* framework (DH 2001b), food and nutrition were identified by patients as a fundamental area of care that is frequently unsatisfactory within the NHS.

Good nutritional care, adequate hydration and enjoyable mealtimes can dramatically improve the general health and well-being of patients who are unable to feed themselves, and can be particularly relevant to older people (Nutrition Summit Stakeholder Group and DH 2007). Unfortunately, it is evident that assistance with meals for those that require it does not always occur. The 2006 inpatient survey undertaken by the Healthcare Commission identified that of those patients who said they needed help to eat their meals, 18% said they did not get enough help and 21% said that they only got enough help sometimes (Healthcare Commission 2007).

Clinical benchmarking (DH 2001b) and clinical initiatives such as protected mealtimes aim to address common problems that patients experience whilst in hospital. Box 8.1 outlines the benchmark for food and nutrition, identifying specific factors that need to be considered when reviewing service provision, in order to promote better practice. The Department of Health and the Nutrition Summit Stakeholder Group have worked together to produce an action plan based on the 10 key characteristics of good nutritional care in hospitals. These are outlined in Box 8.2.

Modification of diet

Practical information on modification of diet can be found in the Royal Marsden Hospital Patient Information Series *Eating Well When You Have Cancer – A Guide for Cancer Patients* (Royal Marsden NHS Trust 2002), *Diet and Cancer* (MCS 2009) and *Have You Got a Small Appetite?* (NAGE, n.d.). See also Table 8.5.

Dietary supplements

If patients are unable to meet their nutritional requirements with food alone then they may require appropriate supple-

---

> **Box 8.2** Ten key characteristics of good nutritional care in hospitals
>
> - All patients are screened on admission to identify the patients who are malnourished or at risk of becoming malnourished. All patients are re-screened weekly.
> - All patients have a care plan which identifies their nutritional care needs and how they are to be met.
> - The hospital includes specific guidance on food services and nutritional care in its Clinical Governance arrangements.
> - Patients are involved in the planning and monitoring arrangements for food service provision.
> - The ward implements Protected Mealtimes to provide an environment conducive to patients enjoying and being able to eat their food.
> - All staff have the appropriate skills and competencies needed to ensure that patients' nutritional needs are met. All staff receive regular training on nutritional care and management.
> - Hospital facilities are designed to be flexible and patient centred with the aim of providing and delivering an excellent experience of food service and nutritional care 24 hours a day, every day.
> - The hospital has a policy for food service and nutritional care which is patient centred and performance managed in line with home country governance frameworks.
> - Food service and nutritional care are delivered to the patient safely.
> - The hospital supports a multidisciplinary approach to nutritional care and values the contribution of all staff groups working in partnership with patients and users.

mentation using dietary supplements. These may be used to improve an inadequate diet or as a sole source of nutrition if taken in sufficient quantity.

Sip feeds

These come in a range of flavours, both sweet and savoury, and are presented as a powder in a packet or ready prepared in a can, bottle or carton. Sip feeds contain whole protein, hydrolysed fat and carbohydrates. Most are called 'complete feeds' since they provide all protein, vitamins, minerals and trace elements to meet requirements if a prescribed volume is taken (Thomas and Bishop 2007). Others may be aimed at specific needs, for example high protein.

Energy supplements

Carbohydrates

Glucose polymers in powder or liquid form contain approximately 350 kcal (1442 kJ) per 100 g and 187–299 kcal (770–1232 kJ) per 100 mL respectively. Powdered glucose polymer is virtually tasteless and may be added to anything in which it will dissolve, for example milk and other drinks, soup, cereals and milk pudding; liquid glucose polymers may be fruit flavoured or

Table 8.5 Suggestions for modification of diet

Eating difficulty	Dietary modification
Anorexia	Serve small meals and snacks, for example twice-daily snack options
	Make food look attractive with garnish
	Fortify foods with butter, cream or cheese to increase energy content of meals
	Use alcohol, steroids, megestrol acetate or medroxyprogesterone as an appetite stimulant
	Encourage food that patient prefers
	Offer nourishing drinks between meals. In hospital consider a 'cocktail' drinks round
Sore mouth	Offer foods that are soft and easy to eat
	Avoid dry foods that require chewing
	Avoid citrus fruits and drinks
	Avoid salt and spicy foods
	Allow hot food to cool before eating
Dysphagia	Offer foods that are soft and serve with additional sauce or gravy
	Some foods may need to be blended: make sure food is served attractively
	Supplement the diet with nourishing drinks between meals
Nausea and vomiting	Have cold foods in preference to hot as these emit less odour
	Keep away from cooking smells
	Sip fizzy, glucose-containing drinks
	Eat small frequent meals and snacks that are high in carbohydrate (e.g. biscuits and toast)
	Try ginger drinks and ginger biscuits
Early satiety	Eat small, frequent meals. In hospital access an 'out-of-hours' meal service
	Avoid high-fat foods which delay gastric emptying
	Avoid drinking large quantities when eating
	Use prokinetics, for example metoclopramide, to encourage gastric emptying

neutral (Thomas and Bishop 2007). Such supplements would be used to increase the energy content of the diet.

Fat

Fat may be in the form of long-chain triglycerides (LCT) or medium-chain triglycerides (MCT) and comes as a liquid which can be added to food and drinks. These oils provide 416–772 kcal (1714–3181 kJ) per 100 mL: the oils with a lower energy value are presented in the form of an emulsion and those with a higher energy value are presented as pure oil (Thomas and Bishop 2007).

Mixed fat and glucose polymer solutions and powders are available and provide 150 kcal per 100 mL or 486 kcal per 100 g, depending on the relative proportion of fat and carbohydrates in the product.

Products containing MCT are used in preference to those containing LCT where a patient suffers from GI impairment causing malabsorption. Patients require specific advice about their use to ensure that they are introduced into the diet slowly and GI tolerance is assessed (Thomas and Bishop 2007).

Always check with the manufacturer for the exact energy content of products.

Note: products containing a glucose polymer are unsuitable for patients with diabetes mellitus.

Protein supplements

These come in the form of a powder and provide 55–90 g protein per 100 g. Protein supplement powders may be added to any food or drink in which they will dissolve, for example milk, fruit juice, soup, milk pudding.

Energy and protein supplements are not used in isolation as these would not provide an adequate nutritional intake. They are used in conjunction with sip feeds and a modified diet. The detailed nutritional compositions of dietary supplements are available from the manufacturers.

Vitamin and mineral supplements

When dietary intake is poor a vitamin and mineral supplement may be required. This can often be given as a one-a-day tablet supplement that provides 100% of the dietary reference values. Care should be taken to avoid unbalanced supplements or those containing amounts larger than the dietary reference value (FSA and Expert Group on Vitamins and Minerals 2003). Excessive doses of vitamins and minerals may be harmful, particularly as some vitamins and minerals are not excreted by the body when taken in amounts exceeding requirements. Additionally, vitamins and minerals may interact with medication to influence its efficacy; for example, vitamin K may influence anticoagulants such as warfarin.

Anticipated patient outcomes

It is anticipated that feeding an adult will ensure safe delivery of the meal, in a comfortable environment which the patient feels is a pleasurable and positive experience, promoting adequate nutritional care.

Legal and professional issues

Protected Mealtimes should be in place on the wards, whereby all non-essential clinical activities have been discontinued and a calm environment exists (Age Concern 2006). The use of Protected Mealtimes within hospitals is strongly encouraged by the National Patient Safety Agency which encourages trusts to have an appropriate policy in place to monitor its implementation on the wards and to have a structure in place to report patients missing meals via the local risk management system (NPSA 2007a).

Preprocedural considerations

Sufficient staff need to be available to support those who need help. Patients who require assistance should be identified through screening and a discreet signal should be evident to identify that further assistance is required, for example a red tray, a coloured serviette or a red sticker (Bradley and Rees 2003).

Assessment and recording tools

Food record charts can provide the essential information that forms the basis of a nutritional assessment and help to determine subsequent nutritional care. They are therefore a valuable resource for dietitians, nurses and ultimately the patient (Freeman 2002). They can be used to assess whether the patient is eating and drinking enough, thereby enabling action to be taken to encourage intake in those who have a reduced dietary intake.

The objective is to quantify the amount of food and drink consumed by a patient over an agreed time period and, although open to error, it has been demonstrated that this type of record keeping provides more accurate information than methods involving recall (Kroke *et al.* 1999). In hospital, a patient's intake frequently changes as a result of disease, symptoms, medication and unfamiliar surroundings and food availability. It is frequently not evident how much a patient is eating, particularly on busy wards with regular staff changes.

All screening, including food charts, should be linked to a care plan and documented in the patient's notes (Freeman 2002, NPSA 2009). If there is noted weight loss, concerns expressed by staff or from relatives regarding the patient's nutritional intake, particularly where there are difficulties observed with eating and drinking, close monitoring of oral intake is essential. The only exception to this is when a patient is receiving palliative care and it has been clarified with the clinical team that active nutritional support is not appropriate.

Food charts should be available on all wards and should be simple to complete. It is often preferable to include on the chart household measures such as tablespoons, slice of bread or hospital portions, to assist with the speed of completion.

Training should be given on how the chart should be completed and preferably should be undertaken by the dietitian or the specialist nutrition nurse, as this will facilitate understanding of the rationale and continuity of recording and improve accuracy. Charts need to be carefully completed over a minimum and consecutive 2 or 3 day period or longer if requested by the dietitian. Some research suggests that information should be collected over at least 7 days in order to estimate protein and energy intake to within ±10% (Bingham 1987).

Specific patient preparations

Before commencing assistance, please discuss this with the patient in order that they understand and consent to assistance being provided. When verbal communication is not possible, non-verbal agreement needs to be obtained wherever possible. Try to engage the patient in the feeding process and interpret and record any preferences or dislikes they may express regarding the meal process.

Make sure the patient has the opportunity to visit the bathroom and wash hands or clean their hands with an antiseptic wipe and to undertake any appropriate mouthcare prior to eating. Establish whether any medication is to be administered prior to or after feeding which will facilitate the feeding and digestive process. Individual symptoms should be assessed; for example, if patients are nauseous they may benefit from the prescribing of antiemetics or prokinetic agents. Patients who have pancreatic insufficiency may require pancreatic enzyme replacements. All drugs should be correctly prescribed on the drug chart. The timing in relation to feeding is important and antiemetics should be given approximately 30 minutes prior to meal service. Any special equipment, such as cutlery or non-slip mats, that is required for assisting the patient with the meal should be provided. This may require referral to an occupational therapist for an assessment.

Procedure guideline 8.9 Feeding an adult patient

Essential equipment

- A clean table or tray
- Equipment required to assist the patient such as adequate drinking water, adapted cups, cutlery and napkin
- A chair for the nurse or carer to sit with the patient

Preprocedure

Action	Rationale
1 Ensure the patient is comfortable, that is, they have an empty bladder, clean hands, clean mouth and if applicable clean dentures. Ensure that there are no unpleasant sights or smells that would put the patient off eating	To make the mealtime a pleasant experience (Age Concern 2006, E).
2 Ensure that the patient is sitting upright in a supported midline position, preferably at a table.	To facilitate swallowing and protect the airway. E
3 Protect the patient's clothing with a napkin.	To maintain dignity and cleanliness. E

Procedure

4 Assist the patient to take appropriate portions of food at the correct temperature but encourage self-feeding. Tailor the size of each mouthful to the individual patient.	To make the mealtime a pleasant experience. To ensure that swallowing is not compromised if the patient feels that they must hurry with the meal (Samuels and Chadwick 2006, E).
5 Allow the patient to chew and swallow foods before the next mouthful. Avoid hovering with the next spoonful.	To maintain the dignity of the patient. E
6 Avoid asking questions when the patient is eating, but check between mouthfuls that the food is suitable and that the patient is able to continue with the meal.	To reduce the risk of aspirating, which may be increased if speaking whilst eating. E
7 Use the napkin to remove particles of food or drink from the patient's face.	To maintain dignity and cleanliness. E
8 Ask the patient when they wish to have a drink. Assist the patient to take a sip. Support the glass or cup gently so that the flow of liquid is controlled or use a straw if this is helpful. Take care with hot drinks to avoid offering these when too hot to drink.	To give the opportunity for the patient to swallow. Hot liquids may scald the patient. E
9 If the food appears too dry, ask the patient if they would like some additional gravy or sauce added to the dish.	To facilitate chewing and swallowing (Wright *et al.* 2008, E).
10 Observe patient for coughing, choking, wet or gurgly voice, nasal regurgitation or effortful swallow. See Table 8.6 for details of problems that may be experienced by patients.	May indicate aspiration, laryngeal penetration or weakness in muscles required for swallowing (Leslie *et al.* 2003, E).
11 Encourage the patient to take as much food as they feel able to eat, but do not press if they indicate that they have eaten enough.	To improve nutritional intake but also maintain patient dignity and choice (Wright *et al.* 2008, E).

Postprocedure

12 After the meal assist the patient to meet hygiene needs, for example, wash hands and face and clean teeth.	To maintain cleanliness and dignity. E

359

Table 8.6 Difficulties that may be experienced by patients during eating and drinking and their potential implications

Difficulty experienced	Implications
Coughing and choking during and after eating and/or drinking	Indicates laryngeal penetration or aspiration (Smith Hammond 2008)
Wet or gurgly voice quality	Indicates laryngeal penetration or aspiration (Leslie *et al.* 2003b)
Drooling/excess oral secretions	Indicates less frequent swallowing and is associated with dysphagia (Langmore *et al.* 1998)
Nasal regurgitation	Indicates impaired velopalatal seal (Leslie *et al.* 2003b)
Food/drink pooling in mouth	Indicates lack of oral sensation from intraoral flaps or may be a sign of cognitive impairment (Logemann 1998)
Swallow is effortful	May indicate weakness in muscles required for swallowing (Logemann *et al.* 2008)
Respiration rate on eating/drinking is increased	Increased respiration rate may be associated with risk of aspiration (Leslie *et al.* 2003b)
Signs of recurrent chest infections and pyrexia	This may indicate aspiration pneumonia as a consequence of dysphagia (Leslie *et al.* 2003b)
Patient report of swallowing problems	Patients can be very accurate in self-diagnosis of dysphagia (Pauloski *et al.* 2002)
Patient reports food sticking	Patients can be very accurate in self-diagnosis of dysphagia (Pauloski *et al.* 2002)
Additional time required to eat a meal	Taking a long time to eat may indicate dysphagia (Leslie *et al.* 2003b)
Avoidance of certain foods	Patients will avoid food items that they find difficult to swallow (Leslie *et al.* 2003b)
Weight loss	Patients may eat less due to difficulty swallowing (Leslie *et al.* 2003b)
Poor oral hygiene	Aspiration of secretions in those with poor oral hygiene may result in aspiration pneumonia (Langmore 2001)

Postprocedural considerations
Education of patient and relevant others

It is important that volunteers, family members or visitors who wish to assist the patient with feeding are familiar with and trained in the processes listed in Procedure guideline 8.9 (NPSA 2009). This is to ensure that the family is confident and can safely and effectively assist the patient.

Documentation

It is essential that the plate is not removed before wastage has been recorded and this is relayed to the ward catering staff prior to meal service commencement. If the patient has not managed a reasonable amount of their meal, this needs to be addressed later in the afternoon or evening. It is also important to ascertain whose responsibility it is for completion of the charts to avoid confusion, that is, nurse, healthcare assistant, ward catering staff or patient, as this will vary across institutions. These charts can be used by the dietitian or healthcare professional to effectively assess the patient's meal pattern and nutrition intake. Some patients may be able to complete the record themselves if given guidance on what is required.

Difficulties arise when the food chart data are not accurately completed or reviewed, during which time malnutrition and its consequences continue, rather than being quickly identified and addressed.

If there is strong concern about the quantity of food that has been consumed by the patient, this must also be verbally relayed to the nurse in charge, ward dietitian and possibly the clinician.

Nutritional management of patients with dysphagia

Definition

Dysphagia is an impairment of swallowing that may involve any structures from the lips to the gastric cardia (Leslie *et al.* 2003).

Evidence-based approaches
Rationale
Indications

Patients who are at high risk of dysphagia are summarized in Box 8.3.

Goals of clinical assessment

Some patients who are eating and drinking may experience dysphagia. It is important to correctly ascertain the presence of dysphagia and the factors contributing to its

361

Box 8.3 Patient groups at high risk of dysphagia

- Head and neck cancer patients undergoing surgery and/ or radiotherapy/chemoradiotherapy. The risk of dysphagia is increased with multimodal therapy. Side-effects from treatment may affect swallow function, such as xerostomia (dry mouth), odynophagia (pain on swallowing), thick oral secretions, nausea, candidiasis, taste changes, mucositis, fatigue, fibrosis and trismus (reduced mouth opening). Nutritional support with enteral tube feeding may be required.
- Patients with neurological involvement including brain tumours or metastases, other co-morbid neurological disorders, for example cerebrovascular accident, multiple sclerosis, motor neurone disease, Parkinson's disease, myasthenia gravis. Such patients may also have cognitive or behavioural issues which can affect their mood, motivation, feeding and appetite.
- Patients with lung cancer and vocal cord paralysis and respiratory disorders such as chronic obstructive pulmonary disease, including mechanically ventilated patients.
- Tracheostomy patients may present with swallowing problems although frequently their medical diagnosis is the primary cause of dysphagia.
- Gastrointestinal patients may present with oropharyngeal or oesophageal dysphagia.
- Any other patient with significant generalized weakness or other co-morbidities, including palliative care patients.
- Patients with psychogenic dysphagia.
- Laryngectomy patients and particularly pharyngolaryngectomy and pharyngolaryngo-oesophageal patients. Some patients may experience dysphagia due to altered anatomy after surgery.

(Donzelli *et al.* 2005, Leder and Ross 2000, Lewin *et al.* 2001, Roe 2005, Roe *et al.* 2007, Royal College of Speech and Language Therapists 2006)

---

possible aetiology. Such patients may be at risk of aspiration and subsequent chest infections and therefore require a referral to a speech and language therapist for a full assessment (Gaziano 2002). Patients require a nutritional assessment from a dietitian with consideration of possible enteral tube feeding if the patient is unable to maintain an adequate nutritional intake or is at risk of aspiration. A suitable swallowing rehabilitation programme should be developed.

Principles of care

Care will be influenced by the timing of patient referral dependent on their disease and treatment status. Management of the dysphagic patient will be tailored to individual needs and they will require regular reviews to ensure that intervention and management decisions remain appropriate. The nature of the dysphagia may persist, recur or worsen depending on the patient's treatment or disease. Treatment options may include normal diet with specifically targeted

therapy techniques, modified diet, combination of alternative feeding and limited oral intake or nil by mouth. Close liaison between the nursing staff, dietitians and members of the MDT is essential. The SLT may recommend that the patient adopts certain head postures or uses swallow techniques to reduce the risk of aspiration or eliminate discomfort. Exercises or swallow techniques may be given to the patient to rehabilitate their swallow (Lazarus *et al.* 2002, Lewin *et al.* 2001, Logemann *et al.* 1997). It is important for nurses to participate in educational programmes for patients and carers in order to improve awareness of the implications of dysphagia. The nurses may be required to supervise patients with oral intake and encourage their participation with regard to therapy exercises.

Methods of assessment
Clinical swallow assessment

In any patient presenting with a new onset of dysphagia, a medical review is necessary as this may be the first indicator of recurrence of cancer or a new tumour. A subsequent specialist speech and language therapy (SLT) referral is then necessary. The SLT will take a full comprehensive case history including subjective reports, medical, physical and mental status. Surgical and/or oncological details will be determined, including where the patient is on the pathway, for example preoperative, postoperative, on treatment or palliative care. Oromotor examination to assess the oral structures is required for swallowing, including cranial nerves and adequate sensation (Figure 8.4). Food and drink trials may be carried out by the SLT.

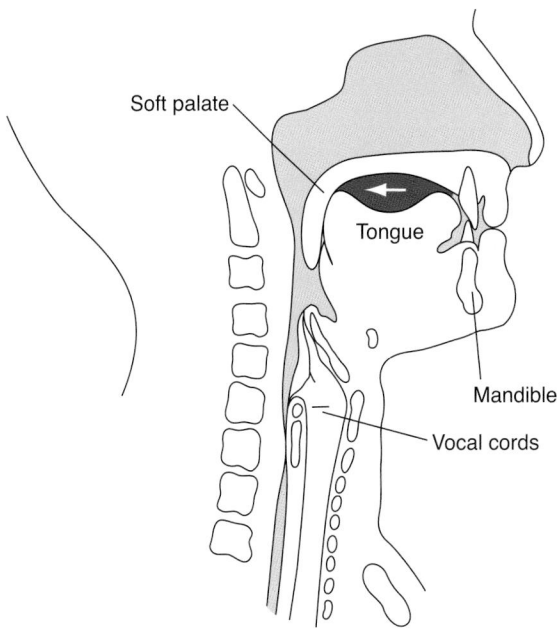

Soft palate

Tongue

Mandible

Vocal cords

Figure 8.4 Oral stage of swallowing.

Following an initial assessment, the SLT may recommend objective/instrumental assessments to evaluate the nature and extent of any swallowing disorder and also plan rehabilitation. Videofluoroscopy (modified barium swallow) takes place in the X-ray department and involves use of radio-opaque contrast mixed with food (Leslie *et al.* 2003). Fibreoptic endoscopic evaluation of swallowing (FEES) (Langmore 2001) involves use of an endoscope passed transnasally allowing a view of the swallow process whilst a patient eats and drinks. These instrumental assessments must be chosen on an individual patient basis, in conjunction with the specialist SLT.

Anticipated patient outcomes

Early identification of dysphagia and appropriate management is an essential part of patient care. Appropriate management aims to reduce the incidence of aspiration, the risk of aspiration pneumonia and to help maintain adequate nutrition. If it is not addressed appropriately it can lead to malnutrition, weight loss and dehydration, aspiration and aspiration pneumonia, low mood and reduced quality of life (Gaziano 2002). Ultimately it may result in increased length of hospital stay (Low *et al.* 2001).

Enteral tube feeding

Definition

Enteral tube feeding refers to the delivery of a nutritionally complete feed (containing protein, fat, carbohydrate, vitamins, minerals, fluid and possibly dietary fibre) directly into the gastrointestinal tract via a tube. The tube is usually placed into the stomach, duodenum or jejunum via either the nose or direct percutaneous route (NCCAC 2006).

Related theory

Enteral feeding tubes allow direct access to the gastrointestinal tract for the purposes of feeding. A nasogastric or nasojejunal tube is placed via the nose and passed down the oesophagus with the feeding tip ending in the stomach (gastric) or small intestine (jejunum) respectively. A gastrostomy tube is placed directly into the stomach allowing infusion of nutrients into the stomach or, alternatively, such tubes may have a jejunal extension passing through the pylorus, allowing feeding into the jejunum (small intestine). A jejunostomy tube allows direct access to the jejunum for feeding. The choice of appropriate tube should be based on the method of insertion and the associated risks, length of time feeding is required, function of the gastrointestinal tract, the physical condition of the patient and body image issues relating to the visibility of the feeding tube, after discussion with the patient. The feeding regimen, care of the tube and stoma will depend on the enteral feeding tube inserted.

Evidence-based approaches
Rationale

While the majority of patients will be able to meet their nutritional requirements orally, there is a group of individuals who will require enteral tube feeding either in the short term or on a more permanent basis.

The primary aim of enteral tube feeding is to:

- avoid further loss of bodyweight
- correct significant nutritional deficiencies
- rehydrate the patient
- stop the related deterioration of quality of life of the patient due to inadequate oral nutritional intake (Loser *et al.* 2005).

Indications

Indications for enteral tube feeding are as follows:

- patient is unable to meet nutritional needs through oral intake alone
- the gastrointestinal tract is accessible and functioning
- it is anticipated that intestinal absorptive function will meet all nutritional needs.

(NCCAC 2006)

Preprocedural considerations
Equipment: types of enteral feed tubes
Nasogastric/nasoduodenal/nasojejunal

Nasogastric feeding is the most commonly used enteral tube feed and is suitable for short-term feeding, that is, 2–4 weeks (NCCAC 2006). Fine-bore feeding tubes should be used whenever possible as these are more comfortable for the patient than wide-bore tubes. They are less likely to cause complications such as rhinitis, oesophageal irritation and gastritis (Payne-James *et al.* 2001). Polyurethane or silicone tubes are preferable to polyvinylchloride (PVC) as they withstand gastric acid and can stay in position longer than the 10–14-day lifespan of the PVC tube (Payne-James *et al.* 2001).

Gastrostomy

A gastrostomy may be more appropriate than a nasogastric tube where medium- or long-term feeding is anticipated. It avoids delays in feeding and discomfort associated with tube displacement (NCCAC 2006). It is suitable for patients who are undergoing radical or hyperfractionated radiotherapy to the neck or children with solid tumours. They will require long-term enteral feeding because the treatment is intensive and prolonged.

A gastrostomy tube may be placed endoscopically (percutaneous endoscopically placed gastrostomy; PEG) or radiologically (radiologically inserted gastrostomy; RIG). They are made from polyurethane or silicone and are therefore suitable for short- or long-term feeding. A flange, flexible dome, inflated balloon or pigtail sits within the stomach and holds the tube in position.

For long-term feeding (i.e. longer than 1 month), a gastrostomy tube may be replaced with a button which is made from silicone. The entry site for feeding is flush with the skin, making it neat and less obvious than a gastrostomy tube. This is more cosmetically acceptable, especially for teenagers or patients who are physically active, but does require a certain amount of manual dexterity from the patient (Thomas and Bishop 2007). The button is held in place by a balloon or dome inside the stomach (Griffiths 1996).

Percutaneous endoscopically placed gastrostomy tubes may be placed while the patient is sedated, thereby avoiding the risks associated with general anaesthesia. However, patients who have compromised airways may require general anaesthesia and appropriate consideration for maintenance of the airway (see Chapter 10).

Certain groups of patients are not suitable for endoscopy; in these cases a RIG can be used. They are indicated for oesophageal patients with bulky tumours where it would be difficult to pass an endoscope and also for head and neck patients whose airway would be obstructed by an endoscope. There is also documented risk of the endoscope seeding the tumour to the gastrostomy site when it pulls the tube past a bulky tumour although this is a rare complication (Pickhardt *et al.* 2002).

Jejunostomy

A jejunostomy is preferable to a gastrostomy if a patient has undergone upper GI surgery or has severe delayed gastric emptying; in some cases it can be used to feed a patient with pyloric obstruction (Thomas and Bishop 2007). Fine-bore feeding jejunostomy tubes may be inserted with the use of a jejunostomy kit, which consists of a needle-fine catheter. The use of needles and an introducer wire allows a fine-bore polyurethane catheter to be inserted into a loop of jejunum. Alternatively, some gastrostomy tubes allow the passage of a fine-bore tube through the pylorus and into the jejunum. A double-lumen tube allows aspiration of stomach contents whilst feed is administered into the small intestine.

Enteral feeding equipment

The administration of enteral feeds may be as a bolus, intermittent or continuous infusion, via gravity drip or pump assisted (Table 8.7). There are many enteral feeding pumps available which vary in their flow rates from 1 to 300 mL per hour. The following systems may be used for feeding via a pump or gravity drip.

- Feed is decanted into plastic bottles or PVC bags. The administration set may be an integral part of the bag or may be supplied separately. The feed is sterile until opened and decanting feed into reservoirs will increase

Table 8.7 Methods of administering enteral feeds

Feeding regimen	Advantages	Disadvantages
Continuous feeding via a pump	■ Easily controlled rate ■ Reduction of GI complications	■ Patient connected to the feed for majority of the day ■ May limit patient's mobility
Intermittent feeding via gravity or a pump	■ Periods of time free of feeding ■ Flexible feeding routine ■ May be easier than managing a pump for some patients	■ May have an increased risk of GI symptoms, for example early satiety ■ Difficult if outside carers are involved with the feed
Bolus feeding	■ May reduce time connected to feed ■ Very easy ■ Minimum equipment required	■ May have an increased risk of GI symptoms ■ May be time consuming

the risk of contamination of the feed from handling (Payne-James *et al.* 2001). Generally this method is only used for feeds that require reconstitution with water. Malnourished and immunocompromised patients are particularly at risk from contamination and infection so this method of administration should be avoided where possible.

- The 'ready-to-hang' system has a glass bottle, plastic bottle or pack attached directly to the administration set. The bottles and packs are available in different types of feeds and sizes for flexibility. This is a closed sterile system which has been shown to be successful in preventing exogenous bacterial contamination (Payne-James *et al.* 2001).

Enteral feeds

Commercially prepared feeds should be used for nasogastric, gastrostomy or jejunostomy feeding. Available in liquid or powder form, they have the advantage of being of known composition and are sterile when packaged.

Whole protein/polymeric feeds

These contain protein, hydrolysed fat and carbohydrate and so require digestion. They may provide 1.0–1.5 kcal/mL (see manufacturer's specifications). As the energy density of the feed increases, so does the osmolarity. Hyperosmolar feeds tend to draw water into the lumen of the gut from the bloodstream and can contribute to diarrhoea if given too rapidly. Fibre may be beneficial for maintaining gut ecology and function, rather than promoting bowel transit time (Thomas and Bishop 2007).

Feeds containing medium chain triglycerides (MCT)

In some whole-protein feeds a proportion of the fat or LCT may be replaced with MCT. The feed often has a lower osmolarity and is therefore less likely to draw fluid from the plasma into the gut lumen. MCT are transported via the portal vein rather than the lymphatic system. These feeds are suitable for patients with fat malabsorption and maybe steatorrhoea (Cummings 2000).

Chemically defined/elemental feeds

These contain free amino acids, short-chain peptides or a combination of both as the nitrogen source. They are often low in fat or may contain some fat as MCT. Glucose polymers provide the main energy source. These feeds require little or no digestion and are suitable for those patients with impaired GI function (Thomas and Bishop 2007). They are hyperosmolar and low in residue.

Special application feeds

These feeds have altered nutrients for particular clinical conditions. Low-protein and -mineral feeds may be used for patients with liver or renal failure. High-fat, low-carbohydrate feeds may be used for ventilated patients because less carbon dioxide is produced per calorie intake compared with a low-fat, high-carbohydrate feed. Very high-energy and protein feeds may be used where nutritional requirements are exceptionally high, for example burns, severe sepsis. These feeds contain approximately double the amount of energy and protein compared to standard whole-protein feeds.

Paediatric feeds

These are designed for children 1–12 years old and/or 8–45 kg in weight. The protein, vitamin and mineral profile is suitable for children. Generally they are lower in osmolarity than adult feeds. The whole-protein/polymeric feeds are based on cow's milk but are lactose free. Some of these feeds may contain dietary fibre. These feeds provide 1.0–1.5 kcal/mL for children who require additional energy and protein in a smaller volume. Protein hydrolysate feeds and elemental feeds are used in conditions such as food allergies or malabsorption. Some specialist centres use these feeds for enteral feeding during bone marrow transplants as children may have malabsorption caused by gut mucositis. The osmolarity of these feeds is higher than whole-protein feeds. They need to be introduced carefully (Thomas and Bishop 2007).

Immune-modulating feeds

There is evidence to show that the addition of glutamine, arginine or omega-3 fatty acids, if given preoperatively, may benefit postsurgical GI patients by reducing the risk of postoperative infections. These specialized liquids may be given pre- or postoperatively (Braga *et al.* 2002, Weimann *et al.* 2006).

Up-to-date information on the exact composition of dietary supplements and enteral feeds can be obtained from the manufacturers.

Enteral tube insertion

Evidence-based approaches
Rationale

It is essential that the position of the nasogastric tube is confirmed prior to feeding to ensure that it has been placed safely in the gastrointestinal tract and has not been inadvertently placed in the lungs. A wire introducer is provided with many of the fine-bore tubes to aid intubation.

Indications

- Patients who require short-term enteral tube feeding (2–4 weeks) as a sole source of nutrition or for supplementary feeding.
- *Indications for insertion without using an introducer:* it is recommended that a nasogastric tube designed for feeding purposes be used wherever possible, for example fine-bore feeding tube, rather than a Ryle's tube, without an introducer, which is used for drainage of gastric contents.

Contraindications

- Patients who require long-term enteral tube feeding in whom it may be more appropriate to use a gastrostomy tube.
- Patients with coagulation disorders should have blood clotting checked by the medical team and appropriate blood products administered if required prior to insertion.

Anticipated patient outcomes

The patient has a nasogastric tube inserted comfortably and safely. The position is checked and it is confirmed that the tube is placed in the stomach.

Legal and professional issues

Those passing the nasogastric tube should have achieved competencies set by the local trust. The procedure should be compliant with the National Patient Safety Agency (NPSA) recommendations, that is, only using syringes that are compatible with enteral feeding tubes (NPSA 2007b).

Preprocedural considerations
Specific patient preparations

The planned procedure should be discussed with the patient so they are aware of the rationale for insertion of a nasogastric tube. Verbal consent for the procedure must be obtained from the patient.

Prior to performing this procedure, the patient's medical and nursing notes should be consulted to check for potential complications. For example, anatomical alterations due to surgery, such as a flap repair, or the presence of a cancerous tumour can prevent a clear passage for the nasogastric tube, resulting in pain and discomfort for the patient and further complications. The assessment of the patient and consent obtained should be clearly documented.

Social and psychological impact

For some patients a nasogastric tube can be distressing. This is not only due to physical discomfort but also people's perceptions of their body image, particularly as this type of

---

Procedure guideline 8.10 **Nasogastric intubation with tubes using an introducer**

Essential equipment

- Clinically clean tray
- Fine-bore radio-opaque nasogastric tube
- Introducer for tube
- Receiver
- Sterile water
- 50 mL enteral syringe

- Hypoallergenic tape
- Adhesive patch if available
- Glass of water
- Lubricating jelly
- CE marked-indicator strips with pH range of 0–6 or 1–11 with gradations of 0.5

Preprocedure

Action	Rationale
1 Explain and discuss the procedure with the patient.	To ensure that the patient understands the procedure and gives his/her valid consent (NMC 2008b, C).
2 Arrange a signal by which the patient can communicate if they want the nurse to stop, for example by raising their hand.	The patient is often less frightened if they feel that they have some control over the procedure. E
3 Assist the patient to sit in a semi-upright position in the bed or chair. Support the patient's head with pillows. *Note:* The head should not be tilted backwards or forwards (Rollins 1997).	To allow for easy passage of the tube. This position enables easy swallowing and ensures that the epiglottis is not obstructing the oesophagus. E
4 Select the appropriate distance mark on the tube by measuring the distance on the tube from the patient's earlobe to the bridge of the nose plus the distance from the earlobe to the bottom of the xiphisternum (the NEX measurement) (see Action Figures 4a, 4b).	To ensure that the appropriate length of tube is passed into the stomach (NPSA 2011, C).
5 Wash hands with bactericidal soap and water or bactericidal alcohol handrub, and assemble the equipment required.	Hands must be cleansed before and after patient contact to minimize cross-infection (Fraise and Bradley 2009, E).
6 Follow manufacturer's instructions to prepare the tube, for example injecting sterile water down the tube and lubricating the proximal end of the tube with lubricating jelly.	Contact with water activates the coating inside the tube and on the tip. This lubricates the tube, assisting its passage through the nasopharynx and allowing easy withdrawal of the introducer. E

Procedure

7 Check that the nostrils are patent by asking the patient to sniff with one nostril closed. Repeat with the other nostril.	To identify any obstructions liable to prevent intubation. E

(Continued)

Procedure guideline 8.10 *(Continued)*

8 Insert the rounded end of the tube into the clearer nostril and slide it backwards and inwards along the floor of the nose to the nasopharynx. If any obstruction is felt, withdraw the tube and try again in a slightly different direction or use the other nostril.	To facilitate the passage of the tube by following the natural anatomy of the nose. E
9 As the tube passes down into the nasopharynx, unless swallowing is contraindicated, ask the patient to start swallowing and sipping water.	To focus the patient's attention on something other than the tube. A swallowing action closes the glottis and the cricopharyngeal sphincter opens, enabling the tube to pass into the oesophagus (Groher 1997, E).
10 Advance the tube through the pharynx as the patient swallows until the predetermined mark has been reached (NEX measurement). If the patient shows signs of distress, for example gasping or cyanosis, remove the tube immediately.	The tube may have accidentally been passed down the trachea instead of the pharynx. Distress may indicate that the tube is in the bronchus. However, absence of distress is not sufficient for detecting a misplaced tube (NPSA 2005, C; NPSA 2011, C).
11 Remove the introducer by using gentle traction. If it is difficult to remove, then remove the tube as well.	If the introducer sticks in the tube, this may indicate that the tube is in the bronchus. E
12 Secure the tape to the nostril with adherent dressing tape, for example Elastoplast, or an adhesive nasogastric stabilization/securing device (Burns *et al.* 1995). Alternatively Tegaderm/Deoderm can be applied to the cheek and then covered in Mepore to secure the nasogastric tube; this can help to prevent skin irritation. A hypoallergenic tape should be used if an allergy is present.	To hold the tube in place. To ensure patient comfort. E

Postprocedure

13 Measure the part of the visible tube from tip of nose and record this and the NEX measurement in care plan. Mark the tube at the exit site with a permanent marker pen (nares).	To provide a record to assist in detecting movement of the tube (Metheny and Titler 2001; NPSA 2011, C).
14 Check the position of the tube to confirm that it is in the stomach by using the following methods.	Feeding via the tube must not begin until the correct position of the tube has been confirmed (NPSA 2011, C). To confirm placement of radio-opaque nasogastric tube.

First line test method: pH paper

Aspirate 0.5–1 mL of stomach contents and test pH on indicator strips (NPSA 2011, C; Rollins 1997). When aspirating fluid for pH testing, wait at least 1 hour after a feed or medication has been administered (either orally or via the tube). Before aspirating, flush the tube with 20 mL of air to clear other substances (Metheny *et al.* 1993). A pH level of between 1 and 5.5 is unlikely to be pulmonary aspirates and it is considered appropriate to proceed to feed through the tube (Metheny and Meert 2004, NPSA 2011).

Indicator strips should have gradations of 0.5 or paper with a range of 0–6 or 1–11 to distinguish between gastric acid and bronchial secretions (NPSA 2011, C).

To prove an accurate test result because the feed or medication may raise the pH of the stomach.

If a pH of 6.0 or above is obtained or there is doubt over the result in the range of pH 5–6 then feeding **must not** commence until a second competent person checks the reading or retests. The nasogastric tube may need to be repositioned or checked with an X-ray.

There is an increased risk of the nasogastric tube being incorrectly placed (NPSA 2011, C).

Second line test method: X-ray confirmation

Take an X-ray of chest and upper abdomen.

X-ray of radio-opaque tubes is the most accurate confirmation of position and is the method of choice in patients with altered anatomy, those who are aspirating or are unconscious with no gag reflex (NPSA 2011, C).

15 The following methods **must not** be used to test the position of a nasogastric feeding tube: auscultation (introducing air into the nasogastric tube and checking for a bubbling sound via a stethoscope, also known as the 'whoosh test'), use of litmus paper or absence of respiratory distress.

These tests are not accurate or reliable as a method of checking the position of a nasogastric tube as they have been shown to give false-positive results (Metheny and Meert 2004, E; NPSA 2011, C).

16 Document the tip position in the patient's notes.

To record the position (NMC 2009, C).

Action Figure 4a Measuring for a nasogastric tube: measure from patient's ear lobe to bridge of nose.

Action Figure 4b Measuring for a nasogastric tube: measure from ear lobe to bottom of xiphisternum.

Procedure guideline 8.11 Nasogastric intubation with tubes without using an introducer, for example, a Ryle's tube

Essential equipment

- Clinically clean tray
- Nasogastric tube that has been stored in a deep freeze for at least half an hour before the procedure is to begin, to ensure a rigid tube that will allow for easy passage
- Receiver
- Topical gauze
- Lubricating jelly

- Hypoallergenic tape
- CE marked-indicator strips with pH range of 0–6 or 1–11 with gradations of 0.5
- 50 mL enteral syringe
- Spigot
- Glass of water

(Continued)

Procedure guideline 8.11 *(Continued)*

Preprocedure

Action	Rationale
1 Explain and discuss the procedure with the patient.	To ensure that the patient understands the procedure and gives their valid consent (NMC 2008b, C).
2 Arrange a signal by which the patient can communicate if they want the nurse to stop, for example by raising their hand.	The patient is often less frightened if they feel that they have some control over the procedure. E
3 Assist the patient to sit in a semi-upright position in the bed or chair. Support the patient's head with pillows. *Note:* The head should not be tilted backwards or forwards (Rollins 1997).	To allow for easy passage of the tube. This position enables easy swallowing and ensures that the epiglottis is not obstructing the oesophagus. E
4 Mark the distance to which the tube is to be passed by measuring the distance on the tube from the patient's earlobe to the bridge of the nose plus the distance from the earlobe to the bottom of the xiphisternum (the NEX measurement).	To indicate the length of tube required for entry into the stomach (NPSA 2011, C).
5 Wash hands with bactericidal soap and water or bactericidal alcohol handrub, and assemble the equipment required.	Hands must be cleansed before and after patient contact to minimize cross-infection (Fraise and Bradley 2009, E).

Procedure

6 Check the nostrils are patent by asking the patient to sniff with one nostril closed. Repeat with the other nostril.	To identify any obstructions liable to prevent intubation. E
7 Lubricate about 15–20 cm of the tube with a thin coat of lubricating jelly that has been placed on a topical swab.	To reduce the friction between the mucous membranes and the tube. E
8 Insert the proximal end of the tube into the clearer nostril and slide it backwards and inwards along the floor of the nose to the nasopharynx. If an obstruction is felt, withdraw the tube and try again in a slightly different direction or use the other nostril.	To facilitate the passage of the tube by following the natural anatomy of the nose. E
9 As the tube passes down into the nasopharynx, ask the patient to start swallowing and sipping water, enabling the tube to pass into the oesophagus.	To focus the patient's attention on something other than the tube. The swallowing action closes the glottis and the cricopharyngeal sphincter opens, enabling the tube to pass into the oesophagus (Groher 1997, R5).
10 Advance the tube through the pharynx as the patient swallows until the tape-marked tube reaches the point of entry into the external nares (NEX measurement). If the patient shows signs of distress, for example gasping or cyanosis, remove the tube immediately.	Distress may indicate that the tube is in the bronchus. However, absence of distress is insufficient for detecting a misplaced tube (NPSA 2005, C; NPSA 2011, C).
11 Secure the tube to the nostril with adherent dressing tape, for example Elastoplast, or an adhesive nasogastric stabilization/securing device (Burns *et al.* 1995). If this is contraindicated, a hypoallergenic tape should be used. An adhesive patch (if available) will secure the tube to the cheek.	To hold the tube in place. To ensure patient comfort. E

Postprocedure

12 Check the position of the tube to confirm that it is in the stomach by using the following methods.

To confirm placement of radio-opaque nasogastric tube.

First line test method: pH paper

Aspirate 0.5–1 mL of stomach contents and test pH on indicator strips (NPSA 2011, C; Rollins 1997). When aspirating fluid for pH testing, wait at least 1 hour after a feed or medication has been administered (either orally or via the tube). Before aspirating, flush tube with 20 mL of air to clear other substances (Metheny et al. 1993). A pH level of between 1 and 5.5 is unlikely to be pulmonary aspirates and it is considered appropriate to proceed to feed through the tube (Metheny and Meert 2004, NPSA 2011).

Indicator strips should have gradations of 0.5 or paper with a range of 0–6 or 1–11 to distinguish between gastric acid and bronchial secretions (NPSA 2011, C). To prove an accurate test result because the feed or medication may raise the pH of the stomach. Wait at least 1 hour before aspirating to enable the feed or medication to be absorbed, otherwise an inaccurate test will be obtained (NPSA 2011, C).

If a pH of 6.0 or above is obtained or there is doubt over the result in the range of pH 5–6 then feeding **must not** commence until a second person checks the reading or retests. The nasogastric tube may need to be repositioned or checked with an X-ray.

There is an increased risk of the nasogastric tube being incorrectly placed (NPSA 2011, C).

Second line test method: X-ray confirmation

Take an X-ray of chest and upper abdomen.

X-ray of radio-opaque tubes is the most accurate confirmation of position and is the method of choice in patients with altered anatomy, those who are aspirating or are unconscious with no gag reflex (NPSA 2011, C).

13 The following methods **must not** be used to test the position of a nasogastric feeding tube: auscultation (introducing air into the nasogastric tube and checking for a bubbling sound via a stethoscope, also known as the 'whoosh test'), use of litmus paper or absence of respiratory distress.

These tests are not accurate or reliable as a method of checking the position of a nasogastric tube as they have been shown to give false-positive results (Metheny and Meert 2004, NPSA 2011, C).

14 Document the NEX measurement, length of visible portion from tip of nose and tip position in the patient's notes.

To record the position (NMC 2009, C).

Problem-solving table 8.3 Prevention and resolution (Procedure guidelines 8.10 and 8.11)

Problem	Cause	Prevention	Action
Unable to obtain aspirate from nasogastric tube	Tip of tube is not sitting in gastric contents, is against the stomach wall or is not advanced sufficiently into the stomach	Measure the tube correctly as described in Action 4	Follow the NPSA flowchart (NPSA 2011) 1 Turn patient onto their side 2 Inject 10–20 mL air into the tube using a 50 mL syringe 3 Wait 15–30 minutes. Advance or withdraw tube by 10–20 cm 4 Try aspirating again
pH of greater than 5.5 is obtained	The nasogastric tube may be placed in the lungs or patient is on acid-inhibiting medication and this may contribute to a higher gastric pH	Check pH of gastric aspirate about the time of administration of acid-inhibiting medication when gastric pH is likely to be at its lowest	Check patient's medication and check the position of the tube at the appropriate time

(Continued)

Problem-solving table 8.3 (*Continued*)

Problem	Cause	Prevention	Action
pH of greater than 5.5 is obtained despite following recommendation about acid-inhibiting medication	The nasogastric tube may be placed in the lungs	Check medication	If initial confirmation cannot be obtained from pH aspirate then tube must be X-rayed as it may be in the lungs
Initial correct placement is confirmed but subsequent measurements are unable to obtain a pH of less than 5.5	The following may have happened 1 The nasogastric tube has become displaced 2 Acid-inhibiting medication is causing pH to be above 5.5 3 Feed/food is influencing pH of stomach contents	Follow NPSA guidance on checking the position of the nasogastric tube. This involves additional actions including advancing the tube 10–20 cm and rechecking. Leave for 1 hour and then aspirate and check again	Undertake risk assessment and document action. The nasogastric tube may need to be repositioned and rechecked with an X-ray
Unable to place the nasogastric tube	The patient has altered anatomy The patient is distressed/ not compliant with the procedure		The nasogastric tube should be placed under X-ray guidance or via endoscopy

feeding tube is highly visible. Some people find that they limit their social activity due to embarrassment, which can lead to feelings of isolation. Others see it as a reminder of ill health which can have an impact on mood. These issues should be discussed with the patient prior to tube insertion. If necessary, the patient should be referred for specialist psychological care.

Postprocedural considerations
Immediate care

The position of the nasogastric tube must be checked at initial placement and again prior to the administration of all medication or feed. Failure to confirm the position of the tube in the stomach can lead to the administration of fluid, medication or feed directly into the lungs, resulting in aspiration pneumonia (Figure 8.5).

The position of the nasogastric tube can be checked using two methods.

- *Testing of gastric aspirate with pH indicator paper.* The use of pH to check the position of the tube is based on an understanding of the pH of body fluids, particularly gastric contents, and the pH scale (see Box 8.4). All patients who do not require an X-ray should have the position of the tube checked with syringed aspirate of gastric content. This should have a pH less than 5.5 (NPSA 2011).
- *Chest X-ray.* A chest X-ray must be used to confirm the position of the tube in high-risk groups such as patients with oesophageal or head and neck tumours, those who have impaired swallowing or who are unconscious, because they are at higher risk of misplacement of the nasogastric tube.

In accordance with NPSA (2011) guidance, the following methods should **not** be used to confirm the position of a feeding tube.

- Auscultation of air insufflated through the feeding tube ('whoosh test').
- Testing the pH of the aspirate using blue litmus paper.
- Interpreting the absence of respiratory distress as an indicator of the correct positioning.
- Monitoring bubbling at the end of the tube.
- Observing the appearance of feeding tube aspirate.

In addition to the initial confirmation, the tube should be checked on a daily basis (see Procedure guideline 8.10).

When the nasogastric tube is confirmed to be in the stomach, a mark should be made on the tube at the exit site from the nostril with a permanent marker pen. The length of tube visible from the exit of the nostril to the end of the tube should be measured in centimetres and recorded along with the NEX measurement. This is to help detect if the nasogastric tube has become displaced. See Figure 8.6 for an X-radiograph of a correctly inserted nasogastric tube, Figure 8.7 for information on the test precision and test risk when checking the position of a nasogastric tube, and Figure 8.8 for checks when using pH indicator sticks.

Ongoing care

Once the nasogastric tube has been confirmed to be in the stomach, feeding may commence. The tube should be kept patent by regular flushing before and after feed and medication. Preferably only liquid medication should be used as tablets may block the lumen of the tube (BAPEN 2003b).

- Estimate NEX measurement. (Place exit port of tube at tip of nose. Extend tube to earlobe, and then to xiphisternum.)
- Insert fully radio-opaque nasogastric tube for feeding (follow manufacturer's instructions for insertion)
- Confirm and document secured NEX measurement
- Aspirate with a syringe using gentle suction

Aspirate obtained?

YES

NO

Try each of these techniques to help gain aspirate:
- If possible, turn adult onto left side
- Inject 10–20 ml air into the tube using a 50 ml syringe
- Wait for 15–30 minutes before aspirating again
- Advance or withdraw tube by 10–20 cm
- Give mouth care to patients who are nil by mouth (stimulates gastric secretion of acid)
- Do not use water to flush

Test aspirate on CE marked pH indicator paper for use on human gastric aspirate

Aspirate obtained?

YES

NO

Proceed to X-ray: ensure reason for X-ray documented on request form

pH between 1 and 5.5

pH NOT between 1 and 5.5

Competent clinician (with evidence of training) to document confirmation of nasogastric tube position in stomach

PROCEED TO FEED or USE TUBE

Record result in notes and subsequently on bedside documentation before each feed/medication/flush

YES

NO

DO NOT FEED or USE TUBE

Consider re-siting tube or call for senior advice

A pH of between 1 and 5.5 is reliable confirmation that the tube is not in the lung, however it does not confirm gastric placement as there is a small chance the tube tip may sit in the oesophagus where it carries a higher risk of aspiration. If this is any concern, the patient should proceed to X-ray in order to confirm tube position.

Where pH readings fall between 5 and 6 it is recommended that a second competent person checks the reading or re-tests.

Figure 8.5 Decision tree for nasogastric tube placement checks in adults (NPSA 2011). Used with permission of the NPSA. For updates see www.npsa.nhs-uk.

Tablets should only be crushed if no alternative liquid preparation is available. Always check with a pharmacist as some medication should not be crushed – see Procedure guideline 8.16.

The position of the tube must be checked with pH testing and recorded on a chart kept at the patients bedside (NPSA 2011):

- before administering each feed
- before giving medication
- following episodes of vomiting, retching or coughing as it is likely the tube may be displaced
- following evidence of tube displacement (e.g. the tube appears visibly longer).

If a pH of below 5.5 is not obtained then it is highly likely that the tube has become displaced. The medical team should be contacted as the tube may need to be replaced. For further details on checking nasogastric tubes, please refer to the full NPSA guidance or local policy.

Education of patient and relevant others

If appropriate, the patient may be taught how to check the position of the nasogastric tube. They should be made aware that if they feel the tube has moved, it must not be used for feeding until its position has been confirmed by one of the methods described.

Box 8.4 The clinical importance of the pH scale

The pH scale

The pH scale is a convenient way of recording large ranges of hydrogen ion concentrations without using the cumbersome numbers that are needed to describe the actual concentrations. That is why each step **down** the scale is a 10-fold **increase** (or a 10-fold **decrease** if going **upscale**) in the acidity. This means that stomach contents of pH 5 have 10 times as much acidity as has lung fluid of pH 6. Not knowing this could place your patient in harm's way.

The midpoint of the scale is 7. This number is related directly to the actual concentration of hydrogen ions in water, which is one ten-millionth units per litre – an extremely small number. One ten-millionth is the same as one divided by 10^7. So a liquid of pH 6 has one-millionth units per litre, that is, 1 divided by 10^6, and has 10 times the concentration of hydrogen ions as does pure water. This example shows why as the pH decreases the hydrogen ion concentration, and thus the acidity, increase. For example lemon juice and vinegar are acidic with a pH of 2.2 and 3 respectively whereas bleach is alkaline with a low concentration of hydrogen ions and a pH of 11.

In the body, the pH of cells, body fluids and organs is usually tightly controlled in a process called *acid–base homoeostasis*. Without this careful regulation of pH or *buffering*, the normal body chemistry cannot take place successfully and illness or in extreme cases death can occur.

The pH of blood is slightly basic with a value of 7.4, whereas gastric acid can range from 5.5 to the highly acidic 0.7 and pancreatic secretions are measured at 8.1. When the pH in the body decreases, that is becomes more acidic, *acidosis* can occur, leading to symptoms such as shortness of breath, muscular seizure and coma.

pH also influences the structure and function of many enzymes in living systems. These enzymes usually only work satisfactorily within narrow pH ranges. Thus pepsin, a stomach enzyme, works best at pH 2. In the duodenum, trypsin functions best at around pH 7.5–8.0. Generally, most human cell enzymes work best in a slightly alkaline medium of about 7.4.

Keeping the cellular pH at the correct level is very important and in the case of *unregulated diabetes,* high blood sugar levels occur, leading to acidic conditions that rapidly destroy enzymes and cells. Consequently regular blood sugar monitoring is crucial for diabetics.

In living systems, pH is therefore more than just a measure of hydrogen ion concentration as it is critical to life and the many biochemical reactions that have to take place to maintain a person in optimum health.

372

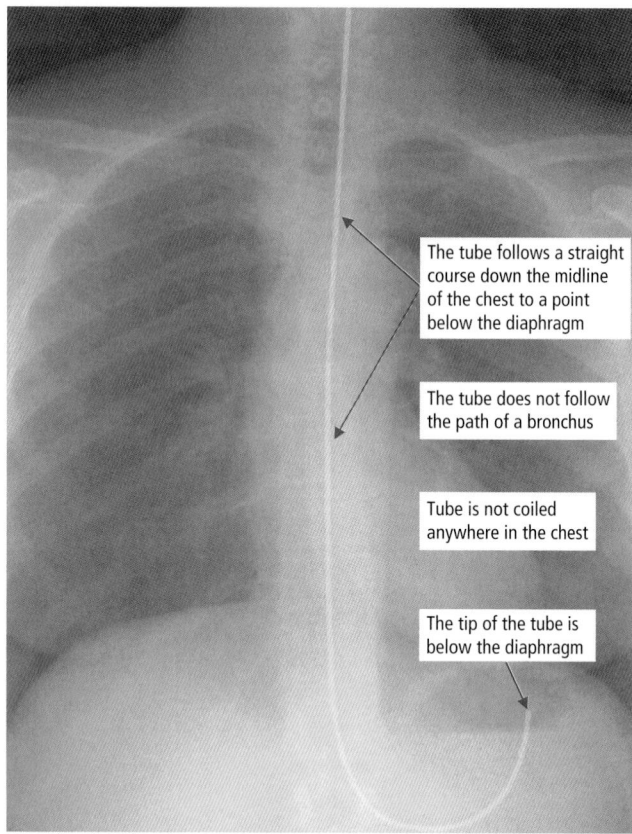

The tube follows a straight course down the midline of the chest to a point below the diaphragm

The tube does not follow the path of a bronchus

Tube is not coiled anywhere in the chest

The tip of the tube is below the diaphragm

Figure 8.6 X-radiograph of a correctly inserted nasogastric tube. Reproduced with permission from PPSA (2006) and ECRI. ECRI Institute is an independent not-for-profit healthcare research organisation and is a Collaborating Centre of the World Health Organisation. www.ecri.org.uk © ECRI Institute 2010.

Figure 8.7 Test precision and test risk: the connection. Reproduced from the training materials 'Positioning naso-gastric feeding tubes' jointly developed for publication by the ECRI Institute and the Royal Marsden Hospital NHS Foundation Trust.

Figure 8.8 Four key checks when using the pH tests. Reproduced from the training materials 'Positioning naso-gastric feeding tubes' jointly developed for publication by the ECRI Institute and the Royal Marsden Hospital NHS Foundation Trust.

Complications
Nasal erosion

Prolonged nasogastric feeding or use of a wide-bore tube can lead to nasal erosion (Ripamonti and Mercadante 2004). In this case it is advised that the tube is removed and replaced in the opposite nostril. If feeding is to be long term then a gastrostomy/jejunostomy should be considered.

Displacement of tube

A tube can accidentally be pulled out, particularly if a patient is restless or distressed. It can also be coughed or vomited out of place. In this situation it is advised that the position of the tube should be checked. If it is not possible to confirm that the nasogastric tube remains within the stomach then it should be removed and a new tube placed (NPSA 2011).

Enteral tube care

Evidence-based approaches
Percutaneous endoscopically placed gastrostomy (PEG) tube care

The first change of dressing should be performed 24 hours after PEG placement or earlier if indicated, for example the site is bleeding (Loser et al. 2005). Until granulation of the stoma canal has taken place, the dressing should be changed daily using aseptic technique. The wound should be inspected for bleeding, erythema, secretion, induration, allergic skin reaction, and so on (Loser et al. 2005). This will help maintain skin integrity and detect any problems early, for example infection, skin breakdown.

Radiologically inserted gastrostomy (RIG) tube care

After 24 hours and during initial daily change of dressing, the wound should be inspected and skin changes should be carefully noted. The site should be checked for bleeding, erythema, secretion or allergic skin reaction. For the first 10 days after the gastrostomy has been inserted, the site should be checked daily to ascertain skin integrity and detect any problems early, for example infection, skin breakdown. Most forms of local infection can be readily treated by cleaning the stoma site using aseptic technique and daily change of dressings (Loser et al. 2005). Antibiotics may be required in some instances. This procedure should be done by a nurse in hospital or suitably trained individual in the community (e.g. district or practice nurse, general practitioner).

Jejunostomy feeding tube care

Care of the exit site should be performed daily to maintain skin integrity and detect any problems early, for example infection, skin breakdown. Most forms of local infection can be readily treated by cleaning the stoma site using aseptic technique and daily change of dressings (Loser *et al.* 2005). Antibiotics may be required in some instances.

Preprocedural considerations

Prior to performing this procedure, the patient's medical and nursing notes should be consulted to identify tube placement date and method, and any infection control issues. The endoscopist's instructions should be noted, including any specific detail with regard to post placement care, for example suture removal, tube rotation, dressing changes.

Procedure guideline 8.12 Percutaneous endoscopically placed gastrostomy (PEG) tube care

Essential equipment

- Sterile procedure pack containing gallipot, low-linting gauze
- Dressing (absorbent, for example Lyofoam)
- 0.9% sodium chloride solution

Preprocedure

Action	Rationale
1 Explain and discuss the procedure with the patient.	To ensure that the patient understands the procedure and gives their valid consent (NMC 2008b, C).

Procedure

2 Remove postprocedural dressing if in place. Observe peristomal skin and stoma site for signs of infection, erythema, irritation or excoriation. Observe tube and consider how it is being kept in place, and note the presence of any sutures, external fixation plates, clamps or balloon ports.	To gain access to stoma site. To detect complications early and instigate appropriate treatment (Lynch and Fang 2004, R5). To minimize the risk of accidental displacement of tube. E
3 Note the number of the measuring guide on the tube closest to the end of the external fixation device. Loosen the tube from the fixation device and ease fixation device away from the abdomen. The external fixation plate should be subjected to very low traction, without tension, to maintain contact of the stomach with the abdominal wall.	To ensure gastrostomy tube is reattached to the fixation device in the correct position (Loser *et al.* 2005, C).
4 Clean the stoma site with a sterile solution such as 0.9% sodium chloride using an aseptic technique. Use a circular outward motion. Using low-linting gauze, dry the area thoroughly.	To minimize the risk of cross-infection (Fraise and Bradley 2009, E) (see Chapter 3, Procedure guideline 3.9). To ensure stoma site is thoroughly cleaned (Lynch and Fang 2004, R5).
5 Rotate the gastrostomy tube 360°.	To prevent the tube adhering to the sides of the stoma tract (Bumpers *et al.* 2003, R4).
6 Gently push the external fixation device against the abdomen, checking the measurement guide.	To enable the gastrostomy tube to be reattached to the fixation device. E

7	Gently but firmly pull the gastrostomy tube and attach to the fixation device. The numbered position mark at the gastrostomy exit site will be noted in the medical and nursing notes. The fixation device should remain at the same length, so that gentle traction on the tube allows 0.5 cm give but no more for the first 14 days if the patient is not receiving chemotherapy.	To ensure that the tube is correctly secured. E
	If they are receiving chemotherapy or have known delayed wound healing, it is advisable to continue with the same gentle traction for 3–4 weeks.	As wound healing may be impaired in chemotherapy or malnutrition. E
8	Ensure the correct point on the measuring guide on the tube is placed closest to the end of the fixation device.	To ensure that the tube is correctly secured. If the patient gains weight the external fixation device should be released slightly to prevent pressure necrosis of the stoma site (Loser *et al.* 2005, C).

Postprocedure

9	The dry dressing should be replaced daily using aseptic technique until the stoma site has no erythema or exudates or any other signs of infection. Most forms of infection can be readily treated by means of antiseptic measures and daily change of dressing using aseptic techniques (Loser *et al.* 2005). Do not replace the dressing with an occlusive type. If the patient complains of pain/discomfort, administer analgesia. If this is persistent, liaise with medical team and/or request a gastroenterology review.	To encourage wound healing. To prevent air getting to the stoma as this may cause infection (Lynch and Fang 2004, R5) or abdominal discomfort.
10	**Do not** use bulky dressings, particularly under the external fixation device.	To prevent increasing the pressure on the internal retention disc or retention balloon and increasing the risk of tissue necrosis and ulceration occurring in the stomach (Nutricia Clinical Care 1996, C).

375

Problem-solving table 8.4 Prevention and resolution (Procedure guideline 8.12)

Problem	Cause	Prevention	Action
Displaced bumper (PEG)	Excessive tension being applied to tube, either when moving external fixator or by overtightening	Support the tube beneath the fixator when moving	Liaise with medical team
Tube failure	Prolonged use of clamp without moving faulty tube	Regular tube care and review Change position of clamp regularly	Liaise with medical team to arrange replacement
Tube blockage	Inadequate tube flushing or overuse for administering meds	Regular tube flushing Avoid/minimize use of tube for medications	See Procedure guideline 8.17

Procedure guideline 8.13 Radiologically inserted gastrostomy (RIG) tube care

Essential equipment

- Sterile procedure pack containing gallipot, low-linting gauze
- Dressing (absorbent, e.g. Lyofoam)
- Sterile 0.9% sodium chloride

Preprocedure

Action	Rationale
1 Explain and discuss the procedure with the patient.	To ensure that the patient understands the procedure and gives their valid consent (NMC 2008b, C).

Procedure

2 Remove postprocedural dressing if in place. Observe peristomal skin and stoma site for signs of infection, erythema, irritation or excoriation.	To gain access to stoma site. To detect complications early and instigate appropriate treatment (Lynch and Fang 2004, R5).
3 Observe tube and consider how it is being kept in place, and note the presence of any sutures, external fixation plates, clamps or balloon ports.	To minimize the risk of accidental displacement of tube. E
4 Check that the T-fasteners are intact. These will stay in place for 10–14 days after RIG insertion. The timing should be checked with the radiologist if no instructions given.	To stabilize the stomach against the abdominal wall and allow the tract to form without complications (Cook (UK) Limited 2007, C).
5 Clean the stoma site with sterile solution such as 0.9% sodium chloride using a circular outward motion.	To minimize the risk of cross-infection and ensure stoma site is thoroughly cleaned (Fraise and Bradley 2009, E; Lynch and Fang 2004, R5) (see Chapter 3, Procedure guideline 3.9).
6 Use low-linting gauze to dry the area thoroughly. Take care not to wet any cotton pads on the T-fasteners.	To ensure stoma site is thoroughly dried (Lynch and Fang 2004, R5).
7 Remove the T-fasteners 10–14 days after insertion and secure fixation plate 1–2 cm away from the skin (if applicable). Refer to manufacturer's guideline's as to whether the tube should be rotated.	To prevent the RIG tube moving into the stomach (Cook (UK) Limited 2007, C).
8 Secure the tube to the skin with hypoallergenic tape. Do not secure near the stoma site.	To prevent the weight of the tube pulling on the exit site. Tape near the stoma site will make it difficult to clean. E
9 Advise the patient not to use moisturizing creams or talcum powder.	To prevent infection and/or irritation to the skin. E

Postprocedure

10 After T-fasteners have been removed, do not cover the gastrostomy site with a new dressing unless there is a heavy discharge or leakage from the stoma site.	To encourage wound healing. E

Procedure guideline 8.14 Jejunostomy feeding tube care

Essential equipment

- Sterile procedure pack containing gallipot, low-linting gauze
- Sterile 0.9% sodium chloride

Preprocedure

Action	Rationale
1 Explain and discuss the procedure with the patient.	To ensure that the patient understands the procedure and gives their valid consent (NMC 2008b, C).

Procedure

2 Remove postprocedural dressing if in place. Observe peristomal skin and stoma for signs of infection, erythema, irritation or excoriation. Observe tube and consider how it is being kept in place, and note the presence of any sutures or external fixation plates.	To gain access to stoma site. To detect complications early and instigate appropriate treatment (Lynch and Fang 2004, R5). To minimize the risk of accidental displacement of tube. E
3 Clean the stoma site with sterile solution such as 0.9% sodium chloride using a circular outward motion.	To minimize the risk of cross-infection and ensure stoma site is thoroughly cleaned (Fraise and Bradley 2009, E; Lynch and Fang 2004, R5) (see Chapter 3, Procedure guideline 3.9).
4 Use low-linting gauze to dry the area thoroughly.	To ensure stoma site is thoroughly dry (Lynch and Fang 2004, R5).
5 Secure the jejunostomy tube to the skin with hypoallergenic tape. The site may be covered with a dry dressing or left uncovered.	To prevent the weight of the tube pulling on the exit site. E

377

Local policy and guidelines (where available) should be identified and followed.

Postprocedural considerations
Immediate care

Local protocols should specify the observations to be taken in the immediate postoperative recovery period. These should include frequency and observation of blood pressure, pulse, respiration and pain score in addition to checks of the stoma site for bleeding, leakage of gastric contents or tube displacement (NPSA 2010). If the patient is complaining of pain or there are signs of peritonitis or tube displacement, contact the medical team immediately. Peritonitis manifests as abdominal pain, fever and a raised white cell count in the initial days after placement. Transient external leakage of the stomach contents from the puncture canal can indicate a likelihood that internal leakage is also occurring (NPSA 2010).

If there is pain on feeding, prolonged or severe pain post procedure or fresh bleeding, or external leakage of gastric contents then the feed should be stopped immediately. The patient should be reviewed by a senior clinician and the following considered: CT scan, contrast study or surgical review (NPSA 2010).

Additional complications that may occur in the immediate period after gastrostomy insertion include aspiration pneumonia, haemorrhage and wound infection. Colonic perforation is rare but may occur during the procedure and is likely to lead to peritonitis.

All assessment and care given should be clearly documented, including details of any observations noted and dressings used. The timing of future assessments should be planned to ensure that relevant aspects of care are followed up; for example, if a swab is taken to ascertain whether there is an infection, this needs to be followed up to monitor the stoma site and in order to act on the results of microbiology culture.

The patient should be advised not to use moisturizing creams or talcum powder around the stoma site. The grease in creams can cause the external retention device to slip, allowing movement of the tube and increasing the risk of hypergranulation, leakage and infection. Creams and talcs can affect the tube material, causing it to stretch or leak (Nutricia Clinical Care 1996). Patients should be taught how to carry out this procedure themselves.

Once the stoma site has healed (approximately 10 days post insertion), it is no longer necessary to perform an aseptic technique. A socially clean procedure using soap and water to clean the stoma site should be adopted. The tube tip should be cleaned daily using water and a small brush (Loser *et al.* 2005).

Where the enteral feeding tube has been placed to allow nutritional support, the patient's feeding regimen should be checked. If there is no feeding regimen, liaise with dietetic staff as needed or contact the medical team.

Ongoing care

To reduce the risk of tube blockage, the patient's medication should be reviewed where the tube is required for drug administration. Liaise with both medical team and pharmacist to discuss the patient's prescription and alternative routes/medication.

Education of patient and relevant others

The need for patient and/or carer teaching should be considered in patients with newly inserted enteral feeding tubes and discharge planning should be initiated.

Complications
Infection

Infection can occur at the time of placement or be due to inappropriate site care, particularly prior to tract maturation. Patients who are immunocompromised may be at increased risk of infection. Initial care after insertion should be carried out using aseptic technique during the daily dressing change until the tract is fully mature. If there are any sign of reddened skin or infection then a swab should be taken and sent off for microbiology culture and sensitivity. Appropriate antibiotic prescribing may be required depending on the condition of the stoma site and the microbiology results from the swab (Loser *et al.* 2005).

Pain or discomfort post insertion

If the patient experiences pain or discomfort following insertion of the tube, they should be assessed using an appropriate pain scale. Analgesia should be prescribed and administered. The site should be observed regularly for signs of infection.

Pressure necrosis

Excessive tightening of the external fixator device may cause pressure necrosis around the stoma site. The external fixator should be adjusted whilst the patient is sitting up, where possible. If the external fixator is adjusted whilst the patient is lying down then it is necessary to ensure that it is applied 1–2 cm from the skin surface.

The stoma site should be reviewed regularly and the patient and carer taught how to adjust and reposition the external fixator. This is particularly important if the patient has gained weight as this may cause pressure on the fixator.

Hypergranulation

Excess movement of the enteral feeding tube within the tract may stimulate the growth of granulation tissue. Ensure that the fixation plate is firm but not too tight on the abdomen to minimize movement of the tube. If the tube does not have an external fixator plate then consider placing one to stop excessive movement of the tube.

Buried bumper

In enteral feeding tubes that have a bumper as the retention device, the retention bumper may become buried in the intestinal wall. The external fixator should be released and the tube pushed in approximately 2 inches and rotated fully both clockwise and anticlockwise.

Peristomal leakage

It is important to examine the tube site for causes of peristomal leakage. Contributory factors may be delayed gastric emptying, buried bumper and infection. Ensure correct management of the stoma area, including checking the internal balloon weekly if this is the method of tube retention. Regular gastric decompression may help if there is delayed gastric emptying. Consider skin care and use protective cream or spray if necessary. Liaise with medical colleagues and consider the need for antacid medication to reduce skin excoriation.

Pneumoperitoneum

This is a known complication of the insertion procedure when air is present in the abdominal cavity. The patient's medical team must be contacted immediately if the patient is complaining of increased pain or pyrexia or has signs of an acute abdomen.

Administration of enteral tube feed

Preprocedural considerations

Prior to using enteral feeding tubes for medication or feed administration, it is vital to know where in the gastrointestinal tract the tube tip lies. This may be difficult in patients who have tubes placed in other organs or where there is little visible difference externally between gastrostomy, gastrojejunostomy or jejunostomy tubes. Where available, the tube size, type, insertion date and method should be clearly documented. If this information is unavailable, the tube should be aspirated and the pH used to differentiate between gastric or small bowel placement. If there are sutures securing the external fixator to the patient's abdomen, these should not be removed until it has been confirmed that they are not required to keep the tube in position.

Procedure guideline 8.15 Enteral feeding tubes: administration of feed

Essential equipment

- 50 mL enteral or catheter-tipped syringe
- Commercial ready-to-hang feed

Optional equipment

- Tap water or sterile water (for jejunostomy tubes or for patients who are immunosuppressed) (NICE 2003). Water should be fresh and kept covered

Preprocedure

Action	Rationale
1 Explain and discuss the procedure with the patient.	To ensure that the patient understands the procedure and gives their valid consent (NMC 2008b, C).

Procedure

2 Check the date on the feed container.	To ensure that the feed has not passed its expiry date. E
3 Shake the feed container gently.	To ensure the feed is evenly dispersed therefore reducing the risk of blocking the giving set. E
4 Take a new giving set from a sealed package and ensure that the roller clamp/tap is closed.	To avoid accidental spillage of feed from end of administration set. E
5 Screw the giving set tightly onto the feed container.	In order to pierce the seal on the container and maintain a sealed system (Matlow et al. 2006, C).
6 Hang the container upside down from the hook on a drip stand.	To avoid backflow of intestinal contents into the feed container (Matlow et al. 2006, C).
7 Open the roller clamp/tap and prime the feed to the end of the giving set. (Follow instructions for individual pump.)	This ensures that air is not fed into the stomach when feeding commences. E
8 Feed the giving set into the pump as directed by the manufacturer's instructions.	To connect the giving set to the pump device. E
9 Set the rate of the feed as directed by the manufacturer's instructions and according to the patient's feeding regimen.	To ensure the correct rate of feed is administered. E
10 Set the dose of the feed as directed by the manufacturer's instructions and according to the patient's feeding regimen.	To ensure that the correct dose of feed is administered. E
11 Flush the feeding tube with a minimum of 30 mL of water or sterile water in an enteral syringe by attaching to the end of the feeding tube. Depress the plunger on the syringe slowly.	To ensure the patency of the feeding tube (BAPEN 2003b, C).
12 Remove the end cover from the giving set and connect to the feeding tube.	To ensure that the feed is delivered via the enteral feeding tube. E
13 Set the rate of the feeding pump and commence administration of feed.	To ensure that the feed is delivered via the enteral feeding tube. E

Postprocedure

14 Document the time that the feed commenced and the rate of administration.	To ensure accurate documentation of nutritional and fluid intake (NMC 2009, C).
15 Dispose of any equipment that is no longer required.	To reduce the chance of equipment being re-used and to reduce cross-contamination with new equipment. E

Problem-solving table 8.5 Prevention and resolution (Procedure guideline 8.15)

Problem	Cause	Prevention	Action
Pump alarms with 'occlusion' or 'empty'	The feed may have finished There may be a blockage in the giving set or feeding tube	Ensure the feed container was shaken well before feeding Ensure the giving set was not bent when feeding was commenced Ensure that the roller clamp/tap is fully open Flush the feeding tube as directed before commencing	Straighten any kinks in the giving set Ensure that the giving set is fixed correctly around the rotor Open the roller clamp/tap fully Check that the feeding tube is not blocked. Disconnect from the feeding tube and run the feed into a container; if feed runs and there is no alarm, this indicates that the pump is working properly and the feeding tube is probably blocked
Pump alarms with 'low battery'	This indicates that the pump battery needs to be recharged and that there is approximately 30 minutes of power remaining	Keep pump plugged in and charged	Connect to the mains power and continue to feed
Unable to prime giving set	The roller clamp/tap may not be fully open There may be a fault with the giving set If a drip chamber is present then feed may not have run into this	Ensure that the roller clamp/tap is fully open when beginning to prime the giving set	Open the roller clamp/tap fully Squeeze some feed into the drip chamber if applicable Try with a new giving set
Continuous audio alarm and all visual displays go blank	The pump may require servicing	Ensure it is serviced regularly	Send to equipment library or manufacturers for servicing

Postprocedural considerations

Immediate care

As soon as the feed commences, check that it appears to be running without problems and is at the correct rate. Monitor this regularly throughout the feed administration.

Monitor the patient for signs of nausea/abdominal discomfort within the first hour and every 2–4 hours during feed administration. This may not be possible if the feed is given overnight and the patient is asleep.

Ongoing care

If appropriate, the patient should be taught how to follow the procedure of setting up the enteral feeding equipment.

They should be confident with the maintenance of the equipment and be aware of how to troubleshoot.

Complications

Aspiration

This may occur due to regurgitation of feed, poor gastric emptying or incorrect placement of a nasogastric tube. The risk of this can be reduced by:

- the use of prokinetics which encourage gastric emptying, for example metoclopramide
- checking the position of the tube before feeding
- ensuring the patient has their head at a 45° angle during feeding. If the patient is in bed then this can be achieved through raising the head of the bed and ensuring the patient has sufficient pillows for support.

Nausea and vomiting

This could be caused by a number of factors. It could be related to disease or a side-effect of treatment or a medication such as antibiotics or analgesia. A combination of poor gastric emptying and rapid infusion rates could also stimulate nausea and vomiting. Nausea and vomiting can be better controlled through the use of antiemetics, a reduction in the infusion rate or a change from bolus to intermittent feeding.

Diarrhoea

This could be a result of:

- medications such as antibiotics, chemotherapy or laxatives
- radiotherapy to the abdomen or pelvis
- disease or treatment, for example pancreatic insufficiency, bile acid malabsorption
- gut infection, for example *Clostridium difficile*.

Antidiarrhoeal agents could be used if a person is experiencing diarrhoea as a side-effect of medication. If possible, an alternative medication should be found that does not cause diarrhoea. In the case of antibiotics, these should be stopped as soon as possible. When the diarrhoea is disease related, the underlying problem should be treated, that is, if a person has pancreatic insufficiency they should be provided with a pancreatic enzyme supplement.

Avoiding microbiological contamination of the feed or equipment will help to reduce the risk of diarrhoea. This will involve keeping the equipment clean and, when feeding, maintaining a sealed system.

A stool sample should be sent to check for any gut infection. If the sample is found to be positive then the infection should be treated appropriately.

Constipation

Constipation could be caused by inadequate fluid intake, immobility, bowel obstruction or the use of opiates or other medications causing gut stasis.

Methods to improve symptoms of constipation include:

- checking fluid balance and increasing fluid intake if necessary
- providing laxatives/bulking agents

- if possible, encouraging mobility
- if in bowel obstruction, discontinuing enteral feeding.

Abdominal distension

This could be caused by poor gastric emptying, rapid infusion of feed, constipation or diarrhoea. Possible ways to improve distension include:

- gastric motility agents
- reducing the rate of infusion
- encouraging mobility if possible
- treating constipation or diarrhoea.

Blocked tube

Blockage can be a result of inadequate flushing or failure to flush the feeding tube or administration of inappropriate medications via the tube. For ways to unblock a feeding tube refer to Procedure guideline 8.17.

Enteral feeding tubes: administration of medication

Evidence-based approaches
Rationale
Indications

- Patients requiring medications who are not able to take oral preparations due to dysphasia.

Contraindications

- Not all medications can be administered through an enteral tube due to risk of blockage.
- If the medication has an enteric coating it should not be crushed.
- Some medications such as cytotoxic chemotherapy may be harmful to the administrator and advice from a pharmacist is required.
- If a number of different medications are required always administer separately. Do not mix medications unless advised to do so by a pharmacist.

Procedure guideline 8.16 Enteral feeding tubes: administration of medication

Essential equipment

- 50 mL enteral syringe
- Mortar and pestle or tablet crusher if tablets are being administered (BAPEN 2003a)

Optional equipment

- Tap water or sterile water (for jejunostomy tubes or for patients who are immunosuppressed) (NICE 2003). Water should be fresh and kept covered

(Continued)

Procedure guideline 8.16 *(Continued)*

Preprocedure

Action	Rationale
1 Check whether patient can take medication orally, whether medication is necessary or if it can be temporarily suspended.	If patient can take medication orally this reduces the risk of tube blockage (BAPEN 2003b, C).
2 Consider whether an alternative route can be used, for example buccal, transdermal, topical, rectal or subcutaneous.	If patient can take medication via an alternative route this reduces the risk of tube blockage (BAPEN 2003b, C).
3 Check drug is absorbed from the site of delivery.	Some drugs may not be absorbed directly from the jejunum (BAPEN 2003b, C).
4 Clean hands with bactericidal soap and water or alcoholic handgel. Put on non-sterile gloves.	To minimize cross-infection and protect the practitioner from gastric/intestinal contents (Fraise and Bradley 2009, E).

Procedure

5 Stop the enteral feed and flush the tube with at least 30 mL of water (sterile water for jejunostomy administration), using an enteral syringe.	To clear the tube of enteral feed as this may cause a blockage or interact with medications. Sterile water should be used for jejunostomy tubes as the water is bypassing the protective acidic environment of the stomach. E

Where there is an absolute contraindication for medicine to be taken with feed:

6 Stop the feed 1–2 hours before and 2 hours after administration (this will depend on the drug), for example for phenytoin administration, stop feed 2 hours before and 2 hours after.	To avoid interaction with enteral feed. E
7 Consult with the dietitian to prescribe a suitable feeding regimen.	To ensure that the patient's nutritional requirements are met in the time available around medicine administration (BAPEN 2003b, C).
8 Prior to preparation, check with the pharmacist which medicines should never be crushed.	Some medications are not designed to be crushed. These include: **(a)** modified-release tablets: absorption will be altered by crushing, possibly causing toxic side-effects **(b)** enteric-coated tablets: the coating is designed to protect the drug against gastric acid **(c)** cytotoxic medicines: this will risk exposing the practitioner to the drug (BNF 2011, C).
9 Prepare each medication to be given separately. Volumes greater than 10 mL may be drawn up in a 50 mL syringe and administered via the tube. For small volumes (less than 10 mL) follow step 12. **Either** **Soluble tablets:** dissolve in 10–15 mL water. **Or** **Liquids:** shake well. For thick liquids mix with an equal volume of water. **Or** **Tablets:** crush using a mortar and pestle or tablet crusher and mix with 10–15 mL water.	To avoid interaction between different medications and to ensure solubility (BAPEN 2003b, C).

10 Never add medication directly to the enteral feed.	To avoid interaction between medicines and feed (BAPEN 2003b, C).
11 Administer the medication through the tube via a 50 mL syringe. Rinse the tablet crusher or mortar with 10 mL water, draw up in a 50 mL syringe, and flush this through the tube.	To ensure the whole dose is administered (BAPEN 2003b, C).
12 If volumes of less than 10 mL are required, the dose should be measured in a 10 mL oral syringe. The plunger of a 50 mL syringe should be removed and the 50 mL syringe connected with the enteral tube. The dose should then be administered into the barrel of the 50 mL syringe and the 10 mL syringe rinsed with water, which should also be administered via the barrel of the 50 mL syringe.	To ensure the whole dose is administered (BAPEN 2003b, C).
13 If more than one medicine is to be administered, flush between drugs with at least 10 mL of water to ensure that the drug is cleared from the tube.	To avoid interactions between medicines (BAPEN 2003b, C).
14 Flush the tube with at least 30 mL water following the administration of the last drug.	To avoid medicines blocking the enteral tube (BAPEN 2003b, C).
15 If the patient is on fluid restriction or for a paediatric patient, consult the dietitian and pharmacist about the quantity of water to be given before and after medication.	To ensure that the patient does not exceed their fluid restriction or requirements (BAPEN 2003b, C).

Postprocedure

16 Record the administration on the prescription chart.	To maintain accurate records (NMC 2008c, C; NMC 2009, C).

Problem-solving table 8.6 Prevention and resolution (Procedure guideline 8.16)

Problem	Cause	Prevention	Action
Tube became blocked with medication	Medication had not been administered in the correct composition and/or the tube was not flushed adequately	Ensure that the guidance from the pharmacist is followed correctly Ensure that the tube is flushed before and after administration	See Procedure guideline 8.17 on how to unblock a feeding tube
Unable to administer required medication	It is in a form that cannot be crushed or dissolved	Ensure that the pharmacist and medical team are aware that all medications need to be administered via an enteral tube	Contact the medical team or pharmacist to seek advice on an alternative medication

Postprocedural considerations

Immediate care

The tube patency should be checked to ensure that the medication has not caused a blockage. This could be done by flushing the tube.

The patient should be monitored to ensure that there are no side-effects of the medication administered.

Ongoing care

In order to avoid complications and ensure optimal nutritional status, it is important to monitor the following in patients on enteral tube feeds:

- oral intake
- bodyweight
- urea and electrolytes

- blood glucose
- full blood count
- fluid balance
- tolerance to feed, for example nausea, fullness and bowel activity
- quantity of feed taken
- care of tube
- care of stoma site (where appropriate).

Education of the patient and relevant others

If the patient is going home with the enteral tube in place, it should be ensured that the patient is educated and confident with administering their medication. If this is not possible then the patient should be referred to a healthcare professional, such as a district nurse, who can undertake this aspect of care.

Home enteral feeding

Some patients who are established on tube feeding in hospital also require enteral tube feeding at home. A multidisciplinary approach is needed for a successful discharge, usually involving a dietitian, doctor, ward nurse, community nurse and general practitioner. The patient's circumstances and the ability of the patient or carers to manage the feed must be considered when discharge is being planned. Adequate time should be allowed in the hospital setting for

patients to become fully accustomed to the techniques of feed administration and care of the feeding tube, prior to discharge home. Patients should also be given written information to reinforce the education they receive prior to discharge (BAPEN 2003a).

Support in the form of the general practitioner, community nurse and community dietetic services should be established before discharge. A multidisciplinary discharge meeting may be of benefit to both the patient and the professionals involved. Many of the commercial feed companies organize for the patient's feed and equipment to be delivered to their home, after consultation with the local community services (BAPEN 2003a). The hospital or community dietitian can arrange this. Early notification of discharge is essential as it usually takes a minimum of 7 days to set this up.

Termination of enteral tube feeding

It is important to ensure that an individual is able to meet their nutritional requirements orally prior to termination of the feed. Ideally, the feeds should be reduced gradually, according to the dietary intake (BAPEN 1999). It may be useful to maintain an overnight feed while the patient is establishing oral intake.

Enteral feeding tubes: unblocking

Enteral feeding tubes may become blocked. See Procedure guideline 8.17 for unblocking.

Procedure guideline 8.17 Enteral feeding tubes: unblocking

Essential equipment

- 50 mL enteral syringe
- Tap water or sterile water (for jejunostomy tubes or for patients who are immunosuppressed) (NICE 2003). Water should be fresh and kept covered
- To obtain lukewarm water (40–45°C), put three-quarters of a cup (120 mL) of cold drinking tap water (sterile water for jejunostomy and for immunosuppressed patients) into a plastic cup and add a quarter of a cup (40 mL) of boiling water from the water still

Optional equipment

- Sterile water (for jejunostomy tubes)

Preprocedure

Action	Rationale
1 Always flush the enteral tube before and after administration of feed and medication with at least 30 mL of water (sterile water for jejunostomy and for immunosuppressed patients).	To avoid the tube blocking. Sterile water should be used for jejunostomy tubes as the water is bypassing the protective acidic environment of the stomach. E
2 Examine the tube for kinks.	To ensure that this is not the cause of the blockage (Pickering 2004, E).

Procedure

3 Draw up 30 mL of water in a 50 mL enteral syringe and attempt to flush/withdraw fluid from the tube.	To dissolve any medication or soften any feed plugs in the tube. To prevent hot water being administered via the feeding tube (BAPEN 2003b, C).
4 Flush tube only with 50 mL water.	To remove blockage and acidic fluids such as carbonated drinks that may cause feed to clot (BAPEN 2003b, C).
5 If tube is still blocked, consider use of a proprietary product designed to unblock tube. Follow manufacturer's instructions.	To break down plug. Such products contain digestive enzymes which may break down a protein plug but they may not unblock a tube blocked with medication (manufacturer's recommendation, C).
6 If all of the above are unsuccessful then the enteral tube will need to be replaced.	To ensure continued enteral access for the administration of feed, fluids and medication. E

Postprocedure

7 Document the procedure in the patient's notes.	To record that the tube was unblocked (NMC 2009, C).

385

Problem-solving table 8.7 Prevention and resolution (Procedure guideline 8.17)

Problem	Cause	Prevention	Action
Cracked/split tube	Too much pressure applied whilst flushing tube	Avoid too much pressure whilst flushing tube and take care with a syringe smaller than 50 mL	If tube cracks or splits then it must be replaced

Parenteral nutrition

Definition

Parenteral nutrition (PN) is the direct infusion into a vein of solutions containing the essential nutrients in quantities to meet all the daily needs of the patient (Furst *et al*. 2001).

Related theory

The basic components of a PN regimen are provided by solutions including the following.

- *Amino acids (nitrogen source).* Commercially available solutions provide both essential amino acids, usually in proportions to meet requirements, and non-essential amino acids, such as alanine and glycine. They may also contain conditionally essential amino acids such as glutamine for use in critical care (Goeters *et al*. 2002, Jian *et al*. 1999, Mertes *et al*. 2000).
- *Glucose (carbohydrate energy source).* Glucose is the carbohydrate source of choice. It provides 3.75 kcal/g (15.5 kJ/g) and usually provides 50% of non-nitrogen energy.
- *Fat emulsion (fat energy source).* Fat generates 9 kcal/g (37 kJ/g) and its inclusion in PN is necessary to provide essential fatty acids. Fat usually provides 50% of non-nitrogen energy. Nitrogen:non-nitrogen energy is usually provided in the ratio of 1:150–200. An insufficient energy supply from carbohydrate and fat will encourage the use of nitrogen for energy.
- *Electrolytes*, for example sodium, potassium, calcium, magnesium and phosphate.
- *Vitamins and minerals.* Both water-soluble and fat-soluble vitamins are required as part of a standard bag.
- *Trace elements*, for example zinc, copper, chromium, selenium (Thomas and Bishop 2007).

Evidence-based approaches
Rationale

Parenteral nutrition should only be used when it is not possible to meet nutritional requirements via the gastrointestinal tract. PN is an invasive and relatively expensive form of nutrition support and, in inexperienced hands, can be associated with risks from catheter placement, catheter infections, thrombosis and metabolic disturbance. Careful consideration is therefore needed when deciding to whom, when and how this form of nutrition support should be given. It should be planned and managed by healthcare professionals with the relevant expertise. Whenever possible, patients should be aware of why this form of nutrition support is needed and its potential risks and benefits.

Parenteral nutrition may be used in combination with enteral nutrition where some gut function is present but this is insufficient to meet nutritional requirements, for example in intestinal failure where the patient can eat but absorptive capacity may be insufficient to maintain nutritional status.

Indications

The indications for parenteral nutrition are:

- failure of gut function (e.g. with obstruction, ileus, dysmotility, fistulae, surgical resection or severe malabsorption) to a degree that definitely prevents adequate gastrointestinal absorption of nutrients
- the consequent intestinal failure has either persisted for several days (e.g. >5 days) or is likely to persist for many days (e.g. 5 days or longer) before significant improvement.
(Bozzetti *et al.*, 2009, Braga *et al.* 2009, NCCAC 2006)

Examples of the use of PN include for patients with prolonged gastrointestinal ileus, intractable vomiting, multiorgan failure where requirements cannot be met by the enteral route and proximal high-output fistula.

Contraindications

If the gut can be used or an attempt to use it has not yet been considered, then PN should be withheld pending the outcome of using the enteral system. PN should also not be used if the perceived risk to the patient outweighs the benefits anticipated (NCCAC 2006).

Contents of parenteral nutrition

Parenteral nutrition provides nutrients in a form that can be used directly by the body when they are infused intravenously. Nitrogen (protein) is provided as free amino acids in a ratio designed to meet requirements for essential amino acids. Specific amino acid profiles may be used for some disease states. Energy is usually provided from carbohydrate and fat. Carbohydrate is present as glucose and fat is provided as a lipid emulsion providing essential fatty acids. The lipid source may be provided by long-chain and/or medium-chain triglycerides with different manufacturers using various lipid blends. Fluid, electrolytes, vitamins, minerals and trace elements are also provided by parenteral nutrition.

Choice of a parenteral nutrition regimen

Parenteral nutrition is usually administered from a single infusion container in which all the requirements for a 24-hour feed are premixed. Such infusions are available as standard ready-prepared bags that require the addition of vitamins, minerals and trace elements or individual bags may be made to a particular prescription and purchased from a compounding unit.

The regimen for a particular patient should be formulated according to their needs for energy and nitrogen. The majority of commercial vitamin and mineral preparations aim to meet both short- and long-term requirements although appropriate monitoring is required to ensure that nutritional requirements are met in the longer term as clinically indicated by the monitoring guidelines. Standard PN regimens may be suitable for some patients who require short-term nutritional support or do not appear to have excessively altered nutritional requirements.

The choice of such regimens depends on the patient's bodyweight and nutritional requirements. To allow for the possible need to vary the constituents of the infusion in response to changes in the patient's electrolyte or nutritional requirements, PN solutions should be ordered daily. Once compounded, most PN preparations last up to 7 days (Weinstein and Plumer 2007) and need to be stored in a refrigerator. However, some triple-chamber PN bags can be stored at ambient temperatures and require mixing prior to administration. These bags generally require the addition of vitamins, minerals and trace elements under aseptic conditions.

Parenteral nutrition should be introduced slowly in the seriously ill or injured, with no more than 50% of requirements given in the first 24–48 hours due to the risk of refeeding syndrome (NCCAC 2006).

Methods of administration

The traditional method of access is via a central venous catheter. Central venous access is required because PN solutions are hyperosmolar and there is a risk of thrombophlebitis associated with feeding into peripheral veins (Springhouse 2002, Wilson and Jordan 2001). However, it has been shown that with care and attention, peripheral veins can be used to provide short-term peripheral PN (NCCAC 2006). This would be via a midline or a peripheral cannula. For the administration of PN, the device should be placed in the largest vein possible, usually in the forearm away from a joint, with rotation of the site every 48–72 hours (Shaw 2008). For insertion see Chapter 18.

A skin-tunnelled catheter is the catheter of choice for long-term nutrition but peripherally inserted central cannulas (PICCs) or non-tunnelled central venous catheters can also be used in the short term. The number of lumens will depend on the patient's peripheral venous access and the number of additional therapies required. It is recommended that the minimum number of lumens is used but if additional intravenous access is required then a double- or triple-lumen catheter should be inserted and then one lumen should be dedicated for use with PN. If using a single-lumen device, routine blood sampling and additional infusions should be carried out independently, using a separate cannula if necessary (Davidson 2005).

For setting up an infusion, see Chapter 16 (Procedure guideline 16.23).

Postprocedural considerations

Ongoing care

Administration sets should always be changed every 24 hours (Pratt *et al.* 2007, Springhouse 2002, Wilson and Jordan 2001). Existing injection sites on the administration set should never be used for giving additional medications as PN is incompatible with numerous medications. Drugs may bind to the nutrients or the PN bag, reducing their availability. If any additional medications, blood products or central venous pressure (CVP) readings are required then they should be given or taken via a separate lumen or via a peripheral device (Mirtallo *et al.* 2004).

A volumetric infusion pump must be used to ensure accurate delivery of PN. No bag should be used for longer than 24 hours (Springhouse 2002, Wilson and Jordan 2001).

If the infusion must be discontinued, the catheter should be flushed to maintain patency. The risk of infection increases if the infusion is disconnected from the central venous device; therefore, it is not advisable to disconnect PN until the whole daily requirement has been administered (Pratt *et al.* 2007).

During intravenous feeding, monitoring is necessary to detect and minimize complications. Once feeding is established and the patient is biochemically stable then the frequency of monitoring may be reduced if the clinical condition of the patient permits (see Table 8.8). Additional patient monitoring such as 24-hour urine collection for urinary urea, nitrogen and checking serum trace element levels may be carried out where indicated, for example in severe malnutrition or when PN is used for prolonged periods of time (Weinstein and Plumer 2007).

Home parenteral nutrition

There are a few indications for home PN. It may be necessary in patients who have complete intestinal failure or insufficient functioning bowel to maintain an adequate nutritional status via the enteral route, for example short bowel syndrome due to Crohn's disease or radiation enteritis.

This is a complicated and specialist treatment, requiring 24-hour access to advice and support, and should be co-ordinated through a specialist centre.

No patient should be considered for home PN without a multidisciplinary discussion of the patient and the formulation of a clear management plan. If continuation of hospital-initiated PN is considered essential, the implications must be discussed with the multiprofessional team, including the medical consultant, dietetics, pharmacy, IV therapy team, complex discharge co-ordinator and patient.

There is national guidance on the training, provision and appropriate support for such patients, which should be consulted prior to any discharge of patients receiving PN (BAPEN 2003a, NHS National Commissioning Group 2008). However, in England there are plans to develop a national clinical network of expert regional units to provide support for patients requiring home PN to ensure that their needs are met appropriately (NHS 2009). Patients require an extensive period of specialized training to manage PN in the home environment and this should be undertaken by such units and clinical teams.

It is important that all members of the multidisciplinary team, including the dietitian, nurse, doctor, pharmacist, catering department and community services, are involved in the patient's nutritional care to ensure a thorough and co-ordinated approach to nutritional management (BAPEN 2003a, NCCAC 2006).

Termination of parenteral nutrition

Parenteral nutrition should not be terminated until oral or enteral tube feeding is well established (NCCAC 2006, Weinstein and Plumer 2007). PN should be weaned off to half rate before stopping, to prevent rebound hypoglycaemia, as well as to ensure adequate nutritional intake via an alternative route. It is important that all members of the multidisciplinary team are involved in the decision to terminate PN and that enteral intake is monitored sufficiently.

Complications

Metabolic complications should be detected by appropriate monitoring. Some of the more common complications are as follows.

Fluid overload

This may occur when other blood products and fluids are given concurrently. It may be possible to reduce the volume of a 24-hour bag of PN while maintaining the nutritional content. A pharmacist and dietitian can advise on the feasibility of creating such regimens.

Hyperglycaemia

This may occur due to stress-induced insulin resistance or carbohydrate overload. A simultaneous sliding scale insulin infusion may be required. Failure to recognize hyperglycaemia may result in osmotic diuresis.

Hypoglycaemia

Abrupt cessation of PN may result in a rebound hypoglycaemia. A reduction in infusion to half the rate prior to stopping the infusion may help prevent this occurring.

Azotaemia

Raised plasma urea may indicate renal dysfunction or dehydration. Alterations in the nitrogen and non-protein energy content of the PN may be required, or an increase in fluid input (Payne-James *et al.* 2001).

387

Table 8.8 Monitoring in nutrition support

Parameter	Frequency of monitoring	Rationale	Interpretation
Catheter entry site	Daily	Signs of infection/inflammation	Interpret with knowledge of infection control
Skin over position of catheter tip	Daily	Signs of thrombophlebitis	
General condition	Daily	To check tolerance of feed and that feed and route continue to be appropriate	
Temperature/blood pressure	Daily, then as needed	Sign of infection, fluid balance	
Sodium, potassium, urea, creatinine	Baseline, then daily until stable, then 1–2 times a week	Assessment of renal function, fluid status	Interpret with knowledge of fluid balance and medication
			Urinary sodium may be helpful in complex cases with gastrointestinal fluid loss
Glucose	Baseline, then 1–2 times daily until stable (more if needed), then weekly	Glucose intolerance is common	Good glycaemic control is necessary
Magnesium, phosphate	Baseline, then daily if risk of refeeding syndrome, then three times a week until stable, then weekly	Depletion is common and under-recognized	Low concentrations indicate poor status
Liver function tests	Baseline, then twice weekly until stable, then weekly	Abnormalities common during PN	Complex. May be due to sepsis, other disease or nutritional intake
Calcium, albumin	Baseline, then weekly	Low or high levels may occur	Correct measured serum calcium concentration for albumin
			Hypocalcaemia may be secondary to magnesium deficiency
			Low albumin reflects disease not protein status
C-reactive protein	Baseline, then 2 or 3 times a week until stable	Assists interpretation of protein, trace element and vitamin results	To assess the presence of an acute-phase reaction
			The trend of results is important
Zinc, copper	Baseline, then every 2–4 weeks depending on results	Deficiency is common, especially with increased losses	People most at risk when anabolic
			Zinc decreases and copper increases in acute-phase reaction
Selenium	Baseline if risk of depletion, further testing depending on this	Deficiency is likely in severe illness and sepsis, or long-term nutrition support	Decreases in acute-phase reaction
			Long-term status better assessed by glutathione peroxidase
Full blood count	Baseline, then 1 or 2 times a week until stable, then weekly	Anaemia due to iron or folate deficiency is common	Effects of sepsis may be important
Iron, ferritin	Baseline, then every 3–6 months	Iron deficiency is common in long-term PN	Iron status is difficult to assess in acute-phase reaction
			Iron decreases, while ferritin increases
Folate, vitamin B_{12}	Baseline then every 2–4 weeks	Iron deficiency is common	Serum folate/B_{12} sufficient with full blood count
Manganese	Every 3–6 months if on home PN	Excess provision to be avoided, more likely in liver disease	Red blood cell or whole blood better measure of excess than plasma
Vitamin D	Six monthly if on long-term PN	Low levels if housebound	Requires normal kidney function for effect
Bone densitometry	On starting home PN, then every 2 years	Diagnosis of metabolic bone disease	Together with lab tests for metabolic bone disease

Adapted from NCCAC (2006), pp. 23–25.

Hypophosphataemia

This is associated with excessive glucose infusion and the refeeding syndrome in malnourished patients (NCCAC 2006, Solomon and Kirby 1990). It is necessary to correct phosphate levels by providing additional phosphate prior to feeding. Phosphate levels should be monitored daily at the start of feeding.

Other complications such as metabolic acidosis, electrolyte disturbances, hypernatraemia, hypokalaemia and hypomagnesaemia may require a review of the PN solution, rate of administration, additional fluids, blood products and drugs.

Transfusion of blood and blood components

Definition

Blood transfusion is the administration of a blood component- or plasma-derived product to the patient (Gray *et al.* 2007). Blood is a raw material from which different therapeutic products are made (McClelland 2007).

Anatomy and physiology
ABO blood groups and rhesus types

In 1901, Landsteiner discovered that human blood groups existed and developed the ABO system which marked the start of safe blood transfusion (Bishop 2008). There are four principal blood groups: A, B, AB and O. Each group relates to the presence or absence of surface antigens on the red blood cells and antibodies in the serum which dictate blood compatibility (Table 8.9).

People with the blood group **AB** have red cells with A and B surface antigens, but they do not have any anti-A or anti-B immunoglobulin M (IgM) antibodies in their serum. Therefore, they are able to receive blood from any group, but can only donate to other people from group AB.

People with group **O** red cells do not have either A or B surface antigens but they do have anti-A and anti-B IgM antibodies in their serum. They are only able to receive blood from group O, but can donate to A, B, O and AB groups.

People with group **A** red cells have type A surface antigens, and they have anti-B IgM antibodies in their serum. They are only able to receive blood from groups **A** or **O** and can only donate blood to people from A and AB groups.

People with group **B** red cells have type B surface antigens and they have anti-A IgM antibodies in their serum. They are therefore only able to receive blood from groups **B** or **O** and can only donate blood to people from B and AB groups.

In addition to the ABO system, the rhesus (Rh) system was discovered in 1940; again, these are surface antigens and they are another essential system used in transfusion therapy (Mollison *et al.* 1997). The Rh D antigen is the most immunogenic of the Rh antigens (Porth 2005). However, many other red cell antigens exist and exposure to them may stimulate the development of corresponding antibodies (McClelland 2007).

Related theory
Blood group incompatibility

The transfusion of ABO incompatible red cells can lead to intravascular haemolysis where the recipient's IgM antibodies bind to the corresponding surface antigens of the transfused cells (McClelland 2007). Complement activation results in lysis of the transfused cells and the haemoglobin that is released precipitates renal failure, with the fragments of the lysed cells activating the clotting pathways, which in turn leads to the development of disseminated intravascular coagulation (DIC) (Mollison *et al.* 1997). Transfusion of rhesus-positive cells to a rhesus-negative individual will result in immunization and the appearance of anti-D antibodies (Hoffbrand *et al.* 2006). However, on any subsequent exposure extravascular haemolysis occurs when rhesus antibody-coated red cells are destroyed by macrophages in the liver and spleen (McClelland 2007).

A patient's rhesus status is of particular importance in pregnancy as haemolytic disease of the newborn (HDN) can occur when the mother is rhesus negative and the developing foetus is rhesus positive as exposure to foetal blood can stimulate anti-D activation in the mother, which in turn can cross the placenta, causing haemolysis (McClelland 2007).

Blood groups in haemopoietic stem cell transplantation

The human leucocyte antigen (HLA) is used to determine compatibility for organ transplantation, including bone

389

Table 8.9 Blood group compatibility

Group	Antigens	IgM antibodies	Compatible donor for	Compatible recipient of
A	A	Anti B	A	A
			AB	O
B	B	Anti A	B	B
			AB	O
AB	A and B	None	AB	A
				B
				AB
				O
O	None	Anti A	A	O
		Anti B	B	
			AB	
			O	

marrow and peripheral blood stem cells. However, because ABO blood groups and HLA tissue types are determined genetically, it is not uncommon to find a suitable HLA donor who is ABO and/or rhesus incompatible with the recipient. In such circumstances, major transfusion reactions can be avoided by red cell and/or plasma depletion of the donor cells in the laboratory before reinfusion (Mollison *et al.* 1997). Occasionally, if the recipient has a very high titre of anti-A or anti-B lytic antibody and the donor marrow or peripheral blood stem cells are blood group A, B or AB, then plasmapheresis of the recipient may be performed to lower the titre of this antibody to safe limits. This is necessary because it is not possible to remove all the red cells from the donor product and those remaining may cause a major transfusion reaction in this situation (Mollison *et al.* 1997).

Evidence-based approaches

The transfusion of blood components is a complex multi-step process involving personnel from diverse backgrounds with differing levels of knowledge and understanding. Errors made in the process of transfusion present a significant risk to patients.

Although there is little evidence to support the efficacy for set procedures to manage this risk, current professional opinion has been provided by the British Committee for Standards in Haematology (BCSH) in collaboration with the Royal College of Nursing (RCN) and the Royal College of Surgeons of England (RCS) (BCSH 1999, Gray and Illingworth 2005). As a result of this guidance, every hospital should have a policy in place for the administration of blood and blood components including identification of the patient, blood sampling, special blood requirement requests, processing of blood samples, the storage, collection and transportation of blood products, administration of blood products and the care and monitoring of the transfused patient. Furthermore, hospitals are also required to manage and report any adverse events or near misses, with a statutory requirement to hold a record of every step of the transfusion process including the final fate of each blood product for 30 years (James 2005). Only staff authorized to do so should be involved at any stage in the transfusion process.

Nurses in the UK are normally the healthcare professionals ultimately responsible for the bedside check and arguably have the final opportunity to prevent errors occurring when patients receive blood transfusions (Wilkinson and Wilkinson 2001). Errors in the requesting, collection and administration of blood components (red cells, platelets and plasma concentrates) lead to significant risks for patients. Since its launch in 1996, the Serious Hazards of Transfusion (SHOT) scheme has continually shown that 'wrong blood into patient' episodes are a frequently reported transfusion hazard. These wrong blood incidents are mainly due to human error arising from misidentification of the patient during blood sampling, blood component collection and delivery or administration which can lead to life-threatening haemolytic transfusion reactions and other significant morbidity (BCSH 2009).

The National Comparative Audits (NCA) of bedside transfusion practice in England and North Wales (2003, 2005 and 2009) show that patients continue to be placed at risk of avoidable complications of transfusion through misidentification and inadequate monitoring of the patient.

Rationale

Blood transfusion is an essential part of modern medicine and healthcare. However, it should be prescribed only to treat conditions associated with significant morbidity or mortality that cannot be prevented or managed by other means (WHO 2005).

Recent publications and legislation have created greater awareness of the need to continue to improve transfusion practice in many ways. Blood and blood products are no longer regarded as safe unlimited resources. There are risks inherent in transfusion practice and therefore unnecessary exposure to blood products should be avoided. This is of particular importance for patients who may only have one transfusion in their lifetime, such as surgical patients. Therefore, these patients should only receive a transfusion when it is absolutely necessary. Furthermore, the appropriate use of products is essential for the conservation of blood supplies. Regularly updated guidance on the safe appropriate use of blood and blood products is now available online at www.transfusionguidelines.org.uk and these should be consulted in collaboration with local hospital and blood transfusion service guidelines.

Indications

Anaemia is defined as a haemoglobin concentration in blood that is below the expected value, when age, gender, pregnancy and certain environmental factors, such as altitude, are taken into consideration. In general, anaemia is a consequence of one or more of the following generic causes:

- increased loss of red blood cells
- decreased production of red blood cells
- increased destruction of red blood cells
- increased demand of red blood cells
- increased production of abnormal red blood cells,

which may be due to nutritional deficits, blood loss, kidney disease, medication or chronic diseases (Fields and Meyers 2006, Moftah 2005).

A minimum transfusion trigger has not been well established because of the variability of patient co-morbidities and anaemia tolerance. Evidence suggests that most patients can safely tolerate anaemia of 7 g/dL of Hb in the absence of active bleeding (Tolich 2008). However, surveys of the UK population show that most blood recipients are relatively elderly; many will have cardiovascular disease and may be less tolerant of low haemoglobin levels than younger, fitter patients. A low transfusion threshold may therefore be unwise, as older patients may also be at greater risk of congestive cardiac failure due to volume overload when blood and other fluids are infused (Blood Safety and Quality Regulations 2005, McClelland 2007).

Blood donation and testing

All blood donated in the UK is given voluntarily. The successful selection of a donor must protect them from any harm that may be caused by the donation process and also protect the possible recipient of products derived from the donor's blood. Donors of blood for therapeutic use should be in good health; if there is any doubt about their suitability, the donation should be deferred and they should be fully assessed by a designated medical officer. All donors of blood or its components (via apheresis) should be assessed in accordance with the Joint UKBTS/NIBSC Professional Advisory Committee (JPAC) donor selection guidelines (JPAC 2007). The assessment of fitness to donate includes a questionnaire relating to general health, lifestyle, past medical history and medication. Donation may be temporarily or permanently deferred for a variety of reasons including cardiovascular disease, central nervous system diseases, malignancy and some infectious diseases, all of which are detailed in the JPAC (2007) guidelines. Donors are also screened for risk of exposure to transmissible infectious diseases, and specific guidance is provided for donors receiving therapeutic drugs.

Prevention of transmission of infection is determined by donor selection criteria and laboratory testing. In the UK, all blood donations are tested for infections which could be passed on to the recipient. However, concern about transfusion-related variant Creutzfeldt–Jakob disease (vCJD) transmission is now supported by clinical evidence (Ludlam and Turner 2006) and, despite continuing research, a screening test for preclinical human infection has yet to be developed (Brown 2005). Therefore, donor exclusion criteria remain an important precautionary measure (Cervenakova and Brown 2004). When a donor has been successfully screened, they must validate the information they have provided and record that they have given consent to proceed.

Autologous donation

Since the 1980s there has been interest in autologous donation (blood and blood components collected from an individual and intended solely for subsequent autologous transfusion to that same individual) (Blood Safety and Quality Regulations 2005). This has largely been attributed to high-profile infection risks: human immunodeficiency virus (HIV), hepatitis C and more recently vCJD (James and Harrison 2002). However, autologous donation is not risk free, with 28 cases of adverse events being reported to SHOT in 2008, the majority of which arose through cell salvage events. Autologous donation is contraindicated in certain circumstances. Furthermore, there has been significant concern about the efficacy of some methods (Carless et al. 2004, Henry et al. 2002). Three principal methods of autologous donation exist.

Preoperative autologous donation (PAD)

This requires the patients to donate up to four units of blood whilst simultaneously taking iron supplements in the month preceding surgery. However, the efficacy of this method has been questioned by systematic review (Henry et al. 2002) and is only indicated in very specific circumstances such as patients with very rare blood types, patients donating bone marrow and fit patients who have a significant fear of receiving allogeneic blood products such that it is preventing them from seeking necessary surgery (James 2004).

Acute normovolaemic haemodilution (ANH)

This involves the donation of up to three units of blood immediately prior to surgery. The patient is then given crystalloids to dilute the circulating volume. This method is only indicated for surgery where considerable blood loss is expected on the principle that the number of red cells lost will be reduced and the patient's autologous whole blood can be returned after surgery; however, little evidence exists to support the efficacy of ANH (Harrison 2004).

Intraoperative cell salvage (ICS)

Blood loss during surgery is collected, anticoagulated, filtered and held in a sterile reservoir. The collected blood is then processed, washed and suspended in saline for return. Although ICS is not without risks such as embolism, bacterial contamination and enhanced inflammatory responses through reinfusion of inflammatory mediators (Harrison 2004), it has been recommended as the most effective form of autologous transfusion to assist in the conservation of blood supplies (James 2004). Trials in orthopaedic surgery indicate that salvage can reduce the proportion of patients who receive allogeneic red cell transfusions. Results in cardiac surgery trials have also shown a slight reduction in the use of allogeneic red cell transfusions (McClelland 2007).

The 2008 SHOT report recorded 28 cases of reported adverse events, 25 from ICS and three from postoperative cell salvage (PCS). There were five hypotensive reactions reported from ICS, but no major mortality or morbidity.

Monitoring of patients receiving autologous transfusion is as important as it is for those receiving allogeneic transfusion (SHOT 2008).

Blood component donation

Donors of blood components by automated apheresis are subject to the same selection criteria used for donating whole blood and any exception to this must be decided by a designated medical officer. Apheresis can be used to collect plasma, red cells and platelets. Leucopheresis procedures are used for the collection of granulocytes, lymphocytes and peripheral blood progenerator cells (James 2005).

391

Appropriate use of donated blood components

Donated blood components are a precious gift; they are not a limitless resource and must be used appropriately. The BCSH has guidelines in place for the use of red cell, platelet, fresh frozen plasma, cryoprecipitate and cryo-supernatant transfusions, available on the BCSH website www.bcshguidelines.com.

The decision to transfuse must be based on a thorough clinical assessment of the patient and their individual needs. Each blood component should only be given after careful consideration, when there is valid clinical indication or when there are no alternative treatment options available (Oldham *et al.* 2009).

Blood and blood products have varying shelf-lives and storage requirements. The range of products currently available, indications for use and recommendations for administration are listed in Table 8.10.

Anticipated patient outcomes

Blood component transfusion can be a life-saving and life-enhancing treatment when used appropriately and when patients are cared for safely and by knowledgeable, skilled practitioners (Oldham *et al.* 2009).

Legal and professional issues
Blood safety and quality in the UK

Approximately 3.4 million blood products are administered in the UK every year (Gray and Illingworth 2005). The transfusion of blood and its components is usually safe and uneventful; however, there are associated risks and there have been significant developments over recent years to improve the quality and safety of transfusion practice in the UK. The Blood Safety and Quality Regulations came into effect in February 2005 and were fully implemented on 8 November 2005. These Regulations cover the collecting, testing, processing, storing and distributing of blood and blood components (Blood Safety and Quality Regulations 2005). The official government agency with jurisdiction for these regulations is the Medicines and Healthcare Products Regulatory Agency (MHRA).

The principal requirements of these Regulations in relation to transfusion practice are as follows.

- *Traceability:* whereby hospitals must have a system to record and retain information on the fate of each unit of blood/blood component for a period of 30 years.
- *Haemovigilance:* an organized surveillance procedure relating to serious adverse or unexpected events or reactions. The reporting of such events can be done via the online Serious Adverse Blood Reactions and Events (SABRE) system which is maintained by the Medical Device Adverse Incident Reporting Centre. This will usually be done by a designated member of laboratory staff and therefore clinical staff must ensure that all incident reporting is conducted in line with hospital policy.

The MHRA defines such events as follows.

- A **serious adverse event** is defined as an unintended occurrence associated with the collection, testing, processing, storage and distribution of blood or blood components that might lead to death or life-threatening, disabling or incapacitating conditions for patients or which results in, or prolongs, hospitalization or morbidity.
- A **serious adverse reaction** is defined as an unintended response in a donor or in a patient associated with the collection or transfusion of blood components that is fatal, life-threatening, disabling or incapacitating, or which results in or prolongs hospitalization or morbidity.

(MHRA 2005)

Prior to these regulations, Better Blood Transfusion initiatives aimed to ensure that such guidance became an integral part of NHS care, making blood transfusion safer, ensuring that all blood used in clinical practice is necessary and improving the information both patients and the public receive about blood transfusion (DH 2007). Therefore it is a key requirement that all staff involved in the process of transfusion maintain their awareness of all appropriate guidance.

Competencies

The transfusion of any blood product carries with it the potential of reaction and risk (SHOT 2005). All staff involved in the transfusion of blood and/or blood products must have the knowledge and skills to ensure the process is completed safely. Therefore, the nurse caring for those receiving transfusion therapy must do so within his or her sphere of competence, always acting to minimize risk to the patient (NMC 2008a).

Practitioners must understand the theory and reasoning behind the necessity to follow the correct transfusion procedures and practices (Pirie and Gray 2007). In November 2006, the NPSA, the Chief Medical Officer's National Blood Transfusion Committee (NBTC) and SHOT, working in collaboration, developed strategies aimed at ensuring that blood transfusions are carried out safely, and issued the Safer Practice Notice (SPN) No. 14, *Right Patient, Right Blood*. One of the key action points in this notice was for all NHS and independent sector organizations involved in administering blood transfusions to develop and implement an action plan for competency-based training and assessments for all staff involved in blood transfusions. The current guideline is for all staff involved in the blood transfusion process to have completed their initial competency assessments by November 2010 (BCSH 2009, Blood Safety snd Quality Regulations 2005).

There are three key principles which underpin every stage of the blood component transfusion process:

- patient identification
- documentation
- communication (BCSH 2009).

Table 8.10 Blood and blood products used for transfusion

Type	Description	Indications	Cross-matching	Shelf life	Average infusion time	Technique	Special considerations
Red cells in optimal additive solutions (SAGM)[a]	Red cells with plasma removed: 100 mL additive fluid used as replacement to give optimal red cell preservation; haematocrit 60–65% leuco-depleted	Correction of anaemia	ABO and Rh compatible (not necessarily identical)	35 days at 2–6°C	1–2 hours/unit. Transfusion to be completed within 4 hours of component's removal from storage	Give via a blood administration set	If more than half blood volume is replaced with red cells in SAGM, use of FFP should be considered to replace clotting factors
Washed red blood cells	Red cells centrifuged and re-suspended twice in 0.9% sodium chloride leuco-depleted	Correction of anaemia where patient may react to plasma components, for example in IgA deficiency	As above	Prepared by non-sterile process, therefore to be used within 24 hours	1–2 hours/unit	As above	–
Frozen red blood cells	Red cells of very rare phenotype leuco-depleted	To treat patients with very rare antibody	As above	Stored frozen cells: 3 years. Use within 12 hours of thawing	2–3 hours/unit	As above	–
White blood cells (buffy coat or aphereseed granulocytes)[b]	Mainly granulocytes obtained by leucophoresis or by 'creaming off' the white blood cell layer from fresh blood	To treat patients with life-threatening granulocytopenia	As above	24 hours after preparation. Stored at room temperature	60–90 minutes/unit	Administer via a blood administration set	White blood cell infusion induces fever, may cause hypotension, rigors and confusion. Treat symptoms and reassure patient Preparation is always irradiated to prevent initiation of transfusion-associated graft-versus-host disease (TA-GVHD). *Do not* give to patients receiving amphotericin B. Indications for granulocyte transfusions should be when possible benefits are thought to outweigh considerable hazards of the treatment option (Brozovis *et al.*, 1998)
Platelets[a]	Platelets in 200–300 mL plasma. May be pooled from 5 donors or aphereseed from a single donor leuco-depleted	To treat thrombocytopenia	No cross-matching necessary	Up to 7 days after collection. Storage is at 22°C, with continuous gentle agitation	20–30 minutes/unit	Administration using a platelet administration set. Use a new set for each transfusion. Do not use micro-aggregate filters	General guide to use: 1 Count less than 10×10^9/L 2 Count $10–20 \times 10^9$/L with haemorrhage and/or persistent pyrexia 3 Count $20–50 \times 10^9$/L in special cases or pre-invasive procedure

(Continued)

Table 8.10 (*Continued*)

Type	Description	Indications	Cross-matching	Shelf life	Average infusion time	Technique	Special considerations
Fresh frozen plasma	Citrated plasma separated from whole blood	To treat a deficiency in clotting factors due to dilution effects, consumption (in DIC), liver failure or overdose of coumarin anticoagulant	No cross-matching necessary	2 years at −30°C. Once thawed, kept at 4°C, to be used as soon as possible but within 24 hours	15–45 minutes/unit (approx. 250 mL)	Administer rapidly via a blood administration set	FFP should be considered if patient has received more than half their blood volume in red cells, to prevent dilutional hypocoagulability
Albumin 4.5% (HAS)	Solution of albumin from pooled plasma in a buffered, stabilized 0.9% sodium chloride diluent. Supplied in 250 mL or 500 mL bottle	To treat hypovolaemic shock or hypoproteinaemia due to burns, trauma, surgery or infection. Sourced outside UK to reduce risk of transmission of vCJD	Unnecessary. Not blood group specific	5 years at room temperature Kept in dark	30–60 minutes/unit	Administer via a standard solution administration set	The solution should be crystal clear with no deposits
Albumin 20% (HAS)	Heat-treated, aqueous, chemically processed fraction of pooled plasma	To treat hypovolaemic shock or hypoproteinaemia due to burns, trauma, surgery or infection. To maintain appropriate electrolyte balance	Unnecessary	5 years at room temperature Kept in dark	30–60 minutes/unit	Administer via a blood administration set undiluted or diluted with 0.9% sodium chloride or 5% glucose solution. Slower administration is advised if a cardiac disorder is present to avoid gross fluid shift	The solution should be crystal clear with no deposits

394

Cryoprecipitate	Cold-insoluble portion of plasma recovered from FFP: rich in factor VIII, von Willebrand's factor and fibrinogen. Available as single packs (20–40 mL) or 5 units pooled (120–140 mL)	To control bleeding disorders due to lack of factor VIII or fibrinogen, for example haemophilia, von Willebrand's disease, DIC	No cross-matching necessary	2 years at –30°C. Use immediately after thawing	15–30 minutes via infusion, 10–15 minutes via intravenous push	Administer rapidly via syringe or blood administration set
Cryo-depleted plasma	FFP with cryoprecipitate removed	Useful in treating thrombotic thrombocytopenic purpura: patients are plasma-exchanged daily to reduce circulating von Willebrand's factor	No cross-matching necessary	2 years at –30°C. Once thawed, kept at 4°C, to be used as soon as possible but within 24 hours	Time varies on machine average ±2.5 hours	Via apheresis machine

[a]Most commonly used blood products.
[b]See leucocyte depletion.

Consent

Providing the patient with information before a procedure and ascertaining that the patient understands the procedure and has consented to it is the responsibility of the healthcare professional carrying out the procedure as well as those prescribing it (NMC 2008b). Although blood components may not be prescribed as they are not medicinal products (Green and Pirie 2009), a blood component transfusion must be treated as any prescribed medicine, that is, patients (or guardian) must be informed of the indication for the transfusion, advised of the risks and benefits, of alternatives to blood transfusion including autologous transfusion (BCSH 1999), be given the opportunity to ask questions and have the right to refuse to receive it in accordance with local and national guidance (NMC 2008b, RCN 2006). One of the key objectives of the HSC 2007/001 Better Blood Transfusion was to improve information provided to patients and to ensure that those who are likely to receive a blood transfusion will be well informed of their choices. There are a number of information leaflets issued by the NHS Blood and Transplant Service for both patients and healthcare professionals.

The issue of consent for blood transfusion is currently being considered by the Advisory Committee on the Safety of Blood, Tissues and Organs (SaBTO). Patients have the right to refuse transfusion and to be treated with respect. Staff must be sensitive to individual patient needs, acknowledging their values, beliefs and cultural background and exploring alternative treatments if appropriate and available (Oldham *et al.* 2009). There is increasing public concern about blood transfusion safety and the need to accommodate some patients' religious beliefs (John *et al.* 2008).

Jehovah's Witnesses and blood transfusion

The role of blood in Jehovah's Witnesses' spiritual belief is based on scripture and followers are usually well informed on both their beliefs and their rights. Many Jehovah's Witnesses carry information with them regarding any objection and therefore the need to ensure informed consent is very important. Staff caring for patients must ensure that decisions to consent to or refuse treatment are respected and recorded appropriately (McClelland 2007). Furthermore, in individual circumstances, practitioners should endeavour to consider non-blood or autologous methods as described previously, where appropriate (McClelland 2007).

Blood product request

The details on the blood component request form and the sample tube are the only direct contact between the clinical area and the blood transfusion laboratory. The accuracy and completeness of this information are therefore of vital importance (BCSH 2009). Incorrect or inadequate patient identification leading to a sample for blood grouping being taken from, or labelled for, the wrong patient may result in

fatal ABO incompatible transfusions (SHOT annual reports 1996–2007). Inadequately or mislabelled samples are up to 40 times more likely to contain blood from the wrong patient (BCSH 2009).

The collection of the blood sample from the patient and the subsequent labelling of the sample tube should be performed as a continuous, uninterrupted event at the patient's (bed)side, involving one patient and one member of staff only (BCSH 2009).

The Chief Medical Officer's National Blood Transfusion Committee for England and North Wales has produced a standardized 'Indication Codes' for transfusion which may be incorporated into the request process (BCSH 2009).

Preprocedural considerations

Equipment
Intravenous access

Blood components may be administered through peripheral cannulas or via a central venous access device. Where possible, one lumen should be reserved for the taking of blood specimens and blood component administration for the duration of therapy.

Administration sets

All blood components must be transfused through a sterile blood component administration set with an integral mesh filter (170–200 micron). Blood administration sets should be changed at least every 12 hours or after every second unit for a continuing transfusion (Gray and Illingworth 2005); please refer to local guidance. Administration sets used for blood components must be changed immediately upon suspected contamination or when the integrity of the product or system has been compromised. Platelets and plasma components may be administered through a normal blood administration set or through a platelet or cryoprecipitate set. Platelets should never be administered through an administration set that has previously been used for red cell transfusion or other blood component as this may cause aggregation of platelets in the administration set (McClelland 2007). Administration sets used for blood components must be changed using aseptic technique and observing universal precautions, in line with manufacturer's instructions (RCN 2010).

Infusion devices

Either gravity or electronic infusion devices may be used for the administration of blood components. There are a variety of electronic infusion devices available and it is therefore essential that individuals using any type of infusion device are competent in their use. Only blood component administration sets compatible with the infusion device should be used. Rapid infusion devices that are CE marked may be used when large volumes have to be infused rapidly. Typically, devices can infuse from 6 to 30 litres an hour and usually incorporate a blood-warming device (BCSH 2009, McClelland 2007).

Blood-warming devices

The warming of blood and blood products is generally not recommended as it is of limited benefit and can be dangerous. Blood warmers are only indicated when:

- massive, rapid transfusion could result in cooling of cardiac tissue, causing potentially fatal dysrhythmia (McClelland 2007). If the rate of transfusion is greater than 100 mL per minute, blood-warming devices should be used (McClelland 2007)
- transfusion is required by patients with cold agglutination disease (Gray and Illingworth 2005)
- exchange transfusion is indicated in the newborn (Weinstein and Plumer 2007)
- thawing of cryopreserved stem cells prior to transfusion (blood or marrow).

Both water baths and dry heat blood warmers are available. However, whichever device is chosen, the temperature should be maintained below 38°C. Warming in excess of this can cause haemolysis of red cells and can denature proteins and increase the risk of bacterial infection. Blood warmers must always be used and maintained according to the manufacturer's guidelines. Blood products must *never* be warmed by improvisation, such as putting the pack into hot water, in a microwave or on a radiator, as uncontrolled heating can damage the contents of the pack (Gray and Illingworth 2005, McClelland 2007). The use of water baths also increases the risk of bacterial contamination. Therefore certain safety measures must be adhered to.

- Water baths must be drained after each use and must be stored dry and empty.
- The blood warmer should be drained after each use and must be stored dry and empty.
- When needed, they should be refilled with sterile water.
- A protective sterile over-bag to thaw blood and blood products reduces the entry of contaminants through microscopic punctures or breaks in the seal.
- The product should be used immediately after it has been thawed.

All devices should be serviced as per hospital health and safety policies, MHRA and manufacturers' guidelines.

Specific patient preparations

In 2007 the NPSA issued a Safer Practice Notice No. 24, *Standardising Wristbands Improves Patient Safety*, stating that only the following core identifiers should be used on patients' identification bands:

- last name
- first name
- date of birth
- NHS number.

Patients should have their identification confirmed on admission to the unit and one wristband attached to their wrist. If a wristband is removed for any reason, for example to gain intravenous access via a cannula, it is the responsibility of the person removing it to ensure that a correctly completed wristband is then reapplied.

The nurse must ensure that the patient has been informed of the proposed transfusion and has had an opportunity to raise any concerns, understands the risks and benefits of the transfusion and has agreed to and is available for the transfusion. Pretransfusion/baseline observations including blood pressure, temperature, pulse and respiratory rate must be undertaken and documented and checked that they are within acceptable parameters and that there is patent venous access prior to administering the transfusion.

Pretransfusion/bedside check

While professional accountability must be taken at every stage by the personnel involved, the final barrier to wrong blood administration is at the bedside. The final link is ensuring the right patient receives the right blood and it is therefore essential that the check is performed thoroughly prior to the transfusion of each component (Oldham *et al.* 2009).

To ensure that each blood component is used to its full advantage, local hospital policy should be followed with regard to correct handling and storage, transportation and administration of blood components. If unused, the component should be returned to the transfusion laboratory as quickly as possible to maximize the opportunity for it to be used for another patient.

The written order for the blood component must be checked to ensure that it is correctly completed and to ensure that it contains the following information.

- Patient core identifiers.
- Date (and time if appropriate) the blood component is required.
- Type of blood component to be administered.
- Any clinical special transfusion requirements, for example irradiated, CMV seronegative, blood warmer.
- Volume or number of units to be transfused (exact number in mL for paediatric transfusions).
- Time over which each unit is to be transfused (exact rate or length of time over which the specified volume is to be transfused for paediatric transfusions).
- Any special instructions, for example concomitant drugs required, such as diuretics.
- Signature of the 'prescriber'.

Procedure guideline 8.18 Blood product request

Essential equipment

- Blood request form

Procedure

Action	Rationale
1 The following information must be completed on the request form. (a) First name (b) Surname (c) Date of birth (d) Gender (e) Hospital identification number (f) Ward or department	Full demographics are required to minimize the risk of patients with the same or similar names being given the incorrect blood component (McClelland 2007, C; SNBTS 2004, C). Details on the request form must match the enclosed blood sample. Discrepant samples should not be processed (James 2005, C).
2 Complete the following clinical information. (a) Diagnosis (b) Reason for request; this should include details of any surgical procedure (c) Number and type of components requested (d) Any special requirements such as irradiated, CMV negative (e) If group and screen only (f) Date and time required	Enables laboratory staff to assess need against the surgical blood ordering schedule (E). Some vulnerable patient groups may have a fatal reaction to wrongly transfused non-irradiated or CMV-positive products (McClelland 2007, C). Negative and positive status should always be written in full and not as + or – as they may get defaced and be incorrectly processed (SNBTS 2004, C). This allows laboratory staff to plan ahead for complex cross-matches to ensure the required products are available at the correct time (SNBTS 2004, C).
3 Each request should also include: (a) the name of the doctor/nurse requesting the products (b) the name and signature of the person who has taken the blood sample	Every step of the transfusion must be fully traceable and the record held for 30 years (James 2005, C).
4 The following information can also be included if it is available in the patient's clinical record. (a) Patient's blood group (b) Presence of known antibodies (c) Date of last transfusion	This information is useful to laboratory staff (E). Negative and positive should always be written in full and not as + or – as they may get defaced and be incorrectly processed (SNBTS 2004, C).

Procedure guideline 8.19 Blood sampling: pretransfusion

Essential equipment

- Antimicrobial skin cleanser – the recommended solution is 0.5% chlorhexidine in 70% alcohol
- Needle/winged infusion device
- Appropriate tubes for blood sample collection
- Gauze
- Hypoallergenic tape
- Non-sterile, well-fitting gloves
- Sharps container

Preprocedure

Action	Rationale
1 Explain and discuss the procedure with the patient.	To ensure that the patient understands the procedure and gives their valid consent (NMC 2008b, C).
2 Take pretransfusion blood from one patient at a time.	To ensure that samples from different patients are not confused which can have fatal consequences and to minimize this risk (SHOT 2008, C).
3 Check all packaging before opening and preparing the equipment.	To ensure there has been no contamination and all equipment is in date. E

Procedure

4 Before taking the sample, ask the patient to state their first name, surname and date of birth. Cross-check these details against the blood request form.	To ensure that the sample obtained corresponds with the request (BCSH 2009, C).
5 Check these details against the patient's identity wristband.	To ensure that the patient is positively identified before obtaining a blood sample (BCSH 2009, C).
6 Check the patient's hospital number on the wristband against that on the blood request form.	To ensure that the sample obtained corresponds with the request (BCSH 2009, C).
7 Obtain the blood sample by direct venepuncture or via central venous access device, in the appropriate tube (see Chapter 11).	To ensure the correct procedure is followed and an adequate sample is obtained. E

Postprocedure

6 Hand-write the sample tube clearly and accurately, ensuring all names are spelled correctly. This should only be done once the sample has been successfully obtained and should be done at patient's (bed)side. (a) First name (b) Surname (c) Date of birth (d) Gender (e) Hospital identification number (f) Ward or department (g) Date	To ensure the sample is labelled with the correct patient details. BCSH guidelines do not recommend the use of addressograph (BCSH 1999, C). Blood tubes should never be completed in advance as this has been identified as a major cause of patient identification errors (SNBTS 2004, C).

Procedure guideline 8.20 Blood components: collection and delivery to the clinical area

Removal of blood components from their storage location continues to be identified as a major source of error in the transfusion process (BCSH 2009). Only those staff who are authorized, trained and competent may remove blood components from storage. A guide to the necessary elements of blood pack labelling is shown in Figure 8.9.

Essential equipment

- Documentation containing the patient's three core identifiers – full name, date of birth and hospital number/unique identifying number – must be held by the person removing the component from storage

Preprocedure

Action	Rationale
1 Check that the reason for the transfusion has been documented in the patient notes.	To ensure the transfusion is appropriate and necessary (BCSH 2009, C).

(Continued)

Compatibility label or tie-on tag

The compatibility label is generated in the hospital transfusion laboratory. It is attached to the blood bag and contains the following patient information: *Surname, First Name(s), Date of Birth, Gender, Hospital Number/Patient Identification Number, Hospital* and *Ward*.
The *blood group*, *component type* and *date requested* are also included on the label. The *unique donation number* is printed on the compatibility label; this number must match exactly with the number on the blood bag label.

Unique donation number

This is the unique number assigned to each blood donation by the transfusion service and allows follow-up from donor to patient. From April 2001 all donations bear the new 14 digit (ISBT 128) donation number.
The unique donation number on the blood bag must match exactly the number on the compatibility label.

Cautionary notes

This section of the label gives instructions on storage conditions and the checking procedures you are required to undertake when administering a blood component. It also includes information on the component type and volume.

Blood group

Shows the blood group of the component.

This does not have to be identical with the patient's blood group but must be compatible.

Group O patients must receive group O red cells.

Expiry date

The expiry date must be checked – do not use any component that is beyond the expiry date.

Special requirements

This shows the special features of the donation, e.g. CMV negative.

Figure 8.9 Blood pack labelling

Procedure guideline 8.20 (*Continued*)

2 Check that there is a valid written order for the administration of the component including special requirements – CMV negative or irradiated components.	To ensure the selected component meets the patient's individual requirements (BCSH 2009, C).
3 Check the patient is aware of and has 'consented' to the procedure.	To ensure the patient is fully informed (BCSH 2009, C).
4 Check the patient is available.	To avoid delays once the component has been removed from storage. E
5 Take baseline observations to include blood pressure, temperature, pulse and respiratory rate.	To ensure that any transfusion reaction can be immediately identified, due to changes in baseline (BCSH 2009, C), and managed appropriately (SNBTS 2004, C).
6 Check the patient has patent venous access.	To avoid any delay in commencement of the transfusion and adhere to 'cold chain' requirements (BCSH 2009, C).
7 Check the patient is wearing an identification wristband.	To avoid delays in confirming patient identity (BCSH 2009, C).

Procedure

8 Where possible, the same person who will administer the component should collect from storage.	To minimize the number of people involved in the process (BCSH 2009, C).
9 Remove the component (using electronic or manual method) from storage in accordance with trust policy.	To ensure that only authorized, trained and competent staff may collect blood components (BCSH 2009, C).
10 Remove one component at a time, unless rapid transportation of large quantities is needed or if blood is being transported to remote areas in specifically designed validated blood transport containers.	To ensure components are stored in the appropriate conditions. E
11 Check the component at the point of removal for correct patient-identifying details. A visual inspection of the component should also be performed to check the expiry date and any signs of leakage, clumping or discoloration.	In order to minimize the risk of incorrectly administering the component to the wrong patient (BCSH 2009, C). Expired or damaged products must not be used (McClelland 2007, E).
12 Deliver the component to the clinical area where an appropriately trained and competent member of staff should check that the correct blood has been delivered.	To ensure the correct component has been received for the patient, to comply with traceability and cold chain requirements (BCSH 2009, C).

401

Procedure guideline 8.21 **Blood component administration**

Essential equipment

- Written order for blood component transfusion
- Blood administration administration set with 170–200 μm macroaggregate filter

Preprocedure

Action	Rationale
1 Check that the component has been correctly prescribed, including any special requirements such as irradiated or CMV-negative blood, and if the patient requires any other medications, for example diuretic, premedication.	To prevent Incorrect Blood Component Transfused (IBCT) error: ABO incompatibility or non-irradiated CMV-positive products may cause a fatal reaction if transfused (McClelland 2007, C). Negative and positive status should always be written in full and not as + or – as they may get defaced and be incorrectly processed. E

(*Continued*)

Procedure guideline 8.21 (*Continued*)

2 Check that the patient's baseline vital signs, temperature, pulse, blood pressure and respirations have been recorded.	To ensure that any transfusion reaction can be immediately identified, due to changes in baseline (E), and managed appropriately (SNBTS 2004, C).
3 Conduct a visual inspection of the component to be used for signs of clumping, discoloration, damage or leaks.	Expired or damaged products must not be used (McClelland 2007, E).
4 If there are any discrepancies at this point do not proceed until they have been resolved.	To ensure an IBCT event does not occur. E
5 Positively identify the patient by asking them to state the following information. (a) First name (b) Surname (c) Date of birth	This is the final check of identity which must be performed next to the patient prior to transfusion and is absolutely vital in minimizing the risk of IBCT errors (BCSH 2009, C; SNBTS 2004, C).
6 Check the details given against the patient's nameband and the patient details on the blood component.	To minimize the risk of error (SNBTS 2004, C).
7 Check that the information on the compatibility label matches the details on the blood component, checking expiry date, unique component donation number, blood group on the component label against the laboratory-produced label. Check special requirements have been met. If there are any interruptions during this checking procedure, the entire process should be restarted from the beginning.	To minimize the risk of error (BCSH 2009, C; SNBTS 2004, C).
8 If there are any discrepancies at this point do not proceed until they have been resolved.	To ensure an IBCT event does not occur (SHOT 2008, C).

Procedure

9 Prime the set with blood unless there are concerns about patency of the device, then prime with 0.9% sodium chloride.	Other agents may damage the product components and precipitate transfusion complications (SNBTS 2004, C), for example dextrose should never be used to prime a set or flush the blood administration set following a transfusion as this can cause haemolysis (SNBTS 2004, C).
10 Set up infusion via a volumetric infusion pump if appropriate. Check the infusion pump and settings prior to use.	To ensure the pump is in working order (BCSH 2009, C). Some older infusion pumps can damage the red cells. Blood administration sets for specific infusion pumps must always be used. If none are available the standard blood administration set should be used via gravity and the rate monitored as necessary. E
11 Set the desired infusion rate as indicated by the blood component being used and the patient's condition. **Either** *Red cell administration* can range from 5–10 minutes in acute blood loss to the maximum time of 4 hours (from the time the component is removed from storage) in elderly patients (SNBTS 2004). **Or**	The rate of administration is indicated by the patient's clinical condition (SNBTS 2004, C; Weinstein and Plumer 2007, E). Dictated by current guidelines (SNBTS 2004, C).

Platelets, fresh frozen plasma and cryoprecipitate should be transfused over 30–60 minutes and must be completed within 4 hours of puncturing the blood component.

12	Sign the written order 'prescription' as the person administering the component. The unique component donation number, the date and start time should be recorded in the patient's clinical notes.	To ensure documentation and traceability requirements are met (BCSH 2009, C).
13	Fifteen minutes after the commencement of each component, take and record patient observations – blood pressure, temperature, pulse and respiratory rate	Adverse reactions will often occur during the first 15 minutes of transfusion (Gray and Illingworth 2005, C). Complaints of serious anxiety, transfusion site pain, loin pain, backache, fever, skin flushing or urticaria could be indicative of a serious transfusion reaction (McClelland 2007, E). In such cases the transfusion should be stopped immediately and urgent medical advice sought (SNBTS 2004, C).
14	Observe and monitor the patient throughout the transfusion episode. If there are any concerns, undertake additional observations as appropriate.	To monitor for any adverse reactions (McClelland 2007, E).
15	Record the finish time of each unit. All units must be completed within 4 hours of removal from storage.	Continuation of a transfusion beyond 4 hours increases the risk of transfusion reaction and complications (BCSH 2009, C).
16	Take and record the patient's observations on completion of each unit, ensuring that post-transfusion observations are performed within 60 minutes of completion of the unit.	To ensure the patient's progress is recorded and acts as a baseline for subsequent units (BCSH 2009, C).

Postprocedure

17	Record the time the transfusion finished and the volume of the component transfused on the patient's fluid balance chart.	To ensure an accurate record of fluid is maintained as fluid balance monitoring can identify fluid overload in at-risk patients (Weinstein and Plumer 2007, E).
18	Carefully file all transfusion documentation in the patient's clinical record. In line with local policy, return information on the final fate of each blood component to the hospital laboratory manager.	To ensure the transfusion episode has been recorded, maintaining the clinical record for patient safety. To comply with Statutory Instrument No. 50, Blood Safety and Quality Regulations (2005, C), where the final fate of all blood components must be held for a duration of 30 years.
19	Return any unused blood components to the laboratory promptly.	Unused components may be reallocated if returned in time. Refer to local guidelines. E
20	Keep all empty blood component bags in the clinical area until the transfusion is completed. Once the transfusion is completed, dispose of in clinical waste.	To ensure transfused bags are available in the event of incident investigation (SNBTS 2004, C).
21	For patients receiving ongoing transfusion support, the blood administration set should be changed at least every 12 hours, or after every second unit transfused. Dispose of used set in clinical waste: refer to local guidelines/protocols.	Minimize risk from bacterial contamination (BCSH 2009, C; McClelland 2007, E; SNBTS 2004, E).

Problem-solving table 8.8 **Prevention and resolution (Procedure guidelines 8.18, 8.19, 8.20 and 8.21)**

Problem	Cause	Prevention	Resolution
Unable to collect patient information	Unknown unconscious patient	Do not transfuse unless clinically essential	Assign unique hospital identification number to all requests and samples
	Major incident	Do not transfuse unless clinically essential	Use unique major incident identification number for all requests and samples
	Patient unable to communicate verbally	Follow hospital policy for identification of patients unable to confirm identity verbally. Consider the introduction of photo identification card	Confirm identity with a relative or second member of staff (SNBTS 2004)
		Ensure interpreting services are available if appropriate	
Patient does not have a nameband	Nameband has been removed or is no longer legible	**Always** follow local policy and **never** use secondary identifiers such as bed numbers, notes or request forms that the patient may be carrying (BCSH 1999). If a person removes a patient's identification band, they are then responsible for ensuring that this is replaced	All inpatients are required to wear a nameband; therefore, replace nameband and reconfirm identity (NPSA 2005, RCN 2005)
	Patient is in an outpatient setting	Follow hospital policy for the identification of patients	Ensure patient has a correctly completed identification wristband prior to commencing a transfusion
Unable to obtain verbal confirmation	Patient unconscious	Ensure hospital policy for the identification of unconscious patients is followed	Confirm identity with a relative or second member of staff or use unique patient identifier
Patient unable to communicate verbally	Due to disease or language barrier	Follow hospital policy for the identification of patients unable to confirm their identity verbally. Consider the introduction of photo identification cards. Ensure interpreting services are available if appropriate	Confirm identity with a relative or second member of staff (SNBTS 2004). Always follow local policy and never use secondary identifiers such as bed numbers, notes or request forms that the patient may be carrying (BCSH 1999)
Infusion slows or stops	Venous spasm due to cold infusion	Apply a heat pad prior to the transfusion to reduce venous spasm	Apply warm compress to dilate the vein and increase the blood flow

Problem	Cause	Prevention	Resolution
	Occlusion	Check patency prior to administration. Always use a pulsatile flush ending with a positive pressure flush	Flush gently with 0.9% sodium chloride and resume infusion. If occlusion persists, consider resiting cannula. For a central venous access device occlusion, see Chapter 18
Elevation in temperature after commencing a unit of blood with no other symptoms. Temperature falls if the blood is slowed/stopped	Pyrogenic reaction	Take history to identify whether patient has had a reaction previously	Observe the patient's temperature, pulse and blood pressure during the transfusion as indicated. If the patient has received multiple transfusions or has previous history, ensure that appropriate medication is prescribed before commencing transfusions

405

Postprocedural considerations

Immediate care

The patient should be asked to inform a member of staff of any symptoms which may indicate a transfusion-related adverse event, such as feeling anxious, rigors (shivering), flushing, pain or shortness of breath. The patient should be cared for where they can be visually observed and should be shown how to use the nurse call system. The patient should have vital signs monitored as indicated in the Procedure guidelines: however, it may be necessary to take additional observations if clinically indicated, such as if the patient complains of feeling unwell or they develop signs of a transfusion reaction (Gray and Illingworth 2005).

Many drugs may cause a pyretic hypersensitivity reaction (BNF 2011). There is at present insufficient evidence to allow guidance on the co-administration of drugs with red blood cell transfusion. A lack of clinical reporting of reactions in patients cannot be taken to indicate safe practice: adverse reactions may be attributed to other causes, subclinical haemolysis or agglutination may occur undetected and serious adverse effects may be masked by pre-existing illness in the patient (Murdock et al. 2009).

Ongoing care

On completion of a blood transfusion episode, observations to include blood pressure, temperature, pulse and respiratory rate should be taken and recorded. The patient's records should be updated to confirm that the transfusion has taken place, including the volume transfused, whether the transfusion achieved the desired effect (either post-transfusion increment rates or an improvement in the patient's symptoms) and the details of any reactions to the transfusion. If intravenous fluids are prescribed to follow the transfusion, these should be administered through a new administration set appropriate for that infusion. The traceability documentation confirming the fate of the component should be returned to the laboratory (Blood Safety and Quality Regulations 2005).

The SHOT report (2008) emphasizes that, on occasion, transfusion reactions can occur many hours and sometimes days after the transfusion is completed. Therefore, for patients receiving a transfusion as a day case, it is important to ensure that they are counselled on the possibility of later adverse reactions and that they have access to clinical advice at all times. The BCSH recommends that day-case and short-stay patients are issued with a contact card facilitating 24-hour access to appropriate clinical advice, similar to the scheme used for patients receiving chemotherapy treatments on an outpatient basis (BCSH 2009).

Complications

Transfusion-associated graft-versus-host disease (TA-GVHD)

Although rare, TA-GVHD is a serious complication for recipients and is often fatal. TA-GVHD is usually caused by an IBCT incident where non-irradiated blood components containing immunocompetent T lymphocytes are given to severely immunocompromised recipients. The donor T lymphocytes engraft and multiply, reacting against the recipient's 'foreign' tissue, causing a graft-versus-host reaction (Davies and Williamson 1998). It is not commonly associated with fresh frozen plasma (FFP) or cryoprecipitate. Onset occurs 1–2 weeks after transfusion and the condition is predominantly fatal (McClelland 2007). Irradiation

(25 gray) of blood and blood products, to inactivate T lymphocytes (McClelland 2007), is essential in the prevention of TA-GVHD and is especially important in the following recipients:

- foetuses receiving intrauterine transfusions
- patients undergoing or who have undergone blood or bone marrow progenitor cell transplantation
- immunocompromised recipients.

Bacterial infections

Contamination of blood and blood products can occur during donation, collection, processing, storage and administration. Despite strict guidelines and procedures, the risk of contamination remains. Most common contaminating organisms are skin contaminants such as staphylococci, diphtheroids and micrococci, which enter the blood at the time of venesection (Barbara and Contreras 2009, Provan et al. 2009). Bacterial contamination can lead to severe septic reaction.

Viral infections

Viruses transmissible via blood transfusions can be either plasma borne or cell associated (Barbara and Contreras 2009, Williamson et al. 1999). Plasma-borne viruses include hepatitis B, hepatitis C, hepatitis A (rarely), serum parvovirus B19, and human immunodeficiency viruses (HIV-1 and HIV-2). Cell-associated viruses include cytomegalovirus (CMV), Epstein–Barr virus, human T cell leukaemia/lymphoma viruses (HTLV-1/HTLV-2) and HIV-1/HIV-2.

Human T cell leukaemia/lymphoma virus type 1 (HTLV-1)

Human T cell leukaemia/lymphoma virus type 1 is an oncogenic retrovirus, associated with the white cells that cause adult T cell leukaemia, and is connected with several degenerative neuromuscular syndromes. The enzyme-linked immunosorbent assay (ELISA) has been recommended because of concerns relating to the transmission of the virus via blood transfusion, and the associated long incubation period of adult T cell leukaemia. In the UK all blood is tested for HTLV (JPAC 2005).

Cytomegalovirus (CMV)

Cytomegalovirus is classified as part of the herpes family and hence has the ability to establish latent infection with reactivation during periods of immunosuppression (Barbara and Contreras 1998, Louis and Heslop 2009). Approximately 50% of the population in the UK has antibodies to CMV. Therefore it is recognized that the virus may be transmitted by transfusion. Although it poses little threat to immunologically competent recipients, CMV infection in vulnerable patient groups can cause significant morbidity

and mortality. For example, CMV pneumonitis carries an 85% mortality rate in blood and bone marrow transplant recipients (Mollison et al. 1997). Screening of donors and the use of CMV-seronegative or leucocyte-depleted blood and blood products are seen as essential for neonates and immunocompromised recipients who have tested negative to CMV (Louis and Heslop 2009).

Hepatitis B virus (HBV)

Screening for hepatitis B surface antigen (HBsAg) in donor blood is mandatory as it is estimated that there are now more than 325,000 people in the UK with chronic hepatitis B and, allowing for factors such as under-reporting, the figure may be even higher (Hepatitis B Foundation UK 2007).

Hepatitis C virus (HCV)

Screening for hepatitis C using the ELISA is mandatory in the UK. Hepatitis C is transmitted primarily via contact with blood or blood products (Friedman 2001).

Human immunodeficiency virus (HIV-1 and HIV-2)

The human immunodeficiency virus is a retrovirus that infects and kills helper T cells, also known as CD4-positive lymphocytes. Transmission of the virus can be via most blood products including red cells, platelets, FFP, and factor VIII and IX concentrates. These viruses are not known to be transmitted in albumin, immunoglobulins or antithrombin III products (Barbara and Contreras 2009). The retrovirus invades cells and slowly destroys the immune system, rendering the individual susceptible to opportunistic infections. Since 1983, when it was recognized that the virus could be transmitted via transfusion, actions have been developed to safeguard blood supplies from transmitting the virus that caused acquired immune deficiency syndrome (AIDS). These include the careful screening of donors and the testing of donated blood.

Other infective agents

Parasites

Plasmodium falciparum is the most dangerous of the human malarial parasites (Barbara and Contreras 2009). Prevention is maintained by questioning donors about foreign travel, in particular those who have visited areas where the disease is prevalent (Bishop 2008).

Prion diseases

Known as transmissible spongiform encephalopathies (TSEs), these are a rare group of conditions which cause progressive neurodegeneration in humans and some animal species (Box 8.5). Prion diseases are believed to be caused by the presence of an abnormal form of a cellular protein

Prion diseases in animal species
- Scrapie, a disease of sheep.
- Bovine spongiform encephalopathy (BSE).
- Feline spongiform encephalopathy (FSE).
- Chronic wasting disease of deer, mule and elk.

Prion diseases in humans
- Sporadic: classic Creutzfeldt–Jakob disease (CJD).
- Inherited: CJD, Gerstmann–Sträussler–Scheinker disease, fatal familial insomnia (FFI).
- Acquired: kuru, vCJD.

(Aguzzi and Collinge 1997, Barbara and Contreras 2009, Vamvakas 1999). These abnormal proteins have an altered cellular shape, and become infectious and multiply by converting normal cellular protein to the irregular form. This irregular form is resistant to digestion and breakdown and, once accumulation occurs, can result in the formation of plaque in brain tissue. Transmission is thought to be by direct contact with infected brain or lymphoreticular tissue (Aguzzi and Collinge 1997, Barbara and Contreras 2009, Vamvakas 1999).

There is evidence to suggest that in TSEs, of which vCJD is one, leucocytes, particularly lymphocytes, are the key cells in the transportation of the putative infectious agent to the brain (Aguzzi and Collinge 1997, Bradley 1999). There were a total of 163 deaths in cases of definite or probable vCJD in the UK up to 31 December 2007. A further three probable cases were alive on 31 December 2007. Analysis of the incidence of vCJD onsets and deaths from January 1994 to December 2007 indicates that a peak has passed. While this is an encouraging finding, the incidence of vCJD may increase again, particularly if different genetic subgroups with longer incubation periods exist (National CJD Surveillance Unit 2008).

In many developed countries, blood undergoes universal leucodepletion for a number of reasons: to reduce the risk of transmission of vCJD, to remove leucocyte-associated viruses such as CMV and to reduce other complications of transfusions related to white cell content (Contreras and Navarrete 2009).

Sepsis

Sepsis occurs when bacteria enter the blood or blood product that is to be infused. Bacteria can enter at any point from the time of collection, during storage through to administration to the patient. Organisms implicated in transfusion-related sepsis include Gram-negative *Pseudomonas*, *Yersinia* and *Flavobacterium* (Provan *et al.* 2009). Septic reactions usually present with a fever, tachycardia and/or hypotension, and can lead rapidly to systemic inflammatory response syndrome (SIRS) (Porth 2005). This is a serious life-threatening condition, sometimes referred to as septic shock, and requires urgent medical attention.

Transfusion-related acute lung injury (TRALI)

Transfusion-related acute lung injury is most frequently associated with plasma-rich products such as whole blood, platelets and FFP (Federico 2009). TRALI is usually caused by anti-leucocyte antibodies reacting against donor leucocytes. This reaction can result in 'leucoagglutination'. Leucoagglutinins can in turn become trapped in the pulmonary microvasculature, causing severe respiratory distress without evidence of circulatory overload or cardiac failure (Contreras and Navarrete 2009). TRALI presents with a rapid onset of breathlessness, a non-productive cough, distress, chills or fever, cyanosis, hypotension and coma. A chest X-ray will show bilateral nodular infiltrates in a characteristic 'bat wing' presentation (McClelland 2007).

Transfusion-related acute lung injury is usually treated as any adult respiratory distress syndrome (ARDS) and therefore patients who develop TRALI may require ventilatory support (SNBTS 2004) and should be treated as an emergency. Diuretics should not be administered as patients are generally hypotensive and hypovolaemic. Although the symptoms resemble ARDS, TRALI is self-limiting and with most patients improving over a 4-day period, without long-term consequences (Federico 2009). As TRALI is donor related, it is essential that cases are reported to the blood transfusion services so that donors can be contacted and removed from the donor panel (McClelland 2007).

Transfusion-related immune modulation

The infusion of foreign antigen during a packed red blood cell (PRBC) transfusion induces a non-specific immunosuppression, which is known as transfusion-associated immunomodulation. Allogeneic plasma components, white blood cells, fibrin and accumulants from the storage process have all been implicated (Englesbe *et al.* 2005).

Urticaria

This uncommon reaction is caused by the recipient reacting to protein in the donor plasma (Davies and Williamson 1998). Urticaria is characterized by localized oedematous plaques, hives and itching and is usually mediated by histamines (Porth 2005). Therefore urticarial reactions usually respond well to antihistamines and they should be administered once the patient has been assessed and antihistamine therapy has been prescribed (SNBTS 2004). The infusion can then be recommenced; however, if symptoms return, the infusion should be discontinued.

Transfusion reactions

In November 1996 the SHOT scheme was launched. This voluntary and anonymized reporting scheme collects data from participating hospitals across the UK and Ireland. The purpose of SHOT is to collect data on the serious morbidity related to the transfusion of blood and blood products.

These data have since been utilized to inform education programmes, policy development and guideline development, ultimately improving hospital transfusion practice (SNBTS 2004).

Although the Blood Safety and Quality Regulations 2005 have now made the reporting of such events via SABRE mandatory, the SHOT scheme remains active and important and has presented yearly retrospective reports of data collected since its inception. These data demonstrate improved performance in recognizing reporting of transfusion-related incidents and continue to generate key recommendations to improve all transfusion practice (SNBTS 2004). Despite significant improvement in the reduction of risk from transfusion-transmitted infection, human error which results in an IBCT – the transfusion of a blood product that is not suitable for or not intended for the recipient – remains the greatest risk to patients (SNBTS 2004). Figures from the 2008 SHOT report confirm 262 cases in this category.

The prompt management of any adverse transfusion reaction can reduce associated morbidity and can be life saving. Therefore staff caring for patients receiving transfused products must be fully familiar with the immediate management of any suspected reaction. However, specialist advice should always be sought for the diagnosis and ongoing management of transfusion reactions, such as haemolytic, anaphylactic and septic reactions (McClelland 2007, SNBTS 2004).

Minor transfusion reactions

It should always be remembered that the symptoms of a 'minor' transfusion reaction may be the prelude to a major, life-threatening reaction. It is essential that staff take any transfusion reaction seriously. Symptomatic patients should have their vital signs monitored closely and they should be clearly observable. Patients with persistent or deteriorating symptoms should always be managed as a major reaction and urgent medical and specialist support should be sought (McClelland 2007, SNBTS 2004).

Allergic and anaphylactic reactions are more common and more severe with transfusion of FFP and platelets than with red blood cells (Domen and Hoeltge 2003).

Symptoms of minor reactions include a temperature rise of up to 1.5°C, rash without systemic disturbance and moderate tachycardia without hypotension (SNBTS 2004). Such reactions may be caused by an immunological reaction to components of the blood product. Whilst it may be possible to manage such symptoms and continue with the transfusion, the following action should always be taken (Contreras and Navarrete 2009).

- Stop the transfusion and inform the responsible medical team.
- Confirm the patient's identity and re-check their details against the product compatibility label.
- Antihistamines should be considered for skin rashes or urticarial itch.
- Antipyretic agents can be considered for mild fever.

It may be possible to continue with the transfusion at a reduced rate once the patient's symptoms are controlled; however, it may be necessary to increase the frequency of observations until the transfusion is completed. Some patients who have regular transfusions may experience recurrent febrile reactions and may benefit from an antipyretic premedication. *Note*: aspirin and other non-steroidal anti-inflammatory drugs (NSAIDs) are contraindicated in patients with a thrombocytopenia or coagulopathy (BNF 2011).

Major transfusion reactions

Major transfusion reactions include anaphylaxis, haemolysis and sepsis and may present as a fever of >38.5°C, tachycardia ± hypotension. In such circumstances a severe reaction should always be considered and the transfusion should be stopped until a specialist assessment has been conducted (Box 8.6).

Care should be taken when returning the blood product to the laboratory, to ensure that the product does not leak and that no needles remain attached.

Any further products being held locally for the patient should also be returned to the hospital transfusion laboratory for assessment. The events surrounding the reaction should be clearly documented and reported in the following ways.

- Record the adverse event in the patient's clinical record.
- Complete a detailed incident form as per local policy.
- Follow local, regional and national criteria for reporting via SABRE and SHOT.

Box 8.6 Initial management of a suspected transfusion reaction

- Stop the transfusion and seek urgent medical help.
- Initiate appropriate emergency procedures, for example call resuscitation team.
- Depending on venous access, withdraw the contents of the lumen being used and disconnect the blood product.
- Keep venous access patent.
- Confirm the patient's identity and re-check their details against the product compatibility label.
- Keep the patient and relative informed of all progress and reassure as indicated.
- Initiate close and frequent observations of temperature, pulse, blood pressure, fluid balance.
- Inform the transfusion laboratory and seek the urgent advice of the haematologist for further management.
- Return the transfused product to the laboratory with new blood samples (10 mL clotted and 5 mL ethylenediamine tetra-acetic acid (EDTA)) from the patient's opposite arm (SNBTS 2004) with a completed transfusion reaction notification form (if available) or note the patient's details, the nature and timing of the reaction and details of the component transfused.

408

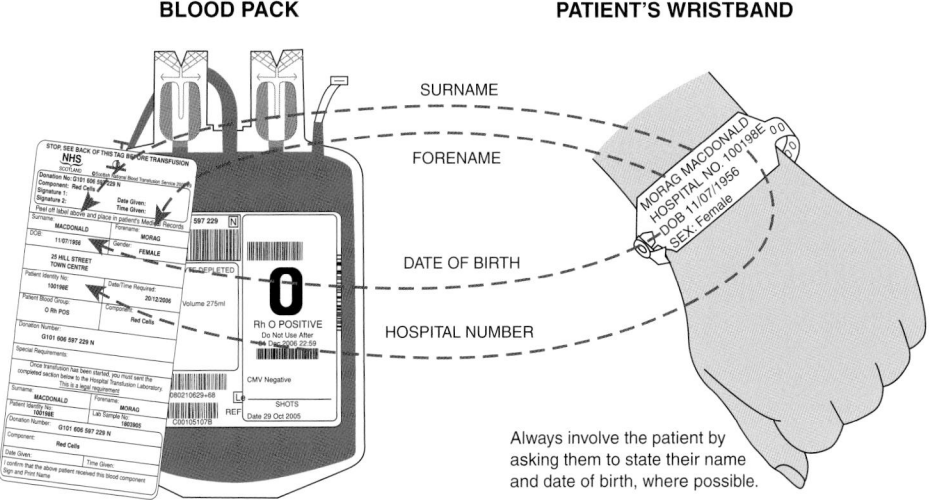

BLOOD PACK   **PATIENT'S WRISTBAND**

SURNAME

FORENAME

DATE OF BIRTH

HOSPITAL NUMBER

Always involve the patient by
asking them to state their name
and date of birth, where possible.

Figure 8.10   Check the compatability label or tie-on-tag against the patient's wristband.

Acute haemolytic reactions

These are usually directly related to ABO incompatibilities due to an IBCT where antigen/antibody reactions occur when the recipient's antibodies react with surface antigens on the donor red cells. This reaction causes a cascade of events within the recipient. Such reaction can present with chills/rigors, facial flushing, pain/oozing at cannula site, burning along the vein, chest pain, lumbar or flank pain, or shock (Gillespie and Hillyer 2001, McClelland 2007). Patients may express a feeling of anxiety or doom, which may be associated with cytokine activity. Haemolytic shock can occur after only a few millilitres of blood have been infused. Treatment is often vigorous to reverse hypotension, aid adequate renal perfusion and renal flow to reduce potential damage to renal tubules, and appropriate therapy for DIC reactions (Provan *et al.* 2009). It is important to remember that most acute haemolytic reactions are preventable as they are usually caused by clerical or checking errors at the bedside, and as this is the final check before administration, it presents the last opportunity to identify and avert an error, thus emphasizing the importance of the final check before transfusion (McClelland 2007) (Figure 8.10).

Acute anaphylactic reactions

These are rare and usually occur after only a few millilitres of blood or plasma have been infused (Weinstein and Plumer 2007) and present with bronchial spasm, respiratory distress, abdominal cramps, shock and potential loss of consciousness.

Circulatory overload (transfusion-associated circulatory overload [TACO])

Circulatory overload can occur when blood or any of its components are infused rapidly or administered to a patient with an increased plasma volume, causing hypervolaemia.

Patients at risk are those with renal or cardiac deficiencies, the young and elderly (Weinstein and Plumer 2007). Patients with signs of cardiac failure should receive their transfusion slowly with diuretic support (McClelland 2007). The need for concomitant drugs such as diuretics should always be assessed before commencing treatment (SNBTS 2004).

Febrile non-haemolytic reactions

These reactions are due to an immunological response to the transfusion of cellular components such as donor leucocytes. Specific patient groups are at risk of greater sensitization to leucocytes, for example, critically ill patients, those receiving anticancer therapies or patients requiring multiple transfusion therapy (Williamson *et al.* 1999). Such reactions present with a mild fever (up to 1.5°C), rash without systemic disturbance and moderate tachycardia without hypotension (SNBTS 2004).

Hypothermia

Infusing large quantities of cold blood rapidly can cause hypothermia. Patients likely to suffer from this reaction are those who have suffered massive blood loss due to trauma, haemorrhage, clotting disorders or thrombocytopenia (McClelland 2007). Such reactions present with alteration in vital signs, and development of pallor and chills.

Delayed effects

These reactions may occur days, months or even years after transfusion.

Delayed haemolytic reactions

These reactions are caused when immune antibodies react to a foreign antigen. Reactions are classified as primary or secondary. A *primary* reaction is often mild, occurring days or weeks after initial transfusion, and may be indicated by no clinical alteration in haemoglobin following transfusion therapy (Cook 1997a). *Secondary* reactions occur with re-exposure to the same antigen, and on rare occasions may be associated with ABO incompatibilities (Cook 1997a). The patient may present with a fever, mild jaundice and unexplained decrease in haemoglobin value and may require antiglobulin testing (McClelland 2007).

Hyperkalaemia

Hyperkalaemia is a rare complication associated with trauma and the subsequent infusion of large quantities of blood. Potassium is known to leak out of red cells during storage, thereby increasing circulatory levels in recipients receiving blood products (Cook 1997b). The process is exacerbated if products are kept too long at room temperature or gamma irradiated (Davies and Williamson 1998). From starting the infusion to completion, the infusion should take

a maximum of 4 hours (McClelland 2007). The patient may present with irritability, anxiety, abdominal cramps, diarrhoea and weakness in the extremities (Cook 1997b). The patient's medical team should be contacted to assess the patient.

Iron overload

Patients who are dependent on frequent transfusion, such as those with thalassaemic, sickle cell and other transfusion-dependent disorders, can become overloaded with iron (McClelland 2007). A unit of red blood cells contains 250 mg iron, which the body is unable to excrete, and as a result patients receiving large volumes of blood are at risk of iron overload (Davies and Williamson 1998). This can result in poor growth, pigment changes, hepatic cirrhosis, hypoparathyroidism, diabetes, arrhythmia, cardiac failure and death. Chelation therapy through the use of desferrioxamine, which induces iron excretion, is used to minimize the accumulation of iron (BNF 2011).

Websites and useful addresses

www.bda.uk.com/resources/Delivering_Nutritional_Care_through_Food_Beverage_Services.pdf

www.bapen.org.uk/ofnsh/OrganizationOfNutritionalSupportWithinHospitals.pdf

www.npsa.nhs.uk/nrls/improvingpatientsafety/cleaning-and-nutrition/nutrition/good-nutritional-care-in-hospitals/nutrition-fact-sheets

www.npsa.nhs.uk/nrls/improvingpatientsafety/cleaning-and-nutrition/nutrition/good-nutritional-care-in-hospitals/nutrition-fact-sheets

www.dh.gov.uk/en/Publicationsandstatistics/Publications/PublicationsPolicyAndGuidance/DH_079931

www.scie.org.uk/publications/guides/guide15/mealtimes

www.bapen.org.uk/pdfs/nsw/nsw07_report.pdf

www.bapen.org.uk/pdfs/nsw/nsw07_report.pdf

www.ageconcern.org.uk/AgeConcern/Hungry_to_be_Heard_August_2006.pdf

ww.dh.gov.uk/en/Publicationsandstatistics/Publications/PublicationsPolicyAndGuidance/DH_079931

www.dh.gov.uk/en/SocialCare/Socialcarereform/Dignityincare/

www.dh.gov.uk/PolicyandGuidance/HealthandSocialCareTopics/SpecialisedServices

www.espen.org/espenguidelines.html

www.nice.org.uk/nicemedia/pdf/cg032fullguideline.pdf

www.bcshguidelines.com

www.hospital.blood.co.uk

www.mhra.gov.uk

www.shotuk.org

www.transfusionguidelines.org.uk

Age Concern
Telephone: 0800 00 99 66
Website: www.ageuk.org.uk

Patients on Intravenous and Nasogastric Nutrition Therapy (PINNT)
Telephone: 01202 481 625
Website: www.pinnt.com

PINNT is a support group for patients receiving parenteral or enteral nutrition therapy.

References

Adam, S.K. and Osborne, S. (2005) *Critical Care Nursing: Science and Practice*, 2nd edn. Oxford University Press, Oxford.

Age Concern (2006) *Hungry to be Heard*. Age Concern, London. www.ageconcern.org.uk/AgeConcern/Documents/Hungry_to_be_Heard_August_2006.pdf.

Aguzzi, A. and Collinge, J. (1997) Post-exposure prophylaxis after accidental prion inoculation. *Lancet*, **350** (9090), 1519–1520.

Ainslie, P.N., Campbell, I.T., Frayn, K.N. *et al.* (2002) Energy balance, metabolism, hydration, and performance during strenuous hill walking: the effect of age. *Journal of Applied Physiology*, **93** (2), 714–723.

Alexander, M.F., Fawcett, J.N. and Runciman, P.J. (2000) *Nursing Practice: Hospital and Home: the Adult*, 2nd edn. Churchill Livingstone, Edinburgh.

BAPEN (1999) *Current Perspectives on Enteral Nutrition in Adults*. British Association for Parenteral and Enteral Nutrition, Maidenhead.

BAPEN (2003a) *Malnutrition Universal Screeening Tool 'Must' Report*. British Association for Parenteral and Enteral Nutrition, Maidenhead.

BAPEN (2003b) *Tube Feeding and Your Medicines: A Guide for Patients and Carers*. British Association for Parenteral and Enteral Nutrition, Maidenhead.

BAPEN (2009) *Nutrition Screening Survey in the UK in 2008. Hospitals, Care Homes and Mental Health Units. A Report by the BAPEN*. British Association for Parenteral and Enteral Nutrition, Maidenhead. www.bapen.org.uk/pdfs/nsw/nsw_report2008-09.pdf.

Baraz, S., Parvardeh, S., Mohammadi, E. and Broumand, B. (2009) Dietary and fluid compliance: an educational intervention for patients having haemodialysis. *Journal of Advanced Nursing*, **66** (1), 60–68.

Barbara, J.A.J. and Contreras, M. (2009) Infectious complications of blood transfusion: bacteria and parasites. In: Contreras, M. (ed) *ABC of Transfusion*, 4th edn. Blackwell Publishing, Oxford. pp. 69–73.

Battezzati, A., Bertoli, S., Testolin, C. and Testolin, G. (2003) Body composition assessment: an indispensable tool for disease management. *Acta Diabetologica*, **40** (Suppl 1), S151–S153.

Bauer, J., Capra, S. and Ferguson, M. (2002) Use of scored patient-generated subjective global assessment (PG-SGA) as a nutritional assessment tool in patients with cancer. *European Journal of Clinical Nutrition*, **56** (8), 779–785.

Baumberger-Henry, M. (2008) *Quick Look Nursing: Fluids and Electrolytes*, 2nd edn Jones and Barlett, Sudbury, MA.

BCSH (2009) *Guideline on the Administration of Blood Components*. British Society of Haematology, London. www.bcshguidelines.com/pdf/Admin_blood_components050110.pdf.

BCSH, RCN, RCS (1999) The administration of blood components and the management of transfused patients. *Transfusion Medicine*, **9**, 227–238.

Bedogni, G., Borghi, A. and Battistini, N. (2003) Body water distribution and disease. *Acta Diabetologica*, **40** (Suppl 1), S200–S202.

Bedogni, G., Brambilla, A., Bellentani, S. and Tiribelli, C. (2006) The assessment of body composition in health and disease. *Human Ecology*, **14**, 21–25.

Bingham, S.A. (1987) The dietary assessment of individuals: methods, accuracy, new techniques and recommendations. *Nutrition Abstracts and Reviews*, **57**, 705–742.

Bishop, E. (2008) Blood transfusion therapy. In: Dougherty L. and Lamb J. (eds) *Intravenous Therapy in Nursing Practice*, 2nd edn. Blackwell Publishing, Oxford. pp. 377–394.

Blood Safety and Quality Regulations (2005) *SI 2005/50*. Stationery Office, London. www.opsi.gov.uk/si/si2005/20050050.htm.

BNF (2011) *British National Formulary*. BMJ Group and RPS Publishing, London.

Bodger, K. and Heatley, R.V. (2001) The immune system and nutrition support. In: Payne-James, J., Grimble, G. and D.B.A., Silk (eds) *Artificial Nutrition Support in Clinical Practice*. Greenwich Medical Media, London, pp. 137–148.

Bozzetti, F. (2001) Nutrition support in patients with cancer. In: Payne-James, J., Grimble, G. and D.B.A., Silk (eds) *Artificial Nutrition Support in Clinical Practice*. Greenwich Medical Media, London, pp. 639–680.

Bozzetti, F., Arends, J., Lundholm, K. *et al.* (2009) ESPEN guidelines on parenteral nutrition: non-surgical oncology. *Clinical Nutrition*, **28** (4), 445–454.

Bradley, L. and Rees, C. (2003) Reducing nutritional risk in hospital: the red tray. *Nursing Standard*, **17** (26), 33–37.

Bradley, R. (1999) BSE transmission studies with particular reference to blood. *Developments in Biological Standardization*, **99**, 35–40.

Braga, M., Gianotti, L., Vignali, A. and Carlo, V.D. (2002) Preoperative oral arginine and n-3 fatty acid supplementation improves the immunometabolic host response and outcome after colorectal resection for cancer. *Surgery*, **132** (5), 805–814.

Braga, M., Ljungqvist, O., Soeters, P. *et al.* (2009) ESPEN guidelines on parenteral nutrition: surgery. *Clinical Nutrition*, **28** (4), 378–386.

Brown, P. (2005) Blood infectivity, processing and screening tests in transmissible spongiform encephalopathy. *Vox sanguinis*, **89** (2), 63–70.

Bryant, H. (2007) Dehydration in older people: assessment and management. *Emergency Nurse*, **15** (4), 22–26.

Bumpers, H.L., Collure, D.W., Best, I.M. *et al.* (2003) Unusual complications of long–term percutaneous gastrostomy tubes. *Journal of Gastrointestinal Surgery*, **7** (7), 917–920.

Burnham, R. and Barton, S. (2001) The role of the nutrition support team. In: Payne-James, J., Grimble, G. and D.B.A., Silk (eds) *Artificial Nutrition Support in Clinical Practice*. Greenwich Medical Media, London, pp. 241–253.

Callum, K.G., Gray, A.J.G., Hoile, R.W. *et al.* (1999) *Extremes of Age: The 1999 Report of the National Confidential Enquiry in Perioperative Deaths*. National Confidential Enquiry into Perioperative Deaths, London. www.ncepod.org.uk/pdf/1999/99full.pdf.

Carless, P., Moxey, A., O'Connell, D. and Henry, D. (2004) Autologous transfusion techniques: a systematic review of their efficacy. *Tranfusion Medicine*, **14** (2), 123–144.

Casey, G. (2004) Oedema: causes, physiology and nursing management. *Nursing Standard*, **18** (51), 45–51.

Cervenakova, L. and Brown, P. (2004) Advances in screening test development for transmissible spongiform encephalopathies. *Expert Review of Anti-Infective Therapy*, **2** (6), 873–880.

Chung, L.H., Chong, S. and French, P. (2002) The efficiency of fluid balance charting: an evidence-based management project. *Journal of Nursing Management*, **10** (2), 103–113.

Committee on Medical Aspects of Food Policy (COMA) and DH (1991) *Dietary Reference Values for Food Energy and Nutrients for the United Kingdom: Report of the Panel on Dietary Reference Values of the Committee on Medical Aspects of Food Policy*. HMSO, London.

Contreras, M. and Navarrete, C. (2009) Immunological complications of blood transfusion. In: Contreras, M. (ed) *ABC of Transfusion*, 4th edn. Blackwell Publishing, Oxford. pp. 61–68.

Council of Europe (2003) *Food and Nutritional Care in Hospitals: How to Prevent Undernutrition*. Council of Europe, Paris.

Cook, L.S. (1997a) Blood transfusion reactions involving an immune response. *Journal of Intravenous Nursing*, **20** (1), 5–14.

Cook, L.S. (1997b) Nonimmune transfusion reactions: when type-and-cross match aren't enough. *Journal of Intravenous Nursing*, **20** (1), 15–22.

Cook, N.F., Deeny, P. and Thompson, K. (2004) Management of fluid and hydration in patients with acute subarachnoid haemorrhage – an action research project. *Journal of Clinical Nursing*, **13** (7), 835–849.

Cook (UK) Limited (2007) *Radiologically inserted gastrostomy and gastrojejunostomy*. Monroe House, Letchworth, Herts.

Cummings, J.H. (2000) Nutritional management of diseases of the gut. In: Garrow, J.S., James W.P.T. and Ralph A. (eds) *Human Nutrition and Dietetics*, 10th edn. Churchill Livingstone, Edinburgh. pp. 547–573.

411

Davidson, A. (2005) Management and effects of parenteral nutrition. *Nursing Times*, **101** (42), 28–31.

Davies, S.C. and Williamson, L.M. (1998) Transfusion of red cells. In: Contreras, M. (ed) *ABC of Transfusion*, 4th edn. Blackwell Publishing, Oxford. pp. 10–17.

DH (2001a) *National Service Framework for Older People*. Department of Health, London.

DH (2001b) *The Essence of Care: Patient-Focused Benchmarking for Health Care Practitioners*. Department of Health, London.

DH (2007) *Better Blood Tranfusion: Safe and Appropriate Use of Blood: HSC 2007/001*. Department of Health, London. www.dh.gov.uk/prod_consum_dh/groups/dh_digitalassets/documents/digitalasset/dh_080803.pdf.

Domen, R.E. and Hoeltge, G.A. (2003) Allergic transfusion reactions: an evaluation of 273 consecutive reactions. *Archives of Pathology and Laboratory Medicine*, **127** (3), 316–320.

Donzelli, J., Brady, S., Wesling, M. and Theisen, M. (2005) Effects of the removal of the tracheotomy tube on swallowing during the fiberoptic endoscopic exam of the swallow (FEES). *Dysphagia*, **20** (4), 283–289.

Durnin, J.V. and Womersley, J. (1974) Body fat assessed from total body density and its estimation from skinfold thickness: measurements on 481 men and women aged from 16 to 72 years. *British Journal of Nutrition*, **32** (1), 77–97.

Edwards, S.L. (2000) Fluid overload and monitoring indices. *Professional Nurse*, **15** (9), 568–572.

Ekberg, O., Hamdy, S., Woisard, V. *et al.* (2002) Social and psychological burden of dysphagia: its impact on diagnosis and treatment. *Dysphagia*, **17** (2), 139–146.

Elebute, M., Stanworth, S. and Navarrete, C. (2009) Platelet and granulocyte transfusions. In: Contreras, M. (ed) *ABC of Transfusion*, 4th edn. Blackwell Publishing, Oxford, pp. 22–26.

Elia, M. (2001) Metabolic response to starvation, injury and sepsis. In: Payne-James, J., Grimble, G. and D.B.A., Silk (eds) *Artificial Nutrition Support in Clinical Practice*. Greenwich Medical Media, London, pp. 1–24.

Englesbe, M.J., Pelletier, S.J., Diehl, K.M. *et al.* (2005) Transfusions in surgical patients. *Journal of the American College of Surgeons*, **200** (2), 249–254.

Epstein, O., Solomons, N.B. and Robins, A. (2003) *Clinical Examination*, 3rd edn. Mosby, Edinburgh.

Federico, A. (2009) Transfusion-related acute lung injury. *Journal of Perianesthesia Nursing*, **24** (1), 35–37.

Fields, R.C. and Meyers, B.F. (2006) The effects of perioperative blood transfusion on morbidity and mortality after esophagectomy. *Thoracic Surgery Clinics*, **16** (1), 75–86.

Flanagan, J., Melillo, K.D., Abdallah, L. and Remington, R. (2007) Interpreting laboratory values in the rehabilitation setting. *Rehabilitation Nursing*, **32** (2), 77–84.

Fraise, A.P. and Bradley, T. (eds) (2009) *Ayliffe's Control of Healthcare-associated Infection: A Practical Handbook*, 5th edn. Hodder Arnold, London.

Freeman, L. (2002) Food record charts. *Nursing Times*, **98** (34), 53–54.

Friedman, D. (2001) Hepatitis. In: Hillyer, C.D. (ed) *Handbook of Transfusion Medicine*. Academic, San Diego, pp. 275–284.

FSA and Expert Group on Vitamins and Minerals (2003) *Safe Upper Levels for Vitamins and Minerals*. Food Standards Agency, London. www.food.gov.uk/multimedia/pdfs/vitmin2003.pdf.

Furst, P., Kuhn, K.S. and Stehle, P. (2001) Parenteral nutrition substrates. In: Payne-James, J., Grimble, G. and Silk, D. (eds) *Artificial Nutrition Support in Clinical Practice*, 2nd edn. Greenwich Medical Media, London, pp. 401–434.

Gaziano, J.E. (2002) Evaluation and management of oropharyngeal dysphagia in head and neck cancer. *Cancer Control*, **9** (5), 400–409.

Geissler, C. and Powers, H. (2005) *Human Nutrition*, 11th edn. Elsevier Churchill Livingstone, Edinburgh.

Gidden, F. and Shenkin, A. (2000) Laboratory support of the clinical nutrition service. *Clinical Chemistry and Laboratory Medicine*, **38** (8), 693–714.

Gillespie, T.W. and Hillyer, D. (2001) Granulocytes. In: Hillyer, C.D. (ed) *Handbook of Transfusion Medicine*. Academic, San Diego, pp. 63–68.

Goertz, S. (2006) Gauging fluid balance with osmolality. *Nursing*, **36** (10), 70–71.

Goeters, C., Wenn, A., Mertes, N. *et al.* (2002) Parenteral L-alanyl-L-glutamine improves 6-month outcome in critically ill patients. *Critical Care Medicine*, **30** (9), 2032–2037.

Gray, A. and Illingworth, J. (2005) *Right Blood, Right Patient, Right Time: RCN Guidance for Improving Transfusion Practice*. Royal College of Nursing, London. www.rcn.org.uk/__data/assets/pdf_file/0009/78615/002306.pdf.

Gray, A., Hearnshaw, K., Izatt, C. *et al.* (2007) Safe transfusion of blood and blood components. *Nursing Standard*, **21** (51), 40–47.

Green, J. and Pirie, L. (2009) *A Framework to Support Nurses and Midwives Making the Clinical Decision and Providing the Written Instruction for Blood Component Transfusion*. UK Blood Transfusion Services, London. www.transfusionguidelines.org.uk/docs/pdfs/BTFramework-final010909.pdf.

Griffiths, M. (1996) Single-stage percutaneous gastrostomy button insertion: a leap forward. *Journal of Parenteral and Enteral Nutrition*, **20** (3), 237–239.

Groher, M.E. (1997) *Dysphagia: Diagnosis and Management*, 3rd edn. Butterworth-Heinemann, Boston.

Harrison, J. (2004) Getting your own back – an update on autologous transfusion. *Blood Matters*, **16**, 7–9. www.blood.co.uk/pdf/publications/blood_matters_16.pdf.

Haskal, R. (2007) Current issues for nurse practitioners: hyponatremia. *Journal of the American Academy of Nurse Practitioners*, **19** (11), 563–579.

Healthcare Commission (2007) *Patient Survey Report 2007*. Healthcare Commission, London. www.nnuh.nhs.uk/viewdoc.asp?ID=329&t=TrustDoc.

Henry, D.A., Carless, P.A., Moxey, A.J. *et al.* (2002) Pre-operative autologous donation for minimising perioperative allogeneic blood transfusion. *Cochrane Database Syst Rev*, (2), CD003602.

Hepatitis B Foundation UK (2007) *Rising Curve: Chronic Hepatitis B Infection in the UK*. www.hepb.org.uk/information/resrources/rising-curve-chronic-hepatitis-b-infection-in-the-uk/.

Hoffbrand, A.V., Moss, P.A.H. and Pettit, J.E. (2006) *Essential Haematology*, 5th edn. Blackwell Publishing, Oxford.

Horgan, G.W. and Stubbs, J. (2003) Predicting basal metabolic rate in the obese is difficult. *European Journal of Clinical Nutrition*, **57** (2), 335–340.

James, V. (2004) *A National Blood Conservation Strategy for NBTC and NBS: Report from the Working Party Autologous Transfusion and the Working Party on Alternatives to Transfusion of the NBS Sub-group on Appropriate use of Blood*. National Blood Service, London. www.dh.gov.uk/prod_consum_dh/groups/dh_digitalassets/@dh/@en/documents/digitalasset/dh_4089513.pdf.

James, V. (2005) *Guidelines for the Blood Transfusion Services in the United Kingdom*, 7th edn. Stationery Office, London.

James, V. and Harrison, J. (2002) The pros and cons of predeposit autologous donation and transfusion. *Blood Matters*, (11), 4–5. www.blood.co.uk/pdf/publications/blood_matters_11.pdf.

412

Janssen, I., Heymsfield, S.B., Baumgartner, R.N. and Ross, R. (2000) Estimation of skeletal muscle mass by bioelectrical impedance analysis. *Journal of Applied Physiology*, **89** (2), 465–471.

Jevon, P. (2010) How to ensure patient observations lead to effective management of oliguria. *Nursing Times*, **106** (7), 18–19.

Jevon, P. and Ewens, B. (2007) *Monitoring the Critically Ill Patient*, 2nd edn. Blackwell, Oxford.

Jian, Z.M., Cao, J.D., Zhu, X.G. *et al.* (1999) The impact of alanyl-glutamine on clinical safety, nitrogen balance, intestinal permeability, and clinical outcome in postoperative patients: a randomized, double-blind, controlled study of 120 patients. *Journal of Parenteral and Enteral Nutrition*, **23** (5 Suppl), S62–S66.

John, T., Rodeman, R. and Colvin, R. (2008) Blood conservation in a congenital cardiac surgery program. *AORN Journal*, **87** (6), 1180–1186.

JPAC (Joint UKBTS/NIBSC Professional Advisory Committee) (2007) *JPAC Donor Selection Guidelines*. www.transfusion-guidelines.org.uk.

King's Fund Research Summary (2005) *Sustainable Food and The NHS*. www.kingsfund.org.uk/publications/kings_fund_publications/sustainable_food.html.

Kondrup, J., Allison, S.P., Elia, M. *et al.* (2003) ESPEN guidelines for nutrition screening 2002. *Clinical Nutrition*, **22** (4), 415–421.

Kroke, A., Klipstein-Grobusch, K., Voss, S. *et al.* (1999) Validation of a self-administered food-frequency questionnaire administered in the European Prospective Investigation into Cancer and Nutrition (EPIC) Study: comparison of energy, protein, and macronutrient intakes estimated with the doubly labeled water, urinary nitrogen, and repeated 24-h dietary recall methods. *American Journal of Clinical Nutrition*, **70** (4), 439–447.

Kyle, U.G., Bosaeus, I., de Lorenzo, A.D. *et al.* (2004) Bioelectrical impedance analysis – part II: utilization in clinical practice. *Clinical Nutrition*, **23** (6), 1430–1453.

Langmore, S.E. (2001) *Endoscopic Evaluation and Treatment of Swallowing Disorders*. Thieme, New York.

Langmore, S.E., Terpenning, M.S., Schork, A. *et al.* (1998) Predictors of aspiration pneumonia: how important is dysphagia? *Dysphagia*, **13** (2), 69–81.

Lazarus, C., Logemann, J.A., Song, C.W. *et al.* (2002) Effects of voluntary maneuvers on tongue base function for swallowing. *Folia Phoniatrica et Logopaedica*, **54** (4), 171–176.

Leder, S.B. and Ross, D.A. (2000) Investigation of the causal relationship between tracheotomy and aspiration in the acute care setting. *The Laryngoscope*, **110** (4), 641–644.

Leslie, P., Carding, P.N. and Wilson, J.A. (2003) Investigation and management of chronic dysphagia. *British Medical Journal (Clinical Research)*, **326** (7386), 433–436.

Levi, R. (2005) Nursing care to prevent dehydration in older adults. *Australian Nursing Journal*, **13** (3), 21–23.

Lewin, J.S., Hebert, T.M., Putnam, J.B. Jr. and DuBrow, R.A. (2001) Experience with the chin tuck maneuver in postesophagectomy aspirators. *Dysphagia*, **16** (3), 216–219.

Logemann, J.A. (1998) *Evaluation and Treatment of Swallowing Disorders*, 2nd edn. Pro-Ed, Austin, TX.

Logemann, J.A., Pauloski, B.R., Rademaker, A.W. and Colangelo, L.A. (1997) Super-supraglottic swallow in irradiated head and neck cancer patients. *Head Neck*, **19** (6), 535–540.

Logemann, J.A., Pauloski, B.R., Rademaker, A.W. *et al.* (2008) Swallowing disorders in the first year after radiation and chemoradiation. *Head Neck*, **30** (2), 148–158.

Loser, C., Aschl, G., Hebuterne, X. *et al.* (2005) ESPEN guidelines on artificial enteral nutrition – percutaneous endoscopic gastrostomy (PEG). *Clinical Nutrition*, **24** (5), 848–861.

Louis, C.U. and Heslop, H.E. (2009) Viral infections. In: Treleaven, J. and Barrett, A.J. (eds) *Hematopoietic Stem Cell Transplanta-tion in Clinical Practice*. Churchill Livingstone, Edinburgh, pp. 423–426.

Low, J., Wyles, C., Wilkinson, T. and Sainsbury, R. (2001) The effect of compliance on clinical outcomes for patients with dysphagia on videofluoroscopy. *Dysphagia*, **16** (2), 123–127.

Ludlam, C.A. and Turner, M.L. (2006) Managing the risk of transmission of variant Creutzfeldt Jakob disease by blood products. *British Journal of Haematology*, **132** (1), 13–24.

Lynch, C.R. and Fang, J.C. (2004) Prevention and management of complications of percutaneous endoscopic gastrostomy (PEG) tubes. *Practical Gastroenterology*, **28** (11), 66–76.

Marieb, E.N. and Hoehn, K. (2010) *Human Anatomy and Physiology*, 8th edn. Benjamin Cummings, San Francisco.

Matlow, A., Jacobson, M., Wray, R. *et al.* (2006) Enteral tube hub as a reservoir for transmissible enteric bacteria. *American Journal of Infection Control*, **34** (3), 131–133.

McCabe, D., Ashford, J., Wheeler-Hegland, K. *et al.* (2009) Evidence-based systematic review: oropharyngeal dysphagia behavioral treatments. Part IV – impact of dysphagia treatment on individuals' postcancer treatments. *Journal of Rehabilitation Research and Development*, **46** (2), 205–214.

McClelland, D.B.L. (2007) *Handbook of Transfusion Medicine*. Stationery Office, London.

MCS (2009) *Diet and Cancer: A Practical Guide to Living with and After Cancer*, 11th edn. Macmillan Cancer Support, London.

Mentes, J. (2006) Oral hydration in older adults: greater awareness is needed in preventing, recognizing, and treating dehydration. *American Journal of Nursing*, **106** (6), 40–49.

Mertes, N., Schulzki, C., Goeters, C. *et al.* (2000) Cost containment through L-alanyl-L-glutamine supplemented total parenteral nutrition after major abdominal surgery: a prospective randomized double-blind controlled study. *Clinical Nutrition*, **19** (6), 395–401.

Metheny, N.A. and Meert, K.L. (2004) Monitoring feeding tube placement. *Nutrition in Clinical Practice*, **19** (5), 487–495.

Metheny, N.A. and Titler, M.G. (2001) Assessing placement of feeding tubes. *American Journal of Nursing*, **101** (5), 36–45; quiz 45–46.

Metheny, N., Reed, L., Wiersema, L. *et al.* (1993) Effectiveness of pH measurements in predicting feeding tube placement: an update. *Nursing Research*, **42** (6), 324–331.

Mirtallo, J., Canada, T., Johnson, D. *et al.* (2004) Safe practices for parenteral nutrition. *Journal of Parenteral and Enteral Nutrition*, **28** (6), S39–S70.

Moftah, F. (2005) Blood transfusion and alternatives in elderly, malignancy and chronic disease. *Hematology*, **10** (Suppl 1), 82–85.

Mollison, P.L., Engelfriet, C.P. and Contreras, M. (1997) *Blood Transfusion in Clinical Medicine*, 10th edn. Blackwell Science, Oxford.

Mooney, G.P. (2007) Fluid balance. *Nursing Times*. www.nursingtimes.net/nursing-practice-clinical-research/fluid-balance/199391.article.

Murdock, J., Watson, D., Doree, C.J. *et al.* (2009) Drugs and blood transfusions: dogma- or evidence-based practice? *Transfusion Medicine*, **19** (1), 6–15.

NAGE (n.d.) *Have You Got a Small Appetite?* Nutrition Advisory Group for Elderly People of the British Dietetic Association, Rotherham.

National CJD Surveillance Unit (2008) *16th Annual Report*. www.cjd.ed.ac.uk/.

NCCAC (2006) *Nutrition Support for Adults: Oral Nutrition, Enteral Support, Enteral Tube Feeding and Parenteral Nutrition: Methods, Evidence and Guidance*. National Collaborating

413

Centre for Acute Care, London. www.nice.org.uk/nicemedia/pdf/cg032fullguideline.pdf.

Newman, L.A., Vieira, F., Schwiezer, V. *et al.* (1998) Eating and weight changes following chemoradiation therapy for advanced head and neck cancer. *Archives of Otolaryngology, Head and Neck Surgery*, **124** (5), 589–592.

NHS (2009) *A Strategic Framework for Intestinal Failure and Home Parenteral Nutrition Services for Adults in England: Implementation Plan: version 2*. National Health Service, National Commissioning Group for Highly Specialised Services, London. www.ncg.nhs.uk/index.php/key-documents/intestinal-failure-and-home-parenteral-nutrition/.

NHS National Commissioning Group for Highly Specialised Services (2008) *A Strategic Framework for Intestinal Failure and Home Parenteral Nutrition Services for Adults in England*. www.specialisedcommissioning.nhs.uk/index.php/key-documents/intestinal-failure-and-home-parenteral-nutrition/.

NICE (2003) *Infection Control: Prevention of Healthcare-Associated Infection in Primary and Community Care: NICE Clinical Guideline 2*. National Institute for Health and Clinical Excellence, London. www.nice.org.uk/nicemedia/live/10922/29117/29117.pdf.

NICE (2007) *Acutely Ill Patients in Hospital: Recognition of and Response to Acute Illness in Adults in Hospital: NICE Clinical Guideline 50*. National Institute for Health and Clinical Excellence, London. www.nice.org.uk/nicemedia/live/10893/28816/28816.pdf.

NMC (2008a) *The Code: Standards of Conduct, Performance and Ethics for Nurses and Midwives*. Nursing and Midwifery Council, London.

NMC (2008b) *Consent*. Nursing and Midwifery Council, London www.nmc-uk.org/Nurses-and-midwives/Advice-by-topic/A/Advice/Consent.

NMC (2008c) *Standards for Medicines Management*. Nursing and Midwifery Council, London.

NMC (2009) *Record Keeping: Guidance for Nurses and Midwives*. Nursing and Midwifery Council, London.

NPSA (2005) *Reducing the Harm Caused by Misplaced Nasogastric Feeding Tubes: Patient Safety Alert 5*. National Patient Safety Agency, London. www.nrls.npsa.nhs.uk/resources/?entryid45=59794.

NPSA (2007a) *Protected Mealtimes Review: Findings and Recommendations Report*. National Patient Safety Agency, London. www.nrls.npsa.nhs.uk/resources/?entryid45=59806.

NPSA (2007b) *Promoting Safer Measurement and Administration of Oral Liquid Medicines. Patient Briefing Alert*. National Patient Safety Agency, London. www.nrls.npsa.nhs.uk/resources/?entryid45=59808.

NPSA (2009) *10 Key Charateristics of Good Nutritional Care: All Staff Volunteers have the Appropriate Skills and Competencies Needed to Ensure that the Nutritional and Fluid Needs of People Using Care Services are Met. All Staff/Volunteers Receive Regular Training on Nutritional Care and Management: Nutrition Fact Sheet 8*. National Patient Safety Agency, London. www.nrls.npsa.nhs.uk/resources/?EntryId45=59865.

NPSA (2010) *Early Detection of Complications after Gastrostomy: Rapid Response Report: NPSA/2010/RRR010*. National Patient Safety Agency, London. www.nrls.npsa.nhs.uk/resources/?EntryId45=73457.

NPSA (2011) *Reducing the Harm Caused by Misplaced Nasogastric Feeding Tubes in Adults, Children and Infants: Patient Safety Alert NPSA/2011/PSA002*. National Patient Safety Agency, London. www.nrls.npsa.nhs.uk/resources/?entryid45=129640

Nutricia Clinical Care (1996) *The Flocare Gastrostomy Range: A Guide to Professional Care*. Nutricia Clinical Care, Trowbridge.

Nutrition Summit Stakeholder Group and DH (2007) *Improving Nutritional Care: A Joint Action Plan from the Department of Health and Nutrition Summit Stakeholders*. Department of Health, London. www.dh.gov.uk/prod_consum_dh/groups/dh_digitalassets/@dh/@en/documents/digitalasset/dh_079932.pdf.

Oldham, J., Sinclair, L. and Hendry, C. (2009) Right patient, right blood, right care: safe transfusion practice. *British Journal of Nursing*, **18** (5), 312, 314, 316–320.

Pauloski, B.R., Rademaker, A.W., Logemann, J.A. *et al.* (2002) Swallow function and perception of dysphagia in patients with head and neck cancer. *Head Neck*, **24** (6), 555–565.

Payne-James, J., Grimble, G. and Silk, D. (2001) Enteral nutrition: tubes and techniques of delivery. In: Payne-James, J., Grimble, G. and D.B.A., Silk (eds) *Artificial Nutrition Support in Clinical Practice*. Greenwich Medical Media, London, pp. 281–302.

Pennington, C.R. (1997) Disease and malnutrition in British hospitals. *Proceedings of the Nutrition Society*, **56** (1B), 393–407.

Perel, P. and Roberts, I. (2007) Colloids versus crystalloids for fluid resuscitation in critically ill patients. *Cochrane Database of Systematic Reviews*, (4), CD000567.

Pickering, K. (2003) The administration of drugs via enteral feeding tubes. *Nursing Times*, **99** (46), 46–49.

Pickhardt, P.J., Rohrmann, C.A. Jr. and Cossentino, M.J. (2002) Stomal metastases complicating percutaneous endoscopic gastrostomy: CT findings and the argument for radiologic tube placement. *American Journal of Roentgenology*, **179** (3), 735–739.

Pirie, E.S. and Gray, M.A. (2007) Exploring the assessors' and nurses' experience of formal assessment of clinical competency in the administration of blood components. *Nurse Education in Practice*, **7** (4), 215–227.

Porth, C. (2005) *Pathophysiology: Concepts of Altered Health States*, 7th edn. Lippincott Williams and Wilkins, Philadelphia, PA.

Powell-Tuck, J., Gosling, P., Lobo, D.N. *et al.* (2009) *British Consensus Guidelines on Intravenous Fluid Therapy For Adult Surgical Patients*. British Association for Parenteral and Enteral Nutrition, Maidenhead.

PPSA (2006) *Confirming feeding tube placement: old habits die hard*. Pennsylvania Patient Safety Authority, USA. www.patientsafetyauthority.org/ADVISORIES/AdvisoryLibrary/2006/Dec3(4)/page23.aspx.

Pratt, R.J., Pellowe, C.M., Wilson, J.A. *et al.* (2007) Epic2: National evidence-based guidelines for preventing healthcare-associated infections in NHS hospitals in England. *Journal of Hospital Infection*, **65** (Suppl 1), S1–S64.

Provan, D., Singer, C.R.J., Baglin, T. and Dokal, I. (2009) *Oxford Handbook of Clinical Haematology*, 3rd edn. Oxford University Press, Oxford.

RCN (2006) *Right Blood, Right Patient, Right Time*. Royal College of Nursing, London.

RCN (2010) *Standards for Infusion Therapy*, 3rd edn. Royal College of Nursing, London.

Reid, J., Robb, E., Stone, D. *et al.* (2004) Improving the monitoring and assessment of fluid balance. *Nursing Times*, **100** (20), 36–39.

Reilly, H.M. (1996) Screening for nutritional risk. *Proceedings of the Nutrition Society*, **55** (3), 841–853.

Resuscitation Council (2005) *Resuscitation Guidelines 2005*. Resuscitation Council, London. www.resus.org.uk/pages/guide.htm.

Ripamonti, C. and Mercadante, S. (2004) How to use octreotide for malignant bowel obstruction. *Journal of Supportive Oncology*, **2** (4), 357–364.

Roe, J. (2005) Oropharyngeal dysphagia in advanced non-head and neck malignancy. *European Journal of Palliative Care*, **12** (6), 229–233.

414

Roe, J.W., Leslie, P. and Drinnan, M.J. (2007) Oropharyngeal dysphagia: the experience of patients with non-head and neck cancers receiving specialist palliative care. *Palliative Medicine*, **21** (7), 567–574.

Rollins, H. (1997) A nose for trouble. *Nursing Times*, **93** (49), 66–67.

Roubenoff, R. and Kehayias, J.J. (1991) The meaning and measurement of lean body mass. *Nutrition Reviews*, **49** (6), 163–175.

Royal College of Speech and Language Therapists (2006) *Communicating Quality 3*. Royal College of Speech and Language Therapists, London.

Royal Marsden NHS Trust (2002) *Eating Well When you Have Cancer – A Guide for Cancer Patients*. Royal Marsden NHS Trust, London.

Samuels, R. and Chadwick, D.D. (2006) Predictors of asphyxiation risk in adults with intellectual disabilities and dysphagia. *Journal of Intellectual Disability Research*, **50** (Pt 5), 362–370.

Scales, K. and Pilsworth, J. (2008) The importance of fluid balance in clinical practice. *Nursing Standard*, **22** (47), 50–57.

Schofield, W.N. (1985) Predicting basal metabolic rate, new standards and review of previous work. *Human Nutrition, Clinical Nutrition*, **39** (Suppl 1), 5–41.

Shaw, C. (2008) Parenteral nutrition. In: Dougherty, L. and Lamb, J. (eds) *Intravenous Therapy in Nursing Practice*, 2nd edn. Blackwell, Oxford.

Shaw, V. and Lawson, M. (2007) Nutritional assessment, dietary requirements and feed supplementation. In: Shaw, V. and Lawson, M. (eds) *Clinical Paediatric Dietetics*, 3rd edn. Blackwell, Oxford, pp. 3–20.

Shenkin, A. (2001) Adult micronutrient requirements. In: Payne-James, J., Grimble, G. and D.B.A., Silk (eds) *Artificial Nutrition Support in Clinical Practice*. Greenwich Medical Media, London, pp. 193–212.

Sheppard, M. and Wright, M.M.B.A. (2006) *Principles and Practice of High Dependency Nursing*, 2nd edn. Baillière Tindall, Edinburgh.

SHOT (2005) *Annual Report 2005*. Serious Hazards of Transfusion, London.

SHOT (2008) *Annual Report 2008*. Serious Hazards of Transfusion, London.

Smith Hammond, C. (2008) Cough and aspiration of food and liquids due to oral pharyngeal dysphagia. *Lung*, **186** (Suppl 1), S35–S40.

SNBTS (2004) *Better Blood Transfusion Level 1: Safe Transfusion Practice : Self-Directed Learning Pack*. Effective Use of Blood Group, Scottish National Blood Transfusion Service, Edinburgh. www.learnbloodtransfusion.org.uk/Level_1_SDL.pdf.

Solomon, S.M. and Kirby, D.F. (1990) The refeeding syndrome: a review. *Journal of Parenteral and Enteral Nutrition*, **14** (1), 90–97.

Sorkin, J.D., Muller, D.C. and Andres, R. (1999) Longitudinal change in height of men and women: implications for interpretation of the body mass index: the Baltimore longitudinal study of aging. *American Journal of Epidemiology*, **150** (9), 969–977.

Springhouse (2002) Parenteral nutrition. In: *I.V. Therapy Made Incredibly Easy*, 2nd edn. Lippincott Williams and Wilkins, Philadelphia, PA, pp. 269–302.

Sumnall, R. (2007) Fluid management and diuretic therapy in acute renal failure. *Nursing in Critical Care*, **12** (1), 27–33.

Thomas, B. and Bishop, J. (2007) *Manual of Dietetic Practice*, 4th edn. Blackwell, Oxford.

Thomas, M.L. (2007) Strategies for achieving transfusion independence in myelodysplastic syndromes. *European Journal of Oncology Nursing*, **11** (2), 151–158.

Todorovic, V.E. and Micklewright, A. (eds) (2004) *A Pocket Guide to Clinical Nutrition*, 3rd edn. Parenteral and Enteral Nutrition Group of the British Dietetic Association, London.

Tolich, D.J. (2008) Alternatives to blood transfusion. *Journal of Infusion Nursing*, **31** (1), 46–51.

Urden, L.D., Stacy, K.M., Lough, M.E. and Thelan, L.A.T. (eds) (2002) *Thelan's Critical Care Nursing: Diagnosis and Management*, 4th edn. Mosby, St. Louis, MO.

Vamvakas, E.C. (1999) Risk of transmission of Creutzfeldt–Jakob disease by transfusion of blood, plasma, and plasma derivatives. *Journal of Clinical Apheresis*, **14** (3), 135–143.

Van Loan, M.D. (2003) Body composition in disease: what can we measure and how can we measure it? *Acta Diabetologica*, **40** (Suppl 1), S154–S157.

Van Wissen, K. and Breton, C. (2004) Perioperative influences on fluid distribution. *Medsurg Nursing*, **13** (5), 304–311.

Weimann, A., Braga, M., Harsanyi, L. *et al.* (2006) ESPEN guidelines on enteral nutrition: surgery including organ transplantation. *Clinical Nutrition*, **25** (2), 224–244.

Weinstein, S.M. and Plumer, A.L. (eds) (2007) *Plumer's Principles and Practice of Intravenous Therapy*, 8th edn. Lippincott Williams and Wilkins, Philadelphia, PA.

WHO (2005) *The clinical use of blood*. WHO/BTS/99.2. http://whqlibdoc.who.int/hq/2001/a72894.pdf.

Wilkinson, J. and Wilkinson, C. (2001) Administration of blood transfusions to adults in general hospital settings: a review of the literature. *Journal of Clinical Nursing*, **10** (2), 161–170.

Williamson, L.M., Lowe, S., Love, E. *et al.* (1999) *Serious Hazards of Transfusion*. SHOT, Manchester. www.shotuk.org/wp-content/uploads/2010/04/SHOT-Report-1997--98.pdf.

Wilson, J.M. and Jordan, N.L. (2001) Parenteral nutrition. In: Hankins, J. (ed) *Infusion Therapy in Clinical Practice*, 2nd edn. W.B. Saunders, St. Louis, pp. 209–247.

Wright, L., Cotter, D. and Hickson, M. (2008) The effectiveness of targeted feeding assistance to improve the nutritional intake of elderly dysphagic patients in hospital. *Journal of Human Nutrition and Dietetics*, **21** (6), 555–562.

415

The Royal Marsden Hospital Manual of Clinical Nursing Procedures, Eighth Edition. Edited by Lisa Dougherty and Sara Lister.
© 2011 The Royal Marsden Hospital. Published 2011 by Blackwell Publishing Ltd.

Overview

The aim of this chapter is to present the many varied procedures that contribute towards the comfort of patients at all times. This ranges from the very specific procedures that are involved in pain management to those that promote comfort from a wider perspective, such as personal hygiene. In ensuring patient comfort, it is necessary to consider aspects of any procedure from the preplanning stage to the return of the patient to their preprocedure position.

Comfort will mean different things to different patients. It may involve being in a relaxed state free from pain, disappointment or perhaps satisfaction or physical well-being provided by another person. For the nurse, aspects of care to be considered include discussions prior to undertaking the procedure, gaining consent, ensuring pain control and maintaining privacy and dignity, offering mouthcare as well as paying attention to the patient's immediate environment.

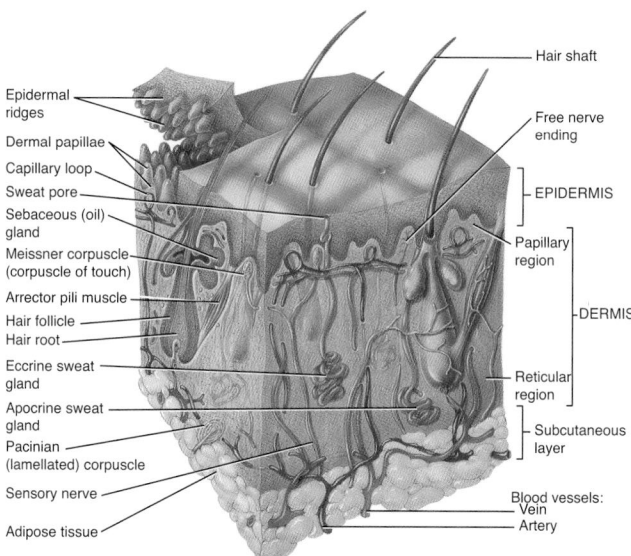

Figure 9.1 Skin and subcutaneous layer. Reproduced from Tortora and Derrickson (2009).

Personal hygiene

Definition

Good 'personal hygiene is imperative for individuals' health and wellbeing' (Pegram *et al.* 2007, p.356). It is the physical act of cleaning the body to ensure that the skin, hair and nails are maintained in an optimum condition (DH 2001).

Anatomy and physiology

Skin

A definition of healthy skin is that it is fulfilling all of its functions, so an individual's quality of life is not adversely affected (Penzer and Finch 2001). Being the largest organ of the body, maintaining the skin's integrity is essential to the prevention of infection and the promotion of both physical and psychological health. The skin has several functions (Burr and Penzer 2005):

- regulation of temperature
- physical and immunological protection
- excretion and preservation of water balance
- sensory perception
- psychosocial: how the individual is perceived, and their own perceptions of their body image.

The skin is made up of three layers: epidermis, dermis and deep subcutaneous layer (Figure 9.1).

Epidermis

The epidermis is the outer coating of the skin and contains no blood vessels or nerve endings. The cells on the sur-

face are gradually shed and replaced by new cells which have developed from the deeper layers; this process takes approximately 28 days. The epidermis has hairs, sweat glands and the ducts of sebaceous glands passing through it. It provides an efficient natural barrier (Burr and Penzer 2005).

Dermis

The dermis is the thicker layer which contains blood and lymph vessels, nerve fibres, sweat and sebaceous glands. It is made up of white fibrous tissue and yellow elastic fibres which give the skin its toughness and elasticity. It provides the epidermis with structural and nutritional support (Holloway and Jones 2005).

Subcutaneous layer

The subcutaneous layer contains the deep fat cells (areolar and adipose tissue) and provides heat regulation for the body. It is also the support structure for the outer layers of the skin (Tortora and Derrickson 2009). Maintaining skin integrity, through good personal hygiene, will allow this complex system to provide an efficient natural barrier to the external environment.

It is important to remember that the skin is a changing organ, affected by internal and external factors, temperature, air humidity and age (Burr and Penzer 2005). It has a great ability to adapt to changes in the environment and stimuli but will be affected by ill health and immobility (McLoughlin 2005). Its integrity, continuity and cleanliness are essential to maintaining its physiological functions.

The ageing process can adversely affect the skin structure. Skin tissue becomes thin and less elastic and resistant to trauma and shearing forces. The blood supply is reduced as cells are replaced more slowly, which adversely affects healing. Transmission of stimuli from sensory receptors slows and can lead to damage. The production of natural oils declines and can lead to dry skin which increases the risk of infection and tissue breakdown (Penzer and Finch 2001). Hence extra care should be taken when washing and drying elderly patients; nursing interventions can protect and restore the skin's natural barrier (Ersser et al. 2005).

Evidence-based approaches

Personal cleanliness is a fundamental value in society. Often, when patients become unwell they depend on nurses to assist them with meeting their personal hygiene needs. When this occurs, it is important that the nurse observes and assesses the patient's needs on an individual basis.

Hygiene is a personal entity and everyone will have their own individual requirements and standards of cleanliness. In this way, 'nurses must take care not to impose their own norms on patients and clients and should respect their autonomy in decisions concerning care' (Spiller 1992, p.431). Within the assessment, the patient's religious and cultural beliefs should be taken into account and incorporated into care. Personal hygiene is individual to that person and is also based on family influences, peer groups, economic and social factors (Cooper 1994).

In Western culture, privacy is of the utmost importance and considered to be a basic human right. However, in some religions like Islam, modesty is crucial and can be challenging to manage in the hospital setting (Hollins 2009). Patients may feel a great deal of embarrassment having to depend on another person to help them with this extremely private act. It is therefore surprising to find that so little reference is made to these elements in the literature. However, in the clinical situation the best person to refer to is the patient; this will encourage open honest communication between the patient and nurse (Pegram et al. 2007).

Florence Nightingale (1859) first noted the importance of good personal hygiene and the essential role nurses have in maintaining this, to prevent infection and increase well-being. Since then, nursing models have provided a conceptual framework for nursing practice and all make some reference to meeting patients' hygiene needs. Roper et al. (1981) adapted Henderson's original concept of nursing (Henderson 1966) to develop a model reflecting the activities of daily living. Another example was given by Orem (1980) who focused on the ability of the patient to self-care and who refers to the universal self-care requisites of the skin, nail and hair condition and the patterns of standard hygiene. Gordon (1994) discusses formulation of nursing diagnosis. Following assessment, clusters of actual or potential health problems are established; specific diagnoses are used to describe these. Clinical knowledge is then applied, to provide problem-solving activities to achieve a set outcome.

The nurse's role is continued provision of appropriate levels of cleanliness (Young 1991), which promotes 'comfort, safety and well-being' for the patient and should be carried out with skill and knowledge (Whiting 1999, p.339). Frequently, the time taken to attend to personal hygiene will provide ample opportunity for communication. Wilson states:

> … a bed bath facilitates listening and enables the nurse to pick up cues to a patient's anxieties and fears. It provides the time and opportunity for the nurse to offer support and encouragement when difficult situations have to be confronted, solutions sought and decisions made …
>
> (Wilson 1986, p.81)

This also focuses on the nurse's ability to be with the patient as well as providing for the patient (Campbell 1984) and is part of the essence of nursing care (Kitson 1999).

It is during the delivery of personal hygiene that the nurse is able to demonstrate a wide range of skills such as assessment, communication, observation and caring for the patient. This can be the most significant social interaction of the day for the patient, as the nurse develops a deeper understanding of the patient's personality and needs, providing a personal bond between the nurse and patient (Hector and Touhy 1997). This relationship offers the nurse an opportunity to encourage the patient to reclaim autonomy and independence within this care need through participation, which can increase patients' feelings of self-worth and dignity.

Healthcare assistants with a recognized qualification such as a National Vocational Qualification (NVQ) can complement the role of the qualified nurse in the implementation of planned care. It is vital that health professionals share their knowledge and any changes identified during procedures; personal feedback and documentation are good vehicles for this.

Comfort, cleanliness, availability of washing facilities, privacy and assistance from nurses were expressed as being important in providing hygiene care by patients in a recent ward audit (unpublished) at the Royal Marsden Hospital. The prevention of infection is also pertinent and will be referred to, as is patient education and health promotion.

Within the activity, opportunities may arise for the patient to discuss issues, concerns or fears that they may have regarding admission, treatment, discharge planning or prognosis. This will help to build a therapeutic relationship and highlight health and social care needs.

The world of nursing is ever changing, and there is a risk that activities such as attending to the personal hygiene of patients may become devalued or just another routine (Voegeli 2008). The literature supports the enhanced quality of care for patients, when hygiene needs are attended to by qualified/experienced practitioners (Carr-Hill et al. 1992).

Personal hygiene is considered part of the essence of care that nurses should never treat as ritualistic.

Principles of care

Skin care is particularly important to prevent the colonization of Gram-positive and -negative micro-organisms on the skin, which if permitted to colonize lead to healthcare-associated infection (Parker 2004). By implementing simple personal hygiene measures, the risk of infection can be reduced.

An initial assessment of the skin using observational skills is essential to ascertain the skin's general condition, colour, texture, smell and temperature (Penzer and Finch 2001). To accurately observe and assess changes in the skin, an understanding of the structure, function and factors that cause disruption is essential, to enable identification of those at increased risk (Ersser *et al.* 2005).

Factors that may influence the appearance of the tissue are as follows.

- *Nutritional and hydration state*: imbalances will cause loss of elasticity and drying of the skin. Oedema will cause stretching and thinning of the skin (Potter and Perry 1995).
- *Incontinence*: the presence of urine and/or faeces on the skin increases the normal pH of 4.0–5.5 and makes the skin wet, which increase the risks of tissue breakdown and infection (Ersser *et al.* 2005).
- *Age, health and mobility status of the individual*: for example, the presence of pressure ulcers (Smoker 1999, Stockton and Flynn 2009).
- *Treatment therapies*: for example, radiotherapy (skin may become moist and cracked), chemotherapy (some cytotoxic agents such as methotrexate can cause erythematous rashes), and continuous infusions of 5-fluorouracil (5-FU) can cause a condition called palmar–plantar erythrodysaesthesia syndrome, which presents with cracking and epidermal sloughing of the palms and soles (Lokich and Moore 1984). A low platelet count can lead to an increased risk of bruising and a decrease in the white blood cells can influence the rate of healing. Steroids may cause the skin to become papery and fragile.
- *Any concurrent conditions*: for example, eczema, psoriasis, diabetes or stress, can affect the ability of skin to maintain its integrity (Holloway and Jones 2005).

Box 9.1 lists the specific considerations for skin care.

Methods of perineal/perianal care

When the nurse is performing care of the perineal and/or perianal area, it is important that informed consent is sought and privacy maintained as the patient may be embarrassed or humiliated. It is important for the nurse and patient to engage in a two-way process where agreement is given for the nurse to provide care (DH 2001).

Box 9.1 Specific areas for skin consideration

- *Frail and papery skin* should prompt the nurse to take extra care in the bathing process. Patients need to be involved in their care plans, ensuring that correct and or preferred lotions are used; this will maintain the integrity of the skin and prevent the skin from being compromised.
- *Areas of red skin*. If redness is noted, wound prevention measures need to be implemented to prevent sores and ulcers from developing. These include good pressure-relieving positioning and repositioning and the use of barrier products in the form of creams, ointments and films (Voegeli 2008).
- *Open wounds*. When open wounds are present, such as pressure ulcers, abrasions or cuts, preventive measures such as pressure-relieving mattresses should be used to prevent further breakdown (Philips and Buttery 2009) and dressings such as hydrocolloids used where appropriate to promote wound healing (Bouza *et al.* 2005).
- *Intravenous devices and drains*. Frequently, patients have intravenous devices and wound drains inserted as part of their therapy and these should be handled with care to prevent the introduction of infection or the 'pulling' of the tubes.

Meticulous care with these areas is vital, especially for those people who may be prone to infection. Problems can arise from treatment modalities; for example, radiotherapy can cause fistulas, diarrhoea, constipation and urinary tract infections. Vigilance with cleanliness can prevent some of these problems or reduce their severity. Whenever possible, patients should be encouraged and assisted to perform this care themselves (Haisfield-Wolfe 1998).

Ideally, perineal hygiene should be attended to after the general bath or, at the very least, the water and wipes should be changed and cleaned once utilized due to the large colonies of bacteria that tend to live in or around this area (Gooch 1989, Gould 1994). It is generally acknowledged that soap and lotions administered incorrectly to the perineum/perianal area can cause irritation and infection (Ersser *et al.* 2005, Holloway and Jones 2005). Many nurses will use soap or a similar chemical derivative in order to promote thorough cleaning, but frequently lack of knowledge can lead to further problems, especially if all the soap is not removed; this can lead to discomfort for the patient if this area is not treated sensitively (Lindell and Olsson 1989).

Methods for hair care

The way a person feels is often related to their appearance, and hair condition and style is usually pertinent to this. Hair care can be complex and so it should be planned and delivered to the patient's personal preferences.

Washing the hair of a bed-bound patient can be challenging, but there are several ways to manage this. To wash a patient's hair, move the patient to the top of the bed and position their head so that it is supported over the end. The patient's condition must always be assessed before performing this task as it would not be appropriate for patients with head and neck or spinal injuries. Shampooing frequency depends on the patient's well-being and their hair condition. Referral to a hairdresser may be appropriate.

Grooming the hair provides an ideal opportunity to observe for dandruff, psoriasis, flaky skin and head lice. Head lice are extremely infectious so it is imperative to treat the hair with a medicated shampoo as soon as possible. Hospital policy/protocol should be followed regarding the disposal of infected linen. Towel drying of hair should occur and hairdryers can be used with the consent of the patient (NMC 2008a). However, use of a hairdryer may not be appropriate if patient has had recent alopecia (loss of hair) due to chemotherapy. Hairdryers should be checked for safety in accordance with local policy. In the oncology setting, chemotherapy is an established treatment and some cytotoxic drugs can cause alopecia. The patient's physical, psychological and social needs can be affected by the loss of hair. Special care and skilled advice are required regarding the adjustment to hair loss. Referral to the hospital surgical appliance officer is appropriate to discuss the choice and fitting of a wig. A shampoo with a neutral pH is recommended for patients who are at risk of alopecia.

Care of the beard and moustache is also important. Excess food can often become lodged here so regular grooming is essential for hygiene and comfort purposes. Beard trimmers can be used as appropriate.

Methods for care of the nails and feet

The feet and nails require special care in order to avoid pain and infection. Poor toe nail condition can affect mobility and compromise independence which can increase length of hospital stay (NHS 2004). Finger and toe nails should be kept short and neat; nail clippers are recommended for the trimming of nails and emery boards for filing to prevent jagged edges (Malkin and Berridge 2009). Patients with visual impairment or dexterity problems and those with learning disabilities may require assistance with the trimming and filing of nails. Consideration should be given to the patient's medical history; for example, do they have peripheral neuropathy, diabetes, peripheral vascular disease, necrosis or infection? If so, additional care should be given and advice sought from a chiropodist and the patient's doctor (Malkin and Berridge 2009).

Specialist foot care advice from a chiropodist can be useful. Chronic diseases such as diabetes and the long-term use of steroids can result in problems such as pressure ulcers, breakdown of the skin integrity and delays in the healing process. Special attention should be paid to cleaning the feet and in between the toes to avoid any fungal infection (Geraghty 2005). Powders and creams are available that help with the treatment of infections and odour management, for example miconazole nitrate 2% for fungal infections (BNF 2011).

Methods for care of the ears and nose

Lack of attention to cleaning the ears and nose can lead to impairment of the senses. Usually these small organs require minimal care but observation for a build-up of wax in the ears and deposits in the nose is essential to maintain patency. The outer ear can be cleaned with cotton wool or gauze and warm water (Alexander et al. 2007).

Patients undergoing enteral feeding and/or oxygen therapy should have regular nasal care to avoid excessive drying and excoriating of the delicate air passages. Gentle cleaning of the nasal mucosa with wool/gauze and water is recommended. Coating the area with a thin water-based lubricant to prevent discomfort can be beneficial, but petroleum jelly is not recommended as a nasal skin barrier when oxygen therapy is in progress as it is highly flammable. These interventions will remove debris and maintain a moist environment (Geraghty 2005).

Patients who have had piercing to the ears or nose will require cleaning of the holes to avoid the risk of infection. Gently cleaning around the pierced area with cotton wool/gauze and warm water and then towel drying is recommended. Observe for inflammation or oozing; if this occurs, inform the patient and doctor and seek permission from the patient to remove the device.

Legal and professional issues
Benchmarking

Benchmarking is a valid framework by which nurses can establish and share best practice throughout the work environment. Three benchmarks – hygiene, self-care and privacy and dignity – cited in the *Essence of Care* (DH 2001), are important to consider when reviewing patient hygiene and the care needs should be carried out to an uncompromising standard (Geraghty 2005) (Box 9.2).

Preprocedural considerations
Non-pharmacological support
Soap

Persistent use of some soaps can alter the pH of the skin and remove the natural oils, leading to drying and cracking (Smoker 1999), which provide an ideal environment for bacteria to multiply (Holloway and Jones 2005). According to Ersser et al. (2005), patients with dry skin have a 2.5-fold greater likelihood of skin breakdown. In addition, patients may like to use moisturizers and this should be respected. Care should be taken with skinfolds and crevices, paying

421

Box 9.2 *Essence of Care* benchmarking standards for hygiene, self-care and privacy and dignity

- All patients are assessed to identify the advice and/or assistance required in maintaining and promoting their individual personal hygiene.
- Planned care is negotiated with patients and/or their carers and is based on assessment of their individual needs.
- Patients have access to an environment that is safe and acceptable to the individual.
- Patients are expected to supply their own toiletries but single-use toiletries are provided until they can supply their own.
- Patients have access to the level of assistance that they require to meet their individual personal hygiene needs.

(DH 2001).

Box 9.3 Religion-specific considerations related to personal hygiene

- Those following *Islam* must perform ablution (*wudhu*, to use the Islamic term) before the daily prayer, which is the formal washing of the face, hands and forearms, and so on. One of the criteria for cleanliness is washing after the use of the lavatory. Any traces of urine or faeces must be eliminated by washing with running water, at least. The use of toilet tissues for cleaning is not sufficient. With such emphasis on washing and personal hygiene, adhering to the practical teaching of Islam on washing would enhance personal hygiene for the individual and therefore reduce the chance of disease and sickness individually and subsequently for the whole society.
- *Hindus* also place importance on washing before prayer; they believe the left hand should dominate in this process and therefore do not eat with the left hand as it is deemed unclean.
- *Sikhs* place great importance on not shaving or cutting hair, choosing to comb their hair twice a day and wash regularly. Male Sikhs wear their hair underneath a turban as a sign of respect for God.

particular attention to thorough drying of the areas and observing for any breaks in the skin. It is recommended that the skin is patted and not rubbed, to reduce damage caused by friction (Ersser *et al.* 2005).

Emollient therapy

Current evidence recommends a move away from the traditional washing using soap and water, and recent research demonstrates that surfactants found in soap are irritant to the skin (Voegeli 2008). Penzer and Finch (2001) and Burr and Penzer (2005) recommend the use of emollient therapy for washing and moisturizing to seal the skin. In a literature review of hygiene practices, the use of soap and water remained common practice but several studies suggest that skin cleansers, for example emollient creams, followed by moisturizing may be less likely to disrupt the skin barrier and have a therapeutic benefit (Ersser *et al.* 2005). These products allow the patient to have a more active role in their own care, as the products can be left within reach and the patient can initiate the activity without the need to access running water (Collins and Hampton 2003).

Prepackaged cloths

Prepackaged cloths impregnated with cleanser and moisturizers are a cost-effective and evidence-based alternative to soap and water (Sheppard and Brenner 2000). They require no rinsing and are as effective at cleansing and more skin preserving than soap and water (Byers *et al.* 1995).

Skin care consists of four main areas: cleansing, hydrating/moisturizing, protection and replenishing (Voegeli 2008). Individual care actions often address more than one area at once, for example washing with water-based aqueous cream and water will cleanse and moisturize the skin.

Cultural and religious factors

The nurse must respect and consider the patient's cultural and religious factors, while maintaining privacy and dignity at all times; for example, some people prefer to sit under running water as opposed to sitting in a bath (Hollins 2009, Sampson 1982). Some religions do not allow hair washing or brushing, while others may require the hair to be covered by a turban. Similarly, in some countries facial hair is significant and should never be removed without the patient's/relatives' consent. Always establish any preferences before beginning care (Hollins 2009) (Box 9.3).

Clothing

Effort should be made to encourage and empower patients to dress in their own clothing during the day, where possible, and in their own nightwear to sleep. This increases independence and well-being, encourages normality and promotes dignity. If the patient is too unwell or does not have their own clothing, hospital provision should be made available to protect their modesty (Wilson 2006).

Bed bathing

Before commencing this procedure, read the patient's care plan, manual handling documentation and risk assessment to gain knowledge of safe practice. Prior to each part of the procedure, explain and obtain agreement from the patient (NMC 2008a). Planned care is negotiated with the patient and is based on assessment of their individual needs. Planned care should be documented and changed according to the patient's/carer's needs on a daily basis. Prior to commencing each step, the patient should be offered the opportunity to participate if able to, to encourage dignity, independence and autonomy.

Privacy and dignity must be maintained throughout, doors and curtains kept closed and only opened when absolutely necessary, with the patient's permission.

Procedure guideline 9.1 Bed bathing a patient

Essential equipment

- Disposable apron
- Non-sterile gloves
- Clean bedlinen
- Bath towels
- Laundry skip, applying local guidelines for soiled and/or infected linen
- Flannels, preferably disposable wipes
- Toiletries, as preferred by patient
- Comb/brush
- Equipment for oral hygiene
- Clean clothes
- Clean wash bowl

Optional equipment

- Antiembolic stockings
- Razor
- Scissors/nail clippers
- Emery boards
- Manual handling equipment
- Urinal, bedpan or commode

Preprocedure

Action	Rationale
1 Assess and plan care with the patient and family/friend as suitable. Note personal preferences, addressing religious and cultural beliefs; offer analgesia as appropriate.	To plan care and encourage participation and independence (Hollins 2009, C; NMC 2008b, E,C; Pegram *et al.* 2007, E).
2 Clear the area of any obstacles, ensure the environment is warm and draw curtains/close doors to guarantee privacy and dignity.	To maintain comfort and a safe environment and promote privacy and dignity (NMC 2008b, C).
3 Offer patient the opportunity to use a urinal, bedpan or commode.	To reduce any disruption to procedure and prevent any discomfort (NMC 2008b, C).
4 Collect all equipment by the bedside.	To minimize time away from patient during procedure. Disposable flannels are preferable as this reduces the risk of infection. To meet patient preference during procedure (NMC 2008b, C).
5 Ensure wash bowl is cleaned with hot soapy water before use, fill bowl with warm water, check temperature with patient and adjust if necessary.	To minimize cross-infection (Fraise and Bradley 2009, E; Parker 2004, C). To promote patient comfort. E
6 Ensure the area is safe; check that the bed brakes are on and adjust the bed to an appropriate height.	To prevent the bed moving unexpectedly and to avoid poor manual handling techniques (Pegram *et al.* 2007, E).
7 Wash hands; use disposable gloves and aprons in accordance with local guidelines.	To minimize risk of cross-infection (Fraise and Bradley 2009, E; Parker 2004, C).

Procedure

8 Assist the patient with the removal of clothing, wristwatches and any other items of personal property. Cover patient with bath towel or fleece and fold back bedclothes, incorporating appropriate manual handing procedures.	To maintain privacy and dignity, body temperature (NMC 2008b, C), and safety (Pegram *et al.* 2007, C).
9 Ask patient whether they use soap on their face; wash, rinse and dry face and neck, with a gentle wipe around and inside the outer ears.	To promote cleanliness and independence (NMC 2008b, C, E).

(Continued)

423

Procedure guideline 9.1 *(Continued)*

10 Assist male patients with facial shaving, apply chosen shaving foam/soap. Ensure skin is taut; begin shaving from cheeks down to neck in short strokes. Rinse razor as required. Change water and rinse face with clean water (or use electric shaver).	To promote positive body image (NMC 2008b, C).
11 Wash, rinse and pat dry top half of body, starting with the side furthest away from you. Care needs to be taken not to wet drains/dressings and IV devices. Apply toiletries as required.	To promote patient well-being and cleanliness and reduce the risk of cross-infection (NMC 2008b, C).
12 Change the water and your disposable gloves. Inform the patient that you are going to wash around the genitalia, gain verbal consent from the patient or ask the patient if they wish to wash this area themselves. Using a separate flannel or wipe, wash around the area and then dry it. Remove gloves, dispose as per hospital policy. When washing this area, remember that female patients wash from the front to back. Male patients should draw back the foreskin, if uncircumcised, when washing the penis. If there is an indwelling catheter, put on clean gloves and wash the tubing, moving the disposable cloth down the tube away from the genitalia area, then dry tubing and remove gloves as per hospital policy. (Patients may prefer to do this themselves.)	To reduce risk of infection and to maintain a safe environment (NMC 2008b, C; Pegram *et al.* 2007, C).
13 Ensure the patient is covered and has nurse call bell within easy reach. Change water and gloves.	To maintain cleanliness, preserving dignity and privacy (NMC 2008b, C).
14 Remove antiembolic stocking if present. Wash legs, rinse and pat dry, starting with the side furthest away from you. If necessary, request assistance from colleagues. Assess the need for possible chiropody referral. Re-fit antiembolic stocking as necessary, measuring according to local policy. Request assistance as necessary to roll patient, wash back and then, using disposable flannel, wash sacral area, observing pressure areas. Cover areas that are not being washed. Return patient onto their back, ensuring they are covered. Apply toiletries as required.	To prevent venous emboli and to prevent and treat pressure ulcers, ensuring appropriate referrals are made (NMC 2008b, C).
15 Inspect finger and toe nails, clean under nails using nail file. Cut or clip finger nails to top level of finger, edges can be shaped using an emery board. Toe nails should be cut/clipped straight across. Note any area of skin dryness, inflammation, calluses.	To enhance positive body image and patient comfort and reduce risk of infection (NMC 2008b, C).
16 If the patient is to remain in bed, replace clothes and change bottom sheet whilst the patient is being turned. Care should be taken to prevent shaking the sheets and allowing particles to enter the atmosphere. Contact with your clothing must be avoided so the linen should be placed directly into the linen skip. Ensure a minimum of two nurses are present during this procedure.	To reduce unnecessary activity for patient and nurse. To prevent any bacteria from the sheet entering the atmosphere and surrounding environment (Parker 2004, C; Pegram *et al.* 2007, C). To maintain safety of patient and safe manual handling, following risk assessment (NMC 2008b, C).
17 Provide appropriate equipment, and assist patient if required, to brush teeth and/or rinse mouth.	To maintain good oral hygiene and prevent infection (Fraise and Bradley 2009, E; Parker 2004, C).

424

18	Dry and comb patient's hair as desired.	To enhance patient comfort, and to promote positive body image (NMC 2008b, C).
19	Remake top bedclothes.	
20	Help patient to sit or lie in desired position.	To enhance patient comfort and reduce risk of pressure area breakdown (NMC 2008b, C).
21	Remove equipment from bedside; replace patient's possessions in their appropriate place. Place locker, bedside table and call bell within reach.	To maintain a safe environment and promote patient independence (NMC 2008b, C).
22	Remove apron and gloves and dispose of them according to local regulations.	To prevent cross-infection (Pratt *et al.* 2001, C).
23	Wash hands, using alcohol-based handwash.	To prevent cross-infection (Fraise and Bradley 2009, E).

Postprocedure

24	Document any changes in planned care.	To provide recorded documentation of care and aid communication to the multiprofessional team (NMC 2009, C).

Eye care

Definition

Eye care is the process of assessing, cleaning and/or irrigating the eye, including the instillation of prescribed ocular preparations where applicable; patient education is also included (Stollery *et al.* 2005, Watkinson and Seewoodhary 2007).

Anatomy and physiology

The eye consists of three main parts: the orbit, the globe (eyeball) and the extrinsic structures.

The orbit

The orbit or socket is formed by seven bones of the skull and is lined with fat; it supports and protects the globe and its accessory structures (blood vessels and nerves) and provides attachments for the ocular muscles (Stollery *et al.* 2005).

The globe

The globe is approximately 2.5 cm in diameter and can be divided into three layers (Figure 9.2).

- The outer layer or fibrous tunic is composed of the transparent cornea and the white sclera. The primary function of the outer layer, in particular the sclera, is protective and it gives shape to the eyeball. The cornea functions as a refracting and protective membrane through which light rays pass on their route to the retina (Watkinson and Seewoodhary 2007).

- The middle layer or vascular tunic comprises the choroid, ciliary body and iris; the globe's vascular supply is provided by the choroid.

- The inner layer or nervous tunic is composed of the retina, which contains the light-sensitive cells called the rods and cones and is responsible for converting light rays into electrical signals that are transmitted to the brain via the optic nerve. This area contains the macula lutea, also known as the yellow spot. The central fovea, the

Figure 9.2 Horizontal section through the eyeball at the level of the optic nerve. Optic axis and axis of eyeball are included.

Figure 9.3 The anterior cavity in front of the lens is incompletely divided into anterior chamber (anterior to iris) and posterior chamber (behind iris), which are continuous through the pupil. Aqueous humour, which fills the cavity, is formed by ciliary processes and reabsorbed into the venous blood by the canal of Schlemm.

area of highest visual acuity, is also located here, as is the blind spot, the area of no visual field (Watkinson and Seewoodhary 2007).

The globe – internally

The globe is divided into two chambers by the lens (see Figure 9.3): the anterior cavity, anterior to the lens, and the vitreous chamber, posterior to the lens. The anterior cavity is divided into the anterior chamber and the posterior chamber by the iris. It contains a clear, watery fluid called the aqueous humour. The vitreous chamber is filled with a jelly-like substance called the vitreous body or vitreous humour. Together, these two fluid-filled cavities help maintain the shape of the eyeball and the intraocular pressure (Tortora and Derrickson 2009).

The aqueous humour is continuously secreted by the ciliary process (a part of the ciliary body) located behind the iris. This fluid then permeates the posterior chamber, passing between the lens and the iris, and flows through the pupil into the anterior chamber. From the anterior chamber, the aqueous humour drains into the scleral venous sinus (canal of Schlemm) and is absorbed back into the bloodstream (Figure 9.2).

The aqueous humour is the principal source of nutrients and waste removal for the lens and cornea, as these structures have no direct blood supply. If the outflow of aqueous humour is blocked, excessive intraocular pressure may develop, leading to the disease process known as glaucoma. This excess pressure can cause degeneration of the retina, which may result in blindness (Lee 2006). The vitreous humour is a clear gelatinous substance which fills the vitreous chamber, which, unlike the aqueous humour, is produced during fetal development and is never replaced (Tortora and Derrickson 2009).

Extrinsic structures

Extrinsic structures of the eye protect the globe from external injury (Stollery *et al.* 2005).

- *Eyelashes*: protect the eye from debris.
- *Eyebrows*: prevent moisture, in particular sweat, from flowing into the eye.
- *Eyelids*: the eyelid is made up of complex muscles for eye movement, glands for tear and oil production that serve as a cleansing mechanism against dirt and foreign objects, and sensitive nerves for defence (Watkinson and Seewoodhary 2007).
- *Lacrimal (tear) apparatus*: tears are produced in the lacrimal glands located at the upper, outer edge of the eye. They are excreted onto the upper surface of the globe and wash over the ocular surface by the action of blinking. The function of tears is to clean, moisten and lubricate the ocular surface and eyelids. Tears also provide antisepsis as they contain an enzyme called lysozyme that is able to rupture the cell membranes of some bacteria, leading to their lysis and death (Forrester 2002). The tears collect in the nasal canthus (inner, medial aspect of the eye) from where they drain into the upper and lower lacrimal puncti which drain into the lacrimal sac. From here, the tears pass into the nasolacrimal duct and empty into the nasal cavity (Figure 9.4) (Marieb 2001, Tortora and Derrickson 2009).

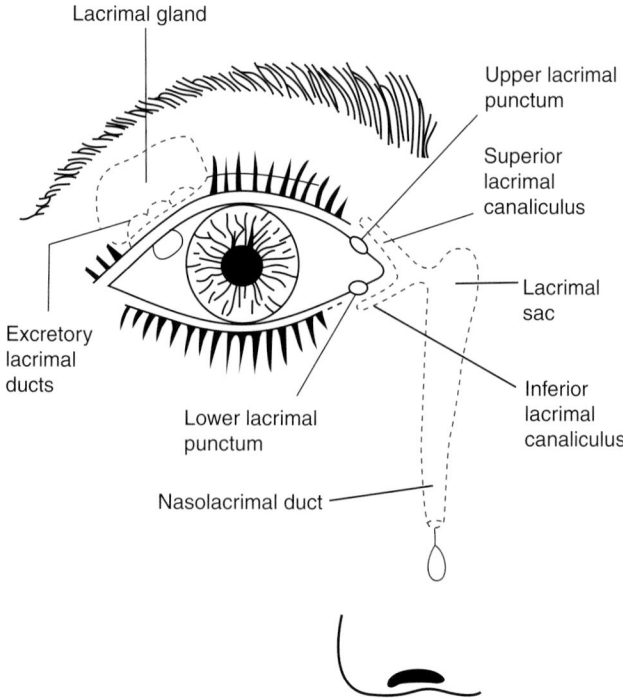

Figure 9.4 Lacrimal apparatus.

Optic nerve

The optic nerve, which is responsible for vision (cranial nerve II), exits the eye to the side of the macula lutea at an area called the optic disc (see Figure 9.2). This area is sometimes referred to as the anatomical blind spot. The optic nerve passes from the orbit through the optic foramen and into the brain. The two separate optic nerves meet at the optic chiasma and some optic nerve fibres cross over here to the opposite side of the brain. The nerves then continue along the optic tracts and terminate in the thalamus. From there, projections extend to the visual areas in the occipital lobe of the cerebral cortex (Tortora and Derrickson 2009) (Figure 9.5).

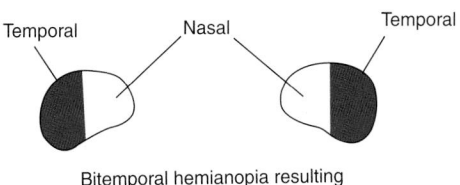

Bitemporal hemianopia resulting from lesion in chiasma

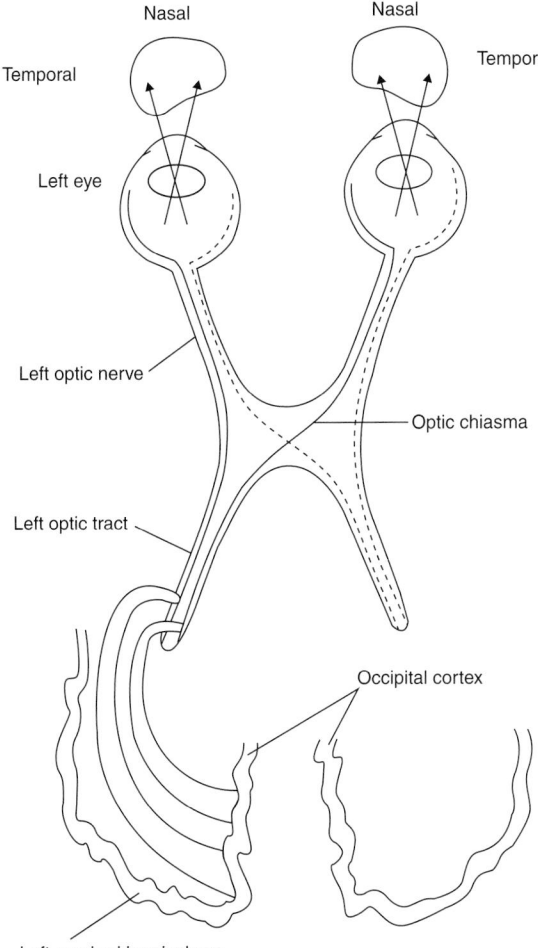

Figure 9.5 Visual pathways and visual fields.

Box 9.4 Effects of ageing on the eye

Anatomical changes

- The retro-orbital fat atrophies.
- Eyelid tissues become weak.
- The levator muscle weakens, causing the eyelid to droop which can occlude the upper visual field.

Physiological changes

- Presbyopia: the distance from which print can be read increases.
- Reduced flexibility of the lens means it can no longer change shape to focus on close objects quickly.
- Cataracts: the lens become dense and yellow, affecting colour perceptions; it can become so dense that the lens proteins precipitate, creating a halo effect around bright lights.
- Night vision reduces.
- Diminished central vision caused by cells within the retina dying.
- Dry eyes from reduced tear production.

(Holman *et al.* 2005, Nigam and Knight 2008)

427

An additional blind spot, or area of depressed vision called a scotoma, may be indicative of a brain tumour. For example, in pituitary gland tumours it is common to develop bilateral defects in the field of vision due to invasion of the optic chiasm (Goodman and Wickham 2005).

The ageing process

The eye changes with age. This process can start in the third decade of life, with most anatomical and physiological changes becoming more prevalent the older a person becomes (Nigam and Knight 2008) (Boxes 9.4 and 9.5).

Box 9.5 Eye conditions common in the older population

- *Glaucoma*: the optic nerve is damaged by increased pressure in the eye, resulting in reduced visual field and pain.
- *Cataract*: as explained in Box 9.4.
- *Diabetic retinopathy*: blood vessels connected to the retina are damaged by the disease and sight becomes blurred and patchy, and can be totally lost.
- *Age-related macular degeneration*: a chronic disorder of the macula cells in the centre of the retina, a highly sensitive area responsible for detailed central vision. As this degenerates, central vision declines which can lead to blindness.

(Holman *et al.* 2005, Watkinson and Seewoodhary 2007)

Related theory

Sight provides us with important sensory input to enable self-care and pleasurable activities such as reading. 'Early detection of changes in the eye is important to enable effective treatment and prevent long-term problems and even blindness (Holman *et al.* 2005, p.37).

Reduced vision or blindness can make the hospital environment very unwelcoming. When caring for patients with eye problems, it is essential to promote a safe, secure environment, where the person is supported and encouraged to communicate their needs effectively.

Evidence-based approaches
Rationale
Indications

Eye care may be necessary under the following circumstances.

- After eye surgery to prevent postoperative complications.
- To relieve pain and discomfort.
- To prevent or treat infection.
- To prevent or treat injury to the eye, for example to remove sharp objects.
- For eye tests such as refraction.
- For screening to detect disease such as glaucoma.
- To treat existing problems such as conjunctivitis.
- To detect drug-induced toxicity at an early stage.
- To maintain contact lenses and care for false eye prostheses.
- To optimize the eye's visual function, especially with age-related degeneration.
  (Boyd-Monk 2005, Cunningham and Gould 1998, Stollery *et al.* 2005, Watkinson and Seewoodhary 2007)

These problems may be experienced in isolation or in combination.

Eye care includes patient education of the eye and surrounding structures as well as health promotion and safety advice to promote quality of life (Watkinson and Seewoodhary 2007).

Principles of care

Eye care is performed to maintain healthy eyes through keeping them moist and infection free. The eye is an important organ and inadequate techniques may lead to the transmission of infection from one eye to the other or the development of irreversible damage to the eye which could lead to loss of sight (Ashurst 1997, Cunningham and Gould 1998). If an infection is present the infected eye should be cleaned and/or treated last to prevent transmission of infection to the uninfected eye (Holman *et al.* 2005).

A clean technique should be used for eye care procedures and an aseptic technique, if deemed necessary, for vulnerable exposed eyes or to reduce the risk of infection (Alexander *et al.* 2007).

The eye area must be treated gently and unnecessary pressure must be avoided, especially to the globe (Alexander *et al.* 2007). Low-linting swabs are generally used; lint from swabs can become detached and scratch the cornea so it is recommended where possible to use lint-free swabs (Woodrow 2006). The fluids most commonly used for eye care procedures are sterile 0.9% sodium chloride or sterile water for irrigation. Sterile 0.9% sodium chloride can irritate and sting the sensitive eye area so where possible it is recommended that sterile water is used (Woodrow 2006).

If able, and after appropriate instruction, patients should be encouraged to carry out eye care procedures themselves. However, in the case of postoperative, physically limited or unconscious patients, it is often the nurse who is responsible for eye care.

Consideration should always be given to patients' sight aids, such as glasses and contact lenses (Holman *et al.* 2005). Assistance may be required to help clean these aids and advice regarding the most appropriate method should be sought, preferably from the patient.

For all procedures which involve removal or insertion of contact lenses or prosthetic eyes, the patient should be encouraged to do this themselves as they will have developed their own particular methods. However, the nurse must observe as the patient may still need education to improve upon their technique. Advice regarding the ideal method of removal and insertion should be sought from the local ophthalmology service or the nursing team in the ophthalmology unit.

Methods of eye assessment

Before beginning any eye care procedure, the eye and surrounding structures should be examined and assessed and then re-examined and reassessed after the intervention. Begin by examining the eye closed, looking carefully at the eyelids, noting any bruising, spasms, inflammation, discharge or crusting (Holman *et al.* 2005). Look for signs that the eyelids are closed properly, as an inability to close completely could indicate the presence of a cyst or lump that would require further investigation and reporting to the patient's doctor.

Ask the patient to open their eyes and, using a pen torch, look for abnormalities in the conjunctiva such as inflammation, redness or the presence of a discharge; the eye should be clear of clouding and redness (Alexander *et al.* 2007). Ask the patient whether they are experiencing any pain or photophobia. Any abnormalities need to be reported to the patient's doctor immediately, as eye complications can develop quickly. Any changes should also be documented (Alexander *et al.* 2007, Holman *et al.* 2005, NMC 2009).

Methods of eye swabbing

Eye swabbing is performed to clear the outer eye structures of foreign bodies, including discharges, which could be infected matter. The swab should be moistened with sterile water for irrigation and lightly wiped over the eyelid from the nose outward. This process should be repeated with clean gauze until the area is clean of discharge or encrustation.

Methods of eye irrigation

Eye irrigation is usually performed to remove foreign bodies or caustic substances from the eye, for example domestic cleaning agents or medications, particularly cytotoxic material; it should be performed as soon as possible to minimize damage (Stollery *et al.* 2005). The procedure is also used for preoperative preparation or to remove infected material.

Using the least volume of sterile water for irrigation necessary will reduce the likelihood of deeper corneal damage which can be a side-effect of the corrosive chemicals due to water's hypotonic nature (Kuckelkorn *et al.* 2002). The volume required will vary depending on the degree of contamination; copious amounts are needed for corrosive chemicals and smaller volumes for removal of eye secretions. The solution may be directed to the area affected by using intravenous tubing. To avoid physical damage, the tubing should be held approximately 2.5 cm from the eye (Stollery *et al.* 2005) and directed to the inner canthus.

Care of contact lenses

Contact lenses are thin, curved discs made of hard or soft plastic or a combination of both. Hard contact lenses are made of a rigid plastic that does not absorb water or saline solutions and can be worn for a maximum of 12–14 hours continuously. Soft contact lenses are more pliable, retain more water and so can be worn for up to 30 days and cleaned once weekly. Ill-fitting lenses may reduce the tear film between lens and cornea, which may result in oxygen deprivation of the cornea, leading to corneal oedema and blurred vision. Further damage to the corneal epithelial cells may lead to corneal abrasion and pain. Gas-permeable lenses are a combination of both hard and soft plastic; these permit oxygen to reach the cornea, providing greater comfort, and can be left in for several days (Olver and Cassidy 2005).

Most people look after their own contact lenses. Cleaning and storage solutions depend on the type of lenses used; manufacturers provide specific instructions for the care of their products. They should be stored in a container with slots for right (R) and left (L) eye, so they can be worn in the correct eye. Seriously ill patients should have their lenses removed and stored correctly until they can reinsert them. Contact lenses are stored in a sterile solution when they are not in the eye; this helps to lubricate the lens and enable it to glide over the cornea, reducing the risk of injury.

Artificial eyes

These are made of glass or plastic; some are permanently implanted. Most people who have artificial eyes care for them themselves. If the patient is unable to do this, it is recommended that the eye is removed once daily for cleaning; the patient will be able to advise how they would like this done (Alexander *et al.* 2007). However, if they are unable to do so, advice should be sought from the local ophthalmology service or the nursing team in the ophthalmology unit.

Preprocedural considerations

Light source

A good light source such as a minor procedure light or bright lamp is necessary to enable careful assessment of the eyes and to avoid damage to the delicate structures.

Position of light source

The light source should be positioned above and behind the nurse. It should never be allowed to shine directly into the patient's eyes, as this will be extremely uncomfortable for the patient (Shaw 2006).

Position of patient

The patient should be sitting or lying with their head tilted backwards and chin pointing upwards. This allows for easy access to the eyes and is usually a good position for patient comfort and compliance (Stollery *et al.* 2005).

429

Procedure guideline 9.2 Eye swabbing

Essential equipment

- Sterile dressing pack
- Sterile low-linting or lint-free swabs
- Sterile water for irrigation
- Light source

Optional equipment

- Sterile/non-sterile powder-free gloves

Preprocedure

Action	Rationale
1 Explain and discuss the procedure with the patient. Ask the patient to explain how their eyes feel, if they are able to.	To ensure that the patient understands the procedure and gives their valid consent (NMC 2008a, C). To have a baseline understanding of current problems or changes the patient is experiencing (NMC 2008b, C).

(Continued)

Procedure guideline 9.2 *(Continued)*

2 Assist the patient into the correct position:	The patient needs to be discouraged from flinching or making unexpected movements and so should be in the most comfortable, pain-free position possible at the start of the procedure (Shaw 2006, R5).
(a) Head well supported and tilted back	To enable access and assessment of the eyes. E
(b) Preferably the patient should be in bed or lying on a couch.	To enable patient comfort. E
3 Ensure an adequate light source, taking care not to dazzle the patient.	To enable maximum observation of the eyes without causing the patient harm or discomfort (Shaw 2006, R5).
4 Wash hands thoroughly using bactericidal soap and water or alcohol handrub, then dry hands.	To reduce the risk of cross-infection (Fraise and Bradley 2009, E).

Procedure

5 Always treat the uninfected or uninflamed eye first.	To reduce the risk of cross-infection (Fraise and Bradley 2009, E).
6 Always bathe lids with the eyes closed first.	To reduce the risk of damaging the cornea and to remove any crusted discharge. E
7 Ask the patient to look up and, using a slightly moistened swab, gently swab the lower lid from the inner canthus outwards. Use an aseptic technique for the damaged or postoperative eye.	If the swab is too wet, the solution will run down the patient's cheek. This increases the risk of cross-infection and causes the patient discomfort. Swabbing from the nasal corner outwards avoids the risk of swabbing discharge into the lacrimal punctum, or even across the bridge of the nose into the other eye. Aseptic technique reduces the risk of cross-infection (Fraise and Bradley 2009, E).
8 Ensure that the edge of the swab is not above the lid margin.	To avoid touching the sensitive cornea. E
9 Using a new swab each time, repeat the procedure until all the discharge has been removed.	To reduce risk of cross-infection (Fraise and Bradley 2009, E).
10 Gently swab the upper lid by slightly everting the lid margin and asking the patient to look down. Swab from the nasal corner outwards and use a new swab each time until all discharge has been removed.	To effectively remove any foreign material from the eye. E To reduce the risk of cross-infection (Fraise and Bradley 2009, E).
11 Once both eyelids have been cleaned and dried, make the patient comfortable.	To ensure patient comfort. E
12 Remove and dispose of equipment.	To keep area clean and reduce risk of cross-infection (Fraise and Bradley 2009, E).
13 Wash hands.	To reduce the risk of cross-infection (Fraise and Bradley 2009, E).

Postprocedure

14 Discuss with the patient any changes post procedure; report any adverse effects to the patient's doctor. Record the procedure in the appropriate documents.	To monitor effectiveness of procedure, trends and fluctuations (NMC 2009, C).

Procedure guideline 9.3 Eye irrigation

Essential equipment

- Sterile dressing pack
- Sterile water for irrigation (in an emergency, tap water may be used)
- Receiver
- Towel
- Plastic cape
- Irrigating flask
- Warm water in a bowl to warm irrigating fluid to tepid temperature
- Low-linting or lint-free swabs
- Light source

Optional equipment

- Anaesthetic drops
- Sterile/non-sterile powder-free gloves

Preprocedure

Action	Rationale
1 Explain and discuss the procedure with the patient. Ask the patient to explain how their eyes feel, if they are able to.	To ensure that the patient understands the procedure and gives their valid consent (NMC 2008a, C). To have a baseline understanding of current problems or changes the patient is experiencing. E
2 Instil anaesthetic drops if required (see Chapter 16, Procedure guideline 16.9).	To avoid any discomfort (Marsden 2006, R5).
3 Prepare the irrigation fluid to the appropriate temperature by placing in bowl of water until warmed.	Tepid fluid will be more comfortable for the patient. The solution should be poured across the inner aspect of the nurse's wrist to test the temperature. E
4 Assist the patient into the appropriate position, with their head comfortably supported with chin almost horizontal and the head inclined to the side of the eye to be treated.	To avoid the solution running either over the nose into the other eye, to avoid cross-infection, or out of the affected eye and down the side of the cheek (Fraise and Bradley 2009, E). To reduce risk of cross-infection (Fraise and Bradley 2009, E). To prevent washing the discharge down the lacrimal duct or across the cheek. E
5 Wash hands using bactericidal soap and water or alcohol handrub, and dry.	To reduce the risk of cross-infection (Fraise and Bradley 2009, E).

Procedure

Action	Rationale
6 If possible, remove any contact lens (see Procedure guidelines 9.6 and 9.7).	To ensure no reservoir of chemical remains in the eye (Marsden 2006, R5).
7 If there is any discharge proceed as for eye swabbing (see Procedure guideline 9.2).	To remove any infected material. E
8 Ask the patient to hold the receiver against the cheek below the eye being irrigated.	To collect irrigation fluid as it runs away from the eye. E
9 Position the towel and plastic cape.	To protect the patient's clothing. E
10 Hold the patient's eyelids apart, using your first and second fingers, against the orbital ridge.	The patient will be unable to hold the eye open once irrigation commences. E
11 Do not press on the eyeball.	To avoid causing the patient discomfort or pain (Alexander *et al.* 2007, C).
12 Warn the patient that the flow of solution is going to start and pour a little onto the cheek first.	To allow time to adjust to the feeling of water flow. E

(Continued)

431

Procedure guideline 9.3 (*Continued*)

13	Direct the flow of the fluid from the nasal corner outwards (see Action Figure 13).	To wash away from the lacrimal punctum and prevent contaminating other eye. E
14	Ask the patient to look up, down and to either side while irrigating.	To ensure that the whole area, including fornices, is irrigated (Stollery *et al.* 2005, E).
15	Evert upper and lower lids whilst irrigating.	To ensure complete removal of any foreign body. E
16	Keep the flow of irrigation fluid constant.	To ensure swift removal of any foreign body (Marsden 2006, R5).
17	When the eye has been thoroughly irrigated, ask the patient to close the eyes and use a new swab to dry the lids.	For patient comfort. E
18	Take the receiver from the patient and dry the cheek.	To prevent spillage of receiver contents and promote patient comfort. E
19	Make the patient comfortable.	

Postprocedure

20	Remove and dispose of equipment.	To keep area clean and reduce risk of cross-infection (Fraise and Bradley 2009, E).
21	Wash hands with bactericidal soap and water.	To reduce the risk of cross-infection (Fraise and Bradley 2009, E).
22	Complete the patient's recording chart and other hospital and/or legally required documents.	To maintain accurate records. To provide a point of reference in the event of any queries. To prevent any duplication of treatment (NMC 2009, C).
23	Discuss with the patient any changes post procedure; report any adverse effects to the patient's doctor.	To monitor effectiveness of procedure, trends and fluctuations (NMC 2009, C).

432

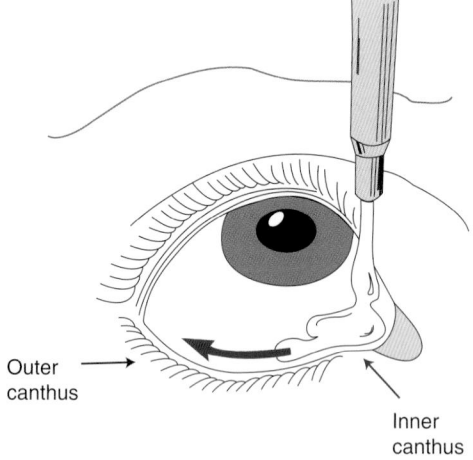

Outer canthus

Inner canthus

Action Figure 13   Irrigation of the eye from inner to outer canthus.

Procedure guideline 9.4 Artificial eye care: insertion

Essential equipment

- Sterile dressing pack
- Sterile water for irrigation
- Low-linting or lint-free swabs

Optional equipment

- Sterile/non-sterile powder-free gloves
- Extractor

Preprocedure

Action	Rationale
1 Explain and discuss the procedure with the patient.	To ensure that the patient understands the procedure and gives their consent (NMC 2008a, C).
2 Wash hands thoroughly using bactericidal soap and water or alcohol handrub.	To reduce the risk of cross-infection (Fraise and Bradley 2009, E).

Procedure

3 Wearing gloves and with the dominant hand, gently lift up the upper eyelid and pull down the lower eyelid. With the other hand, hold the prosthesis between the thumb and index finger and gently insert it.	To minimize patient discomfort and ensure correct insertion. E

Postprocedure

4 Remove and dispose of equipment.	To keep area clean and reduce risk of cross-infection (Fraise and Bradley 2009, E).
5 Wash hands with bactericidal soap and water.	To reduce the risk of cross-infection (Fraise and Bradley 2009, E).
6 Complete the patient's recording chart and other hospital and/or legally required documents.	To maintain accurate records. To provide a point of reference in the event of any queries. To prevent any duplication of treatment (NMC 2009, C).

433

Procedure guideline 9.5 Artificial eye care: removal

Essential equipment

- Sterile dressing pack
- Sterile water for irrigation
- Low-linting or lint-free swabs

Optional equipment

- Sterile/non-sterile powder-free gloves
- Extractor

Preprocedure

Action	Rationale
1 Explain and discuss the procedure with the patient.	To ensure that the patient understands the procedure and gives their consent (NMC 2008a, C).
2 Wash hands thoroughly using bactericidal soap and water or alcohol handrub.	To reduce the risk of cross-infection (Fraise and Bradley 2009, E).

Procedure

3 Wearing gloves and with the dominant hand, gently pull the eyelid downwards and exert slight pressure below the eyelid to overcome the suction, enabling the prosthesis to be removed (see Action Figure 3). An extractor may be necessary to gently lever the eye out.	To minimize patient discomfort and trauma to the area (Alexander et al. 2007, C, E).

(Continued)

Procedure guideline 9.5 *(Continued)*

4 Rinse and drain the eye socket with sterile water for irrigation.	To remove any loose debris and to minimize damage caused by touch. E
5 Clean the eye with sterile water for irrigation.	To prevent the build-up of debris and to reduce the risk of infection (Fraise and Bradley 2009, E).

Postprocedure

6 Remove and dispose of equipment.	To keep area clean and reduce risk of cross-infection (Fraise and Bradley 2009, E).
7 Wash hands with bactericidal soap and water.	To reduce the risk of cross-infection (Fraise and Bradley 2009, E).
8 Complete the patient's recording chart and other hospital and/or legally required documents.	To maintain accurate records. To provide a point of reference in the event of any queries. To prevent any duplication of treatment (NMC 2009, C).

(a)　　　　　　　　　　　　(b)

Action Figure 3　Removing an artificial eye.

Procedure guideline 9.6　Contact lens removal: hard lenses

Essential equipment

- Sterile dressing pack
- Contact lens solution
- Low-linting or lint-free swabs

Optional equipment

- Sterile/non-sterile powder-free gloves

Preprocedure

Action	Rationale
1 Explain and discuss the procedure with the patient.	To ensure that the patient understands the procedure and gives their consent (NMC 2008a, C).
2 Wash hands thoroughly using bactericidal soap or alcohol handrub.	To reduce the risk of cross-infection (Fraise and Bradley 2009, E).

Procedure

3 Using thumb and forefinger, separate the eyelids. Keeping the eyelid stationary, place the index finger on the lens. Gently move the lens to one side of the cornea and pull away (see Action Figure 3).	To minimize corneal trauma (Stollery *et al.* 2005, R5).

4 Store lenses in the appropriate solution as recommended by the manufacturer and ensure lenses are placed in the correct left and right storage pots.	To prevent deterioration and contamination (Stollery *et al.* 2005, R5).
5 Refer to manufacturer's instructions for further storage information, particularly if patient will not be using the lenses for a lengthy period of time.	To prevent deterioration of lens and growth of organisms. E

Postprocedure

6 Remove and dispose of equipment.	To keep area clean and reduce risk of cross-infection (Fraise and Bradley 2009, E).
7 Wash hands with bactericidal soap and water.	To reduce the risk of cross-infection (Fraise and Bradley 2009, E).
8 Complete the patient's recording chart and other hospital and/or legally required documents.	To maintain accurate records. To provide a point of reference in the event of any queries. To prevent any duplication of treatment (NMC 2009, C).

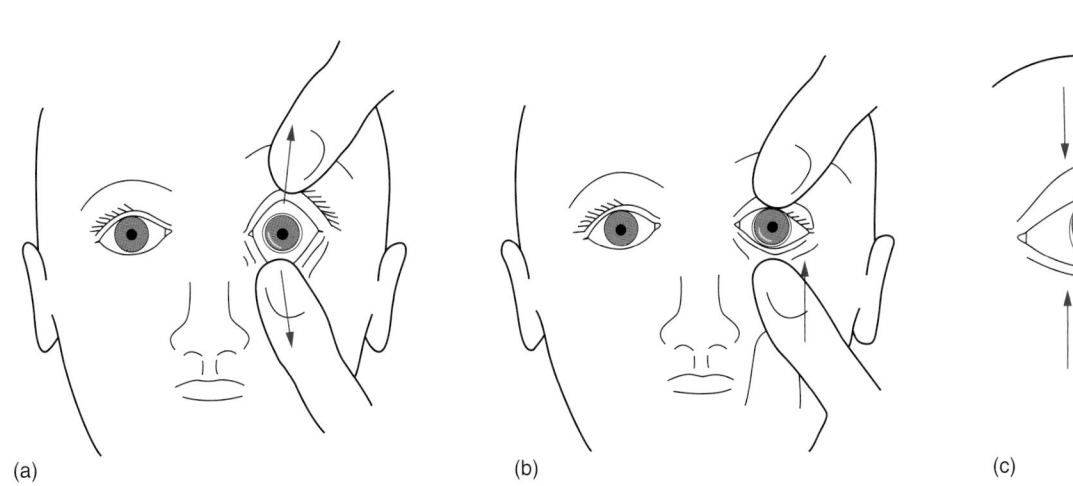

(a)　　　　　　　(b)　　　　　　　(c)

Action Figure 3　Removing hard contact lenses.

Procedure guideline 9.7 Contact lens removal: soft lenses

Essential equipment

- Sterile dressing pack
- Contact lens solution
- Low-linting or lint-free swabs

Optional equipment

- Sterile/non-sterile powder-free gloves

Preprocedure

Action	**Rationale**
1 Explain and discuss the procedure with the patient.	To ensure that the patient understands the procedure and gives their consent (NMC 2008a, C).
2 Wash hands thoroughly using bactericidal soap.	To reduce the risk of cross-infection (Fraise and Bradley 2009, E).

(Continued)

435

Procedure guideline 9.7 *(Continued)*

Procedure

3 Wearing gloves, gently pinch the lens between the thumb and index finger (see Action Figure 3).	To encourage the lens to fold together, allowing air to enter underneath the lens for easy removal. E
4 Store lenses in the appropriate solution as recommended by the manufacturer and ensure lenses are placed in the correct left and right storage pots.	To prevent deterioration and contamination (Stollery *et al.* 2005, E).
5 Refer to manufacturer's instructions for further storage information, particularly if patient will not be using the lenses for a lengthy period of time.	To prevent deterioration and growth of organisms. E
6 Make the patient comfortable.	

Postprocedure

7 Remove and dispose of equipment.	To keep area clean and reduce risk of cross-infection (Fraise and Bradley 2009, E).
8 Wash hands with bactericidal soap and water.	To reduce the risk of cross-infection (Fraise and Bradley 2009, E).
9 Complete the patient's recording chart and other hospital and/or legally required documents.	To maintain accurate records. To provide a point of reference in the event of any queries. To prevent any duplication of treatment (NMC 2009, C).

(a) (b)

Action Figure 3 (a) Moving a soft lens down the interior part of the sclera. (b) Removing a soft lens by pinching it between the pads of the thumb and index finger.

Ear care

Definition

Ear care encompasses the assessment and cleaning of the ears, including the instillation of prescribed ear drops. The monitoring and maintenance of hearing and patient education are also included.

Anatomy and physiology

The ears capture sounds for hearing and maintain balance for equilibrium (Nigam and Knight 2008). The ear has three parts: external, middle and inner (Figure 9.6).

External ear

The external ear is a protective funnel made up of the cartilaginous pinna and external acoustic canal and the eardrum

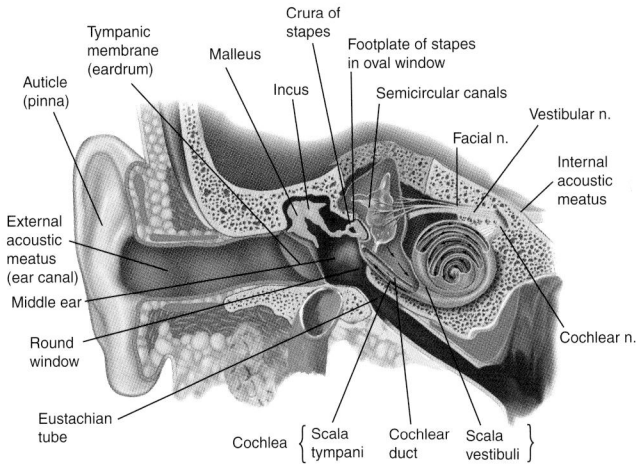

Figure 9.6 Internal structure of the ear.

(Figure 9.6). The external acoustic canal is lined with small hairs and next to it lie the ceruminous glands which produce cerumen or ear wax. The amalgamation of cerumen and hairs prevents foreign objects from entering the ear. As the cerumen dries, it usually falls out of the ear canal but in some circumstances the wax can become impacted (Tortora and Derrickson 2009).

The pinna collects sound waves and delivers them via the external acoustic canal to the tympanic membrane or eardrum which vibrates in harmony (Nigam and Knight 2008, Richardson 2007). The eardrum separates the external and middle ear; it has a slight cone shape and the pointed end sits within the inner ear to assist the funnelling of sounds.

Middle ear

The middle ear is an air-filled chamber. It contains the three smallest bones in the body, the malleus, incus and stapes, collectively known as the auditory ossicles. To one side, it has a thin bony partition that holds two small membrane-covered apertures which are the oval and round windows (Tortora and Derrickson 2009). The auditory ossicles receive vibrations from the tympanic membrane. Vibrations are passed on to the oval window and through to the cochlea in the inner ear; within this process the sound waves are magnified (Alexander *et al.* 2007, Richardson 2007).

At the bottom of the chamber lies the eustachian tube which connects to the nasopharynx and regulates the pressure in the ear. It is usually closed but yawning or swallowing briefly opens it, allowing air to enter or leave until the pressure in the middle ear equalizes to that of external air pressure (Richardson 2007). When the pressures are equalized, the tympanic membrane vibrates freely as the sound waves hit it. However, if the pressures are not balanced, the individual may experience pain, hearing impairment, tinnitius and vertigo (Tortora and Derrickson 2009).

Inner ear

The inner ear is very small and includes the organ of Corti, which is situated inside the snail-shaped cochlea, the three semi-circular canals and vestibular apparatus (see Figure 9.6).

The organ of Corti is the organ for hearing. It is fluid-filled and has a membranous layer that connects to the end of the auditory nerve; the membrane is covered in tiny cells with hair-like projections (Alexander *et al.* 2007). Sound waves travel through the fluid and are distributed to the hair cells. At this point the sound waves change to impulses which pass along the auditory nerve to the brainstem and cortex, where they are interpreted as sound.

The semi-circular canals and vestibular apparatus maintain balance. These canals are highly sensitive; they contain fluid and hair cells that recognize when the head moves and send signals to the brain to maintain equilibrium. The brain interprets these messages along with visual input from the eyes (Nigam and Knight 2008). Adjustments to the muscles and joints are made in response to the information received (Tortora and Derrickson 2009).

If the inner ear structures are damaged, the patient may develop permanent vertigo or hearing loss (Pullen 2006).

Ear wax impaction

Ear wax (cerumen) is a waxy secretion of glands within the auditory canal, combined with skin scales and hair. Ear wax impaction is the biggest cause of ear problems; thousands of people in the UK have ear wax removed every week (Aung and Mulley 2002) (Box 9.6).

The symptoms of ear wax impaction are:

- dull hearing
- tinnitus
- disturbed balance (Alexander *et al.* 2007).

Related theory

Hearing is important for effective communication and balance and these can be affected by poor ear hygiene; for example, using cotton buds to clean the ears can result in ear wax impaction.

Hearing loss can develop over time and become less noticeable to the individual and those close to them, as they

---

Box 9.6 Individuals prone to ear wax impaction

- Older people.
- Those with learning disabilities.
- Narrow ear canals.
- Hearing aid users.
- Those with a hereditary history.
- Those who use cotton buds to clean the ear as this causes the wax to be pushed further down the canal and can cause injury to the surface of the canal.

(Aung and Mulley 2002, Harkin 2008, Kraszewski 2008)

---

find alternative ways to cope. It is imperative that nurses notice poor communications, such as patients not recalling being spoken to or feeling frustrated when communicating with others, and that they then investigate this (Harkin 2005). Nurses need to be aware of how ear problems occur so they are able to explore these with patients and their relatives, to identify problems early and provide appropriate patient education. All findings should be documented and handed over to the patient's doctor for further investigation such as hearing assessment.

Evidence-based approaches

After bathing or showering, the outer ear should be dried with tissue or alcohol-free wipes; nothing should be put into the ear to dry it (Harkin 2008). The ear canal is self-cleaning through jaw movement and epithelial migration action which moves wax and debris up to the outer ear skin (Harkin 2008).

Rationale
Indications

Ear care may be necessary under the following circumstances.

- To relieve pain and discomfort, including tinnitus.
- To prevent or treat infection.
- To prevent loss of hearing.
- To prevent vertigo.
- To prevent or treat injury.
- To detect disease at an early stage.
- Ear care also includes patient education and health and safety advice.

(Harkin 2008)

Contraindications

Ear care can cause:

- otitis media
- trauma to the external meatus
- tinnitus
- deafness
- perforation of the tympanic membrane.

Special care should be taken to avoid damage to the aural cavity and eardrum.

Principles of care
Assessment

Before proceeding with any form of invasive ear care, it is important to undertake careful examination of the ear, taking note of any discharge, redness or swelling, and the amount and texture of any ear wax present, as this will give an indication of the general health of the ear. A small

amount of wax should be found in the ear canal. Its absence may be a sign of a dry skin condition, infection or excessive cleaning that has interfered with the normal wax production (Harkin 2008).

The nurse should discuss with the patient their current level of hearing and after the procedure they should ask the patient if there are any changes so as to monitor the effectiveness of the intervention.

Consideration should always be given to a patient's hearing aids and assistance given to help clean these. Advice regarding the most appropriate method should be sought, preferably from the patient.

Patient education should be provided when required to help the patient maintain healthy ears, hearing and balance.

Irrigation of the inner ear is sometimes necessary to remove foreign bodies from inside the ear or to clear excessive build-up of ear wax (cerumen) (Harkin 2007).

Methods of ear wax softener use

Due to the invasive nature of ear irrigation, it is advised that the patient first tries using wax softeners such as olive oil, which may avoid the need for irrigation (Kraszewski 2008). A typical treatment regime for ear wax softening is 2–3 drops of olive oil into the ear over a 5-day period (Aung and Mulley 2002).

Methods of ear irrigation

An electric oral jet irrigator fitted with a special ear irrigator tip is recommended for ear irrigation as the water pressure can be controlled more precisely, along with the direction of the water (Aung and Mulley 2002). The water temperature should be 37°; if too hot or cold, it can cause dizziness or vertigo (Aung and Mulley 2002). The traditional method of irrigation uses a metal water-filled, hand-held syringe but due to the high risk of infection and trauma to the ear, this is no longer recommended practice (Harkin 2008).

Ear irrigation is an invasive procedure that requires good understanding of the anatomy and physiology of the ear and competence with the procedure (Kraszewski 2008). The procedure is undertaken to remove impacted wax which can cause:

- some degree of hearing loss
- earache
- itchiness in the ear
- reflex cough
- dizziness
- vertigo
- tinnitus
- hearing impairment, which can cause frustration, stress, social isolation, paranoia and depression.

(Aung and Mulley 2002, p.27)

438

Ear irrigation is not recommended in the following circumstances.

- Perforated eardrums.
- Middle ear infection in the previous 6 weeks.
- Mucus discharge.
- *In situ* grommet.
- Cleft palate.
- Acute otitis externa with pain and tenderness to the pinna.
- History of ear surgery.

(Aung and Mulley 2002, Harkin 2007)

The potential adverse effects of this procedure are:

- perforated eardrums
- otitis externa
- damage to the canal
- pain
- deafness
- vertigo
- tinnitus.

(Aung and Mulley 2002)

If irrigation is unsuccessful, further interventions may be necessary, possibly in the form of removal of the wax under direct vision using suction, forceps or probes (Aung and Mulley 2002).

Preprocedural considerations
Specific patient preparations

The patient and nurse should be sitting at the same height to examine the outer ear and pinna (Harkin 2008). Any alteration to the appearance of the ear must be reported to the doctor. Ask the patient to tilt the ear to be treated up to allow the ear drops to reach the middle and inner ears.

Position of light source

A good light source such as a bull's eye lamp and head mirror or an operating lamp positioned above and behind the nurse is necessary prior to commencing ear care procedures to enable careful assessment of the ears and to avoid damage to the delicate structures (Alexander *et al.* 2007).

Mouth care

Definition

Mouth care is the care given to the oral mucosa, lips, teeth and gums in order to promote health and prevent or treat disease. It involves assessment, correct care and patient education to promote independence (Hahn and Jones 2000). Good oral hygiene is essential as poor oral health can affect a patient's ability to eat or taste food, affect verbal and non-verbal communication, limit self-confidence and desire to interact with others and cause pain and infection, in some cases leading to life-threatening illness (Malkin 2009).

Anatomy and physiology
Structure of the oral cavity

The mouth consists of the vestibule and the oral cavity (Figure 9.7). The vestibule is the space between the lips and cheeks on the outside and the teeth and gingivae (gums) on the inside. The palate forms the roof of the oral cavity with the base of the tongue forming the floor of the mouth. It is bordered by the alveolar arches, teeth and gums at either side (Cooley 2002). The lips and cheeks are formed of skeletal muscle; the inner part of the cheeks is known as the buccal mucosa and consists of columnar epithelium. The lips are involved in speech and facial expression and keep food within the oral cavity. The cheeks control the location of food as the teeth break it down.

Teeth

Teeth are formed of the crown (the visible part) and the root. The crown is covered in enamel, a hard, dense material which cannot repair itself once damaged. Below the enamel cap, the tooth is formed of a bonelike material called dentine. This extends into the root and surrounds the pulp cavity, which contains nerve fibres, blood vessels and connective tissue. When the pulp cavity extends into the root, it is known as the root canal. Teeth are embedded in alveoli (sockets) in the maxilla and mandible and are held in place by periodontal ligaments and a substance known as cementum. Teeth are important in breaking down and grinding food and are also involved in producing sounds in speech (Marieb 2001).

439

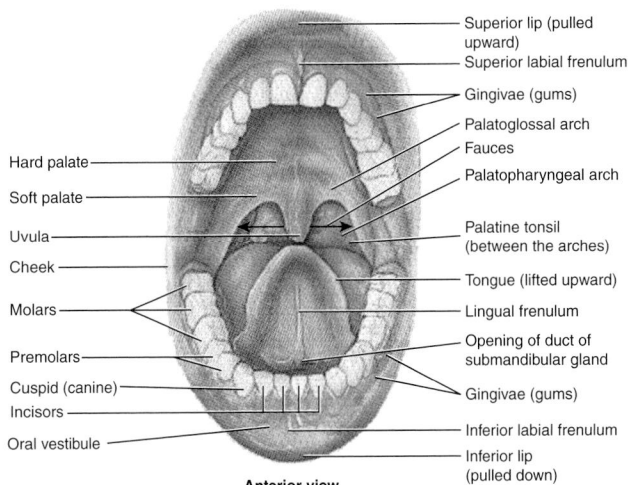

Figure 9.7 Structures of the mouth (oral cavity). Reproduced from Tortora and Derrickson (2009).

Tongue

The tongue is a muscular structure extending from its tip (apex) to the posterior attachment in the oropharynx. It houses taste buds and is involved in taste, forming food into a bolus and pushing it to the back of the mouth for swallowing. It is also involved in the articulation of sounds in speech.

Palate

The palate consists of the hard palate anteriorly and the soft palate which is a muscular structure leading to the palatoglossal arches and the uvula. The hard and soft palates are involved in mastication, swallowing and production of speech (Lockhart and Resick 2006).

Saliva

Saliva is produced by the parotid glands (in front of the ears), which produce saliva rich in amylase, the submandibular glands (in the lower part of the floor of the mouth), which produce mucinous saliva, the sublingual glands (in the floor of the mouth between the side of the tongue and the teeth), producing viscous saliva, and many minor salivary glands throughout the oral cavity (Hahn and Jones 2000). One litre of saliva can be produced daily, consisting of mainly water with electrolytes, amylase, proteins such as mucin, lysozyme and IgA and metabolic wastes (Lockhart and Resick 2006). Saliva is slightly acidic and can act as a buffer. It is also important in mastication, taste and speech. It acts as a defence against infection by physically washing debris off teeth and its proteins also have an antibacterial action (Hahn and Jones 2000).

Related theory
Dental decay

Dental decay begins with the formation of a biofilm known as plaque which is made up of sugar, bacteria and other debris on the teeth. Tooth enamel can be damaged due to bacterial action, resulting in a drop in pH around the tooth. Once there is damage to the enamel then the inner dentine can also decay (Cooley 2002). Areas of decay in teeth are known as caries. Plaque can be physically removed by brushing and flossing teeth. If it is not regularly removed, it can harden to form calculus (tartar) which requires dental treatment for removal. Calculus can also disrupt the seal between the gingiva and the tooth, resulting in red, swollen and bleeding gums (gingivitis). This inflammation can progress to the formation of deep pockets of infection, damaging the teeth and underlying bone (periodontitis) (Marieb 2001). Smoking is known to be a risk factor for periodontitis and other factors such as xerostomia can also increase the risk of such problems.

Box 9.7 Causes of a dry mouth

- Many common drugs can cause dry mouth, including analgesic agents and antidepressants.
- Oxygen, due to its drying effect.
- Mouth breathing.
- Poor appetite.
- Anxiety and depression.
- Radiotherapy to the head and neck can affect the salivary glands; this may be irreversible.
- Chemotherapy, which normally resolves over time
- Diseases such as Sjögren's syndrome.

(Maher 2004)

Xerostomia

Xerostomia is the subjective sensation of dry mouth, which does not always correlate to a reduction in saliva production (Maher 2004). It can be associated with thickened saliva, discomfort which may be burning in nature and difficulty eating or speaking (Davies 2005b). A variety of causes are known (Box 9.7).

Where possible, the cause should be treated; sips of water normally only relieve the problem briefly. Artificial saliva may be helpful and mucin-based salivary substitutes are most effective, available in gel and spray forms. Production of saliva may be stimulated by use of sugar-free chewing gum but acidic sweets should be avoided as they may cause discomfort and increase the risk of dental caries (Davies 2000). Salivary stimulants such as pilocarpine can also be useful. Studies have also demonstrated that acupuncture can be helpful (Davies 2005b).

Patients with xerostomia must pay careful attention to oral hygiene as they are at greatly increased risk of oral complications such as caries and periodontitis due to loss of the protective effect of saliva (Maher 2004).

Oral mucositis

Mucositis is inflammation of the mucous membranes of the oral cavity and gastrointestinal tract (Eilers and Million 2007). The terms 'oral mucositis' and 'stomatitis' refer to inflammation of the oral cavity. Chemotherapy and radiotherapy affect the ability of cells to reproduce and particularly affect areas which have a rapid proliferation rate such as the alimentary tract (Beck 2004). The surface epithelial layer in the oral mucosa is replaced every 7–14 days which means that the oral mucosa is particularly vulnerable to the direct effect of cell death following chemotherapy and subsequent indirect effects of treatment, such as neutropenia and thrombo cytopenia, which can affect healing and vulnerability to infection (Cooley 2002, Otto 2001). The incidence of moderate to severe oral mucositis can be up to 100% in patients receiving radiotherapy to the head and neck (Peterson *et al.* 2009). For patients receiving standard-dose chemotherapy regimens, the incidence varies from 3% to 14% while up to 75% of patients having high-dose chemotherapy as conditioning prior to haematopoietic stem cell transplantation can experience moderate to severe oral mucositis (Peterson *et al.* 2009).

Mucositis is now better understood as a complex process whereby intracellular changes and reactions occur before damage to the mucosa is apparent (Sonis *et al.* 2004). The impact on the patient is that symptoms such as altered sensation or taste and pain may be experienced before there are obvious changes to the mucosa. This can progress to painful lesions or large ulcerated areas. Good nursing care is essential for the patient's well-being and comfort (Eilers and Million 2007). A variety of agents have been used to prevent and treat oral mucositis, with mixed results. Several systematic reviews have been carried out and recommendations formulated (Barasch *et al.* 2006, Clarkson *et al.* 2007a, Keefe *et al.* 2007, Rubenstein *et al.* 2004, Worthington *et al.* 2007).

Evidence-based approaches

Principles of care

The aims of oral care are to:

- keep the oral mucosa and lips clean, soft, moist and intact
- keep natural teeth free from plaque and debris
- maintain denture hygiene and prevent disease related to dentures
- prevent oral infection
- prevent oral discomfort
- maintain the mouth in a state of normal function (Jones 1998).

Box 9.8 lists the recommendations for maintaining oral health.

Within a variety of care settings, patients can find themselves at risk of poor oral health. Patients in particular need of assistance or extra care include those with the following problems.

- Patients who are nil by mouth (including unconscious or ventilated patients).
- Patients who mouth breathe (including those on oxygen therapy or with a nasogastric tube).
- Cancer patients receiving radiotherapy to the head and neck or chemotherapy which can directly affect the oral cavity or result in reduced immunity to infection.
- Patients having oral surgery or who have traumatic injury to the head and neck.
- Older patients.
- Patients with diabetes.
- Patients unable to maintain their own oral hygiene due to physical disability or psychological disorders which could affect motivation.

Box 9.8 Factors that maintain good oral health

- Eating a healthy diet, particularly limiting sugary foods and drinks to reduce the build-up of plaque (this includes sugar-containing medicines).
- Stop smoking; it is known to increase the risk of gum disease and oral cancers.
- Limit alcohol consumption; high intake is a known risk factor for oral cancers.
- Have regular dental check-ups.
- Brush teeth for 2 minutes at least twice daily with a fluoride toothpaste and use floss or an interdental brush to clean areas that are hard to reach.
- Look for signs of oral disease; consult a dentist if anything unusual is seen.
- Take care in activities such as contact sports where facial injuries can occur.

(DH 2005)

- Patients with clotting disorders.
- Patients taking medication which have dry mouth or gum overgrowth as side-effects.

(Potter and Griffin Perry 2003)

There is a variety of evidence available to support practice, ranging from Cochrane reviews to expert opinion. At the very least, each patient should have a thorough assessment of the oral cavity.

Legal and professional issues

Nurses should provide a high standard of care to patients, based on the best evidence available, ensuring they have the necessary skills (NMC 2008b). Numerous studies have found that nurses feel they lack knowledge and training about providing oral care (Southern 2007). Although a number of training tools are available, the provision of adequate training before and after registration requires further attention (Doyle and Dalton 2008, NHSQIS 2004). As is the case for all procedures, a full explanation must be given to the patient and consent obtained (NMC 2008a).

Preprocedural considerations

Equipment

Toothbrush

The toothbrush is recognized as being the most effective means of removing plaque and debris from the teeth and gums. A small-headed, medium-textured brush is most effective at reaching all areas of the mouth. A gentle scrubbing action is recommended, using small movements with gentle

441

pressure for 2 minutes (Sweeney 2005). The brush should be placed at a 45° angle against the teeth and overlaying the gum edge to allow cleaning of the gingival margin (Jones 1998). Powered toothbrushes have been shown to be as effective as manual toothbrushes and may be easier for patients with limited dexterity to use (Robinson *et al.* 2005). Aids such as foam handles can also be obtained from the occupational therapist to make a manual toothbrush easier to hold. The toothbrush should be allowed to air dry to reduce bacterial contamination and changed every 3 months or sooner if worn (Hahn and Jones 2000). For patients with a sore mouth, a soft or baby toothbrush can be used. A pea-sized amount of fluoride toothpaste should be used; fluoride is known to have an anti-caries activity and can reduce dentine sensitivity. If toothpaste is too abrasive for a patient whose mouth is painful, water alone can be used (Sweeney 2005).

Foam sticks

The foam stick is one of the most common pieces of equipment used in hospital to provide oral care although it is well known that less plaque is removed than with a toothbrush, particularly from less obvious areas of the teeth (Pearson and Hutton 2002). The foam stick should only be used on patients who cannot tolerate use of a toothbrush, such as those with painful or bleeding mouths. Foam sticks can be used with chlorhexidine rather than plain water for an antibacterial effect (Huskinson and Lloyd 2009). Care should be taken that the foam head is securely attached to avoid risk of accidental aspiration (Malkin 2009).

Interdental cleaning

The use of dental floss or other equipment is recommended to clean areas between the teeth which may be difficult to reach with a toothbrush (Huskinson and Lloyd 2009). There is currently limited evidence of the efficacy of flossing although it is generally believed to be beneficial (Berchier *et al.* 2008). A variety of equipment is available such as dental floss, dental tape, wood sticks or interdental brushes. For patients who have limited dexterity, this may be difficult or impossible to carry out. Similarly, in patients with painful mouths or bleeding gums, this type of equipment could cause further discomfort or bleeding and should be avoided.

Oral irrigation devices such as the WaterPik® can also be used for interdental cleaning. Oral irrigation involves a jet of water being used to remove debris and plaque and can be useful for people who find it difficult to use dental floss or tape such as those with braces. A systematic review of oral irrigation has shown a positive tendency but no overall benefit in reducing plaque over use of a toothbrush alone (Husseini *et al.* 2008).

Assessment and recording tools

The mouth should be assessed as part of the initial nursing assessment and should be reassessed regularly thereafter (DH 2001, NHSQIS 2004). Frequency of assessment is often based on clinical judgement rather than evidence.

For patients at high risk of changes to the condition of the mouth, such as those receiving high-dose chemotherapy, assessment should be carried out daily (Quinn *et al.* 2008). For elderly patients receiving long-term care, it has been recommended that reassessment takes place monthly (NHSQIS 2004). For certain patients, such as those receiving high-dose chemotherapy or radiotherapy to the head and neck, an assessment by a dentist is recommended prior to starting treatment.

The use of an oral assessment tool is recommended to ensure consistency between assessors and to monitor changes. A number of tools have been devised for different patient groups. Tools such as the WHO scale (WHO 1979) or the Oral Assessment Guide (OAG) (Eilers *et al.* 1988) are commonly used in assessing patients receiving anticancer treatments. Numerous other tools exist to assess oral mucositis, although some lack evidence of validity and reliability. Use of a validated tool is recommended (DH 2001). Several tools have also been designed to meet the needs of elderly patients and those with dementia (Kayser-Jones *et al.* 1995, Roberts 2001). The ideal assessment tool should measure:

- functional changes, for example ability to talk or eat
- physical changes, for example presence of ulcerated areas
- subjective changes, for example pain or dryness.

The ideal tool has not yet been developed and it may be necessary to use a combination of tools to make a thorough assessment. Patient education to encourage self-assessment is also recommended (Quinn *et al.* 2008).

Good assessment is vital before a care plan can be formulated. Assessment should include visual inspection and obtaining a history from the patient. Many factors should be considered when carrying out a full oral assessment (Box 9.9).

Inspection should be undertaken in good light, gloves should be worn, a pen torch should be available, and any

---

Box 9.9 Factors to consider when carrying out an oral assessment

- Usual oral hygiene practice and frequency.
- Regularity of dental visits.
- Oral discomfort or pain.
- Dry mouth.
- Difficulty chewing.
- Difficulty swallowing.
- Difficulty speaking.
- Halitosis (malodorous breath).
- Drooling.
- Presence of dentures and normal care routine.
- Current or past dental problems.
- Other risk factors, for example diabetes, steroid treatment, smoking, alcohol intake, altered nutritional status.

(Davies 2005a, Malkin 2009)

dentures or plates should be removed. It is helpful to have a set order in which areas are examined so nothing is missed. The following areas should be inspected.

- *The lips*: are they dry, cracked or bleeding?
- *The upper and lower labial sulci (inner part of the lip towards the vestibule)*: the lip should be retracted with a gloved finger or tongue depressor.
- *The buccal mucosa on the right and left sides*: is it intact, soft, moist, coated, ulcerated or inflamed?
- *The dorsal surface of the tongue (ask the patient to stick out the tongue)*: is it dry, coated or ulcerated?
- *The ventral surface of the tongue (ask the patient to lift the tongue up and move it from side to side)*: can the patient move it normally?
- *The floor of the mouth should also be inspected*: is the normal saliva pool present, is the saliva watery?
- *The hard and soft palate*: are they intact, ulcerated or red?
- *The gums*: are they inflamed or bleeding?
- *The teeth*: are they present, cared for, loose or stained, is debris present?

(Davies 2005a, Hahn and Jones 2000)

Pharmacological support

The choice of an oral care agent will be dependent on the aim of care. The agent may be used to remove debris and plaque, prevent superimposed infection, alleviate pain, provide comfort, stop bleeding, provide lubrication or treat specific problems (Dickinson and Porter 2006). A wide variety of agents are available and choice should be determined by the individual needs of the patient and the particular clinical situation together with a detailed nursing assessment. There is ongoing debate on the efficacy of agents presently available and there remains insufficient evidence to clearly state the best agents to use in the clinical setting.

Chlorhexidine gluconate

Chlorhexidine gluconate is an effective antibacterial and antiplaque agent. For the patient who is unable to use a toothbrush, it can provide a chemical method of stopping plaque build-up. As chlorhexidine is released from tissues for up to 12 hours, it only needs to be used twice daily. Chlorhexidine does not remove plaque which is already present so brushing of teeth should continue as far as possible (Sweeney 2005). It is also available as a gel formulation which may be useful for those requiring a non-foaming alternative to toothpaste (patients at risk of aspiration or with swallowing difficulties). Chlorhexidine has not been shown to be effective in preventing oral mucositis in patients with head and neck cancers undergoing radiotherapy or in treating oral mucositis in patients receiving chemotherapy although it may be used as part of an oral protocol for its antiplaque and antibacterial action (Barasch *et al.* 2006, Rubenstein *et al.* 2004).

Artificial saliva

Saliva substitutes which are mucin based are more effective than those which are carboxymethylcellulose based for relieving dry mouth (xerostomia) (Davies 2005b). Recommendations are to use several sprays around the mouth, to use the tongue to spread the artificial saliva around the mouth and to use it at least prior to meals and at any other time when the mouth feels dry (Davies 2000).

Coating agents

Several agents have been used to coat the oral mucosa and they are thought to have a protective effect although there is limited evidence to support their use. Sucralfate has not been shown to be effective in preventing or treating chemotherapy- or radiotherapy-associated oral mucositis (Clarkson *et al.* 2007a, Worthington *et al.* 2007a).

Other agents

Several other treatments have been found to be useful in prevention of oral mucositis related to chemotherapy. Palifermin is a recombinant form of human keratinocyte growth factor which stimulates cell growth in the alimentary tract. In trials it has been found to have an effect in preventing oral mucositis in haemato-oncology patients having high-dose chemotherapy and total body irradiation with autologous stem cell transplantation and its use is recommended by the Multinational Association of Supportive Care in Cancer and the International Society for Oral Oncology (MASCC/ISOO) (Keefe *et al.* 2007).

The use of oral cryotherapy, in which ice chips are placed in the mouth during the administration of chemotherapy and for up to 30 minutes afterwards, is recommended for patients receiving 5-fluorouracil and edatrexate chemotherapy (Rubenstein *et al.* 2004). Oral cryotherapy for an hour is recommended for patients receiving high-dose melphalan as it can reduce the severity of mucositis (Keefe *et al.* 2007). Cryotherapy is thought to work by causing vasoconstriction, resulting in reduced delivery of the chemotherapy agent to the tissues in the mouth. Whilst it is a simple procedure, it can be uncomfortable for patients who may be unable to tolerate it for long periods and is only effective for chemotherapy drugs with a short half-life (Aisa *et al.* 2005).

Other agents for which there is limited evidence include allopurinol, benzydamine mouthwash, used to prevent oral mucositis in patients undergoing head and neck radiotherapy, and calcium phosphate mouthwash (Keefe *et al.* 2007, Worthington *et al.* 2007a).

Analgesic agents

For patients with oral mucositis, it is unclear if analgesic agents used topically are effective. There is evidence that systemic opioids are effective, and both continuous infusion and patient-controlled analgesia (PCA) using morphine

443

have been used in patients receiving high-dose chemotherapy and stem cell transplantation. Patients using PCA have been found to use less opioid in total (Clarkson *et al.* 2007a, Rubenstein *et al.* 2004).

Antifungal agents

Colonization of the mouth with yeast occurs in one-third of the population. In patients receiving steroids or antibiotics, the balance of oral flora can be altered and oral candidosis can occur. Predisposing factors also include xerostomia and the presence of dentures. Topical treatment is normally effective using an antifungal oral suspension or lozenges (Finlay and Davies 2005). In patients having anticancer treatment, the use of prophylactic topical antifungal treatments has been investigated. These have not been shown to be useful in preventing oral *Candida* and partly or fully absorbed antifungal agents such as fluconazole or miconazole are recommended (Clarkson *et al.* 2007b).

Contraindicated agents

A number of agents widely used in the past have been found to have detrimental effects and are no longer recommended. Glycerine and lemon swabs have been used for dry mouth but the acid content can damage tooth enamel and the overall effect is to increase oral dryness (Hahn and Jones 2000). Hydrogen peroxide is also not recommended as it can cause mucosal abnormalities (Berry *et al.* 2007).

Non-pharmacological support
Fluoride

Fluoride helps to prevent and arrest tooth decay, especially radiation caries, demineralization and decalcification. High-dose fluoride toothpaste may be recommended for patients with xerostomia (NHSQIS 2004).

Commercial mouthwash

Over-the-counter mouthwashes are not generally recommended. Many have a high alcohol content which can cause stinging, particularly for patients with sensitive mouths (Milligan *et al.* 2001).

Bland rinses

Several agents have been used to rinse the mouth, moisten the mucosa and loosen and remove debris. Normal saline has been recommended by a number of authors as part of a patient's oral care. This relatively cheap and generally well-tolerated solution can alleviate discomfort although it is not effective at removing heavy amounts of debris (Milligan *et al.* 2001). Patients with mucositis can benefit from frequent rinsing of the mouth with warm normal saline to remove debris without causing irritation (Meechan 2005). The use of water has also been suggested to rinse the mouth after meals to

remove debris (Sweeney 2005). Its use in critical care has been discouraged due to risk of infection in vulnerable patients, but sterile water may be an alternative (Berry *et al.* 2007). Sodium bicarbonate has been used in some centres although there is some evidence that patients find it unpleasant to taste and that it can alter pH in the mouth, predisposing to bacterial growth (Wood 2004).

Specific patient preparations
Patients with dentures

Patients with dentures should be encouraged or assisted to remove and clean the denture at least daily. The denture should be cleaned over a towel or a water-filled sink to reduce the risk of damage if it is dropped. It should be brushed with a large toothbrush, denture brush or personal nailbrush and soap and water or denture cleaner. It should be rinsed with water before being replaced in the mouth. Denture wearers are at risk of fungal infections developing under the denture and spreading to the hard palate and should be advised to remove and soak the denture ideally overnight or at least for 1 hour. The denture should be soaked in a solution of dilute sodium hypochlorite (1 part Milton® to 80 parts water). If the denture has metal parts or if infection is present, chlorhexidine 0.2% can be used to disinfect the denture (Sweeney 2005). The denture should be rinsed well before reinsertion. It should be marked with the wearer's name and the storage container should also be marked and should be either disposable or able to be sterilized (Chalmers and Pearson 2005). Denture wearers should also clean any remaining teeth and the gums and tongue with a soft toothbrush and fluoride toothpaste. They should also have regular dental check-ups as ill-fitting dentures can cause ulcers or irritation (Clay 2000, Duffin 2008).

Patients needing assistance

A variety of patient groups may need assistance. Patients with mental illness or learning disabilities may need encouragement or assistance to maintain their oral hygiene (Doyle and Dalton 2008, Griffiths *et al.* 2000). Patients with conditions affecting mobility, sight or dexterity may find it difficult to carry out oral hygiene without assistance. Practical aids such as using a mirror and sitting down rather than standing can aid independence. Use of a foam handle aid to make the toothbrush easier to hold or a pump action toothpaste can also help (Holman *et al.* 2005). Privacy is essential to maintain the patient's dignity. Older patients may be at risk of oral problems due to a natural decline in salivary gland function, wear and tear of teeth, and taking medication with side-effects which can cause oral problems such as dry mouth, taste changes or increased risk of infection (Chalmers and Pearson 2005, Clay 2000, Fitzpatrick 2000). Regular assessment and assistance with maintaining oral hygiene are recommended (NHSQIS 2004). For the patient who needs assistance, it is recommended that the carer stands behind or to the side of the patient and supports the lower jaw (Sweeney 2005).

Unconscious patients

Unconscious patients require particular interventions to maintain oral hygiene and comfort. For patients who are close to death, there is a lack of evidence relating to oral care and the focus should be on patient comfort. Any interventions causing distress should be stopped; mouthcare can be offered 1–2 hourly but should be decided based on the individual's needs (Sweeney 2005). Gentle cleaning with a soft toothbrush or foam stick is recommended and a lubricant should be applied to the lips (Dahlin 2004). In critically ill patients who are unconscious and requiring mechanical ventilation, management is different (Box 9.10).

It is well known that aspiration of oropharyngeal flora can cause bacterial pneumonia (Li *et al*. 2000). Ventilator-associated pneumonia (VAP) is a serious complication which can occur in up to a quarter of ventilated patients and has a mortality of up to 50% (Berry *et al*. 2007). In critically ill patients the mouth can become colonized within 48 hours of admission to hospital with bacteria that tend to be more virulent than those normally found in the mouth (Grap *et al*. 2003). The oropharynx can become colonized, as can an artificial airway. This can allow pathogens to travel to the respiratory tract, resulting in pneumonia (Cutler and Davis

---

Box 9.10 Recommendations for oral care in critically ill patients

- Daily assessment.
- Oral care 2–4 hourly.
- Brushing with a small-headed soft toothbrush and fluoride toothpaste.
- Cleaning the mouth with foam sticks and chlorhexidine mouthwash or gel for patients for whom a toothbrush would be unsuitable, for example bleeding, severe ulcers.
- Use of suction to prevent aspiration.

(Abidia 2007, Stiefel *et al*. 2000)

2005). It is well recognized that good oral care is essential in critically ill patients to reduce the incidence of VAP. Other contributing factors to poor oral health in this group of patients include dry mouth related to use of oxygen, mouth breathing and the patient being nil by mouth. The presence of tubes or securing tapes can make it difficult to view and clean the oral cavity.

Further research is needed in this area as there is a lack of trial-based evidence to support practice (Munro and Grap 2004).

Procedure guideline 9.8 Mouth care

Essential equipment

- Small torch
- Plastic cups
- Mouthwash or cleaning solutions
- Appropriate equipment for cleaning
- Clean receiver or bowl
- Paper tissues/gauze

- Wooden spatula
- Small-headed, soft toothbrush
- Toothpaste
- Non-sterile disposable gloves
- Denture pot

Preprocedure

Action	Rationale
1 Explain and discuss the procedure with the patient. When possible, encourage patients to carry out their own oral care.	To ensure that the patient understands the procedure and gives their valid consent (NMC 2008a, C). To enable patients to gain confidence in managing their own symptom management (DH 2005, C).
2 Wash hands with bactericidal soap and water and dry with paper towel or use alcohol handrub. Put on disposable gloves.	To reduce the risk of cross-infection (Fraise and Bradley 2009, E).

Procedure

3 Prepare solutions required.	Solutions must always be prepared immediately before use to maximize their efficacy and minimize the risk of microbial contamination (Fraise and Bradley 2009, E).

(Continued)

Procedure guideline 9.8 *(Continued)*

4 If the patient cannot remove their own dentures, remove the lower denture first.	The lower denture should be removed first to avoid the risk of aspiration (Sweeney 2005, R5).
(a) *Lower denture*: grasp it in the middle and lift it, rotating it gently to remove from the mouth, and place in denture pot.	
(b) *Upper denture*: remove the upper denture by grasping firmly in the middle and tilting the denture forward while putting pressure on the front teeth to break the seal with the palate. Rotate the denture from side to side to remove it from the mouth and place in denture pot.	Removal of dentures is necessary for cleaning of underlying tissues (Sweeney 2005, R5).
5 Carry out oral assessment using an oral assessment tool.	Provides baseline to enable monitoring of mucosal changes and evaluate response to treatment and care (Eilers *et al.* 1988, R5; Sonis *et al.* 2004, R5).
6 Inspect the patient's mouth, including teeth, with the aid of a torch, spatula and gauze, paying special attention to the lips, buccal mucosa, lateral and ventral surfaces of the tongue, floor of the mouth and the soft palate. Ask the patient if they have any of the following: taste changes, change in saliva production and composition, oral discomfort or difficulty swallowing.	The mouth is examined for changes in condition with respect to moisture, cleanliness, infected or bleeding areas, ulcers, and so on. These areas are known to be more susceptible to cytoxic damage (Sonis *et al.* 2004, R5). To assess nutritional deficits, salivary changes and pain secondary to oral changes (Sonis *et al.* 2004, R5).
7 Using a soft, small toothbrush and toothpaste (or foam stick if the gingiva is damaged or susceptible to bleeding), brush the patient's natural teeth, gums and tongue. Stand behind or to the side of the patient and support the lower jaw with your free hand.	To remove adherent materials from the teeth, tongue and gum surfaces (Beck 2004, E). Brushing stimulates gingival tissues to maintain tone and prevent circulatory stasis (Clay 2000, E; Pearson and Hutton 2002, R1b). Foam stick reduces possibility of trauma (Cooley 2002, E).
8 Hold the brush against the teeth with the bristles at a 45° angle. The tips of the outer bristles should rest against and penetrate under the gingival sulcus. Then move the bristles back and forth using horizontal or circular strokes and a vibrating motion (bass sulcular technique), from the sulcus to the crowns of the teeth. Repeat until all teeth surfaces have been cleaned. Clean the biting surfaces by moving the toothbrush back and forth over them in short strokes and brush tongue to remove any debris.	Brushing loosens and removes debris trapped on and between the teeth and gums (DH 2005, C). This reduces the growth medium for pathogenic organisms and minimizes the risk of plaque formation and dental caries (Beck 2004, E; Clay 2000, E; Pearson and Hutton 2002, R1b). Foam sticks are ineffective for this (Beck 2004, E).
9 Give a beaker of water to the patient. Encourage patient to rinse the mouth vigorously then void contents into a receiver. Paper tissues should be to hand to dry any spillage of water.	Rinsing removes loosened debris and toothpaste and makes the mouth taste fresher (Beck 2004, E).
10 If the patient is unable to rinse and void, use a rinsed toothbrush to clean the teeth and moistened foam sticks to wipe the gums and oral mucosa. Foam sticks should be used with a rotating action so that most of the surface is utilized.	To remove debris as effectively as possible (Beck 2004, E; Sonis *et al.* 2004, R5).
11 Apply several sprays of artificial saliva to the mouth if appropriate and/or suitable lubricant to dry lips.	To increase the patient's feeling of comfort and well-being and prevent further tissue damage (Davies 2000, R1b).

446

12 Clean the patient's dentures on all surfaces with a denture brush or toothbrush and soap and water or denture cleaner. Check the dentures for cracks, sharp edges and missing teeth. Rinse them well and return them to the patient.	Cleaning dentures removes accumulated food debris which could be broken down by salivary enzymes to products which irritate and cause inflammation of the adjacent mucosal tissue (Sweeney 2005, R5).
13 Dentures should be removed for at least 1 hour but ideally overnight and placed in a suitable cleaning solution.	Dentures can easily become colonized by bacteria. Soaking can disinfect the denture, discouraging bacterial growth (Clay 2000, E; Sweeney 2005, R2b).
14 Floss teeth (unless contraindicated, for example clotting abnormality, thrombocytopenia) once in 24 hours using lightly waxed floss. To floss the upper teeth, use your thumb and index finger to stretch the floss and wrap one end of floss around the third finger of each hand. Move the floss up and down between the teeth from the tops of the crowns to the gum and along the gum lines wherever possible. To floss the lower teeth, use the index fingers to stretch the floss.	Flossing helps to remove debris between teeth. Flossing when patient has abnormal clotting or low platelets may lead to bleeding and predispose the oral mucosa to infection (Clay 2000, E; Beck 2004, E).
15 Discard remaining mouthwash solutions.	To prevent infection (Fraise and Bradley 2009, E).
16 Clean the toothbrush and allow it to air dry.	To prevent the risk of contamination (Jones 1998, E).

Postprocedure

17 Ensure the patient is comfortable.	
18 Wash hands with soap and water and dry with paper towel or use alcohol handrub.	To reduce the risk of cross-infection (Fraise and Bradley 2009, E).

Problem-solving table 9.1 Prevention and resolution (Procedure guideline 9.8)

Problem	Cause	Prevention	Action
Dry mouth (xerostomia)	Oxygen therapy, mouth breathing, nil by mouth	Humidified oxygen	Swabbing the mouth with moistened foam stick or encouraging the patient to rinse the mouth with water and spit it out
Dry mouth (xerostomia)	Salivary gland hypofunction due to disease, drugs or side-effects of radiotherapy or chemotherapy	Not always possible to prevent	Good oral hygiene to prevent complications, use of salivary stimulants, for example chewing gum, pilocarpine or saliva substitutes
Patient unable to tolerate toothbrush	Pain, for example post surgery. Mucositis	Consider anaesthetic mouth spray or mouthwash before mouth care. Give regular and/or prn analgesia	Use foam sticks and chlorhexidine 0.2% to clean the patient's teeth, gums and mucosa; 0.9% sodium chloride rinse can be used if the patient cannot tolerate any form of oral care
Toothbrush inappropriate or ineffective	Infected stomatis. Accumulation of dried mucus, new lesions, blood or debris	As above	As above and take a swab of any infected areas for culture before giving mouth care

Pain

Pain is a universal human experience. It is the third most common reason why people visit their General Practitioner. Treating the disease or condition that causes pain often resolves the problem. However, on other occasions treatment is not totally successful (e.g. diabetic neuropathy) and sometimes the cause of the pain is not entirely clear (e.g. pain following surgery, low back pain). Pain then persists.

Chronic pain is defined as an unpleasant sensory and emotional experience associated with actual or potential tissue damage, or described in terms of such damage. Statistics show that nearly one in seven people suffer from chronic pain and 20% have suffered for more than 20 years. It is hardly surprising that people suffering from chronic pain consult their doctor up to five times more frequently than others and that this results in nearly 5 million GP appointments a year.

Two-thirds of chronic pain sufferers surveyed in the UK reported inadequate pain control with only 16% saying they had seen a pain specialist. Despite the fact that many patients want more effective management and better understanding of their pain, 70% were very satisfied with the doctor who treats their pain.

(British Pain Society and Royal College of Physicians 2004)

Definition

Pain is difficult to define due to the complexity of its anatomical and physiological foundations, the experience and perceptions of each individual person and the social and cultural meanings of pain (Paz and Seymour 2008). It is not a simple sensation but a complex phenomenon, having both a physical and an affective (emotional) component. To reflect this, the International Association for the Study of Pain (IASP) (1994) published the following definition of pain: 'An unpleasant sensory and emotional experience associated with actual or potential tissue damage, or described in terms of such damage'. Pain is subjective and another favoured definition for use in clinical practice, proposed originally by McCaffrey (1968) and cited in McCaffrey (2000, p.2), is: 'Pain is whatever the experiencing person says it is, existing whenever the experiencing person says it does'.

Related theory

Many factors influence the expression of pain and may be associated with the patient, the nurse or the clinical environment (organizational aspects) (Carr and Mann 2000). Pain can have many dimensions including physical, psychological, spiritual and sociocultural.

There are several ways to categorize the types of pain that occur, for example, acute or chronic, nociceptive (somatic or visceral) or neuropathic. It is increasingly recognized that acute and chronic pain may represent a continuum rather than being distinct separate entities (Macintyre *et al.* 2010) and may combine different pain mechanisms and vary in duration.

Acute pain

The IASP has defined acute pain as: 'Pain of recent onset and probable limited duration. It usually has an identifiable temporal and causal relationship to injury or disease' (Ready and Edwards 1992, p.1). Acute pain is produced by a wide range of physiological processes, and includes inflammatory, neuropathic, sympathetically maintained, visceral and cancer pain (Walker *et al.* 2006). Acute pain serves a purpose by alerting the individual to a problem and acting as a warning of tissue damage or potential tissue damage. If left untreated, it may result in severe consequences; for example, not seeking help for acute abdominal pain may result in emergency care such as appendicitis progressing to peritonitis. Acute pain is short-term pain of less than 12 weeks' duration (British Pain Society 2008). It occurs in response to any type of injury to the body and resolves when the injury heals.

Chronic pain

Chronic pain is usually prolonged and defined as pain that exists for more than 3 months, lasting beyond the usual course of the acute disease or expected time of healing (IASP 1996). It is often associated with major changes in personality, lifestyle and functional ability (Foley 2004). Chronic pain occurs as a result of both cancer and non-malignant chronic conditions such as neuropathic, musculoskeletal and chronic postoperative pain syndromes.

The term 'breakthrough pain' is widely used. Within the medical literature, other terms are used in the description of breakthrough pain including episodic pain, exacerbation of pain, pain flare, transient pain and transitory pain (Colleau 1999).

The ethos of this section will be based on acute and chronic pain management in cancer and palliative care patients. Many of the principles are transferable to other pain situations.

Anatomy and physiology

Pain mechanisms (anatomy and physiology) are usually described in terms of nociceptive pain or neuropathic pain. As with acute and chronic pain, it may be common for pain to be both nociceptive and neuropathic in origin rather than purely one or the other.

448

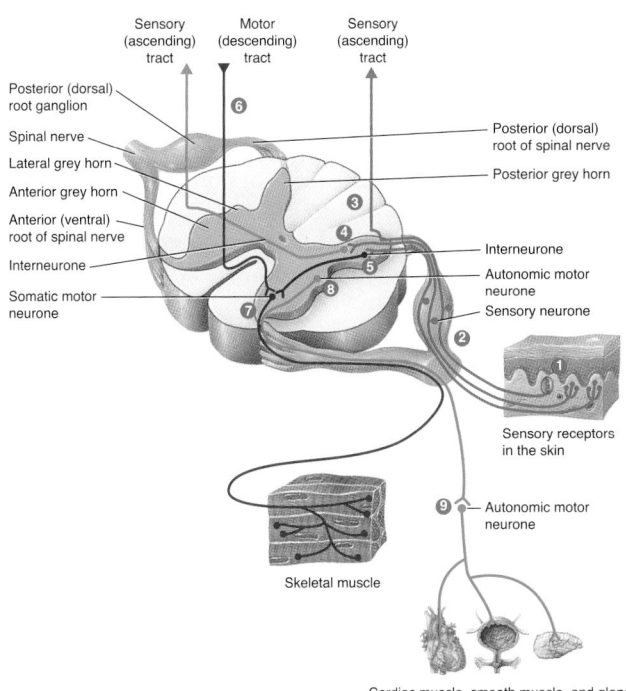

Figure 9.8 Processing of sensory input and motor output by the spinal cord. Reproduced from Tortora and Derrickson (2009).

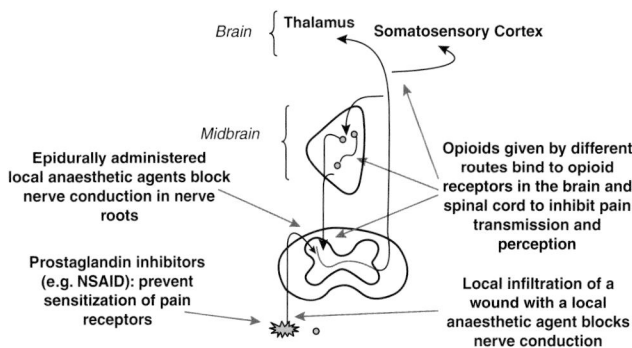

Figure 9.9 The pain pathway showing key sites for particular analgesic interventions.

Nociceptive pain

Nociceptive pain is the 'normal' pain pathway that occurs in response to tissue injury or damage (Figure 9.8). It consists of four components: transduction, transmission, perception and modulation. Nociceptors are free nerve endings found at the end of pain neurones. They are found in skin and subcutaneous tissue, muscle, visceral organs, tendons, fascia, joint capsules and arterial walls (Godfrey 2005). Nociceptors respond to noxious thermal stimuli (heat and cold) and mechanical stimuli (stretching, compression, infiltration) and to the chemical mediators released as part of the inflammatory response to tissue injury. These chemical mediators include prostaglandins, bradykinin, substance P, serotonin and adenosine. As a result of this stimulation process, an action potential is generated in the nerve (*transduction*).

The pain signal is then transmitted along the peripheral nervous system (A delta and C fibres) to the central nervous system, arriving at the dorsal horn of the spinal cord. Neurotransmitters are released to allow the pain signal to be transmitted from the endings of the peripheral nerves to the nociceptors in the dorsal horn. The message is then transmitted to the brain where perception of the pain occurs (*transmission*). *Perception* is the end-result of the neuronal activity of pain transmission. The perception of pain includes behavioural, psychological and emotional components as well as physiological processes.

Modulation occurs when the transmission of pain impulses in the spinal cord is changed or inhibited. Modulatory influences on pain perception are complex, involving a gat-

ing system which is linked to a descending modulatory pathway. Modulation can occur as a result of a natural release of inhibitory neurotransmitter chemicals that inhibit transmission of pain impulses and therefore produce analgesia. Other interventions, including distraction, relaxation, sense of well-being, heat/cold therapy, massage and TENS, can also help to modulate pain perception. Analgesic medications work by inhibiting some of the chemicals involved in pain transduction and transmission and thus modulating pain perception (Figure 9.9). Pain signals can also be increased by certain factors such as anxiety, fear and low mood/depression.

Neuropathic pain

Neuropathic pain is not pain that originates as part of 'normal' pain pathways. It has been described as pain related to abnormal processing within the nervous system (Mann 2008). Nerve injury or dysfunction can be caused by a range of conditions such as infection, trauma, metabolic disorder, chemotherapy, surgery, radiation, neurotoxins, nerve compression, joint degeneration, tumour infiltration and malnutrition (Mann 2008).

The mechanisms by which neuropathic pain is generated and maintained are not fully understood but the following theories are currently thought to contribute.

- Damage or abnormalities in the nerves change the way that nerves communicate with each other.
- Pain receptors require less stimulation to initiate pain signals both in peripheral nerves and the central nervous system, where it is often referred to as central sensitization.
- Pain transmission is altered from its normal sequence.
- There may be an increase in the release of chemical neurotransmitters.
- There can be increased and chaotic firing of nerves.
- Damaged nerves spontaneously generate impulses in the absence of any stimulation.
- The descending inhibitory systems may also be reduced or lost.

These mechanisms result in increased activity or transmission of pain signals despite less input from the peripheral

449

nervous system. Pain can be spontaneous, may be triggered by non-painful stimulus such as touch (allodynia), may be an exaggerated pain response (hyperalgesia) and patients may also experience non-painful sensations such as pins and needles and tingling (paraesthesias).

Evidence-based approaches
Rationale for effective acute pain control

There are several reasons why pain needs to be well controlled following surgery, not least that patients have a right to expect adequate treatment of pain and that all members of the healthcare team have an ethical obligation to provide it (Audit Commission 1997). It is now known that undertreatment of acute pain coupled with the physiological response to surgery, known as the stress response, can have a number of adverse consequences (Macintyre and Schug 2007).

Pain can have long-lasting effects on the central nervous system, leaving an 'imprint' if pain is poorly controlled which may mean that future episodes of pain are difficult to control (Carr 2007). Uncontrolled pain can lead to increased anxiety, fear, sleeplessness and muscle tension which further exacerbate pain. It can delay the recovery process by hindering mobilization and deep breathing, which increases the risk of a patient developing a deep vein thrombosis, chest infection or pressure ulcer. Pain can also lead to significant delays in gastric emptying and a reduction in intestinal motility (Macintyre and Schug 2007). With severe pain, activity of the sympathetic nervous system and the neuroendocrine 'stress response' causes platelet activation, changes in regional blood flow and stress on the heart. These can lead to impaired wound healing and myocardial ischaemia (Macintyre and Schug 2007). There is evidence to suggest that in the long term, poorly controlled acute pain may lead to the development of chronic pain. Perkins and Kehlet (2000) established that moderate to severe acute postoperative pain was a predictor for developing chronic pain after breast surgery, thoracic surgery and hernia repair.

Methods of pain assessment

Assessment is a key step in the process of managing pain. The aim of assessment is to identify all the factors, physical and non-physical, that affect the patient's perception of pain. A comprehensive clinical assessment is essential to gain a thorough understanding of the patient's pain, select an appropriate analgesic therapy, evaluate the effectiveness of interventions and modify therapy according to the patient's response.

Acute pain assessment for surgical patients

For surgical pain to be controlled effectively, pain must be assessed regularly and systematically. The process of pain assessment begins before surgery and continues through to discharge.

A number of psychosocial factors can influence pain. Pain is an individual, multifactorial experience influenced by previous pain events, beliefs about pain and pain management, anxiety, mood and culture (Macintyre *et al.* 2010). Patients may be anxious about the outcome of the surgery or how pain will be controlled, particularly if they have bad memories of previous pain experiences (Audit Commission 1997, Carr and Mann 2000). Anxiety in turn exacerbates pain by increasing muscle tension. Providing patients with appropriate support and information to address these concerns can reduce both anxiety and postoperative pain (Audit Commission 1997, Kalkman *et al.* 2003).

Assessment of pre-existing pain

Patients who have been taking regular opioid analgesics for a pre-existing chronic pain problem may require higher doses of analgesia to manage an acute pain episode (Lewis and Williams 2005, Macintyre 2001, Mehta and Langford 2006). It is therefore important to take a history of pre-existing pain and analgesic use so that appropriate analgesic measures can be planned in advance of surgery. This is particularly important for opioid-tolerant patients irrespective of whether opioid tolerance is due to analgesic therapy or recreational opioid drug use (Box 9.11).

Assessment of location and intensity of pain

Location
Many complex surgical procedures involve more than one incision site and the nature and extent of pain at each site may vary. A careful assessment of the location and type of pain is required, because each pain problem may respond to different pain management techniques. Pain location may also help to determine why pain is exacerbated by certain movements or positions (Anderson and Cleeland 2003).

Box 9.11 Key points for managing acute pain in opioid-dependent patients

- Good communication: patients at risk should be identified at preassessment and effective communication maintained between preassessment staff, recovery staff and anaesthetist/pain service.
- Formalization of peri- and postoperative pain management plan.
- Use of adjuvant drugs and regional analgesia peri- and postoperatively to spare opioid use.
- Physical dependence requires baseline preoperative opioids to be maintained to prevent acute withdrawal symptoms.
- Postoperative opioid requirements may vary depending on the effects of surgery.

(Bourne 2008)

Intensity

As part of the assessment process, it is important to assess the intensity of pain. Only then can the effects of any intervention be evaluated and care modified as appropriate. The simplest techniques for pain measurement involve the use of a verbal rating scale, numerical rating scale or visual analogue scale. Patients are asked to match pain intensity to the scale. Three principles apply to the use of these scales.

■ The patient must be involved in scoring their own pain intensity. It provides the patient with an opportunity to express their pain intensity and also what it means to them and the effect it has on their lives. This is important because healthcare professionals frequently underestimate the intensity of a patient's pain and effectiveness of pain relief (Drayer et al. 1999, Idvall et al. 2002, Loveman and Gale 2000).
■ Pain intensity assessment should incorporate different components of pain. This should include assessment of static (rest) pain and dynamic pain (on sitting, coughing or moving the affected part). For example, in a postoperative patient this is important to prevent complications of delayed recovery such as chest infections and emboli (deep vein thrombosis, pulmonary embolism) and to determine if analgesia is adequate for return of normal function (Hobbs and Hodgkinson 2003, Macintyre and Schug 2007).
■ It is important to remember that a complete picture of a patient's pain cannot be derived solely from the use of a pain scale (Lawler 1997). Ongoing communication with the patient is required to uncover and manage any psychosocial factors that may be affecting the patient's pain experience.

Chronic pain assessment

The prevalence of chronic pain is approximated at being between 30% and 50% amongst patients with cancer who are undergoing active treatment for a solid tumour and between 70% and 90% among those patients with advanced disease (Portenoy and Lesage 1999). For example, approximately two-thirds of advanced cancer patients will also complain of anorexia, one-half will have a symptomatic dry mouth and constipation, and one-third will suffer nausea, vomiting, insomnia, dyspnoea, cough or oedema (Donnelly and Walsh 1995).

It is clear from these figures that chronic pain assessment cannot be seen in isolation; identification of all related symptoms is of equal importance as they will contribute to a lowered pain threshold (the lowest stimulus intensity at which a person perceives pain) and impaired pain tolerance (the greatest stimulus intensity causing pain that a person is prepared to tolerate) (Grond et al. 1996). Furthermore, chronic cancer pain is often multifactorial. Adequate pain assessment requires a comprehensive evaluation of all factors that play a significant role in the cancer pain experience (Zaza and Baine 2002).

A diagnosis of cancer does not necessarily mean that the malignant process is the cause of the pain. Pain in chronic cancer may be:

■ caused by the cancer itself
■ caused by treatment
■ associated with debilitating disease, such as a pressure ulcer
■ unrelated to either the disease or the treatment, such as headache (Twycross and Wilcock 2001).

It is imperative to ascertain the patient's current level of anxiety and depression and to understand each patient's own understanding of the meaning of pain (Foley 2004). The cause of each pain should therefore be identified carefully; many pains unrelated to the cancer will respond to specific treatment. If the pain is due to the cancer, then it is important to determine the precise mechanism of pain because treatment will vary accordingly. Patients with cancer may experience a range of psychological and spiritual problems that extend far beyond the experience of physical pain (Paz and Seymour 2008).

The concept of total pain reminds practitioners that pain is a deeply personal experience and that one of the greatest challenges is for nurses to be able to facilitate the expression for each individual of that particular pain (Krishnasamy 2008). Pain assessment needs to acknowledge these facts and particular attention must be paid to factors that will modulate pain sensitivity (Table 9.1).

Assessment in vulnerable and older adults

Pain assessment in vulnerable adults, for example those with cognitive impairment or dementia, and older adults may require careful consideration. Older adult patients may be reluctant to report pain due to previous bad experiences with healthcare services, anxieties about the potential cause of the pain, stoic attitudes ('put up with pain', 'don't make a fuss') and also have concerns about side-effects of analgesic medications. These issues create barriers to effective assessment

Table 9.1 Factors affecting pain sensitivity

Sensitivity increased	Sensitivity lowered
Discomfort	Relief of symptoms
Insomnia	Sleep
Fatigue	Rest
Anxiety	Sympathy
Fear	Understanding
Anger	Companionship
Sadness	Diversional activity
Depression	Reduction in anxiety
Boredom	Elevation of mood

451

and management of pain and need to be explored and strategies developed to overcome them.

Preprocedural considerations

Assessment and recording tools

Accurate pain assessment is a prerequisite of effective control and is an essential component of nursing care. In the assessment process, the nurse gathers information from the patient that allows an understanding of the patient's experience and its effect on their life. The information obtained guides the nurse in planning and evaluating strategies for care. Pain is rarely static; therefore, its assessment is not a one-time process but is ongoing.

Pain assessment can be difficult to achieve. For example, the tendency suggested by both research and clinical practice is for the patient not to report any pain or to do so inadequately or inaccurately, minimizing the pain experience (McCaffery and Beebe 1989). Nurses are influenced by a number of variables when assessing the amount of pain a patient is suffering (Kitson 1994). Pargeon and Hailey (1999) demonstrated that healthcare providers usually over- or underestimate a patient's pain. It has also been suggested that nurses do not possess sufficient knowledge to care for patients in pain (Drayer et al. 1999, McCaffery and Ferrell 1997). A survey of over 3000 nurses (McCaffery and Robinson 2002) demonstrated that nurse education has improved confidence in the pain assessment process but that further education continues to be required in the pharmacology of pain medications and addressing nurses' fears of opioid addiction and respiratory depression, which continue to contribute to the undertreatment of pain.

A variety of pain assessment tools exist which can be used to assist nurses to assess pain and plan nursing care. They enable pain to be successfully assessed and monitored (McCaffery and Beebe 1989, Twycross et al. 1996, Walker et al. 1987) and improve communication between staff and patients (Raiman 1986). Higginson (1998, p.150) notes that: 'Taking assessments directly from the patient is the most valid way of collecting information on their quality of life'. Encouraging patients to take an active role in their pain assessment by using pain tools helps to increase their confidence and makes them feel part of the pain management process.

Some degree of caution, however, must be exercised with the use of pain assessment tools. The nurse must be careful to select the tool that is most appropriate for a particular type of pain experience (Box 9.12). For example, it would not be appropriate to use a pain assessment tool that had been designed for use with patients with chronic pain to assess postoperative pain. Furthermore, pain tools should not be used totally indiscriminately. Walker et al. (1987) found that pain tools appeared to have little value in cases of unresolved or intractable pain.

The use of pain assessment tools for acute pain has been shown both to increase the effectiveness of nursing inter-

---

Box 9.12 Most commonly used pain assessment tools

The most commonly used pain assessment tools meet the following criteria (Fitzpatrick et al. 1998).

- *Simplicity*: ease of understanding for all patient groups.
- *Reliability*: reliability of the tool when used in similar patient groups; results are reproducible and consistent.
- *Valid*: the tool measures the patient's perception of pain.
- *Sensitivity*: sensitivity of the tool to the patient's pain.
- *Accuracy*: accurate and precise recording of data.
- *Interpretable*: meaningful pain scores or data are produced.
- *Feasiblity/practicality*: the degree of effort involved in using the tool is acceptable; a practical tool is more likely to be used by patients.

---

ventions and to improve the management of pain (Harmer and Davies 1998, Scott 1994). Several pain assessment tools are available. Verbal descriptor scales (VDS) are based on numerically ranked words such as 'none', 'mild', 'moderate', 'severe' and 'very severe' for assessing both pain intensity and response to analgesia. Numerical rating scales (NRS) have both written and verbal forms. The written forms are either a vertical or a horizontal line with '0', indicating no pain, located on one extremity of the line and '10', indicating severe pain, at the other extremity. This type of scale is easily used as a verbal scale of 0–10 if patients are unable to see or focus on a written scale. Although originally published as a line with a scale of 0–10, there are many versions of it (Flaherty 1996). Since many of these scales focus on assessing the intensity of pain, it is important that nurses remember to combine their use of these tools with an assessment of the patient's psychosocial needs.

For practical purposes, a combined pain assessment and observation chart is frequently used in the postoperative period. The Royal Marsden Hospital Postoperative Observation and Pain Assessment Chart is one example of these (Figure 9.10). The patient's assessment of their pain is recorded on the numerical rating pain scale at the bottom of the chart at the same time that other observations are carried out (usually 2–4 hourly but more frequently if pain is not controlled).

Other pain assessment tools have been developed to capture the multidimensional nature of pain. These specifically measure several features of the pain experience, including the location and intensity of pain, pattern of pain over time, the effect of pain on the patient's daily function and activities, the effect on the patient's mood and the ability to interact and socialize with others. Examples of these include the McGill Pain Questionnaire (MPQ) (Melzack 1975) and the Brief Pain Inventory (BPI) (Cleeland 1991). These are more commonly used in chronic pain assessment.

Patient Name: _____ Hosp. No.: _____ C.U./Consultant: _____

POST OPERATIVE OBSERVATION AND PAIN ASSESSMENT CHART

Date																		
Time																		

The Royal Marsden NHS Trust

Temp
40°C
39°C
38°C
37°C
36°C
35°C

B L O O D
P R E S S U R E
P U L S E

220- / -220
210- / -210
200- / -200
190- / -190
180- / -180
170- / -170
160- / -160
150- / -150
140- / -140
130- / -130
120- / -120
110- / -110
100- / -100
95- / -95
90- / -90
85- / -85
80- / -80
75- / -75
70- / -70
65- / -65
60- / -60
55- / -55
50- / -50
45- / -45
40- / -40
35- / -35
30- / -30
25- / -25
20- / -20

Oxygen Saturation If on oxygen add amount	
Respiratory rate	
Sedation Score	
Hourly Rate of Epidural/IV Infusion	
S/C Analgesia Continuous (C), Intermittent (I)	
PCA Accumulative Total	
Height of Epidural Block	
Nausea and Vomiting	
Bowels	
CVP	
Drain	1
	2
	3
Pain Score (0–10)	At Rest
	On Movement

Figure 9.10 The Royal Marsden Hospital NHS Foundation Trust, Postoperative Observation and Pain Assessment Chart.

The Royal Marsden NHS Trust
Patient Held Pain Chart

Surname:

Who completed the assessment:
(specify if nurse or family member helped)

First name:

Date of this assessment:

Instructions for use:

1. This chart is for you to complete (you may want your family or a nurse to help you).

2. Work through the questions in section 1 and 2 of the chart. Do ask for help if you are not clear about any of the questions.

3. When you get to section 3 use the instructions at the top of the sheet to help you keep an ongoing record of your pain and the effect of any pain treatments.

Please keep this chart with you because the nurses and doctors who are looking after you will use it to help manage your pain(s).

Section 1: Where is your pain?

Please draw on the body outlines below to show where you feel pain. Label each site A, B, C, etc. or use a different colour

Section 2: Questions about your pain

How would you describe your pain(s) at the site(s) you drew on the body diagram? (e.g. aching, tender, sharp, shooting, burning).

What helps reduce your pain(s) at each site? (e.g. specific drugs, activities or treatments such as massage).

What makes your pain worse at each site? (e.g. specific activity or heat/cold).

How often do you get pain at each site? (e.g. all the time or at different times during the day).

How do you feel when you are in pain and how has it changed your daily activities? (e.g. moving, sleeping).

Section 3: Scoring and recording your pain scores

Pain Scores	
0	= No pain
1–4	= Mild pain
5–6	= Moderate pain
7–9	= Severe pain
10	= Worst pain imaginable

Instructions for scoring and recording pain scores

1) In the column marked Pain scores use the scoring system shown here to record your pain score(s) at each site (see columns A, B, C, etc.) where you feel pain.
2) Score your pain at regular intervals. Do this before your pain treatments (e.g. analgesics/pain medicines, massage) and 30–45 minutes afterwards so that you can see if they have helped.

Figure 9.11 The Royal Marsden Hospital NHS Foundation Trust, Patient-Held Pain Chart.

Neuropathic pain may require a specific assessment tool. Patients may describe spontaneous pain (arising without detectable stimulation) and evoked pain (abnormal responses to stimuli) (Bennett 2001). The Leeds Assessment of Neuropathic Symptoms and Signs (LANSS) pain scale (Bennett 2001) was developed to more accurately assess this type of pain.

The Royal Marsden Hospital NHS Foundation Trust currently uses a patient-held pain tool for patients with chronic cancer pain (Figure 9.11).

In adults with no or mild cognitive impairment, both numerical rating scales (0–10) and verbal descriptor rating scales (no pain, mild, moderate or severe pain) are both reliable and valid for patients' self-report of pain intensity. Older or vulnerable adults with moderate to severe cognitive/communication impairment may be able to use pictorial rating scales such as the Pain Thermometer or the Faces Pain Scale (Royal College of Physicians, British Geriatric Society and British Pain Society 2007). For patients with dementia or who may be unable to vocalize, an observational tool that assesses pain behaviours may need to be considered, such as the Abbey Scale (Royal College of Physicians, British Geriatric Society and British Pain Society 2007).

Procedure guideline 9.9 Pain assessment and education of patients prior to surgery

1 If patient has had previous surgery, ask for details of:
   (a) Previous and current pain control methods (pharmacological and non-pharmacological)
   (b) Effectiveness of these methods
   (c) Experience of side-effects, such as nausea and vomiting.

2 Assess patient for pre-existing long-term pain problems. Obtain information on:
   (a) Pain type, location and intensity
   (b) Use of analgesics.

3 Check patient suitability for various pain control methods, for example renal function, clotting abnormalities, dexterity, visual impairment.

4 Liaise with multidisciplinary team and patient to select most appropriate pain control method(s).

5 Explain and discuss with patient:
   (a) How pain will be assessed and the use of a pain scale
   (b) How pain will be controlled
   (c) Goals for pain control at rest and on movement.

6 Provide patient with written information about pain control.

7 Where appropriate, demonstrate the use of pain control methods before surgery.

8 Document information in nursing and care plan.

Procedure guideline 9.10 Pain assessment chart: chronic pain recording

Esential equipment

- Copy of a pain assessment chart (Figure 9.11)

Preprocedure

Action	Rationale
1 Explain the purpose of using the chart to the patient.	To ensure that the patient understands the procedure and gives their valid consent and co-operation (NMC 2008a, C; Witt-Sherman et al. 2004, R4).

(Continued)

Procedure guideline 9.10 *(Continued)*

Procedure

2 Encourage the patient, where appropriate, to identify pain themselves.	The body outline (see Figure 9.11) is a vehicle for the patient to describe their own pain experience (Witt-Sherman *et al.* 2004, R4).
3 When it is necessary for the nurse to complete the chart, ensure that the patient's own description of their pain is recorded.	To reduce the risk of misinterpretation. E
4 (a) Record any factors that influence the intensity of the pain, for example activities or interventions that reduce or increase the pain such as distractions or a heat pad. (b) Record whether or not the patient is pain free at night, at rest or on movement. (c) Record frequency of pain, what helps to relieve the pain, what makes the pain worse and how the patient feels when they are in pain.	Ascertaining how and when the patient experiences pain enables the nurse to plan realistic goals. For example, relieving the patient's pain during the night and while they are at rest is usually easier to achieve than relief from pain on movement (Davis and McVicker 2000, E). To ascertain an understanding of the experience of pain for the patient (Twycross and Wilcock 2001, R5).
5 Index each site (A–D; see Figure 9.11) in whatever way seems most appropriate, for example shading or colouring of areas or arrows to indicate shooting pains.	This enables individual pain sites to be located (Witt-Sherman *et al.* 2004, R4).
6 Give each pain site a numerical value according to the key to pain intensity or the pain scale and note time recorded.	To indicate the intensity of the pain at each site (Turk and Okifuji 1999, E).
7 Record any analgesia given and note route and dose.	To monitor efficacy of prescribed analgesia (Twycross and Wilcock 2001, R5).

Postprocedure

8 Record any significant activities that are likely to influence the patient's pain.	Extra pharmacological or non-pharmacological interventions might be indicated (Disorbio *et al.* 2006, E; Turk and Okifuji 1999, E).

Fixed times for reviewing the pain have been omitted intentionally to allow for flexibility. It is suggested that, initially, the patient's pain is reviewed by the patient and nurse every 4 hours. When a patient's level of pain has stabilized, recordings may be made less frequently, for example 12-hourly or daily. The chart should be discontinued if a patient's pain becomes totally controlled.

Pain management

Evidence-based approaches
Management of chronic pain

The control of pain is directed by the 'analgesic ladder', which was presented by the World Health Organization (WHO) in 1996 (Figure 9.12). Pharmacological intervention begins on the first step of the ladder and proceeds upwards as and when the pain reaches a higher level and the current analgesia is no longer effective. Analgesia should be administered 'around the clock' (ATC) to enable chronic persistent pain to be controlled.

It is important to remember that the patient will experience different types of pain due to different aetiological and physiological changes. It is important to make an assessment of each pain separately, since the pain may need to be managed in a different manner and one analgesic intervention will rarely be sufficient. Often the best practice is to combine the baseline analgesia with an appropriate adjuvant treatment in order to achieve maximum pain control (Table 9.2). It is also important to utilize non-pharmacological interventions at all stages of the treatment plan.

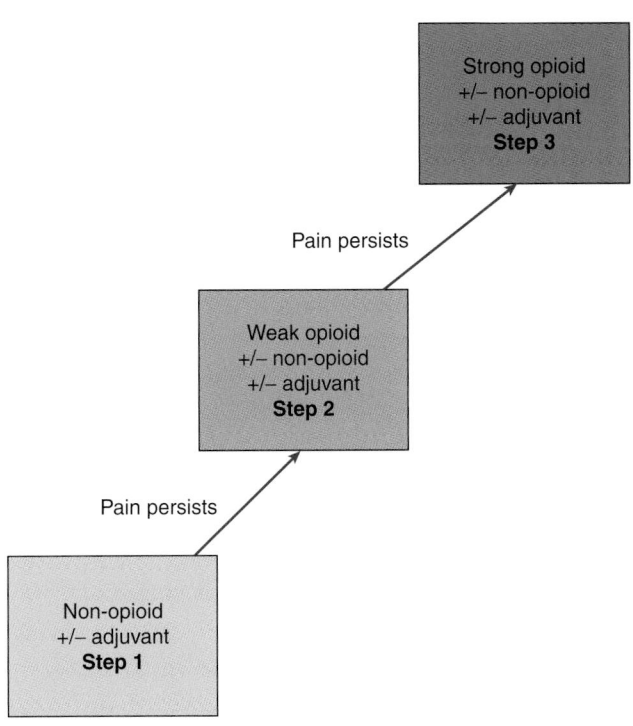

Figure 9.12 The analgesic ladder.

Oral administration of therapeutic interventions may not always be appropriate. In chronic cancer pain the European Association of Palliative Care (EAPC) recommends that if patients can no longer manage the oral route, the preferred alternative route is subcutaneous, which is simple and less painful than the intramuscular route (Hanks *et al.* 2001). In rare circumstances when rapid titration of analgesia is required, the intravenous route may also be used if patients have established intravenous access.

Accurate ongoing assessment is imperative for efficient and effective pain control.

Management of acute pain following surgery

Since nurses, surgeons, anaesthetists, pain specialists, pharmacists and physiotherapists are all involved in the management of surgical pain, teamwork is essential. Professionals must reach clear agreement as to their individual roles so that patients receive the best possible care from preadmission through to discharge (Audit Commission 1997).

A wide variety of pharmacological and non-pharmacological techniques are available for the management of surgical pain. The following basic principles apply to their use (Box 9.13).

457

Table 9.2 The use of adjuvant drugs (co-analgesics)

Type	Use	Examples
NSAIDs	Bone pain	Diclofenac
	Muscular pain	Naproxen
	Inflammation	Ibuprofen
	Visceral pain	
Steroids	Pressure	Dexametasone
	Bone pain	Prednisolone
	Inflammation	
	Raised intracranial pressure	
Tricyclic antidepressants	Neuropathic pain	Amitriptyline
Anticonvulsants		Sodium valproate
		Carbamazepine
		Gabapentin
		Pregabalin
Antibiotics	Infection	Flucloxacillin
		Trimethoprim
Benzodiazepines	Anxiety	Diazepam
		Clonazepam
Antispasmodics	Spasms	Baclofen
Bisphosphonates	Bone pain	Sodium clodronate
		Disodium pamidronate
		Zoledronic acid

Box 9.13 Principles of surgical pain management

- Tailor the treatments to:
  (a) meet individual needs
  (b) prevent pain, rather than allowing it to become established.
- Whenever possible, choose the simplest and safest techniques to achieve the desired level of pain relief (McQuay *et al.* 1997).
- Use the WHO analgesic ladder (see Figure 9.12) to select the most appropriate analgesics for mild, moderate and severe acute pain.
- Choose the most appropriate route for giving analgesia.
- Combine techniques to provide balanced analgesia and enhance overall pain control (Kehlet 1997).
- Ensure patients receive regular antiemetics to control postoperative nausea and vomiting. Vomiting increases muscle tension and exacerbates pain.

Methods of pain management

Using the WHO analgesic ladder

The analgesic ladder was designed as a framework for the management of chronic pain (see Figure 9.12). There are several drugs available to manage chronic pain and the analgesic ladder allows the flexibility to choose from the range according to the patient's requirements and tolerance (Hanks *et al.* 2001). For acute pain management, the WHO ladder can be used as a guide in reverse, starting at step 3 for immediate postoperative pain and moving down through step 2 and then step 1 as postoperative pain improves.

Step 1: non-opioid drugs

Examples of non-opioid drugs include paracetamol, aspirin and NSAIDs that are effective for mild to moderate pain. These drugs are especially effective for musculoskeletal and visceral pain (Twycross and Wilcock 2001).

Step 2: opioids for mild to moderate pain

Examples of opioids for mild to moderate pain include codeine, dihydrocodeine, tramadol and low-dose oxycodone (steps 2 and 3). These drugs are used when adequate pain management is not achieved with the use of non-opioids and are usually used in combination formulations. It is not recommended to administer another analgesic from the same group if the drug being used is not controlling the pain. Uncontrolled pain needs to be assessed and managed with the titration of an opioid by moving up the ladder. The exception to this would be if the patient was experiencing intolerable side-effects on the weak opioid and an alternative drug might be beneficial.

In recent studies tramadol has been recognized as being efficacious in the management of chronic cancer pain of moderate severity (Davis *et al.* 2005). It is uncertain whether tramadol is more effective in neuropathic pain

than other opioids for mild to moderate pain; one report suggests a reduction in allodynia (pain from stimuli which are not normally painful) (Sindrup and Jensen 1999, Twycross and Wilcock 2001). Nurses should be aware that circumstantial reports suggest that tramadol lowers seizure threshold, and therefore care needs to be taken in those patients who have a history of epilepsy, as well as any other medications that may contribute to the lowering of the seizure threshold, for example tricyclic antidepressants and selective serotonin reuptake inhibitors (SSRIs) (Twycross and Wilcock 2001). Few patients with severe pain will achieve a satisfactory level of pain control with tramadol. It is available in immediate and modified-release preparations.

Step 3: opioids for moderate to severe pain

Examples of opioids for moderate to severe pain include morphine, oxycodone, fentanyl, diamorphine, methadone, buprenorphine, hydromorphone and alfentanil.

Breakthrough analgesia

Breakthrough pain refers to a transitory exacerbation of pain experienced by the patient who has relatively stable and adequately controlled background pain (Portenoy *et al.* 2004). There should not be a time limit on this type of prescription because it would need to be given when and if the patient demonstrated any signs of discomfort or pain (with the exception of renal failure where dosages would need to be limited).

Rescue doses are calculated on a 4-hour equivalence; for example, if a patient was prescribed 60 mg MXL (a modified form of morphine given once a day), the equivalent rescue dose would be 10 mg of the immediate-release formulation. If several rescue doses are required within a 24-hour period, then the background analgesia (modified-release preparation) would have to be increased (McMillan 2001). However, it is important to recognize the classifications of breakthrough pain, as increasing the background dose will not always be indicated. Increasing the background preparation for pain that only occurs at certain times or is related to a specific event, such as a patient attending for radiotherapy, can result in a patient experiencing side-effects as the medication is needed for a specific time only.

Breakthrough pain can be classified as follows.

- Spontaneous pain: this type of pain occurs unexpectedly.
- Incident pain: this pain is related to specific events and can be classified into four categories (Davies 2006).
  1 Volitional pain is precipitated by a voluntary act, for example walking.
  2 Non-volitional pain is precipitated by an involuntary act, for example coughing.
  3 Procedural is a type of pain related to a therapeutic intervention, for example wound dressing.
  4 End-of-dose failure is related to analgesic dosing (declining analgesic levels).

The ideal treatment for breakthrough pain is an analgesic with good efficacy, a rapid onset and short duration of action, and which causes minimal adverse effects. In order to try and deliver more effective treatment, various routes of administration have been explored including the transmucosal routes (Zeppetella 2009). These are discussed below.

Methods of drug delivery

Oral analgesia

Oral opioids are used less frequently in the immediate postoperative period because many patients may be nil by mouth or on restricted oral intake for a period of time. Often this route is used if patients require strong analgesics following discontinuation of epidural or intravenous analgesia. Morphine is an ideal oral preparation because it is available as a tablet (Sevredol) or an elixir (Oramorph). Oxycodone can be given as second-line opioid treatment if patients are allergic/sensitive to or fail to respond to morphine.

Intravenous analgesia

Continuous intravenous infusions of opioids such as morphine, diamorphine and fentanyl are effective for controlling pain in the immediate postoperative period. Their use is often restricted to critical care units where patients can be closely monitored because of the potential risk of respiratory depression (Macintyre and Schug 2007). Compared with PCA, continuous infusions of opioids for acute pain management in a general ward setting resulted in a fivefold increase in the incidence of respiratory depression (Schug and Torrie 1993).

Patient-controlled analgesia is an alternative and safer technique for giving intravenous opioids (usually morphine, diamorphine, fentanyl or oxycodone) in the ward environment (Sidebotham et al. 1997). With PCA, patients self-administer intermittent doses of opioids, by using an infusion pump and timing device. When in pain, the patient presses a button connected to the pump and a set dose of opioid is delivered (usually intravenously but it may also be given subcutaneously) to the patient (Macintyre and Schug 2007). For more information about the PCA pump, please see Chapter 16.

There are a number of advantages of using PCA.

- PCA is more likely to maintain reasonably constant blood concentrations of the opioid within the analgesic corridor. This is the blood level where analgesia is achieved without significant side-effects. The flexibility of PCA helps to overcome the wide interpatient variation in opioid requirements (Macintyre and Schug 2007).
- PCA allows patients to titrate analgesia against daily variations in the pain stimulus (Tye and Gell-Walker 2000). By using a PCA pump, patients can administer analgesia as soon as pain occurs and titrate the dose of analgesia according to increases and decreases in the pain stimulus. This is particularly helpful for controlling more intense pain during movement.

Box 9.14 Patients for whom PCA is inappropriate

- Those who are unable to activate the PCA device due to problems with dexterity or visual impairment.
- Those who are unable to understand the concept of PCA, particularly the very young or patients who are confused.
- Those who do not wish to take responsibility for their pain control.

(Tye and Gell-Walker 2000)

- PCA prevents delays in patients receiving analgesics (Chumbley et al. 2002).

Whilst PCA may be very effective for controlling pain for a number of patients undergoing surgery (Macintyre and Schug 2007), it is not suitable for the groups listed in Box 9.14.

Epidural analgesia

Epidural analgesia refers to the provision of pain relief by continuous administration of analgesic pharmacological agents (usually low concentrations of local anaesthetics and opioids) into the epidural space via an indwelling catheter (Macintyre et al. 2010). Giving analgesia epidurally is a particularly valuable technique for the prevention of postoperative pain in patients undergoing major thoracic, abdominal and lower limb surgery, and can sometimes be used to manage the pain associated with trauma. Commonly used opioids for epidural analgesia include fentanyl and diamorphine (Wheatley et al. 2001). Combinations of low concentrations of local anaesthetic agents and opioids have been shown to provide consistently superior pain relief compared with either drug alone (Macintyre and Schug 2007).

Subcutaneous analgesia

Opioids are often given subcutaneously to manage chronic cancer pain. More recently, there has been an increase in the use of subcutaneous opioids for postoperative pain control. Both PCA and nurse-administered opioid injections of morphine, diamorphine or oxycodone via an indwelling subcutaneous cannula have been used successfully to manage postoperative pain (Vijayan 1997). An advantage of giving analgesia subcutaneously is that it avoids the problems associated with maintaining intravenous access.

Intramuscular analgesia

Until the early 1990s, regular 3–4-hourly intramuscular injections of opioids such as pethidine and morphine were routinely used for the management of postoperative pain. Because alternative techniques such as PCA and epidural analgesia are now available, intramuscular analgesia is used less frequently. Some useful algorithms have been developed to give guidance on titrating intramuscular analgesia (Harmer and Davies 1998, Macintyre and Schug 2007). Absorption via this route may be impaired in conditions of poor perfusion (e.g. in hypovolaemia, shock, hypothermia or immobility). This may lead to inadequate early analgesia (the drug cannot be absorbed properly and reach the systemic circulation and forms a drug depot) and late absorption of the drug depot (where the drug has remained in the muscular tissue and is absorbed only once perfusion is restored) (Macintyre *et al.* 2010).

Nasal analgesia

It is suggested that the nasal route may be effective for a number of opioids (Hanks *et al.* 2004). Nasal diamorphine spray has been shown to provide effective pain relief in accident and emergency departments in children and teenagers who are experiencing acute pain. This approach is being investigated in adult cancer patients with acute, episodic pain (Hanks *et al.* 2004).

Preprocedural considerations
Pharmacological support
Non-opioid analgesics

Paracetamol and paracetamol combinations
The use of non-opioid analgesics such as paracetamol or paracetamol combined with a weak opioid such as codeine is recommended for managing pain following minor surgical procedures or when the pain following major surgery begins to subside (McQuay *et al.* 1997). Paracetamol can also be given rectally if the oral route is contraindicated. An intravenous preparation of paracetamol is now available and can provide effective analgesia after surgical procedures (Romsing *et al.* 2002). It is more effective and of faster onset than the same dose given enterally. The use of the intravenous form should be limited to patients in whom the enteral route cannot be used.

Paracetamol taken in the correct dose of not more than 4 g per day is relatively free of side-effects. When used in combination with codeine preparations, the most frequent side-effect is constipation.

Non-steroidal anti-inflammatory drugs
Non-steroidal anti-inflammatory drugs (NSAIDs) have been shown to provide better pain relief than paracetamol combinations for acute pain (McQuay *et al.* 1997). These drugs can be used alone or in combination with both opioid and non-opioid analgesics. Two commonly used NSAIDs are diclofenac, which can be administered by the oral, parenteral, enteral or rectal route, and ibuprofen, which is available only as an oral or enteral preparation. The disadvantage of both of these is that often side-effects such as coagulation problems, renal impairment and gastrointestinal disturbances limit their use. Newer COX-2 -specific NSAIDs have the advantage that they have similar analgesia and anti-inflammatory effects (Reicin *et al.* 2001) but have no effect on platelets or the gastric mucosa (Rowbotham 2000). As a result, coagulation problems and gastrointestinal irritation are likely to be significantly reduced. However, recently several of these drugs have been withdrawn from the market due to long-term cardiovascular side-effects and it will take time for newer products with an improved safety profile to re-establish themselves in practice (Macintyre *et al.* 2010).

Opioid analgesics

Opioids are the first-line treatment for pain that follows major surgery (Macintyre and Jarvis 1996) and can also be prescribed for cancer and non-cancer related chronic pain. Opioid doses need to be titrated carefully to achieve pain relief to suit each individual patient while minimizing any unwanted side-effects (McQuay *et al.* 1997).

A number of opioids are used for controlling pain following surgery. These include morphine, diamorphine, fentanyl and oxycodone. The most common routes of opioid administration are intravenous, epidural, subcutaneous, intramuscular or oral.

Evidence for the concept of opioid rotation when patients have intolerable opioid-related side-effects originates from cancer pain studies (Quigley 2004) but it may be a useful strategy to consider in the management of acute pain as well.

Opioids for mild to moderate pain
Tramadol
Another opioid for mild to moderate pain, which has been shown to be an effective analgesic for postoperative pain, is tramadol (McQuay and Moore 1998, Reicin *et al.* 2001). Although tramadol does have some side-effects, which include nausea and dizziness, it is free of NSAID side-effects and causes less constipation than codeine preparations and opioids (Bamigbade and Langford 1998). The combination of tramadol with paracetamol is more effective than either of the two components administered alone (McQuay and Edwards 2003).

Codeine phosphate
Codeine is metabolized by the hepatic cytochrome CYP2D6 to morphine. Approximately 7% of Caucasians and 1–3% of the Asian population are poor CYP2D6 metabolizers and therefore do not experience effective analgesia with codeine.

Codeine is available in tablet and syrup formulations. Doses of 30–60 mg po qds are generally prescribed to a maximum of 240 mg/24 h. It is also available in combination preparations with a non-opioid. The combination preparations are available in varying strengths of codeine and paracetamol, including co-codamol 8 mg/500 mg, 15 mg/500 mg and 30 mg/500 mg.

Opioids for moderate to severe pain

Morphine

A large amount of information and research is available concerning morphine and therefore it tends to be the drug of choice within this category (Hanks *et al.* 2001, 2004). It is available in oral, rectal, parenteral and intraspinal preparations. A recent study of 43 European palliative care units showed that morphine was the most frequently used opioid for moderate to severe pain, with over 50% of patients taking oral or parenteral preparations (Klepstad *et al.* 2005).

All strong opioids require careful titration from an expert practitioner. It is better to begin with a small dose, usually one that is equivalent to the previous medication, and increase gradually in conjunction with careful assessment of its effectiveness (Hanks *et al.* 2001). Titration begins with the immediate-release form which is available in tablet (Sevredol) or elixir (Oramorph) preparations, and once pain control is achieved the patient can be converted to a modified-release preparation that acts over a 12- or 24-hour period (Zomorph or MXL respectively).

Breakthrough analgesia is administered using the equivalent 4-hourly dose of the immediate-release form. This dose can be given as required (hourly) and subsequent adjustments can be made to the modified form if the patient is requiring more than three breakthrough doses in a 24-hour period (Hanks *et al.* 2001).

Patients should be informed of potential side-effects such as constipation, nausea and increased sleepiness, in order to allay any fear. The patient should also be told that nausea and drowsiness are transitory and normally improve within 48 hours, but that constipation can be an ongoing problem and it is recommended that a laxative should be prescribed at the same time as the opioid is started. It is recommended that the most effective laxative for this group of patients is a combination of both a softening and a stimulating laxative (Davis *et al.* 2005).

Patients often have many concerns about commencing strong drugs such as morphine. Frequent fears centre around addiction and believing that its use signifies the terminal phase of the illness (McQuay 1999). Time should be taken to reassure patients and their families and provide verbal and written information.

Although morphine is still considered to be the opioid drug of choice for moderate to severe pain (Hanks *et al.* 2001), alternative opioids allow the practitioner to carefully assess the patient on an individual basis and select the most appropriate opioid to use.

Durogesic (fentanyl)

Fentanyl is a strong opioid, available in a patch, which is recommended in patients who have stable pain requirements. Transdermal patches are available in doses of 12, 25, 50, 75. It is reported to have an improved side-effect profile in comparison to morphine (Ahmedzai and Brooks 1997), although some patients experience nausea and mild drowsiness (BMA/Royal Pharmaceutical Society of Great Britain 2008) and occasionally patients may develop a reaction to the adhesive in the patch (Ling 1997). Use of the patch has increased because it allows the patient freedom from taking tablets.

Changing of the patch is recommended every 3 days, and steady plasma levels are reported to be reached after 8–16 hours (Zech *et al.* 1994), although in some patients it may be necessary to change it more frequently. The patch should be applied to skin that is free from excess hair and any form of irritation and should not be applied to irradiated areas. It is advisable to change the location on the body to avoid an adverse skin reaction. Occasionally difficulties arise relating to the titration of the patch as each patch is equivalent to a range of morphine (Table 9.3).

Fentanyl is also available in parenteral preparations. If the dose required is too large a volume to use in the syringe driver, then alfentanil may be a useful alternative (Dickman *et al.* 2002).

Table 9.3 Recommended conversion doses from morphine to a fentanyl patch

Morphine dose in 24 hours (mg)	Four-hourly morphine dose (mg)	Fentanyl TTS (µg/h)
<50	2.5–5	12
50–134	5–20	25
135–224	25–35	50
225–314	40–50	75
315–404	55–65	100
405–494	70–80	125
495–584	85–95	150
585–674	100–115	175
675–764	115–125	200
765–854	130–140	225
855–944	145–155	250
945–1034	160–170	275
1035–1124	175–190	300

Palladone (hydromorphone)

Palladone (hydromorphone) is mostly used when patients experience unacceptable drowsiness with morphine. It is similar to morphine in its pharmacokinetic profile and it is approximately 5.0–7.5 times more potent than morphine. It is available in immediate-release and sustained-release preparations and titration occurs in the same manner as morphine (Hays et al. 1994).

The side-effects are similar to those of morphine (Ellershaw 1998).

Methadone

Methadone is a synthetic opioid developed more than 40 years ago (Riley 2006). It is available in oral, rectal and parenteral preparations. There has been some reluctance amongst professionals to use methadone, which arose from the difficulties experienced in titrating the drug due to its long half-life (15 hours) that caused accumulation to occur, especially in the elderly (Gannon 1997). There are different methods of achieving effective titration (Gannon 1997); for example, one regimen is to calculate one-tenth of the total daily dose of morphine (maximum starting dose must not exceed 30 mg). Administer the methadone to the patient on an as-required basis but not within 3 hours of the last fixed dose. The total dose required over a 24-hour period is calculated after 5–6 days, divided and given as a two or three times daily regimen and this avoids the build-up of methadone within the body (Morley and Makin 1998). Titration is recommended within a hospital setting to ensure accurate administration. This can be difficult for patients because they have to experience pain before they are administered a dose of methadone in the titration period.

Methadone can be a cheap, effective alternative to morphine if titration is supervised by the specialist pain or palliative care team (Gardner-Nix 1996).

It is particularly useful in patients with renal failure. Morphine is excreted via the kidneys and if renal failure occurs, this may lead to the patient experiencing severe drowsiness as a result of accumulation of morphine metabolites (Gannon 1997). Methadone is lipid soluble and is metabolized mainly in the liver. About half of the drug and its metabolites are excreted by the intestines and half by the kidneys.

Oxycodone

Oxycodone is available as an immediate- or modified-release preparation and titration should occur in the same way as morphine. Oxycodone is a useful opioid as an alternative to morphine (Riley 2006). It has similar properties to morphine and can be administered orally, rectally and parenterally. Oxycodone has similar side-effects and it is usually given 4–6 hourly. Oxycodone has an analgesic potency of 1.5–2.0 times higher than morphine. It has similar side-effects to morphine, although oxycodone has been found to cause less nausea (Heiskanen and Kalso

1997) and significantly less itchiness (Mucci-LoRusso et al. 1998).

Targinact

This drug is a combination of modified-release oxycodone and naloxone. The aim of the combination of these medications is to prevent the potential negative effects on bowel function. It is suggested that approximately 97% of the naloxone is eliminated by first-pass metabolism in the healthy liver, preventing it from significantly affecting analgesic effects (Vondrackova et al. 2008).

Diamorphine

Diamorphine is used parenterally in a syringe driver pump for the control of moderate to severe pain when patients are unable to take the oral form of morphine. It is calculated by dividing the total daily dose of oral morphine by three. Breakthrough doses are calculated by dividing the 24-hour dose of diamorphine by six and administering on an as-required basis (Hanks et al. 2004). A recent problem with the supply of diamorphine nationally has resulted in centres using morphine sulphate or an alternative opioid as a substitute.

Alfentanil

Alfentanil is also a useful alternative to diamorphine and is used for those patients who have renal impairment. The onset of action is rapid owing to a more rapid blood–brain equilibration. It is 10 times more potent than diamorphine (i.e. diamorphine 10 mg = alfentanil 1 mg). The breakthrough dose can be calculated as one-tenth of the 24-hour dose as opposed to the usual one-sixth. For example, 1 mg of alfentanil over 24 hours will require a breakthrough dose of alfentanil 0.1 mg.

Buprenorphine

Buprenorphine is an alternative strong opioid available in a patch form. The patch has similar advantages to fentanyl but does not contain a reservoir of the drug. Instead it is contained in a matrix form with effective levels of the drug being reached within 24 hours. Titration is recommended with an alternative opioid initially and then transfer to the patch when stable requirements have been reached. A lower dose patch (Butrans) is available in strengths of 5, 10 and 20 μg/h that should be worn continuously by the patient for 7 days. The higher dose patch (Transtec) of 35, 52.5 and 70 μg/h is now licensed to be used up to 96 hours or twice weekly for patient convenience. Conversion is based on the chart supplied by the pharmaceutical company which demonstrates equivalent doses. Buprenorphine is also available as a sublingual tablet, which is titrated from 200 to 800 μg 6-hourly. Conversion is based on multiplying the total daily dose of buprenorphine by 100 to give the total daily dose of morphine (i.e. 200 μg buprenorphine/8-hourly = 600 μg buprenorphine/24 hours = 60 mg morphine/24 hours) (Budd 2002).

Opioids approved for oral transmucosal administration

Oral transmucosal fentanyl citrate (Actiq)

Licensed for the management of breakthrough pain in patients who are already on an established maintenance dose of opioid for cancer pain, oral transmucosal fentanyl citrate (OTFC) is a lozenge which is rubbed against the oral mucosa on the side of the cheek which leads to the lozenge being dissolved by the saliva. The advantage of OTFC is its fast onset via the buccal mucosa (5–15 minutes) and its short duration (up to 2 hours). It is available in a range of doses (200–1600 µg) but there is no direct relation between the baseline analgesia and the breakthrough dose. Titration can be difficult and lengthy as the recommended starting dose is 200 µg with titration upwards (Portenoy et al. 1999). It is recommended that the lozenge be removed from the mouth if the pain subsides before it has completely dissolved. The lozenge should not be reused but should be dissolved under running hot water.

Fentanyl buccal tablet (Effentora)

This is a newly licensed medication for the treatment of breakthrough pain in adults with cancer who are already receiving a maintenance opioid for chronic cancer. Patients receiving maintenance opioid therapy are those who are taking at least 60 mg of oral morphine daily, at least 25 µg of transdermal fentanyl per hour, at least 30 mg of oxycodone daily, at least 8 mg of oral hydromorphone daily or an equi-analgesic dose of another opioid for a week or longer. This buccal tablet is available in 100, 200, 400, 600 and 800 µg. It is placed on the oral mucosa above the third upper molar which leads to the tablet being dissolved by the saliva. It usually takes 15–25 minutes for the tablet to dissolve. It is recommended that if the tablet has not completely dissolved within 30 minutes then the remainder of the tablet should be swallowed with water as it is thought that the tablet will then only be likely to consist of inactive properties rather than active fentanyl (Darwish et al. 2007).

Abstral is an oral transmucosal delivery formulation of fentanyl citrate, indicated for the management of breakthrough pain in patients using opioid therapy for chronic cancer pain (Rauch et al. 2009). The tablet is administered sublingually and it rapidly disintegrates, ensuring the fentanyl dissolves quickly. Abstral is available in six dosing strengths: 100, 200, 300, 400, 600 and 800 µg fentanyl citrate.

Adjuvant drugs (co-analgesics)

Adjuvant drugs are a miscellaneous group whose primary indication is for conditions other than pain which may, however, relieve pain in specific circumstances (Twycross and Wilcock 2001). Examples of this category include NSAIDs, steroids, antibiotics, antidepressants, antiepileptics, N-methyl-D-aspartate (NMDA) receptor channel blockers, antispasmodics and muscle relaxants (Twycross and Wilcock 2001).

The WHO analgesic ladder recommends the use of these drugs in combination with non-opioids, opioids for mild to moderate pain and opioids for moderate to severe pain (see Figure 9.12).

Nitrous oxide (Entonox)

Inhaled nitrous oxide provides analgesia that is short acting and works quickly. It has a special role in managing pain associated with wound dressings and drain removal (see Entonox administration).

Local anaesthetics

In addition to epidural analgesia, local anaesthetics may be used to block individual or groups of peripheral nerves during surgical procedures and to infiltrate surgical wounds at the end of an operation (Carroll and Bowsher 1993). Occasionally these techniques may be used to extend the duration of postoperative analgesia beyond the finite period that a single injection technique provides (Macintyre et al. 2010). Techniques include regular intermittent bolus doses or continuous infusions of local anaesthetic.

A topical preparation (patch) containing local anaesthetic is also available to manage acute or chronic neuropathic pain in areas of intact skin with hypersensitivity.

Cannabis

Studies are currently taking place to examine the potential benefits of using cannabis for the management of chronic conditions, for example multiple sclerosis and cancer. Good-quality research is sparse (Wall et al. 2001) but there are a number of studies that allude to its benefits in managing chronic pain, spasticity and muscle spasms (Consroe et al. 1997, Martyn et al. 1995).

Anaesthetic interventions

Sometimes it is difficult to attain and maintain adequate pain control without significant side-effects and it is in situations such as this that anaesthetic interventions may be of benefit.

Effective control can be achieved by epidural or intrathecal (spinal) infusions:

- as single injections for simple nerve blocks, or
- regional nerve blocks which target individual nerves, plexi or ganglia (Hicks and Simpson 2004).

Examples include managing pelvic pain and postradiation brachial plexopathy.

These interventions can be useful, but careful consideration and assessment must take place to ensure that any potential side-effects are discussed with the patient (anaesthetic interventions may severely limit the patient's activities) and that future planning is addressed with the patient

463

and family as an epidural/intrathecal infusion may limit discharge options for the patient who is dying.

Non-pharmacological methods of managing pain

Optimal pain control is more likely to be achieved by combining non-pharmacological techniques with pharmacological techniques. Despite the lack of research evidence to support the effectiveness of many non-pharmacological techniques, their benefits to patients and families should not be underestimated.

Psychological interventions

A number of simple psychological interventions can improve a patient's pain control by:

- reducing anxiety, stress and muscle tension
- distraction (distraction plays a role in pain management by pushing awareness of pain out of central cognition)
- increasing control and pain-coping mechanisms
- improving general well-being.

Some simple interventions include the following.

Creating trusting therapeutic relationships

By creating trusting relationships with patients, nurses are instrumental in reducing anxiety and helping patients to cope with pain (Carr and Mann 2000). Nurses can help to create a trusting relationship by:

- listening to the patient
- believing the patient's pain experience (Seers 1996)
- acting as a patient advocate
- providing patients with appropriate physical and emotional support.

The use of gentle humour

Pasero (1998) suggests that many patients find gentle humour an effective way of coping with pain. Humour may be particularly helpful prior to a painful procedure as it can have a lasting effect. In the clinical setting, humorous tapes, books and videos can be made available for patient use.

Information/education

Patient information/education can make all the difference between effective and ineffective pain relief. Information/ education helps to reduce anxiety (Hayward 1975, Taylor 2001) and enables patients to make informed decisions about their care. Patients should be given specific information about why pain control is important, what to expect in terms of pain relief, how they can participate in their management and what to do if pain is not controlled. Some caution is required, however, because not all patients respond positively to the same level of information. Patients with high levels of anxiety may find that detailed information

---

Box 9.15 Simple relaxation technique script

Please note that breathing during this technique should be normal for the patient in their present condition.

1. Loosen any tight clothing and position yourself comfortably, either lying or sitting. Have your arms and legs uncrossed. Ensure your back and head are well supported.
2. Allow both your hands to rest on your abdomen, one on top of the other. It may be helpful to place a pillow on your lap for your hands to rest on.
3. Gently allow your eyes to close. Breathe normally in and out through your nose if you find this comfortable.
4. As you breathe in, be aware of your abdomen rising gently under your hands (do not force this movement).
5. As you breathe out, be aware of your abdomen relaxing under your hands.
6. Let your shoulders relax and drop down.
7. Let your jaw relax.
8. Now keep your attention softly focused on the rise and fall of your abdomen as this movement follows each breath.
9. Repeat steps 4–8 for between 3 and 5 minutes or longer if appropriate.

During the exercise

As you become aware of any thoughts that arise, let them go and just bring your attention back to the rise and fall of the abdomen. If you are still having difficulty focusing on the technique, try saying the following phrases: 'I am relaxed' or 'I feel calm'.

To finish the exercise

Now slowly become aware of your surroundings, stretch out your fingers and toes, gently open your eyes and come back to the room.

---

can increase their anxiety and influence their pain control. To avoid this, patients can be given a choice of whether or not they receive simple or detailed information (Mitchell 1997).

Relaxation

Whilst scientific evidence for the effectiveness of relaxation techniques is limited (Carroll and Seers 1998, Seers and Carroll 1998), a number of studies have shown benefits for patients experiencing pain (Good et al. 1999, Lang et al. 2000, Sloman et al. 1994). Payne (1995) describes several relaxation techniques ranging from simple breathing techniques to progressive muscle relaxation and more complex techniques. One simple relaxation technique script that has been adapted for use at the Royal Marsden Hospital is outlined in Box 9.15. This technique can be taught to patients and used during painful procedures or at times when the patient feels anxious or stressed. Patients should be encouraged to practise the technique to gain mastery.

Music

The use of taped music in the healthcare setting can also provide relaxation and distraction from pain (Beck 1991, Good 1996, Heiser *et al.* 1997). Setting up a library of taped music (e.g. easy listening, classical) and having personal stereos available for patient use is a simple way to provide patients with relaxing music.

Art

Art therapies have also been used to assist the patient in moving the focus of attention away from the physical sensation of pain to other aspects of the person (Trauger-Querry and Haghighi 1999). The skills of an art therapist are required to ensure the successful use of this intervention.

Physical interventions

In addition to psychological interventions, a number of physical interventions can be helpful in reducing pain.

Comfort measures

Simple comfort measures such as careful body positioning (for example, supporting a painful arm on a pillow) and the use of soft and therapeutic mattresses (Ballard 1997) can help to improve patient comfort and pain control.

Exercise

Both passive and active physical exercises may benefit patients by increasing range of motion (Feine and Lund 1997), preventing joint stiffness and muscle wasting which may further compound pain problems. Exercise should always be tailored to the patient's tolerance and stamina. A simple exercise regimen which is practised regularly and supervised by a therapist can help patients feel better and more in control as well as having benefits in terms of pain relief.

Rest

In addition to exercise, teaching patients to rest comfortably in any position when in pain is a meaningful action and the base from which a person can learn to move more easily (O'Connor and Webb 2002). A person with a terminal illness may experience restriction of movement and neuromuscular pain with increased tension. For these patients, learning to rest and letting go of any tension can be helpful.

Transcutaneous electrical nerve stimulation

Transcutaneous electrical nerve stimulation (TENS) (Figure 9.13) is thought to work by sending a weak electrical current through the skin to stimulate the sensory nerve endings. Depending on the stimulation parameters used, TENS is thought to modulate pain impulses by closing the gate to pain transmission within the spinal cord by stimulating the release of natural pain-relieving chemicals in the brain and spinal cord (King 1999).

To date, there is limited scientific evidence for the effectiveness of TENS. Despite this, many healthcare professionals

Figure 9.13 TENS machine.

use TENS for a variety of chronic pain conditions and support the view that this is a useful form of analgesia (Walsh 1997). In contrast, TENS has not been found to improve the control of acute pain following surgery (McQuay *et al.* 1997).

Acupuncture

This involves placing fine solid needles into the skin at acupoints or trigger points (Figure 9.14). Although the exact mechanism of action is unknown, acupuncture is believed to work in part by stimulating release of the body's own natural opioids. Although there is also limited scientific evidence for the pain-relieving effects of acupuncture, largely due to the poorly controlled studies (Ezzo *et al.* 2000), it is used widely and has an important role in pain management.

Heat therapies

For decades superficial heat therapy has been used to relieve a variety of muscular and joint pains, including arthritis,

Figure 9.14 An increasing number of hospital pain clinics now offer acupuncture as a treatment for chronic pain. © istockphoto.com/Håvard Sæbø.

back pain and period pain. There is much anecdotal and some scientific evidence to support the usefulness of heat as an adjunct to other pain treatments (Akin *et al.* 2001, Nadler *et al.* 2002, Robinson *et al.* 2002).

Heat works by:

- stimulating thermoreceptors in the skin and deeper tissues, thereby reducing the sensitivity to pain by closing the gating system in the spinal cord
- reducing muscle spasm
- reducing the viscosity of synovial fluid which alleviates painful stiffness during movement and increases joint range (Carr and Mann 2000).

In the home environment people use a variety of different methods for applying heat therapies, such as warm baths, hot water bottles, wheat-based heat packs and electrical heating pads. In the hospital setting, caution is required with this equipment as it does not reach health and safety standards (no even and regular temperature distribution) and there have been incidences of serious burns (Barillo *et al.* 2000). Carr and Mann (2000) note that heat therapy should not be used immediately following tissue damage as it will increase swelling. The Medicines and Healthcare Products Regulatory Agency (MHRA 2005) has documented evidence of burns caused by using heat patches or packs and therefore urges caution in their use and also recommends regular checking of skin throughout therapy.

Cold therapies

Cold therapies can also be used to stimulate nerves and modulate pain (Carr and Mann 2000). Cold may be particularly valuable following an acute bruising injury where it can help to reduce inflammation and limit further damage. Cold can be applied in the form of crushed ice or gel-filled cold packs which should be wrapped in a towel to protect the skin from an ice burn.

Postprocedural considerations

Education of patient
Opioids and driving

In 2004, an article in the journal *Palliative Medicine* offered guidance for professionals on the advice they should offer to patients who were taking opioids and driving. One of the contributors to the guidance was the medical advisor to the Driver and Vehicle Licensing Agency (DVLA) (Pease *et al.* 2004).

(a) A patient should not drive:
- for 5 days after starting or changing the dose of the recommended opioid
- if they feel sleepy
- after drinking alcohol or taking strong opioids which have not been recommended by the doctor or non-medical prescriber, for example cannabis
- on days when additional breakthrough medication of an opioid has been taken.

(b) Patients can restart driving:
- after 5 days starting or changing the dose of the recommended opioid and if the patient does not feel sleepy. But the patient:
  - should make the first trip short
  - should drive on roads that the patient is familiar with
  - should drive at a time when the traffic is not too busy
  - should be accompanied by an experienced driver as this may be helpful.

(c) Patients do not need to inform the DVLA about starting an opioid but may need to inform them of other aspects relating to their illness. The patient should be encouraged to inform their insurance company about their current state of health and current medications.

Complications
The use of opioids in renal failure

Renal failure can cause significant and dangerous side-effects due to the accumulation of the drug. Basic guidelines for pain management in renal failure include the following.

- Reduce analgesia dose and/or dose frequency (6-hourly instead of 4-hourly).
- Select a more appropriate drug (non-renally excreted).
- Avoid modified-release preparations.
- Seek advice from a specialist pain/palliative care team and/or pharmacist (Farrell and Rich 2000).

Epidural and intrathecal analgesia

Definition

The term 'spinal analgesia' refers to both the epidural and intrathecal route (Day 2001, Sloan 2004). The spinal cord rests in a medium of cerebrospinal fluid (CSF), which is contained by the protective membrane of the dura mater. Analgesics applied outside the dura mater are termed epidural analgesia, and medications given into the CSF are termed intrathecal analgesia (Sloan 2004).

Anatomy and physiology

The spinal cord (Figures 9.15 and 9.16) is covered by the meninges; the *pia mater* is closely applied to the cord and the *arachnoid mater* lies closely with the outer, tough covering of the *dura mater* (Behar *et al.* 2007). The epidural space lies outside all three membranes, encasing the spinal cord between the spinal dura and ligamentum flavum. The contents of the epidural space include a rich venous plexus, spinal arterioles, lymphatics and extradural fat.

The intrathecal space (often also termed the subarachnoid space) lies between the arachnoid mater and pia mater and contains the CSF (Chapman and Day 2001).

(a)

POSTERIOR

ANTERIOR

(b)

Figure 9.15 Gross anatomy of the spinal cord. (a) Anterior view and transverse section through spinal cord. (b) Transverse section of the spinal cord within a cervical vertebra. Reproduced from Tortora and Derrickson (2009).

There are 31 pairs of spinal nerves of varying size. These nerves pass out through the intervertebral foramina between each vertebra (Chapman and Day 2001). There are two main groups of nerve fibres.

- *Myelinated*: myelin is a thin, fatty sheath which protects and insulates the nerve fibres and prevents impulses from being transmitted to adjacent fibres.

- *Unmyelinated*: delicate fibres, more susceptible to hypoxia and toxins than myelinated fibres.

The spinal nerves are composed of a posterior and anterior root, which join to form the nerve.

- *Posterior root*: transmits ascending sensory impulses from the periphery to the spinal cord.

468

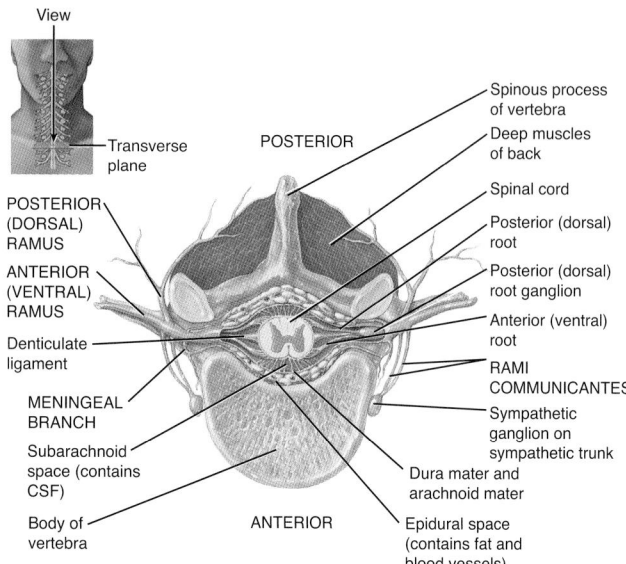

Figure 9.16 Branches of a typical spinal nerve, shown in cross-section through the thoracic portion of the spinal cord: transverse section. Reproduced from Tortora and Derrickson (2009).

- *Anterior root*: transmits descending motor impulses from the spinal cord to the periphery by means of its corresponding spinal nerve.
(Chapman and Day 2001, Day 2001, Urdan *et al.* 2006)

Specific skin surface areas are supplied/innervated by each of the spinal nerves. These skin areas are known as dermatomes (McCaffery and Pasero 1999) (Figure 9.17).

Evidence-based approaches

Epidural analgesia is the administration of analgesics (local anaesthetics and opioids with or without adjuvants such as corticosteroids and clonidine) into the epidural space via an indwelling catheter (Macintyre *et al.* 2010). This technique enables analgesics to be injected close to the spinal cord and spinal nerves where they exert a powerful analgesic effect. It is one of the most effective techniques available for the management of acute pain (Macintyre and Schug 2007, Wheatley *et al.* 2001).

Intrathecal analgesia is the administration of analgesic drugs directly into the CSF in the intrathecal space (Urdan *et al.* 2006). The intrathecal space is also referred to as the subarachnoid space. Analgesic drugs given via this route are 10 times as potent as those given into the epidural space so doses given are much smaller.

The use of drugs via either of these routes can cause both a loss of sensation (anaesthesia) and a loss of pain (analgesia).

Rationale

There are three main advantages to using epidural or intrathecal analgesia.

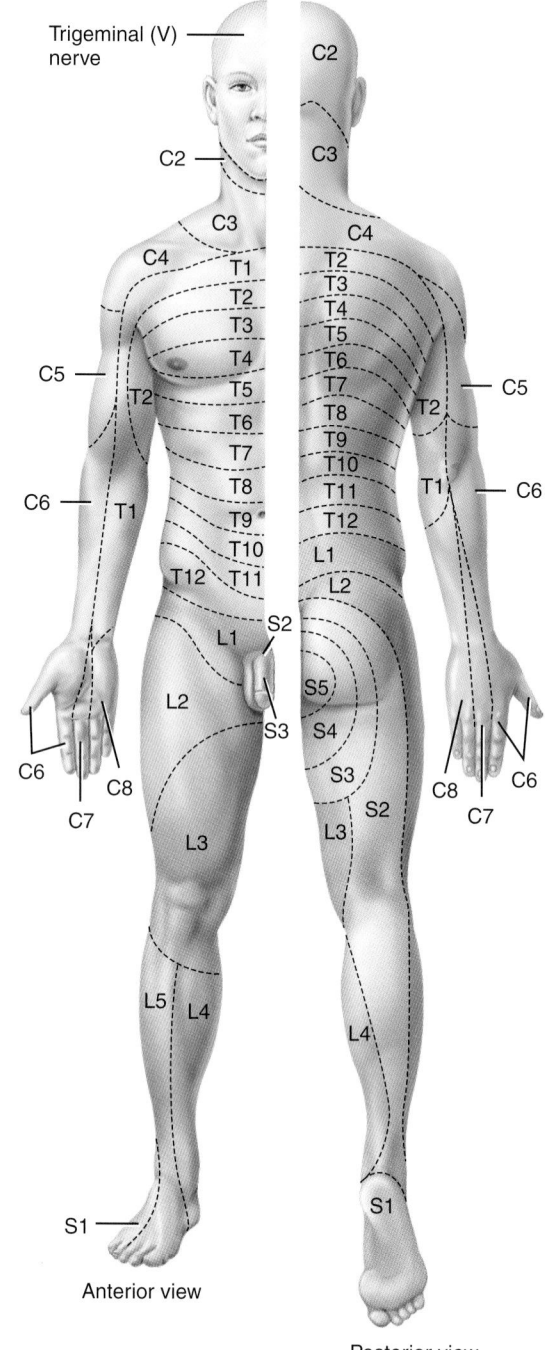

Figure 9.17 Distribution of dermatomes. Reproduced from Tortora and Derrickson (2009).

- It has the potential to provide effective dynamic pain relief for many patients (Wheatley *et al.* 2001).
- The combination of local anaesthetic agents with opioids has a synergistic action that allows the concentration of each drug to be reduced. This limits the unwanted side-effects of each drug (Fotiadis *et al.* 2004).
- There is also evidence that the use of epidural analgesia may reduce the stress response to surgery or trauma,

thereby reducing morbidity, recovery time and hospital stay (Kehlet 1997).

Indications

- Provision of analgesia during labour.
- As an alternative to general anaesthesia, for example in severe respiratory disease or for patients with malignant hyperthermia.
- Provision of postoperative analgesia. Epidural analgesia has been used since the late 1940s as a method of controlling postoperative pain (Chapman and Day 2001).
- Provision of analgesia for pain resulting from trauma, for example fractured ribs, which may result in respiratory impairment due to pain on breathing.
- Management of chronic intractable pain in patients with chronic or cancer-related pain who experience the following:
  - unacceptable side-effects with systemic opioids
  - unsuccessful treatment with opioids via other routes despite escalating doses
  - severe neuropathic pain due to tumour invasion or compression of nerves (Day 2001, Mercadante 1999, Smitt *et al.* 1998).
- To relieve muscle spasm and pain resulting from lumbar cord pressure due to disc protrusion or local oedema and inflammation.

For cancer patients who do not obtain pain relief from treatment with opioids administered orally, rectally, by injection or continuous infusion, there is evidence that both epidural and intrathecal analgesia can be effective (Ballantyne and Carwood 2005). Intrathecal analgesia can either be delivered via an external infusion pump or can be part of a fully implantable reservoir system (Dickson 2004).

Contraindications

These may be absolute or relative.

Absolute
- Patients with coagulation defects, which may result in haematoma formation and spinal cord compression, for example iatrogenic (anticoagulated patient) or congenital (haemophiliacs), or thrombocytopenia due to disease or as the result of anticancer treatment (Horlocker and Wedel 1998).
- Local sepsis at the site of proposed epidural or intrathecal injection; the result might be meningitis or epidural abscess formation.
- Proven allergy to the intended drug.
- Unstable spinal fracture.
- Patient refusal to consent to the procedure.

Relative
- Unstable cardiovascular system.
- Spinal deformity.

- Raised intracranial pressure (a risk of herniation if a dural tap occurs).
- Certain neurological conditions, for example multiple sclerosis, where an epidural may result in an exacerbation of the disease (Hall 2000).
- Unavailability of staff trained in the management of epidural or intrathecal analgesia (Macintyre and Schug 2007). Hall (2000) notes that staff managing patients with epidural or intrathecal analgesia should have undertaken a period of formal training to care for patients safely and competently.

Methods of administration

Continuous infusion

Continuous infusions of epidural drugs are the most effective way of providing dynamic pain relief after major surgical procedures (Kehlet and Holte 2001). Continuous infusions of intrathecal analgesic drugs have been shown to be effective in the management of chronic intractable pain (Ballantyne and Carwood 2005). Continuous infusions can be given by either a syringe pump or a designated infusion pump system. The effectiveness of this method of administering drugs is dependent on a number of factors including the combination of drugs used, the position of the spinal catheter at a level appropriate to the site of surgery or pain (Weetman and Allison 2006) and the volume of the local anaesthetic agent infused (Chapman and Day 2001, Hall 2000).

Patient-controlled epidural analgesia

The use of patient-controlled epidural analgesia (PCEA) has gained popularity in recent years because it enables patients to control their analgesia. For patients with postoperative or chronic pain, PCEA is used more effectively in combination with a low-dose background infusion (Wheatley *et al.* 2001). This ensures a baseline level of analgesia which can then be supplemented by the patient when required.

Bolus injections

Bolus injections of opioids and local anaesthetic agents are used infrequently to manage postoperative pain but are more commonly used for managing labour pain (Grond *et al.* 2000). This procedure is usually performed by the doctor. However, bolus doses of low-dose concentrations may be given by nursing or midwifery staff as part of an advanced practice role, according to local policy. This should follow an agreed period of education and supervised practice, which must be documented.

This is a clean aseptic procedure. Most epidural/intrathecal infusion pumps allow a bolus dose to be programmed and delivered from the pump. This prevents the administration line and bacterial filter from being accessed and thus minimizes the risk of introducing infection. Intrathecal bolus doses are usually only given by the doctor.

Classes of epidural and intrathecal drugs and mechanism of action

Three classes of drugs are commonly used to provide epidural or intrathecal analgesia: opioids, local anaesthetic agents and adjuvant drugs such as corticosteroids and clonidine.

Opioids

Whilst a number of different opioids have been used for epidural and intrathecal analgesia, two of the most commonly used are diamorphine and fentanyl (Bannon *et al.* 2001, Cook *et al.* 1997, Romer and Russell 1998). When either of these opioids is injected into the *epidural* space, part of the opioid dose:

- crosses the dura and arachnoid membrane and enters the CSF. From the CSF a proportion of the drug is taken up into the spinal cord and reaches the opioid receptors in the spinal cord. Once bound to the opioid receptors, this results in blocking of pain impulses
- enters the systemic circulation and contributes to analgesia
- binds to the epidural fat and does not contribute to analgesia.

When opioids are placed directly into the CSF in the intrathecal space, they attach directly to the opioid spinal cord receptor sites (Urdan *et al.* 2006).

Fentanyl differs from diamorphine in that it is more lipid soluble. This means that it passes more easily into the CSF, gaining faster access to the opioid receptors and having a more rapid onset of action. Fentanyl also has a shorter duration of action (1–4 hours) as opposed to diamorphine (6–12 hours) (Macintyre and Schug 2007).

Local anaesthetic drugs

Commonly used local anaesthetic agents include bupivacaine, levobupivacaine and ropivacaine. These drugs gain access to the nerve roots and the spinal cord by crossing the dura and subarachnoid membranes (Macintyre and Schug 2007). They inhibit pain transmission by blocking sodium ion channels which are involved in the propagation of electrical impulses along the spinal nerves.

The dose of a local anaesthetic agent will also determine which nerves are blocked. Low concentrations of bupivacaine (e.g. 0.100–0.125%) preferentially block nerve impulses in the smallest diameter nerve fibres, which include the pain and temperature sensory fibres. As the larger diameter motor fibres are less likely to be blocked with concentrations of 0.100–0.125% bupivacaine, the incidence of leg weakness is reduced and the patient is able to mobilize.

Adjuvant drugs

Corticosteroids

Although not licensed for epidural or intrathecal use, corticosteroid injections are often used to relieve pain caused by inflammatory irritation of nerve roots (Papagelopoulos *et al.* 2001).

Clonidine

Clonidine is a mixed alpha-adrenergic agonist. Although its exact mechanism of action is unknown, clonidine is believed to enhance analgesia provided by spinal opioids and local anaesthetic drugs (Smith and Elliott 2001). Clonidine has a specific role in the management of neuropathic pain in patients with advanced cancer (Mercadante 1999).

Drugs and doses for the management of intractable chronic and cancer pain

Epidural/intrathecal infusions of local anaesthetic–opioid combinations are frequently used for the management of intractable chronic and cancer pain. The most commonly used opioids are morphine, diamorphine and fentanyl. Although there is a lack of consensus over the method of converting from a systemic to an epidural/intrathecal opioid, Mercadante (1999) recommends that if converting from oral morphine, a starting dose of roughly 10% of the oral opioid should be given epidurally and then titrated to effect. For example, if a patient was receiving a total daily dose of 180 mg morphine sulphate orally, this would convert to a total daily dose of 18 mg of morphine via the epidural route. Stevens and Ghazi (2000) recommend that the intrathecal dose should be 10% of the calculated epidural dose. Thus, in the above example the intrathecal dose would be the epidural dose (18 mg) divided by 10 which would convert to a total daily dose of 1.8 mg of morphine via the intrathecal route.

Legal and professional issues

There should be formal induction courses and regular updates for doctors, nurses, theatre and recovery staff who will be responsible for supervising patients receiving continuous epidural analgesia (Royal College of Anaesthetists 2004). The acute pain service or a clearly designated consultant anaesthetist from the anaesthesia department will be responsible for the immediate supervision of patients receiving epidural infusions. The National Patient Safety Agency (NPSA 2007) recommends that in addition to routine training and regular updates, additional training occurs when changes are made to protocols, medicine products or medical devices. Routine training should include a programme to help healthcare staff gain competence and confidence in using infusion devices used to deliver epidural/intrathecal analgesia, a theoretical understanding of how the drugs work, and the monitoring required to detect both drug- and procedure-related side-effects and complications (Box 9.16).

Preprocedural considerations
Equipment

Epidurals are inserted using:

- a Tuohy needle (a bevelled curved tip needle to reduce the risk of accidental dural puncture, with 1 cm length markings, either 16 G or 18 G)

Box 9.16 Example of competency role development profile for epidural analgesia for acute pain. Intended learning outcomes and elements of practitioner competency

Knowledge and understanding

You are expected to possess knowledge and understanding of the following.

- The normal anatomy of the spinal cord.
- The physiology of pain and measures of pain management.
- Education and information needs of the patient/family/carer with regard to the implications of having an epidural, to ensure valid consent is given.
- Contraindications for epidural analgesia.
- Infection control considerations before, during and after insertion of an epidural.
- Principles of epidural care and management including side-effects and complications of epidural insertion and epidural analgesia.
- Observations required during the administration of epidural analgesia and the rationale for the frequency of:
  - respiratory rate/sedation levels
  - cardiovascular status
  - temperature
  - epidural site
  - dermatomal blockade
  - pain assessment.
- The standard prescription for epidural analgesia for acute pain management.
- Deviations from the standard prescription available and situations in which they may be used.
- Pharmacology of epidurally administered local anaesthetics and opioids and their side-effects.
- The optimum infusion rate.
- When to stop and remove an epidural catheter.
- Implications of anticoagulant therapy prior to removing the epidural catheter.
- Considerations for analgesia once epidural analgesia is stopped.

Skills

You are expected to possess the following skills.

- Ability to care for the patient before, during and immediately after epidural insertion.
- Ability to check the epidural site; frequency of checks and what problems to look for.
- How to redress the epidural site and frequency of epidural site dressing changes.
- How to assess pain and the frequency of assessment.
- How to carry out a dermatomal blockade assessment and where to document it.
- Ability to change epidural infusion rate.
- Ability to change epidural infusion bag and awareness of the frequency of infusion bag changes.
- Ability to change and prime the infusion administration set and awareness of the frequency of change.
- Ability to deal with equipment problems:
  - proximal occlusion alarm
  - distal occlusion alarm
  - cassette not fitted
  - low battery.
- Ability to deal with administration problems:
  - catheter disconnection from bacterial filter
  - catheter occlusion
  - catheter leakage
  - the patient still has pain
  - side-effects of analgesia
  - complications of epidural catheter insertion.
- Procedure for removing an epidural catheter.
- Safe disposal of unused epidural infusion bags after discontinuing therapy.

- an epidural catheter (a relatively stiff catheter made of polyamide, length 1000 mm with clear blue markings completely embedded in the catheter material)
- a bacterial filter (filters provide an additional degree of safety and control to prevent bacterial infections. Minimal dead space enables accurate dosing. A high pressure resistance up to 7 bar enhances safety during manual injection)
- connector (to ensure safe catheter fixation)
- loss of resistance device (to aid clear identification of the epidural space).

The equipment often comes in prepared sterile disposable epidural trays or packs (Parizkova and George 2009).

Dressings

The dressing over the epidural/intrathecal exit site needs to fulfil the following three functions.

- To help secure the epidural/intrathecal catheter.
- To minimize the risk of infection.
- To allow observation of the site without disturbing the dressing.

A transparent moisture-responsive occlusive dressing (e.g. Tegaderm™ or Opsite IV 3000™) fulfils these functions. Opsite IV 3000™ has been found to perform well as an epidural catheter fixation product (Lawler and Anderson 2002). The epidural/intrathecal site should be inspected daily and the dressing changed at least once weekly or more frequently if there is any serous discharge from the site (see Procedure guideline 9.16).

Pharmacological support
Combination of drugs used

Epidural or intrathecal infusions of local anaesthetic and opioid combinations are commonly used in the UK (Baker *et al.* 2004, Wheatley *et al.* 2001). The rationale behind their combined use is based on the observation that better analgesia is achieved with lower doses of each drug, therefore minimizing drug-related side-effects produced by higher concentrations (Curatolo *et al.* 1998, Fotiadis *et al.* 2004). Although the solutions used will vary with the clinical situation, common combinations of fentanyl. The use of premixed bags is recommended to minimize medication errors involving the epidural/intrathecal route (NPSA 2007).

Specific patient preparation

Patients undergoing epidural/intrathecal analgesia should always have a venous access device *in situ* before the procedure. This is because, although rare, a reaction to the opioid or local anaesthetic solution (e.g. respiratory depression or sympathetic blockade) may require immediate access to the venous system. The procedure should be performed in a clinical area with access to full resuscitation equipment.

Patient information and consent prior to using epidural/intrathecal analgesia for intractable chronic or cancer pain

The following issues should be addressed with the patient, family and primary healthcare team prior to using epidural/intrathecal analgesia for intractable chronic or cancer pain.

- *Drug-related side-effects*: the concentration of analgesics needed to provide sufficient analgesia for patients

Table 9.4 Optimal catheter location for different surgical sites

Surgical site	Catheter location
Thoracic	T6–T9
Upper abdominal	T7–T10
Lower abdominal	T9–L1
Hip/knee	L1–L4

with chronic cancer pain is often higher than the concentrations used postoperatively. As a result, drug-related side-effects such as motor weakness and urinary retention can occur. Some patients find these side-effects unacceptable and may prefer to avoid epidural/intrathecal analgesia altogether. Therefore, a discussion must take place with the patient and family to ensure that they are aware of these potential side-effects and are willing to continue with epidural/intrathecal analgesia (Wallace 2002).

- *Increased time in hospital*: the patient should also be informed that they will need to spend a period of time in hospital following insertion of the catheter, to allow for dose adjustment and ensure that side-effects are minimized and optimum pain management achieved.

Position of epidural or intrathecal catheter

Local anaesthetic drugs block nerve fibres at spinal segments adjacent to their site of administration. To ensure the local anaesthetic agent spreads to the dermatomes or nerves supplying the area of pain (e.g. the surgical site or the pain location caused by a tumour), the tip of the spinal catheter should be placed within the mid-dermatomal distribution of the pain site (Table 9.4). This achieves optimal analgesia using the least amount of drugs. If the catheter is placed below the dermatomes supplying the pain site then analgesia is likely to be inadequate (Macintyre and Schug 2007).

Procedure guideline 9.11 Epidural/intrathecal catheter insertion

Essential equipment

- Chlorhexidine 0.5% in 70% alcohol
- Local anaesthetic
- Selection of needles and syringes
- Sterile dressing pack
- Facemask
- Tuohy needle or assorted gauge lumbar puncture needles
- Sodium chloride 0.9% 10 mL ampoules

- Epidural/intrathecal catheter
- Bacterial filter
- Moisture-responsive transparent dressing and dressing tape to secure catheter (Cousins *et al.* 2003)

Preprocedure

Action	Rationale
1 Explain and discuss the procedure with the patient. If the intention is to provide postoperative analgesia then explanation and consent should have been discussed the day before surgery.	To ensure that the patient understands the procedure and gives their valid consent (NMC 2008a, C) and to ensure patient has time to assess information and ask questions.
2 Assist the patient into the required position: **Either lying:** ■ Patient should be lying comfortably on a firm surface. ■ Position pillow under patient's head. ■ On side with knees drawn up to the abdomen and clasped by the hands. ■ Support the patient in this position.	To allow identification of the spinal processes and intervertebral discs (Brown 1999, E).
Or sitting: Patient sits on firm surface with arms resting on a table, and with the head resting on the arms.	To ensure maximal widening of the intervertebral spaces which will provide easy access to the epidural/intrathecal space (Brown 1999, E).
3 Support, encourage and observe the patient throughout the procedure.	As the procedure takes place behind the patient, reassurance is very important (Chapman and Day 2001, E).
4 Assist the doctor as required. The doctor will proceed as follows.	

Procedure

5 Clean the skin with alcohol-based solution (e.g. chlorhexidine in 70% isopropyl alcohol).	To clean skin and minimize risk of contamination (Hebl 2006, R5; Kinirons *et al.* 2001, R1b).
6 Identify the area to be punctured and inject the skin and subcutaneous layers with local anaesthetic.	To ensure the spinal catheter is inserted at the correct level to provide analgesia and numb the skin prior to insertion of the Tuohy needle (Brown 1999, E).
7 Introduce Tuohy or spinal needles, usually between the identified vertebrae.	To access the epidural or intrathecal space (Brown 1999, E).
8 Ensure epidural/intrathecal space has been entered.	To prevent anaesthesia being given directly into spinal cord or intravenously by means of the dural veins (Brown 1999, E).
9 Inject test dose of drug (may be performed).	To ensure the position of the needle (Brown 1999, E).
10 Thread spinal catheter through barrel of Tuohy needle.	To facilitate intermittent topping up of anaesthesia and to allow greater control (Brown 1999, E).
11 Attach the bacterial filter.	To prevent injection of contaminants into spinal space (Brown 1999, E).
12 Apply transparent occlusive dressing and tape to the catheter insertion site.	To prevent the catheter being dislodged, to aid visibility and minimize contamination of the site (Baker *et al.* 2004, E).
13 Inject solution into epidural/intrathecal space via catheter.	To provide anaesthesia and analgesia (Brown 1999, E).

(Continued)

Procedure guideline 9.11 (*Continued*)

Postprocedure

14 Position the patient post procedure according to the doctor's instructions, tilting if appropriate.	To ensure spread of solution to provide optimum effect (Brown 1999, E).
15 Take vital signs observations of blood pressure, pulse, respiratory rate and sedation score as dictated by the anaesthetist in the immediate postinsertion period. After this, refer to local guidelines for frequency of observations required (see Box 9.17).	To monitor for signs of hypotension and respiratory depression (Weetman and Allison 2006, E).
16 Make the patient comfortable. Usually the patient is nursed flat for the first 3–6 hours, then slowly elevated into a sitting position. Bedclothes should not constrict the feet.	To ensure that any CSF leak is minimized and to prevent the patient developing a headache. To prevent the development of footdrop due to motor and sensory alterations caused by local anaesthetics. E
17 Assess pain regularly using a visual analogue scale or pain chart if appropriate. Observe the patient's movements and facial expressions. Discuss insufficient or ineffective analgesia with the anaesthetist.	To ensure optimal pain management and that the patient is involved in their pain management (Macintyre and Schug 2007, E).

Box 9.17 Example of frequency of monitoring after epidural insertion and for the duration of therapy

In the Critical Care Unit (CCU) or recovery room

Continuous monitoring of respiratory and cardiovascular function (record 4-hourly observations on epidural analgesia prescription and observation chart in addition to CCU chart).

In the ward

Record observations on epidural analgesia prescription and observation chart.

On return from CCU

- At least **2 hourly** recording of respiratory rate, sedation level (0 awake, 1 dozing intermittently, 2 asleep (rousable), 3 asleep (difficult to rouse)), peripheral tissue oxygen saturation (using the pulse oximeter), pulse and blood pressure **for the first 12 hours.**
- If recordings of the above observations and the epidural infusion rate remain stable, the frequency of observations can then be **reduced to every 2–4 hours**.
- Record the temperature **4 hourly**.

On return from recovery directly to the ward

- ½ **hourly** recording of respiratory rate, sedation level (0 awake, 1 dozing intermittently, 2 asleep (rousable), 3 asleep (difficult to rouse)), peripheral tissue oxygen saturation, pulse and blood pressure **for 2 hours.**
- If recordings are stable and the epidural rate remains stable, the frequency of observations can be reduced to **2 hourly for 24 hours.**
- If recordings and the epidural rate remain stable, the frequency can then be reduced to **2–4 hourly** until the epidural infusion is stopped.

These observations must be carried out even if the patient is asleep.

If the epidural infusion rate is increased the observations should be recorded ½ **hourly for 2 hours after each change in rate** as this may increase the risk of respiratory depression or hypotension. If the observations remain stable then the frequency of observation can be recorded at the same level as prior to the rate change.

Procedure guideline 9.12 Epidural/intrathecal analgesia top-up (bolus)

Essential equipment

- Antiseptic cleaning agent
- Syringes and needles
- Drug prescribed

- Water or 0.9% sodium chloride for injection as necessary
- Patient's prescription chart
- Sterile hub or bung

Preprocedure

Action	Rationale
1 Wash hands with soap and water or bactericidal handrub.	To reduce the risk of cross-infection (Preston 2005, C).
2 Check the drug to be administered and diluents, according to policy.	To ensure the correct drug, amount and concentration are administered to the correct patient (NMC 2008b, C).
3 Draw up the drug as per local policy.	To maintain safe practice in medicines management (NMC 2008b, C).
4 Check patient's nameband against prescription.	To ensure the correct drug, amount and concentration is administered to the correct patient (NMC 2008b, C).

Procedure

5 Clean the access portal of the bacterial filter.	To prevent the introduction of contaminants and micro-organisms into the epidural space. E
6 Inject drug as prescribed.	To give the drug to the patient. E
7 Monitor blood pressure, pulse and respirations at least every 5 minutes for 30–45 minutes.	To monitor for signs of hypotension and respiratory depression (side-effects of local anaesthetic and opioid drugs) (Coniam and Mendham 2005, C).

Postprocedure

8 Dispose of the equipment appropriately.	To prevent injury to patients, staff and to comply with medicines management policy (NMC 2008b, C).
9 Document the bolus dose administration in the medical and nursing records.	To aid communication and dissemination of information between members of the multidisciplinary team (NMC 2009, C).

Procedure guideline 9.13 Epidural/intrathecal sensory blockade: assessment

Essential equipment

- Ice or single use proprietary cold pack OR
- Ethanol spray

- These can be discarded after each test to reduce cross-infection risk
- Copy of a dermatome distribution figure or chart (see Figure 9.17)

Preprocedure

Action	Rationale
1 Explain and discuss the procedure with the patient. Obtain informed verbal consent from the patient.	To ensure that the patient understands the procedure and gives their valid consent (NMC 2008a, C) and to ensure patient has time to assess information and ask questions (NMC 2008a, C).

(Continued)

Procedure guideline 9.13 *(Continued)*

Procedure

2 Explain to the patient that they need to report: ■ If the temperature of the ice/cold changes or becomes warmer ■ If they cannot feel the ice/cold sensation at all.	This will indicate the dermatome level at which the epidural/intrathecal analgesia is working.
3 Remove any clothing that may restrict the assessment.	The ice or spray needs to be applied directly to the skin to undertake the assessment.
4 Test the ice/cold pack or spray on an area of the body that should not be affected by the epidural/ intrathecal infusion (the face or the back of the hand).	To ensure the patient can feel the cold sensation.
5 Starting at the top of the chest (just above nipple level), place the ice/cold pack/spray above the incision or level of pain and ask the patient if this feels as cold as when placed on the test area. Continue this procedure down the torso and the legs if appropriate for the level of epidural/intrathecal analgesia and on the right and left of the body.	

Postprocedure

6 Document at what level the patient can detect a change as per the dermatome chart (see Figure 9.17).

Problem-solving table 9.2 **Prevention and resolution (Procedure guidelines 9.11, 9.12, and 9.13)**

Problem	Cause	Prevention	Suggested action
Headache	Dural puncture	Expertise of practitioner inserting the epidural	Bedrest: headache will be less severe if patient lies flat. Replacement fluids either intravenously or orally to encourage formation of CSF. Administer analgesics for headache. If headache does not settle, contact the anaesthetic team who may consider an epidural blood patch to seal the puncture (Gaiser 2006)
Sedation and respiratory depression (opioid toxicity) Circumoral tingling and numbness, twitching, convulsions and apnoea (local anaesthetic toxicity)	If catheter migrates into a blood vessel, signs of opioid or local anaesthetic toxicity can occur	Expertise of practitioner inserting the epidural Careful monitoring of the patient to detect early symptoms	Stop epidural infusion Contact pain/anaesthetic team or summon emergency assistance. Treat the patient for complications of opioid or local anaesthetic overdose If necessary, support ventilation (Chapman and Day 2001)

Problem	Cause	Prevention	Suggested action
Apnoea, profound hypotension and unconsciousness	If an epidural catheter migrates from the epidural space into the intrathecal space to the CSF, the analgesic solution may reach as high as the cranial subarachnoid space. If this occurs the respiratory muscles are paralysed together with the cranial nerves, resulting in apnoea, profound hypotension and unconsciousness. This is because intrathecal doses are calculated as one-tenth of the epidural dose and migration from the epidural space to the intrathecal space leads to a drug overdose	Expertise of practitioner inserting the epidural Careful monitoring of the patient to detect early symptoms	Stop epidural infusion Summon emergency assistance Prepare emergency equipment to support respiration and ventilate lungs Prepare emergency drugs and intravenous fluids and administer as directed Prepare equipment for intubation
Back pain and tenderness and nerve root pain with sensory and motor weakness.	Epidural haematoma	Assessment of coagulation status before insertion and removal of the epidural/intrathecal catheter	Urgent neurological assessment
			Computed tomography (CT) or magnetic resonance imaging (MRI) scan to accurately diagnose if there is nerve or spinal cord compression. If a haematoma is diagnosed prepare patient for urgent surgery (Chapman and Day 2001)
			To avoid haematoma on removal of epidural in patients treated with prophylactic anticoagulants, see guidelines for timing of removal
Back pain and tenderness May have redness and purulent discharge from catheter exit site May also develop nerve root signs with neuropathic pain and sensory/motor weakness	Epidural abscess	Maintain aseptic technique when accessing the epidural/intrathecal analgesic system Monitor temperature regularly and check insertion site for evidence of infection	If the epidural catheter is still in situ, remove and send tip off for culture and sensitivity Treat with antibiotics Carry out CT or MRI scan and refer for urgent neurosurgery to prevent paraplegia (Chapman and Day 2001)

477

(Continued)

Problem-solving table 9.2 (*Continued*)

Problem	Cause	Prevention	Suggested action
Headaches, fever, neck stiffness, photophobia	Meningitis	Maintain asceptic technique when accessing the epidural/intrathecal analgesic system Monitor temperature regularly	Assist anaesthetist/doctor to obtain CSF sample for microbiology analysis. Initiate antibiotic therapy as per hospital policy Non-pharmacological measures for symptom management, for example dim lights If the infection does not respond to antibiotics it may be necessary to remove the catheter and convert back to systemic analgesia until meningitis has resolved (Mercadante 1999)
Pain, paraesthesia, numbness in lower extremities that may progress to paresis	Intrathecal catheter granuloma (an inflammatory mass that forms around the catheter tip)	In long-term therapy an intrathecal may be preferable to epidural to minimize the development of a granuloma due to the presence of the CSF	MRI scan to diagnose the problem. Stop infusion (granulomas may resolve on their own once the infusion is stopped (Du Pen 2005))

Procedure guideline 9.14 **Epidural/intrathecal catheter removal**

Essential equipment

- Dressing pack
- Skin cleaning agent, for example chlorhexidine 0.5% in 70% alcohol
- Alcohol handrub
- Specimen container (if epidural catheter needs to be sent for bacterial culture)
- Occlusive dressing

Preprocedure

Action	Rationale
1 Explain and discuss the procedure with the patient.	To ensure the patient understands the procedure and gives their valid consent (NMC 2008a, C).
2 Wash hands with bactericidal soap and water or bactericidal alcohol handrub.	To minimize cross-infection (Preston 2005, C).
3 Open dressing pack.	

Procedure

4 Wash hands and remove tape and dressing from catheter insertion site.	To minimize risk of cross-infection (Preston 2005, C).
5 Gently, in one swift movement, remove the catheter. Check that the catheter is intact. This can be done by observing that the tip of the catheter is marked blue and that the 1 cm marks along the length of the catheter are all intact.	To ensure the catheter is removed intact with the minimum of discomfort to the patient. E

6	Clean around the catheter exit site using skin cleaning agent.	To minimize contamination of site by micro-organisms. E
7	Apply an occlusive dressing and leave *in situ* for 24 hours.	To prevent inadvertent access of micro-organisms along the tract. E

Postprocedure

8 The epidural/intrathecal tip may be sent for culture and sensitivity if infection is suspected, or according to local policy.

9 Document that the catheter was removed intact in nursing notes.

Procedure guideline 9.15 Epidural/intrathecal infusion: setting up and utilizing an ambulatory pump

This is a clean aseptic technique.

Equipment

- Pump

Procedure

Action	Rationale
1 Check the prescribed drugs and diluent against the prescription. If not dispensed in infusion bags prepared aseptically in a special unit, specific local arrangements should be agreed between anaesthetists, pharmacists and ward/theatre/recovery staff for the preparation of the solution.	To ensure correct infusion is ready to connect. Except in special circumstances, the solutions should be prepared aseptically in a special unit (Royal College of Anaesthetists 2004, C).
2 Attach relevant extension set; apply drug information label. Recheck against prescription.	Clear labelling must be used to distinguish solutions for epidural/intrathecal infusion from all other infusions (Royal College of Anaesthetists 2004, C).
3 Check patency of epidural/intrathecal catheter as described in local policy or guidelines.	To ensure the catheter is in the correct position. E
4 Insert the extension set into the pump and prime the extension set, following the manufacturer's instructions for use of the pump.	To ensure the set is free from air when the infusion is commenced, thus minimizing the risk of air entering the catheter. E
5 Open the sterile bacterial filter using a non-touch technique.	To minimize the risk of introducing any contaminants and micro-organisms into the epidural/intrathecal space via the filter. E
6 Attach the extension set to the bacterial filter and start the pump.	To ensure the pump is working and the drugs are being delivered. E
7 Place pump and infusion bag into the lock box or 'carry bag/pouch', ensuring that the tubing is not kinked.	To ensure comfort for the patient and to avoid obstruction to the infusion. E

Procedure guideline 9.16 Epidural/intrathecal exit site dressing change

Essential equipment

- Sterile dressing pack
- Skin cleaning agent, for example chlorhexidine in 70% alcohol
- Transparent occlusive dressing

Preprocedure

Action	Rationale
1 Explain and discuss the procedure with the patient.	To ensure that the patient understands the procedure and gives their valid consent (NMC 2008a, C).
2 Wash hands with soap and water. Clean trolley (or plastic tray in the community) with chlorhexidine in 70% alcohol with a paper towel.	To minimize cross-infection (Preston 2005, C). To provide a clean working surface (Parker 2004, E).
3 Position the patient comfortably on their side or sitting forward so that the site is easily accessible without undue exposure of the patient.	To maintain the patient's dignity and comfort. This is especially important when carers are attending to an area that is not visible to the patient (Chapman and Day 2001, E).
4 Prepare trolley or tray with sterile field and cleaning solution.	To minimize risk of infection and ensure equipment is available (Preston 2005, C).

Procedure

5 Remove old dressing and place in disposable bag.	To prevent cross-infection (Fraise and Bradley 2009, E).
6 Wash hands with bactericidal handrub.	To minimize the risk of microbial contamination (Fraise and Bradley 2009, E).
7 Observe site for any signs of infection such as redness, swelling or purulent discharge. If any of these are present contact the hospital anaesthetic/pain team for advice.	To ensure careful monitoring of site to minimize the chance of any infection (Royal College of Anaesthetists 2004, C).
8 Clean site with skin-cleaning agent (chlorhexidine in 70% alcohol).	To minimize the risk of infection (Hebl 2006, R5; Kinirons *et al.* 2001, R1b; Mimoz *et al.* 1999, R1b).
9 Apply transparent occlusive dressing over the whole area.	To anchor the epidural/intrathecal catheter, minimize the risk of infection and allow observation of the epidural/intrathecal site (Burns *et al.* 2001, R1b; Royse *et al.* 2006, E).
10 Ensure that the patient is comfortable.	

Postprocedure

11 Dispose of all material in the clinical waste bag.	To prevent environmental contamination (Preston 2005, C).
12 Wash hands with soap and water.	To reduce the risk of cross-infection (Preston 2005, C).

Procedure guideline 9.17 Discharge planning for patients with epidural/intrathecal catheter *in situ* for chronic cancer pain

An epidural/intrathecal infusion should not be seen as a barrier to the patient leaving hospital. Patients can be safely managed in the community provided the following areas are addressed.

Procedure

Action	Rationale
1 Convert patient's infusion to one that requires the minimum of changing, such as an infusion bag and ambulatory pump rather than a 20 mL syringe and syringe driver.	This will reduce the workload of the patient/family or district nurse and also minimizes the number of interruptions to the patient circuit, thus minimizing the chance of microbial contamination. E
2 Ensure that the patient will not be alone at home.	Epidural/intrathecal catheters can obstruct, become dislodged and the battery can fail on the device; most patients need immediate reassurance and practical help in these situations (Day 2001, E).
3 Arrange preparation of epidural/intrathecal drug infusion bags, usually in batches to provide enough delivery for 1 week. This can be arranged at the cancer centre or the referring hospital if they have the appropriate pharmaceutical arrangements.	Pharmacy reconstitution ensures aseptic preparation, thus minimizing the chance of microbial contamination, and reduces the workload and anxiety for family/district nurse. It should also be noted that epidural/intrathecal infusions may contain a combination of drugs and pharmacy reconstitution may help to reduce preparation error. E
4 Discuss how the infusion bags will be collected each week; they cannot be posted because they contain controlled drugs.	The method of collection needs to be discussed at an early stage with the family/district nurse to ensure continuity of infusion bag delivery and avoid any anxiety or delay to discharge. E
5 The patient/family should be provided with the following equipment to take home. (a) Spare battery. (b) Bottle of bactericidal handrub. (c) Bottle of chlorhexidine in 70% alcohol. (d) Sterile gauze. (e) Syringes and needles. (f) 0.9% Sodium chloride for injection. (g) One spare bacterial filter and screw connector. (h) One week's supply of reconstituted epidural/intrathecal infusion bags. (i) Written advice re contact numbers/troubleshooting and prescription.	To ensure that the first week of therapy continues smoothly.
6 Patient/family and district nurse/general practitioner should be taught and trained in the following areas. (a) Setting up the infusion. (b) The functions of the ambulatory device, including alarms and visual displays. (c) Loading the administration set into the pump and priming the set. (d) Observation of the epidural/intrathecal site for signs and symptoms which would indicate an infection, for example redness, tenderness, swelling, leakage or pus.	To reduce anxiety and increase patient comfort and trust. E To ensure that the patient/family and community team feel confident: (i) in using the infusion pump; (ii) in troubleshooting pump problems; (iii) about where to seek help if they experience any problems. E

481

(Continued)

Procedure guideline 9.17 *(Continued)*

(e) The prescribed therapy for breakthrough pain.
(f) Troubleshooting (see Problem-solving table 9.3).
(g) The procedure for obtaining medical/nursing help locally or at the cancer centre 24 hourly and every day of the week.
(h) Dressing of the epidural/intrathecal site.

7 Arrange any appropriate follow-up. This will be determined by the clinical status of the patient.	Patient may not return to the hospital for follow-up unless there are any problems if the intent is to move the patient's care to the community team, for example, in the terminal phase of illness when the patient may wish to be at home. However, contact with the community team should be maintained to ensure any problems with the epidural/intrathecal system are dealt with swiftly. E

Problem-solving table 9.3 **Prevention and resolution (Procedure guidelines 9.14, 9.15, 9.16 and 9.17)**

Problem	Cause	Prevention	Suggested action
Ambulatory pump auditory alarm	Battery failure is most likely	Only use batteries when ambulatory. Plug machine into mains power source when at rest	Stop pump, remove old and replace with new battery; ensure battery is fitted up snugly to connections. Turn on pump and ensure light indicator is flashing
	Catheter occlusion	Ensure catheter is kept free of obstruction or kinking	Check the catheter and administration set for any kinking or occlusion by equipment. If there is no evidence then stop pump, draw up 0.9% sodium chloride and flush catheter. If catheter clears, reattach pump, press start and ensure light indicator is flashing. If catheter is still obstructed and will not flush, phone cancer centre/general practitioner
Sudden acute pain	Catheter obstruction; catheter movement; change in pathology		Check the catheter for any obvious problems which can be quickly resolved such as catheter disconnection. If the catheter has blocked or migrated outwards, stop the infusion pump and give the patient a breakthrough dose of analgesia orally or subcutaneously. Inform general practitioner and/or hospital anaesthetic/pain team as soon as possible. If the patient has had an exacerbation of pain due to disease progression, follow advice from hospital team (the infusion rate may require titrating or the concentration of drugs may need to be changed)

Problem	Cause	Prevention	Suggested action
Increasing pain and leaking noted on patient's clothes	Disconnection of epidural/ intrathecal catheter from filter. Patient movement: typically turning in bed at night	Use a fixation device or adhesive tape to secure the catheter to the skin to minimize risk of disconnection from friction and pulling on the catheter	Stop the pump. Wrap the disconnected end of the catheter in a piece of sterile gauze and contact the district nursing/ hospital team for advice Suggested procedure for district nursing/ hospital team (Langevin *et al.* 1996): ■ Clean approximately 15 cm of the disconnected catheter with chlorhexidine in 70% alcohol. Allow to air dry completely ■ Using sterile scissors, cut the cleaned catheter 10 cm away from the contaminated end ■ Insert the cleaned end of catheter into a sterile screw connector and catheter filter ■ Change the epidural/intrathecal infusion extension set and recommence infusion
Redness, swelling or leakage of discoloured fluid from site	Infection or local irritation at site from skin interaction with the plastic catheter	Maintain aseptic technique when accessing the epidural/intrathecal analgesic system Monitor temperature regularly	Contact general practitioner and hospital anaesthetic/pain team. If infection is suspected, the patient should be started on antibiotics to prevent spread of any infection into the epidural space. It may be necessary to remove the catheter if the patient has a temperature, there is pus at the exit site or if the patient has back pain

483

Postprocedural considerations

Immediate care

Volume of infusion

As the volume of local anaesthetic agent influences the number of spinal nerves that are blocked, it is important to maintain the hourly infusion rate at a volume which keeps the appropriate nerves blocked (Chapman and Day 2001, Hall 2000).

Monitoring the patient

Effectiveness of blockade

The spinal nerves supply specific areas of skin known as dermatomes (see Figure 9.17). Sensitivity to changes in temperature (such as the cold of ice) along the sensory dermatome can be used to assess the level of epidural/intrathecal block. This level should be checked to ensure that the epidural/intrathecal is providing pain relief by covering the area of the site of pain, but is also necessary to maintain safety during the administration of epidural/intrathecal infusions. If the sensory block is too high (above T4) then there is an increased risk of respiratory and cardiac symptoms as a result of the local anaesthetic effects on nerves at this level, and if it is too dense it will cause unnecessary motor blockade.

Ongoing care

When caring for a patient receiving epidural or intrathecal analgesia, it is important to monitor the patient for the following:

■ drug-related side-effects
■ pain intensity
■ signs of complications due to the epidural or intrathecal procedure (see Problem-solving table 9.2)
■ equipment-related problems, such as the epidural/intrathecal catheter or the infusion pump (see Problem-solving table 9.3).

Drug-related side-effects

There are a number of drug-related side-effects associated with epidural/intrathecal opioids and local anaesthetic agents.

Opioids

- *Respiratory depression*: this is due to the action of opioids on the respiratory centre. Respiratory depression may occur at two different time intervals.
  - *Early*: usually within 2 hours of the opioid injection. This may occur if high blood levels of the opioid follow absorption from the epidural space into the systemic circulation (Macintyre and Schug 2007).
  - *Late*: this may not be seen for 6–12 hours after an opioid is given. It results from rostral migration of the drug in the CSF to the brainstem and respiratory centre (Macintyre and Schug 2007). This is less likely to occur with lipid-soluble opioids such as fentanyl.
- *Sedation*: although there may be many different causes of sedation, epidural/intrathecal opioids can cause sedation owing to their effect on the central nervous system. Opioid-induced sedation is often an early warning sign of respiratory depression.
- *Nausea and vomiting*: nausea and vomiting is caused by the action of opioids on the vomiting centre in the brainstem and stimulation of the chemoreceptor trigger zone in the fourth ventricle of the brain.
- *Pruritus*: although the exact mechanism is unknown, pruritus is presumed to be centrally mediated and a consequence of activation of opioid receptors in the spinal cord (Sands *et al.* 1998).
- *Urinary retention*: this is due to opioid inhibition of the micturition reflex which is evoked by increases in bladder volume.

Local anaesthetic agents

- *Hypotension*: this can be caused by two mechanisms. Firstly, local anaesthetic agents can spread outside the epidural/intrathecal space, blocking the sympathetic nerves. This results in peripheral vasodilation and hypotension. It is most likely to occur if a bolus dose of local anaesthetic agent (e.g. 10 mL of 0.25% bupivacaine) is given to improve pain control (Macintyre and Schug 2007). Secondly, if the local anaesthetic agent spreads above the T4 dermatome (nipple line), the cardio-accelerator nerves may become blocked, leading to bradycardia and hypotension (Macintyre and Schug 2007).
- *Motor blockade*: this will depend on the concentration and total dose of local anaesthetic agent used and the position of the epidural/intrathecal catheter (Hall 2000). Motor blockade occurs when the local anaesthetic agent blocks the larger diameter motor nerves. Leg weakness will occur if the motor nerves supplying the legs are blocked.
- *Urinary retention*: as with epidural/intrathecal opioids, blockade of the nerves supplying the bladder sphincter can cause urinary retention.

Routine monitoring of the patient for these side-effects must be carried out to facilitate early management. The patient's blood pressure, respiratory rate and peripheral tissue oxygenation should be monitored continuously initially and then according to local policy and as the patient's condition dictates.

For guidance on managing the side-effects associated with epidural/intrathecal opioids and local anaesthetic agents, see Table 9.5.

Assessment of pain for patients with epidural analgesia

Pain should be assessed (at rest and on movement) at the same time that the patient's routine observations are carried out. Simple numerical (e.g. 0–10 where 0 is no pain and 10 is the worst pain imaginable) or verbal rating scales (e.g. none, mild, moderate, severe, or very severe) can be used.

Inadequate postoperative pain management can lead to physiological complications (respiratory, cardiovascular, gastrointestinal and endocrine systems) and adverse effects (behavioural, such as reduced mobility, and psychological, such as increased anxiety and reduced mood) (Macintyre and Schug 2007). Thus, when patients are assessed the practitioner should ensure the patient can take a deep breath and cough and mobilize with a minimal level of pain to reduce the impact of the physiological, behavioural and psychological effects of undertreated acute pain.

When used for chronic pain management, the aim of epidural/intrathecal analgesia is to improve the overall quality of life of the patient. Although it is acceptable to use simple pain assessment rating scales, a more in-depth pain assessment scale may be used such as the BPI (Cleeland 1991).

Equipment and prescription safety checks

When a patient is receiving a continuous infusion of epidural/intrathecal analgesia it is advisable to carry out the safety checks given in Table 9.6 at least once per shift.

Removal of epidural/intrathecal catheter

Before an epidural/intrathecal catheter is removed, it is essential to consider the clotting status of the patient's blood. If the patient is fully anticoagulated a clotting profile must be performed and advice sought from the medical staff as to when the catheter can be removed. If the patient is receiving a prophylactic anticoagulant the following guidelines are recommended (Horlocker and Wedel 1998, Rowlingson and Hanson 2005, Vandermeulen *et al.* 1994).

Low-dose low molecular weight heparin

If this is given once daily, the epidural/intrathecal catheter should be removed at least 12 hours after the last injection and several hours prior to the next dose. The timing will depend on the manufacturer's recommended guidelines; for example, for Tinzaparin (Leo Laboratories Ltd) it is recommended that epidural or spinal catheters are removed a minimum of 4 hours before the next dose.

Unfractionated heparin

The epidural/intrathecal catheter should be removed following local guidelines and the advice of the anaesthetic/pain management team.

Table 9.5 Epidural/intrathecal infusions of local anaesthetic agents and opioids: management of side-effects

Problem	Cause	Suggested action
Respiratory depression	Increasing age Elderly patients are more susceptible to the side-effects of opioids due to age-related alterations in the distribution, metabolism and excretion of drugs	If respiratory rate falls to 8 breaths a minute or below: **(a)** Stop the epidural/intrathecal infusion **(b)** Summon emergency assistance **(c)** Commence oxygen via facemask and encourage the patient to take deep breaths **(d)** Review current analgesic prescription and consider reducing opioid and local anaesthetic doses before resuming the infusion (Macintyre *et al.* 2010)
	Concurrent use of systemic opioids or sedatives Patients receiving opioids by epidural/intrathecal infusion should not be given opioids by any other route unless given in the palliative care setting for breakthrough pain	**1** Stop the epidural/intrathecal infusion **2** Stay with the patient and monitor respiratory rate, sedation score and peripheral tissue oxygenation (using a pulse oximeter) continuously **3** Commence oxygen therapy **4** Consider giving naloxone if prescribed by anaesthetist or patient unrousable and naloxone already prescribed (when utilized for acute pain management) **5** Review analgesia: stop any other opioids prescribed and consider changing parameters of epidural/intrathecal infusion (McCaffery and Pasero 1999)
Sedation: *Mild:* patient drowsy but easy to rouse *Severe:* patient difficult to rouse	See Respiratory depression	**1** If patient has mild sedation, consider reducing the rate of the infusion or the dose of opioid or taking the opioid out of the infusion **2** If patient is difficult to rouse and opioid toxicity/overdose is suspected, follow management for respiratory depression
Hypotension	Patients with hypovolaemia Patients with a high thoracic epidural in whom the concentration of local anaesthetic agent and volume of infusion cause blockade of the cardio-accelerator nerves	If blood pressure falls suddenly: **(a)** Stop the epidural/intrathecal infusion **(b)** Summon emergency assistance **(c)** Administer oxygen via facemask or nasal cannula **(d)** Stay with the patient and monitor blood pressure at 5-minute intervals **(e)** Ensure polyfusor of Haemaccel or Gelofusine is readily available and use if prescribed by the anaesthetist **(f)** Vasoconstrictor agents such as ephedrine or metaraminol may need to be given by the anaesthetic team if hypotension does not respond to a fluid challenge of Haemaccel or Gelofusine (Macintyre and Schug 2007)
Motor blockade	More likely to occur when higher concentrations of local anaesthetic agents are given by continuous infusion If a high concentration of a local anaesthetic agent is administered via a low lumbar epidural/intrathecal catheter then the lumbar motor nerves are likely to be blocked, causing leg weakness	Do not attempt to mobilize patient if leg weakness is evident Contact pain or anaesthetic team for advice: reducing the concentration of the local anaesthetic agent or the rate of the epidural/intrathecal infusion may help to resolve this problem (Pasero and McCaffrey 1999)

485

(Continued)

Table 9.5 (*Continued*)

Nausea and vomiting	Previous episodes of nausea and vomiting with opioids	Regular administration of antiemetics
	Exacerbated by low blood pressure	Treat other causes, for example low blood pressure
		Consider use of non-pharmacological methods (e.g. stimulation of the P6 acupressure point)
Pruritus (usually more marked over the face, chest and abdomen)	Previous pruritus with opioids	Administer an antihistamine such as chlorpheniramine (may be contraindicated in patients who are becoming increasingly sedated) or a small dose of naloxone (administer with caution as this can easily reverse analgesia)
		If pruritus does not resolve, consider switching to another opioid or removing the opioid from the infusion (McCaffery and Pasero 1999)
Urinary retention	More likely to occur if opioids and local anaesthetic agents are infused in combination	Catheterize patient

Ongoing care for patients with intractable chronic and cancer pain

Monitoring after insertion

For the first 24 hours after epidural/intrathecal insertion, the patient should be monitored for signs of drug-related side-effects or uncontrolled pain. Intravenous access should be maintained for at least 24 hours so that emergency drugs and fluids can be given if necessary.

After 24 hours, providing the patient's condition is stable, routine monitoring of respiratory rate and cardiac function is not usually required unless indicated clinically by the patient's condition or by local policy guidelines. This allows monitoring for patient safety immediately post insertion whilst minimizing invasive procedures in patients with chronic pain problems. Ongoing assessment of pain and observation for any signs of infection (temperature monitoring and observation of the catheter exit site) should be continued for the duration of epidural/intrathecal analgesia.

Minimizing infection

Infection is a complication with long-term epidural or intrathecal analgesia.

Tunnelling the epidural/intrathecal catheter

To minimize the risk of a serious infection (e.g. epidural abscess, meningitis), it is common to tunnel the epidural/intrathecal catheter during insertion. This reduces the speed at which a local infection can spread along the catheter before reaching the epidural/intrathecal space (Baker *et al.* 2004). Once a local infection is suspected at the tunnelled site, treatment with antibiotics should be prompt to prevent a systemic infection. See Complications specific to intrathecal analgesia, Meningitis.

Epidural/intrathecal bacterial filter changes during longer term infusions

De Cicco *et al.* (1995) found that the use of bacterial filters during prolonged epidural catheterization maintained an unmodified antimicrobial function for more than 60 days when perfused with reduced volumes of drugs. It is recommended that bacterial filters should only be changed every 4–6 weeks unless blocked (De Cicco *et al.* 1995, Mercadente 1999). More frequent filter changes have been associated with an increased risk of microbial colonization as a direct result of the manipulations (De Cicco *et al.* 1995).

Table 9.6 Epidural/intrathecal analgesia: safety checklist

Checklist	Rationale
Check the prescription and rate of the epidural/intrathecal infusion	To ensure epidural/intrathecal drugs are being administered correctly
Check the epidural/intrathecal infusion/syringe pump extension set is connected to the epidural catheter and not to any other access device	To ensure drugs are administered via the correct route
Check the bacterial filter is securely attached to the epidural/intrathecal catheter	To prevent accidental disconnection of the catheter from the filter
Check that the dressing over the epidural/intrathecal catheter exit site is secure	To prevent catheter dislodgement and minimize the risk of contamination of the catheter site

Discharge planning

If it is anticipated that the patient will go home with a continuous epidural or intrathecal infusion, the patient's general practitioner and community nursing team should be consulted at the outset to determine whether they are willing to be involved and/or trained in the management of epidural/intrathecal analgesia care.

Arrangements should also be made with the primary healthcare team for the provision of a suitable epidural/intrathecal pump and the supply of reconstituted syringes/infusion bags. Primary care teams, patients and their families will need to be trained and supplied with the appropriate equipment, drugs, catheter filters, information about the infusion pump, how to identify a catheter-related or systemic infection and what to do if pain occurs or complications arise. Contact numbers must be available in case specialist advice is needed.

Complications

If pain is not controlled and the infusion has already been titrated according to hospital guidelines, the pain/anaesthetic team should be contacted for advice after checking the following.

- The catheter is still *in situ*.
- The catheter is still connected to the bacterial filter.
- There are no leaks within the system.
- The height of the epidural/intrathecal block. This will indicate whether the block has fallen below the upper limit of the incision or pain site. To check the height of the block, use a small piece of ice or cold solution (ethyl alcohol). Start at the top of the chest above the patient's incision or pain site. Gently dab the ice (or apply the cold solution) down each side of the patient's body (one side and then the other). Use a dermatome map to assess the upper and lower limits of where the sensation changes (see Figure 9.17).

If the height of the block has fallen below the upper limit of the incision or pain site, the pain/anaesthetic team may undertake the following: give the patient a bolus dose of local anaesthetic agent to re-establish the block and reposition the epidural catheter. If either of these fails, other methods of analgesia need to be considered.

Haematoma

An epidural haematoma can arise from trauma to an epidural blood vessel during catheter insertion or removal. Although the incidence of a haematoma occurring is extremely rare, particular care must be taken in patients receiving thromboprophylaxis (see Procedure guideline 9.14). Initial symptoms include back pain and tenderness. As the haematoma expands to compress the nerve roots or the spinal cord, this proceeds to sensorimotor weakness (Chapman and Day 2001).

Abscess formation

Wheatley *et al.* (2001) note that infection can be introduced into the epidural space from an exogenous source via contaminated equipment or drugs or from an endogenous source, leading to bacteraemia which seeds to the insertion site or catheter tip. Alternatively, the catheter can act as a wick through which the infection tracks down from the entry site on the skin to the epidural/intrathecal space. Symptoms include back pain and tenderness accompanied by redness with a purulent discharge from the catheter exit site (Day 2001).

Complications specific to epidural analgesia
Dural puncture

This usually occurs when the dura mater is inadvertently punctured during the placement of the epidural catheter. The incidence of a dural puncture arising during placement of the catheter is approximately 0.32–1.23% (Wheatley *et al.* 2001). The main symptom is a headache, which arises from leakage of CSF through the dura.

Catheter migration

Catheter migration is extremely rare, occurring in less than 0.2% of patients (Wheatley *et al.* 2001). The catheter may migrate into either a blood vessel or the CSF. If it migrates into a blood vessel, opioid or local anaesthetic toxicity will occur. Opioid toxicity results in sedation and respiratory depression. Local anaesthetic toxicity results in circumoral tingling, numbness, twitching, convulsions and apnoea (Pasero and McCaffrey 1999). If the catheter migrates into the CSF, the epidural opioids and local anaesthetic agents may reach as high as the cranial subarachnoid space. If this occurs the respiratory muscles are paralysed together with the cranial nerves, resulting in apnoea, profound hypotension and unconsciousness (Macintyre and Schug 2007).

Complications specific to intrathecal analgesia
Meningitis

Meningitis is a rare complication of intrathecal analgesia. The epidural route is often considered safer as the intact dura serves as an effective barrier to the spread of infection to the subarachnoid space. In fact, similar infection rates are reported with both intrathecal and epidural administration (Mercadante 1999). The incidence of major infections varies widely but is reported by Ballantyne and Carwood (2005) as zero and as approximately 5% by Sloan (2004) for epidural and intrathecal therapy with external pump systems. If the patient presents with headaches, fever, neck stiffness or photophobia, they must be reviewed as a matter of urgency by the medical/anaesthetic team, as if meningitis is suspected

CSF samples can be obtained and sent to microbiology for analysis, and antibiotic therapy initiated promptly (Baker *et al.* 2004, Day 2001).

Entonox administration

Definition

Entonox (BOC 1995), a gaseous mixture of 50% nitrous oxide (N_2O) and 50% oxygen (O_2), is a patient-controlled, inhaled analgesic which is used for the short-term relief of acute pain (Stannard and Booth 1998). Nitrous oxide is a colourless, sweet-smelling gas with powerful analgesic properties, supplied in premixed cylinders (Bruce and Franck 2000). The gas is inhaled and self-administered by the patient using a demand valve system attached to a facemask or a mouthpiece. The nitrous oxide component of the gas acts as a powerful analgesic producing similar physiological effects to opioids (Gillman and Lichtigfeld 1994), whilst the oxygen component has an antihypoxic effect (Faddy and Garlick 2005) and ensures good cerebral perfusion and enhanced recovery (Peate and Lancaster 2000).

Related theory

Although the exact mechanism of nitrous oxide is unknown, its effects take place within the pain centres of the brain and spinal cord and are related to the release of endogenous neurotransmitters such as opioid peptides and serotonin and the activation of certain opioid receptors (Fang *et al.* 1997, Gillman and Lichtigfeld 1998). N-methyl-D-aspartate (NMDA) receptor currents are inhibited by nitrous oxide and it is known that these receptors are involved with many central nervous system pathways (Jevtovic-Todorovic *et al.* 1998). The release of these neurotransmitters is thought to activate descending pain pathways which modulate pain transmission in the spinal cord (Maze and Fujinaga 2000). Pulmonary transfer of nitrous oxide is rapid, with onset of effect in seconds and full analgesic effect within 1–2 minutes. It is also rapidly eliminated from the blood, via the lungs, when inhalation ceases (Trojan *et al.* 1997).

Evidence-based approaches
Rationale

There are several advantages to using Entonox.

- As the gas is inhaled, it is painless when compared to systemic methods of administering analgesia (such as injections).
- It has a rapid onset of effect.
- The side-effects are few and are self-limiting as the gas is self-administered.
- It does not depress respiratory or cardiovascular function when used as directed.

- Effects wear off rapidly, usually within 5 minutes.
- The patient is in full control, which can reduce anxiety (BOC 2001).

Because of these properties, Entonox is an ideal agent for short-term pain relief following injury or trauma and during therapeutic and investigative procedures. It is used in a variety of settings including accident and emergency (O'Sullivan and Benger 2003), obstetrics (Rosen 2002), paediatrics (Bruce and Franck 2000, Pickup and Pagdin 2001), endoscopy/biopsy procedures (Forbes and Collins 2000, Manikandan *et al.* 2003) and the ambulance service.

Indications

- Wound and burn dressing, wound debridement and suturing.
- Normal labour.
- Changing or removing of packs and drains.
- Removal of sutures from sensitive areas, for example the vulva.
- Invasive procedures such as catheterization and sigmoidoscopy.
- Removal of radioactive intracavity gynaecological applicators.
- Altering the position of a patient who experiences incident pain.
- Manual evacuation of the bowel in severe constipation.
- Acute trauma, for example applying orthopaedic traction following pathological fracture, reduction of joint dislocation.
- Physiotherapy procedures, particularly postoperatively.

Contraindications

Entonox should not be used with any of the following conditions.

- Maxillofacial injuries (BOC 2000), as the patient may not be able to hold the mask tightly to the face or use the mouthpiece adequately. There is a risk of causing further damage to facial wounds and there may also be a significant risk of blood inhalation.
- Head injuries with impairment of consciousness.
- Heavily sedated patients, as they would be unable to breathe in the Entonox on demand and to potentiate sedation further may be hazardous.
- Intoxicated patients, as drowsiness and aspiration would be a hazard in the event of vomiting.
- Any condition in which gas is entrapped within a body and where its expansion may be dangerous such as:
  - Pneumothorax (artificial, traumatic or spontaneous)
  - Air embolism
  - Severe bullous emphysema
  - Abdominal distension or bowel obstruction
  - Decompression sickness or following a recent dive
  - Following air encephalography

- During myringoplasty
- In patients who have received recent intraocular injection of gas (BOC 2009).
- The nitrous oxide constituent of Entonox passes into any air-filled cavity within the body faster than nitrogen passes out. As the gas expands this is likely to result in a build-up of tension, which will increase the patient's symptoms.

■ Laryngectomy patients, as they will be unable to use the apparatus.

■ Temperatures of below –6°C as the gases separate (BOC 1995). If this occurs the cylinders will initially deliver a high concentration of oxygen but will eventually deliver nearly pure nitrous oxide.

Use during pregnancy and lactation

It has been suggested that prolonged exposure to high levels of nitrous oxide may affect a woman's ability to become pregnant (Axelsson *et al.* 1996). Mild skeletal teratogenic changes have been observed in pregnant rat embryos when the dam (pregnant mother) has been exposed to high levels of nitrous oxide during the period of organogenesis. However, no increased incidence of fetal malformation has been discovered in eight epidemiological studies and case reports in humans (BOC 2009). No published material shows that nitrous oxide is toxic to the human fetus. Therefore, there is no absolute contraindication to its use in the first 16 weeks of pregnancy.

There are no known adverse effects to using Entonox during the breast-feeding period (BOC 2009).

Principles of care
Cautions

Prior to Entonox use, consideration should be given to the following.

■ The high level of oxygen (50%) in Entonox may depress respiration in patients who have chronic obstructive pulmonary disease and are carbon dioxide (CO_2) retainers.

■ Entonox should not be used as a replacement for intravenous analgesia or general anaesthesia in procedures requiring increased levels of medical intervention.

■ If Entonox is used as the sole analgesic/sedative agent, the British Oxygen Company (BOC) 2009 data sheet recommends that driving or operating complex machinery is not recommended until:
- the healthcare professional has judged that the patient has returned to normal mental status (Entonox can cause psychotropic effects)
- the patient feels they are competent to drive after the relevant procedure is completed
- at least 30 minutes has elapsed after the administration of Entonox has ceased.

■ Additional care is needed when Entonox is administered to a patient who has been given concomitant medication.

Legal and professional issues

Healthcare professionals involved in the assessment, administration and continuing care of patients receiving Entonox should have undergone training to do so. They should be able to demonstrate knowledge of the properties of the gas, precautions to be taken, actions in the event of an emergency and the correct operating procedures for equipment. It is important that staff are given appropriate theoretical and practical training (BOC 1998; Peate and Lancaster 2000). This can be supplied by BOC Medical and certificated.

Prescribing of Entonox

In a number of healthcare settings, nurses, midwives and physiotherapists may be able to administer Entonox without a written prescription from a doctor providing there is a local patient group direction to allow this. Where this is the case, Entonox can be used more readily and time is not wasted waiting for a medical prescription. Non-medical prescribers who have completed the relevant training as an independent prescriber may also prescribe Entonox if this is within their area of competence.

Preprocedural considerations
Equipment
Cylinders

Entonox cylinders are available from the BOC in a variety of sizes. All cylinders have blue and white markings on their shoulder (Figure 9.18). The lightweight smaller cylinders have the following advantages.

■ They are easier to carry.
■ They have a live contents gauge.
■ Changing an empty cylinder is simple because it is not necessary to fit a regulator or use a cylinder key.

The smaller size cylinders tend to be used in ambulances and by midwives for their portability in home births. Some clinical areas may have piped Entonox, such as accident and emergency departments, high-dependency units and critical care units. The larger cylinders which require a trolley to move them around are more suitable for ward areas.

Demand apparatus

There are a number of different companies that supply the demand apparatus for self-administered Entonox use. Examples of these include the Ease demand valve (Sabre Medical) and the Carnet single patient use demand valve (Figure 9.19).

Bacterial filters and mouthpieces/facemasks

Because Entonox equipment is a potential source of cross-infection, bacterial filters (single-use only) should be fitted between the facemask or mouthpiece and demand valve if

489

Figure 9.18 Entonox CD-size cyclinder. Courtesy of BOC Healthcare.

Figure 9.19 Example of a demand valve apparatus. Courtesy of BOC Healthcare.

the demand valve is not for single use (Chilvers and Weisz 2000). Facemasks and mouthpieces must also be single-use only and disposable once therapy ceases. Local policies must also be followed for the cleaning/sterilization of non-disposable equipment between patient use.

Assessment

The patient's ability to administer Entonox safely and effectively (particularly the very young or old) must be assessed prior to use. Patients should be able to:

- understand the instructions for Entonox use
- hold the demand valve to self-administer the gas
- inhale the gas through the mask or mouthpiece whilst breathing normally (patients who have impaired lung function may not be able to inhale the gas sufficiently to provide adequate analgesia).

Pharmacological support

Entonox is designed for self-administration by the patient. This method of administration makes use of a demand unit which safeguards the patient from excess inhalation of Entonox. The demand unit ensures that gas can be obtained only by the patient inhaling from the mouthpiece or mask and producing a negative pressure. The gas flow stops when the patient stops inhaling and removes the mouthpiece or mask from their face. Thus patients are able to self-regulate the dose of Entonox (a method of patient-controlled analgesia). Therefore, the patient must hold the mask firmly over the face or mouthpiece to the lips to produce an airtight fit and breathe in before the gas will flow. Expired gases escape by the expiratory valve on the handpiece. It is essential to adhere to this method of self-administration as it is then impossible for patients to overdose themselves because, if they become drowsy, they will relax their grip on the handset and the gas flow will cease when no negative pressure is applied. However, should inhalation continue, light anaesthesia supervenes and the mask drops away as the patient relaxes. Entonox may be self-regulated, but additionally may be administered by attendant medical personnel trained in its use, for example within obstetric/accident and emergency units, and accident ambulances.

Entonox has an oxygen content two-and-a-half times that of air and is therefore a good way of giving extra oxygen as well as providing analgesia.

Duration and frequency of administration

The duration and frequency of Entonox administration should always be tailored to individual patient needs. Because prolonged exposure to Entonox causes inactivation of vitamin B_{12}, impaired folate metabolism and pernicious anaemia (BOC 2009), it is recommended that:

- Entonox is used on a short-term rather than a long-term basis

- it should not be used for more than a total of 24 hours, or more frequently than once every 4 days (BOC 2009)
- if daily use is required for more than 4 days, this should be accompanied by close supervision and haematologi-cal monitoring (blood tests) to check for changes in red and white blood cells (BOC 2009). Consideration should also be given to the administration of B_{12} and folate supplements.

Procedure guideline 9.18 Entonox administration

Essential equipment

- Entonox cylinder and head
- Facemask and/or mouthpiece
- Sterile bacterial filter
- Method of documentation

Preprocedure

Action	Rationale
1 Explain and discuss the procedure with the patient.	To ensure that the patient understands the procedure and gives their valid consent (NMC 2008a, C).
	To reduce patient anxiety (Royal College of Anaesthetists 2006, C).
	To ensure the patient has no underlying medical problems that contraindicate the use of Entonox (BOC 2009, C).

Procedure

2 Turn on the Entonox supply from the cylinder.	To ascertain whether there is any Entonox in the cylinder (BOC 1999, C).
3 Examine the gauge to determine how much gas is in the cylinder.	To ensure an adequate supply of gas throughout the procedure (BOC 1999, C).
4 Ensure that the patient is in as comfortable a position as possible.	To promote patient comfort (BOC 1999, C).
5 Demonstrate how to use the apparatus by holding the mask tightly to your face, replacing the mask/mouth-piece that you have used. Explain to the patient that when they breathe in and out regularly and deeply, a hissing sound will be heard, indicating that the gas is being inhaled.	To ensure that the patient understands what to do and what to expect before any painful procedure commences (BOC 1999, C).
6 Allow the patient to practise using the apparatus.	To enable the patient to adopt the correct technique and for the nurse to observe the analgesic effect of the gas before the procedure commences (BOC 1999, C).
7 Encourage the patient to breathe gas in and out for at least 2 minutes before commencing any painful procedure.	To allow sufficient time for an adequate circulatory level of nitrous oxide to provide analgesia. When the patient inhales, gas enters first the lungs then the pulmonary and systemic circulations. It takes 1–2 minutes to build up reasonable concentrations of nitrous oxide in the brain (BOC 1999, C).
8 During the procedure encourage the patient to breathe in and out regularly and deeply.	To maintain adequate circulatory levels, thus providing adequate analgesia (BOC 1999, C).
9 Evaluate the effectiveness of Entonox with the patient throughout and following the procedure, by verbal questioning and encouraging the patient to self-assess the analgesic effect.	To establish whether the Entonox has been a useful anal-gesic for the procedure. This should then be documented to assist any subsequent procedures, for example dress-ing changes (BOC 1999, C).

491

(Continued)

Procedure guideline 9.18 (*Continued*)

10	At the end of the procedure observe the patient every 5–10 minutes until the effects of the gas have worn off. Observe the patient for up to 30 minutes.	Some patients may feel a transient drowsiness or giddiness and should be discouraged from getting out of bed until these effects have worn off. It is rare for the patient to experience transient amnesia (BOC 1999, C).

Postprocedure

11	Turn off the Entonox supply from the cylinder.	To avoid potential seepage of gas from the apparatus (BOC 1999, C).
12	Depress the diaphragm under the demand valve.	To remove residual gas from tubing (BOC 1999, C).
13	Follow local policies/guidelines for the cleaning and sterilization of expiratory valve and tubing, and facemask (or disposal if single use). Filters and mouthpieces should be discarded after use.	To reduce the risk of cross-infection (BOC 1999, C).
14	Record the administration on appropriate documentation.	To promote continuity of care, maintain accurate records and provide a point of reference in the event of any queries (BOC 1999, C; NMC 2005, C).

Problem-solving table 9.4 **Prevention and resolution (Procedure guideline 9.18)**

Problem	Cause	Prevention	Suggested action
Patient not experiencing adequate analgesic effect	Entonox cylinder empty. Apparatus not properly connected	Check before procedure commences	Change to a full cylinder
	Patient not inhaling deeply enough (BOC 2000)	Education of patient prior to starting procedure	Encourage the patient to breathe in until a hissing noise can be heard from the cylinder. Reassess suitability of patient for Entonox use. The patient may not be strong enough to inhale deeply or may have reduced lung capacity
	Patient inhaling pure oxygen, that is, cylinder has been stored below −6°C and nitrous oxide has liquified and settled at the bottom of the cylinder	All cylinders should be stored horizontally at a temperature of 10°C or above for 24 hours before use (BOC 1995)	Initially safe, but later the patient may inhale pure nitrous oxide and be asphyxiated. Discontinue the procedure. Ensure adequate warming of the cylinder and inversion of the cylinder to remix the gases adequately
	Not enough time has been allowed for nitrous oxide to exert its analgesic effect	Allow at least 2 minutes of Entonox use before commencing the procedure	Stop procedure. Allow 2 minutes of Entonox use. Re-start procedure

Problem	Cause	Prevention	Suggested action
Patient experiences generalized muscle rigidity	Hyperventilation during inhalation (BOC 2000)	Education of patient prior to starting procedure	Discontinue Entonox and allow the patient to recover. Explain the procedure again, stressing deep and regular inspiration. Use a mouthpiece in place of a mask
Patient unable to tolerate a mask	Smell of rubber, feeling of claustrophobia	Assess patient preference to use either mask or mouthpiece before Entonox use	Use a mouthpiece in place of a mask
Patient feels nauseated, drowsy or giddy	Effect of nitrous oxide accumulation (BOC 2000)	None	Discontinue Entonox administration: the effect will then rapidly disappear. Re-start Entonox use; if the same effect occurs stop using Entonox and use alternative analgesia
Patient afraid to use Entonox	Associates gases with previous hospital procedures, for example anaesthesia before surgery (BOC 2000)	Assess suitability of patient for Entonox use. Address fear and anxiety issues before starting Entonox use	Reassure patient and reiterate instructions for use and short-term effects

493

Complications

Events such as euphoria, disorientation, sedation, nausea, vomiting, dizziness and generalized tingling are commonly described. These events are generally minor and rapidly reversible (BOC 2009).

Inappropriate inhalation of Entonox will ultimately result in unconsciousness, passing through stages of increasing light-headedness and intoxication. The treatment is removal to fresh air, mouth-to-mouth resuscitation and, if necessary, the use of an oxygen resuscitator (BOC 1995).

Abdominal paracentesis

Definition

Abdominal paracentesis is a technique used to drain a pathological collection of ascitic fluid from the abdomen (Campbell 2001). This technique is performed to help diagnose the cause of ascites (diagnostic paracentesis) or to relieve the discomfort associated with this condition (therapeutic paracentesis) (McGibbon *et al.* 2007).

Anatomy and physiology

The peritoneum is a semi-permeable serous membrane consisting of two separate layers: the parietal layer and the visceral layer. The parietal layer covers the abdominal and pelvic walls and the undersurface of the diaphragm. The visceral layer lines and supports the abdominal organs and the parietal peritoneum (Figure 9.20). The space between the parietal and visceral layers is known as the peritoneal cavity (Thibodeau and Patton 2007). The normal peritoneal cavity has a small amount of free fluid of approximately 50 mL (McGibbon *et al.* 2007).

In a healthy individual fluid is produced from the capillaries lining the peritoneal cavity and is drained by lymphatic vessels under the diaphragm. The fluid is collected by the right lymphatic duct which drains into the vena cava. The peritoneum forms the largest serous membrane in the body (Tortora and Derrickson 2009). However, in patients with malignant ascites, this balance of production and drainage is disrupted and ascitic fluid collects in the peritoneal cavity (Box 9.18).

Related theory

Ascites can be caused by non-malignant conditions such as cirrhosis of the liver, advanced congestive heart failure and chronic pericarditis and nephrotic syndrome. Cirrhosis of the liver is the most common cause of ascites and in this clinical condition the development of ascites indicates a poor prognosis (Hou and Sanyal 2009, Sargent 2006).

Malignant conditions such as metastatic cancer of the ovary, stomach, colon or breast can also cause ascites. The

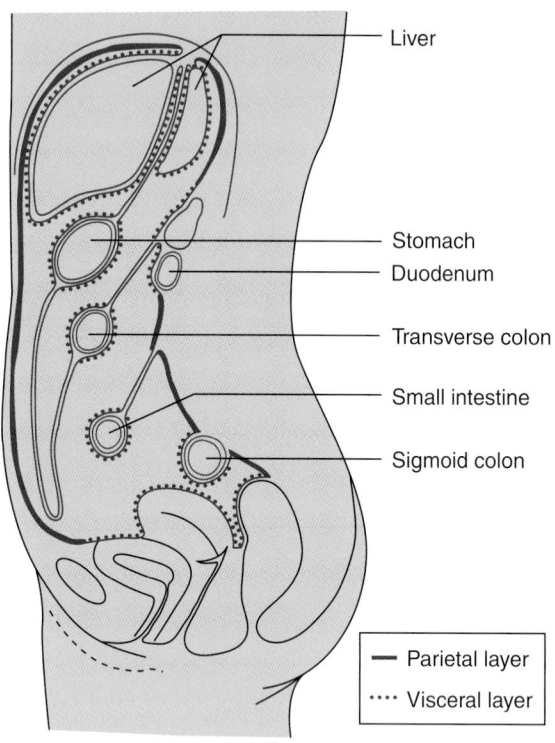

Liver

Stomach
Duodenum

Transverse colon

Small intestine

Sigmoid colon

— Parietal layer
···· Visceral layer

Figure 9.20 Peritoneum of female in lateral view.

494

incidence of ascites in patients with cancer is not well re-corded but it is known to occur in many different cancer types (Cope 2005). Malignant ascites accounts for about 10% of ascites, of which 34–54% are from ovarian cancers (Winkelman 2004). It should be noted that in about one-third of patients with cancer, ascites has a non-malignant cause (Hosttetter *et al.* 2005). In patients with advanced cancer, malignant ascites is the most likely diagnosis of an abdominal fluid collection and often reflects end-stage

---

Box 9.18 Functions of the peritoneum

- The peritoneum is a serous membrane that enables the abdominal contents to glide over each other without friction.
- It forms a partial or complete cover for the abdominal organs.
- It forms ligaments and mesenteries which help to keep the organs in position.
- The mesenteries contain fat and act as a store for the body.
- The mesenteries can move to engulf areas of inflamma-tion and this prevents the spread of infection.
- It has the power to absorb fluids and exchange electro-lytes.

(Thibodeau and Patton 2007, Tortora and Derrickson 2009).

---

disease. However, in some cases such as ovarian cancer and lymphoma, ascites can be an early presentation and efforts to obtain tumour shrinkage and prolongation of survival should be undertaken (Marincola and Schwartzentruber 2001). If a definitive diagnosis is needed to establish cause to aid staging and possible surgical intervention then a peri-toneal tap and analysis of fluid will be useful (Marincola and Schwartzentruber 2001).

The pathogenesis of ascites differs depending on its pri-mary related factors. Cirrhotic ascites is more recently believed to be related to portal hypertension (Hou and Sanyal 2009, Lee and Grap 2008). The increased pres-sure occurs due to fibrosis and scarring of the liver from chronic liver disease, causing obstruction to venous flow (Whiteman and McCormick 2005). In the case of heart failure and constrictive pericarditis, the heart loses its ability to pump blood and this causes a back-up of blood and increases pressure into the portal venous system, leading to portal hypertension and ascites (Lee and Grap 2008).

The pathogenesis of malignant ascites is not as well un-derstood as non-cancer related ascites is (Seike *et al.* 2007) but cytokines, mechanical obstruction and hormonal influ-ence are thought to be related. Cytokines such as vascular endothelial growth factor (VEGF) and vascular perme-ability factor (VPF) regulate vascular permeability. The obstruction of lymphatic drainage by the disseminating malignant cells in the peritoneal cavity reduces absorption of peritoneal exudates (Seike *et al.* 2007). This reduction activates the renin-angiotensin-aldosterone system and leads to sodium retention, which then further exacerbates the ascites. Lee and Grap (2008) explain that in peritoneal carcinomatosis, tumour cells line the peritoneal cavity and produce a protein-like fluid. Extracellular fluid is drawn into the cavity due to increased oncotic pressure of the peritoneal fluid. Fluid also develops in liver metastases and hepatocellular cancer due to portal hypertension. Portal hypertension develops when stenosis or occlusion of the portal vein occurs by thrombosis or tumour nodules (Lee and Grap 2008).

Ascites is often accompanied by debilitating symptoms as large amounts of fluid collect in the peritoneal cavity, causing an increase in intra-abdominal pressure and re-sulting in pressure on internal structures. The fluid accu-mulation may occur over several weeks or rapidly over a few days (Lee and Grap 2008). Symptoms initially include vague abdominal discomfort, which can go on to affect the respiratory and gastrointestinal systems, depending on the amount of fluid present. Pressure on the diaphragm decreases the intrathoracic space and causes shortness of breath. Gastric pressure may cause anorexia, indigestion or hiatus hernia. Intestinal pressure may result in consti-pation, bowel obstruction or decreased bladder capacity. Patients also become increasingly fatigued, finding simple daily tasks difficult (Winkelman 2004). Additionally, body image can be affected even when minimal distension is present.

Cytological confirmation of malignant cells is difficult with only a 50% chance of success (Fentiman 2002).

Evidence-based approaches

Rationale

There is much debate about whether it is safe to drain large volumes of fluid rapidly from the abdomen. One concern is that profound hypotension may follow because of the sudden release of intra-abdominal pressure and consequent possible vasodilation (Lee *et al.* 2000). However, following a local study and literature search, Stephenson and Gilbert (2002) suggest that up to 5 litres of fluid may be safely drained over a few hours. They also state that it is not necessary to drain the abdomen until dry. McNamara (2000) supports this by pointing out that the maximum relief of symptoms may be achieved after the initial few litres are drained. This is further supported by Moorsom (2001) who suggests that several litres can be drained on free flow over 1 hour.

It is generally not necessary to have intravenous fluid or albumin replacement. However, patients with ascites who have large tumours, cirrhosis of the liver or renal impairment may require slower drainage of fluid and possible fluid replacement, depending on their clinical condition. Abdominal and peritoneal tumours can cause ascites to develop independently of the circulatory system and therefore hypotension is not usually seen as the ascites is drained (Klee 2004).

A small study has shown that the success of blind paracentesis is directly related to the amount of fluid present (44% with 300 mL and 78% with 500 mL) (McGibbon *et al.* 2007). The literature suggests the use of ultrasound-guided paracentesis to confirm the presence of ascites and also to identify the best site to perform paracentesis, particularly when a small amount of fluid is present (McGibbon *et al.* 2007).

Indications

- To obtain a specimen of fluid for analysis for diagnostic purposes (diagnostic paracentesis).
- To relieve the symptoms associated with ascites, both physical and psychological (therapeutic paracentesis).
- To administer substances such as cytotoxic drugs (e.g. bleomycin, cisplatin) or other agents into the peritoneal cavity, to achieve regression of serosal deposits responsible for fluid formation (Hosttetter *et al.* 2005).

Contraindications

- *Relative contraindications*: pregnancy, severe bowel distension and previous extensive abdominal or pelvic surgery (McGibbon *et al.* 2007). When relative contraindications are present paracentesis without the assistance of ultrasound (blind paracentesis) is not recommended (McGibbon *et al.* 2007).
- *Absolute contraindication*: clinically evident fibrinolysis or disseminated intravascular coagulation (McGibbon *et al.* 2007).

Preparatory investigations

The patient's clinical condition and purpose of the procedure must be taken into account when deciding what investigations are necessary but most preprocedure investigations include a blood screen and ultrasound examination. To keep intrusion to a minimum for palliative patients, fewer investigations may be performed. Blood is usually checked for full blood picture, urea and electrolytes, creatinine, liver function test, plasma proteins and coagulation screen (Hewish 2006). In the case of a diagnostic paracentesis, the ascitic fluid should be analysed for cell count, bacterial culture, total protein and albumin (Hou and Sanyal 2009).

Methods of managing ascites

Interventions used to treat ascites range from an aggressive approach to a purely palliative approach. There have been few definitive studies that have evaluated the different approaches in the treatment of malignant ascites (Hosttetter *et al.* 2005). While paracentesis is effective, ascites recurs, requiring repeated procedures. This fact imposes a further burden on patients and their families (Mercadante *et al.* 2008). Treatment for ascites may include use of diuretics, paracentesis, diet low in sodium, instillation of peritoneal agents or the insertion of long-term catheters. However, the literature available is mostly generated from studies with patients suffering from acute or chronic liver failure; this should be taken into account when managing patients with non-malignant ascites.

- *Paracentesis*: the most common way of managing ascites as it has an immediate effect in 90% of cases (Campbell 2001, Marincola and Schwartzentruber 2001).
- *Sodium-restricted diet*: the amount of fluid retained in the body depends on the balance between sodium ingested in the diet and sodium excreted in the urine. A reduced sodium intake of 2 g/day is considered a realistic goal (Sargent 2006).
- *Diuretics*: useful mainly in cirrhotic-type ascites. This may be used for malignant ascites together with a restriction of salt and fluid intake, and has been found to be effective in about one-third of patients (Hosttetter *et al.* 2005). Additionally, it appears to be more effective for management of patients with small-volume ascites (only diagnosed by ultrasound). Spironolactone is the diuretic of choice (Hou and Sanyal 2009). The most effective way of monitoring the fluid loss is by weighing the patient daily (Sargent 2006).
- *Instillation of intraperitoneal agents*: cytotoxics, sclerosants and biological substances have been tried in an

495

attempt to control the recurrence of ascites. To date, intraperitoneal agents have not been proven, unequivocally, to have a greater beneficial effect than the use of diuretics (Fentiman 2002).

■ *Long-term catheters*:
  – **Peritoneovenous shunt**: generally used in patients with long-term prognosis. These shunts drain ascitic fluid into the superior vena cava and require a general anaesthesia for insertion (Mamada *et al.* 2007, Seike *et al.* 2007).
  – **PleurX drain**: tunnelled catheter placed under ultrasound and fluoroscopic guidance. This device is associated with low rates of serious adverse clinical events, catheter failure, discomfort and electrolyte imbalance (Courtney *et al.* 2008). Additionally, it may allow patients to avoid spending added time in hospital for repeated paracentesis.
  – **Peritoneal port-catheter**: similar but larger than central venous access ports in order to make access easier and to decrease possible catheter occlusion (Ozkan *et al.* 2007). Very limited number of studies supporting its use.

Anticipated patient outcomes

Nursing and medical care of patients with malignant abdominal ascites should be aimed at improving quality of life by relieving suffering caused by the symptoms (Cope 2005). Each patient should be carefully assessed with consideration of their individual circumstances, maintaining respect for their wish to have or not have interventional treatment (Campbell 2001).

Legal and professional issues
Competencies

The procedure is performed by a doctor or a trained practitioner in paracentesis assisted by a nurse throughout. In most cases medical professionals do not require specific training in paracentesis as learning occurs throughout their career. However, there is recognized training which all professionals wishing to perform paracentesis are expected to complete.

Preprocedural considerations
Equipment

The equipment should be prepared by the health professional performing the paracentesis or by a colleague familiar with the technique. The essential equipment includes a sterile abdominal paracentesis set, a sterile dressing pack, a sterile receiver, a sterile specimen pot, a local anaesthetic, needles and syringes, chlorhexidine 0.5% in 70% alcohol, an adhesive dressing, a large sterile drainage bag or container, gate clamps and sterile gloves.

Nurses should describe the equipment to be used during paracentesis to the patient. This may be more relevant when looking after a patient undergoing the procedure for the first time to whom the size of the catheter used may be very impressive.

Assessment and recording tools

A detailed and consistent nursing assessment is important when caring for patients requiring paracentesis. Nurses should pay particular attention to the cause of the ascites and the frequency with which the procedure is occurring. For some patients the provision of information about counselling and other support strategies is of great benefit as recurrent ascites can be linked with poor prognosis in an oncology setting. The involvement of the palliative care team can at this stage be indicated. In cases of ascites secondary to cirrhosis, nurses should pay special attention to unresolved issues surrounding alcohol abuse, offering support and information to the patient and family.

In preparation for the paracentesis, nurses should measure the patient's girth around the umbilicus and check the patient's weight before the procedure. The same chart should be used to record all subsequent measurements so a comparison can be made.

Pharmacological support

Reassurance about the use of local anaesthetics is essential as patients are often anxious about this being a painful procedure. For a number of patients muscle relaxants may be of benefit prior to the procedure.

Non-pharmacological support

Nurses should enquire about the patient's fears and concerns regarding paracentesis. For some patients, music or relaxation tapes, physical relaxation and visualization techniques are of great benefit so a referral to these services should be considered, if available.

Specific patient preparation
Education

Nursing interventions for patients undergoing abdominal paracentesis include education about the nature of the procedure, what results can realistically be expected, and the risks and benefits. Information should also be given about postprocedure care of the puncture site and about the importance of diet and fluid intake to replace proteins and fluid lost in the ascitic fluid. It is essential that the patient, family and carer are involved in the discussion so that an informed and joint decision may be made in order to achieve the best possible outcome.

Procedure guideline 9.19 **Abdominal paracentesis**

Essential equipment

Sterile abdominal paracentesis set containing forceps, scalpel blade and blade holder, swabs, towels, suturing equipment, trocar and cannula (or other approved catheter and introducer), connector to attach to the cannula and guide fluid into the container.

- Sterile dressing pack
- Sterile receiver
- Sterile specimen pots
- Local anaesthetic
- Needles and syringes
- Chlorhexidine 0.5% in 70% alcohol
- Adhesive dressing
- Large sterile drainage bag or container (with connector if appropriate to attach to cannula)
- Gate clamps
- Sterile gloves

Optional equipment

- Weighing scales
- Tape measure

Preprocedure

Action	Rationale
1 Explain and discuss the procedure with the patient.	To ensure that the patient is involved in the decision and understands the procedure, the agreed aim, the risks and benefits. Informed consent may then be obtained (Campbell 2001, R5; Cope 2005, R5; NMC 2008a, C).
2 Ask the patient to empty their bladder.	If the bladder is full there is a chance of it being punctured when the trocar is introduced (McGibbon et al. 2007, E).
3 Weigh patient before procedure and record.	To assess weight changes and the fluid loss. E
4 Ensure privacy.	To maintain dignity (DH 2006, C).
5 Measure patient's girth around umbilicus before procedure and record. Mark the position.	This provides an indication of fluid shift and how much fluid has reaccumulated. E
6 Lie the patient supine in bed with the head raised 45–50 cm with a backrest.	Normally the pressure in the peritoneal cavity is no greater than atmospheric pressure, but when fluid is present, pressure becomes greater than atmospheric pressure. This position will aid gravity in the removal of fluid and the fluid will drain of its own accord until the pressure is equalized. E

Procedure

7 Prepare the abdomen aseptically and drape with sterile towels. Administer local anaesthetic.	To reduce the risk of local and/or systemic infection. The peritoneal cavity is normally sterile (Fraise and Bradley 2009, E; Lee et al. 2000, R5).
8 Once the anaesthetic has taken effect, the doctor will make an incision into the skin of abdomen (the position may have been marked previously in radiology following ultrasound).	To minimize pain during the procedure and thus maximize patient comfort and facilitate co-operation. E
9 The trocar and cannula are inserted via the incision.	

(Continued)

Procedure guideline 9.19 *(Continued)*

10 The trocar is removed and disposed of in a sharps container.	
11 A closed drainage system is attached to the cannula using a connector if appropriate. A secure dry dressing should be applied to ensure the drain site is protected and taped firmly in position.	A sterile container with a non-return valve is necessary to maintain sterility. To reduce local and/or systemic infection. E
12 Ascitic fluid is collected from the cannula with a syringe (20–100 mL as instructed by the doctor) and sent for cytology.	If necessary, in order to diagnose the cause of ascites (Fentiman 2002; Hosttetter *et al.* 2005, R5).
13 If the cannula is to remain in position, sutures may be inserted adjacent to the cannula and looped around it to prevent it becoming dislodged and to prevent local trauma to the patient.	To ensure cannula remains *in situ*. To reduce risk of trauma to the patient. E

Postprocedure

14 Monitor the patient's blood pressure, pulse and respirations and observe the rate and nature of the drainage. A clamp should be available on the tubing to reduce the flow of fluid if necessary.	To observe for signs of shock and/or infection and to ensure unobstructed drainage. E
15 Monitor the patient's fluid balance.	After removal of large amounts of peritoneal fluid, fluid moves from the vascular space and reaccumulates in the peritoneal cavity. Ascitic fluid contains protein in addition to sodium and potassium. Problems of dehydration and electrolyte imbalance may be present. E
16 Drainage of fluid may be free flowing up to 5 litres unless adverse symptoms present. Alternatively, drainage may be controlled at 2 litres every 4 hours.	If patient shows adverse signs then clamp drain, inform medical team and reopen after medical intervention and advice (Stephenson and Gilbert 2002, R3b).
17 Weigh patient after procedure and record.	To assess weight changes and fluid loss. E
18 Measure patient's girth around umbilicus after procedure and record.	This provides an indication of fluid shift and how much fluid has reaccumulated. E

Problem-solving table 9.5 Prevention and resolution (Procedure guideline 9.19)

Problem	Cause	Prevention	Suggested action
Patient exhibits shock	Major circulatory shift of fluid or sudden release of intra-abdominal pressure, vasodilation and subsequent lowering of blood pressure	Monitor blood pressure and consider administration of intravenous fluid if volumes larger than 5 litres are expected to drain	Clamp the drainage tube with a gate clamp to prevent further fluid loss. Record the patient's vital signs. Refer to the medical staff for immediate intervention

Problem	Cause	Prevention	Suggested action
Cessation of drainage of ascitic fluid	Abdomen is empty of ascitic fluid		Check the total output of ascitic fluid given on the patient's fluid balance chart. Measure the patient's girth; compare this measurement with the preabdominal paracentesis measurement. Suggest to medical staff that the cannula should be removed. Discontinue the drainage system
	Patient's position is inhibiting drainage	Teach patient to avoid exerting pressure on the drainage tubing	Change the patient's position, that is, move the patient upright or onto their side to encourage flow by gravity. Encourage patient to mobilize
	The ascitic fluid has clotted in the drainage system	Keep drainage bag on a stand and lower than the puncture site to facilitate drainage by gravity	'Milk' the tubing. If this is unsuccessful, change the drainage system aseptically. Refer to the medical staff
Cannula becomes dislodged	Ineffective sutures or trauma at the puncture site	Collaborate with medical staff when putting suture or alternatively apply secure dressing. Tube is taped to the skin further down to prevent pulling with movement at the puncture site	Apply a secure dry dressing. Reassure patient. Inform the medical staff
Pain	Pressure of ascites or position of drain	Offer analgesia 30 minutes prior to procedure. Apply dressing, allowing enough padding around the puncture site but avoiding drain movement within abdomen	Identify cause. Anchor drain securely to avoid pulling at insertion site or movement within abdomen. Assist patient with repositioning. Administer appropriate prescribed analgesic, monitor the patient's response and inform medical staff

499

Postprocedural considerations

Immediate care

Observations must be carried out every half an hour for 2 hours and hourly for 4 hours to detect early signs of shock, cardiovascular compromise and infection so that medical staff can be informed and action can be taken promptly. Drainage of the fluid must be monitored regularly, volumes recorded on a fluid balance chart and blockages detected and managed. Patients may require assistance to move and position themselves, and may experience pain, requiring careful repositioning or appropriate analgesia. The drain should be taken out when the desired amount of fluid has been removed; this can take up to 2 days.

Ongoing care

The patient's renal function should be checked following this procedure to ensure that any signs of dehydration or pre-renal failure are treated as early as possible.

Education of patient and relevant others

Patients should be informed that leakage following removal of drain may happen and should be reported promptly.

Complications

- *Bleeding*: manifest as either an abdominal wall haematoma or a haemoperitoneum. The risk of requiring a transfusion following paracentesis is less than 1% (McGibbon *et al.* 2007).
- *Local infection or peritonitis*: there is the theoretical risk of introducing infection into the ascitic fluid, which can be minimized by the use of sterile technique. A swab from the site of the cannula should be obtained for culture review and a dry dressing applied.
- *Bowel or bladder perforation*: this risk is decreased by ensuring the patient has an empty bladder and avoiding areas of scarring where there may be underlying adherent bowel.

Compression therapy in the management of lymphoedema

Definition

Lymphoedema is defined as a chronic oedema caused by a failure of the lymphatic drainage system (International Society of Lymphology 2003).

Anatomy and physiology

The lymphatic system works closely with the cardiovascular system to maintain fluid balance within the body. The cardiovascular system transports nutrients and oxygen to the body's cells via blood vessels. As the blood flows through the vessels, nutrients and water pass into the spaces between the cells, known as the interstitial spaces, to form interstitial fluid (CREST 2008).

The lymphatic system moves this interstitial fluid, now known as 'lymph', via a network of superficial and deep lymphatic vessels in a unidirectional flow towards the two main ducts, the thoracic duct and the right lymphatic duct, before emptying back into the venous system.

Lymph drainage commences with the superficial vessels, called initial lymphatics, which are found in the connective tissue spaces. Movement of lymph in the initial lymphatics is dependent upon muscle activity and changes in tissue pressure (Stanton *et al.* 2000). The larger, deeper lymph vessels act as collecting vessels and contain smooth muscle and valves enabling them to contract and propel lymph in a unidirectional flow. Lymph nodes are situated in groups within the larger lymph vessels and act as filters to collect and destroy bacteria and viruses.

The balance between tissue fluid formation and reabsorption is dependent upon pressures across the capillary wall, known as Starling's forces. Any change can affect fluid levels in the tissues and result in the appearance of oedema (Mortimer 2003a).

Dependency or gravitational oedema is commonly seen in the immobile patient when a failure to activate the muscle pump causes an increase in capillary filtration and reduced lymph drainage in the dependent limb (Mortimer 2003a). Swelling can also occur in chronic venous disease of the lower limbs as a result of lymph drainage failure and increased capillary filtration (Mortimer 2003a). A reduction in the drainage routes of the lymphatic system can occur following cancer-related treatment in lymph node areas and oedema can appear in the adjacent limb or truncal quadrant of the body.

In summary, the lymphatic system has the following main functions.

- To regulate homoeostasis by returning large molecules to the circulation and draining excess fluid from the interstitium.
- To dispose of unwanted cellular byproducts.
- To defend the body from infection by absorbing microorganisms and generating an autoimmune response when necessary.

Related theory

The oedema occurs because the lymphatics are reduced in number, obstructed, obliterated or simply fail to function (Browse 2003). Tissue swelling then appears due to the failure of lymph drainage (Mortimer 2003a). Primary lymphoedema occurs when there is an abnormality in the lymphatic system and is classified according to the time of onset (Kinmouth 1982). Secondary lymphoedema arises from the influence of an external factor affecting the function of the lymphatic system and most commonly occurs following treatment for cancer involving the removal or irradiation of lymph node areas. Other causes of secondary lymphoedema include infection, inflammation and trauma to the lymphatic channels or vessels (Keeley 2000).

Lymphoedema is most commonly seen in cancer patients as a result of damage to lymph nodes following surgery and/or radiotherapy, but it can also occur as a result of local tumour obstruction in lymph node areas. The reported incidence of lymphoedema following cancer treatment varies between studies. In breast cancer patients, the prevalence of chronic arm oedema is reported as being between 12% and 60% and in patients treated for gynaecological cancers, it is between 28% and 47% (Lymphoedema Framework 2006c). The incidence of lymphoedema increases with time and 70–80% of patients with long-term lymphoedema present within 12 months of treatment (National Breast and Ovarian Cancer Centre 2008).

Lymphoedema can affect any part of the body including the face and head, but it most commonly affects a limb. The swelling can have physical, psychological and psychosocial implications for the patient and is associated with a number of complications arising from its development (Towers *et al.* 2008). Limb heaviness may lead to impaired function, reduced mobility and musculoskeletal problems (Tobin *et al.* 1993, Woods 1993). Skin and tissue changes develop with increased lymph stasis in the oedematous limb and give rise to the characteristic deepened skinfolds and skin thickening and over time, complex skin conditions can occur (Lymphoedema Framework 2006b). There is an increased risk of local and systemic infection as a result of poor lymph drainage and recurrent acute inflammatory episodes are common (Mortimer 2003b).

Compression therapy in the management of lymphoedema involves the use of compression garments or low-stretch bandages (Asmussen and Strossenreuther 2003, Partsch and Mosti 2008) and is the mainstay of conservative management for lymphoedema.

Evidence-based approaches

Rationale

Compression therapy initiates physiological effects within the arterial, venous and lymphatic systems (Hafner *et al.* 2000) in order to:

- ensure that lymphatic fluid in the tissues travels through the lymphatic channels towards the root of the limb
- reduce the formation of excess tissue fluid and decrease lymphatic load
- contain the tissues of the swollen limb and help to maintain a normal shape to the limb
- increase blood flow in the microcirculation and initiate a softening of fibrotic tissue
- maximize the effect of the muscle pump (Partsch 2003).

The type of material from which the bandages or garments are made can determine the degree of pressure exerted on the tissues below (Partsch *et al.* 2008), although the level of pressure achieved is also dependent upon a complex combination of other factors including the size and shape of the limb and the activity of the wearer (Clark 2003).

Inelastic and low-stretch bandages are indicated when the lymphoedema is moderate to severe and the limb has swollen out of shape (Williams and Keller 2005). They are also effective when fibrosis of the subcutaneous tissues is present, due to the massaging effect on the tissues caused by the low resting pressures and high working pressures (Foldi *et al.* 2005).

Elastic compression garments are usually used when the lymphoedema is mild and uncomplicated and to maintain the reduced size of a swollen limb after the use of low-stretch bandages (Lymphoedema Framework 2006a).

Principles of care

Compression therapy in the management of lymphoedema can be approached in two phases: the intensive phase and the maintenance phase (Hopkins 2008).

The intensive phase of treatment is a short period of therapist-led treatment usually planned over a 2–3-week period in which specific aims are identified, discussed and agreed between the patient and the therapist. Depending upon the oedema present, however, the treatment may be planned over a longer or shorter time frame. During the intensive or reduction phase of treatment, short-stretch, inelastic bandages are applied to the swollen limb each day and left in place for a period of 23 hours as part of a multilayer system to provide a semi-rigid encasement to the limb (Lymphoedema Framework 2006e). This aspect of treatment is usually combined with other elements of treatment including:

- a skincare regimen to minimize the risks of infection
- specific exercises to promote lymph drainage
- manual lymphatic drainage (MLD) administered by a specially trained therapist to stimulate lymph drainage (Lymphoedema Framework 2006e).

During the maintenance phase, the concept of self-care is promoted to encourage the patient to become independent in the long-term management and control of their swelling. Elastic compression garments are worn for a period of time each day and the therapist evaluates progress at regular intervals to ensure that the garments remain appropriate and that any problems can be identified at an early stage (Lymphoedema Framework 2006a). This aspect of treatment is also combined with other elements of treatment including:

- a skincare regimen to minimize the risks of infection
- specific exercises to promote lymph drainage
- simple lymphatic drainage (SLD), taught to the patient by a therapist to stimulate normal draining lymphatics (British Lymphology Society 2001).

Not all patients will follow both phases of treatment, and many may only need to follow the maintenance phase. The decision concerning the most appropriate phase of treatment for the patient should be made by a skilled therapist taking the patient's wishes into consideration.

Assessment of the patient with lymphoedema and calculation of limb volume

Evidence-based approaches

Rationale

When the use of compression therapy is being considered, a full and careful assessment will highlight the patient's main problems and any co-existing complications. This information is then used to set realistic treatment goals and to determine the most suitable approach to compression therapy treatment. Clinical and physical indications determined during a full assessment of the patient will facilitate the most appropriate choice of compression therapy for the individual patient. A number of treatments are used in combination during the management of lymphoedema and their

501

Figures 9.21 Mild, uncomplicated lymphoedema of the arm.

prior to the use of compression therapy. Palpation of the pedal pulses alone is an unreliable predictor of adequate arterial supply. The measurement of the Ankle to Brachial Pressure Index (ABPI) is recommended if there is any doubt about the patient's peripheral arterial status (Lymphoedema Framework 2006d, Woods 2007a). If patients have a history of diabetes or cardiac failure, a medical assessment should also be completed prior to the commencement of treatment with close supervision followed during its progress (Eagle 2001).

- *Physical assessment*: to determine the cause of the swelling and any symptoms or complicating factors. This includes the cause and extent of the oedema, an assessment of the skin condition and limb shape, the patient's disease status and the presence of any pain or altered sensations within the limb (Woods 2007a). The patient's ability to follow a treatment plan, including compression therapy, should also be assessed.

- Figure 9.21 is an example of mild, uncomplicated lymphoedema of the arm and Figure 9.22 is an example of severe, uncomplicated lymphoedema of the arm.

- *Psychosocial assessment*: to determine the influence of the swelling upon the patient's life. This includes the influence upon limb function and mobility, employment, hobbies, activities and personal roles (Lymphoedema Framework 2006d, Woods 2007a).

choice and usefulness can be determined by the therapist and patient at the time of assessment. The experience of living with lymphoedema as a long-term chronic condition is a unique experience for each patient and can have an impact on many areas of the individual's life (Towers *et al.* 2008). The physical and psychological effects are not short-lived and enormous motivation and perseverance coupled with adaptation are demanded in order to achieve control or reduction of the swelling (Mason 2000).

Clarifying the influence of the lymphoedema on the patient's lifestyle, occupation and chosen social activities will help to identify patient-focused problem areas that may require adjustment. By gaining an understanding of the impact that the swelling may be having upon personal feelings and emotions, relevant supportive strategies can be identified (Woods 2007a).

Principles of care

Assessment should include the following elements.

- *Details of the patient's medical history*: to determine whether compression therapy can be used safely. Arterial insufficiency of the lower limb must always be excluded

Figure 9.22 Severe, uncomplicated lymphoedema of the arm.

- *Psychological assessment*: to determine the effect of the swelling on the patient. This includes an assessment of the effect of the lymphoedema upon relationships, personal concerns and fears (Lymphoedema Framework 2006d, Woods 2007a).
- *Problem identification*: to determine actual and potential patient-focused problem areas combined with patient strengths and preferences.

Assessment should also include the following.

- *Planning*: to improve problems and utilize patient strengths. The healthcare professional should work in partnership with the patient to enable them to take appropriate action in order to manage their lymphoedema and work towards long-term control. Planning should focus on the patient's objectives so that immediate problems can be addressed. Long- and short-term goals can then be identified and agreed with the patient.
- *Implementation*: to determine the appropriateness of interventions and modify where required. An individualized, holistic approach will incorporate education and support, particularly if personal changes are required to minimize the risk of complications developing. Success will be achieved when the patient possesses positive motivational factors and is an active participant in the management of their lymphoedema (Mason 2000).
- *Evaluation*: to assess progress, modify and stop the intervention if necessary. In order to evaluate the outcome of a plan of treatment, suitable outcome indicators are required (Jenns 2000). No standardized method of evaluating the outcome of a plan of treatment has been determined but the measurement of limb volume using surface measurement is the most frequently used means of assessing response to treatment in lymphoedema management (Jenns 2000). The effect of treatment on the patient's psychological and psychosocial well-being should, however, also be monitored, and this is frequently achieved in a more subjective manner where the patient's views are sought (Woods 2002).

Methods of measuring limb volume

A frequently used method of establishing alterations in limb size and shape is the circumferential measurement of limb size (Stanton *et al.* 2000). This can be established by recording and comparing measurements taken of both limbs with a tape measure positioned at fixed points on a limb, usually the wrist and 10 cm above and below the point of the elbow (olecranon process) or 15 cm above and below the superior pole of the patella (Piller 1999). Although this method is easy and quick to complete, its use is primarily to track broad changes in limb circumference only and the method is prone to error if the tape measure is not positioned in the same place on each consecutive occasion.

A more accurate method of assessing response to treatment is the measurement of limb volume (Figure 9.23).

Figure 9.23 Measurement of limb volume.

Multiple circumferential measurements taken of both limbs at 4 cm intervals and applied to the formula for the volume of a cylinder provide a reliable method of determining the size of the limb and a useful, objective means of determining response to treatment. This is the most widely used method of establishing limb volume (Lymphoedema Framework 2006d, Taylor *et al.* 2006). Reproducibility is accurate if care is taken with the procedure and a standard format for the recording of the measurements is used (Woods 2007b).

A variety of methods to measure limb volume have been used.

- Volume measured by water displacement (Bernas *et al.* 1996, Engler and Sweat 1962, Kettle *et al.* 1958).
- Volume measured using an optoelectronic device (Stanton *et al.* 1997).
- Volume calculated from circumferential measurements (Sitzia 1995).

Each of these methods has advantages and disadvantages. However, the calculation of limb volume from circumferential measurements, taken with a tape measure, is uncomplicated and inexpensive (Table 9.7).

Preprocedural considerations

The sequential circumferential measurement of a limb for the calculation of limb volume should not be confused with simple limb measurements used in the choice of compression garment for a patient. These are recorded at set points on the limb and used to guide the therapist in choosing the correct size garment for the patient.

The principles in Table 9.8 should be considered when using surface measurements in order to calculate limb volume (Woods 2007b).

503

Table 9.7 Using limb volume measurements

Indications	Contraindications
To determine the total excess volume of the swollen limb compared to the patient's contralateral normal limb	In palliative care, the tracking of limb volume changes in a limb may not be appropriate and simple circumferential limb measurements can provide an alternative means of assessment
To establish the distribution of the swelling along the limb	In the presence of infection or open wounds
To provide information to assist in the choice of compression therapy (Woods 2007a)	To detect early lymphoedema. Consideration should be given to other symptoms including patterns of transient swelling and any sensation changes (Stanton et al. 2006)
To provide an objective method of determining response to treatment by indicating: ■ changes in the size and shape of the limb over time ■ changes in the excess volume ■ the distribution of any volume loss or gain in the limb (Sitzia 1995)	

Table 9.8 Points for consideration when calculating limb volume

Action	Rationale
Ensure that the same position is used for the same patient each time the limb is measured	The position of the limb will affect the measurements taken because the degree to which muscles are flexed or relaxed will influence the shape and size of the limb
The limb should be marked afresh on each measuring occasion with a washable ink, even when measuring on consecutive days	Any increase or decrease in limb volume will influence the position of the marks on the limb
Tension should not be exerted on the tape measure during measuring	If tension is applied it will vary between measurers and recordings will not be consistent
The tape measure should be positioned so that it is horizontal around the limb, taking care to ensure that it is not pulled tightly	To minimize inaccuracies in measurement
The same number of measurements should be taken on both limbs each time measurements are taken	The normal limb acts as a control in patients with unilateral swelling
The starting point for the taking of measurements should be clearly identified by measuring and clearly recording the distance from the tip of the middle finger to the wrist	This starting point on the wrist should be used each time
A standard format for the recording of measurements should be adopted	To ensure that key points can be referred to

504

Procedure guideline 9.20 **Compression therapy: limb volume calculation: lower limbs**

Essential equipment

■ Ruler, preferably 30 cm or longer
■ Tape measure; avoid those made from fabric which tends to stretch
■ Washable skin marker for marking the limb
■ Record chart and pen

Preprocedure

Action	Rationale
1 Explain and discuss the proposed procedure with the patient.	To ensure that the patient understands the procedure and gives their valid consent (NMC 2008a, C).
2 Place the patient in a sitting position with the legs outstretched horizontally, preferably on a firm couch with adjustable height.	To ensure the lower limbs are relaxed and supported and the adjustable height means that the measurer can work without straining their back. E

Procedure

Action	Rationale
3 Standing on the outside of the leg, ask the patient to flex the foot to a right angle. Measure the distance from the base of the heel to the ankle, along the inside of the leg; mark the ankle, allowing at least 2 cm of leg to lie below the mark, and record the distance on the chart.	To establish and clearly record a reproducible fixed starting point for all subsequent measurements (Badger 1993, C). Note: the marks represent a point midway through each cylinder segment, they do not represent the base of the cylinder, therefore at least half the segment (i.e. 2 cm) must lie below the mark.
4 Ask the patient to relax the foot. From the starting point, using a ruler, mark the inside of the leg at 4 cm intervals along the length of the leg up to the groin.	Reducing the limb to 4 cm segments improves the accuracy of measurement since these segments resemble a cylinder more closely than does the whole limb. The formula used here assumes that the measurements are 4 cm apart (Sitzia 1995, R5).
5 Place the tape measure around the limb and measure the circumference at each marked point, recording the measurement on the chart. Make sure that the tape lies smoothly around the relaxed limb and that it does not lie at an angle. (Decide at the outset whether the tape is to be placed above, below or on the mark and keep to the same position every time.)	Ensuring that there are no gaps between the limb and the tape and that the procedure is the same each time reduces error (Aslem *et al.* 1996, R3b).
6 Repeat the process on the other leg, whether or not it is swollen.	If only one limb is affected the normal limb acts as the patient's own control (Piller 1999, R5).
7 If desired, a circumference measurement may be taken of the foot but this is not included in the calculation of volume.	The foot cannot be considered to be a cylinder and it is therefore inappropriate to include it in the calculation of volume (Taylor *et al.* 2006, R5).

Postprocedure

Action	Rationale
8 Ensure that the same number of measurements are made and clearly recorded on the record sheet for each leg.	Accurate documentation will ensure accuracy during limb volume calculation for each limb (Badger 1993, E).
9 Remove the marks from the patient's skin using warm water and a mild soap preparation.	Removing the marks maintains patient dignity. Mild soap ensures that the skin is not irritated

Procedure guideline 9.21 Compression therapy: limb volume calculation: upper limbs

Essential equipment

- Ruler, preferably 30 cm or longer
- Tape measure; avoid those made from fabric which tends to stretch
- Washable skin marker for marking the limb
- Record chart and pen

Preprocedure

Action	Rationale
1 Explain and discuss the proposed procedure with the patient.	To ensure that the patient understands the procedure and gives their valid consent (NMC 2008a, C).
2 Sit the patient in a chair with the arms extended in front and resting on the back of a chair. The arms should be as close to an angle of 90° to the body as possible.	To ensure the arms are supported and accessible at a standard height. Changing the angle of the arms to the body will result in changes in the measurements (Boland and Adams 1998, R5).
3 If only one arm is swollen, start with the unaffected arm.	

(Continued)

Procedure guideline 9.21 (*Continued*)

Procedure

4 Measure the distance from the tip of the middle finger to the wrist. Mark the wrist, allowing at least 2 cm above the ulnar styloid, and note down the distance.	To establish and clearly record a reproducible fixed starting point for all subsequent measurements (Badger 1993, E). Note: The marks represent a point midway through each cylinder segment, they do not represent the base of the cylinder, therefore at least half the segment (i.e. 2 cm) must lie below the mark.
5 From the starting point, using a ruler, mark along the ulnar aspect of the arm at 4 cm intervals up to the axilla.	Reducing the limb to 4 cm segments improves the accuracy of measurement since these segments resemble a cylinder more closely than does the whole limb (Sitzia 1995, R5).
6 Place the tape measure around the limb and measure the circumference at each marked point, recording each measurement on the chart. Make sure that the tape lies smoothly around the relaxed limb and that it does not lie at an angle. Decide at the outset whether the tape is to be placed above, below or on the mark and keep to the same position every time.	Ensuring that there are no gaps between the limb and the tape and that the procedure is the same each time reduces error (Aslem *et al.* 1996, R3b).
7 Repeat the process on the other arm.	If only one limb is affected, the normal limb acts as the patient's own control (Piller 1999, R5).
8 If desired, a circumference measurement may be taken of the hand but this is not included in the calculation of volume.	The hand cannot be considered to be a cylinder and it is therefore inappropriate to include it in the calculation (Taylor *et al.* 2006, R5).
9 Ensure that the same number of measurements are made and clearly recorded on the record sheet for each arm.	Accurate documentation will ensure accuracy during limb volume calculation for each limb (Badger 1993, E).

Postprocedure

10 Remove the marks from the patient's skin using warm water and a mild soap preparation.	Removing the marks maintains patient dignity. Mild soap ensures that the skin is not irritated.

Problem-solving table 9.6 Prevention and resolution (Procedure guidelines 9.20 and 9.21)

Problem	Cause	Prevention	Action
The tape measure will not lie evenly on the surface of the skin because of the shape of the limb and development of deepened skinfolds	The effect of the lymphoedema on the tissues and the distribution of swelling	The limb shape can be artificially corrected	Wrap the limb in cling film to create a more cylindrical shape. Mark the cling film and measure at these points
Loose areas of skin, making it difficult to place the tape measure smoothly around the limb	Age-related loss of skin turgor or weight loss causing excess skin	The limb shape can be artificially corrected	Elevation of the limb distributes the excess skin and a more accurate measurement of the limb can be gained

Problem	Cause	Prevention	Action
Limited range of movement of upper limb, making limb positioning difficult	Brachial plexopathy	Work within the patient's ability	Position the limb comfortably and seek assistance if necessary to support the limb
Skin lesions, open wounds, pain or tenderness resulting in the omission of some measuring points and inaccurate calculation of limb volume	Measurements cannot be taken where there is a breach of skin integrity or pain	Carefully examine the skin for breaks in skin integrity prior to measuring and check that the patient is comfortable so that action can be taken if necessary	Cover any open wounds with cling film to ensure measurements can be taken in the required place. Avoid pulling the measuring tape tightly to avoid trauma to the area

Postprocedural considerations

Once measurement of both limbs has been completed, a number of formulas may be used to calculate the limb volume of each limb (Badger 1993, Sitzia 1995).

The formula for the volume of a cylinder (Box 9.19) considers the limb as a series of cylinders, each with a height of 4 cm. In order to calculate the volume of the limb, each measurement needs to be converted into a volume for that segment of the cylinder and then totalled. This is illustrated in Table 9.9.

The volume difference between the limbs is then usually expressed as a percentage. The calculation for this is shown in Box 9.20.

Compression bandaging

Definition

Short-stretch, inelastic bandages are used during the intensive or reduction phase of treatment for lymphoedema.

Table 9.9 Calculating the total limb volume of a limb using the formula in Box 9.19

Circumference measurement	C^2/π (3.14)	Volume of each cylinder in mL
18.4	=	107.7
19.1	=	116.1
21	=	140.3
23.2	=	171.3
24.9	=	197.3
25.7	=	210.2
26.6	=	225.2
29.6	=	278.8
30.3	=	292.2
31.7	=	319.8
32.7	=	340.3
33.5	=	357.2
Total volume	=	**2757**

Box 9.19 Procedure for calculating volume from circumferences

The formula for calculating the volume of a cylinder is $\frac{\text{circumference}^2}{\pi}$. The formula must be applied to each circumference measurement ($circ_1$, $circ_2$, . . . , $circ_n$) in order to calculate the volume of each segment; the volumes are then totalled to give the total limb volume.

So $\left(\dfrac{circ_1 \times circ_1}{3.1415}\right) + \left(\dfrac{circ_2 \times circ_2}{3.1415}\right) + \left(\dfrac{circ_3 \times circ_3}{3.1415}\right) + ...etc.$

Use of a programmable calculator will speed up the process of calculation.

Box 9.20 Calculating the volume difference between the limbs as a percentage

Limb volume totals

Swollen limb volume

2757

Unaffected limb volume

2459

Difference between the limbs

298

Divide 100 by the unaffected limb volume (2459) and multiply by the volume difference (298), i.e.: 100/2459 × 298 = 12.11

The swollen limb is 12% bigger than the normal limb

Related theory

The bandages used in compression therapy are termed short-stretch bandages with a high resistance to stretch. When applied to a limb, they provide the limb with a firm external encasement. During joint movement and muscular contraction of the limb, pressure against the firm external encasement leads to a temporary increase in pressure within the tissues, known as working pressure (Osbourne 2007). This produces a massaging effect on the tissues below to stimulate lymph drainage (Hopkins 2008). Conversely, when the muscle is inactive during rest, short-stretch bandages support the tissues and provide a relatively low resting pressure. This ensures that the patient remains comfortable and encourages compliance with the planned course of treatment (Williams 2002).

Long-stretch bandages with a high degree of elasticity are unsuitable in the management of lymphoedema. These bandages exert a high working and high resting pressure on the tissues of the limb and can be uncomfortable when left in place for long periods of time.

The pressure exerted by the short-stretch bandage on the limb is influenced by a number of factors.

- *The circumference of the limb*: the highest pressure is achieved where the limb is narrowest (Clark 2003). When a bandage is applied to a limb of normal proportions, therefore, the highest pressure will be achieved at the ankle or wrist, with graduated, reducing pressure along the length of the limb as the circumference increases (Todd 2000). Limbs that are thin and areas where there are bony prominences will need careful protection to avoid high pressure on these exposed areas which can lead to skin or tissue damage (Hafner *et al.* 2000).
- *The number of layers*: every bandage is applied with a degree of overlap. Several layers applied over each other increase the pressure applied to the limb (Partsch *et al.* 2008).
- *The components of the bandage system*: the use of padding and foam beneath the bandages increases the sub-bandage pressure and stiffness of the assembled bandage (Partsch *et al.* 2008).

Evidence-based approaches

Rationale

Indications

- *Large limbs*: elastic compression garments used on large swollen limbs may be ineffective due to the difficulties of applying sufficient tension to compress the limb (Badger *et al.* 2000, Stillwell 1973).
- *Mis-shapen limbs*: elastic compression garments will promote the development of deep skinfolds if the limb is awkwardly shaped (Todd 2000). Foam or soft padding placed under short-stretch bandages will smooth out the folds and restore normal shape to the limb (see Figures 9.24 and 9.25 for examples of a mis-shapen limb before and after bandaging).

Figure 9.24 Example of a mis-shapen limb before bandaging.

- *Severe lymphoedema*: large limbs with long-standing oedema require high pressures to break down tissue fibrosis. Short-stretch bandages provide a low resting and high working pressure which promotes a softening of hardened tissues (Lymphoedema Framework 2006e).
- *Lymphorrhoea*: the leakage of lymph fluid from the skin responds readily to external pressure provided by short-stretch bandages (Jenns 2000).
- *Damaged or fragile skin*: elastic compression garments can cause damage to fragile skin. Short-stretch bandages should be used until the skin condition improves (Jenns 2000).

Contraindications

Short-stretch bandages should not be used where there is:

- arterial disease; tissue ischaemia can occur
- infection in the swollen limb; pain may occur
- uncontrolled cardiac failure; fluid overload can occur
- deep vein thrombosis; anticoagulation therapy should be commenced prior to the use of bandages
- physical or psychological unsuitability of the patient to comply with treatment (Todd 2000).

Figure 9.25 Example of a mis-shapen limb after bandaging.

Principles to be followed in multilayer bandaging

Short-stretch, inelastic bandages should always be used. These are available in a range of widths and provide a low resting pressure to the swollen limb when the muscle is inactive and a high working pressure during activity when the muscle is pumping against the resistance created by the bandage (Todd 2000).

For bandaging to be effective, the following principles must be considered.

- *An even pressure should be provided around the circumference of the limb.* Where the limb shape is irregular or distorted by swelling, an even profile can be achieved with the use of padding or foam to add bulk to an area where shape requires correcting (Williams and Keller 2005).
- *The pressure from the bandages must be graduated along the length of the limb to ensure that the most pressure is achieved distally and the least proximally.* Graduated pressure will be achieved naturally in a regularly shaped limb where the circumference of the wrist or ankle is smaller than the circumference of the root of the limb.

Graduated pressure can also be achieved by selecting the correct bandage width for the size of the limb and controlling the amount of bandage tension and overlap used (Todd 2000). Moderate tension only should be used and the bandages should never be stretched to their maximum length.

- *The pressure applied to the limb should be adequate to counter the limb circumference.* Greater pressure is required when the circumference of the limb is large. This can be achieved by using more than one layer of bandages and selecting the correct width of bandage for the circumference of the limb (Todd 2000).
- *The bandages should be left in place day and night and removed once every 24 hours.* This enables skin hygiene to be attended to and the condition of the skin to be checked. Reapplication of the bandages then ensures that effective compression is maintained on the changing limb shape (Damstra *et al.* 2008).
- *The bandages should be comfortable for the patient and removed at any time if they cause any pain, numbness or discoloration (blueness) in the fingers or toes.* This may indicate a variety of causes, including too great a compression on the limb. A satisfactory outcome of treatment should be achieved within 2–3 weeks. More advanced stages of lymphoedema may require up to 4–6 weeks of treatment. The patient may then begin the maintenance phase of treatment where containment hosiery is fitted.

Palliative care

Compression bandaging can be versatile and extremely useful in the palliative care setting when volume reduction may be unrealistic or not indicated and the emphasis is on optimizing the patient's quality of life.

The burden of treatment should not exceed the benefit to be gained from providing support and comfort to a limb with a low level of pressure using a modified technique of bandaging designed around the patient's needs. The therapist should have expertise to apply the correct degree of pressure to the limb and avoid forcing fluid into adjacent areas (Todd 2009). The bandages can be left in place for 2–3 days and should not prevent the patient from maintaining full movement in their bandaged limb (Woods 2000).

Legal and professional issues

Compression bandaging should only be carried out by a skilled therapist with the necessary skills and experience to apply bandages to the swollen limb (Lymphoedema Framework 2006e), ensuring that pressure is graduated towards the root of the limb and evenly applied. Poor technique can lead to serious consequences with damage to the skin and tissues if the bandages are incorrectly or inappropriately applied (Feben 2003, RCN 1998, Thomas and Nelson 1998). The therapist has a professional responsibility to ensure the safety of the patient and should therefore always ensure that the arterial status of the patient is known and that there are no contraindications to the use of low-stretch compression bandages.

Studies by Taylor *et al.* (2000), Hafner *et al.* (2000) and Feben (2003) emphasize the importance of training for therapists to ensure that safe, effective pressure is applied to the limb during the use of short-stretch bandages. Appropriate courses are available for therapists throughout the UK.

Preprocedural considerations

If there is any concern regarding the patient's arterial blood flow, an ABPI should be measured using a hand-held Doppler before undertaking any compression therapy. An ABPI reading of 0.8 or below should be referred for medical opinion (Lymphoedema Framework 2006d).

Specific patient preparations

The bandaging materials used on a swollen limb can be bulky and patients will therefore require appropriate information and advice concerning suitable loose-fitting, easily applied clothing and, if the leg is being bandaged, appropriate wide-opening footwear, which will accommodate the bulk of the bandages during the course of treatment.

As the bandages are worn for 23 hours a day, the timing of appointments for the bandages to be replaced will need to consider opportunities to attend to personal hygiene, travel arrangements and accommodate family and work commitments. The bandages can be removed at home before the appointment to allow for personal hygiene but it is advisable for the patient to wear a suitable compression garment on the journey to the appointment. It is not recommended that patients drive themselves in a car to or from appointments. The bandages will mean that the affected limb will be bulkier than usual, making reaction times slower. Safety can therefore be compromised. If the patient chooses to drive, they must be advised to check with their motor insurance company before doing so.

Activities of daily living may have to be adapted because of the bulk of the bandages and the therapist should discuss and outline with the patient an appropriate exercise regimen to be followed during the course of treatment, to ensure that maximum effectiveness is gained from the course of bandaging. Verbal information given should be supported by written information and include details of what the patient should do if problems develop with the bandages and whom to contact (Williams and Keller 2005).

Procedure guideline 9.22 Compression bandaging (standard multilayer): bandaging an arm and the fingers

Essential equipment

- Tubular stockinette: this can be purchased in a long roll and a length cut to suit the limb size. Different widths are available
- Light retention bandages: 6 and 10 cm to bandage digits and to hold foam padding in place
- Synthetic orthopaedic padding rolls: 6 cm rolls to pad and reshape the limb
- Sheet of low-density foam to cut to shape and pad out uneven areas

- Low-stretch bandages, 6 and 8 cm. A variety of widths are required to suit the shape of the limb
- Tape

Preprocedure

Action	Rationale
1 Explain and discuss the procedure with the patient.	To ensure that the patient understands the procedure and gives their valid consent (NMC 2008a, C).
2 If possible, the patient should be seated in a chair with the limb relaxed and supported on the back of a chair or appropriate limb support. The therapist should be positioned in front of the patient.	To ensure the comfort of both the patient and therapist and that the skin and muscles are positioned correctly to avoid inappropriate areas of pressure. C
3 The swollen limb should be clean and well moisturized with a bland cream (e.g. E45) before being bandaged.	To promote skin hygiene and integrity. C

Procedure

4 Cut a length of tubular stockinette long enough to fit the patient's arm. Cut a small hole for the thumb and slip over the patient's arm.	To protect the skin from chafing and from any sensitivity caused by the synthetic materials of the padding and foam (Williams and Keller 2005, E).
5 The fingers must be bandaged (see Action Figure 5a). Using a narrow light retention bandage, anchor the bandage loosely at the wrist and bring across the back of the hand to the thumb. Bandage around the thumb from the tip downwards (start at the level of the nail bed). Do not pull the bandage tight but go gently and firmly. Take the bandage under the wrist and back over the back of the hand to the index finger (see Action Figure 5b). Again, bandage from the nail bed down to the webs of the finger. Repeat the same procedure for all fingers. Finish by tucking in the end of the bandage (see Action Figure 5c).	To reduce or prevent swelling (Williams and Keller 2005, E).
6 Check the colour and temperature of the tips of the fingers.	To ensure that the blood supply is not compromised (Partsch 2003, E).
7 Check that the patient can move the fingers and make a fist.	To check that the bandage is not too tight (Partsch 2003, E).
8 Using the roll of padding, cover the hand in a figure of eight, padding out the palm and back of the hand (see Action Figure 8).	Padding out the hand ensures even pressure distribution and protects the bony areas of the hand (Williams and Keller 2005, E).
9 Continue the padding up to the axilla, doubling it over at the elbow.	Doubling it over at the elbow crease protects the delicate skin at the elbow (Foldi *et al.* 2003, E).
10 Foam can be used to even out any exaggerated contours of the limb. The foam should be cut to fit the length and circumference of the arm from the wrist to axilla. The foam can be cut into two pieces, one for the lower and one for the upper arm, with no gap at elbow.	To protect the elbow joint and provide a smooth, even profile on which to bandage (Williams and Keller 2005, E). The foam also ensures a more even distribution of pressure and softens the lymphostatic fibrosis (Foldi *et al.* 2003, E). It can also be used as a 'brake' to prevent the bandage from slipping (Foldi *et al.* 2003, E).
11 Wrap the foam around the arm, securing with a light retention bandage. Finish by tucking in the end of the bandage (see Action Figure 11).	
12 Take a 6 cm compression bandage and start by anchoring it loosely at the wrist. Advise the patient to hold their fingers apart whilst the hand is bandaged and take the bandage across the dorsum of the hand to wrap it twice around the hand close to the base of the fingers. Continue bandaging the hand firmly in a figure of eight until all of the hand is covered (see Action Figure 12). Continue the rest of the bandage up the forearm in a spiral, covering half of the bandage with each turn. Keep the bandage as smooth as possible.	The bandage width must relate to the circumference of the limb with the narrowest bandage used on the smallest circumference (Thomas 2003, R5).
13 Take an 8 or 10 cm bandage and, starting at the wrist, bandage in a spiral, still covering half of the bandage with each turn, up to the top of the arm (see Action Figure 13).	Two layers are used on the forearm to ensure that pressure is highest distally (Thomas 2003, R5).

511

(Continued)

Procedure guideline 9.22 *(Continued)*

14 A top layer of bandages can be applied in a spiral.	Applying a top layer can even out and maintain optimal pressure.
15 Secure the end of the bandage with tape.	Tape is used instead of fastening clips due to risk of injury (Foldi *et al.* 2003, E)

Postprocedure

16 Once again, check the colour and sensations of the finger tips and check that the patient can move all joints.	To check that the blood flow is not compromised (Partsch 2003, E).
17 Remind the patient to use the limb as normally as possible, to exercise as advised and to remove the bandages if any pain, tingling or numbness is experienced.	To ensure good lymph flow and to prevent complications developing (Partsch 2003, E).
18 Record the details of the procedure followed in the patient's relevant documentation.	To maintain accurate records and provide a point of reference for subsequent treatment (NMC 2005, C).

(a)

Action Figure 5(a) Bandaging swollen fingers.

(b)

Action Figure 5(b) Bandage is taken under wrist, back over hand, to index finger.

(c)

Action Figure 5(c) Finished bandage.

Action Figure 8 Palm and back of hand are padded out.

Action Figure 12 Hand is bandaged firmly in a figure of eight using a 6 cm compression bandage.

Action Figure 11 Foam is wrapped around arm and secured with a light retention bandage.

Action Figure 13 Starting at wrist, an 8 or 10 cm bandage is used to cover to the top of the arm, in a spiral fashion.

Procedure guideline 9.23 Compression bandaging (standard multilayer): bandaging a leg and the toes

Essential equipment

- Tubular stockinette: this can be purchased in a long roll and a length cut to suit the limb size. Different widths are available
- Light retention bandages: 4 cm width to bandage the toes, 6 cm or 10 cm to hold foam in place
- Synthetic orthopaedic padding rolls: 6 cm, 10 cm and 12 cm width rolls to pad and reshape the limb
- Sheet of low-density foam to cut to shape and pad out uneven areas

- Low-stretch compression bandages, 8, 10 and 12 cm. A variety of widths are required to suit the shape of the limb
- Tape
- Scissors

(Continued)

Procedure guideline 9.23 (*Continued*)

Preprocedure

Action	Rationale
1 Explain and discuss the procedure with the patient.	To ensure that the patient understands the procedure and gives their valid consent (NMC 2008a, C).
2 If possible, the patient should be seated upright on a bed or treatment couch. Raise the bed or couch to a comfortable height.	To ensure the comfort of both the patient and nurse. C
3 The swollen limb should be clean and well moisturized with a bland cream (e.g. E45) before being bandaged.	To promote skin hygiene and integrity. C

Procedure

4 Cut a length of tubular stockinette long enough to fit the patient's leg. Slip over the leg.	To protect the skin from chafing (Williams and Keller 2005, E).
5 If the toes are swollen or have a tendency to swell, they must be bandaged. The little toe can be omitted. Using a narrow light retention bandage, anchor the bandage around the foot and bring across the top of the foot to the big toe (see Action Figure 5a). Bandage around the toe from the tip downwards (start at the level of the nail bed). Do not pull the bandage tight, but gently and firmly. Take the bandage under the foot and back over the top of the foot to the next toe (see Action Figure 5b). Repeat the same procedure for each toe that needs to be bandaged. Finish by tucking in the end of the bandage (see Action Figure 5c).	To reduce or prevent swelling (Lymphoedema Framework 2006e, Williams and Keller 2005, E). To prevent friction to and around the little toe (Williams and Keller 2005, E).
6 Cut the foam into pads to fit over the dorsum of the foot, around the ankle and behind the knee (see Action Figures 6a, b).	To protect bony prominences and joint flexures (Williams and Keller 2005, E).
7 Secure the pads firmly in place with light retention bandages.	
8 Using foam and padding, even out any exaggerated contours of the limb.	To create a smooth profile on which to apply the bandages (Williams and Keller 2005, E).
9 Using a 10 cm roll of padding, apply firmly in a spiral up the leg, starting around the foot. Use the 20 cm padding over the thigh (see Action Figure 9).	To protect the skin and create a smooth profile on which to bandage (Lymphoedema Framework 2006e, Williams and Keller 2005, E).
10 Take an 8 cm compression bandage and start by anchoring it loosely at the ankle. Advise the patient to hold their foot at a 90° angle whilst it is bandaged and take the bandage across the dorsum of the foot to wrap it around the foot close to the base of the toes (see Action Figure 10). Continue bandaging the foot firmly, forming a figure of eight to cover the heel and ankle without leaving any gaps. Any surplus bandage should be taken up the leg in a spiral.	To avoid constriction at the ankle. Fluid will accumulate in any unbandaged areas (Williams and Keller 2005, E).
11 Using a 10 cm bandage, continue from where the first bandage finished, using a spiral up the leg and covering half of the bandage with each turn. Remember to bandage firmly. Use the widest bandage over the thigh. Secure the end of the last bandage with tape.	The bandage width must relate to the circumference of the limb with the narrowest bandage used on the smallest circumference (Thomas 2003, R5).

514

| 12 Apply a second layer of bandage, from ankle to thigh, using a figure of eight. Secure the end with tape (see Action Figure 12). | To keep the bandages in place and provide additional pressure along the length of the leg (Williams and Keller 2005, E). |

Postprocedure

13 Check the colour and temperature of the patient's toes. It may be difficult for the patient to flex the knee at first but this should get easier as the bandages loosen slightly.	To check that the blood flow is not compromised (Partsch 2003, E).
14 Remind the patient to use the limb as normally as possible, to exercise as advised and to remove the bandages if any pain, tingling or numbness is experienced.	To ensure good lymph flow and to prevent complications developing (Partsch 2003, E).
15 Record the details of the procedure in the relevant patient documentation.	To maintain accurate records and provide a point of reference for subsequent treatment (NMC 2005, C).

(a)   (b)   (c)

Action Figure 5 **(a)** A narrow light retention bandage is anchored around the foot and brought across the foot to the big toe. **(b)** The toes are bandaged in turn from the nail bed along the length of the toe. **(c)** The bandage is taken under the foot and back over the top of the foot to bandage the next toe.

(a)   (b)

Action Figure 6 **(a)** Foam is used to cover the dorsum of the foot and around the ankle. **(b)** A foam pad is bandaged into position behind the knee.

Procedure guideline 9.23 (*Continued*)

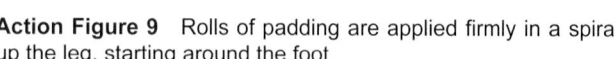

Action Figure 9 Rolls of padding are applied firmly in a spiral up the leg, starting around the foot.

Action Figure 10 Bandaging the foot using an 8 cm compression bandage and starting close to the toes.

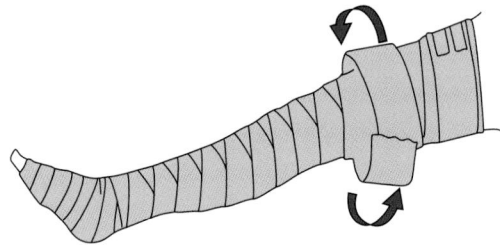

Action Figure 12 Applying a second layer of bandage, from ankle to thigh.

Problem-solving table 9.7 **Prevention and resolution (Procedure guidelines 9.22 and 9.23)**

Problem	Cause	Prevention	Action
Patient becomes breathless	An unknown cardiac pathology may lead to fluid overload as the lymphatic fluid moves from the swollen limb		Medical attention should be sought immediately if the patient becomes breathless during compression bandaging. Compression bandaging should be stopped until the patient's condition is stabilized

Problem	Cause	Prevention	Action
Pain, discomfort, numbness and/or tingling of digits when bandages are in place	Incorrect pressure gradient	Ensure patient gives feedback throughout the procedure Observe the skin each day for signs of inflammation where excess pressure may have been applied	Check the pressure gradient after each bandage application, ensure overlap of bandages is even along the length of the limb. Feel the pressure of the bandages regularly to ensure the consistency of the gradient
Pain and tenderness over bony prominences noted when the bandages are removed, for example wrist and ankle	Inadequate padding over bony prominences	Careful assessment of the limb shape prior to application of bandages	Use foam and padding to protect bony prominences and even out shape of limb
Skin irritation developing in sensitive areas, for example elbow crease and popliteal crease, during the course of bandaging	Areas of excess movement resulting in friction from the bandages	Ensure there are no skin allergies to the materials being used	Use appropriate moisturizer for patient. Protect limb with Tubifast. Use extra padding in areas of sensitivity
Poor compliance with bandaging causing premature removal of bandages each day	Lack of information given to patient Lifestyle commitments	Ensure patient is given appropriate information verbally and in writing prior to commencement of treatment	Explore the problems the patient is experiencing. Explain the procedure thoroughly and its intended benefits
Congestion developing at the root of limb during bandaging	Too much pressure throughout the limb causing an overload of fluid at root of limb		Reduce pressure of bandage throughout limb. Teach SLD. Carry out MLD

517

Postprocedural considerations

Immediate care

Evaluation of each stage of the bandaging procedure is essential to ensure that the bandage and padding have been used appropriately and correctly. This ensures that the best results are being achieved and that resources are being used to the maximum.

The process of evaluation must be thorough and should include the following.

- *Continuous attention to the colour of the digits.* Too much pressure will result in compromised circulation.
- *Continuous attention to the sensations experienced in the bandaged limb.* The bandages should not cause pain, numbness or tingling.
- *The shape of the limb.* A cylindrical contour should be achieved with the use of soft foam and padding.
- *The overlap of the bandages.* This should be even and consistent with no gaps in the bandages.
- *The pressure achieved.* This should feel even to the patient and there should be no creases in the bandages.

Layers should be used appropriately (Todd 2000). The therapist should feel the bandages regularly during the procedure to ensure the consistency of the gradient.

Ongoing care

The patient should feel comfortable and be able to move their limb. Information should be given concerning when and how to remove the bandages if necessary. The patient should be made aware that if the bandages do have to be removed, a compression garment must be worn until their next appointment. It is vital that the patient reports any concerns to the therapist at each visit.

Compression garments

Definition

Elastic compression garments are used in the long-term management of lymphoedema. Patients are required to wear their garments on a daily basis with most patients wearing their garments all day and removing them at night. For some patients, their treatment plan may include the flexibility to wear the garment just for exertive activities or for a few hours each day, depending upon their needs.

Evidence-based approaches

Rationale

Choosing the correct garment for the patient can be a difficult decision which should always follow a detailed assessment of the patient (Eagle 2001) and should only be undertaken by a healthcare professional with knowledge and appropriate skills to ensure patient safety.

The size of the required garment can be determined by following the manufacturer's individual size chart and recording three or four circumferential measurements at set points along the length of the limb. It is important to remember that size charts provide a guide only and the patient's evaluation of the comfort of the fitted garment is essential. An alternative style, larger or smaller size may be required.

Indications

- Mild, uncomplicated, swelling with a normal limb shape (Lymphoedema Framework 2006a).
- The maintenance of limb shape and size following a course of intensive therapy (Lymphoedema Framework 2006a).
- A limb volume less than 20% of the opposite limb if the shape of the limb has been preserved (Badger *et al.* 2000).
- To control swelling and provide support in the palliative treatment of oedema (Woods 2000).

Contraindications

- *Arterial disease*: blood supply may be further compromised (Doherty *et al.* 2006).
- *Acute heart failure*: symptoms may be exacerbated (Doherty *et al.* 2006).
- *Distortion of limb shape*: the garment will not fit (Lymphoedema Framework 2006a).
- *Skinfolds*: the garment will cause ridges and a tourniquet effect to the limb (Lymphoedema Framework 2006a).
- *Open wounds*: the garment will become soiled and pose an infection risk.
- *Fragile skin*: application and removal of the garment may cause further damage to the skin (Doherty *et al.* 2006).
- *Lymphorrhoea*: the garment will become wet and may cause skin excoriation (Doherty *et al.* 2006).
- *An acute infective episode (cellulitis)*: application and removal of the garment may be painful and cause damage to the friable skin (Lymphoedema Framework 2006a).
- *Severe peripheral neuropathy*: the patient will not be able to tell if the garment is causing damage to the skin (Lymphoedema Framework 2006a).

Legal and professional issues

It is important to acknowledge that different classifications of compression exist which are determined by testing methods, yarn specification, compression gradient and garment durability (Clark and Krimmel 2006). In the UK, elastic compression garments are available in the British Standard BS 6612, French Standard ASQUAL and German Standard RAL-GZ 387:2000. Each Standard adopts different testing techniques to determine the degree of pressure measured at the ankle when the garment is in place and the pressure range used to define the compression class of the garment differs between each of these Standards (Clark and Krimmel 2006). The compression levels used are generally higher than those used to treat venous disease and are classified according to the pressure exerted at the ankle by the garment. Table 9.10 outlines the indications for compression garments and the suggested compression classification.

A wide range of elastic compression garments for the treatment of lymphoedema are now available on the drug tariff, making it easier for patients to establish a long-term supply of their garments.

Preprocedural considerations

A number of factors need to be taken into consideration before deciding to fit a patient with an elastic compression garment. The patient should be motivated and compliant with the use of garments and have the physical skills to apply and remove the garment safely. A full physical assessment of the patient will determine the condition of the skin and tissues and the shape and size of the limb in order to determine the style, size and appropriate compression class of the garment suitable for the patient.

Equipment

Elastic compression garments apply an external force to the limb which pulls in to exert pressure on the tissues below (Eagle 2001). The pressure can be sustained over long periods of time during both activity and inactivity of the limb, providing a high working pressure whilst the muscle is active and a high resting pressure during inactivity of the muscle at rest (Todd 2000).

The use of elastic compression garments:

- increases interstitial tissue pressure and reduces production of lymph
- promotes lymph movement along superficial and deep lymphatics
- increases lymph reabsorption (Lymphoedema Framework 2006a)
- provides an external counterforce during activity which enhances muscle pump action (Todd 2000).

A wide range of garments are available which differ in construction, compression class and style, in addition to size and colour.

Table 9.10 Compression classes and indications for their use

Indications	Suggested compression level
Mild lymphoedema ■ Excess limb volume <20% ■ No shape distortion ■ Maintenance ■ Palliation	Class I LOW COMPRESSION British Standard: 14–21 mmHg French Standard: 10–15 mmHg German Standard: 18–21 mmHg
Moderate lymphoedema ■ Excess limb volume 20–40% ■ Mild shape distortion ■ Maintenance	Class 2 MEDIUM COMPRESSION British Standard: 18–24 mmHg French Standard: 15–20 mmHg German Standard: 22–32 mmHg
Severe lymphoedema ■ Excess limb volume >40% ■ Moderate shape distortion ■ Fibrosed tissues ■ Skin changes; hyperkeratosis and papillomatosis	Class 3 HIGH COMPRESSION British Standard: 25–35 mmHg French Standard: 22–32 mmHg German Standard: 34–46 mmHg

■ *Construction*: garments are manufactured as either round knit or flat knit. Round-knit garments are produced in one piece from synthetic fibres and are readily available in a variety of sizes 'off the shelf' to accommodate the needs of most patients. Whilst more cosmetically acceptable to patients, these garments have a tendency to roll or gather in areas along the limb, if the limb is mis-shaped (Linnitt and Davies 2007). They are more suitable therefore for patients with mild lymphoedema whose limbs have maintained a regular shape. Some round-knit garments are manufactured with inelastic materials, creating a stiffer garment. The pressure under these garments will be higher whilst the muscle is active. Flat-knit garments are manufactured from one piece of material sewn together with a seam. The shape can be adjusted during manufacture to suit patients' specific needs and the provision of accurate measurements before manufacture ensures a good fit. Flat-knit garments offer the highest working pressure relative to their resting pressure and are more suitable for patients with moderate to severe lymphoedema (Linnitt and Davies 2007).

■ *Compression class*: the degree of pressure exerted by the garment on the surface of the skin it surrounds determines its compression class (Asmussen and Strossenreuther 2003). The highest compression provided by a garment when fitted can be found at the wrist or the ankle. The compression is then graduated along the length of the limb to encourage movement of the fluid out of the limb.

■ *Style*: all areas influenced by swelling must be contained within the compression garment or further swelling will develop. The patient should be instructed concerning the application, removal and care of the garment to ensure that maximum effectiveness is achieved through its use. The patient's ability must be taken into account when choosing a garment as a high degree of dexterity and strength may be required during its application and removal and this may be impractical for the patient (Todd 2000).

■ *Size*: the correct garment is one that fits well and is comfortable for the patient with no loose pockets of material where swelling can develop and no areas of constriction where a tourniquet effect can occur. The manufacturer's guidance for choosing the correct size is based on simple limb measurements and particular attention should be given to the fit at the ankle or wrist where high levels of compression can occur (Todd 2000).

The application of elastic garments can be greatly eased by the wearing of household rubber gloves during application, which facilitate control of the garment and prevent damage to its fabric. Application aids (see Table 9.11) are also available commercially and may assist some patients who experience difficulties. Any moisturizing cream should be applied at night-time rather than in the morning before putting the garment on. A very fine layer of talcum powder applied to hot sticky skin can ease application. If this is the first time that the patient has worn elastic compression garments, the therapist should explain to the patient that the feeling of pressure may seem strange for the first few hours, but that it should not cause pain in the limb or numbness in the digits or toes.

Table 9.11 Application aids

Aid	Description	Supplier
Acti glide	An application to allow open or closed toe compression stockings to glide onto leg	Activa www.activahealthcare.co.uk
Easy off	Aid for taking off leg stockings which reduces bending	Mediven www.mediuk.co.uk
Easy pad	A rectangular piece of non-slip foam to assist with the application of compression garments	Juzo www.juzo.com
Easyslide	A limb-shaped slide sheet designed to ensure easy application of the garment with the right amount of pressure	Credenhill www.credenhill.co.uk
Foot slide	A shaped piece of silky material to assist with the application of open toe compression garments over the foot	Supplied with most compression stockings
Medi Butler	A specially designed metal frame which holds the garment in place so that the foot or hand can slide into it. The frame has handles which are used to pull the garment up the limb	Mediven www.mediuk.co.uk
Mediven 2 in 1	A limb-shaped slide sheet that assists with the donning and doffing of garments	Mediven www.mediuk.co.uk
Rubber gloves	Cotton-lined rubber gloves to provide a better grip on garments to assist in donning and doffing	Widely available in retail shops and also through Haddenham Healthcare www.hadhealth.com
Sleeve on	A metal applicator with a suction pad to secure the applicator to a firm surface during the application and removal of garments	Haddenham Healthcare www.hadhealth.com
Slide On Stocking (SOS)	Metal frame designed to hold the garment in place so that the foot can slide into it	Sigvaris www.sigvaris.com

Procedure guideline 9.24 Elastic compression garments: application to the leg

Essential equipment

- Appropriate application aids if required (see Table 9.11)
- A compression garment which is appropriate for the patient's lymphoedema

Preprocedure

Action	Rationale
1 Explain and discuss the procedure with the patient.	To ensure that the patient understands the procedure and gives their valid consent (NMC 2008a, C).
2 If possible, position the patient seated upright on a bed or couch and raise the height to a comfortable level.	To ensure the comfort of both the patient and nurse.

Procedure

3 Turn the stocking inside-out to the heel.	This makes it easier to ease the stocking up. E
4 Pull the foot of the stocking over the patient's foot.	
5 Turn the rest of the stocking back over the foot and up the leg.	To prevent a tourniquet effect developing at the ankle and to enable the stocking to be eased up the leg. E
6 Ask the patient to keep the leg straight and if possible to push against the nurse.	To ensure that a good grip can be gained on the stocking. E

7 Starting at the foot, gradually ease the stocking into place over the heel and up the leg a bit at a time, until it is in its final position.	Since it is the material of the stocking that provides the pressure, it must be distributed evenly to ensure an even distribution of pressure (Juzo 2006, C).
8 Do not pull from the top.	This will cause the stocking top to become overstretched and will lead to an uneven distribution of the stocking material (Juzo 2006, C).
9 Once the stocking is in place, check that there are no creases or wrinkles, particularly around the joints.	Wrinkles cause chafing of the skin and constricting bands of pressure. E

Postprocedure

10 Check that the patient finds the stocking comfortable and ask that any feelings of pain, tingling or numbness be reported. Check the toes for any visible signs of altered circulation.	Pain, tingling or numbness indicates that the stocking has been either inappropriately applied or fitted. E
11 To remove the stocking, peel it off the limb from the top downwards. Do not roll it down.	Rolling the stocking can result in tight bands of material forming, which are difficult to move. E
12 Document the manufacturer, style and size of garment that the patient has been provided with.	To maintain accurate records (NMC 2009).

521

Procedure guideline 9.25 Elastic compression garments: application to the arm

Essential equipment

- Appropriate application aids if required (see Table 9.11)
- A compression garment which is appropriate for the patient's lymphoedema

Preprocedure

Action

1 Explain and discuss the procedure with the patient.

Rationale

To ensure that the patient understands the procedure and gives their valid consent (NMC 2008a, C).

2 The patient may be seated or standing.

Procedure

3 Turn the sleeve inside-out to the wrist. Pull over the patient's hand. *Note*: if a glove or separate handpiece is worn, always put the sleeve on *after* the glove or handpiece.	To avoid increasing swelling in the hand. E
4 Turn the rest of the sleeve back over the hand and up the arm.	To prevent a tourniquet effect developing at the wrist and to enable the sleeve to be eased up the arm. E
5 Ask the patient to grip something stable, such as a towel rail or the back of a chair.	This steadies the arm and gives the patient something to pull against. E
6 Working from the hand or wrist, gradually ease the sleeve up the arm.	Since it is the material that provides the pressure, it must be evenly distributed to ensure an even distribution of pressure. C
7 Do not pull up from the top.	To prevent the top becoming overstretched which will result in an uneven distribution of pressure. C
8 Once the sleeve is in place, check that there are no creases or wrinkles, particularly around the joints.	Wrinkles and creases cause chafing of the skin and constricting bands of pressure. E

(Continued)

Procedure guideline 9.25 (*Continued*)

Postprocedure

9	Check that the patient finds the sleeve comfortable and ask that any signs of pain, tingling or numbness be reported. Check the fingers for any visible signs of altered circulation.	Pain, tingling or numbness indicate that the sleeve has been either inappropriately applied or fitted. E
10	To remove the sleeve, peel it off the limb from the top. Do not roll it down.	Rolling the sleeve down can lead to tight bands of material forming which are difficult to move. E
11	Document the manufacturer, style and size of garment that the patient has been provided with.	To maintain accurate records (NMC 2009).

Problem-solving table 9.8 Prevention and resolution (Procedure guidelines 9.24 and 9.25)

Problem	Cause	Prevention	Action
Wrinkling of the garment along the length of the limb	Poor application and positioning of the garment	Supply written instructions with diagrams/pictures concerning the application and removal of the garment	Demonstrate application and removal of the garment and observe the patient's technique when the garment is provided. The use of donning aids may be required
Slippage of garment during wear	Poorly fitting garment	Ensure the correct measurements are taken to guide the therapist in the selection of the correctly sized garment	Review size of garment. Consider the use of a grip top or skin glue to minimize slippage at the top of the garment
Change of sensation in the limb during wear of the garment	Garment too tight	Ensure the correct measurements are taken to guide the therapist in the selection of the correctly sized garment	Assess for other possible reasons for a change in sensation, e.g. musculoskeletal or circulatory impairment Review the size of garment and consider alternative garments
Skin sensitivity or reaction when wearing compression garment	Possible allergic reaction to the material of the garment	Check the patient's allergy status prior to fitting a garment	Treat any allergy appropriately. Remove the garment until skin reaction clears. A cotton Tubifast lining can be worn underneath the garment to protect the skin. An alternative garment may be required
Poor compliance with use of the garment	Limited information given to patient with regard to the importance of wearing garment. Lifestyle commitments	Ensure the patient is given sufficient information to become compliant with treatment	Explore the problems the patient is experiencing. Explain the purpose of the garments thoroughly and the intended benefits
Swelling extending beyond the edge of the garment: fingers or toes, upper thigh or upper arm	Inappropriate style of garment for the patient's needs	Thorough assessment to establish the history and extent of swelling	If fingers or toes are swollen use a compression glove or toe caps. If upper thigh or upper arm is swollen, garment must extend into the adjacent truncal quadrant

Postprocedural considerations

Immediate care

Evaluate the overall fit of the garment. There should be an even pressure throughout the garment, with no areas of loose-fitting material. The garment should be comfortable so that the patient can use their limb without restriction.

Ongoing care

The shape and size of the limb may change due to an increase in swelling. This can cause the garment to become ill fitting and cause trauma or damage to the skin. Compression garments should be checked regularly to ensure they remain appropriate in size, style and fit.

Education of patient and relevant others

- Ensure the patient knows for how long the garment needs to be worn each day. As each patient is different, the therapist should advise appropriately. Ideally garments should be worn during waking hours and removed at night (Jenns 2000).
- Advise the patient on the care of the garment. The garment should be washed after every wear at 40°C. Hand washing is also acceptable. A biological detergent can be used but fabric softener should be avoided. The garment should be air dried and not tumble dried.
- Advise the patient about how to acquire replacement or additional garments. These can either be supplied by the clinic or, if available, obtained on drug tariff from the patient's doctor. It is advisable that the garments are replaced every 6 months.

Websites

British Lymphology Society: www.thebls.com
Lymphoedema Support Network:
www.lymphoedema.org/lsn
Lymphoedema Association of Australia:
www.lymphoedema.org.au
Lymphedema People: www.lymphedemapeople.com
National Lymphoedema Network: www.lymphnet.org

References

Abidia, R.F. (2007) Oral care in the intensive care unit: a review. *Journal of Contemporary Dental Practice*, **8** (1), 1–8.

Ahmedzai, S. and Brooks, D. (1997) Transdermal fentanyl versus sustained-release oral morphine in cancer pain: preference, efficacy, and quality of life. The TTS-Fentanyl Comparative Trial Group. *Journal of Pain and Symptom Management*, **13** (5), 254–261.

Aisa, Y., Mori, T., Kudo, M. *et al.* (2005) Oral cryotherapy for the prevention of high-dose melphalan-induced stomatitis in allogeneic hematopoietic stem cell transplant recipients. *Supportive Care in Cancer*, **13**, 266–269.

Akin, M.D., Weingand, K.W., Hengehold, D.A., Goodale, M.B., Hinkle, R.T. and Smith, R.P. (2001) Continuous low-level topical heat in the treatment of dysmenorrhea. *Obstetrics and Gynecology*, **97** (3), 343–349.

Alexander, M., Fawcett, J. and Runciman, P. (2007) *Nursing Practice: Hospital and Home*, 3rd edn. Churchill Livingstone, London.

Anderson, K.O. and Cleeland, C.S. (2003) The assessment of cancer pain, in *Cancer Pain: Assessment and Management* (eds E. Bruera and R.K. Portenoy). Cambridge University Press, Cambridge, pp.51–66.

Ashurst, S. (1997) Nursing care of the mechanically ventilated patient in ITU: 1. *British Journal of Nursing*, **6** (8), 447–454.

Aslem, M., Tierney, S. and Grace, P. (1996) Swollen leg or just big? *European Journal of Lymphology*, **6** (Suppl), 21.

Asmussen, P. and Strossenreuther, R. (2003) Compression therapy, in *Textbook of Lymphology for Physicians and Lymphoedema Therapists* (eds. M. Foldi, E. Foldi and S. Kubik). Urban Fischer, Munich, Germany, pp. 527–588.

Audit Commission for Local Authorities and the National Health Service in England and Wales (1997) *Anaesthesia Under Examination: The Efficiency and Effectiveness of Anaesthesia and Pain Relief Services in England and Wales*. Audit Commission Publications, Abingdon.

Aung, T. and Mulley, G.P. (2002) Removal of ear wax. *BMJ*, **325** (7354), 27.

Axelsson, G., Ahlborg Jr, G. and Bodin, L. (1996) Shift work, nitrous oxide exposure, and spontaneous abortion among Swedish midwives. *Occupational and Environmental Medicine*, **53** (6), 374–378.

Badger, C. (1993) Guidelines for the calculation of limb volume based on surface measurements. *British Lymphology Interest Group Newsletter*, Issue 7, Sir Michael Sobell House, Oxford.

Badger, C., Peacock, J. and Mortimer, P. (2000) A randomised, controlled parallel-group clinical trial comparing multilayer bandaging followed by hosiery versus hosiery alone in the treatment of patients with lymphoedema of the limb. *Cancer*, **88** (12), 2832–2837.

Baker, L., Lee, M., Regnard, C., Crack, L. and Callin, S. (2004) Evolving spinal analgesia practice in palliative care. *Palliative Medicine*, **18** (6), 507–515.

Ballantyne, J.C. and Carwood, C.M. (2005) Comparative efficacy of epidural, subarachnoid, and intracerebroventricular opioids in patients with pain due to cancer. *Cochrane Database of Systematic Reviews*, 1, CD005178.

Ballard, K. (1997) Pressure-relief mattresses and patient comfort. *Professional Nurse*, **13** (1), 27–32.

Bamigbade, T.A. and Langford, R.M. (1998) Tramadol hydrochloride: an overview of current use. *Hospital Medicine*, **59** (5), 373–376.

Bannon, L., Alexander-Williams, M. and Lutman, D. (2001) A national survey of epidural practice. *Anaesthesia*, **56** (10), 1021.

Barasch, A., Elad, S., Altman, A. *et al.* (2006) Antimicrobials, mucosal coating agents, anesthetics, analgesics, and nutritional supplements for alimentary tract mucositis. *Supportive Care in Cancer*, **14**, 528–532.

Barillo, D.J., Coffey, E.C., Shirani, K.Z. and Goodwin, C.W. (2000) Burns caused by medical therapy. *Journal of Burn Care and Rehabilitation*, **21** (3), 269–273.

Beck, S. (1991) The therapeutic use of music for cancer-related pain. *Oncology Nursing Forum*, **18** (8), 1327–1337.

Beck, S. (2004) Mucositis, in *Cancer Symptom Management Third Edition* (eds C.H. Yarbro, M.H. Frogge and M. Goodman). Jones and Bartlett, Sudbury, MA, pp. 276–292.

Becket, G., Galandi, D. and Blum, H.E. (2006) Malignant ascites: systematic review and guideline for treatment. *European Journal of Cancer*, **42**, 589–597.

Behar, J.M., Gogalniceanu, P. and Bromley, L. (2007) Anaesthesia: regional anaesthesia. *Student BMJ*, **15**, 186–189.

Bennett, M. (2001) The LANSS Pain Scale: the Leeds assessment of neuropathic symptoms and signs. *Pain*, **92** (1-2), 147–157.

Berchier, C.E., Slot, D.E., Haps, S. and van der Weijden, G.A. (2008) The efficacy of dental floss in addition to a toothbrush on plaque and parameters of gingival inflammation: a systematic review. *International Journal of Dental Hygiene*, **6**, 265–279.

Bernas, M., Witte, M. and Witte, C. (1996) Limb volume measurements in lymphoedema. *Lymphology*, **29** (Suppl), 199–202.

Berry, A.M., Davidson, P.M., Masters, J. and Rolls, K. (2007) Systematic literature review of oral hygiene practices for intensive care patients receiving mechanical ventilation. *American Journal of Critical Care*, **16** (6), 552–562.

BMA/Royal Pharmaceutical Society of Great Britain (2008) *British National Formulary*. Pharmaceutical Press, Oxford.

BNF (2011) *British National Formulary*. BMJ Group and RPS Publishing, London.

BOC (1995) *BOC Gases Data Sheet: Entonox*. BOC Group, Manchester.

BOC (1998) *Entonox: The Non-Invasive Patient Controlled Analgesia: Suggested Protocol Document*. BOC Group, Manchester.

BOC (2000) *Entonox: Controlled Pain Relief Reference Guide*. BOC Medical, Manchester.

BOC (2001) *Entonox: Controlled Pain Relief*. BOC Medical, Manchester.

BOC (2009) *Summary of Product Characteristics*. *Entonox*. BOC Ltd, Guildford, Surrey.

Boland, R. and Adams, R. (1998) The effects of arm elevation and overnight head-up tilt on forearms and hand volume. *Journal of Hand Therapy*, **11**, 180–90.

Bourne, N. (2008) Managing acute pain in opioid tolerant patients. *Journal of Perioperative Practice*, **18** (11), 498–503.

Bouza, C., Saz, Z., Munoz, A. and Amate, J.M. (2005) Efficacy of advanced dressings in the treatment of pressure ulcers: a systematic review. *Journal of Wound Care*, **14** (5), 193–199.

Boyd-Monk, H. (2005) Bringing common EYE emergencies into focus. *Nursing*, **35** (12), 46–51.

British Lymphology Society (2001) *Guidelines for the Use of Manual Lymphatic Drainage and Simple Lymphatic Drainage in Lymphoedema*. British Lymphology Society, Cheltenham.

British Pain Society (2008) *FAQ's*. British Pain Society, London. www.britishpainsociety.org/media_faq.htm.

British Pain Society and Royal College of Physicians (2004) *A Practical Guide to the Provision of Chronic Pain Services for Adults in Primary Care*. British Pain Society and Royal College of Physicians, London.

Brown, D.L. (1999) *Atlas of Regional Anesthesia*, 2nd edn. Saunders, Philadelphia.

Browse, N. (2003) Aetiology and classifications of lymphoedema, in *Diseases of the Lymphatics* (eds N. Browse, K. Burn and P. Mortimer). Arnold Publishers, London, pp. 151–156.

Bruce, E. and Franck, L. (2000) Self-administered nitrous oxide (ENTONOX) for the management of procedural pain. *Paediatric Nursing*, **12** (7), 15–20.

Budd, K. (2002) *Evidence-based Medicine in Practice. Bupranorphine: A Review*. Haywood Medical, Newmarket.

Burns, S.M., Cowa, C.M., Barclay, P.M. and Wilkes, R.G. (2001) Intrapartum epidural catheter migration: a comparative study of three dressing applications. *British Journal of Anaesthesia*, **86** (4), 565–567.

Burr, S. and Penzer, R. (2005) Promoting skin health. *Nursing Standard*, **19** (36), 57–65.

Byers, P.H., Ryan, P.A., Regan, M. B., Shields, A. and Carta, S.G. (1995) Effects of incontinence care cleansing regimens on skin integrity. *Journal of Wound, Ostomy, and Continence Nursing*, **22** (4), 187–192.

Campbell, A.V. (1984) Nursing, nurturing and sexism, in *Moderated Love: A Theology of Professional Care*. Society for Promoting Christain Knowledge, London, pp.34–51.

Campbell, C. (2001) Controlling malignant ascites. *European Journal of Palliative Care*, **8** (5), 187–90.

Carr, E. (2007) Barriers to effective pain management. *Journal of Perioperative Practice*, **17** (5), 200–203, 206–208.

Carr, E. and Mann, E.M. (2000) Recognising the barriers to effective pain relief, in *Pain: Creative Approaches to Effective Management*. Palgrave Macmillan, Basingstoke, pp.109–129.

Carr-Hill, R., Dixon, P., Gibbs, I. *et al.* (1992) *Skill Mix and the Effectiveness of Nursing Care*. University of York, Centre for Health Economics, York.

Carroll, D. and Bowsher, D. (1993) *Pain: Management and Nursing Care*. Butterworth-Heinemann, Oxford.

Carroll, D. and Seers, K. (1998) Relaxation for the relief of chronic pain: a systematic review. *Journal of Advanced Nursing*, **27** (3), 476–487.

Chalmers, J. and Pearson, A. (2005) Oral hygiene care for residents with dementia: a literature review. *Journal of Advanced Nursing*, **52** (4), 410–419.

Chapman, S. and Day, R. (2001) Spinal anatomy and the use of epidurals. *Professional Nurse*, **16** (6), 1174–1177.

Chilvers, R.J. and Weisz, M. (2000) Entonox equipment as a potential source of cross-infection. *Anaesthesia*, **55** (2), 176–179.

Chumbley, G.M., Hall, G.M. and Salmon, P. (2002) Patient-controlled analgesia: what information does the patient want? *Journal of Advanced Nursing*, **39** (5), 459–471.

Clark, M. (2003) Compression bandages: principles and definitions, in *EWMA Position Statement: Understanding Compression Therapy* (eds S. Caine, C. Moffatt and S. Thomas). Medical Education Partnership, pp.5–7.

Clark, M. and Krimmel, G. (2006) Lymphoedema and the construction and classification of compression hosiery, in *Lymphoedema Framework: Template for Practice Compression Hosiery in Lymphoedema*. Medical Educational Partnership, London, pp. 2–4.

Clarkson, J.E., Worthington, H.V. and Eden, T.O.B. (2007a) Interventions for treating oral mucositis for patients with cancer receiving treatment. *Cochrane Database of Systematic Reviews*, 2, CD001973.

Clarkson, J.E., Worthington, H.V. and Eden, T.O.B. (2007b) Interventions for preventing oral candidiasis for patients with cancer receiving treatment. *Cochrane Database of Systematic Reviews*, 1, CD003807.

Clay, M. (2000) Oral health in older people. *Nursing Older People*, **12** (7), 21–26.

Cleeland, C.S. (1991) *The Brief Pain Inventory*. www.mdanderson.org/education-and-research/departments-programs-and-labs/departments-and-divisions/symptom-research/symptom-assessment-tools/BPI_UserGuide.pdf.

Colleau, S.M. (1999) The significance of breakthrough pain in cancer. *Cancer Pain Release*, **12** (4), 1–4.

Collins, F. and Hampton, S. (2003) The cost-effective use of Bag-Bath: a new concept in patient hygiene. *British Journal of Nursing*, **12** (16), 984, 986–990.

Coniam, S.W. and Mendham, J. (2005) Management of acute pain: principles and practice, in *Principles of Pain Management for Anaesthetists*. Hodder Arnold, London, pp.74–75.

Consroe, P., Musty, R., Rein, J., Tillery, W. and Pertwee, R. (1997) The perceived effects of smoked cannabis on patients with multiple sclerosis. *European Neurology*, **38** (1), 44–48.

Cook, T.M., Eaton, J.M. and Goodwin, A.P. (1997) Epidural analgesia following upper abdominal surgery: United Kingdom practice. *Acta Anaesthesiologica Scandinavica*, **41** (1 Pt 1), 18–24.

Cooley, C. (2002) Oral health: basic or essential care? *Cancer Nursing Practice*, **1** (3), 33–39.

Cooper, C. (1994) Hygiene and the client, in *Knowledge to Care* (eds C.A. McMahon and J.Harding). Blackwell Scientific, Oxford.

Cope, D. (2005) Malignant effusions and edema, in *Cancer Nursing Principles and Practice*, 6th edn (eds C. Yarbro, M. Frogge and M. Goodman). Jones and Bartlett, Sudbury, MA, pp. 826–840.

Courtney, A., Nemcerk, A., Rosenberg, S. *et al.* (2008) Prospective evaluation of the PleurX catheter when used to treat recurrent ascites associated with malignancy. *Journal of Vascular and Interventional Radiology*, **19**, 1723–1731.

Cousins, K., Duggan, G., Panizza, N., Tinnelly, K., Vojkovic, S. and White, K. (2003) Intrathecal catheters: developing consistency in filter use and dressings in Perth, Australia. *International Journal of Palliative Nursing*, **9** (7), 308–314.

CREST (2008) *Guidelines for the Diagnosis, Assessment and Management of Lymphoedema*, Northern Ireland Lymphoedema Network, Belfast. www.crestni.org.uk.

Cunningham, C. and Gould, D. (1998) Eyecare for the sedated patient undergoing mechanical ventilation: the use of evidence-based care. *International Journal of Nursing Studies*, **35** (1-2), 32–40.

Curatolo, M., Petersen-Felix, S., Scaramozzino, P. and Zbinden, A.M. (1998) Epidural fentanyl, adrenaline and clonidine as adjuvants to local anaesthetics for surgical analgesia: meta-analyses of analgesia and side-effects. *Acta Anaesthesiologica Scandinavica*, **42** (8), 910–920.

Cutler, C.J. and Davis, N. (2005) Improving oral care in patients receiving mechanical ventilation. *American Journal of Critical Care*, **14**, 389–394.

Dahlin, C. (2004) Oral complications at the end of life. *American Journal of Nursing*, **104** (7), 40–47.

Damstra, R., Brouwer, E. and Partsch, H. (2008) Controlled, comparative study of relation between volume changes and interface pressure under short-stretch bandages in leg lymphoedema patients. *Dermatologic Surgery*, **34** (6), 773–779.

Darwish, M., Kirby, M. and Giang, J.D. (2007) Effect of buccal dwell time on the pharmacokinetic profile of fentanyl buccal tablet. *Expert Opinion in Pharmacotherapy*, **8**, 2011–2016.

Davies, A. (2000) A comparison of artificial saliva and chewing gum in the management of xerostomia in patients with advanced cancer. *Palliative Medicine*, **14**, 197–203.

Davies, A. (2005a) Oral assessment, in *Oral Care in Advanced Disease* (eds A. Davies and I. Finlay). Oxford University Press, Oxford, pp. 7–19.

Davies, A. (2005b) Salivary gland dysfunction, in *Oral Care in Advanced Disease* (eds A. Davies and I. Finlay). Oxford University Press, Oxford, pp. 97–113.

Davies, A. (2006) *Cancer-Related Breakthrough Pain*. Oxford University Press, Oxford.

Davis, M.P., Glare, P. and Hardy, J. (2005) *Opioids in Cancer Pain*. Oxford University Press, Oxford.

Davis, B.D. and McVicker, A. (2000) Issues in effective pain control: from assessment to management. *International Journal of Palliative Nursing*, **6** (4), 162–169.

Day, R. (2001) The use of epidural and intrathecal analgesia in palliative care. *International Journal of Palliative Care*, **7** (8), 369–374.

De Cicco, M., Matovic, M., Castellani, G.T. *et al.* (1995) Time-dependent efficacy of bacterial filters and infection risk in long-term epidural catheterization. *Anesthesiology*, **82** (3), 765–771.

DH (2001) *The Essence of Care: Patient Focussed Benchmarking for Healthcare Professionals*. HMSO, London.

DH (2005) *Choosing Better Oral Health: An Oral Health Plan for England*. Department of Health, London.

DH (2006) About dignity in care. www.dh.gov.uk/PolicyAndGuidance/HealthAndSocialCareTopics/SocialCare/DignityInCare/DignityInCare–Article.

Dickinson, L. and Porter, H. (2006) Oral care, in *Nursing in Haematological Oncology*, 2nd edn (ed. M. Grundy). Baillière Tindall, Philadelphia, pp. 371–385.

Dickman, A., Littlewood, C. and Varga, J. (2002) Drug information, in *The Syringe Driver: Continuous Subcutaneous Infusions in Palliative Care* (eds A. Dickman, C. Littlewood and J. Varga). Oxford University Press, Oxford, pp.11–58.

Dickson, D. (2004) Risks and benefits of long-term intrathecal analgesia. *Anaesthesia*, **59** (7), 633–635.

Doherty, D., Morgan, P. and Moffatt, C. (2006) Role of hosiery in lower limb lymphoedema, in *Lymphoedema Framework; Template for Practice: Compression Hosiery in Lymphoedema*. Medical Educational Partnership, London, pp. 10–21.

Disorbio JM, Bruns D, Barolat G (2006) Assessment and treatment of chronic pain. A physicians guide to a biopsychosocial approach. *Practical PAIN MANAGEMENT March 2006*. accessed 17.9.10 www.healthpsych.com/articles/biopsychosocial_tx.pdf

Donnelly, S. and Walsh, D. (1995) The symptoms of advanced cancer. *Seminars in Oncology*, **22** (2 Suppl 3), 67–72.

Doyle, S. and Dalton, C. (2008) Developing clinical guidelines on promoting oral health: an action research approach. *Learning Disability Practice*, **11** (2), 12–15.

Drayer, R.A., Henderson, J. and Reidenberg, M. (1999) Barriers to better pain control in hospitalized patients. *Journal of Pain and Symptom Management*, **17** (6), 434–440.

Duffin, C. (2008) Brushing up on oral hygiene. *Nursing Older People*, **20** (2), 14–16.

Du Pen, A. (2005) Care and management of intrathecal and epidural catheters. *Journal of Infusion Nursing*, **28** (6), 377–381.

Eagle, M. (2001) Compression bandaging. *Nursing Standard*, **15** (38), 47–52.

Eilers, J. and Million, R. (2007) Prevention and management of oral mucositis in patients with cancer. *Seminars in Oncology Nursing*, **23** (3), 201–212.

Eilers, J., Berger, A.M. and Petersen, M.C. (1988) Development, testing, and application of the oral assessment guide. *Oncology Nursing Forum*, **15** (3), 325–330.

Ellershaw, J. (1998) Hydromorphone: a new alternative to morphine. *Prescriber*, **9** (4), 21–27.

Engler, H. and Sweat, R. (1962) Volumetric arm measurements: techniques and results. *American Surgeon*, **28**, 465–468.

Ersser, S.J., Getliffe, K., Voegeli, D. and Regan, S. (2005) A critical review of the inter-relationship between skin vulnerability and urinary incontinence and related nursing intervention. *International Journal of Nursing Studies*, **42** (7), 823–835.

Ezzo, J., Berman, B., Hadhazy, V.A. *et al.* (2000) Is acupuncture effective for the treatment of chronic pain? A systematic review. *Pain*, **86** (3), 217–225.

Faddy, S.C. and Garlick, S.R. (2005) A systematic review of the safety of analgesia with 50% nitrous oxide: can lay responders use analgesic gases in the prehospital setting? *Emergency Medicine Journal*, **22** (12), 901–906.

Fang, F., Guo, T.Z., Davies, M.F. and Maze, M. (1997) Opiate receptors in the periaqueductal gray mediate analgesic effect of nitrous oxide in rats. *European Journal of Pharmacology*, **336** (2-3), 137–141.

Farrell, A. and Rich, A. (2000) Analgesic use in patients with renal failure. *European Journal of Palliative Care*, **7** (6), 201–205.

525

Feben, K. (2003) How effective is training in compression bandaging technique? *British Journal of Community Nursing*, 8 (2), 80–84.

Feine, J.S. and Lund, J.P. (1997) An assessment of the efficacy of physical therapy and physical modalities for the control of chronic musculoskeletal pain. *Pain*, 71 (1), 5–23.

Fentiman, I. (2002) Serous effusions, in *Oxford Textbook of Oncology*, 2nd edn. (eds R.L. Souhami, I. Tannock, P. Hohenberger and J.C. Horiot). Oxford University Press, Oxford, pp. 887–895.

Finlay, I. and Davies, A. (2005) Fungal infections, in *Oral Care in Advanced Disease* (eds A. Davies and I. Finlay). Oxford University Press, Oxford, pp. 55–71.

Fitzpatrick, J. (2000) Oral health needs of dependent older people: responsibilities of nurses and care staff. *Journal of Advanced Nursing*, 32 (6), 1325–1332.

Fitzpatrick, R., Davey, C., Buxton, M.J. and Jones, D.R. (1998) Evaluating patient-based outcome measures for use in clinical trials. *Health Technology Assessment*, 2 (14), i–iv, 1–74. www.hta.ac.uk/execsumm/summ214.shtml.

Flaherty, S.A. (1996) Pain measurement tools for clinical practice and research. *AANA Journal*, 64 (2), 133–140.

Foldi, M., Foldi, E. and Kubik, S. (2003) Compression therapy, in *Textbook of Lymphology for Physicians and Lymphoedema Therapists* (eds M. Foldi, E. Foldi and S. Kubik). Urban Fischer, Munich, Germany, pp. 567–587.

Foldi, E., Junger, M. and Partsch, H. (2005) The science of lymphoedema bandaging, in *European Wound Management Association (EWMA) Focus Document: Lymphoedema Bandaging in Practice*. Medical Educational Partnership, London, pp. 2–4.

Foley, K. (2004) Pain assessment and cancer pain syndromes, in *Oxford Textbook of Palliative Medicine*, 3rd edn (ed. D. Doyle). Oxford University Press, Oxford, pp. 298–316.

Forbes, G.M. and Collins, B.J. (2000) Nitrous oxide for colonoscopy: a randomized controlled study. *Gastrointestinal Endoscopy*, 51 (3), 271–278.

Forrester, J.V. (2002) *The Eye: Basic Sciences in Practice*, 2nd edn. W.B. Saunders, Edinburgh.

Fotiadis, R.J., Badvie, S., Weston, M.D. and Allen-Mersh, T.G. (2004) Epidural analgesia in gastrointestinal surgery. *British Journal of Surgery*, 91 (7), 828–41.

Fraise, A.P. and Bradley, T. (eds) (2009) *Ayliffe's Control of Healthcare-associated Infection: A Practical Handbook*, 5th edn. Hodder Arnold, London.

Friedewald, V.E., Kornman, K.S., Beck, J.D. *et al.* (2009) The American Journal of Cardiology and Journal of Periodontology editors' consensus: periodontitis and atherosclerotic cardiovascular disease. *Journal of Periodontology*, 80 (7), 1021–1032.

Gaiser, R. (2006) Postdural puncture headache. *Current Opinion in Anaesthesiology*, 19 (3), 249–253.

Gannon, C. (1997) Clinical management. The use of methadone in the care of the dying. *European Journal of Palliative Care*, 4 (5), 152–159.

Gardner-Nix, J.S. (1996) Oral methadone for managing chronic nonmalignant pain. *Journal of Pain and Symptom Management*, 11 (5), 321–328.

Geraghty, M. (2005) Nursing the unconscious patient. *Nursing Standard*, 20 (1), 54–64.

Gillman, M.A. and Lichtigfeld, F.J. (1994) Pharmacology of psychotropic analgesic nitrous oxide as a multipotent opioid agonist. *International Journal of Neuroscience*, 76 (1–2), 5–12.

Gillman, M.A. and Lichtigfeld, F.J. (1998) Clinical role and mechanisms of action of analgesic nitrous oxide. *International Journal of Neuroscience*, 93 (1–2), 55–62.

Godfrey, H. (2005) Understanding pain, part 1: physiology of pain. *British Journal of Nursing*, 14 (16), 846–852.

Gooch, J. (1989) Skin hygiene. *Professional Nurse*, 5 (1), 13–18.

Good, M. (1996) Effects of relaxation and music on postoperative pain: a review. *Journal of Advanced Nursing*, 24 (5), 905–914.

Good, M., Stanton-Hicks, M., Grass, J.A. *et al.* (1999) Relief of postoperative pain with jaw relaxation, music and their combination. *Pain*, 81 (1–2), 163–172.

Goodman, M. and Wickham, R. (2005) Endocrine malignancies, in *Cancer Nursing: Principles and Practice*, 6th edn (eds C.H. Yarbro, M. Goodman and M.H. Frogge). Jones and Bartlett, Sudbury, MA, pp. 1215–1243.

Gordon, M. (1994) *Nursing Diagnosis: Process and Application*, 3rd edn. Mosby, St Louis, MO.

Gould, D. (1994) Helping the patient with personal hygiene. *Nursing Standard*, 8 (34), 30–32.

Grap, M.J., Munro, C.L., Ashtiani, B. and Bryant, S. (2003) Oral care interventions in critical care: frequency and documentation. *American Journal of Critical Care*, 12 (2), 113–118.

Griffiths, J., Jones, V., Leeman, I. *et al.* (2000) *Oral Health Care for People with Mental Health Problems Guidelines and Recommendations*. British Society for Disability and Oral Health, Gosforth.

Grond, S., Zech, D., Diefenbach, C., Radbruch, L. and Lehmann, K.A. (1996) Assessment of cancer pain: a prospective evaluation in 2266 cancer patients referred to a pain service. *Pain*, 64 (1), 107–114.

Grond, S., Meuser, T., Stute, P. and Gohring, U.J. (2000) Epidural analgesia for labour pain: a review of availability, current practices and influence on labour. *International Journal of Acute Pain Management*, 3 (1), 31–43.

Hafner, J., Luthi, W., Holger-Hanssle, H. *et al.* (2000) Instruction of compression therapy by means of interface pressure measurement. *Dermatological Surgery*, 26, 481–487.

Hahn, M. and Jones, A. (2000) *Head and Neck Nursing*. Churchill Livingstone, London.

Haisfield-Wolfe, M.E. (1998) Providing effective perineal-rectal skin care to patients with cancer. *Oncology Nursing Forum*, 25 (3), 472.

Hall, J. (2000) Epidural analgesia management. *Nursing Times*, 96 (28), 38–40.

Hanks, G.W., Conno, F., Cherny, N. *et al.* (2001) Morphine and alternative opioids in cancer pain: the EAPC recommendations. *British Journal of Cancer*, 84 (5), 587–593.

Hanks, G., Cherny, N. and Fallon, M. (2004) Opioid analgesic therapy, in *Oxford Textbook of Palliative Medicine*, 3rd edn (ed. D. Doyle). Oxford University Press, Oxford, pp.316–342.

Harkin, H. (2005) A nurse-led ear care clinic: sharing knowledge and improving patient care. *British Journal of Nursing*, 14 (5), 250–254.

Harkin, H. (2007) Ear Care Adivce. www.entnursing.com/earcareadvice.htm.

Harkin, H. (2008) Guidance Document in Ear Care. www.earcarecentre.com/protocols.htm.

Harmer, M. and Davies, K.A. (1998) The effect of education, assessment and a standardised prescription on postoperative pain management. The value of clinical audit in the establishment of acute pain services. *Anaesthesia*, 53 (5), 424–430.

Hays, H., Hagen, N., Thirlwell, M. *et al.* (1994) Comparative clinical efficacy and safety of immediate release and controlled release hydromorphone for chronic severe cancer pain. *Cancer*, 74 (6), 1808–1816.

Hayward, J. (1975) *Information: A Prescription Against Pain*. Royal College of Nursing, London.

Hebl, J.R. (2006) The importance and implications of aseptic techniques during regional anesthesia. *Regional Anesthesia and Pain Medicine*, 31 (4), 311–323.

Hector, L.M. and Touhy, T.A. (1997) The history of the bath: from art to task? Reflections for the future. *Journal of Gerontological Nursing*, **23** (5), 7–15.

Heiser, R.M., Chiles, K., Fudge, M. and Gray, S.E. (1997) The use of music during the immediate postoperative recovery period. *AORN Journal*, **65** (4), 777–778, 781–785.

Heiskanen, T. and Kalso, E. (1997) Controlled-release oxycodone and morphine in cancer related pain. *Pain*, **73** (1), 37–45.

Henderson, V. (1966) *The Nature of Nursing; A Definition and Its Implications for Practice, Research, and Education*. Macmillan, New York.

Hewish, P. (2006) Ascites tapping. www.patient.co.uk/showdoc/40002410/.

Hicks, F. and Simpson, K.H. (2004) Regional nerve blocks, in *Nerve Blocks in Palliative Care* (eds F. Hicks and K.H. Simpson). Oxford University Press, Oxford, pp.53–55.

Higginson, I.J. (1998) Can professionals improve their assessments? *Journal of Pain and Symptom Management*, **15** (3), 149–150.

Hobbs, G.J. and Hodgkinson, V. (2003) Assessment, measurement, history and examination, in *Acute Pain* (eds D.J. Rowbotham and P.E. Macintyre). Arnold, London, pp.93–112.

Hollins, S. (2009) *Religions, Cultures and Healthcare*, 2nd edn. Radcliffe Publishing, Oxford.

Holloway, S. and Jones, V. (2005) The importance of skin care and assessment. *British Journal of Nursing*, **14** (22), 1172–1176.

Holman, C., Roberts, S. and Nicol, M. (2005) Promoting oral hygiene. *Nursing Older People*, **16** (10), 37–38.

Hopkins, A. (2008) Compression therapy for lymphoedema. *Practice Nursing*, **19** (10), 497–503.

Horlocker, T.T. and Wedel, D.J. (1998) Spinal and epidural blockade and perioperative low molecular weight heparin: smooth sailing on the Titanic. *Anesthesia and Analgesia*, **86** (6), 1153–1156.

Hosttetter, R., Marincola, F. and Schwartzentruber, D. (2005). Malignant ascites, in *Cancer Principles and Practice of Oncology*, 7th edn (eds V. Devita, S. Hellman and S. Rosenberg). Lippincott Williams and Wilkins, Philadelphia, pp. 2392–2398.

Hou, W. and Sanyal, A.J. (2009) Ascites: diagnosis and management. *Medical Clinics of North America*, **93** (4), 801–817.

Huskinson, W. and Lloyd, H. (2009) Oral health in hospitalised patients: assessment and hygiene. *Nursing Standard*, **23** (36), 43–47.

Husseini, A., Slot, D.E. and van der Weijden, G.A. (2008) The efficacy of oral irrigation in addition to a toothbrush on plaque and the clinical parameters of periodontal inflammation: a review. *International Journal of Dental Hygiene*, **6**, 304–314.

Idvall, E., Hamrin, E., Sjostrom, B. and Unosson, M. (2002) Patient and nurse assessment of quality of care in postoperative pain management. *Quality and Safety in Health Care*, **11** (4), 327–334.

IASP (1994) IASP pain terminology. www.iasp-pain.org/terms.

IASP (1996) Classification of chronic pain. *Pain*, **3** (Suppl), 51–226.

International Society of Lymphology (2003) The diagnosis and treatment of peripheral lymphoedema. *Consensus Document of the International Society of Lymphology*, **36** (2), 84–91.

Jenns, K. (2000) Management strategies, in *Lymphoedema* (eds R. Twycross, K. Jenns and J. Todd). Radcliffe Medical Press, Oxford, pp. 97–117.

Jevtovic-Todorovic, V., Todorovic, S.M. and Mennerick, S. (1998) Nitrous oxide (laughing gas) is an NMDA antagonist, neuroprotectant and neurotoxin. *Nature Medicine*, **4**, 460–463.

Jones, C.V. (1998) The importance of oral hygiene in nutritional support. *British Journal of Nursing*, **7** (2), 74–83.

Juzo (2006) *Application of Compression Stockings*. Juzo UK, Dundee, Scotland.

Kalkman, C.J., Visser, K., Moen, J. *et al.* (2003) Preoperative prediction of severe postoperative pain. *Pain*, **105** (3), 415–423.

Kayser-Jones, J., Bird, W.F., Paul, S.M. *et al.* (1995) An instrument to assess the oral health status of nursing home residents. *Gerontologist*, **35** (6), 814–824.

Keefe, D.M., Schubert, M.M., Elting, L.S. *et al.* (2007) Updated clinical practice guidelines for the prevention and treatment of mucositis. *Cancer*, **109** (5), 820–831.

Keeley, V. (2000) Clasification of lymphoedema, in *Lymphoedema* (eds R. Twycross, K. Jenns and J. Todd). Radcliffe Medical Press, Oxford, pp. 22–43.

Kehlet, H. (1997) Multimodal approach to control postoperative pathophysiology and rehabilitation. *British Journal of Anaesthesia*, **78** (5), 606–617.

Kehlet, H. and Holte, K. (2001) Effect of postoperative analgesia on surgical outcome. *British Journal of Anaesthesia*, **87** (1), 62–72.

Kettle, J., Rundle, F. and Oddie, T. (1958) Measurement of upper limb volumes: a clinical method. *Australia and New Zealand Journal of Surgery*, **27**, 263–70.

King, A. (1999) *King's Guide to TENS for Health Professionals: A Health Professionals' Guide to Transcutaneous Electrical Nerve Stimulation for the Treatment of Pain*. www.alanking.net/books.html.

Kinirons, B., Mimoz, O., Lafendi, L., Naas, T., Meunier, J. and Nordmann, P. (2001) Chlorhexidine versus povidone iodine in preventing colonization of continuous epidural catheters in children: a randomized, controlled trial. *Anesthesiology*, **94** (2), 239–244.

Kinmouth, J. (1982) *The Lymphatics*, 2nd edn. Arnold, London.

Kitson, A. (1994) Post-operative pain management: a literature review. *Journal of Clinical Nursing*, **3** (1), 7–18.

Kitson, A. (1999) The essence of nursing. *Nursing Standard*, **13** (23), 42–46.

Klee, M. (2004) Symptom control info. www.symptomcontrol.com/88.0.html.

Klepstad, P., Kaasa, S., Cherny, N., Hanks, G. and de Conno, F. (2005) Pain and pain treatments in European palliative care units. A cross sectional survey from the European Association for Palliative Care Research Network. *Palliative Medicine*, **19** (6), 477–484.

Kouraklis, G. (2002) Post-operative drainage in patients with malignant ascites: a safe method. *Journal of Surgical Oncology*, **79**, 124–125.

Kraszewski, S. (2008) Safe and effective ear irrigation. *Nursing Standard*, **22** (43), 45–48.

Krishnasamy, M. (2008) Pain, in *Cancer Nursing: Care in Context*, 2nd edn (eds J. Corner and C.D. Bailey). Blackwell, Oxford, pp.449–461.

Kuckelkorn, R., Schrage, N., Keller, G. and Redbrake, C. (2002) Emergency treatment of chemical and thermal eye burns. *Acta Ophthalmologica Scandinavica*, **80** (1), 4–10.

Lang, E.V., Benotsch, E.G., Fick, L.J. *et al.* (2000) Adjunctive non-pharmacological analgesia for invasive medical procedures: a randomised trial. *Lancet*, **355** (9214), 1486–1490.

Langevin, P.B., Gravenstein, N., Langevin, S.O. and Gulig, P.A. (1996) Epidural catheter reconnection: safe and unsafe practice. *Anesthesiology*, **85** (4), 883–888.

Lawler, K. (1997) Pain assessment. *Professional Nurse*, **13** (1 Suppl), S5–8.

Lawler, K. and Anderson, T. (2002) Regional trial of five epidural fixation products and a commonly used control. *Pain Network Newsletter*, **Spring**, 6–8.

Lee, A. (2006) The angle and aqueous, in *Ophthalmic Care* (ed. J. Marsden). Wiley, Chichester, pp. 420–460.

Lee, A., Lau, T.N. and Yeong, K.Y. (2000) Indwelling catheters for the management of malignant ascites. *Supportive Care in Cancer*, **8** (6), 493–499.

527

Lee, L. and Grap, M.J. (2008) Care and management of the patient with ascites. *Medsurg Nursing*, **17** (6), 376–381.

Lewis, N.L. and Williams, J.E. (2005) Acute pain management in patients receiving opioids for chronic and cancer pain. *Contining Education in Anaesthesia and Critical Care Pain*, **5** (4), 127–129.

Li, X., Kolltveit, K.M., Tronstad, L. and Olsen, I. (2000) Systemic disease caused by oral infection. *Clinical Microbiology Reviews*, **13** (4), 547–558.

Lindell, M.E. and Olsson, H.M. (1989) Lack of care givers' knowledge causes unnecessary suffering in elderly patients. *Journal of Advanced Nursing*, **14** (11), 976–979.

Ling, J. (1997) The use of transdermal fentanyl in palliative care. *International Journal of Palliative Nursing*, **3**(2), 65–68.

Linnitt, N. and Davies, R. (2007) Fundamentals of compression in the management of lymphoedema. *British Journal of Nursing*, **16** (10), 588–592.

Lockhart, J.S. and Resick, L.K. (2006) Anatomy and physiology, in *Head and Neck Cancer* (eds L.K. Clarke and M.J. Dropkin). Oncology Nursing Society, Pittsburgh, PA.

Lokich, J.J. and Moore, C. (1984) Chemotherapy-associated palmar-plantar erythrodysesthesia syndrome. *Annals of Internal Medicine*, **101** (6), 798–799.

Loveman, E. and Gale, A. (2000) Factors influencing nurses' inferences about patient pain. *British Journal of Nursing*, **9** (6), 334–337.

Lymphoedema Framework (2006a) Compression garments, in *Best Practice for the Management of Lymphoedema, International Consensus*. Medical Educational Partnership, London, pp. 39–46.

Lymphoedema Framework (2006b) Skin care and cellulitis/erysipelas, in *Best Practice for the Management of Lymphoedema, International Consensus*. Medical Educational Partnership, London, pp. 24–28.

Lymphoedema Framework (2006c) Introduction, in *Best Practice for the Management of Lymphoedema*, International Consensus. Medical Educational Partnership (MEP) Ltd, London, pp. 1–2.

Lymphoedema Framework (2006d) Assessment, in *Best Practice for the Management of Lymphoedema, International Consensus*. Medical Educational Partnership, London, pp. 6–14.

Lymphoedema Framework (2006e) Multi-layer inelastic lymphoedema bandaging, in *Best Practice for the Management of Lymphoedema, International Consensus*. Medical Educational Partnership, London, pp. 32–38.

Macintyre, P.E. (2001) Safety and efficacy of patient-controlled analgesia. *British Journal of Anaesthesia*, **87** (1), 36–46.

Macintyre, P.E. and Jarvis, D.A. (1996) Age is the best predictor of postoperative morphine requirements. *Pain*, **64** (2), 357–364.

Macintyre, P.E. and Schug, S.A. (2007) *Acute Pain Management: A Practical Guide*. Elsevier Saunders, Edinburgh.

Macintyre, P.E., Schug, S.A., Scott, D.A. *et al.*, for the Working Group of the Australian and New Zealand College of Anaesthetists and Faculty of Pain Medicine (2010) *Acute Pain Management: Scientific Evidence*, 3rd edn. ANZCA and FPM, Melbourne.

Maher, K. (2004) Xerostomia, in *Cancer Symptom Management*, 3rd edn (eds C.H. Yarbro, M.H. Frogge and M. Goodman). Jones and Bartlett, Sudbury, MA.

Malkin, B. (2009) The important of patients' oral health and nurses' role in assessing and maintaining it. *Nursing Times*, **105** (17), 19–23.

Malkin, B. and Berridge, P. (2009) Guidance on maintaining personal hygiene in nail care. *Nursing Standard*, **23** (41), 35–38.

Mamada, Y., Yoshida, H., Taniai, N. *et al.* (2007) Peritoneovenous shunts for palliation of malignant ascites. *Journal of Nippon Medical School*, **74** (5), 355–358.

Manikandan, R., Srirangam, S.J., Brown, S.C.W., O'Reilly, P.H. and Collins, G.N. (2003) Nitrous oxide vs periprostatic nerve block with 1% lidocaine during transrectal ultrasound guided biopsy of the prostate: a prospective, randomized, controlled trial. *Journal of Urology*, **170** (5), 1881–1883.

Mann, E. (2008) Neuropathic pain: could nurses become more involved? *British Journal of Nursing*, **17** (19), 1208–1213.

Marieb, E. (2001) *Human Anatomy and Physiology*, 5th edn. Benjamin Cummings, Boston.

Marincola, F.M. and Schwartzentruber, D.J. (2001) *Cancer Principles and Practice of Oncology*, 6th edn. Lippincott, Williams and Wilkins, Philadelphia, pp. 2745–2752.

Marsden, J. (2006) The care of patients presenting with acute problems, in *Ophthalmic Care* (ed.J.Marsden). Whurr, Chichester, pp. 209–252.

Martyn, C.N., Illis, L.S. and Thom, J. (1995) Nabilone in the treatment of multiple sclerosis. *Lancet*, **345** (8949), 579.

Mason, W. (2000) Exploring rehabilitation within lymphoedema management. *International Journal of Palliative Nursing*, **6** (6), 265–273.

Maze, M. and Fujinaga, M. (2000) Recent advances in understanding the actions and toxicity of nitrous oxide. *Anaesthesia*, **55** (4), 311–314.

McCaffery, M. and Beebe, A. (1989) Perspectives on pain, in *Pain: Clinical Manual for Nursing Practice* (eds M. McCaffery and A. Beebe). Mosby, St Louis, MO, pp. 1–5.

McCaffery, M. and Ferrell, B.R. (1997) Nurses' knowledge of pain assessment and management: how much progress have we made? *Journal of Pain and Symptom Management*, **14** (3), 175–188.

McCaffery, M. and Pasero, C. (1999) *Pain Clinical Manual*, 2nd edn. Mosby, St Louis, MO.

McCaffery, M. and Robinson, E.S. (2002) Your patient is in pain – here's how you respond. *Nursing*, **32** (10), 36–45.

McCaffrey, R. (1968) *Nursing Practice Theories Relating to Cognition, Bodily Pain and Man Environment*. University of California Los Angeles, Los Angeles, CA.

McCaffrey, R. (2000) *Nursing Management of the Patient with Pain*, 3rd edn. Lippincott, Philadelphia.

McGibbon, A., Chen, G.I., Peltekian, K.M. and van Zanten, S.V. (2007) An evidence-based manual for abdominal paracentesis. *Digestive Diseases and Sciences*, **52** (12), 3307–3315.

McLoughlin, C. (2005) A guide to wash creams. *Professional Nurse*, **20** (6), 46–47.

McMillan, C. (2001) Breakthrough pain: assessment and management in cancer patients. *British Journal of Nursing*, **10** (13), 860–866.

McNamara, P. (2000) Paracentesis – an effective method of symptom control in the palliative care setting? *Palliative Medicine*, **14**, 62–64.

McQuay, H. and Edwards, J. (2003) Meta-analysis of single dose oral tramadol plus acetaminophen in acute postoperative pain. *European Journal of Anaesthesiology*, **28** (Suppl), 19–22.

McQuay, H. (1999) Opioids in pain management. *Lancet*, **353** (9171), 2229–2232.

McQuay, H.J. and Moore, R.A. (1998) Oral tramadol versus placebo, codeine and combination analgesics, in *An Evidence-Based Resource for Pain Relief* (eds H.J. McQuay and R.A. Moore). Oxford University Press, Oxford, pp. 138–146.

McQuay, H., Moore, A. and Justins, D. (1997) Treating acute pain in hospital. *BMJ*, **314** (7093), 1531–1535.

Meechan, J. (2005) Oral pain, in *Oral Care in Advanced Disease* (eds A. Davies and I. Finlay). Oxford University Press, Oxford, pp. 133–143.

Mehta, V. and Langford, R.M. (2006) Acute pain management for opioid dependent patients. *Anaesthesia*, **61** (3), 269–276.

Melzack, R. (1975) The McGill Pain Questionnaire: major properties and scoring methods. *Pain*, **1** (3), 277–299.

Mercadante, S. (1999) Problems of long-term spinal opioid treatment in advanced cancer patients. *Pain*, **79** (1), 1–13.

Mercadante, S., Intravia, G., Ferrera, P. *et al.* (2008) Peritoneal catheter for continuous drainage of ascites in advanced cancer patients. *Supportive Care in Cancer*, **16**, 976–978.

MHRA (2005) Medical Device Alert Ref. MDA/2005/027. Heat patches or heat packs intended for pain relief. Medicines and Healthcare products Regulatory Agency, London.

Milligan, S., McGill, M., Sweeney, M.P. and Malarkey, C. (2001) Oral care for people with advanced cancer: an evidence-based protocol. *International Journal of Palliative Nursing*, **7** (9), 418–426.

Mimoz, O., Karim, A., Mercat, A. *et al.* (1999) Chlorhexidine compared with povidone-iodine as skin preparation before blood culture. A randomized, controlled trial. *Annals of Internal Medicine*, **131** (11), 834–837.

Mitchell, M. (1997) Patients' perceptions of pre-operative preparation for day surgery. *Journal of Advanced Nursing*, **26** (2), 356–363.

Moorsom, D. (2001) Paracentesis in a home care setting. *Palliative Medicine*, **15**, 169–170. PubMed CrossRef.

Morley, J.S. and Makin, M.K. (1998) The use of methadone in cancer pain poorly responsive to other opioids. *Pain Reviews*, **5** (1), 51–59.

Mortimer, P. (2003a) Differential diagnosis of chronic swelling of the limbs, in *Diseases of the Lymphatics* (eds N. Browse, K. Burn and P. Mortimer). Arnold Publishers, London, pp. 157–166.

Mortimer, P. (2003b) Principles of medical and physical treatment, in *Diseases of the Lymphatics* (eds N. Browse, K. Burn and P. Mortimer). Arnold Publishers, London, pp. 167–178.

Mucci-LoRusso, P., Berman, B.S., Silberstein, P.T. *et al.* (1998) Controlled-release oxycodone compared with controlled-release morphine in the treatment of cancer pain: a randomized, double-blind, parallel-group study. *European Journal of Pain*, **2** (3), 239–249.

Munro, C.L. and Grap, M.J. (2004) Oral health and care in the intensive care unit: state of the science. *American Journal of Critical Care*, **13** (1), 25–33.

Nadler, S.F., Steiner, D.J., Erasala, G.N. *et al.* (2002) Continuous low-level heat wrap therapy provides more efficacy than Ibuprofen and acetaminophen for acute low back pain. *Spine*, **27** (10), 1012–1017.

National Breast and Ovarian Cancer Centre (2008) *Review of Research Evidence on Secondary Lymphoedema: Incidence, Prevention, Risk Factors and Treatment*. National Breast and Ovarian Cancer Centre, New South Wales, Australia.

National Health Service (2004) *10 High Impact Changes for Service Improvement and Delivery*. Stationery Office, London.

NHS Quality Improvement Scotland (2004) *Working with Dependent Older People to Achieve Good Oral Health*. NHSQIS, Edinburgh.

Nigam, Y. and Knight, J. (2008) Exploring the anatomy and physiology of ageing. Part 6 – the eye and ear. *Nursing Times*, **104** (36), 22–23.

Nightingale, F. (1859) *Notes on Nursing – What It Is and What It Is Not*. Churchill Livingstone, London.

NMC (2008a) *Consent*. Nursing and Midwifery Council, London. www.nmc-uk.org/Nurses-and-midwives/Advice-by-topic/A/Advice/Consent.

NMC (2008b) *The Code: Standards of Conduct, Performance and Ethics for Nurses and Midwives*. Nursing and Midwifery Council, London.

NMC (2009) *Record Keeping: Guidance for Nurses and Midwives*. Nursing and Midwifery Council, London.

NPSA (2007) *The Fifth Report from the Patient Safety Observatory, Safety Care for the Acutely Ill Patient: Learning from Incidents*. National Patient Safety Agency, London. www.nrls.npsa.nhs.uk/resources/?entryid45=59828.

O'Connor, M. and Webb, R. (2002) Learning to rest when in pain. *European Journal of Palliative Care*, **9** (2), 68–72.

Olver, J. and Cassidy, L. (2005) *Ophthalmology at a Glance*. Blackwell Science, Oxford.

Orem, D.E. (1980) *Nursing: Concepts of Practice*, 2nd edn. McGraw-Hill, New York.

Osbourne, K. (2007) Principles of below and above knee inelastic multi-layer bandaging. *Chronic Oedema Wounds UK Supplement*, **3** (2), 29–34.

O'Sullivan, I. and Benger, J. (2003) Nitrous oxide in emergency medicine. *Emergency Medicine Journal*, **20** (3), 214–217.

Otto, S. (2001) *Oncology Nursing*, 4th edn. Mosby, St Louis, MO.

Ozkan, O., Akinci, D., Gocmen, R. *et al.* (2007) Percutaneous placement of peritoneal port-catheter in patients with malignant ascites. *Cardiovascular and Interventional Radiology*, **30** (2), 232–236.

Papagelopoulos, P.J., Petrou, H.G., Triantafyllidis, P.G. *et al.* (2001) Treatment of lumbosacral radicular pain with epidural steroid injections. *Orthopedics*, **24** (2), 145–149.

Pargeon, K.L. and Hailey, B.J. (1999) Barriers to effective cancer pain management: a review of the literature. *Journal of Pain and Symptom Management*, **18** (5), 358–368.

Parizkova, B. and George, S. (2009) Regional anaesthesia and analgesia, Part 2: central neural blockade, in *Perioperative Pain Management* (ed F. Cox). Wiley-Blackwell, Oxford.

Parker, L. (2004) Infection control: maintaining the personal hygiene of patients and staff. *British Journal of Nursing*, **13** (4), 474–478.

Partsch, H. (2003) Understanding the pathophysiological effects of compression, in *European Wound Management Association (EWMA) Position Document. Understanding Compression Therapy* (eds S. Caine, C. Moffatt and S. Thomas). Medical Educational Partnership, London, pp. 2–7.

Partsch, H. and Mosti, G. (2008) Thigh compression. *Phlebology*, **23** (6), 252–258.

Partsch, H., Clark, M., Mosti, G. *et al.* (2008) Classification of compression bandages: practical aspects. *Dermatological Surgery*, **34** (5), 600–609.

Pasero, C. (1998) Pain control – is laughter the best medicine? *American Journal of Nursing*, **98** (12), 12–14.

Payne, R.A. (1995) *Relaxation Techniques: A Practical Handbook for the Health Care Professional*. Churchill Livingstone, Edinburgh.

Paz, S. and Seymour, J.E. (2008) Pain theories, evaluation and management, in *Palliative Care Nursing: Principles and Evidence for Practice*. 2nd edn (eds S. Payne J. Seymour and C. Ingleton). Open University Press, Maidenhead, pp. 252–289.

Pearson, L.S. and Hutton, J.L. (2002) A controlled trial to compare the ability of foam swabs and toothbrushes to remove dental plaque. *Journal of Advanced Nursing*, **39** (5), 480–489.

Pease, N., Taylor, H. and Major, H. (2004) Strong painkillers and driving. *Palliative Medicine*, **18**, 663–668.

Peate, I. and Lancaster, J. (2000) Safe use of medical gases in the clinical setting: practical tips. *British Journal of Nursing*, **9** (4), 231–237.

Pegram, A., Bloomfield, J. and Jones, A. (2007) Clinical skills: bed bathing and personal hygiene needs of patients. *British Journal of Nursing*, **16** (6), 356–358.

Penzer, R. and Finch, M. (2001) Promoting healthy skin in older people. *Nursing Standard*, **15** (34), 46–52.

529

Perkins, F.M. and Kehlet, H. (2000) Chronic pain as an outcome of surgery. A review of predictive factors. *Anesthesiology*, **93** (4), 1123–1133.

Peterson, D.E., Bensadoun, R.-J. and Roila, F. (2009) Management of oral and gastrointestinal mucositis: ESMO clinical recommendations. *Annals of Oncology*, **20** (Suppl 4), iv174–iv177.

Philips, L. and Buttery, J. (2009) *Exploring Pressure Ulcer Prevalence and Preventative Care. Nursing Times*, 16, 105.

Pickup, S. and Pagdin, J. (2000) Procedural pain: Entonox can help. *Paediatric Nursing*, **12** (10), 33–37.

Piller, N. (1999) Gaining an accurate assessment of the stages of lymphoedema subsequent to cancer: the role of objective and subjective information, when to make measurements and their optimal use. *European Journal of Lymphology*, **7** (25), 1–9.

Portenoy, R.K. and Lesage, P. (1999) Management of cancer pain. *Lancet*, **353** (9165), 1695–1700.

Portenoy, R.K., Payne, R., Coluzzi, P. *et al.* (1999) Oral transmucosal fentanyl citrate (OTFC) for the treatment of breakthrough pain in cancer patients: a controlled dose titration study. *Pain*, **79** (2–3), 303–312.

Portenoy, R.K., Forbes, K., Lussier, D. and Hanks, G. (2004) Difficult pain problems: an integrated approach. In: *Oxford Textbook of Palliative Medicine* (ed. D. Doyle). Oxford University Press, Oxford, pp. 316–336.

Potter, P.A. and Griffin Perry, A. (2003) *Basic Nursing Essentials for Practice*, 5th edn. Mosby, St Louis, MO.

Potter, P.A. and Perry, G. (1995) *Basic Nursing Theory and Practice*. Mosby, London.

Pratt, R.J., Pellowe, C., Loveday, H. *et al.* (2001) Guidelines for preventing infections associated with the insertion and maintenance of short-term indwelling urethral catheters in acute care. *Journal of Hospital Infection*, **47**(Supplement), S39–46.

Preston, R.M. (2005) Aseptic technique: evidence-based approach for patient safety. *British Journal of Nursing*, **14** (10), 540–542, 544–546.

Pullen, R.L. Jr. (2006) Spin control: caring for a patient with inner ear disease. *Nursing*, **36** (5), 48–51.

Quigley, C. (2004) Opioid switching to improve pain relief and drug tolerability. *Cochrane Database of Systematic Reviews*, 3, CD004847.

Quinn, B., Potting, C.M.J., Stone, R. *et al.* (2008) Guidelines for the assessment of oral mucositis in adult chemotherapy, radiotherapy and haematopoietic stem cell transplant patients. *European Journal of Cancer*, **44**, 61–72.

Raiman, J. (1986) Coping with pain. Pain relief – a two-way process. *Nursing Times*, **82** (15), 24–28.

RCN (1998) *Clinical Practice Guidelines: The Management of Patients with Venous Leg Ulcers*. RCN Publishing, Harrow.

Rauch, R.L., Tark, M., Reyes, E. *et al.* (2009) Efficacy and long term tolerability of sublingual fentanyl oral disintegrating tablet in the treatment of breakthrough cancer pain. *Current Medical Research and Opinion*, **25** (12), 2877–2885.

Ready, L. and Edwards, W. (1992) *Management of Acute Pain: A Practical Guide*. IASP Publications, Seattle, WA.

Reicin, A., Brown, J., Jove, M. *et al.* (2001) Efficacy of single-dose and multidose rofecoxib in the treatment of post-orthopedic surgery pain. *American Journal of Orthopedics*, **30** (1), 40–48.

Richardson, M. (2007) Hearing and balance: The outer and middle ear. *Nursing Times*, **103** (38) 24–25.

Riley, J. (2006) An overview of opioids in palliative care. *European Journal of Palliative Care*, **13** (6), 230–233.

Roberts, J. (2001) Oral assessment and intervention. *Nursing Older People*, **13** (7), 14–16.

Robinson, P., Deacon, S.A., Deer, C. *et al.* (2005) Manual versus powered toothbrushing for oral health. *Cochrane Database of Systematic Reviews*, 2, CD002281.

Romer, H.C. and Russell, G.N. (1998) A survey of the practice of thoracic epidural analgesia in the United Kingdom. *Anaesthesia*, **53** (10), 1016–1022.

Romsing, J., Moiniche, S. and Dahl, J.B. (2002) Rectal and parenteral paracetamol, and paracetamol in combination with NSAIDs, for postoperative analgesia. *British Journal of Anaesthesia*, **88** (2), 215–226.

Roper, N., Logan, W.W. and Tierney, A.J. (1981) *Learning to Use the Process of Nursing*. Churchill Livingstone, Edinburgh.

Rosen, M.A. (2002) Nitrous oxide for relief of labor pain: a systematic review. *American Journal of Obstetrics and Gynecology*, **186** (5 suppl.), S110–S126.

Ross, J. and Wilson, K. (2001) *Anatomy and Physiology in Health and Illness*. Churchill Livingstone, Edinburgh.

Rowbotham, D.J. (2000) Non-steroidal anti-inflammatory drugs and paracetamol, in *Chronic Pain* (ed. D.J. Rowbotham). Martin Dunitz, London, pp. 19–26.

Rowlingson, J.C. and Hanson, P.B. (2005) Neuraxial anesthesia and low-molecular-weight heparin prophylaxis in major orthopedic surgery in the wake of the latest American Society of Regional Analgesia Guidelines. *Anesthesia and Analgesia*, **100**, 1482–1488.

Royal College of Anaesthetists (2004) *Good Practice in the Management of Continuous Epidural Analgesia in the Hospital Setting*. Royal College of Anaesthetists, London,

Royal College of Anaesthetists (2006) Section 1 Key issues in developing new materials, in *Raising the Standard: Information for Patients*, 2nd edn. Royal College of Anaesthetists, London, pp. 14–29.

Royal College of Physicians, British Geriatric Society and British Pain Society (2007) *The Assessment of Pain in Older People: National Guidelines*. Royal College of Physicians, London.

Royse, C.F., Hall, J. and Royse, A.G. (2006) The 'mesentery' dressing for epidural catheter fixation. *Anaesthesia*, **61** (7), 713.

Rubenstein, E.B., Peterson, D.E., Schubert, M., *et al.* (2004) Clinical practice guidelines for the prevention and treatment of cancer therapy-induced oral and gastrointestinal mucositis. *Cancer*, **100** (S9), 2026–2046.

Sampson, A.C.M. (1982) *The Neglected Ethic: Cultural and Religious Factors in the Care of Patients*. McGraw-Hill, London.

Sands, R., Yarussi, A. and de Leon-Casasola, D. (1998) Complications and side-effects associated with epidural bupivacaine/morphine analgesia. *Acute Pain*, **1** (2), 43–50.

Sargent, S. (2006) Management of patients with advanced liver cirrhosis. *Nursing Standard*, **21** (11), 48–56.

Schug, S.A. and Torrie, J.J. (1993) Safety assessment of postoperative pain management by an acute pain service. *Pain*, **55** (3), 387–391.

Scott, I.E. (1994) Effectiveness of documented assessment of postoperative pain. *British Journal of Nursing*, **3** (10), 494–501.

Seers, K. (1996) The patients' experiences of their chronic nonmalignant pain. *Journal of Advanced Nursing*, **24** (6), 1160–1168.

Seers, K. and Carroll, D. (1998) Relaxation techniques for acute pain management: a systematic review. *Journal of Advanced Nursing*, **27** (3), 466–475.

Seike, M., Maetani, I. and Sakai, Y. (2007) Treatment of malignant ascites in patients with advanced cancer: peritoneovenous shunt versus paracentesis. *Journal of Gastroenterology Hepatololgy*, **22** (12), 2161–2166.

Shaw, M.E. (2006) Examination of the eye, in *Ophthalmic Care* (ed. J. Marsden). Wiley, Chichester, pp. 66–84.

Sheppard, C.M. and Brenner, P.S. (2000) The effects of bathing and skin care practices on skin quality and satisfaction with an

530

innovative product. *Journal of Gerontological Nursing*, **26** (10), 36–45.

Sidebotham, D., Dijkhuizen, M.R. and Schug, S.A. (1997) The safety and utilization of patient-controlled analgesia. *Journal of Pain and Symptom Management*, **14** (4), 202–209.

Sindrup, S.H. and Jensen, T.S. (1999) Efficacy of pharmacological treatments of neuropathic pain: an update and effect related to mechanism of drug action. *Pain*, **83** (3), 389–400.

Sitzia, J. (1995) Volume measurement in lymphoedema treatment: examination of the formulae. *European Journal of Cancer Care*, **4**, 11–16.

Sloan, P.A. (2004) The evolving role of interventional pain management in oncology. *Journal of Supportive Oncology*, **2** (6), 491–500, 503.

Sloman, R., Brown, P., Aldana, E. and Chee, E. (1994) The use of relaxation for the promotion of comfort and pain relief in persons with advanced cancer. *Contemporary Nurse*, **3** (1), 6–12.

Smith, H. and Elliott, J. (2001) Alpha(2) receptors and agonists in pain management. *Current Opinion in Anaesthesiology*, **14** (5), 513–518.

Smitt, P.S., Tsafka, A., Teng-van de Zande, F. *et al.* (1998) Outcome and complications of epidural analgesia in patients with chronic cancer pain. *Cancer*, **83** (9), 2015–2022.

Smoker, A. (1999) Skin care in old age. *Nursing Standard*, **13** (48), 47–53.

Sonis, S.T., Elting, L.S., Keefe, D. *et al.* (2004) Perspectives on cancer therapy-induced mucosal injury. *Cancer*, **100** (S9), 1995–2024.

Southern, H. (2007) Oral care in cancer nursing: nurses' knowledge and education. *Journal of Advanced Nursing*, **57** (6), 631–638.

Spiller, J. (1992) For whose sake – patient or nurse? Ritual practices in patient washing. *Professional Nurse*, **7** (7), 431–434.

Stannard, C.F. and Booth, S. (1998) Management of pain following trauma, in *Churchill's Pocket Book of Pain*. Churchill Livingstone, Edinburgh, p. 178.

Stanton, A., Northfield, J., Holroyd, B. *et al.* (1997) Validation of an optoelectronic limb volumeter (Perometer). *Lymphology*, **30**, 77–97.

Stanton, A., Badger, C. and Sitzia, J. (2000) Non-invasive assessment of the lymphoedematous limb. *Lymphology*, **33**, 122–135.

Stanton, A., Modi, S., Mellor, R. *et al.* (2006) Diagnosing breast cancer related lymphoedema of the arm. *Journal of Lymphoedema*, **1** (1) 12–15.

Stephenson, J. and Gilbert, J. (2002) The development of clinical guidelines on paracentesis for ascites related to malignancy. *Palliative Medicine*, **16**, 213–18.

Stevens, R.A. and Ghazi, S.M. (2000) Routes of opioid analgesic therapy in the management of cancer pain. *Cancer Control*, **7** (2), 132–141.

Stiefel, K.A., Damron, S., Sowers, N.J. and Velez, L. (2000) Improving oral hygiene for the seriously ill patient: implementing research-based practice. *Medsurg Nursing*, **9** (1), 40–46.

Stillwell, G. (1973) The Law of Laplace: some clinical applications. *Mayo Clinic Proceedings*, **48**, 863–869.

Stockton, L. and Flynn, M. (2009) Sitting and pressure ulcers. 1: Risk factors, self-repositioning and other interventions. *Nursing Times*, **105** (24), 12–14.

Stollery, R., Shaw, M.E. and Lee, A. (2005) *Ophthalmic Nursing*, 3rd edn. Blackwell, Oxford.

Sweeney, P. (2005) Oral hygiene, in *Oral Care in Advanced Disease* (eds A. Davies and I. Finlay). Oxford University Press, Oxford, pp. 23–35.

Taylor, H. (2001) The importance of providing good patient information. *Professional Nurse*, **17** (1), 34–36.

Taylor, A., Tayler, J. and Said, S.(2000) Using a bandage pressure monitor as an aid in improving bandaging skills. *Journal of Wound Care*, **7** (3), 131–133.

Taylor, R., Jayasinghe, U., Koelmeyer, L. *et al.* (2006) Reliability and validity of arm volume measurements for assessment of lymphoedema. *Physical Therapy*, **86** (2), 205–214.

Thibodeau, G. and Patton, K. (2007) Anatomy of the digestive system, in *Anatomy and Physiology*, 6th edn (eds G. Thibodeau and K. Patton). Mosby, St. Louis, MO, pp. 925–960.

Thomas, S. (2003) The use of the Laplace equation in the calculation of sub-bandage pressure. *European Wound Management Association Journal*, **3** (1), 21–23.

Thomas, S. and Nelson, A. (1998) Graduated external compression in the treatment of venous disease, in *Compression Therapy: A Complete Guide* EMAP Healthcare, London, pp. 1–4.

Tobin, M., Lacey, H., Meyer, L. and Mortimer, P. (1993) The psychological morbidity of breast cancer related arm swelling. *Cancer*, **72** (11), 3348–3352.

Todd, J. (2000) Containment in the management of lymphoedema, in *Lymphoedema* (eds R. Twycross, K. Jenns and J. Todd). Radcliffe Medical Press, Oxford, pp. 165–202.

Todd, M. (2009) Managing lymphoedema in palliative care patients. *British Journal of Nursing*, **18** (8), 466–472.

Tortora, G.J. and Derrickson, B.H. (2009) *Principles of Anatomy and Physiology*, 12th edn. John Wiley, Hoboken, NJ.

Towers A., Carnevale, F. and Baker, M. (2008) The psychosocial effects of cancer-related lymphedema. *Journal of Palliative Care*, **24** (3), 134–143.

Trauger-Querry, B. and Haghighi, K.R. (1999) Balancing the focus: art and music therapy for pain control and symptom management in hospice care. *Hospice Journal*, **14** (1), 25–38.

Trojan, J., Saunders, B.P., Woloshynowych, M., Debinsky, H.S. and Williams, C.B. (1997) Immediate recovery of psychomotor function after patient-administered nitrous oxide/oxygen inhalation for colonoscopy. *Endoscopy*, **29** (1), 17–22.

Turk, D.C. and Okifuji, A. (1999) Assessment of patients' reporting of pain: an integrated perspective. *Lancet*, **353** (9166), 1784–1788.

Twycross, R.G. and Wilcock, A. (2001) *Symptom Management in Advanced Cancer*, 3rd edn. Radcliffe Medical, Abingdon.

Twycross, R., Harcourt, J. and Bergl, S. (1996) A survey of pain in patients with advanced cancer. *Journal of Pain and Symptom Management*, **12** (5), 273–282.

Tye, T. and Gell-Walker, V. (2000) Patient-controlled analgesia. *Nursing Times*, **96** (25), 38–39.

UKCCSG-PONF Mouth Care Group (2006) *Mouth Care for Children and Young People with Cancer: Evidence-based Guidelines*. United Kingdom Children's Cancer Study Group, Manchester.

Urdan, L.D., Stacy, K.M. and Lough, M.E. (2006) Pain and pain management, in *Thelan's Critical Care Nursing Diagnosis and Management*. Mosby Elsevier, St Louis, MO.

Vandermeulen, E.P., van Aken, H. and Vermylen, J. (1994) Anticoagulants and spinal-epidural anesthesia. *Anesthesia and Analgesia*, **79** (6), 1165–1177.

Vijayan, R. (1997) Subcutaneous morphine – a simple technique for postoperative analgesia. *Acute Pain*, **1** (1), 21–26.

Voegeli, D. (2008) Care or harm: exploring essential components in skin care regimens. *British Journal of Nursing*, **17** (1), 24–30.

Vondrackova, D., Leyendecker, P., Meissner, W. *et al.* (2008) Analgesic efficacy and safety of oxycodone in combination with naloxone as prolonged release tablets in patients with moderate to severe chronic pain. *Journal of Pain*, **9** (12), 1144–1154.

Walker, S.M., Macintyre, P.E., Visser, E. and Scott, D. (2006) Acute pain management: current best evidence provides guide for improved practice. *Pain Medicine*, **7** (1), 3–5.

531

Walker, V., Dicks, B. and Webb, P. (1987) Pain assessment charts in the management of chronic cancer pain. *Palliative Medicine*, **1** (2), 111–116.

Wall, J., Davis, S. and Ridgway, S. (2001) Cannabis: its therapeutic use. *Nursing Standard*, **16** (10), 39–44.

Wallace, M.S. (2002) Treatment options for refractory pain: the role of intrathecal therapy. *Neurology*, **59** (5 Suppl 2), S18–24.

Walsh, D. (1997) Review of clinical studies on TENS, in *TENS: Clinical Applications and Related Theory* (eds D.M. Walsh and E.T. McAdams). Churchill Livingstone, New York, pp. 83–101.

Watkinson, S. and Seewoodhary, R. (2007) Common conditions and practical considerations in eye care. *Nursing Standard*, **21** (44), 42–47.

Weetman, C. and Allison, W. (2006) Use of epidural analgesia in postoperative pain management. *Nursing Standard*, **20** (44), 54–64.

Wheatley, R.G., Schug, S.A. and Watson, D. (2001) Safety and efficacy of postoperative epidural analgesia. *British Journal of Anaesthesia*, **87** (1), 47–61.

Whiteman, K. and McCormick, C. (2005) When your patient is in liver failure. *Nursing*, **35**, 58–63.

Whiting, L.S. (1999) Maintaining patients' personal hygiene. *Professional Nurse*, **14** (5), 338–340.

WHO (1979) *Handbook for Reporting Results of Cancer Treatment*, vol. **48**. World Health Organization, Geneva, pp. 15–22.

Williams, A. (2002) A clinical audit of Actico cohesive short-stretch bandages. *Journal of Clinical Nursing*, **20**, 4–10.

Williams, A. and Keller, M. (2005) Practical guidance on lymphoedema bandaging of the upper and lower limbs, in *European Wound Management Association (EWMA) Focus Document: Lymphoedema Bandaging in Practice*. Medical Educational Partnership, London, pp. 10–14.

Wilson, D. (2006) Giving patients a choice of what to wear in hospital. *Nursing Times*, **102** (20), 29–31.

Wilson, M. (1986) Personal cleanliness. *Nursing (Lond)*, **3** (2), 80–81.

Winkelman, L.M. (2004) Malignant ascites, in *Cancer Symptom Management*, 3rd edn (eds C. Yarbo, M. Frogge and M. Goodman). Jones and Bartlett, Sudbury, MA, pp. 401–19.

Witt-Sherman, D., Matzo, M., Paice, J. *et al.* (2004) Learning pain assessment and management. A goal of the end-of-life nursing education consortium. *Journal of Continuing Education in Nursing*, **35** (3), 107–120.

Wood, A. (2004) Mouth care and ritualistic practice. *Cancer Nursing Practice*, **3** (4), 34–39.

Woodrow, P. (2006) *Intensive Care Nursing: A Framework for Practice*, 2nd edn. Routledge, London.

Woods, M. (1993) Patients' perceptions of breast-cancer related lymphoedema. *European Journal of Cancer Care*, **2**, 125–128.

Woods, M. (2000) Lymphoedema, in *Stepping into Palliative Care: A Handbook for Community Professionals* (ed. J. Cooper). Radcliffe Medical Press, Oxford, pp. 81–88.

Woods, M. (2002) Using philosophy, knowledge and theory to assess a patient with lymphoedema. *International Journal of Palliative Nursing*, **8** (4), 176–181.

Woods, M. (2007a) A framework for the assessment of a patients with lymphoedema, in *Lymphoedema Care* (ed. M. Woods). Blackwell, Oxford, pp. 55–66.

Woods, M. (2007b) Identifying secondary lymphoedema, in *Lymphoedema Care* (ed. M. Woods). Blackwell, Oxford, pp. 37–54.

Worthington, H.V., Clarkson, J.E. and Eden, TOB. (2007a) Interventions for preventing oral mucositis for patients with cancer receiving treatment. *Cochrane Database of Systematic Reviews*, **4**, CD000978.

Worthington, H.V., Clarkson, J.E. and Eden, T.O.B. (2007b) Interventions for treating oral candidiasis for patients with cancer receiving treatment. *Cochrane Database of Systematic Reviews*, **2**, CD001972.

Young, L. (1991) Community care: the clean fight. *Nursing Standard*, **5** (35), 54–55.

Zaza, C. and Baine, N. (2002) Cancer pain and psychosocial factors: a critical review of the literature. *Journal of Pain and Symptom Management*, **24** (5), 526–542.

Zech, D., Lehmann, A. and Ground, S. (1994) A new treatment option for chronic cancer pain. *European Journal of Palliative Care*, **1** (1), 26–30.

Zeppetella, G. (2009) Oral transmucosal opioids, in *Cancer Related Breakthrough Pain* (ed. A. Davies). Oxford University Press, Oxford.

Respiratory care

The Royal Marsden Hospital Manual of Clinical Nursing Procedures, Eighth Edition. Edited by Lisa Dougherty and Sara Lister.
© 2011 The Royal Marsden Hospital. Published 2011 by Blackwell Publishing Ltd.

Overview

This chapter explains the nursing management and assessment of patients with respiratory problems. Administration of oxygen therapy, managing patients with chest drains and tracheostomies, counselling patients regarding smoking cessation and performing cardiopulmonary resuscitation (CPR) will be discussed.

Respiratory therapy

Definitions

The principle of respiratory therapy is the application of pharmacological and non-pharmacological means to improve breathing and therefore improve gaseous exchange. This will include an assessment of the cause of the impaired breathing, reversal of causes where possible and therapies to optimize respiratory function (Shelledy and Mikles 2002).

Anatomy and physiology

See also Chapter 13.

The respiratory system is a complex system that is responsible for the efficient exchange of the respiratory gases, primarily oxygen and carbon dioxide. The respiratory system is responsible for ensuring a continuous optimum supply of oxygen to the tissues and the elimination of carbon dioxide during expiration. Four separate functions are necessary to achieve optimal respiration (Marieb et al. 2010).

1 *Pulmonary ventilation*: adequate breathing and movement of air in and out of the lungs, ensuring a fresh supply of oxygen to the alveoli.
2 *External respiration*: ensuring adequate gas exchange, oxygen uptake and carbon dioxide unloading between the blood and the alveoli of the lungs.
3 *Transport of respiratory gases*: moving oxygen and carbon dioxide between the lungs and the body tissues. Transport is affected by the cardiovascular system and uses the blood as a carrying mechanism.
4 *Cellular respiration*: oxygen delivery and carbon dioxide uptake between the systemic blood and tissue cells.

The respiratory system is composed of the following structures.

- The two respiratory centres in the medulla oblongata and pons of the brain.
- The nose, mouth and connecting airways.
- The trachea, main bronchus, bronchioles and alveoli.
- The respiratory muscles: the diaphragm and the intercostal muscles.
- The respiratory nerves: the subphrenic nerve and the intercostal nerves.
- The bone structure of the thorax: the ribs, vertebrae and sternum.
- The lung parenchyma.
- The pleura.

Alteration, damage or blockage to any of the structures listed above may result in either respiratory impairment or respiratory failure. It is essential when considering respiratory function to remember the close association and dependence between the cardiovascular, neurological, musculo-skeletal and respiratory systems.

Tissue oxygenation

All the cells of the body require a continuous supply of oxygen to ensure growth and repair of tissues and optimum metabolism. Oxygen is drawn into the body through the nose and mouth; it then travels down the trachea and into the smaller airways and alveoli of the lungs. Once it has reached the alveoli, oxygen in solution is able to transfer into the network of capillaries and from there travels via the venous network to all cells of the body. This tissue oxygenation is known as cellular oxygenation. Low oxygen levels are called hypoxia. In low oxygen conditions, anaerobic cellular oxygenation will occur, generating the waste product lactic acid. If the low oxygen state is allowed to continue lactic acid will accumulate, leading to a metabolic acidosis and cell death (Berne 2004, Bersten et al. 2009, Guyton and Hall 2006, Hess 2000, Kumar and Clark 2009, Marieb et al. 2010, Pierson 2000, Tortora and Derrickson 2009, West 2008).

There are three components to oxygenation: oxygen uptake, oxygen transportation and oxygen utilization. *Oxygen uptake* is the process of extracting oxygen from the environment. *Oxygen transportation* is the mechanism by which the uptake of oxygen results in the delivery of oxygen to the cells. *Oxygen utilization* is the metabolic need for molecular oxygen by the cells of the body (Marieb et al. 2010, Tortora and Derrickson 2009).

In order for oxygenation to take place there needs to be an adequate cardiac output.

Oxygen uptake

The air that we breathe in during normal conditions from the atmosphere is composed of the following gases:

- oxygen 21%
- carbon dioxide 0.03%
- nitrogen 79%
- rare gases 0.003%.

Inspired air at sea level has a total atmospheric pressure of 760 mmHg. According to Dalton's Law, where there is a mixture of gases, each gas exerts its own pressure as if there were no other gases present. The pressure of an individual gas in a mixture is called the partial pressure and is denoted as P, which is then followed by the type of gas, so that the partial pressure of oxygen is written PO_2 (Tortora and Derrickson 2009).

- Oxygen $0.21 \times 760 = 159$ mmHg (21 kPa).
- Carbon dioxide $0.03 \times 760 = 22.8$ mmHg (3.0 kPa).
- Nitrogen $0.79 \times 760 = 600$ mmHg (80 kPa).

The partial pressure of gases controls the movement of oxygen and carbon dioxide through the body between the atmosphere and the lungs, the lungs and the blood and finally the blood and the cells.

Gaseous exchange

Movement of gases is by diffusion. Diffusion is the movement of gas molecules from an area of relatively high partial pressure to one of lower partial pressure (Tortora and Derrickson 2009).

Diffusion of oxygen takes place from the alveolus into the pulmonary capillaries and movement of carbon dioxide from the capillary into the alveolus. From the alveolus, the oxygen diffuses from the capillaries into the tissues and mitochondria of the cells (Figure 10.1).

The alveolar oxygen partial pressure is higher than the arterial oxygen partial pressure in order to push the oxygen through the alveolar membrane into the interstitial spaces and from there into the pulmonary capillaries. Oxygen continues to diffuse from the capillaries into the tissues then to the mitochondria of the cells for metabolism (Berne 2004, Bersten *et al.* 2009, Carpenter 1991, Esmond 2001, Guyton and Hall 2006, Marieb *et al.* 2010, Pierce 1995, Tortora and Derrickson 2009).

As inspired air enters the respiratory tract, it encounters water vapour present in the upper airways which warms and humidifies it. Water vapour exerts its own partial pressure of 47 mmHg. The partial pressure of the water vapour must be subtracted from the total atmospheric pressure to give a corrected atmospheric pressure and partial pressure of each gas (Carpenter 1991, Marieb *et al.* 2010).

- Corrected total atmospheric pressure $760 - 47 = 713$ mmHg.
- Oxygen $0.21 \times 713 = 150$ mmHg (20 kPa).
- Carbon dioxide $0.03 \times 713 = 21$ mmHg (2.8 kPa).

As oxygen continues to pass down the respiratory tract to the alveolus, it encounters carbon dioxide leaving the respiratory tract which also exerts a partial pressure, equal to 40 mmHg. This in turn must be subtracted to determine the correct values. Oxygen has a corrected value of $150 - 40 = 110 - 100$ mmHg ($14.6 - 13.3$ kPa).

Oxygen transportation

Oxygen is carried in the blood in two ways.

- *Dissolved in the plasma (serum)*: only 2–3% is carried in this way as oxygen is not very soluble (Ahrens and

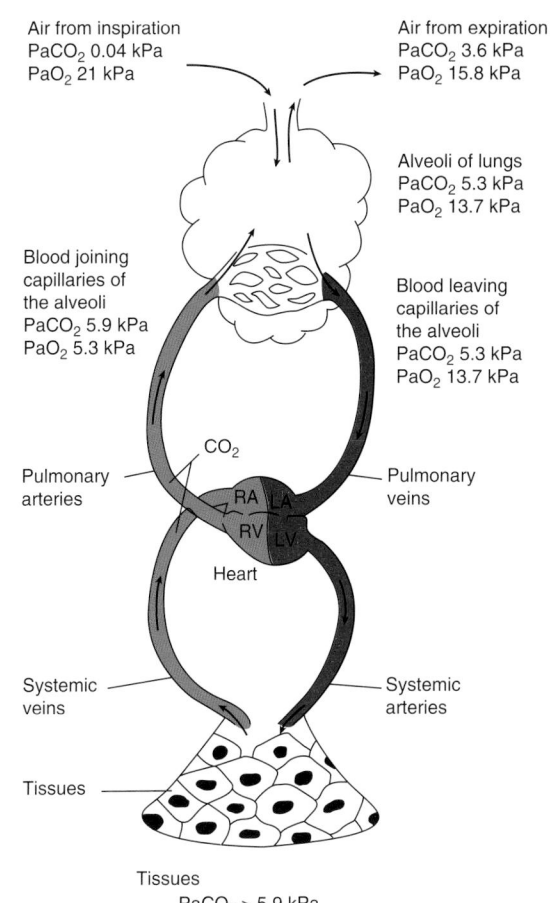

Figure 10.1 Gas movement in the body is facilitated by partial pressure differences. Top of figure illustrates pressure gradients that facilitate oxygen and carbon dioxide exchange in the lungs. Bottom of figure shows pressure gradients that facilitate gas movements from systemic capillaries to tissues.

Tucker 1999, Marieb *et al.* 2010). This is measured as the PaO_2. There is 0.003 mL of blood for each 1 mmHg partial pressure oxygen. At 100 mmHg partial pressure, only 0.3 mL of oxygen would be carried per 100 mL of plasma.

- *Bound to haemoglobin in the red blood cells*: 95–98% of oxygen is carried in this way and is measured as the percentage of oxygen saturated (SaO_2). Each gram of haemoglobin can carry 1.34 mL of oxygen per 100 mL blood.

Haemoglobin is composed of haem (iron) and globulin (protein). Each haemoglobin molecule has four binding sites, each able to carry one molecule of oxygen. A haemoglobin molecule is said to be fully saturated with oxygen when all four haem sites are attached to oxygen. When fewer than four are attached the haemoglobin is said to be partially saturated.

The bond between haemoglobin and oxygen is affected by various physiological factors that shift the oxygen

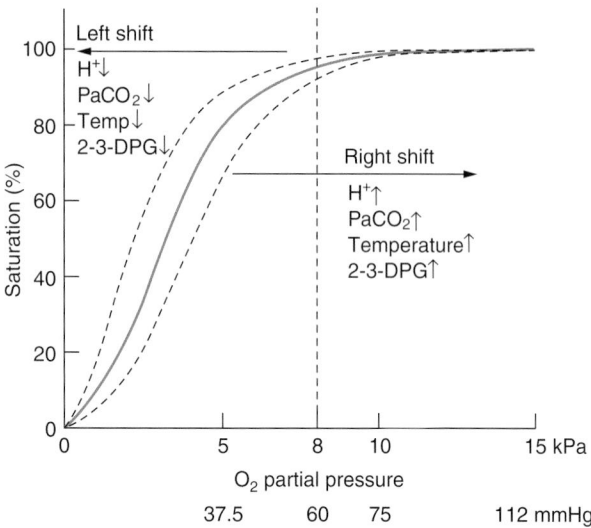

Figure 10.2 Oxyhaemoglobin dissociation curve. With a PaO_2 of 8 kPa and more, saturations will remain high (flat portion of curve). NB: The middle red line is the normal position of the curve.

dissociation curve to the right or left (Figure 10.2) (Marieb *et al.* 2010, Tortora and Derrickson 2009).

Oxyhaemoglobin curve shift to the right

When a shift occurs to the right there is reduced binding of oxygen to haemoglobin and oxygen is given up more easily to the tissues. The saturation will be lower (Pierson 2000).

Factors that cause the curve to shift to the right are an increase in:

- body temperature due to infection, sepsis
- hydrogen ion content (acidaemia), known as the Bohr effect, due to infection, sepsis or other shock conditions
- carbon dioxide due to sepsis, pulmonary disease, postoperatively
- 2-3-DPG (an enzyme found in the red blood cells that affects haemoglobin and oxygen binding).

Oxyhaemoglobin curve shift to the left

When a shift occurs to the left there is an increase in the binding of oxygen to the haemoglobin, oxygen is given up less easily to the tissues and cellular hypoxia can occur (Pierson 2000).

Factors that cause the curve to shift to the left are a decrease in:

- body temperature due to exposure, near drowning, trauma
- hydrogen ion content (alkalaemia)
- carbon dioxide
- 2-3-DPG.

Oxygen utilization

The relationship between the PaO_2 and the SaO_2 is represented as the oxygen dissociation curve. Oxygen uptake in the lungs is shown by the upper flat part of the curve. When the PaO_2 is between 8.0 and 13.3 kPa (60–100 mmHg), the haemoglobin is 90% or more saturated with oxygen. At this point of the curve, large changes in the PaO_2 lead to small changes in the SaO_2 of haemoglobin, because the haemoglobin is almost completely saturated. Release of oxygen to the tissues is shown by the lower part of the curve. There is easy removal of oxygen from the haemoglobin for use by the cells. It is at this part of the curve that small changes in the PaO_2 cause major changes in the SaO_2. This is important clinically (Carpenter 1991, Guyton and Hall 2006, Hess 2000).

A patient's oxygen level must be kept at 8.5 kPa or above (60 mmHg). Below this level, desaturation can occur at a rapid rate, resulting in tissue hypoxia and cell death (Marieb *et al.* 2010).

Oxygen consumption

At rest the normal oxygen consumption is approximately 200–250 mL/min. As the available oxygen per minute in a normal man is about 700 mL, this means there is an oxygen reserve of 450–500 mL/min. Factors that increase the consumption of oxygen include fever, sepsis, shivering, restlessness and increased metabolism (Bersten *et al.* 2009). It is difficult to say at which absolute level oxygen therapy is necessary, as each situation should be judged by the requirements for oxygen and the availability of oxygen. Therefore, all the above information needs to be taken into account together with the measurement of the arterial blood gases.

Generally, additional oxygen will be required when the PaO_2 has fallen to 8.5 kPa (60 mmHg) or less (Bersten *et al.* 2009).

Carbon dioxide excretion

The second function of the respiratory system is to excrete carbonic acid from the lungs during expiration. The normal level of carbon dioxide in the blood is 3.5–5.3 kPa. Carbon dioxide has a direct effect on the respiratory centre in the brain. As the carbon dioxide level rises and diffuses from the blood into the cerebrospinal fluid (CSF), it is hydrated and carbonic acid is formed. The acid then dissociates and hydrogen ions are liberated and as there are no proteins in the CSF to buffer the hydrogen ions, the pH of the CSF falls, which excites the central chemoreceptors and the respiratory rate is increased (Marieb *et al.* 2010).

Evidence-based approaches

Respiratory assessment

Once information about the person's past medical history has been obtained, one of the most reliable and important assessments is to closely observe and talk to the patient. During this time a patient's smoking status should be ascertained and, if appropriate, their smoking habits and the benefits of stopping should be discussed. For smoking cessation, brief interventions typically take about 5–10 minutes and may include one or more of the following.

- Simple opportunistic advice to stop.
- Assessment of patient's desire to stop.
- Offer of pharmacotherapy and/or behavioural support.
- Provision of self-help material and referral to more intensive support such as the NHS Stop Smoking Services.

Normal respiration is effortless and almost unconscious and the person can eat, drink and speak in full sentences without appearing breathless. Essential first steps in respiratory assessment are therefore to observe the person's breathing for the following.

- Ease and comfort.
- Rate.
- Pattern.
- Position the patient has adopted; for example, does the patient need to sit at 90° upright to breathe effectively?
- Rate and ease of breathing during speaking or movement.
- General colour and appearance: is there any evidence of greyness, cyanosis, pallor, sweating?
- Additional audible breath sounds: wheezing or stridor?

Having rapidly made this assessment, other essential assessments are a chest X-ray and arterial blood gas, and a computed tomography (CT) scan or ventilation/perfusion (V/Q) scan may also be necessary (see Chapter 13).

Having made a comprehensive assessment, the immediate cause of respiratory insufficiency should be corrected where possible. It is important to recognize that this may result from interruption to any part of respiration; for example, the patient may be in severe pain and appropriate pain management may improve their respiratory function, or conversely an opioid overdose may result in decreased or absent respiration and the antidote to the opioid will then need to be given. There may be a mechanical obstruction to respiration, such as an infective obstruction like epiglottitis, and the treatment is therefore directed at treating the infection whilst also oxygenating the patient.

Respiratory therapy therefore covers a wide area and will include any manipulation or management of alteration to any part of the respiratory tree. It may include pharmacological management including pain management, antidotes to drug toxicity, support and guidance on smoking cessation, antimicrobials for infections of the respiratory tract, respiratory stimulants, surgery to repair a ruptured diaphragm or to manage trauma, the insertion of a tracheostomy or chest drains, or a thoracoabdominal shunt for superior vena cava obstruction. Finally, positioning and physiotherapy play a major role in improving respiratory function.

Any person who is unable to maintain tissue oxygenation will need to receive supplemental oxygen until they are able to manage again on room air. This oxygen may be delivered in different ways depending on the severity of the condition and the level of hypoxia.

Oxygen therapy

Definition

Oxygen therapy is the administration of oxygen at concentrations greater than that in ambient air with the intention of treating or preventing the symptoms and manifestations of hypoxia.

Evidence-based approaches
Rationale
Indications

- Respiratory failure, of which there are two types, is characterized by problems with some or all of the four functions listed earlier Guyton and Hall 2006, Marieb et al. 2010, Tortora and Derrickson 2009).
  - Type 1, referred to as hypoxaemic respiratory failure (failure to oxygenate the tissues). The PaO_2 is <8 kPa (60 mmHg) while the carbon dioxide (PCO_2) is normal or low. Common causes include infectious conditions, pneumonia, pulmonary oedema and adult respiratory distress syndrome.
  - Type 2, referred to as hypercapnic (raised carbon dioxide) or respiratory pump failure. Alveolar ventilation is insufficient to excrete carbon dioxide accompanied by hypoxaemia (deficiency of oxygen in the arterial blood). The PCO_2 is >6 kPa (45 mmHg). Common causes include chronic obstructive pulmonary disease (COPD), chest wall deformities, drug overdose and chest injury.
- Acute myocardial infarction.
- Cardiac failure.
- Shock – haemorrhagic, bacteraemic and cardiogenic.
- Conditions in which there is a reduced ability to transport oxygen, for example anaemia.
- During anaesthesia.
- Postoperatively.
- Sleep apnoea.
- Severe pain.
- Asthma.
- Pulmonary embolus.
- Conditions that affect the neuromuscular control of breathing such as muscular dystrophy, Guillain–Barré.
- Severe trauma affecting the diaphragm, ribs, lungs or trachea.
- Tension pneumothorax.
- Pleural effusion.

537

Contraindications

No specific contraindications to oxygen therapy exist, but the following precautions or possible contraindications need to be considered.

- With increased PaO_2 ventilatory depression may occur in spontaneously breathing patients with elevated $PaCO_2$.
- With high flow of fractional inspired oxygen (FiO_2), absorption atelectasis, oxygen toxicity and/or depression of ciliary and/or leucocytic function may occur.
- Supplemental oxygen should be administered with caution to patients suffering from paraquat poisoning and those receiving bleomycin.
- During laser bronchoscopy, minimal levels of supplemental oxygen should be used to avoid intratracheal ignition.
- Fire hazard is increased in the presence of increased oxygen concentrations.
- Bacterial contamination associated with certain nebulization and humidification systems is a possible hazard (Kallstrom 2002).

Anticipated patient outcomes

Outcome is determined by clinical and physiological assessment to establish adequacy of the patient response to oxygen therapy.

Legal and professional issues

Competencies

Nursing staff must be trained to adequately administer oxygen therapy and their competency assessed. They should check and document that a device is being used appropriately and the flow is as prescribed and appropriate for the patient's needs. Nursing and physiotherapy staff may assess patients, initiate and monitor oxygen delivery systems within the prescribed parameters, except in emergencies when oxygen should be given first and documented later (NPSA 2009).

Preprocedural considerations

Before commencing oxygen therapy, it is essential that it should be prescribed. This should be in the form of parameters, for example 28–40% to keep saturations (sats) >92%. This will allow nursing staff to alter the oxygen setting to achieve the target saturations without requiring a change to the prescription on each occasion, as well as individualizing treatment to meet the patient's needs. The only exception to this situation is during immediate management of critical illness or emergency situations when oxygen should be given irrespective of it being formally prescribed (O'Driscoll et al. 2008). Regular pulse oximetry monitoring must be available in all clinical environments where oxygen may be administered. Oxygen therapy will need to be adjusted to achieve target saturations rather than giving a fixed dose to

all patients with the same disease. Nurses can make these adjustments without requiring a change to the prescription on each occasion. Most oxygen therapy will be from nasal cannulas rather than masks and will not be given to patients who are not hypoxaemic (except during critical illness).

Equipment

Oxygen is an odourless, tasteless, colourless, transparent gas that is slightly heavier than air. Oxygen supports combustion so there is always a danger of fire when oxygen is being used. The following safety measures should be remembered.

- Oil or grease around oxygen connections should be avoided.
- Alcohol, ether and other inflammatory liquids should be used with caution in the vicinity of oxygen.
- No electrical device must be used in or near an oxygen tent.
- Oxygen cylinders should be kept secure in an upright position and away from heat.
- There must be no smoking in the vicinity of oxygen.
- A fire extinguisher should be readily available.
- Care should be taken with high concentrations of oxygen when using the defibrillator in a cardiorespiratory arrest, or during elective cardioversion.

All oxygen delivery systems should be checked at least once per day. Care should be taken to avoid interruption of oxygen therapy in situations including ambulation or transport for procedures.

Oxygen delivery

Any oxygen delivery system will include these basic components.

- *Oxygen supply*, from either a piped supply or a portable cylinder. All medical gas cylinders have to conform to a standardized colour coding: oxygen cylinders are black with a white shoulder and are labelled 'Oxygen' or 'O_2'. Since 2004, small portable oxygen cylinders have been in use: these are totally white and are a C-size cylinder.
- A *reduction gauge*: to reduce the pressure to atmospheric pressure.
- *Flowmeter*: a device that controls the flow of oxygen in litres per minute.
- *Tubing*: disposable tubing of varying diameter and length.
- *Mechanism for delivery*: a mask or nasal cannulas.
- *Humidifier*: to warm and moisten the oxygen before administration.
- *Water trap* if humidifier in use.

Nasal cannulas

Nasal cannulas (Figure 10.3) consist of two plastic prongs that are inserted inside the anterior nares and supported on a light frame. Advantages to the patient are that they may seem

Figure 10.3 Nasal cannulas.

Figure 10.4 Simple semi-rigid plastic mask.

less claustrophobic and do not interfere with eating, drinking and communication (Fell and Boehm 1998). Nasal cannulas provide an alternative to a mask, but can be used only where the patient requires a low percentage of oxygen and are usually used with flow rates of 1–4 litres of oxygen per minute and provide approximately 28–35% oxygen (Table 10.1). They cannot be attached satisfactorily to an external humidification device but in many cases the oxygen will be humidified as it passes through the nasal passages into the trachea (Marieb *et al.* 2010). They are generally well tolerated and are useful postoperatively or where the patient requires minimal support and are also used in the chronic setting where a patient at home requires long-term oxygen therapy.

Simple semi-rigid plastic masks

Simple semi-rigid plastic masks (Figure 10.4) are low-flow masks which entrain the air from the atmosphere and therefore are able to deliver a variable oxygen percentage (anything from 21% to 60%) (Table 10.2). Large discrepancies between the delivered FiO_2 and the actual amount received by the patient will occur, dependent on the patient's rate and depth of breathing. These masks are useful for patients who need a higher percentage of oxygen temporarily whilst the cause for their hypoxia is treated. This type of mask may be worn for hours or several days, but they should be used in conjunction with a humidifier if used for more than 12 hours. If the patient requires 60% added oxygen or more,

this is the threshold for requiring more invasive respiratory support and expert help should be sought (NICE 2007).

Partial rebreathing masks

These are similar to the simple semi-rigid plastic masks with the addition of a reservoir bag, which allows the oxygen delivered to increase beyond 60%. During inspiration, the patient draws air and oxygen from the mask, bag and through the holes in the side of the mask. When the patient expires, the initial one-third of the expired gases will flow back into the reservoir bag. The expired gas is rich in oxygen and contains very little carbon dioxide. The patient is able to breathe the previously expired gas along with the oxygen from the source (Ball 2000).

Note: if the oxygen flow is too low, the carbon dioxide can accumulate in the reservoir bag and fail to meet the patient's requirements, resulting in an increase in carbon dioxide (Pierce 1995). This device should only be used in the presence of expert nursing and medical support and usually during emergency intervention or before more invasive ventilatory therapy is instituted.

Non-rebreathing mask

The semi-rigid mask (Figure 10.5) has the addition of a reservoir bag with a one-way valve between the reservoir bag and mask, preventing accumulation of expired gases in the reservoir bag and retention of carbon dioxide (Pierce 1995). Oxygen delivery of greater than 80% can be achieved (Ball 2000).

539

Table 10.1 Oxygen flow rates for nasal cannulas

Oxygen flow rate (L/min)	% Oxygen delivered
1	24
2	28
3	32
4	36
5	40
6	44

Table 10.2 Approximate oxygen concentration related to flow rates of semi-rigid masks

Oxygen flow rate (L/min)	% Oxygen delivered
2	24
4	35
6	50
8	55
10	60
12	65
15	70

Figure 10.5   Non-rebreathing mask.

Fixed performance masks or high-flow masks (Venturi-type masks)

With fixed performance masks (Figure 10.6) it is possible to achieve an unvarying mixture of gases and a known concentration of oxygen using the high air flow oxygen enrichment principle (Table 10.3). These masks derive their name from the Venturi barrel in which a relatively low flow rate of oxygen is forced through a narrow jet. There are side holes in the barrel and this jet allows the air to be drawn in at a high rate. As the mixture of gas created is at a flow rate above that of inspiration, the mixture will be constant (Foss 1990). There are many Venturi-type masks available, but the larger-capacity masks are the most accurate and therefore the safest when a known concentration of oxygen is required or when efficient elimination of carbon dioxide is essential, for example, to provide respiratory therapy for the patient with chronic respiratory disease (Fell and Boehm 1998).

Tracheostomy mask

Tracheostomy masks perform in a similar way to the simple semi-rigid plastic facemask. The mask is placed over the tracheostomy tube or stoma.

Figure 10.6   High-flow mask with Venturi barrel.

Table 10.3 Fixed performance mask oxygen flow rates

Oxygen flow rate (L/min)	% Oxygen delivered
2	24
6	31
8	35
10	40
15	60

T-piece circuit

The T-piece circuit is a simple, large-bore, non-rebreathing circuit which is attached directly to an endotracheal or tracheostomy tube (Figure 10.7B). Humidified oxygen is delivered through one part of the T and expired gases leave through the other part. This device may be used as part of the weaning process when a patient has been ventilated previously by a mechanical ventilator (Bersten *et al.* 2009).

Figure 10.7   (A) Oxygen analyser. (B) T-piece. (C) Oxygen (elephant) tubing. (D) Warm bath humidifier. (E) Flow generator oxygen and air drager bellows.

Assessment and recording tools

Clinical assessment including but not limited to cardiac, pulmonary and neurological status is essential. Observations for respiratory rate, oxygen saturation, heart rate and blood pressure need to be recorded on observation charts as well as documenting the oxygen flow rate and method of delivery, for example mask or nasal cannulas. Other assessment methods include arterial blood gas sampling within a critical care environment or for a patient with acute deterioration (NICE 2007).

Pharmacological support

Oxygen cylinders and equipment may be ordered from the pharmacy whilst other medical equipment comes from external sources via stores and needs to be ordered before stocks run out to ensure ready availability in the event of an emergency. Nebulizers and broncholitic agents may improve respiratory status.

Domiciliary oxygen and portable oxygen

Some patients are so disabled by chronic respiratory disease that they require continual supplementary oxygen at home. Low-flow oxygen given over a period of time improves the prognosis of some patients (Benditt 2000).

Long-term oxygen may be prescribed for treatment of COPD, cystic fibrosis, interstitial lung disease, neuromuscular and skeletal disorders, pulmonary hypertension and palliation in lung cancer. It may be provided in the form of cylinders. The problem with this is that the cylinders need changing frequently. Oxygen condensers (concentrators) are far more economical than cylinders. A condenser consists of a compressor powered by electricity. The condenser works by drawing in room air that is passed through a bacterial filter and a sieve bed. The sieve bed contains zeolite which has an affinity with nitrogen and when under pressure works by removing nitrogen and other gases, concentrating oxygen and delivering it through a meter at the front of the compressor.

The oxygen can be delivered to the patient by nasal cannulas or mask (Esmond 2001).

Liquid oxygen

The use of liquid oxygen in a portable cylinder has been developed for portable oxygen delivery. The patient is provided with a large tank in their own home from which smaller cylinders can be filled.

Specific patient preparations

Oxygen delivery to the patient should be explained, including what equipment is to be used (such as a mask or nasal cannula) and the importance of keeping the apparatus in place. The patient should know of the flammability of oxygen and the dangers of any naked flames/lit cigarettes in their immediate vicinity. The nurse should instruct the patient to notify him or her of increasing distress, air hunger, nausea, anxiety, dry nasal passages or 'sore throat' (due to drying).

541

Procedure guideline 10.1 Oxygen therapy

Essential equipment

- Piped/wall oxygen and medical air
- Oxygen flow meter/regulator
- Oxygen cylinders for transport of patients
- Ambu-bag for emergencies
- Nasal cannulas
- Selection of oxygen masks
- Oxygen tubing, varying lengths and types
- Oxygen analysers

Optional equipment

- Non-invasive equipment in non-critical care areas (essential within critical care environments)
- High-flow O_2 and medical air mixers for use in HDU setting
- Humidification equipment
- Cold water bubble humidifiers

Medicinal products

- Asthma inhalers or nebulizers
- Oxygen as prescribed for patient
- Nicotine patches to aid smoking cessation

Preprocedure

Action	Rationale
1 Assess the patient's condition and level of oxygen therapy required, e.g. facemask, humidified oxygenation, nasal cannulas.	To ensure that the appropriate method for delivery of oxygen is chosen to suit the patient's condition (O'Driscoll et al. 2008, C).

(Continued)

Procedure guideline 10.1 (*Continued*)

2 Explain to the patient why they require oxygen therapy and the benefits and problems thereof.	To minimize apprehension and anxiety and improve understanding of treatment. E
3 Attach oxygen tubing to the correct port on the wall oxygen or cylinder, and not to the medical air port.	To ensure proper oxygen delivery and prevent hypoxia if connected to medical air port (NPSA 2007, C).
Procedure	
4 Set oxygen flowmeter to required setting (L/min) and check oxygen is flowing through system by using fingertips.	To ensure system is working properly. E
5 **Either:** *Apply a nasal cannula* by gently placing the nasal prongs of the cannula into the patient's nostrils, draping the tubing over the patient's ears and sliding the fit connector up under the chin to hold the tubing securely in place. **Or:** *Apply an oxygen mask* by placing the mask over the patient's mouth and nose, then pull the elastic strap over the head and adjust the strap on both sides to secure the mask in a position that seals it against the face.	To ensure the mask or cannula is applied correctly to enable the patient to receive the oxygen. E
Postprocedure	
6 Check that the patient is comfortable.	To ensure patient comfort. E
7 Record that oxygen therapy has been commenced, time and flow rate.	To maintain accurate records (NMC 2009, C).

Problem-solving table 10.1 Prevention and resolution (Procedure guideline 10.1)

Problem	Cause	Prevention	Suggested action
Maintenance of airway	Position of patient Airway secretions	Provide pillows to support patient Elevate head of bed Demonstrate to patient orthopnoeic position Provide sputum pot for expectoration Saline nebulizers if prescribed to loosen secretions	Position patient preferably sitting up at an angle of greater than 45° Encourage patient to cough and expectorate if able or remove secretions by suction if patient unable to do so
Maintenance of adequate oxygenation	Inadequate oxygen delivery, patient's condition deteriorating More breathless Oxygen saturation decreased Deteriorating blood gases	Increased frequency and recording of cardiovascular observations and respiration rate Attach pulse oximeter Use of MEWS scoring	Assess level of oxygen support required by assessing previous medical history and current respiratory assessment. Increase oxygen delivery using the lowest percentage of oxygen to achieve the individual goal for the patient
Dry mouth	Oxygen therapy can lead to a dry mouth	Provide regular mouthcare or artificial saliva if prescribed	Add humidification to the circuit (see Procedure guideline 10.2). Give regular mouthcare

Problem	Cause	Prevention	Suggested action
Nasal cannulas or mask discomfort	Position or use of cannulas and oxygen mask	Use appropriate size mask	Ensure correct placement and that the patient is comfortable. Cut off tip of cannulas that protrude into nares to a comfortable length
Intolerance of oxygen therapy	Fear and anxiety Confusion Hypoxia	Explain need for therapy and benefit it will have Allow patients to express their fears/concerns Encourage relatives/carers to stay with patient	Assess patient for change. Ensure continual reassurance given to patient. Ensure patient remains orientated to the environment and oxygen device. If intolerant of mask, nasal cannulas may be tolerated. If hypoxic, oxygen may need to be increased
Inability to communicate	Mask makes communication difficult; patient may not hear carer and nurse may not hear patient	Provide patient with non-verbal means of communication, either pen and paper or symbol board	Assist patient to move around bed area if not able to go far. Mobilize patient with portable oxygen cylinder if appropriate
Inability to maintain personal hygiene	Immobility On bed rest Mask restricting independence	Provide patient with hygiene wipes or offer assistance if unable to meet own hygiene needs	Provide reassurance for patient to remain independent where able. Allow them to carry out their own hygiene if able or help patient with hygiene if not
Inability to maintain safe environment	Detachment of oxygen from flowmeter Kinked or looped oxygen tubing Mask removed by patient	Pulse oximeter with audible alarm	Ensure oxygen attached to flowmeter. Check patient regularly. Ensure no kinks or loops arise. Ensure patient is attached to oxygen

543

Postprocedural considerations

Immediate care

Consider talking to the patient and the family with regard to assisting patient if they remove the mask for a drink, how to put the mask back on and possible psychological issues regarding feeling claustrophobic with the mask, and the reasons for oxygen therapy. Document what percentage of oxygen was commenced and the patient's related observations, and continue to monitor the patient's respiratory status.

Ongoing care

For patients requiring oxygen therapy for more than 24 hours, humidification should be commenced to protect airway defences (Carroll 1997, Ward and Park 2000) as well as general comfort of the patient. Mobilizing patients sitting out in chairs rather than lying or even sitting up in bed will help prevent atelectasis and aid removal of secretions. Ensuring that postoperative patients have effective pain relief will allow for early ambulation, as well as deep breathing and other basic exercises which will help prevent postoperative atelectasis or possible chest infections (Shelledy and Mikles 2002). Preoperative education from physiotherapists and nursing staff about the benefits of these exercises and reinforcement postopera-

tively will also be of benefit. Accurate and frequent monitoring of vital signs and recording of observations as well as oxygen concentration and flow rates administered to the patient in conjunction with a Modified Early Warning System (MEWS) score allows for early identification and referral of patients at risk of deterioration (NICE 2007).

Documentation

Baseline vital signs and oxygen flow rates or concentrations administered as well as the patient's response to therapy must be recorded (NICE 2007).

Education of patient and relevant others

Patients should be educated regarding the necessity of keeping their oxygen masks on, and ambulatory patients must recommence oxygen with the help of nurses after mobilizing.

Before sending a patient home on oxygen, healthcare providers must be sure the patient and family members understand the dangers of smoking in an oxygen-enriched environment. An increased amount of oxygen in the environment increases the speed at which things burn once a fire starts. Oxygen can saturate clothing, fabric, hair, beards and anything in the area. Even flame-retardant clothing can burn when the oxygen content increases. It is important to keep all flames and heat sources away from oxygen containers and oxygen systems. Patients should be advised never to smoke or light a match while using oxygen or allow others in the same room to do so. Patients should also be advised not to smoke in bed. Every home should have at least one working smoke detector on every level and near all bedrooms. As many people on home oxygen therapy have limited mobility, home sprinkler systems can add an extra layer of protection (www.fireservice.co.uk/safety/smokealarms.php). They also need to inform their home and car insurers that oxygen therapy will be used, as well as the local Fire Brigade. They should also be reassured that a full written package of training on safe use and storage of equipment will be provided by the contractor supplying their home oxygen.

Nurses in primary and community care should advise everyone who smokes to try to stop and refer them to an intensive support service (for example, NHS Stop Smoking Services). If they are unwilling or unable to accept this referral they should be offered pharmacotherapy, in line with NICE guidance, and additional support. Nurses who are trained NHS Stop Smoking counsellors may 'refer' to themselves where appropriate. The smoking status of those who are not ready to stop should be recorded and reviewed with the individual once a year, where possible. The NICE recommendations include the following advice.

- Ask patients who smoke how interested they are in stopping.
- If they want to stop, refer them to an intensive support service such as NHS Stop Smoking Services.
- If they are unwilling or unable to accept a referral, offer a stop smoking aid (for example, nicotine replacement therapy (NRT), varenicline or bupropion).
- A range of NHS agencies can offer advice and support on how to stop smoking.
- Monitoring systems should be set up so that health professionals know whether or not their patients smoke (NICE 2006).

Complications

Carbon dioxide narcosis

Carbon dioxide is the chemical that most directly influences respiration by its effect on the efficiency of alveolar ventilation. The normal partial pressure of carbon dioxide in the blood is 4.0–6.0 kPa (30–45 mmHg). When this level rises, the pH of the CSF drops which in turn causes excitation of the central chemoreceptors, and hyperventilation occurs (Marieb *et al.* 2010).

In people who always retain carbon dioxide and are therefore usually hypercapnic because of chronic pulmonary disease such as chronic bronchitis, the chemoreceptors are no longer sensitive to a raised level of carbon dioxide. In these cases the falling PaO_2 becomes the principal respiratory stimulus (the hypoxic drive) (Marieb *et al.* 2010). There-

fore, if a high level of supplementary oxygen was delivered to such patients in non-emergency situations severe respiratory depression would ensue and ultimately unconsciousness and death. The Resuscitation Council UK and British Thoracic Society advise the administration of high-flow oxygen during an acute respiratory distress or arrest situation. Start with 15 litres of oxygen per minute and wean down to the flow rate required to maintain adequate peripheral saturations of 94–98% (BTS 2008).

Oxygen toxicity

Pulmonary toxicity following prolonged higher percentages of oxygen therapy is recognized clinically, but there is still much to be learnt about the condition. The degree of injury is related to the length of time of exposure and percentage of oxygen to which the individual is exposed. The pattern is one of decreasing lung compliance as a result of a sequence of events, tracheal bronchial inflammation, haemorrhagic interstitial and intra-alveolar oedema, leading ultimately to fibrosis (Bersten *et al.* 2009, Pierce 1995, Pierson 2000).

Where possible, long periods (i.e. 24 hours or more) of oxygen therapy above 50% should be avoided (Bryan-Brown and Dracup 2000, Cooper 2002).

Retrolental fibroplasia

Retrolental fibroplasia is a disease affecting premature babies that weigh under 1200 g (about 28 weeks' gestation) if they are exposed to high concentrations of oxygen within the first 3–4 weeks of life. It appears that the oxygen stimulates immature blood vessels in the eye to vasoconstrict and obliterate, which results in neovascularization, accompanied by haemorrhage, fibrosis and then retinal detachment and blindness (Bersten *et al.* 2009, Pierce 1995).

Humidification

Definitions

Humidity is the amount of water vapour present in a gas. The terms used to define humidity are absolute humidity, maximum capacity and relative humidity. Absolute humidity is the mass of water vapour that a given volume of gas can carry at a set temperature. When a gas is at its maximum capacity, it is said to be fully saturated. Relative humidity is the ratio of the absolute humidity to the maximum capacity. The warmer the gas, the more vapour it can hold but if the temperature of the gas falls, water held as vapour will condense out of the gas into the surrounding atmosphere.

Anatomy and physiology

The respiratory tract is lined with ciliated epithelial cells that secrete mucus. Each cell has about 200 hair-like structures known as cilia, whose role is to remove unwanted mucus and secretions. Less than optimal humidification results in the slowing of the mucociliary transport system and pooling of mucus in the lower airways. Pooling of mucus may obstruct a small airway, restricting gas exchange. Pools of mucus also provide an ideal site for bacterial colonization. If less than optimal humidification continues, cell damage occurs and gas conditioning moves deeper into the lung (Estes and Meduri 1995).

Related theory

Normal room air has an approximate temperature of 22°C with a relative humidity of 50% and a water content of 10 mgH$_2$O. For effective gas exchange to occur in the lungs, the air would need to be at a temperature of 37°C with 100% humidity and a water content of 44 mgH$_2$O per litre by the time it reaches the bifurcation in the trachea, which is referred to as the isothermic point. When the temperature falls below 37°C and humidity falls below 100%, several changes take place in the airways. With a drop in temperature and humidity, the mucus that collects in the airways thickens and movement of the cilia is reduced. If there is no improvement the mucus will become thicker and immobile; the cilia will also lose their mobility so clearance of all secretions will stop and infection can set in (Marieb *et al.* 2008).

If there is a continuing lack of humidity further damage occurs. The cilia can break off, causing damage to the mucosal lining of the respiratory tract. The isothermic point of saturation moves from the bifurcation of the trachea to a lower point in the lungs, resulting in further damage which can lead to collapse of the alveoli, decrease in lung function and hypoxaemia (Carroll 1997, Fell and Boehm 1998, Ward and Park 2000).

Evidence-based approaches

Many devices can be used to supply humidification; the best of these will fulfil the following requirements.

- The inspired gas must be delivered to the trachea at a room temperature of 32–36°C with 100% humidity and should have a water content of 33–43 g/m^3 (Bersten *et al.* 2009).
- The set temperature should remain constant; humidification and temperature should not be affected by large ranges of flow.
- The device should have a safety and alarm system to guard against overheating, overhydration and electric shocks.
- It is important that the appliance should not increase resistance or affect the compliance of respiration.
- It is essential that whichever device is selected, wide-bore tubing (elephant tubing) is used to allow efficient formation of water vapour (Figure 10.7C).

Rationale

Inhalation of oxygen used during respiratory therapy, which is a dry gas, can cause evaporation of water from the respiratory tract and lead to the damage of mucosal lining if humidification is not provided. In patients who are intubated or have a tracheostomy, the natural pathway of humidification is bypassed (Wilson 1996).

Indications

- Used for mechanical ventilation and non-invasive ventilation such as continuous positive airway pressure (CPAP)/non-invasive positive end expiration (NIPEE).

Contraindications

- There are no contraindications to humidification, though the device chosen will depend upon type of oxygen therapy, tenacity of secretions, and the patient's clinical condition (i.e. mechanical ventilation, self-ventilating at home, etc.).
- Humidification should not be used for patients requiring open system (mask) ventilation when 'droplet contact' isolation precautions are required.

Anticipated patient outcomes

The provision of adequate humidification of gases enabling clearance of secretions, a reduction in the tenacity of secretions, and improved gas exchange. The patient's airway is to remain patent at all times.

Preprocedural considerations
Equipment
Heat and moisture exchanger (HME)

During ventilatory humidification an HME performs the function of the nose and pharynx in conditioning the inspired air. It retains heat and moisture in the expired air and returns them to the patient in the next inspired breath. Many HMEs contain a bacterial filter. The HME consists of spun, pleated, highly thermal conductive material. It is also known as an artificial or 'Swedish' nose (Figure 10.8). It can be used in a self-ventilating patient with a tracheostomy who is being weaned from oxygen (Figure 10.9). It can also be used in ventilated patients, inserted between the patient's airway and the ventilator circuit.

Cold water bubble humidifier

This device delivers partially humidified oxygen at about 50% relative humidity. Gas is either forced across or bubbled through water at room temperature (Figure 10.10). This method is not advised as it is inefficient (Bersten *et al.* 2009).

Figure 10.8   Swedish nose.

Water bath humidifiers

With these devices, inspired gas is forced over or through a heated reservoir of water (Figure 10.7D). To achieve an adequate humidity for the patient, the water bath must reach a set temperature. The gas will then cool as it moves down the breathing circuit to the patient, and a relative humidity of 100% will be reached. Hot water bath humidifiers

Figure 10.10   Cold water bubble humidifier.

Figure 10.9   Heat and moisture exchanger.

are therefore very efficient and useful for humidification for immobile patients, particularly if they are receiving mechanical ventilatory support. However, they have four main disadvantages.

- Danger of overheating and causing damage to the trachea.
- Their efficiency can alter with changes in gas flow rate, surface area and the water temperature.
- Condensation and collection of water in the oxygen delivery tubes.
- The possibility of microcontamination of stagnant water (Tinker and Zapol 1992).

Aerosol generators

These devices are not governed by temperature, but provide microdroplets of water suspended in the gas (Bersten *et al.* 2009). The gas provided through aerosol devices can be very highly saturated with water. There are three main types of aerosol humidifier.

- Gas-drive nebulizer
- Mechanical (spinning disc) nebulizer
- Ultrasonic nebulizer

These devices are useful for the spontaneously breathing patient with chronic chest disease.

Procedure guideline 10.2 Humidification for respiratory therapy

Various humidifiers exist. Select the system most appropriate for the patient.

Essential equipment

- Bath humidifier
- Heating equipment
- Oxygen (elephant) tubing (Figure 10.7C)
- Oxygen analyser (Figure 10.7A)
- Sterile H_2O bottle or bag depending on type of humidifier used

Preprocedure

Action	Rationale
1 Discuss with patient's doctor the choice of system to be used.	To ensure the most appropriate device is selected to meet the patient's needs. E
2 Explain to patient the reason for use of the humidifier and how it works.	To enable the patient to understand what is happening and to able to tolerate the humidification. E

Procedure

3 Prepare the device to be used (although some circuits are ready prepared with humidifier). (a) Prepare humidifier and circuit.	To ensure the circuit is in working condition and patent to oxygen flow. E
(b) Attach humidifier/wide-bore oxygen tubing: ensure minimal length of tubing, water trap and mask.	Connecting all equipment to oxygen and mask and ensuring all connections are secure. E
4 Once circuit is set up, run the system to check it is functioning correctly and the circuit is intact and check oxygen delivered through oxygen analyser.	To ensure that oxygen is being delivered through the circuit as set. E To ensure the system is humidifying the oxygen and that no leaks exist (MDA 2000, C).
5 If the hot water system is in use, check it is running within recommended temperature range and attach to patient.	To ensure no damage to the patient's lungs if temperature above range. E
6 Check water is present in water source of system; do not allow to run dry.	To aid adequate delivery of humidity to the patient and prevent damage to the humidifier. E
7 Position the circuit tubing below the patient.	To ensure collection of humidity in the circuit is able to drain into the water trap or circuit rather than into the patient. E
8 Ask the patient if they find the humidification comfortable.	To ensure patient comfort. E

Postprocedure

9 Monitor the running of the system.	To ensure the system is functioning adequately and delivering humidity (MDA 2000, C).
10 Reassure the patient as they may find the system noisy and the excessive moisture in the circuit difficult to cope with.	To allow patient to adjust to the feel of the mask, preventing anxiety and panic at the initial increase of work of breathing (Moser and Chung 2003, C).
11 Assess the tenacity of secretions on a regular basis, and document all findings.	To assess how effective the choice of humidification device has been (E). This will enable the same care to be carried on or an alternative method to be evaluated. Documentation is imperative to the multidisciplinary approach to allow for ongoing best practice (Woodrow 2002, E).
12 Change the humidification and circuit on a weekly basis, and document.	To prevent contamination of equipment and minimize the risk of infection (Demers 2002, E).

547

Problem-solving table 10.2 Prevention and resolution (Procedure guideline 10.2)

Problem	Cause	Prevention	Suggested action
Potential blockage of humidifier	Kinking of oxygen tubing or secretions in humidification filter	Change filter 4–6 hourly or more frequently for patients with copious secretions Administer saline nebulizers if prescribed to loosen secretions Check tubing not kinked underneath the patient	Encourage patient to cough and expectorate if able or remove secretions by suction if patient unable to do so Ensure tubing is not too long which would allow kinking

Complications

Possible contamination of water in humidification if tubing collects water and it is reintroduced into the humidification chamber. This chamber provides the perfect environment for contaminants to grow as it is moist and warm (Demers 2002).

Continuous positive airway pressure

Definition

Continuous positive airway pressure (CPAP) therapy is the maintenance of a positive airway pressure greater than ambient pressure throughout inspiration and expiration. It can be delivered through a facemask, nasal mask or mouthpiece, or through an endotracheal or tracheostomy tube (Bersten *et al.* 2009).

Related theory

Use of the CPAP circuit dates back at least to 1912, when Bunnell used a primitive circuit during thoracic surgery. The first recorded use in intensive care was by Poulton and Oxon in 1936. In the 1940s increased interest in CPAP was prompted by research into respiratory support in high altitude flying. Further developments occurred in the 1950s and 1960s, and in 1976 Greenbaum *et al.* reported the use of CPAP with a facemask in adult respiratory distress syndrome. In 1972 Williamson and Modell successfully used CPAP for selected spontaneously breathing patients with acute respiratory failure. For treatment of acute pulmonary oedema, CPAP alone is very effective (Gorini *et al.* 2004, Gray *et al.* 2009, Nehyba 2007).

Non-invasive ventilation

Non-invasive ventilation refers to mechanical ventilatory support applied without an artificial airway (endotracheal tube or tracheostomy). It can be delivered to the patient via a nasal or facemask. The patient must be conscious and co-operative

for this type of ventilation to be effective. It is particularly useful in patients with chronic respiratory disease.

- In restrictive pulmonary disease, for example muscular dystrophy.
- In progressive neuromuscular disease, for example motor neurone disease.
- In obstructive pulmonary disease, for example COPD, bronchiectasis, cystic fibrosis.
- In nocturnal hypoventilation.
- In patients with acute exacerbation of chronic respiratory disease.
- In patients in whom endotracheal intubation and ventilation may not be considered appropriate or where difficulties may be anticipated in weaning a patient from a ventilator.

Non-invasive ventilators generally fall into two categories (Esmond 2001):

- pressure preset machines
- volume preset machines.

Mechanical ventilation

A mechanical ventilator is a device used to replace or assist breathing in order for satisfactory gas exchange to take place. The decision to ventilate a patient will be made after careful clinical examination, including assessment of respiratory mechanics, oxygenation and ventilation.

Ventilators are able to control tidal volume, respiratory rate, time of inspiration against time of expiration, inspired flow rate and inspired oxygen concentration (Bersten *et al.* 2009, Hinds and Watson 2008, Pierce 1995, West 2008).

Ventilators are divided into two main categories: negative pressure and positive pressure.

Negative pressure ventilators

These devices are now rarely used. They mimic normal breathing (negative pressure) and are known as iron lungs. The patient is enclosed in an airtight tank and a negative pressure is created by a separate pump which causes the

548

alveolar pressure to fall within the lungs so a pressure gradient results, with air flowing into the lungs along the pressure gradient in order for ventilation to take place. An adaptation from the tank ventilator is the cuirass shell, which surrounds the thorax and abdomen and works on the same principle. The rare use of these devices would be in patients with chronic respiratory failure (neuromuscular disease, skeletal deformity or sleep-related respiratory problems).

Positive pressure ventilators

These devices provide a satisfactory gas exchange when inflating the lungs with a positive pressure via an endotracheal tube or tracheostomy.

Positive pressure ventilators have four main functions to perform during each respiratory cycle.

- Inflate the lungs.
- Cycle from inspiration to expiration.
- Allow expiration to take place.
- Cycle from expiration to inspiration.

They have a driving mechanism and can cycle from one phase of the respiratory cycle to another by a preset pressure, preset time or preset volume.

Varying modes of ventilation can be used.

- Intermittent mandatory ventilation (IMV).
- Pressure support.
- Pressure control.
- Simulated intermittent mandatory ventilation (SIMV).
- Continuous positive airway pressure (CPAP).

Hyperbaric respiratory therapy

Hyperbaric respiratory therapy is used mainly in the treatment of carbon monoxide poisoning, burns, gas gangrene, skin lesions, soft tissue injury, decompression sickness (the bends) and multiple sclerosis. The therapy is designed to give 100% oxygen at a range of pressures greater than atmospheric pressure. Oxygen is dissolved in the plasma, increasing the oxygen tension in the tissues (Bersten *et al.* 2009).

Evidence-based approaches

The aim of CPAP therapy is to improve gas exchange (oxygen and carbon dioxide) within the lungs and improve the work of breathing. CPAP is able to do this by:

- *Increasing the functional residual capacity* (FRC), which is the amount of gas left in the lungs at the end of normal expiration available for pulmonary gas exchange. In acute lung injury where gaseous exchange is severely inhibited, CPAP increases the FRC by improving ventilation in poorly or non-ventilated alveoli (Miller and Semple 1991).
- *Improving the ventilation/perfusion ratio.* Decreased intrapulmonary shunting with hypoxia could cause ventilation to the lungs to be reduced or blood flow to them

impaired. Intrapulmonary shunting can then occur with underventilation of the lungs. CPAP helps to decrease the intrapulmonary shunting by improving the ventilation-to-perfusion mismatch (Lenique *et al.* 1997).
- *Improved lung compliance (elasticity) of the lungs.* In respiratory failure the lungs become much stiffer and less compliant and breathing can become more difficult. Reduction in lung volume below a certain level results in airway collapse and underventilation. The pressure required to overcome this can be achieved by CPAP.
- *Increasing lung volume (alveolar volume)* for gaseous exchange to take place. The factors above enable the work of breathing to be reduced plus a decrease in the percentage of oxygen that might be required.

Rationale

Continuous positive airway pressure is the maintenance of a positive pressure throughout the whole respiratory cycle when breathing spontaneously. CPAP provides an additional therapy between conventional oxygen therapy and controlled ventilation. It helps prevent atelectasis, reduce the work of breathing and eliminate or reduce hypoxia whilst allowing the normalization of the FRC (Ashurst 1995, Place 1997, Romand and Donald 1995).

Indications

Continuous positive airway pressure is usually commenced to improve lung expansion. CPAP is also indicated in the the presence of clinically significant pulmonary atelectasis when other forms of therapy, such as incentive spirometry, chest physiotherapy and deep breathing exercises, have been unsuccessful.

- Acute respiratory failure.
- Hypercapnic acute respiratory failure.
- Acute exacerbation of COPD.
- Postextubation difficulty.
- Weaning difficulties.
- Postsurgical respiratory failure.
- Thoracic wall deformities.
- Cystic fibrosis.
- Status asthmaticus.
- Acute respiratory failure in obesity hypoventilation syndrome.
- Chronic respiratory failure.
- Immunocompromised patients.
- Patients 'not for intubation'.
- Hypoxaemic acute respiratory failure (Ram *et al.* 2004).

Contraindications

- Recurrent pneumothoraces/untreated pneumothorax – may contribute to barotraumas.
- Severe postoperative pulmonary air leak.
- Central apnoea.
- Epistaxis.

Figure 10.11 CPAP mask and helmet.

- Any condition where an elevated intracranial pressure is undesirable or where reduction in cerebral blood flow is inappropriate (Kolbitsch *et al*. 2000).
- Any situation where there is already significant lung overdistension.
- Unstable facial fractures, extensive facial surgery or lacerations and facial burns.
- Laryngeal trauma, recent tracheal anastomosis.
- Recent ear, nose and throat surgery.
- Basilar skull fracture – at risk of pneumocephalus.

Note: The last four contraindications listed are specific to mask CPAP and not necessarily to helmet CPAP) (Kolbitsch *et al*. 2000).

Methods of delivering CPAP

Continuous positive airway pressure can be delivered by mask or helmet as illustrated in Figure 10.11.

Anticipated patient outcomes

- Ability to wean patient off CPAP mask and improvement of respiratory status with lower oxygen requirements.
- For lung expansion therapy, a minimum delivered tidal volume of at least one-third of the predicted inspiratory capacity (IC) (1/3 × 50 mL/kg) has been suggested. This corresponds to approximately 1200 mL in a 70 kg adult patient (Shelledy & Mikles 2002).
- An increase in peak flow.
- Cough more effective with treatment and secretion clearance enhanced as a consequence of deep breathing and coughing.

- Chest radiograph improved.
- Breath sounds improved (Sorenson and Shelledy 2003).

Legal and professional issues

Competencies

Close and thorough clinical assessment is of paramount importance when caring for a patient receiving CPAP or non-invasive ventilation (NIV). Physiological monitoring is not a substitute for clinical assessment and observation of the patient on the ventilator should be carried out regularly. Therefore nursing staff caring for patients requiring CPAP ventilation would need to be trained in advanced respiratory care or work in areas such as the HDU or CCU setting (Kinnear 2002).

Preprocedural considerations

Care of patients with CPAP should be provided in HDU or CCU settings with cardiac and respiratory monitoring equipment. CPAP should be considered only with a co-operative patient who can control their airway and secretions with an adequate cough reflex. The patient should be able to co-ordinate breathing with the ventilator and breathe unaided for several minutes if CPAP is delivered via a ventilator (Sorenson and Shelledy 2003).

Equipment

- Flow generator with variable flow such as Whisper Flo. A means of generating a flow of pressurized breathable gas at variable rates and oxygen concentrations.
- CPAP mask (two-port type) or CPAP helmet with securing straps (see Figure 10.11).
- Bacterial-viral filter (*not* an HME) (see Figure 10.12). Provides protection against various types of particles including bacteria, viruses and water droplets. The filter helps protect the patient, the equipment and the breathing circuit from contamination.
- Aerosol tubing.
- Oxygen analyser and T-piece (see Figure 10.7).
- CPAP positive end-expiratory pressure (PEEP) valve of prescribed level (Figure 10.13).

Figure 10.12 Bacterial-viral filter.

Figure 10.13   CPAP valves.

- Higher rated CPAP valve (+20 cmH₂O) (Figure 10.13) and T-piece (if using Whisper Flo device).
- Warm bath (heated wire) humidifier (Figure 10.7D). Warms and humidifies inspired gas to core temperature and 100% relative humidity, which maximizes mucociliary clearance and prevents inflammatory reactions while sustaining airway patency and lung compliance (Williams *et al*. 1996.) (If humidifier is used a patient section and 1 litre bag of water for inhalation will be required.) In some departments a complete circuit is available with all of the disposable items provided in one kit.

Assessment and recording tools

While on CPAP it is essential to monitor the patient's cardiovascular status, respiratory rate, pulse oximetery and fluid balance at least hourly as well as regular arterial blood gas (ABG) sampling.

Clinical features that should be assessed are:

- chest wall movement
- co-ordination of respiratory effort with the ventilator
- accessory muscle recruitment
- general assessment – patient sweating/clammy/dyspnoeic
- auscultation of the chest
- patient comfort
- neurological status – signs of confusion/tiredness.

The patient receiving NIV or CPAP should be fully monitored:

- heart rate and rhythm
- respiratory rate
- blood pressure
- oxygen saturation measured by pulse oximetry (SpO₂).

It has been reported that oxygen levels improve rapidly on NIV so it is important to measure SpO₂ continuously in the first 24 hours, aiming to keep it >95% with supplemental O₂ (Kinnear 2002, Sorenson and Shelledy 2003). All the above observations need to be documented on the observation chart or HDU observation chart as applicable.

Pharmacological support

Diuretics may be given if pulmonary oedema is present. In some extreme cases small doses of anxiolytics may be given to combat the distress caused by CPAP therapy. This will require increased levels of monitoring to ensure patient safety (Allison 1991, Keen 2000, Lenique *et al*. 1997).

Non-pharmacological support

In some patients the presence of a relative, nurse or healthcare assistant may alleviate the distress caused by CPAP.

Specific patient preparations
Education

Continuous positive airway pressure can cause distress to patients due especially to the tight-fitting mask, while the hood can seem claustrophobic. If possible, a clear and concise description of how the therapy works should be provided either verbally or via an information leaflet. As with any procedure, consent needs to be gained before treatment can commence. Allow time for the patient to express any concerns/fears they have regarding treatment. Acutely hypoxic patients may not comprehend the relevance of the therapy and so it should be explained to their relative/carer so they can reassure the patient (DH 2002, Moser and Chung 2003).

551

Procedure guideline 10.3 Continuous positive airway pressure

Essential equipment

- Drager bellows or similar high-flow oxygen delivery system (see Figure 10.7)
- Compressed air supply
- CPAP helmet or mask
- CPAP circuit
- Humidification system (mask only) with temperature control

- Flowmeter
- Oxygen analyser
- Pulse oximetry
- Nasogastric tube
- Urinary catheter

(Continued)

Procedure guideline 10.3 (*Continued*)

Preprocedure

Action	Rationale
1 Assess patient's conscious level.	To obtain a baseline and to be able to assess for change in condition (see Chapter 13). E
2 Explain the principles of CPAP to the patient and family and demonstrate the system to them. Observe and record the following:	To gain consent, minimize anxiety, increase knowledge and aid in patient compliance. E
(a) Patient's respiratory function	To obtain a baseline of respiratory function. E
(b) Respiratory rate	To observe for any change in respiratory function. E
(c) Work of breathing	A reduction in level of consciousness or altered mental status may indicate hypoxaemia. E
(d) Colour, skin, and mental status	
(e) Tissue oxygen saturation (SaO_2).	
3 Decide whether it is appropriate to insert an arterial cannula.	In order to monitor the acid/base balance. E
4 Observe and record the patient's cardiovascular function, including:	To obtain a baseline in order to assess any change in conditions (see Chapter 13). E
(a) Heart rate	
(b) Blood pressure	
(c) Temperature	
(d) Central venous pressure (if patient has a central venous access device).	
5 Assess fluid balance:	To obtain a baseline of fluid balance.
(a) Input	To enable assessment of dehydration or fluid overload (Keen 2000, C).
(b) Output	
(c) Accumulative balance	
(d) Overall fluid balance	
(e) Daily weight.	
6 Assess patient's level of anxiety and compliance with treatment (the patient's ability to cope with the treatment).	To enable an assessment to be made and an evaluation of the suitability of CPAP therapy. E

Procedure

7 Set up CPAP circuit.	
8 Ensure patient is in a comfortable position, sitting up in bed at a 45° angle or more or in a chair well supported by a pillow.	To promote comfort and aid lung expansion and breathing (Fell and Boehm 1998, C).
9 Explain to patient how the helmet or mask is to be applied.	To relieve anxiety and to reassure patient. E To aid patient's compliance with CPAP. E
10 Apply helmet/mask gently, applying pressure as the patient adapts to the tight-fitting mask. Hold mask until patient is comfortable and settled.	To relieve anxiety and to reassure patient. E To aid patient's compliance with CPAP. E
11 Once the patient is settled with mask/helmet, apply the head strap or shoulder straps. Ensure mask/helmet and head strap are comfortable for the patient; alter position as required.	To retain mask in place and aid patient comfort (Keilty and Bott 1992, E).
12 Ensure a good seal and that no leaks are present.	To ensure a tight seal in order that the system functions optimally (Greenbaum *et al.* 1976, C).

| 13 | Apply tissue protective dressing around vulnerable pressure points: nose, ears, back of head and neck. | To alleviate pressure and prevent tissue breakdown. E |

Postprocedure

14	Give further explanation to family/next of kin of how CPAP works and the importance of their presence and participation in communication.	To relieve anxiety and support and reassure family and patient. E
15	Reassure the patient constantly.	To relieve patient anxiety and promote co-operation. E
16	Discuss with doctor use of medication that might aid the patient in compliance with CPAP therapy and administer as necessary.	Prophylactic administration of small doses of anxiolytic can aid compliance with CPAP therapy (Kinnear 2002, C).
17	Continue observation of vital signs and work of breathing. If patient is tiring, notify doctor.	To prevent acute respiratory deterioration or to inform doctors in a timely manner in order to intubate the patient to avoid a respiratory arrest situation (NICE 2007, C).
18	Continuing documenting MEWS score in order to flag up deterioration quickly.	To prevent acute respiratory deterioration or to inform doctors in a timely manner in order to intubate the patient to avoid a respiratory arrest situation (NICE 2007, C).

Problem-solving table 10.3 Prevention and resolution (Procedure guideline 10.3)

Problem	Cause	Prevention	Suggested action
Maintenance of airway	Deteriorating respiratory function Physical tiring	Use of MEWS scoring to identify deterioration	Regular monitoring of respiratory function including skin colour, breathing pattern, respiratory rate, oxygen saturation, blood gases Discuss changes with medical or anaesthetic staff
Inability to eat	Gastric distension due to CPAP Loss of appetite Difficulty in eating; distress caused by respiratory status and CPAP Nausea and vomiting	Provide small but regular easily managed (soft) oral diet or supplement drinks	Encourage diet and oral supplementary fluids. If unable to take orally, refer to dietitian as an alternative method of feeding may be considered, for example enteral feeding via nasogastric or jejunal tube, or intravenous feeding (TPN). Administer antiemetic. Encourage and reassure patient
Aspiration, if unable to maintain own airway	Inability to maintain own airway Continuous pressure from CPAP system Insufflation of air	Seek SALT assessment Keep NBM and insert nasogastric tube Insert nasopharyngeal tube (Figure 10.14)	Observe and assess patient closely. After discussion with medical staff, a nasogastric tube may be inserted to reduce gastric distension
Dry mouth	CPAP system utilizes a very high oxygen flow which has a drying effect	Provide adequate oral hydration	Carry out regular mouthcare (see Chapter 9). Give patient regular sips of water, ice to suck or drinks as patient is able to take. Humidify, as in CPAP circuit

(Continued)

Problem-solving table 10.3 (*Continued*)

Problem	Cause	Prevention	Suggested action
Eyes (only applies to facemask CPAP): Dry Sore Conjunctival oedema	Mask: air leak High-flow oxygen Facial pressure from mask causing oedema	Protect eyes from drying out Use correct size of mask/helmet for patient	Ensure mask/helmet is well sealed with no leaks Apply pressure-relieving padding around mask Apply regular eyecare (see Chapter 9) Adjust mask to facial contour Alter and position mask as comfortable Position padding around the head-strap to relieve pressure
Mask/helmet incorrectly sealed	Incorrect size of mask or helmet	Use appropriate size mask/helmet	Alter mask/helmet position to correct and ensure comfort Ensure mask/helmet is correct size Alter position to ensure correct seal
Non-compliance with CPAP equipment	Anxiety	Calm informative communication	Inform patient of any changes taking place. Communicate with the patient's family, keep them informed and involve them in care and communication with patient Inform doctor of patient's anxiety level Administer prescribed anxiolytic agent if required
Helmet not inflating or patient finding it difficult to breath with mask	Disconnection of tubing Not connected to piped oxygen	Switch on all audible alarms on equipment Clarify alarm parameters with medical/senior nursing staff Keep bed space tidy and free from clutter If possible, ensure bed space is close to/visible from nurse station	Ensure nurse present with patient at all times. Observe patient and CPAP system closely to ensure equipment is working optimally and there is no failure of the system
Inability to communicate effectively Feelings of isolation	Mask/helmet restriction	Provide means of non-verbal communication Ask relative/carer/HCA to stay with patient	Reassure patient and ensure they are comfortable Encourage patient to communicate and explain how they can use letterboard to do so Reassure patient

Postprocedural considerations

Immediate care

It is important to maintain a high level of monitoring while encouraging the patient to maintain good lung expansion by sitting upright and expectorating as required (Keen 2000). CPAP can cause the oral mucosa to dry out with prolonged use, leading to an increased risk of infection, so it is essential that regular mouthcare is provided to prevent this occurring. Regular ABG sampling can be used to assess the effectiveness of the treatment as well as guiding any changes required to either oxygen concentration or PEEP. As with all patients requiring an increased level of support, an accurate fluid balance chart should be maintained to ensure that fluid overload does not occur.

Figure 10.14 Nasopharyngeal airway and safety pin.

Ongoing care

See Box 10.1.

Documentation

Document all the vital signs and monitoring as well as the patient's response to CPAP or NIV treatment.

Education of patient and relevant others

It is worth discussing with the patient and family/carer that intermittent use of CPAP is sometimes beneficial and that if it is required again, this does not necessarily indicate deterioration.

Complications

With any circuit that includes the use of positive end-expiratory pressure (PEEP), there is the possibility of reduction in

---

Box 10.1 Continual monitoring of patients requiring CPAP ventilation

- Oxygen flow setting, concentration administered, PEEP used.
- Pulse rate and rhythm from ECG if available.
- Sputum production: quantity, colour, consistency.
- Skin colour.
- Blood pressure.
- Intracranial pressure for patients who have neurological deficit.

- Respiratory rate.
- Patient subjective response to therapy: pain, discomfort, dyspnoea.
- Neurological status and level of consciousness.
- Breath sounds.
- O$_2$ saturation.
- Chest X-ray.

(Sorenson and Shelledy 2003)

---

cardiac output. However, spontaneous ventilation decreases both the incidence and severity of this complication (Bersten *et al.* 2009). There is also a risk of vomiting and aspiration of gastric insufflation (blowing of air causing gastric distension), although this is minimized when used in awake patients or by the insertion of an oro/nasogastric tube (Schumaker *et al.* 1996). Patients requiring CPAP should ideally be in a HDU setting so a higher level of observations can be maintained. Regular checks on skin integrity should be carried out to ensure that the tight-fitting facemask required for CPAP is not compromising the skin integrity of vulnerable areas on the bridge of the nose and over the ears (Keen 2000).

Chest drains

Definitions

A chest drain is a length of tubing, made of clear, rigid yet pliable plastic, which may have a radiopaque strip incorporated into it that enables X-ray detection. It has a proximal and distal end. The proximal end is inserted into the pleura and has a number of holes, which facilitate drainage. The distal end is connected to the drainage system (Marieb *et al.* 2008) (Figure 10.15).

Anatomy and physiology

Each lung is surrounded by a double membrane called the pleura. The outer membrane is the parietal pleura; this is

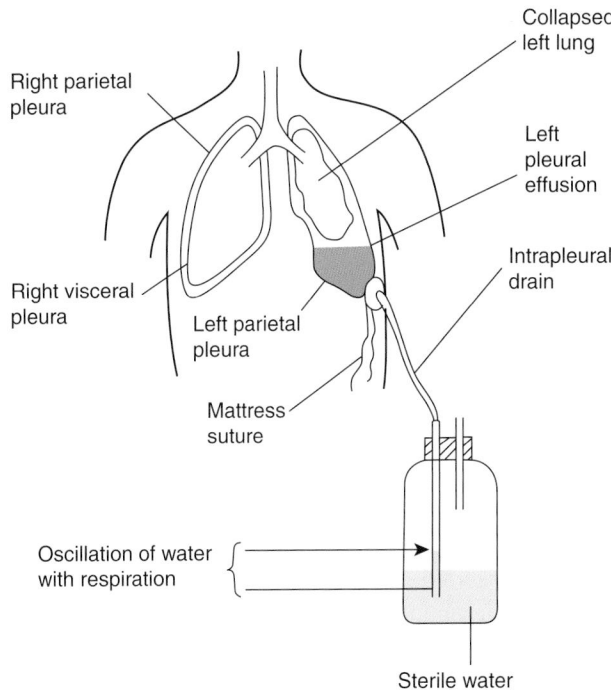

Figure 10.15 A chest drain and underwater seal bottle are used to drain a left pleural effusion.

555

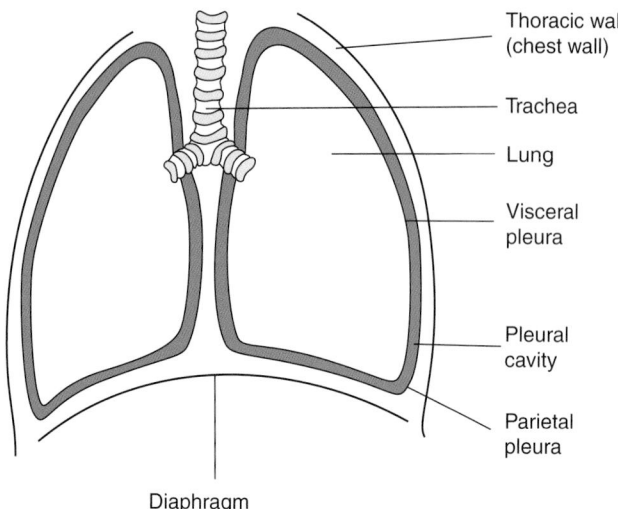

- Thoracic wall (chest wall)
- Trachea
- Lung
- Visceral pleura
- Pleural cavity
- Parietal pleura

Diaphragm

Figure 10.16 Relationship between pleural membranes, chest wall and lungs.

556

attached to the thoracic (chest) wall and contains nerve receptors which detect pain. The inner membrane is the visceral pleura and this adheres to the lung, covering the lung fissures, hilar bronchi and vessels (Figure 10.16). The pleurae are thin, serous and porous, which allows for movement of interstitial fluid across these membranes (Berne 2004, Guyton and Hall 2006, Marieb *et al.* 2008, Tortora and Derrickson 2009).

Pleural space

A space exists between the parietal and visceral pleura commonly known as the pleural space, cavity or potential space. Approximately 3–5 mL of serous fluid produced by the pleurae fills this space, enabling the pleurae to move in unison with the chest wall on inspiration. In addition, the serous fluid enables the membranes to be held closely together by surface tension forces. A careful balance is required to control the amount of fluid present in the pleural space. This balance is maintained by the oncotic pressure across the pleurae and lymphatic drainage. Approximately 1–2 litres of fluid move across the pleural space each day (Urden *et al.* 2006).

The natural recoil tendency of the lungs during breathing causes them to try and collapse, so a negative pressure is required on the outside of the lungs to keep them expanded. This is provided by the pleurae. During respiration, the intrapleural pressure will vary. Before inspiration, the pressure within the pleural space is equal to $-5\,cmH_2O$. During inspiration, there is a decrease in the intrapleural pressure due to the diaphragm being drawn down and outward with expansion of the chest. The pressure falls to $-7.5\,cmH_2O$, and this results in air being drawn in for gaseous exchange (Marieb *et al.* 2008). During expiration, the lung returns to its preinspiratory state by elastic

recoil, with collapse of the chest wall and diaphragm and the exhalation of gas, resulting in a subsequent rise in the intrapleural pressure to $-4\,cmH_2O$. If there is loss of the normal negative pressure, partial or total lung collapse can occur, which can then lead to a reduction in the capacity of the lung available for effective gaseous exchange (Berne 2004, Guyton and Hall 2006, Marieb *et al.* 2008, Tortora and Derrickson 2009).

Related theory

Chest drains are inserted to drain air (pneumothorax) or fluid (haemothorax, pleural effusion or empyema) from the lungs and the management of the chest drain depends on the reason for insertion. As a rule, chest drains inserted for pneumothorax should never be clamped. Chest drains inserted for a pleural effusion need intermittent clamping to

---

Box 10.2 Signs and symptoms of pleural effusions

Dyspnoea

- Dyspnoea is the most common clinical symptom at presentation.
- It indicates a large effusion (usually not <500 mL).
- It is reported to occur in 50% of patients with malignant pleural effusions.
- However, other factors (e.g. underlying lung disease, cardiac dysfunction and anaemia) also may contribute to the development of dyspnoea.

Chest pain

1 Chest pain may be mild or severe; it typically is described as sharp or stabbing, is exacerbated with deep inspiration, and is pleuritic.
2 Pain may be localized to the chest wall or referred to the ipsilateral shoulder or upper abdomen (frequently seen with malignant mesothelioma), usually because of diaphragmatic involvement.
3 It often diminishes in intensity as the pleural effusion increases in size.
4 Chest pain signifies pleural irritation, which can aid in the diagnosis of the cause of the effusion, since most transudative effusions do not cause direct pleural irritation (Maskell and Butland 2003).

Other signs and symptoms (associated more closely with the underlying disease process)

- Increasing lower extremity oedema, orthopnoea and paroxysmal nocturnal dyspnoea all may occur with congestive heart failure.
- Night sweats, fever, haemoptysis and weight loss may occur with TB.
- An acute febrile episode, purulent sputum production and pleuritic chest pain may occur in patients with an effusion associated with aerobic bacterial pneumonia (Maskell and Butland 2003).

Box 10.3 Signs and symptoms of pneumothorax

- Predominant symptom is acute pleuritic chest pain, restlessness, anxiety.
- Dyspnoea results from pulmonary compression.
- Symptoms are proportional to the size of the pneumothorax.
- Also depend on the degree of pulmonary reserve.
- Physical signs include:
  - tachypnoea
  - absent or diminished breath sounds on affected side
  - subcutaneous emphysema
  - decreased tactile and vocal fremitus.
- In a tension pneumothorax:
  - the patient is hypotensive with acute respiratory distress
  - the trachea may be shifted away from the affected side, causing asymmetrical chest expansion
  - there is hyper-resonance (tympany) to percussion on affected side
  - neck veins may be engorged
  - there is progressive cyanosis.
- Diagnosis can be confirmed with a chest X-ray (Bowman 2009).

Box 10.4 Transudative pleural effusion

Can be caused by:

- congestive heart failure (most common transudative effusion)
- hepatic cirrhosis with and without ascites
- nephrotic syndrome
- peritoneal dialysis/continuous ambulatory peritoneal dialysis
- hypoproteinemia (e.g. severe starvation)
- superior vena cava obstruction (Maskell and Butland 2003).

control the amount of fluid drained off in one go to prevent haemodynamic instability (Laws *et al.* 2003). Patients may present with various signs and symptoms of pleural effusions (Box 10.2) and of pneumothorax (Box 10.3).

Pleural effusion

This is defined as an excessive amount of fluid in the pleural space (Kumar and Clark 2009). The fluid can be composed of malignant cells or result from an accumulation of lymph in the pleural space (chylothorax) (Kozer and Adams 2005). An effusion occurs as a result of trauma, carcinoma, heart failure, hypoproteinaemia or pneumonia. Pleural effusions occur when an imbalance in pressure allows the flow of fluid into the pleural space to exceed its absorption (Chernecky and Shelton 2001). Drainage of large pleural effusions should be controlled by periodically clamping the drain. Draining too much fluid off the lungs may cause re-expansion pulmonary oedema, so it is suggested that no more than 500 mL/h and a maximum of 1–2 litres of pleural effusion per day are drained. If the patient's blood pressure drops suddenly then the nurse would need to inform the doctors, clamp the drain, continue frequent observations and consider intravenous fluid challenge to prevent further loss of volume resulting in subsequent hypotension (Laws *et al.* 2003).

Pleural effusions are classified into transudates and exudates.

A *transudative pleural effusion* occurs when the balance of hydrostatic forces influencing the formation and absorption of pleural fluid is altered to favour pleural fluid accu-

mulation. The permeability of the capillaries to proteins is normal (Maskell and Butland 2003).

In contrast, an *exudative pleural effusion* develops when the pleural surface and/or the local capillary permeability are altered (Maskell and Butland 2003). There are many causes of transudates and exudates as illustrated in Box 10.4 and Box 10.5.

Pneumothorax

This can be defined as air in the pleural cavity (Kumar and Clark 2009). When the integrity of either pleural layer is breached, air can enter the pleural cavity, causing the lung to collapse down towards the hilum (Gallon 1998). Many procedures performed in an intensive care or emergency setting can result in an iatrogenic pneumothorax and tension pneumothorax. Examples of these procedures include

Box 10.5 Exudative pleural effusion

Can be caused by:

- *malignant disorders* – metastatic disease to the pleura or lungs, primary lung cancer, mesothelioma, Kaposi's sarcoma, lymphoma, leukaemia
- *infectious diseases* – bacterial, fungal, parasitic and viral infections; infection with atypical organisms such as *Mycoplasma*, Rickettsiae, *Chlamydia*, *Legionella*
- *GI diseases and conditions* – pancreatic disease, Whipple's disease, intra-abdominal abscess, oesophageal perforation, abdominal surgery, diaphragmatic hernia
- *collagen vascular diseases* – rheumatoid arthritis, systemic lupus erythematosus, benign asbestos effusion
- *Meigs syndrome* – benign solid ovarian neoplasm associated with ascites and pleural effusion
- *drug-induced primary pleural disease* – nitrofurantoin, amiodarone, procarbazine, methotrexate, bleomycin, metronidazole
- *injury after cardiac surgery (Dressler's syndrome)* – injury reported after cardiac surgery, pacemaker implantation, myocardial infarction, blunt chest trauma, angioplasty (Maskell and Butland 2003).

incorrect chest tube insertion, mechanical ventilation therapy, central venous cannulation, cardiopulmonary resuscitation, hyperbaric oxygen therapy, needle, transbronchial or transthoracic lung biopsy, liver biopsy or surgery, and neck surgery (Bowman 2009).

Spontaneous pneumothorax

Spontaneous pneumothorax is a collection of air or gas in the chest that causes the lung to collapse (NLM 2010). Spontaneous pneumothorax can occur as a result of trauma, surgery, central venous catheter insertion, during positive pressure ventilation, and in those individuals with lung conditions, for example asthma, chronic bronchitis, tuberculosis, pneumonia or carcinoma of the lung due to the mechanical and physiological processes of these conditions (NLM 2010). If left untreated, a spontaneous pneumothorax can become a tension pneumothorax.

Tension pneumothorax

A tension pneumothorax is a complete collapse of the lung. It occurs when air enters but does not leave the space around the lung (pleural space). It is a life-threatening emergency that requires immediate treatment (NLM 2010).

Haemothorax

Haemothorax is a collection of blood in the space between the chest wall and the lung (the pleural cavity), usually the result of chest injury, trauma to the heart, lungs or major vessels or in a patient who has bled on anticoagulant therapy (NLM 2010).

Haemopneumothorax

Haemothorax may also be associated with pneumothorax. Depending on the amount of blood or air in the pleural cavity, a collapsed lung can lead to respiratory and haemodynamic failure (NLM 2010).

Empyema

This is defined as pus in the pleural space. Its main causes include rupture of an abscess of the lung, following pneumonia, pulmonary tuberculosis, or an infection following thoracic surgery (Kumar and Clark 2009).

Chylothorax

Chylothorax is a milky white fluid from a pleural space, usually resulting from disruption of the thoracic duct or its tributaries. This fluid contains a high level of triglyceride (>110 mg/dL), an essential feature for its diagnosis. More than 50% of chylothorax is due to malignancy, and lymphoma accounts for 75%, followed by lung carcinoma (Maskell and Butland 2003).

Neoplastic disease causes 13–40% of all pleural effusions. Pleural effusion develops in nearly half of all patients with metastatic cancer. The most common tumours that cause malignant pleural effusions are adenocarcinoma and other carcinomas of the lung, breast cancer, lymphoma and leukaemia. These malignancies, combined, account for approximately 75% of all malignant pleural effusions. Other relatively common malignancies associated with pleural effusion are ovarian carcinoma, stomach cancer and sarcomas (including melanoma) (Maskell and Butland 2003).

Evidence-based approaches

Chest drains may be used in patients with collapsed lungs, malignancies, chest trauma or after surgery. Inserting chest drains is a common procedure, which may be carried out in general wards provided adequate monitoring is available. Most are planned, but some may need to be done as emergencies. When chest drains are not inserted properly, the procedure may result in the puncture of major organs such as heart, lungs, liver and spleen (NPSA 2008). The National Patient Safety Agency (NPSA) highlighted the risk associated with chest drain insertion to all healthcare professionals in their report of May 2008. The major causes for injury or harm with insertion of chest drains as highlighted by the NPSA and Medicines and Healthcare Products Regulatory Authority (MHRA) are:

- lack of supervision of junior doctors and lack of experience of clinicians inserting chest drains
- failure to follow manufacturer's instructions
- the site of insertion and poor positioning
- excessive insertion of dilator
- anatomical anomalies and the patient's clinical condition
- inadequate imaging
- lack of knowledge of existing clinical guidelines (NPSA 2008).

Purse-string sutures should not be used as they pull a linear wound into a tight circular shape which causes pain for the patient and leaves an unsightly scar, so mattress sutures (Figure 10.17) should be used to secure chest drains (Laws *et al.* 2003).

Rationale

Any abnormal collection of fluid or air in the pleural space can compress the lung, causing it to collapse either partially or fully, which can seriously compromise ventilation and the mechanics of breathing (Allibone 2003). Chest or intrapleural drainage is a method used to remove the collection of air, fluid, pus or blood from the pleural space in order to restore normal lung expansion and function (Hyde *et al.* 1997, McMahon-Parkes 1997). The type of drainage equipment generally depends on the purpose of chest drain insertion.

A pneumothorax should always have an underwater seal bottle attached to it as bubbling in the bottle is an indication

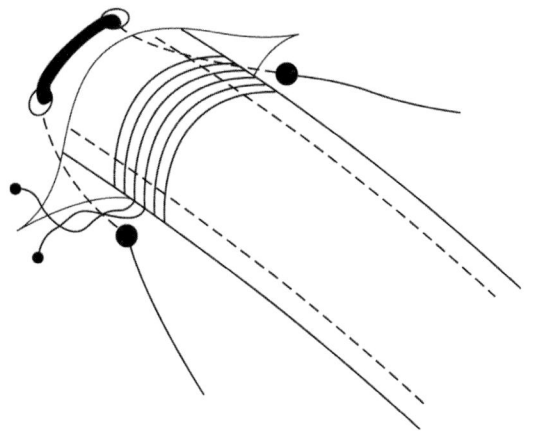

Figure 10.17 Mattress sutures.

of air still in the pleural cavity. If bubbling reduces and then stops, it may indicate that the lung is reinflated. Mostly pleural effusions may be attached to ambulatory chest drainage bags with Heimlich flutter valves which aid early mobilization of patients (Laws *et al.* 2003).

Indications

Indications for chest drain insertion.

- Pneumothorax:
  - in any ventilated patient
  - tension pneumothorax after initial needle relief
  - persistent or recurrent pneumothorax after simple aspiration
  - large secondary spontaneous pneumothorax in patients over 50 years.
- Malignant pleural effusion.
- Empyema and complicated parapneumonic pleural effusion.
- Traumatic haemopneumothorax.
- Postoperative, for example thoracotomy, oesophagectomy, cardiac surgery (Laws *et al.* 2003).
- Drainage of pleural effusions.
- Drainage of chyle (lipids drained by the lymphatic system) (Adam and Osborne 2005, Maskell and Butland 2003).

Contraindications

- Lung densely adhered to chest wall throughout in a hemithorax is an absolute contraindication.
- Differential diagnosis between pneumothorax and bullous lung disease needs to be investigated.
- Drainage of post-pneumonectomy space only after consultation with cardiothoracic surgeon.
- Abnormal blood clotting screen or low platelet count; it is good practice to correct any coagulopathy or thrombocytopenia prior to chest drain insertion.
- Warfarin should be stopped and time allowed for its effects to resolve (Laws *et al.* 2003).

Principles of care

- To maintain sterility of the chest drainage system and avoid introduction of bacteria into the intrapleural space.
- To keep the system patent.
- To keep the system upright and airtight (Kirkwood 2002).
- To monitor the patient's vital signs and amount of drainage and report any changes in breathing or vital signs.

Methods of chest drain insertion

The NPSA (2008) strongly advises the use of ultrasound guidance when inserting a chest drain for fluid removal to prevent injury to adjacent organs. Wherever possible, the drain should be inserted under direct ultrasound guidance, preferably in the radiology department. If not possible, portable ultrasound equipment must be used at the patient's bedside during insertion. Doctors must be competent in the use of the equipment and should be supervised if not experienced.

Legal and professional issues

The current recommendations of the NPSA and BTS (Laws *et al.* 2003) are that:

- chest drains are only inserted by staff with relevant competencies and adequate supervision
- ultrasound guidance is strongly advised when inserting a drain for fluid
- clinical guidelines are followed and staff made aware of the risks
- a lead is identified for training of all staff involved in chest drain insertion
- written evidence of consent is obtained from patients before the procedure, wherever possible
- local incident data relating to chest drains are reviewed and staff encouraged to report further incidents (NPSA 2008).

Consent

Prior to commencing chest tube insertion, the procedure should be explained fully to the patient and consent recorded in accordance with national guidelines. The General Medical Council (GMC) guidelines for consent state that it is the responsibility of the doctor carrying out a procedure, or an appropriately trained individual with sufficient knowledge of a procedure, to explain its nature and the risks associated with it (Laws *et al.* 2003). Written evidence of consent is obtained from patients before the procedure, wherever possible, and documented in the patient's notes.

Competencies

The NPSA alert (2008) highlights the need for training for medical staff who insert chest drains. However, nursing staff need to ensure they are familiar with chest drain management by attending training in their individual hospitals and keeping up to date with NPSA alerts and national guidelines for chest drain management.

Preprocedural considerations

Equipment

Drain size

The size of tube used is dependent on the reason for drainage. As no large randomized trials comparing small- and large-bore tubes have been performed, the optimum size of drainage catheter remains controversial (Laws *et al.* 2003).

In the past the use of a large-bore drain was recommended to prevent the blockage of chest drains, particularly by thick malignant or infected fluid (Hyde *et al.* 1997). However, currently the majority of physicians prefer to use smaller catheters (10–14 French (F)) and some smaller studies have shown that these are often as effective as larger bore tubes (Clementsen *et al.* 1998, Patz 1998). Small-bore drains are more comfortable and better tolerated by the patient (Laws *et al.* 2003).

Drainage systems

Prepacked drainage systems are now available for drainage of pneumothoraces, haemothoraces or pleural effusions. The bottle has a screwtop with two ports. One port has the underwater length of tubing attached. The second port has a shorter length of tubing attached which acts as the venting end and is exposed to air or could be attached to a suction unit. Venting prevents the build-up of pressure in the chest drainage system, which in turn aids evacuation of air or fluid from the lungs (McMahon-Parkes 1997) (Figure 10.18).

The underwater seal occurs when there is adequate water in the bottle, usually 500 mL. The distal end of the chest drain is then attached to the underwater seal port of the chest drain bottle and immersed 2.5 cm below the level of the water. Incoming air bubbles through the water, which acts as a one-way valve and prevents the backflow of air into the intrapleural space (McMahon-Parkes 1997).

For more complicated pneumothoraces or haemothoraces, a plastic multi-chamber system incorporates the one-bottle system into one unit. There are three chambers: the first is for drainage, the second chamber is the underwater seal and the third chamber is the vacuum or suction control. When this system is set up, water is placed in the water seal chamber to the indicated mark, and also placed in the suction control chamber to the required level (Pierce 1995) (Figure 10.19).

Assessment and recording tools

Some hospitals have chest drain-specific charts in order to document swinging or fluctuating, bubbling and draining on a half-hourly or less frequent basis (Laws *et al.* 2003).

Pharmacological support

On insertion of a chest drain, tissue damage occurs and this activates nerve fibres surrounding the insertion site (Gray 2000, Hilton 2004). While the drain is in place, the nerve fibres or tissue cannot heal. Therefore, the patient will experience pain throughout the insertion procedure and after the drain has been inserted (Tomlinson and Treasure 1997). Inadequate pain control can cause the patient to breathe ineffectively and the patient may try to avoid coughing, resulting in complications such as chest infections (Gray 2000). Risk can be reduced by chest physiotherapy from

Figure 10.18   One-bottle system.

Figure 10.19   Underwater chest drainage system. (A) Venting/suction port. (B) Port to patient. (C) Water level.

a physiotherapist (Gray 2000). In a study by Luketich *et al.* (1998), 50% of patients experience pain levels of 9–10 on a scale of 0–10, with 10 being most pain imaginable. Therefore, prior to inserting an intrapleural drain, unless contraindicated, premedication such as benzodiazepine or an opioid should be administered as prescribed (Laws *et al.* 2003). A comprehensive plan for pain control involving the patient and healthcare professionals should be produced. Pain management should cover all stages of the intrapleural drainage process (Gray 2000):

■ insertion
■ management of the chest drain during the drainage process
■ removal of the chest drain.

Current protocols for the management of pain include patient-controlled analgesia, paravertebral blocks, non-steroidal anti-inflammatory drugs or transcutaneous electrical nerve stimulation (Allibone 2005).

Specific patient preparations

The patient's vital signs must be recorded prior to the procedure (Laws *et al.* 2003). Before insertion of a chest drain, the patient should have a chest X-ray reviewed by the doctor. The chest X-ray will confirm the site of the pneumothorax or effusion to be drained.

Patients who are receiving anticoagulation therapy or who have platelet abnormalities should have appropriate haematological investigations (international normalized ratio (INR) or activated partial thromboplastin ratio (APTR)) to ascertain whether correction is required prior to insertion of the drain (Tang *et al.* 2002). If the INR or APTR is too high, bleeding could occur if left untreated.

Chest drains are usually inserted in the chest, in an area which is known as the 'triangle of safety' (Figure 10.20).

Figure 10.20   Triangle of safety. Reproduced from Laws *et al.* (2003), with permission from BMJ Publishing Group Ltd.

This is the triangle bordered by the anterior border of the latissimus dorsi, the lateral border of the pectoralis major muscle, a line superior to the horizontal level of the nipple, and an apex below the axilla (Laws *et al.* 2003). Once the drain has been placed in any position within the 'triangle of safety', re-expansion of the lung occurs. However, in cases of intrapleural adhesions or localized collection of pus or fluids, the doctor will need to position the tip of the drain to assist drainage (Hyde *et al.* 1997, Tang *et al.* 2002).

Education

Nurses need to be aware of new guidelines related to chest drain management and ensure that junior staff are aware of updates and new techniques (Laws *et al.* 2003, NPSA 2008).

Procedure guideline 10.4 Chest drain: insertion

Essential equipment

■ Sterile gloves and gown
■ Sterile chest drain pack, containing gallipot, disposable towel, forceps
■ Skin antiseptic solution, for example iodine or chlorhexidine gluconate 0.5% in 70% alcohol
■ Sterile drapes
■ Gauze swabs
■ A selection of syringes (10 mL × 2) and needles (21–25 gauge)
■ Scalpel and blade
■ Suture (e.g. Mersilk 2.0)
■ Instrument for blunt dissection (e.g. curved clamp)
■ Guidewire with dilators in most Seldinger drain packs (Figure 10.21)
■ Chest tube, for example Seldinger drain or trocar chest drain (Figure 10.22)
■ Connecting tubing
■ Closed drainage system (including sterile water 1 litre if underwater seal bottle is being used):
  ■ Chest drain bottle and tubing (Figure 10.19)
  ■ Ambulatory chest drain bag with Heimlich flutter valve (Figure 10.23)

(Continued)

Procedure guideline 10.4 (*Continued*)

- Occlusive dressing
- Chest drain clamps × 2

Optional equipment

- Low vacuum suction pump if required (high volume, low pressure suction adaptor) (Figure 10.24)

Medicinal products

- Local anaesthetic such as lidocaine 1 or 2% (up to 3 mg/kg) is usually infiltrated. Higher doses may result in toxic levels (Laws *et al.* 2003)

Preprocedure

Action	Rationale
1 Cleanse hands with alcohol handrub. Hands to be cleansed before and after each patient contact.	To minimize the risk of infection (Fraise and Bradley 2009, E).
2 Explain and discuss the procedure with the patient.	To ensure the patient understands why and how the procedure is to be performed and gives their valid consent (Laws *et al.* 2003, C; NMC 2008b, C).
3 Administer analgesia prior to procedure, after discussion with the doctor about the type and route of administration. The analgesia should be given at least half an hour before the procedure.	To minimize any pain during the procedure and to ensure the patient is pain free and able to co-operate (Laws *et al.* 2003, C).
4 Administer sedation on doctor's instruction, if considered appropriate, for example for an anxious patient.	To relieve anxiety and allow the patient to relax and co-operate, and to enable the procedure to proceed. E
5 Cleanse hands with alcohol handrub.	To minimize the risk of infection (Fraise and Bradley 2009, E).
6 Prepare trolley, placing equipment on bottom shelf. Take to patient's bedside.	To ensure all equipment is available. E
7 Prime the underwater seal system with sufficient sterile water to cover the drainage tube. Cleanse hands with alcohol handrub.	This prevents backflow of air or fluid into the pleural space, and marks the initial water level to allow measurement of subsequent drainage (Adam and Osborne 2005, E).
8 Assist doctor in setting up sterile procedure pack.	To minimize risk of infection and to have equipment ready. E
9 Check the correct side of chest for drain insertion on chest X-ray.	To ensure drainage of correct side by checking the chest X-ray (O'Connor and Morgan 2005, E).
10 Position patient in preparation for the procedure. The patient may be positioned flat on the bed with the arm on the affected side placed behind their head away from the chest wall or abducted to 90°. If patient is able to sit upright, they can be positioned resting over a table supported by a pillow.	To facilitate insertion of the intrapleural drain. To aid patient comfort (Hyde *et al.* 1997, E). To prevent injury to adjacent organs (Laws *et al.* 2003, C).

Procedure

11 Observe the patient throughout procedure, with attention to respiratory status including colour, respiratory rate, respiratory pattern, equal movement of chest and peripheral tissue oxygen saturations.	To look for any change in the patient's condition and report to the doctor, to ensure appropriate intervention, for example oxygen therapy (Laws *et al.* 2003, C).
Observe patient for any change to the cardiovascular system by alterations in heart rate or blood pressure.	To look for any change in the patient's condition and report to the doctor, to ensure appropriate intervention (Allibone 2003, E).
12 Communicate with the patient during the procedure and explain what is happening at each stage.	By communicating throughout, the patient feels involved and informed (Laws *et al.* 2003, C).

The following steps would be performed by the doctor or clinician inserting the drain.

13	The doctor will wash their hands with an antiseptic detergent and apply sterile gloves and a gown. Strict aseptic technique is to be adhered to.	To minimize risk of infection (Fraise and Bradley 2009, E).
14	The area for planned insertion of the drain will be cleaned with chlorhexidine gluconate 0.5% in alcohol and allowed to air dry.	To minimize risk of infection (Fraise and Bradley 2009, E).
15	Local anaesthetic will be injected into the skin and deeper tissue (intercostal muscle and parietal pleura) along proposed insertion site.	To minimize the feeling of pain on drain insertion (Gray 2000, P).
16	Wait 2–3 min for local anaesthetic to take effect.	To ensure local anaesthetic has been effective. E
17	An incision is then made with a scalpel to enable the chest drain to be inserted.	To aid and ease the movement of the drain into the correct position. E
18	A finger may then be manoeuvred through to the parietal pleura to guide the drain into place, between the parietal and visceral pleurae in the pleural space for large-bore chest tubes (Miller and Harvey 1993).	To aid the drain into the correct position. E Exploration with a finger is felt to be unnecessary for the elective medical insertion of medium or small-sized chest tubes (Laws *et al*. 2003, C).
19	The drain is then clamped using two clamps until connected to the drainage system.	To prevent further lung collapse and entry of air (Laws *et al*. 2003, C).
20	Connect the distal end of the drain to the drainage system and ensure that it is well supported and secured.	To allow for inflation of the lung or drainage of fluid, to ensure there is no movement of drain and that it remains in the correct position (Allibone 2003, E).
21	The proximal end of the drain is secured and sutured in place with a mattress stitch. Unclamp chest drains.	To secure drain in position. Purse-string stitches should no longer be used as they cause pain and unsightly scarring (Laws *et al*. 2003, C).
22	Clean the site and apply a dressing of gauze, then an occlusive dressing over the gauze.	To ensure site is well covered and sealed (Laws *et al*. 2003, C). To reduce risk of infection (Fraise and Bradley 2009, E).

Postprocedure

23	Send patient for chest X-ray.	To ensure the correct position of the drain and to ensure that the lung has reinflated (Laws *et al*. 2003, C).
24	Check the drain is well secured.	To prevent movement or accidental disconnection of drain (Laws *et al*. 2003, C).
25	Monitor if there is bubbling/swinging of water in the bottle/tubing or drainage fluid and check there are no leaks around the site or any loose connections within the drainage system.	To ensure there is no occlusion or leak which will prevent re-expansion of the lung or drainage of the fluid (Laws *et al*. 2003, C).
26	Record any bubbling, swinging and drainage on observation and fluid balance charts.	To keep an accurate record of type of drainage on fluid balance chart (Laws *et al*. 2003, C; NMC 2009, C).
27	Ensure patient comfort following the procedure. Return the patient to an elevated position sitting in bed, well supported by pillows, and give further analgesia if required.	To ensure patient comfort in order to aid recovery and breathing (Allibone 2003, E).
28	Dispose of waste appropriately.	To reduce risk of sharps injury and cross-infection (DH 2005, C; Fraise and Bradley 2009, E).
29	Cleanse hands with alcohol handrub.	Hands to be cleansed before and after each patient contact (Fraise and Bradley 2009, E).

Figure 10.21   Seldinger drain.

Figure 10.22   Trocar drainage tube.

Procedure guideline 10.5 Chest drainage: suction

Essential equipment

- High-volume and low-pressure suction unit (different to normal wall suction units on wards) (see Figure 10.24)
- 1–2 metres of suction tubing

Preprocedure

Action	Rationale
1 Cleanse hands with alcohol handrub.	To minimize the risk of infection (Fraise and Bradley 2009, E).
2 Communicate with the patient during the application of suction and explain what is happening at each stage.	To keep the patient fully informed. To enable the patient to feel reassured (Laws *et al.* 2003, C).
3 Discuss analgesia management with the patient. Give analgesia to the patient as prescribed.	To ensure patient comfort (Gray 2000, P).

Procedure

4 Prepare the suction unit, which should be low-vacuum suction (bedside suction units are high volume and therefore not suitable), for use with single chamber underwater seal drain bottles and check equipment is working properly and suction can be maintained to the doctor's prescribed pressure.	To maintain safety, ensuring the suction is set at low pressure (Laws *et al.* 2003, C).
5 Connect venting or suction port (see Figure 10.18) to the suction unit, as directed by the medical team. Adjust the suction to required level prescribed, usually –5 cmH$_2$O (Adam and Osborne 2005) or to a level that is tolerable for the patient.	To ensure patient comfort and to ensure suction is applied. E Higher volumes of suction may injure lung tissue (Kirkwood 2002, E).
6 Position patient to aid comfort, ensuring the patient is pain free and relaxed.	To aid breathing for lung expansion. To aid patient comfort (Gray 2000, E).
7 Monitor chest drainage and record amount.	To maintain patient safety by observing level of suction and amount of fluid drained (Allibone 2003, E).
8 Ask patient to inform staff if they need to mobilize and ensure suction is disconnected from patient and reconnected when patient is back in bed.	To prevent pneumothorax, as air connot escape from the bottle. E

Figure 10.23 Ambulatory chest drainage bag with Heimlich flutter valve. (a) Tube connection to patient. (b) Air vent (green). (c) 50 mL syringe filled with air.

Figure 10.24 High-volume, low-suction unit (thoracic suction adaptor).

Procedure guideline 10.6 Chest drain: priming ambulatory chest drain bag

Essential equipment

- Ambulatory chest drainage bag
- 50 mL syringe

Procedure

Procedure	
1 To prime the bag, use the 50 mL syringe to inject air through the drainage tube by inserting the syringe nozzle into the drainage tube (see Figure 10.23). Then draw back on the syringe and resistance should be felt, if there is resistance it means the Heimlich flutter valve is working.	The ambulatory bag MUST be primed prior to use to ensure that the Heimlich flutter valve is working (Choi *et al.* 2007, E).
2 Air will pass through the flutter valve which can be confirmed visually by observing the valve 'leaves' open when air moves through and then close spontaneously and the bag inflating slightly.	This ensures that the Heimlich flutter valve is working. It acts as a one-way valve preventing air from entering the chest cavity when the drain is emptied (Graham *et al.* 1992, R1).

Procedure guideline 10.7 Chest drain: changing the bottle

Essential equipment

- Cleaning solution, for example chlorhexidine in 70% alcohol
- Non-sterile gloves
- Tape
- Sterile chest drain bottle
- 1 litre sterile water bottle
- Chest drain non-toothed clamps × 2
- Procedure pack

(Continued)

Procedure guideline 10.7 *(Continued)*

Preprocedure

Action	Rationale
1 Cleanse hands with alcohol handrub.	Hands to be cleansed before and after each patient contact (Fraise and Bradley 2009, C).
2 Explain and discuss the procedure with the patient.	To ensure the patient is well prepared, and to ensure their co-operation and consent (Laws *et al.* 2003, C; NMC 2008b, C).
3 Cleanse hands with alcohol rub and fill new chest drain bottle to water fill line or until drainage tube is submerged in water.	To prevent infection and to prevent reflux of air or fluid into the lungs, and to create a water seal (Kirkwood 2002, E).

Procedure

4 Undo the taping around the tubing which secures chest drain to chest drain bottle tubing.	In order to disconnect the chest drain tube from the chest drain bottle tube (Kirkwood 2002, E).
5 Clamp the tubing close to the chest wall with two clamps for the shortest time needed to change the bottles.	To prevent air entering the chest cavity and causing a pneumothorax (Laws *et al.* 2003, C). Clamping the drain for long periods of time may increase the risk of pneumothorax (Laws *et al.* 2003, C).
6 Observe patient's breathing and respiratory status during the procedure.	To identify any respiratory deterioration early and report any abnormalities to medical team (Allibone 2005, E).
7 Clean tubing at the connection and remove full bottle and tubing and connect new bottle and tubing to clamped chest tube.	To prevent infection entering system during disconnection and connection of tubing (Fraise and Bradley 2009, E).
8 Ensure a secure connection, unclamp and tape using H-shaped securing tape (see Figure 10.25).	To prevent bottle from falling over or disconnection causing air to re-enter the pleural cavity (Allibone 2005, E).
9 Ensure drain bottle is secure by attaching it to bed or put on a stand on the floor.	To prevent it being knocked over. E
10 Cleanse hands with alcohol rub.	Hands to be cleansed before and after each patient contact (Fraise and Bradley 2009, E).
11 Document new bottle on fluid balance chart and in nursing documentation.	To keep accurate record of amounts drained (Allibone 2005, E; Laws *et al.* 2003; NMC 2009, C).
12 Observe patient for any changes in respiratory status as per previous instructions.	To identify any respiratory deterioration early and report any abnormalities to the medical team (Allibone 2005, E).

Procedure guideline 10.8 Chest drain: removal

Two nurses/assistants are required to facilitate safe removal of a chest drain. One is required to tie the suture and seal the site, and the other to remove the drain.

Essential equipment

- Sterile dressings pack containing gallipot, gauze, sterile towel
- Cleaning solution, for example 0.9% sodium chloride
- Non-sterile gloves
- Stitch cutter
- Sterile dressing
- Tape

Preprocedure

Action	Rationale
1 Cleanse hands with alcohol handrub.	Hands to be cleansed before and after each patient contact (Fraise and Bradley 2009, E).
2 Prepare patient for removal of the drain. Explain and discuss each step of the procedure with the patient.	To ensure the patient is well prepared, and to ensure their co-operation and consent (Laws *et al.* 2003, C; NMC 2008b, C).
3 Encourage patient to practise breathing exercises, as these are required to help with the procedure. The patient should be instructed to take two deep breaths in and out and on the third breath to hold the breath in and perform the Valsalva manoeuvre. It is on this breath that the drain will be removed, that is, end of inspiration (Adam and Osborne 2005).	To prepare the patient and encourage co-operation. E To allow the patient to practise the breathing exercises. E To prevent the entry of air that can occur due to a negative intrathoracic pressure (Allibone 2005, E; Tomlinson and Treasure 1997, E).
4 In order to reduce the complication of recurrent pneumothorax, the Valsalva manoeuvre can be used. This requires patients to hold their breath and to bear down or try to breathe out against a closed glottis (Allibone 2005).	This increases the intrathoracic pressure, which reduces the possibility of air re-entering the pleural space through the drain site (Allibone 2005, E; Laws *et al.* 2003, C).
5 Administer analgesia prior to procedure after discussion with doctor about the type and route of administration. The analgesia should be given at least half an hour before the procedure.	To minimize any pain during the procedure and to ensure the patient is pain free and able to co-operate (Gray 2000, P).
6 Administer sedation on doctor's instruction, if considered appropriate, for example for an anxious patient.	To relieve anxiety and allow the patient to relax and co-operate and to enable the procedure to go ahead. E
7 Discontinue suction if in use and disconnect from venting/suction port.	To prevent a tension pneumothorax (Laws *et al.* 2003, C).
8 Cleanse hands with alcohol handrub.	Hands need to be cleansed before and after each patient contact (Fraise and Bradley 2009, E).
9 Prepare trolley for procedure.	To ensure everything is ready to perform the procedure. E
10 Assist or set up the sterile procedure pack.	To minimize risk of infection and to have equipment ready (Fraise and Bradley 2009, E).

Procedure

Action	Rationale
11 Position patient comfortably.	To aid patient comfort. E
12 Clamping of chest drain prior to removal is not necessary.	Unnecessary clamping increases risk of pneumothorax (Adam and Osborne 2005, Laws *et al.* 2003 C).
13 Place protective pad underneath the patient and drain.	To absorb any ooze from the drain. To reduce risk of contamination of the patient and bed clothing. E
14 Cleanse hands with alcohol handrub before touching the drain or dressing.	To reduce risk of infection (Fraise and Bradley 2009, E).
15 Remove dressing from around drain site, examine sutures present: (a) tube retaining suture (anchor suture) and (b) mattress suture; expose the ends of these sutures.	To prepare for drain removal and check what type of suture is present so that the suture can be used to form an airtight seal when the drain is removed (Adam and Osborne 2005, E).
16 Both assistants for the procedure must wash their hands with an antiseptic solution such as chlorhexidine gluconate 4% w/v skin cleanser, undertaking a full surgical scrub, and apply gloves.	To reduce risk of infection (Fraise and Bradley 2009, E).

(Continued)

Procedure guideline 10.8 (*Continued*)

17	First nurse/assistant prepares mattress suture and loosens ends ready to tie the suture when the drain is removed.	To prepare for drain removal. E
18	Second nurse/assistant prepares and cuts the anchor suture and ensures the drain is mobile and ready to remove.	To prepare for drain removal. E
19	Second nurse/assistant asks the patient to start deep breathing exercises: to take three deep breaths then hold their breath on the third one and bear down (Valsalva manoeuvre) while the drain is pulled out steadily and smoothly.	To aid in drain removal. Deep breathing exercises can help to prevent a tension pneumothorax. During full inspiration and Valsalva manoeuvre the intrathoracic pressure is increased, thus preventing air flowing into the intrathoracic cavity. If a drain is removed too quickly or without due care, a pneumothorax can occur due to rupture of the pleura (Laws *et al.* 2003, C).
20	First nurse/assistant will then tie the mattress suture securely to the skin.	To form an airtight seal and prevent air entry and formation of a pneumothorax (Laws *et al.* 2003, C).

Postprocedure

21	Ask the patient to breathe normally after tube is removed.	To assess if there is any air escaping from suture site. E
22	Clean around site with 0.9% sodium chloride and apply an occlusive dressing, such as gauze soaked in flexible collodion or petroleum gauze under waterproof strapping.	To clean site, form an airtight seal and prevent air entry. E To prevent an air leak if drain puncture site is not closed properly (Adam and Osborne 2005, E).
23	Ensure that the patient is sitting upright, and support with pillows.	To ensure patient comfort and aid respiration (Allibone 2005, E).
24	Dispose of waste appropriately.	To ensure safety and reduce risk of infection (DH 2005, C; Fraise and Bradley 2009, E).
25	Document removal on fluid chart and in nursing notes.	To provide a point of reference for any queries. E
26	A chest X-ray should be performed approximately 2 hours post removal unless acute deterioration.	To check that a pneumothorax has not recurred (O'Connor and Morgan 2005, R5).
27	Both the patient and the drain site should be monitored closely (Allibone 2005). Inform doctor of any changes in patient's breathing, tachycardia or other vital signs. Record vital signs on observation charts including respiration rate and oxygen saturation levels.	To observe for signs of respiratory distress secondary to reaccumulation of fluid/air in pleural cavity (Allibone 2005, E).
28	Cleanse hands with alcohol handrub.	Hands need to be cleansed before and after each patient contact (Fraise and Bradley 2009, E).

Problem-solving table 10.4 Prevention and resolution (Procedure guidelines 10.4, 10.5, 10.6, 10.7 and 10.8)

Problem	Cause	Prevention	Suggested action
Lack of drainage	Kinking, looping or pressure on the tubing may cause reflux of fluid into the intrapleural space or may impede drainage, causing blocking of the intrapleural drain	Ensure tubing is tailored for patient. If patient is able to, involve them in the care of the drain, such as ensuring tubing is not kinked when sitting out in the chair or moving in the bed	Check the system and straighten tubing as required. Secure the tubing to prevent a recurrence of the problem

Problem	Cause	Prevention	Suggested action
Fluid in drain not swinging	Drain occluded due to position or occlusion	Ensure drain is secured and regularly check site for kinking of tubing	Check no loops or kinks present in tubing. Lift drain, not higher than the patient's chest, to see if the obstruction will clear. Seek medical advice as the drain may need replacing
Fluid in drain not bubbling as expected to	Drain occluded or not correctly positioned	Check tubing regularly	Check no loops or kinks in the tubing. Lift tubing to see if it will clear
Continuous bubbling in chest drain bottle	Air leak in system	Check bottle for bubbling and swinging and check integrity of bottle regularly. Ensure all connections are secure	Check system for loose connections in tubing or around drainage unit. If no leak present in the drainage tubing, the leak may be present in the lung. Inform doctor. Prepare chest drain insertion pack
Leakage from drain site	Bleeding or infection	Check site regularly during the day	Remove the dressing and observe the site. Inform doctor, take swab. Clean and redress site. Discuss with medical team regarding prescription of antibiotic therapy
Drainage from around drain site	As a result of the insertion procedure. Incomplete closure with sutures. Infected insertion site	Ensure aseptic technique when dealing with wound. Keep wound clean and dry, check puncture site regularly	Observe drain site, amount and type of drainage. Inform doctor. Take swab from site. Prepare suture pack to be available if required. Discuss with medical team regarding prescription of antibiotic therapy
Accidental disconnection of the drainage tubing from the intrapleural drain	Connections not secure	Tape the connections together by using 'H' dressing which allows nurse to visualize connection site	Apply a clamp to the drain immediately in order to avoid air entering the pleural space. Re-establish the connection as soon as possible in order to re-establish drainage. Ask patient to cough gently to aid air removal. If necessary, use a clean, sterile drainage tube; tubing may have been contaminated when it became disconnected. Report to the doctor, who may wish to X-ray

Record the incident in the relevant records. The patient may have been upset by the incident and will need reassurance |
Intrapleural drain falls out	Drain not secure	Check suture site and dressings daily, ensure anchor stitch is still intact. Apply omental tag dressing to prevent accidental fall-out	Pull the mattress suture immediately to close the wound. Cover the wound with an occlusive sterile dressing. Check the patient's vital signs. Inform a doctor. The objective is to minimize the amount of air entering the pleural space. The drain will probably need reinserting. Prepare chest drain insertion pack. Reassure the patient with appropriate explanations
Poor arm movement	Restriction of arm movement due to position of drain	Explain the need for arm exercises and involve physiotherapy team in mobilizing	Encourage movement of limb to keep mobile. Adjust analgesia as required
Pain	Drain pulling at site	Use omental tag and other dressings to ensure drain does not pull at site	Try repositioning tubing, so that it is not dragging or irritating skin. Give analgesia as prescribed

569

Problem-solving table 10.4 (*Continued*)

Problem	Cause	Prevention	Suggested action
Restricted mobility of patient	Due to position of drain and attachment to the drainage unit. Due to pain at site of insertion	Work in liaison with physiotherapist. Encourage patient to move in bed and change position	Explore with the patient the movement that is possible and aid them where help is required. Offer patient regular analgesia as prescribed and record pain score. Encourage mobility, aid patient to sit in chair

Postprocedural considerations

Immediate care

The nurse should check the patient's vital signs including respiratory rate, temperature, oxygen saturation, heart rate, blood pressure and, if appropriate, arterial blood gases and pain score. The nurse should observe the patient closely for changes in breathing rate or pattern or drop in blood pressure if a large pleural effusion has been drained, as it might drain quite quickly and could cause a significant drop in blood pressure. The drains and connections should be checked to ensure that they are secure and the drain tubing is not kinked. The bottle should always be below the chest drain entry site and monitored for bubbling in the case of a pneumothorax (which indicates air still present in the pleura) and swinging (which indicates the drain is patent). If the patient has a pleural effusion, the amount of fluid drained should be monitored and the amount of fluid drained should be no more than 500 mL/h at a time, as it may induce re-expansion pulmonary oedema. The rate of drainage should be slowed down if the patient's blood pressure drops, by clamping the drain intermittently. The drain should be unclamped if the patient becomes short of breath or experiences dyspnoea, and the doctors and critical care outreach team should be informed of any changes in the patient's condition. A bubbling drain should never be clamped, even for a transfer, and the nurse must be satisfied that the patient is safe for transfer to the X-ray department with the chest drain placed below the chest insertion site.

Securing the drain

The British Thoracic Society (Laws *et al.* 2003) advises that purse-string stitches should not be used as they cause pain by changing a linear wound into a circular one and leave an unsightly scar. Only large- and medium-bore drains require suturing; small-gauge chest tubes do not usually require suturing. The suture material should be strong and non-absorbable to prevent breaking, such as silk (Laws *et al.* 2003). Ensure the drain is secured to the skin to prevent pulling out of sutures with an appropriate self-adhesive securement device such as a Statlock (Moureau and Iannucci 2003) or omental tag (Laws *et al.* 2003).

Dressing the insertion site

A simple dry dressing (low-linting gauze) should be applied around the drain and secured with adhesive tape during drainage and after removal of drain (Tang *et al.* 2002). Heavy strapping should be avoided as it can restrict chest movement. Dressings during the drainage procedure should be kept clean and dry and not removed until the drain is ready for removal (Avery 2000, Tang *et al.* 1999).

Ongoing care
Maintenance of drainage systems

When the drain is attached to the drainage bottle bubbling or swinging should be observed; this indicates that air is being evacuated from the pleural space. As the lung reinflates, the bubbling should decrease. If bubbling continues, a leak may be present in the patient's lung. Causes of air leaks include:

- air in chest from a pneumothorax
- an eyelet from chest tube outside the chest wall
- blocked drain may cause an air leak at puncture site
- inadequate drain size
- poor tube connections
- poor seal around the entry site to the lung (Kirkwood 2002).

The presence of an air leak should be assessed. Bubbling can occur in the underwater seal compartment. If bubbling occurs when the patient coughs, this would usually indicate that the leak is only minor. However, continuous bubbling would indicate a serious air leak in the system. The drain and tube should be inspected thoroughly down to the level of the underwater seal to eliminate any external problems such as loose tubing connections or poor seal around the drain at the insertion site. A chest X-ray should also be ordered to establish the position of the drain. Air leaks should be treated with caution and prompt action is required (such as referral to a specialist respiratory physician).

Tubing should be tailored to suit the patient's needs, allowing room to manoeuvre but preventing coiling and looping (Avery 2000, Hyde *et al.* 1997, Kirkwood 2002). Loops, coiling and kinks in the tubing can cause build-up of the pleural effusion, impaired gas exchange and infection as well as impeding drainage (Gordon *et al.* 1997, Kirkwood 2002) so regular inspection of tubing should be carried out.

Figure 10.25   H-shaped securing tape.

There is debate about recommendations on taping the connection between the chest drainage bottle and drainage tubes (Avery 2000, Godden and Hiley 1998), as the nurse may not be able to see if the connections have parted beneath the tape (Adam and Osborne 2005); however, without any additional method of security, such as tape, there is a risk of the drainage tubing becoming disconnected (Allibone 2005). Using an 'H'-shaped securing tape either side of the joined tubing connections is often undertaken in clinical practice (Figure 10.25).

An omental tag of tape can be used which allows the tube to lie a little away from the chest wall to prevent tube kinking and tension at the insertion site (Laws *et al.* 2003).

Report any pyrexia and monitor site for signs of infection. Continue with monitoring of vital signs, drainage type and amount. Offer patient regular analgesia as prescribed and keep accurate pain score documentation.

Suction and its use

The addition of suction to the drainage system increases the negative pressure, enhancing lung re-expansion. A high-volume, low-pressure suction unit should be applied to single chamber chest drain bottle (Hyde *et al.* 1997, Tang *et al.* 2002), using pressure in the range of 5–15 kPa. The suction pressure should only be increased if the patient's pain is controlled and if the patient tolerates the increase. Once suction has been discontinued, the tubing to the underwater seal should be disconnected, otherwise this could cause positive pressure and may precipitate a tension pneumothorax (Tang *et al.* 2002). The suction unit should be cleaned by wiping it with a damp cloth and a mild disinfectant solution. Most suction units are fitted with a disposable air filter capsule, between the vacuum connector and the filter capsule mount. The filter prevents cross-infection and should be changed after each patient. Ambulatory chest drainage bags connot be attached to suction. Advanced multi-chamber chest drain bottles have built-in suction control and require high flow suction adaptors to facilitate suction levels. Manufacturer's instructions must be followed.

Stripping/milking of chest drains

Milking and stripping of chest tubes to keep tubing patent increases the negative pressure in the intrathoracic cavity to -100 to -400 cmH$_2$O and so it seems that milking or stripping of chest tubes on a routine basis should be avoided as it may harm the tissue in the intrathoracic cavity (Kirkwood 2002). If a chest drain becomes occluded or blocked, the tubing needs to be replaced rather than milking or stripping (Avery 2000).

Clamping of chest drains

The British Thoracic Society guidelines (Laws *et al.* 2003, Miller and Harvey 1993) discourage clamping of chest drains as this can prevent air leaving the pleural space. This in turn can cause a pneumothorax which could progress to a life-threatening tension pneumothorax. A bubbling chest drain should never be clamped. There is also no need to clamp tubing when mobilizing or transporting patients to other departments as this may also cause a tension pneumothorax (Henry *et al.* 2003, Hyde *et al.* 1997). When changing the bottle system, it is necessary to clamp the drain for the shortest period of time possible and during this process, the patient should be under close observation for any signs of deterioration in breathing (Brandt *et al.* 1994).

In cases of pneumothorax, the chest drain, which usually shows bubbling in the chest drain bottle, should not be clamped at the time of its removal (Laws *et al.* 2003). The only time a non-bubbling chest drain should be momentarily clamped is in the event of disconnection, if there is damage to the drainage bottle, to locate a leak in the drainage system or to control the amount of drainage for a pleural effusion (Allibone 2005, Avery 2000, Henry *et al.* 2003, Laws *et al.* 2003).

Chest drain removal

If a patient has had a pneumothorax, the chest drain should not be clamped at the time of its removal (Laws *et al.* 2003). The chest drain should be removed either while the patient is asked to perform a Valsalva manoeuvre or during expiration with a brisk firm movement while an assistant ties the mattress suture to close the wound (Laws *et al.* 2003). The Valsalva manoeuvre (asking the patient to hold their breath while trying to exhale out against a closed glottis, or bear down) increases the intrathoracic pressure which prevents air from entering the thoracic cavity on removal of the drain (Avery 2000, McMahon-Parkes 1997).

The decision to remove a drain is usually made by a medical practitioner based on the following criteria.

- Absence of an air leak into the chest drain bottle, usually noted when the patient exhales forcibly or coughs. When a patient is ventilated with positive pressure this will coincide with the expiration.
- Re-expansion of lung following previous discontinuation of any suction when there should be no air leak or drainage.
- The volume of fluid draining into the chest drain is minimal. Guidelines on what is minimal vary but less than 10 mL/h per drain has been suggested (Higgins 2006).

- There is no evidence of respiratory compromise or failure.
- There is no coagulation deficit or increased risk of bleeding (check latest coagulation results prior to removal).
- In many cases radiological evidence of the absence of air or fluid accumulation will be required before removal.

Advice should be sought from a medical practitioner if there is any doubt as to whether to remove a chest drain (Higgins 2006).

Documentation

Document clearly in the patient's notes and keep an accurate record of type and amount of drainage on relevant nursing observation or fluid balance charts. Document whether the drain is swinging or bubbling or draining and if suction is used and the level of suction used. Document if the drain is clamped to manage the amount of fluid drained for pleural effusion and ensure vital signs are documented at the same time as clamping to ensure early management of any problems. Record vital signs and pain score at least 4 hourly.

Education of patient and relevant others

If the patient is able to, encourage them to take care that the chest drain bottle does not fall over and the tubing is not kinked or pulling. Also teach the patient to ensure that the drain is not lifted above the insertion site and to continue to mobilize if possible; suggest mobility exercises to prevent sore and stiff shoulders. If the patient is not able to assist then ensure that nursing staff continue frequent monitoring of drain and tubing and insertion site and assist the patient in arm movements.

Complications

- Incorrect placement (extrapleural, intrapulmonary, subdiaphragmatic).
- Puncturing of adjacent organs: lung, stomach, spleen, liver, heart and great vessels.
- Pulmonary laceration (haemorrhage, fistula).
- Pneumothorax.
- Bleeding from:
  - local incision, intercostal vessels
  - lung
  - internal mammary artery (with anterior placement)
  - great vessels (rare)
- Infection: empyema.
- Mechanical (kinking, luminal obstruction) which may cause a pneumothorax.
- Surgical emphysema.
- Re-expansion pulmonary oedema, if large amounts of fluid are drained from a pleural effusion over a short period of time (Laws *et al.* 2003).

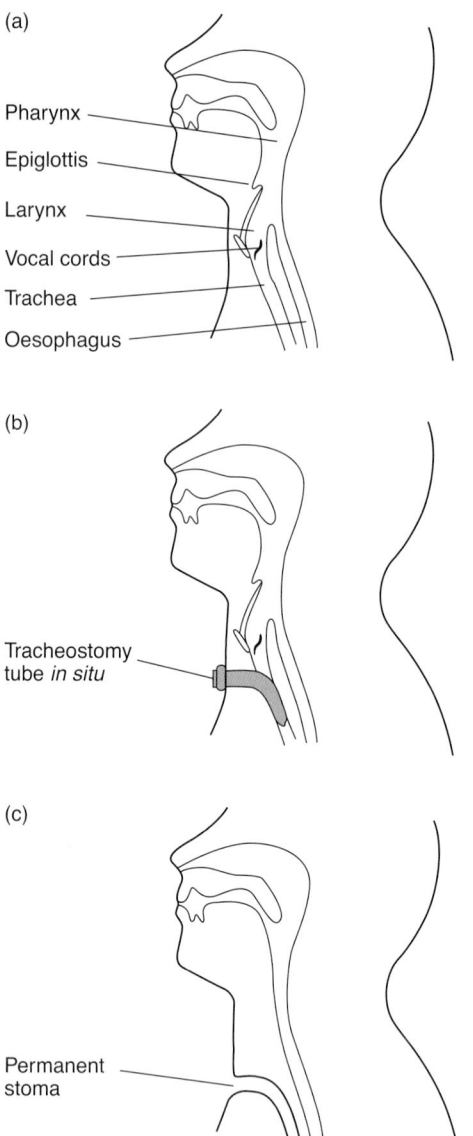

Figure 10.26 (a) Anatomy of the head and neck. (b) Temporary tracheostomy. (c) Permanent tracheostomy.

Tracheostomy and laryngectomy care

Definition

A tracheostomy is the surgical creation of an opening (stoma) into the trachea through the neck (Figure 10.26a). The opening is usually made at the level of the second or third cartilaginous ring (Woodrow 2002) and is kept patent with a tracheostomy tube, curved to accommodate the anatomy of the trachea. When a total laryngectomy (the surgical removal of the larynx) is performed, a permanent stoma is formed by stitching the end of the trachea to the skin of the neck (Woodrow 2002).

Anatomy and physiology

Figure 10.26a shows the anatomy of the neck. The larynx, situated at the top of the trachea, houses the vocal cords and is the point of transition between the upper and lower airways (Epstein 2009). It is made up of nine cartilage segments, the largest of which is called the thyroid cartilage. Inferior to this is the cricoid cartilage which attaches to the large cylindrical tube/elastic structure known as the trachea. This is usually approximately 11 cm long and is made up of rigid cartilage anteriorly and a posterior membranous portion (Epstein 2009). The trachea then divides at the carina to form the right and left mainstem bronchi of the lungs.

Related theory

The exact location of the stoma will be determined on an individual basis according to the patient's neck and rationale for tracheostomy. Low stomas (i.e. beyond the third tracheal ring) increase the risk of bleeding from the brachiocephalic trunk, and a tracheostomy that is too close to the cricoid has an increased risk of subglottic stenosis, a condition that is difficult to treat (De Leyn *et al.* 2007).

Types of tracheostomy

A *temporary tracheostomy* usually refers to stomas formed as an elective procedure at the time of major surgery (such as a total glossectomy) (Prior and Russell 2004) (Figure 10.26b), although percutaneous techniques, performed by the bedside in intensive care units, are becoming commonplace (ICS 2008).

A *permanent tracheostomy* is the creation of a tracheostomy following a total laryngectomy (Prior and Russell 2004) (Figure 10.26c). The larynx is removed and the trachea is sutured in position to form a permanent stoma, known as a laryngectomy stoma (Clotworthy 2006a). The patient will breathe through this stoma for the remainder of their life. As a result, there is no connection between the nasal passages and the trachea (Edgtton-Winn and Wright 2005).

Percutaneous tracheostomy

The percutanous method most commonly used is known as percutaneous dilatational tracheostomy (PDT) (De Leyn *et al.* 2007), enabling the pretracheal tissues to be incised under local anaesthesia. A sheath is inserted into the trachea between the cricoid and the first tracheal ring or between the first and second rings. The trachea is progressively dilated with a series of conical dilators, which are slipped over a guidewire, ready for a tracheostomy tube to be inserted. Now frequently performed in the critical care setting as an early intervention post initiation of mechanical ventilation, the procedure takes less time and requires fewer resources, such as theatres and surgeons, resulting in fewer costs, than a surgical tracheostomy (Patel and Matta 2004). Another potential benefit of percutaneous tracheostomy is more rapid stomal closure and smaller scar formation once the tracheostomy tube has been removed (Patel and Matta 2004).

Surgical

Elective surgical tracheostomy is ideally performed in the operating theatre under general anaesthetic, although it can be performed under local anaesthetic (De Leyn *et al.* 2007). A horizontal incision is made halfway between the sternal notch and the cricoid cartilage (Price 2004a). The strap muscles are divided and the thyroid isthmus is retracted/divided, enabling the trachea to be exposed and the tracheal cartilages to be counted. The tracheostomy should be sited over the second and third or third and fourth tracheal cartilages (Price 2004a).

Mini-tracheostomy

Unlike the previous two techniques, which enable oxygen therapy and mechanical ventilation, this method is used only when frequent aspiration of airway secretions is required. The procedure is also referred to as a cricothyroidotomy (De Leyn *et al.* 2007). The cricothyroid ligament is incised, enabling a small endotracheal tube or a mini-tracheostomy tube to be inserted (Price 2004b). The mini-tracheostomy tube has a small internal diameter, of often only 4 mm. This technique can also be used in an emergency to alleviate upper airway obstruction.

Evidence-based approaches

Rationale

Indications

There are four main indications for tracheostomy.

- To enable the aspiration of tracheobronchial secretions (e.g. excessive secretions/ poor cough).
- To maintain the airway (e.g. upper airway obstruction) (ICS 2008).
- To protect the airway (e.g. bulbar palsy) (ICS 2008).
- For long-term mechanical ventilation and to aid weaning off mechanical ventilation.

Contraindications

The only absolute contraindications for tracheostomy are severe localized sepsis/skin infection, uncontrollable coagulopathy (ICS 2008) or prior major neck surgery which completely obscures the anatomy (De Leyn *et al.* 2007).

Legal and professional issues

Competencies

The most common problems associated with tracheostomy, in both general wards and critical care, are related to obstruction or displacement (ICS 2008). All hospitals or

573

community settings should have a procedure for managing such situations and all staff involved in the care of the patient must be both aware of the procedure and appropriately trained in either managing the situation or supporting additional staff. At all times if there is any doubt about the appropriate care that needs to be given or the management of a situation, call for more senior or emergency help, according to local policy, as soon as possible.

Having emergency equipment readily available is paramount at all times for all types of altered airways (see Preprocedural considerations for equipment required). All staff caring for the patient should also know the type of tube in place at any one time; this and details of all care provided should be clearly documented.

Managing difficult situations with a tracheostomy is stressful for both the patient and staff, so prevention is always better than cure. All procedures should be undertaken only after approved training, supervised practice and competency assessment, and carried out in accordance with local policies and protocols.

Preprocedural considerations

Equipment

The following should always be at the bedside, during transfers or accessible if the patient is self-caring or ambulant.

- Operational oxygen with tracheostomy mask available.
- Operational suction, checked each shift, with a selection of suction catheters present.
- Sterile water (Serra 2000) can be used to help clear suction tubing of secretions after suctioning has been performed.
- Non-powdered latex-free gloves, aprons and eye protection (Day *et al.* 2002).
- Two spare cuffed tracheostomy tubes, one the same size as the patient is wearing, the other a size smaller, in case of an emergency tracheostomy tube change (Serra 2000, Tamburri 2000).
- One 10 mL syringe to inflate cuff.
- Tracheal dilators and artery forceps (ICS 2008) (Figure 10.27).

Figure 10.27 Tracheal dilator.

Figure 10.28 Cuff pressure manometer.

- Spare soft neck ties or tape.
- Suture cutter and lubricating gel.
- Cuff pressure manometer (Serra 2000) (Figure 10.28).
- Readily available rebreathe bag and resuscitation equipment (ICS 2008).

It can be useful to have the above equipment in a small 'tracheostomy box' that can remain by the patient's bedside or move with the patient during transfer.

When caring for the patient who has undergone a total laryngectomy, the equipment listed above should always be by the bedside, and in addition the following equipment is recommended.

- Tilley's forceps: these are angled forceps that can be used to remove crusts or plugs of mucus from in and around the stoma.
- Pen torch (or access to a light source).
- Micropore or Elastoplast tape for those patients with a tracheo-oesophageal puncture, to ensure that the catheter keeping the puncture patent is secured firmly with tape or a suture (see Chapter 5, Communication for an individual with a laryngectomy, for specific information on surgical voice restoration).

Similar to the 'tracheostomy box', it may be useful to have a 'laryngectomy box' readily available by the bedside and for transfers.

Tracheostomy tubes

Tracheostomy tubes are made of either metal or plastic, and therefore vary considerably in rigidity, durability and kink resistance (ICS 2008). Most tubes manufactured now are dual cannula tracheostomies and are inherently safer and most commonly preferred, particularly for use in acute settings. The outer tube maintains the patency of the airway while the inner tube, which fits snugly inside the outer tube, can be removed for cleaning without disturbing the stoma site. The major advantage of an inner cannula is that it allows immediate relief of life-threatening airway obstruction in the event of blockage of a tracheostomy tube with clots or tenacious secretions. Disposable inner tubes are now available; these single-use items are quicker to use (Dropkin 1996) and minimize cross-infection as no cleaning is required.

The majority of tracheostomy tubes are manufactured from plastics of varying types, some that become softer at body temperature (e.g. polyvinyl chloride construction). Some also have a high-volume, low-pressure cuff which distributes the pressure evenly on the tracheal wall and aims to minimize the risk of tracheal ulceration, necrosis and/or stenosis at the cuff site (ICS 2008, Russell 2004). The cuff when inflated provides a seal between the tube and tracheal wall, enabling effective ventilation and protection of the lower respiratory tract against aspiration (Russell 2004).

Most tubes are sized according to their internal diameter in millimetres, varying also in their length and shape. The size and style of the tube chosen will depend upon the size of the trachea and the needs of the individual patient (Bond *et al.* 2003, Lewarski 2005, Serra 2000). It is essential that all staff caring for a patient with a tracheostomy know the type of tube in place at any one time, and that this information is readily available and clearly documented in the patient's notes (ICS 2008).

A selection of tube types and commonly seen tubes is described below.

Cuffed tracheostomy tubes

Portex® blue line and Portex® blue line Ultra® cuffed tracheostomy tubes

These are single-use tracheostomy tubes constructed of siliconized polyvinyl chloride with an introducer and inflatable cuff of 'high-volume/low-pressure' design (Figure 10.29). They are softer and more pliable and are often used when percutaneous tracheostomy is performed in the critical care setting. The cuff pressure should be monitored regularly. Once the stoma is well-formed, after about 7–10 days and depending on the patient's specific weaning needs, the Portex® tube may be replaced by a more suitable, sturdier tube such as a Shiley® tube (Hess 2005).

Shiley® cuffed tracheostomy tube

This is a plastic tube with an introducer and one inner tube (Figure 10.30a). The inner tube has the universal 15 mm extension at its upper aspect to facilitate connection to other equipment. The outer tube has an inflatable cuff to

Figure 10.29 Portex cuffed tube.

give an airtight seal and facilitate ventilation and prevention of aspiration. Shiley® tubes are often used in the immediate postoperative phase, that is, at 24–72 hours. As with all cuffed tracheostomies, the internal cuff pressure should not exceed 25 cmH₂O (ICS 2008) and should be monitored on a regular basis. The cuff should be deflated to remove the tube (to prevent mucosal damage and allow the tube to be removed safely) when the patient is eating and drinking, or when a speaking valve or decannulation plug is *in situ* (ICS 2008). Failure to deflate the cuff when a speaking valve or plug is in place will result in complete occlusion of the patient's airway.

Cuffless tracheostomy tubes

Shiley® cuffless tracheostomy tube

This is a plastic tube with an introducer and two inner tubes (Figure 10.30b). One inner tube has an extension known as a 15 mm hub or adaptor at its upper aspect. The majority of tracheostomy tubes used in the hospital setting have the universally sized 15 mm hub to allow attachment to speaking valves and other equipment (Russell 2004). The other tube has no 15 mm hub extension and is less obtrusive and suitable for those patients not requiring attachment to other equipment (Russell 2004).

A cuffless Shiley® tube is usually used for the following reasons.

- To keep the tracheostomy tract patent if the patient is going to have further surgery.
- In place of a metal tracheostomy tube if the patient is going to have radiotherapy to the neck area (Prior and Russell 2004). Keeping the metal tube *in situ* during radiotherapy can cause reactions due to interference of the metal with the radiotherapy beam and leads to an

(a)

(b)

(c)

(d)

Figure 10.30 (a) Shiley cuffed tube. (b) Shiley plain tube. Courtesy of Tyco Healthcare. (c) Shiley plain fenestrated tube. (d) Shiley cuffed fenestrated tube. Courtesy of Tyco Healthcare.

increased dose being given to the underlying stoma and surrounding skin (Prior and Russell 2004).

■ For a laryngectomy patient who has a benign or malignant stenosis of the trachea and requires a longer tube than the regular length laryngectomy tube to keep the stenosis patent.

Fenestrated tracheostomy tubes
Shiley® fenestrated cuffless tube

The Shiley fenestrated cuffless tube (Figure 10.30c) is a plastic tube with an introducer and three inner tubes. One inner tube has no hub jutting out, is less obtrusive and is suitable for those patients not requiring attachment to other equipment (Russell 2004). The other two inner tubes have the universal 15 mm extension at the upper aspect to facilitate connection to other apparatus, and one of these (with a green coloured hub) also has a fenestration midway down the tube (the clear or white hubbed inner has no fenestrations down the side and sits flush with the outer tube). This is to encourage the passage of air and secretions into the oral and nasal passages. It is useful when attempting to encourage a return to normal function following long-term use of a temporary tracheostomy, for example enabling the patient to communicate verbally. Fenestrated tubes are not recommended for use following percutaneous tracheostomy or when patients are requiring mechanical ventilation due to a risk of surgical emphysema (ICS 2008).

A fenestrated tube is the most suitable for phonation and weaning. A cap (known as a decannulation plug–see Figure 10.36) is placed onto the tube, occluding the artificial airway. This enables air flow through as well as around the tracheostomy tube, allowing the patient to breathe via the oral and nasal passages again. The cap can be left *in situ* for certain periods of time until the patient can tolerate the tube occluded continuously for an uninterrupted period of time. The Intensive Care Society (ICS 2008) states that this period of time should be a *minimum of 4 hours* uninterrupted, though common practice is 24 hours in ward environments. Once this has occurred, removal of the entire tube, known as decannulation, can be considered (Harkin 2004, Serra 2000). The decannulation procedure should ideally take place in the morning, during normal working hours, to ensure that a specialist assessment can be sought if the patient requires tracheostomy tube reinsertion (Harkin 2004).

Shiley® fenestrated cuffed tube

This tube is very similar to the cuffless fenestrated tube although it has an outer cuff to facilitate ventilation and

Figure 10.31 Kapitex Tracheotwist cuffed fenestrated tube.

Figure 10.32 Portex Blue-Line 'Suctionaid' tracheostomy tube.

protect against aspiration, and only two inner tubes (Figure 10.30d). Both inner tubes have the universal 15 mm extension at the upper aspect to facilitate connection to other apparatus, and one of these (with a green coloured hub) also has a fenestration midway down the tube. The outer tube also has a fenestration in the middle of the cannula, again to encourage a return to normal function. The fenestrated tube can also be occluded with a cap, to assess the patient's oral and nasal airway, first ensuring that the *cuff has been completely deflated* and that the fenestrated inner tube is *in situ*. This tube is particularly useful for weaning patients who require both periods of cuff inflation (to protect the airway) and cuff deflation (to enable a speaking valve to be used) (Russell 2004).

Specialist function tubes

Kapitex Tracheotwist® fenestrated tube

This is a plastic tube with an introducer and two inner tubes (Figure 10.31). One of these inner tubes has an extension at its upper end to facilitate connection to other apparatus. The other inner tube has a fenestration midway down the tube, while the outer tube also has a fenestration consisting of a series of small holes. This helps to reduce the risk of granulation tissue growing through the fenestration. The neck plate or flange moves in a vertical and horizontal direction, enabling the plate to move as the patient moves. An inner tube with integrated speaking valve can be ordered separately.

Portex® Blue Line Ultra® 'Suctionaid' (Figure 10.32) and Tracheotwist® 306 tracheostomy tubes

These are specialist tracheostomy tubes that have a facility for aspiration of subglottic secretions. They are mostly used for the prevention of ventilator-associated pneumonia (VAP) in critically ill patients, although they are now also indicated for use in patients with conditions such as bulbar palsy who are unable to effectively clear secretions accumulating above the tracheostomy tube. Suction should not be applied continuously due to the risk of laryngeal injury (ICS 2008).

Metal tubes

Jackson® silver tracheostomy tube

This is a silver tube with an introducer and inner tube (Figure 10.33a). The inner tube is locked in position by a small catch on the outer tube and may be removed and cleaned as necessary without disturbing the outer tube.

Negus® silver tracheostomy tube

This is a silver tracheostomy tube with an introducer and a choice of inner tubes, with and without speaking valves (Figure 10.33b). The outer tube does not have a safety catch so the inner tube can at times be coughed out inadvertently.

Additional tracheostomy supplies

Speaking valves

These are plastic devices with two-way valves that fit onto the 15 mm hub of the fenestrated inner tube. Distinction should be made between open and closed position valves.

- The open position speaking valve (e.g. Rusch® valve) (Figure 10.34) is open by default and closes with positive pressure (expiration) which diverts air through the upper airways past the vocal cords, thus allowing production of a voice.
- The closed position speaking valve (e.g. Passy Muir® valve) (Figure 10.35) is closed by default and requires negative pressure (i.e. the patient's inspiratory effort) to open. Once expiration starts, it closes, causing air to be diverted as described above. This type of valve can be used in ventilator circuits, always with cuff deflation, for patients who are mechanically ventilated.

If a non-fenestrated cuffed tube is in place, the cuff should always be deflated before a speaking valve is fitted as the patient will not be able to exhale (Clotworthy 2006b). Ordinarily, practitioners will also consider changing a non-fenestrated tube for a fenestrated tube (double lumen, with fenestrated inner tube). This will allow air to be diverted through the fenestrations of the tube in addition to air already diverted around the tube to the upper airways.

577

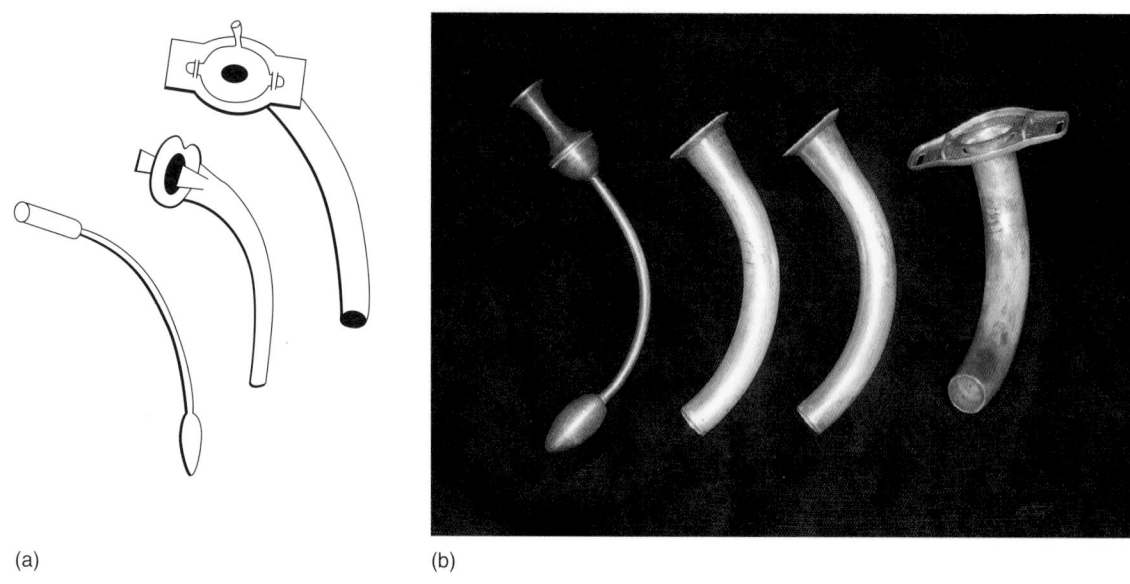

(a)   (b)

Figure 10.33   (a) Jackson silver tube. (b) Negus silver tube.

If a non-fenestrated tube is in place, depending on the size of the tracheostomy tube and the diameter of the patient's trachea, sufficient air may not be diverted past the cuff. This will result in pressure building up because the patient will not be able to breathe out and the valve will not be tolerated. In this case it will be necessary for a complete outer tube change to a fenestrated tube.

However, anecdotal evidence from practice (often in critical care environments) would suggest that in some instances cuff deflation alone (without changing a non-fenestrated tube for a fenestrated tube) may be sufficient to allow air diversion past the cuff through the upper airways as described above. It is important that each individual case is considered carefully and that practitioners weigh up the

potential discomfort and distress a complete tracheostomy tube change may cause against the potential risks of fitting a speaking valve on a non-fenestrated tube. It is therefore imperative that when a speaking valve is used for the first time, the patient is carefully monitored for any signs of respiratory distress. If the patient experiences difficulty in breathing, an inability to vocalize or they begin to sound wheezy or stridulous, the speaking valve should be removed immediately and the patient reassessed (ICS 2008).

Decannulation plug

This is a small plastic plug which fits into the outer fenestrated tube (Figure 10.36). It is used to encourage patients to divert air around the tube past and into the nose and mouth before removal of the tracheostomy tube as described previously. Alternatively, a small plastic plug (Kapitex®) or a blind hub (Shiley®) can be fitted into or over the inner fenestrated tube. This is particularly useful for patients who are still producing tenacious secretions as the plug or hub can be removed to enable the inner tube to be cleaned (Harkin 2004).

Figure 10.34   Rusch speaking valve.

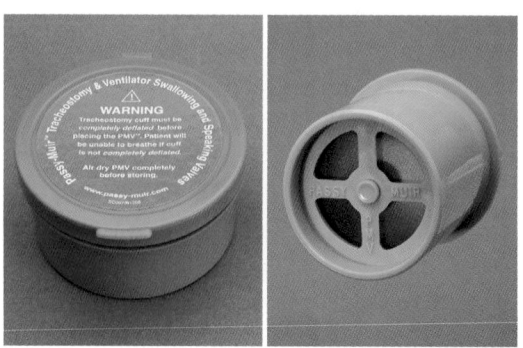

Figure 10.35   Passy Muir valve.

Figure 10.36   Decannulation plug.

Laryngectomy tubes

Patients who have undergone a total laryngectomy may require a cuffed tracheostomy tube for the first 24–48 hours. The tube stents the often oedematous stoma and the inflated cuff prevents blood-stained secretions from entering the lungs. During the immediate postoperative phase, the decision on whether a tube is required and which type is made by the surgeon (Clotworthy 2006a). For those patients with no tube in place, the nurse must be extremely vigilant, assessing the bare stoma frequently to ensure that it is not at risk of stenosis. A stenosed stoma will restrict the patient's breathing, hinder the removal of secretions and prevent the insertion of a cuffed tube in an emergency situation. Stoma size should be sufficiently large, ideally 20–25 mm in diameter (Rhys Evans *et al.* 2003), in order to insert a size 6 or above Shiley tracheostomy tube or

equivalent. In the longer term, many patients no longer require a tube of any type.

Colledge® silver laryngectomy tube
This is a silver laryngectomy tube with an introducer (Figure 10.37a). It is often used to dilate a laryngectomy stoma which has stenosed. These tubes can be cleaned, autoclaved and reused.

Shiley® laryngectomy tube
This is a plastic tube with an introducer and inner tube (Figure 10.37b). The inner tube has the universal 15 mm hub enabling attachment to other equipment. It is shorter in length than a tracheostomy tube, thereby conforming to the slightly shorter trachea in the patient who has undergone a total laryngectomy. The inner tube may be removed and cleaned frequently without disturbing the outer tube. It is sometimes worn postoperatively while the stoma is healing to help facilitate a 'neater' shaped stoma.

Shaw® silver laryngectomy tube
This is a silver laryngectomy tube with an introducer and an inner tube beyond both lower and upper aspects of the outer tube (Figure 10.37c). Thus pressure dressings may be

579

(a)

(b)

(c)

(d)

(e)

Figure 10.37   (a) Colledge silver tube. (b) Shiley laryngectomy tube. (c) Shaw laryngectomy tube. (d) Stoma button. (e) Laryngectomy tube.

secured without occluding the stoma. The silver catch on the outer tube keeps the inner tube in position.

Stoma button

This is a soft silastic 'button' (Figure 10.37d). It may be used in place of a laryngectomy tube. It is very light and comfortable to wear and can be used in conjunction with a Blom-Singer speaking valve. In order to facilitate the use of the Blom-Singer speaking valve, a diamond-shape is cut out of the silastic (see Chapter 5, Communication for an individual with a laryngectomy for specific information on surgical voice restoration).

Silastic laryngectomy tube

This is a slightly opaque silastic tube which is longer in length in comparison to the stoma button. It is available in 36 and 55 mm lengths and in a variety of different sizes (Figure 10.37e). It is most suitable for patients who experience a degree of stenosis further down the trachea (see Chapter 5, Communication for an individual with a laryngectomy, for further information).

Specific patient preparations

Care of the patient with a tracheostomy requires a multidisciplinary approach. Patients may have issues with pain and discomfort, swallowing, speech, mobility and general care. Speech and language therapists will play a pivotal role in the assessment and management of the patient's impaired swallowing and speech. Specialized physiotherapists are skilled in mobilization rehabilitation (see Chapter 7 for information regarding mobilization of the patient with a tracheostomy), humidification techniques and general care for tracheostomies. Patients may have difficulty with an altered body image and need psychological support not only from the team closely involved in their care but also potentially from a formal psychological support team. Other key support teams include rehabilitation teams (for rehabilitation, relaxation and occupational therapy), critical care outreach teams (particularly for newly formed stomas in the ward environment and/or the deteriorating patient with airway difficulties), anaesthetists in the event of an airway emergency, discharge co-ordinators and community teams for patients with airways who are going home.

Humidification

Constant humidification is required while a new stoma adapts to the outside environment. Humidification also prevents the formation of crusts which are liable to obstruct the airway.

Humidification can be provided for patients requiring low rate (1–5 L/min) oxygen therapy by using a disposable nebulizer set with sterile 0.9% sodium chloride (approximately 5 mL), attached to the oxygen supply and setting the gas rate for the liquid to form into humidification droplets. The nebulizer is administered using a specific tracheostomy mask (Figure 10.38) rather than via the nose and mouth, as is usual practice. Local policy will

Figure 10.38 Tracheostomy mask.

determine frequency which may need to be every 4–6 hours or more frequently in patients with more tenacious secretions. 0.9% sodium chloride nebulizers can also be given using air instead of oxygen if the patient is not on oxygen therapy. Patients requiring continual high concentrations of oxygen ($\geq$28%) require humidification via a heated circuit where possible or a cold water Venturi humidified system at all other times (see Figure 10.10). Patients no longer requiring oxygen therapy can receive humidification in the form of a HME and a patient with a laryngectomy stoma can effectively humidify using laryngeal stoma protectors that combine protection along with humidification, for example: Laryngofoam, Buchanan bib, Romet.

Humidification of a tracheostomy is important to prevent drying of the airway which impairs mucus and cilia function resulting in thickened airway secretions. Devices such as HME filters or a Trachphone (Figure 10.39), which also has an integral speaking valve and oxygen port, may be used for tracheostomy patients (Woodrow 2002).

Education

Patient education is paramount to providing quality care. In the initial postoperative/postprocedural phase, this may be purely to aid comfort and relaxation, explaining and stressing the rationale and importance of suctioning, positioning, and how to strengthen cough. This will involve a multidisciplinary approach with all members of the team educating, supporting and providing comfort throughout all interventions.

For patients with long-term tracheostomy needs, early education is vital. Supporting an individual with a tracheostomy of any type requires an understanding of the impact the tracheostomy tube has on the patient's airway and knowing how to manage potential complications (Serra 2000). In order to support and teach the patient and/or their carer, staff must confirm whether the tube serves as the primary airway (i.e. a permanent stoma) or if the patient has a functioning upper airway (Bowers and Scase 2007).

Patient education will come from various sources but primarily the clinical nurse specialists, nursing staff, physiotherapists and community nursing teams will play pivotal roles. Education will be both practical (i.e. through demonstration with their own tracheostomy, possibly utilizing mirrors) or through the use of posters and pictures. Practical tracheal

Figure 10.39 Trachphone.

suctioning on a specialized mannequin and examining the tracheostomy tubes can also be beneficial (Woodrow 2002).

Tracheostomy: dressing change

Evidence-based approaches

A tracheostomy is a surgical opening into the trachea and hence a potential route of infection, so the area should be kept clean. Tracheostomies can also cause damage to the surrounding tissues through pressure and the presence of irritant secretions (Woodrow 2002), necessitating regular inspection and appropriate care of the area to prevent tissue damage and wound breakdown. Changing the dressing will ensure that the surrounding skin remains clean, dry and free from irritation and infection (Edgtton-Winn and Wright 2005).

Rationale
Indications

In some patients, dressing may not be indicated as it creates an ideal environment for bacterial colonization (Higgins 2009).

The decision to dress a tracheostomy should be based on clinical need, although a thorough assessment of the stoma is indicated for all patients with altered airways (i.e. tracheostomy or laryngectomy). The dressing around the tracheostomy tube can be renewed without removing the tube which should be done twice a day or more frequently if necessary (Serra 2000).

Contraindications

Occasionally a surgical team may request that the original dressing remain intact for a period of time, usually 24–48 hours. There may be an increased risk of bleeding associated with the stoma formation and in this instance the dressing should not be changed until consultation with the surgeon has occurred.

Principles of care

Changing the tracheostomy dressing always requires two people (Woodrow 2002): one to secure the tracheostomy and the other to assess and dress the stoma site. When assessing the wound, if infection is suspected, that is, the area is reddened, excoriated, painful, discoloured or exudate is present, a microbiology swab should be sent for culture (Higgins 2009, ICS 2008, Woodrow 2002).

The stoma should be cleaned thoroughly with 0.9% sodium chloride (Woodrow 2002) and an appropriate dressing applied where indicated. This should be a foam dressing, usually manufactured with a cross-shaped incision to fit around the tracheostomy tube (Woodrow 2002). A moisturizing cream, such as E45, can be applied twice daily to the stoma once the tracheostomy tube and associated dressing are removed. For those patients with secretions that tend to accumulate around the stoma, a Cavilon wand can be used to prevent the skin becoming red and excoriated (Hampton 1998).

Stoma sutures (secured to the flange of the tracheostomy tube) are removed on day 7 (day 7–10 if the tracheostomy has been inserted using a percutaneous technique). If the patient has previously received external beam radiotherapy to the neck, stoma sutures are removed on day 10.

581

Procedure guideline 10.9 Tracheostomy: dressing change

This procedures requires two nurses. One is required to hold the tracheostomy in place, and the other to change the dressing.

Essential equipment

- Sterile dressing pack
- Tracheostomy dressing or keyhole dressing
- Cleaning solution, such as 0.9% sodium chloride
- Tracheostomy securing tapes
- Bactericidal alcohol handrub

Medicinal products

- Review a possible need for analgesia

(Continued)

Procedure guideline 10.9 (*Continued*)

Preprocedure

Action	Rationale
1 Explain and discuss the procedure with the patient.	To ensure that the patient understands the procedure and gives their valid consent (NMC 2008b, C).
2 Screen the bed or cubicle.	To ensure the patient's privacy. E
3 Wash hands using bactericidal soap and water or bactericidal alcohol handrub, and prepare the dressing tray or trolley.	To minimize the risk of infection (Fraise and Bradley 2009, E).
4 Perform the procedure using aseptic technique.	To minimize the risk of infection. E

Procedure

5 Remove the soiled dressing from around the tube, clean around the stoma with 0.9% sodium chloride using low-linting gauze.	To reduce the risk of dressing fragments entering the altered airway (Russell 2005, E) and to remove secretions and any crusts.
6 Replace with a tracheostomy dressing or a comfortable foam-backed keyhole dressing (Action Figure 6).	To ensure the patient's comfort. E To avoid pressure from the tube (Scase 2004, E).
7 Renew tracheostomy tapes, checking that 1–2 fingers can be placed between the tapes and neck.	To secure the tube. E To ensure that the tapes are not too tight (Woodrow 2002, E; Scase 2004, E) or too loose, thus decreasing the chance of necrosis caused by excessive pressure from the tapes (Serra 2000, E).

Postprocedure

8 Monitor patient closely for changes in respiratory rate and pattern of breathing, pulse, dyspnoea.	Any procedure to the tracheostomy if not managed correctly may lead to possible dislodgement of tube or secretions, leading to respiratory deterioration or distress. E

Action Figure 6 Sterile tracheostomy dressing or tracheostomy/keyhole dressing.

Tracheostomy: suctioning

Evidence-based approaches

Rationale

An effective cough requires the closure of the glottis, then the reopening of the glottis once an adequate intrathoracic pressure is achieved. When a tracheostomy is *in situ* the mechanism of closing the glottis is compromised, so the patient's ability to remove secretions is reduced as they are unable to generate the high flows required for coughing. In addition to this, the natural mechanisms of warming and humidifying the gases are lost, altering the consistency of secretions. Secretions become thick and dry, inhibiting mucociliary transport (Higgins 2009), leading to a potential blocking of the tracheostomy tube. Tracheal suction is an essential component of managing secretions, maintaining respiratory function and a patent airway.

Indications

The use of routine suctioning should be avoided and careful assessment of the patient's respiratory function should be carried out instead. Inspection, auscultation, percussion and palpation will help to determine the following (Hough 2001, Pryor and Prasad 2008).

- The patient's ability to clear their own secretions.
- Location of any secretions.
- Whether these secretions could be reached by the catheter.
- How detrimental these secretions might be for the patient.

The presence of prominent audible secretions, visible secretions, decreased oxygenation or diminished breath sounds during the assessment would indicate a need for suction (Ireton 2007).

Contraindications

Tracheal suction is an essential component of care for all patients with artificial airways. Most contraindications are relative to the patient's risk of developing adverse reactions or worsening clinical condition as a result of the procedure. Hence choosing to not suction in order to avoid a potential side-effect may sometimes be more harmful to the patient.

However, despite its necessity, suction may be painful and distressing to the patient and can also be complicated by hypoxaemia, bradycardia and cardiovascular compromise (particularly in patients with autonomic dysfunction such as spinal injuries), alveolar collapse, tracheal mucosal damage, bleeding, and the introduction of infection (Higgins 2009, ICS 2008).

Principles of care

Infection risk

Universal precautions must be used at all times when suctioning; this includes wearing aprons, gloves and eye protection. Both the caregiver and patient are at risk of infection when suctioning is performed and in order to minimize this, examination gloves should be worn and an aseptic technique should be used, decontaminating hands with an alcohol handrub before and after the suction procedure (DH and NHSMA 2005). Suction catheters (see Figure 10.58) are for single use only and should be disposed of after each suction.

Method of suctioning

Shallow suctioning, where the catheter is inserted to a pre-measured depth not beyond the distal end of the tracheostomy tube, is preferred to deep suctioning, in which the suction catheter is inserted until resistance is met. Deep suctioning should be avoided as it is associated with increased risks of mucosal damage, inflammation (De Leyn *et al.* 2007) and bleeding, subsequently increasing the risk of airway occlusion. Always suction with the inner tube *in situ* and change to a non-fenestrated inner tube before the procedure. The instillation of 0.9% sodium chloride to 'aid' suctioning is not recommended (Celik and Kanan 2006, ICS 2008).

Anticipated patient outcomes

Suctioning can cause distress, is uncomfortable and is associated with airway changes and cardiovascular instability, and should therefore only be performed when indicated and not at fixed intervals. Frequency should be determined on an individual patient basis and suctioning should aim to clear airway secretions when the patient is not able to, ensuring airway patency and patient safety at all times.

Preprocedural considerations

Equipment

Suction catheter size and suction pressure

Choosing the correct suction catheter size depends on the size of the tracheostomy tube. As a guide, the diameter of the suction catheter should not exceed one-half of the internal diameter of the tracheostomy tube (Griggs 1998, Hough 2001).

The following formula can be used to determine the correct size catheter.

Suction catheter size (Fg) = $2 \times$ (size of tracheostomy tube $- 2$)

For example: 8.00 mm ID tube: $2 \times (8 - 2) = 12$ Fg (ICS 2008)

Removable cap

Black line

Catheter

T piece

Irrigation port

Lock–unlock
control valve

4.0mm (12F)

Kimberly-Clark

Suction
connection

Protective
catheter sleeve

Figure 10.40 Components of a closed-circuit catheter. The control valve locks the vacuum on or off. The catheter is protected inside an airtight sleeve. A T-piece connects the device to the tracheal tube. The irrigation port allows saline instillation for irrigating the patient's airway or for cleaning the catheter.

The incorrect choice of catheter, poor technique and the use of an excessively high suction pressure may all lead to mucosal trauma. The lowest possible vacuum pressure should be used, ≤100–120 mmHg (13–16 kPa), to minimize atelectasis (ICS 2008) and mucosal damage.

Within a critical care setting, a closed-circuit suction system is an alternative method to the open suction system for patients being mechanically ventilated. This closed system has the catheter sealed in a protective plastic sleeve, which is connected permanently into a standard ventilator circuit, thus preventing the catheter becoming contaminated (Figure 10.40). This also reduces the number of times the patient is disconnected from the ventilator, avoiding further hypoxia and cross-infection. Patients who are immunosuppressed, actively infectious patients or those who require high levels of PEEP may in particular benefit from a closed unit (Billau 2004).

Procedure guideline 10.10 Tracheostomy: suctioning a patient

Essential equipment

- Suction source (wall or portable), collection container and tubing, changed every 24 hours to prevent growth of bacteria (Billau 2004)
- Disposable plastic apron
- Eye protection, for example goggles
- Bactericidal alcohol handrub

- Sterile suction catheters (assorted sizes according to tube size)
- A selection of non-sterile, powder-free, clean boxed gloves
- Sterile bottled water (labelled 'suction' with opening date), changed every 24 hours to prevent the growth of bacteria (Billau 2004)

Preprocedure

Action	Rationale
1 If secretions are tenacious, consider using, as prescribed, 2 hourly or more frequently 0.9% sterile sodium chloride nebulizers or other mucolytic agents such as nebulized acetylcysteine.	Suctioning may not be as effective if the secretions become too tenacious or dry. Anecdotal evidence through practice suggests that frequent 0.9% sterile sodium chloride or acetylcysteine nebulizers may assist in loosening dry and thick secretions. E

2	Explain procedure to patient and ensure upright position if possible. If the patient is able to perform their own suction, self-suction should be taught. This is not appropriate in critical care settings.	To obtain the patient's co-operation and to help them relax. E The procedure is unpleasant and can be frightening for the patient (Billau 2004, E). Reassurance is vital. E Self-control of the patient's suction is preferable with long-term stomas, if the patient is able to manage it. E
3	If a patient has a fenestrated outer tube, ensure that a plain inner tube is *in situ*, rather than a fenestrated inner tube (Russell 2005).	Suction via a fenestrated inner tube allows a catheter to pass through the fenestration and cause trauma to the tracheal wall (Billau 2004, E).

Procedure

4	Wash hands with bactericidal soap and water or bactericidal alcohol handrub, and put on a disposable plastic apron, disposable gloves and eye protection.	To minimize the risk of cross-infection. E Gloves minimize the risk of infection transfer to the catheter or from the sputum to the nurse's hands (Fraise and Bradley 2009, E). Some patients may accidentally cough directly ahead at the nurse; standing to one side with tissues at the patient's tracheostomy minimizes this risk. E
5	If patient is oxygen dependent, hyperoxygenate for a period of 3 minutes.	To minimize the risk of acute hypoxia (Billau 2004, E).
6	Ensure that the suction pressure is set to the appropriate level.	Recommended suction pressure is ≤100–120 mmHg (13–16 kPa) to minimize atelectasis (ICS 2008, C).
7	Select the correct size catheter. As a guide, the diameter of the suction catheter should not exceed one-half of the internal diameter of the tracheostomy tube (Griggs 1998, Hough 2001). The following formula can be used to determine the correct size catheter: Suction catheter size (Fg) = 2 × (size of tracheostomy tube − 2) For example: 8.00 mm ID tube: 2 × (8 − 2) = 12 Fg (ICS 2008).	This ensures that hypoxia does not occur while suctioning: the larger the volume, the greater the bore of the tube. E Incorrect choice of catheter size can cause mucosal damage. E A tube with a too small diameter may not be able to remove thick secretion. E
8	Open the end of the suction catheter pack and use the pack to attach the catheter to the suction tubing. Keep the rest of the catheter in the sterile packet. Use an aseptic technique throughout.	To reduce the risk of transferring infection from hands to the catheter and to keep the catheter as clean as possible. E
9	An additional clean, disposable glove can be used on the dominant hand at this stage.	To facilitate easy disposal of the suction catheter after suction. E
10	Remove the catheter from the sleeve and introduce the catheter to about one-third of its length or approximately 10–15 cm (ICS 2008) or until the patient coughs. If resistance is felt, withdraw catheter approximately 1 cm before applying suction by placing the thumb over the suction port control and slowly withdraw the remainder of the catheter (Dean 1997, Wood 1998).	Gentleness is essential; damage to the tracheal mucosa can lead to trauma and respiratory infection. E The catheter should go no further than the carina to prevent trauma. R The catheter is inserted with the suction off to reduce the risk of trauma (Clotworthy 2006c, C).
11	Do not suction the patient for more than 10 seconds (ICS 2008).	Prolonged suctioning may result in acute hypoxia, cardiac arrhythmias (Day *et al.* 2002, C), mucosal trauma, infection and the patient experiencing a feeling of choking.
12	Wrap catheter around dominant hand, then pull back glove over soiled catheter, thus containing catheter in glove, then discard.	Catheters are used only once to reduce the risk of introducing infection. E
13	If the patient is oxygen dependent, reapply oxygen immediately.	To prevent hypoxia. E

585

Procedure guideline 10.10 *(Continued)*

14 Rinse the suction tubing by dipping its end into the sterile water bottle and applying suction until the solution has rinsed the tubing through.	To loosen secretions that have adhered to the inside of the tube. E
15 If the patient requires further suction, repeat the above actions using new gloves and a new catheter. Allow the patient sufficient time to recover between each suction (Billau 2004), particularly if oxygen saturation is low or if patient coughs several times during the procedure. The patient should be observed throughout the procedure.	To ensure general condition is stable. E
16 Repeat the suction until the airway is clear. No more than three suction passes should be made during any one suction episode (Day 2000, Glass and Grap 1995) unless in emergency such as tube occlusion (Nelson 1999).	To minimize the risk of hypoxaemia (Day 2000, E).

Postprocedure

17 Where appropriate, reconnect the patient to oxygen within 10 seconds post suctioning.	To minimize the risk of hypoxaemia (Day 2000, E).
18 Observe patient's respiratory rate and pattern, oxygen saturations, heart rate and work of breathing closely over the following 15 minutes. Observe for signs of bleeding.	Suctioning can be complicated by hypoxaemia, bradycardia, tracheal mucosal damage and bleeding (ICS 2008, C).

Complications

Hypoxia

The act of suctioning reduces vital lung volume from the lungs and upper airways. Each suctioning procedure should last no longer than 10 seconds to decrease the risk of trauma, hypoxia and other side-effects (ICS 2008). Ventilator disconnection or the removal of the oxygen supply will also add to the risk of hypoxia prior to suctioning. Within a critical care setting, this risk can be avoided by hyperoxygenating the lungs with 100% oxygen, either manually or via a ventilator (Glass and Grap 1995, Hough 2001), which should be considered for all patients with high oxygen requirements.

Cardiac arrhythmias

Arrhythmias may be brought about by the onset of hypoxaemia or a vagal reflex instigated by tracheal stimulation by the catheter (MacIntyre and Branson 2009).

Raised intracranial pressure

This may occur if the suction catheter causes excessive tracheal stimulation and results in coughing and an increase in the patient's intrathoracic pressure, both of which compromise cerebral venous drainage (Pryor and Prasad 2008).

Tracheostomy: changing the inner cannula

Evidence-based approaches
Rationale

Tracheostomy tubes with an inner cannula are inherently safer and are now usual practice. Changing the inner cannula regularly allows for visual inspection of secretions, aiding the decision about humidification requirements and reducing the risk of airway occlusion.

Indications

- If a dual-cannula tracheostomy is in use it should always be inspected for patency.

Contraindications

- Only tracheostomy tubes manufactured with a dual inner cannula should be used.
- Care must be taken when considering inspecting and/or changing an inner cannula. Preoxygenation and/or suction may be necessary prior to the procedure so patient stability must be considered.

Principles of care

The inner cannula should be removed, inspected and when necessary changed at regular intervals, the frequency of inspection being determined by the volume and tenacity of the patient's secretions (ICS 2008). In the immediate post-operative phase it may be necessary to change the inner cannula half hourly. Any nurse starting a span of duty should perform a baseline assessment of the airway tube and inner cannula to check, on the type and amount of secretions and the need for humidification (Rhys Evans *et al.* 2003).

Procedure guideline 10.11 Tracheostomy: inner cannula change

Essential equipment

- Sterile dressing pack
- Cleaning solution, such as 0.9% sodium chloride
- Disposable plastic apron, powder-free gloves and eye protection
- Bactericidal alcohol handrub
- Inner cannula of the same size as the tracheostomy tube that is *in situ*

Preprocedure

Action	Rationale
1 Explain and discuss the procedure with the patient.	To ensure that the patient understands the procedure and gives their valid consent (NMC 2008b, C).
2 Ensure the emergency trolley is readily available if required. Inform staff what procedure will be taking place if help required.	In event of difficulty replacing airway. E To ensure that all staff aware that airway is to be changed so in the event of difficulties, staff are available to assist. E
3 Preoxygenate the patient if known to desaturate by increasing the oxygen delivered according to the patient's need to ensure oxygen saturations greater than 95%.	As oxygen mask will be removed for the changing and cleaning or disposing of the inner cannula, the patient will be without additional oxygen for a short period of time and may desaturate (ICS 2008 C).
4 Wash hands using bactericidal soap and water or bactericidal alcohol handrub, and prepare a dressing trolley.	To minimize the risk of infection (Fraise and Bradley 2009, E).
5 Screen the patient's bed.	To ensure the patient's privacy. E

Procedure

Action	Rationale
6 Perform the procedure using clean technique.	To minimize the risk of contamination. E
7 Assist the patient to sit in a semi-recumbent position (Clotworthy 2006d) with the neck extended.	To ensure the patient's comfort and to maintain a patent airway. Extending the neck will make removal and insertion of the tube easier (Clotworthy 2006d, C).
8 Remove the dressing pack from its outer wrappings.	To reduce the risk of cross-infection (Fraise and Bradley 2009, E).
9 Put on a disposable plastic apron and eye protection, for example goggles.	Some patients may accidentally cough directly ahead at the nurse; standing to one side and wearing a disposable apron and eye protection will minimize transfer of secretions on to the nurse. E
10 Clean hands with bactericidal alcohol handrub.	To minimize the risk of infection (Fraise and Bradley 2009, E).
11 Put on clean disposable plastic gloves.	Gloves minimize the risk of infection from the sputum to the nurse's hands (Fraise and Bradley 2009, E).
12 Remove the inner cannula and if disposable, dispose in clinical waste bag. If non-disposable, clean cannula with sterile 0.9% sodium chloride and dry thoroughly. Do not leave the inner cannula to soak.	To minimize the risk of infection (Fraise and Bradley 2009, E). Soaking tubes could result in the absorption of the solution into the material, causing irritation to the trachea (ICS 2008, C) as well as bacterial colonization in stagnant cleaning solution.

587

Procedure guideline 10.11 *(Continued)*

13 Place the new inner tube in position and ensure it is secured in a 'locked' position.	To re-establish airway and prevent cannula from dislodging. E
14 Ensure that the patient is comfortable.	To ensure patient comfort. E
15 Clear away the trolley and equipment.	To remove equipment appropriately. E

Postprocedure

16 Observe patient's respiratory rate and pattern, oxygen saturations, heart rate and work of breathing closely over the following 15 minutes. Observe for signs of bleeding.	Changing a tube is potentially hazardous (ICS 2008, C) and may cause respiratory distress in patients. The insertion of a new tube may cause new bleeding of surrounding tissues. E
17 Document the time when you changed the inner cannula and the type of secretions the patient has, and the size of the tracheostomy tube. Thicker secretions or old blood will require more frequent changes to prevent occlusion of the inner cannula.	To ensure all staff are aware of the tube size and type. (NMC 2009, C). To ensure all staff are aware of the need for and frequency of inner cannula changes. E

Tracheostomy: tube change

Definition

The most critical event after formation of a tracheostomy is the first tube change, although many other aspects of care of these tubes are critical (e.g. suctioning, hygiene, humidity, emergency preparedness). Tube change is a risk because of a possible loss of the airway. The exact period of time to wait before the first postoperative change varies, because time is needed to allow a tract between the skin and the trachea to develop. Therefore around 5 days is usually accepted (Johnson *et al.* 2010).

Evidence-based approaches

Rationale

Indications

- Minimizing risk of postoperative infection and granulation tissue formation around the tube.
- Verifying the formation of a stable tract to allow nursing staff to perform changes.
- Changing from a non-fenestrated to a fenestrated tracheostomy tube to facilitate weaning and communication with tracheostomy speaking valve.

- Downsizing the tracheostomy tube if the patient is clinically improving (MacIntyre and Branson 2009).

Contraindications

- Changing a tracheostomy tube too soon after formation (generally <5 days); this increases likelihood of entry into a false passage as the tract may not have healed adequately.
- Poor visualization of tracheostomy tract and inadequate lighting, exposure, and lack of emergency equipment.
- Performer inexperience without availability of staff versed in airway management.
- Patients with extremely high ventilator settings, which increase the risk of decannulation.
- Patient non-co-operation without ancillary support (Johnson *et al.* 2010).

The Council of the Intensive Care Society recommends that the first tracheostomy tube change should not be performed within 72 hours for surgical tracheostomies, and not before 3–5 (though ideally 7–10) days following a percutaneous tracheostomy to allow the stoma track to establish (ICS 2008).

Procedure guideline 10.12 Tracheostomy: tube change

Essential equipment

- Sterile dressing pack
- Tracheostomy foam-based dressing or keyhole dressing
- Tracheostomy securing tapes or ties
- Cleaning solution, such as 0.9% sodium chloride

- Barrier cream
- Lubricating gel
- Disposable plastic apron, powder-free gloves and eye protection
- Bactericidal alcohol handrub
- New tracheostomy tube for insertion

Preprocedure

Action	Rationale
1 Explain and discuss the procedure with the patient.	To ensure that the patient understands the procedure and gives their valid consent (NMC 2008b, C).
2 Ensure the emergency trolley is readily available. Inform staff what procedure will be taking place in case help is required.	In event of difficulty replacing airway. E To ensure that all staff are aware that airway is to be changed so in the event of difficulties, staff are available to assist. E
3 Recheck suction and oxygen supply, ensure spare tubes, dilators and all emergency equipment are readily available.	To ensure patient safety in the event of inability to secure airway with new tube. E
4 Wash hands using bactericidal soap and water or bactericidal alcohol handrub, and prepare a dressing trolley.	To minimize the risk of infection (Fraise and Bradley 2009, E).
5 Screen the patient's bed.	To ensure the patient's privacy. E

Procedure

Action	Rationale
6 Perform the procedure using clean technique. Always perform the procedure in hospital with a second, appropriately trained, person.	To minimize the risk of contamination. E To ensure patient safety at all times. E
7 Assist the patient to sit in a semi-recumbent position (Clotworthy 2006d) with the neck extended.	To ensure the patient's comfort and to maintain a patent airway. Extending the neck will make removal and insertion of the tube easier (Clotworthy 2006d, C).
8 Remove the dressing pack from its outer wrappings and open the tracheostomy dressing.	To reduce the risk of cross-infection (Fraise and Bradley 2009, E).
9 Put on a disposable plastic apron and eye protection, for example goggles.	Some patients may accidentally cough directly ahead at the nurse; standing to one side and wearing a disposable apron and eye protection will minimize transfer of secretions on to the nurse. E
10 Clean hands with bactericidal alcohol handrub.	To minimize the risk of infection (Fraise and Bradley 2009, E).
11 Put on clean disposable plastic gloves.	Gloves minimize the risk of infection from the sputum to the nurse's hands (Fraise and Bradley 2009, E).
12 If the new tracheostomy is cuffed, check the cuff by inflating it with air (according to manufacturer's instructions) then fully deflate the cuff.	To check for air leaks and spontaneous deflation (Clotworthy 2006d, C).
13 Insert the introducer or obturator of the new tube, checking that it can be easily removed.	To become familiar with removing the introducer or obturator prior to insertion (Clotworthy 2006d, C).
14 Lubricate the new tube sparingly with a lubricating jelly and place on the sterile dressing surface.	To facilitate insertion and maintain sterility. E
15 Thread the new tapes or ties through the slit on one of the flanges by untying one side of the old ties.	To ensure the ties are ready to secure as soon as the tube is inserted. Most ties now are made of Velcro and are comfortable to wear and easy to adjust. E
16 If the old tube is cuffed slowly deflate the cuff, suctioning patient if required.	Pooled secretions above the cuff may enter the lungs when the cuff is deflated (Clotworthy 2006d, C).
17 Gently remove the soiled tube from the patient's neck while asking the patient to breathe out.	Conscious expiration relaxes the patient and reduces the risk of coughing. Coughing can result in unwanted closure of the tracheostomy. E

(Continued)

Procedure guideline 10.12 (*Continued*)

18 Quickly clean around the stoma with 0.9% sodium chloride and dry gently. Apply barrier cream with topical swabs (an aqueous cream may be used if the patient is having the site irradiated).	Provide care efficiently so as to not prolong the time the patient is without a formal airway and/or oxygen. To remove superficial organisms and crusts. Skin around the stoma is at risk of breakdown due to the constant presence of moisture in this area (Serra 2000, C). Meticulous skin care is therefore essential in order to prevent infection. Creams containing metallic compounds must not be used on irradiated skin as metal will worsen any skin reaction (Prior and Russell 2004, C).
19 Insert a clean tube with introducer in place, using an 'up and over' action.	Introduction of the tube is less traumatic if directed along the contour of the trachea. E
20 Remove the introducer immediately.	The patient cannot breathe while the introducer is in place. E
21 Place the inner tube in position.	The inner tube can be changed as necessary when the outer tube is in position, thus minimizing the risk of trauma to trachea and stoma. E The quantity of secretions present will determine the frequency with which the inner tube is changed. E
22 Secure the second tape on the other side of the tracheostomy flange. Ensure the tapes are secure with a space from skin to tie of 1–2 fingers only.	To secure the tube while at the same time ensuring that it will not cause discomfort to the patient. E
23 Remove gloves and ask the patient to breathe out onto the palm of your hand.	Flow of air will be felt if the tube is in the correct position. E
24 With new gloves on, put the tracheostomy dressing around the tube.	To prevent abrasion of the patient's skin by the tube. E
25 Ensure that the patient is comfortable.	The procedure can be traumatic for some patients, resulting in coughing and even discomfort. It is important for the nurse to stay with the patient until coughing has resolved, provide reassurance and administer analgesia where appropriate. E
26 Clear away the trolley and equipment.	To ensure removal of equipment. E
27 Dispose of all single-use tracheostomy tubes immediately in contaminated waste. For long-term reusable tubes, clean the soiled tube with sterile water or in line with the manufacturer's recommendations. If the tube is very soiled then use sodium bicarbonate to remove debris. The tube must be rinsed thoroughly and stored dry at the patient's bedside. Plastic tubes should not be soaked in solutions.	Most new tracheostomy tubes are single use with disposable equipment to prevent infection. To remove debris that may occlude the tube and/or become a source of infection. E Soaking tubes could result in the absorption of the solution into the material, causing irritation to the trachea. E

Postprocedure

28 Observe patient's respiratory rate and pattern, oxygen saturations, heart rate and work of breathing closely over the following 15 minutes. Observe for signs of bleeding.	Changing a tube is potentially hazardous (ICS 2008, C) and may cause respiratory distress in patients. The insertion of a new tube may cause new bleeding of surrounding tissues. E
29 Document the new tube size and type.	To ensure all staff are aware of the tube size and type (NMC 2009, C).

Problem-solving table 10.5 **Prevention and resolution (Procedure guidelines 10.9, 10.10, 10.11, and 10.12)**

Problem	Cause	Prevention	Suggested action
Profuse tracheal secretions	Local reaction to tracheostomy tube	Maintain euvolaemia with adequate and not excessive hydration. Hyoscine can be considered by clinicians to aid in the reduction of excessive secretions following the immediate postoperative phase when excessive secretions are common	Suction frequently, for example every 1–2 hours, or on clinical need
Lumen of tracheostomy tube occluded	Tenacious mucus in tube	Frequent suction as required and regular inner tube changes. Humidify airways. Encourage coughing to clear secretions from within the tube	Change the inner tube. Use 0.9% sodium chloride nebulizers, HMEs and suction. Continue to change the inner tube regularly, for example 1–3-hourly
	Dried blood and mucus in the tube, especially in the postoperative period	As above	Provide humidification (see Procedure guideline 10.2). Humidification, administering air if there is no need for oxygen
Tracheostomy tube dislodged accidentally	Tapes/ties not secured adequately. Tracheostomy tube not secured adequately by staff during moving and handling of patient	Ensure tapes secure at all times with 1–2 finger spaces maximum between skin and tapes/ties. Educate patient and staff about safe mobilization of patients with tracheostomy	Insert spare tube. This should be clean and ready at the bedside (Serra 2000) (emergency box) *Note:* tracheal dilators must be kept at the bedside of patients with tracheostomies (Serra 2000)
Unable to insert clean tracheostomy tube during tube change	Unpredicted shape or angle of stoma	Emergency equipment with spare tubes, lubricant, tracheostomy dilators should always be readily available before tube change. Always perform procedure with a second person when in hospital setting. Only perform if skilled and trained in performing a tube change. Know and understand local policy for emergency management before undertaking the procedure	Remain calm since an outward appearance of distress may cause the patient to panic and lose confidence. Lubricate the tube well and attempt to reinsert at various angles. If unsuccessful, attempt to insert a smaller-size tracheostomy tube. If this is impossible, keep the tracheostomy tract open using tracheal dilators and inform the doctor
	Tracheal stenosis due to patient coughing, patient being very anxious or because the tube has been left out too long		Insert a smaller-size tracheostomy tube. If insertion still proves difficult, do not leave the patient but ask for a tube to be brought to the bed. Keep the tracheostomy patent with tracheal dilators if stenosis is pronounced until the tube is reinserted

(*Continued*)

Problem-solving table 10.5 *(Continued)*

Problem	Cause	Prevention	Suggested action
Tracheal bleeding following or during change of the tube	Trauma due to suction or to the tube being changed. Presence of tumour Granulation tissue forming in fenestration of tube	Ensure emergency equipment including artery forceps available before procedure	Change the tube as planned if bleeding is minimal. For profuse bleeding, insert a cuffed tube and inflate the cuff (Clotworthy 2006d). Inform the doctor. Perform tracheal suction to remove the blood from the trachea
Infection	Nature of surgery and condition of patient often predispose to infection	Ensure dressings are changed when soiled and universal infection precautions are adhered to	Encourage the patient to cough up secretions and/or suction regularly. Change the tube and clean the stoma area frequently, for example 4-hourly. Protect permanent stomas with a bib or gauze. Following result of sputum specimen, commence appropriate antibiotics as needed

Postprocedural considerations

Documentation

All interventions and care given should be clearly documented in the patient's notes once performed. It is essential that all staff caring for a patient with a tracheostomy know the type of tube in place at any one time, and that this information is readily available and clearly documented in the patient's notes (ICS 2008). As discussed, the use of care plans and bundles may aid in standardizing documentation of patients with a tracheostomy, though this should comply with local policy at all times.

Cardiopulmonary resuscitation

Definition

The term cardiac arrest implies a sudden interruption of cardiac output. It may be reversible with appropriate treatment (Handley 2004). The patient will collapse, lose consciousness, stop breathing and will be pulseless (Jevon 2001, Paradis 2007).

The four arrhythmias that cause cardiac arrest are:

- asystole
- ventricular fibrillation (VF)
- pulseless ventricular tachycardia (VT)
- pulseless electrical activity (PEA).

For the purposes of resuscitation guidelines, these rhythms are divided into two groups by their treatment:

- VF and pulseless VT, which require defibrillation.
- non-VF/VT, which do not require defibrillation (Resuscitation Council 2010b).

Resuscitation is the emergency treatment of any condition in which the brain fails to receive enough oxygen.

Anatomy and physiology

The heart

The heart is made up of four chambers: two upper atria and two lower ventricles (Fig 13.5, Conduction system of the heart). The right atrium receives deoxygenated blood via the venous circulation. From the right atrium, blood flows into the right ventricle which pumps it into the lungs via the pulmonary arteries. Carbon dioxide is released and oxygen is absorbed. This blood is oxygenated and returns to the heart via the pulmonary veins that empty into the left atrium. The blood then passes into the left ventricle which pumps it into the aorta and arterial circulation (Waugh and Grant 2010).

The atrioventricular septum completely separates the right and left sides of the heart. From shortly after birth, the two sides of the heart never directly communicate. Blood travels from right side to left side via the lungs only. However, the chambers themselves work together. The two atria contract simultaneously, and the two ventricles contract simultaneously (Waugh and Grant 2010).

To prevent backflow of blood, the heart has valves. The atrioventricular (AV) valves are between the atria and ventricles. The right AV valve between the right atrium and right ventricle is also called the tricuspid valve because it consists of three cusps. The left AV valve between the left atrium and ventricle is called the bicuspid as it has two cusps. Both arteries that emerge from the heart have a valve to prevent blood from flowing back into the heart – the semi-lunar (SL) valves. The pulmonary SL valve lies where the pulmonary trunk leaves the right ventricle and the aortic SL valve is situated at the opening between the aorta and left ventricle. The valves open and close in response to pressure changes as the heart contracts and relaxes (Moran 2010, Tortora and Derrickson 2009).

Cardiac conduction system

This pathway is made up of the:

- sinoatrial (SA) node
- AV node
- bundle of His
- left and right bundle branches
- Purkinje fibres.

The SA node is the natural pacemaker of the heart. It releases electrical stimuli at a regular rate, which will vary depending on whether the body is at rest or in action. As each stimulus passes through the myocardial cells of the atria, it creates a wave of contraction which spreads rapidly through both atria.

The rapidity of atrial contraction is such that around 100 million myocardial cells contract in less than one-third of a second; this is so fast it appears instantaneous.

When the electrical stimulus from the SA node reaches the AV node, it is delayed briefly so that the contracting atria have enough time to pump all the blood into the ventricles. Once the atria are empty of blood, the valves between the atria and ventricles close. At this point the atria begin to refill and the electrical stimulus passes through the AV node, through the bundle of His, along the left and right bundle branches and the Purkinje fibres. In this way all the cells in the ventricles receive an electrical stimulus causing them to contract (Becker 2007).

Around 400 million myocardial cells that make up the ventricles contract in less than one-third of a second. As the ventricles contract, the right ventricle pumps blood to the lungs where carbon dioxide is released and oxygen is absorbed, whilst the left ventricle pumps blood into the aorta from where it passes into the coronary and arterial circulation.

At this point the ventricles are empty, the atria are full and the valves between them are closed. The SA node is about to release another electrical stimulus and the process is about to repeat itself. However, there is a third section to this process. The SA node and AV node contain only one stimulus. Therefore every time the nodes release a stimulus, they must recharge before they can do it again.

In the heart, the SA node recharges whilst the atria are refilling, and the AV node recharges when the ventricles are refilling. This means there is no need for a pause in heart function. Again, this process takes less than one-third of a second. (The times given for the three different stages are based on a heart rate of 60 beats per minute, or 1 beat per second.)

The term used for the release of an electrical stimulus is 'depolarization', and the term for recharging is 'repolarization'.

So, the three stages of a single heart beat are:

- atrial depolarization
- ventricular depolarization
- atrial and ventricular repolarization (Moran 2010, Tortora and Derrickson 2009).

Related theory

Potentially reversible causes of a cardiopulmonary arrest

During cardiac arrest, potential causes or aggravating factors for which specific treatment exists should be considered. For ease of memory, there are eight common causes of arrest, four of which begin with the letter H and four with the letter T.

- Hypoxia.
- Hypovolaemia.
- Hypothermia.
- Hypo/hyperkalaemia.
- Thromboembolism.
- Tension pneumothorax.
- Tamponade.
- Toxicity (metabolic or drug induced) (Resuscitation Council 2010b).

Hypoxia

There are many reasons why a patient may become severely hypoxic, the most common being the following.

- Acute respiratory failure.
- Airway difficulties.
- Acute lung injury.
- Severe anaemia.
- Neuromuscular disorders.

For healthy cell metabolism, the body requires a constant supply of oxygen. When this is interrupted for more than 3 minutes in most situations (except when there is severe hypothermia), cell death occurs, followed by lactic acidosis and very rapidly a cardiorespiratory arrest. The risk of hypoxia is minimized by ensuring that the patient's lungs are ventilated adequately with 100% oxygen (Resuscitation Council 2010b).

Hypovolaemia

Hypovolaemia in adults that results in PEA is usually due to severe blood loss. While it is not the nurse's role to make a medical diagnosis, they may be aware of significant factors in the history of a patient that may have led to PEA.

The most common causes of severe blood loss are:

- trauma
- surgical procedure
- gastrointestinal mucosa erosion
- oesophageal varices
- peripheral vessel erosion (by tumour usually)
- clotting abnormality.

Note: blood loss, although usually overt, can be covert such as a gastrointestinal bleed which may only become apparent when the patient collapses.

The treatment for hypovolaemia is identifying and stopping the source of fluid or blood loss, and replacing the circulating volume with the appropriate fluid. Fluid resuscitation is normally started with a crystalloid, for example 0.9% sodium chloride, and/or colloid, for example Gelofusin (depending on local protocols); there is no evidence that colloids are more effective than crystalloids. Blood is likely to be required rapidly if the blood loss exceeds 1500–2000 mL in an adult (Perel *et al.* 2007, Resuscitation Council 2010b).

Hypothermia

Hypothermia should be suspected in any submersion or immersion injury. During a prolonged resuscitation attempt, a patient who was normothermic at the onset of cardiac arrest may become hypothermic (Resuscitation Council 2010b). A low-reading thermometer should be used if available. Resuscitation in the presence of hypothermia may be prolonged.

Hypo/hyperkalaemia and other metabolic disorders

Because potassium is so closely linked with muscle and nerve excitation, any imbalance will affect both the nervous conduction and the muscular working of the heart. Therefore a severe rise or fall in potassium can cause arrest arrhythmias. The causes of hypokalaemia are:

- gastrointestinal fluid losses
- urinary fluid loss
- drugs that affect cellular potassium, for example antifungal agents such as amphotericin.

The immediate treatment for hypokalaemia that has resulted in an arrest is to give concentrated infusions of potassium while carefully monitoring the serial potassium measurements. Most intensive care unit (ICU)/Accident and Emergency (A&E) departments and coronary care units (CCUs) will have an arterial blood gas analyser that enables the potassium to be measured in 1 minute.

The patients who are most at risk of hyperkalaemia are those with renal failure or Addison's disease. The immediate treatment for hyperkalaemia is to give intravenous calcium. This has the effect of protecting the myocardium during the cardiac arrest. If the patient is successfully resuscitated it will be essential to monitor their serum potassium and if it remains high, to commence therapy to lower or remove the potassium (Resuscitation Council 2006).

Thromboembolism

The most common cause of thromboembolic or mechanical circulatory obstruction is a massive pulmonary embolus. Options for definitive treatment include thrombolysis or, if available, cardiopulmonary bypass and operative removal of the clot (Resuscitation Council 2010b).

Tension pneumothorax

A tension pneumothorax is the sudden collapse of a lung, usually under pressure, which results in a severe change in intrathoracic pressure and cessation of the heart as a pump (Bersten *et al.* 2009). The most common causes are:

- trauma
- acute lung injury
- mechanical ventilation of the newborn.

The immediate treatment is the insertion of a large-bore cannula into the second intercostal space at the midclavicular line of the affected side (Resuscitation Council 2010b). Arrangements should be made for the insertion of a formal chest tube and underwater seal drain (see Procedure guideline 10.4).

Tamponade

This is where there is an acute effusion of fluid in the pericardial space and as it enlarges, the heart is splinted and finally cannot beat. The fluid is usually blood but can be malignant or infected fluid (Dolan and Preston 2006). The most common cause for a sudden tamponade is trauma. The immediate treatment is the insertion of a catheter or surgical drainage of the fluid. After drainage, the cause of the tamponade should be sought and corrected where possible, for example with appropriate antibiotic therapy for a bacterial aetiology or surgical repair of a myocardial laceration (Shoemaker 2000).

Toxicity: poisoning and drug intoxication

Poisoning rarely leads to cardiac arrest but it is a leading cause of death in patients less than 40 years old. Self-poisoning with therapeutic or recreational drugs is the main reason for hospital admission (Resuscitation Council 2010b). There are few specific therapeutic measures for poisons that are useful in the immediate situation. The emphasis must be on intensive supportive therapy, with correction of hypoxia, acid/base balance and electrolyte disorders. Specialist help can be obtained by telephoning one of the regional National Poisons Information Service Centres (Resuscitation Council 2010b).

Evidence-based approaches

Sudden death as a result of cardiac arrest is responsible for 60% of ischaemic heart disease deaths across Europe

(Resuscitation Council 2010b). Survival to hospital discharge is cited as 10.7% of all types of cardiac arrest with survival being higher (21.2%) in ventricular fibrillation arrests (Resuscitation Council 2010b).

Changes to adult basic life support (BLS) guidelines have been made to reflect the importance highlighted by performing high quality chest compressions. The rescuer should reduce the number and duration of pauses during chest compressions (Resuscitation Council 2010b).

Cardiopulmonary resuscitation guidelines in the UK are researched and implemented by the Resuscitation Council UK, and BLS and ALS guidelines are changed according to their recommendations. Although the Resuscitation Council guidelines of 2000 recommended immediate defibrillation for all shockable rhythms, evidence indicates that a period of CPR before defibrillation may improve survival after prolonged collapse (>5 min) (Wik *et al.* 2003). The duration of collapse is frequently difficult to estimate accurately, so CPR should be given before attempted defibrillation outside hospital, unless the arrest is witnessed by a healthcare professional or an automated external defibrillator (AED) is being used (Resuscitation Council 2010b).

In contrast, there is no evidence to support or refute the use of CPR before defibrillation for in-hospital cardiac arrest. For this reason, after in-hospital VF/VT cardiac arrest, a shock should be given as soon as possible (Resuscitation Council 2010b). Continuing good-quality CPR may improve the amplitude and frequency of fine VF and improve the chance of successful defibrillation to a perfusing rhythm, as fine VF is difficult to distinguish from asystole and very unlikely to be shocked successfully.

Rationale

The basic technique involves a rapid simple assessment of the patient followed by the basic life support (BLS) resuscitation. The first international consensus evidence-based guidelines on resuscitation were published in 2000 (AHA/ILCOR, 2010, Shuster *et al.* 2010). These guidelines were reviewed in 2004/05 by the International Liaison Committee on Resuscitation and published in 2005 (AHA/ILCOR 2010). These internationally agreed guidelines based on research and audit now form the basis for the European resuscitation guidelines (Baskett *et al.* 2005) as well as the UK resuscitation guidelines (Resuscitation Council 2010b).

Changes to Resuscitation Council UK guidelines suggest that the rescuer should not stop to check the patient or discontinue CPR unless the person starts to show signs of regaining consciousness, such as coughing, opening eyes, speaking or moving purposefully and starts to breathe normally (Resuscitation Council 2010b).

Indications

- The patient is unconscious, has absent or agonal (gasping) respirations and has no pulse (Perkins *et al.* 2005). Other clinical features such as pupil size, cyanosis and pallor are unreliable and so the practitioner should not waste time looking for them (Skinner and Vincent 1997).

Contraindications

- Do not attempt resuscitation orders (DNAR) (Box 10.6).
- If the environment is going to place the rescuer at risk, do not attempt resuscitation until environment secured.

Principles of care

Failure of the circulation for 3–4 minutes will lead to irreversible cerebral damage (Docherty and Hall 2002). BLS acts to slow down the deterioration of the brain and the heart until defibrillation and/or advanced life support (ALS) can be provided (Resuscitation Council 2010b).

Assessment

There are two stages of assessment.

- An immediate assessment by the rescuer to ensure that CPR may safely proceed (i.e. checking there is no immediate danger to the rescuer from any hazard, for example electrical power supply).
- Assessment by the rescuer of the likelihood of injury sustained by the patient, particularly injury to the cervical spine. Although there may be no external evidence of injury, the immediate situation may provide the necessary evidence. For example, trauma to the cervical spine should be suspected in an accelerating/decelerating injury such as a road traffic accident with a motorbike travelling at speed.

Once these two aspects have been assessed, the patient's level of consciousness should be checked by gently shaking his shoulders and asking loudly if he is all right (Figure 10.41). If there is no response, the rescuer should commence the BLS assessment (Figure 10.42) immediately.

Figure 10.41   Initial verbal assessment.

Box 10.6 Decision making: do not attempt resuscitation (DNAR)

In an attempt to reduce the number of futile resuscitation attempts, many hospitals have introduced formal DNAR policies, which can be applied to individual patients in specific circumstances. Healthcare professionals must be able to show that their decisions relating to CPR are compatible with the human rights set out in the Human Rights Act 1998 implemented on 2 October 2000 (e.g. the right to life, the right to be free from inhuman or degrading treatment and freedom of expression) (BMA 2000, BMA *et al.* 2002). The following guidelines are based on those provided in a joint statement by the British Medical Association (BMA), the Royal College of Nursing (RCN) and the Resuscitation Council UK (BMA *et al.* 2002). (*Note*: where no decision has been made and the express wishes of the patient are unknown, CPR should be performed without delay.)

- Sensitive advance discussion between experienced medical/nursing staff and patients regarding attempting CPR should be encouraged but not forced. Where patients lack competence to participate, people close to them can be helpful in reflecting their views. (*Note*: in England, Wales and Northern Ireland, no person is legally entitled to give consent to medical treatment on behalf of another adult.) Information about CPR needs to be realistic. Written information explaining CPR should be available for patients and those close to them to read. The BMA, in liaison with the Resuscitation Council UK, RCN and Age Concern England, has published an information leaflet that may help patients and families to discuss DNAR with medical and nursing staff (BMA *et al.* 2002).
- Patients are entitled to refuse CPR even when there is a reasonable chance of success.
- Some patients may ask that no DNAR order be made. Patients cannot demand treatment which the healthcare team judges to be inappropriate, but all efforts should be made to accommodate their wishes and preferences.
- An advance DNAR order should only be made after consideration of the likely clinical outcome, the patient's wishes and the patient's human rights. It should be considered on an individual patient basis where:
  - attempting CPR will not start the patient's heart and breathing
  - there is no benefit in restarting the patient's heart and breathing
  - the expected benefit is outweighed by the burdens (Resuscitation Council 2010b).
- The overall responsibility for decisions about CPR and DNAR orders rests with the consultant in charge of the patient's care. Issues should, however, be discussed with other members of the healthcare team, the patient and people close to the patient where appropriate.
- There are exceptional cases where resuscitation discussions with a patient may be inappropriate, for example where senior members of the medical and nursing team consider that CPR would be futile and that such a discussion would cause the patient unnecessary distress and anguish. This could apply to patients in the terminal phase of their illness.
- The most senior members of the medical and nursing team available should clearly document any decisions made about CPR in the patient's medical and nursing notes. The decision should be dated and the reasons for it given. This information must be communicated to all other relevant healthcare professionals. Unless it is against the wishes of the patient, their family should also be informed.
- The DNAR order should be reviewed on each admission or in light of changes in the patient's condition (BMA *et al.* 2002).
- Finally, it should be noted that a DNAR order applies only to CPR and should not reduce the standard of medical or nursing care.

Note: if the arrest is witnessed or monitored, and a defibrillator is not immediately to hand, a single precordial thump should be administered. If delivered within 30 seconds after cardiac arrest, a sharp blow with a closed fist on the patient's sternum may convert VF back to a perfusing rhythm (Resuscitation Council 2010b).

Defibrillation

Defibrillation causes a simultaneous depolarization of the myocardium and aims to restore normal rhythm to the heart. This is the definitive treatment for VF and pulseless VT. It has been suggested that 80–90% of adults who collapse because of non-traumatic cardiac arrest are found to be in VF when first attached to a monitor (Varon *et al.* 1998). In hospital, cardiac arrest is more likely to present as non-VF/VT, in other words asystole or PEA. Early defibrillation is a vital link in the chain of survival and developments in public access defibrillation and first responder defibrillation by ward nurses in hospitals are focusing firmly on this link. Delay in defibrillation decreases the chances of success by 7–10% each minute (Robertson *et al.* 1998). Nurses are often first on the scene at a cardiac arrest, highlighting the obvious need for nurse-led defibrillation at ward level. While not all nurses are trained in defibrillation, they should understand why it is necessary and how it is done and be able to assist in an emergency (Austin and Snow 2000). Resuscitation guidelines suggest asking for an automated external defibrillator (AED), if one is available, as it can be used safely and effectively without previous training (Resuscitation Council 2010b). The aim of an effective defibrillation strategy is to reduce the preshock pause to less than 5 seconds by planning ahead and continuing cardiac compressions during charging, and using a very brief safety check (Resuscitation Council 2010b).

Method of basic life support

Basic life support is sometimes known as the 'ABC'.

Figure 10.44   The recovery position.

Figure 10.42   Basic life support algorithm. Courtesy of Resuscitation Council (2010b).

Airway

The rescuer should look in the mouth and remove any visible obstruction (leave well-fitting dentures in place). The most likely obstruction in an unconscious person is the tongue. The head tilt/chin lift manoeuvre (Figure 10.43), which removes the tongue from occluding the oropharynx, is an effective method of opening an airway and relieving obstruction in 80% of patients (Simmons 2002).

Note: if there is any suspicion of cervical spine injury, try to avoid head tilt.

Breathing

Keeping the airway open, the rescuer should look, listen and feel for breathing (more than an occasional gasp or weak attempts at breathing) for up to 10 seconds. If the patient is breathing they should be turned into the recovery position (Figure 10.44). If the adult patient is not breathing and

Figure 10.43   Head tilt/chin lift manoeuvre.

there is no suspicion of trauma or drowning, an immediate call for the cardiac arrest team should be made. It should be noted that in 40% of cases a person who has arrested still has agonal (gasping) respirations and these can be mistaken for normal breaths (Hauff *et al.* 2003).

Artificial ventilation must then be commenced and maintained. If there are no aids to ventilation available then direct mouth-to-mouth ventilation should be used. There have been isolated reports of infections such as tuberculosis (TB) and severe acute respiratory distress syndrome (SARS) following mouth-to-mouth ventilation but never transmission of HIV. There is no evidence to quantify the degree of risk to the rescuer by performing mouth-to-mouth ventilation but, as it is widely acknowledged that there is reluctance by some people in spite of the lack of evidence, an allowance has been made for them to only perform chest compressions (Resuscitation Council 2010b). The recommended length for each breath is now 1 second (Resuscitation Council 2010b). When cardiac arrest occurs in hospital, the Resuscitation Council recommends the use of adjuncts such as the pocket mask or the bag mask unit. These can be used to avoid direct person-to-person contact and some devices may reduce the risk of cross-infection between patient and rescuer (Resuscitation Council 2010b). In 2005, in recognition of the concern about providing mouth-to-mouth resuscitation, the guidelines changed and the BLS algorithm now starts with chest compressions and then proceeds to two breaths (Resuscitation Council 2010b).

One of the most easily learnt aids is the 'mouth-to-facemask' method (Figure 10.45) in which a ventilation mask with a one-way valve and an oxygen attachment port is used. The mask directs the patient's exhaled air and any fluid away from the rescuer and the oxygen port allows attachment of oxygen with enrichment up to 45%.

If the operator is skilled in airway management, an Ambubag and mask may be used. When the bag is attached to

597

Figure 10.47   Carotid pulse check.

Figure 10.45   Mask with one-way valve over patient's nose and mouth and rescuer giving breath. Used with permission from Moule and Albarran (2009).

num (Figure 10.48). The rescuer should position themselves vertically above the patient with arms straight and elbows locked. The sternum should be pressed down to depress it by 5–6 cm. This should be repeated at a rate of about 100–120 times a minute. After 30 compressions two rescue breaths are given, continuing compressions and rescue breaths in a ratio of 30:2 (Resuscitation Council 2010b). There is evidence that chest compressions are often interrupted and that this is associated with a reduction in the chance of survival. New adult advanced life support guidelines (Resuscitation Council 2010b) suggest an increased emphasis on the importance of minimal interuption in high quality chest compressions throughout any ALS intervention, therefore, chest compressions are now continued while a defibrillator is charging, which will minimize the pre-shock pause. It is therefore imperative that interruptions to chest compressions are minimized by effective co-ordination between rescuers (Eftestol *et al.* 2002, van Alem *et al.* 2003, Resuscitation Council 2010b).

oxygen, high levels, of up to 85%, can be obtained. However, it should be emphasized that to manipulate the head tilt, and hold on a facemask while squeezing a bag is a procedure that requires practice and is most safely achieved by two people, one holding the mask and one squeezing the bag (Hodgetts and Castle 1999, Resuscitation Council 2010b) (Figure 10.46).

The most effective method of airway management is to use an endotracheal tube, thus enabling the application of 100% oxygen (Resuscitation Council 2010b, Robertson *et al.* 1998). This method of airway management is included in the advanced life support (ALS) algorithm.

Circulation

Circulation is assessed by looking for any signs of movement, including swallowing or breathing. If trained to do so, a check should also be made for the carotid pulse (Figure 10.47) for up to 10 seconds. If no circulation is detected, it must be maintained by compressions. The correct place to compress is in the centre of the lower half of the ster-

Legal and professional issues

All members of the healthcare professions who attempt resuscitation will be expected to employ the highest professional standard of care, in line with their level of training. In general, there are two means by which the risk of personal

Figure 10.46   Two people using Ambu-bag and mask. Used with permission from Moule and Albarran (2009).

Figure 10.48   Correct positioning of hands for external compressions.

liability may be minimized. The first is by good practice and the second is by taking out adequate indemnity insurance (NMC 2008a, Resuscitation Council 2010a). To ensure best practice, make sure that regular updates for BLS and if appropriate ALS training are maintained.

The Resuscitation Council (UK) guidelines state that if rescuers are not able, or are unwilling, to give rescue breaths, they should give chest compressions alone (Resuscitation Council 2010b).

Whenever CPR is carried out (outside the hospital setting), particularly on an unknown victim, there is some risk of cross-infection, associated particularly with giving rescue breaths. Normally, this risk is very small and has to be set against the inevitability that a person in cardiac arrest will die if no assistance is given.

Competencies

Cardiopulmonary resuscitation standards and training

The Resuscitation Council UK (RCUK), formed in 1981, aims to promote the education of lay and professional personnel in the most effective methods of resuscitation appropriate to their needs. In its report *CPR Guidance for Clinical Practice and Training in Hospitals* (Resuscitation Council 2004), the Council made a number of recommendations relating to the provision of a resuscitation service in hospital.

- *Resuscitation committee.* This should comprise medical and nursing staff who advise on the role and composition of the cardiac arrest team, resuscitation equipment and resuscitation training equipment.
- *Resuscitation Training Officer* (RTO), who should be responsible for training in resuscitation, equipment maintenance and the auditing of resuscitation/clinical trials.
- *Resuscitation training.* Hospital staff should receive at least annual resuscitation training appropriate to their level and role. Medical and nursing staff should receive basic resuscitation training and should be encouraged to recognize patients who are at risk of having a cardiac arrest and call for appropriate help early. This is the most effective method of improving outcome (Jevon 2002). All medical staff should have advanced resuscitation training and senior nurses and doctors working in acute specialities (CCU, ITU, A&E) should hold a valid RCUK ALS certificate.
- *Cardiac arrest team.* Each hospital should have a team of approximately five people including a minimum of two doctors (physician and anaesthetist), an ALS-trained nurse, the RTO and a porter when possible. Clear procedures should be available for calling the cardiac arrest team. The Resuscitation Council has recommended the development of a medical emergency team which recognizes patients at risk of having a cardiac arrest and initiates the most appropriate clinical intervention to prevent it (Jevon 2002). The development of Track and Trigger systems and MEWS (modified early warning sys-

Figure 10.49 In-hospital resuscitation algorithm. CPR, cardiopulmonary resuscitation; IV, intravenous. Courtesy of Resuscitation Council (2010b).

tem) alerts nurses to when a patient is deteriorating so that they can initiate interventions and early referral to critical care outreach teams or medical emergency teams (DH 2000, NICE 2007). Hospital staff are often trained in BLS techniques (see Figure 10.41) that are more appropriate for the single lay rescuer in an out-of-hospital environment. These new guidelines are aimed primarily at healthcare professionals who are first to respond to an in-hospital cardiac arrest (Figure 10.49). Some of the guidelines are also applicable to healthcare professionals in other clinical settings (Resuscitation Council 2004).

Preprocedural considerations

Equipment

All hospital wards and appropriate departments, for example theatre, computed tomography (CT) scanning, should have a standardized cardiac arrest trolley or box. Resuscitation equipment should be checked on a daily basis (Resuscitation Council 2010b) by the staff on the wards or clinical areas responsible for it, and a record of this check should be maintained (see Procedure guideline 10.13). Defibrillators should also be standardized. The use of AEDs or shock advisory defibrillators is recommended to reduce mortality from cardiac arrests related to ischaemic heart disease (Jevon 2002). Bossaert (1997) recommends that defibrillation should be a basic skill requirement of all nurses.

Training should be provided in the use of AEDs but if there is no trained individual present when a cardiac arrest occurs, the Resuscitation Council (UK) advises that an untrained individual should attempt AED defibrillation. The administration of a defibrillatory shock should not be delayed by waiting for more highly trained personnel to arrive. The same principle should apply to individuals

599

Figure 10.50 Placement of defibrillation pads attached to defibrillator on patient's chest.

whose period of qualification has expired (Resuscitation Council 2010b).

Placement of paddles or self-adhesive electrodes

The right paddle or electrode should be placed to the right of the sternum below the clavicle and the left paddle vertically in the midaxillary line approximately level with the position V6 used in electrocardiogram (ECG) monitoring (see Figure 10.50).

Safe defibrillation practice

Defibrillation in an environment where high flows of oxygen are present could represent a danger to patients and rescuers. It is therefore essential to ensure that oxygen tubing and equipment are moved away from the chest when defibrillation is performed. Using adhesive electrodes to deliver the shock as opposed to paddles may also minimize the danger (Resuscitation Council 2010b).

A *pocket mask with oxygen port* (Figure 10.51) may be used as an adjunct to administer mouth-to-mask ventilation for a patient with respiratory arrest. The patient should be in the supine position with the head in the sniffing position (head tilt, chin lift – see Figure 10.43). Apply the mask to the patient's face using the thumbs of both hands.

Figure 10.51 Pocket mask with oxygen port.

Lift the jaw into the mask with the remaining fingers by exerting pressure behind the angles of the jaw (jaw thrust). Blow through the inspiratory valve and watch the chest rise. Stop inflation and allow the chest to fall before blowing in the second breath.

A *self-inflating resuscitation bag* with oxygen reservoir and tubing (Figure 10.52) may be used to administer high inspired oxygen concentrations to a patient and can be connected to a facemask, laryngeal mask or tracheal mask. As the bag is squeezed, the contents are delivered to the patient's lungs and on release, the expired gas is diverted to the atmosphere via a one-way valve and the bag then refills automatically via an inlet at the opposite end. Used alone, the bag-valve apparatus ventilates the patient's lungs with ambient air only (FiO_2: 0.21), which can be increased to around 45% by attaching oxygen tubing and increasing the flow to 5–6 L/min directly to the bag adjacent to the air intake. If a reservoir system is attached and the oxygen flow is increased to 10 L/min, an inspired oxygen concentration of approximately 85% can be achieved (Resuscitation Council 2010b).

An *oropharyngeal or Guedel airway* is a curved plastic tube, flanged and reinforced at the oral end with a flattened shape to ensure that it fits neatly between the tongue and the hard palate. It is used to overcome backward tongue displacement in an unconscious patient. Guedel airways

Figure 10.52 Self-inflating resuscitation bag with oxygen reservoir.

Figure 10.53 Measure the Guedel airway from the corner of the mouth to the angle of the jaw. Used with permission from Moule and Albarran (2009).

Figure 10.54 Insert the Guedel airway in an upside down position to the junction of the hard and soft palate. Used with permission from Moule and Albarran (2009).

Figure 10.55 Rotate the Guedel airway 180° once you have reached the junction of the hard and soft palate. Used with permission from Moule and Albarran (2009).

Figure 10.56 Insert the Guedel airway until it lies in the oropharynx. Used with permission from Moule and Albarran (2009).

come in sizes 2, 3 and 4, for small, medium and large adults respectively. Choosing the right size is done by measuring the Guedel airway from the corner of the mouth to the angle of the jaw/mandible, as indicated in Figure 10.53.

The technique for insertion of an oropharyngeal airway in the unconscious patient is as follows.

- Open the patient's mouth and ensure, by looking into the mouth, that there is no foreign material that may be pushed into the larynx.
- Insert the airway into the mouth in the 'upside-down' position as far as the junction of the hard and soft palate and then rotate the airway through 180° (Figures 10.54, 10.55, 10.56). Then insert the airway until it lies in the oropharynx. This rotation technique minimizes the chance of pushing the tongue backwards and downwards which would further obstruct the airway (Resuscitation Council 2010b).

Use of the incorrect size oropharyngeal airway may result in trauma, laryngospasm and/or worsening of the airway obstruction.

Suction equipment such as a wide-bore suction end (Yankauer sucker – Figure 10.57) should be used to remove liquid (blood, saliva and gastric contents) from the upper airway. This is done best under direct vision during intubation but should not result in any delay in achieving a definitive airway. If tracheal suction is necessary, it should be as brief as possible and preceded and followed by ventilation with 100% oxygen.

Endotracheal suction catheters (Figure 10.58) are used to clear secretions from endotracheal or tracheostomy tubes or laryngeal airway masks (Hallstrom *et al.* 2000, Resuscitation Council 2010b).

A *laryngeal mask airway* (LMA) (size 4) or Combitube (small) consists of a wide-bore tube with an elliptical inflated cuff designed to seal around the laryngeal opening. It is easier to ventilate a patient using bag-valve-LMA ventilation than using bag-valve-facemask ventilation, because of difficulty of ensuring no air leak on the facemask, especially if there is only one person available to ventilate the patient. The LMA is a reliable and safe device and has a high success rate, after a short period of training (Figure 10.59) (Hallstrom *et al.* 2000, Resuscitation Council 2010b).

Figure 10.57   Yankauer sucker.

Figure 10.59   Laryngeal mask airway.

Figure 10.58   Endotracheal/tracheostomy suction catheter.

Figure 10.60   Magill forceps.

A *Magill forceps* (Figure 10.60) is a curved forceps which can be used by the anaesthetist for a difficult intubation and to help introduce an endotracheal tube during intubation (Figure 10.61). Tracheal intubation is considered to be superior to other advanced techniques of airway management because the airway is reliably isolated from foreign material in the oropharynx (Hallstrom *et al.* 2000). Extensive training and regular practice are required to acquire and maintain the skills of intubation, and endotracheal tubes (oral, cuffed, sizes 6, 7 and 8) are kept on emergency trolleys and should be sized according to the patient's size and gender.

An *introducer* such as a gum elastic bougie (Figure 10.62) or a semi-rigid stylet is a useful aid to intubation. Water-soluble lubricating jelly is used prior to intubation or insertion of the LMA or nasopharyngeal airway to aid smooth insertion.

A *laryngoscope* (see Figure 10.63) with both curved Macintosh and long blades is used by the anaesthetist to visualize the vocal cords prior to intubation. It consists of a handle with either rechargeable or removable batteries and a light source, which needs to be checked regularly, as well as just before use, and in case of malfunction spare batteries and light sources need to be available (Resuscitation Council 2010b).

Figure 10.61   Endotracheal tubes.

Figure 10.62   Bougie.

Figure 10.63 Laryngoscope handle and blade.

Assessment and recording tools

Decisions relating to CPR ideally should have been documented prior to a cardiac arrest. Every hospital should have a DNAR policy based on national guidelines (BMA *et al.* 2002, Jevon 2001).

During and after a cardiac arrest, all resuscitation attempts should be documented for auditing purposes, ideally using a nationally recognized template such as the Utstein template (recommended for use by the RCUK). If these recommendations are implemented, standards in resuscitation and resuscitation training should improve (Jevon 2002).

Pharmacological support

Only a few drugs are indicated during the immediate management of a cardiac arrest and there is only limited scientific evidence supporting their use. Drugs should be considered only after a sequence of shocks has been delivered (if indicated) and chest compressions and ventilation started (Resuscitation Council 2010b). Central venous access is optimum as it allows for drugs to be delivered rapidly. However, this is dependent on the skills available. If a peripheral intravenous cannula is already in place, it should be used first (Resuscitation Council 2010b). It is also possible to administer drugs using the intraosseous route, which is used commonly in the resuscitation of children.

The drugs used in the treatment of cardiac arrest are as follows.

- *Adrenaline* 1 mg (10 mL of a 1:10,000 solution) given intravenously. The main purpose of adrenaline is to utilize its inotropic effect to maintain coronary and cerebral perfusion during a prolonged resuscitation attempt. It is the first drug used in cardiac arrest of any aetiology. Adrenaline is included in the ALS universal algorithm (Figure 10.64), 1 mg to be given every 3–5 minutes (Resuscitation Council 2005).
- *Atropine* is no longer recommended routinely in patients with asystole or PEA (Resuscitation Council 2010b).
- *Amiodarone* (300 mg in 20 mL) should be considered in VF or pulseless VT. It increases the duration of the action potential in the atrial and ventricular myocardium; thus

Figure 10.64 The advanced life support algorithm for the management of cardiac arrest in adults. CPR, cardiopulmonary resuscitation; ECG, electrocardiogram, PEA, pulseless electrical activity; VF, ventricular fibrillation; VT, ventricular tachycardia. Courtesy of the Resuscitation Council (2010b).

the QT interval is prolonged. In refractory VT or VF following recovery from cardiac arrest, a further 300 mg may be given followed by an infusion of 900 mg over 24 hours (Resuscitation Council 2010b). *Note:* lidocaine can still be considered if amiodarone is not available (Resuscitation Council 2010b).

- *Calcium chloride* (10 mL of 10%) is only given during resuscitation when specifically indicated, that is, for the treatment of PEA caused by hyperkalaemia, hypocalcaemia or overdose of calcium channel-blocking drugs (Resuscitation Council 2010b). Although it plays a vital role in the cellular mechanisms underlying myocardial contraction, there is little data supporting any beneficial action for calcium following most cases of cardiac arrest (Resuscitation Council 2010b).
- *Sodium bicarbonate* 8.4% is only used in prolonged cardiac arrest or according to serial blood gas analyses.

603

Figure 10.65 Mini-jet vial and administration chamber with Luer-Lock connector. Used with permission from Moule and Albarran (2009).

Figure 10.66 Remove caps from both mini-jet vials and administration chamber. Used with permission from Moule and Albarran (2009).

Figure 10.67 Screw mini-jet vial into administration chamber. Used with permission from Moule and Albarran (2009).

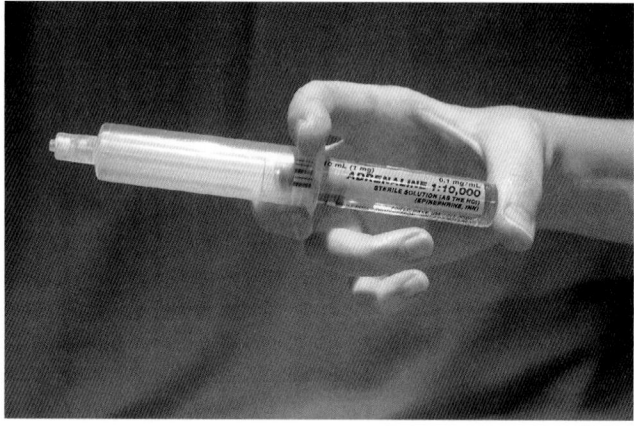

Figure 10.68 Push vial gently to ensure that medication can be administered and connect Luer-Lock to intravenous device and inject entire contents, followed by 0.9% sodium chloride flush. Used with permission from Moule and Albarran (2009).

Potential adverse effects of excessive sodium bicarbonate administration include hypokalaemia, exacerbation of respiratory acidosis and increased affinity of haemoglobin for oxygen. The high concentration of sodium can also exacerbate cerebral oedema. Other adverse effects are increased cardiac irritability and impaired myocardial performance. Sodium bicarbonate is usually given in 25–50 mmol aliquots and repeated as necessary. It can also be given in the special circumstances of tricyclic overdose or hyperkalaemia (Winser 2001).

■ *Magnesium sulphate.* Magnesium (4–8 mmol of 50%) should be given in cardiac arrest where there is a suspicion of hypomagnesaemia as this may precipitate refractory VF/VT (Winser 2001). It is important to recognize torsade de pointes. Many of these patients are hypomagnesaemic and/or hypokalaemic and part of effective treatment (prevention of recurrent episodes) will be giving intravenous magnesium and correction of any other electrolyte abnormality. The normal value for magnesium is 0.8–1.2 mmol/L (Wakeling and Mythen 2000).

Use prefilled syringes (mini-jets) whenever possible for speed and ease of use (Figures 10.65, 10.66, 10.67, 10.68). Drugs should be considered only after chest compressions and ventilation have been started and, where indicated, defibrillation attempted.

Specific patient preparations
Education

Hospital staff should receive at least annual resuscitation training appropriate to their level and role. Medical and nursing staff should receive basic resuscitation training and should be encouraged to recognize patients who are at risk of having a cardiac arrest and call for appropriate help early. MEWS is a track and trigger system which alerts nurses to when a patient is deteriorating in order to initiate interventions and early referral to critical care outreach teams (DH 2000, NICE 2007). This is the most effective method of improving outcome (Jevon 2002). All medical staff should have advanced resuscitation training and senior nurses and doctors working in acute specialties (CCU, ITU, A&E) should hold a valid RCUK ALS certificate. The importance of prevention of cardiac arrest cannot be highlighted enough. Using a structured communication tool, such as Situation, Background, Assessment, Recommendation (SBAR), may help to identify patients at risk in a timely manner (Resuscitation Council 2010b).

Procedure guideline 10.13 Cardiopulmonary resuscitation

Essential equipment

Airway management
- Pocket masks with oxygen port
- Self-inflating resuscitation bag with oxygen reservoir and tubing
- Clear facemasks in sizes 4, 5 and 6
- Oropharyngeal airways in sizes 2, 3 and 4
- Yankauer suckers × 2
- Endotracheal suction catheters × 10
- Laryngeal mask airway (size 4) or Combitube (small)
- Magill forceps
- Endotracheal tubes: oral, cuffed, sizes 6, 7 and 8
- Gum elastic bougie
- Lubricating jelly
- Laryngoscopes × 2: normal and long blades
- Spare laryngoscope bulbs and batteries
- 1 inch ribbon gauze/tape
- Scissors
- Syringe: 20 mL
- Clear oxygen mask with reservoir bag
- Oxygen cylinders × 2 (if no wall oxygen)
- Cylinder key

Circulation equipment:
- Intravenous cannulas: 18 gauge × 3, 14 gauge × 3
- Hypodermic needles: 21 gauge × 10
- Syringes: 2 mL × 6, 5 mL × 6, 10 mL × 6, 20 mL × 6
- Cannula fixing dressings and tapes × 4
- Seldinger wire central venous catheter kits × 2
- 12 gauge non-Seldinger central venous catheter × 2
- Intravenous administration sets × 3
- 0.9% sodium chloride: 1000 mL bags × 2

Optional equipment
- Extra ECG electrodes
- Extra defibrillation gel pads unless using fast patch electrodes
- Clock
- Gloves/goggles/aprons
- A sliding sheet or similar device should be available for safe handling

Medicinal products
Immediately available prefilled syringes of:
- Atropine: 3 mg × 1
- Amiodarone: 300 mg × 1
- Adrenaline: 1 mg (1:10,000) × 4

Other readily available drugs used in CPR:
- Epinephrine (adrenaline): 1 mg (1:10,000) × 4
- Sodium bicarbonate 8.4%: 50 mL × 1
- Calcium chloride 10%: 10 mL × 2
- Lidocaine: 100 mg × 2
- Atropine: 1 mg × 2
- 0.9% sodium chloride: 10 mL ampoules × 10
- Naloxone: 400 g × 2
- Epinephrine/adrenaline 1:1000 × 2
- Amiodarone: 150 mg × 4
- Magnesium sulphate 50% solution: 2 g (4 mL) × 1
- Potassium chloride 40 mmol × 1
- Adenosine: 6 mg × 10
- Hydrocortisone: 200 mg × 1
- Glucose 10%: 500 mL × 1

Preprocedure

Action	Rationale
1 Note time of arrest, if witnessed.	Lack of cerebral perfusion for approximately 3–4 minutes can lead to irreversible brain damage. E

Procedure

2 Give patient precordial thump only in witnessed collapse and in cardiac monitored arrest if defibrillator not immediately available.	This may restore cardiac rhythm, which will give a cardiac output. E. Single precordial thump has low success rate for cardioversion of shockable rhythm (Haman et al. 2009, E).

(Continued)

605

Procedure guideline 10.13 *(Continued)*

3 Summon help. If a second nurse is available, they can call for the cardiac arrest team, bring emergency equipment and screen off the area.	Maintain patient's privacy and dignity. CPR is more effective with two rescuers. One is responsible for inflating the lungs, and the other for chest compressions. Continue until medical help arrives (Resuscitation Council 2010b, C).
4 Lie patient flat on a firm surface/bed. If on a chair, lower the patient to the floor, ensuring that the head is supported.	Effective external cardiac massage can be performed only on a hard surface (Resuscitation Council 2010b, C).
5 If patient is in bed, remove bed head and ensure adequate space between back of bed and wall.	To allow easy access to patient's head in order to facilitate intubation. E
6 Ensure a clear airway. If cervical spine injury is excluded, extend, not hyperextend, the neck (thus lifting the tongue off the posterior wall of the pharynx). This is best achieved by lifting the chin forwards with the finger and thumb of one hand while pressing the forehead backwards with the heel of the other hand (see Figure 10.42). If this fails to establish an airway, there may be obstruction by a foreign body. Try to remove the obstruction if visible. Insert oropharyngeal Guedel airway if you have appropriate training. See Figures 10.53–10.56.	To establish and maintain airway, thus facilitating ventilation (Resuscitation Council 2010b, C).
Do not remove well-fitted dentures.	They help to create a mouth-to-mask seal during ventilation. E
7 Place the heel of one hand in the centre of the sternum and place the other on top, ensuring that the hands are located between the middle and the lower half of the sternum. Ensure that only the heel of the dominant hand is touching the sternum.	To ensure accuracy of external cardiac compression and reduced delay in commencing cardiac compressions (Resuscitation Council 2010b, C).
Place the other hand on top, straighten the elbows and make sure shoulders are directly over the patient's chest.	
The sternum should be depressed sharply by 5–6 cm. The cardiac compressions should be forceful, and sustained at a rate of 100–120 per minute.	This produces a cardiac output by applying direct downward force and compression (Smith 2000, R3).
8 Apply facemask with Ambu-bag over nose and mouth. Compress bag in a rhythmical fashion: the bag should be attached to an oxygen source, 12–15 litres. In order to deliver +85% oxygen, a reservoir may be attached to the Ambu-bag. If, however, oxygen is not immediately available, the Ambu-bag will deliver ambient air.	Room air contains only 21% oxygen. In shock, a low cardiac output, together with ventilation/perfusion mismatch, results in severe hypoxaemia. The importance of providing a high oxygen gradient from mouth to vital cells cannot be exaggerated and so oxygen should be added during CPR as soon as it is available (80–100% is desirable) (Simmons 2002, R3).
9 Maintain cardiac compression and ventilation at a ratio of 30:2. This rate can be achieved effectively by counting out loud 'one and two', and so on. There should be a slight pause to ensure that the delivered breath is sufficient to cause the patient's chest to rise. This must continue until cardiac output returns and the patient has a palpable blood pressure.	Counting aloud will ensure co-ordination of ventilation and compression ratio. To maintain circulation and oxygenation, thus reducing risk of damage to vital organs. E
10 When the cardiac arrest team arrives, it will assume responsibility for the arrest in liaison with the ward staff.	To ensure an effective expert team co-ordinates the resuscitation (Resuscitation Council 2010b, C).
11 Attach patient to ECG monitor using three electrodes or defibrillation patches/paddles.	To obtain adequate ECG signal. Accurate recording of cardiac rhythm will determine the appropriate treatment to be initiated. E

Intubation in CPR

12	Continue to ventilate and oxygenate the patient before intubation.	The risks of cardiac arrhythmias due to hypoxia are decreased (Resuscitation Council 2010b, C).
13	Equipment for intubation should be checked before handing to appropriate medical/nursing staff (a) Suction equipment is operational. (b) The cuff of the endotracheal tube inflates and deflates. (c) The endotracheal tube is well lubricated. (d) That catheter mount with swivel connector is ready for use.	To ensure all equipment is working prior to use. E
14	During intubation, the anaesthetist may request cricoid pressure. This involves compressing the oesophagus between the cricoid ring and the sixth cervical vertebra.	To prevent the risk of regurgitation of gastric contents and the consequent risk of pulmonary aspiration (Resuscitation Council 2010b, C).
15	Recommence ventilation and oxygenation once intubation is completed.	Intubation should interrupt resuscitation only for a maximum of 16 seconds to prevent the occurrence of cerebral anoxia (Handley *et al.* 1997, R3).
16	Once the patient's trachea has been intubated, chest compressions, at a rate of 100–120 per minute, should continue uninterrupted (except for defibrillation and pulse check when indicated) and ventilation should continue at approximately 12 breaths per minute. Compression should continue while the defibrillator is charging.	Uninterrupted compression results in a substantially higher mean coronary perfusion pressure. A pause in chest compressions allows the coronary perfusion pressure to fall. On resuming compressions, there is some delay before the original coronary perfusion pressure is restored (Resuscitation Council 2010b, C). Reducing preshock pause improves time of compression which has a more favourable outcome for patient.

Intravenous access in CPR

17	Venous access must be established through a large vein as soon as possible.	To administer emergency cardiac drugs and fluid replacement (Resuscitation Council 2010b, C).
18	Asepsis should be maintained throughout.	To prevent local and/or systemic infection (Fraise and Bradley 2009, E).
19	The correct rate of infusion is required.	To ensure maximum drug and/or solution effectiveness. E
20	Accurate recording of the administration of solutions infused and drugs added is essential.	To maintain accurate records, provide a point of reference in the event of queries and prevent any duplication of treatment (NMC 2009, C).

Defibrillation

21	Apply pads/paddles to chest. It may be necessary to shave the chest.	To ensure the pads/paddles are applied correctly and make adequate contact which enhances electrical contact (van Alem *et al.* 2003, C).
22	Remove oxygen source at least 1 metre from patient unless intubated.	To reduce the risk of sparks from igniting the oxygen source (Nolan *et al.* 2005, C).
23	The person delivering the shock must ask all members of the resuscitation team to stand clear of the patient.	To ensure that none of the resuscitation team are in contact with the patient or the bed as they may also receive the shock (Perkins and Lockey 2008, C).
24	Deliver single shock to treat VF/ pulseless VT.	To terminate pulseless VT, VF and restart the heart by depolarizing its electrical conduction system and delivering brief measured electrical shocks to the chest wall or the heart muscle itself (Eftestol *et al.* 2002, C; Wik *et al.* 2003, R1).

607

(Continued)

Procedure guideline 10.13 (*Continued*)

Postprocedure

25 Check patient by assessing airway, breathing, circulation, blood pressure and urine output.	To ensure a clear airway, adequate oxygenation and ventilation and aim to maintain normal sinus rhythm and a cardiac output adequate for perfusion of vital organs. To ensure adequacy of ventilation and oxygenation (Perkins and Lockey 2008, C).
26 Check arterial blood gases.	To ensure correction of acid/base balance (Resuscitation Council 2010b, C).
27 Check full blood count, clotting and biochemistry.	To exclude anaemia as a contributor to myocardial ischaemia. A clotting disorder may have contributed to a major haemorrhage. Replacement stored blood for transfusion has fewer clotting factors and the patient may require replacement of clotting factors usually in the form of fresh frozen plasma. E To assess renal function and electrolyte balance (K^+, Mg^{2+} and Ca^{2+}). To ensure normoglycaemia. To commence serial cardiac enzyme assay (Nolan *et al.* 2005, C; Resuscitation Council 2010b, C).
28 Monitor patient's cardiac rhythm and record 12-lead ECG.	Normal sinus rhythm is required for optimum cardiac function (Resuscitation Council 2010b, C). An assessment of whether cardiac arrest has been associated with a myocardial infarction should be made, as the patient may be suitable for coronary angioplasty or thrombolytic therapy (Nolan *et al.* 2005, C).
29 A chest X-ray should be taken.	To establish correct position of tracheal tube, gastric tube and central venous catheter. To exclude left ventricular failure, pulmonary aspiration and pneumothorax. To establish size and shape of heart (Nolan *et al.* 2006, C).
30 Continue respiratory therapy aiming for SaO_2 94–98% for adults.	Hypoxia and hypercarbia both increase the likelihood of a further cardiac arrest (Resuscitation Council 2010b, C).
31 Assess patient's level of consciousness. This can be done by use of the Glasgow Coma Scale. Although this is intended primarily for head injury, it is clinically relevant. It contains five levels of consciousness: (a) Conscious and alert (b) Drowsy but responsive to verbal commands (c) Unconscious but responsive to minimal painful stimuli (d) Unconscious and responsive to deep painful stimuli (e) Unconscious and unresponsive. See Chapter 13.	Once a heart has been resuscitated to a stable rhythm and cardiac output, the organ that influences an individual's survival most significantly is the brain (Resuscitation Council 2010b, C). Initial assessment and regular monitoring will alert the nurse to any changes in function.
32 The patient should be stable prior to any transfer and nursed in the appropriate position, that is semi-Fowler or the recovery position. Avoid nursing supine as this physiologically hinders cardiac output and respiration, unless clinically indicated for patients with acute head or spinal cord injury. Careful explanation and reassurance are vital at all times, particularly if the patient is conscious and aware.	Transferring a patient post arrest may pose risks because of changes in their haemodynamic status. This is due to movement of the trolley – inertia, changes in environment and/or changing equipment, which may impact negatively on the patient's physiological status (Shirley and Bion 2004, E). Nursing a patient in semi-Fowler's position ensures good air entry, and reduces risks for aspiration for patients not contraindicated for head of bed to be elevated (Tablan *et al.* 2004, C).

Problem-solving table 10.6 **Prevention and resolution (Procedure guideline 10.13)**

Problem	Cause	Prevention	Suggested action
Defibrillator not working	Battery pack not charged	Ensure defibrillator is plugged into the mains so battery can recharge	Check defibrillator when doing emergency trolley checks as per hospital policy
No trace when ECG dots or pads are on patient	ECG dots or pads dry Test plug connected to lead	Change ECG dots/pads as they can dry out Ensure that the test plug is not attached	Check expiratory dates of ECG dots/pads when checking emergency trolley/ equipment After emergency trolley checks, ensure that the test plug is no longer attached
Staff unable to use defibrillator	Not had training	Mandatory yearly BLS training for staff who will be present during CPR, and ALS every 3 years for staff who work in specialized areas for example critical care Standardize equipment throughout the hospital	Find a member of staff who is trained in using defibrillator. AED defibrillators should be available as they can be used by people without previous training
Laryngoscope light not working	Laryngoscope handle not charged	Ensure that the laryngoscope handle is charged using rechargeable batteries or new batteries inserted Change laryngoscope light	Check laryngoscope when doing resuscitation equipment checks as per hospital policy If using rechargeable batteries, ensure laryngoscope handle is docked Have spare batteries if not using rechargeable Have spare light bulbs/spare disposable laryngoscope blades on the emergency trolley
Portable suction not working	Battery pack not charged Incorrectly connected tubing	Ensure that suction unit is plugged in so battery can charge Check that tubing correctly connected	Check portable suction is on charge and tubing correctly connected when checking resuscitation equipment as per hospital policy
Emergency drugs missing/expired	Trolley not checked Equipment removed without having been replaced	Have a checklist of the emergency drugs that need to be on the resuscitation trolley	Check drugs and expiry dates when checking resuscitation equipment and resuscitation trolley as per hospital policy and lock trolley for safekeeping of drugs
Equipment missing off resuscitation trolley	Removal of equipment without replacing or returning it	Have a checklist of all equipment needed on resuscitation trolley	Check resuscitation trolley list as per hospital policy. Replace any missing or expired equipment Seal/lock trolley after checks/use Educate all staff not to remove equipment from trolley other than in a cardiac arrest

Postprocedural considerations

Immediate care

Following stabilization of the patient post cardiac or respiratory arrest, consideration should be given to moving them to an appropriate critical care or high-dependency environment. All established monitoring should continue during transfer and the patient should be transferred by individuals capable of monitoring the patient and responding appropriately to any change in the patient's condition, including a further cardiac arrest. A critical care outreach service or designated transfer team, if available, may contribute to the care of the patient during stabilization and transfer (Nolan *et al.* 2006, Resuscitation Council 2010b, Shirley and Bion 2004).

Ongoing care

The patient's haemodynamic status should be continually monitored post resuscitation, as well as observing the patient's level of consciousness, respiration rate and if possible urine output. Monitor blood glucose levels in adults with sustained return of spontaneous circulation (ROSC) after cardiac arrest. Maintaining blood glucose values >10 mmol/L, they should be treated in an HDU/ICU environment, however hypoglycaemia must be avoided (Resuscitation Council 2010b). Documentation of physiological parameters needs to continue and any change in haemodynamic status needs to be reported to the medical team or senior nursing staff attending to the patient prior to transfer to the CCU or HDU.

The Intensive Care Society (UK) has published guidelines for the transport of the critically ill adult (www.ics.ac.uk). These outline the requirements for equipment and personnel when transferring critically ill patients (Nolan *et al.* 2006, Resuscitation Council 2006, Sandroni *et al.* 2007, Shirley and Bion 2004).

Careful explanation and reassurance must be given to the patient before transfer, particularly if the patient is conscious and aware. The patient's relatives will require considerable support and will need to be kept informed of the transfer of their relative and to where. It is important that if the family were not present during the arrest, the appropriate member of the medical team contacts the next of kin and informs them of the arrest and its outcome. If the patient has survived, the next of kin/family will need to know that the patient has been moved to a more appropriate environment for continued monitoring.

Please note: whether the resuscitation attempt was successful or not, the pastoral needs of all those associated with the arrest should not be forgotten (Resuscitation Council 2010b, Sandroni *et al.* 2007).

Documentation

Good record keeping is an integral part of nursing practice, and is essential to the provision of safe and effective care (NMC 2009). There must be documentary evidence of how decisions relating to the patient were made. Accurate recording of the administration of solutions infused and drugs added is essential. All resuscitation attempts should be audited, ideally using a nationally recognized template such as the Utstein template (recommended for use by the Resuscitation Council 2010b). Hospitals should collect data regarding cardiac arrest for the National Cardiac Arrest Audit (NCAA) (Resuscitation Council 2010b).

Education of patient and relevant others

Prevention of cardiac arrest is the most important factor for survival. Education of the patient and relevant others needs to start at first contact with healthcare professionals regarding lifestyle changes, diet, exercise, smoking cessation, and regular check-ups to treat or control any underlying causes such as hypertension and diabetes.

Complications

Some possible complications may arise from cardiopulmonary resuscitation.

- Gastric distension due to bagging too forcefully and/or too quickly, causing air to enter the stomach. A nasogastric tube should be inserted as soon as the airway is secure, to help prevent and manage gastric distension which may cause vomiting and possible aspiration into the lungs.
- Fractured ribs, sternum, punctured lungs can occur as a result of chest compressions. The correct placement of hands during chest compression is vital in helping to prevent fracturing of ribs and sternum.
- Transmission of disease through mouth-to-mouth ventilation. The use of a pocket resuscitation mask with a one-way valve will prevent the transmission of infection from bodily fluids during ventilation (DH 2007).

Websites

British Lung Foundation: www.lunguk.org/

British Thoracic Society: www.brit-thoracic.org.uk

BTS guideline for emergency oxygen use in adult patients: www.brit-thoracic.org.uk/emergencyoxygen)

Intensive Care Society: www.ics.ac.uk/

NPSA Rapid Response Alert May 2008: www.nrls.npsa.nhs.uk

Resuscitation Council UK: www.resus.org.uk

Smoking Cessation Programme Development Group at NICE: www.publichealth.nice.org.uk/page.aspx?o=SmokingCessationPGMain

References

Adam, S.K. and Osborne, S. (2005) *Critical Care Nursing: Science and Practice*, 2nd edn. Oxford University Press, Oxford.

AHA/ILCOR (American Heart Association/International Liaison Committee on Resuscitation) (2000) Guidelines 2000 for CPR and emergency care: an international consensus on science. *Resuscitation*, **46** (1), 73–92, 109–114.

Ahrens, T. and Tucker, K. (1999) Pulse oximetry. *Critical Care Nursing Clinics of North America*, **11** (1), 87–98.

Allibone, L. (2003) Nursing management of chest drains. *Nursing Standard*, **17** (22), 45–54.

Allibone, L. (2005) Principles for inserting and managing chest drains. *Nursing Times*, **101** (42), 45–49.

Allison, R.C. (1991) Initial treatment of pulmonary edema: a physiological approach. *American Journal of the Medical Sciences*, **302** (6), 385–391.

Ashurst, S. (1995) Oxygen therapy. *British Journal of Nursing*, **4** (9), 508–515.

Austin, R. and Snow, A. (2000) Defibrillation, in *Resuscitation: A Guide for Nurses* (ed. A. Cheller). Harcourt, London, pp.141–157.

Avery, S. (2000) Insertion amd management of chest drains. *Nursing Times*, **96** (37), 3–7.

Ball, C. (2000) Optimizing oxygen delivery: haemodynamic workshop. Part 3. *Intensive Care Nursing*, **16**(2), 84–87.

Baskett, P.J., Nolan, J.P., Handley, A., Soar, J., Biarent, D. and Richmond, S. (2005) European Resuscitation Council guidelines for resuscitation 2005. Section 9. Principles of training in resuscitation. *Resuscitation*, **67** (Suppl 1), S181–189.

Becker, D. (2007) Cardiac anatomy and physiology and assessment, in *Critical Care Nursing: Synergy for Optimal Outcomes* (eds R. Kaplow and S.R. Hardin). Jones and Bartlett Publishers, Sudbury, MA, pp. 121–138

Benditt, J.O. (2000) Adverse effects of low-flow oxygen therapy. *Respiratory Care*, **45** (1), 54–61.

Berne, R.M. (2004) *Physiology*, 5th edn. Mosby, St Louis, MO.

Bersten, A.D., Soni, N. and Oh, T.E. (2009) *Oh's Intensive Care Manual*, 6th edn. Butterworth-Heinemann, Oxford.

Billau, C. (2004) Suctioning, in *Tracheostomy: A Multiprofessional Handbook* (eds. C. Russell and B.F. Matta). Cambridge University Press, Cambridge, pp. 157–172.

BMA (2000) *The Impact of the Human Rights Act on Medical Decision-Making*. British Medical Association, London.

BMA, RCN, Resuscitation Council (UK) and Age Concern (2002) *Decisions Relating to Cardiopulmonary Resuscitation: Model Information Leaflet*. British Medical Association, London.

Bond, P., Grant, F., Coltart, L. and Elder, F. (2003) Best practice in the care of patients with a tracheostomy. *Nursing Times*, **99** (30), 24–25.

Bossaert, L.L. (1997) Fibrillation and defibrillation of the heart. *British Journal of Anaesthesia*, **79**(2), 203–213.

Bowers, B. and Scase, C. (2007) Tracheostomy: facilitating successful discharge from hospital to home. *British Journal of Nursing*, **16** (8), 476–479.

Bowman, J.G. (2009) Pneumothorax, tension and traumatic. *Emedicine, Medscape*. http://emedicine.medscape.com/article/827551-treatment.

Brandt, M.L., Luks, F.I., Lacroix, J. *et al.* (1994) The paediatric chest tube. *Clinical Intensive Care: International Journal of Critical and Coronary Care Medicine*, **5** (3), 123–129.

Bryan-Brown, C.W. and Dracup, K. (2000) Too much of a good thing? *American Journal of Critical Care*, **9** (5), 300–303.

BTS (British Thoracic Society) (2008) BTS guideline for emergency oxygen use in adult patients. www.brit-thoracic.org.uk/emergencyoxygen.

Carpenter, K.D. (1991) Oxygen transport in the blood. *Critical Care Nurse*, **11** (9), 20–33.

Carroll, P. (1997) When you want humidity. *RN*, **60** (5), 30–34.

Celik, S.A. and Kanan, N. (2006) A current conflict: use of isotonic sodium chloride solution on endotracheal suctioning in critically ill patients. *Dimensions of Critical Care Nursing: DCCN*, **25** (1), 11–14.

Chernecky, C. and Shelton, B. (2001) Pulmonary complications in patients with cancer: diagnostic and treatment information for the noncritical care nurse. *American Journal of Nursing*, **101** (5), 24A–NaN.

Choi, S.H., Lee, S.W., Hong, S.J., Moon J.A. and Moon, S.W. (2009) Can spontaneous pneumothorax patients be treated by ambulatory care management? *European Journal of Cardiothoracic Surgery*, **31**, 491–495.

Clementsen, P., Evald, T., Grode, G. *et al.* (1998) Treatment of malignant pleural effusion: pleurodesis using a small percutaneous catheter. A prospective randomized study. *Respiratory Medicine*, **92** (3), 593–596.

Clotworthy, N. (2006a) Post-operative care of the patient following a laryngectomy, in *Guidelines for the Care of Patients with Tracheostomy Tubes*. St George's Healthcare NHS Trust, London, pp. 15–16.

Clotworthy, N. (2006b) Tracheostomy tubes, in *Guidelines for the Care of Patients with Tracheostomy Tubes*. St George's Healthcare NHS Trust, London, pp. 9–14.

Clotworthy, N. (2006c) Suctioning, in *Guidelines for the Care of Patients with Tracheostomy Tubes*. St George's Healthcare NHS Trust, London, pp.23–26.

Clotworthy, N. (2006d) Tube changes, in *Guidelines for the Care of Patients with Tracheostomy Tubes*. St George's Healthcare NHS Trust, London, pp.39–42.

Cooper, N. (2002) Oxygen therapy – myths and misconceptions. *Care of the Critically Ill*, **18** (3), 74–77.

Day, T. (2000) Tracheal suctioning: when, why and how. *Nursing Times*, **96** (20), 13–15.

Day, T., Farnell, S. and Wilson-Barnett, J. (2002) Suctioning: a review of current research recommendations. *Intensive Care Nursing*, **18** (2), 79–89.

Dean, B. (1997) Evidence-based suction management in accident and emergency: a vital component of airway care. *Accident and Emergency Nursing*, **5**(2), 92–98.

De Leyn, P., Bedert, L., Delcroix, M. et al. (2007) Tracheotomy: clinical review and guidelines. *European Journal of Cardio-Thoracic Surgery*, **32** (3), 412–421.

Demers, R.R. (2002) Bacterial/viral filtration. Let the breather beware! *Chest*, **120**, 1377–1389.

DH (2000) *Comprehensive Critical Care: A Review of Adult Critical Care Services*. Department of Health, London.

DH (2002) *Critical Care Programme: Weaning and Long-Term Ventilation*. Department of Health, London.

DH (2005) *Hazardous Waste (England) Regulations*. Department of Health, London.

DH (2007) *Pandemic Influenza: Guidance for Infection Control in Hospitals and Primary Care Settings*. Department of Health, London. www.dh.gov.uk.

Docherty, B. and Hall, S. (2002) Basic life support and AED. *Professional Nurse*, **17**(12), 705–706.

Dolan, S. and Preston, N.J. (2006) Malignant effusions, in *Nursing Patients with Cancer: Principles and Practice* (eds N. Kearney and A. Richardson). Elsevier Churchill Livingstone, Edinburgh, pp. 619–632.

Dropkin, M.J. (1996) Nursing research: SOHN's 20-year experience. *Otorhinolaryngology-Head and Neck Nursing*, **14** (3), 14–16.

Edgtton-Winn, M. and Wright, K. (2005) Tracheostomy: a guide to nursing care. *Australian Nursing Journal*, **13** (5), 17–20.

611

Eftestol, T., Sunde, K. and Steen, P.A. (2002) Effects of interrupting precordial compressions on the calculated probability of defibrillation success during out-of-hospital cardiac arrest. *Circulation*, 105 (19), 2270–2273.

Epstein, O. (2009) *Pocket Guide to Clinical Examination*, 4th edn. Mosby, Edinburgh.

Esmond, G. (2001) *Respiratory Nursing*. Baillière Tindall, London.

Estes, R.J. and Meduri, G.U. (1995) The pathogenesis of ventilator-associated pneumonia: I. Mechanisms of bacterial transcolonization and airway inoculation. *Intensive Care Medicine*, 21 (4), 365–383.

Fell, H. and Boehm, M. (1998) Easing the discomfort of oxygen therapy. *Nursing Times*, 94 (38), 56–58.

Foss, M.A. (1990) Oxygen therapy. *Professional Nurse*, 5 (4), 188–190.

Fraise, A.P. and Bradley, T. (eds) (2009) *Ayliffe's Control of Healthcare-associated Infection: A Practical Handbook*, 5th edn. Hodder Arnold, London.

Gallon, A. (1998) Pneumothorax. *Nursing Standard*, 13 (10), 35–39.

Glass, C.A. and Grap, M.J. (1995) Ten tips for safer suctioning. *American Journal of Nursing*, 95 (5), 51–53.

Godden, J. and Hiley, C. (1998) Managing the patient with a chest drain: a review. *Nursing Standard*, 12 (32), 35–39.

Gordon, P.A., Norton, J.M., Guerra, J.M. and Perdue, S.T. (1997) Positioning of chest tubes: effects on pressure and drainage. *American Journal of Critical Care*, 6 (1), 33–38.

Gorini, M., Ginanni, R., Villella, G. et al. (2004) Non-invasive negative and positive pressure ventilation in the treatment of acute on chronic respiratory failure. *Intensive Care Medicine*, 30 (5), 875–881.

Graham, A.N., Cosgrove, A.P., Gibbons, J.R. and McGuigan, J.A. (1992) Randomised clinical trial of chest drainage systems. *Thorax*, 47(6), 461–462.

Gray, A.J., Goodacre, S., Newby, D.E. et al. (2009) A multicentre randomised controlled trial of the use of continuous positive airway pressure and non-invasive positive pressure ventilation in the early treatment of patients presenting to the emergency department with severe acute cardiogenic pulmonary oedema: the 3CPO trial. *Health Technology Assessment*, 13 (33), 1–106.

Gray, E. (2000) Pain management for patients with chest drains. *Nursing Standard*, 14 (23), 40–4.

Greenbaum, D.M., Millen, J.E., Eross, B., Snyder, J.V., Grenvik, A. and Safar, P. (1976) Continuous positive airway pressure without tracheal intubation in spontaneously breathing patients. *Chest*, 69(5), 615–620.

Griggs, A. (1998) Tracheostomy: suctioning and humidification. *Nursing Standard*, 13 (2), 49–53.

Guyton, A.C. and Hall, J.E. (2006) *Textbook of Medical Physiology*, 11th edn. Elsevier Saunders, Philadelphia.

Hallstrom, A., Cobb, L., Johnson, E. and Copass, M. (2000) Cardiopulmonary resuscitation by chest compression alone or with mouth-to-mouth ventilation. *New England Journal of Medicine*, 342, 1546–1553.

Haman, L., Parizek, P. and Vojacek, J. (2009) Precordial thump efficacy in termination of induced ventricular arrhythmias. *Resuscitation*, 80, 14–16.

Hampton, S. (1998) Film subjects win the day. *Nursing Times*, 94 (24), 80–82.

Handley, A.J. (2004) Basic life support, in *ABC of Resuscitation* (eds M. Colqhoun, A. Handley and T. Evans), 4th edn. BMJ Books, London, pp.1–4.

Handley, A.J., Becker, L.B., Allen, M., van Drenth, A., Kramer, E.B. and Montgomery, W.H. (1997) Single rescuer adult basic life support. An advisory statement from the Basic Life Support

Working Group of the International Liaison Committee on Resuscitation (ILCOR). *Resuscitation*, 34(2), 101–108.

Harkin, H. (2004) Decannulation, in *Tracheostomy: A Multiprofessional Handbook* (eds C. Russell and B.F. Matta). Cambridge University Press, Cambridge, pp. 255–268.

Hauff, S.R., Rea, T.D., Culley, L.L. et al. (2003) Factors impeding dispatcher-assisted telephone cardiopulmonary resuscitation. *Annals of Emergency Medicine*, 42 (6), 731–737.

Henry, M., Arnold, T. and Harvey, J. (2003) BTS guidelines for the management of spontaneous pneumothorax. *Thorax*, 58 (Suppl 2), ii39–ii52.

Hess, D. (2000) Detection and monitoring of hypoxemia and oxygen therapy. *Respiratory Care*, 45 (1), 65–80.

Hess, D.R. (2005) Tracheostomy tubes and related appliances. *Respiratory Care*, 50 (4), 497–510.

Higgins, D. (2006) Removal of chest drains. *Nursing Times*, 102 (13), 26–27.

Higgins, D. (2009) Basic nursing principles of caring for patients with a tracheostomy. *Nursing Times*, 105(3), 14–15.

Hilton, P. (2004) Evaluating the treatment options for spontaneous pneumothorax. *Nursing Times*, 100 (28), 32–3.

Hinds, C.J. and Watson, D. (2008) *Intensive Care: A Concise Textbook*, 3rd edn. Saunders, Edinburgh.

Hodgetts, T.J. and Castle, N. (1999) *Resuscitation Rules*. BMJ, London.

Hough, A. (2001) *Physiotherapy in Respiratory Care: An Evidence-Based Approach to Respiratory and Cardiac Management*, 3rd edn. Nelson Thornes, Cheltenham.

Hyde, J., Sykes, T. and Graham, T. (1997) Reducing morbidity from chest drains. *BMJ (Clinical Research ed.)*, 314 (7085), 914–915.

ICS (2008) *Standards for the Care of Adult Patients with a Temporary Tracheostomy*. Intensive Care Society, London. www.ics.ac.uk/intensive_care_professional/standards_and_guidelines/care_of_the_adult_patient_with_a_temporary_tracheostomy_2008.

Ireton, J. (2007) Tracheostomy suction: a protocol for practice. *Paediatric Nursing*, 19 (10), 14–18.

Jevon, P. (2001) Cardiopulmonary resuscitation. Initial assessment. *Nursing Times*, 97 (41), 41–42.

Jevon, P. (2002) Resuscitation in hospital: Resuscitation Council (UK) recommendations. *Nursing Standard*, 16 (33), 41–44.

Johnson, W.A., Pinto, J.M. and Baroody, F.M. (2010) *Tracheostomy Tube Change: Treatment and Medication*. http://emedicine.medscape.com/article/1580576-treatment.

Keen, A. (2000) Continuous positive airway pressure (CPAP) in the intensive care unit – uses and implications for nursing management. *Nursing in Critical Care*, 5 (3), 137–141.

Keilty, S.E.J. and Bott, J. (1992) Continuous positive airways pressure. *Physiotherapy*, 78(2), 90–93.

Kinnear, W. (2002) Non-invasive ventilation in acute respiratory failure. *Thorax*, 57, 192–211.

Kirkwood, P. (2002) Are chest tubes routinely milked, stripped, or suctioned to maintain patency? *Critical Care Nurse*, 22 (4), 70–72.

Kolbitsch, C., Lorenz, I.H., Hormann, C. et al. (2000) The impact of increased mean airway pressure on contrast-enhanced MRI measurement of regional cerebral blood flow (rCBF), regional cerebral blood volume (rCBV), regional mean transit time (rMTT), and regional cerebrovascular resistance (rCVR) in human volunteers. *Human Brain Mapping*, 11 (3), 214–222.

Kozer, R. and Adams, S.D. (2005) Chyclothorax. *Emedicine*. Medscape. http://emedicine.medscape.com/article/172527-overview.

Kumar, P.J. and Clark, M.L. (2009) *Kumar and Clark's Clinical Medicine*, 7th edn. Saunders/Elsevier, Edinburgh.

Laws, D., Neville, E. and Duffy, J. (2003) BTS guidelines for the insertion of a chest drain. *Thorax*, 58 (Suppl 2), ii53–ii59.

612

Lenique, F., Habis, M., Lofaso, F. *et al.* (1997) Ventilatory and he-modynamic effects of continuous positive airway pressure in left heart failure. *American Journal of Respiratory and Critical Care Medicine*, **155** (2), 500–505.

Lewarski, J.S. (2005) Long-term care of the patient with a tracheostomy. *Respiratory Care*, **50** (4), 534–537.

Luketich, J.D., Kiss, M., Hershey, J. *et al.* (1998) Chest tube insertion: a prospective evaluation of pain management. *Clinical Journal of Pain*, 14(2), 152–154.

MacIntyre, N.R. and Branson, R.D. (2009) *Mechanical Ventilation*, 2nd edn. Saunders Elsevier, St Louis, MO.

Marieb, E.N., Kollett, L.S. and Zao, P.Z. (2008) *Human Anatomy and Physiology Laboratory Manual: Main Version*, 8th edn. Pearson Benjamin Cummings, San Francisco.

Marieb, E.N., Hoehn, K. and Hutchinson, M. (2010) *Human Anatomy and Physiology*, 8th edn. Pearson Benjamin Cummings, San Francisco.

Maskell, N.A. and Butland, R.J. (2003) BTS guidelines for the investigation of a unilateral pleural effusion in adults. *Thorax*, **58** (Suppl 2), ii8–ii17.

McMahon-Parkes, K. (1997) Management of pleural drains. *Nursing Times*, **93** (52), 48–52.

MDA (2000) *Continuous Positive Airway Pressure (CPAP) Circuits: Risk of Misassembly*. www.mhra.gov.uk/Publications/Safetywarnings/MedicalDeviceAlerts/Safetynotices/CON008853.

Miller, A.C. and Harvey, J.E. (1993) Guidelines for the management of spontaneous pneumothorax. Standards of Care Committee, British Thoracic Society. *BMJ (Clinical Research ed.)*, **307** (6896), 114–116.

Miller, R.F. and Semple, S.J. (1991) Continuous positive airway pressure ventilation for respiratory failure associated with *Pneumocystis carinii* pneumonia. *Respiratory Medicine*, **85** (2), 133–138.

Moran, G. (2010) *A Beginner's Guide to Normal Heart Function, Sinus Rhythm and Common Cardiac Arrhythmias*. Division of Nursing, University of Nottingham, Nottingham. www.nottingham.ac.uk/nursing/practice/resources/cardiology/introduction/index.php.

Moser, D.K. and Chung, M.L. (2003) Critical care nursing practice regarding patient anxiety assessment and management. *Intensive Care and Critical Care Nursing*, **19** (5), 275–288.

Moule, P. and Albarran, J.W. (eds) (2009) *Practical Resuscitation for Healthcare Professionals*. Blackwell Publishing, Oxford.

Moureau, N. and Iannucci, A.L. (2003) Catheter securement: trends in performance and complications associated with the use of either traditional methods or adhesive anchor devices. *Journal of Vascular Access Devices*, **8** (1), 29–33.

Nehyba, K. (2007) Continuous positive airway pressure ventilation, part 2: indications and contraindications. *British Journal of Cardiac Nursing*, **2** (1), 18–24.

Nelson, L. (1999) Points of friction. *Nursing Times*, **95** (34), 72–75.

NICE (2006) *Brief Interventions and Referral for Smoking Cessation in Primary Care and Other Settings*. National Institute for Health and Clinical Excellence, London.

NICE (2007) *Acutely Ill Patients in Hospital: Recognition of and Response to Acute Illness in Adults in Hospital*. National Institute of Health and Clinical Excellence, London. www.nice.org.uk/nicemedia/pdf/CG50FullGuidance.pdf.

NLM (2010) *MedlinePlus Health Information*. National Library of Medicine, Washington, DC. www.nlm.nih.gov/medlineplus/medlineplus.html.

NMC (2008a) *The Code: Standards of Conduct, Performance and Ethics for Nurses and Midwives*. Nursing and Midwifery Council, London.

NMC (2008b) *Consent*. Nursing and Midwifery Council, London. www.nmc-uk.org/Nurses-and-midwives/Advice-by-topic/A/Advice/Consent/.

NMC (2009) *Record Keeping: Guidance for Nurses and Midwives*. Nursing and Midwifery Council, London.

Nolan, J., Deakin, C.D., Soar, J., Bottiger, B.W. and Smith, G. (2005) European Resuscitation Council guidelines for resuscitation 2005. Section 4. Adult advanced life support. *Resuscitation*, **67** (Suppl 1), S39–86.

Nolan, J., Soar, J., Lockey, A. *et al.* (2006) *Advanced Life Support*, 5th edn. Resuscitation Council (UK), London.

NPSA (2007) *The Fifth Report from the Patient Safety Observatory. Safety Care for the Acutely Ill Patient: Learning from Incidents*. National Patient Safety Agency, London. www.nrls.npsa.nhs.uk/resources/?entryid45=59828.

NPSA (2008) *Chest Drains. Rapid Response Report: Risks Associated with the Insertion of Chest Drains*. National Patient Safety Agency, London.

NPSA (2009) *Rapid Response Report NPSA/2009/RRR006: Oxygen Safety in Hospitals*. National Patient Safety Agency, London.

O'Connor, A.R. and Morgan, W.E. (2005) Radiological review of pneumothorax. *BMJ (Clinical Research Ed.)*, **330**(7506), 1493–1497.

O'Driscoll, B.R., Howard, L.S., Davison, A.G. and British Thoracic Society (2008) BTS guideline for emergency oxygen use in adult patients. *Thorax*, **63** (Suppl VI), 1–73. www.brit-thoracic.org.uk/Portals/0/Clinical%20Information/Emergency%20Oxygen/Emergency%20oxygen%20guideline/THX-63-Suppl_6.pdf.

Paradis, N. (2007) *Cardiac: The Science and Practice of Resuscitation Medicine*, 2nd edn. Cambridge University Press, Cambridge, pp.3–26.

Patel, J. and Matta, B. (2004) Percutaneous dilatational tracheostomy, in *Tracheostomy: A Multiprofessional Handbook* (eds C. Russell and B.F. Matta). Cambridge University Press, Cambridge, pp. 59–68.

Patz, E.F. Jr (1998) Malignant pleural effusions: recent advances and ambulatory sclerotherapy. *Chest*, **113** (1 Suppl), 74S–77S

Peek, G.J., Morcos, S. and Cooper, G. (2000) The pleural cavity. *BMJ (Clinical Research ed.)*, **320** (7245), 1318–1321.

Perel, P., Roberts, I. and Pearson, M. (2007) Colloids versus crystalloids for fluid resuscitation in critically ill patients. *Cochrane Database of Systematic Reviews* 4, CD000567-NaN.

Perkins, G.D. and Lockey, A.S. (2008) Defibrillation – safety versus efficacy. *Resuscitation*, **79**, 1–3.

Perkins, G.D., Stephenson, B., Hulme, J. and Monsieurs, K.G. (2005) Birmingham assessment of breathing study (BABS). *Resuscitation*, **64** (1), 109–113.

Pierce, L.N.B. (1995) *Guide to Mechanical Ventilation and Intensive Respiratory Care*. W.B. Saunders, Philadelphia.

Pierson, D.J. (2000) Pathophysiology and clinical effects of chronic hypoxia. *Respiratory Care*, **45** (1), 39–51.

Place, B. (1997) Using airway pressure. *Nursing Times*, **93** (31), 42–44.

Price, T. (2004a) Surgical tracheostomy, in *Tracheostomy: A Multiprofessional Handbook* (eds C. Russell and B.F. Matta). Cambridge University Press, Cambridge, pp. 35–58.

Price, T. (2004b) What is a tracheostomy? in *Tracheostomy: A Multiprofessional Handbook* (eds C. Russell and B.F. Matta). Cambridge University Press, Cambridge, pp. 29–34.

Prior, T. and Russell, S. (2004) Tracheostomy and head & neck cancer, in *Tracheostomy: A Multiprofessional Handbook* (eds C. Russell and B.F. Matta). Cambridge University Press, Cambridge, pp. 269–283.

Pryor, J.A. and Prasad, S.A. (2008) *Physiotherapy for Respiratory and Cardiac Problems: Adults and Paediatrics*, 4th edn. Churchill Livingstone Elsevier, Edinburgh.

Ram, F.S., Picot, J., Lightowler, J. and Wedzicha, J.A. (2004) Non-invasive positive pressure ventilation for treatment of respira-

613

tory failure due to exacerbations of chronic obstructive pulmonary disease. *Cochrane Database of Systematic Reviews*, 1, CD004104.

Resuscitation Council (2004) *CPR Guidance for Clinical Practice and Training in Hospitals*. Resuscitation Council, London. www.resus.org.uk/pages/standard.pdf.

Resuscitation Council (2006) *Advanced Life Support*, 5th edn. Resuscitation Council, London.

Resuscitation Council (2010a) *Legal Status of Those Who Attempt Resuscitation*. Resuscitation Council, London.

Resuscitation Council (2010b) *Resuscitation Guidelines October 2010*. www.resus.org.uk/page/guidehtm.

Rhys Evans, P.H., Montgomery, P.Q. and Gullane, P.J. (2003) *Principles and Practice of Head and Neck Oncology*. Dunitz, London.

Robertson, C., Steen, P., Adgey, J. *et al.* (1998) The 1998 European Resuscitation Council Guidelines for adult advanced life support. *Resuscitation*, **37** (2), 81–90.

Romand, J.A. and Donald, F. (1995) Physiological effects of continuous positive airway pressure (CPAP) ventilation in the critically ill. *Care of the Critically Ill*, **11** (6), 239–243.

Russell, C. (2004) Tracheostomy tubes, in *Tracheostomy: A Multiprofessional Handbook* (eds C. Russell and B.F. Matta). Cambridge University Press, Cambridge, pp. 85–114.

Russell, C. (2005) Providing the nurse with a guide to tracheostomy care and management. *British Journal of Nursing*, **14** (8), 428–433.

Sandroni, C., Nolan, J., Cavallaro, F. and Antonelli, M. (2007) In-hospital cardiac arrest: incidence, prognosis and possible measures to improve survival. *Intensive Care Medicine*, **33**, 237–245.

Scase, C. (2004) Wound care, in *Tracheostomy: A Multiprofessional Handbook* (eds C. Russell and B.F. Matta). Cambridge University Press, Cambridge, pp.173–186.

Schumaker, W.C., Fink, M.P., Abraham, E. *et al.* (1996) *Textbook of Critical Care*, 5th edn. W.B. Saunders, Philadelphia, pp. 628–952.

Serra, A. (2000) Tracheostomy care. *Nursing Standard*, **14** (42), 45–52.

Shelledy, D.C. and Mikles, S.P. (2002) Patient assessment and respiratory care plan development, in *Critical Thinking in Respiratory Care: A Problem-Based Learning Approach* (eds S.C. Mishoe and M.A. Welch). McGraw-Hill, , New York, pp. 181–234.

Shirley, P.J. and Bion, J.F. (2004) Intra-hospital transport of critically ill patients: minimising risk. *Intensive Care Medicine*, **30**, 1505–1510.

Shoemaker, W.C. (2000) Pericardial tamponade, in *Oxford Textbook of Critical Care* (ed. A. Webb). Oxford University Press, Oxford, pp. 276–279.

Shuster, M., Billi, J.E., Bossaert, L. *et al.* (2010) International consensus on cardiopulmonary resuscitation and emergency cardiovascular care science with treatment recommendations. Part 4: Conflict of interest management before, during and after the 2010 International Consensus Conference on Cardiopulmonary Resuscitation and Emergency Cardiovascular Care Science with Treatment Recommendations. *Resuscitation*, **81**, e41–e47.

Simmons, R. (2002) The airway at risk, in *ABC of Resuscitation* (eds M. Colqhoun, A. Handley and T. Evans), 5th edn. BMJ Books, London, pp.25–31.

Skinner, D.V. and Vincent, R. (1997) *Cardiopulmonary Resuscitation*, 2nd edn. Oxford University Press, Oxford.

Smith, D. (2000) Basic life support, in *Resuscitation: A Guide for Nurses* (ed. A. Cheller). Harcourt, London, pp.65–80.

Sorenson, H.M. and Shelledy, D.C. (2003) AARC clinical practice guideline. Intermittent positive pressure breathing – 2003 revision and update. *Respiratory Care*, **48** (5), 540–546.

Tablan, O.C., Anderson, L.J., Besser, R. *et al.* CDC Healthcare Infection Control Practices Advisory Committee. Guidelines for preventing health care-associated pneumonia, 2003: recommendations of CDC and the Healthcare Infection Control Practices Advisory Committee. *Morbidity and Mortality Weekly Report*, 53(RR-3), 1–36.

Tamburri, L.M. (2000) Care of the patient with a tracheostomy. *Orthopaedic Nursing*, **19** (2), 49–58.

Tang, A., Hooper, T. and Hasan, R. (1999) A regional survey of chest drains: evidence-based practice? *Postgraduate Medical Journal*, **75** (886), 471–474.

Tang, A.T., Velissaris, T.J. and Weeden, D.F. (2002) An evidence-based approach to drainage of the pleural cavity: evaluation of best practice. *Journal of Evaluation in Clinical Practice*, **8** (3), 333–340.

Tinker, J. and Zapol, W.M. (1992) *Care of the Critically Ill Patient*, 2nd edn. Springer-Verlag, New York.

Tomlinson, M.A. and Treasure, T. (1997) Insertion of a chest drain: how to do it. *British Journal of Hospital Medicine*, **58** (6), 248–252.

Tortora, G.J. and Derrickson, B. (2009) *Principles of Anatomy and Physiology*, 12th edn. John Wiley, Hoboken, NJ.

Urden, L.D., Stacy, K.M. and Lough, M.E. (2006) *Thelan's Critical Care Nursing: Diagnosis and Management*, 5th edn. Mosby/Elsevier, St Louis, MO.

Van Alem, A.P., Sanou, B.T. and Koster, R.W. (2003) Interruption of cardiopulmonary resuscitation with the use of the automated external defibrillator in out-of-hospital cardiac arrest. *Annals of Emergency Medicine*, **42** (4), 449–457.

Varon, J., Marik, P.E. and Fromm, R.E. (1998) Cardiopulmonary resuscitation: a review for clinicians. *Resuscitation*, **36** (2), 133–145.

Wakeling, H.G. and Mythen, M.C. (2000) Hypomagnesemia, in *Oxford Textbook of Critical Care* (eds A. Webb *et al.*). Oxford University Press, London, pp.561–564.

Ward, B. and Park, G.R. (2000) Humidification of inspired gases in the critically ill. *Clinical Intensive Care*, **11** (4), 169–176.

Waugh, A. and Grant, A. (2010) *Ross and Wilson's Anatomy and Physiology in Health and Illness*. Churchill Livingstone Elsevier, Edinburgh, pp.77–129.

West, J.B. (2008) *Pulmonary Pathophysiology: The Essentials*, 7th edn. Wolters Kluwer/Lippincott Williams and Wilkins, Philadelphia.

Wik, L., Hansen, T.B., Fylling, F. *et al.* (2003) Delaying defibrillation to give basic cardiopulmonary resuscitation to patients with out-of-hospital ventricular fibrillation: a randomized trial. *JAMA*, **289** (11), 1389–1395.

Williams, R., Rankin, N., Smith, T. *et al.* (1996) Relationship between the humidity and temperature of inspired gas and the function of the airway mucosa. *Critical Care Medicine*, 24, 1920–1929.

Wilson, J. (2006) *Infection Control in Clinical Practice*, 3rd edn. Baillière Tindall/Elsevier, Edinburgh.

Winser, H. (2001) An evidence base for adult resuscitation. *Professional Nurse*, **16** (7), 1210–1213.

Wood, C.J. (1998) Endotracheal suctioning: a literature review. *Intensive Care Nursing*, **14**(3), 124–136.

Woodrow, P. (2002) Managing patients with a tracheostomy in acute care. *Nursing Standard*, **16** (44), 39–46.

Supporting the patient through the diagnostic process

Part three

Interpreting diagnostic tests

Procedure guidelines

The Royal Marsden Hospital Manual of Clinical Nursing Procedures, Eighth Edition. Edited by Lisa Dougherty and Sara Lister.
© 2011 The Royal Marsden Hospital. Published 2011 by Blackwell Publishing Ltd.

Overview

In clinical practice nursing staff are required to instigate, participate or assist in the collection of body fluids and/or specimens for varying purposes. Diagnostic tests are undertaken to aid in diagnosis and treatment of various conditions. This chapter will discuss common diagnostic and microbiological tests encountered in clinical practice.

Diagnostic tests include blood sampling from a vein or from central venous access devices to determine the haematological and biochemical status of patients, lumbar puncture for diagnostic and treatment purposes, liver biopsy, semen collection and cervical swabbing. Depending on the clinical picture, other more invasive diagnostic procedures such as endoscopy or the need for radiological investigations such as X-ray may be required.

Microbiological tests are essential in determining infective organisms in body fluids, compartments or tissues that complicate treatment or that can be implicated in chronic conditions.

Diagnostic tests

Definition

A clinical specimen can be defined as any bodily substance, solid or liquid, that is obtained for the purpose of analysis (Weston 2008). Specimen collection is required when microbiological, biochemical or other laboratory investigations are indicated. The collection of an appropriate specimen for microbiological analysis allows for the isolation and identification of micro-organisms that cause disease, and the determination of antimicrobial sensitivity to guide the appropriate antibiotic treatment.

Related theory

A wide range of methods are available for obtaining cultures and identifying organisms from specimens or swabs. To employ all these tests would be time-consuming and costly, and therefore processing and analysis need to be selective. This is dependent on the type of specimen being processed, the patients' clinical presentations, relevant history, recent or current antimicrobial therapy and investigation required. Based on this information, the microbiology laboratory can select the most appropriate culture media to isolate and identify pathogenic organisms, be they bacterial, viral, fungal or parasitic (Weston 2008). For example, a faecal sample from a patient who also has a history of recent travel would be investigated for organisms not normally looked for in a specimen from a patient without such a history. The sensitivity of the organism to a range of antimicrobials can then be tested to decide on the most appropriate and effective mode of treatment (Higgins 2007).

Box 11.1 Good practice in specimen collection

- Appropriate to the patient's clinical presentation.
- Collected at the right time.
- Collected in a way that minimizes the risk of contamination.
- Collected in a manner that minimizes the health and safety risk to all staff handling the sample.
- Collected using the correct technique, correct equipment and in the correct container.
- Documented clearly, informatively and accurately on the request forms.
- Stored/transported appropriately.

(Higgins 2008)

Evidence-based approaches

Rationale

Successful laboratory diagnosis depends upon the collection of specimens at the appropriate time, using the correct technique and equipment, and transporting them to the designated laboratory safely without delay (Box 11.1). For this to be achieved, it is essential that there is good liaison between medical, nursing, portering and laboratory staff (Mims 2004).

The clinical microbiology laboratory plays a fundamental role in the diagnosis of infection and an increasingly important role in reducing new antibiotic resistance (Woodford et al. 2004). A team approach helps to facilitate more effective infection prevention and control strategies. Close communication between the medical, nursing and laboratory teams is particularly important when unusual infections are suspected or if the patient is immunosuppressed as the infection may be caused by an unusual organism whose identification requires special processing techniques (Thomson 2002).

Indications

Collecting a specimen is often the first crucial step in determining diagnosis and subsequent mode of treatment for patients with suspected infections or to aid in the diagnosis of specific conditions. In other aspects the collection may help determine variation from normal values such as blood sampling or endoscopic findings.

Principles of care

Nursing staff are in a unique position and play a key role within the microbiological process because they often identify the need for microbiological investigations, initiate the collection of specimens and assume responsibility for timely and safe transportation to the laboratory (Higgins 2007). Specimen collection is often the first crucial step in investigations that define the nature of the disease, determine a diagnosis and therefore the mode of treatment.

Methods of investigations

Initial examination

Specimens will be initially examined for clinical variables such as odour, appearance, consistency and turbidity. Foul-smelling, purulent material is suggestive of anaerobic bacteria, cloudy cerebrospinal fluid (CSF) or urine suggests the presence of neutrophils, stool may contain blood or mucus and parasites such as roundworms or tapeworms which are visible to the naked eye (Gould and Brooker 2008).

Direct microscopy

The majority of specimens will then undergo direct microscopic investigation which is valuable as an early indication of the causative organism. High magnification is required to visualize viruses, which are then identified according to their characteristic shapes (Gould and Brooker 2008). Certain parasitic protozoa, such as malaria, are identified by direct microscopy which necessitates the specimen being delivered to the laboratory as quickly as possible whilst the protozoa are mobile and therefore visible (Higgins 2007). In combination with clinical presentations, this may be enough to initiate or change targeted treatments until a more definitive diagnosis is reached (Weston 2008).

Gram staining

Gram staining is a process by which staining substances are added to a sample to differentiate the type of organisms present. Cells with differing properties stain differently in relation to the structure of their cell wall (Mims 2004).

Gram staining allows for the differentiation between Gram-positive bacteria (e.g. *Staphylococcus aureus*), which will stain purple, and Gram-negative bacteria (e.g. *Escherichia coli*), which will stain pink when viewed under the microscope. This can be used to guide the choice of antimicrobial therapy until other investigation methods can provide a definitive identification of pathogenic microorganisms (Mims 2004).

Culture

Depending upon the type of specimen sent to the laboratory and the suspected causative organism, a liquid or solid medium will be selected to enable further identification. Clinical specimens are inoculated onto agar plates or into nutrient broth, then incubated for a certain period of time and observed for growth (Weston 2008). Different species or strains have different growth rates; for example, *Pseudomonas* and *Clostridium* multiply in approximately 10 minutes, *Escherichia coli* has a growth rate of 8 hours whilst *Mycobacterium tuberculosis* takes 18–24 hours to grow (Weston 2008). Growth of bacteria is seen as colonies on the culture media and the size, colour and shape vary according to the type of bacteria identified (Gould and Brooker 2008).

Fungal organisms grow in the same type of media as those used for bacteria, although they generally require an incubation period of 24–48 hours (Higgins 2007). Pathogenic fungi can also be grown on special mycological media, upon which they grow better with less risk of bacterial overgrowth (Mims 2004). Fungi are identified from their characteristic appearance on the surface of the agar and microscopic appearance (Gould and Brooker 2008). The presence of fungi, such as *Candida albicans*, is sometime difficult to interpret because it is commonly present in the upper respiratory, alimentary and female genital tract, and on the skin of healthy people. However, in patients who are immunocompromised this fungus can lead to systemic disease (Garber 2001).

Viruses cannot be cultured outside living cells, although cells grown in nutrient material can be used to culture certain viruses. Their identification is indicated by the characteristic way in which they change the shape of the cell (Gould and Brooker 2008).

Antibiotic sensitivity

Once the pathogenic organism has been identified, it is vital to establish which antibiotics it is sensitive to so the appropriate therapy can be prescribed (Gould and Brooker 2008). The bacteria are inoculated onto a solid media plate and paper discs impregnated with different antibiotics are placed over them and incubated. If the bacteria are sensitive to a particular antibiotic, their growth is inhibited, resulting in a clear zone around the disc.

Serology

Serology is useful in identifying viral infections and bacterial infections with difficult culture organisms and is based upon the host's immunological reaction. Detection of antigens or antibodies in serum, which are activated in response to infection, may suggest that the patient is, or has been, infected (Higgins 2007).

Despite the disadvantage of the test being performed retrospectively, antibody testing is the main method for diagnosing viral infections (Mims 2004). Two serum tests are collected, once at the beginning of the illness and again at 10–14 days, and compared for changes in antibody content. A raised content suggests that the patient's infection is current (Mims 2004).

Histology

Histology is the study of cells and tissues within the body. It also studies how the tissues are arranged to then form organs. The histological focus is on the individual cells' structure and how they are arranged to form the individual organs. The types of tissues that are recognized are epithelial, connective, muscular and nervous (Junqueira and Carneiro 2005).

The tissues are examined under a light microscope where light passes though the tissue components after they have been stained. As most tissues are colourless, they are stained with dyes to enable visualization. An alternative is the electron microscope in which the cells and tissue can be viewed at magnifications of about 120,000 times (Junqueira and Carneiro 2005).

Legal and professional issues

Competencies

In accordance with the NMC's *The Code: Standards of Conduct, Performance and Ethics* (NMC 2008a), the collection of specimens should be undertaken by professionals who are competent and feel confident that they have the knowledge, skill and understanding to do so, following a period of appropriate training and assessment. For microbiological sampling, this will include a knowledge and understanding of the collection, handling and transportation of samples to optimize quality and minimize contamination and inadvertent subversion of the specimen, all of which may have subsequent implications on patient treatment and care.

Consent

The collection of specimens involves invasive procedures and it is therefore essential that practitioners gain consent before beginning any treatment or care (NMC 2008b). Consent is continuous throughout any patient episode and the practitioner must ensure that the patient is kept informed at every stage (Marsden 2007). For specimen collection this includes:

- informing the patient of the rationale for specimen collection
- what the procedure will involve
- ascertaining their level of understanding (especially if they need to be directly involved in the sampling technique)
- how long the results may take to be processed
- how the results will be made available
- information with regard to the implications this may have on their care.

Accurate record keeping and documentation

Good record keeping is an integral part of nursing practice, and it is essential to the provision of safe and effective care (NMC 2009). Accurate, specific and timely documentation of specimen collection should be recorded in the patient notes, care plan or designated record charts/forms such as a microbiological flow chart that details when a specimen was collected, results of analysis, sensitivities or resistance to antimicrobials and changes/modifications to treatment. It is also important to ensure that electronic records are up to

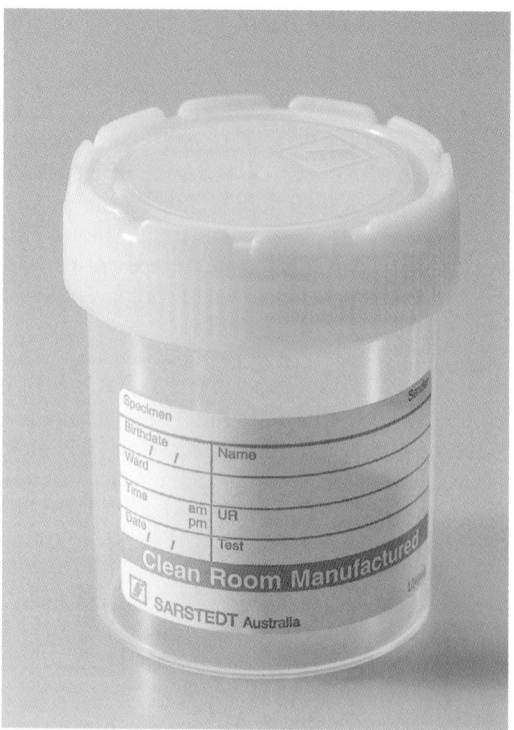

Figure 11.1 Sputum pot.

date. This assists in the communication and dissemination of information between members of the interprofessional healthcare team.

Preprocedural considerations

Equipment

There are a variety of collection equipment/tools designed for the collection of specimens such as sterile pots, swabs and other receptacles (Figures 11.1, 11.2, 11.3 and 11.4). Advice should be sought from the microbiology department about the best type of container for the required investigation (Higgins 2007). It is essential that the specimen and its transport container are appropriate for the type of organism being investigated; for example, bacterial swabs contain a transport medium that is incompatible with viral specimen analysis. Failure to utilize the correct collection method leads to inaccurate results so it is vital that an adequate quantity of material is obtained to allow complete microbiological examination.

Equipment used for transportation

Within healthcare institutions, specimens should be transported in deep-sided trays that are not used for any other purpose, and are disinfected weekly and whenever contaminated (HSE 2003), or robust, leak-proof containers that conform to 'Biological Substances, Category B – UN3373'

Figure 11.2   Various stool pots.

Figure 11.3   Urine pot.

Figure 11.4   Variety of swabs.

regulations (HSE 2005). Specimens that need to be moved outside the hospital must be transported using a triple-packaging system (HSE 2005). This consists of a watertight leak-proof, absorbent primary container, a durable, watertight, leak-proof secondary container and an outer container that complies with 'Biological Substances, Category B – UN 3373' standards (Pankhurst and Coulter 2009). A box for transportation is essential and should carry a warning label for hazardous material. It must be made of smooth impervious material, such as plastic or metal, which will retain liquid and can be easily disinfected and cleaned in the event of a spillage (HSE 2003).

Handling specimens

Specimens should be obtained using safe techniques and practices and practitioners should be aware of the potential physical and infections hazards associated with the collection of diagnostic specimens within the healthcare environment. Standard (Universal) Infection Control Precautions should be adopted by healthcare workers who have direct contact or exposure to the blood, bodily fluids, secretions and excretions of patients (Gould and Brooker 2008). In addition to personal protection, the person collecting the specimen should also be mindful of the collective health and safety of other colleagues/persons who are involved in the handling of samples. Every health authority must ensure that medical, nursing, phlebotomy, portering and any other staff involved in handling specimens are trained to do so (RCN 2005).

In relation to specimen collection, Standard (Universal) Infection Control Precautions should include the following (Tilmouth and Tilmouth 2009).

- Hand hygiene.
- The use of personal protection equipment (PPE).
- Safe sharps management.
- Safe handling, storage and transportation of specimens.
- Waste management.
- Clean environment management.
- Personal and collective management of exposure to body fluids and blood.

621

Selection of PPE should be based upon an assessment of risk to exposure to body fluids (Hairon 2008). As minimum precautions, gloves and aprons should be worn when handling all body fluids. Protective face wear (e.g. goggles, masks and visors) should be worn during any procedure where there is risk of blood, bodily fluid, secretions or excretions splashing into the eyes or face (Gould 2002).

Specimens should be placed in a double, self-sealing bag with one compartment containing the specimen and the other containing the request form. The specimen container used should be appropriate for the purpose and the lid should be securely closed immediately to avoid spillage and contamination. The specimen should not be overfilled and not be externally contaminated by the contents. Any accidental spillages must be cleaned up immediately by staff wearing appropriate protective equipment (HSE 2003).

If a specimen is suspected or known to present an infectious hazard, particularly Hazard Group 3 pathogens (such as hepatitis B or C virus, HIV, *Mycobacterium tuberculosis*), this must be clearly indicated with a 'danger of infection' label on the specimen and the request form to enable those handling the specimen to take appropriate precautions (HSE 2003).

Specimens from patients who have recently been treated with toxic therapy such as gene therapy, cytotoxic drugs, radioactivity or active metabolites need to be handled with caution. Local guidelines on the labelling, bagging and transportation of such samples to the laboratory should be followed. For example, in the case of gene therapy, the specimen must be labelled with a 'biohazard' label, double bagged and transported to the laboratory in a secure box with a fastenable lid.

Selecting specimens

Selecting a specimen that is representative of the disease process is critical to the ability of the laboratory to provide information that is accurate, significant and clinically relevant (Miller 1998). Specimens should only be taken when there are clinical signs of infection (or in the case of specific swabs, such as skin or nasal swabs, as part of an infection screening regimen). Signs of infection such as fever should trigger a careful clinical assessment to ensure that unnecessary tests are avoided and the most useful laboratory samples are obtained to identify therapeutic options (Gould and Brooker 2008). Specimens may also be collected for other diagnostic procedures such as cervical smears, semen collection and lumbar puncture. Tissue sampling may also be indicated during endoscopy or biopsies.

Wherever possible, specimens should be collected before patients are commenced on any treatment such as antibiotics or antiseptics. Treatment with antibiotics before the causative organism has been identified may inhibit its growth, so that it is not easily detected during analysis, yielding a misleading false negative (Weston 2008). If, however, the patient is already receiving such treatment, this must be clearly indicated on the requisition form.

Assessment and recording tools
Request forms

The form should include as much information as possible as this allows the laboratory to select the most appropriate media inoculation for examination and result interpretation (Weston 2008).

Request forms should include the following information.

- Patient's name, date of birth, ward and/or department.
- Hospital number.
- Investigation required so as to avoid indiscriminate specimen analysis which wastes time and money.
- Date and time of specimen collection.
- Type and site of specimen. This should specify the actual anatomical site, such as 'abdominal wound', as this allows the laboratory to differentiate and assess the significance of results based upon the flora normally associated with that site (Miller 1998).
- Diagnosis and relevant clinical information which can help in the interpretation of a sample (Higgins 2007).
- Relevant signs and symptoms.
- Relevant history, for example recent foreign travel.
- Present or recent antimicrobial therapy.
- Whether the patient is immunocompromised as these patients are highly susceptible to opportunistic infections and non-pathogenic organisms (Weston 2008).
- Consultant's name.
- Name and contact details of the doctor requesting the investigation, as it may be necessary to telephone the result before the report is dispatched.
- If a high-risk specimen, it should be labelled with a 'danger of infection' label (HSE 2003).

Communication

For certain specimens that have specific collection techniques or require prompt processing, communication with the laboratory before the sample collection and/or providing information that a sample is being sent to the laboratory can improve efficiency of processing and accuracy of results.

Collecting specimens

The production of high-quality, accurate results which are clinically useful is very much dependent upon the quality of the specimen collection (Higgins 2007). The greater the quantity of material sent for laboratory examination, the greater the chance of isolating a causative organism.

Specimens should be taken as soon as possible after the manifestation of clinical signs and symptoms. The timing of specimen collection is especially important during the acute phase of viral infections. Many viral illnesses have a prodromal phase where multiplication and shedding of the virus are usually at their peak and when the patient is most infective (Mims 2004). This is often before the onset of clinical illness and has often ceased by about day 5 from the onset of symptoms. At this stage, the patient's immune response against the virus has already been mounted and may therefore affect organism isolation (Winter 2005).

Specimens are readily contaminated by poor technique and analysis of such specimens could lead to adverse outcomes such as misdiagnosis, misleading results, extended length of stay or inappropriate therapy (Miller 1998). Therefore, a clean technique must be used to avoid inadvertent contamination of the site of the sample or the specimen itself. Specimens should also be collected in sterile containers with close-fitting lids or with sterile swabs.

Postprocedural considerations

Labelling specimens

Prompt microbiological analysis is only possible if specimens and their accompanying request forms are sent with specific, accurate and complete patient information. Incorrectly or unlabelled specimens will be discarded (HSE 2003).

Samples should include the following information.

- Patient's name, date of birth, ward and/or department.
- Hospital number.
- Date and time of specimen collection.
- Type and site of specimen. This should specify the actual anatomical site such as 'abdominal wound' as this allows the laboratory to differentiate and assess the significance of results based upon the flora normally associated with that site (Miller 1998).
- If a high-risk specimen, it should be labelled with a 'danger of infection' label (HSE 2003).

Transporting specimens

An awareness of the type of organism being investigated and their growth requirements gives the healthcare professional an insight into the correct collection, storage and transportation methods (Table 11.1). Most micro-organisms are also extremely susceptible to environmental fluctuations such as pH, temperature, ultraviolet rays and oxidizing agents (Gould and Brooker 2008). Incorrect or prolonged storage or transportation may result in the organism not surviving

before cultures can be made (Gill *et al.* 2005). Delays in transporting a specimen to the laboratory can compromise the specimen's integrity, leading to false-negative or -positive results, because the sample is no longer representative of the disease process (Higgins 2007).

The sooner a specimen arrives in the laboratory, the greater the chance of organisms being identified. Some pathogens do not survive once they have left the host, whilst normal body flora within the sample may proliferate and overgrow, inhibiting or killing the pathogen (Weston 2008).

If delays are anticipated, samples need to be stored appropriately, depending on the nature of the specimen, until they can be processed. For example, blood cultures need to be incubated at 37°C, whereas swabs must be either refrigerated or kept at ambient temperature, depending on the site from which they were taken.

The transport of clinical specimens must conform to health and safety legislation and regulations, and there are more specific guidelines on the labelling, transport and reception of specimens within clinical laboratories and similar facilities (HSE 2003).

Blood: obtaining samples from a peripheral vein (venepuncture)

Definition

Venepuncture is the procedure of entering a vein with a needle (Weller 2009).

Anatomy and physiology

The superficial veins of the upper limb are most commonly chosen for venepuncture. These veins are numerous and accessible, ensuring that the procedure can be performed safely and with minimum discomfort (Ernst 2005). In adults, veins located on the dorsal portion of the foot may be selected but there is an increased risk of deep vein thrombosis (Garza and Becan-McBride 2010) or tissue necrosis in diabetics (Ernst 2005). Therefore, veins in the lower limbs should be avoided where possible.

Table 11.1 Types of organisms

Organism	Definition
Aerobic	Aerobic bacteria will only grow in the presence of oxygen
Anaerobic	Anaerobic bacteria prefer an atmosphere of reduced oxygen, such as deep in wound bed tissue and facultative anaerobes can grow in either the presence or absence of oxygen
Bacteria	Bacteria are unicellular organisms that multiply and die very rapidly, especially once removed from their optimum environment
Virus	Viruses are intracellular parasites that hijack the genetic material of the host cell, and are therefore unable to multiply outside living cells

Gould and Brooker (2008), Higgins (2007), Winter (2005).

Vein choice

The veins commonly used for venepuncture are those found in the antecubital fossa because they are sizeable veins capable of providing copious and repeated blood specimens (Weinstein and Plumer 2007). However, the venous anatomy of each individual may differ. The main veins of choice are the (Figure 11.5):

- median cubital veins
- cephalic vein
- basilic vein
- metacarpal veins (used only when the others are not accessible).

Median cubital vein

The median cubital vein may not always be visible, but its size and location make it easy to palpate. It is also well supported by subcutaneous tissue, which prevents it from rolling under the needle.

Cephalic vein

On the lateral aspect of the wrist, the cephalic vein rises from the dorsal veins and flows upwards along the radial border of the forearm as the median cephalic, crossing the antecubital fossa as the median cubital vein. Care must be taken to avoid accidental arterial puncture, as this vein crosses the brachial artery. It is also in close proximity to the radial nerve (Dougherty 2008, Masoorli 2002).

Basilic vein

The basilic vein, which has its origins in the ulnar border of the hand and forearm (Marieb and Hoehn 2010), is often overlooked as a site for venepuncture. It may well be prominent but is not well supported by subcutaneous tissue, making it roll easily, which can result in difficult venepuncture. Owing to its position, a haematoma may occur if the patient flexes the arm on removal of the needle, as this squeezes blood from the vein into the surrounding tissues (McCall and Tankersley 2008, Weinstein and Plumer 2007). Care must also be taken to avoid accidental puncture of the median nerve and brachial artery (Garza and Becan-McBride 2010).

Metacarpal veins

The metacarpal veins are easily visualized and palpated. However, the use of these veins is contraindicated in the elderly in whom skin turgor and subcutaneous tissue are diminished (Weinstein and Plumer 2007).

Layers of the vein

Veins consist of three layers: the tunica intima, the tunica media and the tunica adventitia.

Tunica intima

The tunica intima is a smooth endothelial lining, which allows the passage of blood cells. If it becomes damaged, the lining may become roughened, leading to an increased risk of thrombus formation (Weinstein and Plumer 2007). Within this layer are folds of endothelium called valves, which keep blood moving towards the heart by preventing backflow.

(a)

(b)

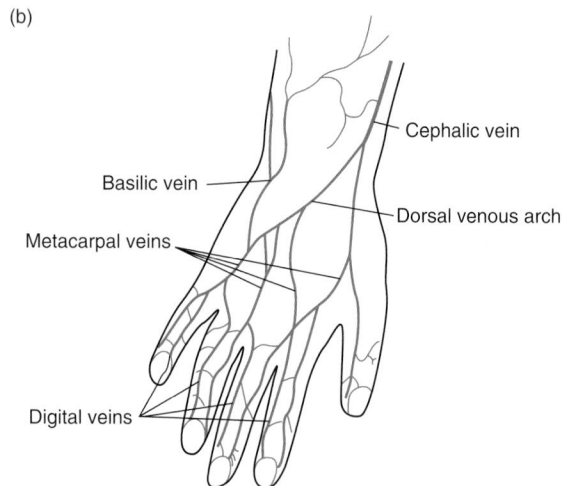

Figure 11.5 (a) Superficial veins of the forearm. (b) Superficial veins of dorsal aspect of the hand. Reproduced with permission from Becton Dickinson and Company.

624

Valves are present in larger vessels and at points of branching and are seen as noticeable bulges in the veins (Weinstein and Plumer 2007). However, when suction is applied during venepuncture, the valve can compress and close the lumen of the vein, thus preventing the withdrawal of blood (Weinstein and Plumer 2007). Therefore, if detected, venepuncture should be performed above the valve in order to facilitate collection of the sample (Weinstein and Plumer 2007).

Tunica media

The tunica media, the middle layer of the vein wall, is composed of muscular tissue and nerve fibres, both vasoconstrictors and vasodilators, which can stimulate the vein to contract or relax. This layer is not as strong or stiff as an artery and therefore veins can distend or collapse as the pressure rises or falls (Waugh *et al.* 2006, Weinstein and Plumer 2007). Stimulation of this layer by a change in temperature, mechanical or chemical stimulation can produce venous spasm, which can make a venepuncture more difficult.

Tunica adventitia

The tunica adventitia is the outer layer and consists of connective tissue, which surrounds and supports the vessel.

Arteries tend to be placed more deeply than veins and can be distinguished by the thicker walls, which do not collapse, the presence of a pulse and the bright red blood. It should be noted that aberrant arteries may be present; these are arteries located superficially in an unusual place (Weinstein and Plumer 2007).

Choosing a vein

The choice of vein must be that which is best for the individual patient. The most prominent vein is not necessarily the most suitable vein for venepuncture (Weinstein and Plumer 2007). There are two stages to locating a vein:

1 visual inspection
2 palpation.

Visual inspection

Visual inspection is the scrutiny of the veins in both arms and is essential prior to choosing a vein. Veins adjacent to foci of infection, bruising and phlebitis should not be considered, owing to the risk of causing more local tissue damage or systemic infection (Dougherty 2008). An oedematous limb should be avoided as there is danger of stasis of lymph, predisposing to such complications as phlebitis and cellulitis (Hoeltke 2006, Smith 1998). Areas of previous venepuncture should be avoided as a build-up of scar tissue can cause difficulty in accessing the vein and can result in pain due to repeated trauma (Hoeltke 2006).

Palpation

Palpation is an important assessment technique, as it determines the location and condition of the vein, distinguishes veins from arteries and tendons, identifies the presence of valves and detects deeper veins (Dougherty 2008). The nurse should always use the same fingers for palpation as this will increase sensitivity and the ability of the nurse to know what they are feeling. The less dominant hand should be used for palpation so that in the event of a missed vein the nurse can repalpate and realign the needle (Hoeltke 2006). The thumb should not be used as it is not as sensitive and has a pulse, which may lead to confusion in distinguishing veins from arteries in the patient (Weinstein and Plumer 2007).

Thrombosed veins feel hard and cord-like, and should be avoided along with tortuous, sclerosed, fibrosed, inflamed or fragile veins, which may be unable to accommodate the device to be used and will result in pain and repeated venepunctures (Dougherty 2008). Use of veins which cross over joints or bony prominences and those with little skin or subcutaneous cover, for example the inner aspect of the wrist, will also subject the patient to more discomfort (Dougherty 2008). Therefore, preference should be given to a vessel that is unused, easily detected by inspection and palpation, patent and healthy. These veins feel soft and bouncy and will refill when depressed (Weinstein and Plumer 2007).

Evidence-based approaches
Rationale
Indications

Venepuncture is carried out for two reasons:

- to obtain a blood sample for diagnostic purposes
- to monitor levels of blood components.

Methods of improving venous access

There are a number of methods of improving venous access.

- *Application of a tourniquet*: this promotes venous distension. The tourniquet should be tight enough to impede venous return but not restrict arterial flow. The tourniquet should be placed about 7–8 cm above the venepuncture site. It may be more comfortable for the patient to position it over a sleeve or paper towel to prevent pinching the skin. The tourniquet should not be left on for longer than 1 minute as this may result in haemoconcentration or pooling of the blood, leading to inaccurate blood results (Hoeltke 2006).
- The patient may be asked to clench the fist and encourage venous distension but should avoid 'pumping' as this action may affect certain blood results, for example potassium (Ernst 2005, Garza and Becan-McBride 2010).
- Lowering the arm below heart level also increases blood supply to the veins.

- Light tapping of the vein may be useful but can be painful and may result in the formation of a haematoma in patients with fragile veins, for example thrombocytopenic patients (Dougherty 2008).
- The use of heat in the form of a warm pack or by immersing the arm in a bowl of warm water for 10 minutes helps to encourage venodilation and venous filling (Lenhardt *et al.* 2002).
- Ointment or patches containing small amounts of glyceryl trinitrate have been used to improve local vasodilation to aid venepuncture (Weinstein and Plumer 2007).

Methods for insertion

Asepsis is vital when performing a venepuncture as the skin is breached and a foreign device is introduced into a sterile circulatory system. The two major sources of microbial contamination are:

- cross-infection from practitioner to patient
- skin flora of the patient.

Good handwashing and drying techniques are essential on the part of the nurse; gloves should be changed between patients (see Chapter 3).

To remove the risk presented by the patient's skin flora, firm and prolonged rubbing with an alcohol-based solution, such as chlorhexidine 0.5% in 70% alcohol, is advised (RCN 2010). This cleaning should continue for about 30 seconds, although some authors state a minimum of 1 minute or longer (Weinstein and Plumer 2007). The area that has been cleaned should then be allowed to dry to: (i) facilitate coagulation of the organisms, thus ensuring disinfection, and (ii) prevent a stinging pain on insertion of the needle due to the alcohol on the end of the needle. The skin must not be touched or the vein repalpated prior to venepuncture.

Legal and professional issues

Venepuncture is one of the most commonly performed invasive procedures (Castledine 1996) and is now routinely being undertaken by nurses (Ernst 2005). In order to perform venepuncture safely, the nurse must have basic knowledge of the following.

- The relevant anatomy and physiology.
- The criteria for choosing both the vein and device to use.
- The potential problems which may be encountered, how to prevent them and necessary interventions.
- The health and safety/risk management of the procedure, as well as the correct disposal of equipment (RCN 2010).

Certain principles, such as adherence to an aseptic technique, must be applied throughout (see Chapter 3). The circulation is a closed sterile system and a venepuncture, however quickly completed, is a breach of this system, providing a means of entry for bacteria.

Nurses must be aware of the physical and psychological comfort of the patient (Hoeltke 2006). They must appreciate the value of adequate explanation and simple measures to prevent the complications of venepuncture, such as haematoma formation, when it is neither a natural nor acceptable consequence of the procedure (Hoeltke 2006).

The number of litigation cases within the healthcare environment has increased in recent years (Garza and Becan-McBride 2010). It is therefore vital that nurses receive accredited and appropriate training, supervision and assessment by an experienced member of staff (RCN 2010). The nurse is then accountable and responsible for ensuring that skills and competence are maintained and knowledge is kept up to date, in order to fulfil the criteria set out in the *The Code* (NMC 2008a).

Preprocedural considerations
Safety of the practitioner

It is recommended that well-fitting gloves are worn during any procedure that involves handling blood and body fluids, particularly venepuncture and cannulation (ICNA 2003, NHS Employers 2007, RCN 2010). This is to prevent contamination of the practitioner from potential blood spills. Whilst it is recognized that gloves will not prevent a needlestick injury, the wiping effect of a glove on a needle may reduce the volume of blood to which the hand is exposed, thereby reducing the volume inoculated and the risk of infection (ICNA 2003, Mitchell Higgs 2002, NAO 2003). However, there is no substitute for good technique and practitioners must always work carefully when performing venepuncture.

A range of safety devices are now available for venepuncture which can reduce the risk of occupational percutaneous injuries amongst healthcare workers, in particular vacuum blood collection systems (Centers for Disease Control and Prevention 1997). Used needles should always be discarded directly into an approved sharps container, without being resheathed (Garza and Becan-McBride 2010, RCN 2010). Specimens from patients with known or suspected infections such as hepatitis or human immunodeficiency virus (HIV) should have a biohazard label attached. The accompanying request forms should be kept separately from the specimen to avoid contamination (HSE 2003). All other non-sharp disposables should be placed in a universal clinical waste bag.

Equipment
Tourniquets

There are several types of tourniquet available. A good-quality, buckle closure, single hand release type is most effective but the choice will depend on availability and operator. Consideration should be given to the type of material and the ability to decontaminate the tourniquet (Golder *et al.* 2000, RCN 2010). Disposable tourniquets are available for single use and should be discarded immediately after use (Warekois *et al.* 2007).

Needles

The intravenous devices commonly used to perform a venepuncture for blood sampling are a straight steel needle and a steel winged infusion device. The optimum gauge to use is 21 swg (standard wire gauge), which measures internal diameter: the smaller the gauge size, the larger the diameter. Standard wire gauge measurement is determined by how many cannulas fit into a tube with an inner diameter of 1 inch (2.5 cm), and uses consecutive numbers from 13 to 24. This enables blood to be withdrawn at a reasonable speed without undue discomfort to the patient or possible damage to the blood cells.

Vacuum systems

A vacuum system consists of a plastic holder which contains or is attached to a double-ended needle or adaptor. It is important to use the correct Luer adaptor to ensure a good connection and avoid blood leakage (Garza and Becan-McBride 2010). The blood tube is vacuumed in order to ensure that the exact amount of blood required is withdrawn when the tube is pushed into the holder. Filling ceases once the tube is full, which removes the need for decanting blood and also reduces blood wastage. The system can also be attached to winged infusion devices (Dougherty 2008).

A number of vacuum systems are available that can be used for taking blood samples. These are simple to use and cost-effective. The manufacturer's instructions should be followed if one of these systems is used. Vacuum systems reduce the risk of healthcare workers being contaminated, because they offer a completely closed system during the process of blood withdrawal and there is no necessity to decant blood into bottles (Dougherty 2008). This makes them the safest method for collecting blood samples.

Blood collection tubes are available in various sizes and have different coloured tops dependent on the type of additives in the tube. The correct volume of blood should be collected into each tube to prevent erroneous results. The expiry dates on the tubes should also be monitored regularly.

Equipment available will depend on local policy (Table 11.2), but with increasing concern about the possibility of contamination to the practitioner, blood collection systems with integrated safety devices are now readily available and should be used wherever possible (Garza and Becan-McBride 2010). However, the nurse must always select the device after assessing the condition and accessibility of the vein.

Pharmacological support

It is important to remember that patients may fear venepuncture and in some cases suffer from severe needle phobia. The use of topical local anaesthetic cream may be beneficial for anxious patients or for venepuncture in children (Weinstein and Plumer 2007). Further information can be found in Chapter 18.

Table 11.2 Choice of intravenous device

Device	Gauge	Advantages	Disadvantages	Use
Needle	21	Cheaper than winged infusion devices. Easy to use with large veins	Rigid. Difficult to manipulate with smaller veins in less conventional sites. May cause more discomfort Venous access only confirmed when sample tube attached	In large, accessible veins in the antecubital fossa When small quantities of blood are to be drawn
Winged infusion device with or without safety shield	21	Flexible due to small needle shaft. Easy to manipulate and insert at any site. Increases the success rate of venepuncture and causes less discomfort (Hefler *et al.* 2004) Usually shows a 'flashback' of blood to indicate a successful venepuncture	More expensive than steel needles The 12–30 cm length of tubing on the device may be caught and dislodge the needle	Veins in sites other than the antecubital fossa When quantities of blood greater than 20 mL are required from any site
	23	Flexible due to small needle shaft. Easy to manipulate and insert at any site. Causes less discomfort. Smaller swg and therefore useful with fragile veins	More expensive than steel needles, plus there can be damage to cells which can cause inaccurate measurements in certain blood samples, for example potassium	Small veins in more painful sites, for example inner aspect of the wrist, especially if measurements are related to plasma and not cellular components

Non-pharmacological support

Patient anxiety about the procedure may result in vasoconstriction. The nurse's manner and approach will also have a direct bearing on the patient's experience (Garza and Becan-McBride 2010). Approaching the patient with a confident manner and giving adequate explanation of the procedure may reduce anxiety. Careful preparation and an unhurried approach will help to relax the patient and this in turn will increase vasodilation (Dougherty 2008, Weinstein and Plumer 2007).

Specific patient preparation

- Injury, disease or treatment, for example amputation, fracture and cerebrovascular accident, may prevent the use of a limb for venepuncture, thereby reducing the venous access. Use of a limb may be contraindicated because of an operation on one side of the body, for example mastectomy and axillary node dissection, as this can lead to impairment of lymphatic drainage, which can influence venous flow regardless of whether there is obvious lymphoedema (Berreth 2010, Cole 2006, Ernst 2005, Hoeltke 2006).
- The age and weight of the patient will also influence choice. Young children have short fine veins, and the elderly have prominent but fragile veins. Care must be taken with fragile veins and the largest vein should be chosen along with the smallest gauge device to reduce the amount of trauma to the vessel. Malnourished patients will often present with friable veins (Dougherty 2008).
- If the patient is in shock or dehydrated there will be poor superficial peripheral access. It may be necessary to take blood after the patient is rehydrated as this will promote venous filling and blood will be obtained more easily (Dougherty 2008).
- Medications can influence the choice of vein in that patients on anticoagulants or steroids or those who are thrombocytopenic tend to have more fragile veins and will be at greater risk of bruising both during venepuncture and on removal of the needle. Therefore choice may be limited by areas of bruising present or the inability to access the vessel without causing bruising (Dougherty 2008).
- The temperature of the environment will influence venous dilation. If the patient is cold, no veins may be evident on first inspection. Application of heat, for example in the form of a warm compress or soaking the arm in warm water, will increase the size and visibility of the veins, thus increasing the likelihood of a successful first attempt (Lenhardt *et al.* 2002, Weinstein and Plumer 2007).
- Venepuncture itself may cause the vein to collapse or go into a spasm. This will produce discomfort and a reduction in blood flow. Careful preparation and choice of vein will reduce the likelihood of this and stroking the vein or applying heat will help resolve it (Dougherty 2008).
- Involving patients in the choice of vein, even if it is simply to choose the non-dominant arm, can increase a feeling of control which in turn helps to relieve anxiety (Hudak 1986).
- The environment is also another important consideration. In the inpatient and outpatient setting, lighting, ventilation, privacy and position must be checked and optimized where possible. This will ensure that the patient and the operator are both comfortable. Having adequate lighting is also beneficial as it illuminates the procedure, ensuring the operator has a good view of the vein and equipment (Dougherty 2008).

Procedure guideline 11.1 Venepuncture

Essential equipment

- Clean tray or receiver
- Tourniquet or sphygmomanometer and cuff
- 21 swg multiple sample needle or 21 swg winged infusion device and multiple sample Luer adaptor
- Plastic tube holder, standard or for blood cultures
- Appropriate vacuumed specimen tubes
- Swab saturated with chlorhexidine in 70% alcohol, or isopropyl alcohol 70%
- Low-linting gauze swabs
- Sterile adhesive plaster or hypoallergenic tape
- Specimen request forms
- Non-sterile, well-fitting gloves
- Plastic apron (optional)
- Sharps bin

Preprocedure

Action	Rationale
1 Approach the patient in a confident manner and explain and discuss the procedure with the patient.	To ensure that the patient understands the procedure and gives their valid consent (NMC 2008b, C).
2 Allow the patient to ask questions and discuss any problems which have arisen previously.	Anxiety results in vasoconstriction; therefore, a patient who is relaxed will have dilated veins, making access easier. E

3 Consult the patient as to any preferences and problems that may have been experienced at previous venepunctures. Check if they have any allergies.	To involve the patient in the treatment. To acquaint the nurse fully with the patient's previous venous history and identify any changes in clinical status, for example mastectomy, as both may influence vein choice (Dougherty 2008, E). To prevent allergic reactions, for example to latex or chlorhexidine (McCall and Tankersley 2008, E).
4 Check that the identity of the patient matches the details on the request form by asking for their full name and date of birth and checking their identification bracelet.	To ensure the sample is taken from the correct patient (NPSA 2007, C; RCN 2010, C).
5 Assemble the equipment necessary for venepuncture.	To ensure that time is not wasted and that the procedure goes smoothly without unnecessary interruptions. E
6 Carefully wash hands using bactericidal soap and water or bactericidal alcohol handrub, and dry before commencement.	To minimize risk of infection (DH 2010; Fraise and Bradley 2009, E).
7 Check hands for any visibly broken skin, and cover with a waterproof dressing.	To minimize the risk of contamination to the practitioner (DH 2010, C; Fraise and Bradley 2009, E).
8 Check all packaging before opening and preparing the equipment on the chosen clean receptacle.	To maintain asepsis throughout and check that no equipment is damaged. E

Procedure

9 Take all the equipment to the patient, exhibiting a competent manner.	To help the patient feel more at ease with the procedure. E
10 Support the chosen limb on a pillow.	To ensure the patient's comfort and facilitate venous access. E
11 Apply a tourniquet to the upper arm on the chosen side, making sure it does not obstruct arterial flow. If the radial pulse cannot be palpated then the tourniquet is too tight (Weinstein and Plumer 2007). The position of the tourniquet may be varied; for example, if a vein in the hand is to be used it may be placed on the forearm. A sphygmomanometer cuff may be used as an alternative.	To dilate the veins by obstructing the venous return (Dougherty 2008, E). To increase the prominence of the veins. E To promote blood flow and therefore distend the veins (Gunwardene and Davenport 1990, E; Lenhardt et al. 2002, R3).
12 If the tourniquet does not improve venous access the following methods can be used. **Either** The arm may be placed in a dependent position. The patient may be asked to clench their fist. **Or** The veins may be tapped gently or stroked. **Or** Remove the tourniquet and apply moist heat, for example a warm compress, soak limb in warm water or, with medical prescription, apply glyceryl trinitrate ointment/patch (Weinstein and Plumer 2007).	To improve venous access (Dougherty 2008, E).
13 Select the vein using the aforementioned criteria (see Action Figure 13).	To prevent haemoconcentration and pooling of the blood (Hoeltke 2006, E).
14 Release the tourniquet.	To ensure patient comfort. E
15 Select the device, based on vein size, site, and so on.	To reduce damage or trauma to the vein (Dougherty 2008, E; RCN 2010, C).

629

(Continued)

Procedure guideline 11.1 *(Continued)*

16 Wash hands with bactericidal soap and water or bactericidal alcohol handrub.	To maintain asepsis, and minimize the risk of infection (DH 2010; Fraise and Bradley 2009, E).
17 Reapply the tourniquet.	To dilate the veins by obstructing the venous return (Dougherty 2008, E).
18 Put on gloves.	To prevent possible contamination of the practitioner (NHS Employers 2007, C).
19 Clean the patient's skin carefully for 30 seconds using an appropriate preparation, for example chlorhexidine in 70% alcohol, and allow to dry. Do not repalpate or touch the skin (see Action Figure 19).	To maintain asepsis and minimize the risk of infection (DH 2010; Fraise and Bradley 2009, E). To prevent pain on insertion (Fraise and Bradley 2009, E; Dougherty 2008, E; RCN 2010, C).
20 Remove the cover from the needle and inspect the device carefully.	To detect faulty equipment, for example bent or barbed needles. If these are present place them in a safe container, record batch details and return to manufacturer (MHRA 2005, C; RCN 2010, C).
21 Anchor the vein by applying manual traction on the skin a few centimetres below the proposed insertion site (see Action Figure 21).	To immobilize the vein. To provide countertension to the vein which will facilitate a smoother needle entry (Dougherty 2008, E).
22 Insert the needle smoothly at an angle of approximately 30°. However, the angle will depend on size and depth of the vein (also see Action Figure 21).	To facilitate a successful, pain-free venepuncture. E
23 Reduce the angle of descent of the needle as soon as a flashback of blood is seen in the tubing of a winged infusion device or when puncture of the vein wall is felt.	To prevent advancing too far through vein wall and causing damage to the vessel. E
24 Slightly advance the needle into the vein, if possible.	To stabilize the device within the vein and prevent it becoming dislodged during withdrawal of blood. E
25 Do not exert any pressure on the needle.	To prevent a puncture occurring through the vein wall. E

26 Withdraw the required amount of blood using a vacuumed blood collection system or syringes (see Action Figure 26). Collect blood samples in the following order:
 	
■ blood culture
■ coagulation
■ serum tube with or without clot activator or gel separator (glass, non-additive tubes can be filled before the coagulation tube)
■ additive tubes such as:
  (a) gel separator tubes (may contain clot activator or heparin)
  (b) heparin tubes
  (c) EDTA
■ all other tubes (Garza and Becan-McBride 2010).
	To minimize the risk of transferring additives from one tube to another and bacterial contamination of blood cultures (manufacturer's guidelines, C).

27 Release the tourniquet. In some instances this may be necessary at the beginning of sampling as inaccurate measurements may be caused by haemostasis, for example when taking blood to assess calcium levels.	To decrease the pressure within the vein. E
28 Remove tube from plastic tube holder.	To prevent blood spillage caused by vacuum in the tube (Campbell *et al.* 1999, E).

29 Pick up a low-linting swab and place it over the puncture point.	To apply pressure. E
30 Remove the needle, but do not apply pressure until the needle has been fully removed.	To prevent pain on removal and damage to the intima of the vein. E
31 Activate safety device, if applicable, and then discard the needle immediately in sharps bin.	To reduce the risk of accidental needlestick injury (NHS Employers 2007, C).
32 Apply digital pressure directly over the puncture site. Pressure should be applied until bleeding has ceased; approximately 1 minute or longer may be required if current disease or treatment interferes with clotting mechanisms.	To stop leakage and haematoma formation. To preserve vein by preventing bruising or haematoma formation. E
33 The patient may apply pressure with the finger but should be discouraged from bending the arm if a vein in the antecubital fossa is used.	To prevent leakage and haematoma formation (Ernst 2005, E).
34 Gently invert the tube at least six times.	To prevent damage to blood cells and to mix with additives (manufacturer's guidelines, C).
35 Label the bottles with the relevant details at the patient's side.	To ensure that the specimens from the right patient are delivered to the laboratory, the requested tests are performed and the results returned to the correct patient's records (NMC 2009, C; NPSA 2007, C).

Postprocedure

36 Inspect the puncture point before applying a dressing.	To check that the puncture point has sealed. E
37 Ascertain whether the patient is allergic to adhesive plaster.	To prevent an allergic skin reaction. E
38 Apply an adhesive plaster or alternative dressing.	To cover the puncture and prevent leakage or contamination. E
39 Ensure that the patient is comfortable.	To ascertain whether patient wishes to rest before leaving (if an outpatient) or whether any other measures need to be taken. E
40 Remove gloves and discard waste, making sure it is placed in the correct containers, for example sharps into a designated receptacle.	To ensure safe disposal and avoid laceration or other injury of staff (Fraise and Bradley 2009, E; DH 2006, C). To prevent reuse of equipment (MDA 2000, C).
41 Follow hospital procedure for collection and transportation of specimens to the laboratory.	To make sure that specimens reach their intended destination. E

631

Action Figure 13   Palpating the vein.

Action Figure 19   Cleaning the skin.

(Continued)

Procedure guideline 11.1 *(Continued)*

Action Figure 21   Anchoring the skin.

Action Figure 26   Attach sample bottle to holder.

Problem-solving table 11.1 Prevention and resolution (Procedure guideline 11.1)

Problem	Cause	Prevention	Suggested action
Pain	Use of vein in sensitive area (e.g. wrist)	Avoid using veins in sensitive areas wherever possible. Use local anaesthetic cream	Complete procedure as quickly as possible
Anxiety	Previous trauma	Minimize the risk of a traumatic venepuncture. Use all methods available to ensure successful venepuncture	Approach patient in a calm and confident manner. Listen to the patient's fears and explain what the procedure involves. Offer patient opportunity to lie down. Suggest use of local anaesthetic cream (Lavery and Ingram 2005)
	Fear of needles		All of the above and perhaps referral to a psychologist if fear is of phobic proportions
Limited venous access	Repeated use of same veins	Use alternative sites if possible	Do not attempt the procedure unless experienced
	Peripheral shutdown	Ensure the room is not cold	Put patient's arm in warm water. Apply glycerol trinitrate patch
	Dehydration		May be necessary to rehydrate patient prior to venepuncture
	Hardened veins (due to scarring and thrombosis)		Do not use these veins as venepuncture will be unsuccessful
	Poor technique/choice of vein or device	Ensure correct device and technique are used	

Problem	Cause	Prevention	Suggested action
Needle inoculation of or contamination to practitioner	Unsafe practice. Incorrect disposal of sharps	Maintain safe practice. Activate safety device if applicable. Ensure sharps are disposed of immediately and safely	Follow accident procedure for sharps injury, for example make site bleed and apply a waterproof dressing. Report and document. An injection of hepatitis B immunoglobulin or triple therapy may be required
Accidental blood spillage	Damaged/faulty equipment	Check equipment prior to use	Report within hospital and/or MHRA
	Reverse vacuum	Use vacuumed plastic blood collection system. Remove blood tube from plastic tube holder before removing needle	Ensure blood is handled and transported correctly
Missed vein	Inadequate anchoring. Poor vein selection. Wrong positioning. Lack of concentration. Poor lighting	Ensure that only properly trained staff perform venepuncture or that those who are training are supervised. Ensure the environment is well lit	Withdraw the needle slightly and realign it, providing the patient is not feeling any discomfort. Ensure all learners are supervised. If the patient is feeling pain, then the needle should be removed immediately
	Difficult venous access		Ask experienced colleague to perform the procedure
Spurt of blood on entry	Bevel tip of needle enters the vein before entire bevel is under the skin; usually occurs when the vein is very superficial		Reassure the patient. Wipe blood away on removal of needle
Blood stops flowing	Through puncture: needle inserted too far	Correct angle	Draw back the needle, but if bruising is evident, then remove the needle immediately and apply pressure
	Contact with valves	Palpate to locate	Withdraw needle slightly to move tip away from valve
	Venous spasm	Results from mechanical irritation and cannot be prevented	Gently massage above the vein or apply heat
	Vein collapse	Use veins with large lumen. Use a smaller device	Release tourniquet, allow veins to refill and retighten tourniquet
	Small vein	Avoid use of small veins wherever possible	May require another venepuncture
	Poor blood flow	Use veins with large lumens	Apply heat above vein

Postprocedural considerations

Immediate care

It is important to ensure that the needle is removed correctly on completion of blood sampling and that the risk of haematoma formation is minimized. Pressure should be applied as the needle is removed from the skin. If pressure is applied too early, it causes the tip of the needle to drag along the intima of the vein, resulting in sharp pain and damage to the lining of the vessel.

The practitioner should ensure that firm pressure is maintained until bleeding has stopped. The patient should also be instructed to keep their arm straight and not bend it as this also increases the risk of bruising (Ernst 2005). A longer period of pressure may be necessary where the patient's blood may take longer to clot, for example, if the patient is receiving anticoagulants or is thrombocytopenic. The practitioner may choose to apply the tourniquet over the venepuncture site to ensure even and constant pressure on the area (Dougherty 2008). Alternatively, they can elevate the arm slightly above the heart to decrease venous pressure (Garza and Becan-McBride 2010).

The practitioner should inspect the site carefully for bleeding or bruising before applying a dressing to the site, and the patient leaving the department. If bruising has occurred the patient should be informed of why this has happened and given instructions for what to do to reduce the bruising and any associated pain. Initially the application of an ice pack may help to soothe and decrease bruising. The application of Hirudoid cream, which is used for the treatment of thrombophlebitis, may be helpful (BNF 2011).

Complications

Complications that may occur when venepuncture is performed include arterial puncture, nerve injury, haematoma, fainting and infection. Careful assessment and preparation will minimize the risks but if they occur then appropriate action should be taken immediately.

Arterial puncture

To prevent an arterial puncture, careful assessment in vein selection is necessary. The nurse should palpate the vessel prior to needle insertion to confirm the absence of a pulse; the angle of insertion should be less than 40° and in the event of a missed vein, blind probing should be avoided.

An arterial puncture can be identified by bright red blood, rapid blood flow and pain. The needle should be removed immediately and pressure applied for 5 minutes by the nurse. A pressure dressing should be applied and the patient should receive verbal and written advice to follow in the event of increased pain, swelling or loss of sensation. No tourniquet or blood pressure cuff should be reapplied to the

arm for 24 hours. The incident should be documented in the patient's notes (Dougherty 2008).

Nerve injury

Careful vein selection and needle insertion should minimize the risk of nerve injury. The angle of insertion should be less than 40° and blind probing should be avoided. In the event of a nerve injury, the patient may complain of a sharp shooting pain, burning or electric shock sensation that radiates down the arm and they may experience numbness/tingling in the fingers. The needle should be removed immediately to prevent further nerve damage. The patient should receive verbal and written advice to follow in the event that the pain/numbness continues for more than a few hours. The incident should be documented in the patient's notes (Dougherty 2008).

Haematoma

Haematoma formation is the most common complication of venepuncture (McCall and Tankersley 2008). A haematoma develops when blood leaks from the vein into the surrounding tissues; it may be caused by the needle penetrating completely through the vein wall, the needle only being partially inserted or insufficient pressure on the site when the needle is removed. If a haematoma develops, the needle should be removed immediately and pressure applied. In the event of a large haematoma developing the nurse can apply an ice pack to relieve pain and swelling. The patient should receive verbal and written advice as a haematoma may lead to a compression injury to the nerve. The incident should be documented in the patient's notes (Dougherty 2008).

Fainting

Fainting may occur during or immediately following venepuncture. The patient may complain of feeling light-headed and appear pale and sweaty. Loss of consciousness may occur suddenly so the nurse should be vigilant throughout the procedure and routinely confirm with the patient that they do not feel unwell or faint. In the event of the patient feeling faint, the nurse should remove the device immediately, apply pressure to the site and encourage the patient to lower the head and breathe deeply. The application of a cold compress to the forehead and increased ventilation (open a window if clinically acceptable) may help to make the patient more comfortable. If the patient suffers a loss of consciousness the nurse should call for assistance and ensure the patient's safety until they recover. The patient should not be allowed to leave the department until fully recovered and be advised not to drive for at least 30 minutes (Garza and Becan-McBride 2005, McCall and Tankersley 2008). The incident should be documented in the patient's notes and the patient advised to inform staff on future occasions.

Infection

Infection at the venepuncture site is a rare occurrence (McCall and Tankersley 2008).

Aseptic technique should be maintained with careful attention to handwashing and skin preparation. The venepuncture site should not be repalpated after cleaning and the site should be covered for 15–20 minutes after the procedure. Infection at the venepuncture site should be reported to a doctor as antibiotics may be required.

Blood sampling from a central venous catheter

Evidence-based approaches

Methods of taking blood samples from a central venous access device

Obtaining blood samples from a central venous access device (CVAD) can lead to inaccurate results, especially coagulation values, if the correct method is not followed to ensure removal of any drug/solution prior to sampling (Frey 2003). A number of methods may be used to withdraw samples and there appears to be no significant difference in laboratory results and no evidence of haemolysis or haemodilution (Adlard 2008, Holmes 1998, RCN 2010).

■ *Discard method*: this is the most commonly used method in the clinical setting (recommended by the Royal Marsden Hospital and demonstrated within Procedure guideline 11.2) where the first 6–10 mL of blood is withdrawn and discarded (Cosca *et al.* 1998, Holmes 1998, Warekois *et al.* 2007). This ensures removal of any heparin or saline solution but may result in excessive blood removal in small children or those requiring multiple samples, for example for pharmacokinetic tests (Adlard 2008, Cosca *et al.* 1998).

■ *Push–pull (mixing) method*: a syringe is attached to the catheter, the catheter is flushed with 0.9% sodium chloride, then 6 mL is withdrawn and pushed back without removing the syringe; this is repeated three times. This removes any residual solution and reduces exposure to blood and there is no blood wastage (Adlard 2008, Holmes 1998). This method supposes that mixing of blood eliminates intravenous fluids and heparin from the catheter lumen (Cosca *et al.* 1998). However, it may be difficult to obtain enough blood to exchange 3–4 times.

■ *Reinfusion method*: this method is performed by taking the first 6 mL of blood, capping off the syringe, taking the samples and then reinfusing the blood first taken (Keller 1994). It does not result in depleted blood volume but there is a risk of blood exposure. The discard syringe could be confused with the specimen sample and there could be contamination or clots in the sample for reinfusion (Frey 2003) and there is a chance of haemolysis with agitation of blood (Frey 2003).

Preprocedural considerations

It is preferable to use the distal lumen of a multilumen catheter when obtaining a sample and where these catheters have different-sized lumens, the largest should be reserved for blood sampling (Dougherty 2006, Gorski *et al.* 2010). However, if a CVAD will not bleed then it may be necessary to take blood from a peripheral vein.

635

Procedure guideline 11.2 Central venous access devices: taking a blood sample for vacuum sampling

Essential equipment

■ Sterile dressing pack
■ Alcohol-based handwash solution
■ Extra 10 mL blood bottle without heparin or sterile 10 mL syringe
■ Vacuum system container holder (shell)
■ Vacuum system adaptor

Medicinal products

■ Appropriate vacuumed blood bottles (*or*)
■ Sterile syringe of appropriate size for sample required
■ Needleless injection cap (as necessary)
■ 10 mL syringe containing 0.9% sodium chloride
■ Flushing solution as per policy
■ 2% chlorhexidine in 70% alcohol swab

Preprocedure

Action	Rationale
1 Explain and discuss the procedure with the patient. Check forms to ascertain sample bottles required and check patient's identity.	To ensure that the patient understands the procedure and gives their valid consent (NMC 2008b, C). To ensure correct bottles are used and blood is taken from correct patient.

(Continued)

Procedure guideline 11.2 (*Continued*)

Procedure

2 Wash hands with bactericidal soap and water or bactericidal alcohol handrub.	To reduce the risk of cross-infection (DH 2010, C).
3 Prepare a tray or trolley and take it to the bedside. Clean hands as above. Open sterile pack and prepare equipment.	To reduce the risk of contamination of contents (DH 2010, C).
4 If intravenous fluid infusion is in progress, switch it off.	To prevent spillage of fluid following disconnection. E
5 Where required, disconnect the administration set from the catheter and cover the end of the set with sterile cap.	To reduce the risk of contaminating the end of the administration set. E
6 Clean hands with a bactericidal alcohol handrub. Put on non-sterile gloves. Clean hub thoroughly with a 2% chlorhexidine in 70% alcohol swab. Allow to dry.	To minimize the risk of introducing infection into the catheter, and prevent contamination of practitioner's hands with blood. To enable disinfection process to be completed (DH 2010, C).
7 Attach vacuum container holder and adaptor via the needleless injection cap and release clamp.	To maintain a closed system and prevent contamination of practitioner or air entry. E
8 Attach extra sample bottle: fill and discard.	To remove blood, heparin and intravenous fluids from the 'dead space' of the catheter. Samples from this 'dead space' are likely to cause inaccuracies in blood tests, because of the risk of contamination of the sample with heparin, sodium chloride or glucose and so on (Cosca *et al.* 1998, R5; Holmes 1998, R4).
9 Attach required sample bottles in correct order of draw for requested specimens.	To obtain sample. It is not necessary to clamp the catheter when changing collection bottles, as the system is not open. E
10 Reclamp catheter and detach vacuum container holder.	To prevent blood loss or air embolism. E
11 Flush with 10 mL 0.9% sodium chloride, using the push–pause method (i.e. 1 mL at a time).	To create turbulence, ensure removal of all blood in the catheter and prevent occlusion (INS 2006, C).
12 Reconnect the administration set, unclamp the catheter and recommence infusion or attach new needleless injection cap. Release clamp and flush catheter through injection cap using the push–pause method and finishing with the positive pressure technique.	To prevent the catheter clotting between uses (Dougherty 2006, E; Moureau 1999, E).
13 Ensure that blood samples have been placed in the correct containers and agitated as necessary to prevent clotting. Label them with patient's name, number, date of birth, and so on, at patient's bedside and send them to the laboratory with the appropriate forms.	To make certain that the specimens, correctly presented and identified, are delivered to the laboratory, enabling the requested tests to be performed and the results returned to the correct patient's records (RCN 2010 C).

Procedure guideline 11.3 Central venous access devices: taking a blood sample for syringe sampling

This may be necessary if the CVAD does not bleed when using a vacuum system, for example silicone PICCs.

Essential equipment

- Sterile dressing pack
- Alcohol-based handwash solution
- Extra 10 mL blood bottle without heparin or sterile 10 mL syringe
- Vacuum system container holder (shell)
- Vacuum system adaptor

- Appropriate vacuumed blood bottles (*or*)
- Sterile syringe of appropriate size for sample required.
- Needleless injection cap (as necessary)
- 2% chlorhexidine in 70% alcohol swab

Medicinal products

- 10 mL syringe containing 0.9% sodium chloride
- Flushing solution as per policy

Preprocedure

Action	Rationale
1 Explain and discuss the procedure with the patient. Check forms to ascertain sample bottles required and check patient's identity.	To ensure that the patient understands the procedure and gives their valid consent (NMC 2008b, C). To ensure correct bottles are used and blood is taken from correct patient. E

Procedure

Action	Rationale
2 Wash hands with bactericidal soap and water or bactericidal alcohol handrub.	To reduce the risk of cross-infection (DH 2010, C).
3 Prepare a tray or trolley and take it to the bedside. Clean hands as above. Open sterile pack and prepare equipment.	To reduce the risk of contamination of contents (DH 2010, C).
4 If intravenous fluid infusion is in progress, switch it off.	To prevent spillage of fluid following disconnection. E
5 Where required, disconnect the administration set from the catheter and cover the end of the set with sterile cap.	To reduce the risk of contaminating the end of the administration set. E
6 Clean hands with a bactericidal alcohol handrub. Put on non-sterile gloves. Clean hub thoroughly with a 2% chlorhexidine in 70% alcohol swab. Allow to dry.	To minimize the risk of introducing infection into the catheter, and prevent contamination of practitioner's hands with blood. To enable disinfection process to be completed (DH 2007c, C).
7 Attach a 10 mL syringe to the needleless injection cap. Release the clamp and withdraw 5–10 mL of blood.	To remove blood, heparin and intravenous fluids from the 'dead space' of the catheter. Samples from this 'dead space' are likely to cause inaccuracies in blood tests (Cosca *et al.* 1998, R5; Holmes 1998, R4).
8 Clamp and remove syringe and discard.	To discard contaminated sample and prevent mixing (Cosca *et al.* 1998, R5; Holmes 1998, R4).
9 Attach a new syringe of appropriate size. Unclamp and withdraw the required amount of blood.	To obtain the sample. E
10 Clamp and detach the syringe.	To prevent blood spillage or air entry. E
11 Decant blood into sample bottles.	To ensure blood is placed into sample bottles as soon as possible. E

(Continued)

Procedure guideline 11.3 (Continued)

12 Flush with 10 mL 0.9% sodium chloride, using the push–pause method (i.e. 1 mL at a time).	To create turbulence, ensure removal of all blood in the catheter and prevent occlusion (INS 2006, C).
13 Reconnect the administration set, unclamp the catheter and recommence infusion or attach new needleless injection cap. Release clamp and flush catheter through injection cap using the push–pause method and finishing with the positive pressure technique.	To prevent the catheter clotting between uses (Dougherty 2006, E: Moureau 1999, E).

Postprocedure

14 Remove gloves and dispose of waste.	To prevent the contamination of others (DH 2010, C).
15 Ensure that blood samples have been placed in the correct containers and agitated as necessary to prevent clotting. Label them with patient's name, number, date of birth, and so on, at patient's bedside and send them to the laboratory with the appropriate forms.	To make certain that the specimens, correctly presented and identified, are delivered to the laboratory, enabling the requested tests to be performed and the results returned to the correct patient's records (RCN 2010, C).

Problem-solving table 11.2 Prevention and resolution (Procedure guidelines 11.2 and 11.3)

Problem	Cause	Prevention	Action
Difficulty may be encountered when taking blood samples	This is more common when the central venous catheter is made of silicone and has been in place for a long period of time. One of the causes is that the tip of the soft catheter lies against the wall of the vessel and the suction required to draw blood brings this into close contact, leading to temporary occlusion. There could also be a collapse of the catheter walls when using the vacuum system which may necessitate the use of syringes to obtain the blood	Tip position in lower superior vena cava or right atrium	Measures to try to dislodge the tip include asking the patient to: (a) cough and breathe deeply (b) roll from side to side (c) raise his/her arms (d) perform the Valsalva manoeuvre, if possible (e) increase general activity, for example walk up and down stairs (Gorski *et al.* 2010)
	The tip of the catheter may be covered in a fibrin sheath, which may result in partial withdrawal occlusion (PWO)		This may be resolved with rapid flushing of the catheter with 0.9% sodium chloride or a dilute solution of heparin. If due to PWO then a fibrinolytic agent may be necessary to remove the fibrin (Mayo 1998)
	Pinch-off syndrome occurs when a CVAD inserted via the percutaneous subclavian site is compressed by the clavicle and first rib and aspirating blood becomes difficult (Andris and Krzywda 1997, Verhage and van Bommel 1999)		Ask patient to lift arm to side. If blood aspiration improves and there is little resistance on flushing, suspect pinch-off and request chest X-ray and cathetergram to check for catheter rupture

Postprocedural considerations

Whichever method is used, once the samples have been taken it is vital that the catheter is adequately flushed with 0.9% sodium chloride followed where appropriate with a heparin solution, to reduce the risk of clot formation and subsequent infection and/or occlusion (Dougherty 2006, RCN 2010).

Arterial sampling

Evidence-based approaches

Arterial punctures

It is worth noting that morbidity associated with arterial cannulation is less than that associated with five or more arterial punctures (Bersten *et al.* 2009) (see Chapter 18). However, arterial punctures are important and useful in the initial and short-term assessment of acid/base balance. Multiple puncture attempts will increase the risk of injury, not only due to the direct trauma but also associated with vasospasm (Lipsitz 2004). If the patient requires repetitive blood sampling it may be more appropriate to admit the patient into a more clinically suitable area where arterial cannulation is possible. This not only minimizes both the distress to the patient and time taken by skilled personnel in obtaining each sample, but reduces the risks associated with multiple punctures.

Preprocedural considerations

Specific patient preparations

Ideally, prior to obtaining any arterial blood gas sample (Figure 11.6), the patient should be in a respiratory steady state for 15–20 minutes. The oxygen should not be titrated,

Figure 11.6 Arterial blood gas sampling.

and if ventilated, suction should not be attempted and ventilation parameters not adjusted (Weinstein and Plumer 2007). Arterial sampling or cannulation is associated with a considerable amount of pain that can be reduced by using local anaesthetic. In an emergency there may be no time for local anaesthetic application but when it is feasible to wait for local anaesthetic to take effect before attempting arterial puncture, studies suggest higher success rates for arterial sampling (Sado and Deakin 2005).

Where a sample is taken from an established arterial cannula, the following volumes of blood should be withdrawn and discarded. This is to ensure that any 0.9% sodium chloride, blood and small emboli from the dead space within the cannula and the three-way tap have been removed. Discarded volumes will vary according to arterial cannula placement due to the length of the arterial cannula.

- Peripheral artery cannula: take 3 mL and discard.
- Femoral artery cannula: take 5 mL and discard.

When using a vacuum system, take one bottle and discard prior to obtaining requested samples.

639

Procedure guideline 11.4 Arterial puncture: radial artery

Essential equipment

- Intravenous sterile dressing pack
- Gloves
- Hypoallergenic tape

- 2% chlorhexidine in 70% alcohol
- Arterial blood gas syringe
- 18 G needle

Preprocedure

Action	Rationale
1 Explain and discuss the procedure with the patient.	To ensure the patient understands the procedure and gives their valid consent (NMC 2008b, C). To minimize anxiety which may distort analysis or exacerbate symptoms. E
2 Check the concentration of oxygen the patient is breathing and body temperature at time of sampling.	Inspired oxygen concentration and temperature parameters are required to interpret arterial blood gases accurately (Weinstein and Plumer 2007, E).

(Continued)

Procedure guideline 11.4 (*Continued*)

3 Check the patient's current coagulation screen, platelet count, medical history and prescription chart for anticoagulation therapy.	To identify possible risk of bleeding and haematoma formation post procedure and, where appropriate, to prevent puncture until coagulation is corrected. E
4 Prepare trolley.	To reduce the risk of cross-infection (DH 2010, C).
5 Wash hands with bactericidal soap and water or bactericidal alcohol handrub.	To reduce the risk of cross-infection (DH 2010, C).

Procedure

6 Perform the Allen test.	To confirm patency of ulnar artery circulation and assess collateral circulation to the hand in the event of radial artery damage, for example thrombosis (White 2003, E).
7 Locate and palpate the radial artery with the middle and index fingers of the non-dominant hand.	To assess maximum pulsation to ensure radial artery is optimum site for successful puncture. The dominant hand will be used to perform puncture (Weinstein and Plumer 2007, E).
8 Inspect and assess the surrounding tissues and anatomical structures.	Check and assess surrounding tissues for excoriation/ infection, poor perfusion or other puncture sites. If any of these are present the site should not be used (Weinstein and Plumer 2007, E).
9 Prepare the patient position: gently extend the wrist over a rolled towel (ask for assistance if required).	To reduce the risk of the patient moving unexpectedly which could result in through puncture (Hudson *et al.* 2006, E; Lipsitz 2004, R5). To flex the hand/foot slightly to facilitate insertion. E
10 Open the pack and equipment onto it. Withdraw the plunger of the syringe 1–2 mL before the puncture.	To reduce blood haemolysis. Arterial pressure causes a brisk pulsatile reflux of blood into the syringe (unless the patient is severely hypotensive) (Weinstein and Plumer 2007, R5).
11 Place a sterile field under the patient's wrist and maintain aseptic technique throughout the procedure.	To minimize the risk of infection (DH 2010, C).
12 Clean site with chlorhexidine in 70% alcohol.	To minimize the risk of infection (DH 2010, C).
13 Administer subcutaneous local anaesthetic.	To minimize pain during the procedure. Local vasodilation effects of the local anaesthetic may reduce vasospasm, making for a successful puncture (Lipsitz 2004, R5).
14 Clean hands with bactericidal skin cleaning solution.	To minimize the risk of infection (DH 2010, C).
15 Apply sterile gloves.	To minimize the risk of infection and prevent contamination of hands with blood (Pratt *et al.* 2007, C).
16 Re-identify the point of maximum pulsation, hold position with index/middle finger.	To guide position of radial artery and aid successful puncture. E

17 Angle the needle 30–45° angle, with the bevel of the needle up just distal to the finger position. Advance needle slowly into the artery until a flashing pulsation is seen in the hub of the needle.	To minimize trauma to the artery. E Rapid insertion may result in a through puncture (White 2003, E). Pulsatile flow indicates access to radial artery. E Arterial pressure causes blood to pulsate spontaneously back into the syringe (Weinstein and Plumer 2007, E).
18 Slowly aspirate by gently pulling the plunger of the arterial gas syringe to a minimum of 0.6 mL of blood for the sample (check recommended amount of blood as directed by manufacturer's guidelines).	To minimize vasospasm. E To ensure optimal volume is obtained in order to ensure an appropriate mix of blood with heparin (see manufacturer's guidelines, C).
19 Withdraw the needle, immediately followed by application of pressure using a low-linting dressing. Promptly return the wrist to the neutral position following sampling.	To prevent haematoma formation and excessive bleeding. E Prolonged hyperextension may be associated with changes in median nerve conduction (Chowet *et al.* 2004, R4).
20 Apply pressure for a minimum of 5 minutes or until no signs of bleeding are observed. Ask for assistance from another nurse if necessary.	To minimize blood loss and to ensure pressure exerted to prevent haematoma and blood loss (RCN 2010, C). Assistance with pressure application enables the sample to be analysed swiftly (Bucher 2001, E).

Postprocedure

21 Dispose of equipment safely.	To prevent contamination of others (DH 2010, C).
22 Expel any air bubbles from the syringe, and cap the arterial syringe and label according to hospital policy.	To keep sample airtight and avoid inaccuracies (White 2003, E).
23 Check puncture site and apply a clean, sterile, low-linting gauze dressing using a non-touch technique. Secure with tape.	To maintain pressure and prevent haematoma formation. E
24 Clearly document rationale for procedure in patient's notes and verbally communicate arterial analysis findings to relevant medical and nursing teams.	To acknowledge accountability for actions and ensure effective comunication. To ensure prompt and appropriate treatment (NMC 2008a, C; NMC 2009, C).

641

Procedure guideline 11.5 Arterial blood gas sampling: arterial cannula

Essential equipment

- Intravenous sterile pack
- 5 mL Luer-Lok syringe
- Gloves

- Arterial blood gas syringe
- 2% chlorhexidine in 70% alcohol
- Bactericidal alcohol handrub

Preprocedure

Action	Rationale
1 Explain and discuss the procedure with the patient.	To ensure the patient understands the procedure and gives their valid consent (NMC 2008b, C).
2 Wash hands with bactericidal soap and water or bactericidal alcohol handrub.	To minimize the risk of cross-infection (DH 2010, C).

(Continued)

Procedure guideline 11.5 (*Continued*)

3 Check the three-way tap is closed to port (see Action Figure 3).	To prevent back-flow of blood and blood spillage. E
4 Clean hands with bactericidal alcohol handrub.	To prevent cross-infection (DH 2010, C).
5 Prepare trolley.	Minimize the risk of cross-infection (DH 2010, C).
6 Press silence button on arterial monitor for duration of sampling.	The continual alarm disturbs both the patient and others in the unit. Alarms of no clinical significance should be minimized (Chambrin 2001, R5).
7 Apply gloves.	To prevent contamination of hands with blood (DH 2010, C).

Procedure

8 Remove cap from three-way tap and clean port with a swab soaked in chlorhexidine in 70% and allow to dry.	To minimize the risk of infection (DH 2010, C).
9 Attach 5 mL Luer-Lok syringe.	To remove saline, old blood and small emboli from the dead space within the cannula. E
10 Turn three-way tap to artery and port (see Action Figure 10).	To prevent contamination of blood with flush solution. E
11 Slowly withdraw appropriate volume of blood.	To prevent the artery going into spasm (Lipsitz 2004, R5).
12 Turn three-way tap diagonally to close off both the artery and flush (see Action Figure 17).	To enable the syringe to be removed without blood loss; to prevent backflow from artery. E
13 Remove 5 mL syringe and discard.	To discard the contaminated sample. E
14 Connect the blood gas syringe.	The gas syringe is open to the artery in order to withdraw the sample. E
15 Turn three-way tap on to artery and port (see Action Figure 10).	To open the syringe directly onto the artery. E
16 Slowly remove the recommended amount of blood (as specified in manufacturer's instructions).	To prevent the artery going into spasm, ensuring the correct volume of blood mixes with the recommended heparin in the gas syringe (Lipsitz 2004, R5).
17 Turn three-way tap diagonally to close off both the artery and flush (see Action Figure 17).	To prevent haemorrhage or blood spillage. E
18 Remove the gas syringe, gently rotate syringe.	Send for analysis, and ensure the blood and heparin contained within the syringe are mixed. E

Postprocedure

19 Turn three-way tap onto flush and port, apply a sterile swab to the port flush squeezing the actuator (see manufacturer's instructions) (see Action Figure 19).	The swab will absorb the blood, preventing contamination (E). Blood is cleared from the port, reducing risk of thrombosis and microemboli (Hazinski 1992, R5).
20 Turn three-way tap onto flush and artery, flush cannula by gently squeezing actuator. As cannula is flushed observe digits for signs of blanching, discoloration or complaints of pain from the patient.	Blood is cleared from the cannula and arterial tubing. E To ensure early recognition of proximal or distal embolism. E
21 Clean port with chlorhexidine in 70% alcohol swab.	To minimize the risk of infection (DH 2010, C).

22 Apply sterile Luer-Lok cap and check it is secure.	To minimize infection and prevent exsanguination (Hart 2006, E).
23 Check pressure infuser cuff is inflated to 300 mmHg.	To prevent backflow of blood into circuit. E
24 Analyse or send to nearest blood gas analyser and document result and report abnormalities.	To obtain result. E

Action Figure 3 Three-way tap: closed to port.

Action Figure 10 Three-way tap: turned to artery and port.

Action Figure 17 Three-way tap: turned diagonally to close off flush, artery and port.

Action Figure 19 Three-way tap: turned to flush and port.

643

Blood tests

Evidence-based approaches
Rationale
Blood tests are routinely collected to:

- confirm disease
- monitor disease
- regulate therapy/treatment.

It is important that the correct blood tube is used for each test. The blood tubes contain special additives relevant to the type of test required, usually indicated by the colour of the tube top. The practitioner should ensure that the correct tube is selected by referring to local hospital guidelines. Correct 'order of draw' should be followed to avoid transferring additive from one bottle to another when filling (Garza and Becan-McBride 2010).

Numerous blood tests are available. Blood samples are sent to various departments within the laboratory, such as haematology, biochemistry and microbiology. Brief outlines

Table 11.3 Haematology

Test	Reference range	Functions/additional information
RBC	Men: 4.5–6.5 × 10^{12}/L Women: 3.9–5.6 × 10^{12}/L	The main function of the RBC is the transport of oxygen and carbon dioxide
Hb	Men: 13.5–17.5 g/dL Women: 11.5–15.5 g/dL	Haemoglobin (Hb) is a protein pigment found within the RBC which carries the oxygen
		Anaemia (deficiency in the number of RBC or in the Hb content) may occur for many reasons. Changes to cell production, deficient dietary intake or blood loss may be relevant and need to be investigated further
WBC	Men: 3.7–9.5 × 10^{9}/L Women: 3.9–11.1 × 10^{9}/L	The function of the WBC is defence against infection
		There are different kinds of WBC: neutrophils, lymphocytes, monocytes, eosinophils and basophils
		Leucopenia is a WBC count lower than 3.7 and is usually associated with the use of cytotoxic drugs
		Leucocytosis (high levels of neutrophils and lymphocytes) occurs as the body's normal response to infection and after surgery
		Leukaemia involves an increased WBC count caused by changes in cell production in the bone marrow. The leukaemic cells enter the blood in increased numbers in an immature state
Platelets	Men: 150–400 × 10^{9}/L Women: 150–400 × 10^{9}/L	Clot formation occurs when platelets and the blood protein fibrin combine
		A patient may be thrombocytopenic (low platelet count) due to drugs/poor production or have a raised count (thrombocytosis) with infection or autoimmune disease
Coagulation/INR	INR range 2–3 (in some cases a range of 3–4.5 is acceptable)	Coagulation occurs to prevent excessive blood loss by the formation of a clot (thrombus). However, a clot that forms in an artery may block the vessel and cause an infarction or ischaemia which can be fatal (Blann 2007)
		Aspirin, warfarin and heparin are three drugs used for the prevention and/or treatment of thrombosis
		It is imperative that patients on warfarin therapy receive regular monitoring to ensure a balance of slowing the clot-forming process and maintaining the ability of the blood to clot (Blann 2007)

of some routine tests are given below. Please refer to specialist reference texts for more detail.

Haematology

The full blood count (FBC) is the most commonly requested blood test (Higgins 2007). The FBC involves monitoring the levels of red blood cells (erythrocytes), white blood cells (leucocytes) and platelets (thrombocytes). Variations to normal values can indicate anaemia, infection and thrombocytopenia (Table 11.3).

Blood transfusion

All patients who require a blood transfusion need to have their blood type confirmed. It is essential that correct patient identification and accurate labelling are maintained. The sample will be screened to determine the ABO and Rh (Rhesus) type. All staff should receive formal documented training in blood transfusion practice. (Refer to Chapter 8.)

Biochemistry

Urea and electrolytes are the most common biochemistry tests requested (Table 11.4).

Liver function tests

There are numerous tests which are used to assess liver function. Additional tests include alkaline phosphatase, gamma-glutamyl transferase (GGT), aspartate aminotransferase (AST) and alanine aminotransferase (ALT).

Microbiology

Various types of sample may be sent to the microbiology laboratory for screening, for example blood, urine, faeces and sputum. Blood tests sent to microbiology may include screening for hepatitis B, hepatitis C and HIV.

Table 11.4 Biochemistry

Test	Reference range	Functions/additional information
Sodium	135–145 mmol/L	The main function of sodium is to maintain extracellular volume (water stored outside the cells), acid/base balance and the transmitting of nerve impulses
		Hypernatraemia (serum sodium >145 mmol/L) may be an indication of dehydration due to fluid loss from diarrhoea, excessive sweating, increased urinary output or a poor oral intake of fluid. An increased salt intake may also cause an elevation
		Hyponatraemia (serum sodium <135 mmol/L) may be indicated in fluid retention (oedema)
Potassium	3.5–5.2 mmol/L	Potassium plays a major role in nerve conduction, muscle function, acid/base balance and osmotic pressure. It has a direct effect on cardiac muscle, influencing cardiac output by helping to control the rate and force of each contraction
		The most common cause of hyperkalaemia (serum potassium >5.2 mmol/L) is chronic renal failure. The kidneys are unable to excrete potassium. The level may be elevated due to an increased intake of potassium supplements during treatment. Tissue cell destruction caused by trauma/cytotoxic therapy may cause a release of potassium from the cells and an elevation in the potassium plasma level. It may also be observed in untreated diabetic ketoacidosis
		Urgent treatment is required as hyperkalaemia may lead to changes in cardiac muscle contraction and cause subsequent cardiac arrest
		The main cause of hypokalaemia (serum potassium <3.5 mmol/L) is the loss of potassium via the kidneys during treatment with thiazide diuretics. Excessive/chronic diarrhoea may also cause a decreased potassium level
Urea	2.5–6.5 mmol/L	Urea is a waste product of metabolism that is transported to the kidneys and excreted as urine. Elevated levels of urea may indicate poor kidney function
Creatinine	55–105 µmol/L	Creatinine is a waste product of metabolism that is transported to the kidneys and excreted as urine. Elevated levels of creatinine may indicate poor kidney function
Calcium	2.20–2.60 mmol/L	Most of the calcium in the body is stored in the bone, but ionized calcium, which circulates in the blood plasma, plays an important role in the transmission of nerve impulses and the functioning of cardiac and skeletal muscle. It is also vital for blood coagulation
		High calcium levels (hypercalcaemia >2.6 mmol/L) can be due to hyperthyroidism, hyperparathyroidism or malignancy. Elevation in calcium levels may cause cardiac arrhythmia, potentially leading to cardiac arrest (Blann 2007)
		Tumour cells can cause excessive production of a protein called parathormone-related polypeptide (PTHrp) which causes a loss of calcium from the bone and an increase in the blood calcium levels. This is a major reason for hypercalcaemia in cancer patients (Higgins 2007)
		Hypocalcaemia (<2.20 mmol/L) is often associated with vitamin D deficiency due to inadequate intake or increased loss due to GI disease. Mild hypocalcaemia may be symptomless but severe hypocalcaemia may cause increased neuromuscular excitability and cardiac arrhythmias. It is also a common feature of chronic renal failure (Higgins 2007)
C-reactive protein (CRP)	<10 mg/L	Elevation in the CRP level can be a useful indication of bacterial infection. CRP is monitored after surgery and for patients who have a high risk of infection. The CRP level can help monitor the severity of inflammation and assist in the diagnosis of conditions such as systemic lupus erythematosus (SLE), ulcerative colitis and Crohn's disease (Higgins 2007)
Albumin	35–50 g/L	Albumin is a protein found in blood plasma which assists in the transport of water-soluble substances and the maintenance of blood plasma volume
Bilirubin	(total) <17 µmol/L	Bilirubin is produced from the breakdown of haemoglobin; it is transported to the liver for excretion in bile. Elevated levels of bilirubin may cause jaundice

Blood cultures

Definition

A blood culture is a specimen of blood obtained from a single venepuncture or CVAD for the purpose of detecting bloodborne organisms (bacteria or fungi) and their associated infections (Lee *et al.* 2007). Inoculation of an aerobic and an anaerobic sample in two separate bottles comprises a set of blood cultures.

Related theory

Blood cultures are an essential part of the management of patients with serious bloodborne infections, enabling the identification of the causative pathogens, antimicrobial susceptibility and treatment guidance (Shore and Sandoe 2008). Bacteraemia and fungaemia are associated with high morbidity and mortality amongst hospitalized patients, particularly those with compromised host defences (Panceri *et al.* 2004). The accurate and timely detection of these remains one of the most important functions of clinical microbiology as early detection has significant diagnostic and prognostic importance (HPA 2008f).

Micro-organisms may be present in the blood intermittently or continuously, depending upon the source of infection (HPA 2008f). The majority of bacteraemias are intermittent, so blood cultures should be taken when there are clinical signs of an infection such as fever, as this is when the concentration of bacteria in the blood is at its highest (Higgins 2007).

Evidence-based approaches

Rationale

Indications

There are many signs and symptoms in the patient which may suggest bacteraemia but clinical judgement is required. The following indicators should be taken into account when assessing a patient for signs of bacteraemia or sepsis which would then indicate the need for blood culture sampling (DH 2010).

- Core temperature out of normal range (>38°C or <36°C).
- Focal signs of infection.
- Abnormal heart rate (raised), blood pressure (low or raised) or respiratory rate (raised).
- Chills or rigors.
- Raised or very low white blood cell count.
- New or worsening confusion/altered levels of consciousness.

Methods of blood culture specimen collection

In recognition of the importance of taking accurate blood cultures, there is now national guidance that implements procedure and policy to improve the quality of blood culture investigations and to reduce the risk of blood sample contamination (DH 2010). Contamination can come from a number of sources: the patient's skin, the equipment used to obtain the sample, the practitioner or the general environment. Failure to use an aseptic technique or careful process procedures when obtaining blood cultures can result in a 'false-positive' result which may lead to extensive diagnostic testing, excessive antibiotic use, prolonged hospitalization and artificially raised incidence rates (Dellinger *et al.* 2008).

In order to optimize the identification of causative organisms, the taking of a peripheral sample is recommended and two sets of cultures should be taken at separate times and from separate sites (DH 2010). In cases of suspected endocarditis, this should be three sets within a 24-hour period. Drawing more than one culture set can help to distinguish true bacteraemia from contaminated cultures (Shafazand and Weinacker 2002). Samples should not be taken from existing peripheral cannulas but if the patient has an existing CVAD a sample can be taken from this following collection of a separate peripheral sample. The femoral vein should be avoided for venepuncture because it is difficult to ensure adequate skin cleansing and disinfection (DH 2010).

Blood cultures should be taken prior to commencing or changing antimicrobial therapy as antibiotics may delay or prevent bacterial growth, causing a falsely negative result (Higgins 2007). However, in accordance with the Surviving Sepsis Campaign, antimicrobial therapy should be started within the first hour of recognition of severe sepsis and blood cultures should be taken before antimicrobial therapy is initiated. This is essential to confirm infection and the responsible pathogens whilst not causing significant delay in antibiotic administration (Dellinger *et al.* 2008). If antibiotic therapy has already been commenced, blood cultures should ideally be taken immediately prior to the next dose, except in paediatric patients (DH 2010).

Legal and professional issues

Competencies

Blood cultures should be collected by practitioners who have been trained in the collection procedure and whose competence in blood culture collection has been assessed (DH 2010). Practitioners must be competent and feel confident that they have the knowledge, skill and understanding to undertake blood culture sampling for microbiological analysis (NMC 2008a).

Preprocedural considerations

Equipment

The use of a needle to decant blood into the culture bottles is now largely redundant due to the wide use of closed, vacuumed blood collection systems (for example, Bio-Merieux BacT/ALERT® system which utilizes either a holder for venous access device sampling or a Luer adaptor safety winged device for peripheral sampling). See Figure 11.7. This reduces the health and safety risk to the healthcare professional and the risk of culture contamination.

Figure 11.7 A vacuumed collection system: two blood culture bottles, Vacutainer holder® and Vacutainer 'butterfly'®.

However, if the use of the needle and syringe method is unavoidable, the needle should not be changed between sample collection and inoculation of blood into the culture bottles (DH 2010). Care should be taken not to under- or overfill the bottles as it is difficult to accurately judge the sample volume with this method (Shore and Sandoe 2008).

Volume of blood culture specimen collection

The volume of blood taken for a culture is also critical to ensure correct blood to liquid culture medium ratio. A false-negative result could occur if an insufficient volume is introduced or if too much blood is introduced, due to the effect of the culture medium in the bottles being diluted (Higgins 2007). The liquid culture medium is a mixture of nutrients that supports microbial growth and inhibits phagocytosis and lysozyme activity (Shore and Sandoe 2008). This helps to determine if there are pathogenic micro-organsims present in the blood. As there are a number of systems in use, the manufacturer's instructions should be followed as to the total volume required for each bottle. Adult patients with clinically significant bacteraemias often have a low number of colony-forming units per millilitre of blood and a minimum of 10 mL per culture bottle is recommended (Dellinger *et al.* 2008).

Non-pharmacological support

Skin preparation products

Poor aseptic technique and skin decontamination can cause contamination of a blood culture with the patient's own skin flora, such as coagulase-negative staphylococci (Weston 2008). A combination of 2% chlorhexidine gluconate in 70% isopropyl alcohol is recommended as being effective for skin antisepsis (DH 2010, Madeo and Barlow 2008, Pratt *et al.* 2007). Chlorhexidine gluconate maintains a persistent antimicrobial function by disrupting the cell membrane and precipitating their contents, whilst the isopropyl alcohol quickly destroys micro-organisms by denaturing cell proteins (Inwood 2007). In order to achieve a reduction and inhibition of the micro-organisms living on the skin, gentle friction is required for 30 seconds and the solution should be allowed to dry to achieve good skin antisepsis and to expose the cracks and fissures of the skin to the solution (Pratt *et al.* 2007).

Central venous access device-related infection

A CVAD presents a high risk of infection with an incidence of bacteraemia of between 4% and 8% (HPA 2008f). When it is suspected that the CVAD is the source of infection, a blood culture sample should ideally be obtained from each lumen of the vascular device, as well as obtaining a peripherally drawn sample (Dellinger *et al.* 2008, DH 2010, Gabriel 2008). Adequate hub cleansing with 2% chlorhexidine in 70% isopropyl alcohol is essential in reducing cross-contamination of the sample (Inwood 2007).

Blood cultures from a CVAD can identify colonization from either the device itself or the bloodstream (Penwarden and Montgomery 2002). To diagnose CVAD-related infections, comparison of the time it takes to achieve a positive result from both central and peripheral cultures is recommended (Catton *et al.* 2005). If a culture from the CVAD is positive much earlier than from the peripheral culture (>2 hours earlier) then it can be assumed that the vascular access device is the source of the infection with up to 96% sensitivity and 92% specificity (Bouza *et al.* 2005). Results of such analysis can guide whether removal of the CVAD is indicated.

Procedure guideline 11.6 Blood cultures: peripheral (winged device collection method)

Essential equipment

- Alcohol-based skin cleaning preparation (2% chlorhexidine in 70% isopropyl alcohol)
- Alcohol-based swab for blood culture bottle decontamination (2% chlorhexidine in 70% isopropyl alcohol)
- A set of blood culture bottles (anaerobic and aerobic)
- Vacuum-assisted collection system (winged device for peripheral cultures)
- Non-sterile gloves
- Gauze swabs
- Appropriate document/form

Preprocedure

Action	Rationale
1 Explain and discuss the procedure with the patient.	To ensure the patient understands the procedure and gives valid consent (NMC 2008b, C).
2 Wash hands with bactericidal soap and water, or decontaminate physically clean hands with alcohol-based handrub. Apply gloves.	To reduce the risk of cross-infection and specimen contamination (DH 2010, C).
3 Clean any visible soiled skin on the patient with soap and water then dry.	To reduce the risk of contamination (DH 2010, C).

(Continued)

Procedure guideline 11.6 (*Continued*)

Procedure

4	Apply a disposable tourniquet and palpate to identify vein.	In preparation for venepuncture. E
5	Clean skin with a 2% chlorhexidine in 70% isopropyl alcohol swab for 30 seconds and allow to dry for 30 seconds. Do not palpate site again after cleaning.	To enable adequate skin antisepsis and decontamination, and to prevent contamination from practitioner's fingers (DH 2010, C; Inwood 2007, C).
6	Remove flip-off caps from culture bottles and clean with 2% chlorhexidine in 70% isopropyl alcohol swab and allow to dry.	To reduce the risk of environmental contamination causing false-positive results (DH 2010, C).
7	Wash and dry hands again or use alcohol handrub and apply clean examination gloves (sterile gloves are not essential).	To decontaminate hands having been in contact with the patient's skin to palpate vein. E
8	Attach winged blood collection set into the appropriate vacuum holder for taking blood cultures. Remove sheath-covering needle at wings and perform venepuncture.	Reduces risk of contamination and health and safety risk to practitioner (DH 2006, C; DH 2010, C).
9	If blood is being taken for other tests, collect the blood culture first. Inoculate the aerobic culture first.	To reduce the risk of contamination of culture bottles after inoculating other blood bottles. E
10	Place adaptor case over blood culture bottle and puncture septum.	To initiate vacuum collection action. E
11	Attach aerobic bottle, hold upright, and use bottle graduation lines to accurately gauge sample volumes (at least 10 mL in each bottle or as recommended by manufacturer). Remove bottle and replace with anaerobic bottle.	To reduce the risk of a false-negative result due to insufficient volume or overdiluted culture medium (Higgins 2007, C).
12	Remove winged device, apply pressure to the venepuncture site and apply appropriate dressing.	To prevent bleeding at the site. E

Postprocedure

13	Discard winged collection set in sharps container.	To reduce risk of sharps injury. E
14	Remove gloves and wash/decontaminate hands.	To ensure correct clinical waste management and reduce risk of cross-infection (DH 2006, C).
15	Label bottles with appropriate patient details, ensuring the barcodes on the bottles are not covered or removed.	To ensure correct patient and sample identity and to aid traceability within the laboratory. E
16	Complete microbiology request form (including relevant information such as indications, site and time of culture).	To maintain accurate records and provide accurate information for laboratory analysis (NMC 2009, C; Weston 2008, E).
17	Arrange prompt delivery to the microbiology laboratory to process immediately (or incubate at 37°C).	To increase the chance of accurate organism identification (Higgins 2007, C).

Procedure guideline 11.7 Blood cultures: central venous access device

Essential equipment

- Alcohol-based skin cleaning preparation (2% chlorhexidine in 70% isopropyl alcohol)
- Alcohol-based swab for blood culture bottle decontamination (2% chlorhexidine in 70% isopropyl alcohol)
- A set of blood culture bottles (anaerobic and aerobic)
- Vacuum-assisted collection system (winged device for peripheral cultures)
- Non-sterile gloves
- Gauze swabs
- Microbiological request form
- Flushing solution

Preprocedure

Action	Rationale
1 Explain and discuss the procedure with the patient.	To ensure the patient understands the procedure and gives valid consent (NMC 2008b, C).
2 Wash hands with bactericidal soap and water, or decontaminate physically clean hands with alcohol-based handrub. Apply gloves.	To reduce the risk of cross-infection and specimen contamination (DH 2010, C).

Procedure

3 Clean each lumen end hub with 2% chlorhexidine in 70% isopropyl alcohol swab and allow to dry for 30 seconds (if continuous infusions running this may not be possible).	To enable adequate antisepsis and decontamination of each lumen (Dellinger et al. 2008, C).
4 Remove flip-off caps from culture bottles and clean with 2% chlorhexidine in 70% isopropyl alcohol swab and allow to dry.	To reduce the risk of environmental contamination causing false-positive results (DH 2010, C).
5 Take and discard at least 10 mL of blood prior to attaching blood culture bottles.	To remove any saline or other drug residue that may be present in the lumen (Dougherty and Lamb 2008, C).
6 If blood is being taken for other tests, collect the blood culture first. Inoculate the aerobic culture first.	To reduce the risk of contamination of culture bottles after inoculating other blood bottles. E
7 Attach vacuum-assisted collection system into hub of CVAD, insert blood culture bottle and puncture septum.	To initiate vacuum collection action. E
8 Attach aerobic bottle, hold upright, and use bottle graduation lines to accurately gauge sample volumes (at least 10 mL in each bottle or as recommended by manufacturer). Remove bottle and replace with anaerobic bottle.	To reduce the risk of a false-negative result due to insufficient volume or overdiluted culture medium (Higgins 2007, C).
9 Repeat steps 4–8 with each lumen if a multi-lumen device is *in situ*.	To accurately determine if the CVAD is the source of infection (Catton et al. 2005, C).
10 Remove and discard vacuumed collection set holder in sharps container.	To reduce risk of sharps injury and ensure correct waste management (DH 2006, C).
11 Flush with 0.9% sodium chloride.	To remove blood from lumen (Dougherty 2008, E).

Postprocedure

12 Remove and dispose of gloves and wash/decontaminate hands.	To ensure correct clinical waste management and reduce risk of cross-infection (DH 2006, C).
13 Label bottles with appropriate patient details, ensuring the barcodes on the bottles are not covered or removed.	To ensure correct patient and sample identity and to aid traceability within the laboratory. E
14 Complete microbiology request form (including relevant information such as indications, site and time of culture).	To maintain accurate records and provide accurate information for laboratory analysis (NMC 2009, C; Weston 2008, E).
15 Arrange prompt delivery to the microbiology laboratory to process immediately (or incubate at 37°C).	To increase the chance of accurate organism identification (Higgins 2007, C).

649

Postprocedural considerations

Immediate care

Blood cultures should be dispatched to the laboratory for immediate process. If cultures cannot be processed immediately they should be incubated at 37°C in order for bacterial growth to begin and to prevent deterioration in pathogenic micro-organism yield (Higgins 2007).

Ongoing care

Decisions on commencing, changing or adding antimicrobial therapy may need to be considered depending upon the patient's condition and history. Drug-resistant micro-organisms have highlighted the need for prudent control of antibiotic prescribing and usage. It is estimated that up to 40% of patients with moderate to severe infections are given unnecessary or inappropriate antibiotics to treat the *in vitro* susceptibility of the pathogen that is subsequently cultured (Johannes 2008). Decisions regarding appropriate choice of empirical therapy as well as the duration and dosage should be made in conjunction with advice from the microbiology team (Tacconelli 2009).

Antimicrobial drug assay

Definition

Therapeutic drug monitoring of blood serum ensures that there are sufficient levels of particular antimicrobial drugs to be therapeutically effective, whilst avoiding potentially toxic excess that may lead to adverse side-effects (Thomson 2004).

Related theory

The majority of drugs used in clinical practice have a wide therapeutic window; that is, the difference between the therapeutic and toxic level is substantial, and quantitative analysis of serum levels is unnecessary. However, there are certain drugs that require monitoring of serum concentration levels due to their narrow therapeutic range where toxicity is associated with persistently high concentrations, whilst therapeutic failure can result from low concentrations (Thomson 2004).

Examples of drugs that need monitoring in clinical practice include lithium, digoxin, theophylline, phenytoin, ciclosporin and certain antibiotics (Higgins 2007). This section will focus on aminoglycoside antibiotics, such as gentamicin and amikacin, and glycopeptide antibiotics such as vancomycin as these are the most commonly monitored antimicrobial assays.

These drugs are excreted almost entirely by glomerular filtration and are potentially nephrotoxic and ototoxic. When aminoglycosides or glycopeptides are used as single modes of treatment, renal toxicity is estimated to be 5–10%, although this can increase to as much as 30% if both are used synergistically (Pannu and Nadim 2008).

- Nephrotoxicity involves the proximal tubules that are capable of regeneration; therefore adverse effects may be reversible over time (Hadaway and Chamallas 2003).
- Ototoxicity causes damage within the neuroepithelial cells of the inner ear, which can cause cochlear damage and/or vestibular impairment. These cells cannot be regenerated so the effects are irreversible (Hammett-Stabler and Johns 1998). Ototoxicity occurs in 0.5–3% of patients and is usually associated with very high serum concentrations of the drugs (Sha 2005).

Aminoglycoside antibiotics

Aminoglycosides such as gentamicin and amikacin are potent antibiotics, which are mainly used against aerobic, Gram-negative bacteria and are often used synergistically against certain Gram-positive organisms (Hammet-Stabler and Johns 1998). Single daily dosing of aminoglycosides is possible because of their rapid 'concentration-dependent' action, which increases both the rate and extent of bacterial cell death (Owens and Shorr 2009). The timing of serum sampling will be determined by the patient's clinical manifestations, particularly renal function. For gentamicin the trough levels should be <1 mg/L (18 hours post dose) and <0.5 mg/L (24 hours post dose). For amikacin the trough level should be <5 mg/L.

Glycopeptide antibiotics

Vancomycin is the glycopeptide antibiotic most widely used for the treatment of serious infections caused by Gram-positive pathogens (Jones 2006). Glycopeptides exhibit 'time-dependent' actions, meaning that their effectiveness increases with the duration of time that the antibiotic serum concentration is above the minimum inhibitory concentration (MIC) of susceptible pathogens (Owens and Shorr 2009).

The use and monitoring of vancomycin have increased due to the emergence of meticillin-resistant *Staphylococcus aureus* (MRSA) but the emergence of vancomycin-resistant MRSA has further complicated its clinical use (Jones 2006).

Determination of serum blood levels of vancomycin depends on the frequency of administration. If given intermittently (usually twice-daily doses), trough levels should be taken at set times, immediately before the administration of the next bolus dose (Jones 2006). The use of the continuous infusion of vancomycin also occurs in clinical practice and it is suggested that this is a less toxic mode of administration (Hadaway and Chamallas 2003). If given intermittently, the trough level should be between 5 and 15 mg/L, whilst continuous infusions aim to maintain serum concentrations at between 15 and 25 mg/L.

Evidence-based approaches

Rationale

The main criterion for monitoring serum drug concentration is to ensure that there is enough drug given for efficacy whilst avoiding concentrations associated with a significant risk of toxicity (Catchpole and Hastings 1995).

Indications

Accurate and timely monitoring of microbial assay levels is indicated in patients receiving intravenous aminoglycoside or glycopeptide antibiotics:

■ to ensure optimum therapeutic range
■ to minimize high serum levels which may cause adverse side-effects of the drugs (particular caution should be exercised in patients who have renal impairment).

Contraindications

The samples should not be taken if there has been insufficient time lapse between dose administration and sample collection.

Principles of care

The initial dosage regimen should be appropriate for the clinical condition being treated, the patient's clinical characteristics (age, weight, renal function and so on) and concomitant drug therapy (Thomson 2004). The timing of the sample and interpretation of the results of analysis need consideration in relation to the dose given and the timing of previous dose administration.

Serum samples can be taken at two different times: the peak or the trough. A peak sample is collected at the drug's highest therapeutic concentration within the dosing period. The postdose peak level timing will vary depending on the drug; ordinarily this is 1 hour after the completion of an infusion, although in the case of vancomycin, which has a slow distribution phase, it is recommended that the sample is taken at least 1–2 hours after the infusion ends (Tobin *et al.* 2002).

Trough levels are measured just prior to the administration of the next dose, that is, at the lowest concentration in the dosing period (Tobin *et al.* 2002). Therefore, trough levels are more commonly used because the level is more representative of how the different variables such as drug absorption and renal function affect the concentration within a predetermined timeframe. The results can then be used to adjust dosages to achieve the optimal response with the minimal toxicity.

Abnormally elevated serum levels may be obtained if the samples are taken from a CVAD through which the drug has been administered. This is more likely when residual drugs remain in the catheter if it has not been flushed correctly following administration of the drug or the first 5–10 mL of blood has not been discarded (Himberger and Himberger 2001). If a multilumen CVAD is *in situ*, a different lumen from the one used to administer the drug should be used to obtain the blood specimen.

Procedure guideline 11.8 Blood sampling: antimicrobial drug assay

Essential equipment

■ Appropriate blood sample bottles
■ Vacuum-assisted collection system
■ Gloves
■ Apron
■ Appropriate documentation/forms

Preprocedure

Action	Rationale
1 Discuss indication for procedure with patient.	To ensure the patient understands the procedure and gives valid consent (NMC 2008b, C).
2 Wash hands with bactericidal soap and water, or decontaminate physically clean hands with alcohol-based handrub. Apply gloves.	To reduce the risk of cross-infection and specimen contamination (Fraise and Bradley 2009, E).

Procedure

3 For trough levels: Following venepuncture, withdraw the volume of blood appropriate to the blood sample bottle using the vacuum-assisted collection system.	To ensure the correct volume of blood is obtained and to reduce the safety risk to practitioner (DH 2006, C; DH 2010, C).
4 Clearly label blood sample bottle and appropriate form with 'pre-drug administration blood'.	To ensure there is no confusion between the pre-drug and post-drug serum level specimens. E

(Continued)

Procedure guideline 11.8 (Continued)

5 Administer intravenous antibiotics as prescribed via the patient's established vascular access device.	To continue with patient's prescribed drug regimen. E
6 If peak level required: Within an allotted time after administration, repeat step 3. Clearly label blood sample bottle and appropriate form with 'post-drug administration blood'.	To allow time for even distribution of the drug through the blood for peak blood levels to be achieved (Jones 2006, E).
7 If CVAD used: The device must be flushed thoroughly before taking the blood sample. Take and discard 3 mL of blood, then attach vacuum-assisted collection system to take drug level sample. Indicate on blood sample bottle and appropriate form that sample is from a CVAD.	To reduce contamination by previously administered therapeutic agents and to allow appropriate interpretation of the results. E

Postprocedure

8 Ensure microbiology request forms are completed correctly including date, exact time and dosage of previously administered dose.	To maintain accurate records and provide accurate information for laboratory analysis (NMC 2009, C; Weston 2008, E).
9 Arrange prompt delivery to the microbiology laboratory.	To allow for prompt analysis and timely adjustments to patient's drug therapy regime if indicated. E

652

Postprocedural considerations

Ongoing care

Changes in dosage regimens will depend upon interpretation of the results by the microbiology, medical and nursing team. Notably high serum drug levels should prompt the microbiology team to telephone a result through to the medical team in charge of the patient's care, especially if this warrants withholding subsequent doses of the drug. A low drug serum level would instigate an increase in the dosage of the drug. Any changes to the drug regime should be communicated and clearly documented on the patient's prescription chart.

Documentation

In accordance with the principles of good record keeping, the date and time of when a trough and/or peak drug assay level is sent to the laboratory should be documented clearly and promptly in the patient's notes, care plan and/or on the patient's drug chart (or antimicrobial flow charts as provided by the pharmacy department) (NMC 2009). This assists in communication and the dissemination of information between members of the interprofessional healthcare team.

Cerebrospinal fluid (CSF) obtained by lumbar puncture

Definition

Lumbar puncture is a medical procedure involving the withdrawal of CSF via a hollow spinal needle inserted into the lumbar subarachnoid space, a technique first described by Quincke (1891). It may be used for either therapeutic or diagnostic purposes (Barker and Chao 2002).

Anatomy and physiology

The spinal cord lies within the spinal column, beginning at the foramen magnum and terminating at a variable level around the first lumbar vertebra although it may be as high as the 12th thoracic vertebra or, rarely, as low as the disc between the second and third lumbar vertebrae (Gruener and Biller 2008) (Figure 11.8). Like the brain, the spinal cord is enclosed and protected by the meninges, that is, the dura mater, arachnoid mater and pia mater (Barker 2002). The dura and arachnoid mater are separated by a potential space known as the subdural space. The arachnoid and pia mater are separated by the subarachnoid space containing

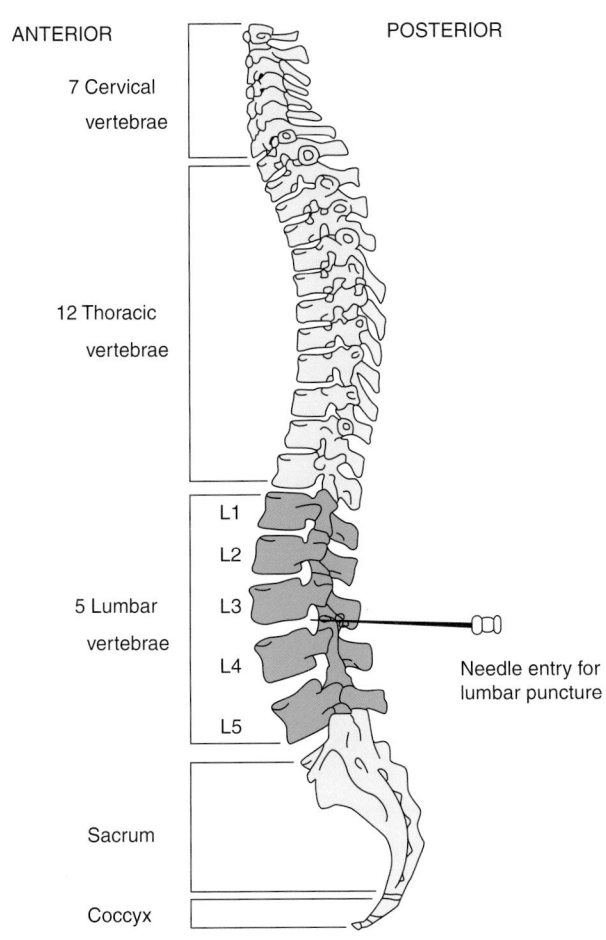

ANTERIOR   POSTERIOR

7 Cervical
vertebrae

12 Thoracic
vertebrae

5 Lumbar   L1
vertebrae   L2
                L3
                L4
                L5

Needle entry for
lumbar puncture

Sacrum

Coccyx

Figure 11.8   Lateral view of spinal column and vertebrae, showing needle entry site for lumbar puncture.

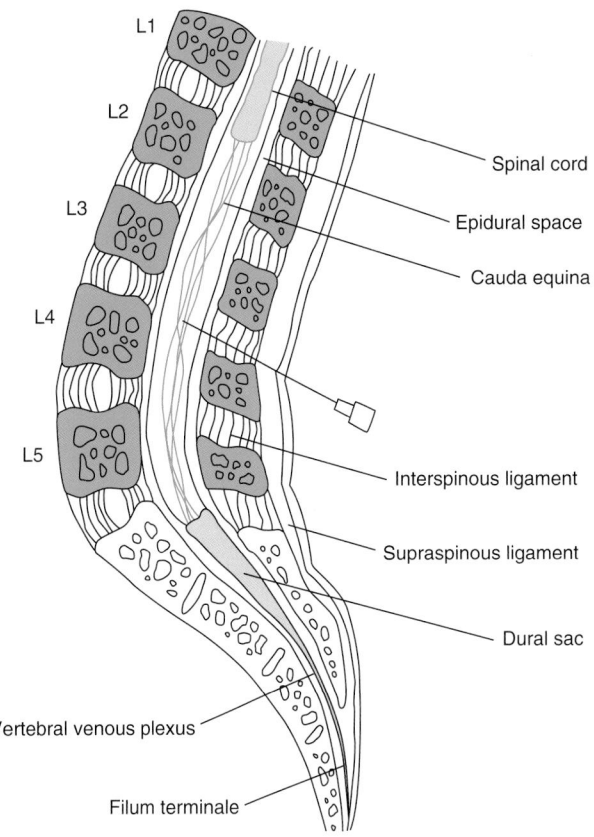

Spinal cord

Epidural space

Cauda equina

Interspinous ligament

Supraspinous ligament

Dural sac

Vertebral venous plexus

Filum terminale

Figure 11.9   Lumbar puncture. Sagittal section through lumbosacral spine. The most common site for lumbar puncture is between L3 and L4 and between L4 and L5 as the spinal cord terminates at L1.

the CSF (Allan 2002). Below the termination of the spinal cord, the subarachnoid space contains CSF, the filum terminale and the cauda equina (the anterior and posterior roots of the lumbar and sacral nerves) (Gruener and Biller 2008). So as to avoid damage to the spinal cord, it is imperative that lumbar puncture is performed at the lowest palpable intervertebral space (Figure 11.9). The higher the space, the greater the risk of spinal cord injury.

The spinal needle will have to pass through the following structures: skin, subcutaneous tissue, supraspinal ligament, interspinous ligament, ligamentum flavum, epidural space, dura mater and arachnoid mater.

Cerebrospinal fluid is formed primarily by filtration and secretion from networks of capillaries, called choroid plexuses, located in the ventricles of the brain. Eventually, absorption takes place through the arachnoid villi, which are finger-like projections of the arachnoid mater that push into the dural venous sinuses. CSF is clear, colourless and slightly alkaline, with a specific gravity of 1.007

(Hickey 2003). In an adult, approximately 500 mL of CSF are produced and reabsorbed each day (Weldon 1998), with 120–150 mL present at one time. CSF constituents include:

■ water
■ mineral salts
■ glucose
■ protein (16–45 mg/dL)
■ urea and creatinine (Hickey 2003).

The functions of CSF include:

■ to act as a shock absorber
■ to carry nutrients to the brain
■ to remove metabolites from the brain
■ to support and protect the brain and spinal cord
■ to keep the brain and spinal cord moist (Hickey 2003).

Related theory
Abnormalities of CSF

A red discoloration of the CSF is indicative of the presence of blood, which is an abnormal finding. If the presence of blood is caused by a traumatic spinal tap, the blood will usually clot and the fluid clears as the procedure continues. If the presence of blood is due to subarachnoid haemorrhage, no clotting will occur (Lindsay and Bone 2004).

Turbid or cloudy CSF is indicative of the presence of a large number of white cells or protein and is an abnormal finding. The causes of such turbidity include infection or the secondary infiltration of the meninges with malignant disease, for example leukaemia or lymphoma (Hoffbrand *et al.* 2006).

The presence of different types of blood cells in the CSF can be diagnostic of a variety of neurological disorders.

- Erythrocytes are indicative of haemorrhage.
- Polymorphonuclear leucocytes are indicative of meningitis or cerebral abcess.
- Monocytes are indicative of a viral or tubercular meningitis or encephalitis.
- Lymphocytes present in larger numbers are indicative of viral meningitis or infiltration of the meninges by malignant disease.
- The presence of leukaemic blast cells is indicative of infiltration of the meninges by leukaemia.
- Viral, bacterial or fungal cultures from the CSF sample are indicative of infection. (Allan 2002, Barker and Chao 2002, Hickey 2003).

Normal CSF pressure falls within a range of 100–150 mmH$_2$O (Lindsay and Bone 2004). Spinal pressure may be raised in the presence of cerebrovascular accident, a space-occupying lesion or bacterial meningitis (Barker and Chao 2002).

Evidence-based approaches
Rationale

A number of tests can be performed on CSF to aid diagnosis (Lindsay and Bone 2004).

- *Culture and sensitivity*. Identifying the presence of microorganisms would confirm the diagnosis of bacterial/fungal meningitis or a cerebral abscess. The isolation of the causative organism would enable the initiation of appropriate antibiotic or antifungal therapy.
- *Virology screening*. Isolation of a causative virus would enable appropriate therapy to be initiated promptly.
- *Serology for syphilis*. Tests include the Wassermann reaction (WR), Venereal Disease Research Laboratory (VDRL) and *Treponema pallidum* immobilization (TPI) tests.
- *Protein*. The total amount of protein in CSF should be 15.45 mg/dL (154.5 µg/mL). Proteins are large molecules which do not readily cross the blood–brain barrier.

There is normally more albumin (80%) than globulin in CSF as albumins are smaller molecules (Fischbach and Dunning 2004). Raised globulin levels are indicative of multiple sclerosis, neurosyphilis, degenerative cord or brain disease. However, raised levels of total protein can be indicative of meningitis, encephalitis, myelitis or the presence of a tumour (Hickey 2003).

- *Cytology*. Central nervous system tumours or secondary meningeal disease tend to shed cells into the CSF, where they float freely. Examination of these cells morphologically after lumbar puncture will determine whether the tumour is malignant or benign (Fischbach and Dunning 2004).

Indications

A lumbar puncture and withdrawal of CSF, with or without the introduction of therapeutic agents, is performed for the following purposes.

- *Diagnosis*: CSF is normally a crystal clear, colourless and sterile liquid which resembles water. Analysis of the CSF for cells not normally present may be made to determine the presence of a pathological process (Price and Madhusudan 2002). In addition, CSF pressure can be measured (Barker and Chao 2002).
- *Introduction of therapeutic agents*: a number of drugs do not cross the blood–brain barrier so in the treatment and prophylaxis of some malignant diseases such as leukaemia and lymphoma, cytotoxic drugs, namely cytarabine, methotrexate and, rarely, thiopeta, may be administered intrathecally (Coward and Cooley 2006, Hoffbrand *et al.* 2006, Scurr *et al.* 2005). Hydrocortisone may also be administered intrathecally.
- *Introduction of spinal anaesthesia for surgery*: spinal anaesthesia, first performed in 1899 by Corning, involves the injection of a local anaesthetic agent such as bupivacaine into the CSF thus producing anaesthesia suitable for operations on the lower body (Yentis *et al.* 2009).
- *Introduction of radiopaque contrast medium*: used to provide radiopaque pictures (myelograms) of the spinal cord (Blows 2002). Myelograms are useful in diagnosing spinal lesions and in helping to plan surgery by isolating the level of the lesion.

Contraindications

The procedure should not be undertaken in the following circumstances.

- In patients in whom raised intracranial pressure (ICP) is suspected or present due to the risk of 'brain herniation' (Belford 2005, Lindsay and Bone 2004).
- In patients with papilloedema, bacterial meningitis or deteriorating neurological symptoms, in whom raised ICP or an intracranial mass is suspected. In this situation, neuroimaging (computed tomography (CT) or magnetic resonance imaging (MRI) scan) should be undertaken prior

to lumbar puncture in order to avoid resultant potentially fatal brainstem compression, herniation or coning (Belford 2005). However, a normal CT scan does not always ensure that it is safe to perform a lumbar puncture so until better non-invasive procedures to monitor ICP become available and are routinely used, the decision to proceed must be left to clinical expertise and judgement (Hickey 2003).

■ Local skin infection may result in meningitis by passage of the bacteria from the skin to the CSF during the procedure (Hickey 2003). Cutaneous or osseous infection at the site of the lumbar puncture may be considered an absolute contraindication (Hickey 2003).

■ In patients who are unable to co-operate or who are too drowsy to give a history. Patient co-operation is essential to carry out a baseline neurological examination and to minimize the potential risk of trauma associated with this procedure (Barker and Chao 2002).

■ In patients who have severe degenerative spinal joint disease. In such cases difficulty will be experienced both in positioning the patient and in accessing between the vertebrae (Hickey 2003).

■ In those patients undergoing anticoagulant therapy or who have coagulopathies or thrombocytopenia (less than 50×10^9/L). These patients are at increased risk of bleeding and therefore coagulopathies and thrombocytopenia must be corrected prior to undertaking lumbar puncture (Lindsay and Bone 2004).

Principles of care

The principles of lumbar puncture are to gain access to the CSF of the patient whilst maintaining sterility and patient comfort throughout the procedure. For patients receiving intrathecal medication, it is essential that the correct agent is given. For diagnostic procedures, it is imperative that accurate measurements are taken and that the sample is handled and labelled correctly. The role of the nurse in caring for a patient undergoing a lumbar puncture procedure may include helping to explain the procedure to the patient, preparing the patient, supporting both patient and physician during the procedure and close follow-up monitoring (Barker and Chao 2002).

Method of lumbar puncture

The patient is positioned either sitting or lying with flexion of the lumbar spine. After cleaning the lumbar area with antiseptic solution, local anaesthetic (usually lidocaine) is infiltrated into the skin at the lowest palpable interspace. The spinal needle is introduced carefully and advanced slowly until there is a perceptible click as the needle tip passes through the dura mater. The stylet of the spinal needle is removed to observe for the free flow of CSF. If a cutting (Quincke type) needle is used, then the cutting edge of the needle should be aligned parallel to the direction of the dural fibres which run vertically. No such precaution is

necessary when using pencil-point (blunt-ended) needles. If opening pressure is to be measured, the patient must be in the lateral position and the manometer should be immediately connected to the hub of the spinal needle. The amount of CSF withdrawn for sampling depends on the investigation required. In practice, approximately 5–10 mL of CSF is usually withdrawn, although investigations for cell count and Gram stain can be performed using 1 mL (Barker and Chao 2002).

Legal and professional issues
Competencies

If a lumbar puncture is being undertaken to administer medication, for example for intrathecal chemotherapy administatration, the practitioner performing the procedure must comply with the national guidance (DH 2008). See Chapter 15.

Preprocedural considerations
Equipment

Enhancements to the design of lumbar puncture needles can confer benefits to the patient in terms of reducing complications and also contribute to reducing drug errors. The newer 'non-cutting' needles such as the Sprotte and Whitacre types cause fewer postdural puncture headaches (PDPH) than the older 'cutting' needles such as the Quincke type (Lavi *et al.* 2006). This is because the vertically aligned dural fibres are split and parted instead of being cut, thus allowing some degree of dural self-sealing. In the same manner, thinner gauge needles create less of a CSF leak and further reduce the occurrence of PDPH (Lambert *et al.* 1997). Needle design is also under review due to a recent NPSA alert regarding the reduction of wrong-drug or wrong-route errors. From 1st April 2011 all needles, syringes and connectors utilized in intrathecal (spinal) boluses or lumbar puncture samples will not be able to connect to any other intravenous device. This will also extend to any epidural, spinal and regional anaesthesia boluses or infusions by 1st April 2013 (NPSA 2009).

Assessment and recording tools

Depending on the patient condition and the reason for the lumbar puncture, various observations and recording tools should be used. As a baseline, the patient's vital signs must be recorded before and after the procedure and documented on an observation chart. If the patient is being investigated for a neurological problem, then the inclusion of preprocedural Glasgow Coma Scale (GCS) assessment is advised. In all cases, neurological observations, including GCS and pupillary response, should be recorded on a specialized neurological observation chart following the procedure. The patient should be monitored for headache and backache and the puncture site should be inspected, particularly if there have been fluctuations in the neurological observations (Hickey 2003).

655

Specific patient preparation

Preparation includes advising the patient to empty their bowels and bladder to ensure comfort during the correct flexed (knee–chest) position that the patient must assume during the procedure. This position is required to increase the space between adjacent vertebral spines to allow for the passage of the needle (Lindsay and Bone 2004).

Skin disinfection is of extreme importance to prevent serious spinal infection. Alcoholic chlorhexidine (0.5%) is the most effective solution in this regard, but must be allowed to air dry completely to prevent the neurotoxic chlorhexidine from coming into contact with neural tissue (Hebl 2006). The potential for neurotoxicity is the reason why preparations of 2% chlorhexidine should be avoided.

Procedure guideline 11.9 Lumbar puncture

Essential equipment

- Antiseptic skin-cleaning agents, for example chlorhexidine in 70% alcohol or isopropyl alcohol
- Selection of needles and syringes
- Sterile gloves
- Sterile dressing pack
- Lumbar puncture needles of assorted sizes
- Disposable manometer

- Three sterile specimen bottles. These should be labelled 1, 2 and 3. The first specimen, which may be bloodstained due to needle trauma, should go into bottle 1. This will assist the laboratory to differentiate between blood due to procedure trauma and that due to subarachnoid haemorrhage
- Plaster dressing

Medicinal products

- Local anaesthetic, for example lidocaine 1%

Preprocedure

Action	Rationale
1 Explain and discuss the procedure with the patient.	To ensure that the patient understands the procedure and gives valid consent (Barker and Chao 2002, E; NMC 2008b, C).
2 Patient should empty their bladder and bowels before procedure.	To ensure comfort (Barker and Chao 2002, Hickey 2003, E).
3 Assist patient into required position on a firm surface. **Either:** *Lying* (see Action Figure 3): ■ One pillow under the patient's head. ■ On side with knees drawn up to the abdomen and clasped by the hands. ■ Support patient to maintain this position. **Or:** *Sitting*: ■ Patient straddles a straight-backed chair so that their back is facing the doctor. ■ Patient folds arms on the back of the chair and rests head on them.	To ensure maximum widening of the intervertebral spaces and thus easier access to the subarachnoid space (Lindsay and Bone 2004, E). To avoid sudden movement by the patient which would produce trauma (Barker and Chao 2002, E). This position may be used for those patients unable to maintain the lying position. It allows more accurate identification of the spinous processes and thus the intervertebral spaces (Barker and Chao 2002, Hickey 2003, E).
4 Continue to support, explain care and observe the patient throughout the procedure.	To facilitate psychological and physical well-being (Barker and Chao 2002, E).

Procedure

5 Wash hands with antibacterial detergent. Put on gloves and apron.	To reduce the risk of contamination and crossinfection (Fraise and Bradley 2009 E; RCN 2005, C).

Assist doctor as required; doctor will proceed to:

6 Clean the skin with the antiseptic cleaning agent.	To ensure the removal of skin flora to minimize the risk of infection (Lindsay and Bone 2004, E).

7 Identify the area to be punctured and infiltrate the skin and subcutaneous layers with local anaesthetic.	To minimize discomfort from the procedure (Barker and Chao 2002, E).
8 Introduce a spinal puncture needle below the second lumbar vertebra and into the subarachnoid space.	This is below the level of the spinal cord but still within the subarachoid space (Lindsay and Bone 2004, E).
9 Ensure that the subarachnoid space has been entered and attach the manometer to the spinal needle, if required.	To obtain a CSF pressure reading (normal pressure is 100–150 mmH$_2$O) (Hickey 2003, E; Lindsay and Bone 2004, E).
10 Obtain the appropriate specimens of CSF (approx. 10 mL) for analysis. Cell count and Gram stain can be performed using 1 mL of fluid.	To establish diagnosis (Hickey, 2003, E).
11 Ensure the specimens are labelled appropriately and sent with the correct forms to the laboratory.	To maintain accurate records and provide accurate information for laboratory analysis (NMC 2009, C; Weston 2008, E).
12 If intrathecal medication is to be instilled, drug and dose must be checked and administered safely according to national guidelines.	To ensure the correct drug and dosage of drug are safely administered (Coward and Cooley 2006, E; DH 2003, C).
13 Withdraw the spinal needle once specimens have been obtained, appropriate pressure measurements taken and intrathecal medication administered.	To minimize the risks of the procedure (Barker and Chao 2002, E).
14 When the needle is withdrawn, apply pressure over the lumbar puncture site using a sterile topical swab.	To maintain asepsis and to stop blood and CSF flow (Hickey 2003, E).
15 When all leakage from the puncture site has ceased, apply a plaster dressing.	To prevent secondary infection (Allan 2002, E; Barker and Chao 2002, E).

Postprocedure

16 Make the patient comfortable. They should lie flat or the head should be tilted slightly downwards. Time to lie flat varies from hospital to hospital, but it is usually around 4 hours if there is no headache.	To avoid headache and decrease the possibility of brainstem herniation (coning) due to a reduction in CSF pressure (Barker and Chao 2002, E; Hickey 2003, E).
17 Remove equipment and dispose of as appropriate.	To prevent the spread of infection and reduce risk of needlestick injury (Allan 2002, E).
18 Record the procedure in the appropriate documents.	To promote continuity of care and provide an accurate record for future reference (Allan 2002, E; NMC 2009, C).
19 Patient should be monitored for the next 24 hours with careful observation of the following:	
■ Leakage from the puncture site	Clear fluid may be a cerebrospinal leak (Barker and Chao 2002, E).
■ Headache	Not unusual following lumbar puncture and may be due to loss of CSF.
■ Backache	As above.
■ Neurological observations/vital signs.	These may indicate signs of change in ICP (Hickey 2003, E). For further information on neurological observations and vital signs, see Chapter 13.
20 Encourage a fluid intake of 2–3 litres in 24 hours.	To replace lost fluid. Patient may have difficulty micturating due to procedure and supine position (Allan 2002, E; Hickey 2003, E).

(Continued)

Iliac crest

Midline

Action Figure 3 Position for lumbar puncture. Head is flexed onto chest and knees are drawn up.

Problem-solving table 11.3 Prevention and resolution (Procedure guideline 11.9)

Problem	Cause	Prevention	Suggested action
Pain down one leg during the procedure	A dorsal nerve root may have been touched by the spinal needle	Make sure the spinal needle is in the midline Advance the needle slowly and stop as soon as CSF is obtained	Inform doctor, who will probably move the needle Reassure patient
Fluctuation of neurological observations: level of consciousness, pulse, respirations, blood pressure or pupillary reaction	Herniation (coning) of the brainstem due to the decrease of ICP. Raised ICP is a contraindication to lumbar puncture	Check that relevant neuroimaging has been reviewed prior to procedure	Observe patient constantly for signs of alteration in ICP. The frequency may be decreased as patient's condition allows. Report any fluctuations in these observations to a doctor immediately (Barker and Chao 2002)

Postprocedural considerations

Immediate care

Patients will usually be nursed flat for a period of up to 4 hours in order to reduce the risk of postspinal headache. There is no evidence that longer periods are useful (Ebinger *et al.* 2004). Follow-up care will include neurological observations, monitoring for issues such as difficulties with voiding, raised temperatures, headaches and discomfort. Analgesia and reassurance may be required (Allan 2002).

Ongoing care

If the procedure has been performed in an outpatient setting, the patient may be discharged home after 1–2 hours but with clear instructions to lie flat in transport and at home, and to report any of the following: leakage from the site, headaches, backaches and neurological symptoms. Backache with leg weakness and bladder disturbance may be caused by a spinal haematoma (cauda equina syndrome) and is usually a surgical emergency (Kennedy *et al.* 2000).

Documentation

The procedure should be documented in the notes along with the record of informed consent. Any problems or immediate complications should be noted along with any treatment required. The sample bottles must be labelled correctly and sent to the laboratory.

Education of patient and relevant others

Patients should be informed about relevant signs of complications and be given verbal and written information prior to discharge. Clear instructions should be given about side-effects and information as to whom to call if side-effects occur.

Complications

Infection

Infection may be inadvertently introduced during the procedure. There is a greater risk in the presence of neutropenia (Hart 2006). Infection may be superficial or deep and may be caused by either skin commensals surviving on the patient or respiratory flora from the person performing the lumbar puncture. Deep infection includes the serious complications of meningitis and spinal abscess and will need urgent intravenous antibiotics after discussion with a microbiologist. Spinal abscess causing nerve root compression may also need urgent neurosurgical decompression. Adequate disinfection of the skin and the use of surgical facemasks will reduce the risk to the patient.

Haemorrhage

Haemorrhage/localized bruising may be caused by a traumatic procedure or in the presence of thrombocytopenia or a coagulopathy (Barker and Chao 2002, Lindsay and Bone 2004). Haematoma formation may also become a surgical emergency if there is nerve root compression.

Herniation

Transtentorial or tonsillar herniation is possible if lumbar puncture is carried out in the presence of raised ICP (Belford 2005). This is a serious and life-threatening complication and so brain imaging studies should be done if raised ICP is suspected. Consultation with a neurologist may also be warranted.

Headache

Frequency of postlumbar puncture headache varies amongst studies and between diagnostic and therapeutic procedures. The following risk factors have been identified: young age, female gender and the presence of headache before or at the time of the lumbar puncture (Evans *et al.* 2000). Less certain risk factors include low Body Mass Index and previous experience of postlumbar puncture headache (Evans *et al.* 2000). Research also suggests that the size of the needle used for the lumbar puncture may contribute to headache and to minimize the risk, a 25 gauge blunt-ended needle is recommended (Connolly 1999, Lambert *et al.* 1997). It is usually relieved by lying flat and, if ordered by the doctor, a mild analgesic (Hickey 2003). Rehydration, pain relief and antiemetic medications can help in milder cases (Ahmed *et al.* 2006) If severe or prolonged, the headache may be treated with an epidural blood patch, usually after referral to an anaesthetist (Gruener and Biller 2008).

Backache

Backache after lumbar puncture may be either due to local bruising from the lumbar puncture needle or from excessive spinal flexion for prolonged periods of time (i.e. during difficult procedures). It does not seem to be affected by different needle sizes nor by repeated attempts to gain CSF (Pan *et al.* 2004). In rare cases, backache may be suggestive of spinal haematoma or abscess, particularly if associated with leg weakness or bladder/bowel disturbance.

Leakage from puncture site

There may be a small amount of bloodstained oozing (Hickey 2003). The presence of clear fluid should be reported immediately to the doctor, especially if accompanied by fluctuation of other symptoms (level of consciousness, motor changes, problems voiding), as it may be a cerebrospinal leak (Barker and Chao 2002).

Arachnoiditis

The combination of intrathecal methotrexate with radiotherapy may cause arachnoiditis (irritation of the meninges), cerebral atrophy and necrotizing encephalopathy (Vasey and Evans 2002). Arachnoiditis has also been reported when administering intrathecal methylprednisolone (Latham *et al.* 1997).

659

Semen collection

Definition

Semen collection may be required for diagnostic and/or therapeutic purposes (Gerris 1999). Common reasons for semen collection include specimen samples to assist in diagnosis of fertility problems and/or conditions and for cryopreservation of semen prior to treatments that may affect fertility, such as the treatment of cancer (NCCWCH and NICE 2004, RCP *et al.* 2007).

Anatomy and physiology

Semen is a mixture of sperm and accessory gland secretions which is the liquid transport medium and nutrient solution that protects and activates sperm. Sperm is a vital component in conception (Marieb and Hoehn 2010).

Components of normal semen

Semen analysis should be compared with the WHO's references as follows.

- Volume: 2.0 mL or more
- Liquefaction time: within 60 minutes

- pH: 7.2 or more
- Sperm concentration: 20 million spermatozoa per mL or more
- Total sperm number: 40 million spermatozoa per ejaculate or more
- Motility: 50% or more motile (grades a* or b**) or 25% or more with progressive motility (grade a) within 60 minutes of ejaculation
- Vitality: 75% or more alive
- White blood cells: fewer than 1 million per mL
- Morphology: 15% or 30%***

*Grade a: Rapid progressive motility (sperm moving swiftly usually in a straight line).
**Grade b: Slow or sluggish progressive motility (may be less linear in progression).
***Currently being reassessed by the WHO.

Related theory

Semen collection is undertaken for various reasons such as fertility treatment and cryopreservation. Azoospermia is the absence of sperm in ejaculated semen. It is the most severe form of male factor infertility with an incidence of approximately 5% of infertile couples. It can arise as a result of an obstructive or mechanical problem or an unobstructive form such as a reduction in sperm production (van Peperstraten *et al.* 2006). In order to identify the quality of semen, a seminal analysis can determine fertility by assessing concentration, motility and the percentage of normal forms (RCP *et al.* 2007). This is compared to the WHO's definition.

Treatment for such conditions may require intracytoplasmic sperm injection (ICSI) or in vitro fertilization (IVF). ICSI is where semen is collected during a surgical procedure. Surgical semen collection may be conducted utilizing different techniques to treat conditions such as severe deficits in semen quality, obstructive azoospermia and unobstructive azoospermia (NCCWCH and NICE 2004). The semen may be retrieved from either the epididymis or the testis dependent on the type of azoospermia (van Peperstraten *et al.* 2006).

Where azoospermia is indicated in the male, couples where the woman is aged between 23 and 39 years at the time of treatment and have been infertile for 3 years should be offered IVF (NCCWCH and NICE 2004). IVF is the process in wich fertilization of an egg or ovum occurs outside the body (NCCWCH and NICE 2004).

Evidence-based approaches

Rationale

This may include collection for assisted reproduction such as intrauterine insemination (IUI) (Boomsma *et al.* 2007), IVF or cryopreservation prior to cancer treatments (NCCWCH and NICE 2004).

Males with mild forms of fertility problems should be offered six cycles of IUI as this increases the chances of successful pregnancy (NCCWCH and NICE 2004).

In order to manage fertility problems after being treated with chemotherapy and/or radiotherapy, cryopreservation of semen may be required (RCP *et al.* 2007). Semen cryopreservation should be offered to men and boys who are preparing for treatments that are likely to make them infertile (NCCWCH and NICE 2004).

Indications

- Fertility treatments.
- Cryopreservation.

Principles of care

Couples who have been having difficulty conceiving should be seen together as decisions made in relation to investigations and treatment may affect both partners. Access to evidence-based information should be made available to ensure informed decisions are made. Information can be given verbally and supplemented with written and/or audio-visual information (NCCWCH and NICE 2004).

Methods of semen collection

Semen collection may be obtained by various methods such as the standard method of masturbation (Gerris 1999) or surgical sperm recovery for ISCI. This section will discuss the standard method of masturbation.

Anticipated patient outcomes

It would be expected that a diagnosis and/or analysis of results in relation to fertility treatments would be available to patients after semen collection had taken place. Cryopreserved semen will give the patient the opportunity to conceive after treatment for fertility-damaging treatment such as chemotherapy and/or radiotherapy.

Legal and professional issues

The collection and storage of semen must be within the domains of the Human Fertilization and Embryology Act (1990).

Consent

During the collection of semen samples it is essential that practitioners gain consent before beginning any treatment or care (NMC 2008b). Consent is continuous throughout any patient episode and the practitioner must ensure that the patient is kept informed at every stage (Marsden 2007). For semen collection this includes:

- informing the patient of the rationale for specimen collection
- what the procedure will involve
- ascertaining their level of understanding (especially if they need to be directly involved in the sampling technique)

- how long the results may take to be processed
- how the results will be made available
- information on how this may affect their care.

Preprocedural considerations

Equipment

A sterile specimen container from the laboratory is required. Container lids must not be waxed cardboard or have plastic or rubber liners to maintain the quality of the sample. Contraceptive condoms are not suitable as the lubricants are spermicidal. Men who are unable to provide a sample on religious or moral grounds may use silastic condoms such as the seminal collection device (Brinsden 2005).

Recording tools

Labelling specimens

Prompt specimen analysis is only possible if specimens and their accompanying request forms are sent with specific, accurate and complete patient information. Incorrectly or unlabelled specimens will be discarded (HSE 2003). The form should include as much information as possible as this allows the laboratory to select the most appropriate media inoculation for examination and result interpretation (Weston 2008). General labelling should be

conducted accurately as discussed at the beginning of the chapter.

Specific patient preparations

It takes between 3 and 4 days for the sperm count to return to normal after ejaculation (Brinsden 2005, NCCWCH and NICE 2004) so patients should be advised that sexual intercourse should not have taken place for 3–4 days prior to semen collection. This will ensure that the semen will have an optimum count and motility (NCCWCH and NICE 2004).

Education

Patients who are to be treated with ICSI should undergo appropriate investigations to determine the diagnosis and enable informed discussion prior to the procedure. This will prepare the patient/couple for the potential implications of treatment. Genetic counselling and testing should be offered to men who have a specific or suspected genetic defect in relation to their infertility (NCCWCH and NICE 2004).

Patients who are undergoing treatments that may lead to infertility should be offered independent counselling to prepare them to cope with the possible physical and psychological implications of the treatment and its side-effects prior to commencing treatment (NCCWCH and NICE 2004, Wo and Viswanathan 2009).

661

Procedure guideline 11.10 Semen collection

Essential equipment

- Private room
- Sterile specimen collection container supplied by laboratory
- Tissues

Preprocedure

Action	Rationale
1 Explain and discuss the procedure with the patient giving clear, comprehensive instructions explaining what should and should not be done. Ask when he last had sexual intercourse.	To ensure the patient understands the procedure and gives valid consent (Brinsden 2005, C; NMC 2008b, C). To ensure the sperm count will be at maximum levels (Brinsden 2005, C).
2 Ensure the patient has a private room.	To ensure privacy for the patient. E

Procedure

3 Instruct the patient to only open the lid prior to ejaculation and replace it immediately after collection.	To minimize microbiological contamination (Brinsden 2005, C).
4 A fresh masturbated specimen must be collected in a sterile container.	To ensure optimum sample is obtained (Brinsden 2005, C).

Postprocedure

5 Complete specimen form and label specimen container (including relevant information such as date and time of collection).	To maintain accurate records and provide accurate information for laboratory analysis (NMC 2009, C; Weston 2008, E).

(Continued)

Procedure guideline 11.10 (*Continued*)

6 Specimens must be transported to the laboratory as quickly as possible, ideally within 1 hour of collection.	To ensure optimum sample is obtained (Brinsden 2005, C).
7 The specimen must be kept at between 25°C and 37°C in a laboratory incubator.	To ensure optimum sample is obtained (Brinsden 2005, C).

Postprocedural considerations

Immediate care

It is important that the patient has information to take away and has a contact number if further questions arise. The patient should be informed of when results are likely to be available and how they will be communicated (NCCWCH and NICE 2004).

Ongoing care

Patients who are undergoing treatments that may lead to infertility should be offered independent counselling to help them cope with the possible physical and psychological implications of the treatment and its side-effects (NCCWCH and NICE 2004).

Cervical uterine smear (pap smear)

Definition

The cervical smear is a test in which a specimen of cellular material is scraped from the cervix. The specimen is then stained and examined under a microscope by a cytologist to identify early cellular changes (Kumar and Clark 2009, Martin 2010).

Anatomy and physiology

The cervix is the narrow neck of the uterus and is located between the vagina and the uterus. It projects into the vagina and the cavity of the cervix is known as the cervical canal. The cervical canal's glands secrete a mucus that blocks the entry of sperm except in the midcycle when a reduction in viscosity allows sperm to pass (Marieb and Hoehn 2010) (Figure 11.10).

Related theory

The intention of a smear test is to collect squamous epithelial cells and some endocervical cells from the transformation zone and squamocolumnar junction of the cervix (see Figure 11.10). The sampling technique must take into consideration that the position of the squamocolumnar junction changes with age, contraception and parity (Higgins 2007, WHO 2006).

Evidence-based approaches

Rationale

The ideal time for obtaining a cervical smear is midcycle if the woman is premenopausal; this prevents contamination from menstrual flow and allows for accuracy of results (Higgins 2007, WHO 2006). It is not ideal to take a cervical smear if a woman is pregnant or immediately postpartum as results obtained can be misleading. Higgins (2007) suggests delaying the procedure for a few months following childbirth; however, the WHO suggests that if a woman is in the target age group and there are concerns about access to screening postpartum, then a cervical smear should be taken after consent is obtained (WHO 2006).

In the UK 80% of cervical smears are taken in the primary care setting and most are taken by practice nurses. Screening is recommended in the UK for all women between the ages of 25 and 65 years and is an investigation to confirm that the cervix is healthy and there are no abnormal changes to the cells; it is not a test for diagnosing cervical cancer (Higgins 2007, NHSCSP 2004).

Indications

- Women between the age of 25 and 64.

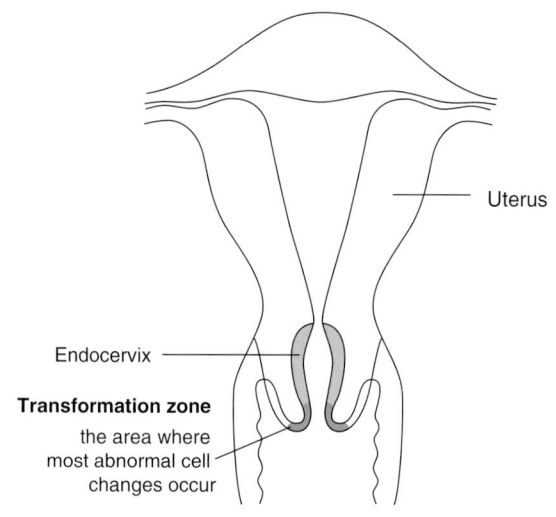

Figure 11.10 The cervix.

Contraindications

- During pregnancy.
- Immediately postpartum.

Method for cervical smears: liquid-based cytology

Liquid-based cytology (LBC) has been used in Europe and the USA since 1996. After extensive clinical trials in 2003 using LBC for cervical smears, the National Institute for Health and Clinical Excellence (NICE) recommended that LBC should replace the conventional cervical smear test by 2008 as part of the NHS cervical screening programmes. The change to LBC for smear taking has resulted in the reduction of reported 'inadequate smears', women's anxieties and the workload for primary care and laboratory personnel (Karnon *et al.* 2004, NHSCSP 2004).

Legal and professional issues

It is advised that the practitioner offers the patient the option of having a chaperone. The chaperone may be a person of the patient's choice who will accompany them throughout the procedure. The decision of the patient in regard to a chaperone should be documented (NMC 2006, RCN 2002). Healthcare professionals conducting cervical smears should also be familiar with national guidance (NHSCSP 2004).

Preprocedural considerations

Equipment

There are several devices which are used in sampling the uterine cervix (Figure 11.11).

- *Vaginal speculum*: this is an instrument used during gynaecological examination to facilitate the visualization of the vagina and cervix. The speculum is introduced via the vagina and its cylinder with a rounded end shape allows easy passage. Once *in situ*, the speculum is opened, holding the vagina open and allowing the health professional to have access to the cervix and perform the cervical smear. Most speculums are now made of plastic and are single use, replacing those formerly made of metal, requiring sterilization after use. There are two categories of speculum: virgin and non-virgin. The latter is available in four sizes: small, medium, large and long. Special attention should be given when selecting a speculum for use in women previously treated with pelvic radiotherapy or postmenopausal.
- *Wooden spatula (Aylesbury spatula)*: a wooden instrument used in smear screening to obtain a cervical sample, i.e. to take a representative cell sample from cervix. It comes in different widths and should be chosen depending upon the condition of the os (NHSCSP 2006). Wooden spatulas are very popular due to their easy and cost-effective use.

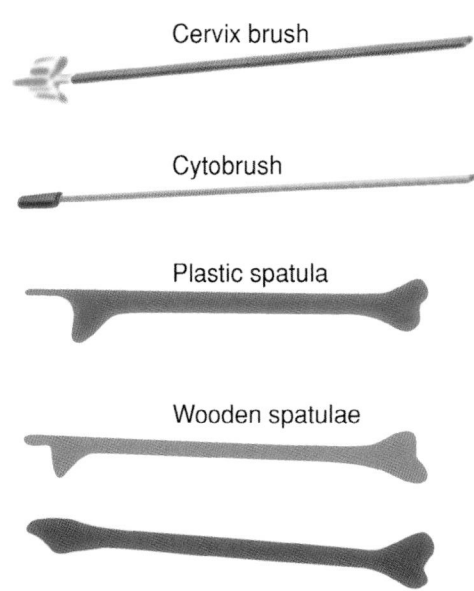

Cervix brush

Cytobrush

Plastic spatula

Wooden spatulae

Figure 11.11   Different types of sampling devices.

- *Cervical broom*: these are plastic broom-shaped tools with a pyramidal arrangement of flexible flat 'teeth'. The longer 'central' tuft fits into the cervical os and must be rotated clockwise through a full circle five times. When used to take a conventional smear, this brush is an adequate and effective sampling device.
- *Endocervical brush*: a plastic instrument used to sample the endocervical canal which should never be used alone (Herzog and Cohn 2001) but always in conjunction with the spatula. The endocervical brush should be used after the spatula and its use is restricted to:
  - where there is difficulty in inserting the spatula into the external os (if the os is narrow or stenosed)
  - when the woman is being followed up for previous borderline nuclear changes in endocervical cells
  - for follow-up in previously treated endocervical glandular abnormality.

The brush should be inserted into the cervical os with the lower bristles remaining visible, and rotated between half and a whole turn to reduce trauma (Insinga *et al.* 2004).

Cotton-tipped swabs are no longer recommended (NHSCSP 2006).

Cervical cytology on samples obtained using conventional smear-taking techniques is the current standard method of screening in the NHS Cervical Screening Programme (NHSCSP).

NICE (2003) has recommended that LBC is used as the primary means of processing samples in the cervical screening programme in England and Wales. It achieves 'cleaner' preparations, which are generally easier to read. Its advantage is a reduction in inadequate samples and there may be gains in reducing borderline results and increasing sensitivity (NHSCSP 2004).

Whichever device is used, once the sample is taken it is vital that the cells collected are transferred onto a glass slide and preserved immediately or placed into the correct vial containing liquid preservative and fixative. Slides must not be placed in a refrigerator (Higgins 2007, NHSCSP 2006).

The environment is also important, with the following equipment required:

- height-adjustable couch
- angle-positioned light source which is ideally free standing for manoeuvrability (NMC 2006).

Non-pharmacological support

The examination must be undertaken in a private room which cannot be entered during the examination. Adequate private changing facilities should also be available that are warm and comfortable. Where possible, face the examination couch away from the door to enhance privacy and dignity for the patient (RCN 2000).

Specific patient preparations

The patient should be given the opportunity to empty her bladder prior to the examination. Ask the patient to undress and explain the position required on the couch. The most common position is prone or alternatively left lateral as it is comfortable and aids in the visualization of the cervix. Once the patient is ready, she should inform the practitioner. A modesty towel or covering should be supplied to enable the patient to partially cover herself (RCN 2000).

Education

Explain the procedure to the patient prior to commencing. It is good practice to offer the patient a demonstration of the speculum and to explain what part will be inserted into the vagina. Any possible side-effects such as spotting post examination should also be discussed prior to commencing the examination (RCN 2000).

Procedure guideline 11.11 Cervical uterine smear using a wooden spatula

Essential equipment

- Alcoholic handrub
- Light source
- An examination couch
- Disposable clean paper couch covers
- Various sized specula (disposable or reusable)
- Disposable clean gloves
- Wooden spatula or sampling device
- A glass slide with frosted edge
- A pencil for labelling slide
- Fixative solution
- Plastic slide container
- Specimen form and plastic specimen bag
- A container of warm water
- Box of tissue paper
- Clinical waste container
- Trolley
- Disposable apron

Optional equipment

- A collecting container for Central Sterile Services (CSS) if reusable instruments are used

Preprocedure

Action	Rationale
1 Discuss benefits and limitations of screening and significance of smear results. Explain the purpose of the procedure and explain what will occur at each step. Document the woman's clinical and screening history, specifically: (a) Date of last menstruation (b) Any abnormal bleeding (c) Any unusual vaginal discharge (d) Contraception (e) Date of last cervical smear (f) Any abnormal smear results (g) Any treatment to the cervix.	To ensure that the woman understands that the procedure involves removing underwear and that the speculum will be inserted into her vagina, and consents to the procedure (NMC 2008b, C). Allows the woman time to ask any questions. E
2 Wash hands before and after the procedure. Place all the equipment required for the procedure on the trolley.	To minimize the risk of infection (Fraise and Bradley 2009, E). To facilitate the efficient taking of the smear. E
3 Close room door or curtains and ask the woman to remove her underwear.	To provide privacy and comfort for the woman. E

Procedure

4 Wash hands with antibacterial detergent and running hand-hot water. Ensure hands are dried with disposable paper hand towels and put on gloves and apron.	To reduce the risk of contamination and cross-infection (Fraise and Bradley 2009, E; RCN 2005, C).
5 Turn the light source on and position at end of examination table.	To provide illumination of the cervix and increase the accuracy of the smear taking (NHSCSP 2004, 2006, C).
6 Assist the woman into a supine position on the couch, with knees drawn up and legs parted. Keep her as covered as possible.	To facilitate easy access of the vaginal speculum and the taking of the cervical smear (NHSCSP 2004, 2006, C; WHO 2006, C).
7 Wash hands thoroughly or use an alcohol-based handrub.	To reduce the risk of contamination (Fraise and Bradley 2009, E).
8 Select the appropriate size speculum, from very small, small, medium, large including a long-bladed narrow speculum if the vagina is long or the cervix is lying posterior. The sterilized speculum can be warmed or cooled using clean tap water.	To promote patient comfort and reduce anxiety (NHSCSP 2006, C). If removed from a sterilizer, speculum may need to be cooled down, if cold then warmed up to reduce patient discomfort. It must be explained to patient that the speculum has been sterilized but the water will not contaminate it. E
9 Apply gloves. Part the labia and holding the speculum blades together sideways, slip the speculum into the vagina.	To insert the speculum and reduce patient discomfort (Fraise and Bradley 2009, E; WHO 2006, C).
10 When the speculum is halfway into the vagina, turn it so that the handle is facing down. If insertion is difficult apply a small amount of water-based lubricant to the sides of the speculum, avoiding the tip.	To promote patient comfort and reduce contamination of the cervix with lubricants (NHSCSP 2006, C).
11 Gently open the blades of the speculum and look for the cervix. It may be necessary to move the speculum up or down until the entire cervix is visible.	To reduce patient discomfort and visualize the cervix (WHO 2006, C).
12 Once the cervix is visible, tighten the screw or lock the speculum in the open position so it remains in place. Adjustment of the light source may be required. Reassure the woman and allow time for her to relax.	To keep the speculum in the correct position and visualize the cervix (WHO 2006, C). To reduce patient discomfort and anxiety. E
13 Take the spatula and insert the long tip into the cervical os; rotate it through 360°.	To ensure an adequate cell sampling is obtained from the transformation zone (Higgins 2007, C; WHO 2006, C).
14 Remove the spatula from the vaginal cavity then smear both sides of the spatula onto the glass slide using straight sweeps.	To ensure maximum collection of cells (WHO 2006, C).
15 Apply fixative immediately. **Either:** Spray fixative used at right angles to the slide and at a distance of 15–20 cm. **Or:** If immersing the slide in 95% ethanol, then leave for 5 minutes, remove from solution and allow to air dry. **Or:** If using 90% ethanol, then leave for 10–15 minutes, remove from solution and allow to air dry. **Or:** If using 'Cytofixx' (95% industrial methylated spirit), apply a few drops to the slide and allow to dry for 5 minutes.	To preserve the specimen and ensure accurate results (Higgins 2007, C; NHSCSP 2006, C; WHO 2006, C).

665

(Continued)

Procedure guideline 11.11 (*Continued*)

16 If there are clinical signs of possible infection then a high vaginal swab is recommended prior to removal of speculum. *(If active infection is present, the cervical smear should be delayed until infection has been treated and resolved.)*	To ensure the swab is taken from the best site (Higgins 2007, C). A charcoal-impregnated swab is recommended if *Trichomonas* species are suspected as these organisms survive longer in this medium (Higgins 2007, C; Mims 2004, R5).
17 Place the swab into the medium.	To ensure specimen is correctly placed in the culture medium to ensure accuracy of results. E
18 Gently pull the speculum out until the blades are clear of the cervix, then close blades and remove speculum, placing in clinical waste bin if disposable or into CSS container if reusable.	To prevent pinching the cervix or vaginal walls and to ensure safe disposal of contaminated equipment (Fraise and Bradley 2009, E; NHSCSP 2006, C; WHO 2006, C).
19 Cover the woman and offer tissue paper to wipe away any excess vaginal discharge.	To ensure dignity and privacy while promoting hygiene and comfort. E

Postprocedure

20 Dispose of the waste into clinical waste receiver.	Safe disposal of clinical waste (DH 2006, C).
21 Assist the woman off the examination table and allow her to dress.	To ensure safety and promote dignity and privacy. E
22 Using a pencil, label the frosted end of the slide with woman's name, clinic number, date of birth and date sample taken. Using a black ballpoint pen, label the vaginal swab.	To ensure patient details are documented correctly on specimen. *Note that ballpoint pens do not work on glass slides*. E
23 Place the slide into transport container.	To prevent the slide from being damaged and ensure safe transportation of specimen to the laboratory for analysis. E
24 Remove gloves and dispose in clinical waste container.	Safe disposal of clinical waste (DH 2006, C).

Procedure guideline 11.12 Cervical uterine smear using liquid-based cytology

Essential equipment

- Alcoholic handrub
- Light source
- An examination couch
- Disposable clean paper couch covers
- Various sized specula (disposable or reusable)
- Disposable clean gloves
- Cervix brush
- A glass slide with frosted edge
- A pencil for labelling slide
- Fixative solution
- Plastic slide container
- Specimen form and plastic specimen bag
- A container of warm water
- Box of tissue paper
- Clinical waste container
- Trolley
- Disposable apron

Preprocedure

Action	Rationale
Please repeat steps 1–3 from Procedure Guideline 11.11	

Procedure

Please repeat steps 4–12 from Procedure Guideline 11.11, then

13 Using the Cervex-Brush®, insert the central bristles into the endocervical canal so that the shorter, outer bristles fully contact the ectocervix.	To ensure accuracy of site sampled (NHSCSP 2004, 2006, C).

14 Using pencil pressure, rotate the brush in a clockwise direction five times. *Note*: the plastic fronds of the brush are bevelled for rotation in a clockwise direction only.	To ensure good contact with the ectocervix and gather a high cellular yield (NHSCSP 2004, 2006, C).
Either:	
Using Thinprep®, using a swirling motion rinse the brush into the fixative vial; then push the brush into the base of the vial at least 10 times, forcing the bristles apart.	Firm pressure is required to ensure the cells do not cling to the brush (NHSCSP 2004, 2006, C).
Inspect the brush for any residual material and remove any remaining material by passing the brush over the edge of the fixative vial.	To ensure a usable amount of cellular material is collected (NHSCSP 2004, 2006, C).
Ensure that the material reaches the liquid. Then tighten the cap so that the material passes the torque line on the vial and give the vial a shake.	To ensure the cellular material reaches the preservative solution (NHSCSP 2004, 2006, C).
Or:	
Using SurePath™, remove head of the brush from the stem and place into the vial of fixative. Then screw lid on tightly and shake the vial. *Note*: it is essential that the sample is placed into the vial immediately in order to achieve fixation.	To ensure that the cells do not cling to the device (NHSCSP 2004, 2006, C). To ensure accurate preservation of cervical material (NHSCSP 2004, 2006, C).
15 Gently pull the speculum out until the blades are clear of the cervix, then close blades and remove speculum, placing in clinical waste bin if disposable or into CSS container if reusable.	To prevent pinching cervix or vaginal walls and ensure safe disposal of contaminated equipment (NHSCSP 2006, E; WHO 2006, C).
16 Cover the woman and offer tissue paper to wipe away any excess vaginal discharge.	To ensure dignity and privacy while promoting hygiene and comfort. E

Postprocedure

17 Remove gloves and dispose of waste in clinical waste receiver.	Safe disposal of clinical waste (DH 2006, C).
18 Assist the woman off the examination table and allow her to dress.	To ensure safety and promote dignity and privacy. E
19 Using a black ballpoint pen, label the vial with woman's name, clinic number and date of birth.	To ensure patient details are documented correctly. E *Note that ballpoint pens do not work on glass slides*. E
20 Place the vial into plastic specimen bag with the correctly labelled specimen form and send to laboratory.	To ensure safe handling and transportation of a biohazard (DH 2006, C).

667

Procedure guideline 11.13 Cervical uterine smear using an endocervical brush

Essential equipment

- Alcoholic handrub
- Light source
- An examination couch
- Disposable clean paper couch covers
- Various sized specula (disposable or reusable)
- Disposable clean gloves
- Wooden spatula or sampling device
- Endocervical brush
- A glass slide with frosted edge

- A pencil for labelling slide
- Fixative solution
- Plastic slide container
- Specimen form and plastic specimen bag
- A container of warm water
- Box of tissue paper
- Clinical waste container
- Trolley
- Disposable apron

(Continued)

Procedure guideline 11.13 (*Continued*)

Optional equipment

- A collecting container for CSS if reusable instruments are used

Preprocedure

Action	Rationale
1 Discuss benefits and limitations of screening and significance of smear results. Explain the purpose of procedure and explain what will occur at each step. Document the woman's clinical and screening history, specifically: (a) Date of last menstruation (b) Any abnormal bleeding (c) Any unusual vaginal discharge (d) Contraception (e) Date of last cervical smear (f) Any abnormal smear results (g) Any treatment to the cervix.	To ensure that the woman understands that the procedure involves removing underwear and that the speculum will be inserted into her vagina, and consents to the procedure (NMC 2008b, C). Allows the woman time to ask any questions. E
2 Wash hands before and after the procedure. Place all the equipment required for the procedure on the trolley.	To minimize the risk of infection (Fraise and Bradley 2009, E). To facilitate the efficient taking of the smear. E
3 Close room door or curtains and ask the woman to remove her underwear.	To provide privacy and comfort for the woman. E

Procedure

4 Wash hands with antibacterial detergent and running hand-hot water. Ensure hands are dried with disposable paper hand towels and apply PPE.	To reduce the risk of contamination and cross-infection (Fraise and Bradley 2009, E; RCN 2005, C).
5 Turn the light source on and position at end of examination table.	To provide illumination of the cervix and increase the accuracy of the smear taking (NHSCSP 2004, 2006, C).
6 Assist the woman into a supine position on the couch, with knees drawn up and legs parted. Keep her as covered as possible.	To facilitate easy access of the vaginal speculum and the taking of the cervical smear (NHSCSP 2004, 2006, C; WHO 2006, C, E).
7 Wash hands thoroughly or use an alcohol-based handrub.	To reduce the risk of contamination (Fraise and Bradley 2009, E).
8 Select the appropriate size speculum, from very small, small, medium, large including a long-bladed narrow speculum if the vagina is long or the cervix is lying posterior. The sterilized speculum can be warmed or cooled using clean tap water.	To promote patient comfort and reduce anxiety (NHSCSP 2006, C). If removed from a sterilizer, speculum may need to be cooled down, if cold then warmed up to reduce patient discomfort. It must be explained to patient that the speculum has been sterilized but the water will not contaminate it. E
9 Apply gloves. Part the labia and holding the speculum blades together sideways, slip the speculum into the vagina.	To insert the speculum and reduce patient discomfort (WHO 2006, C).
10 When the speculum is halfway into the vagina, turn it so that the handle is facing down. If insertion is difficult apply a small amount of water-based lubricant to the sides of the speculum, avoiding the tip.	To promote patient comfort and reduce contamination of the cervix with lubricants (NHSCSP 2006, C).
11 Gently open the blades of the speculum and look for the cervix. It may be necessary to move the speculum up or down until the entire cervix is visible.	To reduce patient discomfort and visualize the cervix (WHO 2006, C).

12 Once the cervix is visible, tighten the screw or lock the speculum in the open position so it remains in place. Adjustment of the light source may be required. Reassure the woman and allow time for her to relax.	To keep the speculum in the correct position and visualize the cervix (WHO 2006, C). To reduce patient discomfort and anxiety. E
13 Take the spatula and insert the long tip into the cervical os; rotate it through 360°.	To ensure an adequate cell sampling is obtained from the transformation zone (Higgins 2007, C; WHO 2006, C).
14 Remove the spatula from the vaginal cavity then smear both sides of the spatula onto the glass slide using straight sweeps.	To ensure maximum collection of cells (WHO 2006, C).
15 Using an endocervical brush in conjunction with a spatula, insert into the cervical os and rotate it through 360° in a clockwise direction. (Laboratories may prefer both spatula and brush samples on the same slide; check with laboratory services.)	To ensure an adequate cell sample is obtained from the endocervical canal (Higgins 2007, C; NHSCSP 2006, C; WHO 2006, C).
16 Remove the brush from the vaginal cavity then gently roll it along the glass slide.	To ensure maximum collection of cells (Higgins 2007, C; NHSCSP 2006, C; WHO 2006, C).
17 Apply fixative immediately. **Either:** Spray fixative is used at right angles to the slide and at a distance of 15–20 cm. **Or:** If immersing the slide in 95% ethanol, then leave for 5 minutes, remove from solution and allow to air dry. **Or:** If using 90% ethanol, then leave for 10–15 minutes, remove from solution and allow to air dry. **Or:** If using 'Cytofixx', apply a few drops to the slide and allow to dry for 5 minutes.	To ensure correct preservation of the specimen and ensure accurate results (Higgins 2007, C; NHSCSP 2006, C; WHO 2006, C).
18 If there are clinical signs of possible infection then a high vaginal swab is recommended prior to removal of speculum. (*If active infection is present, the cervical smear should be delayed until infection has been treated and resolved*.)	To ensure the swab is taken from the best site (Higgins 2007, C). A charcoal-impregnated swab is recommended if *Trichomonas* species are suspected as these organisms survive longer in this medium (Higgins 2007, C; Mims *et al*. 2004, R5).
19 Place the swab into the medium.	To ensure specimen is correctly placed in the culture medium to ensure accuracy of results. E
20 Gently pull the speculum out until the blades are clear of the cervix, then close blades and remove speculum, placing in clinical waste bin if disposable or into CSS container if reusable.	To prevent pinching the cervix or vaginal walls and to ensure safe disposal of contaminated equipment (DH 2006, C; NHSCSP 2006, C; WHO 2006, C).
21 Cover the woman and offer tissue paper to wipe away any excess vaginal discharge.	To ensure dignity and privacy while promoting hygiene and comfort. E

Postprocedure

22 Dispose of the waste into clinical waste receiver.	Safe disposal of clinical waste (DH 2006, C).
23 Assist the woman off the examination table and allow her to dress.	To ensure safety and promote dignity and privacy. E

669

(Continued)

Procedure guideline 11.13 (*Continued*)

24	Using a pencil, label the frosted end of the slide with woman's name, clinic number, date of birth and date sample taken. Using a black ballpoint pen, label the vaginal swab.	To ensure patient details are documented correctly on specimen. *Note that ballpoint pens do not work on glass slides.* E
25	Place the slide into transport container.	To prevent the slide from being damaged and ensure safe transportation of specimen to the laboratory for analysis. E
26	Remove gloves and dispose in clinical waste container.	Safe disposal of clinical waste (DH 2006, C).

Problem-solving table 11.4 Prevention and resolution (Procedure guidelines 11.11, 11.12 and 11.13)

Problem	Cause	Prevention	Action
Inadequate sample	Cervix has not been scraped firmly enough to obtain adequate epithelial cells (WHO 2006)	Ensure adequate pressure to obtain sample	Repeat cervical smear
	Sample on the spatula not completely transferred onto the slide or applied too thinly or thickly (Higgins 2007)	Ensure that the appropriate technique is utilized when transferring sample. Check that the sample has been transferred onto slide adequately before completion of the examination	Repeat cervical smear
	Fixative not applied immediately, allowing the sample to dry and causing the cells to become misshapen (WHO 2006)	Ensure fixative is applied in a timely manner	Repeat cervical smear
	Sample contaminated with lubricants, spermicide or blood (Higgins 2007)	Ensure sample is not contaminated by educating the patient not to use lubricants or spermicide prior to test	Repeat cervical smear
Unable to visualize the cervix	Position of the patient or anatomical position of the cervix	Adequate positioning of the patient	Reposition the patient from the prone to the lateral position. Place a pillow under the buttocks or turn the speculum. Consider assistance from another sample taker or refer to colposcopy clinic if unable to visualize

Postprocedural considerations

Immediate care

Ensure patient modesty is maintained throughout and directly after the examination. To maintain privacy and dignity, the nurse should leave the room while the patient gets undressed and dressed, and advise them to call when ready (RCN 2000).

Ongoing care

The results should be communicated to the patient and appropriate follow-up and/or referral to secondary services arranged where necessary. It is important that the healthcare professional should consider how the patient may react if abnormal results are to be delivered and ensure necessary support (RCN 2000).

Documentation

The nurse should ensure that the request form has been adequately completed and that the samples are also labelled correctly and accurately. If other microbiological tests are conducted, ensure the correct forms are completed and the samples are labelled and document any findings and resulting actions (RCN 2000).

Education of patient and relevant others

It is not unusual for the patient to experience some spotting after the cervical smear. This must be explained to the patient to ensure she is aware and not to worry. The healthcare professional should promote health education programmes and encourage screening to those who are eligible such as accurate information and advice in the prevention of cervical cancer. Patient information leaflets are offered to patients to ensure thay have the appropriate information (RCN 2000).

Specimen collection: swab sampling

Definition

Sterile swabs are commonly used in clinical practice to obtain samples of material from skin and mucous membranes. They are utilized to identify micro-organisms in suspected infection or as part of a screening programme to identify patients who may be carrying pathogens without displaying clinical signs or symptoms (Ferguson 2005). The overall aim is to identify the causative organism and determine the most effective therapy.

Related theory

Rationale

Obtaining a swab is one of the easiest and most unequivocal methods of sampling in clinical practice (Lawrence 1999). Swabbing is aimed at quantitative or qualitative collection of bodily fluid or cutaneous material for the purpose of obtaining a specimen for microbiological analysis (Kingsley 2001). Samples of infected material can be obtained from any accessible part of the body by using a sterile swab tipped with cotton wool or synthetic material (Hampson 2006).

Swabs for screening programmes

Meticillin-resistant *Staphylococcus aureus* is one of the most significant problematic organisms within healthcare (Weston 2008). Colonized and infected patients represent the most important reservoir of MRSA strains within hospitals (HPA 2008b) The transmission of MRSA and the risk of MRSA infection can only be effectively addressed if MRSA carriers are identified and treated to reduce this risk of transmission (DH 2006). These screening control measures guide staff in the protection of patients from MRSA colonization and infection. Active screening of patients for MRSA carriage is performed based on a risk assessment approach to the use of isolation and cohorting facilities (Coia *et al.* 2006).

Obtaining swabs is a key component of an effective MRSA prevention programme and certain patient groups are deemed to be at higher risk of contracting serious MRSA infections: critical care, burns, transplantation, cardiothoracic surgery, orthopaedic surgery, trauma, vascular surgery and renal patients (Coia *et al.* 2006).

The normal habitat of *Staphylococcus aureus*, including MRSA, is human skin, particularly the anterior nares (nose), axilla (armpit) and perineum (groin) (DH 2006). The most commonly sampled site for MRSA screening is the nose, which can detect up to 80% of MRSA-positive patients (DH 2006). If samples from other sites, such as the groin, are included in the screening regime, detection of MRSA-positive patients increases to 100% (DH 2006). Other samples can be taken from the following sites: skin lesions and wounds, invasive line sites and other skin breaks, tracheostomies, catheter specimens of urine (CSU) and sputum from patients with a productive cough (Coia *et al.* 2006). The microbiological request form should clearly indicate that the samples are for MRSA screening to ensure that correct laboratory techniques are used and to avoid potential waste of resources.

Evidence-based approaches

Rationale

Indications

Taking a swab is indicated:

- if there are clinical signs of infection which may manifest as symptoms such as pain, redness, inflammation, heat, pus, odour and so on
- if a patient shows signs of systemic infection or has a pyrexia of unknown origin (PUO)
- as part of a screening programme.

Contraindications

■ As routine use (unless part of a screening regimen).
■ On chronic wounds which will be colonized with skin flora.

Principles of care

Although swabs are relatively simple to use, absorbency of infected material is variable and adequate material collection that is representative of pathogenic changes, for example to wounds, is often dependent upon correct sampling technique (Gould and Brooker 2008). Swab specimens should be collected using an aseptic technique using sterile swabs, with the principal aim of gathering as much material as possible from the site of infection/inflammation. Care should be taken to avoid contamination with anything other than sample material such as surrounding tissue, which will be contaminated with other pathogens such as skin flora (Weston 2008).

If an infected area is producing copious amounts of pus or exudate, a specimen should be aspirated using a sterile syringe because swabs tend to absorb excess overlying exudate, resulting in an inadequate specimen (Gilchrist 2000). If the area to be swabbed is relatively dry, for example nasal or skin swabs, the tip of the swab can be moistened with sterile 0.9% sodium chloride which makes it more absorbent and increases the survival of pathogens (Weston 2008).

Obtaining a swab should be considered in conjunction with a comprehensive nursing assessment. This could include observation of localized infection such as inflammation or discharge from a wound during a dressing change.

Practitioners should know what type of pathogenic micro-organisms they are testing for, for example whether a bacterial or viral infection is suspected, as this will determine which swab is the most appropriate. Advice should be sought from the microbiology laboratory prior to taking a swab to ensure appropriate and resource-effective sampling or specimen collection. For example, whilst viruses cause the majority of throat infections, group A streptococcus is the main bacterial cause of sore throats and therefore if suspected, a swab with bacterial transport medium would need to be used rather than one containing viral transport medium.

Legal and professional issues

Competencies

Obtaining specimens for microbiological analysis is a key component in the patient's assessment and subsequent nursing care. Therefore, practitioners must be competent and feel confident that they have the knowledge, skill and understanding to obtain and correctly process samples for specimen collection (NMC 2008a).

Preprocedural considerations

Equipment

Commercially produced swabs are aseptically packaged in plastic transport tubes which contain either a bacterial or viral transport medium designed to maintain micro-organism viability between sampling and processing (Lawrence and Ameen 1998). If unsure, the practitioner should liaise with the microbiology laboratory to clarify which is the most suitable swab for a particular investigation or type of specimen. See Figure 11.4.

Specific patient preparations

It may be necessary to position the patient in order to obtain the required sample.

Procedure guideline 11.14 Swab sampling: ear

Essential equipment

■ Gloves	■ Sterile swab (with transport medium)
■ Apron	■ Appropriate documentation/form

Preprocedure

Action	Rationale
1 Explain and discuss the procedure with the patient.	To ensure the patient understands the procedure and gives valid consent (NMC 2008b, C).
2 Wash hands with bactericidal soap and water, or decontaminate physically clean hands with alcohol-based handrub. Don apron and gloves.	To reduce the risk of cross-infection and specimen contamination (Fraise and Bradley 2009, E).
3 Ensure no antibiotics or other therapeutic drops have been used in the aural region 3 hours before taking the swab.	To prevent collection of such therapeutic agents which may mask pathogenic organisms and invalidate the specimen (Hampson 2006, E).

Procedure

4 Remove the swab from outer packaging and place at the entrance of the auditory meatus as shown in Action Figure 4. Rotate gently once.	To avoid trauma to the ear and to collect secretions/ suitable specimen material (Mims *et al.* 2004, E).

Postprocedure

5 Remove cap from plastic transport tube.	To avoid contamination of the swab and to maintain the viability of the sampled material during transportation (Ferguson 2005, E; HPA 2008a, C).
6 Remove gloves and apron and wash/decontaminate hands.	To reduce risk of cross-infection (DH 2006, C).
7 Complete microbiology request form (including relevant information such as exact site, nature of specimen and investigation required).	To maintain accurate records and provide accurate information for laboratory analysis (NMC 2009, C; Weston 2008, E).
8 Arrange prompt delivery to the microbiology laboratory or refrigerate at 4–8°C.	To increase the chance of accurate organism identification and to ensure the best possible conditions for laboratory analysis (Higgins 2007, C; HPA 2008c, C).

Pinna
Inner ear
Outer ear
Ear canal
Ear swab
Ear drum
Middle ear
Eustachian tube

Action Figure 4 Area to be swabbed when sampling the outer ear.

673

Procedure guideline 11.15 Swab sampling: eye

Essential equipment

- Gloves
- Apron
- Sterile bacterial or viral swab (with transport medium)
- Appropriate documentation/form

Preprocedure

Action	Rationale
1 Explain and discuss the procedure with the patient.	To ensure the patient understands the procedure and gives valid consent (NMC 2008b, C).
2 Wash hands with bactericidal soap and water, or decontaminate physically clean hands with alcohol-based handrub. Don apron and gloves.	To reduce the risk of cross-infection and specimen contamination (Fraise and Bradley 2009, E).

(Continued)

Procedure guideline 11.15 (*Continued*)

3 Seek advice from the microbiology laboratory as to the correct culture medium and swab required.	Different culture media and swabs are required for bacteria, viruses and chlamydia (Higgins 2007, C).

Procedure

4 Ask patient to look upwards.	To prevent corneal damage (Stollery *et al.* 2005, E).
5 Hold the swab parallel to the cornea and gently rub the conjunctiva in the lower eyelids from nasal side outwards.	To ensure that a swab of the correct site is taken and to avoid contamination by touching the eyelid (Stollery *et al.* 2005, E).
6 *If for chlamydia specimen:* apply slightly more pressure when swabbing	To obtain as many organisms as possible from the follicles and to sweep organisms away from the lower punctum (Stollery *et al.* 2005, E).
7 If both eyes are to be swabbed, label swabs 'right' and 'left' accordingly.	To prevent the wrong swab being placed in the wrong culture medium. E

Postprocedure

8 Remove cap from plastic transport tube.	To avoid contamination of the swab (HPA 2008a, C).
9 Carefully place swab into plastic transport tube, ensuring it is fully immersed in the transport medium. Ensure cap is firmly secured.	To avoid contamination of the swab and to maintain the viability of the sampled material during transportation (Ferguson 2005, E).
10 Remove gloves and apron and wash/decontaminate hands.	To reduce risk of cross-infection (DH 2006, C).
11 Complete microbiology request form (including relevant information such as exact site, nature of specimen and investigation required).	To maintain accurate records and provide accurate information for laboratory analysis (NMC 2009, C; Weston 2008, E).
12 Arrange prompt delivery to the microbiology laboratory.	To increase the chance of accurate organism identification and to ensure the best possible conditions for laboratory analysis (Higgins 2007, C).

674

Procedure guideline 11.16 Swab sampling: nose

Essential equipment

- Gloves
- Apron
- Sterile bacterial or viral swab (with transport medium)
- Appropriate documentation/form

Optional equipment

- 0.9% sodium chloride

Preprocedure

Action	Rationale
1 Explain and discuss the procedure with the patient.	To ensure the patient understands the procedure and gives valid consent (NMC 2008b, C).
2 Wash hands with bactericidal soap and water, or de-contaminate physically clean hands with alcohol-based handrub. Don apron and gloves.	To reduce the risk of cross-infection and specimen contamination (Fraise and Bradley 2009, E).

Procedure

3 Ask patient to tilt head backwards.	To optimize visualization of area to be swabbed (Gould and Brooker 2008, E).
4 Moisten swab with sterile saline.	To prevent discomfort to the patient as the nasal mucosa is normally dry and organisms will adhere more easily to a moist swab (Hampson 2006, C).
5 Insert swab inside the anterior nares with the tip directed upwards and gently rotate (see Action Figure 5).	To ensure that an adequate specimen from the correct site is obtained and to avoid damage to the delicate epithelium (Gould and Brooker 2008, E).
6 Repeat the procedure with the same swab in the other nostril.	To optimize organism collection. E

Postprocedure

7 Remove cap from plastic transport tube.	To avoid contamination of the swab (HPA 2008a, C).
8 Carefully place swab into plastic transport tube, ensuring it is fully immersed in the transport medium. Ensure cap is firmly secured.	To avoid contamination of the swab and to maintain the viability of the sampled material during transportation (Ferguson 2005, E).
9 Provide the patient with a tissue if required.	For patient comfort (Higgins 2008, E).
10 Remove gloves and apron and wash/decontaminate hands.	To reduce risk of cross-infection (DH 2006, C).
11 Complete microbiology request form (including relevant information such as exact site, nature of specimen and investigation required).	To maintain accurate records and provide accurate information for laboratory analysis (NMC 2009, C; Weston 2008, E).
12 *If sample taken for screening:* state clearly on the microbiology request form, for example for MRSA screening.	To ensure only these organisms are being analysed, so the result will only indicate their presence or absence, and sensitivities (HPA 2008d, C).
13 Arrange prompt delivery to the microbiology laboratory.	To increase the chance of accurate organism identification and to ensure the best possible conditions for laboratory analysis (Higgins 2007, C).

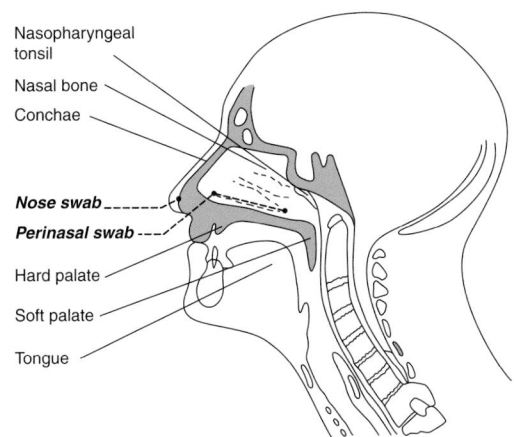

Nasopharyngeal tonsil
Nasal bone
Conchae
Nose swab
Perinasal swab
Hard palate
Soft palate
Tongue

Action Figure 5 Area to be swabbed when sampling the nose.

Procedure guideline 11.17 Swab sampling: penis

Essential equipment

- Gloves
- Apron
- Sterile bacterial or viral swab (with transport medium)
- Appropriate documentation/form

Preprocedure

Action	Rationale
1 Explain and discuss the procedure with the patient.	To ensure the patient understands the procedure and gives valid consent (NMC 2008b, C).
2 Wash hands with bactericidal soap and water, or de-contaminate physically clean hands with alcohol-based handrub. Don apron and gloves.	To reduce the risk of cross-infection and specimen contamination (Fraise and Bradley 2009, E).

Procedure

Action	Rationale
3 The patient should not have passed urine for at least 1 hour.	To ensure a representative sample from the area being swabbed (HPA 2004, C).
4 Retract prepuce.	To obtain maximum visibility of area to be swabbed. E
5 Pass the swab gently through the urethral meatus and rotate gently.	To collect a specimen of discharge or secretions. E

Postprocedure

Action	Rationale
6 Remove cap from plastic transport tube.	To avoid contamination of the swab (HPA 2008a, C).
7 Carefully place swab into plastic transport tube, ensuring it is fully immersed in the transport medium. Ensure cap is firmly secured.	To avoid contamination of the swab and to maintain viability of the sampled material during transportation (Ferguson 2005, E).
8 Remove gloves and apron and wash/decontaminate hands.	To reduce risk of cross-infection (DH 2006, C).
9 Complete microbiology request form (including relevant information such as exact site, nature of specimen and investigation required).	To maintain accurate records and provide accurate information for laboratory analysis (NMC 2009, C; Weston 2008, E).
10 Arrange prompt delivery to the microbiology laboratory (within 4 hours).	To increase the chance of accurate organism identification and to ensure the best possible conditions for laboratory analysis (Higgins 2007, C).

Procedure guideline 11.18 Swab sampling: rectum

Essential equipment

- Gloves
- Apron
- Sterile bacterial or viral swab (with transport medium)
- Appropriate documentation/form

Preprocedure

Action	Rationale
1 Explain and discuss the procedure with the patient.	To ensure the patient understands the procedure and gives valid consent (NMC 2008b, C).

2	Ensure a suitable location in which to carry out the procedure.	To maintain patient privacy and dignity (Gilbert 2006, E).
3	Wash hands with bactericidal soap and water, or decontaminate physically clean hands with alcohol-based handrub. Don apron and gloves.	To reduce the risk of cross-infection and specimen contamination (Fraise and Bradley 2009, E).

Procedure

4	Pass the swab, with care, through the anus into the rectum and rotate gently.	To avoid trauma and to ensure that a rectal, not an anal, sample is obtained. E
5	*If specimen is for suspected threadworm:* take swab from the perianal area.	Threadworms lay their ova on the perianal skin (Mims *et al.* 2004, E).

Postprocedure

6	Remove cap from plastic transport tube.	To avoid contamination of the swab (HPA 2008a, C).
7	Carefully place swab into plastic transport tube, ensuring it is fully immersed in the transport medium. Ensure cap is firmly secured.	To avoid contamination of the swab and to maintain viability of the sampled material during transportation (Ferguson 2005, E).
8	Remove gloves and apron and wash/decontaminate hands.	To reduce risk of cross-infection (DH 2006, C).
9	Complete microbiology request form (including relevant information such as exact site, nature of specimen and investigation required).	To maintain accurate records and provide accurate information for laboratory analysis (NMC 2009, C; Weston 2008, E).
10	Arrange prompt delivery to the microbiology laboratory.	To increase the chance of accurate organism identification and to ensure the best possible conditions for laboratory analysis (Higgins 2007, C).

677

Procedure guideline 11.19 Swab sampling: skin

Essential equipment

- Gloves
- Apron
- Sterile bacterial or viral swab (with transport medium)
- Appropriate documentation/form

Optional equipment

- Scalpel blade/U blade (for trained practitioners only)

Preprocedure

Action	Rationale
1 Explain and discuss the procedure with the patient.	To ensure the patient understands the procedure and gives valid consent (NMC 2008b, C).
2 Wash hands with bactericidal soap and water, or de-contaminate physically clean hands with alcohol-based handrub. Don apron and gloves.	To reduce the risk of cross-infection and specimen contamination (Fraise and Bradley 2009, E).

(Continued)

Procedure guideline 11.19 *(Continued)*

Procedure

3 *For cutaneous sampling (for screening, for example groin)*: moisten swab with sterile saline and roll one swab along the area of skin along the inside of the thighs closest to the genitalia.	Organisms adhere more easily to a moist swab (Hampson 2006, C).
4 *For suspected fungal infection*: skin scrapings should be obtained. Take a scalpel blade and, with the affected area of skin stretched taut between two fingers, gently scrape the skin with a piece of dark paper underneath. Do not cause bleeding.	To identify superficial fungi that inhabit the outer layer of the skin (Mackie 2003, E). To visualize amount of sample and to allow easier transfer. E

Postprocedure

5 **Either:** *For swab specimen:* (a) Remove cap from plastic transport tube. (b) Carefully place swab into plastic transport tube, ensuring it is fully immersed in the transport medium. Ensure cap is firmly secured. **or:** *For skin scrapings:* (a) Transfer scrapings into sterile container.	To avoid contamination of the swab (HPA 2008a, C). To avoid contamination of the swab and to maintain the viability of the sampled material during transportation (Ferguson 2005, E). To allow samples to be processed appropriately in the laboratory. E
6 Remove gloves and apron and wash/decontaminate hands.	To reduce risk of cross-infection (DH 2006, C).
7 Complete microbiology request form (including relevant information such as exact site, nature of specimen and investigation required).	To maintain accurate records and provide accurate information for laboratory analysis (NMC 2009, C; Weston 2008, E).
8 Arrange prompt delivery to the microbiology laboratory (keep at room temperature).	To increase the chance of accurate organism identification and to ensure the best possible conditions for laboratory analysis (Higgins 2007, C).

Procedure guideline 11.20 Swab sampling: throat

Essential equipment

- Gloves
- Apron
- Sterile bacterial or viral swab (with transport medium)
- Appropriate documentation/form
- Tongue spatula
- Light source

Preprocedure

Action	Rationale
1 Explain and discuss the procedure with the patient.	To ensure the patient understands the procedure and gives valid consent (NMC 2008b, C).
2 Wash hands with bactericidal soap and water, or decontaminate physically clean hands with alcohol-based handrub. Don apron and gloves.	To reduce the risk of cross-infection and specimen contamination (Fraise and Bradley 2009, E).

Procedure

3 Ask patient to sit upright facing a strong light, tilt head backwards, open mouth and stick out tongue.	To ensure maximum visibility of the area to be swabbed and avoid contact with the oral mucosa (Gould and Brooker 2008, E).
4 Depress tongue with a spatula.	The procedure may cause the patient to gag. The spatula prevents the tongue moving to the roof of the mouth, which would contaminate the specimen (Rushing 2006, E).
5 Ask patient to say 'Ah'.	To relax the throat muscles and help minimize the gag reflex (Rushing 2006, E).
6 Quickly but gently roll the swab over any area of exudate or inflammation or over the tonsils and posterior pharynx (see Action Figure 6).	To obtain the required sample (Weston 2008, E).
7 Carefully withdraw the swab, avoiding touching any other area of the mouth or tongue.	To prevent contamination of the specimen with the resident flora of the oropharynx (Weston 2008, E).

Postprocedure

8 Remove cap from plastic transport tube.	To avoid contamination of the swab (HPA 2008a, C).
9 Carefully place swab into plastic transport tube, ensuring it is fully immersed in the transport medium. Ensure cap is firmly secured.	To avoid contamination of the swab and maintain the viability of the sampled material during transportation (Ferguson 2005, E).
10 Remove gloves and apron and wash/decontaminate hands.	To reduce risk of cross-infection (DH 2006, C).
11 Complete microbiology request form (including relevant information such as exact site, nature of specimen and investigation required).	To maintain accurate records and provide accurate information for laboratory analysis (NMC 2009, C; Weston 2008, E).
12 Arrange prompt delivery to the microbiology laboratory.	To increase the chance of accurate organism identification and to ensure the best possible conditions for laboratory analysis (Higgins 2007, C).

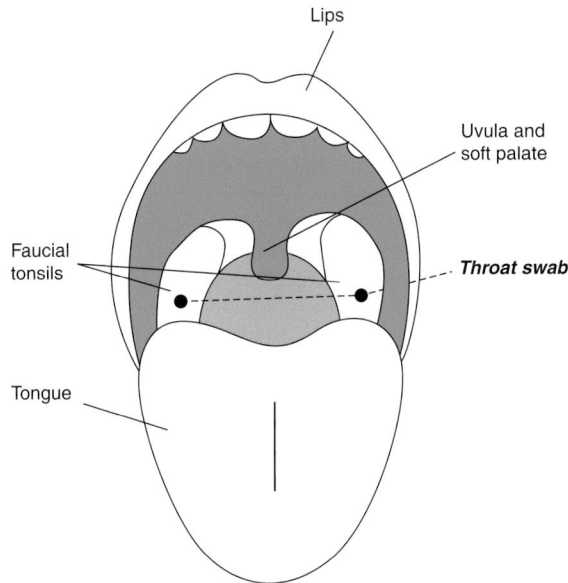

Action Figure 6 Area to be swabbed when sampling the throat.

Procedure guideline 11.21 Swab sampling: vagina

Essential equipment

- Gloves
- Apron
- Sterile bacterial or viral swab (with transport medium)
- Appropriate documentation/form
- Sterile speculum
- Light source

Preprocedure

Action	Rationale
1 Explain and discuss the procedure with the patient.	To ensure the patient understands the procedure and gives valid consent (NMC 2008b, C).
2 Ensure a suitable location in which to carry out the procedure.	To maintain patient privacy and dignity (Gilbert 2006, E).
3 Wash hands with bactericidal soap and water, or de-contaminate physically clean hands with alcohol-based handrub. Don apron and gloves.	To reduce the risk of cross-infection and specimen contamination (Fraise and Bradley 2009, E).
4 Place the patient in a dorsal position supported by a pillow and ask her to bring her heels together, bend her legs and draw her heels towards her bottom.	To ensure patient assumes correct position for the procedure. E

Procedure

5 **Either:** *For low vaginal swab:* (a) Insert the swab into the lower part of the vagina and rotate gently but firmly.	To obtain appropriate sample. E
Or: *For high vaginal swab:* (b) Moisten the speculum with warm water and insert into the vagina to separate the vaginal walls. Wipe away any excess cervical mucus with a cotton swab. Using a sterile swab, sample as high as possible in the vaginal vault. Remove speculum and wipe vagina/vulval area with a tissue.	To ensure maximum visibility of the area to be swabbed and to obtain the appropriate sample (Hampson 2006, E).
6 Allow patient to resume a comfortable position.	To aid patient comfort. E

Postprocedure

7 Remove cap from plastic transport tube.	To avoid contamination of the swab (HPA 2008a, C).
8 Carefully place swab into plastic transport tube, ensuring it is fully immersed in the transport medium. Ensure cap is firmly secured.	To avoid contamination of the swab and to maintain the viability of the sampled material during transportation (HPA 2004, C; Ferguson 2005, E).
9 Remove gloves and apron and wash/decontaminate hands.	To reduce risk of cross-infection (DH 2006, C).
10 Complete microbiology request form (including relevant information such as exact site, nature of specimen and investigation required).	To maintain accurate records and provide accurate information for laboratory analysis (NMC 2009, C; Weston 2008, E).
11 Arrange prompt delivery to the microbiology laboratory (within 4 hours).	To increase the chance of accurate organism identification and to ensure the best possible conditions for laboratory analysis (Higgins 2007, C).

Procedure guideline 11.22 Swab sampling: wound

Essential equipment

- Gloves
- Apron
- Sterile bacterial or viral swab (with transport medium)
- Appropriate documentation/form
- Dressing pack, cleansing solution and dressing (post sampling procedure)

Optional equipment

- 0.9% sodium chloride

Preprocedure

Action	Rationale
1 Explain and discuss the procedure with the patient.	To ensure the patient understands the procedure and gives valid consent (NMC 2008b, C).
2 Wash hands with bactericidal soap and water, or decontaminate physically clean hands with alcohol-based handrub. Don apron and gloves.	To reduce the risk of cross-infection and specimen contamination (Fraise and Bradley 2009, E).
3 Remove current dressing, if applicable.	To expose wound in preparation for swabbing. E
4 Rewash and decontaminate hands. Open sterile dressing pack, decant sterile swab and don sterile gloves.	To reduce the risk of cross-infection (Fraise and Bradley 2009, E) and prepare equipment for sampling.

Procedure

5 Roll swab in a 'zig-zag' motion to cover the entire wound surface whilst simultaneously rotating the swab between the thumb and forefinger.	To maximize collection of micro-organisms within the wound bed (Rushing 2006, C).
6 Use enough pressure to express fluid from within the wound tissue but avoid taking a specimen from exudates or touching the wound margin at the skin.	To gather as much exudate as possible without contaminating the sterile swab with resident skin flora (Kingsley 2001, E).
7 If the wound is dry, the tip of the swab should be moistened with 0.9% sodium chloride.	To make the swab more absorbent and to increase survival of pathogens present prior to culture (Weston 2008, E).
8 If pus is present, it should be aspirated using a sterile syringe and decanted into a sterile specimen pot.	To yield the optimum number of micro-organisms present within the wound (Weston 2008, E).

Postprocedure

9 Remove cap from plastic transport tube.	To avoid contamination of the swab (HPA 2008a, C).
10 Carefully place swab into plastic transport tube, ensuring it is fully immersed in the transport medium. Ensure cap is firmly secured.	To avoid contamination of the swab and to maintain the viability of the sampled material during transportation (Ferguson 2005, E).
11 Redress the wound, if applicable, as per patient care plan.	To redress the wound. E
12 Remove gloves and apron, discard all clinical waste and wash/decontaminate hands.	To reduce risk of cross-infection (DH 2006, C).
13 Complete microbiology request form (including relevant information such as exact site, nature of specimen and investigation required).	To maintain accurate records and provide accurate information for laboratory analysis (NMC 2009, C; Weston 2008, E).
14 Arrange prompt delivery to the microbiology laboratory (keep at room temperature).	To increase the chance of accurate organism identification and to ensure the best possible conditions for laboratory analysis (Higgins 2007, C).

Postprocedural considerations

Immediate care

Specimens may be compromised by incorrect storage and transportation. If not processed immediately, swabs need to be refrigerated or kept at an ambient temperature, depending on where the swab was obtained from, to prevent deterioration of pathogenic micro-organisms (see specific procedure guidelines for exact storage requirements). Advice should be sought from the microbiology laboratory if practitioners are unsure of the storage requirements of the sample.

Documentation

Relevant and detailed information such as clinical presentation, signs and symptoms of infection, and the site and nature of the swab should be indicated on the sample and microbiology request form. This allows the microbiology laboratory to select the most appropriate processing technique and assist in differentiating organisms which would normally be expected at a particular site from those causing infection (Weston 2008).

In accordance with the principles of good record keeping, the date and time of when a swab is sent to the laboratory should be documented clearly and promptly in the patient's notes and care plan (NMC 2009). This should be done alongside documentation of the clinical nursing assessment, particularly in relation to significant findings that have prompted the collection of the sample such as observation of inflammation or discharge at the site. This assists in communication and the dissemination of information between members of the interprofessional healthcare team.

Specimen collection: urine sampling

Definition

Urine samples are intended to identify any organisms causing infection within the urinary tract (Hampson 2006). Urinary tract infections (UTIs) result from the presence and multiplication of bacteria in one or more structures of the urinary tract with associated tissue invasion (HPA 2008g).

Related theory

Protection against infection is normally given by the constant flow of urine and regular bladder emptying, which prevent the colonization of micro-organisms (HPA 2008g). The urethra is colonized with naturally occurring flora but urine proximal to the distal urethra is normally sterile. As urine passes through the urethra some of these micro-organisms are flushed through and normal urine will naturally contain a small number of bacteria. Therefore, the presence of bacteriuria is insignificant in the absence of clinical symptoms of an infection (Weston 2008).

Urinary tract infections account for 19.7% of all overall hospital-acquired infections (DH 2007a). UTIs in adults are common, particularly in women due to the short female urethra and its close proximity to the perineum (HPA 2008g).

Evidence-based approaches

Rationale

Urine sample requests for Microscopy, Culture and Sensitivity (MC&S) constitute the largest single category of specimens examined in microbiological laboratories. The main value of urine culture is to identify bacteria and their sensitivity to antibiotics (Higgins 2007).

Urine sampling should be considered in combination with clinical assessment and urinalysis to avoid unnecessary sample processing which has time and cost implications for the microbiology laboratory (Simerville et al. 2005). A clinical assessment would involve examination of the odour, turbidity and colour, whether there are obvious signs of haematuria and pain particularly around the suprapubic area (Dulczak and Kirk 2005). Urinalysis may reveal a high pH, the presence of blood or positivity to leucocyte esterase (an enzyme released by white blood cells) or nitrite, all of which indicate a high probability of bacteriuria (Higgins 2007).

Indications

Obtaining a urine specimen is indicated:

- when there are clinical signs and symptoms to indicate an UTI
- if there are signs of a systemic infection or in patients with a PUO
- on development of new patient confusion as toxicity from infection can cause alterations in mental status or impairments in cognitive ability (Pellowe 2009).

Principles of care

Urine may be collected using a midstream clean-catch technique or from a catheter using a sterile syringe to access the sample port (Pellatt 2007a). To minimize the contamination of a specimen by bacteria, which may be present on the skin, the perianal region or the external genital tract, good hand and genital hygiene should be encouraged. Therefore, patients should be encouraged to wash their hands prior to collecting a clean-catch midstream urine specimen and to clean around the urethral meatus prior to sample collection (Higgins 2007). The principle for obtaining a midstream collection of urine is that any bacteria present in the urethra are washed away in the first portion of urine voided and therefore the specimen collected more accurately represents the urine in the bladder (Dawson and Whitfield 1996).

Catheter-associated urinary tract infections (CAUTI)

The presence of a urinary catheter, and the duration of its insertion, are contributory factors in the development of a UTI. Some 60% of healthcare-associated UTIs are related to catheter insertion (DH 2007a). For every day the catheter remains *in situ*, the risk of bacteriuria is 5% so that 50% of patients catheterized for longer than 7–10 days will have bacteriuria (Pellowe 2009). Although often asymptomatic, 20–30% of patients with bacteriuria will develop a CAUTI and 1–4% will develop a bacteraemia, which has significant implications for patient morbidity, increased hospital stay and increased cost (Pellowe 2009).

Preprocedural considerations

Equipment

Specimen jars for urine collection must be sterile to ensure no contamination occurs which may lead to an incorrect diagnosis and treatment. The jars must close securely to prevent leakage of the sample. See Figure 11.3.

Specific patient preparations

When collecting a midstream specimen of urine (MSU), the patient must pass a small amount of urine before collecting the specimen. This reduces the risk of contamination of the specimen with naturally occurring micro-organisms/flora within the urethra (Rigby and Gray 2005).

Procedure guideline 11.23 Urine sampling: midstream specimen of urine: male

Essential equipment

- Cleaning solution (e.g. soap and water, 0.9% sodium chloride or disinfectant-free solution)
- Sterile specimen container (with wide opening)
- Gloves
- Apron
- Appropriate documentation/forms

Preprocedure

Action	Rationale
1 Discuss need and indication for procedure with patient.	To obtain valid consent (NMC 2008b, C).
2 Fully explain the steps of the procedure.	The procedure requires the patient to fully understand the procedure in order to avoid inadvertent contamination of specimen and optimize the quality of the sample (Higgins 2008, C).
3 Ensure a suitable, private location.	To maintain patient privacy and dignity (Gilbert 2006, E).

Procedure

4 Ask patient to wash hands with soap and water.	To reduce risk of cross-infection (Fraise and Bradley 2009, E).
5 *If practitioner's assistance required:* wash hands with bactericidal soap or decontaminate physically clean hands with alcohol rub and don apron.	To prevent cross-contamination (Fraise and Bradley 2009, E).
6 Ask patient to retract the foreskin and clean the skin surrounding the urethral meatus with soap and water, 0.9% sodium chloride or a disinfectant-free solution.	To optimize general cleansing and minimize contamination of specimen with other organisms. E Disinfectant solutions may irritate the urethral mucous membrane (Higgins 2007, E).
7 Ask patient to begin voiding first stream of urine (approx. 15–30 mL) into a urinal, toilet or bedpan.	To commence the flow of urine and avoid contamination of specimen with naturally occurring micro-organisms/flora within the urethra (Rigby and Gray 2005, E).
8 Place the wide-necked sterile container into the urine stream without interrupting the flow.	To prevent contamination of specimen and ensure the collection of the midstream of urine which most accurately represents the urine in the bladder (Gilbert 2006, E.)
9 Ask the patient to void his remaining urine into the urinal, toilet or bedpan.	For patient to comfortably continue passing urine. E

(Continued)

Procedure guideline 11.23 (*Continued*)

10	Transfer specimen into sterile universal container.	For despatch to the laboratory. E
11	Allow patient to wash hands.	To maintain personal hygiene. E

Postprocedure

12	Label sample and complete microbiological request form including relevant clinical information, such as signs and symptoms of infection, antibiotic therapy.	To maintain accurate records and provide accurate information for laboratory analysis (NMC 2009, C; Weston 2008, E).
13	Dispatch sample to laboratory immediately (within 2 hours) or refrigerate at 4°C.	To ensure the best possible conditions for microbiological analysis and to prevent micro-organism proliferation (Higgins 2007, C).

Procedure guideline 11.24 Urine sampling: midstream specimen of urine: female

Essential equipment

- Cleaning solution (e.g. soap and water, 0.9% sodium chloride or disinfectant-free solution)
- Sterile specimen container (with wide opening)
- Gloves
- Apron
- Appropriate documentation/forms

Preprocedure

Action	Rationale
1 Discuss need and indication for procedure with patient.	To obtain valid consent (NMC 2008b, C).
2 Fully explain the steps of the procedure.	The procedure requires the patient to fully understand the procedure in order to avoid inadvertent contamination of specimen and optimize the quality of the sample (Higgins 2008, C).
3 Ensure a suitable, private location.	To maintain patient privacy and dignity (Gilbert 2006, E).

Procedure

4 Ask patient to wash hands with soap and water.	To reduce risk of cross-infection (Fraise and Bradley 2009, E).
5 *If practitioner's assistance required:* wash hands with bactericidal soap or decontaminate physically clean hands with alcohol rub and don apron.	To prevent cross-contamination (Fraise and Bradley 2009, E).
6 Ask patient to part the labia and clean the urethral meatus with soap and water, 0.9% sodium chloride or a disinfectant-free solution.	To optimize general cleansing and to minimize other organisms contaminating the specimen. E Disinfectant solutions may irritate the urethral mucous membrane (Higgins 2007, C).
7 Use a separate swab for each wipe and wipe downwards from front to back.	To prevent cross-infection and perianal contamination (Weston 2008, E).
8 Ask patient to begin voiding first stream of urine (approx. 15–30 mL) into a toilet or bedpan whilst separating the labia.	To commence the flow of urine and avoid contamination of specimen with naturally occurring micro-organisms/flora within the urethra (Rigby and Gray 2005, E).

9 Place the wide-necked sterile container into the urine stream without interrupting the flow.	To prevent contamination of specimen and to ensure the collection of the midstream of urine which most accurately represents the urine in the bladder (Gilbert 2006, E).
10 Ask the patient to void her remaining urine into the toilet or bedpan.	For patient to comfortably continue passing urine. E
11 Transfer specimen into sterile universal container.	For dispatch to the laboratory. E
12 Allow patient to wash hands.	To maintain personal hygiene. E

Postprocedure

13 Label sample and complete microbiological request form including relevant clinical information, such as signs and symptoms of infection, antibiotic therapy.	To maintain accurate records and provide accurate information for laboratory analysis (NMC 2009, C; Weston 2008, E).
14 Dispatch sample to laboratory immediately (within 2 hours) or refrigerate at 4°C.	To ensure the best possible conditions for microbiological analysis and to prevent micro-organism proliferation (Higgins 2007, C).

Procedure guideline 11.25 Urine sampling: catheter specimen of urine (CSU)

Essential equipment

685

- Sterile gloves
- Apron
- Syringe (and needle if not a needle-free system)
- Non-traumatic clamps
- Alcohol-based swab
- Universal specimen container
- Appropriate documentation/forms

Optional equipment

- Non-sterile gloves

Preprocedure

Action	Rationale
1 Explain and discuss the procedure with the patient.	To ensure the patient understands the procedure and gives valid consent (NMC 2008b, C).
2 Ensure a suitable, private location.	To maintain patient privacy and dignity (Gilbert 2006, E).
3 Prepare equipment and place on sterile trolley.	To prepare equipment for use. E

Procedure

4 *If no urine visible in catheter tubing*: wash/decontaminate physically clean hands with alcohol rub, don apron and apply non-sterile gloves prior to manipulating the catheter tubing.	To minimize the risk of cross-infection (Pellowe 2009, C).
5 Apply non-traumatic clamp a few centimetres distal to the sampling port.	To ensure sufficient sample has collected to allow for accurate sampling (Higgins 2008, C).

(Continued)

Procedure guideline 11.25 *(Continued)*

6 Wash hands with bactericidal soap and water, or decontaminate physically clean hands with alcohol rub and don sterile gloves.	To prevent cross-contamination (Fraise and Bradley 2009, E).
7 Wipe sampling port with 2% chlorhexidine in 70% isopropyl alcohol and allow drying for 30 seconds.	To decontaminate sampling port and prevent false-positive results (DH 2007a, C).
8 *If using needle and syringe:* using a sterile syringe and needle, insert needle into port at an angle of 45° and aspirate the required amount of urine, then withdraw needle. *Or in a needle-less system:* insert syringe firmly into centre sampling port (according to manufacturer's guidelines), aspirate the required amount of urine and remove syringe.	To enable safe inoculation of urine specimen and to minimize the risk of penetration of the wall of the catheter tubing (Hampson 2006, C) Reduces the risk of sharps injury (DH 2006, C).
9 Transfer an adequate volume of the urine specimen (approx. 10 mL) into a sterile container immediately.	To avoid contamination and to allow for accurate microbiological processing (Gilbert 2006, E).
10 Discard needle and syringe into sharps container.	To prevent the risk of needlestick injury. E
11 Wipe the sampling port with an alcohol wipe and allow to dry.	To reduce contamination of access port and to reduce risk of cross-infection (DH 2007a, C).

Postprocedure

12 Unclamp catheter tubing.	To allow drainage to continue. E
13 Dispose of waste, remove apron and gloves and wash hands.	To ensure correct clinical waste management and reduce risk of cross-infection (DH 2006, C).
14 Label sample and complete microbiological request form including relevant clinical information, such as signs and symptoms of infection, antibiotic therapy.	To maintain accurate records and provide accurate information for laboratory analysis (NMC 2009, C; Weston 2008, E).
15 Dispatch sample to laboratory immediately (within 2 hours) or refrigerate at 4°C.	To ensure the best possible conditions for microbiological analysis and to prevent micro-organism proliferation (Higgins 2007, C).

Procedure guideline 11.26 Urine sampling: sampling from an ileal conduit

Essential equipment

- Sterile trolley
- Sterile dressing pack (with gloves)
- Urinary catheter (not larger than 14 Fr)
- Apron
- Universal specimen container
- Clean stoma appliance
- Appropriate documentation/forms

Preprocedure

Action	Rationale
1 Explain and discuss the procedure with the patient.	To ensure the patient understands the procedure and gives valid consent (NMC 2008b, C).
2 Ensure a suitable, private location.	To maintain patient privacy and dignity (Gilbert 2006, E).
3 Ensure patient is in a comfortable position (sitting up, supported by pillows) and that stoma is easily accessible.	For patient comfort and to allow access to the stoma. E
4 Prepare equipment and place on sterile trolley.	To prepare equipment for use. E

Procedure

5 Wash hands with bactericidal soap and water and dry or decontaminate physically clean hands with alcohol rub. Don non-sterile gloves.	To prevent cross-contamination (Fraise and Bradley 2009, E).
6 Remove the appliance from stoma. Decontaminate hands, apply sterile gloves and place sterile towel/pad under stoma.	To absorb any spillage from the stoma. E
7 Clean around the stoma with sterile water or saline, from the centre outwards.	Cleaning of the area reduces the risk of introducing surface pathogens into the ileal conduit. E
8 Apply gentle skin traction to allow the stoma opening to be more visible.	To avoid catheter coming into contact with external surface of the stoma. E
9 Insert catheter tip gently into the stoma to a depth of 2.5–5 cm only.	Gentle handling reduces the risk of ileal perforation and is more comfortable for the patient. E
10 Allow approximately 10 mL of drain through into a sterile specimen container.	To avoid contamination and to allow for accurate microbiological processing (Gilbert 2006, E).
11 Remove the catheter.	As catheter is no longer required. E
12 Change gloves, attend to stoma and apply new stoma appliance.	To ensure patient comfort. E

Postprocedure

13 Dispose of waste, remove apron and gloves and wash decontaminate hands.	To ensure correct clinical waste management and reduce risk of cross-infection (DH 2006, C).
14 Label sample and complete microbiological request form including relevant clinical information, such as signs and symptoms of infection, antibiotic therapy.	To maintain accurate records and provide accurate information for laboratory analysis (NMC 2009, C; Weston 2008, E).
15 Dispatch sample to laboratory immediately (within 2 hours) or refrigerate at 4°C.	To ensure the best possible conditions for microbiological analysis and to prevent micro-organism proliferation (Higgins 2007, C).

Procedure guideline 11.27 Urine sampling: 24-hour urine collection

Essential equipment

- Clean urine collection containers (e.g. wide-necked pot)
- Large urine containers (with label attached for patient details)
- Appropriate documentation/forms

Optional equipment

- Written patient instruction sheet

Preprocedure

Action	Rationale
1 Discuss need and indication for procedure with patient.	To obtain valid consent (NMC 2008b, C).
2 Fully explain the steps of the procedure, emphasizing the importance of not discarding any urine within the 24-hour period (provide written information if needed).	The procedure requires the patient to fully understand the procedure in order to avoid inadvertent contamination of specimen and optimize the quality of the sample. E

(Continued)

Procedure guideline 11.27 (*Continued*)

Procedure

3 Ask patient to void urine and discard this specimen.	To establish the exact start time of the 24-hour period. E
4 All urine passed in the next 24 hours from this appointed time should be collected in a clean urine collection container.	To ensure the specimen is representative of the variables of altering body chemistry within the 24 hours (Thomson 2002, E).
5 *If catheter in situ:* completely empty catheter bag and hourly chamber (if applicable) or attach new catheter bag. Attach label indicating start time of 24-hour urine collection.	To clearly indicate to all practitioners the 24-hour collection period. E
6 If applicable, transfer urine from collection container into large specimen container.	To ensure specimen is collected in a suitable container for safe transportation to the laboratory. E

Postprocedure

7 Label sample and complete request form.	To maintain accurate records and provide accurate information for laboratory analysis (NMC 2009, C; Weston 2008, E).
8 Dispatch sample to laboratory as soon as possible after completion of the 24-hour period.	To allow accurate laboratory processing and analysis (Higgins 2007, C).

Postprocedural considerations

Immediate care

Urine is a very good culture medium so any bacteria present at the time of collection will continue to multiply in the specimen container. Rapid transport or special measures to ensure preservation of the sample are essential for laboratory diagnosis (Garibaldi 1992). Therefore, specimens should be processed immediately as delays of more than 2 hours at room temperature between collection and examination will yield unreliable results, suggesting falsely raised bacteriuria (Higgins 2007).

Where delays in processing are unavoidable, specimens should be refrigerated at 4°C or a boric acid preservative, which holds the bacterial population steady for 48–96 hours, should be utilized (HPA 2008g).

Specimen collection: faecal sampling

Definition

Faecal specimens are primarily obtained for microbiological analysis to isolate and identify pathogenic bacterial, viral or parasitic organisms suspected of causing gastrointestinal infections or in patients with diarrhoea of potentially infectious aetiology (Higgins 2008). Faecal specimens may also be obtained for other non-microbiological testing to detect the presence of other substances, such as occult blood or as part of the national screening programme for colorectal cancer.

Related theory

There are a number of enteric pathogens normally present within the gastrointestinal (GI) tract, along with resident flora, that play an important role in digestion, and in forming a protective, structural and metabolic barrier against the growth of potentially pathogenic bacteria (Kelly *et al.* 2005). Pathogenic agents that disrupt the balance within the GI tract manifest in symptoms such as prolonged diarrhoea, bloody diarrhoea, nausea, vomiting, abdominal pain and/or fever. Bacteria in faeces are representative of the bacteria present in the GI tract, so the culture of a faecal sample is necessary for identification of GI tract colonization (Lautenbach *et al.* 2005).

Laboratory investigations are requested for bacterial infections such as *Salmonella*, *Campylobacter*, *Shigella* and *Clostridium difficile*, viral infections such as norovirus and rotavirus, and parasitic pathogens such as protozoa, tapeworms and amoebiasis (Weston 2008).

Diarrhoea can be defined as an unusual frequency of bowel actions (>3 times in 24 hours) with the passage of loose, unformed faeces (HPA 2008d). It may be attributable to a variety of bacterial, viral or parasitic pathogens and may be associated with antibiotic use, food or travel-related agents (King 2002). Prompt collection of a faecal sample for microbiological investigation is essential in determining the presence and identification of such agents.

Clostridium difficile

Clostridium difficile (C. diff) is recognized as a major healthcare-acquired infection causing diarrhoea associated with antibiotic use and environmental contamination (DH 2006). It is an anaerobic, Gram-positive bacterium that produces spores that are resistant to many disinfectants and can survive in harsh environmental conditions for prolonged periods (Soyfoo and Shaw 2008). It is recognized as having a significant impact upon patient morbidity and mortality and the signs and symptoms range from mild, self-limiting diarrhoea to severe, life-threatening conditions (DH 2007b). Those most at risk are older patients, immunocompromised patients, and those who have had a recent course of antibiotics.

Antimicrobials, particularly broad-spectrum antibiotics, alter the normal gut flora, allowing *C. diff* to proliferate and become pathogenic in the absence of other organisms (Carney *et al.* 2002). This leads to the production of toxins that irritate and cause mucosal damage of the intestinal tract.

The diagnosis of *C. diff* is through faecal sampling for culture and toxin analysis on patients who develop diarrhoea or who are admitted to healthcare institutions with unexplained diarrhoea.

Evidence-based approaches

Rationale

Timely and accurate identification of patients with infective diarrhoea is crucial in individual management of colonization and within the context of effective infection control management. Obtaining the specimen provides important diagnostic information that can be used to decide how to manage the patient's condition and the mode of treatment (Kyle 2007). Prompt diagnosis can influence aspects of care such as isolation and cohort nursing of infected patients, infection control procedures, environmental decontamination and antibiotic prescribing (DH 2007b).

Indications

Collection of a faecal specimen is indicated:

- to identify an infective agent in the presence of chronic, persistent or extended periods of diarrhoea

- if patients are systemically unwell with symptoms of diarrhoea, nausea and vomiting, pain, abdominal cramps, weight loss and/or fever
- to investigate diarrhoea occurring after foreign travel
- to identify parasites, such as tapeworms (Pellatt 2007b)
- to identify occult (hidden) blood if rectal bleeding is suspected (Pellatt 2007b)
- in the presence of diarrhoea associated with prolonged antibiotic administration
- for symptomatic contacts of individuals with certain organisms (e.g. *E. coli* 0157) where an infection can have serious clinical sequelae (HPA 2008d).

Contraindications

- As routine testing.
- In the absence of diarrhoea in suspected infective colonization.

Principles of care

A sample should be obtained as soon as possible after the onset of symptoms, ideally within the first 48 hours of illness, as the chance of successfully identifying a pathogen diminishes once the acute stage of the illness passes (Weston 2008). The specimen should be obtained using a clean technique in order to avoid inadvertent contamination of the specimen (HPA 2008d).

Preprocedural considerations

Assessment and recording tools

Collecting a faecal sample should be considered in conjunction with a comprehensive nursing assessment. This includes the observation of faeces for colour, presence of blood, consistency and odour (Pellatt 2007b). The most widely used assessment tool is the Bristol Stool Chart (Lewis and Heaton 1997), which categorizes faeces into seven classifications (types) based upon the appearance and consistency. Samples sent to the microbiology laboratory for analysis of suspected *C. difficile* should be classified as Type 6/7 on the Bristol Stool Chart (HPA 2008d).

In addition to other associated symptomology such as vomiting, fever, myalgia or abdominal pain, an accurate history should also include the onset, frequency and duration of diarrhoea, and other information such as history of foreign travel or potential food poisoning.

Procedure guideline 11.28 Faecal sampling

Essential equipment

- A clinically clean bedpan or disposable receiver
- Sterile specimen container (with integrated spoon) (see Figure 11.2)

- Gloves
- Apron
- Appropriate documentation/forms

(Continued)

Procedure guideline 11.28 (*Continued*)

Preprocedure

Action	Rationale
1 Discuss need and indication for procedure with patient.	To ensure the patient understands the procedure and gives valid consent (NMC 2008b, C).
2 Wash hands with bactericidal soap and water, or de-contaminate physically clean hands with alcohol-based handrub. Don apron and gloves.	To reduce the risk of cross-infection and specimen contamination (Fraise and Bradley 2009, E).

Procedure

Action	Rationale
3 Ask patient to defaecate into a clinically clean bedpan or receiver.	To avoid unnecessary contamination from other organisms (Kyle 2007, E).
4 *If the patient has been incontinent:* a sample may be obtained from bedlinen or pads: try to avoid contamination with urine.	Urine would cause contamination of the sample (Higgins 2008, E).
5 Using the integrated 'spoon', scoop enough faecal material to fill a third of the specimen container (or 10–15 mL of liquid stool).	To obtain a suitable amount of specimen for laboratory analysis. E
6 Apply specimen container lid securely.	To prevent risk of spillage. E

Postprocedure

Action	Rationale
7 Dispose of waste, remove apron and gloves, and wash hands with soap and water.	To reduce risk of cross-infection (DH 2006, C). Soap and water must be used as alcohol-based handrubs are ineffective for *C. diff* (DH 2007b, R).
8 Examine the specimen for features such as colour, consistency and odour. Record observations in nursing notes/care plans.	To complete as comprehensive nursing assessment (Pellatt 2007a, C).
9 *In cases of suspected tapeworms:* segments of tapeworm are easily seen in faeces and should be sent to the laboratory for identification.	Unless the head is dislodged, the tapeworm will continue to grow. Laboratory confirmation of the presence of the head is essential (Gould and Brooker 2008, E).
10 Label sample and complete microbiology request form (including relevant information such as onset and duration of diarrhoea, fever or recent foreign travel).	To maintain accurate records and provide accurate information for laboratory analysis (NMC 2009, C; Weston 2008, E).
11 Dispatch sample to the laboratory as soon as possible or refrigerate at 4–8°C and dispatch within 12 hours.	To increase the chance of accurate organism identification and to ensure the best possible conditions for laboratory analysis (Higgins 2007, E).
12 *In cases of suspected amoebic dysentery:* dispatch the sample to the laboratory immediately.	The parasite causing amoebiasis must be identified when mobile and survives for a short period only. Therefore, faeces should remain fresh and warm (Kyle 2007, E).
13 *In cases of prolonged diarrhoea, especially in the presence of a fever:* dispatch the sample to the laboratory immediately.	Due to the risk of *C. diff* and to ensure prompt diagnosis and initiation of appropriate infection control measures (DH 2007b, C).

Postprocedural considerations

Immediate care

A faecal sample should be transported to the laboratory and processed as soon as possible because a number of important pathogens, such as *Shigella*, may not survive changes in pH and temperature once outside the body (HPA 2008d).

If there is an anticipated delay in despatching the sample to the laboratory, it should be refrigerated at 4–8°C and processed within 12 hours (HPA 2008d).

Ongoing care

The result of specimen analysis will determine the patient's ongoing care. The involvement of the microbiology and infection control teams is essential to ensure prudent and safe treatment and nursing care. This should include:

- effective handwashing techniques to minimize the transmission of organisms
- implementation of Standard Precautions (gloves and aprons)
- nursing patients with unexpected or unexplained diarrhoea in isolation *or* cohorted with other infected patients (DH 2007b)
- thorough environmental decontamination (DH 2007b)
- prudent antibiotic prescribing (DH 2007a).

Education of patient and others

Patients should be provided with information and involved in their care as much as they choose to be (NMC 2008a). Confirmation of an infection diagnosis should be relayed to patients and their families alongside information on management strategies (such as antibiotic therapy, the use of PPE, reasons for isolation and visiting restrictions). The provision of written information, such as leaflets, may also prove useful.

Specimen collection: respiratory tract secretion sampling

Definition

Obtaining a specimen from the respiratory tract is important in diagnosing illness, infections and conditions such as tuberculosis and lung cancer (Guest 2008). A sample can be obtained invasively or non-invasively and the correct technique will enable a representative sample to identify respiratory tract pathology and to guide treatment.

Related theory

Excessive respiratory secretions may be due to increased mucus production in cases of infection, impaired mucociliary transport or a weak cough reflex (Hess 2002). Lower airway secretions that are not cleared provide an ideal medium for bacterial growth. Suitable microbiological analysis in diagnosing infection will depend upon (HPA 2008a):

- the adequacy of lower respiratory tract specimens
- avoidance of contamination by upper respiratory tract and oral flora
- use of microscopic techniques and culture methods
- current and recent antimicrobial therapy.

Evidence-based approaches

Rationale

The main aim of sputum/secretion collection is to provide reliable information on the causative agent of bacterial, viral or fungal infection within the respiratory tract and its susceptibility to antibiotics for guiding treatment (Ioanas *et al.* 2001).

Indications

A respiratory tract secretion specimen is indicated:

- when there are clinical signs and symptoms of a chest infection, such as a productive cough, particularly with purulent secretions
- if there are signs of systemic infection or in patients with a PUO.

Methods of non-invasive and semi-invasive sampling

Obtaining a sputum sample

Sputum is a combination of mucus, inflammatory and epithelial cells, and degradation products from the lower respiratory tract (Dulak 2005). It is never free from organisms since material originating from the lower respiratory tract has to pass through the pharynx and the mouth, which have commensal populations of bacteria (Thomson 2002). However, it is important to ensure that material sent to the microbiology laboratory is of sputum rather than a saliva sample, which will contain squamous epithelial cells and be unrepresentative of the underlying pulmonary pathology.

Sputum produced as a result of infection is usually purulent and a good sample can yield a high bacterial load (Weston 2008). For patients who are self-ventilating, co-operative, able to cough and expectorate, and able to follow commands, a sputum sample is a suitable collection method. A sufficient quality of sputum will yield a representative specimen and an early morning specimen is thought to be of the best quality (Weston 2008). In cases of suspected *Mycobacterium tuberculosis*, three sputum specimens need to be collected on consecutive days before the pathogenic organisms can be isolated and appropriate treatment initiated. See Figure 11.1 and Procedure guideline 11.29.

Nasopharyngeal samples

Sampling techniques to obtain specimens from the nasopharynx are semi-invasive but can be used on patients who are self-ventilating. They are indicated in suspected viral infections such as respiratory syncytial virus (RSV), influenza and parainfluenza. The main aim is to collect epithelial cells from the posterior nasopharynx and a sample can be obtained using nasal washing or vacuum-assisted aspiration (see Procedure guideline 11.30).

Invasive sampling techniques

Intubated patients who are unable to clear secretions independently or who require more accurate specimen collection may need a more invasive technique to obtain a sample. Invasive techniques obtain secretions directly from the lower airway and are designed to avoid contamination by upper airway colonization, which may lead to misinterpretation of cultures (Ioanas *et al.* 2001).

691

Vacuum-assisted aspirate via endotracheal tube

Endotracheal suctioning is frequently used as a diagnostic method and for obtaining specimens in intubated patients with suspected pulmonary infection. This technique bypasses the upper respiratory airways and provides an accurate microbiological result. Suctioning aids the clearance of secretions by the application of negative pressure through a sterile flexible suction catheter or a closed suction system. A sterile sputum trap is attached to the suction catheter at one end, whilst the other end is attached to the suction tubing to collect the sample (Figure 11.12).

Bronchoalveolar lavage (BAL)

Bronchoalveolar lavage is a reliable and accurate technique that provides a good diagnostic yield in cases of pulmonary infection, particularly invasive fungal infections (Ioanas *et al.* 2001). It is used to clear secretions and to obtain washings for the retrieval of cellular and non-cellular components of the epithelial surface of the lower respiratory tract (HPA 2008a). It is performed in ventilated patients who will be sedated and paralysed for the procedure to permit effective ventilation and to prevent mucosal damage.

A flexible bronchoscope is inserted through the endotracheal tube (ETT) and advanced distally into a subsegmental bronchus. The area selected for sampling is based upon a correspondent area of infiltration on a chest X-ray or by visualization of a subsegment containing purulent secretions (Ioanas *et al.* 2001). A volume of sterile 0.9% sodium chloride (normally 20–30 mL) is then instilled through a port on the bronchoscope and suctioned back through another port into a sterile sputum trap. The procedure is repeated 3–5 times and the samples are then dispatched to the laboratory for microscopy and microbiological analysis.

Legal and professional issues

Competencies

Practitioners must be competent and feel confident that they have the knowledge, skill and understanding to undertake respiratory tract secretion sampling for microbiological analysis (NMC 2008a). For more advanced skills of specimen collection such as suctioning, the practitioner should receive training and be assessed on their knowledge and understanding of the technique and potential adverse effects that may occur such as hypoxia, cardiovascular instability and mucosal trauma (Thomson 2000). Bronchoalvolar lavage is normally performed by a member of the medical team who has received specialist training and has been deemed competent in the skill.

Preprocedural considerations

Equipment

The use of vacuum-assisted and invasive suctioning techniques requires a comprehensive assessment of clinical

Figure 11.12 Types of vacuum-assisted sputum traps.

indication and safety considerations. These include the following.

- The use of an appropriately sized, single-use, multi-eyed suction catheter which causes less tracheal mucosal trauma (NHSQIS 2007). If suctioning through an ETT, the suction catheter diameter should be half the diameter or less which prevents occlusion of the airway and avoids generation of large negative intrathoracic pressures (Thomson 2000) (see Table 11.5).
- The use of the lowest effective suction pressure that is high enough to clear secretions whilst avoiding trauma to the bronchial mucosa.
- Ensuring suction duration time of <10 seconds to decrease the risk of adverse side-effects (NHSQIS 2007).

Procedures that involve suctioning present a risk of suction-induced hypoxaemia, hypertension, cardiac arrhythmias and other problems that warrant patient monitoring, in particular oxygen saturation and cardiac monitoring (Thomson 2000).

Pharmacological support

Adequate analgesia is a key consideration in ensuring that an effective sputum expectoration technique can be achieved. For example, preprocedural analgesia should be given time to be effective, and wounds need to be supported to maximize inhalation and minimize pain (Guest 2008).

Nebulization of 0.9% sodium chloride and/or mucolytic agents, such as N-acetylcysteine, may need to be administered

Table 11.5 Catheter sizes and suction pressures

Patient age	Catheter size (French)	Suction pressure (mmHg)
Premature infant	6	80–100
Infant	8	80–100
Toddler/preschooler	10	100–120
School age	12	100–120
Adolescent/adult	14	120–150

to help loosen tenacious secretions and to elicit an effective cough (Rajiv 2007).

Non-pharmacological support

Collaboration with the physiotherapy team may assist in obtaining a good-quality sample (Hess 2002). For sputum sampling, physiotherapeutic modalities implemented may include appropriate positioning, active cycle of breathing, deep breathing and effective coughing techniques (HPA 2008a).

Specific patient preparation

Patient position is important in optimizing secretion sampling. Patients should be sat upright or on the edge of the bed, if able, or in a high semi-Fowler position (head elevated to 30–45°) in bed supported by pillows (Dulak 2005).

The quality and quantity of secretion production and mucociliary clearance depend on systemic hydration. Patient hydration can boost sputum production to enable a good sample (Dulak 2005). This can be further enhanced with sufficient airway humidity and nebulization.

Procedure guideline 11.29 Sputum sampling

Essential equipment

- Universal container
- Apron
- Non-sterile gloves
- Eye protection (e.g. goggles/visor)
- Appropriate documentation/form

Optional equipment

- Nebulizer

Preprocedure

Action	Rationale
1 Explain and discuss the procedure with the patient.	To ensure the patient understands the procedure and gives valid consent (NMC 2008b, C).
2 Fully explain the steps of the procedure.	The procedure requires the patient to fully understand and co-operate in order to optimize the quality of the sample (Dulak 2005, E).
3 Position patient upright in a chair or in a semi- or high-Fowler position, supported as necessary with pillows.	For comfort and to facilitate optimum chest/lung expansion. E
4 *If secretions thick/tenacious or having difficulty clearing secretions:* administer nebulization therapy and/or enlist help of the physiotherapist.	To loosen secretions and to assist in techniques that will optimize sputum sample collection (Hess 2002, C).
5 Wash hands with bactericidal soap/decontaminate physically clean hands with alcohol rub. Don apron, gloves and eye protection.	To reduce the risk of cross-infection or splash injury to practitioner and specimen collection (Fraise and Bradley 2009, E).

Procedure

6 Ask patient to take three deep breaths in through their nose, exhale through pursed lips and then force a deep cough.	Deep breathing helps loosen secretions and a deep cough will ensure a lower respiratory tract sample is obtained (Dulack 2005, C).
7 Ask patient to expectorate into a clean container and secure lid.	To prevent contamination. E

Postprocedure

8 Dispose of waste, remove apron, gloves and eye protection and wash/decontaminate hands.	To ensure correct clinical waste management and to reduce the risk of cross-infection (DH 2006, D).
9 Label sample and complete microbiology request form (including relevant information such as indication for sample and current/recent antimicrobial therapy).	To maintain accurate records and provide accurate information for laboratory analysis (NMC 2009, C; Weston 2008, E).
10 Dispatch to the laboratory as soon as possible within 2 hours.	To increase the chance of accurate organism identification (Higgins 2007, C).

693

Procedure guideline 11.30 Nasopharyngeal wash: syringe method

Essential equipment

- Universal container
- 5 mL syringe or wide-bore bladder syringe
- Sterile tubing cut to approximately 2–3″ (e.g. size 8 Fr NG tube or cut off tip from a suction catheter if using a 5 mL syringe)
- 3–5 mL 0.9% sodium chloride

- Viral transport medium (VTM) (if required by laboratory)
- Apron
- Non-sterile gloves
- Eye protection (e.g. goggles/visor)
- Appropriate documentation/form

Preprocedure

Action	Rationale
1 Explain and discuss the procedure with the patient.	To ensure the patient understands the procedure and gives valid consent (NMC 2008b, C).
2 Position patient upright in a chair or in a semi- or high-Fowler position, supported as necessary with pillows.	For comfort and to facilitate optimum specimen collection. E
3 Wash hands with bactericidal soap/decontaminate physically clean hands with alcohol rub. Don apron, gloves and eye protection.	To reduce the risk of cross-infection, splash injury to practitioner and specimen collection (Fraise and Bradley 2009, E).

Procedure

4 Fill syringe with 3–5 mL of 0.9% sodium chloride and attach tubing to syringe tip.	To facilitate instillation of 0.9% sodium chloride high into the patient's nostril. E
5 Ask patient to tilt their head backwards slightly whilst sitting upright.	To promote the flow of 0.9% sodium chloride into the nostril. E
6 Insert tubing into nostril and quickly instil 0.9% sodium chloride into one nostril while holding the second nostril closed.	To facilitate optimal recovery of epithelial cells. E
7 Aspirate fluid while withdrawing and rotating the tube to dislodge cells and secretions. NB: recovery must occur rapidly or instilled fluid will drain down the throat.	To obtain desired nasopharyngeal specimen. E
8 **Either:** Where appropriate, patient may tilt head forward and gently push the fluid out of the nostril into a sterile container. **Or:** *If aspirated*: inject aspirated specimen from syringe into suitable dry, sterile container or one containing viral transport medium, according to virology laboratory requirements.	Patients may find this method more comfortable. E To ensure a good-quality specimen and to prevent cross-contamination. E
9 Repeat procedure with other nostril and inject specimen into the same container (see Action Figure 9).	A combined specimen will promote optimal yield of micro-organisms. E

Postprocedure

10 Remove apron, gloves and eye protection. Dispose of waste, and wash/decontaminate hands.	To ensure correct clinical waste management and to reduce the risk of cross-infection (DH 2006, C).
11 Label sample and complete microbiology request form (including relevant information such as: indication for sample and current/recent antimicrobial therapy).	To maintain accurate records and provide accurate information for laboratory analysis (NMC 2009, C; Weston 2008, E).
12 Dispatch to the laboratory as soon as possible within 2 hours.	To increase the chance of accurate organism identification (Higgins 2007, C).

Action Figure 9   Nasopharyngeal wash: syringe method.

Procedure guideline 11.31 Nasopharyngeal wash: vacuum-assisted aspirate method

Essential equipment

- Suction pump (wall or portable)
- Sterile suction catheter (see Table 11.5 for appropriate size)
- Sterile sputum trap
- Viral transport medium (if required by laboratory)
- Apron
- Sterile gloves
- Eye protection (e.g. goggles/visor)
- Appropriate documentation/form

Preprocedure

Action	Rationale
1 Explain and discuss the procedure with the patient.	To ensure the patient understands the procedure and gives valid consent (NMC 2008b, C).
2 Position patient upright in a chair or in a semi- or high-Fowler position, supported as necessary with pillows.	For comfort and to facilitate optimum specimen collection. E
3 Wash hands with bactericidal soap/decontaminate physically clean hands with alcohol rub. Don apron and eye protection.	To reduce the risk of cross-infection, splash injury to practitioner and specimen collection (Fraise and Bradley 2009, E).

Procedure

Action	Rationale
4 Attach suction tubing to the male adaptor of the specimen trap and attach rubber tubing on the trap to the end of the suction catheter, leaving the packaging on.	To enable correct set-up and to ensure suction catheter remains sterile. E
5 Turn suction on and adjust to correct pressure (see Table 11.5).	To ensure suction pressure is high enough to clear secretions whilst avoiding trauma. E
6 Don sterile glove and remove suction catheter from packaging aseptically.	To prevent cross-contamination of specimen. E
7 Ask patient to tilt their head backwards slightly whilst sitting upright.	To optimize recovery of specimen collection. E
8 Without applying suction, insert catheter into the nostril and direct posteriorly towards the external ear (see Action Figure 8). NB: the depth of insertion necessary to reach the posterior pharynx is equivalent to the distance between the anterior naris and the external ear.	To prevent damage to the nasopharynx and to minimize patient discomfort. E

(Continued)

Procedure guideline 11.31 *(Continued)*

9 Apply suction. Using a rotating movement, slowly withdraw the catheter. NB: catheter should remain in the nasopharynx no longer than 10 seconds.	To prevent damage to the nasopharynx and to obtain desired nasopharyngeal specimen. E
10 Hold trap upright to prevent secretions being suctioned into suction pump.	To prevent the loss of specimen. E
11 Rinse catheter (if necessary) with approximately 20 mL of viral transport medium.	To ensure maximum recovery of epithelial cells and to prevent cross-contamination (Higgins 2007, C).
12 Disconnect suction. Depending on sputum trap type, connect tubing to arm of sputum trap to seal or detach and apply sealable lid.	To ensure specimen container is securely sealed and to prevent cross-contamination. E

Postprocedure

13 Dispose of waste, remove apron, gloves and eye protection and wash/decontaminate hands.	To ensure correct clinical waste management and to reduce the risk of cross-infection (DH 2006, C).
14 Label sample and complete microbiology request form (including relevant information such as: indication for sample and current/recent antimicrobial therapy).	To maintain accurate records and provide accurate information for laboratory analysis (NMC 2009, C; Weston 2008, E).
15 Dispatch to the laboratory as soon as possible within 2 hours.	To increase the chance of accurate organism identification (Higgins 2007, C).

Action Figure 8 Nasopharyngeal wash: vacuum-assisted aspirate method.

Postprocedural considerations

Immediate care

Many organisms responsible for infection of the lower respiratory tract do not survive well outside the host, so specimens should be dispatched to the laboratory immediately and processed within 2 hours (Gould and Brooker 2008). If there is an anticipated delay in despatching the sample to the laboratory, it should be refrigerated at 4–8°C and sent as soon as possible (HPA 2008a).

Documentation

The date and time of when a sputum sample is sent to the laboratory should be documented clearly and promptly in

the patient's notes and care plan (NMC 2009). This should be done alongside documentation in relation to significant findings that have prompted the collection of the sample such as a description of the type and colour of sputum/secretions and method used to obtain the sample.

Specimen collection: pleural fluid

Definition

Specimens of pleural fluid for microbiological analysis are obtained by thoracocentesis to assist in the diagnosis of infection in fluid that has accumulated within the inner and outer (visceral and parietal) layers of the pleural cavity such as parapneumonia, emphyema and tuberculosis (Barnes *et al.* 2005). In the context of microbiological analysis, thoracocentesis is the insertion of a needle into the pleural space to obtain a fluid sample for diagnostic testing (Rushing 2006).

Anatomy and physiology

See Chapter 10.

Related theory

Pleural fluid is generated from pleural vessels as a result of negative intrapleural pressure. It exits via the parietal pleural lymphatic system. Pleural effusions occur when there is an accumulation of fluid within the pleural cavity, which implies either an increased production of fluid that exceeds the capacity of lymphatic removal and/or obstruction of drainage of the pleural space (Pendharkar and Tremblay 2007).

Analysis of pleural effusion fluid is obtained via thoracocentesis, which determines the cause of the effusion. Effusion occurs when factors that influence the formation and absorption of fluid are altered either systematically, for example in cirrhosis or congestive heart failure (transudate effusions), or locally, for example in infection or malignancy (exudate effusions). Pleural fluid in a patient with undiagnosed exudative effusions should be cultured for bacteria (aerobic and anaerobic), mycobacteria and fungi (Barnes *et al.* 2005).

Infection of pleural fluid caused by bacteria, viruses or fungi may originate in the pleura or translocate from another site. Micro-organisms can infiltrate the pleural space by various routes: directly in cases of empyema, primary tuberculous focus rupturing into the pleural cavity, from an adjacent area of pneumonia, thoracic surgery or drainage, chest trauma or by transdiaphragmatic spread from intra-abdominal infection (HPA 2008e).

Pleural fluid is a clear, straw-coloured fluid that contains a small number of white blood cells (WBC) but no red blood cells (RBC) or micro-organsims (HPA 2008e). In cases of suspected infection, it appears cloudy due to the presence of micro-organsims and/or increased WBC (Barnes *et al.* 2005). Differential WBC counts assist further in the diagnosis of infection because increased numbers of neutrophils indicate bacterial infection, whereas an increased number of lymphocytes is indicative of malignancy or tuberculosis (Conner *et al.* 2003). Other changes include decreased glucose levels, increased protein or albumin levels and disturbances in lactate level.

Evidence-based approaches
Rationale

Detection of micro-organsims in fluids that are normally sterile indicates significant infection (HPA 2008e). Pleural fluid may be sent to the microbiology laboratory for bacterial culture to identify the cause of an effusion, isolate pathogenic micro-organisms and establish susceptibility to antimicrobial therapy.

Indications

Obtaining a specimen of pleural fluid is indicated in patients with:

- bacterial pneumonia with radiological suggestion of significant pleural effusions
- systemic infection with pyrexia, severe pleuritic pain and leucocytosis
- suspected tuberculous focus with clinical signs or radiological evidence of significant pleural effusions (HPA 2008e).

Methods of pleural fluid collection

Diagnosis of infection is established by the microbiological analysis of pleural fluid obtained by thoracocentesis using a strict aseptic technique, including meticulous skin antisepsis (Barnes *et al.* 2005).

Following clinical assessment and possible radiological guidance, local anaesthetic is infiltrated into the area of intended thoracocentesis. A needle is advanced superiorly to the ribs to avoid neuromuscular bundle damage and to reduce the risk of causing a pneumothorax (Pendharkar and Tremblay 2007). Fifty to 100 mL of fluid are drawn, transferred into sterile container and sent to the laboratory for analysis.

The samples can initially be observed for characteristics such as colour and turbidity, and Gram stains allow for direct observation of bacteria under a microscope. When bacterial infection of pleural fluid is suspected, a specimen should be drawn and inoculated directly into aerobic and anaerobic blood culture bottles (Pendharkar and Tremblay 2007).

Specimens should be dispatched to the laboratory immediately and liaison with the laboratory is essential to enable efficient processing of the sample. If there are any delays, the sample should be refrigerated at 4°C (HPA 2008e).

Endoscopic investigations

Definition

Occasionally patients will be required to undergo further invasive diagnostic procedures such as an endoscopy. An endoscopy is the direct visual examination of the gastrointestinal tract (Figure 11.13) which may include gastroscopy or colonoscopy. Endoscopy allows the practitioner to evaluate the appearance of the visualized mucosa for the purpose of diagnosis and therapeutic procedures (Smith and Watson 2005).

Gastroscopy

Definition

A gastroscopy or oesophagogastroduodenoscopy (OGD) is a procedure in which a long flexible endoscope is passed

697

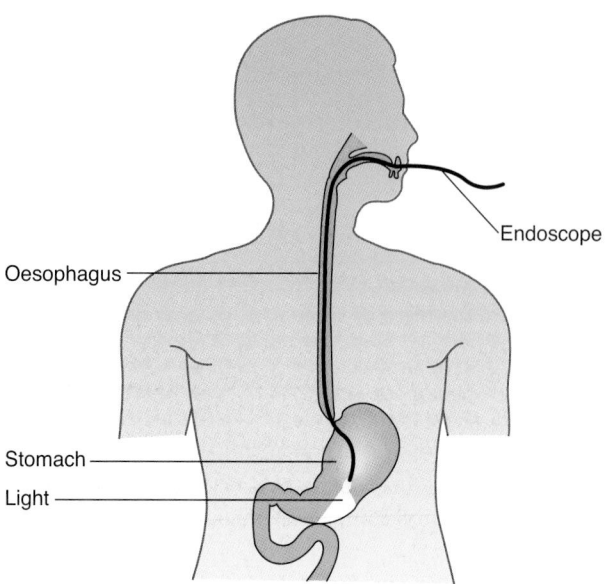

Figure 11.13 Endoscopy. © Cancer Help UK, the patient information website of Cancer Research UK: www.cancerhelp.org.uk. Used with permission.

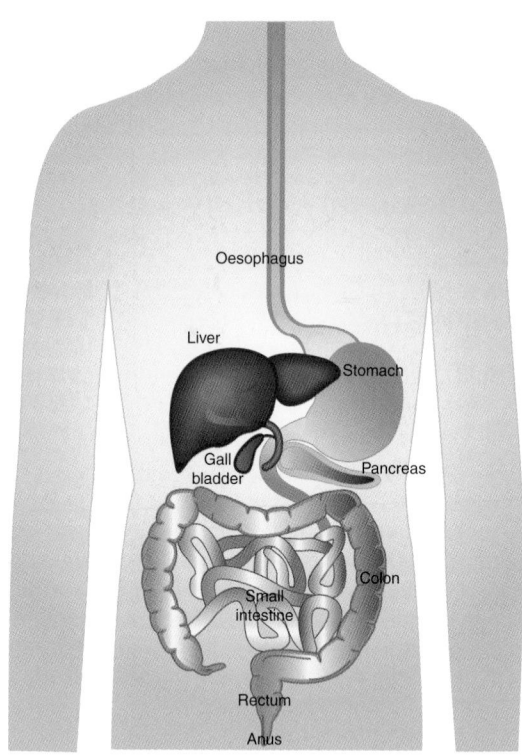

Figure 11.14 Anatomy of the lower gastrointestinal tract.

through the mouth, allowing the doctor or nurse endoscopist to look directly at the lining of the oesophagus, stomach and proximal duodenum. The endoscope is generally less than 10 mm in diameter but a larger scope may be required for therapeutic procedures where suction channels are required (Smith and Watson 2005) (Figure 11.13).

Anatomy and physiology

See Figure 11.14.

Oesophagus

The oesophagus is a muscular thin-walled tube approximately 25 cm long and about 2 cm in diameter. It is located behind the trachea and in front of the vertebral column. There are two sphincters within the oesophagus: the upper or hypopharyngeal sphincter and the lower gastro-oesophageal sphincter. Food passing into the stomach is controlled by the lower sphincter. The oesophagus has three layers, the mucosa, submucosa and the muscularis, with the innermost layer consisting of stratified squamous epithelium (Smith and Watson 2005, Waugh *et al.* 2006).

Stomach

The stomach is located between the oesophagus and the small intestine. It is a J-shaped dilated portion of the alimentary tract. It is also located between the epigastric, umbilical and left hypochondriac regions of the abdomen. It is divided into three regions: the fundus, body and antrum. Distally, the pyloric sphincter is located between the stomach and the duodenum. The stomach has three muscle layers to allow for gastric motility to move the contents adequately whereas

other parts of the alimentary tract only have two muscle layers (Smith and Watson 2005, Waugh *et al.* 2006).

Duodenum

The duodenum is part of the small intestine. It is approximately 25 cm long and 3.5 cm in diameter. It is generally C-shaped and muscular, beginning at the pyloric sphincter of the stomach and joining the jejunum. Both the pancreas and the gall bladder release secretions into the duodenum (Smith and Watson 2005, Waugh *et al.* 2006).

Evidence-based approaches

Rationale

A gastroscopy is undertaken to investigate symptoms originating from the upper GI tract such as reflux and dysphagia. The doctor or nurse endoscopist is able to use direct vision to diagnose, sample and document changes in the upper GI tract.

Indications

- Dysphagia.
- Odynophagia.
- Achalasia.
- Unresponsive reflux disease.
- Gastric and peptic ulcers.
- Haematemesis and melaena.
- Suspected carcinoma.
- Oesophageal or gastric varices.
- Monitoring Barrett's oesophagus disease.

Contraindications

- Fractured base of skull.
- Metastatic adenocarcinoma.
- Some head/neck tumours.
- Symptoms that are functional in origin.

Legal and professional issues

Nurse endoscopists

In some centres nurse endoscopists work alongside medical endoscopists undertaking endoscopy. In 1995 the British Society of Gastroenterology supported the development of non-medical endoscopists. The nurse endoscopist must work within their own professional boundaries and complement the medical endoscopist teams (Smith and Watson 2005). It is essential that all practitioners are adequately trained in the administration of conscious sedation, aware of its side-effects and reversal agents. Clinical units must also limit the possibility of overdose, particularly with midazolam, as highlighted by the NPSA (2008).

Consent

It is essential that informed consent is obtained as previously discussed in this chapter prior to any investigation. This is important as conscious sedation may be utilized during this procedure.

Preprocedural considerations

Equipment

To conduct a gastroscopy, a flexible side- or end-viewing endoscope is required. The endoscope allows visualization of the oesophagus, stomach and proximal duodenum (Smith and Watson 2005). Access to resuscitation equipment is also essential if conscious sedation is going to be administered (BSG 2003).

Assessment and recording tools

A medical and nursing history and assessment must be taken to identify any care needs or concerns that may be significant, in particular, the patient's current drug therapy, drug reactions or allergies, any organ dysfunctions such as cardiac and/or respiratory disease and previous or current illnesses. It is also important to be aware of any coagulopathies as samples of tissue or biopsy may need to be taken during the procedure. This can be pre-empted by reviewing blood results prior to the gastroscopy. A set of observations including temperature, pulse, blood pressure, respiration rate and oxygen saturations should also be taken to identify any preprocedural abnormalities and to provide a baseline. If the patient has diabetes, a blood glucose level should also be checked (BSG 2003, Smith and Watson 2005).

Pharmacological support

Prior to the procedure a local anaesthetic spray may be used on the back of the throat. In some cases conscious sedation may be administered. This technique involves the administration of a benzodiazepine such as midazolam in small doses prescribed by a medical practitioner. Doses must be titrated for elderly patients or those with co-morbidities such as cardiac or renal failure. Oxygen therapy should also be administered for patients at risk or those requiring sedation. Generally 2 litres per minute is adequate for most circumstances to maintain oxygen saturation levels and prevent hypoxaemia (BSG 2003).

Specific patient preparations

The patient must fast for at least 4 hours prior to the gastroscopy to ensure that the stomach is relatively empty. This increases the visual field for the endoscopist and also minimizes the risk of aspiration if the patient vomits. The nurse can also assist by getting the patient to lie on their left side on the trolley (Smith and Watson 2005). If a sedative is used it is essential that the patient is monitored with pulse oximetry and observed for any respiratory depression. Nursing staff can observe and record oxygen saturations and respiratory rate. ECG monitoring may only be required if a patient is at risk of cardiac instability during the procedure (BSG 2003).

Postprocedural considerations

Immediate care

Physiological monitoring must continue in the immediate recovery period. Supplemental oxygen and oxygen saturations may be required especially if a sedative has been used. The patient should avoid drinking or eating for an hour after the use of the throat spray to minimize the risk of aspiration. Once stable, awake and reviewed by the team, the patient may be discharged or transferred to another department.

Ongoing care

It is recommended that patients who have been sedated with an intravenous benzodiazepine do not drive a car, operate machinery, sign legal documents or drink alcohol for 24 hours (BSG 2003). This is irrespective of whether their sedation has been reversed with flumazenil. The patient must be accompanied home if they have been given a sedative. The accompanying adult should stay with the patient for 12 hours at home if they live alone. It is important to remember that aspiration pneumonia may develop hours or days later and the patient should be informed to report any symptoms such as temperatures or breathing difficulty (BSG 2003, Smith and Watson 2005).

Documentation

Any samples should be clearly documented with the appropriate forms as previously discussed in this chapter. All drugs administered, complications and/or findings should be documented.

Complications

Respiratory depression

If oversedation occurs, respiratory function will be affected. It is essential that close monitoring occurs during and after the procedure. A reversal agent may be required such as flumezanil for midazolam (BSG 2003, Smith and Watson 2005).

Perforation

Although rare, it is possible that perforation of the oesophagus, stomach or duodenum may occur. Further medical and/or surgical intervention will be required to manage this potential complication (Putcha and Burdick 2003, Smith and Watson 2005).

Haemorrhage

Where biopsy samples have been taken, this may increase the risk of postprocedural bleeding. Further intervention may be required to stop the bleeding. Patients should be advised to seek medical assistance if there are signs of bleeding which include the presence of fresh blood in the sputum and melaena.

This will be dependent on the specific aetiology of the bleed, for example whether it is from varices when variceal band ligation may be required (SIGN 2008, Smith and Watson 2005).

Colonoscopy

Definition

A colonoscopy is conducted by inserting a colonoscope through the anus into the colon. It provides information regarding the lower GI tract and allows a complete examination of the colon. The colonoscope is similar to the endoscope used in gastroscopy. Its length ranges from 1.2 to 1.8 metres long. It is the most effective method of diagnosing rectal polyps and carcinoma (Smith and Watson 2005, Swan 2005, Taylor et al. 2009).

Anatomy and physiology

The colon is about 1.5 metres long. It begins at the caecum and ends at the rectum and anal canal (Waugh et al. 2006). See Figure 11.14.

Caecum

The caecum is about 8–9 cm long and opens from the ileum and ileocaecal valve (Waugh et al. 2006).

Colon

The colon consists of three parts. The ascending colon runs from the caecum and joins the transverse colon and the hepatic flexure. The transverse colon is in front of the duodenum where it joins the descending colon at the splenic flexure. The descending colon travels down toward the middle of the abdomen where it joins the sigmoid colon which is S-shaped and becomes the rectum (Waugh et al. 2006).

Rectum and anal canal

The rectum is approximately 13 cm long and is a dilated section of the colon. It joins the anal canal which is approximately 3.8 cm long (Waugh et al. 2006).

Evidence-based approaches

Rationale

A colonoscopy is performed to investigate specific symptoms originating from the lower GI tract such as bleeding. The doctor or nurse endoscopist is able to use direct vision to diagnose, sample and document changes in the lower GI tract (Swan 2005, Taylor et al. 2009).

Indications

- Screening of patients with family history of colon cancer, a serious but highly curable malignancy.
- Determining the presence of suspected polyps.
- Monitoring ulcerative colitis.
- Monitoring diverticulosis and diverticulitis.
- Active or occult lower gastrointestinal bleeding.
- Unexplained bleeding or faecal occult blood.
- Abdominal symptoms, such as pain or discomfort, particularly if associated with weight loss or anaemia.
- Chronic diarrhoea, constipation or a change in bowel habits.
- Palliative supportive treatments such as stent insertion.

Contraindications

- Upper gastrointestinal bleeding.
- Inflammatory bowel disease follow-up.
- Acute diarrhoea.

Legal and professional issues

Competencies and consent will be the same as those discussed in the Gastroscopy section.

Preprocedural considerations

Equipment

A colonoscope is a flexible endoscope that allows direct visualization of the rectum and colon (Smith and Watson 2005).

Pharmacological support

Bowel preparation agents, such as senna tablets and Citramag, are given to the patient to take 1 day prior to the colonoscopy to clear the bowel. A sedative and possibly an analgesic are usually administered before the procedure. This involves the administration of a benzodiazepine such as midazolam and an opioid such as fentanyl or pethidine which have been prescribed by a medical practitioner. Doses must be titrated for elderly patients or those with co-morbidities such as cardiac or renal failure. An antispasmodic may also be given. Oxygen therapy should also be administered during sedation. Generally 2 litres per minute is adequate for most circumstances to maintain oxygen saturation levels and prevent hypoxaemia (BSG 2003, Riley 2008, Swan 2005).

Specific patient preparations

To complete a successful colonoscopy, the bowel must be clean so that the physician can clearly view the colon. It is very important that the patient follows all the instructions given for bowel preparation well in advance of the procedure. Without proper preparation, the colonoscopy will not be successful and the test may have to be repeated. If the patient feels nauseated or vomits while taking the bowel preparation, they are advised to wait 30 minutes before drinking more fluid and start with small sips of solution. Some activity such as walking or a few cream crackers may help decrease the nausea (Smith and Watson 2005, Swan 2005).

Two days prior to the endoscopy, specific light foods may be eaten, such as steamed white fish, and others avoided, such as high-fibre foods. On the day before the colonoscopy, breakfast from the approved food groups may be eaten while drinking plenty of clear fluids. On the day of the procedure patients can drink tea/coffee with no milk 4 hours before and water up to 2 hours before (Smith and Watson 2005, Swan 2005).

A medical and nursing history and assessment must be undertaken to identify any care needs or concerns that may be significant. In particular, this should cover the patient's current drug therapy, drug reactions or allergies, any organ dysfunctions such as cardiac and/or respiratory disease, and previous or current illnesses. It is also important to be aware of any coagulopathies as samples of tissue or biopsy may need to be taken during the procedure. This can be pre-empted by reviewing blood results prior to the colonoscopy. A set of observations including temperature, pulse, blood pressure, respiration rate and oxygen saturations should also be taken to identify any preprocedural abnormalities and to provide a baseline. If the patient has diabetes, a blood glucose level should also be checked (BSG 2003, Smith and Watson 2005).

Postprocedural considerations

Immediate care

Physiological monitoring and care post sedation should be the same as those for gastroscopy. However, larger doses of sedative and opioids may have been used so further observation is required. The patient may feel some cramping or a sensation of having gas, but this quickly passes on eating and drinking. Bloating and distension typically occur for about an hour after the examination until the air is expelled. Unless otherwise instructed, the patient may immediately resume a normal diet, but it is generally recommended that the patient waits until the day after the procedure to resume normal activities.

Ongoing care

If a biopsy was taken or a polyp was removed, the patient may notice light rectal bleeding for 1–2 days after the procedure; large amounts of bleeding, the passage of clots or abdominal pain should be reported immediately.

Complications

Perforation

During the procedure the greatest risk or possible complication is bowel perforation. This occurs in 1 in 1000 cases. The nurse monitoring the patient after colonoscopy should be familiar with potential signs and symptoms such as unresolved abdominal pain, rigidity and/or bleeding. If a perforation occurs surgical intervention is likely to be required (Smith and Watson 2005, Swan 2002).

Haemorrhage

On average, haemorrhage occurs in 3 in 1000 procedures but the incidence and complication rates may be higher where a procedure involves a polypectomy. The postprocedure monitoring by the nurse again includes observing for signs and symptoms of bleeding (Smith and Watson 2005, Swan 2002). Depending on the severity of the bleed, it may be managed conservatively or in haemodynamically unstable patients angiography may be required (Farrell and Friedman 2005).

Cystoscopy

Definition

Cystoscopy examines the inside of the urethra and bladder using a cystoscope and is one of the most widely used invasive urological investigations. It gives direct visualization of the urethra and bladder for both males and females but it is especially important in males as the urethra is much more complex (Fillingham and Douglas 2004, Rodgers *et al.* 2006).

Anatomy and physiology

Urethra

The urethra extends from the external urethral orifice to the bladder (Waugh *et al.* 2006).

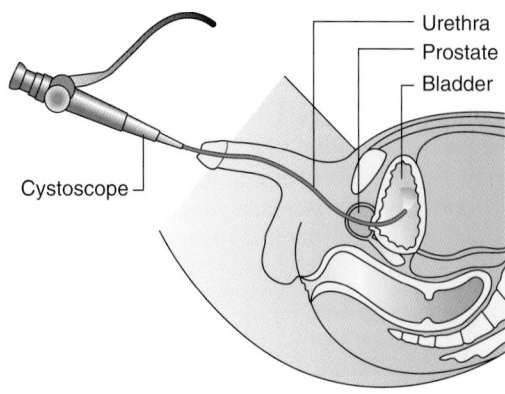

Figure 11.15 Cystoscopy for a man. © Cancer Help UK, the patient information website of Cancer Research UK: www.cancerhelp.org.uk. Used with permission.

Male urethra

The male urethra is approximately 19–20 cm long and provides a common pathway for urine, semen and reproductive organ secretions. The three parts of the male urethra are the prostatic, membranous and spongiose or penile urethra. Originating at the urethral orifice of the bladder, the prostatic urethra passes through the prostate gland (Figure 11.15). The narrowest and shortest part of the urethra is the membranous urethra, originating from the prostate gland and extending to the bulb of the penis. The penile urethra ends at the urethral orifice (Fillingham and Douglas 2004, Waugh *et al.* 2006).

Female urethra

The female urethra is located behind the symphysis pubis and opens at the external urethral orifice (Figure 11.16). It is approximately 4 cm long (Waugh *et al.* 2006).

Evidence-based approaches
Rationale

A cystoscopy is undertaken to gain direct visualization of the urethra and the bladder to aid diagnosis of urological

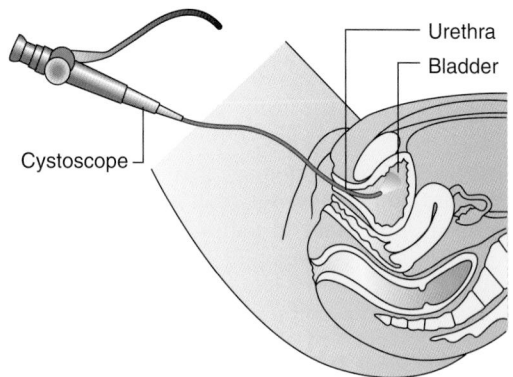

Figure 11.16 Cystoscopy for a woman. © Cancer Help UK, the patient information website of Cancer Research UK: www.cancerhelp.org.uk. Used with permission.

complications and diseases such as bladder cancer (Fillingham and Douglas 2004).

Indications

- Bladder dysfunction.
- Unexplained haematuria.
- Diagnosis of bladder cancer.
- Staging of bladder cancer.
- Obstruction or strictures.
- Dysuria.

Contraindications

- Confirmed urinary tract infection

Preprocedural considerations
Equipment

A cystoscope may be flexible or rigid. A rigid cystoscope is utilized in the operating theatre where the patient is anaesthetized. The flexible cystoscope can be used in the outpatient setting with local anaesthesia. The flexible cystoscope is useful for patients who require more regular examinations for follow-up after bladder cancer treatment (Fillingham and Douglas 2004).

Specific patient preparations

It is essential that the patient does not have a urinary tract infection as the organism that is responsible for the infection may be spread into the bloodstream during the procedure. If the patient is having a general anaesthetic, they will have to fast prior to the procedure, dependent on anaesthetic instruction. Patients undergoing a local anaesthetic can usually eat and drink as normal prior to the procedure. The patient should empty their bladder prior to the procedure (Fillingham and Douglas 2004). It may be necessary for some patients to be treated with antibiotics before the procedure to reduce the risk of infection (AUA 2008).

Postprocedural considerations
Immediate care

Dependent on the type of procedure, recovery will vary. After a general anaesthetic, the patient will be recovered by recovery nursing staff. In the outpatient setting, physiological observations may be required. Nursing staff should monitor for signs of haematuria, infection and excessive pain.

Ongoing care

It is common for the patient to experience some burning sensations whilst passing urine for a few days. It is advised that the patient drink plenty of water post procedure to flush the bladder and reduce the risk of infection. Any signs of excessive bleeding should be reported to the medical team (Fillingham and Douglas 2004).

Complications

Infection

There is a risk of urinary infection in approximately 5% of cystoscopies performed. If an infection were to occur, relevant prescribed antimicrobial therapy may be required (Rodgers *et al.* 2006).

Liver biopsy

Definition

Liver biopsy involves percutaneous puncture using a biopsy needle and removal of a small piece of the liver (Al Knawy and Shiffman 2007).

Anatomy and physiology

The liver is the largest organ in the body. It weighs between 1 and 2.3 kg and is a highly vascular organ. It is incompletely covered by a layer of peritoneum and enclosed in a thin inelastic capsule. There are four lobes in the liver, with the two most obvious ones being the large right lobe and the smaller left lobe which is wedge shaped. The caudate and quadrate lobes are on the posterior surface (Waugh *et al.* 2006).

Functions of the liver

The liver has many functions including:

- carbohydrate metabolism and contributing to maintenance of plasma glucose levels
- fat metabolism
- protein metabolism
- defence against microbes and breakdown of erythrocytes
- detoxification
- inactivation of hormones
- bile secretion
- heat production
- storage of some vitamins, iron, copper and glycogen (Waugh *et al.* 2006).

Evidence-based approaches

Rationale

A liver biopsy is an invaluable tool for diagnosing or monitoring conditions affecting the liver, such as cirrhosis, inflammation or hepatitis of various causes and some metabolic liver disorders (Al Knawy and Shiffman 2007).

Indications

- Diagnosis of cirrhosis.
- Diagnosis of cancer both primary and secondary.
- Miliary tuberculosis.
- Amyloidosis.

Contraindications

- An unco-operative or confused patient.
- Severe purpura.
- Coagulation defects.
- Prolonged clotting time.
- Increased bleeding time.
- Severe jaundice.
- Under 3 years of age.
- Current right lower lobe pneumonia.
- Current pleuritis (Al Knawy and Shiffman 2007).

Methods of liver biopsy

There are a variety of methods for conducting a liver biopsy. A retrospective study by Manolakopoulos *et al.* (2007) found that the ultrasound-assisted approach was as safe as the ultrasound-guided approach and both obtained adequate samples.

Percussion palpation approach

This method is also known as the blind approach where the liver is palpated in order to determine the position required for the liver biopsy.

Image-guided approach

Image guidance may be conducted utilizing ultrasound, computed tomography (CT) or magnetic resonance imaging (MRI) but the preferred method is ultrasound. The ultrasound method utilizes continuous ultrasound or site marking immediately prior to the procedure (Al Knawy and Shiffman 2007).

Ultrasound-assisted approach

The ultrasound is utilized immediately prior to the procedure and a mark is left on the skin indicating the puncture site. It is also known as the 'X' marks the spot technique.

Ultrasound-guided approach

The ultrasound is utilized throughout the procedure where the liver and biopsy needle are viewed in real time (Al Knawy and Shiffman 2007).

Preprocedural considerations

Equipment

Aspiration or suction type needle

There are a few varieties of aspiration or suction type needles such as the Jamshidi, Klatskin and Menghini (Figure 11.17).

703

Figure 11.17 Liver biopsy needles.

The Menghini needle has a retaining device to minimize the risk of the sample being aspirated into the syringe and is the most commonly used. It is 6 cm long and approximately 1.4 mm wide.

Cutting type needles

The Tru-Cut needle utilizes a cutting sheath to obtain the specimen. It is advanced approximately 2–3 cm into the liver and a sample of 12 cm with a diameter of 1 mm is collected.

Pharmacological support

Nursing staff should take a nursing history reviewing social and medical history and determining allergy status. Up to 7 days prior to the procedure, the referring medical team must ensure that a full blood count, clotting screen and biochemistry have been taken. Nursing staff should review bloods as part of their preprocedure assessment. If a patient is currently taking an anticoagulant such as warfarin, a clotting sample must be taken within 24 hours of the procedure. Medications should be reviewed by medical and nursing staff and arrangements made by the medical team for alternative anticoagulant and diabetic medication if necessary. A local anaesthetic such as lidocaine 2% is infiltrated into the area where the biopsy is to be taken. In some cases where the patient is extremely anxious, conscious sedation may be considered; however, management during and after the procedure would include physiological monitoring and recovery as in colonoscopy with conscious sedation (Al Knawy and Shiffman 2007).

Specific patient preparations

A baseline set of physiological observations must be undertaken. If conscious sedation is used the patient must be nil by mouth and they must have patent IV access (Royal College of Radiologists 2006). The patient is usually in the supine position with the right side as close to the edge of the bed as possible. The left side may be supported by a pillow. The patient's right hand is positioned under their head and their head turned to the left. Oxygen therapy may be required if there are pre-existing conditions or when conscious sedation is used.

Postprocedural considerations

Immediate care

Immediately following the procedure the patient must lie on their right side for 3 hours and remain on bed rest for a total of 6 hours. They may be able to go to the toilet after 3 hours. Physiological observations are required every 15 minutes for the first hour, every 30 minutes for the following 2 hours and then the frequency can be reviewed by the registered nurse. Any abnormality must be reported to the medical team immediately. The nurse should also observe the puncture site and abdomen for signs of bleeding and ensure that pain is adequately controlled.

Ongoing care/education

A postprocedure information sheet should be given to the patient identifying possible complications and instructions on what to do if any symptoms occur (Royal College of Radiologists 2006).

Complications

Haemorrhage

An inadvertent puncture of an intrahepatic or extrahepatic blood vessel can lead to haemorrhage manifesting within 4 hours. However, it is normal to lose approximately 5–10 mL of blood from the surface of the liver after the biopsy. Conservative management with blood products may be appropriate but surgical intervention may also be required to treat haemorrhage.

Peritonitis

An inadvertent puncture of the bile duct which consequently results in bile leaking into the peritoneal cavity can lead to peritonitis. Treatment may range from antimicrobial therapy to surgical and/or critical care intervention dependent on the severity.

Pneumothorax

An inadvertent puncture of the pleura can lead to a pneumothorax. If this occurs, urgent medical intervention is required. A formal chest drain may be necessary to relieve the pneumothorax (Denzer *et al.* 2007, Thampanitchawong and Piratvisuth 1999).

Radiological investigations: X-ray

Definition

An X-ray is a short-wavelength electromagnetic radiation that passes through matter and is used in diagnostic radiology and radiotherapy (Martin 2010). Further information can be found in Chapter 14.

Evidence-based approaches
Rationale

The general X-ray department performs a wide range of examinations many of which require no patient preparation in advance, and can often be performed on the day of the request. In accordance with the Ionizing Radiation Regulations (1999), to ensure radiation safety, there is a requirement for radiographers to justify, optimize and limit radiation dosage to a patient.

Indications

Diagnostic X-rays are performed to diagnose medical conditions such as damage to the skeletal structures and organ dysfunction, for example chest X-rays for respiratory complications.

Contraindications

The Ionizing Radiation (Medical Exposure) Regulations (2000) (Regulations 6 and 7) prohibit any medical exposure from being carried out which has not been justified and authorized, and provides an optimization process to ensure that doses arising from exposures are kept as low as reasonably practicable (ALARP).

In accordance with the *Medical and Dental Guidance Notes* (2002) for women known or likely to be pregnant, where the examination has been justified on the basis of clinical urgency and involves irradiation of the abdomen, operators must optimize the technique to minimize irradiation of the foetus (IPEM 2002). Radiography of areas remote from the foetus, for example chest, skull or hand, may be carried out safely at any time during pregnancy as long as good beam collimation and proper shielding equipment are used.

Legal and professional issues

The Ionizing Radiation (Medical Exposure) Regulations (2000) set out the legal roles and responsibilities of all duty holders related to medical exposures to X-rays. See Chapter 14.

In accordance with the Ionizing Radiation (Medical Exposure) Regulations (IR(ME)R) (2000), the completed request form for a medical exposure must be clear and legible and the following information must be supplied.

(a) Unique patient identification – to include at least three identifiers from name, date of birth, hospital number or NHS number.
(b) Sufficient details of the clinical problem to allow the IR(ME)R practitioner to justify the medical exposure, and indication of examination thought to be appropriate.
(c) If applicable, information on the patient's possible pregnancy status.
(d) Signature uniquely identifying the referrer as it is important that the referrer is qualified to order an X-ray.

Blank request cards, pre-signed by a referrer, are a breach of the regulations and any entries on the request form made by others should be checked and initialled by the referrer prior to signing the form.

Preprocedural considerations
Pharmacological support

For some types of X-ray such as the barium swallow or enema, the patient is usually required to drink the contrast or have it administered via an enema and a series of X-ray pictures taken at various intervals. Afterwards the patient will be advised to drink plenty of fluids to clear their system of the contrast as quickly as possible.

Specific patient preparations

The radiology department will inform the patient of any requirements prior to the booked procedure such as being nil by mouth. For most examinations, the patient will be asked to remove some of their clothing and change into a hospital gown, to ensure that no artefacts (any feature in an image which misrepresents the object in the field of view) (McRobbie 2007) are caused in the area of clinical interest on the X-ray image. It is advisable for the patient not to wear jewellery at the time of the appointment as in most cases this will have to be removed, again to prevent the presence of artefacts on the image. For all X-rays the patient will be required to keep still to prevent any blurring of the images. Some procedures are performed on inspiration/expiration, and the patient will be given the appropriate breathing instruction by the operator performing the procedure.

Magnetic resonance imaging (MRI)

Definition

Magnetic resonance imaging provides cross-sectional images of the body. The patient lies inside the bore of a very strong magnet, typically 1.5 tesla. Protons in the body's water molecules spin or 'precess' when exposed to such a strong magnetic field. Radio waves are transmitted into the patient at the same frequency at which the protons are precessing and the patient transmits a signal that is detected by a receiver coil. This signal contains specific information or 'weighting' about the individual tissues that can be mapped to form a two- or three-dimensional image (Weishaupt *et al.* 2006).

Evidence-based approaches
Rationale

Soft tissue structures such as the brain, spinal cord, musculoskeletal system, liver and pelvic structures are particularly well demonstrated using MRI. It is possible to scan the whole body but MRI tends to be a more targeted scan, and they take longer with scan times of 20–60 minutes. MRI does *not* use ionizing radiation and can therefore be used for repeated examinations. The magnetic field is always present so strict safety procedures are necessary to protect staff and patients (Shellock and Spinazzi 2008).

Indications

- Scanning of the brain to assess stroke, tumour, meningeal disease.
- Spinal pathology is particularly well demonstrated, including intervertebral disc pathology, tumour, infarction, spinal dysraphism, infection and degenerative diseases.
- Differentiation and characterization of benign versus malignant pathology in the liver.
- MRI is highly sensitive for imaging of the breast.
- MRI is the gold standard for assessment of pelvic malignancy and pelvic anatomy.

(Royal College of Radiologists 2006, 2007)

Contraindications

Patients with non-MRI compatible implanted devices, such as cardiac pacemakers and cochlear implants, must not be scanned. Other implanted devices, for example stents, must be confirmed as MR safe prior to scanning.

Magnetic resonance imaging tends not to be used for acute trauma or for primary whole-body staging of malignancies, for which CT is the preferred imaging modality.

Preprocedural considerations
Assessment and recording tools

A pre-MRI checklist is undertaken for all patients to identify risks from implanted devices which may be harmful to the patient or may severely degrade the image quality (Shellock and Spinazzi 2008).

Pharmacological support

The patient may require intravenous access for contrast injection, most often of a gadolinium-based contrast agent. This is used to enhance areas of suspected pathology, to define tumour bulk or to improve the efficacy of the scan by delineation or characterization of a pathological process (Runge *et al.* 2009). Claustrophobia can also be an issue and in some cases patients may require an oral sedative to relax them during the procedure. In severe claustrophobia or when scanning young children or individuals with learning difficulties, general anaesthetic may be necessary.

Non-pharmacological support

The scanner is very noisy so it is mandatory that patients are given ear protection during the scan. If the patient feels claustrophobia there are strategies to manage this such as:

- adapting the patient's position
- changing the scanning technique
- using blindfolds or mirrors
- relaxation therapy.

Specific patient preparations

Apart from safety checking, for most scans there is no preparation but for certain body scans the patient may have to abstain from food, but may drink clear (non-caffeine) fluids to ensure their bladder does not fill too quickly, resulting in movement artefacts.

Patients must be able to lie very still, usually lying on their back for significant time periods. Patient comfort is paramount so patients requiring pain relief should continue with pain medication as normal.

Computed tomography (CT)

Definition

Computed tomography images are created when radiation passes through a patient and is absorbed in varying degrees by the body tissue. Multislice data are acquired as a three-dimensional block in a matter of seconds and digitally displayed in coronal, sagittal or axial planes (Fishman and Jeffrey 2004).

Evidence-based approaches
Rationale

Multislice CT has excellent image resolution and is used for diagnosis, staging and monitoring treatment response in the oncology setting, as well as being a research tool. Soft tissues as well as bone and lung anatomy are all seen well on CT scans. Routinely patients are given intravenous contrast medium which perfuses the body tissues and enhances the blood vessels and lesions (Husband and Reznek 2010).

Computed tomography does use radiation but protocols are optimized to give the best image with the lowest dose. Also, the number of body areas scanned and the intervals between scans are closely monitored in accordance with IR(ME)R regulations.

Indications

Computed tomography can image all parts of the body and is used for:

- pretreatment staging
- interval scans to monitor treatment

- follow-up post treatment
- diagnosis and assessment of complications:
  - bowel obstructions and perforation
  - pulmonary embolism
  - stroke, cerebral bleeds
- perfusion CT.

Contraindications

- Pregnancy: CT is not recommended unless clinical benefit outweighs radiation risk.
- Patients with poor renal function or those having iodine therapy may have CT without intravenous contrast.
- Previous CT within short timeframe unless clinically urgent.
- Patients who are unable to lie down in order to pass through the machine (Royal College of Radiologists 2010).

Preprocedural considerations

Assessment and recording tools

Patients complete a questionnaire prior to CT in order to assess their suitability for CT and intravenous (IV) contrast. Intravenous contrast contains iodine, therefore patients with an iodine allergy or previous history of reaction to IV contrast should have a non-IV contrast CT.

Pharmacological support

The patient is cannulated for the intravenous injection of iodine-based contrast medium to enhance the blood vessels and bodily organs. During the injection it is normal for the patient to transiently feel warm over their whole body and to experience a metallic taste at the back of the throat, and some patients feel nauseous. CT examinations such as CT pulmonary angiograms demand contrast to flow at a fast rate and therefore a large gauge cannula (20 G) is required (Thomsen et al. 2009).

Non-pharmacological support

Although CT is a fast imaging technique (5–20 seconds), some patients are very concerned about being claustrophobic during scanning but with kind careful explanation, most patients manage to be scanned.

Specific patient preparations

Patients are prepared for CT by drinking an oral contrast, usually water, which shows the digestive tract. This serves to hydrate the patient which is beneficial post IV contrast and also it acts as a negative contrast agent in the digestive tract. Patients refrain from eating for 2 hours prior to CT in order to allow them to drink easily and to reduce nausea post IV contrast medium (Thomsen et al. 2009).

Patients lie on the CT scan couch and pass through the doughnut-shaped machine. The examination is painless and the majority of patients tolerate the examinations well. Small children require general anaesthetic for CT (Thomsen et al. 2009).

Websites

Diagnostic tests: www.library.wmuh.nhs.uk/pil/diagnostictests.htm
British Infertility Counselling Association: www.bica.net
Cancer Research UK: www.cancerhelp.org.uk
Infertility Network UK: www.infertilitynetworkuk.com
Human Fertilization and Embryology Authority: www.hfea.gov.uk
Macmillan Cancer Support: www.macmillan.org.uk
NHS Cancer Screening Programme publications related to cervical screening: www.cancerscreening.nhs.uk/cervical
NHS information Centre: www.ic.nhs.uk

References

Adlard, K. (2008) Examining the push-pull method of blood sampling from central venous access devices. *Journal of Pediatric Oncology Nursing*, **25** (4), 200–208.
Ahmed, S.V., Jayawarna, C. and Jude, E. (2006) Post lumbar puncture headache: diagnosis and management. *Postgraduate Medical Journal*, **82** (973), 713–716.
Al Knawy, B. and Shiffman, M. (2007) Percutaneous liver biopsy in clinical practice. *Liver International*, **27** (9), 1166–1173.
Allan, D. (2002) Caring for the patient with a disorder of the nervous system. In: Walsh, M. (ed) *Watson's Clinical Nursing and Related Sciences*, 6th edn. Baillière Tindall, Edinburgh, pp. 665–746.
Andris, D.A. and Krzywda, E. A. (1997) Catheter pinch-off syndrome: recognition and management. *Journal of Intravenous Nursing*, **20** (5), 233–237.
AUA (2008) *Best Practice Policy Statement on Urologic Surgery Antimicrobial Prophylaxis*. American Urological Association Education and Research. www.auanet.org/content/media/antimicroprop08.pdf?CFID=2317518&CFTOKEN=12094021&jsessionid=8430364ab2795c3082622c78141f7b19487a.
Barker, E. (2002) Neuroanatomy and physiology of the nervous system, in *Neuroscience Nursing: A Spectrum of Care*, 2nd edn (ed. E.M. Barker), Mosby, St Louis, MO, pp. 3–50.
Barker, E. and Chao, W.P. (2002) Neurodiagnostic and laboratory studies. In: Barker, E.M. (ed) *Neuroscience Nursing: A Spectrum of Care*, 2nd edn. Mosby, St Louis, pp. 99–130.
Barnes, T.W., Olson, E.J., Morgenthaler, T.I. et al. (2005) Low yield of microbiologic studies on pleural fluid specimens. *Chest*, **127** (3), 916–921.
Belford, K. (2005) Central nervous cancers. In: Yarbro, C.H., Frogge, M.H. and Goodman, M. (eds) *Cancer Nursing: Principles and Practice*, 6th edn. Jones and Bartlett, Sudbury, MA, pp. 1089–1136.
Berreth, M. (2010) Minimising the risk of lymphodema: implications for the infusion nurses. *INS Newsline*, **32** (3), 6–7.
Bersten, A.D., Soni, N. and Oh, T.E. (2009) *Oh's Intensive Care Manual*, 6th edn. Butterworth-Heinemann, Oxford.
Blann, A.D. (2007) *Routine Blood Results Explained*, 2nd edn. M and K Update Ltd, Keswick, Cumbria.
Blows, W. (2002) Diagnostic investigations. Part 1. Lumbar puncture. *Nursing Times*, **98** (36), 25–26.
BNF (2011) *British National Formulary*. BMJ Group and RPS Publishing, London.
Boomsma, C.M., Heineman, M.J., Cohlen, B.J. and Farquhar, C. (2007) Semen preparation techniques for intrauterine insemination. *Cochrane Database of Systematic Reviews*, 4, CD004507.

707

Bouza, E., Munoz, P., Burillo, A. *et al.* (2005) The challenge of anticipating catheter tip colonization in major heart surgery patients in the intensive care unit: are surface cultures useful? *Critical Care Medicine*, **33** (9), 1953–1960.

Brinsden, P.R. (2005) *Textbook of In Vitro Fertilization and Assisted Reproduction: the Bourn Hall Guide to Clinical and Laboratory Practice*, 3rd edn. Taylor and Francis, London.

BSG (2003) *Guidelines on Safety and Sedation During Endoscopic Procedures*. British Society of Gastroenterology, London. www.bsg.org.uk/clinical-guidelines/endoscopy/guidelines-on-safety-and-sedation-during-endoscopic-procedures.html.

Bucher, L. (2001) Arterial puncture, in *AACN Procedure Manual for Critical Care* (eds D.J. Lynn-McHale and K.K. Carlson). W.B. Saunders, Philadelphia, pp. 496–502.

Campbell, H., Carrington, M. and Limber, C. (1999) A practice guide to venepuncture and management of complications. *British Journal of Nursing*, **8** (7), 426–431.

Carney, T., Perry, J.D., Ford, M. *et al.* (2002) Evidence for antibiotic induced *Clostridium perfringens* diarrhoea. *Journal of Clinical Pathology*, **55** (3), 240.

Castledine, G. (1996) Nurses' role in peripheral venous cannulation. *British Journal of Nursing*, **5** (20), 1274–1275.

Catchpole, C. and Hastings, J.G. (1995) Measuring pre- and post-dose vancomycin levels – time for a change? *Journal of Medical Microbiology*, **42** (5), 309–311.

Catton, J.A., Dobbins, B.M., Kite, P. *et al.* (2005) In situ diagnosis of intravascular catheter-related bloodstream infection: a comparison of quantitative culture, differential time to positivity, and endoluminal brushing. *Critical Care Medicine*, **33** (4), 787–791.

Centers for Disease Control and Prevention (1997) Evaluation of safety devices for preventing percutaneous injuries among health-care workers during phlebotomy procedures – Minneapolis-St Paul, New York City, and San Francisco, 1993–1995. *JAMA*, **277** (6), 449–450.

Chambrin, M.C. (2001) Alarms in the intensive care unit: how can the number of false alarms be reduced? *Critical Care*, **5** (4), 184–188.

Chowet, A.L., Lopez, J.R., Brock-Utne, J.G. and Jaffe, R.A. (2004) Wrist hyperextension leads to median nerve conduction block: implications for intra-arterial catheter placement. *Anesthesiology*, **100** (2), 287–291.

Coia, J.E., Duckworth, G.J., Edwards, D.I. *et al.* (2006) Guidelines for the control and prevention of meticillin-resistant *Staphylococcus aureus* (MRSA) in healthcare facilities. *Journal of Hospital Infection*, **63** (Suppl 1), S1–S44.

Cole, T. (2006) Risks and benefits of needle use in patients after axillary surgery. *British Journal of Nursing*, **15** (18), 969–979.

Conner, B.D., Lee, Y.C., Branca, P. *et al.* (2003) Variations in pleural fluid WBC count and differential counts with different sample containers and different methods. *Chest*, **123** (4), 1181–1187.

Connolly, M.A. (1999) Clinical snapshot. Postdural puncture headache. *American Journal of Nursing*, **99** (11), 48–49.

Cosca, P.A., Smith, S., Chatfield, S. *et al.* (1998) Reinfusion of discard blood from venous access devices. *Oncology Nursing Form*, **25** (6), 1073–1077.

Coward, M. and Cooley, H.M. (2006) Chemotherapy. In: Kearney, N. and Richardson, A. (eds) *Nursing Patients with Cancer: Principles and Practice*. Elsevier Churchill Livingstone, Edinburgh, pp. 283–302.

Dawson, C. and Whitfield, H. (1996) ABC of urology. Urinary incontinence and urinary infection. *BMJ (Clinical Research)*, **312** (7036), 961–964.

Dellinger, R.P., Levy, M.M., Carlet, J.M. *et al.* (2008) Surviving Sepsis Campaign: international guidelines for management of severe sepsis and septic shock: 2008. *Critical Care Medicine*, **36** (1), 296–327.

Denzer, U., Arnoldy, A., Kanzler, S. *et al.* (2007) Prospective randomized comparison of minilaparoscopy and percutaneous liver biopsy: diagnosis of cirrhosis and complications. *Journal of Clinical Gastroenterology*, **41** (1), 103–110.

DH (2003) *Updated National Guidance on the Safe Administration of Intrathecal Chemotherapy*. HSC 2003/010. Department of Health, London.

DH (2006) *Health Management Memorandum 07-01: Safe Management of Healthcare Waste*. Department of Health, London.

DH (2007a) *Saving Lives: Reducing Infection, Delivering Clean and Safe Health Care. High Impact Intervention no. 6: Urinary Catheter Care Bundle*. Department of Health, London. www.dh.gov.uk/prod_consum_dh/groups/dh_digitalassets/@dh/@en/documents/digitalasset/dh_078125.pdf.

DH (2007b) *Saving Lives: Reducing Infection, Delivering Clean and Safe Health Care. High Impact Intervention no. 7: Care Bundle to Reduce the Risk for Clostridium Difficile*. Department of Health, London. www.dh.gov.uk/prod_consum_dh/groups/dh_digitalassets/@dh/@en/documents/digitalasset/dh_078126.pdf.

DH (2007c) *Saving Lives: Reducing Infection, Delivering Clean and Safe Healthcare. High Impact Intervention no. 1: Central Venous Catheter Care Bundle*. Department of Health, London.

DH (2008) *Updated National Guidance on the Safe Administration of Intrathecal Chemotherapy*. Department of Health, London. www.dh.gov.uk/prod_consum_dh/groups/dh_digitalassets/documents/digitalasset/dh_086844.pdf.

DH (2010) *Clean Safe Care. High Impact Intervention. Taking Blood Cultures: A Summary of Best Practice*. Department of Health, London.

Dougherty, L. (2006) *Central Venous Access Devices: Care and Management*. Blackwell Publishing, Oxford.

Dougherty, L. (2008) Obtaining peripheral venous access. In: Dougherty, L. and Lamb, J. (eds) *Intravenous Therapy in Nursing Practice*, 2nd edn. Blackwell, Oxford, pp. 225–270.

Dougherty, L. and Lamb, J. (eds) (2008) *Intravenous Therapy in Nursing Practice*, 2nd edn. Blackwell, Oxford.

Dulak, S.B. (2005) Sputum sample collection. *RN*, **68** (10), 36ac2–4.

Dulczak, S. and Kirk, J. (2005) Overview of the evaluation, diagnosis, and management of urinary tract infections in infants and children. *Urologic Nursing*, **25** (3), 185–191.

Ebinger, F., Kosel, C., Pietz, J. and Rating, D. (2004) Strict bed rest following lumbar puncture in children and adolescents is of no benefit. *Neurology*, **62** (6), 1003–1005.

Ernst, D.J. (2005) *Applied Phlebotomy*. Lippincott Williams and Wilkins, Philadelphia, PA.

Evans, R.W., Armon, C., Frohman, E.M. and Goodin, D.S. (2000) Assessment: prevention of post-lumbar puncture headaches: report of the therapeutics and technology assessment subcommittee of the American Academy of Neurology. *Neurology*, **55** (7), 909–914.

Farrell, J.J. and Friedman, L.S. (2005) Review article: the management of lower gastrointestinal bleeding. *Alimentary Pharmacology and Therapeutics*, **21** (11), 1281–1298.

Ferguson, A. (2005) Taking a swab. *Nursing Times*, **101** (39), 26–27.

Fillingham, S. and Douglas, J. (2004) *Urological Nursing*, 3rd edn. Baillière Tindall, Edinburgh.

Fischbach, F.T. and Dunning, M.B. (2004) *A Manual of Laboratory and Diagnostic Tests*, 7th edn. Lippincott Williams and Wilkins, Philadelphia, PA.

Fishman, E.K. and Jeffrey, R.B. (2004) *Multidetector CT: Principles, Techniques, and Clinical Applications*. Lippincott Williams and Wilkins, Philadelphia, PA.

Fraise, A.P. and Bradley, T. (eds) (2009) *Ayliffe's Control of Health-care-associated Infection: A Practical Handbook*, 5th edn. Hodder Arnold, London.

Frey, A.M. (2003) Drawing blood samples from vascular access devices. Evidence-based practice. *Journal of Infusion Nursing*, **26** (5), 285–298.

Gabriel, J. (2008) Long term central venous access. In: Dougherty, L. and Lamb, J. (eds) *Intravenous Therapy in Nursing Practice*, 2nd edn. Blackwell, Oxford.

Garber, G. (2001) An overview of fungal infections. *Drugs*, **61** (Suppl 1), 1–12.

Garibaldi, R.A. (1992) Catheter-associated urinary tract infection. *Current Opinion in Infectious Diseases*, **5** (4), 517–523.

Garza, D. and Becan-McBride, K. (2010) *Phlebotomy Handbook: Blood Specimen Collection from Basic to Advanced*, 8th edn. Pearson, Upper Saddle River, NJ.

Gerris, J. (1999) Methods of semen collection not based on masturbation or surgical sperm retrieval. *Human Reproduction Update*, **5** (3), 211–215.

Gilbert, R. (2006) Taking a midstream specimen of urine. *Nursing Times*, **102** (18), 22–23.

Gilchrist, B. (2000) Taking a wound swab. *Nursing Times*, **96** (4 Suppl), 2.

Gill, V., Fedorko, D. and Witebsky, F. (2005) The clinician and the microbiological laboratory. In: Mandell, G.L., Douglas, R.G., Bennett, J.E. and Dolin, R. (eds) *Mandell, Douglas, and Bennett's Principles and Practice of Infectious Diseases*, 6th edn. Elsevier Churchill Livingstone, Philadelphia, PA.

Golder, M., Chan, C.L.H., O'Shea, S. *et al.* (2000) Potential risk of cross-infection during peripheral-venous access by contamination of tourniquets. *Lancet*, **355** (9197), 44.

Gorski, L., Perucca, R. and Hunter, M. (2010) Central venous access devices: care, maintenance, and potential problems. In: Alexander, M., Corrigan, A., Gorski, L. *et al.*(eds) *Infusion Nursing: An Evidence-Based Approach*, 3rd edn. Saunders Elsevier, St Louis, MO, pp. 495–515.

Gould, D. (2002) Preventing cross-infection. *Nursing Times*, **98** (46), 50–51.

Gould, D. and Brooker, C. (2008) *Infection Prevention and Control: Applied Microbiology for Healthcare*, 2nd edn. Palgrave Macmillan, Basingstoke.

Gruener, G. and Biller, J. (2008) Spinal cord anatomy, localization, and overview of spinal cord syndromes. American Academy of Neurology. www.kclj.si/ikn/DEJA/Continuum/MieloRadikulIN pleksopatije/1Spinacordanatomy.pdfw.

Guest, J. (2008) Specimen collection. Part 5 – Obtaining a sputum sample. *Nursing Times*, **104** (21), 26–27.

Gunwardene, R.D. and Davenport, H.T. (1990) Local application of EMLA and glycerol trinitrate ointment before venepuncture. *Anesthesia*, **45**, 52–54.

Hadaway, L. and Chamallas, S.N. (2003) Vancomycin: new perspectives on an old drug. *Journal of Infusion Nursing*, **26** (5), 278–284.

Hairon, N. (2008) Guidelines outline key actions to improve infection control. *Nursing Times*, **104** (36), 19–20.

Hammett-Stabler, C.A. and Johns, T. (1998) Laboratory guidelines for monitoring of antimicrobial drugs. National Academy of Clinical Biochemistry. *Clinical Chemistry*, **44** (5), 1129–1140.

Hampson, G.D. (2006) *Practice Nurse Handbook*, 5th edn. Blackwell, Oxford.

Hart, S. (2006) Prevention of infection. In: Grundy, M.(ed) *Nursing in Haematological Oncology*. 2nd edn. Baillière Tindall Elsevier, Edinburgh, pp. 321–338.

Hazinski, M.F. (1992) *Nursing Care of the Critically Ill Child*, 2nd edn. Mosby Year Book, St Louis, MO.

Hebl, J.R. (2006) The importance and implications of aseptic techniques during regional anesthesia. *Regional Anesthesia and Pain Medicine*, **31** (4), 311–323.

Hefler, L., Grimm, C., Leodolter, S. and Tempfer, C. (2004) To butterfly or to needle: the pilot phase. *Annals of Internal Medicine*, **140** (11), 935–936.

Herzog, T. and Cohn, D. (2001) New innovations in cervical cancer screening. *Clinical Obstetrics and Gynecology*, **44**, 538–549.

Hess, D.R. (2002) The evidence for secreting clearance techniques. *Cardiopulmonary Physical Therapy Journal*, **13** (4), 7–21.

Hickey, J.V. (2003) Cerebrospinal fluids and spinal procedures. In: Hickey, J.V. (ed) *The Clinical Practice of Neurological and Neurosurgical Nursing*, 5th edn. Lippincott Williams and Wilkins, Philadelphia PA, pp. 89–91.

Higgins, C.F. (2007) *Understanding Laboratory Investigations for Nurses and Health Professionals*, 2nd edn. Blackwell, Oxford.

Higgins, D. (2008) Specimen collection. Part 3 – collecting a stool specimen. *Nursing Times*, **104** (19), 22–23.

Himberger, J.R. and Himberger, L.C. (2001) Accuracy of drawing blood through infusing intravenous lines. *Heart and Lung: the Journal of Critical Care*, **30** (1), 66–73.

Hoeltke, L.B. (2006) *The Complete Textbook of Phlebotomy*, 3rd edn. Thomson/Delmar Learning, Clifton Park, NY.

Hoffbrand, A.V., Moss, P.A.H. and Pettit, J.E. (2006) *Essential Haematology*, 5th edn. Blackwell, Oxford.

Holmes, K.R. (1998) Comparison of push-pull versus discard method from central venous catheters for blood testing. *Journal of Intravenous Nursing*, **21** (5), 282–285.

HPA (2004) *Investigation of Genital Tract and Associated Specimens*. National Standard Methods, BSOP 28, Issue 4. Health Protection Agency, London. www.hpa-standardmethods.org.uk/pdf_bacteriology.asp.

HPA (2008a) *Investigation for Bronchovascular Lavage, Sputum and Associated Specimens: BSOP57: Issue 2.3*. Health Protection Agency. www.hpa-standardmethods.org.uk/documents/bsop/pdf/bsop57.pdf.

HPA (2008b) *Investigation for Specimens Screening for MRSA*. Health Protection Agency. www.hpa-standardmethods.org.uk/documents/bsop/pdf/bsop29.pdf.

HPA (2008c) *Investigation of Ear Swabs and Associated Specimens: BSOP1: Issue 8.2*. Health Protection Agency. www.hpa-standardmethods.org.uk/documents/bsop/pdf/bsop1.pdf.

HPA (2008d) *Investigation of Faecal Specimens for Bacterial Pathogens: BSOP 30: Issue 6.1*. Health Protection Agency. www.hpa-standardmethods.org.uk/documents/bsop/pdf/bsop30.pdf.

HPA (2008e) *Investigation of Fluids from Normally Sterile Sites: BSOP 26: Issue 5*. Health Protection Agency. www.hpa-standardmethods.org.uk/documents/bsop/pdf/bsop26.pdf.

HPA (2008f) *Investigation of Intravascular Cannulae and Associated Specimens: BSOP 20: Issue 5*. Health Protection Agency. www.hpa-standardmethods.org.uk/documents/bsop/pdf/bsop20.pdf.

HPA (2008g) *Investigation of Urine: BSOP 41: Issue 7*. Health Protection Agency. www.hpa-standardmethods.org.uk/documents/bsop/pdf/bsop41.pdf.

HSE (2003) *Safe Working and the Prevention of Infection in Clinical Laboratories and Similar Facilities*, 2nd edn. HSE Books, Sudbury.

HSE (2005) *Biological Agents: Managing the Risks in Laboratories and Healthcare Premises*. HSE Books, Sudbury.

Hudak, K. (1986) Compliance in IV therapy. *Journal of the Canadian Intravenous Nurses Association*, **2** (3), 3–8.

Hudson, T.L., Dukes, S.F., Reilly, K. (2006) Use of local anesthesia for arterial punctures. *American Journal of Critical Care*, 15, 595–599.

709

Husband, J.E. and Reznek, R.H. (2010) *Husband and Reznek's Imaging in Oncology*, 3rd edn. Informa Healthcare, London.

ICNA (2003) *Reducing Sharps Injury – Prevention and Risk Management*. Infection Control Nurses Association, London.

INS (2006) Infusion nursing standards of practice. *Journal of Infusion Nursing*, **29** (1 Suppl), S1–92.

Insinga, R.P., Glass, A.G. and Rush, B.B. (2004) Diagnoses and outcomes in cervical cancer screening: a population based study. *American Journal of Obstetrics and Gynecology*, **191**, 105–113.

Inwood, S. (2007) Skin antisepsis: using 2% chlorhexidine gluconate in 70% isopropyl alcohol. *British Journal of Nursing*, **16** (22), 1390, 1392–1394.

Ioanas, M., Ferrer, R., Angrill, J. *et al.* (2001) Microbial investigation in ventilator-associated pneumonia. *European Respiratory Journal*, **17** (4), 791–801.

Ionizing Radiation (Medical Exposure) Regulations (2000) *SI 2000/1059*. Stationery Office, London. www.opsi.gov.uk/si/si2000/20001059.htm.

Ionizing Radiation Regulations (1999) *SI 1999/3232*. Stationery Office, London. www.opsi.gov.uk/si/si1999/19993232.htm.

IPEM (2002) *Medical and Dental Guidance Notes: A Good Practice Guide on All Aspects of Ionising Radiation Protection in the Clinical Environment*. Institute of Physics and Engineering in Medicine, York.

Johannes, R.S. (2008) Epidemiology of early-onset bloodstream infection and implications for treatment. *American Journal of Infection Control*, **36** (10), S171.

Jones, R.N. (2006) Microbiological features of vancomycin in the 21st century: minimum inhibitory concentration creep, bactericidal/static activity, and applied breakpoints to predict clinical outcomes or detect resistant strains. *Clinical Infectious Diseases*, **42** (Suppl 1), S13–S24.

Junqeira, L.C. and Carneiro, J. (2005) *Basic Histology: Text and Atlas*, 11th edn. McGraw-Hill Medical , London.

Karnon, J., Peters, J., Platt, J. *et al.* (2004) Liquid-based cytology in cervical screeening: an updated rapid and systematic review and economic analysis. Executive summary. *Health Technology Assessment*, **8** (20), i–iv, 1–20. www.cancerscreening.nhs.uk/cervical/publications/nhscsp21.pdf.

Keller, C.A. (1994) Method of drawing blood samples through central venous catheters in paediatric patients undergoing bone marrow transplants – results of a national survey. *Oncology Nursing Forum*, **21** (5), 879–884.

Kelly, D., Conway, S. and Aminov, R. (2005) Commensal gut bacteria: mechanisms of immune modulation. *Trends in Immunology*, **26** (6), 326–333.

Kennedy, J.G., Mullett, H.J. and O'Rourke, K. (2000) Cauda equina syndrome. *Current Opinion in Orthopaedics*, **11** (3), 192–195.

King, D. (2002) Determining the cause of diarrhoea. *Nursing Times*, **98** (23), 47–48.

Kingsley, A. (2001) A proactive approach to wound infection. *Nursing Standard*, **15** (30), 50–54, 56, 58.

Kumar, P.J. and Clark, M.L. (2009) *Kumar and Clark's Clinical Medicine*, 7th edn. Saunders/Elsevier, Edinburgh.

Kyle, G. (2007) Bowel care. Part 3 – obtaining a stool sample. *Nursing Times*, **103** (44), 24–25.

Lambert, D.H., Hurley, R.J., Hertwig, L. and Datta, S. (1997) Role of needle gauge and tip configuration in the production of lumbar puncture headache. *Regional Anesthesia*, **22** (1), 66–72.

Latham, J.M., Fraser, R.D., Moore, R.J. *et al.* (1997) The pathologic effects of intrathecal betamethasone. *Spine*, **22** (14), 1558–1562.

Lautenbach, E., Harris, A.D., Perencevich, E.N. *et al.* (2005) Test characteristics of perirectal and rectal swab compared to stool sample for detection of fluoroquinolone-resistant *Escherichia coli* in the gastrointestinal tract. *Antimicrobial Agents and Chemotherapy*, **49** (2), 798–800.

Lavery, I. and Ingram, P. (2005) Venepuncture: best practice. *Nursing Standard*, **19** (49), 55–65.

Lavi, R., Yarnitsky, D., Rowe, J.M. *et al.* (2006) Standard vs atraumatic Whitacre needle for diagnostic lumbar puncture: a randomized trial. *Neurology*, **67** (8), 1492–1494. 10.

Lawrence, J.C. (1999) Swab taking. *Journal of Wound Care*, **8** (5), 251.

Lawrence, J.C. and Ameen, H. (1998) Swabs and other sampling techniques. *Journal of Wound Care*, **7** (5), 232–233.

Lee, A., Mirrett, S., Reller, L.B. and Weinstein, M.P. (2007) Detection of bloodstream infections in adults: how many blood cultures are needed? *Journal of Clinical Microbiology*, **45** (11), 3546–3548.

Lenhardt, R., Seybold, T., Kimberger, O. *et al.* (2002) Local warming and insertion of peripheral venous cannulas: single blinded prospective randomised controlled trial and single blinded randomised crossover trial. *BMJ*, **325** (7361), 409–410.

Lewis, S.J. and Heaton, K.W. (1997) Stool form scale as a useful guide to intestinal transit time. *Scandinavian Journal of Gastroenterology*, **32** (9), 920–924.

Lindsay, K.W. and Bone, I. (2004) *Neurology and Neurosurgery Illustrated*, 4th edn. Churchill Livingstone, Edinburgh.

Lipsitz, E.C. (2004) Cannulation injuries of the radial artery. *American Journal of Critical Care*, **13** (4), 314, 319.

MacKie, R.M. (2003) *Clinical Dermatology*, 5th edn. Oxford University Press, Oxford.

Madeo, M. and Barlow, G. (2008) Reducing blood-culture contamination rates by the use of a 2% chlorhexidine solution applicator in acute admission units. *Journal of Hospital Infection*, **69** (3), 307–309.

Manolakopoulos, S., Triantos, C., Bethanis, S. *et al.* (2007) Ultrasound-guided liver biopsy in real life: comparison of same-day prebiopsy versus real-time ultrasound approach. *Journal of Gastroenterology and Hepatology*, **22** (9), 1490–1493.

Marieb, E.N. and Hoehn, K. (2010) *Human Anatomy and Physiology*, 8th edn. Benjamin Cummings, San Francisco.

Marsden, J. (2007) *An Evidence Base for Ophthalmic Nursing Practice*. John Wiley, Chichester.

Martin, E.A. (2010) *Concise Colour Medical Dictionary*, 5th edn. Oxford University Press, Oxford.

Masoorli, S. (2002) Catheter-related nerve injury: inherent risk of avoidable outcome? *Journal of Vascular Access Devices*, **7** (4), 49.

Mayo, D.J. (1998) Fibrin sheath formation and chemotherapy extravasation: a case report. *Supportive Care in Cancer*, **6** (1), 51–56.

McCall, R.E. and Tankersley, C.M. (2008) *Phlebotomy Essentials*, 4th edn. Lippincott Williams and Wilkins, Philadelphia, PA.

McRobbie, D.W. (2007) *MRI from Picture to Proton*, 2nd edn. Cambridge University Press, Cambridge.

MDA (2000) *Single-Use Medical Devices: Implications and Consequences of Reuse. Device Bulletin 2000, 04*. Department of Health, London.

MHRA (2005) *Alert MDA 2005/01 and Device Bulletin DB 2005 (01): Reporting Adverse Incidents and Disseminating Medical Device Alerts*. Medicines and Healthcare Products Regulatory Agency, London.

Miller, J.M. (1998) The impact of specimen management in microbiology. *Medical Laboratory Observer*, **30** (5), 28–30, 32, 34.

Mims, C.A. (2004) *Medical Microbiology*, 3rd edn. Mosby, Edinburgh.

Mitchell Higgs, N. (2002) Personal protective equipment – improving compliance. All Points Conference, Safer Needles Network, London.

Moureau, N. (1999) Practicing prevention with implanted ports: an overview. *Journal of Vascular Access Devices*, 4 (3), 30–35.

NAO (2003) *A Safer Place to Work: Improving the Management of Health and Safety Risks to Staff in NHS Trusts*. Stationery Office, London. www.nao.org.uk/publications/0203/nhs_health_and_safety.aspx.

NCCWCH and NICE (2004) *Fertility: Assessment and Treatment for People with Fertility Problems*. RCOG Press, London. www.rcog.org.uk/womens-health/clinical-guidance/fertility-assessment-and-treatment-people-fertility-problems.

NHSCSP (2004) *Guidelines on Failsafe Actions for the Follow-up of Cervical Cytology Reports*. NHS Cancer Screening Programme, Sheffield. www.cancerscreening.nhs.uk/cervical/publications/nhscsp21.pdf.

NHSCSP (2006) *An Easy Guide to Cervical Screening*. NHS Cancer Screening Programmes, Sheffield.

NHS Employers (2007) Needlestick injury, in *The Healthy Workplaces Handbook*. NHS Employers, London.

NHSQIS (2007) *Caring for the Patient with a Tracheostomy: Best Practice Statement*. NHS Quality Improvement Scotland, Edinburgh. www.nhshealthquality.org/files/TRACHEOREV_BPS_MAR07.pdf.

NICE (2003) *Guidance on the Use of Liquid-Based Cytology for Cervical Screening*. Technology Appraisal Guidance 69. National Institute for Health and Clinical Excellence, London.

NMC (2008a) *The Code: Standards of Conduct, Performance and Ethics for Nurses and Midwives*. Nursing and Midwifery Council, London. www.nmc-uk.org/aDisplayDocument.aspx?DocumentID=5982.

NMC (2008b) *Consent*. Nursing and Midwifery Council, London. www.nmc-uk.org/Nurses-and-midwives/Advice-by-topic/A/Advice/Consent/.

NMC (2009) *Record Keeping: Guidance for Nurses and Midwives*. Nursing and Midwifery Council, London. www.nmc-uk.org/aDisplayDocument.aspx?DocumentID=6269.

NPSA (2007) *Standardising Wristbands Improves Patient Safety*. Safer Practice Notice 0507. National Patient Safety Agency, London.

NPSA (2008) *Reducing Risk Of Overdose With Midazolam Injection In Adults*. NPSA/2008/RRR011. National Patient Safety Agency, London.

NPSA (2009) *Safer Spinal (Intrathecal), Epidural and Regional Devices: NPSA/2009/PSA004A*. National Patient Safety Agency, London. www.nrls.npsa.nhs.uk.

Owens, R.C. Jr. and Shorr, A.F. (2009) Rational dosing of antimicrobial agents: pharmacokinetic and pharmacodynamic strategies. *American Journal of Health-System Pharmacy*, 66 (12 Suppl 4), S23–S30.

Pan, P.H., Fragneto, R., Moore, C. and Ross, V. (2004) Incidence of postdural puncture headache and backache, and success rate of dural puncture: comparison of two spinal needle designs. *Southern Medical Journal*, 97 (4), 359–363.

Panceri, M.L., Vegni, F.E., Goglio, A. *et al.* (2004) Aetiology and prognosis of bacteraemia in Italy. *Epidemiology and Infection*, 132 (4), 647–654.

Pankhurst, C. and Coulter, W. (2009) *Basic Guide to Infection Prevention and Control in Dentistry*. Wiley-Blackwell, Oxford.

Pannu, N. and Nadim, M.K. (2008) An overview of drug-induced acute kidney injury. *Critical Care Medicine*, 36 (4 Suppl), S216–S223.

Pellatt, G.C. (2007a) Anatomy and physiology of urinary elimination. Part 1. *British Journal of Nursing*, 16 (7), 406–410.

Pellatt, G.C. (2007b) Clinical skills: bowel elimination and management of complications. *British Journal of Nursing*, 16 (6), 351–355.

Pellowe, C. (2009) Using evidence-based guidelines to reduce catheter related urinary tract infections in England. *Journal of Infection Prevention*, 10 (2), 44–49.

Pendharkar, S.R. and Tremblay, A.T. (2007) A diagnostic approach to pleural effusion: guidance on how to identify the cause. *Journal of Respiratory Diseases*, 28 (12), 565.

Penwarden, L.M. and Montgomery, P.G. (2002) Developing a protocol for obtaining blood cultures from central venous catheters and peripheral sites. *Clinical Journal of Oncology Nursing*, 6 (5), 268–270.

Pratt, R., Pellowe, C., Wilson, J. *et al.* (2007) Epic 2: national evidence based guidelines for preventing healthcare-associated infections in NHS hospitals. *European Journal of Hospital Infection*, 65 (S1), S1–S64.

Price, C.G.A. and Madhusudan, S. (2002) Non Hodgkin's lymphoma. In: Price, P. and Sikora, K. (eds) *Treatment of Cancer*, 4th edn. Arnold, London, pp. 977–995.

Putcha, R.V. and Burdick, J.S. (2003) Management of iatrogenic perforation. *Gastroenterology Clinics of North America*, 32 (4), 1289–1309.

Quincke, H. (1891) Verhandlungen des Congresses für Innere Medizin. Zehnter Congress, Wiesbaden, 10, 321–331.

Rajiv, D. (2007) Inhalation therapy in invasive and non-invasive mechanical ventilation. *Current Opinion in Critical Care*, 13 (1), 27–38.

RCN (2000) *Cervical Screening: RCN Guidance for Good Practice*. Royal College of Nursing, London. www.rcn.org.uk/__data/assets/pdf_file/0007/78730/003105.pdf.

RCN (2002) *Chaperoning: The Role of the Nurse and the Rights of Patients*. Royal College of Nursing, London. www.rcn.org.uk/__data/assets/pdf_file/0006/78513/001446.pdf.

RCN (2005) *Good Practice for Infection Prevention and Control*. Royal College of Nursing, London.

RCN (2010) *Standards for Infusion Therapy*, 3rd edn. Royal College of Nursing, London.

RCP, RCR and RCOG (2007) *The Effects of Cancer Treatment on Reproductive Functions: Guidance on Management*. Royal College of Physicians, London. www.rcog.org.uk/files/rcog-corp/uploaded-files/WPREffectCancerReproduction2007.pdf.

Rigby, D. and Gray, K. (2005) Understanding urine testing. *Nursing Times*, 101 (12), 60–62.

Riley, S. (2008) *Colonoscopic Polypectomy and Endoscopic Mucosal Resection: a Practical Guide*. British Society of Gastroenterology, London. www.bsg.org.uk/pdf_word_docs/polypectomy_08.pdf.

Rodgers, M., Nixon, J., Hempel, S. *et al.* (2006) Diagnostic tests and algorithms used in the investigation of haematuria: systematic reviews and economic evaluation. *Health Technology Assessment*, 10 (18). www.hta.ac.uk/1363.

Royal College of Radiologists (2006) *Recommendations for Cross Sectional Imaging in Cancer Management*. Royal College of Radiologists, London.

Royal College of Radiologists (2007) *MBUR6: Royal College of Radiologists Referral Guidelines*, 6th edn. Royal College of Radiologists, London.

Royal College of Radiologists (2010) *Standards for Intravascular Contrast Agent Administration to Adult Patients*. Royal College of Radiologists, London.

Runge, V.M., Nitz, W.R. and Schmeets, S.H. (2009) *The Physics of Clinical MR Taught Through Images*, 2nd edn. Thieme, New York.

Rushing, J. (2006) Assisting with thoracentesis. *Nursing*, 36 (12 Pt.1), 18.

Sado, D.M. and Deakin, C.D. (2005) Local anaesthesia for venous cannulation and arterial blood gas sampling: are doctors using it? *Journal of the Royal Society of Medicine*, 98 (4), 158–160.

711

Scurr, M., Judson, I. and Root, T. (2005) Combination chemotherapy and chemotherapy principles. In: Brighton, D., Johnston, S.R.D. and Wood, M.R.G.N.(eds) *The Royal Marsden Hospital Handbook of Cancer Chemotherapy: A Guide for the Multidisciplinary Team*. Elsevier Churchill Livingstone, Edinburgh, pp. 17–30.

Sha, S. (2005) Physiological and molecular pathology of aminoglycoside ototoxicity. *Volta Review*, **105** (3), 325–335.

Shafazand, S. and Weinacker, A.B. (2002) Blood cultures in the critical care unit: improving utilization and yield. *Chest*, **122** (5), 1727–1736.

Shellock, F.G. and Spinazzi, A. (2008) MRI safety update 2008: part 2, screening patients for MRI. *American Journal of Roentgenology*, **191** (4), 1140–1149.

Shore, A. and Sandoe, J. (2008) Blood cultures. *BMJ*, **16**, 324–325.

SIGN (2008) *Management of Acute Upper and Lower Gastrointestinal Bleeding: A National Guideline*. NHS Quality Improvement Scotland, Edinburgh. www.sign.ac.uk/pdf/sign105.pdf.

Simerville, J.A., Maxted, W.C. and Pahira, J.J. (2005) Urinalysis: a comprehensive review. *American Family Physician*, **71** (6), 1153–1162.

Smith, J. (1998) The practice of venepuncture in lymphoedema. *European Journal of Cancer Care*, 7 (2), 97–99.

Smith, G.D. and Watson, R. (2005) *Gastrointestinal Nursing*, Blackwell, Oxford.

Soyfoo, R. and Shaw, K. (2008) How to cut *Clostridium difficile* infection. *Nursing Times*, **104** (25), 42–44.

Stollery, R., Shaw, M.E. and Lee, A. (2005) *Ophthalmic Nursing*, 3rd edn. Blackwell, Oxford.

Swan, E. (2005) *Colorectal Cancer*. Whurr Publishers, London.

Tacconelli, E. (2009) Antimicrobial use: risk driver of multidrug resistant microorganisms in healthcare settings. *Current Opinion in Infectious Diseases*, **22** (4), 352–358.

Taylor, I., Cutsem, E.V. and Garcia-Aguilar, J. (2009) *Colorectal Disease*, 3rd edn. Health Press, Albuquerque, NM.

Thampanitchawong, P. and Piratvisuth, T. (1999) Liver biopsy: complications and risk factors. *World Journal of Gastroenterology*, 5 (4), 301–304.

Thomsen, H.S., Webb, J.A.W. and Aspelin, P. (eds) (2009) *Contrast Media: Safety Issues and ESUR Guidelines*, 2nd rev edn. Springer, Berlin.

Thomson, A. (2004) Why do therapeutic drug monitoring? *Pharmaceutical Journal*, **273** (7310), 153–155.

Thomson, L. (2000) Tracheal suctioning of adults with an artificial airway. *Best Practice*, 4 (4), 1–7.

Thomson, R. (2002) Use of microbiology laboratory tests in the diagnosis of infectious disease. In: Tan, J.S. (ed) *Expert Guide to Infectious Diseases*. American College of Physicians, American Society of Internal Medicine, Philadelphia.

Tilmouth, T. and Tilmouth, S. (2009) *Safe and Clean Care: Infection Prevention and Control for Health and Social Care Students*. Reflect Press, Exeter.

Tobin, C.M., Darville, J.M., Thomson, A.H. *et al.* (2002) Vancomycin therapeutic drug monitoring: is there a consensus view?

The results of a UK National External Quality Assessment Scheme (UK NEQAS) for Antibiotic Assays questionnaire. *Journal of Antimicrobial Chemotherapy*, **50** (5), 713–718.

Van Peperstraten, A., Proctor, M.L., Johnson, N.P. and Philipson, G. (2006) Techniques for surgical retrieval of sperm prior to ICSI for azoospermia. *Cochrane Database of Systematic Reviews (Online)*, 3, CD002807.

Vasey, P.A. and Evans, J. (2002) Principles of chemotherapy and drug development. In: Price, P. and Sikora, K. (eds) *Treatment of Cancer*. 4th edn. Arnold, London. pp. 103–129.

Verhage, A.H. and van Bommel, E.F.H. (1999) Catheter fracture: an underrecognized and serious condition. *Journal of Vascular Access Devices*, 4 (2), 33–34.

Warekois, R.S., Robinson, R. and Sommer, S.R. (2007) *Phlebotomy: Worktext and Procedures Manual*, 2nd edn. Elsevier Saunders, St Louis, MO.

Waugh, A., Grant, A., Chambers, G. *et al.* (2006) *Ross and Wilson Anatomy and Physiology in Health and Illness*, 10th international edn. Churchill Livingstone, Edinburgh.

Weinstein, S. and Plumer, A.L. (2007) *Plumer's Principles and Practice of Intravenous Therapy*, 8th edn. Lippincott Williams and Wilkins, Philadelphia.

Weishaupt, D., Köchli, V.D. and Marincek, B. (2006) *How does MRI Work? An Introduction to the Physics and Function of Magnetic Resonance Imaging*, 2nd edn. Springer, Berlin.

Weldon, K. (1998) Anatomy and physiology of the nervous system. In: Guerrero, D. (ed) *Neuro-Oncology for Nurses*. Whurr, London, pp. 1–28.

Weller, B.F. and Royal College of Nursing (2009) *Baillière's Nurses' Dictionary*, 23rd edn. Elsevier, Edinburgh.

Weston, D. (2008) *Infection Prevention and Control: Theory and Clinical Practice for Healthcare Professionals*. John Wiley, Chichester.

White, G.C. (2003) *Basic Clinical Lab Competencies for Respiratory Care: An Integrated Approach*, 4th edn. Delmar Publishing, London.

WHO (2006) *Comprehensive Cervical Cancer Control: A Guide to Essential Practice*. World Health Organization, Geneva.

Winter, G. (2005) It's probably a virus. *Practice Nurse*, **30** (3), 26–28.

Wo, J.Y. and Viswanathan, A.N. (2009) Impact of radiotherapy on fertility, pregnancy, and neonatal outcomes in female cancer patients. *International Journal of Radiation Oncology, Biology, Physics*, **73** (5), 1304–1312.

Woodford, E.M., Wilson, K.A. and Marriott, J.F. (2004) Professionals' awareness of operational antibiotic prescribing controls in UK NHS hospitals. *Journal of Hospital Infection*, **58** (3), 193–199.

Yentis, S.M., Hirsch, N. and Smith, G.B. (2009) Spinal anaesthesia, in *Anaesthesia and Intensive Care A-Z: An Encyclopaedia of Principles and Practice*, 4th edn. Churchill Livingstone Elsevier, Edinburgh. pp. 502–505.

712

Haematological procedures

The Royal Marsden Hospital Manual of Clinical Nursing Procedures, Eighth Edition. Edited by Lisa Dougherty and Sara Lister.
© 2011 The Royal Marsden Hospital. Published 2011 by Blackwell Publishing Ltd.

Overview

This chapter provides a review of and guide to procedures commonly undertaken by haematology nurses. Haematological procedures include:

- bone marrow procedures
- apheresis procedures.

Bone marrow procedures

Definitions

1 *Bone marrow procedures* involve the removal of haematopoietic tissue from the medullary cavity of bone. Tissue is removed by either aspiration or biopsy (Perkins 2003). Specific procedures include the following.

- *Aspiration and trephine biopsy* – biopsy of the bone marrow is an indispensable adjunct to the study of diseases of the blood and may be the only way in which a correct diagnosis can be made. Marrow is usually obtained by needle aspiration and percutaneous trephine biopsy. If performed correctly, bone marrow aspiration is simple and safe; it can be repeated many times and performed on outpatients (Lewis *et al.* 2006). Trephine biopsy is a little less simple, but is invaluable in the diagnosis of conditions which yield a 'dry tap' on bone marrow aspiration (e.g. myelofibrosis, infiltrations) or when disrupted architecture of the marrow is an important diagnostic feature (e.g. Hodgkin's disease, lymphoma). It is also performed on outpatients (Lewis *et al.* 2006).

- *Bone marrow harvest* – traditionally bone marrow harvest was the primary method of collecting stem cells in order to facilitate a haematopoietic stem cell transplant (Richardson and Atkinson 2006). The process is similar to that of bone marrow aspiration but multiple aspirations are needed from each posterior iliac crest in order to obtain the necessary volume of stem cells (Henke Yarbro *et al.* 2005). The procedure is performed in the operating room with the donor anaesthetized and this is usually an inpatient procedure (Henke Yarbro *et al.* 2005).

2 *Apheresis* is the generic term applied to blood cell separator procedures which may be used for donor or therapeutic purposes. Cell separators remove whole blood from a patient or donor and separate this into component parts to allow a desired element to be collected, while returning the remainder to the patient or donor (Corbin 2003). Separation of the blood components can be accomplished by filtration, centrifugation or a combination of both. Filtration takes advantage of differences in particle size to separate blood plasma from the cellular elements. Centrifugation uses differences in specific gravity to separate and isolate blood components (Burgstaler 2003). The specific procedures are described according to the blood element being removed (Kaushansky and Williams 2010):

- leucapheresis (white cell depletion)
- thrombocytopheresis (platelet depletion)
- erythrocytapheresis (red cell exchange)
- therapeutic plasmapheresis (plasma exchange).

Anatomy and physiology

Bone marrow

The maturation of blood cells is termed haematopoiesis (Abboud and Lichtman 2009) and takes place in the bone marrow. At 5–9 months of foetal life, the bone marrow, liver and spleen produce the cellular components of blood. At birth the marrow of all bones is involved in haematopoiesis. During childhood, there is some replacement of the haematopoietic tissue (red marrow) with fatty tissue (yellow marrow). In adults, the only sites of haematopoiesis are bones such as the pelvis and sternum (Sieff and Nathan 2000). Yellow marrow has the ability to revert to haematopoietic tissue in certain circumstances such as haemolytic anaemia (Abboud and Lichtman 2009).

Stem cells

All mature blood cells originate from one precursor cell called a stem cell. The stem cell has the ability for unlimited self-renewal (can produce more stem cells) and differentiation (can develop into any of the mature blood cell types) (Figure 12.1).

The self-renewal and differentiation of stem cells are regulated by acidic glycoprotein molecules called haematopoietic growth factors (Traynor 2006). Some growth factors are found naturally in the plasma but others are only detectable following an inflammatory event or other stimulus (Hoffbrand *et al.* 2006). Growth factors include granulocyte-colony stimulating factor (G-CSF), erythropoietin and thrombopoietin (Traynor 2006).

The first step in the differentiation process is a division of the stem cell into two main cell lineages: myeloid and lymphoid. The myeloid progenitor cell divides into red blood cells, platelets, granulocytes (neutrophils, eosinophils and basophils) and monocytes (macrophages). The lymphoid progenitor cell matures into lymphocytes (T and B). Lymphocytes, granulocytes and monocytes are all white cells (Bondurant *et al.* 2009). The main functions of the blood cells and the haematological values for normal adults are listed in Table 12.1.

714

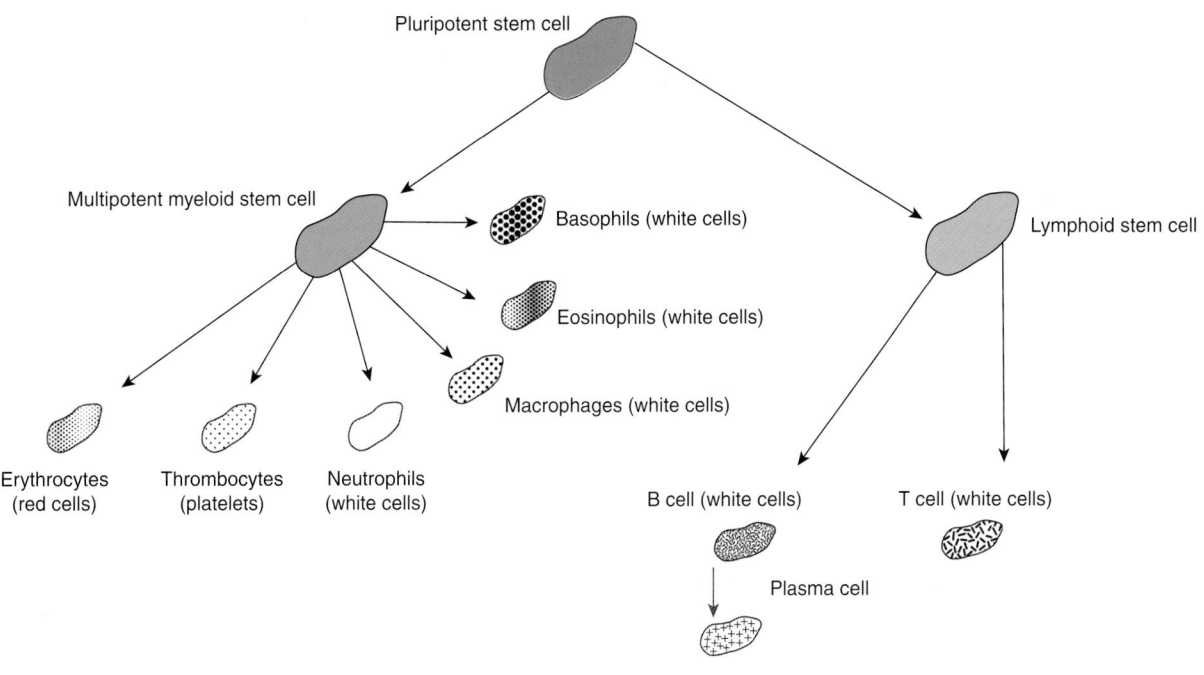

Figure 12.1 The stem cell and the blood cells that arise from it.

Table 12.1 The main function of blood cells and the haematological values for normal adults

Blood cell type and function	Haematological value	Illustration
Red blood cells (erythrocytes) Transport oxygen from the lungs to the tissues and return carbon dioxide from the tissues to be expelled by the lungs	Men: 15 ± 2 g/dL Women: 14 ± 2 g/dL	
Platelets (thrombocytes) The formation of mechanical plugs during the normal haemostatic response to vascular injury	$130–400 \times 10^9$/L	
White blood cells (leucocytes) A group of diverse cells that work together to protect the body from disease and to provide immunity	$7.0 \pm 3.0 \times 10^9$/L	
White blood cell differential *Neutrophil:* Attracted to sites of infection (chemotaxis); ingests micro-organisms (phagocytosis) and destroys them	$2.0–7.0 \times 10^9$/L	

715

(Continued)

Table 12.1 (*Continued*)

Blood cell type and function	Haematological value	Illustration
Eosinophil: Same function as the neutrophil; in addition, helps control parasitic infections; has a role in allergic responses	$0.04\text{--}0.4 \times 10^9/\text{L}$	
Basophil: Has a role in immediate hypersensitivity reactions, allergic and inflammatory responses and in the control of parasitic infections	$0.02\text{--}0.1 \times 10^9/\text{L}$	
T lymphocyte: Attacks cells bearing foreign antigens and antibody-coated cells; can help or suppress B cells (part of cell-mediated immunity) *B lymphocyte:* Matures into a plasma cell, which secretes antibodies (humoral immunity) *Natural killer (NK) lymphocyte:* Attacks foreign cells and tumour cells (part of cell-mediated immunity)	$1.0\text{--}3.0 \times 10^9/\text{L}$	
Monocyte (differentiate to macrophage in tissues): Has a role in chemotaxis, phagocytosis, killing of some micro-organisms (fungi and mycobacteria), release of IL-1 and TNF which stimulate bone marrow stromal cells to produce GM-CSF, G-CSF, M-CSF and IL-6	$0.2\text{--}1.0 \times 10^9/\text{L}$	

Bain (2004), Hoffbrand *et al.* (2001), Hughes-Jones *et al.* (2004), Turgeon (1999), Weatherall (2000)

Plasma

Plasma gives blood its liquid property to allow it to flow through the vascular system. If the cellular components of whole blood were allowed to sediment in a test tube, around 54% of the volume would be the straw-coloured plasma (Traynor 2006). Plasma consists of water, plasma proteins (e.g. fibrinogen, albumin, globulins), electrolytes (e.g. sodium, potassium, chloride) and metabolites (e.g. urea, creatinine, cholesterol). The functions of these elements include clotting, maintaining blood pressure, controlling plasma viscosity, antibody formation and regulating intra/extracellular pressure.

Aspiration and trephine biopsy

Related theory

Examination of the bone marrow usually involves two separate but inter-related specimens. The first is a cytological preparation of bone marrow cells obtained by aspiration of the marrow and a smear of the cells (Perkins 2003). The aspiration specimen is used to assess cell morphology (Longo 2005). The second specimen is a trephine biopsy of the bone and associated marrow, to assess overall marrow architecture, bone marrow cellularity, fibrosis, infections or infiltrative diseases (Longo 2005). Diagnosis and management of many haematological diseases depend on examination of the bone marrow (Perkins 2003).

Evidence-based approaches
Rationale

Before a bone marrow examination is carried out, clear diagnostic goals about the information to be obtained from the procedure should be defined. It should be decided whether any special studies are needed so that all the necessary specimens may be collected and handled correctly (Perkins 2003). Table 12.2 outlines this in more detail.

Table 12.2 Comparison of bone marrow aspiration and trephine biopsy

	Aspiration	Trephine
Site	Posterior/anterior iliac crest or sternum (anterior medial tibial area in children)	Posterior/anterior iliac crest
Result available	1–2 hours	1–7 days (according to decalcification method)
Main indications	Hypoproliferative or unexplained anaemia, leucopenia or thrombocytopenia, suspected leukaemia or myeloma or marrow defect, evaluation of iron stores, work-up of some cases of fever of unknown origin	Performed in addition to aspiration for pancytopenia (aplastic anaemia), metastatic tumour, granulomatous infection (e.g. mycobacteria, brucellosis, histoplasmosis), myelofibrosis, lipid storage disease (e.g. Gaucher's, Niemann–Pick), any case with 'dry tap' on aspiration; evaluation of marrow cellularity
Special tests	Histochemical staining (leukaemias), cytogenetic studies (leukaemias, lymphomas), microbiology (bacterial, mycobacterial, fungal cultures), Prussian blue (iron) stain (assess iron stores, diagnosis of sideroblastic anaemias)	Histochemical staining (e.g. acid phosphatase for metastatic prostate carcinoma), immunoperoxidase staining (e.g. immunoglobulin or cell surface marker detection in multiple myeloma, leukaemia or lymphoma; lysozyme detection in monocytic leukaemia), reticulin staining (increased in myelofibrosis), microbiological staining (e.g. acid-fast staining for mycobacteria)

Hoffbrand *et al.* (2001), Longo (2005), Perkins (2003).

Several sites may be used for bone marrow aspiration and biopsy (Figure 12.2). Normally, only aspirations and not biopsies are done on the sternum because of its small size and proximity to vital organs. The site selected may reflect the normal distribution of bone marrow in relation to the age of the patient. Younger children may have marrow taken from the anterior medial tibial area, whereas adult marrow is best sampled from the sternum at the second intercostal space or from either the anterior or posterior iliac crest area (Perkins 2003). Sternal marrows do not allow a trephine biopsy to be performed, and several possible complications, including haemorrhage and pericardial tamponade, may occur if the inner table of the sternum is penetrated by the needle at areas other than the second intercostal space (Perkins 2003). In contrast, little morbidity is associated with iliac crest aspiration and biopsy, and the posterior iliac crest is the most common site for bone marrow examinations (Figure 12.3). The anterior iliac crest may be used if previous radiation, surgery or patient discomfort does not allow a posterior approach (Perkins 2003).

Indications

There are a number of indications for performing a bone marrow examination. These include (Perkins 2003):

- further work-up of haematological abnormalities observed in the peripheral blood smear
- evaluation of primary bone marrow tumours

717

Posterior iliac crests   Anterior iliac crests   Sternum

Figure 12.2 Common sites for bone marrow examination, arranged in order of preference. Normally, only aspirations and not biopsies are done on the sternum because of its small size and proximity to vital organs.

Ideal location

Figure 12.3 Patient lying in the left lateral position, with the head to the left, exposing the lower back and gluteal region with the right posterior iliac crest palpated.

- staging for bone marrow involvement by metastatic tumours
- assessment of infectious disease processes, including fever of unknown origin
- evaluation of metabolic storage diseases.

Contraindications

- The only absolute reason to avoid performing a bone marrow examination is the presence of coagulation disorders such as haemophilia (unless correctable), which may lead to serious bleeding after the procedure.
- If there is a skin or soft tissue infection over the hip, a different site should be chosen (Goldberg *et al.* 2007).

Principles of care

The procedure should be performed in an aseptic manner with meticulous handwashing to reduce any risk of infection. Any equipment that may cause a needlestick injury must be safely disposed of. Local anaesthetic/general anaesthetic and fasting procedure policies should be followed.

Methods of aspiration and trephine biopsy

- *Aspiration:* an aspirate needle is inserted through the skin into the bone marrow. Once the needle is in the marrow cavity, a syringe is attached and used to aspirate liquid bone marrow (Figure 12.4). This is then spread onto slides (Hoffbrand *et al.* 2006) (Figure 12.5).
- *Trephine:* a trephine needle is inserted and anchored in the bony cortex. The needle is then advanced with a twisting motion and rotated to obtain a solid piece of bone marrow. This piece is then removed along with the needle. A trephine biopsy provides a solid core of bone including marrow and is examined as a histological

Figure 12.4 Aspiration of bone marrow from the marrow cavity

specimen after fixation in formalin, decalcification and sectioning (Hoffbrand *et al.* 2006) (Figure 12.6).

Legal and professional issues

Bone marrow biopsies were traditionally performed by physicians but, more recently, a significant number are being performed by specially trained nurses (Mantik Lewis *et al.* 2004, Ruegg *et al.* 2009). It has long been recognized that with motivated staff and a structured training

(a)

(b)

Figure 12.5 (a) Preparation of aspiration smears. (b) Completed aspiration smear.

718

Figure 12.6 Trephine biopsy sample.

Figure 12.7 From top to bottom: needle guard, sample trap, sample size gauge, trephine biopsy needle with introducer.

programme, it is possible for nurse practitioners to perform the techniques of bone marrow biopsy and obtain specimens of satisfactory quality (Lawson *et al.* 1999). It has also been suggested that this improves the efficiency of a haematology unit and increases the quality of patient care (Lawson *et al.* 1999).

It is common for bone marrow samples to be required for research purposes. These should be collected according to good clinical practice guidelines (MHRA 2009). Other regulations that set standards include the Human Tissue Authority (2009a) *Code of Practice 5: Disposal of Human Tissue.*

The administration of local anaesthetic should be in accordance with a patient group direction or a written prescription.

Competencies

A suitable training package should be available for new practitioners. All practitioners should be assessed by a competent practice facilitator prior to performing procedures on their own. Nurses must always operate within their scope of practice as set out by their profession (NMC 2008b). Learning tools may include competency-based workbooks.

Consent

The practitioner performing the procedure is responsible for providing information prior to the biopsy and obtaining written consent. In the case of paediatric patients, parental consent is required unless the child is over the age of 16 years (NMC 2008a).

Preprocedural considerations

Equipment

Needles with a range of gauges may be used and most have a removable introducer (which prevents plugging of the needle before aspiration) and a stylet that may be used to express the bone marrow biopsy sample. Some models, pri-

marily used for sternal bone marrow aspiration procedures, have adjustable guards that limit the extent of needle penetration (Perkins 2003) (Figure 12.7).

Pharmacological support

In most adult cases, bone marrow biopsies may be carried out with little risk of patient discomfort, provided adequate local anaesthesia is administered. Lidocaine 2% (maximum dose 200 mg) is frequently used (BNF 2011). Patients may describe a 'dragging sensation' during the actual aspiration procedure, even when the site is numb. The duration of the local anaesthetic action is about 90 minutes (BNF 2011).

Apprehensive patients may be given an oral sedative or intravenous conscious sedation before the procedure, but this is usually not necessary (Perkins 2003). If intravenous sedation is used, appropriate resources must be available as per local anaesthetic policy, for example cardiac monitoring, pulse oximetry, oxygen administration, the reversal agent and resuscitation equipment (Provan *et al.* 2009).

This procedure may be more upsetting for paediatric patients and measures to reduce distress include:

- the use of a general anaesthetic
- the application of a thick layer of topical lidocaine 2.5%/prilocaine 2.5% cream under an occlusive dressing to the site selected for cannulation 1–5 hours before the procedure. *Note*: this is not licensed for use in children less than 1 year of age (BMA/PSGB 2009)
- the local infiltration of lidocaine to the bone marrow biopsy site for postoperative pain control. The recommended dose for neonates and children less than 12 years is up to 3 mg/kg (0.3 mL/kg of 1% solution) (BMA/PSGB 2009). If in any doubt, expert advice should be sought.

Non-pharmacological support

Special consideration may also be needed for those who are extremely anxious. Measures include ensuring that the patient has a family member or friend present and complementary therapies such as relaxation, massage and music (Bufalini 2009).

Specific patient preparations

Thrombocytopenia is not a contraindication and bone marrow examination seems to be safe even when thrombocytopenic purpura is present (Lewis *et al.* 2006). However, the nurse must take a history to assess for risk of bleeding (BCSH 2008). This should include details of family history, previous excessive post-traumatic or postsurgical bleeding, liver disease and the use of antithrombotic drugs. If the bleeding history is negative, no further coagulation testing is indicated. If the bleeding history is positive or there is a clear clinical indication (e.g. liver disease), a haematologist should be consulted as to what screening tests are needed and what actions should be taken. Some of these are outlined in the pharmacological support section. If haemorrhage occurs post bone marrow biopsy, the main reasons (in order of frequency) are (Bain 2005):

- diagnosis of a myeloproliferative disorder
- aspirin treatment
- other putative platelet dysfunction.

Questions to determine if the patient's posterior iliac crests have undergone previous radiation, surgery or are affected by soft tissue damage or infection will aid appropriate site selection.

Further assessment should determine if the patient has an allergy to any of the medication, cleaning agents, dressings or equipment to be used.

The need to stop taking antithrombotic drugs prior to the procedure should be discussed with the referring medical team. It is usual practice to stop warfarin 3 days and low molecular weight heparin 24 hours before the procedure. If a patient is on warfarin, a blood test to check the international normalized ratio (INR) should be requested. The result of this should be within the range stipulated by local policy prior to performing the procedure, for example ≤1.5.

Some patients, such as those with multiple myeloma, will require careful positioning due to the infiltration of disease in their bones. These patients may also find bone marrow biopsies more uncomfortable as maintaining the correct position may be difficult. An environment that facilitates the patient's need for privacy and dignity is essential for bone marrow biopsy procedures (NMC 2008a).

Education

The patient's co-operation is essential to ensure the procedure is undertaken safely. All patients should be given access to information and support in a manner that they understand (DH 2005a, NMC 2008a). Written information should be available and patients often access information via the internet at sites such as www.macmillan.org.uk. Consideration must be given to those patients with learning disabilities, language barriers or sensory deficit.

Procedure guideline 12.1 Bone marrow aspiration and trephine biopsy

Essential equipment

- Antiseptic skin cleaning agent (e.g. chlorhexidine gluconate 0.5% in alcohol 70%)
- Sterile dressing pack
- Sterile gloves
- Plastic apron
- Eye protection
- Selection of syringes for bone marrow sampling and administration of local anaesthetic (2, 5 and 10 mL)
- Selection of needles for administration of local anaesthetic (25, 23 and 21 G)
- Marrow aspiration needle and guard
- Trephine biopsy needle
- Cytology slides and coverslips
- Specimen bottles (e.g. plain, formalin, EDTA and heparin)
- Sterile dressing
- Size 11 scalpel

Medicinal products

- Local anaesthetic, for example lidocaine 2%

Preprocedure

Action	Rationale
1 Explain and provide written information about the bone marrow examination.	To ensure the patient is properly informed about the procedure (DH 2005a, C; NMC 2008a, C).

2	Obtain written informed consent.	To enable patients to actively participate in and comply with their treatment (NMC 2008a, C).
3	Check that blood parameters are within safe limits.	To decrease the risk of haemorrhage, which has been identified as the most common and serious adverse event associated with bone marrow examination (Bain 2006, C).
4	Consider oral (e.g. lorazepam) or intravenous (e.g. midazolam) sedation for very anxious patients (Giannoutsos *et al.* 2004).	To ensure that the procedure is performed safely and with minimal distress to the patient. E
5	Prepare the procedure trolley and ensure that all the necessary equipment and specimen containers are readily available.	To ensure the procedure is performed efficiently and that all the necessary specimens are collected and handled correctly (Perkins 2003, C).
6	Ensure patient privacy by drawing the curtains and making use of a sheet or blanket.	An environment that facilitates the patient's need for privacy and dignity is essential for bone marrow biopsy procedures (NMC 2008a, C).
7	Assist the patient into the correct position, which is usually the left or right lateral position with the knees drawn up to the chest.	To access the posterior iliac crest, the most common biopsy site in adults. E

Procedure

8	Wash hands and apply sterile gloves.	To maintain asepsis throughout the procedure to minimize the risk of infection (Fraise and Bradley 2009, E).
9	Reassure and observe the patient throughout the procedure.	To allay anxiety and facilitate the patient's maximum co-operation. P
10	Clean the skin thoroughly at the biopsy site with an antiseptic solution (Perkins 2003), for example chlorhexidine 0.5%, and alcohol solution and allow to dry.	To maintain asepsis throughout the procedure to minimize the risk of infection (Fraise and Bradley 2009, E).
11	Administer local anaesthetic (e.g. lidocaine 2%) intradermally and subcutaneously at the site of the biopsy. Warn the patient that the drug can result in a 'stinging' sensation during administration.	To minimize pain during the procedure (Ruegg *et al.* 2009, R1).
12	Make a small cut in the skin overlying the biopsy site with a scalpel.	To allow for better insertion of the biopsy needle through the skin and to avoid a skin 'plug'. E
13	Insert the aspiration needle through the skin and subcutaneous tissues. Penetrate the marrow cortex 3–10 mm, with a slight rotating motion (Provan *et al.* 2009). Entry of the needle into the bone marrow cavity may be sensed as a slight give.	To access the bone marrow for aspiration. E
14	Remove the introducer, attach a 5 mL syringe to the needle and aspirate a volume of 0.2–2 mL marrow (bloody fluid) (Perkins 2003). Aspiration may cause a very brief, sharp, dragging sensation.	To aspirate liquid bone marrow in order to prepare specimens for further investigation (Hoffbrand *et al.* 2006, C).
15	Smear the marrow quickly onto the cytology slides.	To avoid clotting. E
16	Perform additional aspirations if necessary.	To provide material for flow cytometry, cytogenetics, culture or other special studies as required (Provan *et al.* 2009, C).

721

(Continued)

Procedure guideline 12.1 (*Continued*)

17 Perform the trephine biopsy using the same skin incision if the aspirate has been performed in the iliac crest area. Use a separate biopsy needle, slightly larger than the aspirate needle (Perkins 2003).	In order to minimize the number of skin entry sites. E
18 Advance the trephine needle to penetrate the bone cortex (Provan *et al.* 2009). The biopsy needle may require more pressure to enter the bone because of the larger bore size.	To access the bone for biopsy. E
19 Position the trephine needle away from the area where the aspiration was performed.	To avoid collection of a specimen with extensive artefact induced by the aspiration procedure (Perkins 2003, E).
20 Remove the introducer and use firm hand pressure to advance the needle another 2 cm	To provide a solid core of bone (Provan *et al.* 2009, E).
21 Insert a stylet into the back of the needle.	To give an approximation of the size of the bone core within the needle (Perkins 2003, E).
22 Ensure the length of the trephine specimen is in the range of 1.6–2 cm (Bishop *et al.* 1992, Bain 2001, Campbell *et al.* 2003).	The analysis of the relation between length of trephine and the rate of positivity for neoplasia yielded a minimum adequate length of 1.6 cm before processing (Bishop *et al.* 1992, C).
23 Remove the needle from the bone and use the stylet to express the specimen into the appropriate container (Perkins 2003).	To collect the solid core of bone and marrow to examine as a histological specimen after fixation in formalin, decalcification and sectioning (Hoffbrand *et al.* 2006, C).
24 Apply manual pressure to the site for several minutes until the bleeding stops.	To achieve haemostasis (Perkins 2003, E).
25 Apply a sterile pressure dressing.	To achieve haemostasis and decrease the risk of infection at the biopsy site (Provan *et al.* 2009, E).

Postprocedure

26 Apply pressure bandages and check the site for prolonged bleeding if a patient is thrombocytopenic (Perkins 2003).	To minimize bruising, prevent haematoma and decrease the risk of haemorrhage (Bain 2006, C).
27 Dispose of sharps as per local policy.	To ensure the safe handling and disposal of needles and other sharp instruments and to protect staff, patients and visitors from exposure to bloodborne pathogens (Pratt *et al.* 2007, C).
28 Label specimens as per trust policy and send them to the appropriate laboratory department.	To prevent incorrect diagnosis and disease management through incorrectly labelled specimens (BCSH 1999, C).
29 Record the necessary information in the appropriate documents as per local policy.	To maintain accurate records (NMC 2009, C).
30 Ensure the patient has returned to preprocedure functional status before discharge.	To ensure the safe management and recovery of patients receiving sedation. E
31 Give the patient appropriate aftercare instructions (see Education of patient and relevant others).	To ensure the safe management of patients and to enable them to actively participate in and comply with their treatment (NMC 2008a, C).

Problem-solving table 12.1 Prevention and resolution (Procedure guideline 12.1)

Problem	Cause	Prevention	Action
Anxiety	Fear of pain or anticipatory anxiety due to a previous adverse experience (Lidén *et al.* 2009) Pre-existing pain (Lidén *et al.* 2009) Anxiety about the diagnostic outcome (Lidén *et al.* 2009)	Provide reassurance and support	Answer all questions and consider non-pharmacological support, for example relaxation therapy Consider anxiolytics, for example oral or intravenous benzodiazepines (Perkins 2003)
Difficulty locating posterior iliac crest	An inexperienced practitioner Difficulty in palpating the posterior iliac crest, for example in bariatric patients Altered anatomy, for example multiple myeloma patients who have experienced collapsed vertebrae and loss in height or patients who have had back surgery Patients who are unable to maintain the correct position due to, for example, pre-existing pain	Competency-based learning Guidance and support from an experienced practitioner Elective radiological guided procedure Adequate pain control	Recheck surface landmarks Ask for the assistance of a more experienced practitioner Consider a radiological guided procedure, especially in the case of bariatric patients
Uncontrollable pain	Inadequate administration of local anaesthetic Anticipatory anxiety associated with a previous experience which may augment the experience of pain (Lidén *et al.* 2009) Pre-existing pain related to disease process or co-morbidity	Administer sufficient local anaesthetic and wait for this to take effect Ensure adequate reassurance and support as anxiety may enhance the perception of pain Ensure correct positioning and direct approach Review pain control and consider referral to colleagues in the pain control team for advice	Reassess positioning. It is unusual for the procedure to be unbearably painful if the approach is correct and sufficient local anaesthesia has been used The procedure should be aborted if the pain continues and assistance should be sought Consider sedation for future procedures
No dragging sensation noted by the patient and no marrow obtained	Faulty technique, fibrosis, hyper- or hypocellularity (Humphries 2006)	Ensure correct positioning Ensure guidance and support for new practitioners	Rotate the needle and apply suction again. If no marrow is obtained, another sampling site may be required (Perkins 2003)
No marrow can be aspirated (dry tap)	Faulty technique, fibrosis, hyper- or hypocellularity (Humphries 2006)	Ensure correct positioning Ensure guidance and support for new practitioners	Make touch preparations from the biopsy (trephine roll) (Perkins 2003)

723

Postprocedural considerations

Immediate care

The patient should be advised to lie on their back, exerting pressure downwards on the biopsy site to assist in achieving haemostasis (Bain 2006). The biopsy site should be checked before the patient leaves the department to ensure that there is no bleeding. The patient should not experience any discomfort at the biopsy site immediately after the procedure due to the ongoing action of the local anaesthetic (BNF 2011). The patient should return to preprocedure functional status immediately after the procedure if no sedation has been used. A medical review should be requested if the patient has any unexpected pain or loss of mobility.

Ongoing care

This comprises wound care, pain control and monitoring for signs of infection. This is discussed further in Education of patient and relevant others, as a bone marrow examination is usually an outpatient procedure (Lewis *et al.* 2006).

Documentation

The operator is responsible for documenting the procedure details to ensure accurate records are kept (NMC 2009). These should include:

- the site used and number of puncture sites
- volume and percentage of local anaesthetic
- information about any other medication used
- a list of samples obtained
- any unexpected incidents or adverse events
- dressings and wound care
- follow-up advice and information provided.

Education of patient and relevant others

The patient should be encouraged to contact the hospital if there are any concerns about postprocedural care. Contact telephone numbers and the following advice should be given to patients.

- *Wound care:* the patient should be instructed to check the site frequently and to reapply pressure if the biopsy site does start to ooze. Intermittent application of an ice pack may also help to achieve haemostasis. It is routine practice to advise the patient to keep the dressing dry for 24 hours. The patient may then remove the dressing and wash as normal. Patients are also advised to monitor the biopsy site for any signs of infection such as redness, pain, swelling, failure to heal or exudate (Goldberg *et al.* 2007).
- *Pain:* once the local anaesthetic has worn off, mild discomfort lasting 12–24 hours is common after a bone marrow examination (Goldberg *et al.* 2007). The patient should be advised that this may be dealt with by simple analgesia such as paracetamol (Provan *et al.* 2009).

Complications

Although adverse events after trephine biopsies and bone marrow aspirates are rare, they can have considerable impact on individual patients (Bain 2005).

- *Cardiac tamponade:* the actual risks associated with a sternal puncture are extremely small but penetration of the bone and damage to underlying structures are possible as the sternum is only approximately 1 cm thick in adults (Perkins 2003). The use of a guarded needle helps in preventing too deep an insertion. This is managed with an emergency call to the cardiac arrest team for immediate intervention.

- *Bone fractures:* particularly in small children owing to the pressure exerted. This is managed with analgesia, radiological investigation and referral to the orthopaedic team if indicated.

Bone marrow harvest

Related theory

Collecting haematopoietic stem cells by means of a bone marrow harvest or apheresis is well established in the transplant setting. More recently, transplants have also been facilitated through stem cells obtained from umbilical cords. Cord blood transplantation remains a specialized procedure more relevant for some areas of transplantation than others (Richardson and Atkinson 2006). The protocol for harvesting this alternative source of stem cells is beyond the scope of this chapter.

Evidence-based approaches

Rationale

Every year in the UK about 28,500 people are diagnosed with a haematological malignancy such as leukaemia, lymphoma or myeloma (Leukaemia and Lymphoma Research 2010). A stem cell transplant is one possible treatment option for these diseases (Atkinson 2005). A stem cell transplant aims to replace a patient's own diseased bone marrow with healthy stem cells. Before the patient receives the stem cells, they receive a combination of chemotherapy and radiation to destroy their own bone marrow. The healthy stem cells are collected from a patient when in remission (autologous) or from a donor (allogeneic) (Richardson and Atkinson 2006). The stem cells are then introduced into the patient's bloodstream much in the same manner as a blood transfusion. If the donated stem cells 'engraft', they begin producing normal blood cells (Atkinson 2005). The principles and process of collecting bone marrow apply to both allogeneic and autologous donors.

Indications

Although the use of stem cells collected by apheresis has superseded bone marrow in both the autologous and allogeneic setting in many transplant centres (Richardson and Atkinson 2006), indications for bone marrow include:

- allogeneic donors under the age of 16 years
- allogeneic donors providing cells for a recipient with a non-malignant disorder, for example aplastic anaemia
- donor preference.

Contraindications

Contraindications to donating stem cells by means of bone marrow include:

- a history of back problems
- donors who are unable to undergo a general anaesthetic.

Principles of care

The care of bone marrow donors is guided by a duty of care, encompassing the physical, emotional, psychological, social and spiritual dimensions of well-being (Be the Match Registry 2010). Ethical considerations should be incorporated into local policy and guidelines are available that outline the expected standards of care for unrelated (Hurley and Raffoux 2004) and related (van Walraven *et al.* 2009) donors. The procedure should be performed as a sterile procedure under general anaesthetic and all perioperative principles apply (see Chapter 17). Bone marrow harvests are performed under general anaesthesia because:

- the procedure may last for approximately 1 hour compared with the 15–30 minutes for an aspiration and biopsy
- multiple puncture sites are used
- the procedure may be painful.

Methods for bone marrow harvest

The procedure is undertaken by:

- two trained practitioners to perform the harvest (either two doctors, or a doctor and a nurse)
- one theatre nurse to oversee the equipment, sterile trolley and infusion of bone marrow into the sterile kit
- theatre staff
- an anaesthetist.

Bone marrow is aspirated directly from the marrow with a bone marrow harvest needle and syringe. A volume of 800–1000 mL is aspirated from the posterior iliac crest (in order to acquire sufficient cells per kilogram of the recipient's body weight) (Outhwaite 2000). The marrow is either frozen and stored or given fresh to the recipient (Richardson and Atkinson 2006).

Anticipated patient/donor outcomes

The anticipated outcome from the procedure is to collect a sufficient dose of stem cells in order to facilitate a haematopoietic stem cell transplant. The anticipated outcome for the donor is to:

- remain infection free
- have no nerve, tissue or bone damage
- return to predonation levels of activity within 1 month of the harvest
- adequately manage any pain or discomfort experienced due to the bone marrow harvest.

Legal and professional issues

Standards that regulate bone marrow donation include the Human Tissue Authority (2009c) *Code of Practice 6: Donation of Allogeneic Bone Marrow and Peripheral Blood Stem Cells for Transplantation* and FACT-JACIE's (2008) *International Standards for Cellular Therapy Product Collection, Processing and Administration*.

Competencies

It is a requirement that practitioners performing this procedure have experience and training in bone marrow harvesting (FACT-JACIE 2008). Competence must be demonstrated and documented.

Consent

Before taking consent, donors should be carefully informed about the risks and benefits of the donation procedure in a manner that they understand. Although transplant centres usually have a preference for the source of stem cells, donors should be given a choice whether to donate bone marrow or stem cells by means of apheresis. Consent is an ongoing process and donors have the right to refuse to proceed (FACT-JACIE 2008). They should, however, be warned what the consequences of this would be for the recipient, if they do so after the conditioning regimen for transplant has been commenced.

Children acting as donors require further consideration. Laws and regulations governing minors, acting as a donor for a sick sibling, differ from country to country. Rarely, adult donors with severe developmental or psychological problems rendering them mentally incapable of informed consent are considered as stem cell donors for a relative. These can be either donors who have always been mentally challenged (e.g. Down's syndrome) or those who are suffering from a psychiatric illness. It is advised to first establish whether the aspirant donor would be able to endure the donation procedure (both physically and mentally), before performing tissue type testing (van Walraven *et al.* 2009).

In the United Kingdom, evidence must be documented that the Human Tissue Authority (2009b) *Code of Practice 1: Consent* has been applied. All information should be managed within a strict framework of confidentiality (FACT-JACIE 2008).

Preprocedural considerations

Equipment

Bone marrow harvest needles are usually 11 G with a removable introducer. Harvested bone marrow must be filtered to remove particulate matter prior to final processing and packaging for distribution or transplantation (FACT-JACIE 2008). This process must be performed under sterile conditions in the operating room at the time of harvest or in an appropriate sterile setting in the processing laboratory (FACT-JACIE 2008). Sterile in-line filters are available commercially in a collection set. The filter size may range from coarse (500 μm) to medium (300 μm) to fine (200 μm). All harvested marrow should ultimately pass through a fine filter, while other sizes may only be necessary if the marrow has a large amount of particulate matter (FACT-JACIE 2008).

Pharmacological support

The bone marrow harvest is performed under general anaesthesia and local policy with regard to perioperative care should be followed (see Chapter 17). Local anaesthetic, for example lidocaine 2%, is usually instilled into the harvest sites for postsurgery pain relief. Postoperative pain should be monitored and is usually managed with non-opioids and mild opioids. Iron supplements may be prescribed to facilitate haemoglobin recovery post harvest.

Specific patient/donor preparation

There should be donor evaluation procedures in place to protect the safety of the donor and recipient. All stem cell donors (autologous or allogeneic) should be given a medical examination to confirm they are physically and emotionally fit to undergo anaesthesia and the marrow harvest (Be the Match Registry 2010). The donor's medical history, physical examination and laboratory test results should be performed and documented according to the *International Standards*

for Cellular Therapy Product Collection, Processing and Administration (FACT-JACIE 2008). Both the potential for disease transmission from the donor to the recipient and the risks to the donor from the collection procedure should be assessed (FACT-JACIE 2008). The allogeneic donor's suitability must be documented before the recipient's high-dose therapy has begun.

The psychosocial needs of the donor should be assessed (Blume and Amylon 2004). Key areas for support are: child-care arrangements, transportation, past and present drug and alcohol usage, unique cultural, religious, literacy and language needs and employment issues (Blume and Amylon 2004). An appropriately trained healthcare professional should be available to offer donors counselling, reassurance and support.

Education

It is widely agreed that donors require good-quality information to reduce their anxiety, to enable them to give informed consent and to enable them to actively participate with the donation process (Chapman and Rush 2003, NMC 2008a). An increasing number of people are obtaining information from the internet and may be quite informed (or misinformed) based on the quality of the information they acquire. Transplant facilities and donor registries should develop their own centre-specific information which can be posted on their website or mailed to donors in advance of their first clinic visit to meet some of the education needs (Blume and Amylon 2004).

Procedure guideline 12.2 Bone marrow harvest

Essential equipment

- Skin cleaning agent, for example 2% chlorhexidine solution
- A sterile collection set with transfer packs and in-line filters (e.g. 500 and 200 μm) containing specified anticoagulant, for example ACDA
- 250 mL 0.9% sodium chloride with 50 mL of heparin (1000 units per mL preservative free)
- Two 11 G bone marrow harvest needles flushed with heparinized saline
- 20 mL syringes containing 1 mL of heparinized saline × 6
- Selection of syringes and needles for administration of local anaesthetic
- Dressings
- Sterile gauze
- Sterile drapes
- Two receivers
- Face masks
- Sterile gowns
- Sterile gloves
- Sterile pack containing jug, gallipot, gauze swabs, forceps, towel clips
- Documentation as per accreditation and local policy requirements

Medicinal products

- General anaesthesia (as per local policy)
- Lidocaine 2%

Preprocedure

Action	Rationale
1 Explain and provide written information about the bone marrow harvest.	To ensure the donor is properly informed about the procedure (DH 2005a, C; NMC 2008a, C).
2 Obtain written informed consent.	To enable donors to actively participate in and comply with their treatment (NMC 2008a, C; FACT-JACIE 2008, C; Human Tissue Authority 2009b, C).
3 Ensure that two units of cross-matched, allogeneic packed red cells are available on the day of harvest. These should only be used in exceptional circumstances, for example massive haemorrhage.	To reduce the risks associated with allogeneic blood transfusion (Confer 2004, C).
4 Prepare the sterile procedure trolley and ensure that all the necessary equipment is available.	To ensure the procedure is performed efficiently and that the cells are collected and handled correctly. E
5 Bring the donor into the operating room when anaesthetized and position correctly on the operating table. In adults, this is usually the prone position with hands placed above the head.	To allow marrow to be collected simultaneously from both the left and right posterior iliac crest by two practitioners (Confer 2004, C).
6 Ensure the harvest is performed as a sterile procedure. (a) Don facemasks. (b) Scrub hands meticulously. (c) Don sterile gowns. (d) Don sterile gloves.	To maintain asepsis throughout the procedure to minimize the risk of infection (Fraise and Bradley 2009, E).

Procedure

7 Clean the skin over the posterior iliac crests thoroughly with an antiseptic solution and allow to dry.	To maintain asepsis throughout the procedure to minimize the risk of infection (Fraise and Bradley 2009, E).
8 Place four sterile drapes over the patient to maintain a sterile field. (a) One drape placed above the posterior iliac crests and spread towards the donor's head. (b) One drape placed below the posterior iliac crests and spread towards the donor's feet. (c) Two drapes spread left and right of the harvest site respectively.	To create a sterile field around the harvest site and to maintain asepsis throughout the procedure to minimize the risk of infection (Fraise and Bradley 2009, E).
9 Place two receivers on the sterile towels. (a) One should contain two 11 G harvest needles (flushed with heparinized saline). (b) One should contain six 20 mL syringes (flushed with heparinized saline and drawn up to 1 mL with heparinized saline).	To ensure the harvest equipment is easily accessible. The heparinized saline prevents the marrow from clotting in the syringe. E
10 Locate the posterior iliac spine through palpation (Confer 2004).	To ensure the preferred site for harvest is located. E
11 Insert the harvest needle through the skin and subcutaneous tissues, and penetrate the marrow cortex 3–10 mm, with a slight rotating motion. Entry of the needle into the bone marrow cavity may be sensed as a slight give.	To access the marrow within the bony cortex (Confer 2004, C).
12 Remove the introducer and attach the harvest needle to a 20 mL syringe. Aspirate a volume of 10–20 mL of marrow (bloody fluid) by applying vigorous suction.	To aspirate marrow from the donor. Short, vigorous aspirations are generally thought to produce a higher concentration of marrow cells relative to peripheral blood (Confer 2004, E).

Procedure guideline 12.2 (*Continued*)

13	Place filled syringes in the receiver.	To allow the nurse responsible for transferring the marrow into the sterile collection set to access them. E
14	If using ACDA, the nurse should add 70 mL of ACDA to the main collection bag prior to each harvest of 420 mL.	To prevent any clotting. E
15	Remove the filled syringe from the receiver and dispel any air from the syringe.	To ensure that the correct amount of marrow is aspirated. E
16	Ensure the marrow volume is recorded by a member of the theatre staff.	To keep a running total to ensure that the correct amount of marrow is aspirated. E
17	The nurse should gently add the marrow to the collection bag and gently agitate the collection bag to mix the marrow with the anticoagulant.	To prevent any clotting. E
18	Flush the syringe with heparinized saline (leaving 1 mL in the syringe).	To prevent any clotting. E
19	Return it to the receiver ready for subsequent aspirations.	To ensure the practitioners performing the harvest have a supply of appropriately prepared syringes to perform the aspirations. E
20	Advance the harvest needle several millimetres and repeat the process.	To allow for several aspirations from a single bone puncture as the needle is repeatedly advanced (Confer 2004, C).
21	After a number of aspirations from the same site, replace the introducer and move the position of the harvest needle to another place in the bone approximately 2 cm from the first entry site.	To allow the bone to be entered multiple times through a single skin entry site. A typical collection may involve 70 marrow aspirations obtained through only a few skin punctures. E
22	Once a total of 420 mL of marrow has been collected, open the clips to allow the marrow to pass through the in-line filters (the 500 μm filter and then the 200 μm filter) from the collection bag to the first transfer pack. Then close the two clips prior to adding a second volume of 70 mL of ACDA to the collection bag and beginning bone marrow aspirations for a second transfer pack.	To ensure that transfer packs are not overfilled and that the correct amount of anticoagulant is added to prevent clotting (E) and to remove particulate matter (FACT-JACIE 2008, C).
	The total volume in each bag should approximate 420 mL of marrow and 70 mL of ACDA. If less than 420 mL of marrow is required for subsequent bags, the ACDA should be reduced accordingly to maintain a ratio of 1:7 ACDA:marrow.	To prevent any clotting. E
23	Aspirate a small sample from the first transfer pack when this has been filled.	To allow the adequacy of the collection to be determined by a nucleated cell count (Confer 2004, C).
24	Place the sample in an EDTA specimen container.	This is the preferred medium for nucleated cell count analysis (Confer 2004, C).
25	Label specimen container.	To ensure safe and correct processing of sample (Western Sussex Hospitals NHS Trust 2009, C).
26	Send sample to the laboratory for a white cell count.	To allow the adequacy of the collection to be determined by a nucleated cell count (Confer 2004, C).

27	This process should be repeated for each transfer pack filled.	To allow the adequacy of the entire collection to be determined by a nucleated cell count (Confer 2004, C).
28	Document the number of puncture holes made in the hospital notes.	To facilitate postoperative wound care and to maintain accurate records (NMC 2009, C).
29	The nurse should seal the transfer packs as per local policy, using an approved heat sealer.	To maintain asepsis, minimize the risk of infection and facilitate the safe transport of the cells (Fraise and Bradley 2009, E).
30	The nurse should record the respective volume of bone marrow on the outside of the transfer pack in millilitres, using FACT-JACIE approved labels.	To establish total amount of bone marrow in each bag. E
31	Withdraw the harvest needles from the posterior iliac crest, pack sterile gauze over the left and right harvest sites respectively and maintain digital pressure until the bleeding has stopped.	To achieve haemostasis, minimize leakage and prevent the formation of a haematoma. E
32	Instil lidocaine 2% intradermally into the harvest sites up to the maximum recommended dose.	To help with pain control immediately postoperatively. E

Postprocedure

33	Dispose of sharps as per local policy.	To ensure the safe handling and disposal of needles and other sharp instruments and to protect staff, patients and visitors from exposure to bloodborne pathogens (DH 2005b, C; Pratt *et al.* 2007, C).
34	Inspect the puncture sites for bleeding. Mepore and a pressure dressing may be applied over the sterile gauze.	To achieve haemostasis and decrease the risk of infection at the harvest sites. E
35	Take the donor to the recovery room.	To ensure appropriate postoperative care. E
36	Label each transfer pack as per local policy with FACT-JACIE compliant labels.	To ensure correct management of the product (FACT-JACIE 2008, C).
37	Place the transfer packs in a secondary container (e.g. a zip-type resealable bag) prior to transfer to the appropriate processing facility.	To prevent the loss of a portion of the collection, to minimize the potential of postcollection contamination of the component and to prevent potential spillage of biohazard material in areas where it may pose a risk to employees, visitors or patients (FACT-JACIE 2008, C).
38	Transport the marrow to the appropriate processing facility with the necessary forms and in a FACT-JACIE compliant container.	To allow for cell measurement, storage and/or issue of the marrow. E
39	Record the necessary information in the appropriate documents as per local policy.	To maintain accurate records (NMC 2009, C).
40	Ensure postdonation care is appropriately managed (see Postprocedural considerations).	To ensure the safe management of patients and to enable them to actively participate in and comply with their treatment (NMC 2008a, C).

Problem-solving table 12.2 Prevention and resolution (Procedure guideline 12.2)

Problem	Cause	Prevention	Action
Reactions to the anaesthetic agents and associated morbidity (Rosenmayr *et al.* 2003)	Allergic reactions, hypersensitivity reactions or idiosyncratic reactions (Confer 2004)	Careful preassessment	Instigate urgent treatment and mechanical ventilation as necessary (Confer 2004)
Haemorrhage, which can result in life-threatening blood loss and can also create severe pain from the compression of soft tissues (Confer 2004)	Poor technique Antiplatelet drugs Anticoagulant drugs Coagulopathies	Careful preassessment Experienced practitioners	Pressure dressing Platelet transfusion Correction of clotting derangement Analgesia
Target cell dose not achieved through aspiration from the posterior iliac crests	This may occur if the marrow space of the crest has been compromised by, for example, trauma or radiation (Confer 2004). This is particularly applicable to autologous donors	Careful preassessment Experienced practitioners	Marrow may then also be collected from the anterior iliac crests or the sternum (Confer 2004)

Postprocedural considerations

Immediate care

Immediate postdonation care includes:

- all usual postoperative nursing care measures
- postoperative full blood count
- adequate analgesia and antiemetic cover
- wound and dressing check before discharge.

Documentation

Bone marrow harvests should be strictly regulated within a quality management system with clear standard operating procedures and documentation. Archived documentation should be maintained according to governmental, regulatory or institutional policy, whichever is longer (FACT-JACIE 2008). Due to the strict regulatory nature of bone marrow harvests, a record-keeping system must be in place to ensure the authenticity, integrity and confidentiality of all documents (FACT-JACIE 2008). All nursing records must be clearly maintained to ensure accurate data (NMC 2009).

Education of patient and relevant others

All donors should be informed that it is normal to experience some pain, bruising and stiffness, feel more tired than usual and run a low-grade fever during the first week after donation. Soreness at the collection site usually eases off in around a week with pain relief (Be the Match Registry 2010). Further guidelines to be given to donors post procedure are detailed in Box 12.1.

Furthermore, all donors should receive written instructions to contact the hospital if they experience any of the following symptoms (Be the Match Registry 2010).

- Temperature of 38°C or higher.
- Increased redness, bleeding, swelling, drainage or pain at the collection area.
- Muscle weakness or severe headache within 2 weeks of donation.
- Pain more than 14 days after the donation.

Box 12.1 Guidelines to be given to bone marrow harvest donors post procedure (Be the Match Registry 2010)

- The discomfort at the harvest site should resolve in about 1 week.
- Analgesia should be taken as directed.
- Aspirin should be avoided during the first week after the donation unless instructed by the medical team.
- The harvest site should be checked daily for bleeding or increasing erythema.
- The harvest site should be kept dry the night after the procedure.
- Bandages should be removed 24 hours after surgery, and replaced with an adhesive dressing.
- Some wound drainage is expected.
- Showers rather than baths should be taken for the first 2–3 days to decrease the risk of infection.
- The adhesive dressings should be changed daily after a shower until the wounds have healed.
- If bleeding occurs, firm pressure should be applied for 5 minutes, followed by an ice pack. The patient should be advised that if the bleeding does not stop after 10 minutes of constant direct pressure, to contact the hospital.
- It is common to experience 'hard lumps' at the harvest sites where the needles were inserted. These may take a few weeks to resolve.

Complications

The complications of bone marrow harvests are rare but it remains a significant procedure and not without physical risk or psychological consequences (Blume and Amylon 2004). There is potential for bone, nerve or other tissue damage at the aspiration sites (Rosenmayr *et al.* 2003). Sciatic pain, lasting up to 18 months, has been reported in a related donor (Confer 2004). Other complications include:

- A potential for *infection* at the aspiration sites (Rosenmayr *et al.* 2003). These may occur due to poor practitioner technique or inadequate wound care. Hand decontamination, infection control and wound care policies should be followed as essential preventive measures (Fraise and Bradley 2009). Antibiotics should be used to treat infections if indicated (Confer 2004).
- *Anaemia*, due to the large amount of bone marrow aspirated (Rosenmayr *et al.* 2003). Resultant allogeneic transfusions may cause transfusion reactions, transmit viral infections and, rarely, bacterial infections (Confer 2004). Transfusion practice for bone marrow donation varies depending on the collection physician (see Box 12.2). Discharge medication should include ferrous sulphate.
- *Fatigue* related to procedure-induced anaemia. The severity of anaemia is determined entirely by the donor's preoperative haemoglobin level and the net blood loss. Treatment with transfusion has already been described. Other measures include:
  - a gradual return to work (usually after 1 week)
  - ensuring rest between periods of work
  - avoiding strenuous activity for 3–4 weeks
  - a 1-month follow-up appointment for check-up and repeat full blood count.

Box 12.2 Reported bone marrow harvest transfusion practice

- Units of autologous blood may be collected from donors a few weeks prior to the harvest for transfusion after the procedure. This practice is becoming less common.
- Autologous red cells may be recovered from the collected bone marrow. This process has been successfully applied in child donors without compromising the quality of the marrow donation.
- Administration of erythropoietin (EPO) may also diminish the likelihood of allogeneic blood transfusion. A theoretical concern about pretreatment of donors with EPO is diminished quality of the collected marrow.

(Confer 2004)

In the event of complications, donors should be referred to the medical team, physiotherapist and the wider multidisciplinary team as necessary.

Apheresis

Related theory

Apheresis was introduced in the late 1960s and was innovative as it served to remove the major blood cell constituents or plasma rapidly, while processing large volumes of blood efficiently (Kaushansky and Williams 2010). The earliest procedures were performed on patients with chronic myeloid leukaemia (CML). In these instances, the procedure served to lower the patient's white cell count (Kaushansky and Williams 2010).

With scientific advances, apheresis is no longer only used on patients in order to remove blood components or exchange them for therapeutic purposes and it is now possible to harvest blood components such as stem cells to be used for donation. Stem cells can be 'mobilized' into the peripheral blood following treatment with cytotoxic chemotherapy and/or the administration of the haematopoietic growth factor G-CSF, with or without Plerixafor. The use of stem cells collected by means of apheresis has superseded bone marrow in many transplant centres (Richardson and Atkinson 2006). Exact protocols vary according to underlying disease, treatment regimens, local practice and the type of stem cell donor; for example, cytotoxic chemotherapy and Plerixafor are not used to mobilize stem cells from healthy donors.

Evidence-based approaches

Rationale

Apheresis is used for a number of donor and therapeutic purposes. A therapeutic procedure is when a blood component is removed from a patient to decrease the amount of defective cells or deplete a disease mediator (GambroBCT 2005). A donor procedure is when a blood component (e.g. stem cells, lymphocytes, platelets) is removed to be used for therapeutic purposes (e.g. peripheral blood stem cell transplant, donor lymphocyte infusion, platelet transfusion).

Indications

The American Society for Apheresis (ASFA) Applications Committee reviews and categorizes the indications for therapeutic apheresis every 7 years. It aims to provide uniformity, is as evidence based as possible and provides comprehensive information which could be shared with patients and clinical services requesting the use of therapeutic apheresis (Szczepiorkowski *et al.* 2007). Some apheresis applications and indications are outlined in Table 12.3.

731

Table 12.3 Apheresis applications and indications

Applications	Indications
Therapeutic apheresis	
Plasma exchange:	
Removal of a patient's own plasma and replacement with appropriate fluids, for example albumin, FFP. This is in order to remove disease mediators including: ■ alloantibodies ■ autoimmune antibodies ■ antigen-antibody complexes ■ abnormal or increased amounts of plasma protein ■ very high cholesterol levels ■ high levels of plasma metabolic waste products ■ plasma-bound poisons or drugs	■ Thrombotic thrombocytopenia purpura (TTP) ■ Guillain–Barré syndrome ■ Myasthenia gravis
Red blood cell exchange:	
Removal of large volumes of patient red blood cells and replacement with normal donor red blood cells	■ Sickle cell disease ■ Malaria ■ Babesiosis
Cellular depletion:	
Rapid removal of greatly elevated number of cells from the intravascular space. Decreases the risk associated with vascular stasis, for example: ■ White blood cell depletion ■ Platelet depletion	■ Symptomatic leucocytosis in, for example, a patient newly diagnosed with acute myeloid leukaemia ■ Symptomatic thrombocytosis in a patient with thrombophilia
Photopheresis:	
Use of apheresis technology, light-activated drugs and ultraviolet light to modulate lymphocyte activity	■ Cutaneous T cell lymphoma ■ Pemphigus vulgaris ■ Chronic graft-versus-host disease ■ Acute and chronic graft rejection
Immunoadsorption:	
Removal of a disease mediator from the patient's plasma and the subsequent return of the treated plasma to the patient	■ Immune thrombocytopenic purpura (ITP) ■ Rheumatoid arthritis ■ Platelet refractoriness ■ Haemolytic uraemic syndrome
Dendritic cell collection:	
Removal of dendritic cells in order to manipulate them *in vitro* by providing them with tumour antigen so that they are capable of activating T lymphocytes to fight malignancy	■ Prostate cancer ■ Melanoma ■ Multiple myeloma ■ Small cell lung cancer ■ Renal cell carcinoma ■ Breast cancer
LDL apheresis:	
Selective removal of LDL cholesterol from a patient's plasma through secondary processing	■ Familial hypercholesterolaemia unresponsive to drug therapy

Table 12.3 (*Continued*)

Applications	Indications
Donor apheresis	
Peripheral blood stem cell collection:	
White cell procedure to collect haemopoietic stem cells. The collected stem cells may be used fresh or cryopreserved for both malignant and non-malignant conditions	■ Autologous stem cell collection (patient's own stem cells) ■ Allogeneic stem cell collection (collected from an HLA-matched related or unrelated donor) ■ Syngeneic stem cell collection (collected from the patient's identical twin) ■ Haploidentical stem cell collection (collected from either the mother or father of the patient)
Granulocyte collection:	
White cell procedure to collect granulocytes (neutrophils) from suitable donors	■ Transfuse to neutropenic patients in order to provide adequate numbers of functional neutrophils to fight bacterial, fungal or yeast infections
Lymphocyte collection:	
White cell procedure to collect lymphocytes from a related or unrelated donor for a patient following an allogeneic stem cell transplant (the donor of the graft cells is also the donor of the lymphocytes)	■ Post allogeneic stem cell transplantation in the event of malignancy relapse ■ Non-myeloablative allogeneic stem cell transplant ■ Production of targeted cytotoxic T lymphocytes
Platelet collection:	
Collection of platelets from healthy donors. Primarily the role of the blood transfusion service	■ For patients who, for a multitude of reasons, require a platelet transfusion

Foss (2003), Gambro (2005), Strauss (2003)

Contraindications

Contraindications will depend on the reason for undertaking the procedure, that is, donor or therapeutic.

■ *Donors*: there are strict processes in place that regulate whether an individual may donate a blood component for therapeutic use. These include FACT-JACIE's (2008) *International Standards for Cellular Therapy Product Collection, Processing and Administration* for stem cell and lymphocyte donors and the regulations that national blood services put forward for platelet and granulocyte donors. Contraindications should be stated in the cell separator facility's standard operating procedure manual. An example of a contraindication for allogeneic donors is a diagnosis of human immunodeficiency virus (HIV).

■ *Patients*: it is a medical decision as to whether a patient is fit to proceed with a cell separator procedure for therapeutic reasons. It may be appropriate to undertake a cell separator procedure in a very unwell patient if it is deemed to be a life-saving intervention. For example, some patients with acute myeloid leukaemia present with a high white cell count and are at risk of leucostasis and are therefore referred for white cell depletion. All decisions must be documented in the patient's medical notes.

Principles of care

There has been an increase in the clinical use of cell separators for the treatment of a greater variety of clinical conditions and to collect a greater range of therapeutic products. It is therefore important that careful consideration is given to the likely clinical conditions to be treated, blood products to be collected, the most suitable type of equipment to use and the appropriate training of staff when setting up a cell separator service (BCSH 1998).

The decision to use a cell separator for donor or therapeutic purposes is the responsibility of a medical consultant. In view of the known risks and complications associated with the use of cell separators, appropriately trained medical and nursing staff must be in attendance (BCSH 1998).

Methods for apheresis

The procedure for performing apheresis is complex and differs depending on the system and application. The basic steps in apheresis are:

■ removal of whole blood from a patient or donor into a cell separator
■ addition of an anticoagulant to the blood to prevent clotting in the extracorporeal circuit
■ centrifugation and/or filtration to achieve separation of the blood components
■ removal/collection of the desired blood component
■ return of the rest of the blood to the patient with or without replacement products.

The ability of various techniques and equipment to carry out these basic steps determines collection efficiency and product purity (Burgstaler 2003). Further information can be gained from the respective apheresis operators' manuals.

Anticipated patient/donor outcomes

Anticipated patient/donor outcomes are dependent on the indication for carrying out the procedure. It is anticipated that cell separator procedures do no harm to patients or donors. Local standard operating procedures should be followed to ensure that desired end-points are reached and the efficacy of the procedure is within an expected range, irrespective of the operator.

Legal and professional issues

Other regulations that regulate apheresis, if being used in the field of stem cell transplantation, include the Human Tissue Authority (2009c) *Code of Practice 6: Donation of Allogeneic Bone Marrow and Peripheral Blood Stem Cells for Transplantation* and FACT-JACIE's (2008) *International Standards for Cellular Therapy Product Collection, Processing and Administration.*

Cell separator procedures should only be performed after a written and signed order from the medical team. The administration of any drugs and fluids used should be in accordance with a patient group direction or a written prescription.

Competencies

Apheresis should only be performed by specially trained operators who are deemed competent to work at an advanced level. Nurses must always operate within their scope of practice (NMC 2008b). Training packages should address the theoretical base and clinical skills needed to work as an apheresis nurse and should be carried out in accordance with local standard operating procedures. It is usual for the manufacturers of cell separator machines to offer training days and supply training materials, for example workbooks. This is often supported by work-based learning with a mentor or practice facilitator. Academic modules at university level are offered in some countries. Training should cover the assessment and management of patients and donors (including paediatrics if appropriate) undergoing apheresis, as well as the technology used to carry out the applications. Other training needs, dependent on particular centres, may include:

- principles of basic haematology, coagulation and immunology
- knowledge of the diseases for which apheresis is required
- collection of specific blood components by apheresis
- recognition and treatment of common complications
- validation of procedures and processes within a quality management system
- regulatory, legal and professional issues.

A suitable assessment, designed to determine the level of competence, must be performed and documentation of knowledge and technical ability must be maintained (BCSH 1998). Apheresis nurses must also ensure that their cardiopulmonary resuscitation training is up to date (BCSH 1998).

Consent

The routine of obtaining consent from patients and donors undergoing apheresis represents good clinical practice (MHRA 2009). Clearly written explanatory literature or other forms of information should be available to assist in obtaining informed consent. This should include any drugs or replacement fluids which may be used (BCSH 1998).

If the apheresis procedure is being undertaken as part of a stem cell transplantation procedure, all regulations and principles pertaining to consent apply, as discussed in the Bone marrow harvest section.

Preprocedural considerations

Equipment

Numerous types of cell separator machines are now available, but all operate on either a continuous or intermittent flow principle, allowing for the rapid return of anticoagulated blood (Figure 12.8). These systems consist of a device that will carry out whole-blood separation, normally using a sterile, functionally closed-system, single-use disposable apheresis kit (BCSH 1998) with a citrate or heparin anticoagulant solution. All equipment must conform to relevant safety requirements. Regular servicing should be undertaken according to manufacturers' guidelines with service records kept (BCSH 1998). It is recommended that a service contract exists to ensure that an engineer can be contacted to repair the machine within a stipulated timeframe. Cell separator machines must be regularly cleaned with a suitable decontaminating agent and a standard procedure for

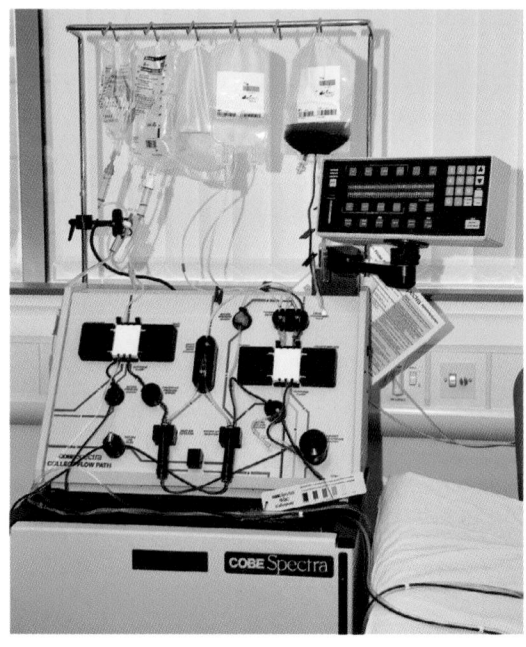

Figure 12.8 Cell separator machines.

Figure 12.9 Peripheral venous access for cell separator procedures.

dealing with blood spillage must be used (BCSH 1998). It is recommended that cell separator facilities undertake a risk assessment and prepare a business continuity plan to manage untoward incidents (FACT-JACIE 2008).

Vascular access

High blood flow rates are required for apheresis, so particular care must be taken over the peripheral venous assessment of patients and donors. A rigid 16 G needle, cannula or equivalent is placed in the antecubital fossa for access and a 20 G cannula or equivalent is sited in a peripheral vein for return. Peripheral access and return are usually sited in opposing arms (Figure 12.9). Side-effects from needle insertion may include pain, bleeding and haematoma. In addition, patients and donors may suffer from needlephobia, resulting in anxiety and vasovagal reactions (Dougherty 2008).

When there is poor venous access, a central venous catheter needs to be placed to undertake the procedure (NHS Blood and Transplant 2010). This has been identified as the greatest risk that patients and donors face (Stroncek et al. 2000). Standard alternatives to peripheral access include rigid percutaneous polyurethane or tunnelled silicone catheters (Pertine et al. 2002). An estimated 1% of central catheter placements are associated with haemorrhage, pneumothorax or infection (Stroncek et al. 2000). These risks are reduced by experienced personnel inserting the catheters with the assistance of ultrasound. In addition, placing the catheters in the femoral vein eliminates the risk of pneumothorax and these types of catheters are well tolerated for a short time (Stroncek et al. 2000). Further information about the general management of venous access devices can be found in Chapter 18.

Assessment and recording tools

It is standard practice to make use of a pre-prepared apheresis worksheet and this should form part of a wider quality management and document control system. Information detailed usually contains at least the information included in Box 12.3.

Pharmacological support

It is good practice to apply a local anaesthetic cream to peripheral venous access sites to minimize pain and discomfort during cannulation. Apprehensive patients may be given an oral sedative to relieve anxiety.

Anticoagulants used to prevent blood clotting in the extracorporeal circuit are usually citrate based; however, heparin is used for some procedures. If a citrate-based anticoagulant is used, it is important that nurses are aware that electrolyte supplements may be needed during the procedure if the patient/donor experiences any signs of citrate toxicity. One example is tetany related to hypocalcaemia. An algorithm of drug management for citrate toxicity should be used to guide staff.

Replacement fluids that may be used during exchange procedures include sodium chloride 0.9%, human albumin solutions, fresh frozen plasma (FFP), cryo-poor FFP and human red cell concentrates.

Predosage of donors with corticosteroids and G-CSF to enhance the yield of granulocyte collections is sometimes undertaken. Records of cumulative doses for each donor must be kept (BCSH 1998).

Granulocyte-colony stimulating factor is routinely used for patients and donors to stimulate haematopoietic stem cell release and improve collection efficiency during stem cell collections by means of apheresis. Recently, Plerixafor has been launched, which enhances the mobilization of stem cells for collection and subsequent autologous transplantation in patients with lymphoma and multiple myeloma whose cells mobilized poorly with G-CSF alone. Plerixafor is an antagonist which blocks stromal cell-derived factor (SDF)-1-alpha to the cellular receptor CXCR4, resulting in stem cell release from bone marrow (National Cancer Institute 2010). An additional application of Plerixafor to a standard G-CSF mobilization regimen may lead to a significant increase in stem cell release (Fruehauf *et al.* 2009). Both G-CSF and Plerixafor should be used in accordance with manufacturer's recommendations and local guidelines.

Nurses working in cell separator facilities with responsibility for patient/donor care must have knowledge of the side-effects of any fluids and drugs used and also any drugs patients may already be taking which may affect the apheresis procedure, for example ACE inhibitors (BCSH 1998).

Non-pharmacological support

An apprehensive patient will experience a sympathetic nervous system response and consequently vasoconstriction. This will diminish blood flow to the cell separator and result in a less efficient procedure. All measures should be taken to reassure and calm patients and provide them with support.

Specific patient/donor preparations

Cell separator procedures can take up to 5 hours and it is important to ensure that patients and donors are as comfortable as possible. Some considerations include the following.

- The positioning of donors and patients on a bed or apheresis chair. Pillows should be used for support as necessary.

- The need to encourage patients and donors to eat and drink as normal; however, care must be taken if there is a need to use the toilet, as it is not usually possible to interrupt the cell separator procedure. This is due to the need to maintain a functionally closed system for sterility purposes.
- Distractions such as access to a television, DVDs, radio, music and reading material.
- The use of a heated blanket at the venous access or return sites to ease any discomfort that may occur due to vasoconstriction.
- Asking if patients and donors would like a friend or family member to accompany them during the procedure. Space constraints usually limit additional visitors.

There should be sufficient space in the cell separator facility to allow staff to operate all equipment without danger to themselves, donors/patients or visitors. The area should also be adequate to allow a cardiac arrest team to operate and resuscitation equipment must be available (FACT-JACIE 2008).

Education

All patients and donors should be given access to information and support in a manner that they understand (DH 2005a; NMC 2008a). Consideration must be given to those patients with learning disabilities, language barriers or sensory deficit.

Procedure guideline 12.3 **Apheresis**

This is a general guide as it is beyond the scope of this chapter to detail each procedure.

Essential equipment
- Cell separator machine
- Disposable tubing set compatible with cell separator machine and application needed, for example white blood cell, therapeutic plasma exchange or red blood cell exchange kit
- For peripheral venous access: a rigid 16 G needle, cannula or equipment for insertion (see Chapter 18)
- For peripheral venous return: 20 G device, for example cannula and equipment for insertion (see Chapter 18)
- For central venous access and return: equipment to access (see Chapter 18)
- Documentation as per local policy and dependent on procedure type
- Apheresis system operator's manual
- Access to patient/donor medical notes/prescription chart

Medicinal products
- Anticoagulant, for example 500 mL ACDA anticoagulant (number of bags needed is usually stipulated by length of procedure)
- 1000 mL 0.9% sodium chloride
- Local anaesthetic cream for venous access if indicated
- Replacement fluids as indicated dependent on the type of procedure, for example sodium chloride 0.9%, human albumin solutions, FFP, cryo-poor FFP and human red cell concentrates
- Electrolyte supplements, for example calcium as per the local policy for the management of citrate toxicity

Preprocedure

Action	Rationale
1 Explain and provide written information about the apheresis procedure.	To ensure the patient or donor is properly informed about the procedure (DH 2005a, C; NMC 2008a, C).
2 Check that written informed consent has been taken and that the patient has a good understanding of the procedure.	To enable patients or donors to actively participate in and comply with their treatment (NMC 2008a, C; FACT-JACIE 2008, C; Human Tissue Authority 2009b, C).
3 Check that all documentation, which may vary according to local policy and also procedure type, is complete.	To maintain accurate records and comply with regulatory policy (FACT-JACIE 2008, C; Human Tissue Authority 2009b, C; NMC 2009, C).
4 Ensure the patient or donor is wearing a wristband correctly labelled with their name, hospital number and date of birth.	To prevent patient safety incidents and near misses relating to missing wristbands or wristbands with incorrect information (NPSA 2005, C).
5 Check that pertinent serological tests have been carried out within the timeframes stipulated by local and/or regulatory policy.	To prevent cross-infection with bloodborne infections (FACT-JACIE 2008, C; Human Tissue Authority 2009b, C).
6 Consider oral sedation (e.g. lorazepam) for very anxious patients.	To ensure that the procedure is performed safely and with minimal distress to the patient. E
7 Document which apheresis machine is being used.	To ensure traceability of procedures and assist in the audit of collection efficiency (FACT-JACIE 2008, C).
8 Obtain and record the patient or donor's biological parameters, for example height, weight and gender, to calculate total blood volume.	To ensure accurate data input and machine settings. E
9 Obtain and record the patient or donor's baseline observations, for example temperature, pulse rate, blood pressure.	Subsequent observations can be compared against the baseline to assist in accurately informing the need for intervention if the patient or donor's condition appears to deteriorate during the procedure. E
10 Check and record pertinent blood results, e.g haemoglobin, haematocrit, platelet count, white cell differential, blood group, electrolytes, plasma viscosity, haemoglobin S, peripheral CD34-positive count and clotting. The blood tests required will differ depending on procedure type. Local policy should be followed.	To ensure accurate data input, machine settings, disease monitoring and patient/donor safety (FACT-JACIE 2008, C; Human Tissue Authority 2009c, C).
11 Ensure solutions and drugs needed for the procedure have been prescribed.	To ensure good medicines management (NMC, 2008c, C).
12 If a central venous catheter placed in the superior vena cava is used, check the catheter tip position prior to use. This should be documented in the medical records after a chest X-ray.	High flow rates are required for apheresis so good venous access is essential (FACT-JACIE 2008, C).
13 Check that the apheresis machine has been cleaned and maintained as per local policy. This must be documented.	Environmental conditions must be controlled for surface contaminates to minimize the risk of contamination or cross-contamination (FACT-JACIE 2008, C).
14 Prepare the procedure trolley and ensure that all the necessary equipment and specimen containers are readily available.	To ensure the procedure is performed efficiently and that all the necessary specimens are collected and handled correctly (Perkins 2003, C).

737

(Continued)

Procedure guideline 12.3 *(Continued)*

15 Visually examine all reagents used for damage or evidence of contamination prior to use. Note the lot numbers and expiry dates of all reagents. Ensure local incident reporting systems are used if any reagents are not suitable for use.	To ensure an effective quality management plan is established and maintained and to minimize the risk of contamination or cross-contamination (FACT-JACIE 2008, C).
16 Select and load the disposable set and reagents. The set will differ depending on what procedure is undertaken and which type of cell separator is used.	To prepare the apheresis machine prior to connecting the patient and to ensure that it is in good working order (Foss 2003, E; Gambro 2005, C; Strauss 2003, C).
17 Prime the disposable tubing set with 0.9% sodium chloride and anticoagulant.	To expel air from the disposable tubing set. E
18 Perform alarm tests and checks.	To prepare the apheresis machine prior to connecting the patient and to ensure that it is in good working order (Foss 2003, E; Gambro 2005, C; Strauss 2003, C).
19 If the apheresis machine alarms during the procedure, refer to the troubleshooting section of the operator's manual and follow the relevant instructions.	To prepare the apheresis machine prior to connecting the patient and to ensure that it is in good working order (Foss 2003, E; Gambro 2005, C; Strauss 2003, C).
20 Enter the patient or donor's biological parameters and pertinent blood results into the apheresis machine as prompted. Amend settings as required by local policy.	To customize and optimize the procedure (Foss 2003, E; Gambro 2005, C; Strauss 2003, C).
21 Document target run results and pertinent information as required by local policy.	To maintain accurate records (NMC 2009, C).
22 Ensure patient privacy by drawing the curtains as per patient preference. A blanket or sheet may be needed if vascular access is via a femoral, percutaneous or tunnelled central venous catheter.	An environment that facilitates the patient's need for privacy and dignity is essential (NMC 2008a, C).
23 Assist the patient into the correct position, which is usually the supine position with arms comfortably rested at their sides. The back of the bed or apheresis chair is usually slightly elevated, but this is guided by patient preference.	To maintain patient comfort and access either peripheral or central venous access devices. E
24 Wash hands and apply gloves. Gloves must be used when handling biological specimens (FACT-JACIE 2008, C).	To maintain asepsis throughout the procedure to minimize the risk of infection (Fraise and Bradley 2009, E).
Procedure	
25 Connect the patient or donor to the apheresis machine via the preselected venous access devices. There must be one lumen for access and one for return of blood. Check that all venous access devices are patent by withdrawing blood and flushing with 10 mL 0.9% sodium chloride. No resistance should be felt.	High flow rates are required for apheresis so good venous access is essential (NHS Blood and Transplant 2010, C).
26 Proceed with the run as per the operator's manual depending on procedure type.	To achieve therapeutic or donation targets (Kaushansky and Williams 2010, C).
27 Monitor the condition of the patient or donor and also the progress of the procedure and intervene as required (see Problem-solving table 12.3 for troubleshooting).	To ensure the procedure runs smoothly and the patient or donor is safely managed. E

28	Dependent on the procedure type, perform a rinseback when the procedure targets have been met. A rinseback is when the cell separator is flushed through with sodium chloride 0.9% to ensure that any blood remaining in the machine is returned to the patient (Burgstaler 2003).	To ensure accurate fluid balance and haemodynamic stability (BCSH 1998, C). For this reason, it is unusual to perform a rinseback in, for example, paediatric cases (where a blood prime has been used) or after red cell exchanges for patients with sickle cell disease (Burgstaler 2003).

Postprocedure

29	If undertaking a donation procedure, permanently seal the product bags, preferably by using a heat sealer. As a contingency, three sealing clips closed by clamp may be used.	To ensure safe handling and protect product from exposure to pathogens (DH 2005b, C; Pratt *et al.* 2007, C).
30	Take any postcollection blood sampling, for example full blood count, from the access device prior to removal.	To monitor cellular loss as a result of the apheresis procedure (Crookston and Simon 2003, C) and to make corrections or give advice as necessary.
31	Disconnect the donor/patient from the machine before unloading the pumps and removing the disposable set from the apheresis machine.	To ensure the safety of the patient/donor. E
32	Dispose of sharps and waste products as per local policy.	To ensure the safe handling and disposal of needles and other sharp instruments and to protect staff, patients and visitors from exposure to bloodborne pathogens (DH 2005b, C; Pratt *et al.* 2007, C).
33	Inspect the cannulation sites for bleeding. A pressure dressing may be applied over sterile gauze.	To achieve haemostasis and decrease the risk of infection. E
34	For donation products, label collection bags and complete documentation for release of products from the collection facility. FACT-JACIE (2008) compliant labels and paperwork must be used.	To ensure correct management of the product (FACT-JACIE 2008, C).
35	Place the collection bags in a secondary container (e.g. a zip-type resealable bag) prior to transfer to the appropriate processing facility (for donation procedures).	To prevent the loss of a portion of the collection, to minimize the potential of postcollection contamination of the component and to prevent potential spillage of biohazard material in areas where it may pose a risk to employees, visitors or patients (FACT-JACIE 2008, C).
36	For donation procedures, transport the collection bags to the appropriate processing facility with the necessary forms and in a FACT-JACIE compliant container.	To allow for cell measurement, storage and/or issue of the donated product. E
37	Record the necessary information in the appropriate documents as per local policy.	To maintain accurate records (NMC 2009, C).
38	Ensure postdonation care is appropriately managed (see Postprocedural considerations).	To ensure the safe management of patients and to enable them to actively participate in and comply with their treatment (NMC 2008a, C).
39	Remove the disposable tubing set from the apheresis machine as per the operator's manual and dispose of it in a hazardous waste container.	To ensure the safe handling and disposal of clinical waste to protect staff, patients and visitors from exposure to bloodborne pathogens (DH 2005b, C; Pratt *et al.* 2007, C).
40	Clean the apheresis machine with a suitable decontaminating agent as per local policy (BCSH 1998).	To protect staff, patients and visitors from exposure to bloodborne pathogens (FACT-JACIE 2008, C).

Problem-solving table 12.3 Prevention and resolution (Procedure guideline 12.3)

Problem	Cause	Prevention	Action
Vascular access, for example high return pressure or low access pressure	Haematoma Kinking in tubing Valves in closed position Vascular inadequacy Needlephobia Vasovagal episode	Careful venous preassessment Central venous catheter insertion Experienced practitioners	Reassurance Check tubing for kinks Check position of valves Reduce inlet flow Adjust or resite access or return devices Central venous catheter insertion
Citrate toxicity	Electrolyte imbalance if citrate formulation is used as anticoagulant	Consider administration of electrolyte supplements (IV or oral), for example calcium Ensure correct anticoagulant rate settings	Decrease flow rate Consider administration of calcium supplements (IV or oral) Pause/stop procedure
Under-anticoagulation which may manifest as clotting or unstable interface	Incorrect biometric measurement Incorrect data input Incorrect settings with a lower AC:inlet ratio than needed	Ensure correct anticoagulant rate settings	Check tubing for kinks Increase AC:inlet ratio Stop procedure
Fluid overload	Cardiac impairment Renal impairment Paediatric patient	Careful preassessment Do not perform a rinseback in the paediatric setting Careful data input	Operate at negative fluid balance Request medical review Stop procedure
Hypotension	Hypovolaemia Paediatric patient Vasovagal episode	Blood prime Careful preassessment Careful data input Reassurance	Operate at positive fluid balance Increase colloid:crystalloid ratio
Chilling	Cold environment Cold replacement fluids	Use blood warmer Ensure adequate climate control	Increase room temperature Provide additional blankets Use blood warmer
Adverse reaction	Allergic reaction to replacement fluids or anticoagulant Incompatible transfusion Septicaemia Anaphylaxis	Careful preassessment Careful monitoring Adherence to blood product administration protocols	Request urgent medical review Instigate treatment as indicated, for example administer antimicrobials, antihistamine, hydrocortisone and emergency treatment Stop procedure

BCSH (1998), Dougherty (2008), Freshwater and Maslin-Prothero (2005), Stroncek *et al.* (2000).

Postprocedural considerations

Immediate care

During the procedure, blood is prevented from clotting in the extracorporeal circuit by a citrate-based anticoagulant. This functions by binding the calcium in the blood and removing it from the clotting cascade. Donors may experience symptoms of hypocalcaemia, such as muscular irritability, tetany, numbness and 'pins and needles' in extremities, light-headedness, nausea and vomiting (Freshwater and Maslin-Prothero 2005). This side-effect is known as citrate toxicity and is controlled by giving the donor calcium supplements or reducing the dose of citrate administered by decreasing the blood flow rate (Stroncek *et al.* 2000).

Different procedures may produce varying haemodynamic effects. Fluid overload may be a problem for patients with cardiac or renal impairment, whereas hypovolaemia may be of concern in the paediatric setting (Crookston and Simon 2003). Blood pressure should be monitored in particular, as hypotension may occur.

With red cell and plasma exchanges, patients may experience transfusion reactions, for example fever, chills and allergic reactions (see Chapter 8).

There is a potential for cellular loss as large volumes of donor or patient blood circulate through the apheresis machine and blood cells are intentionally or incidentally removed. Studies show that individual apheresis procedures produce only modest decreases in circulating blood cell counts, which are not associated with immediate toxicity (Crookston and Simon 2003). Patients with underlying instabilities or those undergoing repeated procedures may need to be supported by blood component transfusion.

Any adverse reaction must be dealt with promptly and must be documented. The patient/donor must have recovered as fully as possible before being allowed to leave the facility (BCSH 1998).

Ongoing care

Patients and donors should be encouraged to rest and take refreshment before leaving the cell separator facility. A full blood count should be taken at the end of the procedure and advice given dependent on the result. For instance, there is a potential for platelet loss during stem cell collections by means of apheresis and patients and donors should be advised to moderate alcohol consumption and avoid strenuous exercise and activities that may put them at risk of bleeding or bruising. The platelet count usually recovers within a few days (Crookston and Simon 2003).

Documentation

Apheresis should be strictly regulated within a quality management system with clear standard operating procedures and documentation. Archived documentation should be maintained according to governmental, regulatory or institutional policy, whichever is longer (FACT-JACIE 2008). Due to the strict regulatory nature of apheresis, a record-keeping system must be in place to ensure the authenticity, integrity and confidentiality of all documents (MHRA 2009). All nursing records must be clearly maintained to ensure accurate data (NMC 2009).

Education of patient/donor and relevant others

If the donor or patient is likely to feel fatigued, it is sensible that someone accompanies them home. Advice needs to be customized to the particular procedure undertaken.

Complications

Overall rates of adverse reactions have decreased significantly over the past two decades. Greater understanding of the physiology of apheresis has guided continued improvements in technology and the potential for untoward effects has been minimized so that most procedures are performed without adverse events. This is especially true of donation procedures, which have become very routine (Crookston and Simon 2003). Caution is in order if cell or plasma removal exceeds current guidelines or if patients have underlying instabilities that predispose them to untoward events (Crookston and Simon 2003).

The use of central venous catheters can be associated with well-described complications and these complications lead to the majority of fatalities associated with apheresis (Stroncek *et al.* 2000). Subclavian and superior vena caval catheters can be associated with perforation, haemothorax, pneumothorax, infection and thrombosis. The use of femoral catheters can be associated with the occurrence of haemorrhage, thrombosis and infection (BCSH 1998). These risks are reduced by experienced personnel inserting the catheters with the assistance of ultrasound (Stroncek *et al.* 2000).

741

Websites

www.anthonynolan.org.uk
www.bcshguidelines.com
www.bsbmt.co.uk
www.blood.co.uk
www.ebmt.co.uk
www.ebmt.org
www.hta.gov.uk
www.jacie.org
www.macmillan.org.uk
www.worldmarrow.org
www.wtail.org.uk/WBMDR.htm

References

Abboud, C. and Lichtman, M. (2009) Structure of the marrow and the hematopoietic microenvironment. In: Lichtman, M. *et al.* (eds) *Williams' Haematology.* McGraw-Hill, London, pp. 29–59.

Atkinson, M. (2005) Communicating news of patients' deaths to unrelated stem cell donors. *Nursing Standard*, **19** (32), 41–47.

Bain, B. (2001) Bone marrow trephine biopsy. *Journal of Clinical Pathology*, **54**, 737–742.

Bain, B. (2004) *A Beginner's Guide to Blood Cells*, 2nd edn. Blackwell Publishing, Boston, MA.

Bain, B. (2005) Bone marrow biopsy morbidity: review of 2003. *Journal of Clinical Pathology*, **58** (4), 406–408.

Bain, B. (2006) Morbidity associated with bone marrow aspiration and trephine biopsy – a review of 2004. *Haematologica*, **91**, 1293–1294.

BCSH (1998) Guidelines for the clinical use of blood cell separators: prepared by the Joint Working Party of the transfusion and clinical haematology task forces of the British Committee for Standards in Haematology. *Clinical and Laboratory Haematology*, **20**, 265–278.

BCSH (1999) The administration of blood and blood components and the management of transfused patients. *Transfusion Medicine*, **9**, 227–238.

BCSH (2008) Guidelines on the assessment of bleeding risk prior to surgery or invasive procedures. www.bcshguidelines.com/pdf/bleeding_risk_guideline.pdf.

Bishop, B., McNally, K. and Harris, M. (1992) Audit of bone marrow trephines. *Journal of Clinical Pathology*, **45**, 1105–1108.

Be the Match Registry (2010) Understanding your commitment. www.marrow.org/JOIN/Understanding_Your_Commitment/index.html.

Blume, K. and Amylon, M. (2004) The evaluation and counselling of candidates for hematopoietic cell transplantation. In: Blume, K., Forman, S. and Appelbaum, F. (eds) *Thomas' Hematopoietic Cell Transplantation*, 3rd edn. Blackwell Publishing, Boston, MA.

BMA/PSGB (2009) *British National Formulary for children*. Lidocaine hydrochloride. http://bnfc.org/bnfc/bnfc/2009/6686.htm?q=%22lidocaine%22.

BNF (2011) *British National Formulary*. BMJ Group and RPS Publishing, London.

Bondurant, M., Mahmud, N. and Rhodes, N. (2009) Origin and development of blood cells. In: Greer, J. *et al.* (eds) *Wintrobe's Clinical Hematology*, 12th edn. Lippincott, Williams and Wilkins, Philadelphia, pp. 79–89.

Bufalini, A. (2009) Role of interactive music in oncological pediatric patients undergoing painful procedures. *Minerva Pediatric*, **61** (4), 379–389.

Burgstaler, E. (2003) Current instrumentation for apheresis. In: McLeod, B., Price, T. and Weinstein, R. (eds) *Apheresis: Principles and Practice*, 2nd edn. AABB Press, Bethesda, MD, pp. 95–130.

Campbell, J., Matthews, J. and Seymour, M. (2003) Optimum trephine length in the assessment of bone marrow involvement in patients with diffuse large cell lymphoma. *Annals of Oncology*, **14**, 273–276.

Chapman, K. and Rush, K. (2003) Patient and family satisfaction with cancer-related information: a review of the literature. *Canadian Oncology Nursing Journal*, **13** (2), 107–116.

Confer, D. (2004) Hematopoietic cell donors. In: Blume, K., Forman, S. and Appelbaum, F. (eds) *Thomas' Hematopoietic Cell Transplantation*, 3rd edn. Blackwell Publishing, Boston, MA, pp. 538–549.

Corbin, F. (2003) Development of apheresis instrumentation. In: McLeod, B., Price, T. and Weinstein, R. (eds) *Apheresis: Principles and Practice*, 2nd edn. AABB Press, Bethesda, MD, pp. 1–27.

Crookston, K. and Simon, T. (2003) Physiology of apheresis. In: McLeod, B., Price, T. and Weinstein, R. (eds) *Apheresis: Principles and Practice*, 2nd edn. AABB Press, Bethesda, MD, pp. 71–93.

DH (2005a) *Creating a Patient-Led NHS – Delivering the NHS Improvement Plan*. Department of Health, London.

DH (2005b) *Hazardous Waste (England) Regulations*. Department of Health, London.

Dougherty, L. (2008) Obtaining peripheral venous access. In: Dougherty, L. and Lamb, J. (eds) *Intravenous Therapy in Nursing Practice*, 2nd edn. Blackwell Publishing, Oxford.

FACT-JACIE (2008) *International Standards for Cellular Therapy Product Collection, Processing and Administration*. FACT-JACIE, Barcelona. www.factwebsite.org/uploadedFiles/News/4th%20Ed.%20Standards%20for%20Web.pdf.

Foss, M. (2003) Photopheresis. In: McLeod, B., Price, T. and Weinstein, R. (eds) *Apheresis: Principles and Practice*, 2nd edn. AABB Press, Bethesda, MD, pp. 623–642.

Fraise, A.P. and Bradley, T. (eds) (2009) *Ayliffe's Control of Healthcare-associated Infection: A Practical Handbook*, 5th edn. Hodder Arnold, London.

Freshwater, D. and Maslin-Prothero, S. (eds) (2005) *Blackwell's Nursing Dictionary*. Blackwell Publishing, Oxford.

Fruehauf, S., Veldwijk, M.R., Seeger, T. *et al.* (2009) A combination of granulocyte-colony-stimulating factor (G-CSF) and plerixafor AMD3100 (plerixafor) mobilizes more primitive peripheral blood progenitor cells than G-CSF alone: results of a European phase II study. *Cytotherapy*, **31**, 1–10.

GambroBCT (2005) *Spectra™ System Therapeutics Reference Book*. GambroBCT, Denver, CO.

Giannoutsos, I., Grech, H., Maboreke, T. and Morgenstern, G. (2004) Performing bone marrow biopsies with or without sedation: a comparison. *Clinical and Laboratory Haematology*, **26** (3), 201–204.

Goldberg, C., Vergidis, D. and Sacher, R. (2007) *Bone Aspiration and Biopsy*. Medscape, New York. emedicine.medscape.com/article/207575-overview#section-author_information.

Henke Yarbro, C., Hansen Frogge, M. and Goodman, M. (2005) *Cancer Nursing: Principles and Practice*, 6th edn. Jones and Bartlett, Sudbury, MA.

Hoffbrand, A.V., Moss, P.A.H. and Pettit, J.E. (2006) *Essential Haematology*, 5th edn. Blackwell Science, Oxford.

Hughes-Jones, N., Wickramasinghe, S. and Hatton, C. (2004) *Lecture Notes on Haematology*, 7th edn. Blackwell Publishing, Oxford.

Human Tissue Authority (2009a) *Code of Practice 5: Disposal of Human Tissue*. www.hta.gov.uk.

Human Tissue Authority (2009b) *Code of Practice 1: Consent*. www.hta.gov.uk.

Human Tissue Authority (2009c) *Code of Practice 6: Donation of Allogeneic Bone Marrow and Peripheral Blood Stem Cells for Transplantation*. www.hta.gov.uk.

Humphries, J. (2006) Dry tap bone marrow aspiration: clinical significance. *American Journal of Hematology*, **35** (4), 247–250.

Hurley, C. and Raffoux, C. (2004) Special report: World Marrow Donor Association: International Standards for unrelated hematopoietic stem cell registries. *Bone Marrow Transplantation*, **34**, 97–101.

Kaushansky, K. and Williams, W.J. (2010) *Williams' Hematology*, 8th edn. McGraw-Hill, New York.

Lawson, S., Aston, S., Baker, L. *et al.* (1999) Trained nurses can obtain satisfactory bone marrow aspirates and trephine biopsies. *Journal of Clinical Pathology*, **52** (2), 154–156.

Leukaemia and Lymphoma Research (2010) Facts about blood cancers. www.beatbloodcancers.org/facts-about-blood-cancers.

Lewis, S.M., Bain, B.J. and Bates, I. (2006) *Dacie and Lewis Practical Haematology*, 10th edn. Churchill Livingstone, London.

Lidén, Y., Landgren, O., Arnér, S. *et al.* (2009) Procedure related pain among adult patients with hematologic malignancies. *Acta Anaesthesiologica Scandinavica*, **53** (3), 354–363.

Longo, D. (2005) Examination of blood smears and bone marrow. In: Kasper, D., Braunwald, E. and Fauci, A. (eds) *Harrison's Manual of Medicine*, 16th edn. McGraw-Hill, New York, pp. 265–267.

Mantik Lewis, S., McLean Heitkemper, M. and Ruff Dirksen, S. (2004) *Medical-Surgical Nursing: Assessment and Management of Clinical Problems*, 6th edn. Mosby, St Louis, MO.

MHRA (2009) Good clinical practice. Medicines and Healthcare products Regulatory Agency, London. www.mhra.gov.uk/Howweregulate/Medicines/Inspectionandstandards/GoodClinicalPractice/index.htm.

National Cancer Institute (2010) NCI drug dictionary. National Cancer Institute, Bethesda, MD. www.cancer.gov.drugdictionary/.

NHS Blood and Transplant (2010) Haematopoietic stem cell transplant services. National Cancer Institute, Bethesda, MD. http://hospital.blood.co.uk/diagnostic_services/stem_cell_immunotherapy_services/collection/index.asp#Ven.

NMC (2008a) *Consent*. Nursing and Midwifery Council, London www.nmc-uk.org/Nurses-and-midwives/Advice-by-topic/A/Advice/Consent.

NMC (2008b) *The Code: Standards of Conduct, Performance and Ethics for Nurses and Midwives*. Nursing and Midwifery Council, London.

NMC (2008c) *Standards for medicine management*. Nursing and Midwifery Council, London.

NMC (2009) *Record Keeping: Guidance for Nurses and Midwives*. Nursing and Midwifery Council, London.

NPSA (2005) *Safer patient identification*. National Patient Safety Agency, London. www.nrls.npsa.nhs.uk/resources/patient-safety-topics/patient-admission-transfer-discharge/?entryid45=59799.

Outhwaite, H. (2000) Blood and marrow transplantation. In: Grundy M. (ed) *Nursing in Haematological Oncology*. Baillière Tindall, Edinburgh, pp. 140–155.

Perkins, S. (2003) Bone marrow examination. In: Greer, J. *et al.* (eds) *Wintrobe's Clinical Hematology*, 11th edn. Lippincott, Williams and Wilkins, Philadelphia, pp. 3–22.

Pertine, B., Razvi, S. and Weinstein, R. (2002) Prospective investigation of a subcutaneous, implantable central venous access device for therapeutic plasma exchange in adults with neurological disorders. *Journal of Clinical Apheresis*, **17** (1), 1–6.

Pratt, R., Pellowe, C.M., Wilson, J.A. *et al.* (2007) Epic 2: National evidence-based guidelines for preventing healthcare-associated infection in NHS hospitals in England. *Journal of Hospital Infection*, **65** (1)(suppl), S2–S12.

Provan, D., Singer, C., Baglin, T. and Dokal, I. (2009) *Oxford Handbook of Clinical Haematology*, 3rd edn. Oxford University Press, Oxford.

Richardson, C. and Atkinson, J. (2006) Blood and marrow transplantation. In: Grundy M. (ed) *Nursing in Haematological Oncology*. Baillière Tindall, Edinburgh, pp. 265–291.

Rosenmayr, A., Hartwell, L. and Egeland, T. (2003) Informed consent – suggested procedures for informed consent for unrelated haematopoietic stem cell donors at various stages of recruitment, donor evaluation, and donor workup. *Bone Marrow Transplantation*, **31**, 539–545.

Ruegg, T., Curran, C. and Lamb, T. (2009) Use of buffered lidocaine in bone marrow biopsies: a randomized, controlled trial. *Oncology Nursing Forum*, **36** (1), 52–60.

Sieff, C. and Nathan, D. (2000) Stem cells and haemopoiesis. In: Ledingham, J. and Warrell, D. (eds) *Concise Oxford Textbook of Medicine*. Oxford University Press, Oxford, pp. 180–183.

Strauss, R. (2003) Granulocyte (neutrophil) transfusion. In: McLeod, B., Price, T. and Weinstein, R. (eds) *Apheresis: Principles and Practice*, 2nd edn. AABB Press, Bethesda, MD, pp. 237–252.

Stroncek, D., Confer, D. and Leitman, S. (2000) Peripheral blood progenitor cells for HPC transplants involving unrelated donors. *Transfusion*, **40**, 731–741.

Szczepiorkowski, Z.M., Bandarenko, N., Kim, H. *et al.* (2007) Guidelines on the use of therapeutic apheresis in clinical practice – evidence-based approach from the Apheresis Applications Committee of the American Society for Apheresis. *Journal of Clinical Apheresis*, **22**, 106–175.

Traynor, B. (2006) Haematopoiesis. In: Grundy M. (ed) *Nursing in Haematological Oncology*. Baillière Tindall, Edinburgh, pp. 3–20.

Turgeon, M.L. (1999) *Clinical Haematology, Theory and Procedures*, 3rd edn. Lippincott, Williams and Wilkins, Philadelphia.

Van Walraven, A., Nicoloso-de Faveri, G., Axdorph-Nygell, U. *et al.* for the WMDA Ethics and Working Groups (2010) Family donor care management: principles and recommendations. *Bone Marrow Transplantation*, **45** (8), 1269–1273.

Weatherall, D. (2000) Haematology. In: Ledingham, J. and Warrell, D. (eds) *Concise Oxford Textbook of Medicine*. Oxford University Press, Oxford, pp. 175–180.

Western Sussex Hospitals NHS Trust (2009) *St Richard's Hospital Pathology User Handbook*. www.rwstgp.org.uk/guidelines/UH-GEN-HANDBK.pdf.

743

Observations

The Royal Marsden Hospital Manual of Clinical Nursing Procedures, Eighth Edition. Edited by Lisa Dougherty and Sara Lister.
© 2011 The Royal Marsden Hospital. Published 2011 by Blackwell Publishing Ltd.

Overview

The following observations will be discussed: pulse, blood pressure, respiration, peak flow, temperature, urinalysis, blood glucose, central venous pressure and neurological observations. For each observation discussed, we provide a definition, the rationale, legal and professional issues, procedural guidelines and a guide to problem solving.

Observations

Definitions

The term 'observation' refers to the physical assessment of a patient, including assessment of wounds, intravenous therapy, wound drains, pain and vital signs collection and specialized assessments such as neurological observations (Zeitz and McCutcheon 2006). 'Vital signs' are traditionally used in the context of the collection of a cluster of physical measures, such as pulse, respiration, temperature and blood pressure, and more recently pulse oximetry.

Evidence-based approaches

Rationale

The taking of patient observations forms a fundamental part of the assessment process. The interpretation of the data from the assessment is vital in determining the level of care a patient requires, providing an intervention or treatment and preventing a patient deteriorating from an otherwise preventable cause (Wheatley 2006) (see Chapter 2).

Indications

Observations are usually undertaken:

- to act as a baseline to help determine the patient's usual range (Bickley and Szilargyi 2009)
- to assist in recognizing if a patient's condition is deteriorating or indeed improving (Kisiel and Perkins 2006).

Principles of care

Adult patients in acute hospital settings should have:

- observations taken when they are admitted or initially assessed
- a clearly documented plan which identifies which observations should be taken and how frequently subsequent observations should be done. This plan should take into consideration:
  - the diagnosis
  - plan for patient's treatment
  - any co-morbidities which may affect their health.
  (NICE 2007b)

All patients in hospital should have their observations taken at least once every 12 hours, unless specified otherwise by senior staff (NICE 2007b).

Methods of measuring and recording observations

To assist with the identification of critically ill patients and those at risk of deterioration, physiological scoring systems were introduced (Wheatley 2006). These include the Modified Early Warning System (MEWS) (see Figure 13.1), medical emergency team (MET) scoring and patient-at-risk team (PART) score (DH 2001, Hodgetts *et al.* 2002). These scoring systems rely on nursing staff performing basic patient observations, that is, respiratory rate, heart rate, blood pressure, temperature and fluid balance (Wheatley 2006) and informing medical staff/outreach team of deviations from normal.

There are many such scores in use although they should be used in conjunction with clinical judgement and a holistic assessment rather than being relied on as an absolute measure of the patient's condition (Critical Care Stakeholders Forum and National Outreach Forum 2007). They are of use in helping ward nurses to improve and focus their recognition of patients who may need further support and monitoring (DH 2000). Critical care outreach teams are available in many hospitals now and where present, they must be informed of any patients who are deteriorating or at risk of deteriorating, so that they can provide support to ward staff and assess the patient (DH 2000).

One tool that has been found to assist with structuring and standardizing communication is the Situation-Background-Assessment-Recommendations (SBAR) tool (see Figure 13.2). SBAR is an easy-to-remember, concrete mechanism useful for framing any conversation, especially critical ones, requiring a clinician's immediate attention and action. It allows for an easy and focused way to set expectations for what will be communicated and how between members of the team, which is essential for developing teamwork and fostering a culture of patient safety (Woodhall 2008).

Anticipated patient outcomes

Physiological observations are extremely important in recognizing if a patient's condition is deteriorating or indeed improving (Kisiel and Perkins 2006).

Legal and professional issues

Nurses are accountable and responsible for providing optimum care for their patients. The Nursing and Midwifery Council's (NMC) *The Code* provides the main source of professional accountability for nurses (NMC 2008a). It is essential that nursing staff objectively examine the information gathered from assessments and observations as well as any information previously recorded (Crouch and Meurier 2005).

MEWS - Early Warning Scoring System

A score of **3 or more** should alert the ward nursing staff that the patient is at **risk of RAPID deterioration.**

Seek **immediate** review by outreach team / medical team / on call team

Critical Care Outreach Service

The outreach team can be contacted for any patient you are worried about, even if they do not fit the above criteria.

Chelsea Out of hours:			Sutton Out of hours:		Step Up Bay:	

Score	3	2	1	0	1	2	3
Pulse		< 40	41 - 50	51 - 100	101 - 110	111 - 130	> 131
Systolic BP	< 70	71 - 80	81 - 100	101 - 149	150 - 199	> 200	
Respiratory rate		< 10		9 - 14	15 - 20	21 - 29	> 30
Temperature		<35	35.1 - 36	36.1 - 37.9	38 - 38.5	> 38.6	
Urine output	< 10 ml/hr	< 0.5 ml/kg/hr					
Neurological response	No response	To painful stimuli	To verbal stimuli	Alert & orientated	Confused / agitated		
GCS				15	14	9 - 13	< 8

Figure 13.1   MEWS – Early Warning Scoring System (DH 2000).

747

For nurses' own professional accountability and for the achievement of safe, effective and proficient care of the patient, it is essential that nurses are able to discuss (using physiological rationale) the potential reasons for the observations they have recorded (Kisiel and Perkins 2006). Professional accountability demands more than nurses just undertaking observations. It is about nurses being able to interpret them and then to take appropriate action (Kisiel and Perkins 2006).

Observations should be taken by staff who have undergone the appropriate training regarding the procedure, not only so that they are able to perform the procedure correctly and accurately but also, crucially, so they are able to act on and understand the clinical relevance of the results (NICE 2007b). The degree of training should be suitable to the level of care which the practitioner is providing (NICE 2007b). However, all staff should have competencies in relation to measuring, monitoring, interpretation and when to respond promptly (NICE 2007b).

Preprocedural considerations

Equipment

All practitioners need to be aware of the strengths and limitations of the devices they are using and need to have adequate training on the use of all equipment. They must ensure that the devices are validated, checked, maintained and recalibrated regularly according to the manufacturer's instructions (NICE 2006). In addition, the use of the device should be within the permitted manufacturer's guidelines.

Prior to the procedure, check when the device was last serviced. All devices, manual or automated, are only accurate if they are working and used correctly. Most trusts have the devices checked annually and the date documented on

Royal Marsden NHS Foundation Trust
SBAR report to Doctor or Outreach Nurse about a critical situation
Hospital Number: **Date:**   **Time:**

<u>Situation</u>
I am calling about <u><patient name and location></u>. Consultant:
The patient's resuscitation status is <u>For Resus?</u>   <u>Not for Resus?</u>
The problem I am calling about is_____.
The patient was admitted with_____.
I have informed_____**the Nurse in Charge.**
        □ I am afraid the patient is going to arrest.
I have just assessed the patient personally:
Observations are: BP_____, Pulse_____, Respirations_____and temperature_____.
Blood Glusose___mmol/l, Potassium_____mmol/l, Magnasium_____mmol/l.
Pain = Site / Duration   Epidural Y/N   or PCA Y/N
I am concerned about the:
        Observation in the red or yellow bands on the observation chart
                □ Blood pressure because it is □ over 150 systolic or □ less than 100 systolic or
                    □ 30 mmHg below usual
                □ Pulse because it is □ over 110 or □ less than 50
                □ Respiration because it is □ less than 9 or □ over 21
                □ Temperature because it is □ less than 36°C or over 38°C
                □ Conscious level / general condition is deteriorating
                □ Urine output is less than 0.5ml/kg/hr
                □ Oxygenation
                □ The MEWS is_____.

<u>Background</u>
The patients mental status is:
                □ Alert and orientated to person, place and time
                □ Confused and □ cooperative or □ non-coperative
                □ Agitated
                □ Lethargic but conversant and able to swallow
                □ Drowsy and no talking clearly and possibly not able to swallow
                □ Comatose □ Eyes closed □ Not responding to stimulation.
The skin is:
                □ Warm and dry
                □ Pale / Clammy
                □ Sweaty
                □ Extremities are cold
                □ Extremities are warm
The patient □ is not or □ is on oxygen.
                □ The patient has been on____(l/min) or (%) oxygen for____minutes (hours)
                □ The oximeter is reading____%
                □ The oximeter does not detect a good pulse and is giving erratic readings
The patient has □ no access □ a peripheral cannula □ a CVAD.

<u>Assessment</u>
                □ I think the problem is_____.
                □ I don't know what the problem is but the patient is deteriorating.
                □ The patient has fallen in the ward

<u>Recommendation</u>
                □ Patient to be seen within the next 30 minutes
                □ Patient to be seen now
                □ Would like approval of my course of action which is_____.
Are any tests needed:
                □ Do you need any tests?_____.
If a change in treatment is ordered then ask:
                □ How often do you want the observations done?
                □ If the patient does not get better when would you want us to call again?

Call initiated by Nurse:_____   To:_____.

Figure 13.2   Situation-Background-Assessment-Recommendations (SBAR) tool.

the device and staff should check this and report when it is due for servicing (Woodrow 2004a).

Postprocedural considerations

Documentation

Adequate training on good record keeping and documentation is essential. The NMC (2009) states that the quality of good record keeping is also a reflection of the standard of the individual's professional practice. All records must be contemporaneous, accurate and unambiguous (Dawes and Durham 2007).

Pulse

Definition

The pulse is a pressure wave that is transmitted through the arterial tree with each heart beat following the alternating expansion and recoil of arteries during each cardiac cycle (Marieb and Hoehn 2010). A pulse can be palpated in any artery that lies close to the surface of the body. The radial artery at the wrist is easily accessible and therefore the radial pulse is frequently used, but there are several other clinically important arterial pulse points, such as the carotid, femoral and brachial plexus (Marieb and Hoehn 2010) (see Figure 13.3).

Anatomy and physiology

In health, the arterial pulse is one of the measurements used to assess the effects of activity, postural changes and emotions on the heart rate. In ill health, the pulse can be used to assess the effects of disease, treatments and response to therapy. Each time the heart beats, it pushes blood through the arteries. The pumping action of the heart causes the walls of the arteries to expand and distend, causing a wave-like sensation which can then be felt as the pulse (Marieb and Hoehn 2010). The pulse is measured by lightly compressing the artery against firm tissue and by counting the number of beats in a minute.

Pulse Points

STRUCTURE	LOCATION	STRUCTURE	LOCATION
Superficial temporal artery	Lateral to orbit of eye.	Femoral artery	Inferior to inguinal ligament.
Facial artery	Mandible (lower jawbone) on a line with the corners of the mouth.	Popliteal artery	Posterior to knee.
		Radial artery	Distal aspect of wrist.
Common carotid artery	Lateral to larynx (voice box).	Dorsal artery of the foot (dorsalis pedis artery)	Superior to instep of foot.
Brachial artery	Medial side of biceps brachii muscle.		

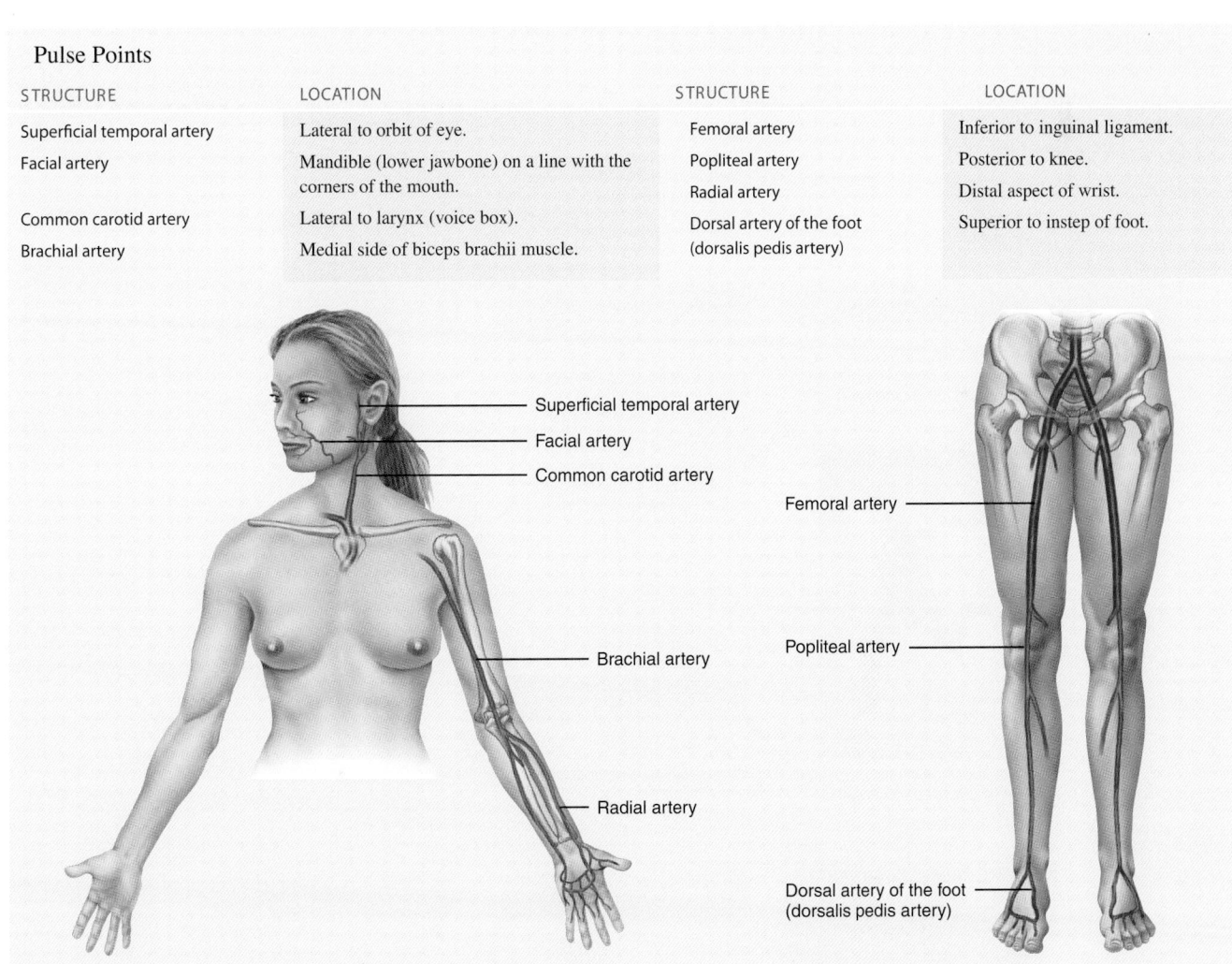

Superficial temporal artery
Facial artery
Common carotid artery
Brachial artery
Radial artery
Femoral artery
Popliteal artery
Dorsal artery of the foot (dorsalis pedis artery)

Figure 13.3 Pulse points. Reproduced from Tortora and Derrickson (2009).

Table 13.1 Normal pulse rates per minute at various ages

Age	Approximate range
1 week–3 months	100–160
3 months–2 years	80–150
2–10 years	70–110
10 years–adult	55–90

The pulse is palpated to note the following:

- rate
- rhythm
- amplitude.

Rate

The normal pulse rate varies in different client groups as age-related changes affect the pulse rate (Weber and Kelley 2003). The approximate range is illustrated in Table 13.1.

The pulse may vary depending on the posture of an individual. For example, the pulse of a healthy man may be around 66 beats per minute when he is lying down; this increases to 70 beats per minute when sitting up and 80 beats per minute when he suddenly stands (Marieb and Hoehn 2010).

The rate of the pulse of an individual with a healthy heart tends to be relatively constant. However, when blood volume drops suddenly or when the heart has been weakened by disease, the stroke volume declines and cardiac output is maintained only by increasing the rate of heart beat.

Cardiac output (CO) is the amount of blood pumped out by each ventricle in 1 minute. It is the product of heart rate (HR) and stroke volume (SV). Stroke volume is defined as the volume of blood pumped out by one ventricle with each beat. Using normal resting values for heart rate (75 beats/minute) and stroke volume (70 mL/beat), the average adult cardiac output can be calculated:

$$CO = HR \times SV = 75 \text{ beats/min} \times 70 \text{ mL/beat}$$
$$= 5250 \text{ mL/min} = 5.25 \text{ L/min (Marieb and Hoehn 2010).}$$

The heart rate and hence pulse rate are influenced by various factors acting through neural, chemical and physically induced homoeostatic mechanisms (see Figure 13.4 for factors that increase cardiac output).

- Neural changes in heart rate are caused by the activation of the sympathetic nervous system which increases heart

Figure 13.4 Factors that increase cardiac output. Reproduced from Tortora and Derrickson (2009).

rate, while parasympathetic activation decreases heart rate (Patton and Thiobodeau 2009).

- Chemical regulation of the heart is affected by hormones (adrenaline and thyroxine) and electrolytes (sodium, potassium and calcium) (Patton and Thiobodeau 2009). High or low levels of electrolytes, particularly potassium, magnesium and calcium, can cause an alteration in the heart's rhythm and rate.
- Other factors that influence heart rate are age, sex, exercise and body temperature (Marieb and Hoehn 2010).

Tachycardia

This is an abnormally fast heart rate, over 100 beats per minute in adults. It may result from an elevated body temperature, stress, certain drugs or heart disease (Marieb and Hoehn 2010). Persistent tachycardia is considered pathological because tachycardia occasionally promotes fibrillation (Marieb and Hoehn 2010).

Bradycardia

This is a heart rate slower than 60 beats per minute (Marieb and Hoehn 2010). It may be the result of a low body temperature, certain drugs or parasympathetic nervous system activation. It is also found in fit athletes when physical and cardiovascular conditioning occurs (Marieb and Hoehn 2010). This results in hypertrophy of the heart with an increase in its stroke volume, leading to a lower resting heart rate but with the same cardiac output (Marieb and Hoehn 2010). If persistent bradycardia occurs in an individual as a result of ill health, this may result in inadequate blood circulation to body tissues. Bradycardia is often a warning of brain oedema after head trauma (Marieb and Hoehn 2010) and is one of the indications of raised intracranial pressure.

Rhythm

The pulse rhythm is the sequence of beats. In health, these are regular. The co-ordinated action of the muscles of the heart in producing a regular heart rhythm is due to the ability of cardiac muscle to contract inherently without nervous control (Marieb and Hoehn 2010). The co-ordinated action of the muscles in the heart results from two physiological factors.

- Gap junctions in the cardiac muscles which form interconnections between adjacent cardiac muscles and allow transmission of nervous impulses from cell to cell (Marieb and Hoehn 2010).
- Specialized nerve-like cardiac cells that form the nodal system. These initiate and distribute impulses throughout the heart, so that the heart beats as one unit (Marieb and Hoehn 2010). The nodal system is composed of the sinoatrial node, atrioventricular node, atrioventricular bundle and the Purkinje fibres.

The sinoatrial node is the pacemaker, initiating each wave of contraction. This sets the rhythm for the heart as a whole (see Figure 13.5). Its characteristic rhythm is called *sinus rhythm*.

In patients younger than 40 years, irregularity may be linked to breathing, when the heart rate increases on inspiration and decreases on expiration. Although this is rarely

751

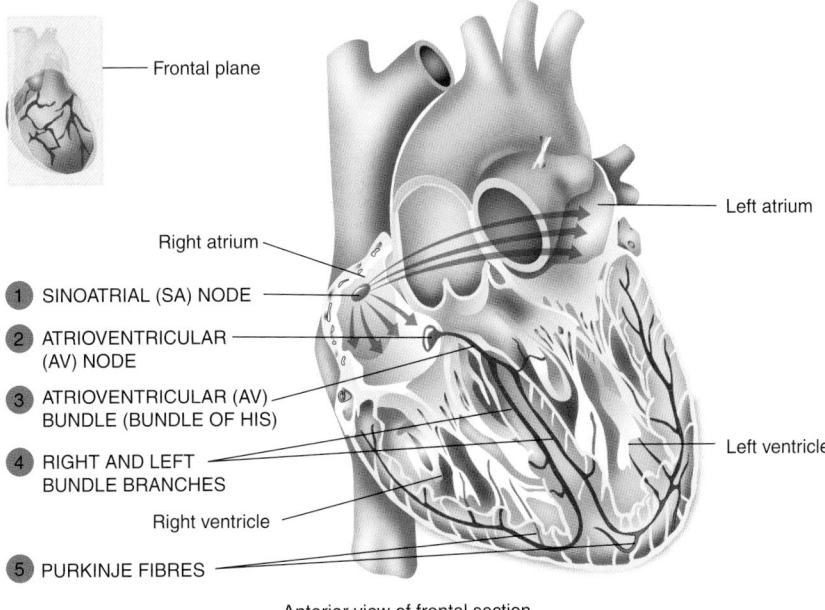

Frontal plane
Left atrium
Right atrium
1 SINOATRIAL (SA) NODE
2 ATRIOVENTRICULAR (AV) NODE
3 ATRIOVENTRICULAR (AV) BUNDLE (BUNDLE OF HIS)
4 RIGHT AND LEFT BUNDLE BRANCHES
Left ventricle
Right ventricle
5 PURKINJE FIBRES

Anterior view of frontal section

Figure 13.5 Conduction system of the heart. Autorhythmic fibres in the SA node, located in the right atrial wall, act as the heart's pacemaker, initiating cardiac action potentials that cause contraction of the heart's chambers. The conduction system ensures that the chambers of the heart contract in a co-ordinated manner. Redrawn from Tortora and Derrickson (2009) with permission.

noticeable in adults (Higgins 2008), it is normal and is known as sinus arrhythmia (Woods *et al.* 2005). Defects in the conduction system of the heart can cause irregular heart rhythms, or arrhythmias, resulting in unco-ordinated contraction of the heart.

Fibrillation

Fibrillation is a condition of rapid and irregular contractions. A fibrillating heart is ineffective as a pump (Marieb and Hoehn 2010).

Atrial fibrillation is a disruption of rhythm in the atrial areas of the heart occurring at extremely rapid and unco-ordinated intervals. The rapid impulses result in the ventricles not being able to respond to every atrial beat and, therefore, the ventricles contract irregularly (Adam and Osborne 2005). The incidence of atrial fibrillation in the general population is approximately 1%, rising to 10% in people aged over 70 years (Goodacre and Irons 2002).

There are many causes of this condition, but the following are the most common:

- ischaemic heart disease
- acute illness
- electrolyte abnormality
- thyrotoxicosis.

Atrial fibrillation can complicate or cause many other medical conditions, including stroke and heart failure (Navas 2003a). If poorly managed, patients are at increased risk of arterial thromboembolism and ischaemic stroke (Jevon 2007). If the patient has a fast ventricular rate some contractions may not be strong enough to transmit a pulse wave that is detectable at the radial artery. In this instance, checking the radial pulse is an unreliable method of assessing ventricular rate. Simultaneous monitoring of the apex beat and radial pulse is advisable in patients with atrial fibrillation, because it will determine the ventricular rate more reliably and identify whether there is an apex beat-radial pulse deficit (Jevon 2007).

This procedure requires two nurses and is described in Assessing gross pulse irregularity.

Ventricular fibrillation is an irregular heart rhythm characterized by chaotic contraction of the ventricles at very rapid rates (Adam and Osborne 2005). Ventricular fibrillation results in cardiac arrest and death if not reversed with defibrillation and the injection of adrenaline. The cause of this condition is often myocardial infarction (MI), electrical shock, acidosis, electrolyte disturbances and hypovolaemia (Resuscitation Council UK 2005).

Body fluids are good conductors of electricity so it is possible through electrocardiography to observe how the currents generated are transmitted through the heart. The electrocardiograph provides a graphic representation and record (electrocardiogram (ECG)) of electrical activity as the heart beats (see Twelve-lead electrocardiogram (ECG)). The ECG makes it possible to identify abnormalities in electrical conduction within the heart. Changes in the pattern or timing of the deflection in the ECG may indicate problems with the heart's conduction system, such as those caused by MI (Marieb and Hoehn 2010). For examples of normal and abnormal ECGs, see Twelve-lead electrocardiogram (ECG).

Amplitude

Amplitude is a reflection of pulse strength and the elasticity of the arterial wall. This varies because of the alternating strong and weak ventricular contractions (Bickley and Szilagyi 2009). The flexibility of the artery of the young adult feels different from the hard artery of the patient suffering from arteriosclerosis. It takes some clinical experience to appreciate the differences in amplitude. However, it is important to be able to recognize major changes such as the faint flickering pulse of the severely hypovolaemic patient or the irregular pulse in cardiac arrhythmias.

Assessing gross pulse irregularity

Paradoxical pulse is a pulse that markedly decreases in amplitude during inspiration. On inspiration, more blood is pooled in the lungs and so decreases the return to the left side of the heart; this affects the consequent stroke volume. A paradoxical pulse is usually regarded as normal, although in conjunction with such features as hypotension and dyspnoea, it may indicate cardiac tamponade (Bickley and Szilagyi 2009), hypovolaemia, severe airway obstruction or tension pneumothorax (Wong 2007).

When there is a gross pulse irregularity, it may be useful to use a stethoscope to assess the apical heart beat. This is done by placing the diaphragm of the stethoscope over the apex of the heart and counting the beats for 60 seconds. A second nurse should record the radial pulse at the same time. The deficit between the two should be noted using, for example, different colours on the patient's chart to indicate the apex and radial rates (Docherty 2002).

Evidence-based approaches

Rationale

The pulse is taken for the following reasons.

- To gather information on the heart rate, pattern of beats (rhythm) and amplitude (strength) of pulse.
- To determine the individual's pulse on admission as a base for comparing future measurements.
- To monitor changes in pulse.

(Marieb and Hoehn 2010)

Indications

Conditions in which a patient's pulse may need careful monitoring are described below.

- Postoperative and critically ill patients require monitoring of the pulse to assess for cardiovascular stability. The patient's pulse should be recorded preoperatively in order to establish a baseline and to make comparisons. Hypovolaemic shock post surgery from the loss of plasma or whole blood results in a decrease in circulatory blood volume. The resulting acceleration in heart rate causes a tachycardia that can be felt in the pulse. The greater the loss in volume, the more thready the pulse is likely to feel.

■ Blood transfusions require careful monitoring of the pulse as an incompatible blood transfusion may lead to a rise in pulse rate (British Committee for Standards in Haematology 1999) (see Chapter 8).

■ Patients with local or systemic infections or inflammatory reactions require monitoring of their pulse to detect sepsis/severe sepsis. This is characterized by a decrease in the mean arterial pressure (MAP) and a rise in pulse rate (Marieb and Hoehn 2010).

■ Patients with cardiovascular conditions require regular assessment of the pulse to monitor their condition and the efficacy of medications.

Methods of pulse measurement
Manual

The pulse is measured by lightly compressing the artery against firm tissue and by counting the number of beats in a minute.

Electronic

Automated electronic equipment such as a pulse oximeter, blood pressure recording devices, 12-lead ECG or continuous cardiac monitoring may be used to determine the pulse. However, even where the patient has continuous ECG monitoring, it is still essential to manually feel for a pulse to determine amplitude and volume and whether the pulse is irregular. In pulseless electrical activity (PEA), normal sinus rhythm is shown on the monitor but a pulse is not palpable (Levine et al. 2008).

Preprocedural considerations
Equipment

Pulse can be measured using a:

■ *stethoscope*: instrument used for listening to internal body sounds, especially from the heart and lung. It consists of a hollow tube, one end of which is placed to the ear of the examiner (Weller 2005) and the other end consists of a diaphragm (disc), used to pick up high-pitched sounds, or bell (hollow cup), used to detect low-pitched sounds (Bickley and Szilagyi 2009)

■ *electronic pulse measurement device* (pulse oximeter): a small electronic device, consisting of a probe which is placed onto the end of a finger to record pulse rate.

Specific patient preparations

Ideally a patient should be at rest for 20 minutes before trying to obtain an accurate pulse. Strenuous activity will result in falsely elevated readings (Rawlings-Anderson and Hunter 2008).

Procedure guideline 13.1 Pulse measurement

Essential equipment

■ A watch that has a second hand
■ Alcohol handrub
■ Observations chart
■ Black pen
■ A stethoscope (if counting the apical beat)
■ Electronic pulse measurement device, for example pulse oximeter, blood pressure measuring device or cardiac monitor

Preprocedure

Action	Rationale
1 Wash hands and dry hands.	To prevent cross-infection (Fraise and Bradley 2009, E).
2 Explain and discuss the procedure with the patient.	To ensure that the patient understands the procedure and gives their valid consent (NMC 2008b, C).

Procedure

3 Where possible, measure the pulse under the same conditions each time.	To ensure continuity and consistency in recording. E
4 Ensure that the patient is comfortable and relaxed. Ideally the patient should refrain from physical activity for 20 minutes.	To ensure that the patient is comfortable. E Strenuous activity will result in falsely elevated readings (Rawlings-Anderson and Hunter 2008, E).

753

(Continued)

Procedure guideline 13.1 *(Continued)*

5 Place the first and second or in addition the third finger along the appropriate artery and apply light pressure until the pulse is felt (see Action Figure 5).	The fingertips are sensitive to touch. Practitioners should be aware that the thumb and forefinger have pulses of their own and therefore these may be mistaken for the patient's pulse (Docherty and Coote 2006, E).
6 Press gently against the peripheral artery being used to record the pulse.	The radial artery is usually used as it is often the most readily accessible (Bickley and Szilagyi 2009, E).
7 The pulse should be counted for 60 seconds.	Sufficient time is required to detect irregularities in rhythm or volume. If the pulse is regular and of good volume subsequent readings may be taken for 30 seconds and then doubled to give beats per minute. If the rhythm or volume changes on subsequent readings then pulse must be taken for 60 seconds (Rawlings-Anderson and Hunter 2008), E).
8 Record the pulse rate on appropriate documentation. Additional factors such as the rhythm, volume and skin condition (dry, sweaty or clammy) may be described in the patient's nursing notes.	To monitor differences and detect trends; any irregularities should be brought to the attention of the appropriate senior nursing and medical teams (NMC 2008a, C). Additional qualitative characteristics of the pulse may aid diagnosis of the patient's condition (Rawlings-Anderson and Hunter 2008), E).

Postprocedure

9 Discuss result and any further action with the patient.	To involve the patient in their care and provide assurance of a normal result or explain the actions to be undertaking in the event of an abnormal result. E, P
10 Wash and dry hands or decontaminate with alcohol handrub.	To prevent cross-infection (Fraise and Bradley 2009, E).

Action Figure 5   Taking a pulse.

Problem-solving table 13.1 Prevention and resolution (Procedure guideline 13.1)

Problem	Cause	Prevention	Action
No pulse palpable	Incorrect positioning of fingers	Refer to Figure 13.3 for palpation sites.	Place 2 or 3 fingers over the appropriate artery and lighty depress against the tissue or bone. Try alternative sites such as brachial or carotid artery.
Absent or faint pulse	Poor perfusion	Assess patient's existing co-morbidities for further information. Identify any causes of hypovolaemia	Inform medical team if the patient is cardiovascularly compromised
	Obstruction, for example clot	Perform a venous thromboembolism (VTE) risk assessment for your patient on admission (NICE 2007a) and ensure appropriate preventive measures in place, for example antiembolism stockings, mechanical devices applying intermittent pneumatic pressure, for example Flowtron, or injections of low molecular weight heparin preparations (Lees and McAuliffe 2010)	Perform a neurovascular assessment, assessing all pulse sites to determine compromised area. Also feel for warmth and sensation and capillary refill to provide further information on the degree of vascular sufficiency
Pulse too fast and irregular to manually palpate	Patient may be in an abnormal rhythm	Haemodynamic assessment, monitoring and maintenance of electrolyte balance	Use electronic recording device. New-onset tachycardia and irregular rhythms should prompt a full set of observations: BP, respiratory rate, oxygen saturation and temperature. It is essential to perform a 12-lead ECG and have this reviewed by a doctor

Postprocedural considerations

Documentation

The pulse should be recorded in the patient's notes on the institution's approved observation chart. The recording should be dated and timed so that the pulse trend may be viewed easily as part of ongoing patient monitoring.

Twelve-lead electrocardiogram (ECG)

Definition

Electrical currents generated and transmitted through the heart also spread throughout the body and can be monitored and amplified with an instrument called an electrocardiogram (Marieb and Hoehn 2010).

A 12-lead ECG is a quick non-invasive way of acquiring data to ascertain information about the electrophysiology of the heart (Marieb and Hoehn 2010). Electrical changes, which take place as the cardiac muscle contracts and relaxes, are recorded on the ECG trace and produce 12 different tracings from different combinations of limb and chest leads (Tortora and Derrickson 2009).

Anatomy and physiology

The starting point of the cardiac electrical cycle is the sinoatrial (SA) node. This is the heart's natural pacemaker, which can create impulses at 60–100 beats per minute. Its ability to spontaneously generate and discharge an electrical impulse is called automaticity (Docherty 2005).

A typical ECG consists of a series of three distinguishable waves called deflection waves (see Figure 13.6). The first wave, the small P wave, lasting about 0.08 seconds,

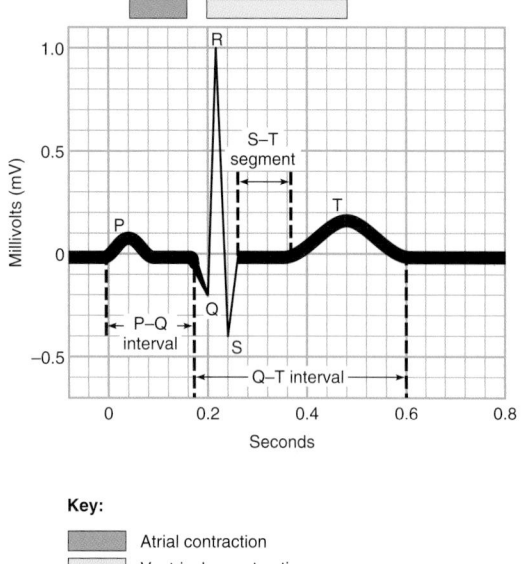

Key:
Atrial contraction
Ventricular contraction

Figure 13.6 Normal electrocardiograms or ECG (lead II). P-wave = arterial depolarization; QRS complex = onset of ventricular depolarization; T-wave = ventricular repolarization. Reproduced from Tortora and Derrickson (2009).

results from movement of the depolarization wave from the SA node through the atria. The impulse travels from the atria to the ventricles via the atrioventricular (AV) node through internodal tracts (Lemery *et al*. 2003): this is the PR interval. From the AV node, the impulse travels down the His–Purkinje system and throughout the ventricles. The septal area contracts before the main ventricle muscle (Tortora and Derrickson 2009), giving rise to a small negatively deflected Q wave on the ECG.

The His–Purkinje system consists of the His bundle, right bundle branch, left bundle branch and Purkinje fibres (Tortora and Derrickson 2009). The Purkinje fibres conduct impulses through the muscle assisting depolarization almost simultaneously (Philip and Kowery 2001), giving rise to the positive R-wave deflection on the ECG, followed by an S-wave as the ECG then detects the right ventricle muscle movement (Docherty 2005). The T-wave illustrates ventricular repolarization, commonly referred to as the resting phase of the ventricles. Sometime a small U-wave preceding the T-wave is noticeable and this represents relaxation of the ventricles (Chummun 2009). Atrial repolarization is not graphically represented on the ECG as it is hidden in the QRS complex (Sharman 2007).

Related theory

The first three leads or views of the heart (leads I, II and III) were introduced in 1902 by Willem Einthoven. Figure 13.7 illustrates the specific arrangement known as the Einthoven triangle together with normal ECG lead tracings (Einthoven 1902). In acute clinical areas where continuous cardiac

monitoring is required, the three limb leads can be placed according to Figure 13.7 and the monitor is set to show lead II as this gives the best picture and is the most accurate atrial monitoring lead (Docherty 2002, Navas 2003b). An ECG lead records the difference in electrical potential between a negative and positive electrode.

Recording a 12-lead ECG requires the connection of two groups of electrodes to the patient.

- Limb leads (I, II, III, aVR, aVL, aVF).
- Chest or precordial leads (generally V1 to V6) (Wilson *et al*. 1944, Noble *et al*. 2010).

The 12-lead ECG is the gold standard for diagnostic purposes and the standard electrode placement is shown in Figure 13.7 and described in Procedure guideline 13.2. However, it should be noted that an alternative positioning of the limb leads on the torso, known as the Mason-Likar 12-lead system, can also be used. The Mason-Likar arrangement is more suitable in acute areas where continuous 12-lead ECG monitoring is required as the waveforms are easily viewed without interference from limb movement (Pelter 2008).

Evidence-based approaches
Rationale

An ECG is performed electively prior to various interventions such as surgery and anticancer chemotherapy. An ECG should also be considered to aid diagnosis during an acute situation, particularly in the presence of chest pain, haemodynamic disturbance or cardiac rhythm changes. Twenty-four hour ambulatory ECG monitoring, also known as 24-hour tape, may be used to record and analyse the patient's heart rhythm. This is useful to capture abnormalities that might be missed with a standard 12-lead ECG and is a specialist test. If required, up to 72 hours of ambulatory ECG monitoring may be recorded.

Legal and professional issues
Competencies

Any healthcare professional who has been trained and assessed as competent can take a 12-lead ECG in line with local hospital policy. However, its analysis and diagnosis are usually undertaken by medical staff or specialist nurses (Sharman 2007).

Preprocedural considerations
Equipment

- *12-lead ECG machine*: consisting of 12 wires which are connected to electrodes fixed to the body. The machine detects and amplifies the electrical impulses that occur at each heart beat and records them on to a paper or computer.
- *ECG paper (25 mm/s style)*: waveforms produced by the heart's electrical current are recorded on graphed ECG

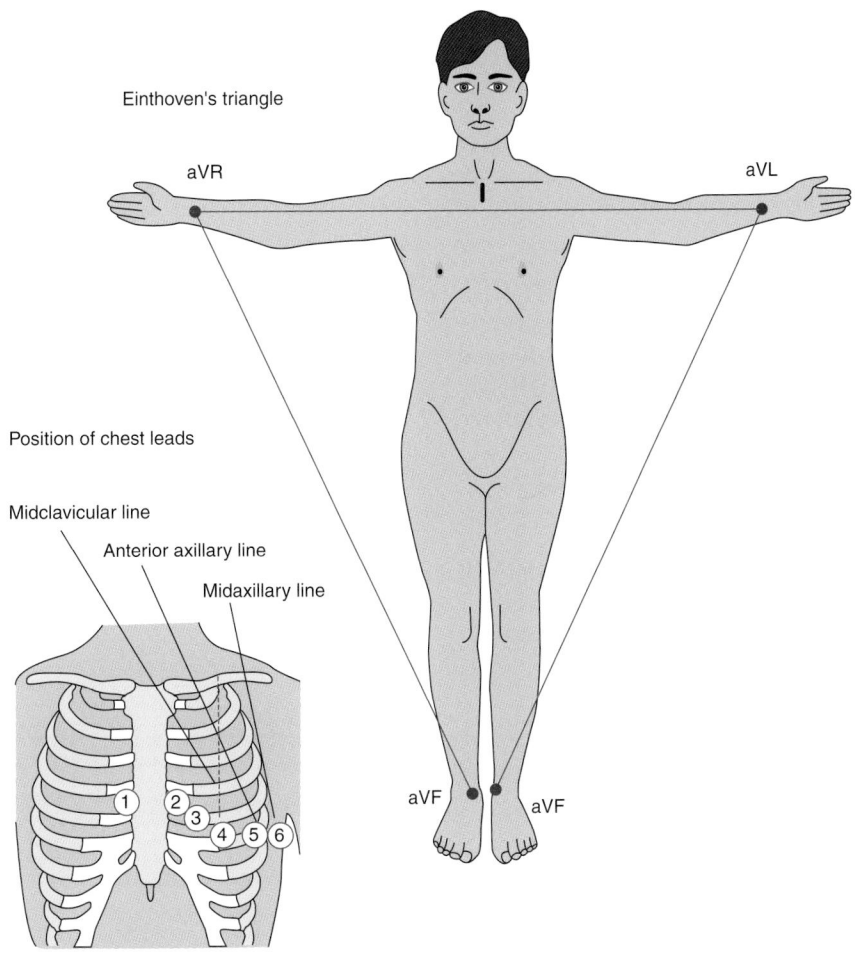

Einthoven's triangle

aVR

aVL

Position of chest leads

Midclavicular line

Anterior axillary line

Midaxillary line

① ② ③ ④ ⑤ ⑥

aVF

aVF

Figure 13.7   Position of electrodes for 12-lead ECG. Redrawn from Metcalf (2000) with permission.

paper by a stylus. ECG paper consists of horizontal and vertical lines forming a grid. A piece of ECG paper is called an ECG strip or tracing. The horizontal axis of the strip represents time. Each small block equals 0.04 second, and five small blocks form a large block, which equals 0.2 second. Five large blocks equal 1 second (5 × 0.2). The ECG strip's vertical axis measures amplitude in millimetres (mm) or electrical volts in millivolts (mV) (Levine *et al.* 2008) (see Figure 13.6).

- *Filter selection*: modern ECG monitors offer multiple filters for signal processing. The most common settings are monitor mode and diagnostic mode. In monitor mode, the low-frequency filter is set at either 0.5 Hz or 1 Hz and the high-frequency filter is set at 40 Hz. This limits artefact for routine cardiac rhythm monitoring. The high-pass filter helps reduce wandering baseline and the low-pass filter helps reduce 50 or 60 Hz power line noise. In diagnostic mode, the high-pass filter is set at 0.05 Hz, which allows accurate ST segments to be recorded. The low-pass filter is set to 40, 100 or 150 Hz. Consequently, the monitor mode ECG display is more filtered than diagnostic mode, because its passband is narrower.

- *12 leads*: in electrocardiography, the word *lead* may refer to either the electrodes attached to the patient or the voltage between two electrodes. The electrodes are attached to the patient's body, usually with sticky circles of thick tape-like material (the electrode is embedded in the centre of this circle), onto which ECG leads clip, using different combinations of electrodes to measure various signals from the heart.

- *Abrasive strips*: can be used to aid electrode contact by gently rubbing over the skin in the position of the electrodes. Gentle friction creates a roughened skin surface without causing cuts, which is helpful in creating a good contact between the electrode and the skin.

- *24–72-hour ambulatory ECG recorder*: a continuous recording of an ECG over a 24–72-hour period, which enables a patient to continue with their daily activities.

Use of filter

The filter should not be used for the initial recording as it will distort the ECG. The Society for Cardiology Science and Technology advises the use of the filter only once other efforts to reduce interference, for example attempts to relax the patient and promote their comfort, have been exhausted (SCST 2006). Use of the filter should be clearly identified on the ECG.

Specific patient preparations

Female patients

Placement of the lateral chest leads (V4, V5 and V6) is by convention under the left breast. Whilst there is emerging evidence to support the positioning of these electrodes over the breast, it is currently insufficient to suggest a change of procedure (SCST 2006).

Dextrocardia

Dextrocardia is used to describe a heart that is located within the right side of the chest rather than the left. It may be associated with the condition situs inversus where all the patient's organs are in a mirror image position.

The following are recommended by the SCST (2006).

Patients with an unknown dextrocardia

The initial ECG recorded in the standard arrangement will show an inverted P-wave in lead I (P-axis >90°) together with poor R-wave progression across the chest leads. If suspected, a second ECG should be recorded with the chest electrodes positioned on the right side of the chest using the same intercostal spacing and anatomical landmarks. This approach will provide a 'true' ECG representation. The limb lead complexes will continue to appear inverted, demonstrating the abnormal location of the heart. However, the repositioned chest leads will now show the appropriate R-wave progression. Both ECGs should be retained for inclusion in the patient's notes.

Patient known to have dextrocardia

The ECG should be recorded with the limb leads in the usual position and the chest lead should be placed across the right side of the chest. Note that swapping of the right and left limb leads will 'normalize' the appearance of the limb leads.

When swapping leads, it is imperative that the ECG is clearly annotated to describe the new positions of the electrodes (for example, V3R, V4R, etc.) to prevent possibility of dextrocardia being overlooked.

If there is difficulty attaching the ECG sticker, see Problem-solving table 13.2.

Procedure guideline 13.2 Electrocardiogram

Essential equipment

- ECG machine with chest and limb leads labelled respectively, for example LA to left arm, V1 to first chest lead
- Disposable electrodes
- Swabs saturated with 70% isopropyl alcohol to cleanse and prepare the skin prior to electrode placement
- Abrasive strips
- Alcohol handrub

Preprocedure

Action	Rationale
1 Wash hands using bactericidal soap and water or bactericidal alcohol handrub, and dry.	To minimize the risk of infection (Fraise and Bradley 2009, E).
2 Explain to the patient that the ECG is to be taken, that it is not a painful procedure and that it will be useful to aid diagnosis.	To ensure that the patient understands the procedure and gives their valid consent (NMC 2008b, C; Roberts 2002, E).
3 Ensure that the patient is comfortably positioned either lying or sitting (preferably in semi-recumbent position). Any variations to standard recording techniques must be highlighted on the trace, for example 'ECG recorded whilst patient in wheelchair'.	To ensure optimal recording and comfort of the patient (Roberts 2002, E). The ECG may vary depending on the patient's position so it is important to note this on the ECG (SCST 2006, C).
4 Clean limb and chest electrode sites (see Figure 13.7). If necessary, prepare skin by clipping hairs or use abrasive strip.	To ensure good grip and therefore good contact between skin and electrode which results in less electrical artefact (Roberts 2002, E). Shaving should be avoided due to the risk of infection if the skin is grazed (Sharman 2007, E) or bleeding if the patient is on anticoagulation therapy (Pelter 2008, E).

Procedure

5 Apply the chest electrodes as described in Figure 13.7. Apply the limb leads proximal to the appropriate wrist and ankle. For advice on placement in females and known cardiac abnormalities please see the Specific patient preparations.	To obtain the ECG recording from vertical and horizontal planes (Roberts 2002, E). Following a standard arrangement ensures consistency between recordings and prevents invalid recordings and false diagnosis (SCST 2006, C).
6 Attach the leads from the ECG machine to the electrodes.	To obtain the ECG recording (Roberts 2002, E).
7 Check that the leads are connected correctly and to the relevant electrode.	To ensure the correct polarity in the ECG recording (Roberts 2002, E).
8 Ensure that the leads are not pulling on the electrodes or lying over each other. Offer the patient a gown or sheet to place over their exposed chest.	To reduce electrical artefact and to obtain a good ECG recording (Roberts 2002, E). To promote patient dignity and reduce anxiety (SCST 2006, C).
9 Ask patient to relax and refrain from movement.	To obtain the optimal recording by the reduction of artefact from muscular movement (Roberts 2002, E; SCST 2006, C).
10 Encourage the patient to breath normally and not to speak while the trace is being taken.	Speaking can alter the recording (Roberts 2002, E).
11 Check that calibration is 10 mm/mV.	To ensure standard recording to aid interpretation. E
12 Commence the recording.	To obtain ECG. E
13 In the case of artefact or poor recording, check electrodes and connections.	To ensure optimal recording (Roberts 2002, E).
14 During the procedure give reassurance to the patient.	To ensure the patient feels informed and reassured (Roberts 2002, E).
15 If necessary, record a rhythm strip utilizing leads II and V1.	To assist with interpretation if there have been any acute rhythm disturbances. Can also ensure steady baseline (Roberts 2002, E).
16 Detach ECG print-out and label with patient's name, hospital number, date and time. File the ECG recording in the appropriate documentation.	To ensure that the ECG is labelled with the correct patient, date and time (NMC 2009, C). To ensure that the recording does not get lost (NMC 2009, C).

Postprocedure

17 Inform patient that the procedure is now finished and help to remove the electrodes.	To ensure that the patient can relax and that the electrodes are removed. E
18 Wash hands using bactericidal soap and water or bactericidal alcohol handrub, and dry.	To minimize the risk of infection (Fraise and Bradley 2009, E).
19 Inform nursing and medical staff that the ECG has been completed and its location.	To enable relevant nursing and medical staff to use the ECG data in their care planning and treatment (NMC 2008a, C).
20 Clean the ECG machine following manufacturer's advice after patient use and return it to its storage place and plug it in to keep the battery fully charged.	The ECG machine forms part of a ward's emergency equipment and should always be available and in good working order with a charged battery for use in an emergency (Metcalfe 2000, E).

Problem-solving table 13.2 Prevention and resolution (Procedure guideline 13.2)

Problem	Cause	Prevention	Action
Unable to turn on the ECG machine	Low battery	Ensure the ECG is left on continuous charge when not in use	The ECG will function once it is connected to a power supply
ECG machine is working but the rhythm display is blank	Loose connection	Carefully store the leads after use to prevent damage	Check that each lead is connected to the electrode clip and that the base of the lead is connected to the ECG machine
	Electrode stickers peel off from the patient's skin	The patient may have used body lotion or the skin may be clammy, making adhesion difficult	Check if the patient has used body lotions; if so, cleanse the electrode sites with soap and water to remove the lotion and allow to dry then reapply new electrode stickers
		The patient's chest may be too hairy which makes adhesion difficult	If the patient has a hairy chest try to push the hair out of the way when applying stickers to make a better contact; sometimes reinforcement with tape is required. If this fails to work, ask the patient for permission to shave off a small amount of hair at the electrode sites, cleanse to remove loose hair, allow to dry and apply new electrode stickers
	The electrode stickers may be intact but there is still no rhythm – is the patient's skin excessively dry and flaky?	Identify underlying causes and severity of dry skin and address them with the MDT as appropriate	With the patient's permission, vigorous but gentle rubbing with soap and water, 2% chlorhexidine wipes or abrasive strips should be performed to remove the superficial dead skin cells. The skin should be allowed to dry and new electrode stickers applied
ECG is printing but some of the views are missing	A loose connection	Good skin preparation and maintenance of the ECG machine	Check that the electrode sticker is intact and follow above suggestions for skin preparation. Check that the leads are all connected properly
ECG is printing but there is interference, making it difficult to interpret safely	Patient movement	Ask the patient not to speak and remain still but breathe normally.	Ensure the patient is not moving or talking and repeat the ECG once the displayed rhythm has stabilized
		The patient may be cold and therefore involuntarily shivering	Once the electrodes are connected, place blankets over the patient to warm them
	Peripheral interference		Place the limb leads more centrally as shown in the Mason-Likar placement (see Figure 13.7) to reduce interference from limb movement

Problem	Cause	Prevention	Action
	General interference/wandering baseline	Poor skin contact with the electrodes, poor electrode placement or thoracic movement (Metcalfe 2000)	Ensure good skin preparation. Ask the patient to take shallow breaths if possible. Check that the leads are properly placed. If necessary, record an additional ECG with the 'filter' function on to limit interference. Write on the ECG that the 'filter' function was used
ECG is working and displays a rhythm but the print-out is blank	Different manufacturer's ECG paper has been loaded	Only use the manufacturer's recommended paper for the ECG machine	Reload using the correct paper
	Internal fault	Ensure manufacturer's recommendations re-maintenance and servicing are followed	Contact in-house engineer or medical device technician or manufacturer for advice

Postprocedural considerations

Immediate care

Any changes on the ECG that might require urgent medical attention should be identified and advice sought from a senior member of staff. If the patient has any cardiac symptoms at the time of recording, such as chest pain or palpitations, then this should be noted on the tracing and brought to the immediate attention of a doctor (SCST 2006). Examples of normal and some important abnormal ECG tracings are shown in Figure 13.8.

Documentation

Once the nurse has recorded the ECG, this should be reviewed by an appropriate member of the medical team,

(a) Normal electrocardiogram (ECG)

(b) First-degree AV block

(c) Atrial fibrillation

(d) Ventricular tachycardia

(e) Ventricular fibrillation

Figure 13.8 Normal and abnormal ECG tracings. Reproduced from Tortora and Derrickson (2009).

usually a doctor. It is good practice for the reviewer to document their interpretation of the ECG directly on to the ECG and to sign and date it. Once reviewed, the ECG should be filed in the patient's medical notes. Nurses should document in the nursing notes when the ECG was recorded, who was asked to review it and the actual time the ECG was reviewed and indicate whether it was normal or, if abnormal, what further action was taken.

Blood pressure

Definition

Blood pressure may be defined as the force of blood inside the blood vessels against the vessel walls (Marieb and Hoehn 2010). Systolic pressure is the peak pressure of the left ventricle contracting and blood entering the aorta, causing it to stretch and therefore in part reflects the function of the left ventricle (Marieb and Hoehn 2010). Diastolic pressure is when the aortic valve closes, blood flows from the aorta into the smaller vessels and the aorta recoils back. This is when the aortic pressure is at its lowest and tends to reflect the resistance of the blood vessels (Marieb and Hoehn 2010).

Related theory

Blood pressure is determined by cardiac output and vascular resistance and can be described as:

$$\underset{\text{(Blood pressure)}}{BP} = \underset{\text{(Cardiac output)}}{CO} \times \underset{\text{(Systemic vascular resistance)}}{SVR}$$

(Woodrow 2004b)

Cardiac output is the volume of blood which flows out of the heart over a specified length of time (Marieb and Hoehn 2010). It is governed by the stroke volume of the heart (the amount of blood pumped out of the ventricles per beat) and the heart rate. The relationship is:

$$\underset{\text{(Cardiac output)}}{CO} = \underset{\text{(Stroke volume)}}{SV} \times \underset{\text{(Heart rate)}}{HR}$$

(Patton and Thiobodeau 2009)

Therefore, if the two equations are combined, blood pressure could be seen as being:

$$BP = SV \times HR \times SVR$$

(Woodrow 2004b)

In theory, anything which alters one of the above components (stroke volume, heart rate and resistance) will therefore produce a change in blood pressure. However, this is not always the case as a drop in one may be compensated for by an increase in the other (Patton and Thiobodeau 2009).

Normal blood pressure

Normal blood pressure ranges between 110–140 mmHg systolic and 70–80 mmHg diastolic at rest (Marieb and Hoehn 2010). However, it varies depending on age (increasing with age), activity and sleep, emotion and positioning (Levick 2010). It also varies depending on the time of day, being at its lowest while we sleep (Levick 2010). Blood pressure therefore reflects individual variations but an abnormal blood pressure should not be assumed to be the individual's norm; rather, it will need to be assessed in relation to their previous results, general condition and other observations.

Hypotension

Hypotension is generally defined in adults as a systolic blood pressure below 100 mmHg (Marieb and Hoehn 2010). A low blood pressure may indicate orthostatic hypotension, that is, sudden drop in blood pressure when the patient rises from a supine or sitting position. This is usually compensated for by the baroreceptor reflex and the sympathetic nervous system but especially in older people, this may not work as efficiently (Marieb and Hoehn 2010). Hypotension can also be a symptom of many other conditions including shock, haemorrhage and malnutrition (Marieb and Hoehn 2010). Hypotension results in reduced tissue perfusion leading to hypoxia and an accumulation of waste products (Foxall 2009).

Hypertension

Hypertension is defined as sustained blood pressure greater than 140/90 mmHg (NICE 2006, Patton and Thiobodeau 2009). It can be either *primary* hypertension, with no single known cause, or *secondary* hypertension related to another factor such as kidney disease (Patton and Thiobodeau 2009). Factors leading to hypertension include gender, genetic factors and age, alongside risk factors such as obesity, lack of exercise, smoking and high caffeine and alcohol intake (Patton and Thiobodeau 2009). If hypertension is sustained, the heart will have an increased workload to maintain circulation; greater stress will be placed on the blood vessel walls and cardiac ischaemia can occur (Foxall 2009).

There are many illnesses and factors which can lead to changes in blood pressure (see Figure 13.9).

Mean arterial pressure

The MAP indicates the average pressure of blood throughout the pulse cycle and thus is a reliable indication of perfusion (Woodrow 2004a). Mathematically, the MAP is derived from the diastolic pressure and the pulse pressure (which is the difference between systolic and diastolic blood pressure). The equation is:

$$MAP = \text{diastolic pressure} + (\text{pulse pressure}/3)$$

(Marieb and Hoehn 2010)

Therefore, a patient with a blood pressure of 123/90 mmHg has a MAP of 101 mmHg. An adequate MAP is usually deemed to be between 65 mmHg (Hinds and Watson 2009) and 70 mmHg (Woodrow 2004a).

762

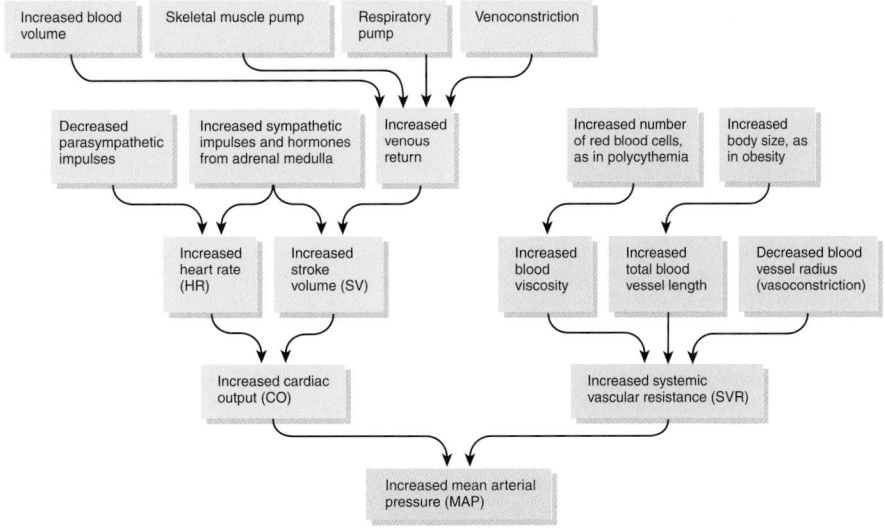

Figure 13.9 Factors that lead to an increase in blood pressure. Changes noted within green boxes increase cardiac output; changes noted within blue boxes increase systemic vascular resistance. Reproduced from Tortora and Derrickson (2009).

Resistance

Resistance is effectively opposition to blood flow (Marieb and Hoehn 2010) and is created by friction between the walls of blood vessels and the blood itself (Patton and Thiobodeau 2009). It is termed peripheral or systemic resistance because most of the resistance occurs in the vessels away from the heart (Marieb and Hoehn 2010). Peripheral resistance varies depending on the degree of vasoconstriction or vasodilation, and the viscosity of blood and the length of the vessels, although the latter two factors generally remain relatively static (Marieb and Hoehn 2010). Arterioles can dilate or contract; when contracted, peripheral resistance increases and blood flow to the tissues decreases, increasing the arterial blood pressure (Patton and Thiobodeau 2009). This can occur systemically, when there is total peripheral resistance, or locally (Patton and Thiobodeau 2009). Blood pressure in the vessels of the cardiovascular system can be seen in Figure 13.10.

Blood pressure control

There are many inter-related physiological mechanisms which control blood pressure.

Hormonal control

Many hormones help to regulate blood pressure, including adrenaline and noradrenaline which are released from the adrenal medullae in response to a drop in blood pressure; these hormones increase cardiac contractility and thus cardiac output (Foxall 2009). Atrial natriuretic peptide (ANP) is a hormone which is produced from the atria of the heart in response to hypertension. It works by inhibiting the renin-angiotensin system, raising the glomerular

filtration rate by causing specific vasodilation, inhibiting sodium reabsorption and causing fluid transfer into the instital space (Levick 2010).

Neural control

When blood pressure increases, the baroreceptors, or stretch receptors, are stimulated and in turn stimulate the cardiac

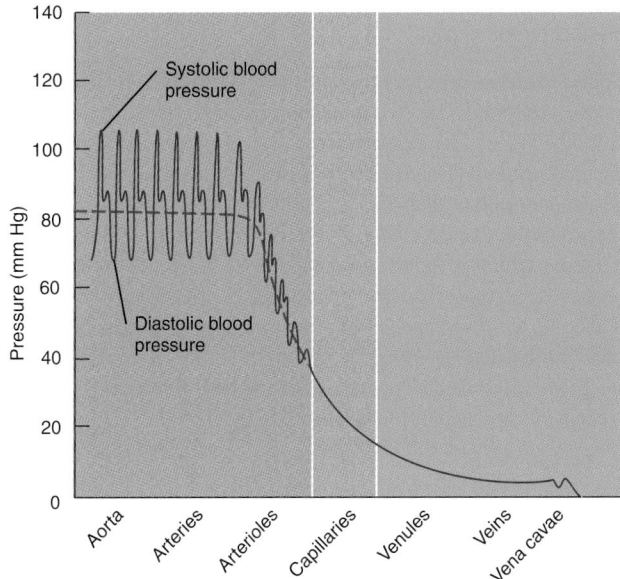

Figure 13.10 Blood pressure in various parts of the cardiovascular system. The dashed line is the mean (average) blood pressure in the aorta, arteries and arterioles. Reproduced from Tortora and Derrickson (2009).

inhibitory centre, reducing sympathetic nerve impulses and increasing parasympathetic nerve impulses (Foxall 2009). This causes a vasodilation and a decrease in cardiac output, thereby reducing the blood pressure (Foxall 2009). Similarly, when blood pressure is low the opposite occurs. This response is termed a reflex arch, continually maintaining homoeostasis (Marieb and Hoehn 2010). Baroreceptors are located in the aortic arch, carotid sinuses and in the walls of most of the large arteries in the thorax and neck (Marieb and Hoehn 2010). Close to these are chemoreceptors which are stimulated when the pH of the blood drops or when the carbon dioxide rises, and when oxygen levels drop significantly, these cause an increase in cardiac output and vasoconstriction, leading to an increase in blood pressure (Marieb and Hoehn 2010).

Renal control

When there is a decrease in blood pressure, adrenaline, increased sympathetic activity and a reduction in the stimulation of stretch receptors stimulate the juxtaglomerular cells within the kidneys to release renin (Levick 2010). This causes angiotensin I to be produced, leading to the production of angiotensin-converting enzyme which converts angiotensin I to angiotensin II (Patton and Thiobodeau 2009). Angiotensin II has a potent effect on blood pressure, causing cardiac output and vasoconstriction to increase, stimulating the production of aldosterone and antidiuretic hormone which leads to the reabsorption of water and sodium and stimulates the thirst receptors (Foxall 2009). This increases the circulatory volume of fluid and thereby blood pressure (Foxall 2009). Similarly, the reverse happens when fluid volume in the circulatory system is high.

Other mechanisms which influence blood pressure

Skeletal muscle contractions and respiration promote venous return of blood to the heart and therefore increase cardiac output. The skeletal muscles contract on movement, compressing the veins and pushing the blood towards the heart, and respiration causes a change in thoracic and abdominal pressure which acts to pump venous blood (Patton and Thiobodeau 2009). A factor which affects stroke volume is Starling's Law of the heart which states that the force of the contraction of the heart is related to how much blood volume is in the heart (Patton and Thiobodeau 2009). The more stretched the muscle fibres are prior to contraction, the stronger the contraction and the greater volume it will pump (Foxall 2009).

Evidence-based approaches

Rationale

Indications

Blood pressure measurements should be taken as follows.

- On admission to a ward, in A&E departments when a decision to admit has been made (NICE 2007b).

- When a patient is transferred to a ward setting from intensive or high-dependency care (NICE 2007b).
- At least once every 12 hours while in hospital (NICE 2007b).
- For patients at risk of, or with known, infections (Chalmers et al. 2008).
- To assess response to interventions put in place to correct the patient's blood pressure (Curran 2009, NICE 2006).
- On patients preoperatively, to establish a baseline, and postoperatively to assess cardiovascular stability.
- Critically or acutely ill patients, or those who are at risk of rapid deterioration, will require close and potentially continuous monitoring.
- Patients who are receiving blood or blood products transfusions, to establish a baseline, during and after the transfusion (McClelland 2007).
- Any patient showing any signs of shock should have frequent monitoring.
- Any patient who is receiving medications which could alter their blood pressure, such as epidurals or anaesthetics.

Contraindications

There are contraindications or times when certain methods of blood pressure measurement should be used with caution.

- Oscillometric blood pressure devices may not be accurate in those with weak or thready pulse or patients with pre-eclampsia (MHRA 2005).
- The brachial artery should not be used to measure blood pressure in those with arteriovenous fistulas (Turner et al. 2008).
- Patients with atrial fibrillation should have auscultatory blood pressure measurements taken, rather than oscillometric, and may require multiple readings (Williams et al. 2004).
- Korotkoff sounds are not dependably audible in children under the age of 1 year, and many children under 5 years (Curran 2009). Therefore, ultrasound, Doppler or oscillometric devices are recommended (O'Brien et al. 2003).
- Patients who have had trauma to the upper arm, previous mastectomy or a forearm amputation should not have blood pressure measured on the affected side at the brachial artery (Turner et al. 2008).
- Oscillometric devices should be used with caution in those with atherosclerosis and/or high or low blood pressures, as they may not measure accurately (Bern et al. 2007).
- The manufacturer's guidance should be sought for contraindications specific to the device used.
- Blood pressure should not be measured on an arm that has had brachial artery surgery or is at risk of lymphoedema (Bickley and Szilagyi 2009).

Methods of measuring blood pressure

There are two main methods of measuring blood pressure – direct and indirect.

Direct

The direct method enables continuous monitoring of the blood pressure and so is commonly used for critically ill patients, for example in intensive care units and theatres (Woodrow 2004a). To do this a cannula is inserted into an artery, most commonly the radial artery, as it is easy to access and monitor (Foxall 2009). The cannula has a transducer attached to it and is attached at the external end to a cardiac monitor where the blood pressure is shown as a waveform; it is also attached to a pressurized flush of solution to prevent blood backflow (Foxall 2009). This method has potential risks of severe haemorrhage, thrombosis and air embolism (Foxall 2009); therefore, it must only be used where patients can be continuously observed (Woodrow 2004a).

Indirect

For indirect blood pressure measurement, either manual auscultatory sphygmomanometers or automated oscillometric devices are used (Bern *et al.* 2007). Oscillometric devices electronically measure blood pressure by measuring the oscillation of air pressure in the cuff, so when the artery begins to pulse it causes a corresponding oscillation of cuff pressure (Levick 2010). Manual auscultatory blood pressure involves occluding the artery by use of a pressurized cuff and then gradually releasing the pressure; when the systolic blood pressure exceeds cuff pressure, blood re-enters the arteries briefly, during systole, enabling a pulse to be palpated and producing vibrations in the artery (Levick 2010). As the cuff pressure descends, the sounds cease as the artery remains open throughout the pulse wave (Kacmerek *et al.* 2005).

Systolic blood pressure is usually defined as being at stage 1 of the Korotkoff sounds and diastolic at stage 5 (Curran

---

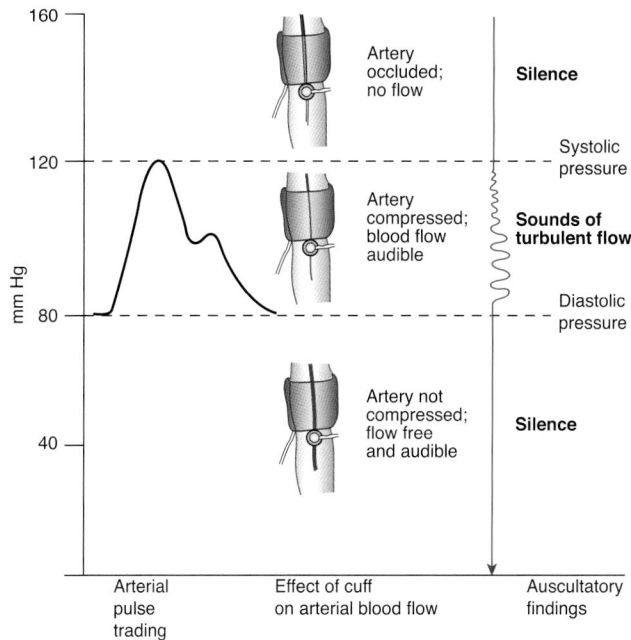

Figure 13.11 Korotkoff sounds. Reproduced from Bickley and Szilagyi (2009).

2009, Marieb and Hoehn 2010, NICE 2006, Patton and Thiobodeau 2009). See Box 13.1 for the Korotkoff sounds and the five phases. However, in some patients the Korotkoff sounds may continue until the cuff is completely deflated; in such cases stage 4 will represent the diastolic blood pressure (Williams *et al.* 2004). The auscultatory gap represents silence between the Korotkoff sounds and may sometimes be present; it is often associated with arterial stiffness, and it is vital not to mistake this for the actual blood pressure (Bickley and Szilagyi 2009). See Figure 13.11 for the Korotkoff sounds.

Alternative sites/methods

Blood pressure measurement at the thigh
There may be some patients for whom brachial artery blood pressure measurement is inappropriate, therefore, alternative sites have to be considered. To measure the blood pressure in the thigh, the patient should be prone with the bladder centred over the posterior popliteal artery and the stethoscope placed over the artery below the cuff (Bickley and Szilagyi 2009). When the appropriate sized cuffs are used, they should give an equal pressure to that in the arm (Bickley and Szilagyi 2009).

Measurement of orthostatic blood pressure
Orthostatic blood pressure measurement may be indicated if the patient has a history of dizziness or syncope on changing position (Lahrmann *et al.* 2006). The patient needs to rest on a bed in the supine position for 10 minutes prior to the initial blood pressure measurement being taken, then

---

Box 13.1 Korotkoff sounds

The sounds heard are called the Korotkoff sounds and have five phases.

1 The first phase is the clear tapping, repetitive sounds which increase in intensity and indicate the systolic pressure.
2 The second phase is murmuring or swishing sounds heard between systolic and diastolic pressures.

Some people may have an auscultatory gap – a disappearance of sounds between the second and third phases.

3 The third phase is sharper and crisper sounds.
4 The fourth phase is the distinct muffling of sounds which may sound soft and blowing.
5 The fifth phase is silence as the cuff pressure drops below the diastolic blood pressure. This disappearance is considered to be the diastolic blood pressure.

(NICE 2006, O'Brien *et al.* 2003)

they should stand upright and have their blood pressure taken again within 3 minutes (Bickley and Szilagyi 2009). While in the standing position, the practitioner should support the patient's arm at the elbow, to maintain it at the correct level and ensure accuracy (O'Brien *et al.* 2003). Orthostatic hypotension is diagnosed if systolic blood pressure drops by at least 20 mmHg or the diastolic blood pressure reduces by at least 10 mmHg within the 3 minutes when the patient is upright (Consensus Committee of the American Autonomic Society and the American Academy of Neurology 1996).

Preprocedural considerations

Equipment

Sphygmomanometers

Sphygmomanometers which are uncalibrated or not working accurately are a cause of potential blood pressure measurement error (Curran 2009). If using a manual sphygmomanometer, check that the dial is set at zero or the mercury level is at zero prior to commencing (O'Brien *et al.* 2003). In addition, follow the manufacturer's recommendations and local policies regarding servicing and care of the device.

Manual mercury sphygmomanometers

The Medicines and Healthcare products Regulatory Agency suggests that manual mercury sphygmomanometers should be gradually phased out and replaced with a dial or electronic manometer due to potential mercury leaks which are hazardous to both the environment and humans (MHRA 2005). Where mercury sphygmomanometers are used, there should be appropriate health and safety guidelines in place to guide staff, they should have access to mercury spillage kits, be trained in their use and be aware of how to dispose of the sphygmomanometers safely (MHRA 2005).

Manual aneroid sphygmomanometers

Aneroid sphygmomanometers measure blood pressure through a lever and bellows system which is more complex than the mercury sphygmomanometer. However, if it is damaged it may become inaccurate (O'Brien *et al.* 2003). If aneroid sphygmomanometers have a dial gauge then there is a need to be aware of the risk of damage with significant errors occurring with the calibration and setting of zero (MHRA 2005). As a result, O'Brien *et al.* (2003) recommend that these devices are serviced every 6 months to ensure accuracy.

Automated oscillometric sphygmomanometers

These devices show blood pressure on an electronic display (MHRA 2005). Some studies have found that the results differ between automated and manual blood pressure devices (Bern *et al.* 2007). Indeed, there are concerns that there is a greater need for validation of the devices so it is recommended that only devices which have passed recognized validation criteria should be used (BHS 2006, MHRA

2005, Stergiou *et al.* 2010, Williams *et al.* 2004). If levels of accuracy and reliability can be achieved then they do have certain advantages:

- many devices combine blood pressure with other observations (O'Brien *et al.* 2003)
- a print-out can be obtained, reducing the risk of bias (O'Brien *et al.* 2003)
- the preference of terminal digits (0 or 5) should be eradicated (O'Brien *et al.* 2003)
- data can be stored on the device (O'Brien *et al.* 2003)
- they enable the setting of alarms (MHRA 2005).

Practitioners must refer to the manufacturer's instructions and be aware of the limitations of the device. If there is any doubt about a measurement then it should be verified by an accurate manual blood pressure reading. Patients who have arrhythmias, hypotension or hypertension or are acutely unwell should have a manual blood pressure taken rather than an automated one.

The cuff

The cuff is made of an inelastic material which encloses an inflatable bladder and encircles the arm. Cuffs that are too small yield a reading that is falsely high and large cuffs give a falsely low reading (Williams *et al.* 2004). In the correct size cuff the bladder should encircle 80% of the patient's arm (Williams *et al.* 2004). Please see Table 13.2 for guidance to blood pressure cuff sizes.

Alternative adult cuffs (width × length, 12 × 35 cm) have been recommended for all adult patients, but can result in problems with over- and undercuffing. The British Hypertension Society recommends that cuff size be selected based on arm circumference (Williams *et al.* 2004).

The inflatable bladder, valve, pump and tubing

In a manual sphygmomanometer, the system used to inflate and deflate the bladder consists of a bulb attached to the bladder with rubber tubing. When the bulb is compressed, air is forced into the bladder; to deflate the bladder there is a release valve (O'Brien *et al.* 2003). The rubber tubes have conventionally been placed so they are inferior to the cuff; however, it is

Table 13.2 Blood pressure cuff sizes for mercury sphygmomanometer, semi-automatic and ambulatory monitors

Indication	Bladder width × length (cm)	Arm circumference (cm)
Small adult/child	12 × 18	<23
Standard adult	12 × 26	<33
Large adult	12 × 40	<50
Adult thigh cuff	20 × 42	<53

Reproduced with permission from Williams *et al.* (2004).

now recommended that they are placed superiorly to prevent them impeding auscultation (O'Brien *et al.* 2003).

The stethoscope

It is recommended that the stethoscope be of high quality with well-fitting earpieces (O'Brien *et al.* 2003). It should be placed over the brachial artery at the antecubital fossa (O'Brien *et al.* 2003). The bell part of the stethoscope may capture the low pitch of the Korotkoff sounds better than the diaphragm but the diaphragm has a larger surface area and is easier to manipulate with one hand (O'Brien *et al.* 2003).

Specific patient preparations

It is important to maintain a standardized environment in which to take the patient's blood pressure (NICE 2006). The patient should be seated (unless thigh or orthostatic blood pressure measurements are required) in a relaxed, quiet, temperate setting (NICE 2006). Their arm should be outstretched and supported, as in unsupported arms diastolic blood pressure may be increased by 10% (O'Brien *et al.* 2003). The brachial artery at the antecubital fossa should be positioned equal to heart level, approximately equal to where the fourth intercostals space meets the sternum (Bickley and Szilagyi 2009).

The patient's back should be supported (Turner *et al.* 2008) and their feet should be on the floor as systolic blood pressure can increase by an average of 6.6 mmHg in people with their legs crossed (van Groningen *et al.* 2008). Blood pressure should be taken after a short period of rest, as slight hypertension on standing and moving is initiated by the baroreceptor reflex (Turner *et al.* 2008). Correct patient positioning can be seen in Figure 13.12.

Blood pressure should initially be measured in both arms as often people have a significant difference in blood pressure measurement between their arms (NICE 2006). Those patients who have a large and persistent disparity may have underlying conditions such as occlusive artery disease

Figure 13.12 Correct blood pressure reading techniques.

(Eguchi *et al.* 2007, O'Brien *et al.* 2003). Differences up to 10 mmHg can be due to random variation (Eguchi *et al.* 2007). The arm with the highest reading should be the one used for subsequent measurements (NICE 2006).

767

Procedure guideline 13.3 **Blood pressure measurement (manual)**

Essential equipment

- A range of cuffs
- Sphygmomanometer, working and calibrated
- Stethoscope
- Chair with arm rest
- Documentation
- Alcohol handrub
- Detergent wipes

Optional equipment

- Pillow if required to provide extra arm support
- If necessary a bed or examination bench, so the patient can have their blood pressure measured lying down

Preprocedure

Action	Rationale
1 Explain to the patient that you need to measure their blood pressure and discuss the procedure.	To ensure that the patient understands the procedure and gives their valid consent (NMC 2008b, **C**).

(Continued)

Procedure guideline 13.3 (*Continued*)

2 Wash hands using bactericidal soap and water or bactericidal alcohol handrub, and dry.	To minimize the risk of infection (Fraise and Bradley 2009, E)
3 Ask the patient if they have any of the following conditions: ■ lymphoedema or are at risk ■ an arteriovenous fistula ■ trauma to their arm ■ brachial artery surgery.	To ensure there are no contraindications to using a particular arm (Bickley and Szilagyi 2009, E; Curran 2009, E; Turner *et al.* 2008, E).
4 Provide a standardized environment which should be relaxed and temperate. The patient needs to be seated comfortably, in a chair with back support, for at least 5 min prior to measuring blood pressure (Bickley and Szilagyi 2009, O'Brien *et al.* 2003, Turner *et al.* 2008).	To enable comparisons to be drawn with prior blood pressure results (NICE 2006, C). Variations in temperature and emotions can alter blood pressure readings (O'Brien *et al.* 2003, E).
5 Ensure the manometer is no more than 1 metre away, vertical and at eye level (O'Brien *et al.* 2003).	If using a mercury manometer, the meniscus should be close to eye level or the angle of vision will mean an inaccurate result will be taken (O'Brien *et al.* 2003, E). With an aneroid scale, the eye level should be equal with the centre of the gauge (O'Brien *et al.* 2003, E).
6 Ensure the cuff is the correct size for the arm. The cuff bladder length should be 80% of the arm circumference and its width 40% (BHS 2006).	Small cuffs give falsely high readings and large cuffs give falsely low readings (Williams *et al.* 2004, E).
7 Check the patient's arm is free from clothing, supported and placed at heart level (midsternal level) (Bickley and Szilagyi 2009, NICE 2006, O'Brien *et al.* 2003). Their legs should be uncrossed with feet flat on the floor (Turner *et al.* 2008). See Figure 13.12.	If the arm is lower than heart level it can lead to falsely high readings, and vice versa (O'Brien *et al.* 2003, E). Diastolic pressure can increase by up to 10% if the arm is unsupported (O'Brien *et al.* 2003, E). Blood pressure results can be falsely high if the patient has their legs crossed (van Groningen *et al.* 2008, R).

Procedure

8 Wrap the cuff of the sphygmomanometer around the arm, with the bladder centred over the artery and superior to the elbow (Marieb and Hoehn 2010, Patton and Thiobodeau 2009). The lower edge of the cuff should be 2–3 cm above the brachial artery pulsation (O'Brien *et al.* 2003).	To obtain an accurate reading (BHS 2006, C), and so that the artery can easily be palpated (NICE 2006, C).
9 Ask the patient to stop talking, eating and so on, during the procedure.	Activity can cause a falsely high blood pressure (BHS 2006, C).
10 Palpate the brachial artery while pumping air into the cuff using the bulb. Once the pulse can no longer be felt rapidly inflate the cuff for further 20–30 mmHg (Bickley and Szilagyi 2009, NICE 2006).	Inflating the cuff to only 20/30 mmHg above the predicted systolic level prevents undue discomfort (Bickley and Szilagyi 2009, E). The brachial pulse is advocated rather than the radial pulse (NICE 2006, C) and doing this locates the correct position for stethoscope placement (Valler-Jones and Wedgbury 2005, E).
11 Deflate the cuff and the point at which the pulse reappears approximates the systolic blood pressure (BHS 2006, NICE 2006, O'Brien *et al.* 2003).	This provides an indication of systolic pressure and can ensure accurate results in those who have an auscultatory gap (Curran 2009, E; BHS 2006, C).
12 Deflate the cuff completely and wait 15–30 seconds (Bickley and Szilagyi 2009).	To allow venous congestion to resolve (O'Brien *et al.* 2003, E).

13 The stethoscope should be firmly, but without too much pressure, placed on bare skin over the brachial artery where the pulse is palpable (O'Brien *et al.* 2003). The bell of the stethoscope may hear the tone of the Korotkoff sounds better (Bickley and Szilagyi 2009). However, the diaphragm has a larger surface area and is easier to hold in place (O'Brien *et al.* 2003).	If the stethoscope is in contact with material it may distort the Korotkoff sounds (O'Brien *et al.* 2003, E). Applying pressure with the stethoscope may partially occlude the artery (O'Brien *et al.* 2003, E).
14 Inflate the cuff again to 20–30 mmHg above the predicted systolic blood pressure (Bickley and Szilagyi 2009, NICE 2006).	To ensure an accurate measurement (NICE 2006, C).
15 Release the air in the cuff slowly (at an approximate rate of 2–3 mmHg per pulsation) until the first tapping sounds are heard (first Korotkoff sound). This is the systolic blood pressure (Patton and Thiobodeau 2009).	The cuff should not be deflated too quickly as this may result in inaccurate readings being taken (O'Brien *et al.* 2003, E).
16 Continue to slowly release the air, listening to the Korotkoff sounds; the point at which the sounds disappear is the best representation of the diastolic blood pressure (fifth Korofkoff sound). Continue to deflate the cuff slowly until you are sure the sounds have disappeared (after another 10–20 mmHg) (Bickley and Szilagyi 2009).	To ensure an accurate diastolic blood pressure and that you note any irregularities such as if the sounds never disappear, or disappear significantly below the fourth Korotkoff sound (Bickley and Szilagyi 2009, E).
17 Once no further sounds can be heard, the cuff should be rapidly deflated (O'Brien *et al.* 2003).	To prevent venous congestion to the arm (O'Brien *et al.* 2003, E).
18 If you need to recheck the blood pressure wait 1–2 min before proceeding (BHS 2006).	Venous congestion may make the Korotkoff sounds less audible (Bickley and Szilagyi 2009, E).

Postprocedure

19 Inform patient that the procedure is now finished.	To reassure the patient. E
20 Wash hands using bactericidal soap and water or bactericidal alcohol handrub, and dry. Clean bell of stethoscope and cuff with detergent wipe (no alcohol).	To minimize the risk of infection (Fraise and Bradley 2009, E).
21 Document fully as soon as the measurement has been taken and compare with previous results (O'Brien *et al.* 2003).	Any interruption in the process may result in the measurement being incorrectly remembered (O'Brien *et al.* 2003, E).

Problem-solving table 13.3 Prevention and resolution (Procedure guideline 13.3)

Problem	Cause	Prevention	Action
The result is unexpectedly low or high	This may be due to poor technique or faulty equipment. It may also be due to the patient being incorrectly positioned or post exercise	Check the sphygmomanometer prior to use to see when it was last serviced. Check all the components for signs of damage. Ensure the patient is correctly positioned, and has rested prior to the procedure	Wait 1–2 min prior to repeating the blood pressure measurement (BHS 2006). If the measurement is still unexpected consider changing devices or asking a colleague to repeat the procedure. If it remains abnormal notify the medical team of the result

(Continued)

Problem-solving table 13.3 (*Continued*)

Problem	Cause	Prevention	Action
On auscultation the Korotkoff sounds disappear after the initial sound, then reappear and then disappear again (Curran 2009)	This is called the auscultatory gap – it may mislead the practitioner into obtaining an incorrect result (Curran 2009)	Palpate the pulse as the cuff is being deflated to gain an approximation of the systolic blood pressure (O'Brien *et al.* 2003)	Document that the patient has an auscultatory gap and ensure other practitioners are aware to prevent future errors (O'Brien *et al.* 2003). Recheck using the correct procedure
On auscultation the Korotkoff sounds are inaudible or very weak	May be due to poor placement of the stethoscope, a noisy environment, venous congestion;or the patient may be in shock (Bickley and Szilagyi 2009, Verrij *et al.* 2009)	Find a quiet environment in which to measure the patient's blood pressure, listen with the bell of the stethoscope rather than the diaphragm, wait for venous congestion to resolve (Bickley and Szilagyi 2009)	If still inaudible ask the patient to elevate their arm overhead for 30 seconds, then bring it back to the correct height to inflate the cuff and measure their blood pressure; this increases the loudness of the sounds (Bickley and Szilagyi 2009, Verrij *et al.* 2009)

Postprocedural considerations

Immediate care

Notify medical staff of an abnormal blood pressure result. As the treatment will depend on what is causing the abnormality, and its severity, it is important that practitioners try to ascertain the possible cause for the physiological change in blood pressure (Kisiel and Perkins 2006). Hypovolaemia will require fluid replacement and, if persistent, then inotropes and other cardiovascular drugs may be necessary (Hinds and Watson 2009). If the hypertension is transient, for example related to anxiety or pain, then it is important to address that issue and monitor the blood pressure until it resolves. However, if the patient is diagnosed as having hypertension they will require drug therapy to control their condition (NICE 2006). To determine the cause of the altered blood pressure more information will be required, including:

- gaining a comprehensive medical history from the patient (Steele and Hardin 2007)
- gaining a full set of observations
- an ECG (Steele and Hardin 2007)
- urinalysis including protein, leucocytes, blood and the osmolality of the urine (Steele and Hardin 2007)
- blood tests for full blood count, urea, creatinine and electrolytes (Steele and Hardin 2007) and fasting blood tests for glucose and lipids (Camm and Bunce 2009)
- a chest X-ray or further radiological investigations may be required (Camm and Bunce 2009)
- a septic screen including blood cultures, sputum specimen, swabs of any wounds or potential sites of infection (Hinds and Watson 2009)
- their current fluid balance (Kisiel and Perkins 2006).

Ongoing care

If the patient is hypertensive and in primary care, they will require at least monthly blood pressure measurement and more frequently if it is accelerated hypertension or there are any further concerns (NICE 2006). Additionally, it will be necessary to give lifestyle advice on, for example, eating healthily, smoking cessation (NICE 2006). If the hypotension is orthostatic then advise the patient to change position slowly so the baroreceptors and sympathetic nervous system have time to adapt the blood pressure to each stage (Marieb and Hoehn 2010).

Documentation

As well as the accurate recording of the blood pressure measurement it is also important to record:

- the position the patient was in
- the arm used, and if both arms were used initially, the pressure of each
- arm circumference and the cuff size used
- if there is an auscultatory gap or any difficulties in obtaining a reading, such as the absence of stage 5
- the state of the patient, for example were they in pain, frightened, and so on
- any medication they are on and when they last took it.
                                                      (O'Brien *et al.* 2003)

When documenting the medication the patient is on, it is important to include not only cardiovascular medication but also other medication which might affect their blood pressure, including tricyclic antidepressants, neuroleptic agents (O'Brien *et al.* 2003), contraceptives, decongestants, NSAIDs and cocaine (Steele and Hardin 2007).

Central venous pressure

Definition

Central venous pressure (CVP) is the pressure of blood returning to or filling the right atrium. CVP is a good approximation of right atrial pressure and a major determinant of right ventricular end-diastolic volume and right ventricular preload (Izakovic 2008). It indicates blood volume, vascular tone and cardiac function (Hudek *et al.* 1998).

Anatomy and physiology

Veins carrying the venous return from the head, neck, arms and upper thorax converge to form the superior vena cava (SVC), while the veins carrying the venous return from the legs, abdomen and lower thorax converge to form the inferior vena cava (IVC) (Scales 2008a). The venae cavae are in continuity with the right atrium and consequently the pressure of the blood in the great veins is essentially the same as the pressure in the right atrium (Magder 2006a). Normal right atrial pressure (RAP) has a range of 1–10 mmHg and the mean pressure is 5 mmHg (Muralidhar 2002). In effect, CVP = RAP (Scales 2010).

Central venous pressure also reflects the filling of the left ventricle (Scales 2008b), because blood flows from the right ventricle, through the pulmonary bed and back to the left side of the heart. An estimation of the filling of the left ventricle is important because the ventricle pumps blood around the systemic system (Scales 2010). The amount of blood in the circulation (intravascular volume) is an important component of CVP and is primarily maintained by controlling the body's fluid balance (Scales and Pilsworth 2008).

Evidence-based approaches

Rationale

Indications

Central venous pressure monitoring is performed in acute and critical care settings to provide additional physiological information to assist with the patient's clinical management (Scales 2010). It is used to monitor and guide fluid therapy in the following situations:

- fluid resuscitation in major trauma
- cardiac surgery
- thoracic surgery
- major abdominal surgery
- to optimize fluid replacement in acute renal failure
- to optimize fluid replacement in sepsis
- to guide fluid replacement in heart failure (Scales 2010).

Central venous pressure monitoring can also be used for diagnostic purposes. It is performed in critical care to assess right heart failure and during cardiac catheterization to aid or confirm diagnosis (Scales 2010).

Table 13.3 Factors that may increase or decrease CVP

Causes of increased CVP	Causes of decreased CVP
Hypervolaemia	Hypovolaemia
Forced exhalation (transient increase)	Septic shock
Being on a ventilator (due to PEEP)	Deep inhalation (transient)
Tension pneumothorax	Increased venous compliance
Pleural effusion	
Heart failure	
Chronic obstructive pulmonary disease or asthma due to straining during exhalation	

Reproduced with permission from Izakovic (2008).

Principles of care

Central venous pressure may be influenced by several factors as identified in Table 13.3.

Central venous pressure monitoring is often misleading if interpreted as an isolated reading. It is subject to varying placement of pressure transducers between healthcare workers (Figg and Nemergut 2009). Despite the limitations of CVP, it is frequently used in acute clinical practice to assess volume status and cardiac preload (Ward *et al.* 2006). Knowledge of a patient's CVP can be helpful in the diagnosis and management of a variety of critical illnesses and injuries including trauma, burns, sepsis, congestive heart failure, cardiogenic shock and traumatic brain injury (Ward *et al.* 2006). In order to obtain maximum benefits, trend measurements over a period of time should be studied and correlated with the patient's clinical status (Udwadia 2005), as a reflection of level of hydration and cardiac function. Clinical observations such as auscultation of breath sounds, heart and respiratory rate, ECG, neck vein distension and urine output are all paramount when interpreting the meaning of the CVP recording (Morton *et al.* 2005). CVP can be more meaningfully interpreted in the light of a measure of cardiac output or a surrogate of cardiac output such as venous oxygen saturation or pulse pressure variations (Magder 2006b). An increase in central venous oxygen saturation can represent an increase in cardiac output (Rivers *et al.* 2001).

Methods of measuring a CVP

The CVP should be measured level with the midpoint of the right atrium, as this is where the blood returning to the heart interacts with cardiac function (Magder 2006b). CVP is usually recorded at the midaxilla identified at a vertical distance 5 cm below the sternal angle, which is where the second rib meets the sternum. This is true whether the patient is supine or sitting up at a 60° angle because the right atrium is anterior in the chest and has a relatively round shape. Thus a 5 cm vertical line from the sternal angle remains in

771

Figure 13.13   Measuring a CVP using a water manometer. Adapted from Edwards and Manley (1998).

the approximate centre of the atrium even when the patient is sitting upright at a 60° angle. This means that patients do not have to be supine for CVP measurements when this reference level is used (Magder 2006b). Note that in critical care units it is more common to use the midthoracic position at the level of the fifth rib as this is easier to teach; however, this should only be used in supine position as the reference position changes in relation to the mid-right atrium with changes in posture (Magder 2006b).

Central venous pressure measurements can be recorded either manually, using a 0.9% sodium chloride manometer set, or electronically, using a transducer. Electronic measurement is most commonly used in the critical care environment. Although there are no direct complications in the actual process of recording CVP, it is noted that the choice of lumen on a central venous catheter could help early detection of catheter migration. Using the proximal lumen to detect early catheter migration out of the blood vessel results in loss of the CVP waveform. This can alert staff and minimize extravasation of fluid or drugs into the pleural or subcutaneous space (Bolton 1997, Davies and Moores 2003). The accuracy of CVP readings from different lumens has been studied by Scott *et al.* (1995) who concluded that pressure differences were small and unlikely to be clinically important.

Zeroing a CVP

Zeroing a CVP is an essential part of measurement. This is a technique used to ensure that the atmospheric pressure at the point of measurement is read as zero. In critical care areas CVPs are usually measured by monitors that can be set to zero electronically once the transducer is placed at right atrial level, with flow from the transducer open to air but closed to the patient (Woodrow 2002). When measuring with water manometers, which are used on the wards, the zero should align with the right atrial level. This is usually checked by a spirit level (see Figure 13.13).

Reading a CVP

After zeroing a manual manometer, the giving set chamber should be filled with fluid nearly to the top. This is done by turning the flow tap to allow fluid, such as 0.9% sodium chloride, to flow into the measuring chamber, while closing the flow to the patient. Care should be taken not to get the air filter at the top wet, as a wet filter will resist air entry and give a falsely raised reading. The tap should then be turned so the fluid flow is stopped and the chamber opened to the patient. Gravity will cause the water level to fall until resistance from the patient's CVP matches the pressure of gravity. However, slight changes in pressure caused by the patient's respiration, usually 1 cm, will make the fluid fall in a swinging pattern, until it oscillates between two figures. The intrathoracic pressure represented by the fluid level in the chamber falls on inspiration so the higher figure should be recorded. CVP can be measured in either millimetres of mercury (mmHg) or centimetres of water (cmH_2O) (Woodrow 2002).

Normal pressures

A normal CVP value should be 5–10 mmHg midaxilla or 0–5 mmHg sternal angle (Henderson 1997), which is 7–14 cmH_2O midaxilla or 0–7 cmH_2O sternal angle. A low CVP usually indicates fluid loss through haemorrhage or excessive diuresis; poor venous return and peripheral vasodilation can also lower the CVP. In some patients there can be a discrepancy between CVP and left-side heart filling pressures. Falsely high CVP can be seen in patients with the following conditions:

- tricuspid valve regurgitation
- congestive cardiac failure
- pulmonary valve stenosis
- pulmonary artery hypertension
- severe pulmonary embolism
- COPD.

(O'Neill and Le Grove 2003)

These patients can have a high CVP measurement yet be hypovolaemic. For this reason, comparing changes in a CVP measurement with a baseline measurement is more beneficial than noting the initial recording (O'Neill and Le Grove 2003). Various other factors such as lumen occlusion/obstruction and user error can also give high CVP readings (Woodrow 2002).

Legal and professional issues
Competencies

Staff with appropriate knowledge and training may undertake CVP readings. As this will involve accessing a central venous device and administering intravenous fluid, local rules regarding intravenous medication administration should be followed. A registered nurse must only perform a CVP reading if they have the appropriate knowledge and training to do so otherwise they should refer to a colleague who is competent in this technique (NMC 2008a).

Preprocedural considerations
Equipment
Manometer

A manometer is a measurement scale for manually determining CVP and the recording is recorded in cmH$_2$O. It requires a specially designed administration set that is attached to the manometer scale and primed with 0.9% sodium chloride. Care should be taken not to wet the filter in the administration set which is situated at the top of the scale, as this may affect the validity of the measurement. A manual manometer should be used in a ward environment where access to electronic continuous cardiac monitoring is not often possible. As the manometer is not used for continuous recordings, there is no issue with maintaining CVC patency therefore the use of a pressure bag is not necessary. The CVC should be flushed with 10 mL of 0.9% sodium chloride after the manometer has been disconnected to ensure patency.

Transducer

In areas where continuous cardiac monitoring is used, for example theatres and intensive care, the CVP may be continuously monitored using an electronic transducer. The transducer is an integral part of the administration set and is connected by cable to a monitor.

Pharmacological support

Intravenous 0.9% sodium chloride (500 mL–1 litre bag) is used to assist with the measurement of CVP reading. It is recommended that the infusion bag should be changed every 24 hours or as per hospital policy. Administration sets should be replaced every 72 hours or as hospital policy states.

Specific patient preparations

Ideally, the patient should lie flat in a supine position to reflect the right atrial pressure. However, many breathless patients cannot tolerate lying supine, so the measurement can also be taken in a semi-recumbent or recumbent position (Hatchett 2000). If the patient is supine an alternative position is via the sternal angle. It is important to use just one method, to promote consistency, as readings from the sternal angle are about 5 cm lower than those taken from the midaxilla (Hatchett 2000, Woodrow 2002). It is vital that the site from which the measurement is being recorded is marked and documented to maintain the continuity and accuracy of the trend of the CVP (Mooney and Comerford 2003).

Education

The patient should be fully informed about the procedure before a CVP measurement is carried out, ensuring that any anxieties or misconceptions are relieved.

773

Procedure guideline 13.4 Central venous pressure measurement

Essential equipment

- Spirit level
- Manometer
- Drip stand
- CVP monitoring intravenous administration set
- 0.9% sodium chloride

Preprocedure

Action	Rationale
1 Explain and discuss the procedure with the patient.	To ensure that the patient understands the procedure and gives their valid consent (NMC 2008b, C).
2 Wash and dry hands.	To maintain infection control and minimize the risk of cross-infection (Fraise and Bradley 2009, E).

(Continued)

Procedure guideline 13.4 (*Continued*)

Procedure

3 Ascertain the point of CVP reading, that is, sternal angle or midaxilla. If the patient agrees, this point should be marked on the patient and noted in the care plan chart for future reference.	CVP must always be read from the same point because the sternal angle reading is about 5 cmH$_2$O higher than the midaxilla reading (Edwards 2000, E).
4 Assist the patient to get into a supine, recumbent or semi-recumbent position to a maximum angle of 45°.	The position of the patient must allow the baseline of the manometer to be level with the patient's right atrium. If the patient is upright or is lying on their side, the right atrium will not be in line with the sternal angle or the midaxilla. However, if it is impossible for the patient to be in any other position, the CVP reading may be recorded with the patient sitting up at a 90° angle, but this must be recorded on the observation chart (Edwards 2000, E).
5 Position the manometer so that the baseline is level with the right atrium.	To obtain an accurate CVP reading, the baseline and the right atrium must be level (Edwards 2000, E).
6 Loosen the securing screw and slide the scale up or down until the baseline zero is lined up with the zero on the arm of the spirit level (see Figure 13.13).	To remove the effect of extraneous pressure and to ensure the baseline is always the same in order to have a single point of reference (Edwards 2000, E).
7 Check that the baseline and right atrium are level by extending the arm of the spirit level to the sternal angle or to the midaxilla. Move the manometer until the bubble is between the parallel lines of the spirit level (see Figure 13.13).	To ensure a more accurate reading (Edwards 2000, E).
8 Care should be taken when flushing the central venous catheter regarding the volume and type of fluid.	To ensure the patency of the catheter and to check for leaks, kinks, blockages, and so on. To ensure that correct solution is used to flush, for example 0.9% sodium chloride or dextrose, and not a solution containing drugs (Edwards 2000, E).
9 Turn off the three-way tap to the patient (see Figure 13.13).	To allow the intravenous fluid to run into the manometer.
10 Allow the manometer to fill slowly.	To avoid: (a) bubbles, which cause inaccurate readings (b) overfilling of, and spillage from, the manometer that would put the patient at risk from infection (Edwards 2000, E).
11 Turn off the three-way tap to the intravenous fluid.	To allow fluid from the manometer to enter the patient's right atrium (Edwards 2000, E).
12 The column of water should fall rapidly.	Indicating patency of the catheter, resulting in an accurate CVP reading (Edwards 2000, E).
13 When the level of fluid in the manometer ceases to drop, and oscillates with the patient's respirations, the reading can be taken.	The pressure of the column of water in the manometer now equals the pressure in the right atrium (Edwards 2000, E).
14 Turn off the three-way tap to the manometer.	To restore infusion via the intravenous catheter (Edwards 2000, E).
15 Readjust the infusion rate.	To ensure correct rate setting. E

Postprocedure

16 Wash and dry hands.	To maintain infection control and minimize the risk of cross-infection (Fraise and Bradley 2009, E).
17 Record the CVP measurement on the appropriate chart. Compare this measurement with the patient's acceptable CVP limits as stated by the medical team.	Acceptable CVP values vary with the patient observations and their overall condition. Deviations from these limits may require urgent medical intervention. E

Problem-solving table 13.4 Prevention and resolution (Procedure guideline 13.4)

Problem	Cause	Prevention	Action
Inaccurate CVP readings	Patient in a position different from that in which the initial reading was taken	Refer to the patient's records to identify the correct position for recording CVP	Position the patient consistently as documented in the patient's records
	Reference point on the patient not observed	Refer to the patient's records to identify the correct reference point, that is, midaxilla or sternal angle	Zero the manometer level with the patient's right atrium and consistently follow the correct reference point as documented in the patient's records
	Faulty pressure reading technique	Only staff competent in intravenous fluid administration and CVP measurement should perform CVP recordings. Inexperienced staff should receive appropriate training and supervision	If the CVP reading is outside the limits deemed acceptable for that patient and it is considered to be an accurate reading, recheck it after 15 or 30 minutes and inform a doctor if unchanged
Elevated CVP	Increased intrathoracic pressure caused by coughing, increased movement or pain	Encourage coughing before taking the reading. Ensure that the patient is comfortable and pain free	Attend to the patient's comfort first
	Lower extremities elevated	Refer to the patient's records to identify the correct position for recording CVP	Position the patient so that they are lying in a supine position
	Patient having intermittent positive-pressure ventilation		Read the CVP at the end-expiratory level (lowest point of fluctuation). This will always be higher than the 'normal' reading
	Anxiety and/or restlessness	Clearly explain the procedure and respond to any concerns the patient expresses	Once the cause of the anxiety or restlessness has been identified take action to reassure patient
	Blood transfusion currently infusing via the CVP catheter	Attach the CVP administration set to a dedicated central venous lumen; use the same one each time and document which lumen is used in the patient's record	Flush the catheter with 0.9% sodium chloride and read again

(Continued)

Problem-solving table 13.4 *(Continued)*

Problem	Cause	Prevention	Action
	Shivering and/or muscular spasm, for example postanaesthetic reaction (see Chapter 17)		Assess the patient's condition, for example pulse, blood pressure, temperature. Check that the patient is warm enough. Inform a doctor
Low CVP reading	Leak in the system or equipment adjusted inaccurately	Carefully assemble the CVP administration system and prime with 0.9% sodium chloride and check for leaks, prior to connection to the central venous access device	Check and readjust the system
	Changing of the patient's position from recumbent to semi-recumbent	Refer to the patient's records to identify the correct position for recording CVP	Repeat the measurement with the patient in the recumbent position
No reading or absent waveform on continuous monitoring	CVC tip migration out of the vein	Ensure dressing is intact and CVC is sutured in place	Exclude other reasons for loss of waveform. Observe site for signs of extravasation – pain, swelling, leakage or erythema. Seek medical advice if extravasation is suspected and follow local extravasation policy
	Occluded CVC lumen	Ensure no kinks	Assess patency, check for blood return and attempt to flush with 0.9% sodium chloride using a 10 mL syringe. Flushing with smaller syringes carries a risk of internal catheter rupture
Blood is back-tracking up the tubing	Pressure bag is not pressurized	Check the pressure indicator on the pressure bag	If low, reinflate to 300 mmHg
	Fluid bag may be empty	Check fluid bag	Replace if empty or low in volume

Postprocedural considerations
Ongoing care

Central venous pressure should be regarded as a trend. Multiple fluid boluses might be necessary before the CVP reaches the target range and the patient is commenced on maintenance fluid infusion. The ability to continuously monitor CVP and therefore the result of fluid challenges is normally reserved for electronically monitored patients in critical care areas.

Respiration and pulse oximetry

Definition

The function of the respiratory system is to ensure that the cells and tissues of the human body have oxygen supplied to them and carbon dioxide removed, in order that they can continue to carry out their functions (Patton and Thiobodeau 2009). Respiration consists of four processes: ventilation; external respiration or gaseous exchange; transport; and internal respiration (Marieb and Hoehn 2010) (see Chapter 10).

Anatomy and physiology

For effective respiration to occur, effective functioning and interaction between the various body systems are required, including the circulatory system, nervous system and musculoskeletal system (Patton and Thiobodeau 2010). The organs and structures of the respiratory system can be split into two groups: the conducting zone and the respiratory zone (Marieb and Hoehn 2010). The conducting zone consists of the respiratory passages through which air passes to get to the area of gaseous exchange, such as the nasal cavity and the bronchi; this area provides conduits through which air can pass and also be warmed, humidified and cleansed (Marieb and Hoehn 2010). The respiratory zone consists of the bronchioles, alveolar ducts, alveoli and the microscopic anatomy which provide the site for gaseous exchange (Marieb and Hoehn 2010). The respiratory muscles (the diaphragm and intercostal muscles) promote ventilation by causing volume and pressure changes within the respiratory system (Marieb and Hoehn 2010).

The mechanism of breathing

The key mechanism of pulmonary ventilation is that changes of volume within the respiratory system lead to changes in pressure and these in turn lead to a flow of gases (Marieb and Hoehn 2010). Indeed, the vital principle of respiration is that the flow of air will always go down a pressure gradient; this means that air will flow from an area of higher pressure to an area of lower pressure (Patton and Thiobodeau 2009). The two main pressures are intrapulmonary, or intra-alveolar, pressure, which varies with breathing but which always eventually is equal to atmospheric pressure (the pressure of gases or air outside the body) (Marieb and Hoehn 2010), and intrapleural pressure, which also varies with breathing but which is generally about 4 mmHg less than the intrapulmonary pressure (Marieb and Hoehn 2010). Boyle's Law describes how at a constant temperature, the pressure of a gas has an inverse relationship to its volume (Patton and Thiobodeau 2009). Therefore, in a larger container the

pressure of gas is less than in a smaller one. The relationship of these pressures can be seen in Figure 13.14.

Inspiration

Inspiration occurs because the phrenic nerve stimulates the diaphragm to flatten and descend; this movement results in the greatest volume change in the lungs (Davies and Moores 2003). The intercostal muscles lift the rib cage and sternum, causing the ribs to broaden outwards and increasing the diameter of the thoracic cavity, both from side to side and front to back (Patton and Thiobodeau 2009). This change in volume of the thoracic cavity causes the volume of the lungs to increase; therefore, according to Boyle's Law the pressure of gas within the lungs is less. This drop in pressure causes air to move in from outside the body, from an area of higher pressure to one of lower pressure (Marieb and Hoehn 2010), thereby causing inspiration.

Expiration

The inspiratory muscles relax, causing the thoracic cavity to return to its normal size, the lungs recoil and this decrease in size compresses the alveoli, causing an increase in intrapulmonary pressures and forcing gases to flow out of the lungs

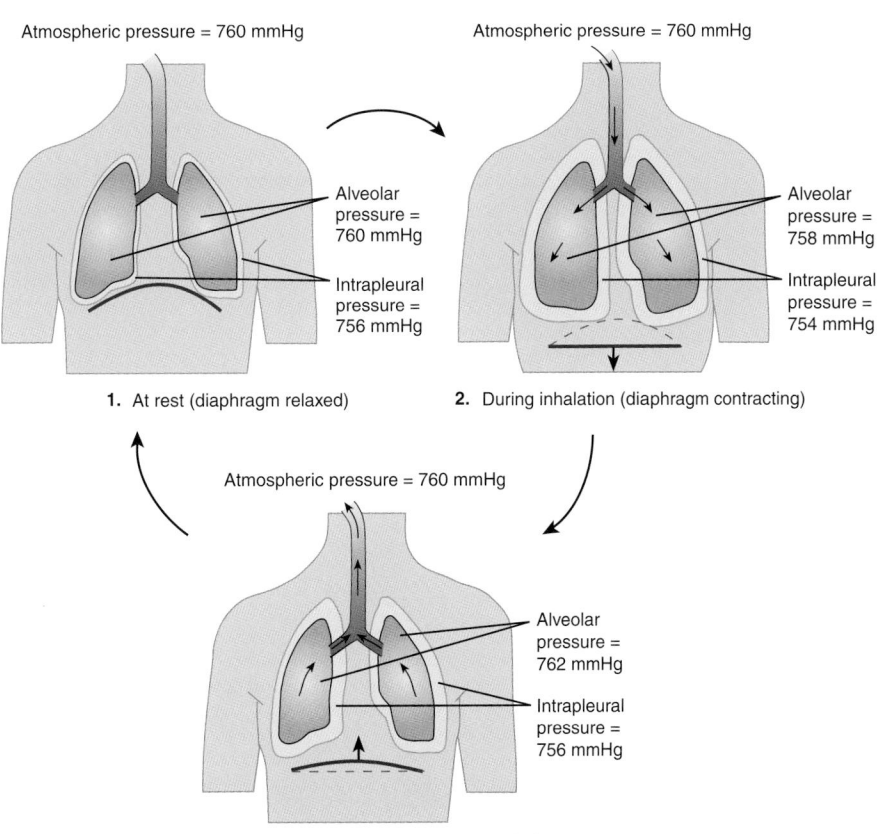

1. At rest (diaphragm relaxed)

2. During inhalation (diaphragm contracting)

3. During exhalation (diaphragm relaxing)

Figure 13.14 Pressure changes in pulmonary ventilation. Reproduced from Tortora and Derrickson (2009).

Sequence of events

Changes in anterior-posterior and superior-inferior dimensions

Changes in lateral dimensions (superior view)

Inspiration

(1) Inspiratory muscles contract (diaphragm descends; rib cage rises).

(2) Thoracic cavity volume increases.

(3) Lungs are stretched; intrapulmonary volume increases.

(4) Intrapulmonary pressure drops (to −1 mm Hg).

(5) Air (gases) flows into lungs down its pressure gradient until intrapulmonary pressure is 0 (equal to atmospheric pressure).

Ribs are elevated and sternum flares as external intercostals contract.

Diaphragm moves inferiorly during contraction.

External intercostals contract.

Expiration

(1) Inspiratory muscles relax (diaphragm rises; rib cage descends due to recoil of costal cartilages).

(2) Thoracic cavity volume decreases.

(2) Elastic lungs recoil passively; intrapulmonary volume decreases.

(4) Intrapulmonary pressure rises (to + 1 mm Hg).

(5) Air (gases) flows out of lungs down its pressure gradient until intrapulmonary pressure is 0.

Ribs and sternum are depressed as external intercostals relax.

Diaphragm moves superiorly as it relaxes.

External intercostals relax.

Figure 13.15 Changes in thoracic volume and sequence of events during inspiration and expiration. The sequence of events in the left column includes volume changes during inspiration (*top*) and expiration (*bottom*). The lateral views in the middle column show changes in the superior-inferior dimension (as the diaphragm alternately contracts and relaxes) and in the interior-posterior dimension (as the external intercostal muscles alternately contract and relax). The superior views of transverse thoracic sections in the right column show lateral dimension changes resulting from alternate contraction and relaxation of the external intercostal muscles. Reproduced from Marieb and Hoehn (2010). Reproduced from Fig. 21.15d, p. 622 from *Human Anatomy*, 3rd edn, by E.N. Marieb and J. Mallatt. © 2001 by Benjamin Cummings. Reprinted by permission of Pearson Education, Inc.

into the atmosphere (Marieb and Hoehn 2010). Therefore, in normal, gentle breathing the process of expiration is largely passive. The mechanism of inspiration and expiration in relation to pulmonary volume can be seen in Figure 13.15.

The accessory muscles

The accessory muscles of the neck (the scalenes and sternocleidomastoid muscles) and the chest (pectoralis minor) can increase the volume of the thoracic cavity and therefore increase the volume of breathing; this can occur during exercise or if the individual is in respiratory distress (Marieb and Hoehn 2010). The muscles of the abdomen and those that cause flexion of the spine are also accessory muscles but aid with expiration (Davies and Moores 2003). When these muscles contract they press the abdominal organs upwards, forcing the diaphragm up, reducing the thoracic volume and causing expiration (Davies and Moores 2003).

Control of respiration
The respiratory centres

Within the medulla are two clusters of neurones which co-ordinate the respiratory system; these are the *dorsal respiratory group* and the *ventral respiratory group* (Marieb and Hoehn 2010). The ventral respiratory group contains neurones that fire during inspiration, stimulating the diaphragm and the intercostal muscles to contract, via the phrenic and intercostal nerves, and other neurones which fire during expiration causing the stimulation to stop so the muscles relax. These neurones deliver our normal respiratory rate (Marieb and Hoehn 2010).

The dorsal respiratory group co-ordinates input from the chemoreceptors and stretch receptors and relays this to the ventral respiratory group to alter respiratory rate as required (Marieb and Hoehn 2010). Chemoreceptors monitor the arterial blood for changes in the partial pressure of carbon dioxide (PCO_2) and pH, but also, to a lesser extent, the partial pressure of oxygen (PO_2) (Patton and Thiobodeau 2009). For more information on the chemical factors which affect respiration please, see Chapter 10.

The pontine respiratory centres also relay impulses to the ventral respiratory group to modify breathing rhythms so that there is a smooth transition from inspiration to expiration and so that breathing can be modified to allow for speech, exercise and sleeping patterns (Marieb and Hoehn 2010). In the higher cortical centres respiration can be altered through factors such as strong emotions, pain and alteration of temperature (Marieb and Hoehn 2010, Patton and Thiobodeau 2009). The cerebral motor cortex yields a degree of voluntary control over breathing; however, this can be over-ridden by the other mechanisms (Patton and Thiobodeau 2009).

Carbon dioxide

Although oxygen is essential for every cell in the body, the body's need to rid itself of carbon dioxide is the most vital

stimulus to respiration in a healthy person (Marieb and Hoehn 2010). The arterial PCO_2 is very closely monitored and balanced and when it increases slightly, it causes the chemoreceptors to be stimulated (Patton and Thiobodeau 2009). Carbon dioxide passes easily from the blood into the cerebrospinal fluid where it forms carbonic acid, releasing hydrogen ions (H^+) (Marieb and Hoehn 2010). This increase of H^+ causes the pH to drop, stimulating the central chemoreceptors, found in the brainstem, to increase the rate and depth of breathing and increasing the amount of carbon dioxide exhaled (Marieb and Hoehn 2010). Similarly, metabolic causes for low pH levels, such as a build-up of lactic acid, will also cause an alteration of respiration (Marieb and Hoehn 2010).

Oxygen

The peripheral chemoreceptors, found in the aortic arch and carotid arteries, are responsible for the sensing the PO_2 in the body (Marieb and Hoehn 2010). Normally, decreasing levels of oxygen only affect respiratory rate by causing the peripheral chemoreceptors to have increased sensitivity to carbon dioxide (Marieb and Hoehn 2010). Arterial PO_2 must drop from the normal level of 100 mmHg to at least 60 mmHg before it stimulates respiratory function; at this point the central receptors become suppressed as a result but the peripheral receptors stimulate the respiratory centres and ventilation is increased (Marieb and Hoehn 2010). This mechanism usually only works as an emergency measure, because the level of oxygen has to drop significantly before stimulation of the chemoreceptors occurs (Patton and Thiobodeau 2009).

Other ways in which respiration is controlled

There are a number of irritant receptors in the lungs which can cause constriction of the air passages, and when stimulated in the bronchi or trachea, a cough is initiated (Marieb and Hoehn 2010). These have a protective mechanism to prevent obstruction or aspiration of food or liquids (Patton and Thiobodeau 2009). There are also stretch receptors present in the conducting passages and the visceral pleura which are stimulated when the lungs inflate; these then signal the respiratory centres to end inspiration (Marieb and Hoehn 2010).

Some of the mechanisms through which breathing is controlled are summarized in Figure 13.16.

Related theory
Respiratory volumes

The quantity of air that is breathed in and out of the lungs varies depending on the condition of inspiration and expiration (Marieb and Hoehn 2010). Therefore, information about the different volumes of the lungs and combinations or respiratory capacities of these various volumes can give an indication about the respiratory condition of the individual (Marieb and Hoehn 2010). A summary of these volumes can be seen in Figure 13.17. See Table 13.4 for a summary of respiratory volumes and capacities for males and females.

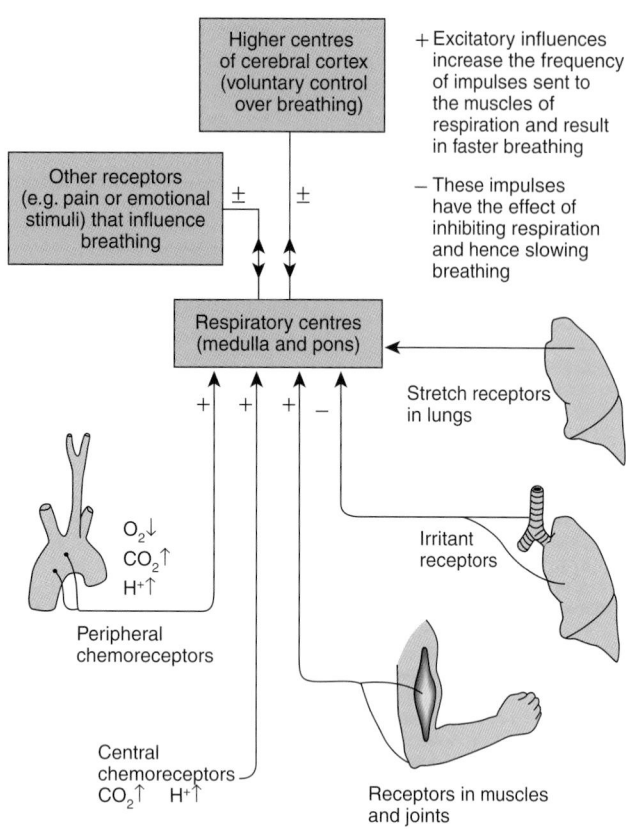

Figure 13.16 Factors influencing rate and depth of breathing.

Legend items shown in figure:

+ Excitatory influences increase the frequency of impulses sent to the muscles of respiration and result in faster breathing

− These impulses have the effect of inhibiting respiration and hence slowing breathing

Gaseous exchange

Gaseous exchange occurs during *external respiration* where oxygen and carbon dioxide diffuse into or out of the blood at the lungs (Marieb and Hoehn 2010). This occurs as there is a flow of gases from areas of higher pressure to areas of lower pressure, so oxygen diffuses from the alveoli into the blood, as the pressure of oxygen in the alveoli is higher than in the blood, and the reverse happens with carbon dioxide (Marieb and Hoehn 2010). *Internal respiration* takes place where the same gases move into or out of the tissues of the body by diffusion, so oxygen moves into the tissues and carbon dioxide moves out of them (Marieb and Hoehn 2010) (see Chapter 10 for further information).

Transport through the blood

1.5% of the oxygen is transported through our blood by being dissolved in the plasma; the other 98.5% is bound to haemoglobin, forming oxyhaemoglobin, and carried in the red blood cells (Marieb and Hoehn 2010). Carbon dioxide is transported in the blood chiefly as a bicarbonate ion within the plasma (70% is transported via this method), 20% is bound to haemoglobin forming carbaminohaemoglobin, and the other 7–10% is dissolved in the plasma (Marieb and Hoehn 2010). This process is summarized in Figure 13.18; see also Chapter 10.

Hypercapnia and hypoxia

Hypercapnia is an elevated level of carbon dioxide level in the blood. Signs include tachypnoea (eventually becoming bradypnoea as it worsens), dyspnoea, tachycardia, hypertension, headaches, vasodilation, drowsiness, sweating and a red colouration (Shelledy 2009). Patients with hypercapnia will require urgent medical attention and close monitoring as hypercapnia will cause a respiratory acidosis (Beachy 2009). Patients with chronic hypercapnia have, at least partially, adapted to the chronically high levels of carbon dioxide, such as those who have COPD; in these patients oxygen therapy needs to be administered with caution (Marieb and Hoehn 2010).

Hypoxia is defined as a low level of oxygen delivery to the tissues and the signs of it include tachypnoea, dyspnoea,

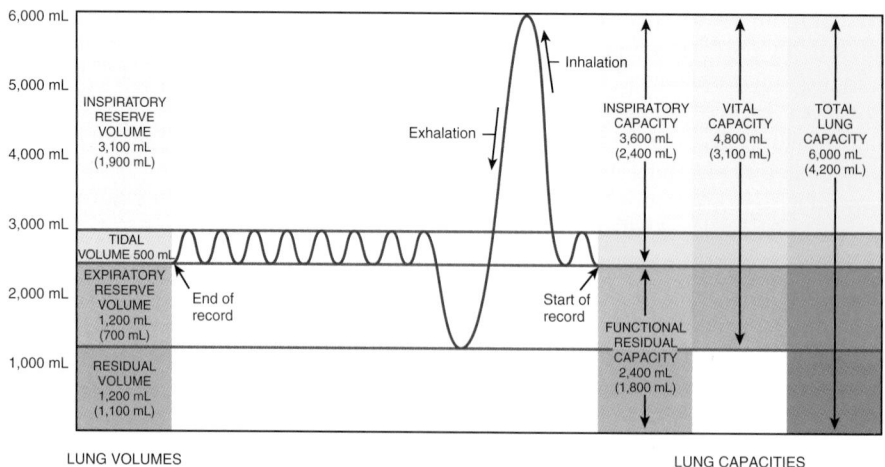

Figure 13.17 Spirogram of lung volumes and capacities. The average values for a healthy average male and female are indicated, with the values for a female in parenthesis. Note that the spirogram is read from right (start of record) to left (end of record). Reproduced from Tortora and Derrickson (2009).

Table 13.4 Summary of respiratory volumes and capacities for males and females

	Measurement	Adult male average value (mL)	Adult female average value (mL)	Description
Respiratory volumes	Tidal volume (TV)	500	500	Amount of air inhaled with each breath under resting conditions
	Inspiratory reserve volume (IRV)	3100	1900	Amount of air that can be forcefully inhaled after a normal tidal volume inhalation
	Expiratory reserve volume (ERV)	1200	700	Amount of air that can be forcefully exhaled after a normal tidal volume exhalation
	Residual volume (RV)	1100	1100	Amount of air remaining in the lungs after a forced exhalation
Respiratory capacities	Total lung capacity (TLC)	6000	4200	Maximum amount of air contained in lungs after a maximum inspiratory effort: $$TLC = TV + IRV + REV + RV$$
	Vital capacity (VC)	4800	3100	Maximum amount of air that can be expired after a maximum inspiratory effort: $$VC = TV + IRV + ERV$$
	Inspiratory capacity (IC)	3600	2400	Maximum amount of air that can be inspired after a normal expiration: $$IC = TV + IRV$$
	Functional residual capacity (FRC)	2400	1800	Volume of air remaining in the lungs after a normal tidal volume expiration: $$FRC = ERV + RV$$

Reproduced from Fig. 22.16, p. 852 from *Human Anatomy & Physiology,* 7th edn, by E.N. Marieb and K. Hoehn. © 2007 by Pearson Education, Inc. Reprinted by permission.

(a) Exchange of O_2 and CO_2 in pulmonary capillaries (external respiration)

(b) Exchange of O_2 and CO_2 in systemic capillaries (internal respiration)

Figure 13.18 Summary of chemical reactions that occur during gas exchange. Reproduced from Tortora and Derrickson (2009).

tachycardia, restlessness and confusion, headache, mild hypertension and pallor (Shelledy 2009). However, in its severe stages the symptoms will worsen leading to slow, irregular breathing, cyanosis, hypotension, altered level of consciousness, blurred vision and eventual respiratory arrest (Shelledy 2009). Hypoxia can have various causes.

- *Anaemic hypoxia*: low red blood cell counts or red blood cells which do not contain enough haemoglobin cannot transport adequate amounts of oxygen.
- *Ischaemic hypoxia*: this is where blood flow to a specific area is inadequate to supply enough oxygen, which can occur as a result of embolism or thrombosis.
- *Histotoxic hypoxia*: there is adequate oxygenation but the cells cannot use the oxygen; this can occur as a result of poisons such as cyanide.
- *Hypoxaemic hypoxia*: there is reduced arterial oxygen as a result of abnormal ventilation or perfusion to the lungs, or breathing air with inadequate amounts of oxygen. Carbon monoxide poisoning can also cause this.

(Marieb and Hoehn 2010)

Evidence-based approaches
Rationale

A thorough respiratory assessment is vital to:

- identify patients who are at risk of deterioration
- commence treatment that may stabilize and improve the patient's condition and outcomes
- help prevent unnecessary admission to critical care or intensive care units.

(Higginson and Jones 2009)

An alteration in the respiratory observations can indicate a severe derangement in a range of body systems, not simply the respiratory system, so it is a vital indicator of morbidity (Cretikos *et al.* 2008). Indeed, respiratory observations are often the first sign to alter in a deteriorating patient so timely, accurate observations, leading to escalation of treatment, could prevent critical events occurring (Goldhill *et al.* 1999, Hunter and Rawlings-Anderson 2008).

Indications

- All patients who are in hospital should have observations taken at the time of their admission or their initial assessment (NICE 2007b).
- When a patient is transferred to a ward setting for intensive or high-dependency care (NICE 2007b).
- At least once every 12 hours while in hospital (NICE 2007b).
- If there is any change or deterioration in the patient's condition (NICE 2007b).
- If the patient is acutely ill or at risk of respiratory deterioration then they will require continuous pulse oximetry and frequent respiratory assessment (Booker 2009, Levine 2007).
- If the patient is receiving oxygen therapy then they will need to be closely monitored to ensure its efficacy (Higginson and Jones 2009).
- Following medical situations including surgery, trauma or infections (Booker 2009, Hunter and Rawlings-Anderson 2008).
- To monitor the patient who is receiving blood or blood product transfusions or intravenous fluids (Hunter and Rawlings-Anderson 2008).
- Any patient who has, or is at risk of, chronic hypercapnia should have close monitoring of their respiratory function (O'Driscoll *et al.* 2008).
- To monitor the patient's response to medications, including opiates and bronchodilators (Hunter and Rawling-Anderson 2008).

Methods of assessing respiration
Airway assessment

It is important to assess whether there is any obstruction to the patient's airway from vomit, foreign bodies or the patient's tongue (Higginson and Jones 2009). In the conscious patient, a way to check for a patent airway is to ask them a question; if they are able to answer normally then their airway is unobscured (Higginson and Jones 2009) (see Chapter 10 for further information).

Breathing assessment

Eupnoea, normal rate and rhythm of breathing, describes unconscious, gentle respiration (Patton and Thiobodeau 2009). It is important to observe the patient and the way they are breathing, including:

- the colour of the patient's skin and mucous membranes, which can show how well perfused and oxygenated they are; look for any cyanosis
- any use of accessory muscles or other respiratory signs
- the rhythm, rate and depth of respiration
- shape and expansion of the chest.

(Higginson and Jones 2009)

Skin colour

Cyanosis is a blue tone to the skin and mucous membranes (Parkman 2007). It can be either central, affecting the lips and oral mucosa, or peripheral, best observed by looking at the patient's nail bed and skin (Simpson 2006). Peripheral cyanosis may be an indication of peripheral perfusion as it can be caused by vasoconstriction, whereas central cyanosis is more indicative of cardiorespiratory insufficiency. However, patients who are anaemic may not be cyanotic as there is insufficient haemoglobin (Moore 2007). Cyanosis is observable when oxygen saturations drop to 85–90% (Moore 2004b). A pale skin tone may indicate that the patient is anaemic or in shock (Bickley and Szilagyi 2009).

Use of accessory muscles

When the patient is in respiratory distress they may use their abdominal, sternomastoid and scalene muscles to increase respiration (Higginson and Jones 2009). To observe these, look at the patient's neck during inspiration to see if there is any contraction of the sternomastoid or other accessory muscles (Bickley and Szilagyi 2009). In addition, some patients may breathe through pursed lips or have nasal flaring (Higginson and Jones 2009).

Rhythm, rate and depth of respiration

The normal respiratory rate is 12–18 breaths per minute with expiration lasting approximately twice as long as inspiration (Higginson and Jones 2009). The rate should be counted for 1 minute to fully assess both the rate and the rhythm (Moore 2004b). Patients with a respiratory rate greater than 24 breaths/min should have frequent observations and be closely monitored; if they also have other physiological alterations, they should receive prompt medical attention, as should all patients with a respiratory rate greater than 27 breaths/min (Cretikos et al. 2008). Respiratory rates which are 8 or less also require urgent medical care (Docherty 2002). Abnormalities in the rate and rhythm of breathing can take various forms, some of which are listed below.

- *Bradypneoa*: breathing which is slower than the normal range; it may indicate respiratory depression or increased intracranial pressure or a diabetic coma (Bickley and Szilagyi 2009, Moore 2004b).
- *Tachypnoea*: breathing which is faster than the normal range and shallow; can indicate a number of conditions including anxiety, pain, restrictive lung disease, cardiac or circulatory problems, or pyrexia (Bickley and Szilagyi 2009, Moore 2004b, Simpson 2006).
- *Dyspnoea*: breathing where the individual is conscious of the effort to breathe and finds it more difficult; when dyspnoea occurs when the patient lies flat, it is termed orthopnoea (Patton and Thiobodeau 2009).
- *Apnoea*: is a temporary cessation of breathing (Patton and Thiobodeau 2009).
- *Biot's breathing*: alternating periods of deep gasping with periods of apnoea, seen in patients with increased intracranial pressure and spinal meningitis (Patton and Thiobodeau 2009, Simpson 2006).
- *Cheyne–Stokes breathing*: alternating periods of deep breathing with periods of apnoea; can have many causes including heart failure or brain damage (Bickley and Szilagyi 2009).
- *Hyperventilation*: this is rapid but deep breathing and can be caused by anxiety, exercise or metabolic acidosis (Bickley and Szilagyi 2009).
- *Hypoventilation*: is shallow and irregular breathing and can be caused by an overdose of certain anaesthetic agents or opiate drugs (Simpson 2006).

Shape and expansion of the chest

This part of the assessment involves looking at the antero-posterior (AP) diameter which may give an indication of underlying respiratory conditions or problems (Higginson and Jones 2009). The AP diameter may change with ageing, and it might also increase in chronic pulmonary disease (Bickley and Szilagyi 2009). As well as observing the shape of the chest wall, it is also important to view the way the chest expands with each breath; when normal, it should be equal and bilateral (Higginson and Jones 2009). Any paradoxical movements should be noted as they can indicate a particular problem with one side of the chest (Higginson and Jones 2009).

Pulse oximetry

This is a continuous and non-invasive monitor which measures the oxygen saturation of the patient (Higginson and Jones 2009). These devices work by measuring the colour of the blood as oxyhaemoglobin is a brighter red than haemoglobin; from this, the device can work out what percentage of the haemoglobin is oxygenated (Davies and Moores 2003). A normal oxygen saturation will range between 95% and 100% (Parkman 2007) but patients with chronic respiratory conditions may have lower oxygen saturations which have become 'normal' for them (Higginson and Jones 2009). Therefore, the patient's doctor should specify what saturation is acceptable for patients with chronic respiratory conditions (Levine 2007).

The British Thoracic Society states that oxygen saturation should be kept at 94–98% for acutely ill adults and 88–92% for those at risk or known to have hypercapnia (O'Driscoll et al. 2008). In patients who are not hypoxic, a sudden drop of greater than 3% of their oxygen saturation should prompt the nurse to check that the device is working correctly and, if so, to undertake further assessment into the patient's condition (O'Driscoll et al. 2008). Arterial blood gases also produce a reading of oxygen saturation, but the use of pulse oximetry may reduce the need for arterial samples to be taken (Simpson 2006).

General condition or distress of the patient

Respiratory assessment also involves assessing the entire patient for other signs or symptoms of respiratory insufficiency; these include assessing the level of consciousness of the patient, how alert and orientated they are and if they appear distressed (Docherty 2002). If the patient can only speak in very short sentences or only a few words without needing to stop to breathe then they are in respiratory distress (Higginson and Jones 2009).

Preprocedural considerations

Equipment

Pulse oximeter

In order to achieve a successful reading, the sensor of the pulse oximeter should be placed in the best location to achieve the reading. Therefore the sensor may be attached to the patient's fingers, ears, toes or nose (Higginson and Jones 2009, Moore 2004a). The sensor contains one red light-emitting diode and one infra-red light-emitting diode, placed opposite a photodetector which measures the light of both frequencies absorbed by oxyhaemoglobin and deoxy-haemoglobin (Moore 2004a). Pulse oximetry does not give an indication of haemoglobin so if the patient is profoundly anaemic then their oxygen saturation may be normal but they may still be hypoxic (Levine 2007).

Pulse oximetry should not be used if there is a risk of light interference from surgical lamps, infra-red warming lamps or even direct sunlight (Adam and Osborne 2005). It should not be used in patients with carbon monoxide poisoning as the device cannot differentiate between carbon monoxide and oxygen. Smoke inhalation causes similar problems so pulse oximetry should be cautiously (Levine 2007).

Specific patient preparations

Positioning of the patient can help ease any respiratory distress and facilitate the assessment and observation of their breathing (Moore 2004b). The patient should be positioned upright, if this is not contraindicated, with their head slightly forward and it may be useful to remove clothing from their thorax to aid with observation of their breathing (Moore 2004b). Positioning can also help to relax the patient and therefore potentially reduce the distress resulting from breathlessness (Gosselink *et al.* 2008). They should be asked to keep still while pulse oximetry is being performed so that an accurate result can be obtained (Hunter and Rawlings-Anderson 2008). If the patient is vasoconstricted or has an occlusion superior to the pulse oximeter sensor then an inaccurate result will be obtained (Levine 2007). If the patient is having a seizure, shivering or moving then pulse oximetry will not be accurate (Levine 2007). Pulse oximetry must not be used on nails with nail polish or on patients who have received dye treatment such as methylene blue, indiocyanine green and indiocarmine (Levine 2007). It should be used in caution with those with arrhythmias, and only be used if there is a correlation between the actual and recorded pulse (Booker 2008).

Procedure guideline 13.5 Respiratory assessment and pulse oximetry

Essential equipment

- Pulse oximeter
- Power source
- Cleaning materials (according to manufacturer's recommendations and local policy)
- Sensor applicable to the chosen site
- Appropriate method of documentation and a pen

Optional equipment

- Variety of sensors available for different sites

Preprocedure

Action	Rationale
1 Wash hands thoroughly with soap and water and dry.	To reduce the risk of cross-contamination (Fraise and Bradley 2009, E; Hunter and Rawlings-Anderson 2008, E).
2 Explain the procedure to the patient, answering any questions they may have, and gain their consent.	Consent must be gained prior to commencing any procedure (NMC 2008b, C).
3 While talking to the patient, assess their respiratory condition including their ability to talk in full sentences, the colour of their skin, whether they appear to be in distress or not, and whether they are alert and orientated.	This initial assessment can give important information about the patient's respiratory function and any potential problems (Higginson and Jones, 2009, E; Wilkins 2009, E).
4 Determine the site to be used to perform pulse oximetry. The site should have a good blood supply, determined by checking it is warm, with a proximal pulse and brisk capillary refill.	The sensor requires a well-perfused area or it will not get strong enough signals to produce a result (Adam and Osborne 2005, E; Levine 2007, E).

5 Ensure that the area to be used is clean and free from dirt, and that the sensor is also clean (Moore 2004a). If using the patient's fingers ensure that all nail polish has been removed.	Dirt or nail polish may interfere with the transmission of the light signals, causing inaccurate results (Moore 2004a, E).
6 Select the correct pulse oximeter sensor for the site which is most appropriate for your patient, dependent on circulation and the manufacturer's instructions.	The correct sensor should be used for each site to ensure good contact and not apply too much pressure (Levine 2007, E).

Procedure

7 Position the sensor securely but do not secure it with tape, unless specifically recommended by the manufacturer (MHRA 2001) (see Action Figure 7). If the pulse oximetry is to be continuous then the site needs to be changed at least every 4 hours.	If it is too tight it may impede the blood flow, leading to i naccurate results and the potential for pressure ulcer formation to the site (Moore 2004a, E).
8 Turn the pulse oximeter on and set the alarms on the device dependent on the patient's condition and within locally agreed limits.	To ensure that it is ready to use (Adam and Osborne 2005, E).
9 Check that the pulse reading on the device corresponds with their actual pulse. Ask the patient not to talk while you palpate their pulse. Once the pulse rate has been obtained, keep your fingers on their wrist and count their respiratory rate for a full minute. One breath is equal to one inspiration and expiration and is done by watching the abdomen or chest wall move in and out. Assess the regularity and depth of breathing, the shape and expansion of the chest, and look for any use of accessory muscles.	Any large deviations in pulse may show that the device is not measuring accurately or is being affected by movement (Levine 2007, E). The patient should ideally not be aware that their respiratory rate is being counted as this may produce inaccurate results (Wilkins 2009, E).

Postprocedure

10 Document results clearly, including the time and date of the reading.	Records must be kept of all assessments made and care provided (NMC 2009, C).
11 Clean the pulse oximeter according to manufacturer's recommendations and local policy.	It may become colonized and be a source of infection to another patient (Woodrow 1999, E).

785

Action Figure 7   Position of an oxygen probe.

Problem-solving table 13.5 Prevention and resolution (Procedure guideline 13.5)

Problem	Cause	Prevention	Action
Movement due to patient having a seizure, shivering or tremors	Movement can affect the accuracy of the reading (Levine 2007)	Try to use a site which is less affected, for example an ear (Levine 2007)	If the finger has been used, compare the pulse rate as given by the oximeter with the palpated radial pulse – if there is a difference then the oxygen saturation reading will not be accurate (Levine 2007). Arterial blood gases may be required to monitor their oxygen saturation, if a saturation cannot be obtained (Levine 2007)
Unexpectedly low result which does not correlate with their clinical condition	The site chosen may not have an adequate blood supply (Adam and Osborne, 2005)	Check for perfusion by palpating for a pulse and checking the area is warm with good capillary refill	Reposition sensor to new site. If it remains low, arterial blood gases may need to be considered (Adam and Osborne 2005)

Postprocedural considerations

Immediate care

Any abnormalities of respiration discovered during the respiratory assessment should prompt rapid action (Higginson and Jones 2009). If there is risk of a compromised airway or respiratory insufficiency/failure then senior nursing and medical assistance, including an anaesthetist, will be required urgently (Docherty 2002). Further information will be needed, including obtaining:

- a history of their current condition and any past medical history, including a list of the medications they are taking (Bickley and Szilagyi 2009)
- a full set of observations including temperature, blood pressure and heart rate (Higginson and Jones 2009).

In addition, other tests may be required depending on the condition of the patient, including the following.

- Arterial blood gases to check for level of carbon dioxide, oxygen level, pH, acid/base balance (Higginson and Jones 2009).
- Sputum collection to assess for an infection or specific diseases such as tuberculosis (Docherty 2002, Simpson 2006).
- Chest X-ray or CT scan (Simpson 2006).
- Blood tests including a full blood count, urea and electrolytes, clotting and cross-match (Docherty 2002).
- Fluid balance to monitor for signs of fluid overload or dehydration (Docherty 2002).

Airway management and administration of oxygen

For further information on this, see Life support and Chapter 10.

Ongoing care

As well as involving senior nurses, the medical team and potentially anaesthestists in the care of the patient, it may also be useful to refer the patient to the physiotherapy team (Docherty 2002).

Documentation

It is vital that all documentation on oxygen saturations should state whether the patient was breathing air or oxygen, and the flow of oxygen and method of administration (O'Driscoll *et al.* 2008). If the oxygen is being given in an emergency situation without a prescription then subsequent documentation must state the rationale for the administration of oxygen and the flow rate (O'Driscoll *et al.* 2008).

Education of patient and relevant others

One of the key focuses of education to patients with respiratory conditions should be to ascertain if they smoke and if they do, to encourage them to stop as smoking cessation can help to improve their prognosis (Tonnesen *et al.* 2007). For more information on this topic see Chapter 10.

Complications

It is recommended that to prevent any tissue damage, the pulse oximeter sensor is not taped in place (unless recommended by the manufacturer) and that the sensor should be resited every 4 hours or more frequently if necessary, depending on the patient's condition and the manufacturer's recommendations (MHRA 2001).

Peak flow

Definition

Peak expiratory flow (PEF) is the maximum flow of air which can be achieved when air is expired with maximum force following maximal inspiration (Quanjer *et al.* 1997).

Anatomy and physiology

The factors which determine PEF are:

- the dimensions of the extra- and intrathoracic airways, including their diameter and compliance
- the force the expiratory muscles generate, which is related to the degree of lung inflation
- the volume of the lungs, which is affected by the stature of the person, and speed and degree of maximal alveolar pressure that the person can reach
- the degree of stretch the lungs have been subjected to previously and the recoil ability of the lung
- the resistance of the instrument used to measure peak expiratory flow.

(Quanjer *et al.* 1997)

Therefore, any condition which alters the above factors could affect PEF. However, a reduction in one of the above factors may be compensated for by an increase in one of the others, meaning that PEF does not alter, therefore potentially underestimating the severity of the condition (Quanjer *et al.* 1997).

Related theory

The most common disorders which affect PEF are those which increase the resistance to air flow in the intrathoracic airways, such as asthma (Quanjer *et al.* 1997). However, PEF may also be impaired by:

- disorders which limit chest movement and respiratory musculoskeletal problems
- obstruction of the extrathoracic airways
- impairment of nerves supplying the respiratory system.

(Quanjer *et al.* 1997)

Peak expiratory flow readings are subject to individual variation depending on the patient's age, gender, ethnic origin and stature (Quanjer *et al.* 1997). Therefore, results need to be compared against normal results for people of the same stature and gender (Figure 13.19) and against any previous results for that individual.

Peak expiratory flow is similar to forced expired volume in 1 second (FEV_1) measurements but the two are not interchangeable and both measure different aspects of lung function (Ruffin 2004). FEV_1 measures the volume of air exhaled during the first second of forced vital capacity (FVC), which occurs when an individual exhales forcefully to their maximum capacity following a deep inspiration (Marieb and Hoehn 2010). FEV_1 is usually 80% of FVC in healthy participants (Marieb and Hoehn 2010). FEV_1 is felt to be more sensitive in detecting mild airway obstruction, and peak expiratory flow is effort dependent and so can have a greater degree of intrasubject variability (Hansen *et al.* 2001). However, both FEV_1 and PEF were found to have similar predictive ability in relation to mortality in patients with COPD, although FEV_1 was found to be a better predictor in patients with asthma (Hansen *et al.* 2001).

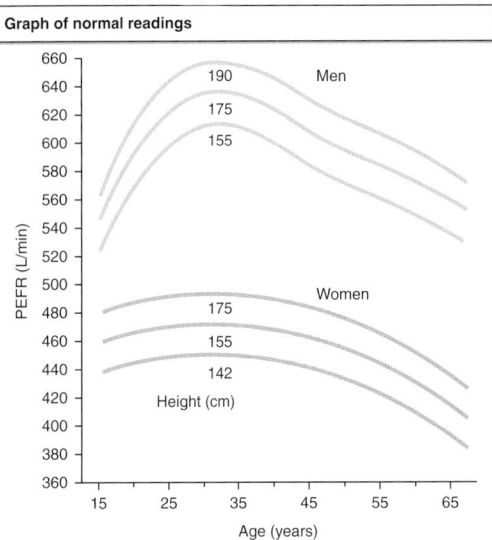

Figure 13.19 Normal peak flow measurements. Reproduced from Kumar and Clarke (2009).

Evidence-based approaches

Rationale

Peak expiratory flow is a simple, objective procedure which can be used to measure the degree of air flow limitation and although it may not give a full representation of lung function, it can monitor efficacy of treatment and progression of the condition (Frew and Holgate 2009).

Indications

Peak expiratory flow can be used to:

- monitor the severity of the condition in patients with chronic severe asthma (Reddel 2006)
- monitor progression of respiratory disease (Frew and Holgate 2009)
- evaluate effectiveness of treatment (Frew and Holgate 2009)
- identify exacerbating factors (Reddel 2006).

Contraindications

Peak expiratory flow should be used with caution as follows.

- Severe air flow obstruction, as included in the measurement, may be air coming from the collapsing airway, yielding an erroneously high result (Quanjer *et al.* 1997).
- If the patient is unable to take a full inspiration, for example if they have a persistent cough, then the results will be inaccurate (Quanjer *et al.* 1997).
- If the procedure itself causes an exacerbation of the air flow limitation, shown by consecutive results producing a reduction in scoring (Quanjer *et al.* 1997).

- Young children may not understand the procedure correctly (Gorelick *et al.* 2004).

Methods for measuring peak flow

Treatment is often based on the PEF measurements so it is vital that they are as accurate as possible, and performed even when the patient is symptom free (Buist *et al.* 2006). Patients need to adhere to the peak flow monitoring regimen as trends can be more important than isolated results (unless the isolated results reflect an exacerbation) (Booker 2009). The patient needs to repeat the procedure three times with the best result of the three being documented (Quanjer *et al.* 1997). Unless the procedure induces an exacerbation, there should be consistency between the three results. If the top two results have a greater disparity than 40 L/min then, as long as the patient is not fatigued, a further two attempts can be made to reach a greater level of consistency (Quanjer *et al.* 1997).

Timing of peak flow readings

While isolated PEF measurement can indicate a restriction in air flow, in general sequential measurements are of more use, displaying trends essential to understanding the severity and progression of the disease (Quanjer *et al.* 1997). However, there may be significant diurnal variations, with the lowest measurements occurring during the night and first thing in the morning (Quanjer *et al.* 1997). Therefore, it is recommended that measurements should be taken on waking, in the afternoon and prior to going to bed and the results documented (Frew and Holgate 2009). If it is suspected that the patient may have restricted air flow due to occupational causes, the patient should take measurements for a minimum of 2 weeks while at work and 2 weeks while not at work to enable a comparison (Frew and Holgate 2009).

Preprocedural considerations

Equipment

The Wright and mini-Wright peak flow meter

The Wright peak flow meter was developed in 1959 and was a portable, simple device for monitoring PEF in the home. It has since been redesigned as the mini-Wright peak flow meter which is commonly in use today (Ruffin 2004). Peak flow is measured by the patient exhaling as quickly and forcefully as possible following maximal inspiration; the maximum expiratory flow is measured and usually occurs early in expiration (Bongers and O'Driscoll 2006). In September 2004 the scales of measurement used on peak flow meters were changed to a new EU scale (Bongers and O'Driscoll 2006). This increased the accuracy of the assessment and enhanced the ability to compare measurements with conventional spirometry (MHRA 2004). Although all new prescriptions of peak flow meters after this time were for the new model, some patients may still have the older one which will read up to 30% higher in the mid-range readings so it is important to check which device they are using; the new model is labelled as 'EN 13826' or 'EU scale' (MHRA 2004). If the patient is unable to use their own meter then multiple patient use meters are available in clinics and hospital; these are valved and have disposable single patient use mouthpieces to prevent infection (Booker 2009).

Spirometers

Spirometers can produce a reading for PEF alongside other lung function measurements such as FVC. However, these results may not be comparable to those obtained using a mini-Wright meter due to both the equipment and technique used. Therefore, the patient should use the same equipment and technique each time to enable comparisons with past results (Bongers and O'Driscoll 2006).

Assessment and recording tools

Recording peak flow measurements on individualized action plans/booklets gives patients a greater degree of control and awareness about when they need to access medical care. The use of these recording tools is strongly advocated (British Thoracic Society/Scottish Intercollegiate Guidelines Network 2009, Gibson *et al.* 2002).

Specific patient preparations

The procedure should be performed when the patient is at rest (unless otherwise specified) and may be performed with them sitting upright or standing as long as their neck is not flexed (Quanjer *et al.* 1997). To increase reliability and enable comparisons to be drawn, it is advisable that they use the same posture each time (Booker 2009).

Education

The practitioner must ensure that the patient is fully informed about how to perform the procedure and performs it accurately, as even small alterations in technique may produce inaccurate results. If the patient has never performed the procedure, then education should be given and they should have the opportunity to have it demonstrated for them and have their own practice attempts (Quanjer *et al.* 1997).

Procedure guideline 13.6 Peak flow reading using a manual peak flow meter

Essential equipment

- Peak flow meter (calibrated and working correctly)
- Disposable mouthpiece
- Peak flow chart to document results on and a pen

Optional equipment

- Other lung function tests including pulse oximetry
- Oxygen mask and oxygen source
- Equipment to give a nebulizer
- Emergency resuscitation equipment

Preprocedure

Action	Rationale
1 Explain the procedure to the patient and obtain consent.	To ensure the patient understands the procedure and gives valid consent (NMC 2008b, C).
2 Ask the patient what their best peak flow measurements have been and what their current peak flow readings are.	This will enable a comparison to be drawn between their current and previous results (British Thoracic Society/Scottish Intercollegiate Guidelines Network 2009, C).
3 Wash and dry hands or use alcohol handrub.	To minimize the spread of cross-infection (Fraise and Bradley 2009, E).
4 Assemble equipment; ask the patient to use their own meter, if it is in good working order. If using a multiple patient use device ensure that it is valved and has disposable single patient use mouthpieces.	As different equipment might have slight variations in results (Bongers and O'Driscoll 2006, E). To prevent cross-infection (Booker 2009, E).
5 Ask the patient to stand or sit upright in whatever position they usually do their peak expiratory flow measurements in. They should be advised not to flex their neck.	So that their maximal lung volume can be reached and so that there is no positional obstruction which could affect the results, and to enable comparisons between results (Booker 2009, E; Quanjer et al. 1997, E).
6 Push needle on the gauge down to zero.	To ensure the results are accurate (Booker 2009, E).

Procedure

7 Ask the patient to hold the peak flow meter horizontally, ensuring their fingers do not impede the gauge.	So that the movement of the needle is not obstructed and can move easily (Booker 2009, E; Frew and Holgate 2009, E).
8 Ask the patient to take a full inspiration to their total lung capacity through their mouth.	To ensure they achieve the greatest measurement (Frew and Holgate 2009, E; Quanjer et al. 1997, E).
9 Ask the patient to immediately place their lips tightly around the mouthpiece. The inspiration should be held for no longer than 2 s at total lung capacity.	To form an air seal and to prevent their tongue and teeth from obstructing it (Booker 2009, E; Quanjer et al. 1997, E).
10 Ask the patient to blow out down the meter in a short sharp 'huff' as forcefully as they can. See Action Figure 10.	This can be very quick and need only take about 1 s, to enable accuracy of results (Booker 2009, E; Quanjer et al. 1997, E).
11 Take a note of the reading. As results may vary, ask them to repeat the process a further 2 times and record the maximum measurement achieved.	To ensure that the best possible result is achieved (Frew and Holgate 2009, E; Quanjer et al. 1997, E).

(Continued)

789

Procedure guideline 13.6 *(Continued)*

Postprocedure

12 Document the readings on the record chart and take further action if necessary.

Records must be kept of all assessments made, treatment or care provided and the outcome of this (NMC 2009, C).

13 Discard the mouthpiece and clean the meter in line with local policies and the manufacturer's recommendation. Wash hands.

To prevent the risk of cross-infection (Fraise and Bradley 2009, E).

Action Figure 10   Manual peak flow meter technique.

Problem-solving table 13.6 Prevention and resolution (Procedure guideline 13.6)

Problem	Cause	Prevention	Action
A higher than expected result is obtained	May be caused by the needle not being pushed back to zero prior to commencement, or by poor technique leading to 'explosive decompression' whereby there is sudden opening of the glottis, or release of the tongue occluding the mouthpiece, or caused by spitting into the mouthpiece (Quanjer *et al.* 1997)	Allow practice runs prior to the procedure and ensure that the individual is educated on technique	Reset the needle back to zero, educate them on the correct technique, and if they appear fatigued, allow them to rest prior to repeating the procedure

Postprocedural considerations
Immediate care

A reduction in peak flow may indicate a life-threatening situation and so should receive urgent medical attention. The treatment provided will be aimed at increasing air flow and oxygenation. Oxygen therapy is usually applied with the aim of keeping oxygen saturations at 94–98% (British Thoracic Society/Scottish Intercollegiate Guidelines Network, 2009). In patients who are known, or suspected, to have hypercapnia, oxygen should be initially administered at 28% via a Venturi mask out of hospital, and in hospital at 24% via a Venturi mask, unless their condition is of such severity to require a greater flow (O'Driscoll *et al.* 2008). However, if their oxygen saturation exceeds 92% then the flow of oxygen should be reduced (O'Driscoll *et al.* 2008). All of these patients will require arterial blood gas samples to be taken at the earliest opportunity to enable their condition to be more thoroughly assessed (O'Driscoll *et al.* 2008). Medication will be used to try and reverse the air flow reduction and this will usually include a combination of inhaled bronchodilators and steroids (British Thoracic Society/Scottish Intercollegiate Guidelines Network 2009).

Ongoing care

It should be noted if the patient had experienced/been in contact with any of the following prior to the exacerbation.

- Cold air.
- Heightened levels of emotion.
- Exposure to allergens.
- Viral infection.
- Inhaled irritants such as pollution or dust.
- Medication or drugs, including anti-inflammatories and beta-adrenoreceptor blocking agents.
- Occupational sensitizers.

(Frew and Holgate 2009)

The patient will probably require other medical tests to assess their condition; these may include chest X-ray, blood and sputum tests (Frew and Holgate 2009).

Education of patient and relevant others

Patient education is vital so that patients can manage their own condition (Buist *et al.* 2006). This will include information on exacerbating factors, smoking cessation and when to access medical help. A Cochrane review found that if patients received education on the self-management of asthma this led to a reduction of patients requiring hospitalization or emergency care for their asthma (Gibson *et al.* 2002).

Temperature

Definition

Body temperature represents the balance between heat production and heat loss (Marieb and Hoehn 2010). All body tissues produce heat depending on how metabolically active they are. When the body is resting, most heat is generated by the heart, liver, brain and endocrine organs (Marieb and Hoehn 2010).

Anatomy and physiology

Core body temperature measurements are taken to assess for deviation from the normal range of 36–37.5°C, to maintain cell metabolic activity. The core body temperature is set and closely regulated by the thermoregulatory centre of the hypothalamus in the brain (Tortora and Derrickson 2009).

Body temperature is a regulated function of the hypothalamus, and is the balance between heat gain (metabolism) and heat loss (respiration). All tissues produce heat as a result of cell metabolism, and this is increased by exercise and activity (Marieb and Hoehn 2010). Humans have the ability through homoeostasis to maintain a constant core temperature in spite of environmental changes. The body core generally has the highest temperature while the skin is the coolest (Figure 13.20). Core temperature reflects the heat of

Figure 13.20 Body core and skin temperature.

arterial blood and represents the balance between the heat generated by body tissues in metabolic activity and that lost through various mechanisms (Marieb and Hoehn 2010).

The hypothalamus comprises a group of neurones in the anterior and posterior portions, referred to as the preoptic area (Tortora and Derrickson 2009), which works as a thermostat (Figure 13.21). A relatively constant temperature is maintained by homoeostasis, which is a constant process of heat gain and heat loss. The body requires stability of its temperature to produce an optimum environment for biochemical and enzymic reactions to maintain cellular function. Body temperature above or below this normal range affects total body function (Marieb and Hoehn 2010). A temperature above 41°C can cause convulsions and a temperature of 43°C renders life unsustainable.

Heat is gained through metabolic activity of the body, especially of the muscles and liver. Heat loss is achieved through the skin by the processes of radiation, convection, conduction and evaporation (Marieb and Hoehn 2010).

Various factors cause fluctuations of temperature.

- The body's circadian rhythms cause daily fluctuations. The body temperature is higher in the evening than in the morning (Marieb and Hoehn 2010). Minor and Waterhouse (1981) recorded a difference of 0.5–1.5°C between morning and evening measurements.

791

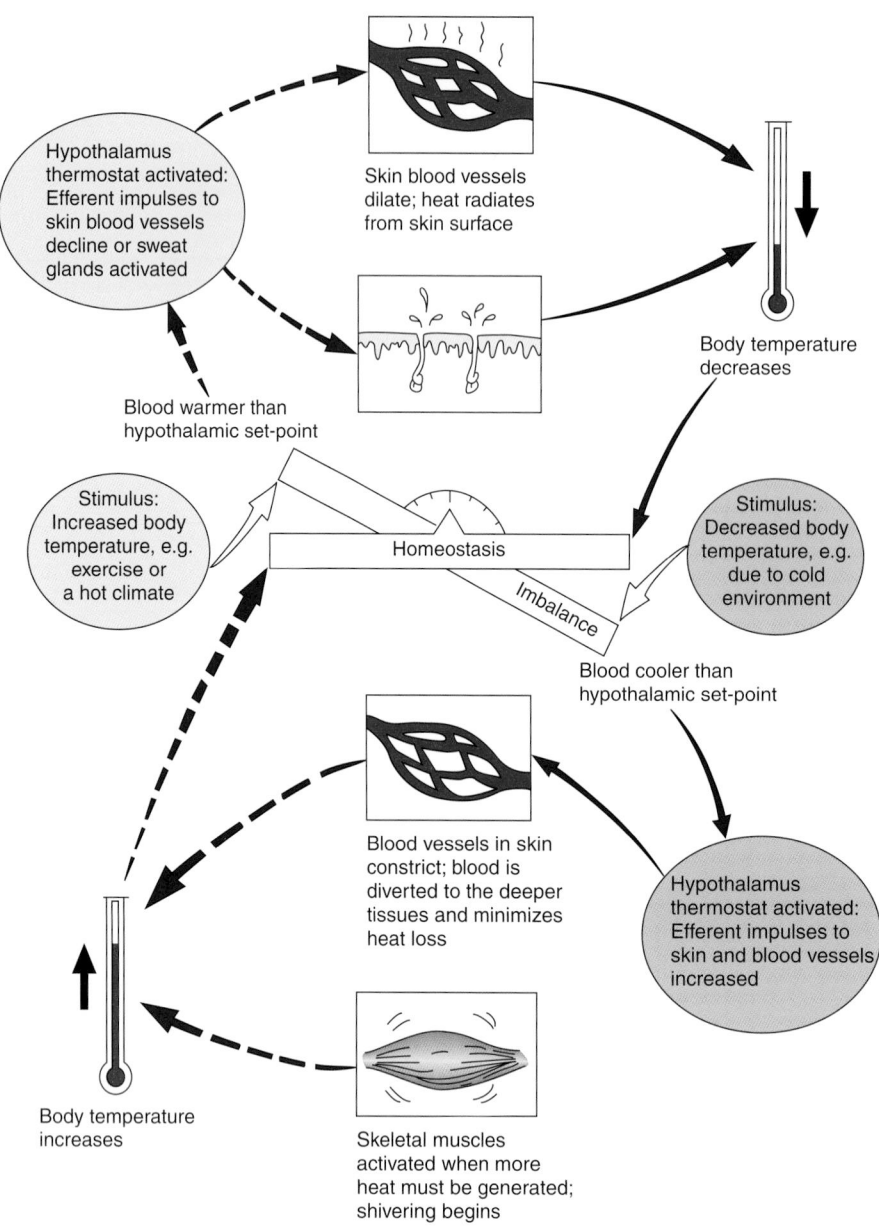

Figure 13.21 Mechanisms of body temperature regulation.

- Ovulation can elevate the body's temperature as it influences the basal metabolic rate (Tortora and Derrickson 2009).
- Exercise and eating cause an elevation in temperature (Marieb and Hoehn 2010).
- Extremes of age affect a person's response to environmental change. While young people will shiver at a temperature of 36°, most people over the age of 80 will not shiver until the body temperature falls to 35.1° (Kenney and Munce 2003). Thermoregulation is inadequate in the newborn and especially in low-birthweight babies. In older people, there is an increased sensitivity to cold and the body temperature is generally lower (Nakamura *et al.* 1997).

Related theory

Hypothermia

Hypothermia is defined as a core temperature of 35°C that causes the metabolic rate to decrease (Trim 2005). Hypothermia may be classified as mild (32–35°C), moderate (28–32°C) and severe (less than 28°C) (Cuddy 2004). This occurs when the body loses more heat and is subsequently unable to maintain homoeostasis (Neno 2005). If the temperature does fall below 35°C, the patient will start to shiver severely (Edwards 1997). However, hypothermia frequently escapes detection due to symptoms being non-specific and an oral thermometer's failure to record in the appropriate range (Marini and Wheeler 2010). It can occur in all ages, although the elderly are at particular risk, and is often multifactorial in origin. It can arise as a result of:

- environmental exposure
- medications that can alter the perception of cold, increase heat loss through vasodilation or inhibit heat generation, for example alcohol, paracetamol
- metabolic conditions, for example hypoglycaemia and adrenal insufficiency
- the exposure of the body and internal organs during surgery and the use of drugs which dampen the vasoconstrictor response (Marini and Wheeler 2010).

Surgical patients having procedures longer than 1 hour have increased disruption to normal homoeostatic mechanisms resulting in a drop in temperature. Complications can include cardiovascular ischaemia, delayed wound healing and increased risk for wound infections and increase in postoperative recovery time (Wagner 2006).

Hyperthermia

Sudden temperature elevations usually indicate infection, making it prudent to perform a directed physical examination and, if indicated, obtain appropriate cultures and institute antibiotics. However, although infection is the most common explanation, several life-threatening non-infectious causes of fever are frequently overlooked (Marini and Wheeler 2010) (Table 13.5).

Fever caused by pyrexia (elevated body temperature) is the result of the internal thermostat resetting to higher levels. This resetting of the thermostat is the result of the action of pyrogens, which are chemical substances now known to be cytokines. Cytokines are chemical mediators, which are involved in cellular immunity (Marieb and Hoehn 2010). They enhance the immune response and are released from white blood cells, injured tissues and macrophages. This causes the hypothalamus to release prostaglandins, which in turn reset the hypothalamic thermostat. The body then promotes heat-producing mechanisms such as vasoconstriction. As a result of vasoconstriction, heat loss from the body surface declines, the skin cools and shivering begins to generate heat. These 'chills' are a sign that body temperature is rising (Marieb and Hoehn 2010) and are often referred to as 'rigors'. A rigor is marked by shivering and the patient complains of feeling cold. The temperature quickly rises as a result of the normal physiological response to cold. This results in the following physiological changes.

Table 13.5 Non-infectious causes of hyperthermia

Agonist drugs	Malignancy
Alcohol withdrawal	Malignant hyperthermia
Anticholinergic drugs	Neuroleptic malignant syndrome
Allergic drug or transfusion reaction	Pheochromocytoma
Autonomic insufficiency	Salicylate intoxication
Crystalline arthritis (gout)	Status epilepticus
Drug allergy	Stroke or central nervous system damage
Heat stroke	Vasculitis hyperthyroidism

- Thermoreceptors in the skin are stimulated, resulting in vasoconstriction. This decreases heat loss through conduction and convection.
- Sweat gland activity is reduced to minimize evaporation.
- Shivering occurs; muscles contract and relax out of sequence with each other, thus generating heat.
- The body increases catecholamine and thyroxine levels, elevating the metabolic rate in an attempt to increase temperature.

(Marieb and Hoehn 2010)

All these changes contribute to a rise in metabolism with an increase in carbon dioxide excretion and the need for oxygen. This leads to an increased respiratory rate. When the body temperature reaches its new 'setpoint' the patient no longer complains of feeling cold, shivering ceases and sweating commences.

There are several grades of pyrexia, and these are described in Table 13.6.

Evidence-based approaches

Rationale

Core body temperature measurements are taken to assess for deviation from the normal range that may indicate disease, deterioration in condition, infection or reaction to treatment.

Body temperature measurement is part of routine care in clinical practice and can influence important decisions regarding tests, diagnosis and treatment (Le Frant *et al.* 2003). Temperature needs to be measured accurately and monitored effectively to enable temperature changes to

793

Table 13.6 Grades of pyrexia

Low-grade pyrexia	Normal to 38°C	Indicative of an inflammatory response due to a mild infection, allergy, disturbance of body tissue by trauma, surgery, malignancy or thrombosis
Moderate to high-grade pyrexia	38–40°C	May be caused by wound, respiratory or urinary tract infections
Hyperpyrexia	40°C and above	May arise because of bacteraemia, damage to the hypothalamus or high environmental temperatures

be detected quickly and any necessary intervention commenced (Watson 1998). Temperature assessment accuracy depends on several factors: measurement technique, device type, body site, healthcare professionals' training and competence. Temperature recording is a core assessment (and reassessment) in nursing practice, but can create clinical issues if not performed appropriately (Docherty 2000).

Indications

Conditions in which a patient's temperature requires careful monitoring include the following.

- Patients with conditions that affect basal metabolic rate, such as disorders of the thyroid gland, require monitoring of body temperature. Hypothyroidism is a condition where an inadequate secretion of hormones from the thyroid gland results in slowing of physical and metabolic activity; thus the individual has a decrease in body temperature. Hyperthyroidism is excessive activity of the thyroid gland; a hypermetabolic condition results, with an increase in all metabolic processes. The patient complains of a low heat tolerance. Thyrotoxic crisis is a sudden increase in thyroid hormones and can cause a hyperpyrexia (Walsh 2002).
- Postoperative and critically ill patients require monitoring of temperature. The patient's temperature should be observed preoperatively in order to make any significant comparisons. In the postoperative period the nurse should observe the patient for hyperthermia or hypothermia as a reaction to the surgical procedures (Wagner 2006).
- Patients with a susceptibility to infection, for example those with a low white blood cell count (less than 1000 cells/mm^3) or those undergoing radiotherapy, chemotherapy or steroid treatment, will require a more frequent observation of temperature. The fluctuation in temperature is influenced by the body's response to pyrogens. Immunocompromised patients are less able to respond to infection. Bacteraemia means a bacterial invasion of the bloodstream. Septic shock is a circulatory collapse as a result of severe infection. Pyrexia may be absent in those who are immunosuppressed or in the elderly (Neno 2005).
- Patients with a systemic or local infection require monitoring of temperature to assess development or regression of infection.
- Pyrexia can occur when patients are receiving a blood transfusion but severe transfusion reactions usually occur within the first 15 minutes of starting (BCSH 1999).

Methods of recording temperature

Traditionally, the mouth, axilla and rectum have been the preferred sites for obtaining temperature readings, due to their accessibility. With the development of new technology the use of the tympanic membrane is increasingly popular, as it is less invasive and provides rapid results (Burke 1996). It has been suggested that tympanic membrane thermometers give a more accurate representation of actual body temperature, as the tympanic membrane lies close to the temperature regulation centre in the hypothalamus and shares the same artery (van Staaij *et al.* 2003).

Oral

To most accurately measure the temperature orally, the thermometer is placed in the posterior sublingual pocket of tissue at the base of the tongue (Torrance and Semple 1998). It is important that the thermometer is placed in this region and not in the area under the front of the tongue, as there may be a temperature difference of up to 1.7°C between these areas. This temperature difference is due to the sublingual pockets being protected from the air currents, which cool the frontal areas (Neff *et al.* 1989). This area is in close proximity to the thermoreceptors which respond rapidly to changes in the core temperature, hence changes in core temperatures are reflected quickly here (Carroll 2000, Stevenson 2004).

Oral temperatures are affected by the temperatures of ingested foods and fluids, smoking and by the muscular activity of chewing. It has been shown that oxygen therapy does not affect the oral temperature reading (Hasler and Cohen 1982, Lim-Levy 1982). A respiratory rate that exceeds 18 breaths per minute, together with a patient who smokes, will also reduce the core temperature values (Knies 2003).

Rectal

The rectal temperature is often higher than the oral temperature because this site is more sheltered from the external environment. Rectal thermometry has been demonstrated in clinical trials to be more accurate than oral or axillary thermometry; however, it is not advocated due to its invasive nature (Trim 2005). While other more precise methods can still detect fever, the rectal method offers greater precision. However, the presence of soft stool may separate the thermometer from the bowel wall and give a false reading, especially if the central temperature is changing rapidly. In infants this method is not recommended as it carries a risk of rectal ulceration or perforation (Jensen *et al.* 1994).

A rectal thermometer should be inserted at least 4 cm in an adult to obtain the most accurate reading.

Axillary

The axilla is considered less desirable than the other sites because of the difficulty in achieving accurate and reliable readings (Evans and Kenkre 2006) as it is not close to major vessels, and skin surface temperatures vary more with changes in temperature of the environment (Woollens 1996). It is usually only used for patients who are unsuitable for, or who cannot tolerate, oral thermometers, for example after general anaesthetic or patients with mouth injuries (Edwards 1997).

To take an axillary temperature reading, the thermometer should be placed in the centre of the armpit, with the patient's arm firmly against the side of the chest. It is important that the same arm is used for each measurement as there is often a variation in temperature between left and right (Heindenreich and Giuffe 1990).

Whichever route is used for temperature measurement, it is important that this is then used consistently, as switching between sites can produce a record that is misleading or difficult to interpret.

Consideration is required when interpreting variations in 4–6 hourly observations, and when taking once-only daily temperatures as the average person experiences circadian rhythms which make their highest body temperature occur in the late afternoon or early evening, that is between 4 pm and 8 pm. The most sensitive time for detecting pyrexias appears to be between 7 pm and 8 pm (Angerami 1980). Samples *et al.* (1985) found the highest temperature between 5 pm and 7 pm. These studies suggest that the most useful time to measure and detect an abnormal temperature would be approximately 6 pm.

Anticipated patient outcomes

To determine the patient's temperature on admission as a baseline for comparison with future measurements and to monitor fluctuations in temperature.

Preprocedural considerations

Temperature can be measured at a number of different sites, using different tools for measurement. When assessing the body temperature it is important to consider the methods and tools used for measurement (Docherty 2006).

The critical issue to consider when using any thermometer is whether you are controlling the factors that affect the accuracy and precision of the measurement. These factors must be addressed when educating staff on the use of different temperature measurement methods. It is therefore important to recall that therapeutic decisions should not be made on the basis of a single vital sign (Bridges 2009).

Equipment

A variety of thermometers are now available, from clinical glass thermometers with oral or rectal bulbs to the electronic sensor thermometer to the tympanic thermometer. Until recently, mercury in glass thermometers continued to be used, even though it had been shown that they were unable to detect temperatures lower than 34.5°C (94°F) or higher than 40.5°C (105°F) (Khorshid *et al.* 2005). The MHRA (2005) advises that, for safety, equipment with mercury should be replaced where possible. Mercury thermometers respond slowly to temperature changes, making use of an electronic device preferable when recording temperature extremes and rapid fluctuations (Marini and Wheeler 2010). Other types of thermometer include those listed by Docherty (2000).

- Single-use plastic-coated strips with heat-sensitive recorders (dots) which change colour to indicate the temperature (record from 35.5 to 40.4°C).
- Digital analogue probe thermometers with plastic disposable sheets (record from 32 to 42°C).
- Invasive thermometers attached to a pulmonary artery catheter (record from 0 to 50°C) (Braun *et al.* 1998, O'Toole 1997).

Tympanic membrane thermometer

Tympanic thermometers are small hand-held devices that have a disposable probe cover that is inserted into the patient's ear canal. The sensor at the end of the probe records the infra-red radiation (IRR) that is emitted by the tympanic membrane, as a result of its warmth, and converts this into a temperature reading presented on a digital screen (Jevon and Jevon 2001). The probe is protected by a disposable cover, which is changed between patients to prevent cross-infection (Gallimore 2004). Van Staaij *et al.* (2003) suggest that tympanic thermometers give a more accurate representation of actual body temperature because the tympanic membrane lies close to the temperature regulation centre in the hypothalamus and shares the same artery.

A common problem with using tympanic thermometers is poor technique leading to inaccurate temperature measurements (Gilbert *et al.* 2002). The placement of the probe to fit snugly within the ear canal (see Figure 13.22) is crucial as differences between the opening of the ear canal and the tympanic membrane can be as much as 2.8°C (Hudek *et al.* 1998). Jevon and Jevon (2001) highlight other causes of false readings, which include dirty or cracked probe lens, incorrect installation of the probe cover and short time intervals between measurements (less than 2–3 minutes).

Specific patient preparations

Asking the patient when they last ate, smoked and had a drink as these may have influences on their temperature.

Figure 13.22 Tympanic membrane thermometer.

Procedure guideline 13.7 Temperature measurement

Essential equipment

- Tympanic membrane thermometer
- Disposable probe covers
- Alcohol handrub

Preprocedure

Action	Rationale
1 Explain and discuss procedure with the patient.	To ensure that the patient understands the procedure and gives their valid consent (NMC 2008b, C).
2 Wash and dry hands.	To minimize the risks of cross-infection and contamination (Fraise and Bradley 2009, E).

Procedure

3 Document which ear is used to ensure consecutive readings.	Anatomical differences between the two ears can result in a difference of up to 1°C (Jevon and Jevon 2001, E).
4 Remove thermometer from the base unit and ensure the lens is clean and not cracked. Use a dry wipe to clean if required.	Alcohol-based wipes should not be used as this can lead to a false low temperature measurement (Jevon and Jevon 2001, E).
5 Place disposable probe cover on the probe tip, ensuring the manufacturer's instructions are followed.	The probe cover protects the tip of the probe and is necessary for the functioning of the instrument (Jevon and Jevon 2001, E).
6 Gently place the probe tip in the ear canal to seal the opening, ensuring a snug fit. See Figure 13.22.	To prevent air at the opening of the ear from entering it, causing a false low temperature measurement (Bayham *et al.* 1996, C; Jevon and Jevon 2001, E).
7 Press and release SCAN button.	To commence the scanning (Bayham *et al.* 1996, C).
8 Remove probe tip from the ear as soon as the thermometer display reads DONE, usually indicated by beeps.	To ensure procedure is carried out for allocated time. Measurement is usually complete within 2 seconds (Bayham *et al.* 1996, C).
9 Read the temperature display and document in the patient's records and compare with previous results.	Any interruption in the process may result in the measurement being incorrectly remembered (O'Brien *et al.* 2003, E). Deviations from normal temperature ranges may result in urgent medical/clinical attention (Jevon and Jevon 2001, E; NMC 2008a, C).

Postprocedure

10 Press RELEASE/EJECT button to discard probe cover into domestic waste bin.	Probe covers are for single use only (Jevon and Jevon 2001, E).
11 Wipe thermometer clean and replace in base unit.	To reduce the risk of cross-infection (Fraise and Bradley 2009, E).

Problem-solving table 13.7 Prevention and resolution (Procedure guideline 13.7)

Problem	Cause	Prevention	Action
Thermometer is not working properly, for example 'error' is showing	The battery may be low	At the first level, the low battery sign is lit and approximately 100 more temperatures may be taken	Replace the battery
If the 'wait' indicator is on	Wait indicator will appear if you attempt to take successive temperatures in too short a period of time	Wait briefly until the 'wait' indicator disappears before taking another temperature	Retry and if still instructing to 'wait', send for repair
'Use new cover' showing even though probe cover has been installed.	Probe cover replaced too quickly	Check that probe cover has been fitted correctly	Press RELEASE/EJECT button and reinstall probe cover

Postprocedural considerations
Immediate care
There are different methods for lowering body temperature. Antipyretics, including paracetamol, can mask the function of the hypothalamus by reducing the temperature while hiding the underlying signs of disease (Cuddy 2004). It is thought that these drugs inhibit the inflammatory action of prostaglandins, affecting the hypothalamus by temporarily resetting the thermostat to normal levels. However, these drugs must be used with caution in patients with established liver disease or a history of gastric bleeding as they can cause gastric irritation and put an increased strain on a diseased liver to break down the drug.

Fanning is of benefit for moderate to high pyrexias. Fanning and tepid sponging are not recommended while the patient's temperature is still rising as this will only make the patient feel colder, cause distress (Sharber 1997) and cause the peripheral thermoreceptors to detect a decrease in temperature that leads the hypothalamus to initiate heat-gaining activities such as shivering and peripheral vasoconstriction (Krikler 1990).

Documentation
Recordings of body temperature are an index of biological function and are a valuable indicator of a patient's health.

Urinalysis

Definition
Urinalysis is the analysis of the volume and physical, chemical and microscopic properties of urine (Tortora and Derrickson 2009) and can provide valuable information about a patient's condition, allowing detection of systemic disease and infection (Bishop 2008).

Anatomy and physiology
Urine is formed in the kidneys, which process approximately 180 litres of blood-derived fluid a day. Approximately 1% of this total actually leaves the body as urine, the rest returns to the circulation (Marieb and Hoehn 2010). Urine formation, and the simultaneous adjustment of blood composition, involves three processes (see Figure 13.23):

- glomerular filtration
- tubular reabsorption
- tubular secretion (Marieb and Hoehn 2010).

Glomerular filtration
This occurs in the glomeruli of the kidney, which act as non-selective filters. Filtration occurs as a result of increased glomerular blood pressure caused by the difference in diameter between afferent and efferent arterioles. The effect is a simple mechanical filter that permits substances smaller than plasma proteins to pass from the glomeruli to the glomerular capsule (Marieb and Hoehn 2010).

Tubular reabsorption
Tubular reabsorption then occurs, removing necessary substances from the filtrate and returning them to the peritubular capillaries. Tubular reabsorption is an active process that requires protein carriers and energy. Substances reabsorbed include nutrients and most ions. It is also a passive process, however, driven by electrochemical gradients. Substances reabsorbed in this way include sodium ions and water. Creatinine and the metabolites of drugs are not reabsorbed because of their size, insolubility or a lack of carriers. Most

797

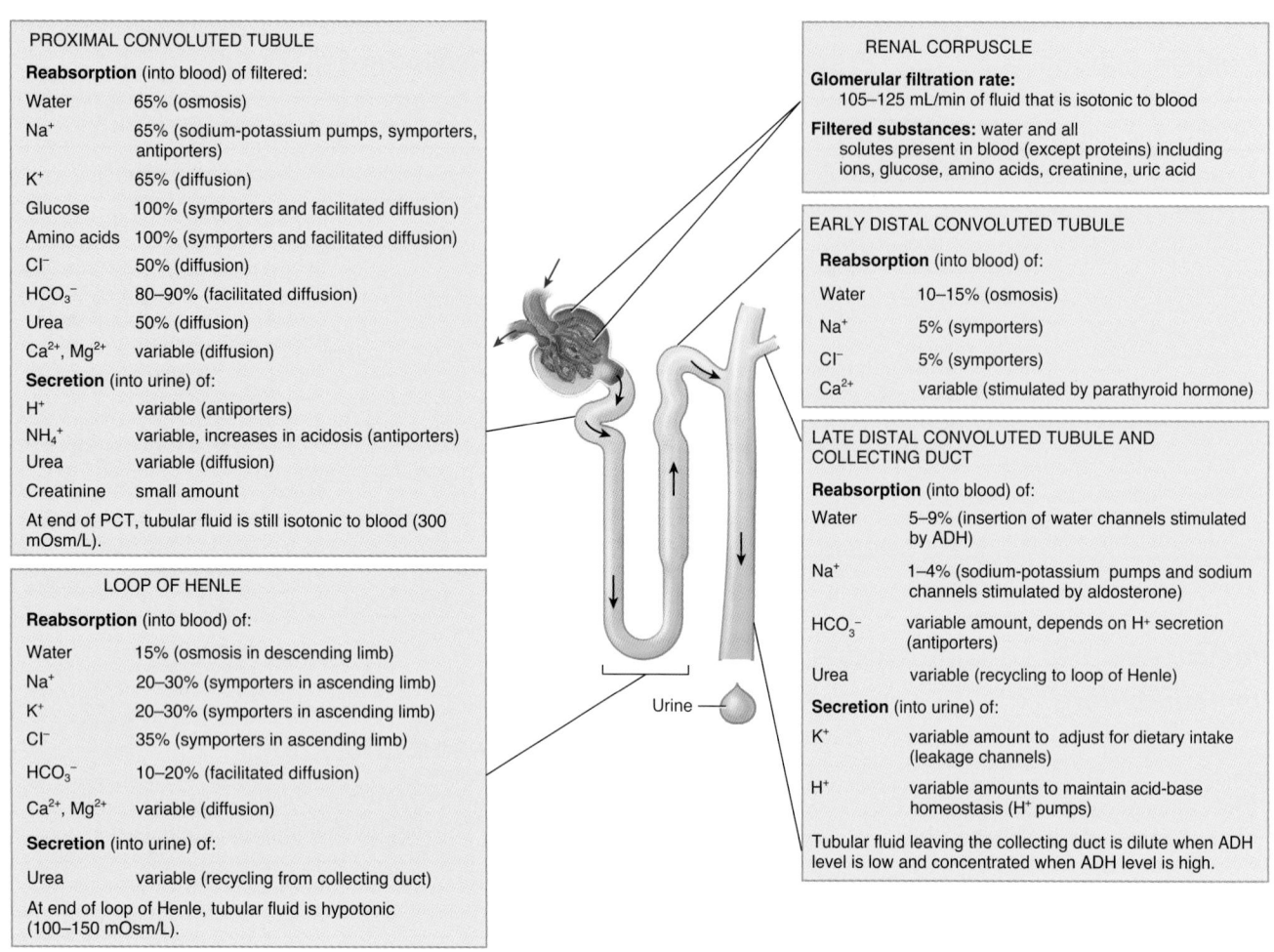

PROXIMAL CONVOLUTED TUBULE

Reabsorption (into blood) of filtered:

Water	65% (osmosis)
Na$^+$	65% (sodium-potassium pumps, symporters, antiporters)
K$^+$	65% (diffusion)
Glucose	100% (symporters and facilitated diffusion)
Amino acids	100% (symporters and facilitated diffusion)
Cl$^-$	50% (diffusion)
HCO$_3^-$	80–90% (facilitated diffusion)
Urea	50% (diffusion)
Ca^{2+}, Mg^{2+}	variable (diffusion)

Secretion (into urine) of:

H$^+$	variable (antiporters)
NH$_4^+$	variable, increases in acidosis (antiporters)
Urea	variable (diffusion)
Creatinine	small amount

At end of PCT, tubular fluid is still isotonic to blood (300 mOsm/L).

LOOP OF HENLE

Reabsorption (into blood) of:

Water	15% (osmosis in descending limb)
Na$^+$	20–30% (symporters in ascending limb)
K$^+$	20–30% (symporters in ascending limb)
Cl$^-$	35% (symporters in ascending limb)
HCO$_3^-$	10–20% (facilitated diffusion)
Ca^{2+}, Mg^{2+}	variable (diffusion)

Secretion (into urine) of:

Urea	variable (recycling from collecting duct)

At end of loop of Henle, tubular fluid is hypotonic (100–150 mOsm/L).

RENAL CORPUSCLE

Glomerular filtration rate:
105–125 mL/min of fluid that is isotonic to blood

Filtered substances: water and all solutes present in blood (except proteins) including ions, glucose, amino acids, creatinine, uric acid

EARLY DISTAL CONVOLUTED TUBULE

Reabsorption (into blood) of:

Water	10–15% (osmosis)
Na$^+$	5% (symporters)
Cl$^-$	5% (symporters)
Ca^{2+}	variable (stimulated by parathyroid hormone)

LATE DISTAL CONVOLUTED TUBULE AND COLLECTING DUCT

Reabsorption (into blood) of:

Water	5–9% (insertion of water channels stimulated by ADH)
Na$^+$	1–4% (sodium-potassium pumps and sodium channels stimulated by aldosterone)
HCO$_3^-$	variable amount, depends on H$^+$ secretion (antiporters)
Urea	variable (recycling to loop of Henle)

Secretion (into urine) of:

K$^+$	variable amount to adjust for dietary intake (leakage channels)
H$^+$	variable amounts to maintain acid-base homeostasis (H$^+$ pumps)

Tubular fluid leaving the collecting duct is dilute when ADH level is low and concentrated when ADH level is high.

Urine

Figure 13.23 Summary of filtration, reabsorption and secretion in the nephron and collecting duct. Reproduced from Tortora and Derrickson (2009).

of the nutrients, 65% of the water and sodium ions, and the majority of actively transported ions are reabsorbed in the proximal convoluted tubules (Marieb and Hoehn 2010).

Reabsorption of additional sodium ions and water occurs in the distal tubules and collecting ducts and is hormonally controlled. Aldosterone increases the reabsorption of sodium, and antidiuretic hormone (ADH) enhances water reabsorption by the collecting ducts (Marieb and Hoehn 2010).

Tubular secretion

Tubular secretion is an active process that is important in eliminating drugs, certain wastes and excess ions and in maintaining the acid/base balance of blood (Marieb and Hoehn 2010).

Regulation of urine concentration and volume occurs in the loop of Henle, where the osmolarity of the filtrate is controlled. As the filtrate flows through the tubules, the permeability of the walls controls how dilute or concentrated the resulting urine will be. In the absence of ADH, dilute urine is formed because the filtrate is not reabsorbed as it passes through the kidneys. As levels of ADH increase, the collecting tubules become more permeable to water, and water moves out of the filtrate back into the blood. Consequently, more concentrated urine is produced, and in smaller amounts (Marieb and Hoehn 2010).

Urine is a clear, straw-coloured fluid. The normal composition of urine includes water, urea, creatinine, sodium, potassium, organic acids, protein, small traces of glucose and cellular components. The colour of urine is due to a pigment called urochrome which is derived from the body's destruction of haemoglobin. The more concentrated urine, the deeper yellow it becomes. An abnormal colour such as pink or brown may result from eating certain foods (beetroot or rhubarb), or may be due to the presence in the urine of bile products or blood (Marieb and Hoehn 2010). Often fresh urine appears turbid (cloudy), indicating that there may be an infection of the urinary tract. The urinary tract is the most common site of bacterial infection. Risk factors for urinary tract infections (UTI) include presence of a urinary catheter, female gender, diabetes and advanced age (Marini and Wheeler 2010). See Figure 13.24 for other UTI predisposing factors.

Age
Underlying
diseases
predisposing
to UTI –
diabetes,
prostatitis,
incontinence

Anatomical
reasons: renal
calculi

Obstructions and
reflux: pregnancy,
bladder stones

Women are more at
risk than men because
of a short urethra

Prostate hypertrophy

Catheterization

Sexual activity

Figure 13.24 Predisposition to UTIs.

Bacteriuria is defined as the presence of bacteria in the urine (Rigby and Gray 2005). Urine specimens are rarely sterile, as a result of contamination with periurethral flora during collection. Infection is distinguished by counting the number of bacteria. Significant bacteriuria is defined as the presence of more than 10^5 organisms per mL of urine in the presence of clinical symptoms (Marini and Wheeler 2010). See Figure 13.25 for illustration of significant bacteriuria.

Fresh urine is slightly aromatic. This can change as a result of disease processes such as diabetes mellitus, when acetone is present in the urine, giving it a fruity smell (Marieb and Hoehn 2010). The composition of urine can change dramatically as a result of disease, and abnormal substances may be present. Urinalysis can identify many of

these substances, and should be part of every physical assessment (Cook 1996, Torrance and Elley 1998).

Evidence-based approaches

Rationale

Urinalysis (urine testing) is commonly undertaken in general practice, being one of a range of assessment and screening procedures, such as new patient registration, screening for diabetes mellitus and testing for infections and pregnancy.

Indications

The composition of urine can change dramatically as a result of disease processes. It may contain red blood cells, glucose, proteins, white blood cells or bile (Marieb and Hoehn 2010). It can reveal diseases that have gone unnoticed because they do not produce striking symptoms, and may also be used in ongoing management of conditions (Higgins, 2008).

- *Screening*: for systemic disease, for example, diabetes mellitus or renal conditions.
- *Diagnosis*: to confirm or exclude suspected conditions, for example urinary tract infection.
- *Management and planning*: to ascertain as a baseline, monitor progress of an existing condition and/or plan programme of care and medication (Wilson 2005).

Methods of urinalysis

Renal clearance refers to the volume of plasma that is cleared of a particular substance in a given time, usually 1 minute. Renal clearance tests are done to determine the glomerular filtration

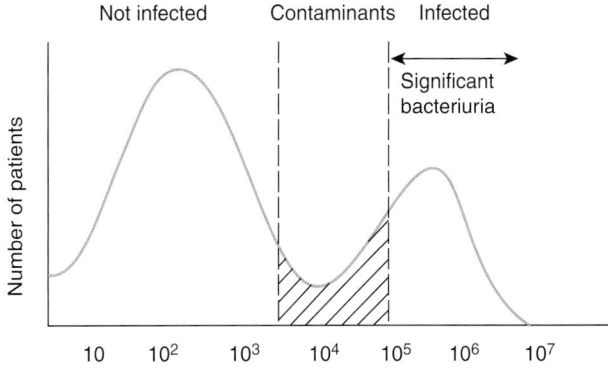

Figure 13.25 Significant bacteriuria. Specimens of urine are rarely sterile. A cut-off point is identified to distinguish true infection (significant bacteriuria) from effects of contamination from surrounding tissues.

Table 13.7 Routine observations of urine: possible indications and plan of action

Observation	Possible indications	Plan of action
Colour		
Green	*Pseudomonas* infection, presence of bilirubin	Culture and microscopy
	Excretion of cytotoxic agents, for example mitomycin, or substances, for example methylene blue	Discard with care
Pink/Red	Blood	Culture and microscopy. If currently receiving chemotherapy, for example ifosfamide, further mesna may need to be given
	Excretion of cytotoxic agents, for example doxorubicin	Discard with care
Orange	Excess urobiliogen, rifampicin	Discard
Yellow	Bilirubin	Discard
Brown	Bilirubin	Discard
Odour		
Fishy	Infection	Culture and microscopy
Sweet smelling	Ketones	Culture and microscopy
Debris		
Cloudy	Infection, stale urine	Culture and microscopy
Sediment	Infection, contamination	Culture and microscopy

Modified from Rigby and Gray (2005) with kind permission from *Nursing Times*.

rate (GFR), which allows us to detect glomerular damage and follow the progress of renal disease (Marieb and Hoehn 2010).

In the microbiology laboratory, urine samples constitute about 40% of the total workload; of these, 70–80% of samples are not infected. This means that much time, energy and finances are wasted on unnecessary sample processing and investigation (Bayer Diagnostics 1997).

Further testing may be necessary, such as culture and sensitivity testing under laboratory conditions, to identify organisms responsible for infection and to determine the most effective treatment (Wilson 2005) (Table 13.7). Twenty-four hour collection is also used to measure substances such as steroids, white cells and electrolytes or to determine urine osmolarity (Tortora and Derrickson 2009).

Before using a reagent strip to analyse a sample of urine, the following observations should be made.

- Colour.
- Clarity.
- Odour.

These properties should be considered with reference to clinical condition, urine output and fluid balance records over the past 24 hours.

The following factors can affect the analysis of results.

- Bilirubin and urobilinogen are relatively unstable compounds when subjected to light and at room temperature, so it is important to use fresh urine to obtain the most accurate result.
- Exposure of unpreserved urine at room temperature for a considerable period of time may result in an increase in micro-organisms in the urine and change in pH.

- Bacterial growth of contaminated organisms in urine may produce a positive blood reaction.
- Urine that is high in alkaline may show false-positive results in respect of presence of protein.
- Glucose in urine may reduce its pH as a result of metabolism of glucose by organisms present in the urine.
- The presence of urea-splitting organisms that convert urea to ammonia may cause urine to become more alkaline.

(Wilson 2005)

Preprocedural considerations

Equipment

Dipstick (reagent) tests

Strips that have been impregnated with chemicals are dipped quickly in urine and read. When dipped in urine, the chemicals react with abnormal substances and change colour. Although dipstick reagents have been primarily used as screening tools for protein or glucose in the urine, more sophisticated reagents are now available. These reagents test for nitrites and leucocyte esterase as indicators of bacterial infection. Leucocyte esterase is an enzyme from neutrophils not normally found in urine and is a marker of infection. Nitrites are produced by the bacterial breakdown of dietary nitrate, which is a waste product of protein metabolism (Rigby and Gray 2005). It is essential to use the strips according to the manufacturer's instructions and be aware of factors that may affect the results, including specific drugs (Table 13.8), the quality of the urine specimen itself and the possibility of false-negative results.

Table 13.8 How drugs may influence the results of reagent sticks

Drug	Reagent test	Effect on the results
Ascorbic acid	Glucose, blood, nitrite	High concentrations may diminish colour
L-Dopa	Glucose	High concentrations may give a false-negative reaction
	Ketones	Atypical colour
Nalidixic acid	Urobilinogen	Atypical colour – probenacid
Phenazopyridine (pyridium)	Protein	May give atypical colour
	Ketones	Coloured metabolites may mask a small reaction
	Urobilinogen, bilirubin	May mimic a positive reaction
	Nitrite	
Rifampicin	Bilirubin	Coloured metabolites may mask a small reaction
Salicylates (aspirin)	Glucose	High doses may give a false-negative reaction

Specific patient preparations
Education

Most patients need advice on hygiene and technique before the procedure to prevent contamination from hands or the genital area (Higgins 2008) and to ensure that the midstream sample is collected correctly. Midstream urine specimens are indicated in adults and children who are continent and can empty their bladder on request (Gilbert 2006).

Procedure guideline 13.8 Urinalysis: reagent strip procedure

Essential equipment

- Non-sterile disposable gloves
- Apron
- Urine dipsticks, that are in date; make sure they have been stored according to the manufacturer's recommendations
- Appropriate urine specimen pot

Preprocedure

Action	Rationale
1 Explain and discuss the procedure with the patient.	To ensure that the patient understands the procedure and gives their valid consent (NMC 2008b, C).
2 If taking the specimen from a urinary catheter it should be collected using an aseptic technique.	To avoid contamination (Fraise and Bradley 2009, E).
3 Wash and dry hands and put on gloves and apron.	To maintain infection control and prevent cross-infection (Fraise and Bradley 2009, E).

Procedure

4 Obtain clean specimen of fresh urine from patient.	Urine that has been stored deteriorates rapidly and can give false results (Bayer Diagnostics 2006, C).
5 Check reagent sticks have been stored in accordance with manufacturer's instructions. This is usually a dark dry place.	Tests may depend on enzymic reaction. To ensure reliable results (Bayer Diagnostics 2006, C).
6 Dip the reagent strip into the urine. The strip should be completely immersed in the urine and then removed immediately. Run edge of strip along the container. This will remove excess urine and prevent mixing of chemicals from adjacent reagent areas.	To remove any excess urine (Bayer Diagnostics 2006, C).

(Continued)

801

Procedure guideline 13.8 *(Continued)*

7 Hold the stick at an angle.	Urine reagent strips should not be held upright when reading them because urine may run from square to square, mixing various reagents (Bayer Diagnostics 2006, C).
8 Wait the required time interval before reading the strip against the colour chart (see Action Figure 8).	The strips must be read at exactly the time interval specified or the reagents will not have time to react, or may be inaccurate (Bayer Diagnostics 2006, C).

Postprocedure

9 Dispose of urine sample appropriately in either sluice or toilet. Dispose of urinalysis stick and gloves in correct wastage bin. Ensure cap to urine reagent strips is replaced immediately and closed tightly.	To ensure strips are in airtight container according to storage guidelines. C
10 Wash and dry hands.	To maintain infection control and prevent cross-infection (Fraise and Bradley 2009, E).
11 Document urinalysis readings and inform medical staff of any abnormal readings.	To allow prompt action if change to treatment plan required (NMC 2009, C).

Action Figure 8 Compare urinalysis results and document results on appropriate forms.

Postprocedural considerations

When sending a urine specimen to the laboratory, check that the laboratory form is completed and that all relevant information is included. Take care not to contaminate the outside of the container or the request forms (Bishop 2008).

Reagent strips are a quick and easy method of testing urine and can provide valuable information about a patient's condition. However, patients should be made aware that further tests and investigations may be required if the urine sample indicates any abnormality (Steggall 2007).

Blood glucose

Definition

Blood glucose is the amount of glucose in the blood (Brooker 2010). See Table 13.9 for normal target ranges,

which are expressed as millimoles per litre (mmol/L) (NICE 2004).

Normally blood glucose levels stay within narrow limits throughout the day: 4–8 mmol/L. But they are higher after meals and usually lowest in the morning.

Anatomy and physiology

Blood glucose is regulated by insulin and glucogon. Insulin is synthesized and secreted from the beta cells within the islets

Table 13.9 Normal target blood glucose ranges

Children ≤18 years of age	Adults >18 years of age
Preprandial blood glucose levels 4–8 mmol/L	Preprandial blood glucose levels 4–7 mmol/L
Postprandial blood glucose levels of less than 10 mmol/L	Postprandial blood glucose levels of less than 9 mmol/L

Reproduced with permission from NICE (2004); www.nice.org.uk/guidance/CG15.

of Langerhans found in the pancreas (Wallymahmed 2007). It is produced in response to high blood glucose levels (i.e. after meals) promoting the uptake and storage of sugar by fat and muscle tissue as glycogen (Crosser and McDowell 2007). Glucagon is secreted by the alpha cells in response to low blood glucose levels and results in the release of stored sugar back into the blood (Wallymahmed 2007). These processes maintain the blood glucose stability within the body (homoeostasis) (Crosser and McDowell 2007).

Diabetes mellitus (DM) is a heterogeneous disorder characterized by chronic hyperglycaemia due to lack of insulin or complete insulin deficiency or the body's resistance to it (Blake and Nathan 2004, WHO 2006). There are two main types of DM: type 1 and type 2. Type 1 is believed to be triggered by an autoimmune process causing destruction of the beta cells in the pancreas, which produce insulin, resulting in complete loss of insulin production. Type 2 diabetes is characterized by a resistance to insulin (Thornton 2009).

People with type 1 or type 2 diabetes will have total or partial disruption to this normal metabolic regulatory system. Type 1 diabetes normally occurs in the younger population (Gillibrand et al. 2009) and means that they will need replacement injected insulin to compensate (Crosser and McDowell 2007). Type 2 diabetes is strongly linked to obesity, age and family history (Gillibrand et al. 2009) but can also be a result of steroid use and pancreatic cancer (Schwab and Porter 2007). Both these can result in hyperglycaemia (high blood glucose) which may cause degenerative changes affecting the kidneys, nerves and eyes (Wallymahmed 2007), resulting in blindness, renal failure and neuropathies. Further complications including coronary artery and peripheral vascular disease, stroke, renal disease, central and peripheral nerve damage, amputations and blindness are also serious consequences of uncontrolled blood glucose (Gillibrand et al. 2009, WHO 2006).

A diagnosis of diabetes can primarily be based on a fasting blood glucose of more than or equal to 7 mmol/L or a random plasma glucose of more than or equal to 11.1 mmol/L accompanied by symptoms associated with diabetes such as polydipsia, polyuria and weight loss (Blake and Nathan 2004, WHO 2006). These features of diabetes do not appear until 80% of beta cells are lost and so it is possible to reverse type 2 diabetes if it is picked up early enough (Schwab and Porter 2007).

Furthermore, during infection, major surgery or critical illness such as sepsis, pancreatitis or respiratory distress, counter-regulatory or stress hormones (adrenaline, noradrenaline, cortisol, growth hormone and glucagon) are released causing significant metabolic alterations. These hormones increase insulin resistance which decreases peripheral intake of glucose and also promotes glucogenesis by stimulating glycogen and fat breakdown, causing hyperglycaemia (Crosser and McDowell 2007). For this reason patients with diabetes may need treatment of insulin or antidiabetic medication during acute illness, in order to replicate this homoeostasis or improve the body's ability to produce insulin or use it.

Hyperglycaemia

Hyperglycaemia is defined as a random blood glucose of more than 11.1 mmol/L (WHO 2006). When insulin is deficient or absent as in type 1 or 2 diabetes, blood glucose levels will remain high after a meal, in times of illness or stress because it is unable to enter most cells (Wallymahmed 2007). Therefore cells are starved of glucose and the body reacts inappropriately by producing stress hormones that cause glycogenolysis (the breakdown of glycogen to release glucose), lipolysis (the breakdown of stored fat into glycerol and fatty acids) and gluconeogenesis (the conversion of glycerol and amino acids into glucose) (D'Hondt 2008, Marieb and Hoehn 2010) (see Figure 13.26).

This causes the blood glucose to rise further which results in a number of signs and symptoms. Water reabsorption in the kidneys becomes inhibited, resulting in frequent, large volumes of urine (polyuria). This will cause the person to feel excessive thirst (polydipsia) and may also result in extreme hunger (polyphagia). Polyuria and polydipsia will cause dehydration, a fall in blood pressure and electrolyte imbalance (Marini and Wheeler 2010). Moreover, the subsequent loss of sodium (hyponatraemia) and potassium (hypokalaemia) leads to muscle cramps, nausea, vomiting and diarrhoea, confusion, blurred vision, lethargy, cardiac events, coma and death.

Despite the excessive glucose in the body, the body cannot utilize it, so the body starts to break down its fat and protein stores for energy, which leads to high levels of fatty acids in the blood (lipidaemia) (Marieb and Hoehn 2010). This can also cause sudden and dramatic weight loss. These fatty acids are converted to ketones. They accumulate in the blood more quickly than they can be excreted or used and cause the blood pH to fall, resulting in ketoacidosis. Ketones will also be present in the urine. If ketoacidosis is allowed to continue it can become life threatening, disrupting all physiological processes, including oxygen transportation and heart activity and depression of the nervous system, leading to coma and death (Marieb and Hoehn 2010).

Reasons for hyperglyceamia include:

- inadequate doses of insulin
- stress
- infection/sepsis
- surgery
- medications, for example steroids
- nutritional support, for example parenteral nutrition (PN) or enteral nutrition.

It has been found that enteral and parenteral feeding contributes to hyperglycaemia in both patients with a diagnosis of diabetes and those without (McNight and Carter 2008). This is particularly true of patients receiving PN which bypasses the gut and therefore the incretin hormones that also help to maintain glucose homoeostasis (McNight and Carter 2008). Hyperglycaemia in response to steroids, for example dexamethasone, is another consideration and some researchers believe that their hypermetabolic action

Organs/tissue involved	Organ/tissue responses to insulin deficiency	Resulting conditions		Signs and symptoms
		In blood	In urine	
	Decreased glucose uptake and utilization	Hyperglycaemia	Glycosuria	
	Glycogenolysis		Osmotic diuresis	Polydipsia (and fatigue, weight loss)
	Protein catabolism and gluconeogenesis			Polyphagia
	Lipolysis and ketogenesis	Lipidaemia and ketoacidosis	Ketonuria	Acetone breath
				Hyperpnoea
			Loss of Na$^+$, K$^+$; electrolyte and acid–base imbalances	Nausea/vomiting/abdominal pain
				Cardiac irregularities
				Central nervous system depression; coma

= Muscle   = Adipose tissue   = Liver

Figure 13.26   Consequences of insulin deficiency.

decreases glucose uptake, increases hepatic glucose production and may directly inhibit insulin release (Delaunay et al. 1997, Ogawa et al. 1992, Wallymahmed 2007). For this reason these patients will need blood glucose monitoring and potential changes to their insulin needs or to temporarily commence insulin.

Hypoglycaemia

Hypoglycaemia is described as a blood glucose level that is unable to meet the metabolic needs of the body (Marini and Wheeler 2010), normally lower than 4 mmol/L (Wallymahmed 2007). Often young, healthy individuals can be asymptomatic during this inadequate level of glucose in the blood but early symptoms can be sweating, tremor, weakness, nervousness, tachycardia and hypertension (Wallymahmed 2007), although these depend on not only the absolute blood glucose but also its rate of decline (Tortora and Derrickson 2009). Severe hypoglycaemia can lead to mental disorientation, convulsions, unconsciousness and death but a blood glucose less than 3 mmol can start to affect the brain.

The most common causes of hypoglycaemia are missed or delayed meals, not eating enough, exercise without carbohydrate compensation, too much glucose-lowering medication (e.g. insulin) and excessive alcohol (Wallymahmed 2007). Other causes could be infection, muscle and fat depletion (e.g. anorexia), diarrhoea and vomiting, hepatic failure due to tumour or cirrhosis, salicylate poisoning, insulin-secreting tumours, ventilation, congestive heart failure, cerebral vascular accident, concurrent medications (beta-blockers, adrenaline) and surgery (D'Hondt 2008, Marini and Wheeler 2010).

Treatment should ideally be the administration of glucose. The route will depend on the consciousness level of the patient, their treatment and their ability to take oral substances (Marini and Wheeler 2010). If they can tolerate an oral or enteral intake they should be given a fast-acting carbohydrate such as 3–6 glucose tablets, 150 mL sugary fizzy drink or 50–100 mL Lucozade followed by a longer acting carbohydrate such as a sandwich or biscuits. If unconscious or unable to take food and drink then they can receive intramuscular glucagon or intravenous dextrose (Wallymahmed 2007). Blood glucose needs to be checked 5–10 minutes after treatment and then as necessary. Diabetic treatment should not be omitted because of a single episode of hypoglycaemia, but if it remains a consistent problem treatment should be reviewed (Wallymahmed 2007).

Evidence-based approaches
Rationale

Blood glucose monitoring provides an accurate indication of how the body is controlling glucose metabolism and provides feedback to guide clinicians and patients about their treatment adjustments in order to achieve optimal glucose control. In the short term it can prevent hypo- and hyperglycaemia and in the long term it can significantly reduce the risk of prolonged, life-threatening microvascular complications (Rizvi and Saunders 2006).

Capillary blood glucose monitoring is preferred due to immediacy of results and its ability to inform us whether blood sugar is high or low, whereas urine testing only indicates instances of high blood sugar (Wallymahmed 2007).

Capillary blood glucose monitoring is also referred to as point-of-care testing (POCT).

Indications

Conditions in which blood glucose monitoring will need to take place include the following.

- To make a diagnosis of diabetes indicated by signs and symptoms of polyuria, polydipsia, weightloss for type 1 or weight gain, family history for type 2 (WHO 2006).
- To monitor and manage the day-to-day treatment of known type 1 and type 2 diabetes (Wallymahmed 2007).
- In acute management of unstable diabetes, that is, evidence of hyperglycaemia, hypoglycaemia, diabetic ketoacidosis, hyperosmolar non-ketonic coma (once severe dehydration is corrected) (Wallymahmed 2007).
- Hospitalized patients with diabetes according to morbidity and treatment, that is, sliding scales, nutritional intake/support (McNight and Carter 2008, Wallymahmed 2007).
- Initial parenteral and enteral nutritional support of all patients (McNight and Carter 2008).
- Patients taking steroids and other drugs that cause raised blood glucose (Schwab and Porter 2007).

Contraindications

The following conditions can affect the accuracy of blood glucose monitoring and it may be necessary to obtain a venous sample for more accurate results (DH 2005).

- Peripheral circulatory failure and severe dehydration, for example diabetic ketoacidosis, hyperosmolor non-ketotic coma, shock, hypotension. These conditions cause peripheral shutdown, which can cause artificially low capillary readings.
- Haematocrit values above 55% may lead to inaccurate levels if the blood glucose level is more than 11 mmol/L.
- Intravenous infusion of ascorbic acid.
- Pre-eclampsia.
- Some renal dialysis treatments.
- Hyperlipidaemia: cholesterol levels above 13 mmol/L may lead to artificially raised capillary blood glucose readings.

Principles of care

Although capillary blood glucose monitoring is an essential part of diabetic management, it can have severe consequences if not done correctly (Wallymahmed 2007). The Department of Health issued a hazard warning in 1987 and a safety notice in 1996 highlighting the need for formal training and strict quality control (DH 1996).

Blood glucose monitoring needs to be performed regularly enough for patterns to be established on which treatment changes can be based (Walker 2004). 'Regularly' will vary in different circumstances and any unusual situation, for example illness, change of daily routine, hospitalization, will affect diabetes control and therefore require more frequent testing (Walker 2004). Generally people with type 1 diabetes will need to test blood glucose several times a day or more depending on treatment while those with type 2 will require less testing due to a lower risk of such great fluctuations in blood glucose levels (Goldie 2008). The following list provides guidance on frequency and timing of blood glucose monitoring depending on the type of diabetes and its treatment.

- *Type 1 diabetes:* four or more times daily; more often in unusual circumstances, for example impaired hypoglycaemia awareness, illness, terminal care.
- *Type 2 diabetes (intensive insulin treatment):* as type 1 diabetes.
- *Type 2 diabetes (conventional insulin):* once per day on once-daily insulin; twice per day on twice-daily insulin.
- *Type 2 diabetes (insulin and oral treatment):* one test a day if on daily insulin or more if control fluctuates.
- *Type 2 diabetes (diet and exercise; metformin +/− glitazone, glitazone +/− metformin):* routine testing not required as low risk of hypoglycaemia.
- *Type 2 diabetes (sulphonylurea alone or in combination with other oral hypoglycaemic agents):* test at least three times a week to detect any unknown hypoglycaemia.

(Owens *et al.* 2004)

In all the above types of diabetes more regular testing will be required in certain circumstances, for example illness, steroid treatment, changes in diet, exercise and routine (Owens *et al.* 2004).

For all patients (irrespective of previous diabetic diagnosis) receiving nutritional support, that is enteral or parenteral feeding, blood glucose levels should be checked once or twice daily (or more if needed) until stable and then weekly (NICE 2008).

Methods of blood glucose testing

Blood glucose testing involves obtaining a drop of capillary blood and putting it on a testing strip that is read by a blood glucose meter (Goldie 2008). Most meters offer the option of using blood from the finger tips, palm of the hand, upper arm, forearm, calf or thigh (Dale 2006). The most commonly used site is the finger tip as the blood from this area responds rapidly to changes in blood glucose level, as does the blood from the palm of the hand, and therefore delivers the most accurate results (Dale 2006, Goldie 2008). However, the finger tips contain nerve endings which can become sore and less sensitive with frequent testing. The outer parts of the finger are less painful to prick and the thumb and forefinger should be used sparingly due to their continual use in apposition (Goldie 2008). It is important to rotate areas used for blood glucose testing to avoid infection from multiple stabbings, areas becoming toughened and to reduce pain (Roche Diagnostics 2004).

Anticipated patient outcomes

There have been several trials investigating the benefits of tight glycaemic control to near normal levels. D'Hondt (2008) refers to three randomized controlled trials in which intensive insulin treatment was used in hospitalized patients. The trials showed that intensive insulin treatment to achieve tight glycaemic control did result in reductions in length of stay, sepsis, dialysis and hospital mortality and morbidity (Furnary *et al.* 2000, Krinsley 2004, van den Berghe *et al.* 2001). Blood glucose testing is integral to achieving this tight control but there is currently no absolute conclusion for the standardization of this treatment (D'Hondt 2008). It does, however, indicate that keeping blood sugar levels as near normal as possible should be the ultimate aim of blood glucose testing.

Legal and professional issues

The DH report (1996) highlights that there must be standardization in training, reliability and quality control for blood glucose testing. In order to achieve this, the following aspects must be considered when selecting monitoring devices.

1 Equipment is designed for use by non-laboratory staff and is suitable for use in the clinical environment.
2 All equipment is compatible and will give reliable results.
3 The biochemistry laboratory is involved in the purchase and maintenance of the equipment. This may involve the purchase of one type of device from one company for the whole hospital, to reduce costs and provide standardization (Lowe 1995).
4 The equipment should be easy to use and the staff should be involved in the choice of device (Hall 2005).
5 The ongoing cost and maintenance of the device need to be considered, including buying strips, control solutions and replacement devices (Hall 2005).
6 Written standard operating procedures should be available and kept with the device.
7 Training is given to the operators of the equipment and records are kept of this. After training, the following learning outcomes should be demonstrated by the operator (MDA 2002):
   – knowledge of the basic principles of measurement and normal ranges
   – the proper use of equipment as stated by the operating instructions
   – the consequences of incorrect use
   – health and safety procedures for the collection of blood samples, that is, to prevent spillage and needlestick injuries
   – the importance of complete documentation
   – use of appropriate calibration and quality control techniques
   – an understanding that blood sugar analysis should only be used as a guide to diagnosis and treatment and decisions should be made formally with laboratory results (DH 1996).

It is a hospital and government directive to keep records of training and quality testing results and the frequency of these quality control tests may vary according to manufacturer or hospital policy (Walker 2004). Independent quality control should be carried out with the collaboration of the biochemistry laboratory and external auditing of quality control should be undertaken, which may be provided by the company providing the equipment.

Preprocedural considerations

Equipment

All equipment should be checked for expiry dates (according to individual hospital trust policy) and successful calibration, and stored according to manufacturer's guidelines.

- *Blood glucose monitor*: a medical device which measures the concentration of glucose in a human blood sample using a blood glucose test strip (Roche Diagnostics 2004).
- *Testing strip*: strip with a small window used to collect a sample of the patient's blood to be inserted into the blood glucose monitor. The strips must be calibrated with the monitor prior to use (Roche Diagnostics 2004)
- *Lancet*: a device used to draw out a small amount of blood from the patient for testing of glucose level. Single-use lancets are used to minimize the risk of cross-infection and accidental needlestick injury and set to the correct depth according to the skin turgor (Roche Diagnostics 2004). Disposable lancets are advisable following an outbreak of hepatitis B in French and US hospitals (DH 1996, Roche Diagnostics 2004).

Specific patient preparations

Patients should be advised to wash their hands prior to testing or the test area should be cleaned with soap and water and then dried. Use of alcohol gel should be avoided to ensure non-contamination of the result. The patient should be encouraged to warm their hands before sampling to encourage blood flow and to obtain an adequate amount of blood to cover the test strip (Dale 2006, Wallymahmed 2007).

Procedure guideline 13.9 Blood glucose monitoring

- Blood glucose monitor
- Test strips
- Control solution
- Single-use safety lancets

- Gloves
- Cotton wool/gauze
- Sharps box

Preprocedure

Action	Rationale
1 Before taking the device to the patient, the monitor needs to be checked for the following: - Testing trips are in date and have not been left exposed to air - The monitor and test strips have been calibrated together - If a new pack of strips is required, the monitor is recalibrated - Internal quality control carried out in accordance to trust guidelines - Result of internal quality control is recorded in equipment log book and signed.	To ensure accuracy of the result and ensure patient safety (Roche Diagnostics 2004, C).
2 Explain procedure to the patient.	The patient should give consent to the procedure. Explanation may allay any fear or anxieties (NMC 2008b, C).

Procedure

Action	Rationale
3 Ask patient to sit or lie down.	To ensure the patient's safety and minimize the risks if they feel faint when blood is taken (Roche Diagnostics 2004, C).
4 Wash hands and put on gloves.	To minimize the risk of cross-infection and contamination (Fraise and Bradley 2009, E).
5 Take a single-use lancet and if it has depth settings, ensure the correct setting is used (most commonly middle one).	To minimize the risk of cross-infection and accidental needlestick injury (Fraise and Bradley 2009, E).
6 Take a blood sample from the side of the finger using the lancet, ensuring that the site of piercing is rotated (see Action Figure 6). Avoid frequent use of index finger and thumb. Other areas may be used if finger or palm of hand unusable. The finger tip may need 'milking' from palm of hand towards finger to gain a large enough droplet of blood.	The side of the finger is less painful and easier to obtain a hanging droplet of blood. Sites are rotated to avoid infection from multiple stabbings, area becoming toughened and to reduce pain (Roche Diagnostics 2004, C).
7 Insert testing strip into blood glucose monitor and apply the blood to the testing strip. Some strips are hydrophilic and are dosed/filled from the side instead of dropping blood directly onto the strip. Ensure that the window on the test strip is entirely covered with blood (see Action Figure 7).	The window on the test strip allows verification of a correctly dosed strip which needs to be covered to ensure accurate results (Blake and Nathan 2004, E; Roche Diagnostics 2004, C).
8 Insert testing strip into blood glucose monitor.	To initiate the process of analysis. E

(Continued)

Procedure guideline 13.9 *(Continued)*

9 Dispose of lancet in a sharps container.	To reduce the risk of needlestick injury (Roche Diagnostics 2004, C).
10 Place gauze over puncture site and monitor for excess bleeding.	To ensure patient safety (Wallymahmed 2007, C).

Postprocedure

11 Once result is obtained (see Action Figure 11), document and sign.	To ensure accuracy (NMC 2009, C; Roche Diagnostics 2004, C).
12 Report any unexpected results.	To ensure appropriate treatment and obtain optimal blood glucose range (Wallymahmed 2007, E).

Action Figure 6   Blood glucose taking: Step 1. Take a blood sample from the side of the finger using a lancet, ensuring that the site of piercing is rotated.

Action Figure 7   Blood glucose taking: Step 2. Insert the test strip into the blood glucose monitor and apply the blood to the test strip. Ensure that the window on the test strip is entirely covered with blood.

Action Figure 11   Blood glucose taking: Step 3. Read the result.

Problem-solving table 13.8 Prevention and resolution (Procedure guideline 13.9)

Problem	Cause	Prevention	Action
Inaccurate results	User error including: ■ inadequate meter calibration ■ failure to code correctly ■ poor meter maintenance ■ incorrect user technique 50% of errors are due to an inadequate amount of blood on the test strip, which can lead to a falsely low reading (Blake and Nathan 2004). Out of date or incorrectly stored test strips are other common errors leading to lower glucose levels	Staff training and education about diabetes are essential in prevention of these errors (D'Hondt 2008)	Contact colleague to repeat test and if error persists, report glucose meter to technician and use another machine

Postprocedural considerations

Immediate care

If a true abnormal blood glucose result is detected then the appropriate action should be taken according to medical advice and hospital policy.

Education of patient and relevant others

Diabetes mellitus is a long-term, often lifelong condition affecting all aspects of a person's life. Ninety-five percent of diabetes care is self-care and all people with type 1 and type 2 diabetes should have access to self-monitoring. The nurse has a role in educating and promoting self-management of diabetes and advising patients on the type and frequency of monitoring based on individual clinical need so that patients can monitor and adjust their own treatment (Diabetes UK 2008). NICE and the Department of Health also recommend that people are given annual updates to ensure they are still able to perform tests accurately and learn about any new developments (DH 2008, NICE 2004, NICE 2008). Healthcare professionals should advocate a healthy lifestyle for patients with diabetes, including regulating blood pressure, low-sugar diet and exercise (NICE 2008).

Neurological observations

Definition

Neurological observations relate to the assessment and evaluation of the integrity and function of an individual's nervous system (Rowley and Fielding 1991).

Anatomy and physiology

The nervous system co-ordinates all body functions, enabling a person to adapt to changes in internal and external environments. It has two main types of neurones: the conducting cells and neuroglia, the supportive cells.

The central nervous system

The central nervous system consists of the brain and spinal cord (Bickley and Szilagyi 2009).

The brain

The brain has four regions: the cerebrum, the diencephalon, the brainstem and the cerebellum. The cerebral hemispheres contain the greatest mass of brain tissue. Each hemisphere is subdivided into frontal, parietal, temporal and occipital lobes, as seen in Figure 13.27.

Each lobe has a particular function.

- The frontal lobe is the primary motor area of the cerebrum which influences personality and abstract reasoning. It also controls the skeletal muscle influencing voluntary movement.
- The parietal lobe is the primary sensory area which integrates the senses of touch and pain.
- The occipital lobe integrates visual stimuli and is primarily responsible for sight.
- The temporal lobe is responsible for olfactory (smell) and auditory (sound) areas (Clark 2005).

The spinal cord

This is a cylindrical mass of nerve tissue encased within the bony vertebral column, extending from the medulla to the first or second lumbar vertebra. It contains important motor and sensory nerve pathways that exit and enter the cord through anterior and posterior nerve roots and spinal and peripheral nerves. The spinal cord also mediates reflex activity of the deep tendon reflexes from the spinal nerves.

Sagittal plane

View

DIENCEPHALON:
Thalamus
Hypothalamus
Pineal gland
(part of
epithalamus)
BRAIN STEM:
Midbrain
Pons
Medulla oblongata
CEREBELLUM
Spinal cord

CEREBRUM

Pituitary gland

POSTERIOR

ANTERIOR

(a) Medial view of sagittal section

CEREBRUM

CEREBELLUM

Spinal cord

DIENCEPHALON:
Thalamus
Hypothalamus
BRAIN STEM:
Midbrain
Pons
Medulla oblongata

(b) Medial view of sagittal section

Figure 13.27   The brain. Reproduced from Tortora and Derrickson (2009).

The spinal cord is divided into five segments: cervical, from C1 to C8; thoracic, from T1 to T12; lumbar, from L1 to L5; sacral, from S1 to S5; and coccygeal (Bickley and Szilagyi 2009) (see Figure 13.28).

The peripheral nervous system

The peripheral nervous system consists of the 12 pairs of cranial nerves and the spinal and peripheral nerves. Most of the peripheral nerves contain both motor and sensory fibres (Bickley and Szilagyi 2009).

The cranial nerves

Twelve pairs of special nerves called cranial nerves emerge within the skull or cranium. Cranial nerves II–XII arise from the diencephalon and the brainstem (see Table 13.10). Cranial nerves I and II are actually fibre tracts emerging from the brain.

Some cranial nerves are limited to general motor or sensory functions, whereas others are specialized, producing smell, vision or hearing (I, II, VIII) (Bickley and Szilagyi 2009).

The peripheral nerves

In addition to cranial nerves, the peripheral nervous system also includes spinal and peripheral nerves that carry impulses to and from the cord. Thirty-one pairs of nerves attach to the spinal cord: eight cervical, 12 thoracic, five lumbar, five sacral and one coccygeal. Most peripheral nerves contain both sensory and motor fibres (Bickley and Szilagyi 2009).

Related theory

Changes in neurological status can be rapid and dramatic or subtle, developing over minutes, hours, days, weeks or even months depending on the insult (Aucken and Crawford

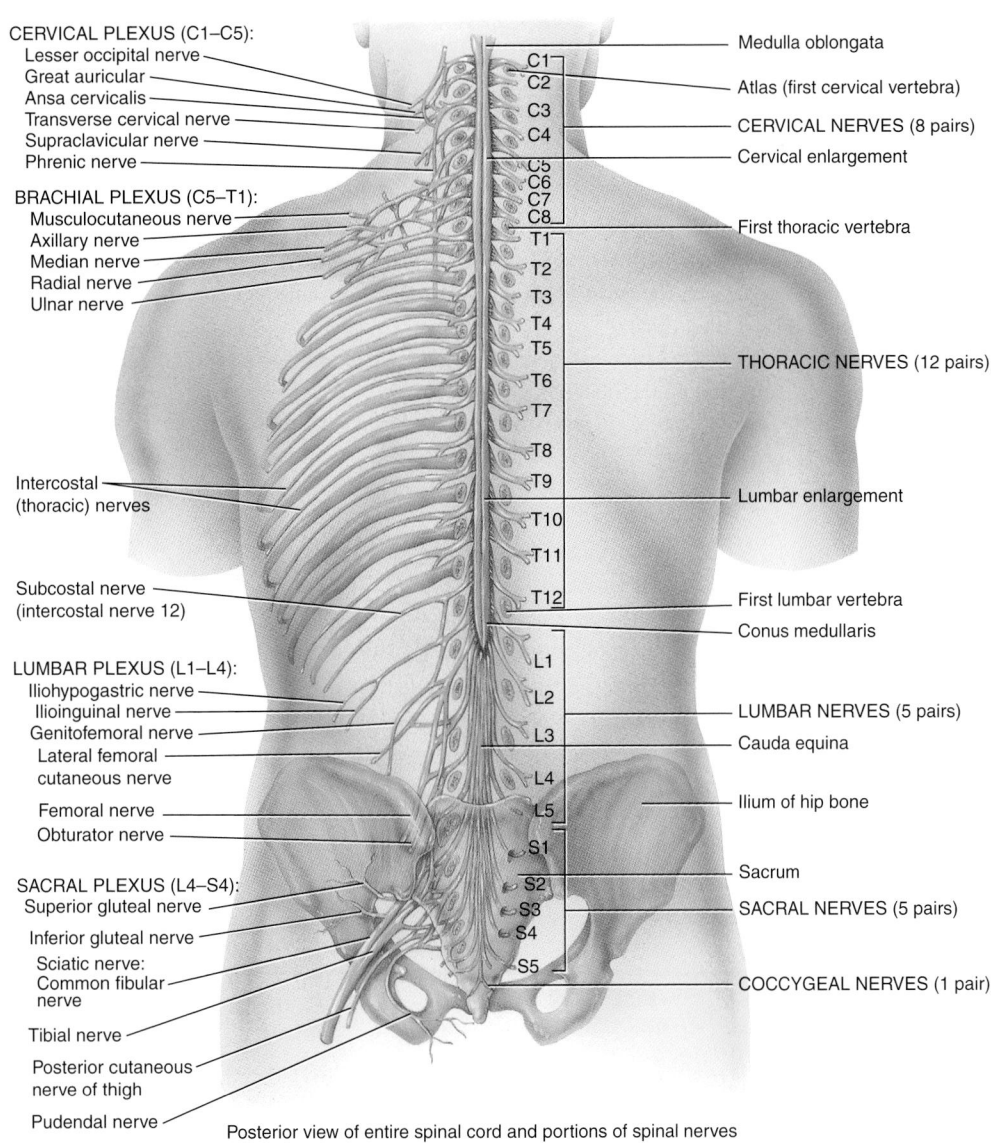

CERVICAL PLEXUS (C1–C5):
Lesser occipital nerve
Great auricular
Ansa cervicalis
Transverse cervical nerve
Supraclavicular nerve
Phrenic nerve

BRACHIAL PLEXUS (C5–T1):
Musculocutaneous nerve
Axillary nerve
Median nerve
Radial nerve
Ulnar nerve

Intercostal
(thoracic) nerves

Subcostal nerve
(intercostal nerve 12)

LUMBAR PLEXUS (L1–L4):
Iliohypogastric nerve
Ilioinguinal nerve
Genitofemoral nerve
Lateral femoral
cutaneous nerve

Femoral nerve
Obturator nerve

SACRAL PLEXUS (L4–S4):
Superior gluteal nerve

Inferior gluteal nerve

Sciatic nerve:
Common fibular
nerve

Tibial nerve

Posterior cutaneous
nerve of thigh

Pudendal nerve

C1
C2
C3
C4
C5
C6
C7
C8
T1
T2
T3
T4
T5
T6
T7
T8
T9
T10
T11
T12
L1
L2
L3
L4
L5
S1
S2
S3
S4
S5

Medulla oblongata

Atlas (first cervical vertebra)

CERVICAL NERVES (8 pairs)

Cervical enlargement

First thoracic vertebra

THORACIC NERVES (12 pairs)

Lumbar enlargement

First lumbar vertebra

Conus medullaris

LUMBAR NERVES (5 pairs)

Cauda equina

Ilium of hip bone

Sacrum

SACRAL NERVES (5 pairs)

COCCYGEAL NERVES (1 pair)

Posterior view of entire spinal cord and portions of spinal nerves

Figure 13.28 External anatomy of the spinal cord and the spinal nerves (posterior view). Reproduced from Tortora and Derrickson (2009).

811

1998). Therefore the frequency of neurological observations will depend upon the patient's condition and the rapidity with which changes are occurring or expected to occur.

Neurological function is assessed by observing five critical areas:

- level of consciousness
- pupillary activity
- motor function
- sensory function
- vital signs.

Level of consciousness

Consciousness is a state of awareness of self and the environment and is dependent upon two components:

- arousability
- awareness.

(Carlson 2002a)

Arousability

This depends on the integrity of the reticular activating system (RAS) (Figure 13.29). The core of nuclei which make up the RAS extends from the brainstem to the thalamic nuclei in the cerebral hemispheres. Thus cognitive ability depends on the ability of the cerebral cortex to permit reciprocal stimulation and conscious behaviour. Consciousness therefore depends on the intactness of the cerebral cortex and the RAS and their ability to communicate effectively (Carlson 2002b, Fairley and McLernon 2005).

Table 13.10 The functions of the cranial nerves

Number	Name	Function
I	Olfactory	Sense of smell
II	Optic	Vision
III	Oculomotor	Pupillary constriction, opening the eye, and most extraocular movements
IV	Trochlear	Downward, inward movement of the eye
VI	Abducens	Lateral deviation of the eye
V	Trigeminal	*Motor* – temporal and masseter muscles (jaw clenching), also lateral movement of the jaw
		Sensory – facial. The nerve has three divisions: (1) ophthalmic, (2) maxillary and (3) mandibular
VII	Facial	*Motor* – facial movements, including those of facial expression, closing the eye, and closing the mouth
		Sensory – taste for salty, sweet, sour and bitter substances on the anterior two-thirds of the tongue
VIII	Acoustic	Hearing (cochlear division) and balance (vestibular division)
IX	Glossopharyngeal	*Motor* – pharynx
		Sensory – posterior portions of the eardrum and ear canal, the pharynx, and the posterior tongue, including taste (salty, sweet, sour, bitter)
X	Vagus	*Motor* – palate, pharynx and larynx
		Sensory – pharynx and larynx
XI	Spinal accessory	*Motor* – the sternomastoid and upper portion of the trapezius
XII	Hypoglossal	*Motor* – tongue

Bickley and Szilagyi (2009).

Awareness

This requires an intact cerebral cortex to interpret sensory input and respond accordingly. This is the content of the consciousness (Bateman 2001, Scherer 1986).

Levels of consciousness may vary and are dependent on the location and extent of any neurological damage (Aucken

and Crawford 1998). Previous and/or co-existing problems should be heeded when noting levels of consciousness, for example deafness, hemiparesis/hemiplegia.

Alterations in level of consciousness can vary from slight to severe changes, indicating the degree of brain dysfunction (Aucken and Crawford 1998). Consciousness ranges on a continuum from alert wakefulness to deep coma with no apparent responsiveness. Therefore, nurses must ensure that families and friends are involved at initial history taking and throughout care so as to chronicle accurately any change in neurological symptoms.

Terms such as 'fully conscious', 'semi-conscious', 'lethargic' or 'stuporous' used to describe levels of consciousness are subjective and open to misinterpretation. Thus, level of consciousness is often measured using the Glasgow Coma Scale (GCS) (see Assessment and recording tools).

Application of painful stimuli

Painful stimuli should be employed only if the patient does not respond to firm and clear commands. It is always important that the least amount of pressure to elicit a response is applied so as to avoid bruising or paining the patient. As such, it should only be undertaken by experienced professionals.

As the ability to localize pain is lost, various responses may be observed when painful stimuli are applied (Carlson

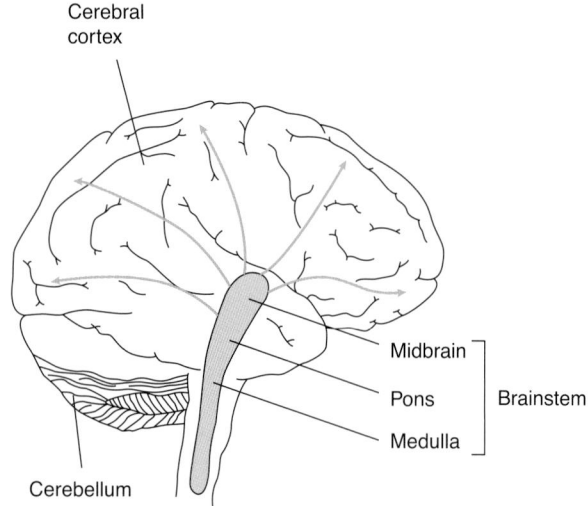

Figure 13.29 Reticular activating system.

2002a). It is important to note, when applying a painful stimulus, that the brain responds to central stimulation and the spine responds first to peripheral stimulation (Aucken and Crawford 1998).

Central stimulation can be applied in the following ways (Aucken and Crawford 1998, Carlson 2002a, Price 2002).

- *Trapezium squeeze*: using the thumb and two fingers, hold 5 cm of the trapezius muscle where the neck meets the shoulder and twist the muscle.
- *Supraorbital pressure*: running a finger along the supraorbital margin, a notch is felt. Applying pressure to the notch causes an ipsilateral (on that side) sinus headache. This method is not to be used if the facial or cranial bones are unstable, facial fractures are suspected, after facial surgery or if the assessor has sharp fingernails.
- *Sternal rub*: using the knuckles of a clenched fist to grind on the centre of the sternum. When applied adequately, marks are left on the skin as sternal tissue is tender and bruises easily. Please note that because of the danger of bruising, this method should not be used for repeated assessment but may be indicated if a decision as to whether to re-scan or alter management, for example proceed to surgery, is necessary.

Peripheral stimulation can be applied in the following way. Place the patient's finger between the assessor's thumb and a pencil or pen. Pressure is gradually increased over a few seconds until the slightest response is seen. Any finger can be used, although the third and fourth fingers are often most sensitive (Frawley 1990). Please note that because of the risk of bruising, pressure should not be applied to the nailbed. It must be remembered that nailbed pressure is a peripheral stimulus and should only be used to assess limbs that have not moved in response to a central stimulus (Aucken and Crawford 1998).

It cannot be overemphasized that the above methods of patient assessment should only be undertaken by appropriately qualified and trained nurses.

Pupillary activity

Careful examination of the reactions of the pupils to light is an important part of neurological assessment (Table 13.11).

The size, shape, equality, reaction to light (both direct and consensual responses, that is, the response from the eye that is not directly exposed to light) and position of the eyes should be noted. Are the eyes deviated upwards or downwards? Are both eyes conjugate (moving together) or dysconjugate (not moving together)? Impaired pupillary accommodation (adjustment of the eye resulting in pupil constriction or dilation) signifies that the midbrain itself may be suffering from pressure exerted by a swelling mass in the brain. Pupillary constriction and dilation are controlled by cranial nerve III (oculomotor) and any changes may indicate pressure on this nerve or brainstem damage (Figure 13.30) (Fuller 2004).

It should be noted that 'normal' visual function depends on a full and conjugate range of eye movements (involving cranial nerves III, IV, VI) in addition to normally functioning optic and oculomotor nerves and an intact visual centre in the occipital cortex (Aucken and Crawford 1998).

Motor function

Damage to any part of the motor nervous system can affect the ability to move. After assessing motor function on one side of the body, the contralateral muscle group should also be evaluated to detect asymmetry. Motor function assessment involves an evaluation of the following.

- Muscle strength.
- Muscle tone.
- Muscle co-ordination.
- Reflexes.
- Abnormal movements.
  (Aucken and Crawford 1998, Fuller 2004)

Muscle strength

This involves testing the patient's muscle strength against the pull of gravity and then against one's own resistance. Changes in motor strength, especially between right and left sides, may indicate imminent neurological failure (Carlson 2002a).

Muscle tone

This involves flexing and extending the patient's limbs on both sides and noting how well such movements are resisted.

Table 13.11 Examination of pupils

Observation	Pupil size	Pupil reactiveness	Possible indication
Pupils equal	Pinpoint	—	Opiates or pontine lesion
	Small	Reactive	Metabolic encephalopathy
	Mid-sized	Fixed	Midbrain lesion
		Reactive	Metabolic lesion
Pupils unequal	Dilated	Unreactive	3rd nerve palsy
	Small	Reactive	Horner's syndrome

Reproduced with permission from Fuller (2004).

813

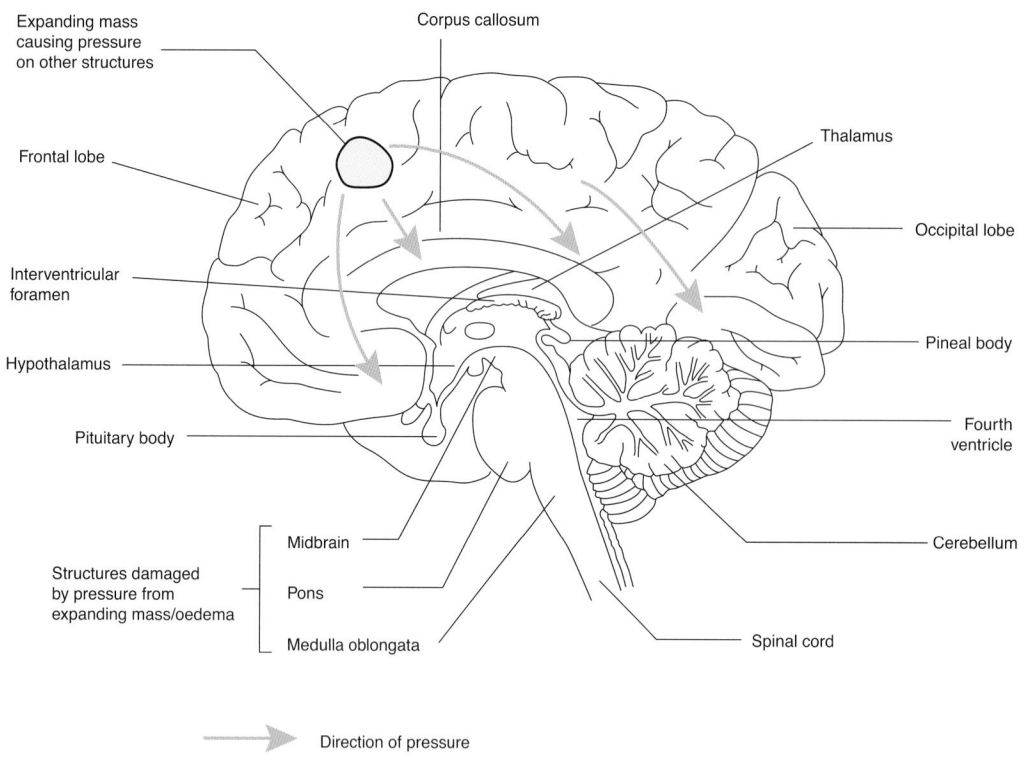

Figure 13.30   Pressure from expanding mass and/or cerebral oedema.

Increased resistance would denote increased muscle tone and vice versa.

Muscle co-ordination

Any disease or injury that involves the cerebellum or basal ganglia will affect co-ordination. Assessment of hand and leg co-ordination can be achieved by testing the rapidity and rhythm of alternating movements and point-to-point movements.

Reflexes

Amongst the most important reflexes are blink, gag and swallow, oculocephalic and plantar.

- *Blink*: this is a protective reflex and can be affected by damage to the Vth cranial nerve (trigeminal) and the VIIth cranial nerve (facial). Absence of the corneal reflex (Vth and VIIth cranial nerves) may result in corneal damage. Facial weakness (VIIth cranial nerve) will affect eye closure.
- *Gag and swallow*: damage to the IXth cranial nerve (glossopharyngeal) and Xth cranial nerve (vagus) may impair protective reflexes. These two cranial nerves are always assessed together as their functions overlap. Muscle innervation of the palate is from the vagus, while sensation is supplied by the glossopharyngeal nerves (Aucken and Crawford 1998, Fuller 2004).

- *Oculocephalic*: this reflex is an eye movement that occurs only in patients with a severely decreased level of consciousness. In conscious patients this reflex is not present. When the reflex is present, the patient's eyes will move in the opposite direction from the side to which the head is turned. However, in patients with absent brainstem reflexes, the eyes will appear to remain stationary in the centre. Assessing this reflex should not be carried out if there is suspected instability of the cervical spine as this reflex can involve head movement which could exacerbate any spinal injury (Aucken and Crawford 1998).
- *Plantar*: abnormalities of plantar reflex will help to locate the anatomical site of the lesion. Upgoing plantar (extension) reflex is termed 'positive Babinski' and indicates an upper motor neurone lesion. It should be noted that in babies under 1 year of age upgoing plantar is normal (Aucken and Crawford 1998).

Abnormal movements

When carrying out neurological observations, any abnormal movements such as seizures, tics and tremors must be noted.

Sensory functions

Constant sensory input enables an individual to alter responses and behaviour to suit the environment. When disease or injury damages the sensory pathways, the sensory responses are always affected. Any assessment of sensory function should include an evaluation of the following.

- Central and peripheral vision.
- Hearing and ability to understand verbal communication.
- Superficial sensations (light touch, pain) and deep sensations (muscle and joint pain, muscle and joint position).
(Carlson 2002a, Fuller 2004)

Visual acuity

The clarity or clearness of vision may be tested with a Snellen chart, which uses decreasing letter size, or newspaper prints, with and without glasses if worn.

Visual fields

Lesions at different points in the visual pathways affect vision (Table 13.12). It should be noted that loss of vision is always described with reference to the visual fields rather than the retinal fields (Weldon 1998).

Vital signs

It is recommended that assessments of vital signs should be made in the following order.

1 Respirations.
2 Temperature.
3 Blood pressure.
4 Pulse.

See relevant sections in this chapter.

Respirations

Of these four vital signs, respiratory patterns give the clearest indication of how the brain is functioning because the complex process of respiration is controlled by more than

Table 13.12 Visual pathways

Defect	Implication
Monocular field defects	Lesion anterior to optic chiasm
Bitemporal field defects	Lesion at the optic chiasm
Homonymous field defects	Lesion behind the optic chiasm
Congruous homonymous field defects	Lesion behind lateral geniculate bodies

Reproduced with permission from Fuller (2004).

one area of the brain. Any disease or injury that affects these areas may produce respiratory changes. The rate, character and pattern of a patient's respiration must be noted. Abnormal respiratory patterns are listed in Table 13.13.

Constant re-evaluation of the patient's ability to maintain and protect their airway is a concern when there is evidence of reduced consciousness or coma (GCS score is less than 8). At this stage, muscles often become flaccid and the use of the recovery position may need to be considered. Patients who have deteriorated may require adjuncts to protect the airway and possibly artificial ventilation (Resuscitation Council 2006). Close working liaison with physiotherapists and speech and language therapists is important to minimize the danger of chest infections.

Temperature

Damage to the hypothalamus, the temperature-regulating centre, may result in grossly fluctuating temperatures (Fairley and McLernon 2005).

Blood pressure, pulse and respirations

Observations of blood pressure, pulse and respirations will provide evidence of increased intracranial pressure. When intracranial pressure is greater than 33 mmHg for even a

Table 13.13 Abnormal respiratory patterns

Type	Pattern	Significance
Cheyne–Stokes	Rhythmic waxing and waning of both rate and depth of respirations, alternating regularly with briefer periods of apnoea. Greater than normal respiration, that is 16–24 breaths per minute	May indicate deep cerebral or cerebellar lesions, usually bilateral; may occur with upper brainstem involvement
Central neurogenic hyperventilation	Sustained, regular, rapid respirations, with forced inspiration and expiration	May indicate a lesion of the low midbrain or upper pons areas of the brainstem
Apneustic	Prolonged inspiration with a pause at full inspiration; there may also be expiratory pauses	May indicate a lesion of the lower pons or upper medulla, hypoglycaemia or drug-induced respiratory depression
Cluster breathing	Clusters of irregular respirations alternating with longer periods of apnoea	May indicate a lesion of lower pons or upper medulla
Ataxic breathing	A completely irregular pattern with random deep and shallow respirations; irregular pauses may also appear	May indicate a lesion of the medulla

815

short time, cerebral blood flow is significantly reduced. The resulting ischaemia stimulates the vasomotor centre, causing systemic blood pressure to rise. The patient becomes bradycardic and the respiratory rate falls. Abnormalities of blood pressure and pulse usually occur late, after the patient's level of consciousness has begun to deteriorate. This change in the blood pressure was first described by Cushing and is known as the Cushing reflex (Carlson 2002b).

Evidence-based approaches

Rationale

Indications

An accurate neurological assessment is essential in planning patient care. The information gained from a neurological assessment can be used in the following ways.

- To aid diagnosis (Douglas *et al.* 2005).
- As a baseline for observations (Crouch and Meurier 2005).
- To determine both subtle and rapid changes in an individual's condition (Crouch and Meurier 2005).
- To monitor neurological status following a neurological procedure (Mooney and Comeford 2003).
- To observe for deterioration and establish the extent of a traumatic head injury (Walsh 2006).
- To detect life-threatening situations (Alcock *et al.* 2002).

Frequency of observations

The frequency and type of neurological observation are matters of much debate (Price 2002). It is therefore not possible to be prescriptive, as the frequency will depend on the underlying pathology and possible consequences. For example, in a patient with a head injury and a skull fracture, there may be bruising to the brain (contusion), cerebral oedema and an extradural haemorrhage which may increase in size. The bruising and oedema may develop over a couple of days and gradually give rise to subtle neurological changes, whilst the extradural haemorrhage can develop very quickly and cause profound neurological changes over a matter of a few hours. Therefore such a patient may require frequent 30-minute GCS observations for the first 6 hours followed by 1–2-hourly observations for a further 48 hours. The nurse must be competent and take appropriate action if changes in the patient's neurological status occur, as well as reporting any subtle signs that may indicate deterioration, for

example if the patient is incontinent, reluctant to eat, drink or initiate interaction. It should never be assumed that difficulty to rouse a patient is due to night-time sleep as even a deeply asleep patient with no focal deficit should respond to pain. Therefore if the patient requires an increased amount of stimulus to achieve the same GCS score, this may also be a pointer to subtle deterioration (Table 13.14) (Aucken and Crawford 1998, Waterhouse 2005).

Preprocedural considerations

Equipment

The following equipment may be used as part of the neurological assessment.

- *Pen torch*: used to assess the reaction of the pupils to light and consensual light reflex (Aucken and Crawford 1998).
- *Tongue depressor*: device used to depress the tongue to allow for examination of mouth and throat (Fuller 2004).
- *Patella hammer*: a tendon hammer used to strike the patella tendon below the knee to assess the deep knee jerk/reflex (Fuller 2004).
- *Neuro tips*: sharp instrument used to apply pressure and test for superficial sensations to pain. Can be replaced by a safety pin or other suitable sharp object (Fuller 2004).
- *Snellen chart*: an eye chart used to measure visual acuity.
- *Ophthalmoscope*: instrument used to examine the eye.

Assessment and recording tools

The initial assessment of a patient should include a history (taken from relatives or friends if appropriate), noting changes in mood, intellect, memory and personality, since these may be indicators of a long-standing problem, for example brain tumour (Belford 2005).

The GCS, first developed by Teasdale and Jennett (1974), is a common way to assess a patient's conscious level. It forms a quick, objective and easily interpreted mode of neurological assessment. The GCS measures arousal, awareness and activity, by assessing three different areas of the patient's behaviour: eye opening, verbal response and motor response (Dawes and Durham 2007).

Each area is allocated a score, enabling objectivity, ease of recording and comparison between recordings. The total sum provides a score out of 15. A score of 15 indicates a fully alert and responsive patient, whereas a score of 3 (the lowest possible score) indicates unconsciousness (Dawes

Table 13.14 Frequency of observations

Category	Frequency	Rationale
All patients diagnosed as suffering from neurological or neurosurgical conditions. Unconscious patients (including ventilated and anaesthetized)	At least 4-hourly, affected by the patient's condition. Frequency indicated by patient's condition	To monitor the condition of the patient so that any necessary action can be instigated. To monitor the condition closely and to detect trends so that appropriate action may be taken

Table 13.15 Scoring activities of the Glasgow Coma Scale. Scores are added, with the highest score 15 indicating full consciousness

Category	Score	Response
Eye opening		
Spontaneous	4	Eyes open spontaneously without stimulation
To speech	3	Eyes open to verbal stimulation (normal, raised or repeated)
To pain	2	Eyes open with painful/noxious stimuli
None	1	No eye opening regardless of level of stimulation
Verbal response		
Orientated	5	Able to give accurate information regarding time, person and place
Confused	4	Able to answer in sentences using correct language but cannot answer orientation questions appropriately
Inappropriate words	3	Uses incomprehensible words in a random or disorganized fashion
Incomprehensible sounds	2	Makes unintelligible sounds, for example moans and groans
None	1	No verbal response despite verbal or other stimuli
Best motor response		
Obeys commands	6	Obeys and can repeat simple commands, for example arm raise
Localizes to pain	5	Purposeful movement to remove painful stimuli
Normal flexion	4	Withdraws extremity from source of pain, for example flexes arm at elbow without wrist rotation in response to painful stimuli
Abnormal flexion	3	Decorticate posturing (flexion of arms, hyperextension of legs) spontaneously or in response to noxious stimuli
Extension	2	Decerebrate posturing (limbs extended and internally rotated) spontaneously or in response to noxious stimuli
None	1	No response to noxious stimuli. Flaccid limbs

Aucken and Crawford (1998), Carlson (2002a).

and Durham 2007). When used consistently, the GCS provides a graphical representation that shows improvement or deterioration of the patient's conscious level at a glance (see Figure 13.31 and Table 13.15).

Assessment of level of consciousness

Assessment using the GCS involves three phases (Teasdale and Jennett 1974).

1 Eye opening.
2 Evaluation of verbal response.
3 Evaluation of motor response.

Evaluation of eye opening

Eye opening indicates that the arousal mechanism in the brain is active. Eye opening may be: spontaneous; to speech, for example spoken name; to painful stimulus; or not at all. Arousal (eye opening) is always the first measurement undertaken when performing the GCS, as without arousal, cognition cannot occur (Aucken and Crawford 1998). It must, however, be remembered that swollen or permanently closed eyes (e.g. after tarsorrhaphy surgery in which the upper and lower eyelids are partially or wholly joined to protect the cornea; Martin 2003) will not open and do not necessarily indicate a falling conscious level.

Evaluation of verbal response

- *Orientated*: the patient is aware of self and environment.
- *Confused*: the patient's responses to questions are incorrect and patient is unaware of self or environment.
- *Inappropriate words*: the patient responds using intelligible words which are unsuitable as responses.
- *Incomprehensible*: the patient may moan and groan without recognizable words.
- *Absent*: the patient does not speak or make sounds at all.

The absence of speech may not always indicate a falling level of consciousness. The patient may not speak English (though they can still speak), may have a tracheostomy or may be dysphasic. The patient may have a motor (expressive) dysphasia, and therefore be able to understand but be unable to find the right word, or a sensory (receptive) dysphasia, being unable to comprehend what is being told to them (Aucken and Crawford 1998, Shah 1999). At times patients with expressive dysphasia may also have receptive problems; therefore it is important to make an early referral to a speech and language therapist. The nurse should also bear in mind that some patients may need a lot of stimulation to maintain their concentration to answer questions,

Figure 13.31   The Glasgow Coma Scale.

even though they can answer them correctly. It is, therefore, important to note the amount of stimulation that the patient required as part of the baseline assessment (Aucken and Crawford 1998). If a patient cannot follow the instruction due to a language barrier or unconsciousness, observe spontaneous movements and note how strong they appear. Then, if necessary, apply painful stimuli.

Evaluation of motor response

To obtain an accurate picture of brain function, motor response is tested by using the upper limbs because responses in the lower limbs reflect spinal function (Aucken and Crawford 1998). The patient should be asked to obey commands; for example, the patient should be asked to squeeze the examiner's hands (both sides) with the best motor response recorded. The nurse should note power in the hands and the patient's ability to release the grip. This is because some patients with cerebral dysfunction, for example those with diffuse brain disease, may show an involuntary grasp reflex where stimulation of the palm of their hand causes them to grip (Aucken and Crawford 1998). If movement is spontaneous, the nurse should note which limbs move, and how, for example whether the movement is purposeful.

Response to painful stimulus may be:

- *localized*: the patient moves the other hand to the site of the stimulus
- *flexor*: the patient's limb flexes away from pain
- *extensor*: the patient's limb extends from pain
- *flaccid*: no motor response at all.
  (Aucken and Crawford 1998, Shah 1999)

Procedure guideline 13.10 Neurological observations and assessment

Essential equipment

- Pen torch
- Thermometer
- Sphygmomanometer
- Tongue depressor

- Patella hammer
- Neuro tips
- Alcohol handrub

Optional equipment

- Low-linting swabs
- Two test tubes

- Snellen chart
- Ophthalmoscope

Preprocedure

Action	Rationale
1 Inform the patient of the procedure, whether conscious or not, and explain and discuss the observations.	Sense of hearing is frequently unimpaired even in unconscious patients. It is important, as far as is possible, that the patient understands the procedure and gives their valid consent (NMC 2008b, C).

Procedure

2 Wash and dry hands.	To minimize the risk of cross contamination (Fraise and Bradley 2009, E).
3 Talk to the patient. Note whether they are alert and giving full attention or restless or lethargic and drowsy. Ask the patient who they are, the correct day, month and year, where they are and to give details about family.	To establish whether the patient's level of consciousness is deteriorating. If the patient is becoming disorientated, changes will occur in this order: (a) disorientation as to time (b) disorientation as to place (c) disorientation as to person (Aucken and Crawford 1998, R5).
4 Ask the patient to squeeze and release your fingers (include both sides of the body) and then to stick out their tongue.	To evaluate motor responses and to ensure that the responses are equal and are not reflexive (Carlson 2002a, R5).
5 If the patient does not respond, apply painful stimuli. Suggested methods have been discussed earlier.	Responses grow less purposeful as the patient's level of consciousness deteriorates. As the condition worsens, the patient may no longer localize pain and respond to it in a purposeful way (Aucken and Crawford 1998, R5).

819

(*Continued*)

Procedure guideline 13.10 *(Continued)*

6 Record the findings precisely, recording the patient's best response. Write exactly what stimulus was used, where it was applied, how much pressure was needed to elicit the response, and how the patient responded.	Vague terms can be easily misinterpreted. Accurate recording will enable continuity of assessment and comply with NMC guidelines (NMC 2009, C).
7 Extend both hands and ask the patient to squeeze your fingers as hard as possible. Compare grip and strength.	To test grip and ascertain strength. Record best arm in GCS chart to reflect best outcome (Carlson 2002a, R5).
8 Darken the room, if necessary, or shield the patient's eyes with your hands.	To enable a better view of the eye. E
9 Ask the patient to open their eyes. If the patient cannot do so, hold the eyelids open and note the size, shape and equality of the pupils.	To assess the size, shape and equality of the pupils as an indication of brain damage. Normal pupils are spherical, usually at mid-position and have a diameter ranging from 2 to 5 mm (Shah 1999, R5).
10 Hold each eyelid open in turn. Move torch towards the patient from the side. Shine it directly into the eye. This should cause the pupil to constrict promptly.	To assess the reaction of the pupils to light. A normal reaction indicates no lesions in the area of the brainstem regulating pupil constriction (Aucken and Crawford 1998, R5).
11 Hold both eyelids open but shine the light into one eye only. The pupil into which the light is not shone should also constrict.	To assess consensual light reflex. Prompt constriction indicates intact connections between the brainstem areas regulating pupil constriction (Scherer 1986, R5).
12 Record unusual eye movements.	To assess cranial nerve damage (Aucken and Crawford 1998, R5).
13 Note the rate, character and pattern of the patient's respirations.	Respirations are controlled by different areas of the brain. When disease or injury affects these areas, respiratory changes may occur (Carlson 2002a, R5).
14 Take and record the patient's temperature at specified intervals.	Damage to the hypothalamus, the temperature-regulating centre in the brain, will be reflected in grossly abnormal temperatures (Fairley and McLernon 2005, R5).
15 Take and record the patient's blood pressure and pulse at specified intervals.	To monitor signs of increased intracranial pressure. Hypertension and bradycardia usually occur late, after the patient's level of consciousness has begun to deteriorate. Call for medical assistance as soon as it is evident that there is a deterioration in the patient's level of consciousness (Scherer 1986, R5; Tortora and Derrickson 2009, R5).
16 Ask the patient to close the eyes and hold the arms straight out in front, with palms upwards, for 20–30 seconds. The weaker limb will 'fall away'.	To show weakness and difference in limbs (Carlson 2002a, R5).
17 Stand in front of the patient and extend your hands. Ask the patient to push and pull against your hands. Ask the patient to lie on their back in bed. Place the patient's leg with knee flexed and foot resting on the bed. Instruct the patient to keep the foot down as you attempt to extend the leg. Then instruct the patient to straighten the leg while you offer resistance.	To test arm strength. If one arm drifts downwards or turns inwards, it may indicate hemiparesis. To test flexion and extension strength in the patient's extremities by having the patient push and pull against your resistance (Carlson 2002a, R5).
18 Flex and extend all the patient's limbs. Note how well the movements are resisted.	To test muscle tone (Carlson 2002a, R5).

19	Ask the patient to pat the thigh as fast as possible. Note whether the movements seem slow or clumsy. Ask the patient to turn the hand over and back several times in succession. Evaluate co-ordination. Ask the patient to touch the back of the fingers with the thumb in sequence rapidly.	To assess hand and arm co-ordination. The dominant hand should perform better (Carlson 2002a, R5).
20	Extend one of your hands towards the patient. Ask the patient to touch your index finger, then their nose, several times in succession. Repeat the test with the patient's eyes closed.	To assess hand and arm co-ordination/cerebellar function (Carlson 2002a, R5).
21	Ask the patient to place a heel on the opposite knee and slide it down the shin to the foot. Check each leg separately.	To assess leg co-ordination (Fuller 2004, R5).
22	Ask the patient to look up or hold the eyelid open. With your hand, approach the eye unexpectedly or touch the eyelashes.	To test the corneal (blink) reflex (Fuller 2004, R5).
23	Ask the patient to open the mouth, and hold down the tongue with a tongue depressor. Touch the back of the pharynx, on each side, with a low-linting swab.	To test the gag reflex (Fuller 2004, R5).
24	Ask the patient to lie on their back in bed. Place your hand under the knee, raise and flex it. Tap the patellar tendon. Note whether the leg responds.	To assess the deep tendon knee-jerk reflex (Fuller 2004, R5).
25	Stroke the lateral aspect of the sole of the patient's foot. If the response is abnormal (Babinski's response), the big toe will dorsiflex and the remaining toes will fan out.	To assess for upper motor neurone lesion (Fuller 2004, R5).
26	Ask the patient to read something aloud. Check each eye separately. If vision is so poor that the patient is unable to read, ask the patient to count your upraised fingers or distinguish light from dark.	To test for visual acuity (Fuller 2004, R5).
27	Occlude one ear with a low-linting swab. Stand a short way from the patient. Whisper numbers into the open ear. Ask for feedback. Repeat for the other ear.	To test hearing and comprehension (Fuller 2004, R5).
28	Ask the patient to close the eyes. Using the point of a Neuro tip (sharp instrument for applying pressure), stroke the skin. Use the blunt end occasionally. Ask patient to tell you what is felt. See if the patient can distinguish between sharp and dull sensations.	To test superficial sensations to pain (Fuller 2004, R5).
29	Ask the patient to close the eyes. Fill two test tubes with water: one warm, one cold. Touch the patient's skin with each test tube and ask patient to distinguish between them.	To test superficial sensations to temperature (Fuller 2004, R5).
30	Stroke a low-linting swab lightly over the patient's skin. Ask the patient to say what they feel.	To test superficial sensations to touch (Fuller 2004, R5).
31	Ask the patient to close the eyes. Hold the tip of one of the patient's fingers between your thumb and index finger. Move it up and down and ask the patient to say in which direction it is moving. Repeat with the other hand. For the legs, hold the big toe.	To test proprioception. (Bickley and Szilagyi 2009, E). *Proprioception* is the receipt of information from muscles and tendons in the labyrinth that enables the brain to determine movements and the position of the body (Tortora and Derrickson 2009, E).

821

(Continued)

Procedure guideline 13.10 (*Continued*)

Postprocedure

Action	Rationale
32 Document the observation recordings on the patient's observation chart, record only what you see and do not be influenced by previous observations.	To ensure adequate records and enable continued care of the patient (NMC 2009, C).
33 Report any abnormal findings to medical staff.	To prevent further deterioration. E
34 Clean the equipment after use.	To prevent cross-infection (Fraise and Bradley 2009, E).

Problem-solving table 13.9 Prevention and resolution (Procedure guideline 13.10)

Problem	Cause	Prevention	Action
Language difficulties or dysphasia	Difficulty making accurate assessment of consciousness	Knowledge of language difficulties	Use of interpreter for language barrier Consideration when taking into account overall assessment process
Patient unable to open eye(s)	Result of swelling	Unable to prevent	Does not necessarily indicate a low or falling conscious level

Postprocedural considerations

Documentation

A validated observation chart is the most common method of monitoring and recording neurological observations. Although the layout may differ from chart to chart, in essence all neurological observation charts measure and record the same clinical information, including the level of consciousness, pupil size and response, motor and sensory response and vital signs (Dawes and Durham 2007).

Observation charts ensure a systematic approach to collecting and analysing essential information regarding a patient's condition. Such charts also act as a means of communication between nurses and other healthcare professionals (Dawes and Durham 2007).

References

Adam, S.K. and Osborne, S. (2005) *Critical Care Nursing: Science and Practice*, 2nd edn. Oxford University Press, Oxford.

Alcock, K., Clancy, M. and Crouch, R. (2002) Physiological observations of patients admitted from A and E. *Nursing Standard*, 16 (34), 33–37.

Angerami, E.L.S. (1980) Epidemiological study of body temperature in patients in a teaching hospital. *International Journal of Nursing Studies*, 17, 91–99.

Aucken, S. and Crawford, B. (1998) Neurological observations, in *Neuro-Oncology for Nurses* (ed. D. Guerrero). Whurr, London, pp. 29–65.

Bateman, D. (2001) Neurological assessment of coma. *Journal of Neurology Neurosurgery and Psychiatry*, 71 (Suppl 1), i13–i17.

Bayer Diagnostics (1997) *Urinary Tract Infection*. Technical Information Bulletin No. 8. Bayer Diagnostics, Newbury.

Bayer Diagnostics (2006) *Your Practical Guide to Urine Analysis*. Bayer Diagnostics, Newbury.

Bayham, E., Fucile, F., McKenzie, N. and O'Hara, O (1996) *Clinical Considerations for Use of First Temp R and First Temp Tympanic Thermometers*, Sherwood Davis and Geck, St Louis, MO.

BCSH (1999) The administration of blood and blood components and the management of transfused patients. *Transfusion Medicine*, 9, 227–238.

Beachy, W. (2009) Acid-base balance, in *Egan's Fundamentals of Respiratory Care*, 9th edn (eds R.L. Wilkins, J.K. Stoller and R.M. Kacmarek). Mosby Elsevier, St Louis, MO.

Belford, K. (2005) Central nervous system cancers, in *Cancer Nursing: Principles and Practice*, 6th edn (eds C. Henke-Yarbro, M. Frogge and M. Goodman). Jones and Bartlett, Sudbury, MA, pp. 1089–1136.

Bern, L., Brandt, M., Mbelu, N. *et al.* (2007) Differences in blood pressure values obtained with automated and manual methods in medical inpatients. *MEDSURG Nursing*, 16 (6), 356–361.

BHS (2006) Factfile 01/2006 – Blood pressure measurement. www.bhsoc.org/bhf_factfiles/bhf_factfile_jan_2006.doc.

Bickley, L.S., and Szilagyi, P.G. (2009) *Bates' Guide to Physical Examination and History Taking*, 10th edn. Lippincott Williams and Wilkins, London.

Bishop, T. (2008) Urine testing. *Practice Nurse*, 35 (12), 18–20.

Blake D.R. and Nathan D.M. (2004) Point-of-care testing for diabetes. *Critical Care Nurse*, 27 (2), 150–161.

Bolton, D. (1997) Extravasation associated with a multilumen central catheter. *Anaesthesia*, 52, 1119.

Booker, R. (2008) Pulse oximetry. *Nursing Standard*, **22** (30), 39–41.

Booker, R. (2009) Interpretation and evaluation of pulmonary function tests. *Nursing Standard*, **23** (39), 46–56.

Bongers, T, and O'Driscoll, B.R. (2006) Effects of equipment and technique on peak flow measurements. *BMC Pulmonary Medicine*, **6** (14), 1–6.

Braun, S.K., Preston, P. and Smith, R.N. (1998) Getting a better read on thermometry. *Registered Nurses*, **61** (3), 57–60.

Bridges, E. (2009) Noninvasive measurements of body temperature in critically ill patients. *Critical Care Nurse*, **29** (3), pp. 94–97.

British Committee for Standards in Haematology (1999) The administration of blood and blood components and the management of the transfused patient. *Transfusion Medicine*, **9**, 227–238.

British Thoracic Society/Scottish Intercollegiate Guidelines Network (2009) *British Guideline on the Management of Asthma: Quick Reference Guide*. British Thoracic Society, London.

Brooker, C. (2010) *Mosby's Dictionary of Medicine, Nursing and Health Professions*. Mosby Elsevier, London.

Buist, A.S., Vollmer, W.M., Wilson, S.R. *et al.* (2006) A randomized clinical trial of peak flow versus symptom monitoring in older patients with asthma. *American Journal of Respiratory and Critical Care Medicine*, **74** (10), 1077–1087.

Burke, K. (1996) The tympanic membrane thermometer in paediatrics: a review of the literature. *Accident and Emergency Nursing*, **4** (4), 190–193.

Camm, A.J. and Bunce, N. (2009) Cardiovascular disease, in *Clinical Medicine*, 7th edn (eds P. Kumar and M. Clarke). Elsevier, London.

Carlson, B.A. (2002a) Neurologic clinical assessment, in *Critical Care Nursing: Diagnosis and Management* (eds L. Urden, K. Stacy and M. Lough), 4th edn. Mosby, St Louis, MO, pp. 645–657.

Carlson, B.A. (2002b) Neurologic anatomy and physiology, in *Critical Care Nursing: Diagnosis and Management*, 4th edn (eds L. Urden, K. Stacy and M. Lough). Mosby, St Louis, MO, pp. 617–44.

Carroll, M. (2000) An evaluation of temperature measurement. *Nursing Standard*, 14 (4), 39–43.

Chalmers, J.D., Singanayagam, A. and Hill, A.T. (2008) Systolic blood pressure is superior to other haemodynamic predictors of outcome in community acquired pneumonia. *Thorax*, **63**, 698–702.

Chummun, H. (2009) Understanding changes in cardiovascular pathophysiology. *British Journal of Nursing*, **18** (6), 359–364.

Clark, R. K. (2005) *Anatomy and Physiology: Understanding the Human Body*. Jones and Bartlett Publishers, London.

Consensus Committee of the American Autonomic Society and the American Academy of Neurology (1996) Consensus statement on the definition of orthostatic hypotension, pure autonomic failure, and multiple system atrophy. *Neurology*, 46 (5), 1470.

Cook, R. (1996) Urinalysis: ensuring accurate urine testing. *Nursing Standard*, 10 (46), 49–55.

Cretikos, M.A., Bellomo, R., Hillman, K. *et al.* (2008) Respiratory rate: the neglected vital sign. *Medical Journal of Australia*, **188** (11), 657–659.

Critical Care Stakeholders Forum and National Outreach Forum (2007) *Clinical Indicators for Critical Care Outreach Services*. www.dh.gov.uk.

Crosser, A. and McDowell, J.R.S. (2007) Nurses' rationale for blood glucose monitoring in critical care. *British Journal of Nursing*, **16** (10), 576–580.

Crouch, A. and Meurier, C. (2005) *Vital Notes for Nurses: Health Assessment*. Blackwell Publishing, Oxford.

Cuddy, M. (2004) The effects of drugs on thermoregulation. *Advanced Practice in Acute Critical Care*, **15** (2), 238–253.

Curran, R. (2009) The vital signs, part 1: blood pressure. *EMS*, **38** (3), 62–66.

Dale, L. (2006) Make a point about alternate site blood glucose sampling. *Nursing*, **36** (2), 52–53.

Davies, A, and Moores, C. (2003) *The Respiratory System*. Churchill Livingstone, London.

Dawes, E. and Durham, L. (2007) Monitoring and recording patients' neurological observations. *Nursing Standard*, **22** (10), 40–45.

Delaunay, F., Khan, A., Cintra, A. *et al.* (1997) Pancreatic beta cells are important targets for diabetogenic effects of glucocorticoids. *Journal of Clinical Investigation*, **100**, 2094–2098.

DH (1996) *Extra-Laboratory Use of Blood Glucose Meters and Test Strips: Contraindications, Training and Advice to Users*. Medical Devices Agency Adverse Incident Centre Safety Notice 9616. Department of Health, London.

DH (2000) *Comprehensive Critical Care: A Review of Adult Critical Care Services*. Department of Health, London.

DH (2001) *The Nursing Contribution to the Provision of a Comprehensive Critical Care for Adults. A Strategic Programme of Action*. Department of Health, London.

DH (2005) *Point of Care Testing. Blood Glucose Meters. Advice for Health Care Professionals*. Department of Health, London. www.mhra.gov.uk.

DH (2005b) *Saving Lives: A Delivery Programme to Reduce Healthcare Associated Infection Including MRSA: Skills for Implementation*. Department of Health, London. www.dh.gov.uk/publications.

DH (2008) *Five Years On: Delivering the Diabetes National Service Framework*. Department of Health, London. www.dh.gov.uk.

D'Hondt, J.N. (2008) Continuous intravenous insulin ready for prime time. *Diabetes Spectrum*, **21** (4), 255–261.

Diabetes UK (2008) Position statements: self-monitoring of blood glucose. www.diabetes.org.uk.

Docherty, B. (2000) Temperature recording. *Professional Nurse*, **16** (3), 943.

Docherty, B. (2002) Cardiorespiratory physical assessment for the acutely ill: 1. *British Journal of Nursing*, **11** (11), 750–758.

Docherty, B. (2005) The arteriovenous system: part one, the anatomy. *Nursing Times*, **101** (34), 28–29.

Docherty, B. (2006) Homeostasis part 3: temperature regulation. *Nursing Times*, **102** (16), 21–21.

Docherty, B. and Coote, S. (2006) Monitoring the pulse as part of the track and trigger. *Nursing Times*, **102** (43), 28–29.

Douglas, G., Nicol, F. and Robertson, C. (2005) *MacLeod's Clinical Examination*, 11th edn. Churchill Livingstone, London.

Edwards, L. and Manley, K.L. (1998) *Care of Adults in Hospital*. Edward Arnold, London.

Edwards S. (1997) Measuring temperature. *Professional Nurse*, **13** (2), 55–57.

Edwards S.L. (2000) Maintaining an adequate circulation, in *Surgical Nursing Advanced Practice* (eds K. Manley and L. Bellman). Churchill Livingstone, London, pp. 507–537.

Eguchi, K., Yacoub, M., Jhalani, J. *et al.* (2007) Consistency of blood pressure differences between the right and left arms. *Archives of Internal Medicine*, **167** (4), 388–393.

Einthoven, W. (1902) Galvanometrische registratie van het menschilijk electrocardiogram, in *Herinneringsbundel* (ed. S.S. Rosenstein). Eduard Ijdo, Leiden.

Evans, J. and Kenkre, J. (2006) Current practice and knowledge of nurses regarding patient temperature measurement. *Journal of Medical Engineering and Technology*, **30** (4), 218–223.

Fairley, S. and McLernon S. (2005) Neurological problems, in *Critical Care Nursing: Science and Practice*, 2nd edn (eds S. Adam and S.Osborne). Oxford University Press, Oxford, pp. 285–327.

Figg, K. and Nemergut, E. (2009) Error in central venous pressure measurement. *Anesthesia and Analgesia*, **108** (4), 1209–1211.

Foxall, F. (2009) *Haemodynamic Monitoring and Manipulation: An Easy Learning Guide*. M & K Publishing, Keswick.

Fraise, A.P. and Bradley, T. (eds) (2009) *Ayliffe's Control of Healthcare-associated Infection: A Practical Handbook*, 5th edn. Hodder Arnold, London.

Frawley, P. (1990) Neurological observations. *Nursing Times*, **86** (35), 29–34.

Frew, A.J., and Holgate, S.T. (2009) Respiratory disease, in *Clinical Medicine*, 7th edn (eds P. Kumar and M. Clarke). Elsevier, London.

Fuller, G. (2004) *Neurological Examinations Made Easy*, 3rd edn. Churchill Livingstone, Edinburgh.

Furnary, A.P., Chaugle, H., Kerr, K.J. and Grunkmeier, G.L. (2000) Postoperative hyperglycaemia prolongs length of stay in diabetic CABG patients. *Circulation*, **102**, 11–556.

Gallimore, D. (2004) Reviewing the effectiveness of tympanic thermometers. *Nursing Times*, **100** (32), 32–35.

Gibson, P.G., Powell, H., Wilson, A. *et al.* (2002) Self-management education and regular practitioner review for adults with asthma. *Cochrane Database of Systematic Reviews*, 1, CD001117.

Gilbert, M., Barton, A.J. and Counsell, C.M. (2002) Comparison of oral and tympanic temperatures in adult surgical patients. *Applied Nursing Research*, **15** (1), 42–47.

Gilbert, R. (2006) Taking a midstream specimen of urine. *Nursing Times*, **102** (18), 22–23.

Gillibrand, W., Holdich, P. and Covill, C. (2009) Managing type 2 diabetes: new policy and interventions. *British Journal of Community Nursing*, **14** (7), 285–291.

Goldhill, D.R., White, S.A. and Sumner, A. (1999) Physiological values and procedures in the 24 h before ICU admission from the ward. *Anaesthesia*, **54** (6), 529–534.

Goldie L. (2008) Insulin injection and blood glucose monitoring. *Practice Nurse*, **36** (2), 11–14.

Goodacre, S. and Irons, R. (2002) ABC of clinical electrocardiography: atrial arrhythmias. *British Medical Journal*, **324**, 594–597.

Gorelick, M.H., Stevens, M.W., Schultz, T. and Scribano, P.V. (2004) Difficulty in obtaining peak expiratory flow measurements in children with acute asthma. *Pediatric Emergency Care*, **20** (1), 22–26.

Gosselink, R., Bott, J., Johnson, M. *et al.* (2008) Physiotherapy for adult patients with critical illness: recommendations of the European Respiratory Society and European Society of Intensive Care Medicine Task Force on Physiotherapy for Critically Ill Patients. *Intensive Care Medicine*, **34** (7), 1188–1199.

Hall G. (2005) Choosing and teaching the use of blood glucose monitors. *Practice Nurse*, **30** (7), 46–50.

Hansen, E.F., Vestbo, J., Phanareth, K. *et al.* (2001) Peak flow as a predictor of overall mortality in asthma and chronic pulmonary disease. *American Journal of Respiratory Critical Care Medicine*, **163**, 690–693.

Hasler, M. and Cohen, J. (1982) The effect of oxygen administration on oral temperature assessment. *Nursing Research*, **31**, 265–268.

Hatchett, R. (2000) Central venous pressure measurement. *Nursing Times*, **96** (15), 49–50.

Heindenreich, T. and Giuffe, M. (1990) Postoperative temperature measurement. *Nursing Research*, **39** (3), 153–155.

Henderson, N. (1997) Central venous lines. *Nursing Standard*, **11** (42), 49–56.

Higgins, D. (2008) Patient assessment part 5 – measuring pulse. *Nursing Times*, **104** (11), 24–25.

Higginson, R, and Jones, B. (2009) Respiratory assessment in critically ill patients: airway and breathing. *British Journal of Nursing*, **18** (8), 456–461.

Hinds, C.J. and Watson, D. (2009) Intensive care medicine, in *Clinical Medicine*, 7th edn (eds P. Kumar and M. Clarke). Elsevier, London.

Hodgetts, T., Kenward, G., Vlackonikolis, I. *et al.* (2002) The identification of risk factors for cardiac arrest and formulation of activation criteria to alert a medical emergency team. *Resuscitation*, **54**, 125–131.

Hudek, C.M., Gallo, B.M. and Morton, P.G. (1998) *Critical Care Nursing: A Holistic Approach*, 7th edn. Lippincott, New York.

Hunter, J., and Rawlings-Anderson, K. (2008) Respiratory assessment. *Nursing Standard*, **22** (41), 41–43.

Izakovic, M. (2008) Central venous pressure – evaluation, interpretation, monitoring, clinical implications. *Bratislavske Lekarske Listy*, **109** (4), 185–187.

Jensen, B.N., Jeppesen, L., Mortensen, B. *et al.* (1994) The superiority of rectal thermometry to oral thermometry with regard to accuracy. *Journal of Advanced Nursing*, **20**, 660–665.

Jevon, P. (2007) Cardiac monitoring part 4 – monitoring the apex beat. *Nursing Times*, **103** (4), 28–29.

Jevon, P. and Jevon, M. (2001) Using a tympanic thermometer. *Nursing Times*, **97** (9), 43–44.

Kacmerek, R.M., Dimas, S. and Mack, C.W. (2005) *The Essentials of Respiratory Care*, 4th edn. Elsevier Mosby, St Louis, MO.

Kenney, W.L, and Munce, T.A. (2003) Invited review: aging and human temperature regulation. *Journal of Applied Physiology*, **95**, 2598–2603.

Khorshid, L., Eser, I., Zaybak, A. and Yapucu, U. (2005) Comparing mercury-in-glass, tympanic and disposable thermometers in measuring body temperature in healthy young people. *Journal of Clinical Nursing*, **14** (4), 496–500.

Kisiel, M. and Perkins, C. (2006) Nursing observations: knowledge to help prevent critical illness. *British Journal of Nursing*, **15** (19), 1052–1056.

Knies, R. (2003) Temperature measurement in acute care: the who, what, where, when, why, and how? www.enw.org/Research-Thermometry.htm.

Krikler, S. (1990) Pyrexia: what to do about temperatures. *Nursing Standard*, **4** (25), 37–38.

Krinsley, J.S. (2004) Effect of an intensive glucose management protocol on the mortality of critically ill adult patients. *Mayo Clinical Proceedings*, **79**, 992–1000.

Kumar, P. and Clarke, M. (2009) *Clinical Medicine*, 7th edn. Elsevier Saunders, London.

Lahrmann, H., Cortelli, P., Hilz, M., Mathias, C. J., Struhal, W. and Tassinari, M. (2006) EFNS guidelines on the diagnosis and management of orthostatic hypotension. *European Journal of Neurology*, 13 (9), 930–936.

Lees, L. and McAuliffe, M. (2010) Venous thromboembolism risk assessments in acute care. *Nursing Standard*, **24** (22), 35–41.

Le Frant, J.Y., Muller, L., de la Coussaye, J. *et al.* (2003) Temperature measurement in intensive care patients: comparison of urinary bladder, oesophageal, rectal, axillary and inguinal methods versus pulmonary artery core method. *Intensive Care Medicine*, **29**, 414–418.

Lemery, R., Guiraudon, G. and Veinot, J. (2003) Anatomic description of Bachmann's bundle and its relation to the atria septum. *American Journal of Cardiology*, **91** (12), 1482–1485.

Levick, J.R. (2010) *An Introduction to Cardiovascular Physiology*, 5th edn. Hodder Arnold, London.

Levine, D. (2007) Respiratory monitoring, in *Critical Care Nursing: Synergy for Optimal Outcomes* (eds R. Kaplow and S.R. Hardin). Jones and Bartlett, London.

Levine, J., Munden, J. and Thompson, G. (2008) *ECG Interpretation Made Incredibly Easy*. Lippincott Williams and Wilkins, London.

Lim-Levy, F. (1982) The effect of oxygen inhalation on oral temperature. *Nursing Research*, **31**, 150–152.

Lowe, L. (1995) Accuracy in ward-based blood glucose monitoring. *Nursing Times*, **91** (13), 44–45.

Magder, S. (2006a) Central venous pressure monitoring. *Current Opinion in Critical Care*, **12** (3), 219–227.

Magder, S. (2006b) Central venous pressure: a useful but no so simple measurement. *Critical Care Medicine*, **34** (8), 2224–2227.

Marieb, E.M. and Hoehn, K. (2010) *Human Anatomy and Physiology*, 8th edn. Pearson Benjamin Cummings, San Francisco.

Marini, J. and Wheeler, A. (2010) *Critical Care Medicine: The Essentials*, 4th edn. Lippincott Williams and Wilkins, Philadelphia.

Martin, E.A. (2003) *Oxford Concise Colour Medical Dictionary*, 3rd edn. Oxford University Press, Oxford.

McClelland, D.B.L. (ed.) (2007) *Handbook of Transfusion Medicine*, 4th edn. Stationery Office, London.

McKnight, K.A. and Carter, L. (2008) From trays to tube feedings: overcoming the challenges of hospital nutrition and glycemic control. *Diabetes Spectrum*, **21** (4), 233–240.

MDA (2002) Self monitoring in type 2 diabetes mellitus: a meta-analysis. *Diabetic Medicine*, **11**, 755–761.

Metcalfe, H. (2000) Recording a 12-lead electrocardiogram – 1. *Nursing Times*, **96** (19), 43–44.

MHRA (2001) Tissue Necrosis Caused by Pulse Oximeter Probes. SN 2001 (08). www.mhra.gov.uk/home.

MHRA (2004) Medical Device ALERT: Peak expiratory flow meter (PFM) all makes. www.mhra.gov.uk/home.

MHRA (2005) Report of the Independent Advisory Group on Blood Pressure Monitoring in Clinical Practice. www.mhra.gov.uk/home.

Minor, D.G. and Waterhouse, J.M. (1981) *Circadian Rhythms and the Human*. Wright, Bristol.

Mooney, G. and Comerford, D. (2003) Neurological observations. *Nursing Times*, **99** (17), 24–25.

Moore, T. (2004a) Pulse oximetry, in *High Dependency Nursing Care: Observation, Intervention and Support* (eds T. Moore and P. Woodrow). Routledge, London.

Moore, T. (2004b) Respiratory assessment, in *High Dependency Nursing Care: Observation, Intervention and Support* (eds T. Moore and P. Woodrow). Routledge, London.

Moore, T. (2007) Respiratory assessment in adults. *Nursing Standard*, **21** (49), 48–56.

Morton, P.G., Tucker, T. and van Rueden, R. (2005) *Critical Care Nursing: A Holistic Approach*, 8th edn. Lippincott Williams and Wilkins, Philadelphia.

Muralidhar, K. (2002) Central venous pressure and pulmonary capillary wedge pressure monitoring. *Indian Journal of Anaesthesia*, **46** (4), 298–303.

Nakamura, K., Tanaka, M., Motohashi, Y. and Maeda, A. (1997) Oral temperatures in the elderly in nursing homes in summer and winter in relation to activities of daily living. *International Journal of Biometerology*, **40** (2), 103–106.

Navas, S. (2003a) Atrial fibrillation: part 2. *Nursing Standard*, **17** (38), 47–54.

Navas, S. (2003b) Atrial fibrillation: part 1. *Nursing Standard*, **17** (37), 45–54.

Neff, J., Ayoub, J., Longman, A. and Noyes, A. (1989) Effect of respiratory rate, respiratory depth, and open versus closed mouth breathing on sublingual temperature. *Research in Nursing and Health*, **12**, 195–202.

Neno, R. (2005) Hypothermia: assessment, treatment and prevention. *Nursing Standard*, **19** (20), 47–52.

NICE (2004) Guidelines for the diagnosis and management of Type 1 diabetes in children, young people and adults. Guideline Number 15. www.nice.org.uk.

NICE (2006) *Hypertension: Management of Hypertension in Adults in Primary Care (a Partial Update of NICE Clinical Guideline 18)*. National Institute for Health and Clinical Excellence, London.

NICE (2007a) *Venous Thromboembolism: Reducing the Risk of Venous Thromboembolism (Deep Vein Thrombosis and Pulmonary Embolism) in Inpatients Undergoing Surgery*. National Institute for Health and Clinical Excellence, London.

NICE (2007b) *Acutely Ill Patients in Hospital: Recognition of and Response to Acute Illness in Adults in Hospital*, National Institute for Health and Clinical Excellence, London.

NICE (2008) Guideline for type 2 diabetes. www.nice.org.uk/CG66.

NMC (2008a) *The Code: Standards of Conduct, Performance and Ethics for Nurses and Midwives*. Nursing and Midwifery Council, London. www.nmc-uk.org.

NMC (2008b) *Consent*. Nursing and Midwifery Council, London. www.nmc-uk.org/Nurses-and-midwives/Advice-by-topic/A/Advice/Consent/.

NMC (2009) *Record Keeping: Guidance for Nurses and Midwives*. Nursing and Midwifery Council, London.

Noble, R., Johnson, R., Thomas, A. and Bass, P. (2010) *The Cardiovascular System: Basic Science and Clinical Conditions*, 2nd edn. Churchill Livingston Elsevier: Edinburgh

O'Brien,E., Asmar, R., Beilin, L. *et al.*, on behalf of the European Society of Hypertension Working Group on Blood Pressure Monitoring (2003) European Society of Hypertension recommendations for conventional, ambulatory and home blood pressure measurement. *Journal of Hypertension*, **21**, 821–848.

O'Driscoll, B.R., Howard, L.S., Davison, A.G., on behalf of the British Thoracic Society (2008) *BTS Guideline for Emergency Oxygen use in Adult Patients*. www.brit-thoracic.org.uk.

Ogawa, A., Johnson, J.H., Ohneda, M. *et al.* (1992) Roles of insulin resistance and beta-cell dysfunction in dexamethasone-induced diabetes. *Journal of Clinical Investigation*, **90**, 497–509.

O'Neill, D. and Le Grove, A. (2003) Monitoring critically ill patients in accident and emergency. *Nursing Times*, **99** (45), 32–35.

O'Toole, S. (1997) Alternatives to mercury thermometers. *Professional Nurse*, **12** (11), 783–786.

Owens D., Barnett A.H., Pickup J. *et al.* (2004) Blood glucose self-monitoring in type 1 and type 2 diabetes: reaching a multidisciplinary consensus. *Diabetes and Primary Care*, **6** (1), 8–16.

Parkman, S. (2007) Respiratory anatomy, physiology and assessment, in *Critical Care Nursing: Synergy for Optimal Outcomes* (eds R. Kaplow and S.R. Hardin). Jones and Bartlett, London.

Patton, K.T. and Thiobodeau, G.A. (2009) *Anatomy and Physiology*, 7th edn. Mosby Elsevier, St Louis, MO.

Pelter, M. (2008) Electrocardiographic monitoring in the medical-surgical setting: clinical implications, bases, lead configurations, and nursing implications. *MEDSURG Nursing*, **17** (6), 421–428.

Philip, J.P. and Kowery, P.R. (2001) *Cardiac Arrhythmia: Mechanisms, Diagnosis and Management*, 2nd edn. Lippincott Williams and Wilkins, Philadelphia.

Price, T. (2002) Painful stimuli and the Glasgow Coma Scale. *Nursing Critical Care*, **7** (1), 17–23.

825

Quanjer, P.H., Lebowitz, M.D., Gregg, I. *et al.* (1997) Peak expiratory flow: conclusions and recommendations of a Working Party of the European Respiratory Society. *European Respiratory Journal*, **10** (24), 2s–8s.

Rawlings-Anderson, K. and Hunter, J. (2008) Monitoring pulse rate. *Nursing Standard*, **22** (31), 41–43.

Reddel, H.K. (2006) Peak flow monitoring in clinical practice and clinical asthma trials. *Current Opinion in Pulmonary Medicine*, **12** (1), 75–81.

Resuscitation Council UK (2005) *Resuscitation Guidelines*. RCUK Publications, London.

Resuscitation Council (UK) (2006) Airway management and ventilation, in *Advanced Life Support*, 5th edn. Resuscitation Council (UK), London, pp. 41–57.

Rigby, D. and Gray, K. (2005) Understanding urine testing. *Nursing Times*, **101** (12), 60–61.

Rivers, E., Nguyen, B., Havstad, S. *et al.* (2001) Early goal-directed therapy in the treatment of severe sepsis and septic shock. *New England Journal of Medicine*, **345**, 1368–1377.

Rizvi A.A. and Saunders M.B. (2006) Assessment and monitoring of glycemic control in primary care: monitoring techniques, record keeping, meter downloads, tests of average glycemia and point of care evaluation. *Journal of American Academy of Nurse Practitioners*, **18**, 11–21.

Roberts, A. (2002) The role of anatomy and physiology in interpreting ECGs. *Nursing Times*, **98** (20), 34–36.

Roche Diagnostics (2004) *Accu-Chem Safe T-Pro Plus: Information Leaflet*. Roche, East Sussex.

Rowley, G. and Fielding, K. (1991) Reliability and accuracy of the Glasgow Coma Scale with experienced and inexperienced users. *Lancet*, **337** (8740), 535–538.

Ruffin, R. (2004) Peak expiratory flow (PEF) monitoring. *Thorax*, **59**, 913.

Samples, F., van Cott, M., Long, C. *et al.* (1985) Circadian rhythms: basis for screening for fever. *Nursing Research*, **34** (6), 377–379.

Scales, K. (2008a) Anatomy and physiology related to intravenous therapy, in *Intravenous Therapy in Nursing Practice*, 2nd edn (eds L. Dougherty and J. Lamb). Blackwell, Oxford.

Scales, K. (2008b) Vascular access in the acute care setting, in *Intravenous Therapy in Nursing Practice*, 2nd edn (eds L. Dougherty and J. Lamb). Blackwell, Oxford.

Scales, K. (2010) Central venous pressure monitoring in clinical practice. *Nursing Standard*, **24** (29), 49–55.

Scales, K. and Pilsworth, J. (2008) The importance of fluid balance in clinical practice. *Nursing Standard*, **22** (47), 50–57.

Scherer, P. (1986) The logic of coma. *American Journal of Nursing*, **86**, 542–549.

Schwab, M. and Porter, M. (2007) Inpatient diabetes mellitus in the oncology setting. *Clinical Journal of Oncology Nursing*, **11** (4), 489–492.

Scott, S., Giuliano, K., Pysznik, E. *et al.* (1995) Influence of port site on central venous pressure measurements from triple-lumen catheters in critically ill adults. *American Journal of Critical Care*, **7**, 60–63.

SCST (2006) Clinical guidelines by consensus recording a standard 12-lead electrocardiogram an approved methodology. Society for Cardiology Science and Technology. www.scst.org.uk.

Shah, S. (1999) Neurological assessment. *Nursing Times*, **13**, 49–56.

Sharber, J. (1997) The efficacy of tepid sponge bathing to reduce fever in young children. *American Journal of Emergency Medicine*, **15** (2), 188–192.

Sharman, J. (2007) Clinical skills: cardiac rhythm recognition and monitoring. *British Journal of Nursing*, **16** (5), 306–311.

Shelledy, D.C. (2009) Initiating and adjusting ventilatory support, in *Egan's Fundamentals of Respiratory Care*, 9th edn (eds R.L. Wilkins, J.K. Stoller and R.M. Kacmarek). Mosby Elsevier, St Louis, MO.

Simpson, H. (2006) Respiratory assessment. *British Journal of Nursing*, **15** (9), 484–488.

Steele, J.R. and Hardin, S.R. (2007) Hypertension, in *Critical Care Nursing: Synergy for Optimal Outcomes* (eds R. Kaplow and S.R. Hardin). Jones and Bartlett, London.

Steggall, M. (2007) Urine samples and urinalysis. *Nursing Standard*, **22** (14), 42–45.

Stergiou, G.S., Karpettas, N., Atkins, N. and O'Brien, E. (2010) European Society of Hypertension International Protocol for the validation of blood pressure monitors: a critical review of its application and rationale for revision. *Blood Pressure Monitoring*, **15** (1), 39–48.

Stevenson, T. (2004) Achieving best practice in routine observation of hospital patients. *Nursing Times*, **100** (30), 34–35.

Teasdale, G. and Jennett, B. (1974) Assessment of coma and impaired consciousness: a practical scale. *Lancet*, **2**, 81–84.

Thornton, H. (2009) Type 1 diabetes, part 1: An introduction. *British Journal of Nursing*, **4** (5), 223–227.

Tonnesen, P., Carrozzi, L., Fagerstrom, K. *et al.* (2007) Smoking cessation in patients with respiratory diseases: a high priority, integral component of therapy. *European Respiratory Journal*, **29**, 390–417.

Torrance, C. and Elley, K. (1998) Urine testing 2 – urinalysis. *Nursing Times*, **94** (5), 1–2.

Torrance, C. and Semple, M. (1998) Recording temperature. *Nursing Times*, **94** (2), 1–2.

Tortora G.J. and Derrickson B. (2009) *Principles of Anatomy and Physiology*, 12th edn. John Wiley, New Jersey.

Trim, J. (2005) Monitoring temperature. *Nursing Times*, **101** (20), 30–31.

Turner, M., Burns, S., Chaney, C. *et al.* (2008) Measuring blood pressure accurately in an ambulatory cardiology clinic setting: do patient position and timing really matter? *MEDSURG Nursing*, **17** (2), 93–98.

Udwadia, F.E. (2005) *Principles of Critical Care*, 2nd edn. Oxford University Press, Oxford.

Valler-Jones, T. and Wedgbury, K. (2005) Measuring blood pressure using the mercury sphygmomanometer. *British Journal of Nursing*, **14** (3), 145–150.

Van Den Berghe, G., Wouters, P., Weekers, F. *et al.* (2001) Intensive insulin therapy in critically ill patients. *New England Journal of Medicine*, **345** (19), 1359–1367.

Van Groningen, L., Adiyaman, A., Elving, L. *et al.* (2008) Which physiological mechanism is responsible for the increase in blood pressure during leg crossing? *Journal of Hypertension*, **26** (3), 433–437.

Van Staaij, B.K., Rovers, M., Schilder, A. and Hoes, A.W. (2003) Accuracy and feasibility of daily infrared tympanic membrane temperature measurements in identification of fever in children. *International Journal of Pediatric Otorhinolaryngology*, **67**, 1091–1097.

Verrij, E.A., Nieuwenhuizen, L. and Bos, W.J.W. (2009) Raising the arm before cuff inflation increases the loudness of Korotkoff sounds. *Blood Pressure Monitoring*, **14** (6), 268–273.

Wagner, D. (2006) Unplanned perioperative hypothermia. *AORN Journal*, **83** (2), 470–476.

Walker, R. (2004) Capillary blood glucose monitoring and its role in diabetes management. *British Journal of Community Nursing*, **9** (10), 438–440.

Wallymahmed, M. (2007) Capillary blood glucose monitoring. *Nursing Standard*, **21** (38), 35–38.

826

Walsh, M. (2002) *Watson's Clinical Nursing and Related Sciences*, 6th edn. Baillière Tindall, London.

Walsh, M. (2006) *Nurse Practitioners: Clinical Skills and Professional Issues*, 2nd edn. Butterworth-Heinemann, Edinburgh.

Ward, K., Tiba, M., Barbee, R. *et al.* (2006) A new noninvasive method to determine central venous pressure. *Resuscitation*, 70, 238–46.

Waterhouse, C. (2005) The Glasgow Coma Scale and other neurological observations. *Nursing Standard*, 19 (33), 56–64.

Watson, R. (1998) Controlling body temperature in adults. *Nursing Standard*, 12 (20), 49–55.

Weber, J. and Kelley, J. (2003) *Health Assessment in Nursing*, 2nd edn. Lippincott Williams and Wilkins, Philadelphia.

Weldon, K. (1998) Neurological observations, in *Neuro-Oncology for Nurses* (ed. D. Guerrero). Whurr, London, pp. 1–28.

Weller, B (2005) *Baillière's Nurses' Dictionary for Nurses and Healthcare Workers*, 24th edn. Elsevier, Edinburgh.

Wheatley, I. (2006) The nursing practice of taking level 1 patient observations. *Intensive and Critical Care Nursing*, 22, 115–121.

WHO (2006) *Definition and Diagnosis of Diabetes Mellitus and Intermediate Hyperglycaemia*. World Health Organization, Geneva. www.who.int/diabetes/publications/en/.

Wilkins, R.L. (2009) Bedside assessment of the patient, in *Egan's Fundamentals of Respiratory Care*, 9th edn (eds R.L. Wilkins, J.K. Stoller and R.M. Kacmarek). Mosby Elsevier, St Louis, MO.

Williams, B., Poulter, N., Brown, M. *et al.* (2004) Guidelines for management of hypertension: report of the fourth working party

of the British Hypertension Society 2004 – BHS IV. *Journal of Human Hyptertension*, 18 (3), 139–185.

Wilson, F., Johnson, F. and Rosenbaum, F. (1944) The precordial electrocardiogram. *American Heart Journal*, 27, 19–85.

Wilson, L.A. (2005) Urinalysis. *Nursing Standard*, 19 (35), 51–54.

Wong, F. (2007) Pulsus paradoxus in ventilated and non-ventilated patients. *Dynamics*, 18 (3), 16–18.

Woodhall, L. (2008) Implementation of the SBAR communication technique in a tertiary centre. *Journal of Emergency Nursing*, 34 (4), 314–317.

Woodrow, P. (1999) Pulse oximetry. *Nursing Standard*, 13 (42), 42–46.

Woodrow, P. (2002) Central venous catheters and central venous pressure. *Nursing Standard*, 16 (26), 45–51.

Woodrow, P. (2004a) Arterial blood pressure monitoring, in *High Dependency Nursing Care: Observation, Intervention and Support* (eds T. Moore and P. Woodrow). Routledge, London.

Woodrow, P. (2004b) Central venous pressure measurement and cardiac studies, in *High Dependency Nursing Care: Observation, Intervention and Support* (eds T. Moore and P. Woodrow). Routledge, London.

Woods, S., Froelicher, E.S., Motzer, S.A. *et al.* (2005) *Cardiac Nursing*, 5th edn. Lippincott Williams and Wilkins, Philadelphia.

Woollens, S. (1996) Temperature measurement devices. *Professional Nurse*, 11 (8), 541–547.

Zietz, K. and McCutcheon, H. (2006) Observations and vital signs: ritual or vital for the monitoring of postoperative patients? *Applied Nursing Research*, 19, 204–211.

Radionuclide investigations and therapy

Procedure guidelines

The Royal Marsden Hospital Manual of Clinical Nursing Procedures, Eighth Edition. Edited by Lisa Dougherty and Sara Lister.
© 2011 The Royal Marsden Hospital. Published 2011 by Blackwell Publishing Ltd.

Overview

Radiation is capable of being beneficial and harmful; it is therefore essential that every effort is made to minimize the harmful effects of diagnostic and therapeutic radiation whilst maximizing its benefits (Darby 1999).

This chapter provides specific detailed information on the principles of nursing care in relation to radioisotopes in the clinical setting. This will enable staff to apply best practice principles when caring for patients, and facilitate the education and support of other healthcare professionals and visitors.

Radiation

Definitions

Radiation occurs when energy is emitted or generated as either waves or particles (known as electromagnetic or particulate radiation). Radioactivity is a natural phenomenon in which unstable atoms emit radiation. In stable atoms ionizing radiation is produced through excitation, ionization and nuclear disintegration. Radiography is the practice of using X-rays to produce an image on film.

Related theory

Every minute of our lives we are exposed to radiation from natural and artificial sources.

Naturally occurring radiation comprises radiation from outer space (cosmic radiation), from the ground and from the air (radon). Small amounts of naturally occurring radiation are also present in the food we eat. Natural radiation accounts for 85.5% of the total radiation received by the UK population. This belongs to a class of radiation known as electromagnetic radiation which transports energy through space in the form of electric and magnetic waves. Electromagnetic radiation is encountered in our day-to-day lives; in fact, life as we know it would not be possible without electromagnetic radiation.

Electromagnetic radiation provides radio and television signals, microwaves, visible light, X-rays and gamma rays; however, it is well known that, as well as providing many benefits, there are potentially serious health effects associated with electromagnetic radiation. The nature of these effects varies depending on which part of the spectrum the radiation belongs to. Radiation may also be encountered in the form of particles, rather than waves; particulate radiation is also capable of producing ionization and can therefore produce biological effects. Radiation particles most commonly used in hospitals are streams of electrons, known as beta radiation.

Artificial sources of radiation including medical exposures, discharges from industrial premises and fall-out from atomic weapons testing make up the remaining 14.5% of the radiation received by the population, with medical exposures being the largest contributor.

Radiation is capable of disrupting the chemical balance in the cell by damaging the DNA. This is caused by the introduction of free radicals, atoms/molecules with unpaired electrons (Health Protection Agency 2010), which may lead to cell death or cancer at some time in the future. Therefore substantial emphasis is placed on reducing the amount of radiation given during medical exposures.

Radiation is used in treating malignant disease and includes X-rays produced artificially by electron bombardment of a metal target; gamma rays (a natural emission in the nuclear decay of radioisotopes), sometimes referred to as 'photon' radiation; and beta particles (capable of ionization). These are distinguishable from electromagnetic radiation by their characteristic of carrying a negative electrical charge; beta particles result when a neutron within the nucleus disintegrates to form a proton and an electron. The electron is ejected from the nucleus, producing beta radiation (IPEM/RCN 2002).

Radiation used in nuclear medicine, in laboratory tests and for certain types of radiotherapy treatments is emitted by radioactive materials. In a process known as radioactive decay, the amount of radiation emitted by radioactive material diminishes continuously over time until the material no longer produces radiation. The time taken for the radioactivity in such a material to be halved is known as the half-life. Different materials have different half-lives ranging from a few seconds or minutes to many years. The majority of radioactive materials used in hospitals have relatively short half-lives and so diminish to insignificant levels within a few hours or a few days (Health Protection Agency 2010).

Radioactive material may be encountered in solid (sealed), liquid or gaseous form (unsealed). Liquid or gaseous radioactive materials have the important advantage that they can be used *in vivo* to study metabolic processes. As radioactive materials emit radiation in all directions, they are usually kept in lead containers for safety.

Ionizing radiation is the term used to describe energetic particles (e.g. alpha, beta) or electromagnetic waves with a wavelength of no more than 100 nanometres because they are capable of producing ions by ejecting electrons from their atoms (DH 2000).

Radioisotopes are measured in becquerels (Bq). A becquerel is the Système International (SI) unit of activity and is 1 disintegration per second:

$$k \text{ (kilo)} = 1 \times 10^3$$
$$M \text{ (mega)} = 1 \times 10^6, \text{ e.g. megabecquerel (MBq)}$$
$$G \text{ (giga)} = 1 \times 10^9$$

The half-life of a radioactive substance is the time taken for it to decay to half its original number of radioactive atoms (Bomford 2002a). The sensitive target appears to be DNA in the nucleus of the cell. The ionizing radiation thus passes through the cells and tissues, and the dose of radiation received is measured in terms of energy absorbed; the unit of absorbed dose is known as a gray:

$$100 \text{ centigray (cGy)} = 1 \text{ gray (Gy)}$$

For the purposes of radiation protection for staff and patients, the dose calculated to the whole body must be known. Whereas the absorbed dose is measured in grays, the dose to the whole body is measured in sieverts. For example, staff over 18 years of age who are not pregnant must wear a monitoring badge to monitor their individual exposure to radiation. There is an annual dose limit of 20 millisieverts (mSv), but the dose to staff should be kept below 6 mSv (DH 2000).

Radiation protection

Evidence-based approaches

Rationale

Radiation protection is based on three principles.

1 *Justification:* no practice should be adopted unless its introduction produces a net benefit.
2 *Optimization:* all exposure shall be as low as reasonably practicable (ALARP).
3 *Limitation:* the dose equivalent to staff and members of the public shall not exceed the dose limits.

Requirements for procedures involving unsealed sources include the following.

■ Those administering radioactive material must hold an approved Administration of Radioactive Substances Advisory Committee (ARSAC) certificate for each radionuclide they intend to use.
■ Administration of therapeutic and diagnostic radioactive substances can only be carried out in centres with appropriate facilities (Cormack *et al.* 1998). Therapeutic unsealed sources generate a significant amount of liquid radioactive waste, from showers and toilets. The amount of radioactive waste that enters the sewage system is governed by local regulations. Multiple holding tank systems can be employed where waste can be held to allow decay to occur before being released into the main waste drainage system (Leung and Nikolic 1998).
■ Risk assessments must be carried out prior to work with ionizing radiation, to ensure risks are properly controlled (Pearson *et al.* 2001).
■ All controlled areas will have warning notices to restrict entry.
■ All controlled and supervised areas have local rules and systems of work, summarizing the arrangements for controlling work with ionizing radiation. The radiation protection supervisor ensures that the local rules are followed.
■ Visitors are restricted. Doses received by relatives/friends of patients undergoing treatment or examination with ionizing radiation are restricted to the doses allowed to members of the public unless they are classified as com-

forters and carers when different rules and restrictions apply.
■ Exposure is controlled by the use of time, distance and shielding.
■ Personal protective clothing including gloves, aprons and overshoes must be used to limit the risk of contamination.
■ Procedures are in place for reporting incidents (RIDDOR 1995).
■ Adequate training is provided and only trained staff are allowed to work unsupervised.
■ No pregnant or breastfeeding staff to enter the controlled area.
■ Quality assurance initiatives have to be undertaken; these include clinical audit of procedures and standards.

Legal and professional issues
Regulations

Radiation regulations are an essential component designed to protect healthcare workers; it is law that all organizations involved in a procedure using ionizing and non-ionizing radiation must adhere to radiation regulations.

The International Commission on Radiological Protection (ICRP) oversees radiation safety. The Health Protection Agency (HPA) has statutory responsibility for advising UK government departments as well as other professional groups such as the Institute of Physics and Engineering in Medicine (IPEM) on radiation protection and regulation.

Box 14.1 describes the legal Acts that all organizations must adhere to when providing diagnostic and therapeutic unsealed and sealed source radioisotopes.

Preprocedural considerations
Controlled area

The entrance to the controlled area must be marked with a warning sign.

Information is displayed to indicate the following.

■ The radioactive material and activity administered.
■ That only essential nursing procedures should be carried out and unnecessary time must not be spent in close proximity to the patient while the sign is displayed.

Appropriate barriers, that is lead shields, should be placed at the entrance to:

■ prevent inadvertent entry by unauthorized personnel
■ reduce radiation exposure to visitors and staff.

Patients treated with unsealed radioactive sources should be confined to their rooms, except for special medical or nursing procedures, when they must be accompanied by suitably trained staff.

Box 14.1 Legal Acts

The Radioactive Substances Act 1993

- Controls the use and disposal of radioactive materials in hospitals and elsewhere, and is enforced by the Environment Agency, via a system of licensing and inspection.

Pregnancy and Work in Diagnostic Imaging, Report of a Joint Working Party of the Royal College of Radiologists and British Institute of Radiology, 1992

- This report provides a summary of present knowledge on radiation effects in the foetus and recommends the steps to be taken when a member of staff declares she is pregnant.

Health and Safety at Work Act 1974

- Provides the umbrella for all safety-related legislation.
- Regulates safety in the workplace.
- Puts the responsibility for safety on the employer, for example the health authority, trust board or chief executive.
- Enforced by inspectors of the Health and Safety Executive who can prosecute for contravention of regulations and serve improvement and enforcement notices.
- Provides for health and safety representatives.

Ionizing Radiations Regulations, SI 3232, 1999

- Regulate all radiation work from dental X-rays to nuclear power stations.
- Cover dose limitation and management systems for radiation safety including Local Rules, appointment of advisers and supervisors.

Approved Code of Practice, 'Work with Ionizing Radiation', 2000

- 'Approved' by the Health and Safety Commission.
- Gives acceptable methods of complying with legal requirements.
- Should be followed unless there is good reason to use alternatives.

Ionizing Radiation (Medical Exposure) Regulations, SI 1059, 2000

- Employers are responsible for the radiation safety of patients.
- Staff must be competent and properly trained to undertake their role in any process which exposes patients to radiation.
- Expert advice must be sought from a medical physicist.
- Patient doses must be justifiable.

Medical and Dental Guidance Notes

- A good practice guide on all aspects of ionizing radiation protection in the clinical environment.
- Practical guide to safe practice.
- No legal status.

832

Figure 14.1 TLD dose meter.

Decon should be available in the controlled area. Decon is an approved solution for neutralizing radiopharmaceuticals in the event of a spillage. The solution should be diluted according to manufacturer's instructions or be available as ready-to-use wipes. Once the spillage area has been initially wiped with absorbent paper/pads, Decon is used to clean the surface. The area is then monitored to check for radiation contamination. The process should be repeated until the contamination has been reduced to a safe level (DH 2000).

Figure 14.2 Hand and foot monitor.

Equipment

Thermoluminescent (TLD) dose meter

TLD dose meters measure a persons exposure to radiation and must be worn at all times when on duty (Figure 14.1). A digital dosimeter should be used when ongoing immediate dose records are required.

Use of contamination monitor

Waste and equipment must be monitored before being removed from controlled areas where patients have received or are receiving unsealed or sealed sources. This monitoring will establish if contamination has occurred or a sealed source is present amongst the items being removed (Hart 2006). Before using a contamination monitor (Figures 14.2 and 14.3), it is important to check that the monitor's batteries are fully charged; the background reading on the monitor must then be noted before undertaking the monitoring. The background must be reasonably low (normally less than 10 counts per second), otherwise it will be difficult to detect small levels of radioactivity present on the item being monitored. If the background reading immediately outside the treatment room is found to be

Figure 14.3 Hand-held monitor.

high it will be necessary to monitor the items further away where the background is lower.

Items should be monitored by passing the monitor's probe over each item, while watching for fluctuations in the count rate. If an item is found to be contaminated (indicated by a sustained increase in count rate), it should either be returned to a safe location in the treatment room or set aside in a designated area while help is sought from the physics department (Bomford 2002a).

Procedure guideline 14.1 Radiation protection: major spillage of radioactive body fluids through incontinence and/or vomiting

Essential equipment

- Absorbent pads/paper
- Gloves
- Overshoes
- Apron and/or gown

Optional equipment

- Decon, an approved solution for neutralizing isotopes

- (COSHH) radiation waste bag
- Radiation warning tape
- Hand-held radiation monitor

Procedure

Action	Rationale
1 Put on the protective clothing found in the spillage kit and immediately cover the spillage with absorbent material.	To absorb contamination and to contain area of spillage (DH 2000, C).
2 Inform the physics department immediately.	So that the physics department can advise on radiation protection as soon as possible, to ensure local policy is adhered to (DH 2000, C).
3 If physics department staff are not immediately available, use a radiation monitor to assess the extent of the spillage.	To define extent of contamination and determine what further measures need to be taken (DH 2000, C).
4 Any waste that cannot be flushed down the toilet or macerated must be placed in a purple polythene bag and the physics staff informed.	To prevent contamination of the environment (DH 2000, C).
5 Follow the advice of the physics department staff in clearing the spillage using the designated spillage kit.	To prevent spread of contamination (DH 2000, C).

Procedure guideline 14.2 Radiation protection: contamination of bare hands by radioactive body fluids

Essential equipment

- Soap and water
- Hand held radiation monitor

Optional equipment

- Decon, an approved solution for neutralizing isotopes

Procedure

Action	Rationale
1 Wash hands in warm soapy water, paying special attention to the areas around the fingernails, between the fingers and on the outer edges of the hands. Continue washing and monitoring hands until contamination is below the permissible limits indicated by local monitoring protocols.	To remove radioactive material from any areas where it might be trapped (HSE 2002, C).
2 If the skin is broken in a contamination accident, wash thoroughly under running water, opening the edges of the cut. This should be continued until physics department staff can demonstrate that no residual radioactivity remains in the wound.	To stimulate bleeding and permit thorough flushing of the cut. E

Procedure guideline 14.3 Radiation protection: death of patient who has received unsealed radioactive source therapy

Essential equipment

- Absorbent pads/paper
- Gloves
- Overshoes
- Apron and/or gown
- (COSHH) radiation waste bag
- Radiation warning tape
- Hand-held radiation monitor

Optional equipment

- Decon, an approved solution for neutralizing isotopes

Procedure

Action	Rationale
1 Inform the physics department immediately.	So that the physics department staff can begin making the necessary arrangements for removal of the body to the mortuary (DH 2000, C).
2 Two nurses wearing gloves, plastic aprons or gown, and overshoes should perform Last Offices. All orifices must be packed carefully. Any vomit, blood, faeces or urine must be cleaned from the body.	To avoid contamination with body fluids. Minimal handling of the body reduces the risk of contamination. E
3 The body should be totally enclosed in a plastic body bag.	To avoid contamination of the porters and the mortuary staff (DH 2000, C).
4 Transfer of the body should be arranged with the physics department.	The physics department will supervise the transfer of the body. E

Procedure guideline 14.4 Radiation protection: cardiac arrest of patient who has received unsealed radioactive source therapy

Essential equipment

- Absorbent pads/paper
- Gloves
- Overshoes
- Apron and/or gown

- (COSHH) radiation waste bag
- Radiation warning tape
- Hand-held radiation monitor

Optional equipment

- Decon, an approved solution for neutralizing isotopes

Procedure

Action	Rationale
1 The switchboard must be told to inform the physics department as soon as possible after alerting the emergency resuscitation team.	So that the physics department can advise on radiation protection as soon as possible (DH 2000, C).
2 Do not use mouth-to-mouth resuscitation. All areas must be supplied with an Ambu-bag for this purpose.	Mouth-to-mouth contact could result in contamination of the resuscitator (DH 2000, C).
3 Overshoes, gloves and apron or gowns must be put on as soon as is practicably possible.	To minimize personal contamination (DH 2000, C; HSE 2002, C).
4 All emergency equipment must be monitored and decontaminated as necessary before being returned to general use.	To prevent contaminated equipment leaving the controlled area (DH 2000, C).

Procedure guideline 14.5 Radiation protection: evacuation due to fire of patients who have received unsealed radioactive source therapy

Procedure

Action	Rationale
1 Every effort should be made to contact the physics department without compromising the patient's safety.	To help in the evacuation of the patients treated with iodine-131 (DH 2000, C).
2 Following evacuation, patients treated with iodine-131 should be kept at a distance from other patients and staff.	To minimize exposure of others to radiation (DH 2000, C).

Postprocedural considerations

Ongoing care

Contamination control

When using unsealed sources, it is important to guard against contamination of both personnel and the hospital environment by the correct use of protective gloves, plastic apron or gowns and overshoes (DH 2000). The patient's body fluids are highly radioactive, especially in the days immediately after iodine-131 has been administered. Any action that is likely to cause contamination of personnel, for example the application of cosmetics, eating, drinking or smoking when the healthcare worker's hands are contaminated with radioactivity, is prohibited.

In an emergency, the safety and medical care of the patient must take precedence over any potential radiation hazards to staff. Written radiation safety instructions must be available in all radiation areas where an emergency may arise. These instructions must contain a detailed description of how to manage a patient in the event of a medical emergency and the action required in other emergency situations, such as fire. The course of action in an emergency procedure depends on local circumstances and the nature of the emergency.

An incident occurring within the first 24 hours of iodine-131 being administered is obviously a greater hazard than a similar incident on the day of discharge. Movement of the patient to other wards or areas, for example X-ray or critical care unit (CCU), must only be undertaken following the physics department's advice.

Incident procedure

If an accident or incident has occurred or if one is suspected, the immediate priority is to ensure the safety of patients, staff and visitors and to take whatever action is practicable to prevent further damage or injury (see Procedure guideline 14.1). As soon as immediate care has been provided, all accidents, untoward incidents and near misses, irrespective of severity, must be reported on an incident report form. Proactive and reactive risk management processes are important. These processes should identify areas of potentially higher risk or allow lessons to be learnt from past incidents and accidents. This will allow the implementation of appropriate action plans to reduce the probability and/or severity of an incident occurring or recurring.

Diagnostic radioisotope procedures (nuclear medicine)

Definition

Nuclear medicine involves the administration of radioactive material in the form of a radiopharmaceutical to patients for diagnosis or therapy (DH 2000). In both cases, the radioactive material is attached to a pharmaceutical chosen according to the organ or system to be investigated or treated. For example, radioactively labelled phosphates will be concentrated in the bone and are therefore used for bone scans, whereas radioactive iodine (given in the form of sodium iodide) concentrates in the thyroid and is used for both imaging and treating various thyroid conditions. A radiopharmaceutical is injected intravenously or given orally prior to a gamma camera scan or as a treatment, when it is referred to as radionuclide therapy.

A radionuclide investigation involves administration of the appropriate radiopharmaceutical and using dynamic imaging or waiting a predetermined time to allow the radiopharmaceutical to be taken up in the organ to be investigated. The patient is then positioned on the camera table, usually lying flat, and is required to keep still during the scan. Movement causes artefacts which reduce diagnostic accuracy. The scan may last 15–60 minutes (Ziessman *et al.* 2006) (Table 14.1).

Evidence-based approaches

Rationale

The important properties that make the radiopharmaceutical useful for diagnostic purposes include:

- the physical half-life
- decay characteristics
- ease of incorporation into radiopharmaceuticals
- availability of radionuclide.

A desirable radionuclide should have a half-life just long enough to allow for preparation, administration and concentration in the region of interest, but short enough for radiation to effectively disappear after the test (Cherry *et al.* 2003). Imaging studies commonly performed in a nuclear medicine department include:

- assessment of structures and/or function of organs
- sites of infection
- presence of tumours.

Common non-imaging studies include investigations into red cell mass and plasma volume, gastrointestinal tract and renal function.

Principles of care

Radiation protection is more complex than for X-ray procedures because, in addition to the external hazard, there is an internal hazard from contamination arising from contact with the radiopharmaceutical itself or with the patient's body fluids.

Once a patient has been given a radioactive material, they become radioactive themselves, how much and for how long depend on the type and amount of radioactive material used. In the case of diagnostic nuclear medicine, the safety of ward staff nursing these patients can be assured by following very simple advice. The advice regarding therapeutic procedures is more detailed and the nuclear medicine department, Radiation Protection Adviser or Supervisor should always discuss procedures with the ward before the patient is treated.

Legal and professional issues

Radiopharmaceuticals are legally categorized as prescription-only medicines (POMs), and, in addition to the standard legislation surrounding the administration of such drugs, are subject to regulations related to their radioactive content. In the UK, a statutory committee called the Administration of Radioactive Substances Advisory Committee (ARSAC) was established to give ionizing radiation advice to health ministers and to manage the certification process for administration of radiopharmaceuticals. This committee issues certificates which authorize individuals to administer radiopharmaceuticals to patients. It also lists the maximum permissible doses of radioactivity that may be administered

Table 14.1 Radionuclide investigations

Investigation/target organ	Radiopharmaceutical	Procedures and clinical interventions
Imaging studies		
Bone scan Used to assess bone function in which malignancy, fractures and diseases such as osteomalacia and Paget's disease can be diagnosed	Technetium (^{99m}Tc) phosphate and phosphonate compounds, including methylene diphosphonate (MDP) and hydroxymethylene diphosphonate (HDP)	Patient to drink 5–6 cups of fluid and to empty bladder regularly while waiting for scan. This is to enhance soft tissue clearance and minimize absorbed radiation dose to the bladder
Renogram (dynamic renal study) Used to assess renal function by monitoring clearance of radiopharmaceutical via kidneys	^{99m}Tc MAG$_3$ Benzoylmercaptoacetyltriglycine ^{99m}Tc DTPA (diethylenetriamine penta-acetic acid)	Patients to drink approximately 600 mL of fluid and to empty bladder prior to scan, which takes approximately 1 hour Intravenous diuretic is to be administered to patient during the scan to diagnose obstructive uropathy (Russell 1998)
Static renal study Used to assess size, shape and position and function of kidneys. Used to diagnose renal scarring in children	^{99m}Tc DMSA (dimercaptosuccinic acid)	No preparation
Perfusion lung scan Used to assess blood supply to alveolar tree. Provides complementary information to a ventilation lung scan Used to diagnose pulmonary embolism	^{99m}Tc MAA (macroaggregated albumin)	Radiopharmaceutical is administered as a slow bolus intravenous injection. Patient to lie supine and breathe deeply while injection is being given. This is to enhance even distribution of MAA through lung capillary bed. If patient is pregnant, administered activity needs to be reduced
Ventilation lung scan Provides complementary information to a perfusion lung scan in diagnosis of pulmonary embolism. Used to assess patency of airways	^{99m}Tc Technegas, ^{99m}Tc aerosol, ^{81m}Kr gas, ^{133}Xe gas	A chest X-ray performed within the preceding 24 hours is required prior to scan, to assist with interpretation of lung scan. Patient breathes the radiopharmaceutical through a special mouthpiece while scan is being performed
Cardiac studies: perfusion imaging Used to assess areas of viable perfused myocardium. This is a two-part test with myocardial perfusion monitored under stress and subsequently at rest. Stress may be exercise or pharmacologically induced. Often performed on patients with suspected coronary artery disease, recent myocardial infarction or those who have undergone coronary artery bypass surgery	^{99m}Tc MIBI, ^{99m}Tc tetrafosmin, ^{201}Tl thallous chloride	Patient needs to be closely monitored during post-exercise period because there is the potential risk of triggering a myocardial infarction after stress This test is usually performed within a cardiology unit with appropriately trained personnel and equipment. Patient is usually kept in the department until they have been assessed by a clinician
Cardiac – left ventricular ejection fraction/ multiple gated acquisition scan Used to evaluate cardiac function in patients prior to and during courses of chemotherapy containing cardiotoxic agents	^{99m}Tc-labelled red blood cells	Current weight of patient is required for calculation of dose of a red bood cell labelling agent, which ensures red blood cells are labelled with required radioactivity This volume calculated is then administered intravenously 20–30 minutes prior to scan. Patient lies supine for 30–40 minutes

(Continued)

Table 14.1 (*Continued*)

Investigation/target organ	Radiopharmaceutical	Procedures and clinical interventions
Thyroid scan May be used to confirm presence of one or more nodules within the thyroid, or to identify functional characteristics of nodule(s)	^{99m}Tc pertechnetate, ^{123}I/^{124}I/^{131}I sodium iodide	Patient to avoid foods containing iodine (including seasalt, seafood, cod liver oil, mineral tablets and kelp) for 3 days prior to test. These foods decrease uptake of radiopharmaceutical within thyroid bed. Patient to discontinue thyroid medication for between 3 days and 3 weeks prior to test, depending on specific instructions given by clinician
Parathyroid scan Used to diagnose parathyroid adenomas in patients with primary hyper-parathyroidism	^{99m}Tc pertechnetate, ^{201}Tl thallous chloride	This is a two-part test, comprising a thyroid scan which is completed prior to the parathyroid scan. Patient should follow instructions for thyroid test
Tumour imaging Used to differentiate between metabolically active tumours and space-occupying lesions, or for the diagnosis of unknown primary tumours	^{18}F FDG 2-fluorodeoxyglucose	Patient to fast for up to 6 hours prior to injection, with only water to be taken. Patients may experience a metallic taste in the mouth immediately after administration. Waiting interval between injection and scan is 30 minutes, scan being performed with a positron emission tomography (PET) camera
Used to diagnose infection and diagnose and stage cancers such as lung, Hodgkin's disease and lymphomas	^{67}Ga gallium citrate	Due to excretion of gallium citrate via the gastrointestinal tract, patients should be given laxatives or encouraged to increase fibre and fluid intake to avoid constipation. There are specific radiation protection precautions to be adhered to
Used to diagnose and assess patients with neuroectodermal tumours including phaeochromocytomas, neuroblastomas, carcinoid, medullary thyroid cancers and paragangliomas	^{123}I mIBG (meta-iodobenzylguanidine)	Patient must take Lugol's iodine or potassium iodide for 2 days prior to and for 3 days after day of administration. mIBG may cause hypertension and is administered slowly over a 10-minute period. On occasions, patients may experience some discomfort at the injection site. This may be relieved by applying heat to the area of discomfort and reducing rate of infusion. For paediatric patients, it is preferable to administer mIBG via a central venous catheter. Some drugs that act on the adrenergic system may interfere with uptake of mIBG
Often used in conjunction with mIBG scans to assist with localization of the primary tumour and sites of metastatic spread in the aforementioned diseases	^{111}In octreotide DTPA-D-Phe-1-octreotide	Patients with insulinoma should have their blood sugar levels monitored before and after injection. An intravenous solution containing glucose should be available in case of hypoglycaemia. Patients should be encouraged to increase fluid and fibre intake to avoid constipation
Sites of infection To identify areas of lymphocyte localization in patients with either acute or chronic inflammatory infections	Labelled white blood cells	50 mL of blood is taken from patient using a 19 G needle. Labelled blood is reinjected after approximately 2 hours, following which patient is scanned later the same day and/or the following day

Table 14.1 (*Continued*)

Investigation/target organ	Radiopharmaceutical	Procedures and clinical interventions
Gastrointestinal tract To determine cause of gastrointestinal bleeding, including Meckel's diverticulum	^{99m}Tc pertechnetate	Patients (usually children) need to fast for 4–6 hours before scan; adults to fast from midnight
Non-imaging studies		
Kidney function Measurement of glomerular filtration rate (GFR) provides an assessment of renal function. Often used in renal transplant patients, in compromised renal function due to long-term use of certain drugs (e.g. ciclosporin) or in patients with systemic lupus erythematosus. Oncology patients often have renal function assessed prior to chemotherapy, particularly if regimen includes platinum-based cytotoxic agents	^{51}Cr EDTA (ethylenediamine tetra-acetic acid)	Renal clearance of administered radiopharmaceutical is assessed from residual radioactivity in blood samples taken from patient at either 3 hours, or at 2, 3 and 4 hours post injection. Patient's height and weight are required to enable GFR to be calculated accurately. It is important that no hydration or blood products are commenced during the test as this may alter results of test
Red cell mass/plasma volume Often used to diagnose polycythaemia vera in patients with cardiovascular disease	^{125}I human serum albumin, ^{51}Cr or ^{99m}Tc-labelled red blood cells	10 mL of blood is taken from patient using a 19 G needle. Labelled blood is reinjected after approximately 1.5 hours, following which patient's blood is taken at 10-minute intervals for 40 minutes. Patient's height and weight are recorded
Sentinel node localization. Sentinel lymph nodes receive drainage from the breasts (Luini *et al.* 2005). By undertaking biopsies of these nodes, the surgeon can predict the cancer status of all nodes in the axillary region. This procedure allows for accurate diagnosis of the patient's cancer status, avoiding unnecessary axillary dissection (Schrenk *et al.* 2005)	^{99m}Tc colloid	0.1–0.2 mL is injected intradermally into the designated area on the breast for location of main sentinel node. Minimum of 1 hour (up to 24 hours) prior to surgical procedure During the procedure all staff must wear their film badges and those handling the specimen must wear finger dosimeters. The theatre door should be labelled with a warning controlled area sign and disposable drapes and gowns should be used. The specimen should be placed in a screw-top container, which is labelled with the radioactive symbol and the details recorded in the log book. The specimen is then stored for 48 hours, after which time it is sent to histopathology in the normal way. The radioactive label is removed in histology after 1 week when the specimen is then considered non-radioactive On completion of the procedure, the used drapes, gown and gloves should be placed in a clinical waste bag and the environment and waste monitored to ensure no contamination is present. Any contaminated items should be marked radioactive and stored in a secure store, until sufficient radioactive decay has occurred. Only then should the warning symbols be removed by the physics department and the waste disposed of in the normal way

839

Henkin (2006), Peter and Gambhir (2004), Ziessman *et al.* (2006).

to adult patients, and appropriately reduced adult doses for children, according to a child's bodyweight or body surface area (Health Protection Agency 2006).

Preprocedural considerations

The patient should be physically and psychologically prepared for the procedure so they understand the procedure and give their informed consent (O'Dwyer *et al.* 2003). The following aspects should be considered prior to the procedure.

- Pregnant women will generally not be scanned. When essential tests must be undertaken, the patient must sign a consent form and receive a reduced dose of radionuclide. This is to avoid unnecessary irradiation to the abdominal/pelvic region which will include the embryo or foetus (Ionizing Radiation Regulations 1999).
- The person accompanying the patient should not be pregnant, or bring young children or babies with them so that unnecessary exposure in the time period immediately after the radionuclide administration can be avoided (DH 2000).
- In women of reproductive age, the possibility of pregnancy must be excluded and the patient asked if her menstrual period is late. Patients receiving iodine-131 or other radioactive agent with a long half-life should not become pregnant for a minimum of 3 months after the procedure (Sharp *et al.* 1998) to ensure that unnecessary irradiation to the abdomen of a woman who may be pregnant is avoided (DH 2000).

- If mothers are breastfeeding then advice from the radiation protection adviser should be sought. Radioactivity can be excreted in breast milk. Therefore breastfeeding may need to be suspended (Health Protection Agency 2006) and the mother encouraged to avoid unnecessary cuddling of the child during this time (DH 2000).
- Provide effective pain control for those patients with pain to ensure they are pain free so that immobility during scan time can be maintained (see Chapter 9).
- If the patient is incontinent, incontinence pads should be worn and universal precautions are to be adopted, to limit the spread of contamination. Disposable gloves and apron should be worn and handwashing performed following patient contact, as these will prevent contamination of staff in close contact with the patient (DH 2000). Urine bags must be emptied regularly to remove the radioactivity from the patient area.
- Debilitated patients may require prolonged close contact. Nursing staff should share the care of these patients, by regular rotation of staff. This will keep doses to staff as low as possible and avoid prolonged exposure to any one member of staff (DH 2000).

Procedure guideline 14.6 Unsealed radioactive sources for diagnostic investigations: patient care

Essential equipment

- Selection of needles and syringes
- Winged infusion device
- Alcohol wipes
- Syringe shield

- Tape and gauze
- Documentation regarding the isotope to be administered
- Radioactive isotope
- Disposable apron and gloves
- TLD finger dose meter
- Film badge

Preprocedure

Action	Rationale
1 Explain and discuss the procedure with the patient, and, if relevant, with the relative accompanying the patient.	To ensure the patient is physically and psychologically prepared for the procedure and understands the procedure and gives their informed consent (O'Dwyer *et al.* 2003, E).
2 Apply the relevant thermoluminescent (TLD) dose meter and film badge.	To measure radiation doses received by member of staff (Ionizing Radiation Regulations 1999, C).
3 Apply disposable gloves and plastic apron.	To reduce the risk of contamination (DH 2000, C).

Procedure

4 Place the empty syringe in a lead syringe shield and attach needle. Place behind the lead body shield.	To reduce exposure to radiation (DH 2000, C).
5 Stand behind lead body shield and draw up the prescribed dose of the radiopharmaceutical.	To reduce exposure to radiation (DH 2000, C).

6 Administer the radionuclide intravenously via winged infusion device (see Chapter 18).	To administer the radionuclide. E
7 Dispose of all used syringes, needles, and winged infusion device in a designated radioactive sharps disposal bin which is stored within a lead shield.	To contain radioactivity and allow safe disposal (Ionizing Radiation Regulations 1999, C).
8 Apply pressure and cover the exit site with gauze and secure with tape.	Prevent any blood loss from skin exit site and possible contamination.
9 Remove disposable gloves and wash hands at end of procedure.	To remove any possible radioactive contamination (DH 2005, R1a; DH 2000, C).

Postprocedure

10 Place a yellow identity bracelet on the wrists of all in-patients and complete information card with the details of when precautions can be discontinued. Give the completed information card to the patient or the nurse accompanying the patient. Sign and complete administration documentation.	The yellow wristband will provide visual warning to inform all healthcare workers of the patient's recent diagnostic investigation. The information card will inform ward staff of restrictions related to managing a patient, as well as when measures that have to be adopted in the event of the patient vomiting or being incontinent can be discontinued (DH 2000, C). The card also states where to obtain help and advice related to the patient's diagnostic investigation. E
11 Monitor hands at end of procedure and before leaving the room.	To check for possible radioactive contamination (DH 2000, C).
12 Monitor the room for radioactive contamination at the end of each day or if contamination may have occurred.	To establish whether contamination has occurred (DH 2000, C).

Postprocedural considerations
Immediate care

Avoid urine, faecal and blood sample collection for laboratories other than nuclear medicine for 24 hours. If collection is unavoidable, a radiation warning sticker must be attached to the specimen and request card, and the specimen taken to the laboratory under the supervision of the physics departmental staff. This is to prevent contamination of the laboratory and its staff, as specimens taken within 24 hours of some scans may contain radioactivity (HSE 2003a, Vialard-Miguel *et al.* 2005).

Ongoing care

Bone marrow and stem cell harvests should be avoided for 24 hours. Advice should be sought from the physics department as cells may contain radioactivity (HSE 2003a, Vialard-Miguel *et al.* 2005). Seek advice from physics staff if the patient is to undergo a procedure in the operating theatre within 24 hours of a scan in order to prevent theatre equipment from becoming contaminated with radioactivity. Place soiled bed linen used within the first 24 hours of certain scans, for example bone scan, within a purple plastic bag and inform the physics departmental staff.

Unsealed source therapy

Definition

Unsealed source therapy or radionuclide therapy uses the same principles as for diagnostic nuclear medicine procedures. There will be a vector (a pharmaceutical that will recognize the tumour or target organ) and an isotope (see Table 14.2). Depending on the half-life of the radiopharmaceutical, the therapy can be given in both the outpatient and inpatient settings.

Evidence-based approaches
Rationale

Unsealed source therapy is complex because, in addition to the external hazard, there is an internal hazard from contamination arising from contact with the radiopharmaceutical itself or with the patient's body fluids.

Once a patient has been given a radioactive material, they become radioactive themselves, how much and for how long being dependent on the type and amount of radioactive material used.

841

Table 14.2 Therapeutic treatments

Radioactive material	In/outpatient	Condition	Route of administration	Notes
Iodine-131 sodium iodide	Out	Thyrotoxicosis	Oral (capsule or drink)	Most radioactive iodine is concentrated in the thyroid, but a substantial amount will be present in the urine and blood. Lesser quantities will be found in the patient's faeces, sweat, saliva and seminal fluid. The patient should receive an instruction card listing the precautions necessary to safeguard others. The patient may be infirm or incontinent and therefore admitted for treatment.
Iodine-131 sodium iodide	In	Thyroid cancer	Oral (capsule or drink)	Large administered dose therefore more significant risks. The patient is usually isolated in a special suite.
Iodine-131 mIBG	In	Neuroblastoma	IV via infusion pump	As above
Strontium-89	Out	Bone metastases	IV	The patient may be admitted to a ward within a short period of time following treatment, for example upon deterioration of condition
Samarium-153	Out	Bone metastases	IV	Patients should be advised to drink plenty of fluids prior to treatment, and urine should be collected for at least 6 hours post treatment.
Indium-111 octreotide	In	GI cancer and neuroendocrine cancer	IV	Patients are always isolated following treatment, often in specially shielded rooms
Rhenium-186	Out	Prostate cancer	IV	
Radium-223	Out	Prostate cancer	IV	

The safety of all staff caring for these patients can be assured by implementing very detailed nuclear medicine and physics protocols and procedures.

Legal and professional issues
Patient preparation and consent

Every therapeutic use of radiation has an inherent risk. Awareness of the risk is essential for all staff who have to obtain informed consent from their patients (Picano 2004). A survey of patients and family members of patients receiving radioactive iodine found that many experienced psychological distress and few received adequate help (Fitch and McGrath 2003). Therefore careful preparation of the patient before the administration of unsealed source therapy is essential.

Patients and relatives should be educated (Skalla *et al.* 2004) about the principles of radiation protection and the procedures with which the patient has to comply while in isolation; this is part of the consent process. Psychosocial and physical needs must be addressed which require a collaborative approach between patients and nurses (Stajduhar *et al.* 2000). It is important to identify potential anxieties before administration while the nurse is able to reassure the patient and is unconstrained by time limits. Fully pre-

pared, knowledgeable patients and visitors are the key to radiation safety and contamination control (Stajduhar *et al.* 2000, Thompson 2001). Incidents and accidents are less likely to occur if the patient fully understands the reasons for the restrictions. The name and telephone number of the 'key worker', usually a clinical nurse specialist, is essential for patients before, during and after treatment with sealed source brachytherapy (DH 2000, NICE 2005).

All patients are required to sign a consent form agreeing to treatment, following a full explanation from the treating clinician. This is to comply with medical, ethical and legal requirements and local hospital policy. Consent is usually obtained in the outpatient clinic before ordering the radioactive material. The patient must also agree to stay in hospital until the physics department advises that the level of radioactivity permits discharge (ICRP 2004).

Preprocedural considerations
Equipment

Equipment should be kept to a minimum. It must be checked to ensure that it is in working order, as maintenance staff will only be allowed into the room in exceptional circumstances.

Bed linen and disposable items (gloves, aprons, over-shoes, cutlery and crockery) should be kept in a utility room or anteroom along with the patient's treatment chart and a radiation monitor.

Protective floor covering

Plastic-backed absorbent paper, kept in place by adhesive tape, is used to retain accidental urine spills or splashes on the floor immediately surrounding the toilet. Each patient is assessed to decide whether further floor covering is necessary; for example, catheterized patients will require floor covering below the catheter bag.

Specific patient preparations

Although the patient will have been assessed in the outpatient department, it is important that they are reassessed on admission for their suitability for treatment. In particular, the needs of a debilitated patient must be assessed to ensure that appropriate nursing care can be provided within the time constraints. A review of a patient who was quadriplegic, doubly incontinent and unable to swallow found that nurses could provide appropriate care whilst following the recommended radiation protection restrictions (Williams

and Woodward 2005). Multidisciplinary co-ordination of care is required in such cases.

Before the administration of unsealed sources, any symptoms of diarrhoea or constipation must be resolved. Diarrhoea could result in contamination of the treatment area. Constipation not only inhibits the elimination of radioactivity but also could obscure radiological investigations, for example scanning. All investigations including blood tests must be undertaken before administration of diagnostic and therapeutic unsealed sources. If essential specimens need to be processed after administration, the specimen and the request card must be labelled with a radiation warning sticker, and the laboratories must follow their standard operating procedures for processing and disposal of these specimens.

Personal items

Nurses should be sensitive to the psychological implications for patients of being labelled 'radioactive' and confined in isolation. Although patients may want to bring some personal belongings with them, they should be advised to keep these to a minimum, as items may become contaminated and need to be stored until radioactivity has decayed. Patients can be supplied with disposable slippers and be asked to wear the hospital nightwear.

Procedure guideline 14.7 Unsealed source therapy: entering and leaving the room of a patient who has received an unsealed radioactive source

Essential equipment

- Gloves
- Apron or gown
- Overshoes
- Clinical waste bag
- Soap and water

Preprocedure

Action	Rationale
1 Collect digital dosimeter, record reading before entering and on leaving room.	Digital dosimeter provides ongoing and immediate indication of the amount of exposure received (Ionizing Radiation Regulations 1999, C).

Procedure

On entering:

2 Put on disposable gloves.	To prevent contamination of the hands (HSE 2002, C).
3 Put on disposable overshoes.	To prevent spread of contamination outside the treatment area (HSE 2002, C).
4 Put on a suitable protective plastic apron or gown:	
(a) Long-sleeved cotton gown, for example for lifting patient	To protect against low levels of contamination, for example from the patient's skin (HSE 2002, C).
(b) Disposable plastic apron, for example for dealing with vomit or incontinence.	To protect against high levels of contamination (HSE 2002, C).

(Continued)

Procedure guideline 14.7 (*Continued*)

5 Plan work before entering the controlled area and then work quickly and efficiently, keeping within the time allowance stated.	To minimize radiation exposure, as consistent with good nursing care (Ionizing Radiation Regulations 1999, C).

On leaving:

6 Remove overshoes, taking care not to touch the shoes worn underneath.	These are removed first while gloves are still being worn to prevent the spread of contamination to hands or the floor outside the room. E
7 Remove the plastic apron, by holding the front of apron and breaking the neck and waist ties.	To prevent transfer of contamination from the gloves onto the uniform below. E
8 Remove gloves by peeling them off the hands, taking care not to touch the outside surfaces with bare hands, and discard them in the clinical waste bag provided.	To prevent transfer of contamination from the gloves' outer surfaces to the hands. E
9 Wash hands thoroughly using soap and water.	To remove any contamination (HSE 2003b, C).

Postprocedure

10 Use the radiation monitor each time when leaving the room and monitor for contamination of the hands, feet and clothing. If contamination has occurred, inform the physics department immediately and follow the decontamination procedure. The physics department will advise if further whole-body monitoring is required.	To ensure that the nurse is not contaminated (Ionizing Radiation Regulations 1999, C).

Procedure guideline 14.8 Unsealed source therapy: iodine-131 (oral capsule/liquid): administration

Essential equipment

- Radioactive source
- Straw
- Water

Preprocedure

Action	Rationale
1 Explain and discuss the procedure with the patient.	To ensure that the patient understands the procedure and gives their valid consent (O'Dwyer *et al.* 2003, R1b).
2 Check that consent, administrative documents, pregnancy status is recorded (must be negative to proceed with procedure).	Safe administration of radiopharmaceutical medicine (DH 2000, C; NMC 2008, C).

Procedure

3 Administer a prophylactic antiemetic 30 minutes before scheduled administration of the dose.	To reduce the risk of nausea and/or vomiting after ingestion of a radioactive source. E
4 Check that the preparation of the room and the patient is complete. Ensure that any surplus items have been removed.	To prevent contamination of extraneous equipment. E
5 Assist the patient to remove dentures/bridges, if dose is administered in liquid form.	To prevent radioactive material being trapped behind dental plates. E

6 Allow the patient to swallow the capsule or drink the iodine-131 through a straw, physically directed by an authorized member of staff.	Drinking through a straw reduces the amount of radioactive material left around the mouth. To comply with ARSAC regulations (Health Protection Agency 2006, C).
7 Offer the patient a cold drink of water to rinse out the mouth and then swallow. Assist the patient to replace dentures.	To remove any iodine-131 from inside the mouth. E

Postprocedure

8 Ensure that the physics staff place the radiation warning sign at the entrance to the therapy room.	To identify the room as a controlled area (DH 2000, C).

Procedure guideline 14.9 Unsealed source therapy: iodine-131 mIBG treatment: patient care

Essential equipment

- A selection of needles and syringes
- Alcohol wipes
- Syringe shields
- Tape and gauze swabs
- Documentation for isotope to be administered

Preprocedure

Action	Rationale
1 Explain and discuss the procedure with patient and/or parents if the patient is a child.	To ensure that the patient and/or parents understand the procedure and give their consent (O'Dwyer *et al.* 2003, R1b).
2 Apply a vital signs monitor with a variable time setting mode to the patient that will be visible to staff from outside the room.	Following the administration of mIBG, a transient rise in blood pressure and pulse may occur (Brophy *et al.* 2004, E).
3 Check that the patient has a patent vascular access device *in situ*, usually a cannula or, for children, a central venous access device.	To ensure administration of mIBG. E

Procedure

4 The nurse or doctor will set up the iodine-131 mIBG infusion and administer as prescribed.	To ensure safe administration of iodine-131 mIBG (DH 2000, C).
5 During the procedure, monitor blood pressure and pulse rate:	
(a) at 5-minute intervals during infusion	To detect and monitor any change to blood pressure and pulse rate. Alter rate according to changes as prescribed by clinician. E
(b) monitor whole-body retention measurements at regular intervals as directed by physics department.	This may vary according to department policies. E

Postprocedural considerations

Ongoing care

Encourage the patient to shower frequently, at least once a day, and to wash their hands thoroughly after each possible contact with bodily fluids, for example cleaning teeth, going to the toilet. The patient should regularly remove any dentures and clean them under running water and remove any contact lenses and rinse in their usual cleaning fluid. All these actions will reduce any radioactivity from the skin or mucous membranes. The nurse should encourage the patient to maintain a fluid intake of between 2 and 3 litres per day to increase the urinary output and elimination of radioactivity from the bladder (Thompson 2001). The patient should have their own personal toilet facilities and flush the toilet twice after use to reduce contamination of others and of the environment as the urine of patients treated with iodine-131 is initially highly radioactive (Thompson 2001). Bedbound patients should be catheterized before the dose is given and the bag emptied every 4–6 hours, or more frequently if necessary to reduce the radiation level in the room. If the patient requires a bedpan or urinal, this item must be kept solely for this patient's use. The bedpan or urinal must be handled carefully and the contents disposed of in the patient's toilet (and flushed twice). The bedpan or urinal may be washed in the bedpan washer but sealed in a plastic bag for the journey to and from the sluice.

If leakage occurs from injection sites, wound sites and so on, the nurse should contact the medical staff and the physics department immediately. Any contact with the dressing should be carried out with long-handled forceps and gloves (HSE 2003a, HSE 2003b). All used linen must be deposited in a special bag provided for this purpose and must be monitored for contamination before going to the laundry.

Collection of laboratory specimens should, if possible, be deferred. If collections are unavoidable, a radiation warning sticker must be attached to the specimen and request card and the specimen delivered to the laboratory following consultations with the physics department in order to reduce the risk of contamination of the laboratory and its staff (Vialard-Miguel *et al.* 2005).

Only disposable crockery and cutlery should be used to present meals to patients as china crockery and cutlery may become contaminated. Uneaten food and disposable cutlery and crockery are disposed of in a macerator and all fruit stones and fish and meat bones should be removed from the diet to prevent blocking the macerator.

Guidance for visitors

Visitors must not enter radiation treatment areas unless special training and arrangements have been agreed in order to minimize the exposure of visitors to radiation (DH 2000). Visiting time during the first day following administration of an unsealed source should be limited as advised by the physicist because the patient is highly radioactive during this period (Ionizing Radiation Regulations 1999). On subsequent days, visiting is unlimited, providing visitors remain outside the room behind the lead screen, the exception being parents of young children who will need to be authorized by the physics department. Physical contact with the patient or bed linen is not allowed as protective clothing is not available to visitors. Children under 16 years of age and pregnant women are discouraged from visiting to ensure that radiation exposure of children and the unborn is kept as low as practicable (DH 2000).

Discharge of patient

A patient should not be discharged from hospital until the radiation activity retained has fallen below recommended levels (DH 2000, Health Protection Agency 2006). This level will depend on several factors, including:

- mode of transport on leaving hospital
- journey time involved

- personal circumstances, for example young children or pregnant women at home.

Patients will be assessed individually for radiation clearance by the physics department before discharge. The treating physician will then be advised of the results of the assessment. Advice will be given to patients on issues such as return to work and visits to public places. On discharge, patients will be given appropriate information in the form of an instruction card carrying details of the precautions to be taken. This card must be signed by the treating clinician or the physics department staff.

It must be emphasized that this card must be carried and the instructions followed until the latest date shown so that, for instance, staff would be alerted should the patient be readmitted to hospital. Additional verbal instructions may be necessary.

Cleaning the treatment room

During occupancy of the treatment room by the patient, cleaning of the room is kept to a minimum and should be supervised by the physics staff. After the patient is discharged, monitoring and any necessary decontamination of the room will be arranged by the physics department, which will inform the relevant personnel when this has been completed. Only then may the room be entered and thoroughly cleaned (DH 2000).

Sealed source therapy

Definition

Radioactive isotopes used as sealed sources for brachytherapy emit both beta and gamma radiation. Brachytherapy is the term used for intracavity treatment where radioisotope sources are placed in pre-existing body cavities, such as the uterine cavity or vagina, or for interstitial treatment where radioisotope sources are inserted directly into the tissues using tubes or needles (Hoskin and Coyle 2005).

Sealed source therapy is complex because of the variation in sources and delivery systems used to administer radiation treatment. The main difference between sealed source and unsealed source treatment is the absence of contaminated bodily fluids. The hazard is therefore external sources.

Related theory

Specific isotopes used to treat malignant tumours

Iodine-125 used in prostate cancer

Seeds of iodine-125 have replaced those of gold-198, with the half-life of iodine-125 approximately 60 days. Some therapists believe that there is a radiobiological advantage to this long half-life in treating slow-growing tumours such as carcinoma of the prostate (Blank *et al.* 2000). The iodine-125 seeds are inserted into the tissue that is to be irradiated, for example the prostate gland, utilizing ultrasound guidance or an image intensifier control; the procedure requires the patient to have a general anaesthetic for the insertion.

As the energy of the gamma-ray emission from iodine-125 is very low compared with that of gold-198, large numbers of seeds are required, which means that more precautions must be taken in order to achieve a regular geometrical arrangement to ensure satisfactory distribution of the dose (Stock *et al.* 2000). Implantation of iodine-125 is now a well-established procedure and an increasing number of patients throughout the world are treated in this manner (Anglesio *et al.* 2005, NICE 2005).

There are known complications from this form of treatment including incontinence, obstructive urinary symptoms, rectal symptoms and sexual dysfunction. The impotence rate has been reported at between 10% and 15%, much lower when compared with 45% of those patients undergoing radical prostatectomy (NICE 2005).

Zelefsky's (2006) study found that quality of life was initially worse during the first 4 weeks following iodine-125 treatment but returned to baseline values 1 year after the implants were inserted; it is therefore important that the patient understands the uncertainties of iodine-125 seed therapy and the possible alternative treatment options. The consent process should ensure that the patient is fully informed of:

- the rationale for the procedure
- the potential side-effects of the procedure
- the alternative options
- the results of the treatment.

It is also important that the patient understands that it is unclear how the procedure affects general health or the chance of the cancer returning in the long term (Wust *et al.* 2004), and that the patient is followed up and monitored (NICE 2005).

Iridium-192 used in head and neck cancer

Iridium-192 is a radioisotope which is used in the form of pins or wires in interstitial therapy (Fung 2002). The half-life is 74.2 days and it is used because of the low energy of its gamma emission compared to caesium, which simplifies radiation protection issues. Iridium-192 is available in the form of a platinum–iridium alloy thin flexible wire. The wires consist of an active platinum–iridium alloy core encased in a sheath of platinum 10 μm thick, which screens out the beta radiation from the iridium-192.

This high-activity source of iridium is used in a high dose-rate remote afterloading system, reducing the amount of radiation to which staff are exposed. Iridium-192 is used under the following circumstances.

- As a treatment for small primary lesions, for example, tongue or breast lesions (Lapeyre *et al.* 2004).

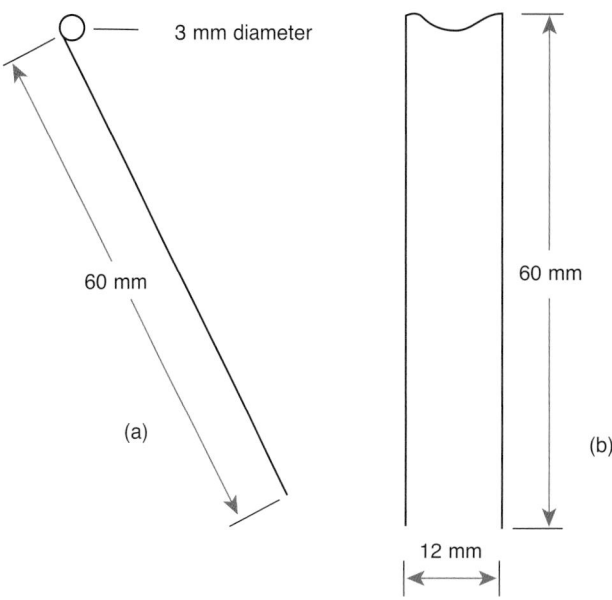

Figure 14.4 Iridium-192 pins. (a) Iridium single pin. (b) Iridium hair pin.

- As a 'boost' dose after external radiotherapy for larger primary tumours or where nodes are also involved (Grabenbauer *et al.* 2001).
- To treat recurrence (Nutting *et al.* 2006).

Iridium-192 hair pin and single pin types of implants are usually used intraorally (see Figure 14.4) and are slotted into tissue using steel guides to obtain accurate alignment. Radiological examination is used to check the position of the guides before the iridium is inserted and the pins are held in place by sutures. Physicists are normally responsible for calculating how long a radioactive implant is to stay in place, which is usually about 6 days depending on the size of the tumour. Removal is carried out in theatre by the clinical oncologist.

Iridium-192 wires are usually used for head and neck, breast, vulva or perineum lesions (see Figure 14.5). Polythene

Figure 14.5 Iridium-192 wire in polythene cannula. Typical assembly in tissue.

Figure 14.6 Interstitial perineal template device.

or metal cannulas are inserted under a general anaesthetic, and in the case of breast lesions, both ends of each tube protrude through the skin. Correct alignment is established often with the aid of a Perspex template which fits over the breast and holds the metal cannulas in the correct alignment or, in the case of vulval or perineal insertions, one end of the tube protrudes. For alignment of the sources to be achieved, a Perspex template and vaginal obturator are used.

Iridium-192 interstitial brachytherapy can be used to treat locally advanced or recurrent tumours. Interstitial brachytherapy is a suitable alternative to standard intracavity brachytherapy where the treatment may be considered unsuitable because the dose distribution may be suboptimal (Agrawal *et al.* 2005).

The device itself consists of two acrylic cylinders and an acrylic template with an array of holes that serve as guides for trocars and a cover plate (Figure 14.6). The cylinders are usually placed in the vagina but can also be used in the rectum for rectal tumours. They are then fastened to the template, so that a fixed geometric relationship amongst the tumour volume and normal structures, that is bladder and rectum, is produced. This ensures that the source placement is preserved throughout the course of the implantation. The iridium wire is then manually afterloaded and held in place with a crimped washer to prevent movement of the source during treatment (see Figure 14.5).

The tiny size of the high-activity iridium-192 source in high dose-rate machines may allow some interstitial brachytherapy to be given as a few treatments of several minutes each, in contrast to the single treatment of many hours' duration which is necessary with low-activity iridium wire (Hart 2006). Clinical oncologists are responsible for calculating how long a radioactive implant should stay in place, which is usually for 3–6 days depending on the size of the tumour. Removal of these implants is usually carried out in the ward area. The procedures deliver a dose that is higher than can be achieved by external beam radiation alone, improving organ preservation rates and reducing side-effects (Karakoyun-Celik *et al.* 2005).

In a study by Budrukkar *et al.* (2001) evaluating the long-term efficacy and safety of transperineal interstitial implants for advanced pelvic malignancy, it was found that treatment offered a 5- and 10-year disease-free survival of 48% for patients aged 45 years and less, and an 80% disease-free survival in patients aged over 45 years.

Nursing care is similar to the care that patients receive for intracavity brachytherapy, with side-effects similar to those seen in 'afterloading' techniques and, according to Syed *et al.* (2002), considered to be acceptable. Late effects of this type of treatment, specifically fistula formation and bowel complications that may require surgery, have been documented (Nag *et al.* 2002).

Caesium-137 used in head and neck cancer and gynaecological cancers

Caesium-137 is a radioisotope that can be used in the form of interstitial implants or in intracavity applicators allowing a highly conformal dose of radioactivity to be delivered directly to the site of the cancer (Karakoyun-Celik *et al.* 2005). The most common malignancies treated by the use of radioactive applicators are tumours of the female genital tract (Kucera *et al.* 2001). Intracavity applicators are used to deliver a high dose to the region of the cervix, the paracervical tissue, the upper part of the vagina and the uterine body. Caesium has a half-life of 30 years and has largely replaced radium as a source for various brachytherapy treatments.

Oral implants of caesium-137 are 'needle-like' implants that are inserted directly into the tissue surrounding the tumour, and are a fairly common treatment for early lesions of the cheek, lip and anterior two-thirds of the tongue (Leborgne *et al.* 2002, Nutting *et al.* 2006). Oral implants have the advantage of allowing preservation of the structure and function of the tongue whilst avoiding the toxicity of external beam radiotherapy to the oral mucosa (Wadsley *et al.* 2003). If there is known or suspected bone involvement, in the mandible for example, the alternative external beam treatment will be given.

Caesium-137 sources (see Figure 14.7) are inserted in theatre under a general anaesthetic and placed individually in a predetermined pattern so that the implant covers the whole growth with a safety margin of at least 1 cm. Each individual needle is positioned by pushers so that its eye, through which silk is threaded, is just visible beneath the mucosal surface. Each silk is then stitched to the tongue with a single suture, and when all the needles have been inserted the silks are counted and gathered together. They are then threaded through a piece of rubber to prevent friction and trauma to the mouth. The silks are then strapped to the cheek to prevent any needle being swallowed should it work loose.

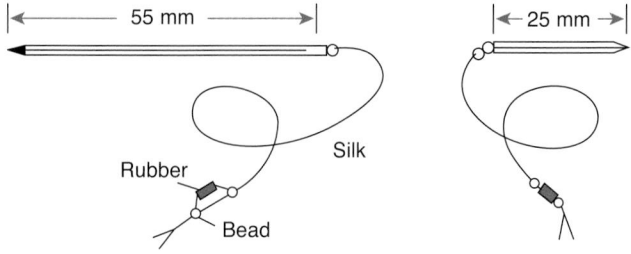

Figure 14.7 Caesium-137 needles.

Small beads are attached to the ends of the threads to facilitate counting the needles. X-rays are always taken to check the positions of the needles and to enable estimation of the dose distribution (Takacsi-Nagy *et al.* 2001).

Evidence-based approaches
Methods of application
Intracavity applicators and interstitial implants

The application of sources varies dependent on the source and delivery method. Small sealed sources inserted into the body may take the form of:

(a) intracavity applicators, where sources are placed in natural cavities and usually held in place by packing
(b) interstitial implants where sources are inserted directly into the tumour-bearing tissue (Hoskin and Coyle 2005).

Intracavity applicators and interstitial implants can be used in three forms.

1. The source is *preloaded in the applicator* before it is placed in the patient for a fixed length of time, for example caesium-137 needles and iridium-192 hair pins.
2. *Permanent insertion* in the case of iodine-125 seeds which, once inserted, would be difficult to remove. The available data show that, except in the case where the patient's partner is pregnant at the time of implantation, no restrictions are required once the patient is discharged home. Written information must be given to the patient on discharge which must include the following.
   i Possibility of triggering certain types of security radiation monitors.
   ii Altered fertility, which is dependent on diagnosis, previous treatment, age, type of brachytherapy offered.
   iii The implant should be discussed if surgery is a possibility in the future.
   iv Specific instruction should be available if the patient dies and cremation is required (ICRP 2005).
   v Whilst an inpatient, all urine must be checked to ensure no seed has become dislodged; if this occurs, the loose seed should be placed in a lead pot with long-handled forceps. Any seed in a catheter bag should also be saved and placed into a lead pot and collected by the Hospital Radiation Protection Service, which is generally the physics department.
3. *Afterloading systems.* The applicator is placed in position and the radioactive source is inserted when the position of the applicator and the condition of the patient are satisfactory. Insertion of the sealed source can be undertaken manually in the case of iridium-192 wires or by remote control in the case of the low dose-rate 'Selectron' and high dose-rate 'micro-Selectron' machines mainly used in the gynaecological setting. The proportions of radioisotope, initially radium and latterly caesium-137, within the intrauterine tube and the vaginal ovoids are calculated to give a constant dose rate to a geometrical *point A* when using different lengths of intrauterine tube and different sizes of vaginal ovoids.

Types of gynaecological brachytherapy applicators

Manchester applicator
Manchester applicators (Figure 14.8a) in their original form were live sources enclosed in intrauterine tubes of varying

Figure 14.8 Gynaecological caesium applicators. Arrangement of brachytherapy sources in the uterus and vagina for treatment of cervical carcinoma. Sources may be active or, more usually these days, afterloaded into applicators along catheters protruding from the vagina. (a) Manchester applicator. (b) Modified Stockholm applicator. (c) Fletcher applicator. (d) Dobbie applicator.

lengths and vaginal applicators (ovoids) of varying sizes. The applicators were inserted under general anaesthetic and held in place by a gauze pack and were modified for either manual or remote afterloading for low dose or high dose rates with the principle of the three applicator system remaining. Removal of the applicators and live sources is carried out on the ward.

Stockholm applicator

For carcinoma of the uterine body or cervix. Usually a uterine tube and two vaginal packets are inserted. Occasionally, if the vaginal vault is small, one packet is omitted or replaced by a vaginal tube. The radioactive material is held in place with a proflavine-soaked gauze pack left in place for approximately 22 hours. Tubes and packets have strings attached for removal and colour-coded beads indicate which should be removed first (Bomford 2002b).

Modified Stockholm applicator

For carcinoma of the uterine body and cervix; it consists of a uterine tube and a square box which connect together by a point and a hole. The vagina is then packed with proflavine-soaked gauze pack and the applicator is left *in situ* for approximately 20 hours, and the box is removed first (Bomford 2002b). See Figure 14.8b.

Fletcher applicator

For carcinoma of the corpus or cervix, with the patient needing to have a fairly capacious vaginal vault. Hollow applicators, a uterine tube and two vaginal ovoids are inserted in theatre and afterloaded with the radioactive sources on the ward by the radiotherapist. The apparatus is held in place with a proflavine pack; long ends project through the vulva so that afterloading can be carried out. No strings are needed for this procedure, with insertions usually left in place for 60–72 hours (Bomford 2002b). See Figure 14.8c.

Dobbie applicator

For irradiation of the whole vagina; this is a Perspex cylindrical applicator, with radioactive sources in the centre and inserted into the vagina and sutured in place to the vulva. Can be used with low or high dose rate sources with strings attached to the applicator for removal (Bomford 2002b). See Figure 14.8d.

Manual afterloading systems for treatment of gynaecological malignancies

The basis of 'afterloading brachytherapy' is that the applicators are placed within the cervix and vaginal fornices and may then be inserted manually or by remote control. The radiation source is only introduced when the applicator's position has been checked as correct by imaging, the patient is comfortable and is in a designated protected environment (Hoskin and Coyle 2005).

These rules ensure that the correct source has been inserted into the correct applicator for the programmed length of time. They also allow the dose rate of brachytherapy to be increased. Classically, the dose rate with the 'Manchester System' was approximately 50 cGy per hour to point A. With modern engineering methods, caesium-137 pellets can be produced which will allow a dose rate of between 150 and 200 cGy per hour to point A. Many systems now use sources that allow a higher than standard dose rate to be delivered, with the added advantage of reducing treatment time for the patient (Kuipers *et al.* 2001).

Manual afterloading systems are now largely being replaced by remote systems, but are still used in a few hospitals where services are still developing. The plastic applicator tubes follow the pattern of the 'Manchester System' with an intrauterine tube and two vaginal ovoids (oval intracavity applicators are inserted into the vagina). The plastic tubes are designed to be disposed of after a single use. The tubes are inserted under general anaesthetic. X-rays are taken to confirm that the 'inactive' sources are in the correct position.

As with the classic 'Manchester System', there are varying lengths of intrauterine tube and sizes of ovoids. With X-ray confirmation and dosimetry calculated, the radioactive caesium-137 sources are introduced using long-handled forceps; once in place, a silver metal cap is screwed over the end of the plastic tube to hold the sources securely. Manual afterloading does not permit the use of high-activity sources for reasons of staff safety and treatment may last many hours or even several days. When treatment is complete, the caps are removed from the tubes and the sources are withdrawn and placed immediately in a lead storage vessel with the plastic applicator tubes then removed.

It is particularly important to observe for displacement or extrusion of the applicator tubes over the long treatment times. It is customary to mark the thigh level with the end of the applicator tubes and to compare this alignment at regular intervals as the treatment progresses and the silver metal caps must be monitored regularly to assess for loosening or displacement (Bomford 2002b).

Remote afterloading

Remote systems have the advantage of complete protection of staff, but the disadvantage of high cost and the need for interlocking mechanisms (Bomford 2002b).

Remote-controlled afterloading machines transfer active sources from a radiation-proof safe to the patient only when it is safe to do so (Hoskin and Coyle 2005). There are two types of delivery machine: a low dose rate (LDR), termed a Selectron, and a high dose rate (HDR) machine termed a micro-Selectron; both are used generally in the treatment of gynaecological cancers and in some cases may also be useful in the treatment of bronchial, oesophageal and other intraluminal carcinomas (Tessa *et al.* 2005, Ung *et al.* 2006).

Low dose rate (LDR) Selectron unit

The Selectron unit comprises a lead-shielded safe containing caesium-137 sources in the form of small spherical pellets, a microprocessor, a keyboard, display unit and printer

Patient

Applicators

Coupling device

Shielding

Remote control
unit

Transfer tubes

Microprocessor,
keyboard,
display,
printer

Selectron
unit

Lead safe
storing
sources

Treatment area

Air and
power supply

Figure 14.9 Selectron unit.

Patients have hollow, lightweight stainless steel applicators positioned in the operating theatre under a general anaesthetic. These are usually modified Manchester or Fletcher type applicators consisting of a uterine tube and two vaginal ovoids held in place with proflavine-soaked vaginal packing. A urinary catheter is inserted in theatre at the same time to reduce urinary retention and the risk of the sources becoming dislodged by the patient when micturating. Accurate positioning of the applicators is confirmed by taking X-rays with dummy sources *in situ* and the optimum source configuration is selected, taking account of individual anatomical variations.

The Selectron unit is then programmed by the physicist. For each treatment channel being used, active source pellets are interspersed with inactive stainless steel spacer pellets to achieve the desired dose distribution (Hoskin and Coyle 2005). The treatment time required to reach the prescribed dose is also entered; with a six-channel Selectron, it is possible to treat two patients with three applicators each simultaneously. The radiotherapist is responsible for connecting the transfer tubes to the applicators, with the transfer tubes led over a bed bracket which supports the weight of the tubes and prevents traction being applied to the applicators inside the patient. If the wrong catheter is connected to the applicator, the system will fail to operate.

Operating the Selectron

Treatment is commenced by activation of the remote control unit when all staff have left the treatment area. While treatment is in progress, it can be interrupted and restarted from the remote control unit by pressing the stop and start buttons. The display panel indicates which channels are being used for treatment and which are unused, with red and green lights respectively. The time of the longest treatment is displayed on the panel and a telephone intercom system allows for communication with the patient without the need to interrupt treatment (Hoskin and Coyle 2005).

Interrupting the treatment is done by pressing the green stop button, which results in the radioactive sources being withdrawn into the Selectron unit and stops the treatment timer. This then allows nursing staff to enter the treatment area in safety and give care to the patient. Pressing the red start button transfers the sources back into the applicators and restarts the treatment timer; the red lights demonstrate that the channels are operating again satisfactorily. The system has built-in safety features so that in the event of a failure in the system, treatment stops automatically and an audible and visual alarm at the remote control unit is instigated. This alerts staff to a problem, indicating whether this is a fault related to the air or power supply, the sources or the timer.

In some hospitals an optional nurse station display unit is installed with similar alarm indicators which emit audible signals when treatment has been interrupted. This helps to prevent treatment being inadvertently interrupted for long periods. The Selectron records all breaks in treatment and this is shown on the print-out from the unit itself together with any programming

851

(see Figure 14.9). Leading from the unit are either three or six flexible plastic transfer tubes corresponding to numbered treatment channels; each tube ends in a fragile plastic catheter which is inserted into the appropriately numbered applicator and secured by a coupling device. The unit has a supply of compressed air and it is air pressure that the system uses to transfer the sources from the safe within the unit to the applicators along the connecting tubes.

Operation of the unit is initiated from a remote-control unit situated outside the protected treatment area (Hoskin and Coyle 2005) and provides an accurate and safe method of radiotherapy treatment for cancers of the cervix, uterus and upper part of the vagina.

The advantages of the LDR Selectron system are as follows.

- Remote afterloading eliminates contact with radioactive material and protects personnel. The unit is switched off each time someone enters the patient's room, and only once all staff leave the room will the unit be switched back on. The unit will automatically return the radioactive pellets into the applicators, and the treatment that was temporarily discontinued will be recommenced (Hart 2006).
- It allows highly accurate dosimetry.
- The activity of the caesium-137 sources is such (up to 1.5 GBq) that treatment times for patients are considerably shorter than with conventional techniques.

or system fault. These appear as an error code and can be identified by reference to the Selectron user's manual.

At the end of the treatment time, all sources will be withdrawn automatically from the applicators back into the Selectron unit. If two patients are being treated simultaneously, termination of the treatment of one patient may be some time before that of the other. This means the timer will register the longer treatment time, but the indicator lights for the channels used for the first patient will have changed from red to green.

Additional safety features include a door switch facility to retract sources immediately if the door to the treatment area is opened when treatment is in progress, and/or Geiger dose meters visible when entering the treatment area and approaching the patient, which indicate when there are radioactive sources either in the patient or in the connecting tubes.

High dose rate (HDR) micro-Selectron unit

The operating principles of the HDR micro-Selectron are similar to those of the LDR Selectron. LDR Selectron applicators are afterloaded with active sources interspersed with inactive spacers to produce the correct isodose pattern. HDR micro-Selectron machines, on the other hand, achieve the desired isodose pattern with a single iridium-192 source which moves within the applicators and stops at preset positions for predetermined dwell times.

The HDR micro-Selectron delivers radiation at approximately 100 times the rate of the LDR Selectron and treatment times are therefore much shorter, with the added advantage of applicators with a smaller diameter which can be put in place under local anaesthetic in the outpatient department. This is a suitable alternative for patients who may not be able to tolerate the demands of LDR (Hoskin and Coyle 2005).

Once in position, the micro-Selectron intracavity applicators are fixed to the treatment couch by means of an adjustable clamp; movement of the applicators is minimal and dosimetry calculations accurately represent actual treatment. In addition, more constant and reproducible geometry of source positioning is possible (Jones *et al.* 1999). Treatment protocols generally consist of two treatments but can involve as many as five. Following explanation and support for the patient, the procedure is carried out under local anaesthetic (Faithfull and Wells 2003); for the first treatment, a urinary catheter is passed and the balloon is inflated with dilute contrast medium. A check X-ray is taken once the applicator tubes are in place to collect information which is fed into the Selectron planning computer to calculate the treatment time (Hoskin and Coyle 2005).

The HDR micro-Selectron follows the same principles for programming and treatment as the LDR Selectron; when treatment is complete, the applicators and catheter are removed and the patient is free to go home after they have passed urine. A case report on patients undergoing treatment with HDR micro-Selectron for gynaecological cancer suggested that they found the experience to be acceptable (Tan *et al.* 2004).

Adequate preparation and information sharing about this treatment are essential, as time spent preparing the patient for brachytherapy treatment makes them better equipped to make informed decisions related to their care (Faithfull and Wells 2003, Wallace *et al.* 2006). Poorly prepared patients are more anxious and less able to follow instructions and can be less tolerant of the implant procedure (Montgomery *et al.* 1999). An assessment of patients' physical and emotional needs must be made prior to each treatment to identify whether any aspect of the treatment is problematic (Faithfull and Wells 2003).

The advantages of HDR micro-Selectron brachytherapy are as follows.

- Shorter treatment time reduces variations in the patient's position and allows more accurate dosimetry (Jones *et al.* 1999).
- Treatment lasts only minutes, minimizing the need for immobilization; this reduces discomfort and the risk of complications associated with bed rest.
- Treatment can be offered on an outpatient basis with a consequent reduction in cost.
- It is an alternative to LDR Selectron and may be more suitable for some patients.
- Complication rates are comparable with low-dose brachytherapy (Wong *et al.* 2003).

Legal and professional issues
Patient preparation and consent

Every therapeutic use of radiation has an inherent risk. Awareness of the risk is essential for all staff who have to obtain informed consent from their patients (Picano 2004).

Information about radiation therapy should be given to patients and carers when therapy is first discussed to allay fears and misconceptions about radiotherapy. Verbal information should be reinforced with written material to prepare the patient, reduce anxiety and promote coping (Faithfull and Wells 2003). A contact name and telephone number of the 'key worker', usually a clinical nurse specialist, are essential for patients before, during and after treatment with sealed source brachytherapy (DH 2000, NICE 2005).

All patients require a thorough nursing assessment to assess their suitability for the treatment, ensuring that they are able to comply with the demands of the treatment and associated radiation protection measures. Any doubt regarding physical or psychological concerns or problems can then be discussed with the patient and their medical team. Prior assessment allows for action to be taken, either to improve the patient's general condition so they are suitable for treatment or to postpone or cancel the radioactive sealed source therapy in favour of a more suitable treatment option (Velji and Fitch 2001). Information for this group is divided into three main categories: (i) disease and treatment; (ii) short- and long-term side-effects from the treatment; and (iii) sexuality and sexual health (Faithfull and White 2008).

Preprocedural considerations for gynaecological brachytherapy

Equipment

Equipment should be kept to a minimum. It must be checked to ensure that it is in working order, as maintenance staff will only be allowed into the room in exceptional circumstances.

Bed linen and disposable items (e.g. gloves, aprons, catheter packs, sanitary towels) should be kept in a utility room or anteroom along with the patient's treatment chart and a radiation monitor.

Specific patient preparations

The patient is usually admitted 12–48 hours before the procedure so that any preanaesthetic investigations may be performed. Full bowel preparation with a low-residue diet will reduce the chance of the patient having a bowel action while the sources are in place to help reduce the risk of sources being dislodged. If patients present with pre-existing diarrhoea on admission caused by previous radiotherapy, then regular antidiarrhoea medication should be prescribed and administered before and during the application of the sources. A full explanation should be given about the method and mode of treatment, possible side-effects, radiation protection issues and obtaining informed consent. The patient should be encouraged to bath before any premedication is administered.

Low dose-rate brachytherapy often follows 5 weeks of external beam radiotherapy (EBRT) to the pelvis (Petereit *et al.* 1998). Patients may embark on treatment already experiencing a number of symptoms which are likely to include radiation-induced enteritis, nausea, fatigue, pain and skin reactions. Management of these symptoms is essential to ensure the safe and effective use of LDR brachytherapy.

Prior to the procedure, patients should also be prepared for the number of applicators to be inserted, dependent on previous treatment. A urinary catheter will be inserted because of the restriction around movement during the treatment. Small but significant aspects to highlight to the patient at this preassessment meeting include the noises made by the Selectron system, especially when sources are being transferred in and out of the applicators, that connection to the Selectron unit is with flexible plastic tubes, and informing all patients that this treatment will only enable them to lie in a semi-recumbent position.

A maximum of two pillows can be used to support the head whilst maintaining the pelvis in roughly the same position, ensuring no significant movement of the applicators. Where practicable, the patient should be closely monitored during treatment by the use of CCTV, telephone and/or intercom access for the patient as well as a nurse call system; all provide further reassurance for patients undergoing this treatment.

Personal items

Nurses should be sensitive to the psychological implications for patients confined in isolation and receiving radiation treatment. Although patients may want to bring some personal belongings with them, they should be advised to keep these to a minimum.

Procedure guideline 14.10 **Sealed source therapy: caesium sources (manual or afterloading): patient care**

853

Essential equipment
- Gloves and apron

Procedure

Action	Rationale
1 On return from theatre, the following should be checked:	
■ Sanitary towel	To contain any blood loss from procedure and observe and record vaginal blood loss. E
■ Disposable pants in position	To secure the position of the sanitary towel. E
■ A urinary catheter is in position and draining urine.	To ensure that urine is draining freely and to accurately monitor urinary output. E
2 Observe any blood loss and/or other discharge from the vagina.	To monitor for haemorrhage, shock and other postoperative complications. E
3 Ensure routine postoperative observations are performed until patient is stable. Continue to monitor temperature, BP and pulse throughout treatment at least 2–4 hourly.	To ensure early detection of possible complications. E

(Continued)

Procedure guideline 14.10 (Continued)

4 Administer prescribed analgesia, antiemetics and antidiarrhoeal agents.	For the patient's comfort and reduction of symptoms that may impact on the safe delivery of treatment using radiation sources. E
5 Encourage oral fluid intake as soon as the patient is allowed to drink. Encourage a fluid intake of 50–100% a day over and above the patient's normal intake.	To ensure adequate hydration. To reduce the risk of urinary tract infection (Beetz 2003, R1a).
6 A low-residue diet may be taken. Liaise with dietitian regarding suitable supplements.	To prevent the stimulation of a bowel action. E
7 The patient must remain in bed in a recumbent or semi-recumbent position while the applicators or implants are in place.	To prevent the applicators becoming dislodged or changing their position in relation to the adjacent internal organs. E
8 Log rolling the patient from side to side is permitted.	To promote comfort, relieve skin of prolonged pressure on any one area, thus reducing pressure sores to at-risk tissue. E

Procedure guideline 14.11 Sealed source therapy: low dose-rate Selectron treatment

Preprocedure

Action	Rationale
1 Ensure written consent has been obtained, checking the patient is prepared to go ahead with the procedure.	To ensure consent has been obtained. To ensure patient fully understands and agrees to the treatment planned and is offered the opportunity to ask any questions or mention any concerns they may still have (Faithfull and Wells 2003, E).
2 Ensure thorough nursing assessment of patient has been undertaken by nursing staff.	To ensure patient is suitable and will comply with treatment restrictions (Gosselin and Waring 2001, E).
3 Ensure full preoperative medical assessment has been undertaken including baseline blood tests (FBC, clotting, U&E and LFT), ECG and chest X-ray.	To ensure patient is fit for treatment. E
4 Administer antidiarrhoeal drugs the night before treatment. Patient to be monitored and if necessary treatment provided for radiation-induced enteritis.	To prevent bowel action during treatment which may dislodge applicators during treatment. E

Procedure

5 Nurse the patient on a pressure-relieving mattress or with a foam wedge under her buttocks or a pillow under her knees to alter position.	To promote comfort and to relieve backache since rolling is not encouraged and in some areas not permitted. E
6 Ensure the plastic transfer tubes are supported securely in the bed bracket, leaving slight slack.	To enable the patient to change position slightly without putting traction on the applicators. E
7 Limit the frequency and duration of interruptions to treatment. Visitors are discouraged unless the patient is markedly distressed.	To prevent unnecessary prolongation of treatment time. E

8 Check patient's physical and psychological condition 2-hourly:	
(a) Temperature, pulse and vaginal loss	To monitor for haemorrhage, shock or other postoperative complications. E
(b) Contents of catheter drainage bag	To ensure urine is draining freely. E
(c) Assist patient to adjust her position.	To promote comfort and relieve prolonged pressure on any one area. To maintain skin integrity and prevent friction. E
9 Check position of applicators. Marking the position of the applicators on the patient's legs can assist in the checking of their position.	To ensure no movement of the applicators has occurred. E
10 Administer prescribed analgesia, antiemetics, antidiarrhoeal and sedative agents as appropriate, observing and evaluating effect.	To promote the patient's comfort and well-being. E
11 Encourage fluid intake as soon as the patient is able to drink.	To ensure adequate hydration and reduce the risk of urinary tract infection and dehydration (Beetz 2003, R1a).
12 Encourage a light, low-residue diet to be taken, appropriate for consuming easily in a lying down position.	To maintain nutritional needs whilst reducing stimulation of a bowel action. E

Postprocedure

13 Perform accurate documentation.	To ensure accurate record keeping (NMC 2009, C).

Procedure guideline 14.12 Sealed source therapy: Selectron applicator removal

Essential equipment

- Gloves
- Plastic apron/gown
- Clinical waste bag
- Clean sanitary pad
- Gauze
- Catheter removal pack including syringe to remove water from catheter, large collecting tray for applicators and CSSD bag for returning applicators and rubber caps for ends of applicators
- Prescription chart
- Pre-removal medications
- Entonox and mask

Preprocedure

Action	**Rationale**
1 Explain and discuss the procedure with the patient.	To ensure that the patient understands the procedure and gives her valid consent (Faithfull and Wells 2003, E).
2 Check treatment has been terminated by:	
(a) Ensuring the appropriate channel lights are green	The applicators should be removed only on completion of treatment. E
(b) Ensuring the time display on the Selectron unit reads zero for the appropriate channels	To ensure that the treatment completed corresponds with the patient. This is essential when delivering treatment via the same machine to two patients at the same time. E
(c) Ensuring the print-out indicates that treatment has stopped for those channels.	

(Continued)

Procedure guideline 14.12 (*Continued*)

3 Check that the closed-circuit television camera is not focused on the patient.	To ensure privacy and dignity. E

Procedure

4 Ensure any pre-removal drugs have been administered.	To allow analgesic and/or sedative medications time to be effective. E
5 Assist the patient into a comfortable position with her knees apart.	To allow access to the applicators. E
6 Uncouple the plastic transfer tubes by rotating the black coupling anticlockwise in the direction of the arrow and very carefully store the tubes on the plastic supporting mantle attached to the Selectron unit.	To prevent the plastic catheter becoming damaged or kinked. E
7 Place rubber caps on the ends of the applicators.	To ensure no fluid or debris is allowed to enter the applicator tubes. E
8 Commence administration of Entonox (see Chapter 9) at least 2 minutes before removal of the applicators if patient has consented to that.	To allow the effect of the gas to become maximal. E
9 Prepare the equipment and put on non-sterile gloves.	This procedure is clinically clean and not aseptic (Rossoff *et al.* 1993, R1b).
10 Remove the vulval dressing pads and any sutures and vaginal packing.	These must be removed before the applicators can be eased out. E
11 Dismantle the applicators by loosening the screws holding them together.	To promote ease of removal. E
12 Remove the uterine tube first ensuring it is taken out complete with its small white flange and then followed by removal of remaining applicators and the ovoids. Check all parts of the equipment used in the procedure are accounted for.	To prevent the flange being left in the patient's vagina. E To ensure no equipment or packing has been left in the patient. E
13 Remove the catheter after balloon has been deflated, provide vulva care and ensure the patient has a clean sanitary pad and a fresh sheet under the patient. Ensure the patient informs the nurse when she has passed urine after catheter removal.	To promote cleanliness and patient comfort. Observe for any bleeding post applicator removal. E To identify any changes to the vulva or surrounding skin areas. E To ensure that there is no urinary retention post catheter removal. E
14 The patient can then be assisted into a comfortable position. Instruct patient to inform the nurse when she requires assistance with personal hygiene as she adjusts to an upright position.	To reassure the patient that the procedure has been completed, that she is no longer receiving radiation treatment and can resume normal activities. E

Postprocedure

15 Applicators are then placed into CSSD return bags and returned to CSSD for cleaning in accordance with local policies.	To ensure correct sterilization and/or disposal. E

Problem-solving table 14.1 Prevention and resolution (Procedure guidelines 14.11 and 14.12)

Problem	Cause	Prevention	Action
Patient removes the applicators herself	Possible causes can be postanaesthetic, infection and/or isolation issues	Clear explanation to the patient about the problems of removing the applicators	Check room for any sources that may have escaped, using contamination monitor; sources that have escaped should be placed in lead pots using long-handled forceps and the physics department notified
			Remove applicators completely if partially removed as per instructions above. In the confused patient this is a two-nurse procedure
Applicator is partially dislodged	Patient may have moved too much or too vigorously	Explanation to patient about amount of movement allowed.	Interrupt treatment and inform physicist and radiotherapist; the applicator may have to be removed as above
Alarm sounding at nurse station	Treatment has been interrupted and inadvertently left off	Check all settings when leaving the patient	Check patient is not requiring any nursing intervention and then check patient is unattended; if unattended, recommence treatment
Sources are not transferred to the applicators	Incorrect coupling or loose connection	Check all connections	Check print-out to identify which channel is at fault; tighten appropriate coupling device. If not resolved, contact physics department
Alarm activated at remote control unit	Failure in the system	Check Selectron is kept maintained	Check the error code on the print-out with the Selectron user's manual
			Rectify as indicated in the manual or seek technical assistance from the physics department
Pellets stuck in the applicator or transfer tubing	A damaged or kinked catheter tubing	Check the catheter tubing prior to use.	A risk assessment to be completed regarding the likelihood of this occurrence (HSE 2003a). Inform the patient of problem and contact physics department and the medical team

Postprocedural considerations

Ongoing care

Discharge of patient

Patients are usually discharged on the day of completion of brachytherapy. All patients must void after removal of applicators and vaginal packing.

Patients can sometimes be unsteady on their feet after prolonged bed rest and may require assistance. They should be informed that normal bowel actions may not return for a day or so; advice on managing diarrhoea or constipation should be given. Light spotting or discharge from the vagina is normal and should be discussed with patients to prevent any unnecessary concerns once at home. If patients experience pain or any more marked bleeding, hospital staff should be contacted immediately. Symptoms of urinary tract infection such as dysuria and/or elevated temperature should also be reported and a plan of care established prior to discharge.

Complications

Early complications include pain, post-treatment fatigue, increased bowel activity, urinary urgency or frequency, dysuria, nocturia, vaginal discharge and perineal irritation (Faithfull and Wells 2003). Severe reactions, although uncommon, can include severe or prolonged proctitis in patients with pre-existing bowel disease and late complications, including bowel and bladder complications, vaginal dryness, vaginal narrowing, vaginal stenosis, dyspareunia, premenopausal symptoms and early menopause (Chen *et al.* 2004, Jefferies *et al.* 2007, Lancaster 2004).

The vaginal canal is included in the radiation field, therefore side-effects from treatment can be significant on the delicate tissue in the vagina. All patients need to be aware of possible complications associated with the treatment causing alteration to the elasticity and lubrication within the vagina, changes in sensation, vaginal stenosis and tissue fibrosis. It is therefore important, as stated earlier, for this patient population to be supported by a clinical nurse specialist to provide supportive care and intervention strategies that have the potential to reduce some of the short- and long-term toxicities associated with this treatment (Jefferies *et al.* 2007, Muscari Lin *et al.* 1999).

Possible interventions

- Women who are sexually active should be advised to continue intimate relations as tolerated with the use of analgesia as required.
- A provision for assessing discomfort and/or pain.
- Provide adequate and appropriate analgesia.
- Allow for radiation reactions to resolve, providing specific information on using vaginal dilators and personal hygiene care (Jefferies *et al.* 2007).
- The lifelong use of vaginal dilators (Jefferies *et al.* 2007).
- The use of water-soluble lubricants to help alleviate the dry mucosa (Muscari Lin *et al.* 1999).
- Short courses of localized hormone therapy to increase natural lubrication (Blake *et al.* 1998).

A review of 107 patients who had received radiotherapy found that advice from healthcare professionals was valuable in managing complications of treatment (Gami *et al.* 2003). Syed *et al.* (2002) completed a 20-year evaluation of the long-term survival and safety of interstitial and intracavity brachytherapy in the treatment of carcinoma of the cervix and found a reasonable chance of cure with acceptable morbidity. Teruya *et al.* (2002) found that all patients included in a retrospective review of HDR micro-Selectron brachytherapy reported vaginal mucosal changes but few complaints regarding sexual functioning.

However, this specific cancer treatment can cause persistent changes to the vagina resulting in considerable distress by compromising sexual activity (Bergmark *et al.* 1999). Patients need to be reassured that many women regain their capacity for sexual activity and enjoyment. Extra support in the form of counselling or psychosexual counselling may facilitate this patient population if difficult issues arise. Follow-up strategies focusing on specific areas such as self-esteem, body image and sexuality can provide a mechanism to identify these specific issues over the longer term (Farrell 2002).

Male partners of women with cancer reported difficulty in knowing how to behave and how to communicate with their partners (Lalos *et al.* 1995). Almost all male partners were given the news of the diagnosis exclusively by their ill partner, which provoked feelings of anger and bitterness (Lalos 1997). Coping improved if the men were integrated in the patient's care from the time the diagnosis of cancer was made (Lalos *et al.* 1995).

Sealed source iodine-125 seeds used in prostate malignancies

Postprocedural considerations
Ongoing care

Seeds are implanted permanently into the tissue and the patient must agree to stay in hospital until the physics team states that the radioactivity is at a legally permissible level for discharge. The urine should be checked with the contamination monitor to ensure that the sources have not been expelled in the urine. If no radioactivity is found, the urine may be disposed of in the usual way.

The morning after implant, a CT scan is performed to check the number of seeds inserted and then the urinary catheter is removed. Once the patient has voided normally they may be discharged. Prophylactic antibiotics are prescribed to prevent infections for 5 days after the implant. Anti-inflammatory medication will also be prescribed to prevent discomfort and swelling.

In the event of an accidental or sudden death within 1 year of the iodine seed implant, burial rather than cremation should be performed. It is also advised that burial should take place up to 3 years after implant. If cremation is planned during the 1–3 years post implant, the crematorium would first have to be told to contact the hospital for advice.

Education of patient

Advise the patient to observe for haematoma under the scrotum and give advice on reporting to medical team. In the first weeks after the implant, the patient may experience dysuria or frequency and they should be advised to drink at least 2 litres of fluid a day and that any haematuria should resolve quickly. It should also be explained that some patients may experience soft stools or some diarrhoea or mucus in the faeces and that generally most of these symptoms disappear within a few days to a week.

The radioactive iodine seeds implanted into the prostate have a very limited range of radiation. This radiation is not harmful to the patient or their family at home and patients can be discharged when clinically stable. However, advice should be given regarding avoiding close contact with small children and pregnant women for the first few months after treatment. Sexual intercourse is possible after treatment but advise the patient to wait for a few weeks after the procedure. If sexual intercourse is planned in the first 2 months after the procedure, patients should use a condom, in case of the rare occurrence when a radioactive seed may be expelled during ejaculation. For the first few occasions, the colour of the ejaculation fluid may be discoloured, ranging from a light red to black.

For the first few weeks after treatment, it may be possible that one or more radioactive seeds may be expelled during urination. For this reason patients should be advised to sit down when using the toilet, rather than use a urinal. Any seeds that are expelled will then be flushed away. Patients must be informed not to touch any loose seeds with their hands but if necessary to use a spoon or a pair of forceps. All other social contact and activities can be resumed, including travelling.

Complications

Although rare, severe treatment-related side-effects cannot be totally excluded.

- Small risk of incontinence (less than 2%).
- *Erectile dysfunction:* occurs in 40–50% of men under the age of 60 and is more common in older men. Its frequency depends on the level of erectile function before treatment. Treatment is available for those men who develop difficulties.

- *Reduced volume of ejaculate:* the prostate is responsible for semen production and radiation treatments cause the relevant glands in the prostate to stop production.
- *Proctitis:* persistent inflammation of the rectum leading to increased urge to open bowels and the passing of mucus. This occurs rarely (in less than 1% patients).

Intraoral sealed sources

Preprocedural considerations

All patients receiving this treatment will have a dental assessment by an oral surgeon and any issues around dental caries, mouth infections and possible dental extractions will be addressed prior to the treatment because of the possible alteration of blood supply being impaired by treatment.

The patient is usually admitted 24 hours before the implant, during which time the nature of the procedure and the implications of having a radioactive source should be explained to the patient. The patient is nursed in a single controlled room away from other patients as per Radiation Protection guidance to keep exposure to staff and other patients and visitors as low as reasonably possible (ALARP). Only staff and visitors authorized to enter the controlled area should go into the room, and written arrangements for entering the room should be contained within the local rules displayed at the door of the room.

Procedure guideline 14.13 Sealed source therapy: insertion of sealed radioactive sources into the oral cavity

Essential equipment
- Lead pot
- Long-handled forceps
- Hand-held radiation monitor
- Shielding
- Disposable gloves
- Overshoes
- Plastic apron and/or gown

Preprocedure

Action	Rationale
1 Before treatment begins, ensure the room is set up appropriately. This includes placing a lead pot and long-handled forceps in the room to hold any dislodged sources.	To reduce unnecessary time spent in the room once patient returns from theatre (Hart 2006, E).
2 Switch on controlled area radiation warning light outside the room and check it is working correctly.	To warn staff, visitors and other patients of the radiation risk and to ensure only trained personnel enter the room (Hart 2006, E).
3 Place radiation warning notice outside patient's room.	To ensure only authorized personnel enter the room. E

(Continued)

Procedure guideline 14.13 *(Continued)*

Procedure

4 A yellow radiation hazard board should accompany the patient back from theatre. This must remain at the bottom of the bed or outside the cubicle until the source is removed.	To alert everybody that the patient has a radioactive source. E
5 Place lead shields in position at the door. All staff entering the room should work behind the lead shield when in close contact with the patient.	To reduce radiation exposure of staff in close contact with the patient (Hart 2006, E).
6 When transferring patients from theatre to ward, the nurse and porter should remain at the head and foot of the bed and at least 120 cm from the centre of the bed in the event of any delay in the transfer.	To minimize the risk of exposure to radiation. E
7 Nursing staff must calculate the time allowed with the patient in any 24-hour period. This time should be written on the yellow warning notice on the bed or cubicle door.	To minimize exposure to radiation (Hart 2006, E).
8 A contamination monitor should be available on the ward.	To monitor radioactivity if a dislodged source is suspected, for example in the bed linen (Hart 2006, E).
9 Whilst one nurse should be responsible for planning the nursing care of the patient, the time spent with the patient should be shared between all suitably trained nurses and all time spent in performing nursing procedures must be kept to a minimum. Only those staff whose presence is necessary should spend time with the patient.	To minimize the risk of overexposure to radiation (Hart 2006, E).
10 Every nurse must wear a radiation badge above the level of the lead shield.	To record the extent of exposure to radiation (Ionizing Radiation Regulations 1999, C).
11 All bed linen and waste materials removed from the patient area should be monitored before being removed from the ward.	To prevent loss of an accidentally dislodged source (Hart 2006, E).
12 If a source becomes dislodged, use the long-handled forceps to put the source into a lead pot. Care should be taken not to damage the source. It must never be handled directly with the fingers.	To minimize the dose of radiation received (Hart 2006, E).
13 Visitors must seek permission each time they wish to enter the room. Visitors must remain at least 120 cm away from the patient. Visitors must always sit behind one of the bed shields. The visit should not last longer than the time shown on the warning notice. No children or pregnant women are allowed to visit.	To minimize the risk of overexposure to radiation (DH 2000, E).
14 When the patient needs to visit another department, for example X-ray, the following must be ensured.	In order that medical care can continue to be provided while the patient is receiving radioactive sealed source therapy. E
(a) That the receiving department is aware of the hazard of exposure to radioactivity.	To allow the appointment to be made when the department is quiet, thus ensuring waiting time is kept to a minimum and to minimize exposure to others (Ionizing Radiation Regulations 1999, C).

(b) One porter and a nurse should accompany the patient in a wheelchair; two porters and a nurse should accompany the patient on a trolley. In the event of any delays, the nurse and porters should remain at the head and foot of the bed and at least 120 cm from the centre of the bed.	To minimize the risk of exposure of staff to radiation. E
(c) A radiation warning hazard sign should accompany the patient.	To warn all staff that the patient has a radioactive source *in situ* (Ionizing Radiation Regulations 1999, C).
(d) Unless the patient is likely to be in the department for a long time, the nurse and porter should stay with the patient.	To ensure time, distance, shielding and segregation restrictions are maintained. E
(e) If the source becomes dislodged during transfer, the porter must ring the switchboard who will send out an emergency call to the physics department. The nurse must ensure the area around the patient is kept clear of other patients, staff and visitors.	To minimize the risk of exposure to radiation. E
(f) A member of staff from the ward should take a lead pot, forceps and a monitor to the nurse who will place the source in the lead pot and monitor the area to ensure it is free of radioactivity.	To contain the radioactive source and minimize the risk of exposure (Hart 2006, E).
(g) The Radiation Protection Adviser and supervisor should be informed of incident.	To evaluate the incident, and to prevent it recurring (DH 2000, C).
15 *In the event of a cardiac arrest*, an Ambu-bag or similar device must be used, and the physics department must be informed immediately.	To minimize exposure. E
16 *In the event of a fire*, the fire policy must be followed. Following evacuation, the appropriate distance between the radioactive patient and other staff should be maintained; help should be sought from the physics department.	To minimize exposure. E
17 *In the event of a patient's death:*	
Either: *Removable sources*: the radiation sources should be removed by the radiotherapist. Inform the physics department.	Remove radioactivity to allow Last Offices to be undertaken as normal. E
Or: *Non-removable sources*: inform the physics department immediately. The body should be placed in a body bag.	In order for the physics department staff to begin making the necessary arrangements for removal of the body to the mortuary. Arrangements would include: segregated refrigerator, warning notices and use of body bag to contain sources if they became dislodged. E
Transfer of the body should be arranged by the physics department.	The physics staff will supervise the transfer of the body. E
18 *In the event of bleeding*: in order to stem bleeding in the vicinity of the implant, apply pressure using at least four thickness dressing pads. The padding should only be compressed for 15 minutes by any single person.	To minimize exposure. E

861

(Continued)

Procedure guideline 14.13 (*Continued*)

19 In the event of a confused or agitated patient, premature removal of sources may be required.	To prevent overexposure to radiation of the nurses attending the patient, as well as to prevent the patient removing or dislodging sources. E
20 Only staff who have received training and have been authorized may enter a controlled area. A list of suitably trained staff should be kept by the domestic and catering managers and by the ward's local Radiation Protection Supervisor. A domestic or catering supervisor should undertake tasks if the ward-based employee is not trained.	To keep all radiation exposure as low as can be reasonably achieved (Ionizing Radiation Regulations 1999, C).
21 Domestic and catering staff should not remove items such as cleaning equipment and crockery until it has been monitored by a nurse and deemed safe.	To prevent sources being removed from the room before it is safe to do so (Hart 2006, E).

Postprocedural considerations

Ongoing care

Mouth care

The patient may have difficulty in swallowing due to soreness and oedema and may be at risk of localized mouth infection (Ionizing Radiation Regulations 1999) so frequent mouth care using a sterile saline solution as a mouthwash is important. Any rinsed solution should be collected in the disposable bowls to check for a dislodged source. Nurses should ensure that the patient has paper tissues and a bowl, crushed ice for the patient to suck and/or soluble aspirin as a mouthwash. Steroids may also be prescribed to help reduce oedema.

A soft, purèed or liquid diet, avoiding spicy and/or hot foods, must be provided to maintain nutritional levels, reduce the complexity of eating when implants are present and further exacerbation of local reactions or soreness from the implants as well as reducing the risk of the patient biting into the source or their tongue. Carbonated drinks can also alleviate dryness caused by the treatment.

Writing equipment must be provided for the patient to reduce the need for oral communication as this can increase soreness and pain, and potentially alter the distribution of the sources. The sources should be checked at regular intervals, for example at the beginning of each shift, to ensure they have not become dislodged. The patient should be confined to the room and only leave when necessary, for example to visit the X-ray department, to minimize the risk of radiation exposure to other people on the ward.

Discharge of the patient

The patient is usually discharged the day after the removal of the implant; the patient should be warned about the painful local reaction that they may experience from cell breakdown and cell death induced by the radiation. In order to minimize the risk of infection or soreness, the patient should be taught oral hygiene and to observe the mouth for any infection (Hoskin and Coyle 2005).

Websites
Ionising Radiation Regulations 1999 (SI 3232): www.legislation.hmso.gov.uk/si/si1999/19993232.htm
Ionising Radiation (Medical Exposure) Regulations 2000 (SI 1059): www.legislation.hmso.gov.uk/si/si2000/20001059.htm
www.doh.gov.uk/irmir.htm
www.legislation.hmso.gov.uk/si/si1999/19993232.htm
legislation.hso.gov.uk/si/si2000/20001059.htm

References

Agrawal, P.P., Singhal, S.S., Neema, J.P. *et al.* (2005) The role of interstitial brachytherapy using template in locally advanced gynecological malignancies. *Gynecologic Oncology,* 99 (1), 169–175.

Anglesio, S., Calamia, E., Fiandra, C. *et al.* (2005) Prostate brachytherapy with iodine-125 seeds: radiation protection issues. *Tumori,* 91 (4), 335–338.

Beetz, R. (2003) Mild dehydration: a risk factor for urinary tract infection? *European Journal of Clinical Nutrition,* 57 (Suppl 2), S52–S58.

Bergmark, K., Avall-Lundqvist, E., Dickman, P.W., Henningsohn, L. and Steineck, G. (1999) Vaginal changes and sexuality in women with a history of cervical cancer. *New England Journal of Medicine,* 340 (18), 1383–1389.

Blake, P.R., Lambert, H.E. and Crawford, R. (1998) *Gynaecological Oncology: A Guide to Clinical Management*, Oxford University Press, Oxford.

Blank, L.E., Gonzalez Gonzalez, D., de Reijke, T. *et al.* (2000) Brachytherapy with transperineal [125]-iodine seeds for localized prostate cancer. *Radiotherapy and Oncology,* 57 (3), 307–313.

Bomford, C.K (2002a) Radiation protection. In: Bomford, C.K. and Kunkler, I.K. (eds) *Walters and Miller Textbook of Radiotherapy*, 6th edn. Churchill Livingstone, Edinburgh, pp. 69–88.

Bomford, C.K. (2002b) Brachytherapy. In: Bomford, C.K. and Kunkler, I.K. (eds) *Walters and Miller Textbook of Radiotherapy*, 6th edn. Churchill Livingstone, Edinburgh, pp. 225–244.

Brophy, P., Schmus, C. and Balistreri, L. (2004) Meeting the nursing challenge in treating children with 131 I-mIBG. *Journal of Paediatric Oncology Nursing*, **21** (1), 9–15.

Budrukkar, A.N., Shrivastava, S.K., Jalali, R. *et al.* (2001) Transperineal low-dose rate iridium-192 interstitial brachytherapy in cervical carcinoma stage IIB. *Strahlentherapie und Onkologie*, **177** (10), 517–524.

Chen, S.W., Liang, J.A., Yang, S.N. *et al.* (2004) Radiation injury to intestine following hysterectomy and adjuvant radiotherapy for cervical cancer. *Gynecologic Oncology*, **95** (1), 208–214.

Cherry, S.R., Sorenson, J.A. and Phelps, M.E. (2003) *Physics in Nuclear Medicine*, 3rd edn. Saunders, Oxford.

Cormack, J., Towson, J.E.C. and Flower, M.A. (1998) Radiation protection and dosimetry in clinical practice. In: Murray, I.P.C. and Ell, P.J. (eds) *Nuclear Medicine in Clinical Diagnosis and Treatment*, 2nd edn. Churchill Livingstone, Edinburgh, pp. 1651–1677.

Darby, S. (1999) Radiation risks. *BMJ*, **319** (7216), 1019–1020.

DH (2000) *Ionising Radiation (Medical Exposure) Regulations No. 1059*. HMSO, London.

DH (2005) *Saving Lives: A Delivery Programme to Reduce Healthcare Associated Infection Including MRSA*. Department of Health, London.

Faithfull, S. and Wells, M. (2003) *Supportive Care in Radiotherapy*. Churchill Livingstone, Edinburgh.

Faithfull, S. and White, I. (2008) Delivering sensitive healthcare information challenging the taboo of women's sexual health after pelvic radiotherapy. *Patient Education and Counseling*, **71** (2), 228–233.

Farrell, E. (2002) Premature menopause. 'I feel like an alien'. *Australian Family Physician*, **31** (5), 419–421.

Fitch, M.I. and McGrath, P.N. (2003) The needs of family members of patients receiving radioactive iodine. *Canadian Oncology Nursing Journal*, **13** (4), 220–231.

Fung, A.Y. (2002) The Syed temporary interstitial iridium gynaecological implant: an inverse planning system. *Physics in Medicine and Biology*, **47** (16), N203–208.

Gami, B., Harrington, K., Blake, P. *et al.* (2003) How patients manage gastrointestinal symptoms after pelvic radiotherapy. *Alimentary Pharmacology and Therapeutics*, **18** (10), 987–994.

Gosselin, T.K. and Waring, J.S. (2001) Nursing management of patients receiving brachytherapy for gynaecologic malignancies. *Clinical Journal of Oncology Nursing*, **5** (2), 59–63.

Grabenbauer, G.G., Rodel, C., Brunner, T. *et al.* (2001) Interstitial brachytherapy with Ir-192 low-dose-rate in the treatment of primary and recurrent cancer of the oral cavity and oropharynx. Review of 318 patients treated between 1985 and 1997. *Strahlentherapie und Onkologie*, **177** (7), 338–344.

Hart, S. (2006) Ionising radiation: promoting safety for patients, visitors and staff. *Nursing Standard*, **20** (47), 47–57.

Health Protection Agency (2006) *Administration of Radioactive Substances Advisory Committee, Guidance Notes*. Health Protection Agency, London.

Health Protection Agency (2010) www.hpa.org.uk/radiation.

Henkin, R.E. (2006) *Nuclear Medicine*, 2nd edn. Mosby, St Louis, MO.

Hod, N., Hagag, P. and Baumer, M. (2005) Differentiated thyroid carcinoma in children and young adults: evaluation of response to treatment. *Clinical Nuclear Medicine*, **30** (6), 387–390.

Hoskin, P. and Coyle, C. (2005) *Radiotherapy in Practice: Brachytherapy*. Oxford University Press, Oxford.

HSE (2002) *Control of Substances Hazardous to Health Regulations (COSHH)*. Health and Safety Executive Books, Norwich.

HSE (2003a) *Five Steps to Risk Assessment*. Health and Safety Executive Books, Norwich.

HSE (2003b) *Safe Working and the Prevention of Infection in Clinical Laboratories and Similar Facilities*. Health and Safety Executive Books, Norwich.

Huang, S., Yang, H. and Zhuang, H. (2006) Initial diagnosis and treatment follow up of neuroblastoma invasion of inferior vena cava with 1-131 mIBG. *Clinical Nuclear Medicine*, **31** (11), 718–720.

ICRP (2004) Release of patients after therapy with unsealed radionuclide. *Annals of the ICRP*, **34** (20), v–vi and 1–79.

ICRP (2005) Radiation safety aspects of brachytherapy for prostate cancer using permanently implanted sources. ICRP Publication 98. *Annals of the ICRP*, **35** (3), iii–vi and 3–50.

Ionizing Radiation Regulations (1999) HMSO, London.

IPEM/RCN (2002) Procedures involving radiation. In: *Ionising Radiation Safety. A Handbook for Nurses*. York Publishing, York, pp. 17–32.

Jefferies, H., Hoy, S., McCahill R. and Crichton, A. (2007) The development of Best Practice guidelines for the use of vaginal dilators following pelvic radiotherapy. *Nursing Times*, **103** (30), 28–29.

Jensen, P.T., Groenvold, M., Klee, M.C. *et al.* (2003) Longitudinal study of sexual function and vaginal changes after radiotherapy for cervical cancer. *International Journal of Radiation Oncology, Biology and Physics*, **56**, 937–949.

Johnson, K.E. (2002) *Preventing Vaginal Stenosis after Pelvic Radiotherapy: Current UK Practice*. 12th International Conference on Cancer Nursing, London.

Jones, B., Pryce, P., Blake, P. and Dale, R. (1999) High dose brachytherapy practice for the treatment of gynaecological cancers in the UK. *British Journal of Radiology*, **72** (856), 371–377.

Juraskova, I., Butow, P., Robertson, R. *et al.* (2003) Post-treatment sexual adjustment following cervical and endometrial cancer: a qualitative insight. *Psycho-Oncology*, **12**, 267–279.

Karakoyun-Celik, O., Norris, C. Jr, Tishler, R. *et al.* (2005) Definitive radiotherapy with interstitial implant boost for squamous cell carcinoma of the tongue base. *Head and Neck*, **27** (5), 353–361.

Kucera, H., Mock, U., Knocke, T. *et al.* (2001) Radiotherapy alone for invasive vaginal cancer: outcome with intracavitary high dose rate brachytherapy versus conventional low dose rate brachytherapy. *Acta Obstetrica et Gynecologica Scandinavica*, **80** (4), 355–360.

Kuipers, T., Hoekstra, C., van 't Riet, A. *et al.* (2001) HDR brachytherapy applied to cervical carcinoma with moderate lateral expansion: modified principles of treatment. *Radiotherapy and Oncology*, **58** (1), 25–30.

Lalos, A. (1997) The impact of diagnosis on cervical and endometrial cancer patients and their spouses. *European Journal of Gynaecological Oncology*, **18** (6), 513–519.

Lalos, A., Jacobsson, L., Lalos, O. and Stendahl, U. (1995) Experiences of the male partner in cervical and endometrial cancer – a prospective interview study. *Journal of Psychosomatic Obstetrics and Gynecology*, **16** (3), 153–165.

Lamb, M.A. (1998) Questions women ask about gynecologic cancer and sexual functioning. *Developments in Supportive Cancer Care*, **2** (1), 11–13.

Lancaster, L. (2004) Preventing vaginal stenosis after brachytherapy for gynaecological cancer: an overview of australian practices. *European Journal of Oncology Nursing*, **8** (1), 30–39.

Lapeyre, M., Bollet, M., Racadot, S. *et al.* (2004) Postoperative brachytherapy alone and combined postoperative radiotherapy and brachytherapy boost for squamous cell carcinoma of the oral cavity, with positive or close margins. *Head and Neck*, **26** (3), 216–223.

Leborgne, F., Leborgne, J.H., Zubizarreta, E. and Mezzera, J. (2002) Cesium-137 needle brachytherapy boosts after external beam irradiation for locally advanced carcinoma of the tongue and floor of the mouth. *Brachytherapy*, **1** (3), 126–130.

Leung, P.M. and Nikolic, M. (1998) Disposal of therapeutic 131-I waste using a multiple holding tank system. *Health Physics*, **75** (3), 315–321.

Liepe, K., Runge, R. and Kotzerke, J. (2005) Systematic radionuclide therapy in pain palliation. *American Journal of Hospice Palliative Care*, **22** (6), 457–464.

Luini, A., Galimberti, V., Gatti, G. *et al.* (2005) The sentinel node biopsy after previous breast surgery: preliminary results on 543 patients treated at the European Institute of Oncology. *Breast Cancer Research and Treatment*, **89** (2), 159–163.

Manger, W.M. (2006a) Diagnosis and management of pheochromocytoma – recent advances and current concepts. *Kidney International Supplement*, **12** (104), S30–S35.

Manger, W.M. (2006b) An overview of pheochromocytoma: history, current concepts, vagaries, and diagnostic challenges. *Annals of the New York Academy of Science*, **1073**, 1–20.

McEwan, A.J. (1998) Palliation of bone pain In: Murray, I.P.C. and Ell, P.J. (eds) *Nuclear Medicine in Clinical Diagnosis and Treatment*, 2nd edn. Churchill Livingstone, Edinburgh, pp. 1083–1100.

McKay, A. (1999) Psychoeducational group increases vaginal dilation for young women and reduces sexual fears for women of all ages with gynaecological carcinaoma treated with radiotherapy. *Canadian Journal of Human Sexuality*, **8** (2), 145–146.

Montgomery, C., Lydon, A. and Lloyd, K. (1999) Psychological distress among cancer patients and informed consent. *Journal of Psychosomatic Research*, **46** (3), 241–245.

Muscari Lin, E., Aikin, J.L. and Good, B.C. (1999) Premature menopause after cancer treatment. *Cancer Practice*, **7** (3), 114–121.

Nag, S. (2004) High dose rate brachytherapy: its clinical applications and treatment guidelines. *Technology in Cancer Research and Treatment*, **3** (3), 269–287.

Nag, S., Yacoub, S., Copeland, L.J. and Fowler, J.M. (2002) Interstitial brachytherapy for salvage treatment of vaginal recurrences in previously unirradiated endometrial cancer patients. *International Journal of Radiation Oncology, Biology, Physics*, **54** (4), 1153–1159.

National Radiation Protection Board 14 (1) www.nrpb.org

NICE (2005) *Low Dose Rate Brachytherapy for Localised Prostate Cancer*. National Institute for Health and Clinical Excellence, London. www.nice.org.uk/IPG132.

NMC (2008) *Standards for Medicines Management*. Nursing and Midwifery Council, London.

NMC (2009) *Record Keeping: Guidance for Nurses and Midwives*. Nursing and Midwifery Council, London.

Nutting, C., Horlock, N., A'Hern, R. *et al.* (2006) Manually afterloaded 192Ir low-dose rate brachytherapy after subtotal excision and flap reconstruction of recurrent cervical lymphadenopathy from head and neck cancer. *Radiotherapy and Oncology*, **80** (1), 39–42.

O'Dwyer, H.M., Lyon, S., Fotheringham, T. and Lee, M. (2003) Informed consent for interventional radiology procedures: a survey detailing current European practice. *Cardiovascular and Interventional Radiology*, **26** (5), 428–433.

Okuyama, C., Ushijima, Y., Kubota, T. *et al.* (2002) Utility of follow up studies using meta-[123-I]iodobenzylguanidine scintig-

raphy for detecting recurrent neuroblastoma. *Nuclear Medicine Communications*, **23** (7), 663–672.

Pacini, F., Capezzone, M., Elisei, R. *et al.* (2002) Diagnostic 131-iodine whole body scan may be avoided in thyroid cancer patients who have undetectable stimulated serum Tg levels after initial treatment. *Journal of Clinical Endocrinology and Metabolism*, **87** (4), 1499–1501.

Pearson, D., Rogers, A.T. and Moss, E. (2001) A generic approach to risk assessment for the Ionising Radiation Regulations 1999. *British Journal of Radiology*, **74** (877), 62–68.

Peter, J.E. and Gambhir, S. (2004) *Nuclear Medicine in Clinical Diagnosis and Treatment*, 3rd edn. Churchill Livingstone, Edinburgh.

Petereit, D.G., Sarkaria, J.N. and Chappell, R.J. (1998) Perioperative morbidity and mortality of high-dose-rate gynecologic brachytherapy. *International Journal of Radiation Oncology, Biology, Physics*, **42** (5), 1025–1031.

Picano, E. (2004) Informed consent and communication of risk from radiological and nuclear medicine examination: how to escape from a communication inferno. *BMJ*, **329** (7470), 849–851.

Preston, D.L., Shimizu, Y., Pierce, D. *et al.* (2003) Studies of mortality of atomic bomb survivors. Report 13: Solid cancer and noncancer disease mortality: 1950–1997. *Radiation Research*, **160** (4), 381–407.

RIDDOR (1995) *The Reporting of Injuries, Diseases and Dangerous Occurrences Regulations*. HMSO, London.

Rossoff, L.J., Lam, S., Hilton, E., Borenstein, M. and Isenberg, H.D. (1993) Is the use of boxed gloves in an intensive care unit safe? *American Journal of Medicine*, **94** (6), 602–607.

Russell, C. (1998) Measurement and interpretation of renal transit times. In: Murray, I.P.C. and Ell, P.J. (eds) *Nuclear Medicine in Clinical Diagnosis and Treatment*, 2nd edn. Churchill Livingstone, Edinburgh, pp. 257–262.

Schrenk, P., Woelfl, S., Bogner, S. *et al.* (2005) The use of sentinel node biopsy in breast cancer patients undergoing skin sparing mastectomy and immediate autologous reconstruction. *Plastic and Reconstructive Surgery*, **116** (5), 1278–1286.

Sharp, C., Shrimpton, J.A. and Bury, R.F. (1998) *Diagnostic Medical Exposures: Advice on Exposure to Ionising Radiation during Pregnancy*. National Radiological Protection Board, Didcot.

Skalla, K.A., Bakitas, M., Furstenberg, C.T., Ahles, T. and Henderson, J.V. (2004) Patients' need for information about cancer therapy. *Oncology Nursing Forum*, **31** (2), 313–319.

So, W.K. and Yuen, J.K. (2006) Evaluation of an educational programme for Chinese women receiving internal radiation for uterine cervical cancer. *Journal of Clinical Nursing*, **15** (3), 358–360.

Stajduhar, K.I., Neithercut, J., Chu, E. *et al.* (2000) Thyroid cancer patients' experience of receiving iodine-131 therapy. *Oncology Nursing Forum*, **27** (8), 1213–1218.

Stock, R.G., Stone, N., Lo, Y. *et al.* (2000) Postimplant dosimetry for 125I prostate implants: definitions and factors affecting outcome. *International Journal of Radiation, Oncology, Biology, Physics*, **48** (3), 899–906.

Syed, A.M., Puthawala, A.A., Abdelaziz, N.N. *et al.* (2002) Long-term results of low-dose-rate interstitial-intracavitary brachytherapy in the treatment of carcinoma of the cervix. *International Journal of Radiation Oncology, Biology, Physics*, **54** (1), 67–78.

Takacsi-Nagy, Z., Oberna, F., Polgar, C. *et al.* (2001) The importance of interstitial radiotherapy in the treatment of the base of tongue tumors: a retrospective analysis. *Neoplasma*, **48** (1), 76–81.

Tan, L.T., Russell, S. and Burgess, L. (2004) Acute toxicity of chemo-radiotherapy for cervical cancer: the Addenbrooke's experience. *Clinical Oncology,* **16** (4), 255–260.

Teruya, Y., Sakumoto, K., Moromizato, H. *et al.* (2002) High-dose intracavitary brachytherapy for carcinoma in situ of the vagina occurring after hysterectomy: a rational prescription of radiation dose. *American Journal of Obstetrics and Gynecology,* **187** (2), 360–364.

Tessa, M., Rotta, P., Ragona, R. *et al.* (2005) Concomitant chemotherapy and external radiotherapy plus brachytherapy for locally advanced esophageal cancer: results of a retrospective multicenter study. *Tumori,* **91** (5), 406–414.

Thompson, M.A. (2001) Radiation safety precautions in the management of the hospitalized 131-I therapy patient. *Nuclear Medicine Technology,* **29** (2), 61–66.

Ung, Y.C., Yu, E., Falkson, C., Haynes, A.E., Stys-Norman, D. and Evans, W.K. (2006) The role of high-dose-rate brachytherapy in the palliation of symptoms in patients with non-small-cell lung cancer: a systematic review. *Brachytherapy,* 5(3), 189–202.

Velji, K. and Fitch, M. (2001) The experience of women receiving brachytherapy for gynecologic cancer. *Oncology Nursing Forum,* **28** (4), 743–751.

Vialard-Miguel, J., Mazere, J., Mora, S. *et al.* (2005) [I131 in blood samples: management in the laboratory.] *Annales de Biologie Clinique (Paris),* **63** (5), 561–565.

Wadsley, J.C., Patel, M., Tomlins, C. *et al.* (2003) Iridium-192 implantation for T1 and T2a carcinoma of the tongue and floor of mouth: retrospective study of the results of treatment at the Royal Berkshire Hospital. *British Journal of Radiology,* **76**, 414–417.

Wallace, K., Fleshner, N., Jewett, M., Basiuk, J. and Crook, J. (2006) Impact of a multi-disciplinary patient education session on accrual to a difficult clinical trial: the Toronto experience with the surgical prostatectomy versus interstitial radiation intervention trial. *Journal of Clinical Oncology,* **24** (25), 4158–4162.

Williams, C.E. and Woodward, A.F. (2005) Management of the hapless patent after radioiodine ablation therapy. Are we being too strict? *Nuclear Medicine Communications,* **26** (10), 925–928.

Wong, F.C., Tung, S.Y., Leung, T.W. *et al.* (2003) Treatment results of high-dose-rate remote afterloading brachytherapy for cervical cancer and retrospective comparison of two regimens. *International Journal of Radiation, Oncology, Biology, Physics,* 55 (5), 1254–1264.

Wust, P., von Borczyskowski, D., Henkel, T. *et al.* (2004) Clinical and physical determinants for toxicity of 125-I seed brachytherapy. *Radiotherapy and Oncology,* **73** (1), 39–48.

Zelefsky, M.J. (2006) Quality of life of patients after permanent prostate brachytherapy in relation to dosimetry. *Urologic Oncology,* **24** (4), 377–378.

Ziessman, H.A., O'Malley, J.P. and Thrall, J.H. (2006) *Nuclear Medicine,* 3rd edn. Mosby, St Louis, MO.

Supporting the patient through treatment

Part four

Cytotoxic therapy

Procedure guidelines

The Royal Marsden Hospital Manual of Clinical Nursing Procedures, Eighth Edition. Edited by Lisa Dougherty and Sara Lister.

Overview

This chapter focuses upon the theoretical and practical aspects of administering chemotherapy. Procedure guidelines are included in the text as well as essential information which is provided in the tables and boxes.

Cytotoxic therapy

Definition

The term 'cytotoxic', literally translated, means 'toxic to cells'. Hence these drugs are those which kill cells (malignant or non-malignant). Chemotherapy works by disrupting cellular growth and causing damage to DNA (Dougherty and Bailey 2008). The aim of chemotherapy is to control disease progression and optimize survival.

Related theory

All proliferating cells (normal cells and cancer cells) go through the same division cycle. The cell cycle is a series of phases through which cells must pass as they replicate (Dougherty and Bailey 2008). The DNA in a parent cell replicates and divides, producing two daughter cells (Schulmeister 2009).

- Following cell division or mitosis (M) (which occurs within an hour), cells enter the first gap or G phase, where cells prepare to synthesize DNA but where synthesis of RNA and protein occurs (Kelland 2005).
- The next phase, called the S phase or synthesis phase, results in the cells doubling their DNA content. Many cytotoxic drugs work by disrupting the genetic codes during DNA synthesis.
- The second gap or G_2 phase is where the cell is preparing for division. DNA synthesis stops whilst RNA synthesis and protein synthesis continue in preparation for mitosis.
- Mitosis occurs in the final stage of the cell cycle, M phase, and can last from 30 to 90 minutes. At the end of this phase, cells either rejoin the cell cycle at G or enter the resting subphase G_0. See Figure 15.1.

Cancer chemotherapy drugs tend to be administered in combination which means that they can act upon different phases of the cell cycle, thus producing maximum cytotoxic effect. There are now many drugs licensed for the treatment of cancer and most of these (with the exception of antihormonal drugs used to treat breast and prostate cancers) target rapidly dividing cells either through the effects on DNA or factors involved in mitosis (Kelland 2005).

Cancer drugs can be classified into the following categories: alkylating agents; antimetabolites; antimicrotubule agents; topoisomerase inhibitors and antihormonal agents. An understanding of the cell cycle is important when considering the use of anticancer drugs because the drugs can either act on the phases of the cell cycle or act independently

Figure 15.1 The cell cycle. Reproduced from Tortora and Derrickson (2009).

of the cell cycle (Kelland 2005). Chemotherapy can be administered as single agents or in combination regimens.

Cytotoxic handling

Evidence-based approaches

Cytotoxic drug handling by nursing, pharmacy and other healthcare professionals is an occupational hazard (Weinstein and Plumer 2007). Cytotoxic drugs have been shown to be mutagenic, teratogenic and carcinogenic when given at therapeutic levels to animals and humans to destroy malignant cells (MARCH 2007, Weinstein and Plumer 2007). Patients may develop secondary cancers as a result of treatment with cytotoxic drugs and while such risks may be acceptable to patients who have a life-threatening illness (Ferguson and Wright 2002), they are not acceptable to personnel involved in the reconstitution and administration of cytotoxic drugs and the handling of waste and spills.

The risk to health associated with exposure is measured by the time, dose and routes of exposure. Since safe levels of exposure to hazardous agents cannot be determined because of the lack of a reliable monitoring method to measure exposure risks, personal protective equipment (PPE) is vital for the protection of healthcare workers (Nixon and Schulmeister 2009). A study in the United Kingdom demonstrated that the use of PPE decreased levels of contamination of the urine samples of nurses and of wipe samples on work surfaces in the clinical environment (Ziegler et al. 2002). Cytotoxic drugs can be absorbed through the skin (although with the majority of the compounds there is little or no absorption through intact skin; the exceptions are those which are lipid soluble) (Weinstein and Plumer 2007) . Skin exposure can be by contact with contaminated equipment used in preparing or administering the drugs or during the handling and disposal of waste. Pethran *et al.* (2003) demonstrated that antineoplastic drugs were found in the urine of nurses and pharmacy personnel who were involved in the handling of cytotoxic drugs.

On the basis of the evidence available at present, risks to personnel involved in the reconstitution and administration of cytotoxic drugs fall into three categories: short-term effects, reproductive risks and systemic effects.

Short-term effects

These are usually caused by direct contact with the skin, eyes and mucous membranes, for example dermatitis, inflammation of mucous membranes, excessive lacrimation, pigmentation, blistering (associated with mustine) and other miscellaneous, allergic reactions (Dranitsaris *et al.* 2005, Weinstein and Plumer 2007).

Reproductive risks

These include menstrual dysfunction following exposure to cytotoxic drugs and infertility (Valanis *et al.* 1997). A number of other experimental studies have suggested that serious long-term effects may result from exposure to cytotoxic drugs during pregnancy. Effects include miscarriages and stillbirths (Valanis *et al.* 1999), chromosomal abnormalities (Harrison 2008), low birthweight and congenital abnormalities (Scheepers *et al.* 1999). However, when analysing the data, consideration needs to be given to the fact that most of the studies were conducted in the 1980s or based on staff exposure data from that time. During that period, PPE and safe working practices were not well established and therefore these data do not reflect current working practices (MARCH 2007).

The issue is of high importance to staff, and organizational procedures should be in place to minimize the risk of exposure to all staff at all times. It is suggested that the greatest risk occurs in the first trimester of pregnancy due to rapid cell division and differentiation of the fetus and that the 'use of chemotherapy in the second and third trimester seems to be safe' (Cardonick and Iacobucci 2004, p.289). The Health and Safety Executive has issued guidance for new and expectant mothers and states that because 'a safe level of exposure cannot be determined for these drugs, one should avoid exposure or reduce it to as low a level as possible' (HSE 2003).

Systemic effects

It has been shown that although alterations in cell structure have been detected, they appear to be transient and at a low level. It has yet to be demonstrated whether these changes in cell structure are harmful and whether this level of mutagenesis can be equated with more serious consequences. There are also many limitations in testing blood and urine due to the range of agents which cannot be detected, low levels of drugs and metabolites and reduced sensitivity of the tests (Ferguson and Wright 2002). This has led to difficulties when offering staff monitoring and surveillance and it is less common to do extensive biological testing as there are no data

to support a cause and effect in cell structure. Therefore, the 'emphasis should be on clear guidelines to reduce occupational exposure to all staff at all times' (MARCH 2007).

Cytotoxic drugs may also have harmful short- or long-term systemic effects if inhaled or ingested during preparation. These effects include light-headedness, dizziness, nausea, headache, rashes and skin discoloration (Hayden and Goodman 2005).

Legal and professional issues

The hazards of handling cytotoxic drugs are well recognized along with the requirement to adhere to safety measures recommended in order to protect all staff who prepare, administer and handle cytotoxic drugs or waste products. Control of Substances Hazardous to Health (COSHH) Regulations were updated in 2002 (SI 2002). The Health and Safety Executive (HSE 2003) has produced a document on the safe handling of cytotoxic drugs. National evidence-based guidelines have been implemented in an attempt to reduce exposure, provide adequate protective equipment, ensure regular staff monitoring and provide effective written procedures for dealing with preparation, administration, disposal and dealing with spills and accidents. In order to limit exposure, cytotoxic drugs should be prepared only by skilled, knowledgeable and experienced healthcare professionals (Polovich *et al.* 2009, RCN 2010). A full risk assessment under the COSHH Regulations must be made by all departments and wards handling, preparing or administering cytotoxics (SI 2002). The assessment should identify all appropriate procedures for the safety of staff.

Health surveillance

It has been suggested that organizations should provide health surveillance programmes for staff exposed to hazardous drugs and that it should be an integral part of health and safety in the workplace (Nixon and Schulmeister 2009). Some organizations offer yearly health surveillance for staff directly involved in handling cytotoxics on a regular basis, for example certain staff working in pharmacy reconstitution units. Surveillance normally includes physical examinations, blood samples and history of exposure. If no surveillance is offered then a risk assessment focusing upon exposure should be initiated (Box 15.1).

Preprocedural considerations
Equipment

It is vital for healthcare personnel to use PPE whilst handling cytotoxic drugs. This includes consideration of the environment. The most effective means of minimizing the hazard is to arrange for all cytotoxic drugs to be prepared on a named patient basis by trained pharmacy staff in a specially equipped area (Polovich *et al.* 2009). Chemotherapy should be reconstituted in a vertical class II or III biological safety cabinet with laminar flow or an isolator if drugs are prepared on the ward (Ferguson and Wright 2002, Hayden

> **Box 15.1** Employers' obligations regarding safe handling of cytotoxic medications
>
> Employers are obliged to:
> - identify substances that are a hazard to staff and others who may be exposed
> - manage how the drugs should be handled and what to do in the event of a spill or accident
> - ensure that healthcare personnel have access to the ideal environment, protective clothing, policies and procedures, a system of monitoring and recording effects, and any necessary equipment such as spill kits.

and Goodman 2005, Weinstein and Plumer 2007). Cabinets should be situated in a dedicated area with access restricted to trained or supervised personnel.

There is no doubt that the existence of a formal hospital policy for handling cytotoxic drugs has a positive influence on the use of PPE. Minimizing occupational exposure to hazardous drugs, and therefore reducing health risks for personnel, can only be achieved by strict adherence to policies and procedures regarding the safe handling of cytotoxic drugs (Ferguson and Wright 2002, Polovich 2003, Polovich et al. 2009). Protective clothing should always be worn during all types of cytotoxic drug handling. There are minimum requirements for the type and degree of protective clothing which are based on possible exposure and type of environment.

Gloves

Disposable gloves should be worn at all times and appear to be the only type of protective clothing which most practitioners consistently wear when handling cytotoxic drugs. Polovich et al. (2009) state that 94–99% of nurses routinely wear gloves when handling hazardous materials. No type of glove is completely impermeable to every cytotoxic agent and there is no consensus as to which glove material offers the best protection (Gabriel 2008, Hayden and Goodman 2005, Weinstein and Plumer 2007). The key points to consider when selecting gloves are the main factors which affect permeation rates, including glove thickness, lipophilicity, the nature of the solvent in which the cytotoxic drug is dissolved and glove material composition (Ferguson and Wright 2002, Polovich et al. 2009). Using poor-quality low-cost gloves is neither safe nor cost-effective. The risk of allergic reactions to latex and powdered medical gloves has been well documented in recent years. The National Health Service Executive (NHSE) issued a Health Service Circular (HSC) (DH 1999) which recommended that healthcare organizations limit their use of these types of gloves. Powder-free gloves should be used for handling cytotoxic drugs and should be inspected for any defects before use. Gloves should be changed regularly (every 1 hour) during each work session or at the end of a work session and immediately if contaminated with cytotoxic agent or punctured (MARCH 2007, Polovich 2003, Polovich et al. 2009).

The use of gloves made of other material, such as nitrile, provides protection when dealing with a cytotoxic spill. Double gloving is recommended when reconstituting cytotoxic drugs (Polovich 2003, Polovich et al. 2009, Weinstein and Plumer 2007).

Gowns

The literature supports the use of a disposable gown for both reconstitution and administration (MARCH 2007). It has been suggested that a long-sleeved, non-absorbent gown made of a low-linting, low-permeability material such as Tyvek is used (Ferguson and Wright 2002, Weinstein and Plumer 2007). Armlets and plastic aprons can be used as a substitute for long-sleeved gowns during administration (HSE 2003, Polovich et al. 2009).

Goggles

Goggles are used to protect the eyes from splashes and particles; they should fully cover the eyes of the handler. Goggles should meet BS EN 166–8 requirements and be worn whenever reconstituting chemotherapy, where there is a possibility of splashing or dealing with a spill (Ferguson and Wright 2002).

Masks

These should be worn whenever there is a possibility of inhalation or the drug is being prepared in an uncontrolled environment. Masks should conform to BS EN 149:1992 standard. The key factor with regard to respiratory protective equipment is that it fits well and is sealed properly to the wearer's face. A range of different sizes of disposable masks should be made available to healthcare workers (Ferguson and Wright 2002). A suitable dust mask or particulate respirator, such as the 3M 8810, affords the best protection.

Waste disposal

Sharps should be placed in a sharps bin which is compliant with waste management regulations in order to ensure incineration and to prevent laceration and/or inoculation during transit and disposal (DH 2005). Dry waste, intravenous administration sets and other contaminated material should be placed in the appropriate waste disposal bags. The practitioner should wear gloves and an apron when disposing of contaminated waste (DH 2005, Polovich et al. 2009).

Spillage

Spillage is when cytotoxic drugs are accidentally splashed, spilt or leaked onto a surface, equipment or a person's skin or mucous membranes. Procedure guideline 15.1 should be followed when managing a spillage. Prevention is by careful connection of infusions using Luer-Lok equipment to reduce risk of disconnection and spiking infusion bags flat in a plastic tray (and never hanging).

Procedure guideline 15.1 Cytotoxic spillage management

Essential equipment

- Two plastic overshoes
- Two disposable armlets
- Two clinical waste bags
- Two pairs of disposable non-sterile vinyl or nitrile gloves
- Goggles (non-disposable): EN 166–8
- Particulate respirator mask

- Plastic apron
- Gown
- Paper towels
- Plastic bucket
- Copy of spillage procedure

Preprocedure

Action	Rationale
1 Act immediately. Assess the level of exposure of any individual and isolate them from the spill.	Any spillage may become a health hazard (Polovich *et al.* 2009, C).
2 Collect spillage kit.	It contains all necessary equipment (Polovich *et al.* 2009, C).
3 Put on both pairs of gloves, goggles and a gown and then a disposable plastic apron over the gown (see Action Figure 3).	To provide personal protection. E
■ If there is visible powder spill, put on a good-quality particulate respirator mask.	To prevent inhalation of powder. E
■ If spillage is on the floor, put on overshoes.	For protection and to minimize the spread of contamination. E

Procedure

4 Wipe up powder spillage quickly with well-dampened paper towels, starting at the outer edge of the spill area and working in a circular motion towards the middle to contain spill (Weinstein and Plumer 2007), and dispose of the towels as 'high-risk' waste.	To prevent dispersal of powder. To prevent spread of contamination to a wider area. To protect others and ensure safe disposal by incineration (DH 2005, C; Weinstein and Plumer 2007, E).
5 Mop up liquids which have been spilled on a hard surface with paper towels, starting at the outer edge of the spill area and working in a circular motion towards the middle to contain spill (Ferguson and Wright 2002), and dispose of the towels as 'high-risk' waste.	To prevent spread of contamination to a wider area. To protect others and ensure safe disposal by incineration (DH 2005, C).
6 Wash hard surfaces at least twice with copious amounts of cold, soapy water and dry with paper towels. The floor should then be given a routine clean as soon afterwards as possible. If spillage has occurred on a carpet, it will require cleaning as soon as possible.	To remove residual contamination. E
■ If spillage is on clothing, remove it as soon as possible and treat as 'soiled linen'.	To decontaminate clothing without hazard to laundry staff. E
■ If spillage has penetrated clothing, wash contaminated skin liberally with soap and cold water.	To decontaminate skin and prevent drug absorption. E
■ If spillage is on bedlinen, put on gloves and an apron, change it immediately and treat as 'soiled linen'.	To protect the patient and the laundry staff. E
■ If an accident or spillage involving direct skin contact occurs, the area should be washed thoroughly with soapy water as soon as possible. In the event of a cytotoxic splash to the eye, irrigate thoroughly with 0.9% sodium chloride or tap water for at least 15 minutes.	To decontaminate the area and minimize the risk of drug absorption and damage (Weinstein and Plumer 2007, E).

873

(Continued)

Procedure guideline 15.1 (*Continued*)

Postprocedure

7 Any accident or spillage by nursing staff involving direct skin contact with a cytotoxic drug must be reported to the occupational health department and manager as soon as possible after the first aid is performed and appropriate documentation completed (see Box 15.2).

To ensure that details of accidental contact are entered in the nurse's health record, and appropriate follow-up is initiated (Polovich *et al.* 2009, C).

Action Figure 3 Protective clothing for spillage kit.

Box 15.2 Cytotoxic health questionnaires

1 Annual 'cytotoxic health questionnaires' which cover:

  ■ detailed medical history of the individual
  ■ exposure record
  ■ personal protective equipment used
  ■ control measures in place.

2 Symptoms which may be attributed to the effects of harmful levels of cytotoxic drugs, for example headache, dizziness, eye or skin irritation.
3 Six-monthly blood tests are taken, which include full blood count, urea and electrolytes and liver function tests.
4 Six-monthly urinalysis is performed to detect raised protein, presence of glucose, blood and bilirubin and any abnormal cytology.
5 If any abnormalities are present, the individual is referred to the occupational health doctor.

Administration of cytotoxic medications by nurses

Legal and professional issues

The nurse is accountable to the public, employer, patient and the profession. The Nursing and Midwifery Council requires registrants to maintain and develop their knowledge and skill and to obtain help or supervision for any knowledge deficit (NMC 2008a). It is important that the nurse understands the legal responsibilities of administering chemotherapy. Cytotoxic drugs can be administered via a variety of routes but regardless of the route used, there are certain preadministration principles which the nurse should apply. The nurse should remember that the administration of medicines is a collaborative process which involves the nurse, doctor and pharmacist (NMC 2008b). Medicine administration is not solely a mechanistic task – it requires thought and exercising of professional judgement (NMC 2008a). Furthermore, the nurse must operate within the limit of their competence (NMC 2008a). Therefore, cytotoxic drugs should always be administered by a knowledgeable and skilled practitioner.

Competencies

Administering chemotherapy requires extensive knowledge and skill as well as practical experience. In order to provide consistently safe, appropriate and high-quality patient care, the nurse must be assessed as being competent to administer chemotherapy. The National Chemotherapy Advisory Group (NCAG) has recognized the need for chemotherapy to be administered and managed by knowledgeable chemotherapy-trained nurses to ensure quality and safety (NCAG 2009). Individual hospitals and organizations provide educational input along with practical experience in administration of chemotherapy. The NCAG has highlighted the need for high-quality, continual professional development in order to maximize and provide safe and effective care. It also recommends that the National Peer Review Team audits cancer services and that subsequently areas such as nurse chemotherapy competencies should be self-assessed on a yearly basis (NCAG 2009).

National standards for safe administration of chemotherapy have been developed by the Oncology Nursing Society (ONS) in America, the aim of which was to improve patient safety (Jacobson *et al.* 2009). The Royal College of Nursing has produced standards for infusion therapy and states that the nurse managing chemotherapy should have knowledge of and technical expertise in both administration and specific interventions associated with cytotoxic agents and have received education and training (RCN 2010). Standardizing education and practical guidelines for safe administration of chemotherapy reduce the risk of error. Having a comprehensive knowledge and skill base for administering chemotherapy also ensures that the nurse is fit for purpose (NMC 2008b).

Non-medical prescribing of chemotherapy has been developing over the years, with many organizations having nurse-led chemotherapy prescription clinics as part of normal practice. *The Cancer Reform Strategy* (DH 2007) advocated nurse-led chemotherapy services for cancer patients to improve the patient experience and reduce waiting times. Improving efficiency of services for patients was echoed in the NCAG (2009) report which identified the need to improve the patient care experience by ensuring quality and safety. Nurse-led interventions, such as nurse-chemotherapy prescribing, is recognized as enhancing the chemotherapy care pathway.

Consent

Patients have a fundamental and ethical right to determine what happens to their bodies, and consent is central to all aspects of healthcare delivery. When gaining valid consent, the nurse must be sure that the patient is a legally competent person, and gives consent voluntarily after being fully informed of what they are consenting to (NMC 2008c).

Written consent must be obtained before chemotherapy is commenced and every time the patient is changed from one protocol/regimen to another. The standard NHS consent form dictates the amount of information necessary in order to obtain valid consent. For example, if there is a possibility that the patient may require a blood transfusion then the patient and the doctor must sign to state that this has been discussed with the patient. Electronic scanning of consent forms into the patient's medical record is advocated and utilized in many organizations. However, if the organization is not paperless then one copy of the consent form is kept in the medical notes whilst the other is given to the patient (NMC 2008c).

Preprocedural considerations
Specific patient preparations
Provision of information

The provision of patient information is an integral part of the care pathway. The patient should be fully informed of all the possible side-effects of chemotherapy, how to cope with any side-effects at home, types of supportive therapy they may receive, as well as where and how they are to receive the drugs (NCAG 2009, NMC 2008b). Patients should then receive written information, which can be used to reinforce verbal explanation and will enable patients to spend time reading and formulating any questions about treatments (INS 2006, NMC 2008a, van der Molen 2005). The main aim of providing information is to help the patient and their family to gain control, reduce anxiety, improve compliance, develop realistic expectations, promote self-care, enhance participation, and generate feelings of safety and security (van der Molen 2005). The nurse should consider barriers to effective communication, for example hearing difficulties, sight difficulties, culture and language difficulties, and plan realistic interventions in respect of such barriers. Written information about side-effects of the treatment as well as healthcare professional contact numbers should be provided (DH 2007, NCAG 2009). A 24-hour contact number as well as advice on how to deal with emergencies should be included. Many organizations provide patients with chemotherapy alert cards that contain essential information for out-of-hours queries (NCAG 2009).

Ascertaining whether the patient is fit for treatment

There are criteria that have to be confirmed prior to administration of chemotherapy. For example, a full blood count, electrolyte and renal function blood results are essential in order to:

- ensure that the patient is fit enough to receive the treatment; if any of the blood results are too low, then supportive therapy may be prescribed
- calculate the dose of drug, for example in the case of platinum-based drugs, ethylenediaminetetra-acetic acid (EDTA), or if 24-hour urine collection for creatinine is required (Polovich *et al.* 2009).

Box 15.3 The five rights

Nurses should ensure that they have checked the five rights.

- The right patient.
- The right drug chemotherapy regimen (many chemotherapy prescriptions are computer generated to reduce the risk of error).
- The right dose.
- The right time.
- The right route of administration.

(Findlay et al. 2008, NMC 2008b).

Calculating body surface area

This is done by using the patient's height and weight and should be performed every time a cycle or dose of chemotherapy is given. The patient's height and weight should be recorded on the prescription chart, ideally by the person who performed the recording. The surface area is then determined, and this will be used to calculate the dose of chemotherapy drug.

Knowledge of the chemotherapy regimen

Prior to administering chemotherapy in the hospital setting, the NPSA guidance for safer practice should be adhered to, including the use of standardized patient wristbands which contain the core patient identifiers, all of which should be written in black pen (NPSA 2009). The patient's allergy status should be checked by the prescriber and checked again by the nurse prior to the administration of any drug (NMC 2007). Allergy status can be dynamic and therefore should be reconfirmed with the patient prior to any medication being given. The prescription should be signed by the medical practitioner and verified by a pharmacist. Electronic prescribing and the use of computer-generated prescriptions may reduce the risk of medication error. It is recommended that two Registered Nurses check chemotherapy prior to administration. Independent 'double checking' involves the first check of prescription and medication carried out by one nurse and the chart signed as 'first checker'. This can be carried out in the clinical room. The second check is carried out by the nurse who will be administering the chemotherapy, immediately prior to administration beside the patient and signed on completion of the administration (NMC 2008b). See Box 15.3.

Intravenous administration of cytotoxic drugs

Definition

This is the administration of cytotoxic drugs via a peripheral or central vein, which is the route most commonly used.

Evidence-based approaches
Rationale

Intravenous administration enables:

- rapid and reliable delivery of a cytotoxic drug to the tumour site
- rapid dilution of a drug which reduces local irritation and the risk of tissue damage
- accurate titration of drug to achieve desired effect.

Methods of administration

Cytotoxic drugs may be administered as a direct bolus injection (Figure 15.2), a bolus via the side arm of a rapid infusion of 0.9% sodium chloride or a continuous infusion. The choice is dependent on:

- the type of cytotoxic drug, for example etoposide is only given as an infusion
- pharmacological considerations, for example stability, need for dilution
- degree of venous irritation, for example vinorelbine is a highly irritant drug
- whether the drug is a vesicant
- the type of device *in situ* (Gabriel 2008).

The advantage of the bolus injection is that the integrity of the vein and any early signs of extravasation can be observed more easily than during an infusion. However, bolus injections can increase the risk of venous irritation due to the constant contact of the drug with the intima of the vein, resulting in pain, which makes it difficult to differentiate between venous spasm and extravasation (Gabriel 2008). It could also lead to inappropriate rapid administration of the drug (Weinstein and Plumer 2007).

Bolus injections administered via the side arm of a rapid infusion of solution ensure greater dilution of potentially

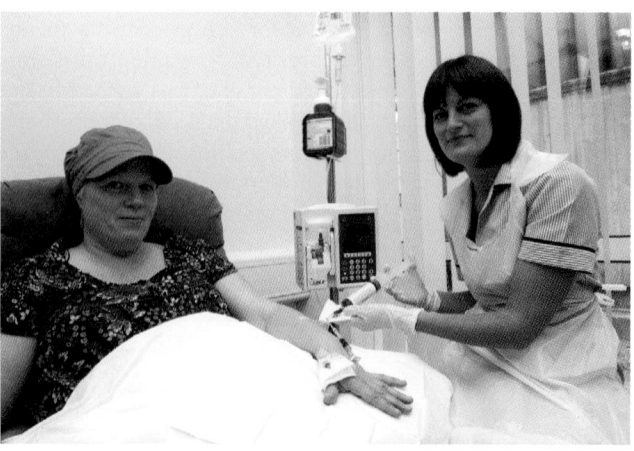

Figure 15.2 Chemotherapy bolus being administered.

Table 15.1 Arguments for using either a large- or small-gauge peripheral vascular access device

Larger	Smaller
Enables irritant drugs to reach general circulation quickly, without irritating peripheral veins	Less chance of puncturing the posterior vein wall
Administration time is decreased and therefore patient does not need to spend as much time in a stressful environment	Less likely to cause trauma and result in scar formation
	Less pain on needle insertion
	Increased blood flow around small needle increases dilution of drug and reduces risk of chemical phlebitis

irritating drugs and enable rapid removal of the drug from the insertion site and smaller vessels. The disadvantages are that a small vein may not allow rapid flow of the infusate and this may result in the drug backing up the tubing, causing the practitioner to clamp the tubing whilst checking for blood return and flow rate of the infusate, therefore interrupting constant observation of the site (Gabriel 2008).

Adding the drug to an infusion bag allows for greater dilution, thus reducing the possibility of chemical irritation. Some drugs may only be administered as infusions owing to the type of side-effects associated with them (e.g. hypotension with etoposide) and long-term continuous infusions, for example 5-fluorouracil (5-FU) may also be necessary to reduce the risk of side-effects such as diarrhoea. Patency and device position cannot be easily assessed and the longer the infusion, the greater the possibility of device dislodgement, extravasation or infiltration and general complications associated with the device (Weinstein and Plumer 2007).

Preprocedural considerations

Equipment

Cytotoxic drugs may be administered via a peripheral cannula or a central venous access device (CVAD). A peripheral cannula is used for bolus injections and short or intermittent infusions of both vesicant and non-vesicant drugs (Table 15.1). However, this device is associated with phlebitis and requires repeated resiting every 72–96 hours (Gabriel 2008, INS 2006, Scales 2005). A central venous catheter is useful for patients with poor venous access, those at high risk of extravasation and for those undergoing long-term, high-dose or continuous infusional chemotherapy (Gabriel 2008, Weinstein and Plumer 2007). These devices are associated with infection and thrombosis (Dougherty 2006a).

For the peripheral route, a cannula may be used. The insertion site of choice should be the large veins of the forearm (cephalic or basilic) as these are easier to access, reduce the risk of chemical phlebitis and result in fewer problems if extravasation should occur (Weinstein and Plumer 2007).

The next area of choice would be the dorsum of the hand, then the wrist. The antecubital fossa should only be used as the last resort as it can limit movement and is associated with problems if extravasation occurs in this area (Gabriel 2008, Weinstein and Plumer 2007). The general rule is to start distally and proceed proximally where possible and also to alternate the arms (Weinstein and Plumer 2007) to ensure that the same veins are not being used and damaged by chemical and mechanical irritation (Scales 2005).

When using the peripheral intravenous route, the following should be adhered to.

- Patency should be checked at the start of administration by achieving a blood return and then flushing with 10 mL of 0.9% sodium chloride to ensure there is no resistance, swelling or pain. Blood return should then be checked after every 2–4 mL of a bolus drug is administered (Gabriel 2008, Weinstein and Plumer 2007).
- The site should be assessed for signs of phlebitis.
- The site should be observed when a bolus injection is administered, particularly if a vesicant drug, for signs of infiltration or extravasation.
- Certain vesicants must not be administered as infusions into a peripheral vein as the risk of extravasation and damage is greater than via the central venous route (Weinstein and Plumer 2007).

In addition, where possible, a new site should be used for vesicants, to ensure the vein is healthy and patent, although this may not always be possible. There are some controversial issues related to peripheral intravenous cytotoxic drug administration (Table 15.2).

Central venous access devices have the advantage of providing a more reliable form of vascular access (Table 15.3). This is because the problems associated with peripheral devices, such as phlebitis, venous irritation and pain, are eliminated as central venous access enables rapid dilution and circulation of the drug. However, extravasation can still occur as a result of catheter tip malposition, catheter malfunction, a damaged catheter, port needle dislodgement or fibrin sheath formation along the length of the catheter, faulty equipment, human error and system problems (Dougherty 2006a, Mayo 1998).

Table 15.2 Controversial issues: use of antecubital fossa

For	Against
Larger veins permit rapid infusion of drug	Mobility is restricted
Larger veins allow irritant drugs to reach general circulation more quickly and with less irritation than small veins	Risk of extravasation is increased if patient tends to be mobile
Easier to palpate and therefore increases successful insertion of device	Early recognition of extravasation is difficult due to the deep veins. This means there is less chance of observing swelling which could go undetected. The patient may also have a delayed reaction to pain
	Damage can result in loss of structure and function, ulceration and fibrosis

Table 15.3 Types of central venous access devices

CVAD	Advantages	Disadvantages	Suggested for
PICC	■ Ease of insertion ■ Ease of removal ■ Ease of access ■ Small catheter gauge	■ Risk of infection and thrombosis ■ Self-care not possible ■ Needs specialist dressing whilst *in situ* ■ Restrictive to ADLs	Short-term (<6 cycles) intermittent IV therapy and slow-rate continuous infusion. for example FEC or continuous 5-FU
Implanted port	■ Low infection risk ■ Low obtrusiveness	■ Surgical insertion/GA ■ Specialist equipment and skills required ■ Surgical removal	Long-term intermittent IV therapy (>6 months), for example trastuzumab
Skin-tunnelled catheter	■ Low infection risk ■ Self-care possible ■ High flow rates	■ Risk of thrombosis ■ Large catheter gauge ■ Surgical removal ■ Restrictive to ADLs	Fluid-intensive and myelosuppressive therapy, for example leukaemic inductions

Procedure guideline 15.2 Cytotoxic therapy: intravenous administration of cytotoxic drugs

Essential equipment

■ Patient prescription chart
■ Patient information literature

Medicinal products

■ Medication(s)

Preprocedure

Action	Rationale
1 Explain and discuss the procedure with the patient. Evaluate the patient's knowledge of cytotoxic therapy. If this knowledge appears to be inadequate, offer an explanation of the use, action, dose and potential side-effects of the drug or drugs involved.	To ensure that the patient understands the procedure and gives their valid consent. The patient has a right to information (NMC 2008c; van der Molen 2005, C).

2 Put on gloves and an apron before commencing the procedure.	To protect the nurse from local contamination of skin or clothing (Polovich 2003, C; Polovich *et al.* 2009, C). *Note*: with careful handling technique, this risk is minimal but splashes can occur when changing syringes or infusion containers. Always change infusion bags over a deep plastic tray to contain any splashes.
3 Prepare necessary equipment for an aseptic administration procedure.	To minimize the risk of local and/or systemic infection (Fraise and Bradley 2009, E). Patients are frequently immunosuppressed and at greater risk of hospital-acquired infection (Weinstein and Plumer 2007, E).
4 Check that the prescription and medication have been first checked by another chemotherapy-competent nurse and then check that all details on the syringe or infusion container are correct when compared with the patient's prescription, before opening the sterile packaging.	To ensure the patient is given the correct drug which has been dispensed for them. To prevent wastage (NMC 2008b, C).
5 Be aware of the immediate effects of the drug.	To observe the patient during administration for any known side-effects. To be prepared to manage any side-effects that occur (NMC 2008b, C).
6 Take the medication and the prescription chart to the patient. Check the patient's identity, drug, dose, route and timing of administration.	To prevent error and comply with professional guidelines (NMC 2008a, C).

Procedure

7 Ensure that an appropriate device has been inserted. Inspect the device site, and consult the patient about sensation around the site.	To detect any problems, for example phlebitis, which would render the device unusable (Dougherty 2006a, E; Lavery and Ingram 2006, E).
8 Check the patency of the vein for blood return and then flush using 0.9% sodium chloride.	To determine whether the vein will accommodate the extra fluid flow and irritant drugs and remain patent (Weinstein and Plumer 2007, E).
9 Ensure the syringe is attached carefully to the needle-free injection site of the administration set, extension set or injection cap.	To prevent disconnection and possible contamination (MARCH 2007, C).
10 Secure a good connection by always using Luer-Lok syringes.	To prevent leakage or separation, which may occur due to pressure during administration, resulting in spray and contamination (MARCH 2007, C).
11 Take care when removing the blind hub, changing syringes, and inserting the administration set spike into the infusion container or changing bags (which must be done with the bag lying flat on a hard surface).	To avoid leakage or splashes and contamination of the nurse or patient. To prevent mis-spiking the bag and puncturing it (MARCH 2007, C).
12 Check the injection site or injection cap at the end of the procedure.	To ensure that there is no leakage (MARCH 2007, C).
13 Act promptly if any contamination of an individual is noted by washing the area with soap and water.	To prevent any local skin reaction (itchiness, redness or inflammation of the skin). To prevent absorption on skin, mucous membranes, and so on (Polovich 2003, C; Polovich *et al.* 2009, C).
14 Administer drugs in the correct order, antiemetics then cytotoxic drugs – that is, vesicants first.	To ensure that those agents likely to cause tissue damage are given when venous integrity is greatest, that is, at the beginning of the administration process (Gabriel 2008, E).

(Continued)

Procedure guideline 15.2 *(Continued)*

15 Ensure the correct administration rate.	To prevent 'speed shock'. To prevent extra pressure and irritation within the vein (Weinstein and Plumer 2007, E).
16 Observe the vein throughout for signs of infiltration or extravasation, for example swelling or leakage at the site of injection. Note the patient's comments about sensation at the site, for example pain.	To detect any problems at the earliest opportunity. To prevent any damage to soft tissue, and to enable the remainder of the drug(s) to be given correctly at another site. To enable prompt treatment to be given, thus minimizing local damage, and possibly preserving venous access for future treatment (Polovich *et al.* 2009). (For further information see Methods for preventing extravasation.)
17 Flush the device with 5–10 mL 0.9% sodium chloride between drugs and after administration.	To prevent drug interaction. To prevent leakage of drug from the puncture site, on removal of the device (Dougherty 2008, E).
18 Be aware of the patient's comfort throughout the procedure.	To minimize trauma to the patient. To involve the patient in treatment and detect any side-effects and/or problems that may then be avoided at the next treatment. E

Postprocedure

19 Record details of the administration in the appropriate documents.	To prevent any duplication of treatment and to provide a point of reference in the event of queries and adhere to professional guidelines (NMC 2009, C).

Complications

See Extravasation of vesicant drugs.

Extravasation of vesicant drugs

Definition

Extravasation literally means 'leaking into the tissues' but it has been linked with vesicants (or blistering agents) to describe a process that requires immediate action if local tissue damage is to be prevented (Polovich *et al.* 2009, Schulmeister 2009). A vesicant is any solution or medication that causes the formation of blisters with subsequent tissue necrosis and may be DNA and non-DNA binding (Hayden and Goodman 2005, Polovich *et al.* 2009).

Related theory

It is important to recognize an extravasation and distinguish it from an infiltration or flare reaction.

Infiltration tends to refer to the leakage of non-vesicant solutions/medications into the surrounding tissues and generally does not cause tissue necrosis but can result in long-term injury due to local inflammatory reactions or by compression of the surrounding tissues (if a large volume infiltrates) which is known as compartment syndrome (Doellman *et al.* 2009, RCN 2010, Schulmeister 2009). Irritants

are drugs capable of causing inflammation and irritation but if they infiltrate, they rarely cause any tissue breakdown (Ferguson and Wright 2002, Polovich *et al.* 2009, Stanley 2002).

Flare reaction is a local inflammatory reaction to an agent manifested by red tracking along the vein or red blotches but without pain (although the area may feel itchy) (Polovich *et al.* 2009). It occurs in 3–6% of patients (How and Brown 1998). It is caused by a venous inflammatory response to histamine release, is characterized by redness and blotchiness and may result in the formation of small wheals, having a similar appearance to a nettle rash. It usually subsides in 30–60 minutes, with 86% resolving within 45 minutes (Hayden and Goodman 2005, How and Brown 1998). Slowing infusion rates may be helpful but it responds well within a few minutes to the application of a topical steroid (Schulmeister 2009, Weinstein and Plumer 2007).

Tissue damage following extravasation of vesicant drugs occurs for a number of reasons.

- Whether the drugs bind to DNA or not:
  - DNA-binding vesicants (e.g. doxorubicin, epirubicin) bind to nucleic acids in the DNA of healthy cells, resulting in cell death. There is then cellular uptake of extracellular substances and this sets up a continuing cycle of tissue damage as the DNA-binding vesicant is retained and recirculated in the tissue, sometimes for a prolonged period of time (Goolsby and Lombardo 2006, Polovich *et al.* 2009, Schulmeister 2009).

– Non-DNA binding vesicants (e.g. paclitaxel, vinca alkaloids) have an indirect rather than a direct effect on the cells. They are eventually metabolized in the tissue and then neutralized (more easily than DNA-binding vesicants) (Polovich *et al.* 2009).

■ The concentration and amount of vesicant drug in the tissue.

■ The location of the extravasation, for example hand, arm.

■ Patient factors, for example older age, co-morbidities.

(Polovich *et al.* 2009, Schulmeister 2009)

Evidence-based approaches

Extravasation is a well-recognized complication of intravenous (IV) chemotherapy administration, but in general is a condition that is often underdiagnosed, undertreated and under-reported (Stanley 2002). The incidence of extravasation is estimated to be between 0.5% and 6.0% of all cytotoxic drug administrations (Goolsby and Lombardo 2006, Kassner 2000, Khan and Holmes 2002, Lawson 2003, Masoorli 2003), with some estimates for peripheral extravasation between 23% and 25% (Roth 2003). CVADs have decreased the incidence of extravasation but it can still occur and the incidence is estimated to be up to 6% with ports (Masoorli 2003). However, whilst the incidence is lower, the severity of the injuries is far greater as detection tends to occur later (Kassner 2000, Polovich *et al.* 2009, Stanley 2002). Even when practitioners have many years of experience, extravasation of vesicant agents can occur and is an extremely stressful event, but is not in itself an act of negligence (Weinstein and Plumer 2007). Early detection and treatment are crucial if the consequences of an untreated or poorly managed extravasation are to be avoided (Box 15.4, Figure 15.3). These may include:

■ blistering (typically occurs 1–2 weeks post extravasation)

■ peeling and sloughing of the skin (about 2 weeks post extravastion)

■ tissue necrosis (2–3 weeks post extravasation) with resulting pain

■ damage to tendons, nerves and joints

■ functional and sensory impairment of affected area such as limb

---

Box 15.4 Considerations for the prevention of extravasation

■ Monitoring the site.
■ Location of the device.
■ Patients at risk.
■ Sequence of drugs.
■ Types of devices.
■ Method of administration.
■ Skill of practitioner.
■ Informing the patient.

Figure 15.3   Extravasation.

■ disfigurement
■ loss of limb or breast.

(Polovich *et al.* 2009)

These can all result in possible hospitalization and plastic surgery, delay in the treatment of disease and psychological distress for the patient.

Before administration of vesicant cytotoxic drugs, the nurse should know which agents are capable of producing tissue necrosis (Table 15.4). If in any doubt, the drug data sheet should be consulted or reference made to a research trial protocol. Drugs should not be reconstituted to give solutions which are higher than the manufacturer's recommended concentration, and the method of administration should be checked, for example infusion, injection.

A variety of vesicant non-cytotoxic agents in frequent use are also capable of causing severe tissue damage if extravasated and damage is usually caused as a result of the

Table 15.4 Examples of vesicant cytotoxic drugs in common use

Group A drugs	Group B drugs
Vinca alkaloids:	Amsacrine
Vinblastine	Carmustine (concentrated solution)
Vindesine	Dacarbazine (concentrated solution)
Vinorelbine	Dactinomycin
Vincristine	Daunorubicin
Vinflunine	Doxorubicin
Paclitaxel	Epirubicin
	Idarubicin
	Amrubicin
	Actinomycin D
	Mitomycin C
	Mechlorethamine
	Streptozocin

Table 15.5 Examples of vesicant non-cytotoxic drugs in common use

Group A drugs	Group B drugs
Calcium chloride	Aciclovir
Calcium gluconate	Amphotericin
Phenytoin	Cefotaxime
Hypertonic solutions, for example sodium chloride >0.9%	Diazepam
	Ganciclovir
Sodium bicarbonate (>5%)	Mannitol
Glucose 50%	Potssium chloride (>40 mmol/L)
	Potassium phosphate
	Thiopental

Box 15.5 Patients at risk of extravasation

- Infants and young children.
- Elderly patients.
- Those who are unable to communicate, for example sedated, unconscious, confused, language issues.
- Those with chronic diseases, for example cancer, peripheral vascular disease, superior vena cava (SVC) syndrome, lymphoedema.
- Those on medications: anticoagulants, steroids.
- Those who have undergone repeated intravenous cannulation/venepuncture.
- Those with fragile veins or who are thrombocytopenic.

(Hayden and Goodman 2005, Polovich *et al.* 2009, Sauerland *et al.* 2006)

pH, osmolarity or vasoconstrictive nature of the drugs. This potential hazard should always be remembered (Table 15.5). The actions listed in this procedure may not be appropriate in all these instances. Drug data sheets should always be checked and the pharmacy department should be consulted if the information is insufficient, regarding action to take if a vesicant drug extravasates. Consideration should be given to the management of mixed vesicant drug extravasation in terms of which drug to treat with which antidote. For example, if drug A and drug B were in the same infusion and they required different antidotes but if drug A would cause more damage than drug B, the correct action would be to use antidote for drug A (How and Brown 1998).

Possible causes of extravasation are shown in Table 15.6.

Methods for preventing extravasation

The nurse's focus should be on safe intravenous technique and implementing strategies to minimize risk (Weinstein and Plumer 2007). This includes the following strategies.

Patients at risk

Patients who are at increased risk of extravasation (Box 15.5) should be observed more closely and cared for with extra caution.

Types of devices

The use of steel needles is associated with a greater risk of extravasation and should be discouraged and a plastic cannula should be used instead (Sauerland *et al.* 2006, Schrijvers 2003, Polovich *et al.* 2009). Vesicants should be given via a newly established cannula wherever possible (Dougherty 2005, Goolsby and Lombardo 2006) and consideration should be given to changing the cannula site after 24 hours (Hayden and Goodman 2005). However, if the fluid runs freely, there is good blood return and there are no signs of erythema, pain or swelling at the site, there is no reason to inflict a second cannulation on the patient (Weinstein and Plumer 2007). Consideration should be given to a CVAD if peripheral access is difficult and a decision-making tool can assist with this.

Location of the device

The most appropriate site for the location of a peripheral cannula is considered to be the forearm (Schrijvers 2003, Weinstein and Plumer 2007). However, a large straight vein over the dorsum of the hand is preferable to a smaller vein in the forearm (Weinstein and Plumer 2007). Siting over joints

Table 15.6 Possible causes of extravasation

Peripheral devices	Central venous access devices
Vein wall puncture or trauma	Perforation of the vein
Dislodgement of the cannula from the vein	Catheter leakage, rupture or fracture
Administration of a vesicant in a vein below a recent venepuncture or cannulation site (<24 hours)	Separation of the catheter from the portal body of an implanted port
	Incomplete insertion of needle into an implanted port
	Needle dislodgement from an implanted port
	Fibrin sheath – leading to backflow of drug along the catheter from the insertion site

Mayo (1998), Polovich *et al.* (2009), Schulmeister (1998).

should be avoided as tissue damage in this area may limit joint movement in the future. It is also recommended that the antecubital fossa should never be used for the administration of vesicants because of the risk of damage to local structures such as nerves and tendons (Gabriel 2008, Hayden and Goodman 2005, Weinstein and Plumer 2007). Avoid venepuncture sites in limbs with impaired circulation, sclerosis, thrombosis or scar formation. Also avoid cannulation below a recent venepuncture site (Goolsby and Lombardo 2006).

Sequence of drugs

Vesicants should be given first (Table 15.7) (Goolsby and Lombardo 2006, Kassner 2000, Hayden and Goodman 2005). Reasons for this include the following.

- Vascular integrity decreases over time.
- Vein is most stable and least irritated at start of treatment.
- Initial assessment of vein patency is most accurate.
- Patient's awareness of changes more acute (Weinstein and Plumer 2007).

Methods of administration

Many vesicants must be given as a slow bolus injection, often via the side arm of a fast-running intravenous infusion of a compatible solution, for example doxorubicin or epirubicin via an infusion of 0.9% sodium chloride. If repeated infusions are to be given then a CVAD may be more appropriate (Stanley 2002, Weinstein and Plumer 2007).

Monitoring the site and early recognition of extravasation

Confirming venous patency by flushing with 0.9% sodium chloride solution with at least 5–10 mL prior to administration of vesicants and frequent monitoring thereafter (Goolsby and Lombardo 2006, Weinstein and Plumer 2007). Checking blood return after every 2–5 mL is recommended but cannot be relied upon as the key sign when giving a bolus

Table 15.7 Drug sequencing – rationale for administering vesicant drugs first or last

Vesicants first	Vesicants last
Vascular integrity decreases over time	Vesicants are irritating and increase vein fragility
Vein is most stable and least irritated at start of treatment	Venous spasm may occur and mask signs of extravasation
Initial assessment of vein patency is most accurate	
Patient's awareness of changes more acute	

Stanley (2002), Weinstein and Plumer (2007).

injection, and monitoring the site every 5–10 minutes for any swelling (Weinstein and Plumer 2007). It is important that the nurse can recognize an extravasation quickly and distinguish it from other local reactions such as flare reaction (Dougherty 2008) (see Table 15.8 and Box 15.6).

Legal and professional issues
Competencies

Nurses are now being named in malpractice allegations, and extravasation injuries are an area for concern (Dougherty 2003, Masoorli 2003, Roth 2003, Weinstein and Plumer 2007). Therefore it is vital that nurses have the correct level of knowledge and skills in order to perform the following:

- correct choice of device and location
- the ability to use the most appropriate vasodilation techniques
- early recognition of extravasation and ability to take prompt action.
  (Dougherty 2008, Goolsby and Lombardo 2006, Sauerland *et al.* 2006, Schrijvers 2003)

Successful cannulation at the first attempt is ideal, as vesicants have been known to seep into tissues at a vein entry site of a previous cannulation (Gault and Challands 1997). This also includes accessing a port as it is vital that the correct selection of needle is made and that the device is secured adequately (Camp-Sorrell 2005).

Consent

Patients should be informed of the potential problems of administering vesicants and the possible consequences of extravasation (Polovich *et al.* 2009, Sauerland *et al.* 2006, Stanley 2002, Weinstein and Plumer 2007). Adequate information given to patients will ensure early recognition and cooperation as patients are the first to notice pain. The patient should be urged to report immediately any change in sensation such as burning or stinging (Goolsby and Lombardo 2006).

Preprocedural considerations
Equipment
Extravasation kits

The use of extravasation kits has been recommended in order to provide immediate management (Hayden and Goodman 2005, Khan and Holmes 2002). Kits should be assembled according to the particular needs of individual institutions. They should be kept in all areas where staff are regularly administering vesicant drugs, so that staff have immediate access to equipment (Gabriel 2008). The kit should be simple, to avoid confusion, but comprehensive enough to meet all reasonable needs (Stanley 2002) (see Procedure guideline 15.3). Instructions should be clear and easy to follow, and the use

Table 15.8 Nursing assessment of extravasation

Assessment parameter	Flare reaction	Venous irritation	Immediate manifestations, i.e. during drug administration	Delayed manifestations, i.e. from 24 hours after extravasation
Pain	None	Aching, throbbing sensation along vein and in the limb	Severe stinging or burning pain (not always present). This can last from minutes to hours and will eventually subside. Occurs during drug administration at the device site and surrounding areas	Can continue following extravasation or start within 48 hours. Pain may intensify over time
Redness	Immediate blotches or tracking along the vein. This will subside within 30–45 minutes with or without treatment (usually steroid cream)	Vein may become red or darkened	Not always present immediately: more likely to see blanching of the skin. As area becomes inflamed, redness will appear around the device site	Later occurrence
Swelling	Unlikely	Unlikely	May occur immediately but may not always be easy to identify immediately	Usually within 48 hours
Blood return	Usually present	Usually present but may require application of heat to improve blood return	Inability to obtain blood return (peripheral or central) but blood return may be present throughout	
Ulceration	Unlikely	Unlikely	Unlikely	Can occur within 48–96 hours but may take 3–4 weeks to develop
Others	Urticaria	None	Change in quality of the infusion or pressure on the syringe	Local tingling and sensory deficits

---

Box 15.6 Signs of extravasation

- The patient complains of burning, stinging pain or any other acute change at the injection site, although this is not always present (Hayden and Goodman 2005, Polovich *et al.* 2009). This should be distinguished from a feeling of cold, which may occur with some drugs, or venous spasm which can be caused by irritation usually accompanied by pain described as an achiness or tightness (Hayden and Goodman 2005). Any change of sensation warrants further investigation (Goolsby and Lombardo 2006).
- Swelling is a common symptom (Polovich *et al.* 2009). Induration or leakage may also occur at the injection site. Swelling may not always be immediately obvious if the patient has the cannula sited in an area of deep subcutaneous fat, in a deep vein or if the leak is via the posterior vein wall (Dougherty 2005).
- Blanching of the skin occurs (Comerford *et al.* 2002). Erythema can occur around the injection site but this is not usually present immediately (Hayden and Goodman 2005). It is important that this is distinguished from a flare reaction (Polovich *et al.* 2009).

- Blood return is one of the most misleading of all signs particularly related to peripheral devices. In peripheral devices, if blood return is sluggish or absent, this may indicate lack of patency or incorrect position of the device. However, if no other signs are apparent, this should not be regarded as an indication of a non-patent vein, as a vein may not bleed back for a number of reasons and extravasation may occur even in the event of good blood return as the device may still be in the vein but the leak may be in the posterior vein wall (Hayden and Goodman 2005). Any change in blood flow should be investigated (Hayden and Goodman 2005, Weinstein and Plumer 2007). In CVADs there should always be blood return and if this is absent, steps should be followed to verify correct tip and needle position or resolve a fibrin sheath (see Figure 15.4).
- A resistance is felt on the plunger of the syringe if drugs are given by bolus (Stanley 2002).
- There is absence of free flow when administration is by infusion, once other reasons have been excluded, for example position (Polovich *et al.* 2009, Stanley 2002).
- Leaking around the IV cannula or implanted port needle (Polovich *et al.* 2009).

Note: one or more of the above may be present. If extravasation is suspected or confirmed, the injection or infusion must be stopped immediately and action must be taken (INS 2006, Polovich *et al.* 2009, Weinstein and Plumer 2007).

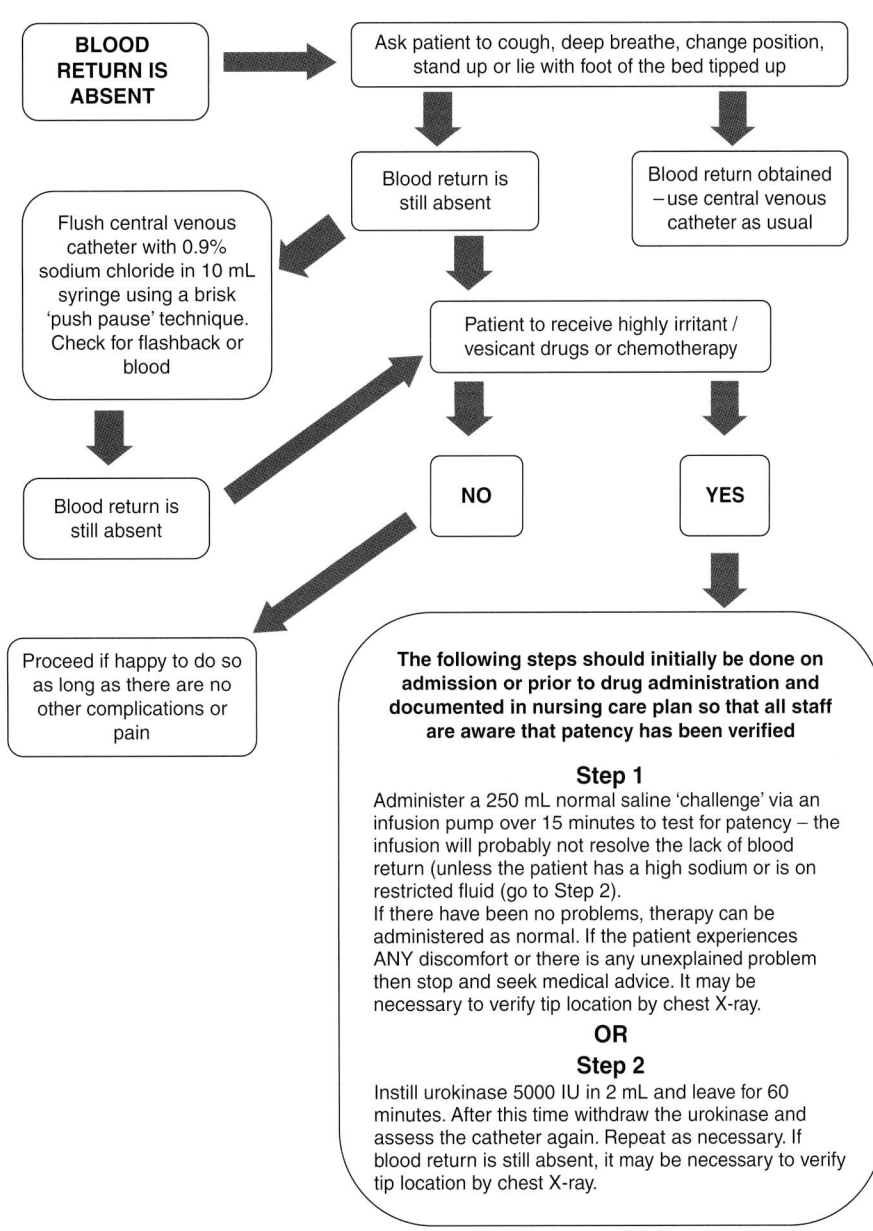

Figure 15.4 Persistent withdrawal occlusion flowchart.

of a flowchart enables staff to follow the management procedure in easy steps (Figure 15.5).

Assessment and recording tools

Decision-making tools have been developed both nationally and locally to address issues related to venous access related to administration of chemotherapy. See Figure 15.6 for an example.

Pharmacological support

A number of 'antidotes' are available but, again, there is a lack of scientific evidence to demonstrate their value and so the role of antidotes is still not clear (Polovich *et al.* 2009). There appear to be two main methods: (i) localize and neutral-

ize (using hyaluronidase) (CP Pharmaceuticals 1999); and (ii) spread and dilute (using an antidote) (Stanley 2002). Administration of injectable antidotes if not via the cannula is by the pincushion technique; that is, instilling small volumes around and over the areas affected using a small-gauge (25) needle towards the centre of a clock face. The procedure causes considerable discomfort to patients and if large areas are to be tackled, analgesia should be considered (Stanley 2002).

Hyaluronidase

This is an enzyme which breaks down hyaluronic acid, a normal component of tissue 'cement', and helps to reduce or prevent tissue damage by allowing rapid (within 10 minutes)

Suspect an extravasation if:

1 Patient complains of burning or stinging pain *or*
2 There is evidence of swelling, induration, leakage at the site *or*
3 There is resistance on plunger of syringe or absence of free flow of infusion *or*
4 There is no blood return (if found in isolation, this should not be regarded as an indication of a non-patent vein)

Stop the injection/infusion
Withdraw as much of the drug as possible
Remove the cannula
Collect the extravasation pack
Consider performing the flush out technique

Group A drugs

Inject 1500 IU hyaluronidase subcutaneously around site.
Apply warm pack to aid absorption of hyaluronidase.
Warm pack to remain in situ for 2–4 hours.

Group B drugs

Apply cold pack to cause vasoconstriction.
Apply cold packs for 15–20 minutes, 3–4 times for at least 24 hours.
However if extravasation is with any of the following category B drugs: mitomycin C; doxorubicin; idarubicin; epirubicin; actinomycin D then:

- draw around area of extravasation with indelible pen
- put on gloves
- apply thin layer of DMSO topically to the marked area using the small plastic spatula in lid of the bottle
- allow it to dry
- apply gauze
- this should be applied within 10–25 minutes.

Consider the administration of dexrazoxane

Elevate the limb

Apply hydrocortisone cream to reduce local inflammation (twice daily)

Where appropriate, apply DMSO every 2 hours on day 1 and then every 6 hours for up to 7 days

Inform medical staff

Document in duplicate – one copy in patient's notes and one to nurse consultant IV therapy and complete a clinical incident form

Give patient a patient information sheet

Figure 15.5 Treatment of extravasation.

diffusion of the extravasated fluid and restoration of tissue permeability within 24–48 hours (Doellman *et al.* 2009, Few 1987). The usual dose is 1500 IU (Bertelli 1995). It should be injected within 1 hour of extravasation, ideally through the intravenous device delivering the enzyme to the same tissue (Gault and Challands 1997, Stanley 2002, Weinstein and Plumer 2007).

Note: Hyaluronidase increases the absorption of local anaesthetic. Therefore, if local anaesthetic has been applied to the area, for example Ametop gel prior to cannulation, within 6 hours of extravasation, then the patient should be monitored for signs and symptoms of systemic anaesthesia such as increased pulse rate and decreased respirations and the doctor informed immediately (BNF 2011).

Corticosteroids

These have long been advocated as a treatment for anthracycline extravasation in reducing inflammatory components, although inflammation is not a prominent feature of tissue necrosis (Camp-Sorrell 1998) and they appear to have little benefit. Data now discourage the use of locally injected steroids, as there is little evidence to support their use (Bertelli 1995, Gault and Challands 1997, Wickham *et al.* 2006). However, given as a cream, they can help to reduce local trauma and irritation (Stanley 2002).

Dimethylsulphoxide (DMSO)

This is a topically applied solvent that may improve systematic absorption of vesicants. It acts as a potent free radical scavenger that rapidly penetrates tissues and prevents DNA damage (Bertelli 1995, Doellman *et al.* 2009). Reports on the clinical use of topical DMSO show it is effective and well tolerated in extravasation (Bertelli 1995). However, this is based on a high dose (99%) and only 50% is easily available in the UK (Stanley 2002). Side-effects from DMSO include itching, erythema, mild burning and a characteristic breath odour (Bertelli 1995).

Dexrazoxane (Savene)

A topoisomerase II catalytic inhibitor, used clinically to minimize the cardiotoxicity of doxorubicin, has been tested in animal models (Langer *et al.* 2006) and a small number of patients for its use in extravasation. It is given IV as soon as possible after the extravasation and it appears to reduce the wound size and duration of tissue damage with anthracyclines. The triple dosage appears to be more effective than a single dose (El-Saghir *et al.* 2004, Langer *et al.* 2000). In two multicentre studies, it was shown that the administration of Savene reduced the need for surgical interventions, and late sequelae such as pain, fibrosis, atrophy and sensory disturbance were judged as mild (Mouridsen *et al.* 2007).

A consensus group (Jackson 2006) developed recommendations for the use of dexrazoxane and these have been further adapted by the European Oncology Nursing Society

Any drug to be delivered by a continuous ambulatory drug delivery system or TPN must be administered via central venous access.

Patient Identification label		Date	
	Regimen		
	Planned length of treatment		

Vein assessment	Yes	No	
Absence of larger palpable veins			Does the patient have accessible peripheral veins of sufficient quality suitable to provide the required level of venous access? Does your team have the necessary skill level to establish peripheral venous access for the patient at every visit?
Extensive oedema / adipose tissue over forearms			
Inadequate venous fill of target veins			
Significant vein wall rigidity			
Significant cellulitis of forearm and/or upper arms			

Vein availability	Yes	No	
Axillary lymph node clearance			Will the patient have accessible peripheral veins available for the proposed term of treatment? (accounting for vein rotation and deterioration)
Upper limb/axilla/SVC venous thrombosis			
Extensive skin lesions - forearms			
Previous CVA			
Thrombo-phlebitis present			

VAD insertion & patency factors	Yes	No	
Fragile skin quality			Is there an increased risk of cannula dislodgement, haematoma formation or thrombo-phlebitis for the patient with peripheral venous access? Is there an increased risk of infection for this patient? e.g. long-term steroid therapy
Decreased platelets < 50 x 10^9/L			
Anticoagulant therapy i.e warfarin, aspirin, LMW heparin			
Anxiety / Needle phobia			

Factors affecting long-term venous access patency	Yes	No	
Vesicant and/or irritant therapy for > 6 cycles			Will the patient be receiving therapy where intensive fluid management will be required? (such as concentrated electrolytes) Is there an increased risk of vein deterioration and thrombo-phlebitis in the patient? Would a skin tunnelled catheter or implanted port offer a lower risk of site infection for the patient?
Anticipated intensive IV therapy, i.e. blood products, electrolyte support, fluid support, multiple antimicrobial therapy			
Expected periods of sustained neutropenia (<0.5 x 10^9/L for > 7 days)			

Co-morbidities that may affect peripheral venous access	Yes	No	
Diabetes			The effects of co-morbidities individual to the patient must be accounted when undertaking a venous access assessment. Would the patient be able to cope with the presence of a CVAD and notify the team appropriately to report adverse events?
Peripheral vascular disease			
Raynaud's phenomenon			
Hypotension			
Other (please state):			
Other (please state):			

887

Practitioner recommended venous access device:	
Comments:	

Patient & practitioner agreed venous access device:	
Comments:	

Figure 15.6 Decision-making tool for vascular access device (Flynn *et al.* 2010).

Figure 15.6 *(Continued)*

(European Oncology Nursing Society 2007) which now recommends the following.

- For anthracycline extravasations resulting from peripheral administration, the site expert or team should be consulted in order to determine whether the use of dexrazoxane is indicated.
- Absolute indications are if the peripherally extravasated volume exceeds 5 mL and in the event of a central venous access device extravasation (Langer 2008).

Granulocyte macrophage-colony stimulating factor

Finally, granulocyte macrophage-colony stimulating factor (GM-CSF) is a growth factor and has been found effective in accelerating wound healing and inducing formation of granulation tissue (El-Saghir *et al.* 2004, Ulutin *et al.* 2000).

Non-pharmacological support
Stopping infusion/injection and aspirating the drug

It appears that most authors are agreed that aspirating as much of the drug as possible, as soon as extravasation is suspected, is beneficial (Polovich *et al.* 2009, Rudolph and Larson 1987, Weinstein and Plumer 2007) and can help lower the concentration of the drug in the area (Goolsby and Lombardo 2006). However, withdrawal is only immediately possible during bolus injections, as an infusion would need to be stopped and a syringe attached in an attempt to aspirate. Aspiration may be successful if extravasation presents as a raised blister, but may be unsuccessful if tissue is soft and soggy (CP Pharmaceuticals 1999, Stanley 2002). It may help to reduce the size of the lesion. In practice, it may achieve little and often distresses the patient (Gault and Challands 1997). The likelihood of withdrawing blood (as suggested by Ignoffo and Friedman (1980) is small and the practitioner may waste valuable time attempting this which could lead to delay in the rest of the management procedure.

Removing the device

Some clinicians advocate that the peripheral vascular access device be left *in situ* in order to instil the antidote via the device and into the affected tissues (Kassner 2000, Stanley 2002, Weinstein and Plumer 2007). However, others recommend that the peripheral device should be removed to prevent any injected solution increasing the size of the affected area (CP Pharmaceuticals 1999, Rudolph and Larson 1987). There appears to be no research evidence to support either practice.

Application of hot or cold packs

Cooling appears to be a better choice, with the exception of the vinca alkaloids and some non-cytotoxic drugs, than warming (Bertelli 1995, CP Pharmaceuticals 1999). Cold causes vasoconstriction, localizing the extravasation and perhaps allowing time for local vascular and lymphatic systems to contain the drug. It should be applied for 15–20 minutes, 3–4 times a day for up to 3 days (CP Pharmaceuticals 1999, Gault and Challands 1997, Polovich *et al.* 2009). Heat promotes healing after the first 24 hours by increasing the blood supply (Polovich *et al.* 2009, Weinstein and Plumer 2007). It also decreases local drug concentration, increasing the blood flow which results in enhanced resolution of pain and reabsorption of local swelling.

Elevation of limb

This is recommended as it minimizes swelling (Rudolph and Larson 1987) and movement should be encouraged to prevent adhesion of damaged areas to underlying tissue (Gabriel 2008). This can be achieved by use of a Bradford sling but this is usually recommended when the extravasation has occurred in the hand.

Surgical techniques

It is now recognized that a plastic surgery consultation should be performed as part of the management procedure in order to remove the tissue containing the drug. Surgical intervention is recommended, especially if the lesion is greater than 2 cm, there is significant residual pain 1–2 weeks after extravasation, or there is minimal healing 2–3 weeks after injury despite local therapeutic measures (Goolsby and Lombardo 2006). A liposuction cannula can be used to aspirate extravasated material and subcutaneous fat or the use of a flush-out technique can remove extravasated drug without resorting to excision and skin grafting.

Flush-out technique

If there is little subcutaneous fat, then the saline flush-out technique is recommended, particularly if done within the first 24 hours (Gault 1993). It has been suggested as a less traumatic and cheaper procedure than surgery. Only appropriately trained doctors or nurses may perform the flush-out technique for superficial peripheral extravasations where there is no visible skin damage or extensive swelling. A number of small stab incisions are made and large volumes of 0.9% sodium chloride are administered which flush out the extravasated drug (Gault and Challands 1997); this is more successful if performed within 24 hours of extravasation (see Procedure guideline 15.4).

Procedure guideline 15.3 **Extravasation management: peripheral cannula**

The procedure detailed was drawn up with the assistance of pharmacist and medical colleagues. It relates specifically to the management of extravasation of a drug from a peripheral cannula.

889

Essential equipment

- Gel packs × 2 : one to be kept in the fridge and one available for heating
  (an electric heating blanket can be used whilst pack is heating)
- 2 mL syringe × 1
- 25 G needles × 2
- Alcohol swabs
- Documentation forms
- Copy of extravasation management procedure
- Patient information leaflet

Medicinal products

- Hyaluronidase 1500 IU/2 mL sterile water
- Hydrocortisone cream 1% 15 g tube × 1
- Savene (dexrazoxane) (optional)

(Continued)

Procedure guideline 15.3 *(Continued)*

Preprocedure

Action	Rationale
1 Explain and discuss the procedure with the patient.	To ensure that the patient understands the procedure and gives their valid consent (NMC 2008c, C).

Procedure

Action	Rationale
2 Stop injection or infusion *immediately,* leaving the cannula in place.	To minimize local injury. To allow aspiration of the drug to be attempted (Polovich *et al.* 2009, C; RCN 2010, C).
3 Aspirate any residual drug from the device and suspected extravasation site.	To minimize local injury by removing as much drug as possible but only attempt if appropriate. Subsequent damage is related to the volume of the extravasation, in addition to other factors (Polovich *et al.* 2009, C; RCN 2010, C).
4 Remove the cannula.	To prevent the device from being used for antidote administration (Rudolph and Larson 1987, E).
5 Consider contacting the extravasation team and whether the flush-out technique would be appropriate (see Figure 15.6).	Flush-out is most effective if undertaken as soon as extravasation is suspected (Gault 1993, E).
6 Collect the extravasation pack and take it to the patient.	It contains all the equipment necessary for managing extravasation (Dougherty 2005, E; Stanley 2002, E).
7 **Either:** *For Group A drugs:* ■ Draw up hyaluronidase 1500 IU in 1 mL water for injection and inject volumes of 0.1–0.2 mL subcutaneously at points of the compass around the circumference of the area of extravasation. ■ Apply warm pack. **Or:** *For Group B drugs (except those listed below):* ■ Apply cold pack or ice instantly. **Or:** If extravasation is with any of the following category B drugs: mitomycin C; doxorubicin; idarubicin; epirubicin; actinomycin D; then: ■ Draw around area of extravasation with indelible pen. ■ Put on gloves.	This is the recommended agent for group A drugs. The warm pack speeds up absorption of the drug by the tissues (Bertelli 1995, E). To localize the area of extravasation, slow cell metabolism and decrease the area of tissue destruction. To reduce local pain (Polovich *et al.* 2009, C). This is the recommended agent for these anthracyclines and helps to reduce local tissue damage (Bertelli 1995, C).
■ Apply thin layer of DMSO topically to the marked area using the small plastic spatula in lid of the bottle. ■ Allow it to dry. ■ Apply gauze. ■ This should be applied within 10–25 minutes. **Or:** If extravasation of doxorubicin, epirubicin, idarubicin or daunarubicin occurs (i.e. 5 mL or more peripherally or any volume a central venous access device) then stop cold pack, do not apply DMSO and contact member of extravasation team to advise on use of dexrazoxane.	Cooling and DMSO interfere with the efficacy of dexrazoxane and it should be administered as soon as possible after extravasation (El Saghir *et al.* 2004, Langer *et al.* 2000).

8 Where possible, elevate the extremity and/or encourage movement.	To minimize swelling and to prevent adhesion of damaged area to underlying tissue, which could result in restriction of movement (Rudolph and Larson 1987, E).

Postprocedure

9 Inform a member of the medical staff at the earliest opportunity and administer any other prescribed antidotes, for example dexrazoxane.	To enable actions differing from agreed policy to be taken if considered in the best interests of the patient. To notify the doctor of the need to prescribe any other drugs. E
10 Apply hydrocortisone cream 1% twice daily, and instruct the patient how to do this. Continue as long as erythema persists.	To reduce local inflammation and promote patient comfort (Stanley 2002, E).
11 Where appropriate, apply DMSO every 2 hours on day 1 and then every 6 hours for up to 7 days (patients will need to have this prescribed as a to take out (TTO) and continue treatment at home where necessary).	To help reduce local tissue damage (Bertelli 1995, E).
12 Heat packs (group A drugs) should be reapplied after initial management for 2–4 hours. Cold packs (group B drugs) should be applied for 15–20 minutes, 3–4 times a day for up to 3 days.	To localize the steroid effect in the area of extravasation. To reduce local pain and promote patient comfort (Bertelli 1995, E).
13 Provide analgesia as required.	To promote patient comfort. To encourage movement of the limb as advised. E
14 Document the following details, in duplicate, on the form provided. (a) Patient's name/number. (b) Ward/unit. (c) Date, time. (d) Signs and symptoms. (e) Cannulation site (on diagram). (f) Drug sequence. (g) Drug administration technique, that is, 'bolus' or infusion. (h) Approximate amount of the drug extravasated. (i) Diameter, length and width of extravasation area. (j) Appearance of the area. (k) Step-by-step management with date and time of each step performed and medical officer notification. (l) Patient's complaints, comments, statements. (m) Indication that patient's information sheet has been given to patient. (n) Follow-up section. (o) Whether photograph was taken. (p) If required, when patient referred to plastic surgeon. (q) Signature of the nurse.	To provide an immediate full record of all details of the incident, which may be referred to if necessary. To provide a baseline for future observation and monitoring of patient's condition. To comply with NMC guidelines (NMC 2009, C; RCN 2010, C; Schulmeister 2009, E; Weinstein and Plumer 2007, E).
15 Explain to the patient that the site may remain sore for several days.	To reduce anxiety and ensure continued co-operation. P, E
16 Observe the area regularly for erythema, induration, blistering or necrosis. *Inpatients*: monitor daily. Where appropriate, take photograph.	To detect any changes at the earliest possible moment (RCN 2010, C).

891

(Continued)

Procedure guideline 15.3 (*Continued*)

17 All patients should receive written information explaining what has occurred, what management has been carried out, what they need to look for at the site and when to report any changes. For example, increased discomfort, peeling or blistering of the skin should be reported immediately.	To detect any changes as early as possible, and allow for a review of future management. This may include referral to a plastic surgeon (Gault and Challands 1997, E; Polovich *et al.* 2009, C; RCN 2010, C).
18 If blistering or tissue breakdown occurs, begin dressing techniques and seek advice regarding wound management.	To minimize the risk of a superimposed infection and sterile increase healing (Naylor 2005, E).
19 Depending on size of lesion, degree of pain, type of drug, refer to plastic surgeon.	To prevent further pain or other complications as chemically induced ulcers rarely heal spontaneously (Dougherty 2005, E; Polovich et al. 2009, C).

Procedure guideline 15.4 Extravasation: performing flush-out following an extravasation

This procedure would commence once the immediate management of extravasation had been performed; that is, stop infusion/injection, aspirate any drug if possible, apply appropriate pack and elevate limb.

Essential equipment

- Eye protection
- Disposable gown
- 20 mL Luer-Lok syringe × 1
- 10 mL Luer-Lok syringe × 1
- 5 mL Luer-Lok syringe × 1
- 25 G needle × 1
- 23 G needle × 3
- Disposable scalpel (size 11)
- Bandage
- Sterile pack (containing gauze, drapes/towels and gallipot)

- Sterile gloves
- Cleaning solution (2% chlorhexidine Chloraprep 3 mL)
- Blunt needle/18 G or 20 G cannula × 4
- Three-way tap with extension set
- Blank labels for syringes
- Solution administration set
- Sterile marker pen
- Plastic-backed towel (e.g. incontinence pad)

Medicinal products

- Lidocaine 1% 10 mL (kept at room temperature)
- Hyaluronidase 1500 IU and 2 mL water for injection
- Mepitel dressing
- 500 mL 0.9% sodium chloride infusion bag
- Bactericidal alcohol handrub
- Bactericidal soap

Preprocedure

Action	Rationale
1 Explain the procedure and reason for performing it to the patient and gain written consent using pre-prepared consent form.	To ensure that the patient understands the procedure and gives their valid consent (NMC 2008c, C).
2 Ascertain what emergency treatment has been carried out, for example was hyaluronidase administered?	To ensure that only required treatment is carried out; for example, if hyaluronidase has been given, no further dose would be administered as this could result in a sensitivity reaction. E
3 Assemble all the equipment necessary for the procedure.	To ensure that time is not wasted and the procedure goes smoothly without any unnecessary interruptions. E

4	Check all packaging before opening and preparing the equipment to be used.	To maintain asepsis throughout and check that no equipment is damaged or out of date (Fraise and Bradley 2009, E).
5	Carefully wash hands using bactericidal soap and water or bactericidal alcohol handrub before commencement and dry.	To minimize the risk of infection (DH 2007, C).
6	Place the patient's arm on the plastic-backed towel.	To prevent leakage of the flushed-out solution and possible contamination of the area with cytotoxic drugs. E
7	Apply disposable gown and eye protection.	To prevent possible contamination of practitioner with cytotoxic drugs. E
8	Open a pack, empty all equipment onto the pack and place a sterile dressing towel under the patient's arm.	To create a sterile working area. E
9	Wash hands using bactericidal soap and water.	To minimize the risk of infection (DH 2007, C; Fraise and Bradley 2009, E).
10	Apply sterile gloves.	To minimise the risk of infection (DH, 2007, C; Fraise and Bradley 2009, E) and prevent contamination of the nurse.
11	Clean skin with 2% chlorhexidine and allow the area to dry.	To maintain asepsis and remove skin flora (DH, 2007, C; Fraise and Bradley 2009, E).

Procedure

12	Draw up 1% lidocaine in 10 mL syringe.	To prepare for infiltration of area. E
13	Mix hyaluronidase with sterile water in a separate 5 mL syringe	To ensure drug is reconstituted correctly (BNF 2011, C).
14	Mark the area of extravasation with a sterile marker where incisions will be made.	To ensure the correct area is treated. E
15	Using a 25 G needle, make a small bleb by inserting the needle intradermally and administering 0.1–2 mL of lidocaine slowly towards the four points of the compass. Allow it to take effect.	To reduce any discomfort to the patient. E
16	Then, using a 23 G needle, infiltrate the marked area with lidocaine subdermally towards the four points of the compass. Check with patient what kind of sensation they can feel, for example sharp or dull, before proceeding.	To ensure administration of anaesthetic to area and to ensure anaesthetic has taken effect. E
17	Attach a 23 G needle to the syringe of hyaluronidase and infiltrate the anaesthetized area at the four points of the compass.	This will facilitate the flush-out by loosening the tissues. E
18	Attach the administration set, three-way tap and extension set to the bag of 0.9% sodium chloride and withdraw 20 mL via the tap.	To prepare the syringe and to enable continued access without having to open the system. E
19	Make at least four incisions at the four points of the compass using a size 11 scalpel by inserting the blade straight down to a depth of no more than 0.5 cm and one small incision to use for insertion of the cannula.	To prepare the area for flushing. The number of incisions will depend on the size of the area to be treated. To reduce risk of damage to tendons or other anatomical structures (Gault 1993, E).
20	Gently press on the area.	This alone may allow the fluid to escape (Gault 1993, E).

893

(Continued)

Procedure guideline 15.4 *(Continued)*

21	Insert the cannula through one of the incisions and push along tissues within marked area.	To free up tissues from skin and to aid advancement of cannula and flush (Gault 1993, E).
22	Remove the stylet and attach the extension set to the cannula.	To facilitate the flushing. E
23	Flush the 0.9% sodium chloride through – it will exit out of the other incision holes. Pat with a sterile gauze swab, massaging and milking the area at the same time. The area will become puffy and swollen – this is normal.	To commence the flushing procedure. To assist with removal of saline (Gault 1993, E).
24	Draw up more 0.9% sodium chloride and repeat procedure using a minimum of 100 mL (up to 500 mL) of 0.9% sodium chloride .	To facilitate the flushing of the drug from the area (Gault 1993, E).
25	If saline does not flow out of one incision, it may be necessary to remove the cannula from the original incision and insert it into another one – a new cannula must then be used.	To ensure all areas are flushed. E

Postprocedure

26	Clean and dry the area although it will continue to leak.	To aid patient comfort. E
27	Apply a Mepitel dressing and a loose bandage (do not wrap tightly).	To reduce the risk of infection and to prevent compression of the skin. E
28	Elevate the limb so that the hand is level with the head.	To aid reduction of oedema. E
29	Discard waste in appropriate containers.	To ensure safe disposal in the correct containers and avoid laceration or injury of other staff. E
30	Document in patient's medical and nursing notes and on flush-out technique form.	To ensure adequate records and enable continued care of the patient (NMC 2009, C).
31	Discuss with medical colleagues re prescribing oral antibiotics (flucloxacillin is recommended for reducing skin pathogens) and if necessary analgesia.	If the patient is neutropenic they may be more at risk of infection. To minimize pain and discomfort. E
32	Refer to plastic surgeon if any problems during procedure or any skin problems.	To ensure rapid access for further management. E
33	Monitor and review within first 24 hours. Have photograph taken if possible.	To observe and document for any skin changes or infection and provide immediate treatment. E
34	Dressing will need to be changed every 48 hours and should remain *in situ* for up to a week. The skin incisions will heal within 1–2 weeks.	To prevent risk of infection. E
35	Ensure patient has details of who and when to contact if any problems once at home and organize for dressing changes with hospital or District Nurses. Inform patient to contact hospital if swelling does not reduce, they have pain or there is any tingling or numbness in the fingers or arm.	To ensure patient receives immediate treatment should there be any problems post procedure. E

Table 15.9 Grading scale for monitoring extravasation

Grade	1	2	3	4	5
Skin colour	Normal	Pink	Red	Blanched area surrounded by red	Blackened
Skin integrity	Unbroken	Blistered	Superficial skin loss	Tissue loss and exposed subcutaneous tissue	Tissue loss and exposed bone/muscle with necrosis/crater
Skin temperature	Normal	Warm	Hot		
Oedema	Absent	Non-pitting	Pitting		
Mobility	Full	Slightly limited	Very limited	Immobile	
Pain	Grade using a scale of 0–10 where 0 = no pain and 10 = worst pain				
Temperature	Normal	Elevated (indicate actual temperature)			

Postprocedural considerations

Ongoing care

Patient follow-up will be dependent upon the patient's needs and the degree of damage. Assessment should include inspection and management of the area of extravasation, skin integrity, presence of pain, other symptoms and mobility and sensation of limb (see Table 15.9). If damage has occurred, it will be affected by the site, amount of drug, concentration of the agent and if it binds to DNA or not (Polovich *et al.* 2009). Blistering may occur within 24 hours (for example, with vinorelbine) or ulceration may occur over a period of days to weeks (for example, with epirubicin) and extravasation wounds may be complicated by tissue ischaemia related to endothelial damage (Naylor 2005). The type of injury will dictate the type of dressing. Assessment of the wound should include position and size of the wound, amount and type of tissue present, amount and type of exudate, and extent and spread of erythema (Naylor 2005). If the flush-out technique has been undertaken then the incisions should be dressed using a dressing that allows the fluid to continue to leak from the site, for example Mepitel.

Documentation

An extravasation must be reported and fully documented as it is an accident and the patient may require follow-up care (NMC 2009, RCN 2010). The ONS lists the key elements of vesicant extravasation documentation (Polovich *et al.* 2009) (see Box 15.7). Information may also be used for statistical purposes, for example collation and analysis using the Green Card scheme devised by St Chad's Hospital, Birmingham (Stanley 2002). Statistics on the incidence, degree, causes and corrective action should be monitored and analysed (INS 2006). Finally, it may be required in case of litigation, which is now on the increase (Doellman *et al.* 2009, Dougherty 2003, Masoorli 2003).

Education of patient and relevant others

Patients should always be informed when an extravasation has occurred and be given an explanation of what has happened and what management has been carried out (McCaffrey Boyle and Engelking 1995). An information sheet should be given to patients with instructions of what symptoms to look out for and when to contact the hospital during the follow-up period (Gabriel 2008).

Complications

If the extravasation is not managed correctly then an injury will result. In certain circumstances, in spite of managing an extravasation, an injury can still result and must be dealt

---

Box 15.7 Key elements of vesicant extravasation documentation

- Date and time the extravasation occurred.
- Type and size of vascular access device.
- Length and gauge of needle (ports only).
- Location of device.
- Details of how patency was established before and during administration (description and quality of blood return).
- Number and location of all cannulation attempts.
- Vesicant administration method, for example bolus, infusion.
- Estimated amount of extravasated drug.
- Symptoms reported by the patient.
- Description of device site, for example swelling, redness and so on.
- Assessment of limb (where applicable) for range of movement.
- Immediate nursing interventions.
- Follow-up interventions.
- Patient information.

with on an individual basis. Following the flush-out technique, it may be necessary to administer prophylactic antibiotics to prevent local infection (although this is rare).

Oral administration of cytotoxic drugs

Definition

The term 'oral anticancer medicine' is used to refer to drugs with direct antitumour activity, administered via the oral route to cancer patients, including traditional cytotoxic chemotherapy (e.g. capecitabine, vinorelbine), small molecule treatments (e.g. imatinib, erlotanib) and other agents such as thalidomide. It does not include hormonal therapies such as tamoxifen or anastrazole (BOPA 2004, NPSA 2008a).

Evidence-based approaches

Rationale

The use of oral anticancer medications, while not new, has increased greatly in recent years. This increase is set to continue, with around 25% of all anticancer drugs in development being oral preparations (Bedell 2003, Szetela and Gibson 2007). This shift to oral anticancer medications has implications for nurses who will focus less on drug administration and more on educating and monitoring patients (Kav et al. 2008, Szetela and Gibson 2007).

There are considerable advantages to administering anticancer medications via the oral route. The primary benefit is one of patient preference. The majority of patients (90%) would prefer to take oral anticancer medications as long as there was no reduced efficacy (Aisner 2007, Barefoot et al. 2009, Sharma and Saltz 2000). Patients prefer oral anticancer medication because of its ease and convenience; it allows them to take their medication in the comfort of their own home and is often associated with fewer or shorter hospital appointments (Barefoot et al. 2009, Bedell 2003, Winkeljohn 2007). Oral anticancer therapy is non-invasive, eliminating the need for intravenous access (Hayden and Goodman 2005, Sharma and Saltz 2000).

Some evidence suggests that oral anticancer therapy is more cost-effective. Although the cost of new oral medications may be high, the staff and equipment costs of IV administration can be greater. Therefore, the overall costs of administrating oral anticancer therapy may be less (Holmberg and Zanni 2005). Oral anticancer medications are also often considered to be less toxic than the other routes of administration (Hayden and Goodman 2005, Holmberg and Zanni 2005). However, this view is not universally accepted (Birner et al. 2006, Sharma and Saltz 2000). Use of the oral route can be beneficial when chronic exposure to a drug is important, for example, cell cycle-specific drugs (Scurr 2005).

There are several disadvantages associated with giving anticancer medications orally. Oral formulations are not

Table 15.10 Time taken for chemotherapy tablets to dissolve/disperse in water

Tablet	Minutes
Busulfan	15
Capecitabine	20
Chlorambucil	20
Cyclophosphamide	25
Mercaptopurine	5
Methotrexate	5
Tioguanine	5

suitable for all patients. While most oral anticancer drugs are absorbed well if the gastrointestinal tract is functioning normally, many factors affecting cancer patients can alter absorption, making the oral route unreliable (Findlay et al. 2008, O'Neill and Twelves 2002). These include primary tumour, GI surgery and concomitant medications. Side-effects of anticancer treatment such as diarrhoea or nausea and vomiting can also affect absorption (Goodin 2007, Hayden and Goodman 2005, Scurr 2005, Sharma and Saltz 2000).

Some patients may experience difficulty swallowing, which making taking tablets or capsules problematic. Crushing or dissolving oral anticancer medications could result in changes to the tablets' disposition and effectiveness, and advice should be sought from an oncology pharmacist (Table 15.10 and Table 15.11).

Patients usually self-administer at home which can result in less monitoring and support from healthcare professionals (Kav et al. 2008). This can lead to poor adherence and under-reporting of side-effects (Barefoot et al. 2009). Patient adherence to anticancer treatment is important in order to maximize the chance of achieving the goals of therapy. However, there is a greater chance of patient non-adherence with oral anticancer medications than with parenteral therapy which tends to be administered under direct supervision in a healthcare setting. Fear of side-effects can lead patients to stop taking or reduce their dose of oral anticancer medications.

Conversely, patients may feel that their oral chemotherapy is not effective enough and increase their doses (Findlay et al.

Table 15.11 Liquids or soft foods suitable for giving with opened chemotherapy capsules

Capsule	Liquid, food
Hydroxycarbamide	Water, jam, honey, lemon curd, yogurt
Lomustine	Water, jam, honey, lemon curd, yogurt
Procarbazine	Milk, jam, honey, lemon curd, yogurt
Temozolomide	Water, fruit juice (not grapefruit juice), apple sauce
Thalidomide	Water (use feed formula for giving down a nasogastric tube), apple sauce, yogurt, ice cream

Table 15.12 Oral anticancer medications

Drug class	Drug	Cancers for which drug is used
Alkylating agent	Busulfan	Leukaemias
	Chlorambucil	Leukaemia, lymphoma
	Cyclophosphamide	Leukaemia, lymphomas, many solid tumours
	Lomustine (CCNU)	Lymphoma
	Melphalan	Myeloma
	Temozolamide	Glioma (brain tumour)
Antimetabolites	Capecitabine	Breast, colorectal, upper GI
	Fludarabine	Leukaemia
	Mercaptopurine	Leukaemia
	Methotrexate	Leukaemia, solid tumours
	Tegafur-uracil	Colorectal cancer
	Tioguanine	Leukaemia
Epipodophyllotoxins	Etoposide	Leukaemia, solid tumours (lung, testicular)
Tyrosine kinase inhibitors	Imatinib	Chronic myeloid leukaemia
	Dasatinib	Chronic myeloid leukaemia
	Lapatinib	Breast cancer
	Erlotanib	Lung cancer
	Gifetinib	Lung cancer
	Nilotinib	Chronic myeloid leukaemia
	Sorafenib	Renal and liver
	Sunitinib	Renal cancer, GIST
Antitumour antibiotics	Idarubicin	Leukaemia
Plant alkaloids	Vinorelbine	Lung and breast
Miscellaneous	Hydroxycarbamide	Leukaemia
	Lenalidomide	Myeloma
	Tretinoin	Leukaemia
	Thalidomide	Myeloma

(Adapted from Williamson 2008)

2008, Ruddy *et al.* 2009). They may continue taking oral anticancer medications despite toxicity because they feel the treatment is helping and do not want it stopped (Szetela and Gibson 2007). Other factors that can affect adherence are the complexity of the treatment regimen, number and type of concomitant medications, cognitive impairment, treatment of asymptomatic disease, lack of insight into disease seriousness, lack of confidence in treatment and poor patient–provider relationships (Barefoot *et al.* 2009, Hartigan 2003, Hayden and Goodman 2005, Holmberg and Zanni 2005, Viele 2007, Winkeljohn 2007) (Table 15.12).

Preprocedural considerations
Specific patient considerations
Education

Patient education and information are known to improve patient adherence and ensure safety (Winkeljohn 2007)

(Box 15.8). Nurses must take an active role in patient education. It is imperative that the nurse ensures that the patient understands the importance of timing and schedule of the medication prescribed and when to stop medication if side-effects become too severe. Teaching should include information about the name of the medication, dosages, what the tablets look like (shape and colour) and how many of each to take. It must also include advice on side-effects and when to call the hospital and emergency contact details. Pretreatment education and the use of oral anticancer medication diary cards can assist the patient to record the doses of medication that have been taken and side-effects experienced (Hartigan 2003, Oakley *et al.* 2010, Winkeljohn 2007) (Box 15.9).

Patients need to be informed of proper safe handling and storage of their medication. Oral anticancer medications need to be stored safely out of reach of children and pets (Griffin 2003). The risk of exposure to those handling oral anticancer medications is unknown. If gloves are not worn,

---

Box 15.8 Procedure for counselling/educating patients on oral anticancer chemotherapy

1 Prior to the **first cycle** of treatment, all patients should be seen and counselled/educated by an appropriately trained pharmacist, pharmacy technician or nurse using the checklist in Box 15.9.

2 Before **every treatment cycle**, all patients should be seen by an appropriately trained pharmacist, pharmacy technician or nurse to ensure that (a) they were seen and counselled/educated as described above on their first cycle of treatment, (b) they had no problems taking their first cycle of treatment, for example they understood how to take their tablets, they had no problems with vomiting, (c) if a dose reduction has been made, the patient is aware why their dose has been changed and how many tablets/capsules they should take.

3 After counselling/educating the patient using the checklist, the pharmacist, pharmacy technician or nurse should sign the counselling section on the oral chemotherapy prescription chart.

---

the potential for skin absorption exists. Therefore, patients should be provided with gloves and advised to wear them when handling oral chemotherapy tablets and taught to use a non-touch approach by tipping the tablets into a plastic medication container (Goodin 2007, Griffin 2003, Polovich *et al.* 2009, Winkeljohn 2007). There is little evidence on the effectiveness of gowns or aprons in oral anticancer medications so generally their use is not necessary (Griffin 2003). However, aprons should be worn when dissolving tablets or handling liquid preparations.

Many tablets are coated and this protects the drug in its inner core. There is no risk of contamination if these coatings remain intact. A small number of tablets are compressed powders, but there appears to be no risk of contamination where there is no free powder visible. Capsules are also not a risk if they have not been opened or broken or have not leaked (Polovich *et al.* 2009). If tablets are crushed, they may release powder which could be inhaled. Therefore if oral chemotherapy agents need to be dissolved, crushed or otherwise manipulated, this ideally should be

---

Box 15.9 Chemotherapy prescription proforma

Patient outcomes

Patients will verbalize an understanding of administration details, storage, safe handling, what to do in the event of missing a dose, vomiting a dose, obtaining supplies and left-over supplies.

Counselling/educating points prior to the first cycle of chemotherapy

1 The patient understands that the medicine has been prescribed only for them and should not be given to anyone else.

2 They understand that the medicine should be stored in a safe place away from children and should not be handled by anyone else (unless it is being given by a carer, see point 3).

3 If a carer is administering the medicine, they are aware that they should not handle the tablets or capsules directly (they should be tipped or pushed out from the blister pack directly into a medicine pot).

4 The patient (or relative/carer) understands how and when to take their medicine (in particular, if there are breaks in treatment, they know when this should be and how long it should be for).

5 The patient understands any specific directions (usually identified by the directorate pharmacist on the proforma) relating to taking their medicine. (If they miss a dose, they should not try and catch up or double the next dose. They should take the next dose as prescribed. Missed doses should be recorded on patient treatment diaries where applicable.)

6 They understand what to do if they vomit a dose. (If they are sick immediately and they can see the tablet whole, then the dose can be repeated 1 hour later. If, however, they are using liquid or opened capsules or they were asked to crush or dissolve tablets, the dose should not be repeated. They should wait and take the next dose as prescribed.)

7 They understand what the side-effects of treatment are and what they should do if they experience them. In particular, they know who they should contact.

8 They know how to obtain further supplies. (All supplies of oral chemotherapy should be obtained from the hospital pharmacy.)

9 They understand what they should do with left-over tablets. (All left-over tablets should be returned to the hospital pharmacy. They should not be disposed of in household refuse or flushed down the toilet.)

10 They understand the role of their GP and the role of the hospital multiprofessional team. (Any side-effects of treatment should be reported to the hospital team. The hospital doctors are responsible for prescribing the chemotherapy.) In case of chest pain during treatment, the patient should contact 999 as an emergency.

11 A factsheet, 'Taking oral chemotherapy', has been given to the patient.

12 They are able to take their medicine in the dosage form supplied.

13 If the patient is unable to swallow tablets or capsules, they have been given the appropriate RMH factsheet entitled 'Crushing oral chemotherapy tablets safely', 'Dissolving oral chemotherapy tablets safely',' Opening oral chemotherapy capsules safely' or 'Giving chemotherapy by mouth or through a feeding tube using a syringe'. (Please refer to pharmacy for provision of suitable factsheet and standard pack containing disposables.)

14 If a patient treatment diary is available, it has been completed by a nurse or pharmacist.

done in a pharmacy (Goodin 2007, Griffin 2003). If patients/carers are required to crush or dissolve their own medication, they must be given verbal and written information on how to do it and provided with the necessary equipment. The risk of exposure does not disappear when drugs are administered. Contamination can still occur through contact with body fluids. Body fluids such as urine should be treated as a biohazard (Griffin 2003). Any visible spillage should be dealt with as previously directed (see Procedure guideline 15.1).

Procedure guideline 15.5 Cytotoxic therapy: education for patients on oral cytotoxic drugs

Essential equipment

- Patient prescription chart
- Patient information literature

Medicinal products

- Medication(s) to be supplied to patient

Preprocedure

Action	Rationale
1 Prior to the first cycle of treatment, check that the appropriate consent procedure has been completed.	To ensure that the patient gives valid informed consent for treatment (NMC 2008c, C).
2 Evaluate the patient's knowledge of the oral anticancer medication(s) being administered. Explain the treatment plan to the patient and/or carer. Teaching should include verbal and up-to-date written information on the use, action, dose and potential side-effects of prescribed oral anticancer medication(s).	To ensure that the patient is fully informed and understands the aim of the treatment and potential adverse effects (DH 2009a, C; NMC 2008b, C; NPSA 2008a, C; van der Molen 2005, E; Viele 2007, E).

Procedure

3 Educate patient and/or carer about oral anticancer treatment, including: (a) How to take their medication(s) (b) What dose to take (c) When to take their medication(s) and any breaks in treatment (d) What to do in the event of omitted doses (e) What to do if they vomit a dose (f) When to seek advice about adverse effects (g) When and who to contact in the event of an emergency (h) Use of PPE, safe handling and storage (i) Disposal of unused oral anticancer medication(s).	To ensure patients understand that they need to take the correct dose for maximum therapeutic effect. To ensure safety of patient and/or carers. In line with national and local policies (BOPA 2004, C; NECN 2008, C).
4 Before supplying oral anticancer medication(s) to patient, consult the prescription chart and ascertain that the following are correct. (a) Medication (b) Dose (c) Route (d) Dates and times of administration (e) Prescription is correct and legible (f) Signature of prescriber	To ensure the patient is given the correct medications(s) and dose via the correct route at the correct times (NMC 2008b, C). To protect the patient from harm (NMC 2008a, C).
5 Check the patient's identity by asking them to state their full name and date of birth. If unable to verbally confirm details then check identity wristband against prescription chart.	To ensure the medication is supplied to the correct patient (NMC 2008a, C; NPSA 2005, C).

899

(Continued)

Procedure guideline 15.5 (*Continued*)

6 Obtain a full medication history from the patient and check for potential allergies and drug interactions with oral anticancer medication(s).	To protect patient from harm (NMC 2008a, C; Szetela and Gibson 2007, C). To prevent unwanted toxicity and therapeutic failure (Goodin 2007, C).
7 Assess patient's ability to take oral anticancer medications in the dosage and form supplied. If any problems with taking medication(s) in prescribed form are identified, provide teaching and written information on crushing or dissolving oral anticancer medication(s) along with any necessary equipment.	To ensure patient can take prescribed treatment (BOPA 2004, C).

Postprocedure

8 Record and sign that medication(s) have been supplied on the appropriate section on the oral chemotherapy prescription chart.	To provide a written record that medication has been supplied to patient (NECN 2008, C; NMC 2009, C).

Postprocedural considerations

Monitoring and follow-up of patients who have been prescribed oral anticancer medication(s) are vital (Oakley *et al.* 2010). All patients should be fully assessed by a healthcare professional with specialist knowledge prior to each cycle. The following should be assessed and recorded.

- Adherence to prescribed therapy and the continued ability of the patient to manage treatment at home (BOPA 2004, Oakley *et al.* 2010).
- Assessment of toxicity, including grade, duration and management (BOPA 2004, NECN 2008, Oakley *et al.* 2010).
- Performance status of patient (Oakley *et al.* 2010).
- Dose modifications and/or cycle delays. Patients and carers need to be fully informed of any alterations to the dose of oral anticancer medication(s) or to the treatment schedule and the reasons for the changes. Ensure that any written instructions on taking medications are updated (BOPA 2004, NECN 2008, Oakley *et al.* 2010).

The use of oral anticancer medication diary cards can assist the patient to record the doses of medication that have been taken and side-effects experienced (Hartigan 2003, Winkeljohn 2007).

Intramuscular and subcutaneous administration of cytotoxic drugs

Definition

This is the administration of cytotoxic drugs by injection into the muscle or subcutaneous tissues. Intramuscular injections deliver medications into the dense part of the muscle fascia, allowing rapid systemic uptake (Hunter 2008). The subcutaneous route is used for slow, sustained absorption of medication (Workman 1999).

Evidence-based approaches
Rationale
Indications

Intramuscular and subcutaneous injections are a useful route:

- when administering therapy in the community
- for patient convenience
- when regular administration is required and journeys to the hospital are impractical, for example younger or elderly patients on maintenance therapy.

It is also useful if venous access is limited, although only small volumes (up to 3 mL) are recommended using this route (Polovich 2003, Polovich *et al.* 2009, Sewell *et al.* 2002). Cytotoxic and biological agents administered in this way include:

- methotrexate
- bleomycin
- cytosine arabinoside
- L-asparaginase
- ifosfamide
- interferon
- colony-stimulating factor.

(Stanley 2002, Weinstein and Plumer 2007)

Contraindications

Reasons for not administering cytotoxic drugs via the IM or SC routes would include the following factors.

- The irritant nature of the drugs and/or tissue damage.
- Incomplete absorption may occur.
- Bleeding as a result of thrombocytopenia.
- Discomfort of regular injections (Polovich 2003, Polovich *et al.* 2009).

Although the volume of drug and diluent handled is less than for the intravenous route, preparation and reconstitution of the agents should be commensurate with the information listed in the safe handling section. The nurse should wear an apron and gloves during administration. Disposal of equipment and spillage should be dealt with in the same way as for any other cytotoxic medication. Where community nurses are to be responsible for administration, they must be supplied with adequate information when the patient is discharged.

Recommendations about administration should be followed carefully, for example deep intramuscular injection using a Z-track technique to prevent leakage onto the skin (Hayden and Goodman 2005) and rotation of sites to prevent local irritation developing. The skin should be cleaned with antiseptic prior to injection (Sansivero and Barton-Burke 2001) and the smallest needle used, the gauge of which will allow passage of the solution to minimize discomfort and scarring (Weinstein and Plumer 2007).

Procedure guideline 15.6 Cytotoxic therapy: intramuscular administration of cytotoxic drugs (Z-track)

Essential equipment

- Alcohol swab
- Needle
- Syringe containing prepared IM medication
- Non-sterile gloves
- Plastic apron

Preprocedure

Action	Rationale
1 Explain and discuss the procedure with the patient.	To ensure that the patient understands the procedure and gives their valid consent (Griffith *et al.* 2003, E; NMC 2008c, C).
2 Consult the patient's prescription sheet, and ascertain the following. (a) Drug. (b) Dose. (c) Date and time of administration. (d) Route and method of administration. (e) Diluent as appropriate. (f) Validity of prescription. (g) Signature of doctor. (h) Allergy status.	To ensure that the patient is given the correct drug in the prescribed dose using the appropriate diluent and by the correct route (NMC 2008a, C; NPSA 2008a, C).

Procedure

3 Assist the patient into the required position.	To allow access to the injection site and to ensure the designated muscle group is flexed and therefore relaxed (Workman 1999, E).
4 Put on apron and gloves.	To ensure that practitioner is protected from possible accidental exposure (MARCH 2007, C).
5 Remove the appropriate garment to expose the injection site.	To gain access for injection (Workman 1999, E).
5 Assess the injection site for signs of inflammation, oedema, infection and skin lesions.	To promote effectiveness of administration. To reduce the risk of infection (Workman 1999, E). To avoid skin lesions and avoid possible trauma to the patient (Elkin *et al.* 2007, E; Workman 1999, E).

(Continued)

Procedure guideline 15.6 *(Continued)*

6 Clean the injection site with a swab saturated with iso-propyl alcohol 70% for 30 seconds and allow to dry for 30 seconds.	To reduce the number of pathogens introduced into the skin by the needle at the time of insertion. To prevent stinging sensation if alcohol is taken into the tissues upon needle entry (Hunter 2008, E; Workman 1999, E).
7 With the non-dominant hand, pull the skin 2–3 cm side-ways or downwards from the injection site.	To displace the underlying subcutaneous tissues to slide over the underlying muscle by 1–2 cm (Hunter 2008, E; Workman 1999, E).
8 Holding the syringe in the dominant hand like a dart, inform the patient and quickly plunge the needle at an angle of 90° into the skin until about 1 cm of the needle is left showing.	To ensure that the needle penetrates the muscle (Hunter 2008, E; Workman 1999, E).
9 Pull back the plunger. If no blood is aspirated, depress the plunger at approximately 1 mL every 10 seconds and inject the drug slowly. If blood appears, withdraw the needle completely, replace it and begin again. Explain to the patient what has occurred.	To confirm that the needle is in the correct position and not in a vein (Workman 1999, E). This allows time for the muscle fibres to expand and absorb the solution (Hunter 2008, E; Workman 1999, E). To prevent pain and ensure even distribution of the drug (Elkin *et al.* 2007, E).
10 Wait 10 seconds before withdrawing the needle.	To allow the medication to diffuse into the tissue (Elkin *et al.* 2007, E; Workman 1999, E).
11 Withdraw the needle rapidly and release the tension on the skin.	This causes the tissues to return to their original position to create a disjointed pathway and seals the injection entry point to prevent medication from seeping into the subcutaneous tissues or from leaking out through the injection site (Hunter 2008).
12 Apply gentle pressure to any bleeding point and then apply a small plaster over the puncture site.	To prevent tissue injury and haematoma formation (Elkin *et al.* 2007, E).

Postprocedure

13 Ensure that all sharps and non-sharps waste are disposed of safely and in accordance with locally approved procedures, for example put sharps into sharps bin and syringes into cytotoxic clinical waste bag.	To ensure safe disposal and to avoid laceration or other injury to staff (DH 2009b, C).
14 Record the administration on appropriate charts.	To maintain accurate records, provide a point of reference in the event of any queries and prevent any duplication of treatment (NMC 2008a, C; NMC 2009, C; NPSA 2008a, C).

Topical application of cytotoxic drugs

Definition

Topical application is the application of cream or ointments containing cytotoxic agents.

Evidence-based approaches

Rationale

Indications

Topical application is only suitable for superficial lesions and has been found to be useful in the treatment of cutaneous malignant lesions, for example cutaneous T-cell lymphomas, basal cell carcinoma, squamous cell carcinoma and Kaposi's sarcoma (Hayden and Goodman 2005).

Principles of care

Topical agents include mustine and 5-FU (Hayden and Goodman 2005). The most widely used is 5% 5-FU cream for the treatment of basal and squamous cell carcinomas, which is usually applied once or twice daily until significant penetration of the damaged or diseased skin can be achieved, and a typical response pattern has been observed. This can take up to 4 weeks when local erythema, blistering and ulceration occur. Once the affected skin starts sloughing, regranulization of normal tissue will begin to occur (Sewell *et al.* 2002).

Procedure guideline 15.7 Cytotoxic therapy: topical application of cytotoxic drugs

Essential equipment

- Clean non-sterile gloves
- Plastic apron
- Applicators
- Sterile topical swabs

Preprocedure

Action	Rationale
1 Explain and discuss the procedure with the patient.	To ensure that the patient understands the procedure and gives their valid consent (Griffith *et al.* 2003, E; NMC 2008c, C).
2 Check the patient's prescription chart against the chemotherapy medication.	To ensure that the patient is given the correct drug and dose (NMC 2008a, C).

Procedure

3 Close room door or curtains if appropriate.	To ensure patient privacy and dignity. E
4 Put on apron and gloves.	To ensure that the practitioner is protected from accidental spillage (MARCH 2007, C).
5 Assist the patient into the required position.	To allow access to the affected area of skin. E
6 Assess the condition of the skin and use aseptic technique if the skin is broken.	To prevent local or systemic infection (DH 2007, C; Fraise and Bradley 2009, E).
7 If the medication is to be rubbed into the skin, the preparation should be placed on a sterile topical swab.	To minimize the risk of cross-infection. To protect the nurse (DH, 2007, C; Fraise and Bradley 2009, E).
8 If the preparation causes staining, advise the patient of this.	To ensure that adequate precautions are taken beforehand and to prevent unwanted stains (NMC 2008b, C).
9 Use a sterile dressing if required	To ensure the ointment remains in place (Chernecky *et al.* 2002, E).

Postprocedure

10 Record the administration on appropriate charts.	To maintain accurate records, provide a point of reference in the event of any queries and prevent any duplication of treatment (NMC 2009, C; NPSA, 2007, C).

Considerations include safe handling when applying the cream by wearing gloves and using low-linting swabs or non-metal applicators (Hayden and Goodman 2005, Weinstein and Plumer 2007). It is important to protect the normal skin and avoid the eyes and other mucous membranes.

Postprocedural considerations

Ongoing care

The affected area should not be washed vigorously during the treatment (Hayden and Goodman 2005). The area should be observed for any adverse reactions such as pain,

pruritus and hyperpigmentation, which may result in discontinuation and subsequent dose reduction.

Intrathecal administration of cytotoxic drugs

Definition

Intrathecal administration is the administration of cytotoxic drugs into the central nervous system (CNS) via the cerebrospinal fluid. This is usually achieved using a lumbar

903

puncture (Hayden and Goodman 2005, Polovich *et al.* 2009, Stanley 2002).

Related theory

Intrathecal administration is only appropriate for a limited number of drugs.

- Thiotepa.
- Cytarabine.
- Methotrexate (Scurr 2005).

The advantage of this route is that it allows the direct access to the CNS of drugs which do not normally cross the blood–brain barrier in sufficient amounts and thus ensures constant levels of the drug in this area. The main disadvantage is that it requires a standard lumbar puncture before the drug can be injected, and this may need to be performed on a daily to weekly basis (Hayden and Goodman 2005, Stanley 2002). Although this can be quick and easy to perform, it can be distressing for the patient, and could even result in CNS trauma and infection. It may also only reach the epidural or subdural spaces and therefore the concentrations in the ventricles may not be therapeutic (Hayden and Goodman 2005). However, central instillation of the drug into the ventricle can be achieved via an Ommaya reservoir (Figure 15.7), which is surgically implanted through the cranium (Hayden and Goodman 2005, Sewell *et al.* 2002, Weinstein and Plumer 2007). It carries more risks but provides permanent access and can be inserted under local or general anaesthetic (Hayden and Goodman 2005, Sansivero and Barton-Burke 2001). Doses of intraventricular drugs tend to be lower than those given intrathecally.

Evidence-based approaches
Rationale
Indications

Intrathecal administration has proved to be of benefit in prophylactic treatment in cases of leukaemias and some lymphomas, where the CNS may provide a sanctuary site for tumour cells not reached during systemic chemotherapy (Hayden and Goodman 2005). It has no place in the treatment of CNS metastases of solid tumours (Stanley 2002).

Principles of care

The preparation of the drug must be performed using aseptic technique to reduce the risk of infection. The drug should be free from preservatives to reduce neurotoxicity. Cerebrospinal fluid removal and volumes of medications should not be more than 2 mL/min.

Legal and professional issues

Chemotherapy administered using this route has the potential to cause great harm (Sewell *et al.* 2002) and has been associated with the deaths of at least 13 patients since 1985. The risks of intrathecal chemotherapy have been well documented in *An Organization with a Memory* (DH 2000) and the government set a target to eliminate the incidents of patients dying or being paralysed by maladministered intrathecal injections by the end of 2001 (DH 2000). Two reports on injection errors (Toft 2001) gave rise to the publication of the national guidance for the safe administration of intrathecal chemotherapy.

Following the publication of the guidance, all UK trusts that undertake to administer intrathecal cytotoxic chemotherapy (ITC) must ensure safe practice guidelines have been introduced and that they are fully compliant with the *Updated National Guidance on the Safe Administration of Intrathecal Chemotherapy* (DH 2008). The key requirements of the guidance are noted in Box 15.10.

The chief executive must identify a 'designated lead' who in turn must ensure the appropriate induction, training and continuing professional development of designated personnel authorized to administer intrathecal chemotherapy. A register of these personnel must be kept along with details of certain competency-based tasks such as prescribing, dispensing, issuing, checking and administration. It is important to keep up to date with relevant safety alerts concerning intrathecal chemotherapy which may be issued by the Department of Health agencies such as the Medicines and Healthcare products Regulatory Agency (MHRA) or National Patient Safety Agency (NPSA). Such reports have highlighted concerns over the risk of neurological injury due to implantable drug pumps for intrathecal therapy (MHRA 2008) and the storage of vinca alkaloid minibags (NPSA 2008b).

Figure 15.7 Ommaya reservoir.

Box 15.10 Summary – requirements of intrathecal guidance

- Only trained, designated personnel whose names are recorded on the appropriate intrathecal register are authorized to prescribe, dispense, check or administer intrathecal chemotherapy.
- All staff involved in the intrathecal chemotherapy process must undertake a formal competency-based induction programme that is appropriate to their role and annual training must be provided for all professional staff to remain on the register.
- Staff involved with intrathecal chemotherapy must use this policy in conjunction with the national guidance HSC 2008/001 and the Rapid Response Report NPSA/2008/RRR004 relating to intravenous vinca alkaloid administration.
- Staff are given an annual date-expiring certificate on satisfactory completion of their training.
- Intrathecal chemotherapy must be prescribed by a consultant, associate specialist, specialist registrar, staff grade or ST3 grade doctor only and they must be on the register.

- Intrathecal chemotherapy drugs must be issued and received by designated staff only. Any such products not used must be returned to pharmacy at the end of the intrathecal chemotherapy session.
- In adults, intravenous drugs must be administered BEFORE intrathecal drugs are issued (or once intravenous continuous infusions have been started).
- Children receiving intrathecal therapy under general anaesthetic will have their intrathecal treatment first in theatre. Intravenous drugs (excluding vinca alkaloids) may be given later in day care or on the ward, but never in theatre.
- Intrathecal chemotherapy should always be administered in a designated area, within normal working hours; out-of-hours administration must only occur in exceptional circumstances.
- Checks must be made by medical, nursing and pharmacy staff at relevant stages throughout the prescribing, preparation and administration process.
- This guidance predominantly relates to treatment given intrathecally, by lumbar puncture (i.e. via spinal injection) but is also relevant to intraventricular chemotherapy (i.e. via injection into the ventricles of the brain).

Procedure guideline 15.8 **Cytotoxic therapy: intraventricular administration of cytotoxic drugs via an intraventricular access device (Ommaya reservoir)**

Essential equipment

- 25 G winged infusion devices or small non-coring needle
- Sterile dressing pack
- Cleaning solution
- Pre-prepared chemotherapy
- Three-way tap

Preprocedure

Action	Procedure
1 Explain and discuss the procedure with the patient.	To ensure that the patient understands the procedure and gives their valid consent (Griffith *et al.* 2003, E; NMC 2008c, C).
2 Consult the patient's prescription sheet, and ascertain the following. (a) Drug. (b) Dose. (c) Date and time of administration. (d) Route and method of administration. (e) Diluent as appropriate. (f) Validity of prescription. (g) Signature of doctor. (h) Allergy status.	To ensure that the patient is given the correct drug in the prescribed dose using the appropriate diluent and by the correct route (NMC 2008a, C; NPSA 2007, C).
3 Position patient comfortably.	To gain access to the site. E

(Continued)

905

Procedure guideline 15.8 (*Continued*)

4 Apply apron and necessary PPE, for example gloves, googles.	To protect the practioner from splashes and spills (HSE 2003, C; MARCH 2007, C; RCN 2010, C).
5 Wash hands with antibacterial soap.	To prevent contamination (Fraise and Bradley 2009, E).
6 Open sterile pack and pour antiseptic liquid into gallipot.	To prepare the area. E
7 Open intrathecal chemotherapy drugs by cutting plastic pack and place on sterile field.	To gain access to chemotherapy. E
8 Open non-coring winged infusion device and connect a three-way tap to the tubing.	To prepare the equipment. E
9 Clean hands with alcohol gel.	To prevent contamination (Fraise and Bradley 2009, E).

Procedure

10 Locate the reservoir by slightly depressing the dome several times. There should be free flow of CSF from the ventricle into the dome.	To ascertain where the reservoir is and that it is functional (RCN 2010, C).
11 Wash hands with antibacterial handwash and put on sterile gloves.	To prevent contamination (Fraise and Bradley 2009, E).
12 Prepare the skin by cleaning the site.	To minimize risk of infection (Fraise and Bradley 2009, E).
13 Using the 25 G needle, access the reservoir and re-move a small amount of CSF equal to the amount of drug to be instilled.	To check free flow of CSF and patency of reservoir (RCN 2010, C).
14 Connect syringe containing chemotherapy to three-way tap and inject slowly. No resistance should be felt.	To maintain a closed system and administer medication (RCN 2010, C).
15 Compress and release dome after all medication is given.	To facilitate medication administration and dispense drug (RCN 2010, C).
16 The reservoir can now be flushed with the CSF removed at start of procedure. Do not flush with 0.9% sodium chloride or heparin.	Flushing is not required as CSF flows freely through the device (RCN 2010, C; West 1998, E).
17 Remove the needle and apply pressure with gauze.	To prevent leakage of CSF or chemotherapy. E
18 Dispose of sharps and syringe in purple lidded sharps container.	To maintain a safe environment. E
19 Once CSF stops leaking, apply a small gauze dressing and tape.	To minimize risk of infection (Fraise and Bradley 2009, E).

Postprocedure

20 Assist patient in repositioning if required.	To maintain comfort. E
21 Dispose of equipment in appropriate waste bags.	To maintain a safe environment. E
22 Wash and dry hands.	To minimize risk of contamination (Fraise and Bradley 2009, E).
23 Document chemotherapy administration on prescription chart.	To maintain records and for continuity of care (NMC 2009, C).
24 Monitor patient for any side-effects of the drugs and check reservoir site for any leaks.	To recognize complications early and report to medical staff (RCN 2010, C).

Postprocedural considerations

It is important that the nurse monitors the patient for signs of discomfort and administers any analgesics required. Vital signs should be recorded regularly, at least every 1–2 hours initially and then 4 hourly. Observations should include signs of infection, headache and raised intercranial pressure (Hayden and Goodman 2005, Scurr *et al.* 2005). For more detail, see section on lumbar puncture in Chapter 11.

Intrapleural instillation of cytotoxic drugs

Definition

Introduction of cytotoxic drugs, or other substances, into the pleural cavity.

Related theory

Pleural effusion is a common complication of malignant disease and may pose a considerable management problem. Instillation should occur following drainage of an effusion to prevent or delay a recurrence caused by malignant cells, as after aspiration alone 60% of patients would present with pleural malignant recurrence (Hayden and Goodman 2005).

The most common neoplasms associated with the development of malignant pleural effusions are those of the:

- breast
- lung
- gastrointestinal tract
- prostate
- ovary (Hayden and Goodman 2005).

Such effusions can be very distressing to the patient, causing progressive discomfort, dyspnoea and death from respiratory insufficiency.

The alteration in normal anatomy due to the pressure of an effusion is illustrated in Figure 15.8. In health, less than 5 mL of transudate fluid is present between the visceral and parietal pleurae. This fluid acts as a lubricant and hydraulic seal (see Chapter 10). Infections and malignancies disrupt this mechanism, often repeatedly. Patients may survive for months or years, therefore effective palliation is important in maintaining or improving their quality of life. Administering chemotherapy via this route may alleviate symptoms and also has the potential for delivering the drugs to a site of poor systemic penetration (Sewell *et al.* 2002). A recent study using intrapleural hypotonic cisplatin for malignant pleural effusion demonstrated encouraging results. Eighty patients were observed during the study, of which 27 (34%) and 39 (49%) achieved a complete response and partial response respectively (Seto *et al.* 2006).

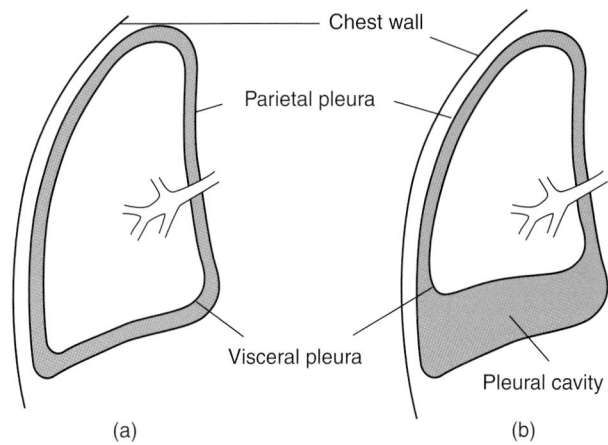

Figure 15.8 Lung anatomy. (a) Normal lung anatomy showing pleura. (b) Lung demonstrating presence of pleural effusion.

Evidence-based approaches
Principles of care

Several methods have been used to treat pleural effusions, including:

- surgical techniques, such as ablation of the pleural space
- radiotherapy
- systemic chemotherapy
- the insertion of a small-bore catheter and installation of a pleural shunt (Sewell *et al.* 2002) to deliver cytotoxic agents.

In addition, instillation of sclerosing agents into the pleural space has been reported to have highly variable success rates of 20–88% (Sewell *et al.* 2002). Cytology may show the presence of tumour cells in effusion fluid, but even when these are absent, instillation of drugs may be effective in preventing recurrence due to the inflammatory reaction which obliterates the pleural space.

Agents used have included talc, radio-active phosphorus, bacille Calmette-Guérin (BCG), tetracycline and, more recently, cytotoxic drugs. The drug most frequently instilled is bleomycin, but others include mitozantrone, doxorubicin, mustine and thiotepa (Hayden and Goodman 2005, Sewell *et al.* 2002).

Preprocedural considerations
Equipment

Improvements in equipment used, for example flexible cannulas or catheters, and lengthening of both the initial drainage period and that following instillation of the drug have contributed to increased patient comfort and greater effectiveness (Hayden and Goodman 2005). The insertion of small-bore percutaneously placed catheters or ports, as well as pleuroperitoneal shunts (Hayden and Goodman 2005), has been found to be useful for recurrent effusions.

Procedure guideline 15.9 Cytotoxic therapy: intrapleural instillation of cytotoxic drugs

Essential equipment

- Sterile chest drain pack containing gallipot, disposable towel, forceps, disposable scalpel and sterile low-linting gauze
- Suture material: silk
- Cleaning solution: chlorhexidine gluconate 0.5% in 70% alcohol
- Sterile gloves and gown
- Syringes: 2 × 10 mL

- Needles: 1 × 21G, 1 × 23G
- Chest drain. Check appropriate size to be used for insertion
- Sterile dressing
- Tape
- Chest drain tubing
- Chest drain bottle
- Chest drain clamps × 2
- Low-vacuum suction pump, if required

Medicinal products

- Local anaesthetic: lidocaine 1%
- Sterile water: 1 litre bottle

Preprocedure

Action	Rationale
1 Explain and discuss the procedure with the patient.	To ensure that the patient understands the procedure and gives their valid consent (NMC 2008c, C).
2 Administer premedication to patients if prescribed.	To relax the patient. E
3 Prepare the required equipment and cytotoxic drug. Wear protective clothing.	To ensure the procedure goes smoothly without interruption. To protect practitioner from exposure (HSE 2003, C).

Procedure

4 Assist the doctor with the instillation and provide support for the patient.	To increase the efficiency of the procedure and reduce discomfort for the patient. E
5 At the end of the instillation, clamp the drainage tube and leave for the desired period.	To prevent backflow of the drug (Weinstein and Plumer 2007, E).
6 Assess the clinical status of the patient and ability to tolerate the desired rotation.	To prevent discomfort the patient may feel and to ensure that the doctor is informed of the patient's inability to comply. E
7 Turn the patient in the following rotation: (a) Left side (b) Supine (c) Right side (d) Prone.	To ensure that the drug coats and washes the pleural cavity completely. E
8 Carry out the rotations as instructed. Examples are as follows. (a) Five minutes in each position, repeated once, equals 20 minutes. (b) Thirty minutes in each position, repeated once, equals 2 hours. (c) One hour in each position equals 4 hours.	As above. E
9 Observe regularly for patient comfort. Administer analgesic as required.	To keep the patient comfortable and free from pain. E
10 Record the patient's respirations and colour at least every 15 minutes for 1 hour, then every hour until stable, then 4 hourly or as frequently as the patient's condition dictates. Record temperature at least 4 hourly.	To ensure there is no change in respiratory function following the procedure. E To observe for pyrexia, a common side-effect that may indicate a developing infection or a reaction to chemotherapy. E Administer antihistamine if required. E

Postprocedure

11	When ready to remove the drain, ensure the patient is in a comfortable position, and is aware of any limitations about movement.	To prevent discomfort or dislodgement of the drainage tube. E
12	Unclamp the chest tube.	To allow drainage of the drug instilled. E
13	Record the colour and amount of fluid drained.	To monitor the immediate effectiveness of therapy (NMC 2009, C).

Postprocedural considerations

Immediate care

The literature recommends that the patient should be turned regularly following instillation of the drug to facilitate its complete distribution over the pleural surfaces. It has been recommended that the timing for turning should be every 10–15 minutes for between 2 and 6 hours (Chaudhary 2007). The rationale for such turning is based on clinical observation and there is a lack of research comparing patients who are turned with those who are not.

Ongoing care

Local pleural pain and inflammation can last for 24–48 hours after instillation. Good symptom management should focus upon emesis control, adequate analgesia and emotional support and chest tube security to ensure patient comfort (Hayden and Goodman 2005).

Intravesical instillation of cytotoxic drugs

Definition

Intravesical instillation is the instillation of cytotoxic drugs directly into the bladder, via a urinary catheter (Dougherty and Bailey 2008).

Related theory

Instillation of cytotoxic agents, and immunotherapy, into the bladder via a urinary catheter has been used for many years in selected cases and has proven to be an effective and simple method of controlling and treating superficial bladder cancer (Scurr 2005). In measurable disease, average response rates are 60%. Approximately 30% of patients experience a complete response. Cytotoxic drugs found to be effective include:

- thiotepa
- mitomycin C
- doxorubicin
- epirubicin
- mitoxantrone
- BCG (Washburn 2007).

Intravesical instillation allows a high concentration of drug to bathe the endothelium, which enables localized treatment of the tumour and limits the systemic absorption so toxicity is reduced. Systemic toxicity is a problem with thiotepa, but otherwise the main problems are local inflammation, pain, burning on urination, frequency and occasional haematuria. The procedure should be performed using an aseptic technique as there is an increased risk of urinary tract infection.

Evidence-based approaches

Rationale

Indications

- Intravesical instillation has been shown to be effective in the treatment of small, multiple, superficial, well-differentiated, non-invasive papillomatous carcinomas, as high drug concentrations can be achieved using this route, because there is limited penetration of the drug into normal and malignant tissue.
- This method is only of benefit when treating small and superficial disease (Scurr 2005).
- It minimizes recurrence in patients with a history of multiple tumours known to readily seed locally (Stanley 2002).
- It also reduces cytotoxic exposure to patients and their carers because excretion of the drug is quicker than when administered systemically (Washburn 2007).

Preprocedural considerations

Specific patient preparations

Instillation first involves the insertion of a urinary catheter, drainage of the bladder, then the instillation of the drug. This usually takes about 50–60 minutes; it is retained for 1–2 hours with frequent movement by the patient to disperse the drug through the bladder (Hayden and Goodman 2005, Sewell et al. 2002). Therapy may be repeated on alternating days for three doses or weekly for varying lengths of time (4–12 weeks).

Procedure guideline 15.10 Cytotoxic therapy: intravesical instillation of cytotoxic drugs

Essential equipment

- Urotainer containing prescribed drug in clinically clean tray (delivered from pharmacy reconstitution unit)
- Sterile gloves
- Disposable apron and eye protection
- Gate clip or equivalent clamp for catheter
- Catheter drainage bag, if catheter is to remain in position
- 10 or 20 mL sterile syringe
- Small dressing pack, that includes a sterile field

Preprocedure

Action	Rationale
1 Explain and discuss the procedure with the patient.	To ensure that the patient understands the procedure and gives their valid consent (NMC 2008c, C).
2 Check the patient's full blood count, as instructed by the medical staff, and inform them of any deficit before administration.	Absorption of the drug through the bladder wall may cause some myelosuppression. However, there are differing opinions as to whether regular checks are necessary. E
3 Check all the details on the container of cytotoxic drug against the patient's prescription chart.	To minimize the risk of error and comply with legal requirements (NMC 2008b, C).
4 Assemble all necessary equipment, including the cytotoxic drug container, and proceed to the patient.	To ensure that the instillation proceeds smoothly and without interruption. E
5 Screen the patient's bed/couch.	To ensure privacy during the procedure. E
6 Check that the patient's identity matches the patient's details on the prescription chart.	To ensure that the correct patient has been identified. To reduce the risk of error (NMC 2008a, C).

Procedure

7 If patient does not have a catheter *in situ*, then pass a catheter (see Chapter 6).	To enable the medication to be administered. E
8 Ensure the bladder is empty of urine.	To prevent dilution of the drug. (Washburn 2007, E)
9 Put on gloves, apron and eye protection.	To protect the nurse from contact with the cytotoxic drugs. With correct technique, the risk of contamination is minimal but splashes can occur (Hayden and Goodman 2005, E).
10 Using aseptic technique and sterile gloves, place a receiver under the end of the catheter to catch any urine and disconnect the drainage bag.	To protect the patient from infection. To protect the nurse from drug spillage. To gain access to the catheter. To prevent urine from soiling the bed. E
11 Remove the cover from the urotainer, connect to the catheter and release the clamp on the urotainer.	To facilitate drug instillation. E
12 Using gravity to create pressure, instil the cytotoxic drug into the bladder. Gentle squeezing may be needed to assist this process.	Rapid instillation would be uncomfortable for the patient, especially if the bladder is small or scarred from previous treatment or disease. E
13 When the correct prescribed volume has been instilled, slide urotainer clamp over filling port.	To prevent drainage of drug from the bladder (Weinstein and Plumer 2007, E).
14 When the drug has been in the bladder for 1 hour, ask the patient to micturate or slide clamp across filling port and place receiver under connectors. Disconnect urotainer and connect new drainage bag.	One hour is the usual time specified for intravesical drugs to ensure the maximum therapeutic effect with minimum toxicity. To prevent contamination of bedlinen (Nixon and Schulmeister 2009). E

Postprocedure

15 If the catheter is to be removed, withdraw the water from the catheter balloon (if appropriate – some catheters do not have a balloon: see Chapter 6) using the sterile syringe and remove the catheter using gentle traction. Dispose of equipment into clinical waste bag and seal.		The catheter may not be required for continued urinary drainage, and may have been inserted to facilitate drug administration, particularly in the outpatient department. The risk of infection is greater if the catheter remains *in situ* (Weinstein and Plumer 2007). E
16 Patient should be made aware that their urine may be cloudy. Instruct the patient to report any discomfort or inability to pass urine immediately to ward staff or general practitioner/district nurse, or to telephone the hospital if anxious.		To detect and resolve any problems at the earliest moment. To reduce anxiety experienced by the patient. E

Problem-solving table 15.1 **Prevention and resolution (Procedure guideline 15.10)**

Problem	Cause	Prevention	Action
No drainage of urine when the catheter is inserted	Bladder is empty or the catheter is in the wrong place, for example in the urethra or in a false track. False tracks may develop after repeated cystoscopy or bladder surgery	Ensure experienced nurses catheterize the patient and check notes for any previous difficulties with insertion or false tracks	Do not inflate the balloon but tape the catheter to the skin to keep it in position. Check when the patient last micturated. Encourage the patient to drink a few glasses of fluid. Do not give the drug until urine flow is seen or correct positioning of the catheter is established. Inform a doctor if no urine has drained during the next 30 minutes
No drainage of urine when catheter unclamped	Blocked with clots or debris	May not be possible to prevent	Check the position of the catheter and bladder lavage performed if necessary
Patient has pain during instillation of the drug or while the drug is in the bladder	Following resection of mucosa, the bladder can become acutely sensitive to irritants, thus causing painful spasm, resulting in possible expulsion of the cytotoxic agent	Administer analgesics pre-procedure Help to keep the patient as calm and comfortable as possible	Allow the drug to drain out and/or stop instillation if the pain is severe. Inform a doctor. Administer Entonox if appropriate (see Chapter 9) and have analgesics prescribed for subsequent administration
Patients may be unable to retain the requisite drug volume in the bladder for the time required	Low bladder capacity; weak sphincter muscles or unstable detrusor muscle causing uncontrolled bladder contractions	May not be able to prevent	The nurse should record the actual duration of the drug in the bladder and inform a doctor if the patient is unable to retain the drug in the bladder
Unable to pass urine following removal of catheter	Anxiety; poor bladder tone or prostatism	Reassure patient and encourge fluids prior to removal	The nurse should provide comfort and reassurance to the patient and encourage the patient to drink fluids

Postprocedural considerations

Education of patient and relevant others

The patient should be provided with information about the amount of movement required, but if an outpatient, the journey home is usually sufficient to coat the bladder mucosa. An increase in oral intake while the treatment is being given will increase the dilution of medication required, ensure that there is sufficient washing out of the bladder and reduce the likelihood of local irritation or difficulty in urination due to debris from the tumour (Hayden and Goodman 2005).

Patients should be instructed in good personal hygiene such as washing hands and genitalia thoroughly after voiding, and the toilet should be flushed at least twice after voiding.

Complications

Haematuria

This can occur within 24–48 hours as a direct consequence of the trauma of catheterization or the loosening of blood clots following cystoscopy by fluid injected into the bladder. The patient needs to be monitored for signs of clot retention, shock, haemorrhage or fluid retention and any complications should be reported to the medical team. The patient should be encouraged to drink plenty of fluids to help reduce the risk of clot formation.

Leakage

Another complication can be leakage from around the catheter following administration of the drug, which may be caused by the catheter slipping out of the bladder or bladder spasm caused by the drug itself. It is therefore important that the nurse checks the position of the catheter regularly and informs the doctor if leakage persists. Any leakage should be washed thoroughly using protective personal equipment. The patient's skin should be protected by wrapping sterile topical swabs around the catheter (Polovich *et al.* 2009).

Intraperitoneal instillation of cytotoxic drugs

Definition

Intraperitoneal administration is the introduction of cytotoxic drugs into the peritoneal cavity following drainage of ascites, to prevent or delay a recurrence.

Related theory

The peritoneal space is semi-permeable, which allows high concentrations of the drugs to be achieved at the site of the tumour throughout the peritoneal space, but with lower concentrations entering the bloodstream, thus reducing the toxicity (Sewell *et al.* 2002). Therefore, increased dosages of drug can be delivered to the tumour site than could be delivered systemically.

Large volumes of fluid containing chemotherapy agents should be administered intermittently. The chemotherapy agents used include:

- cisplatin
- carboplatin
- bleomycin
- paclitaxel
- mitoxantrone
- mitomycin C
- 5-FU (Sewell *et al.* 2002).

Evidence-based approaches

Rationale

Indications

Treatment failures of primary malignant tumours of the colon and rectum as well as ovary occur most frequently as local regional disease. Extensive tumours may be present intra-abdominally without evidence of disease at other sites in the body. In view of this, chemotherapy treatment given intraperitoneally has been shown to be effective in treating locally recurrent ovarian and colon cancer (Hayden and Goodman 2005, Sewell *et al.* 2002).

Methods of accessing the peritoneal space

There are three methods of accessing the peritoneal space.

1 Intermittent placement of a temporary indwelling catheter into the peritoneal cavity. This is used for a short time such as for symptom relief or palliation.
2 Placement of an external catheter such as a Tenckhoff. This is surgically placed through the anterior abdominal wall and the catheter exits through the skin on the abdomen. This is the most widely used method and the Tenckhoff catheter has the advantages of allowing a high flow rate (2 litres in 10–15 minutes) and also allows for manipulation to dislodge fibrin deposits (Hayden and Goodman 2005). Problems include occlusion infection, leakage around the catheter and body image problems.
3 Placement of an implantable peritoneal port. The port is internal with no care required when not accessed and therefore has a lower rate of infection and may be more acceptable to the patient. However, ports tend to provide a slower flow rate than a catheter (Hayden and Goodman 2005).

Procedure guideline 15.11 Cytotoxic therapy: intraperitoneal instillation of cytotoxic drugs

Essential equipment

- Sterile gloves
- Disposable apron and goggles
- Y-tube irrigation set

- Gate clip or equivalent clamp for catheter
- Catheter drainage bag, if catheter is to remain in position
- Small dressing pack, containing sterile field

Medicinal products

- Syringe or infusion bag containing prescribed drug in clinically clean tray (delivered from pharmacy reconstitution unit)

Preprocedure

Action	Rationale
1 Explain and discuss the procedure with the patient.	To ensure that the patient understands the procedure and gives their valid consent (NMC 2008c, C).
2 Administer premedication to patient if prescribed.	To ensure the patient is relaxed during the procedure. E
3 Check all the details on the container of the cytotoxic drug against the patient's prescription chart.	To minimize the risk of error and comply with legal requirements (NMC 2008b, C).
4 Assemble all necessary equipment, including the cytotoxic drug container, and proceed to the patient.	To ensure that the instillation proceeds smoothly and without interruption. E

Procedure

5 Prior to instillation, prewarm infusion to body temperature.	To prevent cramping. (Hayden and Goodman 2005, E; Polovich *et al.* 2009, E).
6 Use a Y-tube irrigation set. The catheter is attached by this Y-tube to a bottle of dialysate and a drainage bag.	To ensure minimum intervention in draining peritoneal cavity. E
7 Instil fluid at prescribed rate, usually 1–2 litres over 10–15 minutes, but can be extended to 30–60 minutes .	To ensure the correct instillation at the correct rate (Hayden and Goodman 2005, E; NMC 2008b, C)
8 Document administration on prescription chart.	To record administration (NMC 2008b, C).
9 Wait prescribed period of time after administration prior to draining off excess fluid. This may be from 1 to 3 hours.	To ensure fluid has coated all parts of peritoneal cavity. E
10 Observe regularly for patient comfort and intervene as appropriate. If the patient experiences any discomfort or pain, administer prescribed analgesia.	To keep patient comfortable and pain free. E
11 Record temperature 4 hourly.	To observe for pyrexia, a common side-effect that may indicate a developing infection or a reaction to chemotherapy. E
12 Unclamp drainage tube and, where necessary, flush port or pump using appropriate flushing solution. The catheter may be removed after drainage is complete.	To allow drainage of drug. E

Postprocedure

13 Record accurate fluid balance.	To maintain accurate records (NMC 2009, C).

913

Problem-solving table 15.2 Prevention and resolution (Procedure guideline 15.11)

Problem	Cause	Prevention	Action
Abdominal pain or discomfort	Peritoneal irritation following placement of catheter Incomplete drainage of the dialysate solution Failure to warm dialysate solution to body temperature Chemical peritonitis resulting from chemotherapeutic agent	Warm the dialysate fluid	Observe for a reaction and treat symptomatically
Leakage from around the catheter following administration of the drug	Peritoneum is not intact or catheter is not entirely within peritoneal cavity	Check that the catheter is in correct place before administration	Strict aseptic technique required. Dressings to be changed frequently. When skin around the catheter has healed, there should be no further leakage

Postprocedural considerations

To ensure safe disposal of waste, it is important that if there is leakage around the drainage site or a drainage bag is attached, nurses must remember that the fluid may still contain the cytotoxic drug and should therefore take the same precautions as when handling any cytotoxic waste.

Complications

General complications of intraperitoneal chemotherapy include respiratory distress, abdominal pain and distension, discomfort and diarrhoea (which all result in increased abdominal pressure) (Polovich *et al.* 2009). Other problems include mechanical difficulties with the catheter (inflow and outflow obstructions), electrolyte imbalance and peritonitis caused by chemical irritation of the peritoneal space, or by infection or both. Commonly, intraperitoneal chemotherapy is usually tolerated well by patients and provides a safe and effective treatment in the management of peritoneal disease (Weinstein and Plumer 2007).

Intra-arterial administration of cytotoxic drugs

Definition

Intra-arterial administration is the delivery of a cytotoxic drug to the tumour site by catheterization of the artery providing the blood supply to the affected organ. This allows a high concentration of drug to be delivered (Weinstein and Plumer 2007).

Related theory

The advantage of the route is that it facilitates the delivery of high concentrations of drug to the primary or secondary tumour mass (Sewell *et al.* 2002). A reduction in systemic circulating levels of drugs has been shown to occur in many circumstances, resulting in a corresponding reduction in side-effects to the patient (Hayden and Goodman 2005). The cytotoxic drugs used vary with the histology and site of the tumour. All of the following have been administered via the intra-arterial route:

- actinomycin D
- BCNU (carmustine)
- bleomycin
- cisplatin
- doxorubicin
- 5-FU
- 5-FUDR
- methotrexate
- melphalan
- mitomycin C
- vincristine (Weinstein and Plumer 2007).

The main disadvantage of this route is that very high levels of drug in a perfused organ may result in excessive tissue damage (Sewell *et al.* 2002).

Evidence-based approaches
Rationale

The tumour site determines which artery will be used to deliver the chemotherapy since it is the artery supplying the tumour which is cannulated. The most common route is the hepatic artery (Weinstein and Plumer 2007).

Indications

Intra-arterial chemotherapy has been used to treat a variety of malignancies at a number of different sites. These include:

- head and neck lesions
- liver metastases from colorectal cancer
- sarcomas/melanomas of upper and lower limb (including isolated limb perfusion)
- carcinoma of the stomach
- carcinoma of the breast
- carcinoma of the cervix.

Methods of infusion

Two main methods are used for infusional chemotherapy; these are termed external and internal arterial infusions.

The external method

Involves radiographic placement of an arterial catheter and attachment to an external infusion pump (Hayden and Goodman 2005). Temporary catheter placement is used for short-term therapies, that is, from hours up to 5 days. Therapy can be given intermittently for several courses. This method is unsuitable for long-term use (6 months or longer) as it is uncomfortable, inconvenient and expensive, although a subcutaneous implanted port increases the patient's comfort and freedom (Hayden and Goodman 2005).

Once the catheter is in place and secured, cytotoxic drugs may be administered by:

- injection, using a syringe
- small-volume infusion, using a syringe pump.
- large-volume infusion, using a volumetric pump.

Internal or implantable methods

Involve the surgical placement of a totally implantable pump and appear to have a lower complication rate than the external method. The catheter is inserted into an appropriate artery and attached to the pump, which is filled with chemotherapy. This approach is more frequently used for colorectal cancer metastases to the liver.

Confirmation that the artery supplies the desired area can be achieved by instillation of yellow fluorescent dye if the tumour site is visible, or contrast medium if an internal organ such as the liver is the target area.

All delivery systems must provide adequate pressure to combat arterial pressure, that is, 300 mmHg (Hayden and Goodman 2005). The majority of infusion pumps meet this requirement. Patient education is very important as the patient may have to maintain the implantable pump and be able to recognize any complications or malfunctions.

Principles of care

The catheter is inserted in theatre or in the X-ray department and its position checked at that time. The catheter is then secured and an occlusive dressing applied. This should *not* be touched as it is essential that the catheter is *not* displaced. A three- or one-way tap is connected to the catheter and it is at this point that all manipulations take place. An extension set should be connected to this at the time of insertion or on return to the ward to prevent unnecessary handling near the skin exit site. The system will consist of catheter/tap/extension set/administration set and infusion device.

Legal and professional issues
Consent

Insertion is an operative procedure and consent must be obtained. Adequate explanation to the patient is essential, especially what to expect on return to the ward.

Procedure guideline 15.12 Intra-arterial administration of cytotoxic drugs

Essential equipment

- Sterile dressing pack
- Infusion pump containing the prescribed drug in a clinically clean tray (delivered from pharmacy reconstitution unit)
- Disposable gown and gloves
- Luer-Lok extension set with clamp
- Three-way tap

Preprocedure

Action	Rationale
1 Explain and discuss the procedure with the patient.	To ensure that the patient understands the procedure and gives their valid consent (Griffith *et al.* 2003, E; NMC 2008c, C).
2 Check the patient's prescription chart.	To ensure that the patient is given the correct drug and dose (NMC 2008a, C).

(Continued)

Procedure guideline 15.12 (*Continued*)

Procedure

3 Close room door or curtains if appropriate.	To ensure patient privacy and dignity. E
4 Assist the patient into the required position.	To allow access to the arterial device. E
5 Check confirmation of patency with medical and radiological team as necessary.	To confirm patency to ensure that the catherter is in the correct position (Hayden and Goodman 2005, E).
6 Use aseptic technique at all manipulations.	To minimize the risk of cross-infection (Hayden and Goodman 2005, E).
7 Attach the medication to the extension set, ensuring that the equipment is securely connected.	To minimize risk of air entry to the device or artery (Hayden and Goodman 2005, E).
8 Administer chemotherapy.	To ensure patient receives therapy as prescribed. E
9 Ensure that the dressing is secure.	To prevent dislodgement of the catheter (Hayden and Goodman 2005, E).

Postprocedure

10 Record the administration on appropriate charts.	To maintain accurate records, provide a point of reference in the event of any queries and prevent any duplication of treatment (NMC 2009, C; NPSA 2008a, C).
11 Observe for signs of bleeding.	To prevent haemorrhage (Hayden and Goodman 2005, E).

Problem-solving table 15.3 Prevention and resolution (Procedure guideline 15.12)

Problem	Cause	Prevention	Action
Displacement of the catheter	Dressing disturbed	Do not disturb the dressing. Ensure that the dressing and all equipment is connected securely and monitor site regularly	If bleeding occurs, pressure should be applied immediately and a member of the medical staff contacted
	Excessive movement by patient	Instruct the patient on amount of movement permitted. Check position daily	.

Postprocedural considerations

Immediate care

The dressing must not be touched but should be observed regularly for signs of bleeding and all Luer-Lok connections should be checked to prevent exsanguination, air embolism or disconnection under pressure. Any bleeding should be reported immediately to the medical staff, including the radiologist (Allwood *et al.* 2002).

Ongoing care

The catheter must be clamped securely or switched off, closing the tap *in situ* before any equipment changes. A positive pressure greater than arterial pressure must be maintained at all times. When chemotherapy is not being infused, the flushing solution must be used to maintain patency. This should be via a syringe or syringe pump during transfer between wards or departments, or via a syringe pump or infusion pump in the ward (when a nurse escort may be necessary). It should be delivered at the minimum rate sufficient to combat arterial pressure and maintain patency, approximately 3–5 mL per hour or 10 drops per minute, depending on the device used. If a specialist delivery system is used, then manufacturer's instructions should be followed.

The position of the catheter may be checked daily by X-ray, which will be performed on the ward. Fluoroscopy and instillation of dye are other methods of confirming position. At the end of treatment, the patency of the arterial catheter should be maintained using an appropriate flushing solution until a decision has been made about removal. Instructions for this and the amount of heparin to be used should be prescribed in advance to enable the nurse to initiate the procedure when appropriate. Before removal, the tap may be switched off and the catheter allowed to clot. The catheter should be removed by a doctor and firm pressure applied for at least 5 minutes or until all bleeding has ceased. A dressing should be applied to the site. Pressure dressings are not indicated if bleeding has ceased as they can obscure the formation of a haematoma.

Education of the patient and relevant others

The patient must be instructed on how often they are allowed to move and mobilize. This may vary depending on the site of the catheter. Assistance may be needed to maintain personal hygiene and relieve pressure in order to prevent the development of pressure ulcers on all points of contact.

Complications
Arterial occlusion and thrombosis

The literature indicates that thrombosis occurs in over 40% of arteries catheterized for over 48 hours. However, this is dependent on the vessel used. Most catheters used for chemotherapy delivery pose no problem and will remain patent for the treatment period. However, a thrombus may embolize, causing vascular insufficiency, distal or central embolism (Weinstein and Plumer 2007). When occlusion occurs due to thrombus formation or spasm, blood flow is usually maintained by the collateral circulation until the vessel recovers. Presence of a pulse and the colour of the area should be checked daily or a Doppler flow meter may be used. Any abnormality should be reported to the medical staff and radiologist. The catheter should be removed by the doctor using firm, steady traction, in an attempt to prevent dislodging any thrombus present. The condition of the patient and the limb/area should be observed carefully at the time that vital signs are measured.

Damage to the artery, arteriovenous fistula, aneurysm formation

The incidence of these is low and the likelihood of problems occurring can be minimized by gentle handling of the catheter and immobilization of the limb/area as soon as appropriate.

Chemical hepatitis and biliary sclerosis

The occurrence of these will be evident from elevated liver enzymes. Therefore, monitoring of liver function tests is important. Any elevation is usually transient.

Exsanguination/air embolism

The seriousness of an air embolus depends on the siting of the arterial catheter and whether it is a direct route to the carotid artery and so to the brain. Luer-Lok connections must be used throughout the pathway. These should be checked at regular intervals, and continuous flow maintained. Care must be taken when changing equipment to prevent blood loss occurring, or air entering the catheter, for example shut off the tap, firm clamping, if necessary.

Infection due to poor aseptic technique

Strict aseptic technique must be maintained for all procedures and manipulations of the arterial catheter (Weinstein and Plumer 2007).

Extravasation of the medication and failure of the medication to reach the target

Although these are both rare, they may occur as a consequence of incorrect placement of catheter. If there is any doubt concerning the placement of the catheter, the doctor and radiologist should be notified as extravasation of the medication may lead to ulceration and necrosis.

Side-effects

The systemic side-effects of chemotherapy vary for every individual and are influenced by the drug or combination of drugs that the patient is receiving (Schulmeister 2009). The essential prerequisite of chemotherapy delivery is a comprehensive medical or nursing assessment of the patient in order to ascertain fitness for treatment. The assessment also allows the determination of response to therapy (i.e. tumour markers) and regulating the dose of drugs in relation to toxicity (Dougherty and Bailey 2008). Using tools such as a Chemotherapy Symptom Assessment Scale (CSAS) can enhance the accuracy of reporting the patient's symptoms whilst receiving chemotherapy, which can have a positive impact upon the nursing and medical interventions offered. Such tools are essentially a patient-held record of symptoms following chemotherapy and reflect the extent to which the symptoms impact upon the daily life of the patient. The patient produces the record at each cycle of chemotherapy and the information is used to plan interventions to suit their individual needs (Brown *et al.* 2001, Dikken 2003).

Bone marrow suppression

Myelosuppression is one of the most common dose-limiting side-effects of chemotherapy (Schulmeister 2009). All chemotherapy has an effect on the bone marrow, resulting in a reduction in white blood cells, red blood cells and platelets. Myelosuppression that causes bleeding or infection can be life-threatening. Colony-stimulating factors (CSFs) enhance granulocyte production and shorten the nadir (the point at which the lowest blood count is reached after chemotherapy) (Schulmeister 2009).

Leucopenia

Leucopenia is classified as a lower than normal amount of white blood cells in the bloodstream. White blood cells are often categorized as granulocytes and agranulocytes. Granulocytes include neutrophils, which have a lifespan of 6 hours to a few days, eosinophils, which have a lifespan of 8–12 days, and basophils, which have a lifespan of a few hours to few days. CSFs such as filgrastim and pegfilgrastim can be used to manage neutropenia, a condition in which the number of neutrophils in the bloodstream is decreased, impairing the body's ability to fight infection (Campbell 2005).

Anaemia

The life of a red blood cell is 120 days. A patient is considered anaemic if the haemoglobin level is lower than 8 g/dL (Weinstein and Plumer 2007). Patients with anaemia may be asymptomatic or may manifest symptoms such as headache, light-headedness, shortness of breath, fatigue, pale skin and nail beds. A blood transfusion will help raise the haemoglobin levels. One unit of red blood cells can raise the haemoglobin by 1 g/dL (Schulmeister 2009). Erythropoietin can be used to stimulate red blood cell production (Weinstein and Plumer 2007).

Thrombocytopenia

Thrombocytopenia is classified as a lower than normal amount of platelets in the bloodstream. A normal range for the platelet count is 150,000–400,000 mm^3. The risk of bleeding increases if the platelet count reduces to 100,000/mm^3 (Schulmeister 2009). Signs and symptoms of bleeding include bruising, petechiae, bleeding from the gums and nose and haemorrhage in the central nervous system or gastrointestinal tract (Dougherty and Bailey 2008). Severe risk of bleeding is considered when the platelet count reaches 20,000/mm^3. Activities that carry a high risk, such as contact sports, should be avoided since they can cause injury and subsequent bleeding. Patients should be encouraged to report signs of spontaneous bruising, nosebleeds, bleeding gums and bloody stools (Weinstein and Plumer 2007). A low platelet count can delay the continuation of chemotherapy. Platelet transfusions can be given in order to manage thrombocytopenia.

Nausea and vomiting

Nausea and vomiting are two of the most common and distressing side-effects of chemotherapy (Schulmeister 2009). Approximately 70–80% of all cancer patients receiving chemotherapy experience vomiting (Weinstein and Plumer 2007). Chemotherapy-induced nausea and vomiting can be described as acute (occurring within 2 hours and lasting up to 24 hours), delayed (occurring 24 hours after chemotherapy administration) and anticipatory (which happens before and during chemotherapy administration, often as a result of conditioning from stimuli associated with the chemotherapy process or environment) (Dougherty and Bailey 2008). Factors predisposing to nausea and vomiting include age and gender, younger patients experience more nausea and vomiting than older patients and more females than males.

Successful management of nausea and vomiting is an approach that combines pharmacological intervention with non-pharmacological strategies. Antiemetic guidelines are available in most treatment centres and antiemetics should be commenced prior to treatment and continued throughout the emetic activity of the chemotherapy drug used (Weinstein and Plumer 2007). Non-pharmacological interventions such as acupressure have been reported to relieve nausea. Acupressure works on the principle of pressure being applied to the P6 (Pericardium) pressure point. The pressure point is located on the inner aspect of the wrist and the pressure band disc is placed three fingers' width from the wrist crease between the two tendons (Figure 15.9). Whilst it has been suggested that nausea can be relieved within the first 24 hours following chemotherapy, the pressure bands do not appear to have any impact upon vomiting (Dougherty and Bailey 2008).

Fatigue

Fatigue has been defined as an overwhelming sense of exhaustion and inability to perform physical or mental work,

Figure 15.9 Sea-bands on wrist.

that is, not relieved by rest (Weinstein and Plumer 2007). It is a common side-effect of chemotherapy (60% of patients) and is often not recognized, reported or treated (Schwartz 2007). Fatigue can also be a result of anaemia, infection, dehydration, electrolyte inbalances and poor nutritional status (Chapter 8). Interventions are focused upon conserving energy, resting or sleeping for short periods of time, and alternating periods of rest with activity in order to build up the body to maintain levels of functionality (Dougherty and Bailey 2008).

Taste changes/anorexia

Patients receiving chemotherapy can experience changes in taste as well as loss of appetite. Foods that the patient is used to eating can taste very different following chemotherapy (Weinstein and Plumer 2007). It is therefore important to ensure that a nutritional assessment forms part of the patient's care plan and that strategies are adopted to maximize nutritional well-being. Many patients complain of a bitter or metallic taste and can be advised to experiment with different flavours and spices, the aim of which is to stimulate the taste buds, making the mouth feel more comfortable (Schulmeister 2009). Plastic utensils can help reduce the metallic taste. Generally, patients find that cold food as opposed to hot is more palatable and that having meals served on glass rather than plastic helps reduce odours (Bernhardson et al. 2009).

Odours from cooking can have a negative impact upon the desire to eat and avoiding areas where food is being prepared is advised. Appetite stimulants can be prescribed if neccessary in an attempt to maintain a healthy diet. Nutritional supplements such as protein drinks, protein powders and soft foods may be required (Schulmeister 2009).

Constipation

Constipation is the passing of hard, dry stools, causing difficulty in defaecation (Weinstein and Plumer 2007). The severity of the problem can range from mild discomfort to paralytic ileus (Schulmeister 2009). There are many causes of constipation including side-effects of medication, hypercalcaemia, dehydration, immobility and dietary deficiencies. Chemotherapy agents such as vinca alkaloids (vincristine, vinblastine) commonly cause constipation secondary to automatic nerve dysfunction (Dougherty and Bailey 2008).

Prevention of constipation should be part of the medical and nursing assessment of the patient and prophylactic laxatives, lubricants or stimulants should be used. Education about prevention interventions is important and the patient should be instructed to increase their dietary intake of fresh fruits, vegetables and fibre. Patients should be encouraged to have 2–3 litres of fluid a day and to avoid cheese, eggs and starches (Weinstein and Plumer 2007). Since physical activity stimulates peristalsis, patients can be encouraged to be as mobile as possible. They should also be encouraged to defaecate immediately upon feeling the urge to do so and not to wait (Weinstein and Plumer 2007). See Chapter 6.

Diarrhoea

The function of the colon is to absorb fluid and when this does not happen, diarrhoea ensues. Diarrhoea is the abnormal passage of three or more loose or watery stools in a 24-hour period and is often accompanied by abdominal cramps (Schulmeister 2009). There are many causes of diarrhoea including postoperative intestinal resection, Clostridium difficile and other intestinal infections. Chemotherapy agents such as 5-fluorouracil, capecitabine, docetaxol, doxorubicin and methotrexate can cause diarrhoea (Dougherty and Bailey 2008).

Nursing interventions should focus on the early detection of the problem and patients should be encouraged to report symptoms promptly. Normal bowel activity should be assessed as well as the frequency of the diarrhoea and the patient's oral intake over a 24-hour period. Patients require a minimum of 2 litres of fluid in a 24-hour period because electrolytes are lost as a consequence of diarrhoea (Schulmeister 2009). Potassium is the most significant electrolyte to be redcued and the patient should be encouraged to eat potassium-rich foods (Weinstein and Plumer 2007). Intravenous fluid replacement as well as antimotility agents can be used in severe cases. A high-calorie, high-protein and low-residue diet is recommended (Dougherty and Bailey 2008). See Chapter 8.

Alopecia

Definition

Chemotherapy-induced alopecia is the temporary loss of all body hair (Dougherty 2005).

Anatomy and physiology

The hair follicle comprises a bulb at the base of the follicle. The actual hair is produced by cells in the hair matrix zone where nutrients and growth factors are provided by the dermal papilla. Keratinocytes in the hair matrix zone begin to rapidly divide and a keratinized hair emerges with a thin outer cuticle and a thin cortex (Janssen 2007). The hair follicle goes through three growth phases. Anagen is a phase of intensive growth and hair shaft production, which may last as long as 7 years. The hair then enters the catagen phase (involution) when the old hair shaft is broken down and a new hair follicle is formed. This lasts 2–3 weeks and is followed by the telogen phase (resting) which lasts 2–3 months and then an intermediate regrowing state starts and new hair follicles are produced.

Chemotherapy affects rapidly growing keratinocytes in the hair matrix zone in anagen hair follicles and a decrease in the diameter of the hair bulb can be seen 4–6 days after administration of a single dose (Olsen 2003). Not all the hair follicles have the same rhythm of cycling and as approximately 90% of hair follicles are in a phase of growth at any given time, the resulting hair loss can be rapid and extensive (Janssen 2007).

Related theory

Alopecia is a common consequence of many chemotherapeutic regimens and is one of the most devastating effects of cancer chemotherapy (Pickard-Holley 1995, Williams *et al.*1999). In a study of breast cancer survivors who completed a psychophysical scaling method, hair loss was ranked in the top five distressful side-effects of chemotherapy (Mulders *et al.* 2008), while Mols *et al.* (2009) found that the hair loss associated with chemotherapy was a source of distress for patients, and was rated in the three most troublesome side-effects of treatment, along with nausea and vomiting. Chemotherapy-induced alopecia adversely affects psychosocial functioning and quality of life (Hesketh *et al.* 2004, Lemieux *et al.* 2008, Rosman 2004). It has been identified as such a devastating prospect that some patients may refuse to accept treatment or choose regimens with less favourable outcomes (Boehmke and Dickerson 2005, Browall *et al.* 2006, Hesketh *et al.* 2004, Rosenblatt 2006, Williams *et al.* 1999). Hair loss can also result in changes to the patient's body image (Freedman 1994, Gallagher 1996, Williams *et al.* 1999) which may not be reversed by the regrowth of hair (Munstedt *et al.* 1997).

Prevention of chemotherapy-induced alopecia

Several techniques have been tested to prevent chemotherapy-induced hair loss, the first being scalp tourniquets. These were used to minimize the contact the drug had with the hair follicles by occluding, using pressure, the superficial blood vessels supplying the scalp (Maxwell 1980). However, while some investigators found scalp tourniquets effective, others reported this method to be time-consuming, uncomfortable or ineffective (Parker 1987). Research findings indicate that scalp hypothermia (cooling) may be simpler, less traumatic and more effective as a means of preventing alopecia when compared with the scalp tourniquet (David and Speechley 1987).

It has been documented that men and women experience similar concerns about body image when they have experienced chemotherapy-induced hair loss, although women tended to speak about hair loss from the head and face (above eyeline) while men spoke of losing hair from wider body surfaces (Hilton *et al.* 2008). Healthcare professionals must therefore be mindful that scalp cooling should be offered to patients as determined by the chemotherapy

regimen and not the gender of the patient (Hilton *et al.* 2008).

In a study in which patients receiving chemotherapy for breast cancer who underwent scalp cooling were given questionnaires to complete before chemotherapy, after 3 weeks of treatment and 6 months after completion, they rated the burden of scalp cooling as low, suggesting that nursing staff must be aware of how distressing the matter of hair loss can be for patients, and scalp cooling should be offered wherever possible (Mols *et al.* 2009). Physicians tend to underestimate the impact of hair loss on patients so it may be up to the nurse to provide information on scalp cooling (Mulders *et al.* 2008, Rosman 2004).

Scalp cooling is a method of preventing chemotherapy-induced alopecia. It works in three ways (Batchelor 2001, Bulow *et al.* 1985).

1 Reducing perfusion of hair follicles by vasoconstriction, thus limiting the amount of exposure of chemotherapy (an intradermal scalp temperature of 30°C decreases scalp blood flow by 25%).
2 Reduced temperature-dependent cellular uptake of chemotherapy.
3 Reduced intrafollicular metabolic rate.

The rationale is based on characteristics of hair growth, the effect of cytotoxic drugs on hair follicles, physiological changes in scalp circulation and pharmacokinetics (Keller and Blausey 1988). Ninety percent of all scalp hair is in an active phase of growth, characterized by significant mitotic activity; this means the hair bulb is especially sensitive to chemotherapeutic agents (Parker 1987). Scalp hypothermia produces changes in the scalp circulation by causing vasoconstriction of superficial vessels. Decreased blood flow to the scalp reduces the amount of the drug reaching the hair follicles and thus minimizes damage to the scalp hair (Kennedy *et al.* 1983, Parker 1987). Its success is also related to the metabolic effects of cooling, that is, slowing the metabolic rate (Bulow *et al.* 1985), and it also appears that the degree of hair loss is temperature dependent.

In order to prevent alopecia, the temperature of the scalp must be reduced to at least 24°C but preferably 22°C (Gregory *et al.* 1982). Caps have to be kept in a freezer in order to reach temperatures of −18 to −20°C (Anderson *et al.* 1981, Giaccone *et al.* 1988, Kennedy *et al.* 1983). Then when the cap is placed on the head, the scalp temperature will drop from 37°C to 23–24°C within the first 15 minutes (Guy *et al.* 1982, Tollenaar *et al.* 1994). This is why a preinjection scalp cooling time of 20–30 minutes is said to be required (Anderson *et al.* 1981, Giaccone *et al.* 1988, Kennedy *et al.* 1983, Middleton *et al.* 1985, Robinson *et al.* 1987, Satterwhite and Zimm 1984). Janssen (2007) studied the link between heat transfer in the human head and the transport of doxorubicin. This led to the development of a population-based computational model for scalp cooling which included doses of doxorubicin of 60–70 mg, lowering skin temperature to 17–18°C, leaving the cap on for the total infusion time plus 1 hour and having a haircut to reduce thermal resistance between head and cap, all of which provided the most effective scalp cooling.

Scalp cooling has been used in an attempt to reduce hair loss with palliative whole-brain radiotherapy. However, a pilot study (Shah *et al.* 2000) found that all patients still lost their hair and there was evidence that the cold cap application increased the dose of radiotherapy to the scalp.

More recently, biological methods of preventing hair loss have focused on promoting hair growth or protecting the hair follicles (Batchelor 2001). For example:

- minoxidil 2% topical solution applied twice a day (Shapiro and Price 1998)
- topical topitriol (Hidalgo *et al.* 1999)
- application of a steroid 5-alpha reductase inhibitor (Uno and Kurata 1993)
- immunosuppressive immunophilin ligands such as ciclosporin (Maurer *et al.* 1997), immunomodulators, AS101 (Sredni *et al.* 1996), CDK2 inhibitors (Davis *et al.* 2001) and P53 (a mediator of cellular response which is essential for chemotherapy-induced hair loss) (Botchkarev *et al.* 2000).

Evidence-based approaches

Rationale

Indications

All patients with solid tumours receiving doxorubicin, epirubicin or docetaxel as a single agent or in combination should be offered scalp cooling.

Contraindications

Scalp cooling should not be offered to patients:

- with haematological disease unless the consultant feels it is appropriate to offer scalp cooling on the basis of quality of life
- receiving drugs that cause hair loss, for example vincristine, where there is no research or evidence of the effectiveness of scalp cooling
- who have already received a first course of chemotherapy which may induce hair loss but who were not offered or declined scalp cooling.

(Dougherty 2005)

Principles of care

Scalp cooling

The effectiveness of scalp cooling has been demonstrated satisfactorily with doxorubicin, epirubicin, docetaxel and paclitaxel (Dean *et al.* 1979, Katsimbri *et al.* 2000, Lemenager *et al.* 1995, Robinson *et al.* 1987). Patients receiving other cytotoxic drugs which may cause alopecia, such as vindesine and vincristine, have undergone the procedure, although there are insufficient data to evaluate its effectiveness with these drugs.

Doxorubin is commonly used in cancer chemotherapy and has a uniquely short half-life of approximately 30 minutes (compared to other drugs, such as cyclophosphamide which has a plasma half-life of over 6 hours) (Priestman 1989). This factor makes prophylactic scalp cooling feasible because it need only be utilized during peak plasma levels (Cline 1984). This is particularly important since doxorubicin results in a consistently high incidence of alopecia (80–90% of all patients), often leading to total hair loss (Dean *et al.* 1983). The involvement of doxorubicin, whether used alone or in combination, is a feature of most of the reported scalp-cooling studies. In some studies, there was less success in maintaining hair with increasing doses of doxorubicin and/or liver metastases (David and Speechley 1987, Dean *et al.* 1983), but this may be resolved by extending the time the cap remains in place following chemotherapy administration.

Scalp cooling has also been used during the administration of epirubicin, as a single agent, with good results (Robinson *et al.* 1987), although doses may influence outcomes (Adams *et al.* 1992). Subsequent studies have investigated combination regimens containing epirubicin and other drugs such as cyclophosphamide and 5-fluorouracil, with results of mild to moderate hair loss. However, when intravenous cyclophosphamide is added to anthracycline, the success rate is reduced from 80% of patients keeping most of their hair to about 50–60% of patients (David and Speechley 1987, Middleton *et al.* 1985). Some authors have therefore concluded that when combinations of cyclophosphamide and anthracyclines are given, scalp cooling has no place at all (Tollenaar *et al.* 1994). The group of drugs known as the taxanes also have the unfortunate side-effect of total alopecia; however, there is now evidence that using scalp cooling in patients receiving docetaxel and paclitaxel can prevent complete hair loss (Katsimbri *et al.* 2000, Lemenager *et al.* 1995, 1997, Macduff *et al.* 2003).

Scalp cooling requires the consultant's permission as the procedure may protect micrometastases in the scalp from chemotherapy, especially where there is the possibility of circulating cancer cells, for example in cases of leukaemia and lymphoma (Witman *et al.* 1981). In spite of this, scalp cooling has been used successfully in patients with relapsed lymphoma (Purohit 1992). Dean *et al.* (1983), drawing on evidence from 7800 women with breast cancer, found that only two experienced recurrence of disease on the scalp, suggesting that the risk of scalp metastases was minimal. They concluded that scalp cooling should not be contraindicated and could be used routinely with a wide variety of solid tumours. Nevertheless, patients with advanced metastatic disease have been found to develop scalp metastases during scalp cooling and Middleton *et al.* (1985) argued strongly against the use of scalp cooling in this group. Other studies have found no scalp metastases at follow-up (Ron *et al.* 1997). Lemieux *et al.* (2008) found the incidence of scalp metastases was low and no case presented as an isolated site of relapse. However, the potential risk of scalp metastases, albeit remote, should be addressed and demands discussion by healthcare professionals and patients (Batchelor 2001, Peck *et al.* 2000).

The issues relating to scalp metastases are controversial. This dilemma, along with the media coverage regarding preventive measures for chemotherapy-induced alopecia (Carr 1998, Kendell 2001), have led some practitioners to question whether scalp cooling should be offered.

Patients have highlighted how they feel about hair loss (Carr 1998) and also the need to provide more comfortable and effective scalp cooling in all cancer units and centres (Wilson 1994). In addition, an extensive review of the literature concluded that scalp cooling was effective and should be offered to all patients for whom it was appropriate (Batchelor 2001, Crowe *et al.* 1998). This was supported by the views of many nurses who felt that the use of scalp cooling with chemotherapy protocols which are associated with hair loss can effectively prevent alopecia and result in improved quality of life for patients (Lemenager 1998). Patients also feel it is worthwhile to undergo scalp cooling regardless of how successful it is (Dougherty 2006b). However, whilst scalp cooling contributes to well-being in successfully scalp-cooled patients, it can cause additional distress when patients lose their hair despite scalp cooling and so additional support may be required for those patients when scalp cooling is not successful (van den Hurk *et al.* 2010).

Limitations of scalp-cooling studies

Despite the large number of studies on scalp cooling, they are difficult to compare with one another, owing to the many variables: different types of scalp-cooling caps, varying methods of applying the caps, different chemotherapy regimens, tools for assessment of hair loss and who performs the assessment. Also sample numbers are often small and few studies are randomized or have a control group (Dougherty 2006b, Grevelman and Breed 2005). This results in difficulties when making decisions related to selection of scalp-cooling systems, discussing the risk of scalp metastases, or even whether to offer scalp cooling at all (Breed 2004, Christodoulou *et al.* 2002, Grevelman and Breed 2005, Randall and Ream 2005).

Anticipated patient outcomes

The success of all these methods of preventing hair loss varies and the amount of hair loss experienced by the patient is dependent on a number of factors.

- Involvement of the liver with metastatic disease leads to elevated plasma levels of doxorubicin for a longer period. Early studies seemed to indicate that extension of the cooling period did not improve the results (Satterwhite and Zimm 1984) but more recent studies are finding that longer cooling times in general improve success rates (Massey 2004).

- Inadequate cooling because of exceptionally thick hair may lead to partial loss. It has been demonstrated that maximum cooling occurs 20 minutes after the cap has been placed in position.
- The weight of the cap (as well as the temperature) may be a factor, as this ensures that the contact is maintained over the complete scalp (Hunt *et al.* 1982).
- Success does not appear to be dose dependent, as was first thought (David and Speechley 1987, Dougherty 2006b).
- It seems likely that when anthracyclines are used in combination with other drugs that cause alopecia (e.g. etoposide and cyclophosphamide), the success rate is not as high as with anthracyclines alone (Middleton *et al.* 1985). It has also been found that the type of anthracycline used will affect success rates as hair loss is greater with doxorubicin and cyclophosphamide than when using epirubicin and cyclophosphamide (Dougherty 2006b).

Legal and professional issues
Consent

Patients must give consent for the procedure but must first be fully informed about the nature and length of the procedure, the chances of success and, where appropriate, the risk of scalp metastases (Peck *et al.* 2000). Scalp cooling can be a long and uncomfortable procedure and should not be offered unless it is beneficial or the patient insists on undergoing the procedure. Patients must also be informed that they may discontinue the procedure at any time if they find it too physically or psychologically traumatic (Tierney 1987) or if they fail to retain hair.

Research shows that scalp cooling can be very distressing (Tierney 1989), although patients still find it a worthwhile procedure to undergo regardless of whether or not it is successful and many would have it again if necessary (Dougherty 1996, 2006b). It has also been shown that the severity and distress associated with hair loss may be less for those who use scalp cooling (Protiere *et al.* 2002).

Preprocedural considerations
Equipment

Most of the studies that used an ice cap method of scalp cooling used a 'home-made' or commercial cap (Anderson *et al.* 1981, David and Speechley 1987, Dean *et al.* 1983, Lemenager *et al.* 1997).

Home-made caps

Initially scalp cooling was achieved using crushed ice in plastic bags (Dean *et al.* 1979). A study of the efficacy of using a moulded prefrozen ice cap hand-made from cryogel bags was conducted at the Royal Marsden Hospital (Anderson *et al.* 1981, David and Speechley 1987).

Cryogel caps

The first commercial cap (Kold Kap) was successful in reducing hair loss, particularly with higher doses of doxorubicin (Dean *et al.* 1983). A three-layer cap (inner cotton, middle cryogel, outer lamb's wool) was also reported to prevent total hair loss (Howard and Stenner 1983). However, Wheelock *et al.* found that most patients suffered from severe hair loss even with the use of the Kold Kap (Wheelock *et al.* 1984). The most recent work has involved the use of cryogel caps such as the Chemocap and Penguin caps, which have been used for patients receiving single agents and combinations of anthracyclines (Christodoulou *et al.* 2002, Katsimbri *et al.* 2000, Peck *et al.* 2000) as well as in the use of docetaxel (Lemenager *et al.* 1995, 1997).

A large (170 patients) randomized study comparing Chemocap with the gelpack method found no statistical difference in efficacy between the two caps but Chemocap was shown to be more comfortable and offered a better fit, as well as being easier to use (Dougherty 2006b).

Scalp-cooling machines

Attempts have been made to produce an alternative type of cap that would improve the effectiveness of scalp cooling, in particular to ensure a sufficiently low and constant reduction in scalp temperature that would endure during the entire procedure. Two types of scalp-cooling machine have been designed.

1 The use of refrigerated air passed over the patient's scalp via a hair-drying helmet was reported to be beneficial in over 50% of patients, with most experiencing no hair loss or slight hair loss and six requiring a wig (Symonds *et al.* 1986). However, other authors found that the system was only successful at lower doses of epirubicin (Adams *et al.* 1992).

2 Refrigerated cooling systems where liquid coolant is pumped via a cap and maintains a more reliable temperature. Guy *et al.* (1982) reported encouraging results when the thermocirculator was first introduced, although Tollenaar *et al.* (1994) found that when used with patients receiving fluorouracil, epirubicin and cyclophosphamide (FEC), there was still a 50% chance of total alopecia occurring. The newer scalp-cooling machines appear to provide a more comfortable and effective system, for example Paxman or Dignitana (Henriksen and Jensen 2003, Massey 2004, Ridderheim *et al.* 2003, Spaeth *et al.* 2008) (Figures 15.10, 15.11).

Figure 15.10 Paxman machine.

Figure 15.11 Dignitana machine.

Procedure guideline 15.13 **Scalp cooling**

Essential equipment

- A scalp-cooling cap, for example Chemocap, or machine, for example Paxman scalp-cooling machine
- Overcap
- Skin protection, for example gauze, cotton wool pads
- Comfortable chair (recliner) or bed
- Extra pillows and blankets as required
- Equipment to wet and condition patient's hair as determined by manufacturer's instructions

Preprocedure

Action	Rationale
1 Before beginning, it is important to explain and discuss the procedure fully with the patient. Explain that the coldest and most uncomfortable time is the first 15 minutes after the cap has been applied. The patient should understand that the scalp cooling can be discontinued at any time and that it will not jeopardize the chemotherapy.	To ensure that the patient understands the procedure and what the success rate is likely to be depending on the type of chemotherapy regimen they are receiving (Dougherty 2006b, R2b). Patients who have undergone scalp cooling highlighted this as important knowledge to share when first undergoing the procedure (Dougherty 2006b, R2b). To ensure that the patient gives their valid consent and knows that if the scalp cooling does not work, they can obtain a wig (NMC 2008c, C).

Procedure

2 Check the cap has been in the freezer for a minimum of 12 hours (temperature –25 to –32°C), or that the machine has been cooled to the recommended temperature.	To ensure the cap is cold enough to be effective (manufacturer's recommendations, C).
3 If necessary wet hair and the place the cap on the patient's head, making sure it fits closely and covers the whole hairline (see Action Figure 3).	To ensure cooling over the head, including all the hair roots. E
4 Apply the overcap to the patient's head (see Action Figure 4).	To ensure even and close contact of the cap to the scalp (Dougherty 2006b, R2b).
5 Place protection in any areas where the cap touches the skin.	To prevent cold injury and improve the patient's comfort. E, P
6 Place a pillow behind the patient's head if required.	To provide support for the patient's head and neck and to reduce the effect of the heaviness of the cap (P; Dougherty 1996, R2b).
7 Offer the patient the use of a blanket.	To provide the patient with some protection against the feeling of cold (P; Dougherty 1996, R2b).
8 Leave the patient for at least 15 minutes before injection of the drug.	To obtain initial cooling of the scalp (Dougherty 2006b, R2b; Hunt et al. 1982, R4; Lemenager et al. 1997, R2b).
9 Administer the drug by intravenous injection as per prescription.	To administer treatment as appropriate. E
10 The cap must be changed after 30 minutes regardless of the stage of administration or, if using a machine, the cap must be on continuously for the recommended times.	To maintain adequate cooling (Dougherty 2006b, R2b; Hunt et al. 1982, R4; Lemenager et al. 1997, R2b).
11 If a drug takes longer than 30 minutes to administer, the cap will need to be changed after 45–60 minutes and then every hour thereafter depending on the type of drug and the temperature of the freezer.	To maintain adequate cooling (Dougherty 2006b, R2b; Janssen 2007, R2b).

12 On completion of the drug (i.e. the one likely to cause alopecia, for example doxorubicin), leave the patient for a further 45 minutes or according to the manufacturer's recommendations.	To maintain cooling until the plasma levels of drug have fallen (Dougherty 2006b, R2b; Hunt *et al.* 1982, R4; Janssen 2007, R2b; Lemenager *et al.* 1997, R2b).
13 When sufficient time has elapsed, remove the cap.	To prevent damage to the scalp and hair. E, P

Postprocedure

14 Encourage the patient to rest, if desired.	To prevent the patient feeling faint when the cap is lifted off the head. P, E
15 Wash or wipe the cap with detergent wipes, dry and store on cardboard insert or according to manufacturer's instructions.	To minimize cross-infection and to maintain shape (DH 2007, C).
16 Ensure the patient is given a patient information booklet on how to care for hair and manage hair loss.	To reinforce verbal information given during procedure. E, P

Action Figure 3 Place the cap on the patient's head, making sure it fits closely and covers the whole hairline.

Action Figure 4 Apply the overcap to the patient's head.

Problem-solving table 15.4 Prevention and resolution (Procedure guideline 15.13)

Problem	Cause	Prevention	Action
Inadequate cooling	Poorly fitting cap. Cap not sufficiently cooled	Select correct size cap for each individual patient Ensure that caps are maintained at correct temperature Follow the procedure correctly	Check that the cap fits and is the correct size and that the hair roots are covered. Ensure the cap is changed at correct times. Check the cap has been cooled to the correct temperature
Excess cooling	Thin hair	Use plenty of gauze between the cap and scalp	Apply more gauze. If it is still painful then discontinue the procedure
Complaints of headache	Weight and coldness of cap	Warn patient of weight and cold sensation. Provide physical support to the neck and shoulders and blankets as required	Provide more support and warmth. Reassure patient that it will ease off as cooling continues
Distressed patient	Claustrophobia	Discuss with patient and allow them to try cap on before starting procedure	Support and reassure the patient. If necessary, remove the cap
	Ice phobia	Discuss with patient and allow them to try cap on before starting procedure	Be aware of this possible problem; encourage the patient to discuss their feelings
Hair loss	Scalp cooling was not successful	Use correct size cap and cool for recommended time	Offer the patient the opportunity to discontinue the scalp cooling. Make arrangements for the patient to see the appliance officer and obtain a wig. Discuss care of hair and scalp and give patient information booklet

Postprocedural considerations

Immediate care

It is important to ensure that if a patient fails to retain hair or decides not to undergo scalp cooling, adequate time is spent helping the patient to adapt to the hair loss physically, psychologically and socially. It is recommended that nursing interventions be directed towards helping the patient and family to adapt to alopecia by using patient education, available resources and supportive listening (Pickard-Holley 1995). This can be partly achieved by ensuring that the patient sees the surgical appliance officer as soon as possible, in order to obtain a wig that can be matched to the patient's desired hair style and colour.

Ongoing care

Advice can be given on hair care such as the type of shampoo. There is a misconception that a mild shampoo such as baby shampoo is best, but this kind of shampoo is alkaline and it is recommended that a neutral pH shampoo be used (Dougherty 2005, 2006b). Using a wide-toothed comb can

prevent pulling on hair but the patient should not be afraid to comb hair daily (Dougherty 2006b). Patients should be advised to avoid anything that can dry out their hair such as using hair dryers, curlers, and so on, or using chemicals such as perming lotions or hair dyes, and should seek advice from a hairdresser. Finally the patient should be given advice about the use of head covering such as hats, turbans and scarves. All verbal information should be reinforced with a hair care information booklet (Batchelor 2001, Pickard-Holley 1995).

Complications

Patients have reported adverse effects during and following treatment such as headaches, claustrophobia, dizziness and ice phobias (Dougherty 2006b, Mols et al. 2009, Rosman 2004). Nurses need to understand the meaning that hair loss has for the patient. Alopecia can cause depression, loss of self-confidence and humiliation: it is a very visible sign of cancer. Patients who have relapsed and are undergoing further chemotherapy which causes alopecia may find the loss of hair a second time to be more devastating (Gallagher 1996).

References

Adams, L., Lawson, N., Maxted, K.J. and Symonds, R.P. (1992) The prevention of hair loss from chemotherapy by the use of cold-air scalp-cooling. *European Journal of Cancer Care,* **1** (5), 16–19.

Aisner, J. (2007) Overview of the changing paradigm in cancer treatment: oral chemotherapy. *American Journal of Health-System Pharmacy,* **64** (9 Suppl 5), S4–S7.

Allwood, M.C., Wright, P. and Stanley, A. (eds) (2002) *The Cytotoxics Handbook,* 4th edn. Radcliff, Oxford.

Anderson, J.E., Hunt, J.M. and Smith, I.E. (1981) Prevention of doxorubicin-induced alopecia by scalp cooling in patients with advanced breast cancer. *BMJ,* **282** (6262), 423–424.

Barefoot, J., Bletcher, C.S. and Emery, R. (2009) Keeping pace with oral chemotherapy. *Oncology Issues,* **24** (3), 36–39.

Batchelor, D. (2001) Hair and cancer chemotherapy: consequences and nursing care – a literature study. *European Journal of Cancer Care,* **10** (3), 147–163.

Bedell, C.H. (2003) A changing paradigm for cancer treatment: the advent of new oral chemotherapy agents. *Clinical Journal of Oncology Nursing,* **7** (6 Suppl), 5–9.

Bernhardson, B., Tishelman, C. and Rutqvist, L.E. (2009) Taste and smell changes in patients receiving cancer chemotherapy: distress, impact on daily life and self care strategies. *Cancer Nursing,* **32** (1), 45–54.

Bertelli, G. (1995) Prevention and management of extravasation of cytotoxic drugs. *Drug Safety,* **12** (4), 245–255.

Birner, A.M., Bedell, M.K., Avery, J.T. and Ernstoff, M.S. (2006) Program to support safe administration of oral chemotherapy. *Journal of Oncology Practice,* **2** (1), 5–6.

BNF (2011) *British National Formulary.* British Medical Association/Pharmaceutical Society of Great Britain, London.

Boehmke, M.M. and Dickerson, S.S. (2005) Symptom, symptom experiences, and symptom distress encountered by women with breast cancer undergoing current treatment modalities. *Cancer Nursing,* **28** (5), 382–389.

BOPA (2004) Position statement on safe practice and the pharmaceutical care of patients receiving oral anticancer chemotherapy, in *British National Formulary.* Pharmaceutical Press, London.

Botchkarev, V.A., Komarova, E.A., Siebenhaar, F. *et al.* (2000) p53 is essential for chemotherapy-induced hair loss. *Cancer Research,* **60** (18), 5002–5006.

Breed, W.P. (2004) What is wrong with the 30-year-old practice of scalp cooling for the prevention of chemotherapy-induced hair loss? *Supportive Care in Cancer,* **12** (1), 3–5.

Browall, M., Gaston-Johansson, F. and Danielson, E. (2006) Postmenopausal women with breast cancer: their experiences of the chemotherapy treatment period. *Cancer Nursing,* **29** (1), 34–42.

Brown, V., Sitzia, J., Richardson, A., Hughes, J., Harrison, H. and Oakley, C. (2001) The development of the Chemotherapy Symptom Assessment Scale (C-SAS): a scale for the routine clinical assessment of the symptom experiences of patients receiving cytotoxic chemotherapy. *International Journal of Nursing Studies,* **38** (5), 497–510.

Bulow, J., Friberg, L., Gaardsting, O. and Hansen, M. (1985) Frontal subcutaneous blood flow, and epi- and subcutaneous temperatures during scalp cooling in normal man. *Scandinavian Journal of Clinical and Laboratory Investigation,* **45** (6), 505–508.

Campbell, K. (2005) Blood cells. Part three–granulocytes and monocytes. *Nursing times,* **101** (42), 26–7.

Camp-Sorrell, D. (1998) Developing extravasation protocols and monitoring outcomes. *Journal of Intravenous Nursing,* **21** (4), 232–239.

Camp-Sorrell, D. (2005) *Oncology Nursing Society Access Device Guidelines: Recommendations for Nursing Practice and Education.* Oncology Nursing Society, Pittsburgh, PA.

Cardonick, E. and Iacobucci, A. (2004) Use of chemotherapy during human pregnancy. *Lancet Oncology,* **5** (5), 283–291.

Carr, K. (1998) How I survived the fall out. *You Magazine, Mail on Sunday,* 10 May, pp. 61–67.

Chaudhary, R.T. (2007) Malignanat pleural, peritoneal and pericardial effusions and meningeal infiltrates, in *Handbook of Cancer Chemotherapy,* 7th edn (ed. R.T. Skeel). Lippincott, Philadelphia.

Christodoulou, C., Klouvas, G., Efstathiou, E. *et al.* (2002) Effectiveness of the MSC cold cap system in the prevention of chemotherapy-induced alopecia. *Oncology,* **62** (2), 97–102.

Cline, B.W. (1984) Prevention of chemotherapy-induced alopecia: a review of the literature. *Cancer Nursing,* **7** (3), 221–228.

Comerford, K., Eggenberger, T. and Robinson, K. (2002) Chemotherapy infusions, in *Intravenous Therapy Made Incredibly Easy.* Springhouse Publishing, Philadelphia.

CP Pharmaceuticals (1999) *How Quickly Could you Act?* CP Pharmaceuticals, Wrexham.

Crowe, M., Kendrick, M. and Woods, S. (1998) *Is Scalp Cooling a Procedure that should be Offered to Patients Recieving Alopecia Induced Chemotherapy for Solid Tumours?* Proceedings of 10th International Conference on Cancer Nursing, Jerusalem.

David, J. and Speechley, V. (1987) Scalp cooling to prevent alopecia. *Nursing Times,* **83** (32), 36–37.

Davis, S.T., Benson, B.G., Bramson, H.N. *et al.* (2001) Prevention of chemotherapy-induced alopecia in rats by CDK inhibitors. *Science,* **291** (5501), 134–137.

Dean, J.C., Salmon, S.E. and Griffith, K.S. (1979) Prevention of doxorubicin-induced hair loss with scalp hypothermia. *New England Journal of Medicine,* **301** (26), 1427–1429.

Dean, J.C., Griffith, K.S., Cetas, T.C. *et al.* (1983) Scalp hypothermia: a comparison of ice packs and the Kold Kap in the prevention of doxorubicin-induced alopecia. *Journal of Clinical Oncology,* **1** (1), 33–37.

DH (1999) *Latex Medical Gloves and Powdered Latex Medical Gloves: Reducing the Risk of Allergic Reaction to Latex and Powdered Medical Gloves,* Department of Health, London. www.dh.gov.uk/prod_consum_dh/groups/dh_digitalassets/@dh/@en/documents/digitalasset/dh_4012106.pdf.

DH (2000) *An Organisation with a Memory.* Department of Health, London. www.dh.gov.uk/prod_consum_dh/groups/dh_digitalassets/@dh/@en/documents/digitalasset/dh_4065086.pdf.

DH (2005) *Hazardous Waste (England) Regulations.* Department of Health, London.

DH (2007) *Cancer Reform Strategy.* Department of Health, London. www.dh.gov.uk/prod_consum_dh/groups/dh_digitalassets/documents/digitalasset/dh_081007.pdf.

DH (2008) Updated National Guidance on the Safe Administration of Intrathecal Chemotherapy. www.dh.gov.uk/prod_consum_dh/groups/dh_digitalassets/documents/digitalasset/dh_086844.pdf.

DH (2009a) *Reference Guide to Consent for Examination or Treatment,* 2nd edn. Department of Health, London. www.dh.gov.uk/en/Publicationsandstatistics/Publications/PublicationsPolicyAndGuidance/DH_103643.

DH (2009b) *The Operating Framework Enabling High Quality Care Throughout the NHS.* Department of Health, London.

Dikken, C. (2003) Benefits of using a chemotherapy symptom assessment scale. *Nursing Times,* **99** (39), 50.

Doellman, D., Hadaway, L., Bowe-Geddes, L.A. *et al.* (2009) Infiltration and extravasation: update on prevention and management. *Journal of Infusion Nursing,* **32** (4), 203–211.

927

Dougherty, L. (1996) Scalp cooling to prevent hair loss in chemotherapy. *Professional Nurse*, 11 (8), 507–509.

Dougherty, L. (2003) The expert witness: working within the legal system of the United Kingdom. *Journal of Vascular Access Devices*, 8 (2), 29–35.

Dougherty, L. (2005) Alopecia, in *The Royal Marsden Hospital Handbook of Cancer Chemotherapy: A Guide for the Multidisciplinary Team* (eds D. Brighton and M. Wood). Elsevier Churchill Livingstone, Edinburgh, pp.197–200.

Dougherty, L. (2006a) *Central Venous Access Devices: Care and Management*. Blackwell Publishing, Oxford.

Dougherty, L. (2006b) Comparing methods to prevent chemotherapy-induced alopecia. *Cancer Nursing Practice*, 5 (6), 25–31.

Dougherty, L. (2008) IV therapy: recognizing the differences between infiltration and extravasation. *British Journal of Nursing*, 17 (14), 896, 898–901.

Dougherty, L. and Bailey, C. (2008) Chemotherapy, in *Cancer Nursing Care in Context* (eds J. Corner and C. Bailey). Wiley-Blackwell, Chichester.

Dranitsaris, G., Johnston, M., Poirier, S. *et al.* (2005) Are health care providers who work with cancer drugs at an increased risk for toxic events? A systematic review and meta-analysis of the literature. *Journal of Oncology Pharmacy Practice*, 11 (2), 69–78.

Elkin, M.K., Perry, A.G. and Potter, P.A. (2007) *Nursing Interventions and Clinical Skills*, 4th edn. Mosby, St Louis, MO.

El-Saghir, N., Otrock, Z., Mufarrij, A. *et al.* (2004) Dexrazoxane for anthracycline extravasation and GM-CSF for skin ulceration and wound healing. *Lancet Oncology*, 5 (5), 320–321.

European Oncology Nursing Society (2007) *Extravasation Guidelines: Guidelines Implementation Toolkit*. European Oncology Nursing Society, Brussels.

Ferguson, L. and Wright, P. (2002) Health and safety aspects of cytotoxics services, in *The Cytotoxics Handbook*, 4th edn (eds M. Allwood and A. Stanley). Radcliffe Medical Press, Oxford, pp.35–62.

Few, B.J. (1987) Hyaluronidase for treating intravenous extravasations. *MCN: The American Journal of Maternal Child Nursing*, 12 (1), 23–24.

Findlay, M., von Minckwitz, G. and Wardley, A. (2008) Effective oral chemotherapy for breast cancer: pillars of strength. *Annals of Oncology*, 19 (2), 212–222.

Flynn, M., Dougherty, L., Freires, M. *et al.* (2010) *Designing and implementing a generic vascular access assessment tool into clinical cancer practice*. Poster presentation, UKONS conference, October 14–18, Manchester.

Fraise, A.P. and Bradley, T. (eds) (2009) *Ayliffe's Control of Healthcare-associated Infection: A Practical Handbook*, 5th edn. Hodder Arnold, London.

Freedman, T.G. (1994) Social and cultural dimensions of hair loss in women treated for breast cancer. *Cancer Nursing*, 17 (4), 334–341.

Gabriel, J. (2008) Safe administration of intravenous cytotoxic drugs, in *Intravenous Therapy in Nursing Practice*, 2nd edn (eds L. Dougherty and J. Lamb). Blackwell Publishing, Oxford, pp.461–494.

Gallagher, J. (1996) *Women's Experiences of Hair Loss Associated with Chemotherapy – Longitudinal Perspective*. 9th International Conference on Cancer Nursing, Brighton.

Gault, D. (1993) Extravasation injuries. *British Journal of Plastic Surgery*, 46 (2), 91–96.

Gault, D. and Challands, J. (1997) Extravasation of drugs. *Anaesthesia Review*, 13, 223–241.

Giaccone, G., Di Giulio, F., Morandini, M.P. and Calciati, A. (1988) Scalp hypothermia in the prevention of doxorubicin-induced hair loss. *Cancer Nursing*, 11 (3), 170–173.

Goodin, S. (2007) Safe Handling of Oral Chemo Agents in Community Settings. www.dh.gov.uk/prod_consum_dh/groups/dh_digitalassets/documents/digitalasset/dh_086844.pdf.

Goolsby, T.V. and Lombardo F.A. (2006) Extravasation of chemotherapeutic agents: prevention and treatment. *Seminars in Oncology*, 33 (1), 139–143.

Gregory, R.P., Cooke, T., Middleton, J. *et al.* (1982) Prevention of doxorubicin-induced alopedia by scalp hypothermia: relation to degree of cooling. *BMJ*, 284 (6330), 1674.

Grevelman, E.G. and Breed, W.P. (2005) Prevention of chemotherapy-induced hair loss by scalp cooling. *Annals of Oncology*, 16 (3), 352–358.

Griffin, E. (2003) Safety considerations and safe handling of oral chemotherapy agents. *Clinical Journal of Oncology Nursing*, 7 (6 Suppl), 25–29.

Griffith, R., Griffiths, H. and Jordan, S. (2003) Administration of medicines. Part 1: The law and nursing. *Nursing Standard*, 18 (2), 47–53.

Guy, R., Shah, S., Parker, H. and Geddes, D. (1982) Scalp cooling by thermocirculator. *Lancet*, 1 (8278), 937–938.

Harrison, B. (2008) Risks of handling cytotoxic drugs: a review, in *The Chemotherapy Source Book*, 4th edn (ed. W.K. Health). Lippincott Williams and Wilkins, Philadelphia, pp.566–582.

Hartigan, K. (2003) Patient education: the cornerstone of successful oral chemotherapy treatment. *Clinical Journal of Oncology Nursing*, 7 (6 Suppl), 21–24.

Hayden, B.K. and Goodman M. (2005) Chemotherapy: principles of administration, in *Cancer Nursing: Principles and Practice*, 6th edn (eds C.H. Yarbro, M.H. Frogge and M. Goodman). Jones and Bartlett, Sudbury, MA, pp.351–411.

Henricksen, T. and Jensen, B.K. (2003) Advanced computerised cold cap for preventing chemothepray induced alopecia. Paper presented at ECCO, Copenhagen, 21–25th September.

Hesketh, P.J., Batchelor, D., Golant, M. *et al.* (2004) Chemotherapy-induced alopecia: psychosocial impact and therapeutic approaches. *Supportive Care in Cancer*, 12 (8), 543–549.

Hidalgo, M., Rinaldi, D., Medina, G. *et al.* (1999) A phase I trial of topical topitriol (calcitriol, 1,25-dihydroxyvitamin D3) to prevent chemotherapy-induced alopecia. *Anti-Cancer Drugs*, 10 (4), 393–395.

Hilton, S., Hunt, K., Emslie, C. *et al.* (2008) Have men been overlooked? A comparison of young men and women's experiences of chemotherapy-induced alopecia. *Psychooncology*, 17 (6), 577–583.

Holmberg, M. and Zanni, G.R. (2005) Bring hope home with oral antineoplastic agents. *Pharmacy Times*, 71 (3), 103–111.

How, C. and Brown, J. (1998) Extravasation of cytotoxic chemotherapy from peripheral veins. *European Journal of Oncology Nursing*, 2 (1), 51–59.

Howard, N. and Stenner, R.W. (1983) An improved "ice-cap" to prevent alopecia caused by adriamycin (doxorubicin). *British Journal of Radiology*, 56 (672), 963–964.

HSE (2003) Safe Handling of Cytotoxic Drugs: HSE Information Sheet MISC615. Health and Safety Executive, Caerphilly. www.hse.gov.uk/pubns/misc615.pdf.

Hunt, J.M., Anderson, J.E. and Smith, I.E. (1982) Scalp hypothermia to prevent adriamycin-induced hair loss. *Cancer Nursing*, 5 (1), 25–31.

Hunter, J. (2008) Intramuscular injection techniques. *Art and Science*, 22 (24), 35–40.

Ignoffo, R.J. and Friedman, M.A. (1980) Therapy of local toxicities caused by extravasation of cancer chemotherapeutic drugs. *Cancer Treatment Reviews*, 7 (1), 17–27.

INS (2006) Infusion nursing standards of practice. *Journal of Infusion Nursing*, 29 (1), Suppl, S1–S92.

Jackson, G. (2006) *Consensus Opinion on the Use of Dexrazoxane (Savene) in the Treatment of Anthracycline Extravasation*. Topotarget, UK.

Jacobson, J., Cummings, C., Galioto, M. *et al.* (2009) American Society of Clinical Oncology/Oncology Nursing Society chemotherapy administration safety standards. *Oncology Nursing Forum*, **36** (6), 651–658.

Janssen, F.P.E.M. (2007) Modelling physiological and biochemical aspects of scalp cooling. Unpublished thesis.

Kassner, E. (2000) Evaluation and treatment of chemotherapy extravasation injuries. *Journal of Pediatric Oncology Nursing*, **17** (3), 135–148.

Katsimbri, P., Bamias, A. and Pavlidis, N. (2000) Prevention of chemotherapy-induced alopecia using an effective scalp cooling system. *European Journal of Cancer*, **36** (6), 766–771.

Kav, S., Johnson, J., Rittenberg, C. *et al.* (2008) Role of the nurse in patient education and follow-up of people receiving oral chemotherapy treatment: an international survey. *Supportive Care in Cancer*, **16** (9), 1075–1083.

Kelland, L. (2005) Cancer cell biology, drug action and resistance, in *The Royal Marsden Hospital Handbook of Cancer Chemotherapy: A Guide for the Multidisciplinary Team* (eds D. Brighton and M. Wood). Elsevier Churchill Livingstone, Edinburgh, pp. 3–15.

Keller, J.F. and Blausey, L.A. (1988) Nursing issues and management in chemotherapy-induced alopecia. *Oncology Nursing Forum*, **15** (5), 603–607.

Kendell, P. (2001) Magic gel that helps cancer patients hold onto their hair. *Dail Mail*, 6 January, p.19.

Kennedy, M., Packard, R., Grant, M. *et al.* (1983) The effects of using Chemocap on occurrence of chemotherapy-induced alopecia. *Oncology Nursing Forum*, **10** (1), 19–24.

Khan, M.S. and Holmes, J.D. (2002) Reducing the morbidity from extravasation injuries. *Annals of Plastic Surgery*, **48** (6), 628–632; discussion 632.

Langer, S. (2008) Treatment of anthracycline extravasation from centrally inserted venous catheters. *Oncology Reviews*, **2** (2), 114–116.

Langer, S.W., Sehested, M. and Jensen, P.B. (2000) Treatment of anthracycline extravasation with dexrazoxane. *Clinical Cancer Research*, **6** (9), 3680–3686.

Langer, S.W., Thougaard, A.V., Sehested, M. and Jensen, P.B. (2006) Treatment of anthracycline extravasation in mice with dexrazoxane with or without DMSO and hydrocortisone. *Cancer Chemotherapy and Pharmacology*, **57** (1), 125–128.

Lavery, I. and Ingram, P. (2006) Prevention of infection in peripheral intravenous devices. *Nursing Standard*, **20** (49), 49–56.

Lawson, T. (2003) A legal perspective on CVC-related extravasation. *Journal of Vascular Access Devices*, **8** (1), 25–27.

Lemenager, M. (1998) Alopecia induced by chemotherapy – a controllable side-effect. *Oncology Nursing Today*, **3** (2), 18–20.

Lemenager, M., Genouville, C., Bessa, E.H. and Bonneterre, J. (1995) Docetaxel-induced alopecia can be prevented. *Lancet*, **346** (8971), 371–372.

Lemenager, M., Lecomte, S., Bonneterre, M.E. *et al.* (1997) Effectiveness of cold cap in the prevention of docetaxel-induced alopecia. *European Journal of Cancer*, **33** (2), 297–300.

Lemieux, J., Maunsell, E. and Provencher, L. (2008) Chemotherapy-induced alopecia and effects on quality of life among women with breast cancer: a literature review. *Psychooncology*, **17** (4), 317–328.

Macduff, C., Mackenzie, T., Hutcheon, A. *et al.* (2003) The effectiveness of scalp cooling in preventing alopecia for patients receiving epirubicin and docetaxel. *European Journal of Cancer Care*, **12** (2), 154–161.

MARCH (2007) Management and awareness of the risks of cytotoxics handling. www.marchguidelines.com.

Masoorli, S. (2003) Extravasation injuries associated with the use of central vascular access devices. *Journal of Vascular Access Devices*, **8** (1), 21–23.

Massey, C.S. (2004) A multicentre study to determine the efficacy and patient acceptability of the Paxman Scalp Cooler to prevent hair loss in patients receiving chemotherapy. *European Journal of Oncology Nursing*, **8** (2), 121–130.

Maurer, M., Handjiski, B. and Paus, R. (1997) Hair growth modulation by topical immunophilin ligands: induction of anagen, inhibition of massive catagen development, and relative protection from chemotherapy-induced alopecia. *American Journal of Pathology*, **150** (4), 1433–1441.

Maxwell, M.B. (1980) Scalp tourniquets for chemotherapy-induced alopecia. *American Journal of Nursing*, **80** (5), 900–903.

Mayo, D.J. (1998) Fibrin sheath formation and chemotherapy extravasation: a case report. *Supportive Care in Cancer*, **6** (1), 51–56.

McCaffrey Boyle, D. and Engelking, C. (1995) Vesicant extravasation: myths and realities. *Oncology Nursing Forum*, **22** (1), 57–67.

MHRA (2008) *Implantable Drug Pumps for Intrathecal Therapy. All Manufacturers: MDA/2008/038.* Medicines and Healthcare products Regulatory Agency, London. www.mhra.gov.uk/Publications/Safetywarnings/MedicalDeviceAlerts/CON018012.

Middleton, J., Franks, D., Buchanan, R.B. *et al.* (1985) Failure of scalp hypothermia to prevent hair loss when cyclophosphamide is added to doxorubicin and vincristine. *Cancer Treatment Reports*, **69** (4), 373–375.

Mols, F., Van Den Hurk, C.J., Vingerhoets, A.J. and Breed, W.P. (2009) Scalp cooling to prevent chemotherapy-induced hair loss: practical and clinical considerations. *Supportive Care in Cancer*, **17** (2), 181–189.

Mouridsen, H.T., Langer, S.W., Buter, J. *et al.* (2007) Treatment of anthracycline extravasation with Savene (dexrazoxane): results from two prospective clinical multicentre studies. *Annals of Oncology*, **18** (3), 546–550.

Mulders, M., Vingerhoets, A. and Breed, W. (2008) The impact of cancer and chemotherapy: perceptual similarities and differences between cancer patients, nurses and physicians. *European Journal of Oncology Nursing*, **12** (2), 97–102.

Munstedt, K., Manthey, N., Sachsse, S. and Vahrson, H. (1997) Changes in self-concept and body image during alopecia induced cancer chemotherapy. *Supportive Care in Cancer*, **5** (2), 139–143.

Naylor, W. (2005) Extravasation of wounds; aetiology and management, in *The Royal Marsden Hospital Handbook of Cancer Chemotherapy: A Guide for the Multidisciplinary Team* (eds D. Brighton and M. Wood). Elsevier Churchill Livingstone, Edinburgh, pp.109–112.

NCAG (2009) *Chemotherapy Services in England: Ensuring Quality and Safety.* National Chemotherapy Advisory Group, London.

NECN (North of England Cancer Network) (2008) *Standards for the Safe Use of Oral Anticancer Medicines.* www.cancernorth.nhs.uk/.../NECNOralAnticancerMedicinePolicyv1.4.pdf.

Nixon, S. and Schulmeister, L. (2009) Safe handling of hazardous drugs: are you protected? *Clinical Journal of Oncology Nursing*, **13** (4), 433–439.

NMC (2008a) *The Code: Standards of Conduct, Performance and Ethics for Nurses and Midwives.* Nursing and Midwifery Council, London. www.nmc-uk.org/aDisplayDocument.aspx?DocumentID=5982.

NMC (2008b) *Standards for Medicines Management.* Nursing and Midwifery Council, London. www.nmc-uk.org/aDisplayDocument.aspx?DocumentID=6978.

NMC (2008c) *Consent.* Nursing and Midwifery Council, London. www.nmc-uk.org/Nurses-and-midwives/Advice-by-topic/A/Advice/Consent/.

NMC (2009) *Record Keeping: Guidance for Nurses and Midwives.* Nursing and Midwifery Council, London.

NPSA (2008a) The National Patient Safety Agency's rapid response report. *Oncology Nursing*, **11** (3), 387–395.

NPSA (2008b) *Vinca Alkaloid Minibags (adult/adolescent units): NPSA/2008/RRR004*. National Patient Safety Agency, London. www.nrls.npsa.nhs.uk/resources/?EntryId45=59890.

NPSA (2009) *Standardising Wristbands Improves Patient Safety*. National Patient Safety Agency, London. www.npsa.nhs.uk.

Oakley, C., Lennan, E., Roe, H. et al., for the UK Oncology Nursing Society (2010) Safe practice and nursing care of patients receiving oral anticancer medicines: a position statement from UKONS. Ecancermedicalscience, 4, article number 117.

Oakley, C., Johnson, J. and Ream, E. (2010) Developing an intervention for cancer patients prescribed oral chemotherapy. *European Journal of Cancer Care*, 19, 21–28.

Olsen, E.A. (2003) Current and novel methods for assessing efficacy of hair growth promoters in pattern hair loss. *Journal of the American Academy of Dermatology*, **48** (2 supplement), 253–262.

O'Neill, V.J. and Twelves, C.J. (2002) Oral cancer treatment: developments in chemotherapy and beyond. *British Journal of Cancer*, 87, 933–937.

Parker, R. (1987) The effectiveness of scalp hypothermia in preventing cyclophosphamide-induced alopecia. *Oncology Nursing Forum*, 14 (6), 49–53.

Peck, H.J., Mitchell, H. and Stewart, A.L. (2000) Evaluating the efficacy of scalp cooling using the Penguin cold cap system to reduce alopecia in patients undergoing chemotherapy for breast cancer. *European Journal of Oncology Nursing*, 4 (4), 246–248.

Pethran, A., Schierl, R., Hauff, K. et al. (2003) Uptake of antineoplastic agents in pharmacy and hospital personnel. Part I: monitoring of urinary concentrations. *International Archives of Occupational and Environmental Health*, 76 (1), 5–10.

Pickard-Holley, S. (1995) The symptom experience of alopecia. *Seminars in Oncology Nursing*, 11 (4), 235–238.

Polovich, M. (2003) *Safe Handling of Hazardous Drugs*, 3rd edn. Oncology Nursing Society, Pittsburgh, PA.

Polovich, M., Whitford, J.M. and Olsen, M. (eds) (2009) *Chemotherapy and Biotherapy Guidelines and Recommendations for Practice*, 3rd edn. Oncology Nursing Society, Pittsburgh, PA.

Priestman, T.J. (1989) *Cancer Chemotherapy: An Introduction*, 3rd edn. Springer-Verlag, London.

Protiere, C., Evans, K., Camerlo, J. et al. (2002) Efficacy and tolerance of a scalp-cooling system for prevention of hair loss and the experience of breast cancer patients treated by adjuvant chemotherapy. *Supportive Care in Cancer*, 10 (7), 529–537.

Purohit, O.P. (1992) A 6 week chemotherapy regimen for relapsed lymphoma efficacy results and the influence of scalp cooling. *Annals of Oncology*, 3 (5 supp), 126.

Randall, J. and Ream, E. (2005) Hair loss with chemotherapy: at a loss over its management? *European Journal of Cancer Care*, 14 (3), 223–231.

RCN (2010) *Standards for Infusion Therapy*. Royal College of Nursing, London.

Ridderheim, M., Bjurberg, M. and Gustavsson, A. (2003) Scalp hypothermia to prevent chemotherapy-induced alopecia is effective and safe: a pilot study of a new digitized scalp-cooling system used in 74 patients. *Supportive Care in Cancer*, 11 (6), 371–377.

Robinson, M.H., Jones, A.C. and Durrant, K.D. (1987) Effectiveness of scalp cooling in reducing alopecia caused by epirubicin treatment of advanced breast cancer. *Cancer Treatment Reports*, 71 (10), 913–914.

Ron, I.G., Kalmus, Y., Kalmus, Z. et al. (1997) Scalp cooling in the prevention of alopecia in patients receiving depilating chemotherapy. *Supportive Care in Cancer*, 5 (2), 136–138.

Rosenblatt, L. (2006) Being the monster: women's narratives of body and self after treatment for breast cancer. *Medical Humanities*, 32 (1), 53–56.

Rosman, S. (2004) Cancer and stigma: experience of patients with chemotherapy-induced alopecia. *Patient Education and Counseling*, 52 (3), 333–339.

Roth, D. (2003) Extravasation injuries of peripheral veins: a basis for litigation. *Journal of Vascular Access Devices*, 8 (1), 13–20.

Ruddy, K., Mayer, E. and Partridge, A. (2009) Patient adherence and persistence with oral anticancer treatment. *CA: Cancer Journal for Clinicians*, **59**, 56–66.

Rudolph, R. and Larson, D.L. (1987) Etiology and treatment of chemotherapeutic agent extravasation injuries: a review. *Journal of Clinical Oncology*, 5 (7), 1116–1126.

Sansivero, G. and Barton-Burke, M. (2001) Chemotherapy administration: general principles for vascular access, in *Cancer Chemotherapy: A Nursing Process Approach*, 3rd edn (eds M. Barton-Burke, G.M. Wilkes and K. Ingwersen). Jones and Bartlett, Sudbury, MA, pp.645–670.

Satterwhite, B. and Zimm, S. (1984) The use of scalp hypothermia in the prevention of doxorubicin-induced hair loss. *Cancer*, 54 (1), 34–37.

Sauerland, C., Engelking, C., Wickham, R. and Corbi, D. (2006) Vesicant extravasation part I: mechanisms, pathogenesis, and nursing care to reduce risk. *Oncology Nursing Forum*, 33 (6), 1134–1142.

Scales, K. (2005) Vascular access: a guide to peripheral venous cannulation. *Nursing Standard*, 19 (49), 48–52.

Scheepers, H.C., van Erp, E.J. and van den Bergh, A.S. (1999) Use of misoprostol in first and second trimester abortion: a review. *Obstetrical and Gynecological Survey*, 54 (9), 592–600.

Schrijvers, D.L. (2003) Extravasation: a dreaded complication of chemotherapy. *Annals of Oncology*, 14 (Suppl 3), iii26–iii30.

Schulmeister, L. (1998) A complication of vascular access device insertion. A case study and review of subsequent legal action. *Journal of Intravenous Nursing*, 21 (4), 197–202.

Schulmeister, L. (2009) Antineoplastic therapy, in *Infusion Therapy and Transfusion Medicine*. S. Karger AG, Basel, pp.366–367.

Schwartz, A.L. (2007) Understanding and treating cancer-related fatigue. *Oncology*, 21 (11 suppl), 30–34.

Scurr, M. (2005) Combination chemotherapy and chemotherapy principles, in *The Royal Marsden Hospital Handbook of Cancer Chemotherapy: A Guide for the Multidisciplinary Team* (eds D. Brighton and M. Wood). Elsevier Churchill Livingstone, Edinburgh, pp. 17–29.

Seto, T., Ushijima, S., Yamamoto, H. et al. (2006) Intrapleural hypotonic cisplatin treatment for malignant pleural effusion in 80 patients with non-small-cell lung cancer: a multi-institutional phase II trial. *British Journal of Cancer*, 95 (6), 717–721.

Sewell, G., Summerhayes, M. and Stanley, A. (2002) Administration of chemotherapy, in *The Cytotoxics Handbook*, 4th edn (eds M. Allwood, A. Stanley and P. Wright). Radcliffe Medical Press, Oxford, pp. 85–115.

Shah, N., Groom, N., Jackson, S. et al. (2000) A pilot study to assess the feasibility of prior scalp cooling with palliative whole brain radiotherapy. *British Journal of Radiology*, 73 (869), 514–516.

Shapiro, J. and Price, V.H. (1998) Hair regrowth. Therapeutic agents. *Dermatologic Clinics*, 16 (2), 341–356.

Sharma, S. and Saltz, L.B. (2000) Oral chemotherapeutic agents for colorectal cancer. *Oncologist*, 5 (2), 99–107.

SI 2002/2677 (2002) *The Control of Substances Hazardous to Health Regulations 2002*. Stationery Office, London. www.opsi.gov.uk/si/si2002/20022677.htm.

Spaëth, D., Luporsi, E., Coudert, B. et al. (2008) Efficacy and safety of cooling helmets for the prevention of chemotherapy induced alopecia: a prospective study of 911 patients. Paper presented at ASCO, Chicago, May 30–June 3.

Sredni, B., Xu, R.H., Albeck, M. *et al.* (1996) The protective role of the immunomodulator AS101 against chemotherapy-induced alopecia studies on human and animal models. *International Journal of Cancer*, **65** (1), 97–103.

Stanley, A. (2002) Managing complications of chemotherapy administration, in *The Cytotoxics Handbook*, 4th edn (eds M. Allwood, A. Stanley and P. Wright). Radcliffe Medical Press, Oxford, pp. 119–192.

Symonds, R.P., McCormick, C.V. and Maxted, K.J. (1986) Adriamycin alopecia prevented by cold air scalp cooling. *American Journal of Clinical Oncology*, **9** (5), 454–457.

Szetela, A.B. and Gibson, D.E. (2007) How the new oral antineoplastics affect nursing practice: capecitabine serves to illustrate. *American Journal of Nursing*, **107** (12), 40–48.

Tierney, A.J. (1987) Preventing chemotherapy-induced alopecia in cancer patients: is scalp cooling worthwhile? *Journal of Advanced Nursing*, **12** (3), 303–310.

Tierney, A.J. (1989) *A Study to Inform Nursing Support of Patients Coping with Chemotherapy for Breast Cancer*. Department of Nursing Studies, University of Edinburgh, Edinburgh.

Toft, B. (2001) External Inquiry into the Adverse Incident that Occurred at Queen's Medical Centre, Nottingham, 4th January 2001. Department of Health, London. www.dh.gov.uk/prod_consum_dh/groups/dh_digitalassets/@dh/@en/documents/digitalasset/dh_4082098.pdf.

Tollenaar, R.A., Liefers, G.J., Repelaer van Driel, O.J. and van de Velde, C.J. (1994) Scalp cooling has no place in the prevention of alopecia in adjuvant chemotherapy for breast cancer. *European Journal of Cancer*, **30A** (10), 1448–1453.

Tortora, G.J. and Derrickson, B. (2009) *Principles of Anatomy and Physiology*, 12th edn. John Wiley, Hoboken, N.J.

Ulutin, H.C., Guden, M., Dede, M. and Pak, Y. (2000) Comparison of granulocyte-colony, stimulating factor and granulocyte macrophage-colony stimulating factor in the treatment of chemotherapy extravasation ulcers. *European Journal of Gynaecological Oncology*, **21** (6), 613–615.

Uno, H. and Kurata, S. (1993) Chemical agents and peptides affect hair growth. *Journal of Investigative Dermatology*, **101** (1 Suppl), 143S–147S.

Valanis, B., Vollmer, W., Labuhn, K. and Glass, A. (1997) Occupational exposure to antineoplastic agents and self-reported infertility among nurses and pharmacists. *Journal of Occupational and Environmental Medicine*, **39** (6), 574–580.

Valanis, B., Vollmer, W.M. and Steele, P. (1999) Occupational exposure to antineoplastic agents: self-reported miscarriages and stillbirths among nurses and pharmacists. *Journal of Occupational and Environmental Medicine*, **41** (8), 632–638.

Van den Hurk, C.J.G., Mols, F., Vingerhoets, J.J.M. and Breed, W.P.M. (2010) Impact of alopecia and scalp cooling on the well being of breast cancer patients. *Psychooncology*, **19** (7), 701–709.

Van der Molen, B. (2005) Patient information and education, in *The Royal Marsden Hospital Handbook of Cancer Chemotherapy: A Guide for the Multidisciplinary Team* (eds D. Brighton and M. Wood). Elsevier Churchill Livingstone, Edinburgh, pp.49–59.

Viele, C.S. (2007) Managing oral chemotherapy: the healthcare practitioner's role. *American Journal of Health-System Pharmacy*, **64** (9 Suppl 5), S25–S32.

Washburn, D.J. (2007) Intravesical antineoplastic therapy following transurethral resection of bladder tumors: nursing implications from the operating room to discharge. *Clinical Journal of Oncology Nursing*, **11** (4), 553–559.

Weinstein, S. and Plumer, A.L. (2007) *Plumer's Principles and Practice of Intravenous Therapy*, 8th edn Lippincott Williams and Wilkins, Philadelphia.

Wheelock, J.B., Myers, M.B., Krebs, H.B. and Goplerud, D.R. (1984) Ineffectiveness of scalp hypothermia in the prevention of alopecia in patients treated with doxorubicin and cisplatin combinations. *Cancer Treatment Reports*, **68** (11), 1387–1388.

Wickham, R., Engelking, C., Sauerland, C. and Corbi, D. (2006) Vesicant extravasation part II: Evidence-based management and continuing controversies. *Oncology Nursing Forum*, **33** (6), 1143–1150.

Williams, J., Wood, C. and Cunningham-Warburton, P. (1999) A narrative study of chemotherapy-induced alopecia. *Oncology Nursing Forum*, **26** (9), 1463–1468.

Williamson, S. (2008) Management of oral anti cancer therapies. *Pharmaceutical Journal*, **281**, 399–402.

Wilson, C. (1994) The ice cap that could help save your hair. *Daily Mail*, September 20th, pp.36–37.

Winkeljohn, D.L. (2007) Oral chemotherapy medications: the need for a nurse's touch. *Clinical Journal of Oncology Nursing*, **11** (6), 793–796.

Witman, G., Cadman, E. and Chen, M. (1981) Misuse of scalp hypothermia. *Cancer Treatment Reports*, **65** (5–6), 507–508.

Workman, B. (1999) Safe injection techniques. *Nursing Standard*, **13** (39), 47–53.

Ziegler, E., Mason, H. and Baxter, P. (2002) Occupational exposure to cytotoxic drugs in two UK oncology wards. *Occupational and Environmental Medicine*, **59** (9), 608–612.

Chapter 16

Medicines management

The Royal Marsden Hospital Manual of Clinical Nursing Procedures, Eighth Edition. Edited by Lisa Dougherty and Sara Lister.
© 2011 The Royal Marsden Hospital. Published 2011 by Blackwell Publishing Ltd.

Overview

This chapter will provide an overview of medicine management and the main routes of administration such as oral and injections. Other routes such as inhalation, topical and vaginal will also be discussed.

Medicines management

Definitions

Medicines management can be defined as the way medicines are selected, procured, delivered, prescribed, administered and reviewed to optimize the contributions that medicines make to producing informed and desired outcomes of patient care (Audit Commission 2001). The Medicines and Healthcare Products Regulatory Agency (MHRA 2004) defines it as the clinical, cost-effective and safe use of medicines to ensure patients get the maximum benefit from the medicines they need, while at the same time minimizing potential harm. The professional role of the nurse in medicines management is the safe handling and administration of medicines, including a responsibility for making sure that patients understand what medicines they are taking and why, as well as the likely side-effects (Luker and Wolfson 1999). Medicinal products are defined, according to the Medicines Act 1968, as, 'substances sold or supplied for administration to humans (or animals) for medicinal purposes' (HMSO 1968), and can be used for treating or preventing disease, making a medical diagnosis or restoring, correcting or modifying physiological functions (Council Directive 65/65/EEC).

Related theory

Pharmacology is a wide-ranging subject which looks at the history of drugs, where they are sourced from, what properties they have, how they are made, what effects they have and how they are processed by the body (Hardman *et al.* 1996).

Pharmacokinetics looks at the absorption, distribution, metabolism and excretion of drugs within the body. When these four factors are considered, with the dose of a drug given, the concentration of drug in the body over a period of time can be determined. Pharmacokinetics is most useful when considered with pharmacodynamics which is the study of the mechanisms of action of drugs and other biochemical and physiological effects (Hardman *et al.* 1996).

The effects of most drugs arise from the way they interact with receptors in the body. The most important type of receptor is a protein receptor. These proteins can be regulatory proteins involved in the mediating effects of neurotransmitters and hormones, enzymes involved in metabolic or regulatory pathways, transport proteins or structural proteins (Hardman *et al.* 1996).

Some drugs do not exert their effect through combination with receptors but by interacting with small molecules that can

be normally or abnormally present in the body; for example, mesna assists in neutralizing the urotoxic metabolites of ifosfamide and cyclophosphamide to reduce the incidence of haemorrhagic cystitis and haematuria (Brock and Pohl 1983).

Evidence-based approaches

Rationale

Indications

Medicines can be administered for the following purposes.

- Diagnostic purposes, for example assessment of liver function.
- Prophylaxis, for example heparin to prevent thrombosis or antibiotics to prevent infection.
- Therapeutic purposes, for example replacement of fluids and vitamins, supportive purposes (to enable other treatments such as anaesthesia), palliation of pain and cure (as in the case of antibiotics).

Contraindications

Whilst there are no contraindications to the overall administration of medications, there will be contraindications for individual medications or patients such as:

- allergic to medication
- medication interactions
- medication given based on patient's condition, for example digoxin, chemotherapy
- certain preparations can only be administered via certain routes.

Methods for the safe and secure handling of medicines

Administration of medicines is an everyday activity that carries great responsibility and is one of the greatest areas of risk in nursing practice (Hand and Barber 2000). However, although it requires clinical decision making by nurses, it is often associated with routinized behaviour because it is carried out so frequently (Armitage and Knapman 2003). Incidents involving medicines were the third largest group of all incidents reported to the National Patient Safety Agency (NPSA) although the majority of the outcomes are of no or low harm (NPSA/NRLS 2009). It seems that nearly half the reports describe incidents with the administration or supply of a medicine in a clinical area (NPSA/NRLS 2009). The NPSA (2007a) has listed the key areas of risk for medication error (Box 16.1).

Incidents involving injectable medicine represented 62% of all reported incidents leading to death or severe harm (NPSA/NRLS 2009). There are seven key actions to improve medication safety (Box 16.2).

The effective and safe prescribing, dispensing and administration of medicines to patients demands a partnership between the various health professionals concerned, that is

---

Box 16.1 Key areas of risk for medication error

- Wrong drug/diluents.
- Calculation errors.
- Level of knowledge.
- Administration to wrong patient.
- Administration via wrong route.
- Unsafe handling/poor aseptic technique.

(NPSA 2007a)

---

doctors, pharmacists and nurses. The revised Duthie Report, *The Safe and Secure of Handling of Medicines: A Team Approach* (RPSGB 2005) defined a medicine as 'all products administered by mouth, applied to the body or introduced into the body for the purpose of treating or preventing disease, diagnosing disease or ascertaining the existence, degree or extent of a physiological condition, contraception, inducing anaesthesia, or otherwise preventing or interfering with the normal operation of a physiological function'. It follows from this definition that infusions or injections of sodium chloride 0.9% and water for injection are included, as are all medicinal products covered by the European Directive on Medicines. This report details how the key principles of compliance with legislation, adherence to guidance and safety of patients and staff should be applied to the management and handling of medicines. In order to achieve this, organizations should have in place Standard Operating Procedures (SOPs) for each activity in the medicines trail, also indicating clear responsibilities, training, competencies and performance standards for each member of staff. Processes for validation, audit and risk assessment of the activities also need to be included.

The activities defined in the medicines trail are:

- prescribing/initiation of treatment
- procurement/acquisition of medicines
- manufacture/manipulation of medicines
- receipt of medicines
- issue to point of use/dispensing or supply
- preparation/manipulation of medicines for administration
- use of medicines/administration

Box 16.2 Seven key actions to improve medication safety

- Increase reporting and learning from medication incidents.
- Implement NPSA safer medication practice recommendations.
- Improve staff skills and competencies.
- Minimize dosing errors.
- Ensure medicines are not omitted.
- Ensure the correct medicines are given to the correct patients.
- Document patients' medicine allergy status.

(NPSA 2007a)

- removal/disposal of surplus/waste medicines from wards and departments
- removal/disposal of surplus/waste medicines or related materials from the hospital.

Principles of care

Prescribing

All medicines administered in hospital must be considered prescription only. This is because administration, whether by a nurse or by a patient to themselves, may only take place in accordance with one or more of the following processes:

- patient-specific direction (PSD)
- patient medicines administration chart may also be called a medicines administration record (MAR)
- patient group directions (PGD)
- Medicines Act exemplar
- standing orders
- homely remedy protocol
- prescription form.

(NMC 2008a, pp. 13–16)

Prescriptions can be handwritten on a chart, a prescription pad or provided electronically. E-prescribing has been defined as the 'utilization of electronic systems to facilitate and enhance the communication of a prescription or medicine order, aiding the choice, administration and supply of a medicine through knowledge and decision support and providing a robust audit trail for the entire medicines uses process' (NHS Connecting for Health 2009). Some of the benefits include:

- prescibers can accurately and clearly enter complete medication orders
- the system can provide relevant patient information, for example allergies
- prescription data can be stored securely and communicated to other members of the healthcare team without the risk of paper records being lost
- pharmacists can access medication orders remotely and check and amend as required
- nurses have clear and legible medication orders
- medication records can be accessed remotely by all healthcare professionals (NHS Connecting for Health 2009) (see Box 16.3).

A growing number of hospitals in the UK have introduced e-prescribing systems. One major motivation for introducing them is to improve the safety of medicines used and reduce the current and unacceptable levels of adverse drug events. In a systematic review, nine of the 13 studies demonstrated a significant reduction in prescribing errors for all or some drug types when electronic prescribing was used (Reckmann *et al.* 2009).

'Verbal orders'

The NMC (2008a) clearly states that a verbal order is not acceptable on its own. 'In exceptional circumstances, where

---

Box 16.3 Benefits of e-prescribing systems

The Connecting for Health programme has outlined the benefits of e-prescribing systems as:

- computerized entry and management of prescriptions
- knowledge support, with immediate access to medicines information, for example British National Formulary
- decision support, aiding the choice of medicines and other therapies, with alerts such as drug interactions
- computerized links between hospital wards/departments and pharmacies
- ultimately, links to other elements of patients' individual care records
- improvements in existing work processes
- a robust audit trail for the entire medicines use process
- a reduction in the risk of medication errors as a result of several factors, including:
  - more legible prescriptions
  - alerts for contraindications, allergic reactions and drug interactions
  - guidance for inexperienced prescribers
  - improved communication between different departments and care settings
  - reduction in paperwork-related problems, for example fewer lost or illegible prescriptions
  - clearer, and more complete, audit trails of medication administration
  - improved formulary guidance and management and appropriate reminders within care pathways.

(www.connectingforhealth.nhs.uk/systemsandservices/eprescribing)

---

the medication (NOT including controlled drugs) has been previously prescribed and the prescriber is unable to issue a new prescription, but where changes to the dose are considered necessary, the use of information technology (such as fax or e-mail) may be used but must confirm any changes to the original prescription' (NMC 2008a, p. 32). This should be followed up by a new prescription confirming the changes, signed by the prescriber within a maximum of 24 hours. The changes must be authorized before the new dosage is administered (NMC 2008a).

Nurse prescribing and patient group directions

As nurses have undertaken increasingly specialized roles, the need for them to have powers to prescribe has become more apparent. The report of the Advisory Committee on Nurse Prescribing (DH 1989) initially recommended a limited nurses' formulary for district nurses and health visitors. The Medicinal Products: Prescription by Nurse, etc. Act (1992) granted the statutory authority for this to occur. The Crown Report (DH 1989) also recommended that doctors and nurses collaborate in drawing up local protocols for the administration of medicines in situations that would benefit specific groups of patients, for example those requiring vaccinations.

The practice of prescribing under group protocols became widespread across the NHS, and they were used to support initiatives such as nurse-led clinics (Laverty *et al.* 1997, Mallett *et al.* 1997). The legality of this practice was then questioned. Section 58 of the Medicines Act (1968) states that 'no one should administer any medication (other than to himself) unless he is the appropriate practitioner or a person who is acting according to directions from an appropriate practitioner'. The terms *direction* and *administration* were open to interpretation and how they were used varied across the country (McHale 2002).

Nurse prescribing was therefore reviewed and two further reports were published:

- *Review of Prescribing, Supply and Administration of Medicines. A Report on the Supply and Administration of Medicines under Group Protocols* (DH 1998)
- *Review of Prescribing, Supply and Administration of Medicines. Final Report* (DH 1999).

The first specifically offered guidance about group protocols, including changing the name to patient group directions (PGD) (see Box 16.4).

The second report looked at the existing arrangements for prescribing, supply and administration of medicines and suggested the introduction of a new form of prescribing to be undertaken by non-medical health professionals (DH 2003a). Independent nurse prescribing was initially allowed from an extremely limited formulary (Shuttleworth 2005). It was then extended a number of times until finally, appropriately qualified nurses were allowed to prescribe from the whole British National Formulary.

- *Independent prescribing*: this allows nurses who are registered as independent prescribers to prescribe any licensed

---

Box 16.4 Patient group directions

The legal definition of a patient group direction is 'a written instruction for the supply and/or administration of a licensed medicine (or medicines) in an identified clinical situation signed by a doctor or dentist and a pharmacist' (NPC 2009). It is drawn up locally by doctors, pharmacists and other appropriate professionals and must be approved by the employer, advised by the relevant professional advisory committee. It applies to groups of patients or other service users who may not be individually identified before presentation for treatment (DH 2004). The Health and Safety Commission (HSC) advised that the majority of medication 'should be prescribed and administered on an individual patient specific basis', but that it is appropriate to use PGDs for the supply and administration of medicines in situations where this offers an advantage for patient care (DH 2000). Shepherd suggests that this means 'where medical staff are either inaccessible or unavailable' (Shepherd 2002b, p. 44). The flowchart in Figure 16.1 aims to assist practitioners in deciding the appropriate system for the prescription, supply or administration of medicines. Using a PGD is not a form of prescribing.

Figure 16.1 Patient group directions (PGDs) flowchart. The diagram takes the practitioner through a logical process that aims to assist in determining if a PGD can be used. With permission, adapted from the national Patient Group Directions (England only) website www.pgd.nhs.uk. Please check the PGD website for the most recent version of this tool and for further resources and guidance relating to PGDs.

medicine (and now unlicensed; DH 2009) for any medical condition (this also includes some controlled drugs) but only within their own level of experience and competence, and acting in accordance with the NMC *Code* (DH 2006, NMC 2008b). Only those who have undergone appropriate training and are registered with the NMC as an independent prescriber can prescribe (NMC 2006a). It must also be considered to be part of that nurse's role.

■ *Supplementary prescribing* has been defined as: 'A voluntary prescribing partnership between an independent prescriber and a supplementary prescriber to implement an agreed patient specific clinical management plan with the patient's agreement' (DH 2003a). Amendments to the Prescription Only Medicines Order and the NHS regulations allowed supplementary prescribing by suitably trained nurses from April 2003. Supplementary prescribers prescribe in partnership with a doctor or dentist (the independent prescriber) and are able to prescribe any medicine, including controlled drugs and unlicensed medicines that are listed in an agreed clinical management plan. The plan is drawn up with the patient's agreement, following diagnosis of the patient by an independent prescriber and following consultation and agreement between the independent and supplementary prescribers.

(DH 2003a, pp. 6 and 7)

The key principles that underpin supplementary prescribing are:

■ the importance of communication between prescribing partners
■ the need for access to shared patient records
■ the patient is treated as a partner in their care and is involved at all stages in decision making, including whether part of their care is delivered via supplementary prescribing (NPC 2003a).

Preparation for both independent nurse prescribing and supplementary prescribing is at least 26 days in length and must follow the standards set out in the NMC *Circular 25/2002* (NMC 2001c). Any preparation must enable independent and supplementary non-medical prescribers to reach the competencies outlined in *Maintaining Competency in Prescribing: An Outline Framework to Help Nurse Prescribers* (NPC 2001), *Maintaining Competency in Prescribing: An Outline Framework to Help Nurse Supplementary Prescribers* (NPC 2003b) and the competences in shared decision making within the Medicines Partnership document (Medicines Partnership Programme 2007).

The addition of prescriptive authority to the nurse role has been a positive way of not only making a service more responsive for service users, but also has helped to meet increasing demands on health services (Bridge *et al.* 2005). Patients are satisfied with nurse prescribing (Latter *et al.* 2005). In 2005 it was estimated that there were 28,000 nurses who were able to prescribe from the limited formulary and 4000 extended prescribers (MHRA 2005). A national survey of

---

Box 16.5 An evaluation of nurse prescribing

■ Most nurse prescribers were confident in their prescribing practice.
■ Most felt extended prescribing had a positive impact on patient care and enabled them to make better use of their skills.
■ Most felt that the limited nurse formulary imposed unhelpful limitations on their practice.
■ Nurses were satisfied with the support received from their medical practitioner.
■ Patients were positive about their experience of nurse prescribing.
■ Doctors were positive about the development of nurse prescribers in their teams.

(Latter *et al.* 2005)

246 nurse prescribers concluded that nurse prescribing is largely successful in both practice and policy terms (Latter *et al.* 2005): this is discussed in more detail in Box 16.5. A range of competencies and skills are required to ensure quality and safe prescribing – the nurse prescriber:

■ identifies main medical condition
■ explores patient's presenting symptoms and their management
■ explores past medical history, current medication, including over-the-counter (OTC), allergies and family history
■ is able to initiate a physical examination
■ is able to request and interepret diagnostic tests.

The evidence is that nurses need greater consistency in the frequency with which they apply these skills (Latter 2008).

Unlicensed and 'off-label' medicines

Under European medicines legislation, a medicinal product placed on the market is required to have a marketing authorization (product licence) granted following demonstration of safety, quality and efficacy. However, member states can put in place arrangements to allow an authorized healthcare professional to gain access to an unlicensed medicine, that is, a medicine that doesn't have a marketing authorization, to meet the special needs of individual patients. In the UK, this occurs via the arrangements for 'specials' manufactured in the UK and the notification scheme for products imported into the UK.

'Specials' can be supplied if there is an order for them, a registered doctor has requested the product and the product will be used for a patient under the care of that doctor and under that doctor's supervision. A 'special' cannot be supplied if an equivalent licensed product is available which will meet the patient's needs. If a 'special' is manufactured in the UK, the manufacturer must hold a manufacturer's (special) licence issued by the MHRA. An unlicensed medicine may also be imported if the importer holds the appropriate wholesaler dealer license or wholesaler dealer import license issued by the MHRA. The importer will need to inform the MHRA on each occasion that they intend to import the product. 'Off label' refers to the use of a medicine outside the terms of its licence.

For herbal medicines, there are three possible regulatory routes by which they can reach the market in the UK: as an unlicensed herbal remedy, as a registered traditional herbal medicine (identified as the product container or packaging will include a nine-digit registration number starting with the letters THR (MHRA 2009) and as a licensed herbal medicine. Unlicensed herbal remedies are the most common route for such medicines to reach the market.

Unlicensed medicines can be prescribed by doctors, dentists and nurse independent prescribers (DH 2009). 'Off-label' medicines can be prescribed by doctors, dentists, independent nurse prescribers, independent pharmacist prescribers and independent optometrist prescribers. The MHRA has published advice for prescribers on the use of unlicensed and off-label medicines due to the responsibility for prescribing such medicines being potentially greater than for licensed products (Box 16.6). Nurse independent prescribers can also mix medicines prior to administration and direct others to mix, for example for use within syringe pumps/drivers (DH 2009).

Finally, the MHRA advises that healthcare professionals have a responsibility to help monitor the safety of medicines in clinical use through submission of suspected adverse drug reactions to the MHRA and CHM via the Yellow Card Scheme (www.yellowcard.gov.uk). Such reporting is equally important for unlicensed medicines or those used off-label as for those that are licensed (MHRA 2009).

Dispensing

Dispensing is defined as 'to label from stock and supply a clinically appropriate medicine to a patient/client/carer usually against a written prescription, for self administration or administration by another professional and to advise on safe and effective use' (NMC 2008a, p. 28). The majority of these activities in hospitals are undertaken by the pharmacy department. They can supply medicines as stock to a ward or for specific patients, either as inpatients or outpatients. Pharmacists are professionally accountable for all decisions to supply a medicine and offer advice. As part of this accountability, they must ensure that if any tasks are to be delegated, they are delegated to persons competent to perform them. Nurses may only dispense in exceptional circumstances (NMC 2008a).

A pharmaceutical assessment of a prescription, which is the point at which pharmacists apply their knowledge to establish the safety, quality, efficacy and perhaps cost-effective use of drug treatments specified by a prescriber, must be performed by a pharmacist and must be carried out on every prescription (RPSGB 2007a). Following this assessment, the assembly of the prescription can be delegated to a pharmacy technician or a pharmacy assistant. Once the prescription is

---

Box 16.6 MHRA advice for prescribers on the use of unlicensed and off-label medicines

- Before prescribing an unlicensed medicine, be satisfied that an alternative, licensed medicine would not meet the patient's needs.
- Before prescribing a medicine off label, be satisfied that such use would better serve the patient's needs than an appropriately licensed alternative.
- Before prescribing an unlicensed medicine or using a medicine off-label:
  - be satisfied that there is a sufficient evidence base and/or experience of using the medicine to show its safety and efficacy
  - take responsibility for prescribing the medicine and for overseeing the patient's care, including monitoring and follow-up
  - record the medicine prescribed and, where common practice is not being followed, the reasons for prescribing this medicine; you may wish to record that you have discussed the issue with the patient.

The MHRA also advises that best practice suggests that:

- you give patients, or those authorizing treatment on their behalf, sufficient information about the proposed treatment, including known serious or common adverse reactions, to enable them to make an informed decision
- where current practice supports the use of a medicine outside the terms of its licence, it may not be necessary to draw attention to the licence when seeking consent. However, it is good practice to give as much information as patients or carers require or which they may see as relevant
- you explain the reasons for prescribing a medicine off label or an unlicensed medicine where there is little evidence to support its use, or where such use of a medicine is innovative.

---

assembled, it will be presented for accuracy checking by a pharmacist or a suitably qualified pharmacy technician.

Many pharmacies have also now adopted practices of one-stop dispensing and robotic dispensing. One-stop dispensing involves the medicine supply for inpatients being supplied in a form ready for discharge. Robotic and automated systems can be used to pick and label medicines in order to reduce errors in these areas (RPSGB 2007a).

Methods for storage of medicines

The report *The Safe and Secure of Handling of Medicines: A Team Approach* (RPSGB 2005) details that the responsibility for establishing and maintaining a system for the security of medicines should be that of the senior pharmacist in the hospital. They should do this in consultation with senior nursing staff and appropriate medical staff. The appointed nurse in charge of the area will have the responsibility of ensuring that this system is followed and that the security of medicines is maintained. The nurse in charge may delegate some of these duties but always remains responsible for this task. The safe and secure handling of medicines on the ward is governed by the following principles.

Security

All drugs should be stored in locked cupboards with separate storage for internal medicines, external medicines, controlled drugs and medicines needing refrigeration or storage in a freezer.

Diagnostic reagents, intravenous and topical agents should also be kept separately in individual storage.

Stability

No medicinal preparation should be stored where it may be subject to substantial variations in temperature, for example not in direct sunlight.

The normal temperature ranges for storage are as follows.

- *Cold storage*: products to be stored between 2°C and 8°C. Refrigerators should be placed in an area where the ambient temperature does not affect the temperature control within it. Most refrigerators will function effectively in an environment of 10–32°C. Refrigerators should have a minimum and maximum thermometer fitted which should be read and reset daily (MHRA 2001).
- *Cool storage*: products that need to be stored in a cool place or between 8°C and 15°C. If these temperatures cannot be achieved, these products should be stored in a fridge provided that temperatures below 8°C do not affect the stability of the product. If lower temperatures do affect the stability, it is recommended that they are stored in an area where the temperature will not exceed 18°C (MHRA 2001).
- *Room temperature*: for products that need to be stored at room temperature or not above 25°C (MHRA 2001).

Containers

The type of container used may have been chosen for specific reasons. Therefore all medicines should be stored in the containers in which they were supplied by pharmacy. Medicinal preparations should never be transferred (in bulk) from one container to another except in the pharmacy.

Stock control

A system of stock rotation must be operated (e.g. first in, first out) to ensure that there is no accumulation of old stocks. Only one pack/container of a named medicine should be in use at any one time. A list of stock medicines to be kept on the ward should be regularly reviewed according to usage figures. The medicines to be held on the ward should be dis-

cussed between the nurse in charge and a pharmacist with relevant medical staff.

Storage requirements of specific preparations

- *Aerosol containers* should not be stored in direct sunlight or over radiators: there is a risk of explosion if they are heated.
- *Creams* may deteriorate rapidly if subjected to extremes of temperature.
- *Eye drops and ointments* may become contaminated with micro-organisms during use and thus pose a danger to the recipient. Therefore in hospitals, eye preparations should be discarded 7 days after they are first opened. For use at home, this limit is extended to 28 days.
- *Mixtures* may have a relatively short shelf-life. Most antibiotic mixtures require refrigerated storage and even then have a shelf-life of only 7–14 days. Always check the label for details.
- *Tablets and capsules* are relatively stable but are susceptible to moisture unless correctly packed. They should be stored only in the containers in which they were supplied by the pharmacy.
- *Vaccines* and similar preparations usually require refrigerated storage and may deteriorate rapidly if exposed to heat.

Patient's own drugs

Patients are encouraged to bring their medication into hospital with them to facilitate a comprehensive medicines reconciliation process. This can also be useful if the organization has a policy of using the patient's own drugs.

These medicines remain the property of the patient and should not be destroyed without prior consent from the patient or their representative. If the patient does agree to the destruction of the medicines, they must be sent to the pharmacy for destruction. If the patient does not want the medicines to be stored in the hospital or sent to pharmacy for destruction, they must be sent home with the patient's representative. These medicines should only be used if they can be positively identified, are of a suitable quality and are labelled according to labelling requirements. They should be stored to the same security standards as other medicine stock on the ward. They should be used for the sole use of the patient whose property they remain (RPSGB 2005).

Methods for preparation

The NMC clearly states that:

> It is unacceptable to prepare substances for injection in advance of their immediate use or to administer medication drawn into a syringe or container by another registrant when not in their presence. An exception of this is an already established infusion which has been instigated by another registrant following the principles set out above, or medication prepared

940

under the direction of a pharmacist from a central intravenous additive service and clearly labelled for that patient/client.

(NMC 2008a, p. 28)

However, the NMC acknowledges that a registrant 'may be required in an emergency to prepare substances for other professionals' (NMC 2008a).

Methods for administration

The nurse is responsible for the administration of drugs by a variety of methods. The NMC *Standards for Medicines Management* emphasizes that this 'is not solely a mechanistic task to be performed in strict compliance with the written prescription of a medical practitioner (now independent supplementary prescriber). It requires thought and the exercise of professional judgement...' (NMC 2008a, p. 6). Shepherd (2002b) maintains that the administration of a medicine is arguably the most common clinical procedure that a nurse will undertake. He goes on to state that it is the manner in which a medicine is administered that determines to some extent whether or not the patient gains any clinical benefit and whether any adverse effect is experienced.

The nurse is accountable for the safe administration of medicines. In order to do this, the nurse requires a thorough knowledge of the principles and their application and a responsible attitude, which ensures that medications are not given without full knowledge of immediate and late effects, toxicities and nursing implications (NMC 2008a). The nurse must also be able to justify any actions taken and be accountable for the action taken (NMC 2008a). If they delegate any of aspects of the administration of a medicinal product, they are also accountable for ensuring that the patient or carer/care assistant is competent to carry out the task (NMC 2008a). In delegating to unregistered practitioners, it is the registered nurse who must apply the principles of administration and they may then delegate the unregistered practitioner to assist the patient in the ingestion or application of the medicinal product (NMC 2008a, p. 31). Student nurses must never administer/supply medicinal products without direct supervision and both student and registered nurse must sign the medication chart or document the administration in the notes (NMC 2008a).

Medicine administration should ensure that the correct patient receives:

- the appropriate medicine
- in the appropriate formulation
- by the appropriate route
- at the appropriate dose
- at the appropriate time
- at the appropriate rate
- for the appropriate duration of therapy
- with the appropriate monitoring to ensure safety and efficacy of therapy
- with the appropriate reporting of adverse drug reactions (Sexton 1999, p. 240).

To achieve this, the nurse must have a sound knowledge of the use, action, usual dose and side-effects of the drugs being administered. Institutional policies and procedures also assist the nurse to administer drugs safely and a sound knowledge of local procedures is essential. Organizational policies therefore need to reflect a culture that encourages disclosure and in which the management of medication errors is viewed as a learning process as opposed to a punitive act (Gladstone 1995, Martin 1994). The NMC states that all errors and incidents require a thorough and careful investigation at a local level, taking full account of the context, circumstances and position of the practitioner involved. Such incidents require a sensitive management and a comprehensive assessment of all the circumstances before a professional and managerial decision is reached on the appropriate way to proceed (NMC 2008a). It must be recognized, however, that errors in drug administration can have traumatic consequences for the individual nurse involved and that disciplinary procedures invoke fear in most nurses (Arndt 1994).

Single or double checking of medicines

Medicines can be prepared and administered by a single qualified nurse or by two nurses checking (known as double checking). There are certain times when double or second checking is required. It is recommended that for the administration of controlled drugs, a secondary signature is required (NMC 2008a). The NMC *Standards for Medicines Management* also states that 'wherever possible two registrants should check medication to be administered intravenously, one of whom should also be the registrant who then administers the intravenous medication' (NMC 2008a, p. 31). Where the administration of a medicine requires complex calculations, it is deemed good practice for a second practitioner (a registered professional) to check the calculation independently to minimize the risk of error (NMC 2008a).

Jarman *et al.*'s (2002) review of 129 nurses, using questionnaires and reviewing incidents, both during double checking and then once single checking had been introduced, demonstrated no increase in drug errors following the change. Single checking provided satisfaction for nurses and more effective use of time and the nurses felt that single checking allowed them more autonomy and that it was more beneficial to patients and enabled them to be more responsive to their needs. Armitage (2008) suggested that double checking is a common but inconsistent process. Athough often seen to be integral to safe practice, it is often sacrificed when there is a shortage of time or staff (Armitage 2008). He listed the issues with double checking as:

- deference to authority
- reduction of responsibility
- auto processing (familiarity)
- lack of time (to check properly)
- solutions (how to do it).

A recent study viewed independent double checking as an alternative. This is when two nurses check a drug independently of each other. In this study nurses were observed during the setting up of ambulatory chemotherapy pumps. When compared with the old system of double checking, the new system showed no significantly statistical difference in reducing errors in dose, rate or documentation but did show a reduction in errors related to patient identification (Savage and Tripp 2008).

Those nurses who wish or need to have their administration supervised will retain the right to do so until such time as all parties agree that the requested level of proficiency has been achieved. The nurse checking the medicine must be able to justify any action taken and be accountable for the action taken. This is in keeping with the principles of *The Code* (NMC 2008b).

Patient identification

Patient misidentification can occur at any stage of a patient's journey and as it is under-reported, its 'true' incidence unknown (Rosenthal 2003). Not identifying the patient correctly can result in the administration of a wrong drug or dose and can sometimes be fatal, such as transfusion of blood to the wrong patient (Schulmeister 2008). The NMC (2008a) is clear that the nurse must be certain of the identity of the patient to whom the medicine is to be administered. The NPSA (2007b) recommended that to avoid misidentification of patients, staff should check the patient's identity using an identification wristband. The NPSA (2007b) issued guidance on the use of wristband for patient identification, which also encompasses the use of wristbands to identify allergy status. It recommends that the NHS should be supporting patients with auto identity technology. Where there are difficulties in clarifying an individual's identity, an up-to-date photograph can be attached to the prescription charts (NMC 2008a). Schulmeister (2008) suggested that one strategy to reduce the risk of patient misidentification would be to instruct patients to show their namebands to nurses rather than passively wait to be asked to see the nameband.

Legal and professional issues

Administration of medicines has been one of the most common clinical procedures undertaken by nurses for at least the past 50 years (Shepherd 2002a). With changes in legal, professional and cultural boundaries in healthcare, the role of the nurse has broadened to one of medicines management. Medicines management and specifically medicines administration require thought and professional judgement (Luker and Wolfson 1999, NMC 2008a). All aspects of a medicine's use must be managed with a multidisciplinary approach to ensure it is supported by a strong evidence base and that the safety and well-being of the patient remain paramount (NMC 2008b, Shepherd 2002a). Nurses are taught how to prepare and administer medication via the common routes

during their basic training. This includes calculation, which is vital as any miscalculation of medication dosage represents a potential threat to both patient safety and clinical effectiveness (Weeks *et al.* 2000). There are now a number of computer-based programmes on infection control and IV therapy, infusion pumps (NHSCLU 2009) and medication dosage calculation problem-solving skills (Weeks *et al.* 2001) which provide knowledge and competency for nurses.

Legislation

Legislative frameworks, government guidelines and professional regulations govern medicines management in the UK. The primary pieces of legislation are the Medicines Act 1968, European Directives and the Misuse of Drugs Act 1971 (HMSO 1971).

The Medicines Act 1968

European Community Council Directives and Regulations and the Medicines Act 1968 (HMSO 1968) regulate the manufacture, distribution and importation of medicines for human use. The Medicines and Health Care Products Regulatory Agency (MHRA) in the UK and the European Medicines Agency (EMEA) are responsible for the licensing procedures for medicinal products. The availability of products is restricted by defining which of the following legal categories they are in:

- prescription-only medicines (POM)
- pharmacy-only medicines (P)
- general sales list medicines (GSL).

Different requirements apply to the sale, supply and labelling of medicines in each category. In hospitals, medicines can be supplied in line with patient-specific directions, from an appropriate practitioner in relation to the medicine, which in most cases will be an instruction on the patient ward drug chart. This written instruction does not need to comply with the requirements specified for prescriptions but does need to relate to a specific patient. The legislation also allows the supply of prescription-only medicines to be made under a PGD. A PGD needs to be signed by a doctor and a pharmacist. The regulations permit certain registered professionals to supply or administer under a PGD.

In addition to the above, there are also a range of exemptions from the regulations which allow certain groups of health professionals to sell, supply and administer particular medicines direct to patients (Applebe and Wingfield 2005, RPSGB 2009).

Complications
Drug interactions

As well as adverse drug reactions and allergic reactions to drugs, consideration should be given to the interactions between drugs.

Table 16.1 Types of pharmacokinetic interactions

Type of interaction	Interaction caused by	Example of when to consider in clinical practice
Drug absorption interactions	Changes in the GI pH Adsorption or chelation in the GI tract Changes in GI motility Induction or inhibition of transporter proteins or malabsorption	Allopurinol and mercaptopurine – allopurinol inhibits xanthane oxidase, an enzyme which metabolizes mercaptopurine to an inactive metabolite, thereby resulting in increased mercaptopurine toxicity such as bone marrow suppression. If used together, the mercaptopurine dose should be decreased to a third of the original dose (Baxter 2008)
Drug distribution interactions	Protein binding or inhibition or induction of drug transporter proteins	Therapeutic drug monitoring as drugs that can be displaced in this way can appear subtherapeutic when monitored but doses would not need to be increased (Baxter 2008)
Drug metabolism interactions	Changes in first-pass metabolism, enzyme induction, enzyme inhibition and genetic factors The hepatic cytochrome P450 enzyme system is the major site of drug metabolism and most drug–drug interactions occur at this site	Grapefruit juice can inhibit the cytochrome P450 isoenzyme CYP3A4, thus reducing the metabolism of calcium channel blockers (Baxter 2008)
Drug excretion interactions	Changes in urinary pH, active renal tubular excretion, renal blood flow and biliary excretion or the enterohepatic shunt	Probenecid and penicillin compete for the same active transport systems in the renal tubules. As a result, probenecid reduces the excretion of penicillin which can lead to penicillin toxicity (Baxter 2008)

A drug interaction occurs when the effect of a particular drug is altered when it is taken with another drug, herbal medicine, food or drink (Baxter 2008). These interactions can result in an increased effect, causing toxicity, or a decreased effect, resulting in a decreased efficacy of the drug. Interactions can be unwanted but in some cases they can be desirable, for example vitamin K is used to oppose the effects of warfarin when toxicity has occurred.

Drug interactions can be divided into pharmacokinetic (Table 16.1) and pharmacodynamic interactions (Table 16.2).

Herbal and complementary medicines have been increasingly used in the UK over recent years and as a result there has been an increase in the reporting of interactions between these agents and conventional drugs. Some of the most common herbal interactions are those involving St John's wort, a popular herbal product used as an antidepressant. Mathijssen et al. (2002) found that St Johns wort (or *Hypericum perforatum*) interacts with irinotecan. Five patients with various types of cancer were given 350 mg/m² irinotecan intravenously with or without 900 mg St Johns wort once a day orally for 18 days. The researchers found that in the presence of St Johns wort the plasma concentrations of the active metabolite of irinotecan decreased by 42% and myelosuppression was worse in the absence of St Johns wort.

Interactions can also occur between drugs and food. Food can have an effect on drugs by changing GI motility or by binding to drugs whilst in GI transit. An example of interactions between food and a drug can be seen with procarbazine and tyramine-containing foods. Tyramine is a chemical present in certain foods that are rich in protein and can interact with monoamine oxidase inhibitors (MAOIs). As procarbazine has mild MAOI properties, it is possible that taking both together could result in a hypertensive reaction which can cause symptoms of raised blood pressure, headache, pounding heart, neck stiffness, sweating, flushing and vomiting. Patients should therefore be advised to avoid tyramine-rich foods such as mature and aged cheeses, yeast

Table 16.2 Types of pharmacodynamic interactions

Type of interaction	Interaction caused by	Example of when to consider in clinical practice
Additive or synergistic interactions	Two drugs have the same pharmacological effect and therefore the results can be additive	Opioids with benzodiazepines causing increased drowsiness (Baxter 2008)
Antagonistic or opposing interactions	Two drugs have opposing activities	Vitamin K and warfarin resulting in the effects of the anticoagulant being opposed (Baxter 2008)

Beijnen and Schellens (2004).

or meat extracts, pickled fish, salami and heavy red wines (Baxter 2008).

Adverse drug reactions

Although we use drugs to diagnose, prevent or treat disease, no drug is administered without risk. However, it is important when choosing a drug treatment that consideration is given to the balance between clinical effect and undesired effects. The World Health Organization definition of adverse drug reactions (ADRs) is 'harmful, unintended reactions to medicines that occur at doses normally used for treatment' (WHO 2008). ADRs can be classified as type A or type B reactions. Type A reactions are pharmacologically predictable and usually dose dependent and therefore reversible by reducing or withdrawing the drug in question. An example of a type A reaction would be antidiabetic drugs causing hypoglycaemia. Type B reactions cannot be related to the pharmacological action of the drug, are not dose related and therefore cannot be controlled by dose reduction. An example of a type B reaction would be anaphylaxis due to penicillins. Type A reactions are more common than type B but type B reactions tend to cause a higher rate of serious illness and mortality (Rawlins and Thompson 1977).

The WHO states that 'ADRs are amongst the leading causes of death in many countries and that in some countries ADR-related costs, such as hospitalization, surgery and lost productivity, exceed the cost of the medications' (WHO 2008). One study found that the median percentage of preventable drug-related admissions to hospital was 3.7% (the range was between 1.4% and 15.4%). The majority (51%) of preventable drug-related admissions involved either antiplatelets (16%), diuretics (16%), non-steroidal anti-inflammatory drugs (11%) or anticoagulants (8%) (Howard *et al.* 2007).

Although the effect of a drug cannot always be predicted, it is important that when a drug is given to a patient, the risk of harm is minimized by ensuring that good-quality medicines are used and that they are safe and effective. Consideration should always be given to predisposing factors

that drugs or a patient may have which could increase the risk of ADRs, including:

- polypharmacy
- age of the patient
- gender
- co-morbidities such as renal disease, race, genetic factors such as G6PD deficiency (some children and adults with G6PD deficiency may develop haemolysis and anaemia if they get a fever or if they take certain medicines (UCL Institute of Child Health 2008))
- allergies
- drug–drug interactions.
  (Koda-Kimble *et al.* 2005, Walker and Edwards 2003)

Pharmacovigilance is an important aspect for all healthcare professionals to consider in order to identify information about potential new hazards related to medicines and prevent harm to patients (MHRA 2010a).

Although medicines are widely tested within clinical trials before they become commercially available, information on patient populations different from those in the trials cannot be provided. The only way for this information to be collected is through careful patient monitoring and further collection of data through postmarketing surveillance. In the UK this information is collected through the Yellow Card Scheme which is run by the MHRA and the Commission on Human Medicines (CHM). The scheme is used to collect information from both health professionals and patients on suspected ADR with prescribed medicines, OTC medicines and herbal medicines. Yellow Cards can be completed by using the MHRA website or by completing a hard copy found in the British National Formulary (BNF), the ABPI Medicines Compendium or in the MIMS Companion.

Allergic reactions

Allergic reactions are specific types of adverse drug reactions. They are immune mediated and can be classified as in Table 16.3.

There are many risk factors that increase the likelihood of having an allergic reaction. These can be split into those

Table 16.3 Types of allergic reactions

Type of reaction	Result of reaction	Example of reaction
Type I – IgE-mediated reactions	Urticaria, angio-oedema, anaphylaxis and bronchospasm	Anaphylaxis from beta-lactam antibiotic
Type II – IgG/M-mediated cytotoxic reaction	Anaemia, cytopenia and thrombocytopenia	Haemolytic anaemia from penicillin
Type III – IgG/M-mediated immune complexes	Vasculitis, lymphadenopathy, fever, arthropathy and rashes Can also be known as serum sickness	Serum sickness from antithymocyte globulin
Type IV – delayed hypersensitivity reactions	Dermatitis, bullous exanthema, maculo-papular and pustular xanthemata	Contact dermatitis from topical antihistamine

Beijnen and Schellens (2004), Riedl and Casillas (2003).

that are specific to the patient and those that are specific to the drug.

The patient-related factors include the following.

- *Immune status*: previous reaction to the same or related compound.
- *Age*: younger adults are more likely to have allergic reactions than infants or the elderly.
- *Gender*: women are more likely than men to suffer cutaneous reactions.
- *Genetic*: atopic predisposition is more likely to result in a severe reaction and genetic polymorphisms may predispose to drug hypersensitivity, for example G6PD deficiency, slow acetylators.
- *Concomitant disease*: viral infections such as HIV and herpes are associated with an increased risk of allergic reactions; cystic fibrosis is associated with an increased risk of allergic reactions to antibiotics, which is though to be due to the prolonged use in this group of patients.

(Mirakian *et al.* 2009)

The drug-related risk factors include the following.

- *Drug chemistry*: some drugs are more likely to cause reactions than others. These are high molecular weight compounds, for example dextran and insulin. Also, drugs that bind to proteins called haptens, forming complexes that can cause an immune response, for example beta-lactam antibiotics.
- *Route of administration*: the topical route is most likely to cause an allergy, with the oral route being least likely. The intramuscular route is more likely than the intravenous route.
- *Dose*: a large single dose is less likely to cause a reaction than prolonged or frequent doses.

(Mirakian *et al.* 2009)

Although the incidence of true allergic drug reactions is low, the potential morbidity and mortality related to these reactions can be high, so it is important that drug allergies are accurately diagnosed and treated. The first step towards an accurate diagnosis is a detailed history (Mirakian *et al.* 2009). Guidance on what information should be collated is detailed in the BSACI drug allergy guidelines which can be found on the website at www.bscaci.com and includes the following.

- Detailed description of reaction:
  - symptom sequence and duration
  - treatment provided
  - outcome.
- Timing of symptoms in relation to drug administration.
- Has the patient had the suspected drug before this course of treatment?
  - How long had the drug(s) been taken before onset of reaction?
  - When was/were the drug(s) stopped?
  - What was the effect?

Box 16.7 Treatment of acute drug reaction

An acute drug reaction must be treated promptly and appropriately.

1. Stop the suspected drug.
2. Treat the reaction.
3. Identify and avoid potential cross-reacting drugs.
4. Record precise details of the reaction and its treatment.
5. Identify a safe alternative. In some cases this may not be possible so where the case is less severe, it may be decided to continue with the medication with suppression of the symptoms with, for example, a corticosteroid and an antihistamine.

Also see Complications of intravenous injections and infusions.

(Mirakian *et al.* 2009)

- Witness description (patient, relative, doctor).
- Is there a photograph of the reaction?
- Illness for which suspected drug was being taken, that is, underlying illness (this may be the cause of the symptoms, rather than the drug).
- List of all drugs taken at the time of the reaction (including regular medication, OTC and 'alternative' remedies).
- Previous history:
  - other drug reactions
  - other allergies
  - other illnesses.

(Mirakian *et al.* 2009)

This guideline also gives details on further investigations which may be required in order to accurately diagnose an allergic reaction (Box 16.7).

In some cases, desensitization may be considered but this is rarely indicated.

In addition to the treatment of drug allergies, it is extremely important that the patient is given information regarding what medication they should avoid. The drugs to avoid should also be recorded clearly in medical records, including paper and electronic records. All inpatients should have their allergy indicated by wearing a red-coloured identity band (NPSA 2007b). Allergic drug reactions should be reported using the Yellow Card Scheme (Mirakian *et al.* 2009).

Self-administration of medicines

Evidence-based approaches

Rationale

The report by the Audit Commission, *A Spoonful of Sugar – Medicines Management in NHS Hospitals* (2001) recommended self-administration of medicines by patients. This

Table 16.4 Examples of levels of supervision for self-administration of medicines

Level of supervision	Role of patient	Role of nurse
Level 1	None	Nurse administers medicine from cabinet
		Key locked in cabinet and nurse uses master
		Nurse signs drug administration chart
Level 2	Patient administers medicine with nurse supervision	Cabinet is opened by nurse
		Nurse supervises patient administration
		Nurse signs drug administration chart
Level 3	Key kept by patient	Nurse must check that the appropriate medication was taken and endorse the chart with an identifier to indicate that the patient is self-administering and their initials
	Patient administers their own medicines	

NPC (2007).

report detailed how studies have shown that only one-half of patients take their medicines properly when they get home. The National Institute for Clinical Excellence (NICE) published Clinical Guideline 76 on medicines adherence (NICE 2009) which states that between a third and a half of medicines that are prescribed for long-term conditions are not used. This non-adherence has quality and cost implications for the NHS due to wasted medicines and readmissions for patients.

The Audit Commission states that self-administration is beneficial to patients because it allows the patient to take medication when they should, for example painkillers when they are in pain and medicines to be taken before and after food. It simplifies the medicine regimen for patients, especially those who take many medicines, as it allows a fuller assessment of the benefits of all the medicines that a patient may be taking. It allows patients to practise taking their medicines in hospital under supervision so that any problems that may arise can be dealt with. It has also been found that patients who had administered their own medications in hospital were more likely to report that their overall care was excellent and that they were satisfied with the discharge process than patients who had not (Deeks and Byatt 2000).

The Healthcare Commission report, *The Best Medicine – The Management of Medicines in Acute and Specialist Trusts* (2007) states that where patients are self-administering, it is important that medicines are stored securely in suitable storage near to the bedside and that procedures and training will need to be in place which should cover the assessment process and the patient's suitability for self-administration. Although, by definition, self-administration of medicines shifts the balance of responsibility for this part of care towards the patient, it in no way diminishes the fundamental professional duty of care. It is therefore essential that local policies, procedures and records are

adequate to ensure that this duty is, and can be shown to be, discharged. The revised Duthie Report (RPSGB 2005) states that any transfer of responsibility should occur on the basis of an assessment of the patient's ability to manage the tasks involved and with the patient's agreement. The patient's agreement should be recorded with the date and time.

The NMC sets out the responsibilities of the nurse regarding the self-administration of medicines which includes viewing the medicines, checking the suitability of use and that they have been prescribed, assessment of the patient, what should be documented and how they should be stored (NMC 2008a).

Assessments of patients for self-administration normally results in the allocation of a level of supervision. Examples of levels of supervision can be seen in Table 16.4.

Even if a patient is self-administering their medication, continual assessment of this aspect of their care while they are in hospital is important. The nurse must continually be aware of the patient's capability to self-administer and the action of the drugs the patient is taking (NPSA 2007c).

Preprocedural considerations

A medicines reconciliation needs to be carried out with the patient and they will be assessed for their ability to self-administer. Any constraint such as physical or visual handicap must be addressed. Changes in performance status may result from the underlying condition or its treatment, and must be allowed for (NMC 2008a, Shepherd 2002a).

If a compliance aid such as a 'dosette' box is to be used, responsibility for filling and labelling the aid, especially whilst used on the ward, must be agreed and documented in local policies (NMC 2008a, Shepherd 2002a).

Procedure guideline 16.1 Medication: self-administration

Essential equipment

- Drugs to be administered
- Recording sheet or book as required by law or hospital policy
- Patient's prescription chart, to check dose, route and so on
- Any protective clothing required by hospital policy for specified drugs, such as antibiotics or cytotoxic drugs (see Chapter 15)

Preprocedure

Action	Rationale
1 Carry out a medicines reconciliation with the patient on admission by reviewing proposed (inpatient) prescription in liaison with the pharmacist and compare with details given by the patient and medicines in their possession. Any differences should be investigated and highlighted with the medical team.	To ensure an accurate record of: all medicines being taken (prescribed or otherwise); dietary supplements, for example multivitamins, herbal remedies, complementary therapies; allergies or hypersensitivities; understanding of current medicines; possible problems with self-administration (Jordan *et al.* 2003, E; NMC 2008a, C; NMC 2009, C; Shepherd 2002b, E; NPSA/NICE 2007, C).
2 Carry out an assessment of the patient's ability to self-administer medication using an assessment form with the criteria in Table 16.5.	Technical patient safety solutions for medicines reconciliation on admission of adults to hospital (NPSA/NICE 2007, C).
3 Consider whether there are any constraints on self-administration and if so, how they might be overcome. Discuss this with appropriate members of the multidisciplinary team.	To promote successful and safe self-administration and ensure that medicines are dispensed and labelled appropriately for the patient's needs (DH 2003b, C; NMC 2008a, C; Shepherd 2002a, E).
4 Following the assessment, a level of supervision will be recommended and entered on the assessment form. The assessment form and the consent will be filed in the nursing notes. For examples of levels see Table 16.4.	To ensure that the correct level of supervsion is selected and communicated to other staff. E

Procedure

5 Discuss with the patient their medication and any problems they may be having with the regimen. Document discussions in the care plan. Teach any special skills required, for example correct use of aerosol inhalers. Reassess whether they need any changes to their levels of supervision, either up or down.	To promote the informed commitment and involvement of patients in their own care, where appropriate. To ensure that treatment is received as intended (NMC 2008a, C; Shepherd 2002b, E).

Postprocedure

6 Check every day that drugs are taken as intended, and that the necessary records are kept.	To ensure that the patient is taking the medication as the nurse continues to take overall responsibility for patient care and well-being. To maintain a record of responsibilities undertaken (NMC 2008a, C; NMC 2008b, C; NMC 2009, C).
7 Monitor changes in the patient's prescription.	To ensure that changes are put into effect promptly; drugs are properly relabelled or redispensed; any discontinued drugs are retrieved from the patient (DH 2003b, C; NMC 2008a, C; Shepherd 2002b, E).
8 Check when drug supplies are expected to run out and make arrangements for resupply. Order drugs to take out (TTO) as far in advance as possible.	To ensure that drugs are represcribed and dispensed in time to allow uninterrupted treatment and to facilitate planned discharge (DH 2003b, C; NMC 2008a, C; Shepherd 2002b, E).
9 Evaluate the effectiveness of the self-administration teaching programme and record any difficulties encountered and interventions made.	To identify further learning and teaching needs and modify care plan accordingly (NMC 2008a, C; NMC 2008b, C; NMC 2009, C; Shepherd 2002b, E).

Table 16.5 Assessment form

Assessment criteria	Rationale
■ Is the patient willing to participate in self-administration after being given information explaining the scheme with associated time to read and understand it?	Patient's agreement should be recorded with a date and time (RPSGB 2005)
■ Has the patient signed a consent form agreeing to self-administration?	Patient's agreement should be recorded with a date and time (RPSGB 2005)
■ Is the patient sufficiently well to take part in the scheme?	Patients who are not well enough or who are undergoing surgery will not be able to self-administer until they have recovered and have been reassessed. If frequent changes of drug or dose are expected, immediate self-administration may be undesirable and/or impractical
■ Is the patient confused, forgetful or disorientated?	Patients who are confused, forgetful or disorientated will need to have their medicines administered by a nurse in the usual way. This may be assessed by asking relatives or carers or by asking specific questions for assessing state of mind
■ Does the patient have a history of drug/alcohol abuse/self-harm?	Patients with this history can self-administer under the supervision of a nurse
■ Does the patient self-administer medicines at home?	Patients who are not responsible for self-administering their medicines in the community will need to have their medicines administered by a nurse in the usual way
■ Can the patient read the labels on the medicines?	These patients can either self-administer with supervision or have their medicines administered by a nurse. Referral can be made to pharmacy around assessment of labels. Can they be given extra large or Braille labels if necessary?
■ Can the patient open the medicine bottles and foil strips?	These patients can either self-administer with supervision or have their medicines administered by a nurse. Referral can be made to pharmacy for assessment and provision of appropriate containers
■ Can the patient open the locker where the medicines are stored while they are in hospital?	Patients who cannot open the locker can self-administer with nurse supervision
■ Does the patient know what their medicines are for, their dosage, instructions and potential side-effects (Shepherd 2002b)?	Patients who don't know this can be allowed to self-administer with nurse supervision. Re-education can take place in order to achieve full self-administration

Postprocedural considerations
Ongoing care

The nurse must monitor for any changes in the patient's prescription and condition. They must check when drugs supplied are expected to run out and ensure that drugs are ordered along with any TTOs. The effectiveness of the self-administration teaching programme must be evaluated (Shepherd 2002b).

Documentation

Particular care with record keeping is needed in the period of gradual transition from nurse administration to self-administration. Any problems encountered must be addressed (NMC 2008a, NMC 2008b, NMC 2009).

The detail and format of the record may vary according to the patient's needs and performance status the complexity of treatment, and local circumstances and policy (NMC 2008a, NMC 2008b, NMC 2009).

Controlled drugs

Definition

Controlled drugs are those drugs that are classified under the Misuse of Drugs Act 1971 and have controls around certain activities related to them, for example diamorphine, morphine, amphetamines, benzodiazepines. The use of controlled drugs in medicine is permitted by the Misuse of Drugs Regulations and related regulations, as detailed in the next section, Legal and professional issues.

Legal and professional issues
Legislation
Medicines Act 1968

The Act and the regulations under it allow midwives to supply and/or administer diamorphine, morphine, pethidine and pentazocine. A number of healthcare professionals are

948

Table 16.6 Legal requirements for the schedules of controlled drugs (CDs)

	Schedule 2 Includes opioids and major stimulants, for example amphetamines	Schedule 3 Includes minor stimulants, temazepam, barbiturates	Schedule 4 part I Includes benzodiazepines	Schedule 4 part II Includes anabolic steroids, growth hormones	Schedule 5 Includes low-dose opioids
Designation	CD	CD No Reg	CD Benz	CD Anab	CD Inv
Safe custody	Yes, except quinalbarbitone	Yes, except certain exemptions listed in the Medicines, Ethics and Practices inc. phenobarbitone	No	No	No
Prescription requirements inc. handwriting requirements	Yes	Yes, except temazepam	No	No	No
Requisitions necessary	Yes	Yes	No	No	No
Records to be kept in CD register	Yes	No	No	No	No
Pharmacist must ascertain the identity of the person collecting the CD	Yes	No	No	No	No
Emergency supplies allowed	No	No, except phenobarbitone for epilepsy	Yes	Yes	Yes
Validity of prescription	28 days	28 days	28 days	28 days	6 months
Maximum duration that can be prescribed	30 days as good practice	30 days as good practice	30 days as good practice	30 days as good practice	

Adapted from DH (2007).

also permitted to supply and/or administer controlled drugs in accordance with a PGD.

Misuse of Drugs Act 1971

For reasons of public safety, the Misuse of Drugs Act (1971) controls the import, export, production, supply, possession and manufacture of controlled drugs to prevent abuse as most are potentially addictive or habit forming. Other regulations of the Act govern safe storage, destruction and supply to known addicts.

Misuse of Drugs (Safe Custody) Regulations 1973

These regulations controlled the storage of controlled drugs. The level of control of storage depends on the premises in which they are being stored.

Misuse of Drugs Regulations 2001

Under these regulations, controlled drugs are classified into five schedules, each representing a different level of control (Table 16.6).

The requirements of the Act as they apply to nurses working in a hospital with a pharmacy department are described in Table 16.7.

Controlled Drugs (Supervision of Management and Use) Regulations 2006

These regulations set out the requirements for certain NHS bodies and independent hospitals to appoint an accountable officer. The duties and responsibilities of the accountable officer are to improve the management and use of controlled drugs. These regulations also allow the periodic inspection of premises.

Misuse of Drugs and Misuse of Drugs (Safe Custody) (Amendment) Regulations 2007

These regulations give accountable officers authority to nominate persons to witness the destruction of controlled drugs within their organization. They also allow operating department practitioners to order, possess and supply controlled drugs.

Table 16.7 Summary of legal requirements for handling of controlled drugs (CDs) as they apply to nurses in hospitals with a pharmacy

	Schedule 1: CDs Home Office licence	Schedule 2: CDs subject to full controls	Schedule 3: CDs with no register entry	Schedule 4: CDs anabolic steroids/benzodiazepines	Schedule 5: CDs needing invoice retention
Drugs in the schedule	Cannabis + derivatives but excluding nabilone, LSD (lysergic acid diethylamide)	Most opioids in common use including: alfentanyl; amphetamines; cocaine; diamorphine; methadone; morphine papaveretum; fentanyl; phenoperidine; pethidine; codeine; dihydrocodeine injections; pentazocine	Minor stimulants; barbiturates (but excluding hexobarbitone, thiopentone); diethylpropion; buprenorphine; temazepam[a]	Part 1: anabolic steroids Part 2: benzodiazepines	Some preparations containing very low strengths of cocaine; codeine; morphine; pholcodine and some other opioids
Ordering	Possession and supply permitted only by special licence from the Secretary of State issued (to a doctor only) for scientific or research purposes	A requisition must be signed in duplicate by the nurse in charge. The requisition must be endorsed to indicate that the drugs have been supplied. Copies should be kept for 2 years	As Schedule 2	No requirement[b]	No requirement[b]
Storage	Must be kept in a suitable locked cupboard to which access is restricted	As Schedule 1	Buprenorphine and diethylpropion: as Schedule 1 drugs. All other drugs. no requirement	No requirement[b]	No requirement[b]
Record keeping	Controlled drug register must be used	As Schedule 1	No requirement	No requirement[b]	No requirement[b]
Prescription	Prescription must include: ■ the name and address of patient ■ the drug, the dose, the form of preparation ■ the total quantity of drug or the total number of dosage units to be supplied. This quantity must be stated in words and figures The prescription must be written indelibly in the prescriber's own handwriting	As Schedule 1	As Schedule 1 except for phenobarbitone (this includes all preparations of phenobarbitone and phenobarbitone sodium). Because of its use as an antiepileptic, it does not need to be written in the prescriber's own handwriting	No requirement[b]	No requirement[b]
Administration to patients	Under special licence only A doctor or dentist or anyone acting on their instructions may administer these drugs to anyone for whom they have been prescribed	A doctor or dentist or anyone acting on their instructions may administer these drugs to anyone for whom they have been prescribed	A doctor or dentist or anyone acting on their instructions may administer these drugs to anyone for whom they have been prescribed	No requirement[b]	No requirement[b]

[a]Temazepam preparations are exempt from record-keeping and prescription requirements, but are subject to storage requirements.

[b]'No requirement' indicates that the Misuse of Drugs Act 1971 imposes no legal requirements additional to those imposed by the Medicines Act 1968 (HMSO 1968).

In addition, they set out changes to the record keeping for controlled drugs, with requirements for recording in the controlled drug register the person (the patient, patient's representative or a healthcare professional) collecting the Schedule 2 controlled drug. If it is a healthcare professional, there is a requirement for the name and address of that person. Records need to be kept regarding whether proof of identity was requested of the patient or the patient's representative and whether this proof of identity was provided. These requirements also changed midazolam from Schedule 4 to Schedule 3.

Implications of the regulations for nursing practice
Accountability and responsibility

The nurse in charge of an area is responsible for the safe and appropriate management of controlled drugs in that area. Certain tasks such as holding of the keys can be delegated to a registered nurse but the overall responsibility remains with the nurse in charge.

Requisition

The nurse in charge of an area is responsible for the requisition of controlled drugs for that area. This task can be delegated to a registered nurse but the overall responsibility remains with that nurse in charge. Orders should be written on suitable stationery and must be signed by an authorized signatory. All those who are authorized to order should have a copy of their signatures kept in pharmacy for validation.

Receipt

When controlled drugs are delivered to the ward they must be handed to an appropriate individual and not left unattended. A registered nurse in charge should check the order against the requisition, including the number ordered and received, and if all is correct they should sign the 'received by' section of the order book (Figure 16.2).

The controlled drug should be entered in the controlled drug register, recording the following information: date, number of requisition, quantity, name, formulation and strength of drug, name and signature of person making the entry, name and signature of witness and the balance in stock. The updated balance should be checked against the controlled drugs physically present and that these are the same. The number of units received should be written in words not figures. The controlled drugs will then be placed in the controlled drug cupboard.

Storage

Controlled drugs should be stored in controlled drug cupboards that conform to British Standard BS2881. If the amount of controlled drugs that are stored is large or in areas where there is not a 24-hour staff presence, a security cabinet that has been evaluated against the SOLD SECURE standard SS304 should be used.

Cupboards should be locked when not in use. The lock must not be common to any other lock in the hospital. Keys must only be available to authorized members of staff and at any time the key holder should be readily identifiable. The cupboard must be dedicated to the storage of controlled drugs. Controlled drugs must be locked away when not in use. There must be arrangements for keeping keys secure, especially in areas that are not operational at all times.

Key holding and access

The nurse in charge is responsible for the controlled drug keys. Key holding may be delegated but the legal responsibility lies with the nurse in charge. The controlled drug keys should be returned to the nurse in charge immediately after use.

For the purpose of stock checking, the key may be handed to an authorized member of pharmacy staff. If keys are lost, the senior nurse, the pharmacy manager and accountable officer must be contacted. Spare keys can be issued to ensure that patient care is not impeded.

68	NAME, FORM OF PREPARATION AND STRENGTH		Morphine Sulphate Injection 10mg / 1 mL						
AMOUNT(S) OBTAINED			AMOUNT(S) ADMINISTERED						
Amount	Date Received	Serial No. of Requisition	Date	Time	Patient's Name	Amount given	Given by (Signature)	Witnessed by (Signature)	STOCK BALANCE
10 amps	26/5/2010	12	26/5/2010	14⁰⁰	Received from Pharmacy				10
			27/5/10	14¹⁵	Mr. John Smith	10 mg			9
			27/5/10	18⁰⁰	Mrs. Daisy Rose	5mg given/5mg wasted			8

Figure 16.2 Controlled drugs order book.

Record keeping

Each ward that holds controlled drugs should keep a record of received and administered controlled drugs in a controlled drug record book. The nurse in charge is responsible for keeping the controlled drug record book up to date and in good order.

The controlled drug record book should have sequentially numbered pages, have a separate page for each drug and strength, entries should be in chronological order and in ink. The entries in the controlled drug record book should be signed by a registered nurse and then witnessed by a second registered nurse. If a second nurse is unavailable, the transaction can be witnessed by another practitioner such as a doctor, pharmacist or pharmacy technician.

When the end of a page is reached, the balance should be transferred to another page. The new number should be written on the bottom of the finished page and as a matter of good practice the transfer should be witnessed. If a mistake is made in the record book, the mistake should be bracketed so that the original entry is still clear and then signed, dated and witnessed by another nurse or registered professional who will also do the same for the correction.

Stock checks and discrepancies

The stock balance entered in the controlled drug record book should be checked against the amounts in the cupboard. In addition, regular stock checks should be carried out by pharmacy. The nurse in charge is responsible for ensuring that the stock checks are carried out. The stock checks should be carried out by two registered nurses. When checking the balance, the record book should be checked against the contents of the cupboard, not the reverse. Packs with unopened tamper-evident seals do not need to be opened during the check and liquid medicines can be checked by visual inspection. A record should be made in the record book that the stock has been checked with words such as 'check of stock level' and a signature of the registered nurse and the witness.

If a discrepancy is found it should be checked that all requisitions have been entered, that all drugs administered have been entered, that items have not been recorded in the wrong place in the record book, that the drugs have not been placed in the wrong cupboard and that the balances have been added correctly. If an error is found, the nurse in charge should make an entry to correct the balance which should be witnessed. If the error cannot be found, the chief pharmacist and the accountable officer should be contacted immediately.

Archiving

Controlled drug record books should be stored for a minimum of 2 years from the date the last entry was made/date of use.

Administration

Any registered practitioner can administer any drug specified as Schedule 2, 3 and 4 provided they are acting in accordance with the directions of an appropriately qualified prescriber (see Prescribing).

Two practitioners must be involved in the administration of controlled drugs, and both practitioners should be present during the whole administration procedure (NMC 2008a). The two practitioners should have clearly defined roles. One should be the checker and the other should take responsibility for taking the drug out of the cupboard, preparing and administering the drug. These roles should not be interchangeable during the procedure as this can result in errors. They should both witness the preparation, the controlled drug being administered and the destruction of any surplus drug. An entry should be made in the controlled drug record book recording the following information:

- the date and time the dose was administered
- the name of the patient
- quantity administered
- the name
- formulation
- the strength being administered
- the name and signature of the person administering
- the name and signature of the witness
- the balance in stock (see procedure).

Return and disposal including part vials

Unused controlled drug stock should be returned to pharmacy. Controlled drugs that are expired should also be returned to pharmacy for safe destruction. An entry should be made in the relevant page of the record book recording the following information:

- date
- reason for return
- name and signature of registered nurse
- name and signature of witness
- quantity removed
- name, form and strength
- the balance remaining.

Disposal of controlled drugs can take place on the ward if a part vial is administered to the patient or if individual doses of controlled drugs were prepared and not administered. If destroying a part vial, the registered nurse should record the amount given and the amount wasted under the administration entry in the record book. The entry and destruction should be witnessed by a registered nurse or other registered professional. If destroying an unused prepared controlled drug, this should also be recorded in the record book and the entry and destruction witnessed by another registered professional.

Stationery

Controlled drug stationery should be stored in a locked cupboard or drawer. Controlled drug stationery will be issued from pharmacy against a written requisition signed by an appropriate member of staff. Only one requisition book should be in use by a ward. If a new record book is started, the stock balance transfer should be witnessed by a registered nurse.

Transport

Controlled drugs should be transferred in a secure, locked or sealed, tamper-evident container.

A person collecting controlled drugs should be aware of safe storage and security and the importance of handing over to an authorized person to obtain a signature. They must also have a valid ID badge.

Supply under PGD

Registered nurses in accident and emergency departments and coronary care units can supply or administer diamorphine for the treatment of cardiac pain in accordance with a PGD.

They can also supply or administer any Schedule 3 or 4 controlled drug in accordance with a PGD (except anabolic steroids in Schedule 4 Part 2 and injectable formulations for the purpose of treating a person who is addicted to a drug).

Prescribing

A supplementary prescriber, when acting in accordance with a clinical management plan, can prescribe a controlled drug provided the controlled drug is included in the clinical management plan. An independent nurse prescriber can prescribe from the list of controlled drugs included in the nurse prescribers' formulary solely for the medical conditions indicated (DH 2007). The controlled drugs most commonly prescribed by nurses between 2007 and 2008 were methadone, buprenophine, diazepam and co-codamol (Care Quality Commission 2009).

In response to seven case reports, published between 2000 and 2005, regarding deaths due to the administration of high-dose (30 mg or greater) morphine or diamorphine to patients who had not previously received doses of opiates, the NPSA released a safer practice notice in 2006, *Ensuring Safer Practice with High Dose Ampoules of Morphine and Diamorphine* (NPSA 2006). In line with this safer practice notice, the following guidance should be adhered to (Box 16.8).

Between 2005 and 2008, 4223 incidents were reported to the NRLS involving opioid medicines and the 'wrong/unclear dose or strength' or 'wrong frequency' of medication. As a result, the NPSA released a Rapid Response Report in July 2008. The guidance shown in Box 16.9 has been given.

Box 16.8 High-dose opiate guidance

- High-strength preparations of morphine or diamorphine (30 mg or above) should be stored in a location separate from lower-strength preparations (10 mg) within the controlled drugs cupboard.
- Awareness should be raised of the similarities of drug packaging, and consider use of alert stickers being attached to high-strength preparations by pharmacy.
- A review of stock levels should be undertaken in all clinical areas where morphine and diamorphine are stored to assess whether high-strength preparations need to be kept on a permanent basis or whether they could be ordered according to specific patient requirements.
- Clear guidance should be provided to ensure that the correct doses of diamorphine and morphine are prepared in the appropriate clinical situation. For example, diamorphine 5 mg and 10 mg ampoules could be used for both bolus administration and patients newly commenced on diamorphine infusions; diamorphine 30 mg ampoules could be reserved for patients already receiving diamorphine infusions and who require higher daily doses.
- Patients should be observed for the first hour after receiving their first dose of diamorphine or morphine injection.
- Naloxone injections should be available in all clinical areas where morphine and diamorphine are stored.

(NPSA 2006)

The NPSA was notified of 498 midazolam patient safety incidents between November 2004 and November 2008 where the dose prescribed or administered to the patient was inappropriate. Three midazolam-related incidents have resulted in death. As a result, the NPSA released a Rapid Response Report in December 2008. The guidance in Box 16.10 has been given.

Box 16.9 Opioid dose/strength guidance

- Confirm any recent opioid dose, formulation, frequency of administration and any other analgesic medicines prescribed for the patient. This may be done, for example, through discussion with the patient or their representative (although not in the case of treatment for addiction), the prescriber or through medication records.
- Where a dose increase is intended, ensure that the calculated dose is safe for the patient (e.g. for oral morphine or oxycodone in adult patients, not normally more than 50% higher than the previous dose).
- Ensure they are familiar with the following characteristics of that medicine and formulation: usual starting dose, frequency of administration, standard dosing increments, symptoms of overdose, common side-effects.

(NPSA 2008a)

Box 16.10 Midazolam guidance

- Ensure that the storage and use of high-strength midazolam (5 mg/mL in 2 mL and 10 mL ampoules, or 2 mg/mL in 5 mL ampoules) are restricted to general anaesthesia, intensive care, palliative medicine and clinical areas/ situations where its use has been formally risk assessed, for example, where syringe drivers are used.
- Ensure that in other clinical areas, storage and use of high-strength midazolam are replaced with low-strength midazolam (1 mg/mL in 2 mL or 5 mL ampoules).
- Review therapeutic protocols to ensure that guidance on use of midazolam is clear and that the risks, particularly for the elderly or frail, are fully assessed.

- Ensure that all healthcare practitioners involved directly or participating in sedation techniques have the necessary knowledge, skills and competences.
- Ensure that stocks of flumazenil are available where midazolam is used and that the use of flumazenil is regularly audited as a marker of excessive dosing of midazolam.
- Ensure that sedation is covered by organizational policy and that overall responsibility is assigned to a senior clinician which, in most cases, will be an anaesthetist.

(NPSA 2008b)

Procedure guideline 16.2 Medication: controlled drug administration

Essential equipment

- Prescription chart
- Controlled drug record book
- Appropriate medication container, for example medicine pot or syringe

Preprocedure

Action	Rationale
1 Consult the patient's prescription chart, checking the name, date of birth, hospital number, allergy status and then ascertain the following: (a) Drug name (generic) (b) Dose (c) Date and time of administration (d) Frequency (e) Route and method of administration	To ensure that the patient is given the correct drug, in the correct formulation, in the prescribed dose using the appropriate diluent and by the correct route (DH 2003b, C; NMC 2008a, C).
(f) Formulation of oral preparation, e.g. modified release, immediate release	To ensure the correct formulation is given as many different formulations are available for the same drug. E
(g) Diluent as appropriate	
(h) Validity of prescription	Ensure prescription is legal (DH 2003b, C).
(i) Legible signature and contact details of prescriber.	To ensure prescription is legal and complies with hospital policy (DH 2003b, C).
(j) Check when the drug was last administered.	To ensure that the patient requires the drug at this time. E

Procedure

2 With the second Registered Nurse, take the keys and open the controlled drug cupboard. Take the ward controlled drug record book that contains the prescribed controlled drug and turn to the relevant page headed with the name and strength of the controlled drug.	To be able to check the stock and to enter the details into the controlled drug record book (DH 2003b, C).
3 With the second Registered Nurse, select the correct drug from the controlled drug cupboard.	To comply with hospital policy and to ensure patient receives the correct medicine (DH 2003b, C; NMC 2008a, C; NPSA 2006, C).
4 With the second Registered Nurse, check the stock level against the last entry in the ward record book.	To comply with hospital policy (DH 2003b, C; NMC 2008a, C; NPSA 2006, C).

5 With the second Registered Nurse, check the appropriate dose and concentration/strength (e.g. 10 mg in 1 mL or 5 mg in 5 mL) and formulation against the prescription chart and remove the dose from the box/bottle and place into an appropriate container, e.g. medicine pot or syringe.	To comply with hospital policy and to ensure patient receives the correct dose and strength of medicine (DH 2003b, C; NMC 2008a, C; NPSA 2006, C).
6 Return the remaining stock to the cupboard and lock the cupboard.	To comply with hospital policy (DH 2003b, C; NMC 2008a, C; NPSA 2006, C).
7 Enter the date, dose, new stock level and the patient's name in the ward record book, ensuring that both you and the second Registered Nurse sign the entry. NB: May require entry into different sections if the dose is to be made up of different doses, e.g. 70 mg = 1 × 50 mg and 2 × 10 mg). If any is wasted then ensure it is documented correctly, e.g. 5 mg given and 5 mg wasted.	To comply with hospital policy (DH 2003b, C; NMC 2008a, C; NPSA 2006, C).
8 With the second Registered Nurse, take the prepared dose to the patient and check the patient's identity by asking them to verbally identify themselves (where possible) and check against the patient's identification wristband. Also ask and check allergy status.	To prevent error and confirm patient's identity (NPSA 2005, C; NPSA 2007b, C).
9 Administer the drug after checking the prescription chart again. If given orally, wait until the patient has swallowed the medication.	To ensure the patient receives the medicines (DH 2003b, C).

Postprocedure

10 Once the drug has been administered, the prescription chart is signed by the nurse responsible for administering the medication and the Registered Nurse who witnessed the administration.	To prevent duplication of treatment. To comply with hospital policy (DH 2003b, C; NMC 2008a, C; NPSA 2006, C). To maintain accurate records, provide a point of reference in the event of any queries and prevent any duplication of treatment (NMC 2008a, C; NMC 2008b, C; NMC 2009, C).
11 The nurse should check the patient after administration to check for effectiveness and/or toxicity.	To ensure that the drug has been effective and to administer a breakthrough dose if necessary. To check that the patient has not experienced any toxicity that may require interventions. E
12 If drug given via a syringe driver/pump, the nurse should return to check the infusion and site and document in the appropriate records.	To ensure that the infusion is infusing at the correct rate and the site is suitable. E

Postprocedural considerations

Ongoing care

Patients should be monitored for signs of adverse effects from opioids and for signs of toxicity.

The most common side-effects are constipation, nausea and vomiting and drowsiness. All patients who are prescribed an opioid regularly should be prescribed laxatives concurrently to prevent constipation. Nausea and vomiting should subside after a few days but patients should be prescribed antiemetics and given reassurance. Drowsiness due to opioids should also subside after a few days so pa-

tients should be given reassurance. (Regnard and Hockley 2004)

The warning signs of toxicity due to opioids are:

- drowsiness
- confusion
- myoclonus
- hallucinations and nightmares
- respiratory depression.

If patients are showing signs of toxicity the opioid dose should be reduced or stopped and as-required opioid pain relief given (Regnard and Hockley 2004). Changing to an alternative opioid can also be considered (Regnard and Hockley 2004).

Naloxone, a specific opioid antagonist, has a high affinity for opioid receptors and reverses the effect of opioid analgesics. It is rarely needed in palliative care but may be needed in the case of opioid-induced respiratory depression (with respiration rate of 8 or below).

Care must be taken not to give naloxone to patients who have opioid-induced drowsiness, confusion or hallucinations that are not life threatening due to the risk of reversing the opioid analgesic effect (Twycross and Wilcock 2007).

Naloxone should be given in stat doses every 2 minutes until respiratory function is satisfactory and doses should be titrated against respiratory function and not consciousness in order to avoid total reversal of the analgesic effect (Twycross and Wilcock 2007). Flumazanil may be required for reversal of midazolam.

Routes of administration

The three basic routes of administration are enteral, parenteral and topical. The enteral route uses the gastrointestinal (GI) tract for absorption of drugs. The parenteral route bypasses the GI tract and is associated with all forms of injections. The topical route also bypasses the GI tract and is associated with drugs that are administered to the skin and mucous membranes (see Table 16.8).

Table 16.8 Advantages and disadvantages of the routes of administration

Route	Advantages	Disadvantages
Oral	Convenient	Compliance
	Easy to administer	Some drugs not suitable for oral route
	Least expensive	May not be able to swallow or take oral medications
Topical	Easy to apply	Can stain clothing
	Local effects	Local irritation
Injections	Absorbed quickly	Invasive
	Avoids GI tract	Pain
		Complications such as infection
		May be difficult to self-administer
Site specific, for example eye, ear, nasal, vaginal, rectal, pulmonary	Often for local effects	Discomfort and embarrassment
		May be difficult to self-administer

Oral administration

Definition

Medication taken either through the mouth that is swallowed by the patient or administered via a feeding tube for example nasogastric, percutaneous endoscopic gastrostomy (PEG) (Snyder 2007).

Oral administration is the most convenient route for drug administration and may result in better compliance (Kelly and Wright 2009). It is the least expensive and is usually the safest. Due to their widespread use, oral drugs are prepared in a variety of dosage forms.

Related theory

Tablets

These come in a great variety of shapes, sizes, colours and types. The formulation may be very simple, presenting as a plain, white, uncoated tablet, or complex, designed with specific therapeutic aims. Sugar coatings are used to improve appearance and palatability. In cases where the drug is a gastric irritant or is broken down by gastric acid, an enteric coating may be used; this is designed to allow the tablet to remain intact in the stomach and to pass unchanged into the small bowel where the coating dissolves and the drug is released and absorbed. Tablets may be formulated specifically to achieve control of the rate of release of drug from the tablet as it passes through the alimentary tract. Terms such as 'sustained-release', 'controlled-release' and 'modified-release' are used by manufacturers to describe these preparations. Tablets may also be formulated specifically to dissolve readily ('soluble' or 'effervescent'), to be chewed or to be held under the tongue ('sublingual') or placed between the gum and inside of the mouth ('buccal'). Unscored or coated tablets should not be crushed or broken, nor should most 'slow-release' or 'sustained-action' tablets, since this can alter the rate of release of drug from the tablet (Smyth 2006).

Capsules

These offer a useful method of formulating drugs which are difficult to make into a tablet or are particularly unpalatable.

The capsule shells are usually made of gelatine and the contents of the capsules may be solid, liquid or of a paste-like consistency. The contents do not cause deterioration of the shell. The shell, however, is attacked by the digestive fluids and the contents are then released. Delayed-release capsule formulations also exist. Gastro-resistant capsules are delayed-release capsules that are intended to resist the gastric fluid and to release their active substance or substances in the intestinal fluid (British Pharmacopoeia 2007). If for any reason the capsule is unpalatable or the patient is unable to take it, the contents should not routinely be removed from the shell without first seeking advice from a pharmacist. Removing contents from the capsule could destroy their properties and cause gastric irritation or premature release of the drug into an incompatible pH (Downie *et al.* 2003).

Lozenges and pastilles

Lozenges and pastilles are solid, single-dose preparations intended to be sucked to obtain a local or systemic effect to the mouth and/or throat (British Pharmacopoeia 2007).

Linctuses, elixirs and mixtures

Linctuses

These are viscous oral liquids that may contain one or more active ingredients; the solution usually contains a high proportion of sucrose. Linctuses are intended for use in the treatment or relief of cough.

Elixirs

These are clear, flavoured oral liquids containing one or more active ingredients dissolved in a vehicle that usually contains a high proportion of sucrose. A vehicle is a substance usually without therapeutic action used as a medium to give bulk for the administration of medicines. If the active drug is sensitive to moisture it may be formulated as a flavoured powder or granulation and then dissolved in water just before use.

Mixtures

Mixtures are usually aqueous preparations, containing one or more drug, which can be in the form of either a solution or a suspension. Mixtures are normally made up when required as they have a shelf-life of 2 weeks from preparation. Suspended drugs may slowly separate on standing but are easily redispersed by shaking which should be done before every use.

Drugs suspended, mixed or dispersed in liquids are often referred to as syrups. However, syrups do not contain active ingredients but are used as a vehicle for medications in order to decrease crystallization, increase solubility and provide aromatic and flavouring properties (British Pharmacopoeia 2007).

Evidence-based approaches

Observational studies suggest that medication administration errors for oral medicine range from 3% to 8% (Ho *et al.* 1997, Taxis *et al.* 1999) but this has been found to be twice as high in mental health patients who have swallowing difficulties (Haw *et al.* 2007). A proportion of these difficulties are due to an aversion to swallowing tablets, the most common cause being dysphagia (Kelly and Wright 2009). Guidance on medicines management related to dysphagia can be found within the NMC *Standards for Medicines Management* (NMC 2008a). When giving medicines to patients with dysphagia, both the patient and the medicine should be reviewed on a regular basis. If they cannot swallow tablets then liquid or dispersible medications should be the first

consideration (Kelly and Wright 2009). If the oral route is not patent then alternative routes should be used.

Covert drug administration

The NMC recognizes that 'this is a complex issue', as covert drug administration involves the fundamental principles of patient and client autonomy and consent to treatment, which are set out in common law and statute and underpinned by the Human Rights Act 1998 (NMC 2008a). The covert administration of medicines should not be confused with the administration of medicines against someone's will, which in itself may not be deceptive, but may be unlawful (NMC 2008a).

Some vulnerable groups of patients, such as those who are confused, may refuse to take medication. Traditionally, in some places, medication has therefore been hidden or disguised in food. The NMC (2001a, 2001b, 2008a) offered the following position statement.

> As a general principle, by disguising medication in food or drink, the patient or client is being led to believe that they are not receiving medication when in fact they are. The registered nurse, midwife or health visitor will need to be sure that what they are doing is in the best interests of the patient or client and be accountable for this decision.

Disguising medication in food and drink is acceptable under exceptional circumstances in which covert administration may be considered to prevent a patient, who is incapable of informed consent, from missing out on essential treatment (NMC 2001b, NMC 2008a). The following principles should be followed when making such a decision.

- The medication must be considered essential for the patient's health and well-being.
- The decision to administer medication covertly should be considered only as a contingency in an emergency, not as regular practice.
- The registered practitioner must make the decision only after discussion and with the support of the multiprofessional team and, if appropriate, the patient's relatives, carers or advocates.
- The pharmacist must be involved in these decisions as adding medication to food or drink can alter its pharmacological properties and thereby affect its performance.
- The decision and action taken must be fully documented in the patient's care plan and regularly reviewed.
- Regular attempts should continue to be made to encourage the patient to take the medication voluntarily (NMC 2001b, NMC 2008a, Treloar *et al.* 2000).

Preprocedural considerations

Equipment

Medicine pots

Medicine pots (Figure 16.3) allow a dosage form to be taken from its original container to allow immediate

957

Figure 16.5 Tablet crusher.

Figure 16.3 Medicine pot.

administration to a patient. The person who removes medication from its original container and places it into a medicine pot must oversee the administration of this medication. This responsibility cannot be transferred to someone else.

Tablet splitters

Commercially available tablet splitters (Figure 16.4) may increase the accuracy of tablet splitting when this activity is necessary. Tablets that are unscored, unusually thick or oddly shaped, sugar coated, enteric coated and sustained-release tablets are not suitable for splitting. Areas for consideration when using a tablet splitter include the following.

- Can the tablets be split? This must always be discussed with the pharmacy department.
- Do patients have the manual dexterity to use a tablet splitter when at home?
- Will splitting the tablets affect patient adherence when they are at home? Will patients skip or double dose rather than split tablets?
- How will the storage of split tablets affect the stability of the tablets? What about the effect of light and air (Marriott and Nation 2002)?

Figure 16.4 Tablet splitter.

Tablet crushers

Tablet crushers (Figure 16.5) can be used when a patient has swallowing difficulties and no alternative dosage form exists. Crushing tablets is usually outside the product licence. The Medicines Act 1968 states that unlicensed medicines can only be authorized by a medical or dental practitioner so if the activity of crushing tablets is going to take place, there should be discussion and agreement between the prescriber and the person who will administer the medicine. Discussion should also take place with the pharmacist to check that the tablet is suitable for crushing and that the efficacy of the medication is not changed as a result. Tablets that are enteric coated, sustained release or chewable cannot be crushed. Areas for consideration when crushing a tablet include the following.

- Can the tablet be crushed? This must always be discussed with the pharmacy department.
- Will crushing make the tablet unpalatable?
- Will crushing the tablet cause any adverse effects for the patient, for example burning of the oral mucosa?
- Will crushing the tablet result in inaccurate dosing (Kelly and Wright 2009)?

When a tablet crusher is used, water should be added to the crushed tablet and the resulting solution drawn up using an oral syringe. The crusher should then be rinsed and the process repeated. Tablet crushers should be rinsed before and after use to prevent cross-contamination with other medicines (Fair and Proctor 2007, Smyth 2006).

When a tablet crusher has been used, it should be opened and washed under running water, dried with a tissue and left to air dry on a tissue or paper towel.

Monitored dosage systems and compliance aids

Monitored dosage systems and compliance aids, for example dosette boxes (Figure 16.6), are designed to help patients remember when to take their medication. They can also let carers know whether patients have taken their medication. The following should be considered when using these systems.

Figure 16.6   Dosette box.

Figure 16.7   Oral syringe (compliant with NPSA guidance).

- They can only be used for tablets and capsules.
- Medicines that are susceptible to moisture should not be put in these systems.
- Light-sensitive medicines should not be put in these systems.
- Medicines that are harmful when handled should not be put in these systems.
- If the patient is on medications that cannot be stored in these systems, precautions should be put in place to ensure that they can cope with two systems.
- If the patient's drug regimen is not stable, consideration should be given to how easy it will be to make changes to the system.
- As-required medication cannot be placed in these systems.
- These systems comply with labelling and leaflet legislation so they must always be dispensed by a pharmacy department (RPSGB 2007b).

Oral syringes

If a syringe is needed to measure and administer an oral dose, an oral syringe (Figure 16.7) that cannot be attached to intravenous catheters or ports should be used. These syringes are purple in colour. All oral syringes containing oral liquid medicines must be labelled by the person who prepared the syringe with the name and strength of the medicine, the patient name and the time it was prepared. Labelling is unecessary if the preparation and administration is one uninterrupted process and the labelled syringe does not leave the hands of the person who prepared it. Only one unlabelled syringe should be handled at any one time (NPSA 2007d).

Specific patient preparations

Before administering oral medication, the nurses should assess for:

- the patient's ability to understand the purpose of the medication being administered
- any medication allergies and hypersensitivities
- nil by mouth status
- the patient's ability to swallow the form of medication
- the patient's cough and gag reflexes
- any contraindications to oral medications including nausea and vomiting, absence of bowel sounds/reduced peristalsis, nasogastric suctioning or any circumstance affecting bowel motility or absorption of medication, for example general anaesthesia, GI surgery, inflammatory bowel disease
- any possibility of drug–drug or drug–food interactions
- any preadministration assessment for specific medications, for example pulse or blood pressure.

(Chernecky *et al.* 2002, Snyder 2007)

Procedure guideline 16.3 Medication: oral drug administration

959

See also Table 16.9

Essential equipment

- Drugs to be administered
- Recording sheet or book as required by law or hospital policy
- Patient's prescription chart, to check dose, route and so on
- Glass of water
- Any protective clothing required by hospital policy for specified drugs, such as antibiotics or cytotoxic drugs, for example gloves (see Chapter 15)
- Medicine container (disposable if possible)

Preprocedure

Action	Rationale
1 Wash hands with bactericidal soap and water or bactericidal alcohol handrub.	To minimize the risk of cross-infection (DH 2007, C; Fraise and Bradley 2009, E).

(Continued)

Procedure guideline 16.3 *(Continued)*

2 Before administering any prescribed drug, check that it is due and has not already been given. Check that the information contained in the prescription chart is complete, correct and legible.	To protect the patient from harm (DH 2003b, C; NMC 2008a, C).
3 Before administering any prescribed drug, consult the patient's prescription chart and ascertain the following: (a) Drug (b) Dose (c) Date and time of administration (d) Route and method of administration (e) Diluent as appropriate (f) Validity of prescription (g) Signature of prescriber (h) The prescription is legible.	To ensure that the patient is given the correct drug in the prescribed dose using the appropriate diluent and by the correct route (DH 2003b, C; NMC 2008a, C). To protect the patient from harm (DH 2003b, C; NMC 2008a, C).

Procedure

4 Select the required medication and check the expiry date.	Treatment with medication that is outside the expiry date is dangerous. Drugs deteriorate with storage. The expiry date indicates when a particular drug is no longer pharmacologically efficacious (DH 2003b, C; NMC 2008a, C).
5 Empty the required dose into a medicine container. Avoid touching the preparation.	To minimize the risk of cross-infection. To minimize the risk of harm to the nurse (DH 2007, C; Fraise and Bradley 2009, E).
6 Take the medication and the prescription chart to the patient. Check the patient's identity by asking the patient to state their full name and date of birth. If the patient is unable to confirm details then check patient identity band against prescription chart.	To ensure that the medication is administered to the correct patient (NPSA 2005, C).
7 Evaluate the patient's knowledge of the medication being offered. If this knowledge appears to be faulty or incorrect, offer an explanation of the use, action, dose and potential side-effects of the drug or drugs involved.	A patient has a right to information about treatment (NMC 2008a, C; NMC 2008b, C).
8 Assist the patient to a sitting position where possible. A side-lying position may also be used if the patient is unable to sit.	To ease swallowing and prevent aspiration (Chernecky *et al.* 2002, E).
9 Make any required assessments such as pulse, BP or respiration.	These are required to ensure the patient is fit enough to receive medication, for example BP before antihypertensives (Chernecky *et al.* 2002, E).
10 Administer the drug as prescribed.	To meet legal requirements and hospital policy (DH 2003b, C; NMC 2008a, C; NMC 2008b, C; NMC 2009, C).
11 Offer a glass of water, if allowed, assisting the patient where necessary.	To facilitate swallowing of the medication (Chernecky *et al.* 2002, E; Jordan *et al.* 2003, E).
12 Stay with the patient until they have swallowed all the medication.	To ensure that medication has been taken on time (Chernecky *et al.* 2002, E).

Postprocedure

13 Record the dose given in the prescription chart and in any other place made necessary by legal requirement or hospital policy.	To meet legal requirements and hospital policy (DH 2003b, C; NMC 2008a, C; NMC 2008b, C; NMC 2009, C).

Table 16.9 Considerations for specific types of administration

Consideration	Rationale
Administer irritant drugs with meals or snacks	To minimize their effect on the gastric mucosa (Jordan *et al.* 2003, Shepherd 2002a)
Administer drugs that interact with food, or that are destroyed in significant proportions by digestive enzymes, between meals or on an empty stomach	To prevent interference with the absorption of the drug (Jordan *et al.* 2003, Shepherd 2002a)
Do not break a tablet unless it is scored and appropriate to do so. Break scored tablets with a file or a tablet cutter. Wash after use	Breaking may cause incorrect dosage, gastrointestinal irritation or destruction of a drug in an incompatible pH. To reduce risk of contamination between tablets (DH 2007, Jordan *et al.* 2003, NMC 2008a, Shepherd 2002a)
Do not interfere with time-release capsules and enteric-coated tablets. Ask patients to swallow these whole and not to chew them	The absorption rate of the drug will be altered (Jordan *et al.* 2003, Perry 2007)
Sublingual tablets must be placed under the tongue and buccal tablets between gum and cheek	To allow for correct absorption (Perry 2007)
When administering liquids to babies and young children, or when an accurately measured dose in multiples of 1 mL is needed for an adult, an oral syringe should be used in preference to a medicine spoon or measure	An oral syringe is much more accurate than a measure or a 5 mL spoon
	Use of a syringe makes administration of the correct dose much easier in an unco-operative child
	Oral syringes are available and are designed to be washable and reused for the same patient. However, in the immuno-compromised patient single use only is recommended. Oral syringes must be clearly labelled for oral or enteral use only (DH 2007, NPSA 2007d)
In babies and children especially, correct use of the syringe is very important. The tip should be gently pushed into and towards the side of the mouth. The contents are then *slowly* discharged towards the inside of the cheek, pausing if necessary to allow the liquid to be swallowed. If children are unco-operative it may help to place the end of the barrel between the teeth	To prevent injury to the mouth and eliminate the danger of choking the patient (Watt 2003)
	To get the dose in and to prevent the patient spitting it out (Watt 2003)
When administering gargling medication, throat irrigations should not be warmer than body temperature	Liquid warmer than body temperature may cause discomfort or damage tissue.

Problem-solving table 16.1 Prevention and resolution (Procedure guideline 16.3)

Problem	Cause	Prevention	Action
Patient vomits when taking or after taking tablets	Patient suffering from nausea and vomiting	Administer antiemetics prior to administration of tablets. These may need to be given via rectal, IM or IV route	If patient vomits immediately after tablet swallowed then it may be given again (maybe after antiemetics). If vomits some time after tablet taken it may depend on type and frequency of medication as to whether it can be retaken. Patients are advised to retake if they can see a whole tablet in vomit
Patient unable to swallow tablets	Patient suffering from dysphagia or has issues swallowing tablets	Discuss with pharmacy regarding availability of medication in liquid form	Discuss with prescriber as to administering the medicine in another form or route

Topical administration

Definition

Medication applied onto the skin and mucous membranes primarily for its local effects, for example creams and ointments (Chernecky et al. 2002, Snyder 2007).

Related theory

Creams

Creams are emulsions of oil and water and are generally well absorbed into the skin. They are usually more cosmetically acceptable than ointments because they are less greasy and easier to apply (BNF 2011). They may be used as a 'base' in which a variety of drugs may be applied for local therapy (BNF 2011).

Ointments

Ointments are greasy preparations, which are normally anhydrous and insoluble in water, and are more occlusive than creams (BNF 2011). They are absorbed more slowly into the skin and leave a greasy residue. They have similar uses to creams and are particularly suitable for dry, scaly lesions (BNF 2011).

Lotions

These are emollient liquid solutions, emulsions or suspensions which may be water or oil based (Snyder 2007).

Pastes

These are semi-solid preparations with adhesive properties and they tend to be thicker than ointment or creams (Snyder 2007).

Wound products

See Chapter 19.

Evidence-based approaches

The risk of serious effects is generally low but systemic effects can occur if the skin is thin, if drug concentration is high or contact is prolonged (Snyder 2007).

Preprocedural considerations

Specific patient preparations

The condition of the affected site should be assessed for altered skin integrity as applying medicines to broken skin could cause them to be absorbed too rapidly, resulting in systemic effects (Chernecky et al. 2002, Snyder 2007). The affected area must be washed and dried before applying the topical medicines where appropriate, unless the prescription directs otherwise.

Procedure guideline 16.4 Medication: topical applications

Essential equipment

- Clean non-sterile gloves
- Sterile topical swabs
- Applicators

Preprocedure

Action	Rationale
1 Explain and discuss the procedure with the patient.	To ensure that the patient understands the procedure and gives their valid consent (Griffith and Jordan 2003, E; NMC 2008b, C; NMC 2008c, C).
2 Check the patient's prescription chart and the patient's identity.	To ensure that the patient is given the correct drug and dose (NMC 2008a, C).

Procedure

3 Assist the patient into the required position.	To allow access to the affected area of skin. E
4 Close room door or curtains if appropriate.	To ensure patient privacy and dignity. E
5 Assess the condition of the skin and use aseptic technique if the skin is broken.	To prevent local or systemic infection (DH 2007, C; Fraise and Bradley 2009, E).
6 If the medication is to be rubbed into the skin, the preparation should be placed on a sterile topical swab.	To minimize the risk of cross-infection. To protect the nurse (DH 2007, C; Fraise and Bradley 2009, E).

Transdermal administration

7 If the preparation causes staining, advise the patient of this.	To ensure that adequate precautions are taken beforehand such as removal of clothing and to prevent stains (NMC 2008b, C).
8 Use a sterile dressing if required.	To ensure the ointment remains in place (Chernecky *et al.* 2002, E).

Postprocedure

9 Record the administration on appropriate charts.	To maintain accurate records, provide a point of reference in the event of any queries and prevent any duplication of treatment (NMC 2008a, C; NMC 2009, C)

Postprocedural considerations

Educate the patient to inform the nurse if there is any itching, skin colour change or signs of a rash following application.

Complications
Local skin reaction

The skin site may appear inflamed and oedema with blistering indicates subacute inflammation or eczema has developed from worsening of skin lesions. Patients may also complain of pruritus and tenderness which could indicate slow or impaired healing and should be referred to the prescriber; alternative therapies may be required (Snyder 2007).

Transdermal administration

Definition

Medication applied to the outermost layer of the skin, the stratum corneum, usually as an adhesive medicated disc that allows the medication to be absorbed at a slow and constant rate in order to produce a systemic effect (Chernecky *et al.* 2002).

Related theory
Conventional transdermal systems

These systems consist of a gel or ointment which is measured and placed directly onto the skin. Drugs that are used in this way include glyceryl trinitrate and oestradiol. Delivering drugs in this way can be messy for patients and can also result in variations of the dose delivered due to the amount applied, the amount of rubbing in of the product, the amount of product transferred onto clothing and so on.

Transdermal patches

A transdermal patch (Figure 16.8) contains a certain amount of drug and delivers it in a quantity which is sufficient to cause the desired pharmacological effect when it crosses the skin and into the systemic system.

Three types of transdermal patch are available.

Adhesive

These are simply designed patches which consist of a drug-containing adhesive and a backing material. These patches do not provide much control over the rate of delivery and in most cases the stratum corneum controls the rate (Hillery *et al.* 2001).

Layered or matrix patches

Layered patches consist of a drug-containing matrix, an adhesive layer and a backing material. The drug-containing matrix controls the release of drug from the system (Hillery *et al.* 2001).

Reservoir

Reservoir patches consist of an enclosed reservoir of drug, a membrane layer, an adhesive layer and a backing material. The membrane layer controls the rate of drug delivery from the reservoir of drug.

Drugs which can be delivered in a transdermal system include fentanyl, hyoscine, nicotine and oestradiol (Hillery *et al.* 2001).

Evidence-based approaches

The advantages of transdermal systems are the avoidance of the presystemic metabolism, the drug effects can be maintained within the therapeutic window for longer which reduces side-effects and maintains constant dosing, there can be improved patient compliance and drug effects can be stopped with the withdrawal of the patch and the avoidance of the first-pass metabolism (Hillery *et al.* 2001). First-pass

Figure 16.8 Transdermal patches.

metabolism occurs when a drug passes through the digestive system and enters the hepatic portal system and the liver before it reaches the rest of the body. The liver metabolizes many drugs, thus reducing their bio-availability before reaching the rest of the circulatory system (Hardman *et al.* 1996).

A disadvantage of transdermal systems is the limited number of drugs for which the system is suitable; for example, drugs have to have a suitable potency to allow them to absorb across the skin and cause an effect. Tolerance-inducing drugs would need a period during which they were not administered, which is not always possible with transdermal systems. In addition, drugs to be used in transdermal systems cannot be irritating to the skin otherwise they would not be tolerated by patients (Hillery *et al.* 2001).

Preprocedural considerations
Specific patient preparations

The condition of the affected site should be assessed for altered skin integrity as applying medicines to broken skin could cause too rapid absorption, resulting in systemic effects (Cherneck *et al.* 2002, Snyder 2007). The affected area must be washed and dried before applying the patch, which should be attached to hairless areas of skin. The upper chest, upper arms and upper back are recommended sites and the distal areas of extermities should be avoided (Chernecky *et al.* 2002). Patches should not be trimmed or cut. Contact with water does not affect the patch (Chernecky *et al.* 2002).

Procedure guideline 16.5 Medication: transdermal applications

Essential equipment

- Transdermal patch

Preprocedure

Action	Rationale
1 Explain and discuss the procedure with the patient.	To ensure that the patient understands the procedure and gives their valid consent (Griffith and Jordan 2003, E; NMC 2008b, C; NMC 2008c, C).
2 Check the patient's prescription chart and patient's identity.	To ensure that the patient is given the correct drug and dose (NMC 2008a, C).

Procedure

3 Close room door or curtains if appropriate.	To ensure patient privacy and dignity. E
4 Assist the patient into the required position.	To allow access to the affected area of skin. E
5 Assess the condition of the skin and do not apply to skin that is oily, burnt, cut or irritated in any way.	To prevent local or systemic effects and to ensure the patch will remain in place (DH 2007, C; Snyder 2007, E).
6 Remove any drug residue from the former site before placing the next patch.	To avoid any skin irritation (Chernecky *et al.* 2002, E).
7 Carefully remove the patch from its protective cover and hold it by the edge without touching the adhesive edges.	To ensure the patch will adhere and the medication dose will not be affected (Snyder 2007, E).
8 Apply the patch immediately, pressing firmly with the palm of the hand for up to 10 seconds, making sure the patch sticks well around the edges.	To ensure adequate adhesion and prevent loss of patch which would result in reduced dose and effectiveness (Snyder 2007, E).
9 Date and initial the patch	To ensure all staff know when it must be changed (Snyder 2007, E).

Postprocedure

10 Record the administration on appropriate charts.	To maintain accurate records, provide a point of reference in the event of any queries and prevent any duplication of treatment (NMC 2008a, C; NMC 2009, C).

Postprocedural considerations

Ongoing care

To avoid skin irritation, the sites of transdermal patches should be rotated (Chernecky *et al.* 2002). After use, the patch still contains substantial quantities of active ingredients which may have harmful effects if they reach the aquatic environment. Hence, after removal, the used patch should be folded in half, adhesive side inwards so that the release membrane is not exposed, placed in the original sachet and then discarded safely out of reach of children. Any used or unused patches should be discarded according to local policy or returned to the pharmacy. Used patches should not be flushed down the toilet or placed in liquid waste disposal systems (www.medicines.org.uk).

Complications

See Topical applications.

Rectal administration

Definition

These are medications administered via the rectum which may exert a local effect on the GI mucosa such as promoting defaecation or systemic effects such as providing analgesia or relieving nausea and vomiting (Chernecky *et al.* 2002, Snyder 2007).

Related theory

Suppositories

Suppositories are solid preparations which may contain one or more drug. The drugs are normally ground or sieved and then dissolved or dispersed into a glyceride-type fatty acid base or a water-soluble one. These suppositories will either melt after insertion into the body or dissolve and mix with the available volume of rectal fluid (Aulton 1988).

Enemas

Enemas are solutions or dispersions of a drug in a small volume of water or oil. These preparations are presented in a small plastic container made of a bulb which contains the drug and an application tube. The bulb can be compressed when the tube has been inserted in the rectum to deliver the drug. Enemas can be difficult for patients to use by themselves compared to suppositories and therefore their use is not as widespread (Aulton 1988).

Evidence-based approaches

The advantages of rectal administration include the following.

- The drug can be administered when the patient is not able to make use of the oral route, for example if the patient is vomiting or is postoperative and therefore either unconscious or unable to ingest via the oral route.
- In some categories of patient it may be easier to use the rectal route than the oral one as it does not require swallowing, for example children, the elderly.
- The drug may be less suited to the oral route, for example the oral route can cause severe local GI side-effects. The drug may not be stable after GI administration or it may have an unacceptable taste which makes it unpalatable via the oral route.
- Rarely cause local irritation or side-effects.
                    (Chernecky *et al.* 2002, Snyder 2007)

The disadvantages of the rectal route include the following.

- Strong feelings against the rectal route by some patients in some countries and also feelings of discomfort and embarrassment.
- There can be slow and incomplete absorption via the rectal route.
- The development of proctitis has been reported with rectal drug administration.
- Contraindicated in patients who have had rectal surgery or have active rectal bleeding.
(Chernecky *et al.* 2002, Downie *et al.* 2003, Snyder 2007)

After a suppository is inserted into the rectum, body temperature melts the suppository so it can be distributed. Proper placement is important to promote retention of the medication until it dissolves and is absorbed into the mucosa (Snyder 2007).

For further information about the administration of rectal medication, see Chapter 6 and Procedure guideline 6.15.

Vaginal administration

Definition

Medications are inserted into the vaginal canal usually for local effects such as treatment of infections (e.g. *Trichomonas* and *Candida* infections) and contraceptive purposes. They are used less commonly for systemic effects (such as oestrogens and progesterones) (Chernecky *et al.* 2002, Snyder 2007).

Related theory

Vaginal preparations can be delivered in a wide variety of dosage forms including pessaries, creams, aerosol foams, gels and tablets (Chernecky *et al.* 2002, Snyder 2007).

Evidence-based approaches

The advantages of the vaginal route include the following.

- The vagina offers a large surface area for drug absorption.

- A rich blood supply ensures a rapid absorption of drug.
- This route can act as an alternative to drugs that cannot be delivered via the oral route (as for suppositories).
- This route can be used when patients cannot take drugs via the oral route (as for suppositories).
- The vaginal route can deliver drug over a controlled period of time, thus avoiding peaks and troughs which result in less toxicity and risk of ineffectiveness.

The disadvantages include the following.

- The route is limited to drugs that are potent molecules and are therefore easily absorbed.
- The vagina can be easily irritated by the use of devices or locally irritating drugs.
- Care must be taken with the use of vaginal devices to ensure they are sterilized and not acting as a growth medium for bacteria.

- The vaginal bio-availability can be affected by hormone levels and can therefore change during menstrual cycles, with age and during pregnancy.
- Leakage can occur with vaginal preparations. This can be alleviated by using the preparation at night.
- This route may not be acceptable to some patients.

(Hillery *et al.* 2001)

Preprocedural considerations
Specific patient preparations

Check patient for any allergies and also whether they have recently given birth or undergone vaginal surgery as this may alter tissue integrity and the level of discomfort. The nurse should also review the patient's willingness and ability to self administer the medication (Chernecky *et al.* 2002; Snyder 2007).

Procedure guideline 16.6 Medication: vaginal administration

Essential equipment

- Disposable gloves
- Topical swabs
- Disposable sanitary pad
- Lubricating jelly
- Prescription chart
- Warm water
- Pen torch

Medicinal products

- Pessary

Preprocedure

Action	Rationale
1 Explain and discuss the procedure with the patient.	To ensure that the patient understands the procedure and gives her valid consent (Griffith and Jordan 2003, E; NMC 2008b, C; NMC 2008c, C).
2 Consult the patient's prescription sheet and ascertain the following: (a) Drug (b) Dose (c) Date and time of administration (d) Route and method of administration (e) Validity of prescription (f) Signature of doctor	To ensure that the patient is given the correct drug in the prescribed dose and by the correct route (NMC 2008a, C).
3 Select the appropriate pessary and check it with the prescription chart.	To ensure that the correct medication is given to the correct patient at the appropriate time (NMC 2008a, C).
Procedure	
4 Close room door or curtains, keeping the patient covered as much as possible.	To ensure patient privacy and dignity. E
5 Assist the patient into the appropriate position, either left lateral with buttocks to the edge of the bed or supine with the knees drawn up and legs parted. May require a light source, e.g. lamp or torch.	To facilitate easy access to the vaginal canal, visualize the external genitalia and vaginal canal and facilitate correct insertion of the pessary (manufacturer's instruction, C; Chernecky *et al.* 2002, E; Snyder 2007, E).

6 Wash hands with bactericidal soap and water or bactericidal alcohol handrub, and put on gloves.	To minimize the risk of cross-infection (DH 2007, C; Fraise and Bradley 2009, E).
7 Clean the area with warm water if necessary.	To remove any previously applied creams (Downie *et al.* 2003, E).
8 Remove the pessary from wrapper and apply lubricating jelly to a topical swab and from the swab on to the pessary. Lubricate gloved index finger of dominant hand.	To facilitate insertion of the pessary and ensure the patient's comfort (manufacturer's instruction, C).
9 With non-dominant gloved hand gently retract labial folds to expose vaginal orifice.	To enable insertion of pessary into correct orifice (Snyder 2007, E).
10 Insert the rounded end of the pessary along the posterior vaginal wall and into the top of the vagina (entire length of finger).	To ensure the pessary is inserted into the correct position to ensure equal distribution of medication (Snyder 2007, E). To ensure that the pessary is retained and that the medication can reach its maximum efficiency (manufacturer's instruction, C; Chernecky *et al.* 2002, E).
11 Wipe away any excess lubricating jelly from the patient's vulval and/or perineal area with a topical swab.	To promote patient comfort (Snyder 2007, E).
12 Make the patient comfortable and explain to her that there may be a small amount of discharge and apply a clean sanitary pad.	To absorb any excess discharge (Snyder 2007, E).

Postprocedure

13 Remove and dispose of gloves safely and in accordance with locally approved procedures.	To ensure safe disposal (DH 2005, C; MHRA 2004, C).
14 Record the administration on appropriate charts.	To maintain accurate records, provide a point of reference in the event of any queries and prevent any duplication of treatment (NMC 2008a, C; NMC 2009, C).

Postprocedural considerations

The patient needs to retain the medication so it is recommended that the medication is administered prior to going to bed or the patient should remain supine for 5–10 minutes after instilling the pessary (Chernecky *et al.* 2002, Snyder 2007). It should be explained to the patient that she may also notice a discharge following administration and that it is nothing to be concerned about.

Pulmonary administration

Definition

'Dosage forms introduced into the body via the lungs in an aerosol form to achieve local effects such as to improve bronchodilation or to improve clearance of pulmonary secretions' (Chernecky *et al.* 2002, Snyder 2007). Systemic effects can also be achieved through the pulmonary route, for example volatile anaesthetics (Hillery *et al.* 2001). Some are inhaled via the mouth, some via the nose and some via nose and mouth (Downie *et al.* 2003).

Related theory

In order for drugs to reach the lungs, they must be delivered in an aerosol form. The aerosol penetrates the lung airways and the deeper passages of the respiratory tract provide a large surface area for drug absorption and the alveolar-capillary network absorbs medication rapidly (Snyder 2007). There are three ways in which this aerosol can be produced: by nebulizer, by pressurized metered dose inhalers and by drug powder inhalers.

■ *Nebulization* involves the passage of air or oxygen driven through a solution of a drug. The resulting fine mist is then inhaled via a facemask (Trounce and Gould 2000). Some antibiotics and bronchodilators may be given in this way (Figure 16.9).

■ *Metered dose inhalers* (MDI) involve a drug being suspended in a propellant in a small hand-held aerosol can in the form of a spray, mist or fine powder. Metered doses can then be delivered from the aerosol by the use of a metering valve within the device which is designed to release a fixed volume, for example ventolin. Steroid medications are often administered by MDI to

967

Figure 16.12   Turbohaler®.

Figure 16.9   Nebulizer.

Figure 16.10   Metered dose inhaler (MDI).

Figure 16.11   Accuhaler®.

treat long-term reactive airway disease (Chernecky *et al.* 2002, Snyder 2007) (Figure 16.10).

- *Dry powder inhalers* (DPI) involve a powder being delivered to the lung via a breath-actuated device. Examples of inhalers in this group are the Accuhaler® (Figure 16.11) and the Turbohaler® (Figure 16.12).

Preprocedural considerations
Equipment
Nebulizer

The advantage of nebulizers is that they can deliver more drug to the lungs than standard inhalers because of the smaller particles that are generated. They also do not require any co-ordination in order to deliver the drug to the lungs. The disadvantages are that they are expensive, they are not easily portable and the delivery of drug can be difficult to control, for example due to loss in the tubing and mouthpiece.

Metered dose inhaler (MDI)

The advantages of MDIs are that they are convenient, can deliver a fixed dose and are inexpensive. The disadvantage

Figure 16.13 Spacer device.

can be the co-ordination needed to use one. In order to be effective, the patient needs to trigger the MDI during a deep slow inhalation and then hold their breath for around 10 seconds. This need for co-ordination between actuation of the dose and inhalation can be removed by using a spacer device (Figure 16.13). The spacer device reduces the speed with which the dose is delivered and the resultant 'cold freon' effect that can occur, which can prevent a patient from continuing to inhale after actuation of the MDI. Spacers are also useful for patients on high-dose inhaled steroids in order to prevent oral candidiasis, children and patients requiring higher doses, and can improve dose delivery to 15% (Downie *et al.* 2003). Spacer devices are designed to be compatible with specific inhalers and therefore care should be taken to ensure the correct spacer device is used.

Medication in MDIs is under pressure and so they should not be punctured or stored near heat or in hot conditions (e.g. patients must be taught not to leave their MDI in a hot car) (Chernecky *et al.* 2002).

Dry powder inhalers (DPI)

Dry powder inhalers are also useful when there are problems with co-ordination. However, they can initiate a cough reflex and patients need to have sufficient breath inhalation to activate the device.

It is also important to remember that because these medications are absorbed rapidly through the pulmonary circulation, most create systemic side-effects (Chernecky *et al.* 2002, Snyder 2007).

Specific patient preparations

Patients who suffer from chronic respiratory disease and require airway management frequently receive inhalational medications. Maximum benefit is obtained only when the correct technique of inhalation is used so it is vital that patients are taught how to use these devices correctly and safely. Periodic checks should be carried out to ensure that efficiency is being maintained. Use of a MDI requires co-ordination during the breathing cycle and impairment of grasp or presence of tremors of the hands interferes with patient ability to depress the canister within the inhaler (Chernecky *et al.* 2002, Snyder 2007). Studies have shown that both adults and children have difficulties with aerosol inhalers and problems include co-ordinating activation and inhalation, too rapid inhalation and too short breaths after inspiration (Hilton 1990). Baseline observations of pulse, respirations and breath sounds should be performed before beginning treatment to use as a comparison during and after treatment (Snyder 2007). Patients who are to receive nebulized medicines should be in a sitting position either in bed or a chair (Downie *et al.* 2003).

Education

Compliance is more likely to be achieved if the patient is well informed. It is the responsibilty of the nurse, doctor and pharamcists to ensure that patients have adequate teaching and demonstration and are monitored at intervals. Downie *et al.* (2003) suggest that the patient should know the following.

- About the disease, the purpose of the therapy, how to recognize and report deterioration in the condition.
- How to use and care for the inhaler.
- The dose to be taken.
- The time interval.
- The maximum number of inhalations which should be taken in 24 hours.

Procedure guideline 16.7 Medication: administration by inhalation using a metered dose inhaler

Essential equipment

- MDI device
- Spacer device

Preprocedure

Action	Rationale
1 Explain and discuss the procedure with the patient.	To ensure that the patient understands the procedure and gives their valid consent (Griffith and Jordan 2003, E; NMC 2008b, C; NMC 2008c, C).

(Continued)

Procedure guideline 16.7 *(Continued)*

2 Correct use of inhalers is essential (see manufacturer's information leaflet) and will be achieved only if this is carefully explained and demonstrated to the patient. If further advice is required, contact the hospital pharmacist.	Incorrect use may result in most of the dose remaining in the mouth and/or being expelled almost immediately. This renders treatment ineffective (Watt 2003, E; manufacturer's instructions, C).

Procedure

3 Sit the patient in an upright position if possible in the bed or a chair.	To permit full expansion of the diaphragm. E
4 Consult the patient's prescription chart, and ascertain the following: (a) Drug (b) Dose (c) Date and time of administration (d) Route and method of administration (e) Diluent as appropriate (f) Validity of prescription (g) Signature of doctor.	To ensure that the patient is given the correct drug in the prescribed dose using the appropriate diluent and by the correct route (NMC 2006b, C).
5 Remove mouthpiece cover from inhaler.	To expose the area for use. E
6 Shake inhaler well for 2–5 seconds.	To ensure mixing of medication in canister (Snyder 2007, E).
7 **Without a spacer device:** Ask patient to take a deep breath and exhale completely, open lips and place inhaler opening 1–2 cm from mouth but not touching the lips. **With a spacer device:** Ask the patient to exhale and then grasp spacer mouthpiece with teeth and lips while holding inhaler.	To avoid rapid influx of inhaled medication and possible irritation of the airway (Snyder 2007, E). To enable the medication to reach the airways instead of hitting the back of the throat (Snyder 2007, E).
8 Ask the patient to tip head back slightly, inhale slowly and deeply through the mouth whilst depressing canister.	To allow medication to be distrubted to airways during inhalation (Snyder 2007, E).
9 Instruct the patient to breathe in slowly for 2–3 seconds and hold their breath for approximately 10 seconds, then to exhale slowly through pursed lips.	To enable aerosol spray to reach deeper branches of airways (Chernecky *et al.* 2002, E; Snyder 2007, E).
10 Instruct the patient to wait 2–5 minutes between puffs and if more than one type of inhaled medication is prescribed, to wait 5–10 minutes between inhalations.	To ensure that the medication has optimum effect and minimal side-effects (Snyder 2007, E).
11 If steroid medication is administered ask the patient to rinse their mouth after the procedure.	To remove any medication residue from oral cavity area to reduce risk of oral yeast infection (Snyder 2007, E).

Postprocedure

12 Clean any equipment used and discard all disposable equipment in appropriate containers.	To minimize the risk of infection (DH 2007c, C; Fraise and Bradley 2009, E).
13 Record the administration on appropriate charts.	To maintain accurate records, provide a point of reference in the event of any queries and prevent any duplication of treatment (NMC 2008a, C; NPSA 2007c, C; NMC 2009, C).

Procedure guideline 16.8 Medication: administration by inhalation using a nebulizer

Essential equipment

- Facemask or mouthpiece
- Nebulizer and tubing

Medicinal products

- Medication required

Preprocedure

Action	Rationale
1 Explain and discuss the procedure with the patient.	To ensure that the patient understands the procedure and gives their valid consent (Griffith and Jordan 2003, E; NMC 2008b, C; NMC 2008c, C).
2 Sit the patient in an upright position if possible in the bed or a chair.	To permit full expansion of the diaphragm. E
3 Consult the patient's prescription chart and ascertain the following: (a) Drug (b) Dose (c) Date and time of administration (d) Route and method of administration (e) Diluent as appropriate (f) Validity of prescription (g) Signature of doctor.	To ensure that the patient is given the correct drug in the prescribed dose using the appropriate diluent and by the correct route (NMC 2006b, C).

Procedure

4 Administer only one drug at a time unless specifically instructed to the contrary.	Several drugs used together may cause undesirable reactions or may inactivate each other (Jordan *et al.* 2003, E).
5 Assemble the nebulizer equipment as per manufacturer's instructions.	To ensure correct administration (manufacturer's instructions, C).
6 Measure any liquid medication with a syringe. Add the prescribed medication and diluent (if needed) to the nebulizer.	To ensure the correct dose (DH 2007, C).
7 Ask the patient to hold the mouthpiece between the lips or apply the facemask and take a slow deep breath.	To promote greater deposition of medication in the airways (Snyder 2007, E).
8 After inspiration, the patient should pause briefly and then exhale.	To ensure correct administration. E
9 Turn on the O_2 and ensure sufficient mist is formed. A minimum flow rate of 6 litres per minute is required. This will deliver 65% of the medication.	To ensure at least 65% of the droplets are of a size which enables drug penetration into the distal airways (Downie *et al.* 2003, E).
10 The patient should continue to breathe as above until all the nebulized medication is completed (0.5 mL will remain in chamber).	To ensure all medication has been received. E
11 Optimal nebulization of 4 mL takes approximately 10 minutes.	To ensure it is effective. E.

Postprocedure

12 Clean any equipment used and/or discard all single use disposable equipment in appropriate containers.	To minimize the risk of infection (DH 2007, C; Fraise and Bradley 2009, E).
13 Record the administration on appropriate charts.	To maintain accurate records, provide a point of reference in the event of any queries and prevent any duplication of treatment (NMC 2008a, C; NMC 2009, C).

971

Postprocedural considerations

If the nebulizer is marked as single use then it must be discarded after each use. However, nebulizers should not be used for single patient use unless clearly indicated by the manufacturer. If it can be reused, then the nebulizer chamber and mask should be washed in hot soapy water, rinsed thoroughly and dried with paper towels to reduce bacterial contamination and also to prevent any build-up of crystallized medication in the nebulizer (Downie *et al.* 2003). Spacer devices should be washed, rinsed and allowed to dry naturally on a weekly basis and replaced after 6–12 months (Downie *et al.* 2003).

Complications

There is a risk of patients developing oral candidiasis when using a MDI. This can be reduced by using a spacer device. Overuse of some inhalers can result in cardiac dysrhythmias and patients may suffer from tachycardia, palpitations, headache, restlessness and insomnia. The doctor should be informed and observations commenced (Snyder 2007).

Ophthalmic administration

Definition

Dosage forms introduced into the eye for local effects, for example, to treat infections, to dilate or constrict the pupil, or to treat eye conditions such as glaucoma (Snyder 2007).

Related theory

The topical route is the most popular way to introduce drugs into the eye in the form of eye drops or eye ointment. Most types of drops are instilled into the inferior fornix, the pocket formed by gently pulling on the lower eyelid as the conjunctiva in this area is less sensitive than that overlying the cornea. Administering medications in this area prevents immediate loss of the drops into the nasolacrimal drainage system.

There are many factors that affect how much of this drug will have an effect on the eye. The eye has a highly selective corneal barrier which can prevent absorption of drug.

It also has a tear film which provides an effective clearance mechanism. When an excess volume of fluid is present in the eye, this fluid will either be spilled onto the cheeks and eyelashes or will enter the nasolacrimal drainage system with a potential for systemic absorption of drug. Drugs also need to be introduced to the eye at a neutral pH, as acidic or alkaline preparations will result in reflex lacrimation which will remove the drug from the eye.

Evidence-based approaches

In order to optimize the effects of topical eye preparations, attempts should be made to ensure that there is proper placement of eye drops and ointments and that the volume applied is kept to a minimum. The number of drops instilled depends on the type of solution used and its purpose. Usually one drop only is ordered and will be sufficient if it is instilled in the correct manner. The exceptions to the 'one drop' rule are as follows.

- *Oil-based solutions*: these are used for lubricating the eyeball. Usually one drop is instilled and repeated as required.
- *Anaesthetic drops*: used to anaesthetize the eye; one drop should be instilled at a time. This is repeated until the drop cannot be felt on the eye.

The dropper should be held as close to the eye as possible without touching the lids or the cornea. This will avoid corneal damage and reduce the risk of cross-infection. If the drop falls from too great a height, it is difficult to control and will be uncomfortable for the patient. The eye should be closed for as long as possible after application, preferably for 1–2 minutes.

Useful properties of eye ointment include:

- longer duration of action than eye drops
- a soothing emollient action
- easy to apply
- long shelf-life (Downie *et al.* 2003).

Ointments are applied to the upper rim of the inferior fornix using a similar technique to eye drops (Figures 16.14, 16.15). A 2 cm line of ointment should be applied from the nasal canthus outwards. Similarly to the instillation of eye drops, the nozzle should be held approximately 2.5 cm

Figure 16.14 How to instil eye drops.

Figure 16.15 How to instil eye ointment.

above the eye to avoid contract with the cornea and eyelids (Aldridge 2010, Alexander *et al.* 2007).

Preprocedural considerations

Equipment

A variety of droppers and bottles are available for the instillation of eye preparations. These include pipettes, bottles incorporating pipettes, plastic bottles with a dropper attachment and single-dose packs. Pipettes are easy to use but need to be dried and sterilized between doses. Plastic bottles can be squeezed and so avoid the need for a pipette and they are also cheaper than glass bottles with a dropper. Each patient should have their own indivdual eye drop container for each eye and single-dose containers should be used for all patients in eye clinics or in accident and emergency departments (BNF 2011).

It is important that eye preparations are sterile before use and attempts are made to reduce microbial contamination. Eye preparations being used at home should be discarded after 4 weeks whereas eye preparations being used in hospital should be discarded after 1 week. If concerns exist around cross-contamination from one eye to another, separate bottles should be issued.

A number of patients experience problems instilling eye medication. This may be due to difficulty aiming eye drops or squeezing the bottle. Aids are available to assist patients with both these problems. Patients will need guidance in how to use any aids (Downie *et al.* 2003).

If patients are going to use more than one eye drop preparation, they may experience overflow and dilution so they should be advised to leave an interval of 5 minutes between the two (BNF 2011). If both drops and ointments are prescribed, the drops should be applied before the ointment as ointment will leave a film on the eye and hamper the the absorption of the medication in drop form (Aldridge 2010).

Pharmacological support

Drugs may be given either systemically or topically to exert an effect on the eye (BNF 2011). However, if given systemically, the prescribing doctor needs to take account of the blood–aqueous barrier which exists within the eye. This barrier is selective in allowing drugs to pass into the intraocular fluids. The permeability of this barrier may increase during inflammatory conditions or following paracentesis – the removal of excess fluid with a needle or cannula (Andrew 2006).

Medications applied topically meet some resistance at the barrier presented by the lacrimal system (tear film barrier). A further barrier is the cornea which is selectively permeable and only allows the passage of water and not drugs. However, corneal resistance may alter if there is damage to the corneal epithelium (Kirkwood 2006). Many drugs will produce a similar effect on both the healthy and diseased eye. Drugs for use in the eye are usually classified according to their action.

Mydriatics and cycloplegics

These drugs cause pupil dilation and produce their effects by paralysing the ciliary muscle, stimulating the dilator muscle of the pupil (Figure 16.16) or by a combination of both. They are used mainly for diagnostic purposes and most have an anticholinergic action. The most commonly used preparations are cyclopentolate hydrochloride, tropicamide and atropine (BNF 2011).

Miotics

These drugs produce their effects by contracting the ciliary muscle and constricting the pupil (Figure 16.17). Miotics help in the drainage of aqueous humour and are used primarily in the treatment of glaucoma. Examples are pilocarpine and carbachol (BNF 2011).

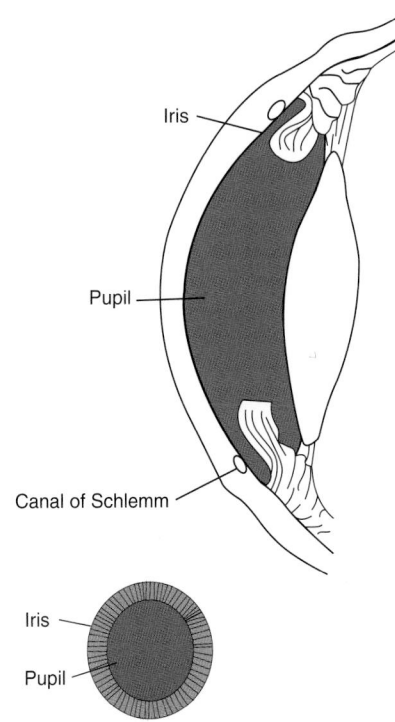

Figure 16.16 Effects of mydriatics.

Dilator pupillae

Constrictor pupillae

Iris

Pupil

Figure 16.17 Effect of miotics.

Local anaesthetics

These render the eye and the inner surfaces of the lids insensitive. They are used before minor surgery, removal of foreign bodies and tonometry (measurement of intraocular pressure). The most widely used eye anaesthetics are oxybuprocaine and amethocaine (BNF 2011).

Anti-inflammatories

Anti-inflammatory drugs include steroids, antihistamines, lodoxamide and sodium cromoglycate. The most commonly used steroid preparations are dexametasone, prednisolone and betametasone (BNF 2011).

Corticosteroid eye drops should be used with caution as they can cause cataract formation or a gradual rise in intraocular pressure in a small percentage of people, particularly if they have a history of glaucoma (Forrester *et al.* 2002).

Antibacterials/antivirals/antifungals

Antibacterials and antivirals can be used for the active treatment of infections or as prophylactic treatment for eye surgery, after removal of a foreign body or following an eye injury. Antibiotic preparations in common use are chloramphenicol, neomycin and framycetin. Aciclovir is the only commonly used antiviral available as an eye preparation although ganciclovir is licensed for the treatment of acute herpetic keratitis (BNF 2011).

Artificial tears

Artificial tears are used when there is a deficiency in natural tear production. This can be due to a disease process, postradiotherapy treatment, as a side-effect of certain drugs or when the eye-blink reflex is absent. These artificial lubricants commonly contain hypromellose or hydroxyethylcellulose (BNF 2011). Additionally, pilocarpine can be given orally. The severity of the problem and the patient's choice will determine the treatment.

Specific patient preparations

The eye to be treated must be ascertained and the unaffected eye should not be dosed. Ascertain if the patient is wearing contact lenses as contact of the medication with the lens can lead to increased drug absoprtion, visual distortion and discolouration of the lens (Chernecky *et al.* 2002). It may be necessary for the patient to remove the lenses and replace them with glasses for the duration of their treatment.

Procedure guideline 16.9 Medication: eye administration

Essential equipment

- Non-sterile powder-free gloves
- Low-linting swabs
- Sterile 0.9% sodium chloride or warm water

Medicinal products

- Eye drops at room temperature

Optional equipment

- Eye swab

Preprocedure

Action	Rationale
1 Explain and discuss the procedure with the patient. Ask the patient to explain how their eyes feel, if they are able to.	To ensure that the patient understands the procedure and gives their valid consent (Griffith and Jordan 2003, E; NMC 2008b, C; NMC 2008c, C). To gain a baseline understanding of current problems or changes the patient is experiencing. E

2 Wash hands and apply gloves.	To reduce the risk of cross-infection (DH 2007, C; Fraise and Bradley 2009, E).

Procedure

3 Ask the patient to sit back with neck slightly hyperextended or lie down.	To ensure a position that allows easy access for medication instillation and to avoid excess running down the patient's cheek (Stollery *et al.* 2005, E). Correct positioning minimizes drainage of eye medication into tear duct (Snyder 2007, E).
4 Consult the patient's prescription chart and ascertain the following: **(a)** Drug **(b)** Dose **(c)** Date and time of administration **(d)** Route and method of administration, including which eye the drops are prescribed for **(e)** Expiry date on bottle **(f)** Validity of prescription **(g)** Signature of doctor.	To ensure that the patient is given the correct drug in the prescribed dose using the appropriate diluent and by the correct route (NMC 2006b, C).
5 If there is any discharge, proceed as for eye swabbing (see Chapter 11). If any crusting or drainage is present around the eye, gently wash away with warm water or 0.9% sodium chloride.	To prevent the introduction of micro-organisms into the lacrimal ducts (Snyder 2007, E).
6 Ask the patient to look at the ceiling and carefully pull the skin below the affected eye using a wet swab to expose the conjunctival sac.	To move the sensitive cornea up and away from the conjunctival sac and reduce stimulation of blink reflex (Snyder 2007, E).
7 Either: Administer the prescribed number of drops holding the eye dropper 1–2 cm above the eye. If the patient blinks or closes their eye, repeat the procedure.	To provide even distribution of medication across the eye (Snyder 2007, E).
Or: Apply a thin stream of ointment along the upper lid margin on the inner conjunctiva from the nasal corner outwards. If there is excess medication on the eyelid, gently wipe it from inner to outer canthus.	To provide even distribution of medication across the eye and reduce the risk of cross-infection, contamination of the tube and trauma to the eye (Fraise and Bradley 2009, E; Snyder 2007, E; Stollery *et al.* 2005, E). To avoid excess ointment irritating the suroounding skin (Stollery *et al.* 2005, E).
8 Ask the patient to close their eyes and keep them closed for 1–2 minutes.	To help distribute medication (Snyder 2007, E; Aldridge 2010, E).
9 Explain to the patient that they may have blurred vision for a few minutes after application.	To ensure the patient understands why they have blurred vision and to refrain from driving or operating machinery until their vision returns to normal (Aldridge 2010, E).

Postprocedure

10 Clean any equipment used and discard all disposable equipment in appropriate containers.	To minimize the risk of infection (DH 2007, C; Fraise and Bradley 2009, E).
11 Record the administration on appropriate charts.	To maintain accurate records, provide a point of reference in the event of any queries and prevent any duplication of treatment (NMC 2008a, C; NMC 2009, C).

Postprocedural considerations

Immediate care

After using any eye medications, any excess medication should be wiped off from inner to outer canthus. If an eye patch is to be worn, it should be secured without putting any pressure on the eye. Patients should be warned not to drive for 1–2 hours after instillation of mydriatics (which dilate the pupil and paralyse the ciliary muscle) (BNF 2011). Patients should be taught how to instil eye medication. If it is difficult for them to do so then it may be necessary for a community nurse to attend and administer the eye medications (Chernecky *et al.* 2002).

Nasal administration

Definition

Medication introduced to the cavity of the nose for local or systemic effects (Aldridge 2010).

Related theory

The nasal passages are lined with highly vascular mucous membranes covered with ciliated epithelium which warms and moistens air and traps dust. Medication can be delivered directly to the nasal cavity to relieve local symptoms such as allergic rhinitis in the form of nasal drops or nasal sprays (Aldridge 2010).

The nasal cavity can also be used to allow the delivery of drugs systemically. Examples include sumatriptan for migraine, desmopressin for the treatment of diabetes insipidus and nocturia and fentanyl for the treatment of breakthrough pain.

Evidence-based approaches

The advantages of the delivery of drugs using the nasal route include the large vascular surface of the nasal cavity which allows rapid absorption, the avoidance of first-pass metabolism, the accessibility of the nose, the ease of administration and the fact that this route can be used when patients are unable to swallow. There are some disadvantages to the nasal route, including the presence of mucus which acts as a barrier to absorption, the mucociliary clearance which reduces the time that drugs are held in the nasal cavity, disorders such as colds that can affect absorption from the nasal cavity, and drugs can have an irritating effect on the nasal cavity.

Preprocedural considerations

Specific patient preparations

The patient should be encouraged to clear their nostrils by blowing or manually cleaning with a tissue or damp cotton bud to ensure that the drug has access to the nasal mucosa (Aldridge 2010).

Procedure guideline 16.10 Medication: nasal drop administration

Essential equipment

- Tissues
- Clean non-sterile gloves

Medicinal product

- Nasal spray or drops

Optional equipment

- Cotton bud

Preprocedure

Action	Rationale
1 Explain and discuss the procedure with the patient.	To ensure that the patient understands the procedure and gives their valid consent (Griffith and Jordan 2003, E; NMC 2008b, C; NMC 2008c, C).
2 Consult the patient's prescription sheet and ascertain the following: (a) Drug (b) Dose (c) Date and time of administration (d) Route and method of administration (e) Validity of prescription (f) Signature of doctor.	To ensure that the patient is given the correct drug in the prescribed dose and by the correct route (NMC 2006b, C).
3 Have paper tissues available.	To wipe away secretions and/or medication. E

Procedure

4	Ask the patient to blow their nose to clear the nasal passages, if appropriate.	To ensure maximum penetration for the medication (Chernecky *et al.* 2002, E).
5	Place the patient in a supine position and hyperextend the patient's neck (unless clinically contraindicated, for example cervical spondylosis).	To obtain a safe optimum position for insertion of the medication. E
6	Wash hands and put on gloves.	To reduce the risk of cross-infection (DH 2007, C; Fraise and Bradley 2009, E).
7	With the non-dominant hand, gently push upward on the end of the patient's nose.	To aid in opening the nostrils. E
8	Avoid touching the external nares with the dropper and instil the drops just inside the nostril of affected side.	To prevent the patient from sneezing. E
9	Ask the patient to sniff back any liquid into the back of the nose or to maintain their position for 2 or 3 minutes.	To ensure full absorption of the medication. E
10	Discard any remaining medication in the dropper into the sink before returning it to the container.	To minimize the risk of cross-infection (Chernecky *et al.* 2002, E; DH 2007, C; Fraise and Bradley 2009, E).
11	Instruct patient not to blow their nose.	To maintain the medication in contact with nasal passages. E
12	Each patient should have their own medication and dropper.	To minimize the risk of cross-infection (DH 2007, C; Fraise and Bradley 2009, E).

Postprocedure

13	Record the administration on appropriate charts.	To maintain accurate records, provide a point of reference in the event of any queries and prevent any duplication of treatment (NMC 2008a, C; NMC 2009, C).

Postprocedural considerations

The patient should be discouraged from sniffing too vigorously post administraton as this can cause 'run-off' of the medication down the nasopharynx. This can cause an unpleasant taste in the throat and affect absorption of the medication (Aldridge 2010).

Otic administration

Definition

Medication introduced into the ear for local effects such as treatment of ear infections and softening of ear wax (cerumen) (Aldridge 2010, Chernecky *et al.* 2002).

Related theory

Drugs administered via this route are intended to have a localized effect and act within the anatomy of the ear and auditory canal (Aldridge 2010). Ear preparations can be presented in the form of drops, sprays, ointments and solutions. Certain factors can affect the absorption or action of drugs in the ear, including ear wax and the acidic environment around the ear skin surface.

Evidence-based approaches

Internal ear structures are very sensitive to temperature extremes and so solutions should be administered at room temperature. When drops are instilled cold, patients may experience vertigo, ataxia or nausea (Chernecky *et al.* 2002, Snyder 2007). Solutions should never be forced into the ear canal as medication administered under pressure can injure the eardrum. The ear drop solution should be labelled for the ear it is intended to treat. The dropper should be held as close to the ear as possile without touching to reduce the risk of cross-infection.

Preprocedural considerations
Specific patient preparations

The nurse should examine the ear, taking note of any discharge, redness, swelling and the amount and texture of

977

any ear wax present as these will give an indication of the general health of the ear (Harkin 2008). The nurse should also discuss with the patient their current level of hearing.

It should be explained to the patient that they must lie still as sudden movements could cause injury from the ear dropper.

Procedure guideline 16.11 Medication: ear drop administration

Essential equipment	Medicinal products
■ Clean non-sterile gloves ■ Tissues	■ Ear drops

Preprocedure

Action	Rationale
1 Explain and discuss the procedure with the patient.	To ensure that the patient understands the procedure and gives their valid consent (Griffith and Jordan 2003, E; NMC 2008b, C; NMC 2008c, C).
2 Consult the patient's prescription chart and ascertain the following: (a) Drug (b) Dose (c) Date and time of administration (d) Route and method of administration (e) Validity of prescription (f) Signature of doctor.	To ensure that the patient is given the correct drug in the prescribed dose using the appropriate diluent and by the correct route (NMC 2008a, C).

Procedure

3 Ask the patient to lie on their side with the ear to be treated uppermost.	To ensure the best position for insertion of the drops. E
4 Warm the drops to body temperature if allowed.	To prevent trauma to the patient (Harkin 2008, E; Snyder 2007, E).
5 Wash hands and apply gloves.	To reduce the risk of cross-infection (DH 2007, C; Fraise and Bradley 2009, E).
6 Pull the cartilaginous part of the pinna backwards and upwards (see Action Figure 6).	To prepare the auditory meatus for instillation of the drops (Harkin 2008, E).
7 If cerumen (ear wax) or drainage occludes outermost portion of the ear canal, wipe out gently with cotton-tipped applicator.	To enable the medication to enter the ear. E
8 Allow the drop(s) to fall in direction of the external canal. The dropper should not touch the ear.	To ensure that the medication reaches the area requiring therapy. E
9 Gently massage over tragus to help work in the drops.	To aid the passge of medication into the ear and prevent escape of medication. E
10 It may be necessary to temporarily place a gauze swab over the ear canal.	To prevent escape of the medication (Chernecky et al. 2002, E).
11 Request the patient to remain in this position for 2–3 minutes.	To allow the medication to reach the eardrum and be absorbed. To prevent escape of the medication (Aldridge, 2010, E; Snyder 2007, E).

Postprocedure

12 Record the administration on appropriate charts.	To maintain accurate records, provide a point of reference in the event of any queries and prevent any duplication of treatment (NMC 2008a, C; NMC 2009, C).

Action Figure 6 Holding ear for ear drops.

Postprocedural considerations

The nurse should ask the patient if there are any changes in order to monitor effectiveness of the intervention. Consideration should also be given to the patient's hearing aids and assistance given to help clean these.

Injections and infusions

Definitions

Injections are sterile solutions, emulsions or suspensions. They are prepared by dissolving, emulsifying or suspending the active ingredient and any added substances in either water for injections or a suitable non-aqueous liquid or in a mixture of these vehicles (British Pharmacopoeia 2007). Box 16.11 lists the types of injections and infusions.

Injections can be described as the act of giving medication by use of a syringe and needle. An infusion is defined as an amount of fluid in excess of 100 mL designated for parenteral infusion because the volume must be administered over a long period of time. However, medications may be given in small volumes (50–100 mL) or over a shorter period (30–60 minutes) (Weinstein and Plumer 2007).

Box 16.11 Types of injections and infusions

- Intradermal injection.
- Subcutaneous injection and infusion.
- Intramuscular injection.
- Intra-arterial injection.
- Intraosseous injection.
- Intra-articular injection.
- Intrathecal injection and infusion.
- Intravenous:
  - bolus injection
  - intermittent and continuous infusion.

Anatomy and physiology

The skin is made up of two layers: the dermis and epidermis. Within the dermis there is the papillary layer (upper dermal region) which contains capillaries, pain and touch receptors. The reticular layer contains blood vessels, sweat and oil glands. Both collagen and elastic fibres are found throughout the dermis. Collagen fibres are responsible for the toughness of the dermis. The skin also has a rich nerve supply (Marieb and Hoehn 2007). There are three types of muscles – skeletal, cardiac and smooth. Skeletal muscles are attached to the body's skeleton and are also known as striated muscle because the fibres appear to be striped (Marieb and Hoehn 2007). For specific muscles used for injections, see intramuscular injection sites.

Evidence-based approaches

Medicines should only be administered by injection when no other route is suitable or available. As injections avoid the GI tract, this is described as parenteral administration. Injections would be administered when the medications might be destroyed by the stomach; rapid first-pass metabolism may be extensive; the drug is not absorbed when given orally; precise control over dosage is required; unable to be given by mouth; achieve high drug plasma levels (Downie *et al.* 2003, Perry 2007). There are disadvantages as injections are invasive, cause pain and discomfort, and can put the patient at risk of infection and, in the case of intravenous injections, infiltration and extravasation.

Methods for injection or infusion

There are a number of routes for injection or infusion. See Box 16.11. The selection may be predetermined, for example intra-arterial, intracardiac injections. The choice of other routes will normally depend on the desired therapeutic effect and the patient's safety and comfort.

Intra-arterial

This special technique allows the delivery of a high concentration of drug to the tissues or organ supplied by a particular artery if the medications are rapidly metabolized or systematically toxic (Downie *et al.* 2003). This route can be used for the administration of chemotherapy and vasodilators and for diagnostic purposes. Injection of drugs into an artery is a rare and hazardous procedure. The introduction of the cannula or catheter must be performed with care as the vessel may go into spasm, causing pain and occlusion. This could result in necrosis of an organ or part of a limb. Injection of irritant chemicals increases the risk of spasm and its sequelae; however, arterial catheterization is occasionally performed when it is desirable to deliver a high concentration of a drug to a tumour mass (see Chapter 18). The most common procedures are catheterization of the hepatic artery and isolated limb perfusion.

Intra-articular

In inflammatory conditions of the joints, corticosteroids are given by intra-articular injection to relieve inflammation and increase joint mobility (Downie *et al.* 2003).

Intraosseous

This route is used for emergency or short-term treatment when access by the vascular route is difficult or cannot be achieved and the patient's condition is considered life threatening (RCN 2010). The preferred sites are the iliac crest or sternum (RCN 2010). Any drug administered intravenously can be administered via the intraosseous route.

Intrathecal

Medications can be administered intrathecally if they have poor lipid solubility and therefore do not pass the blood–brain barrier (Downie *et al.* 2003). Only medication specially prepared for the intrathecal route should be used; doses should be carefully calculated and are usually much smaller than would be given by intramuscular or intravenous injection. Water-soluble antibiotics are administered by the intrathecal route to achieve adequate concentrations in the cerebrospinal fluid (CSF) in the treatment of meningitis. Other medicines administered via this route include antifungal agents, opioids, cytotoxic therapy and radiopaque substances (used in the diagnosis of spinal lesions) (Downie *et al.* 2003) (see Chapters 11 and 15).

Preprocedural considerations

Equipment

Ampoule

Ampoules (Figure 16.18) are single-dose glass containers although plastic ampoules are now used for certain products (Downie *et al.* 2003). They have a wide-ranging capacity and are sealed by heat fusion to exclude any contamination. They have a thin wall which allows rupture of the glass to expose the contents of liquid or powder. There is a narrow constriction leading to the neck which is often marked with

Figure 16.18 Ampoules.

a white ring which indicates the place where the neck can be snapped off (Downie *et al.* 2003). Ampoule opening devices of various designs are available. They are available in several sizes from 1 to 20 mL (Perry 2007).

Vials

Vials (Figure 16.19) are glass containers which have a rubber closure which can be penetrated to allow the addition of a vehicle to dissolve powder contents and to allow the withdrawal of a dose via the needle. The exposed rubber surface is usually covered by a protective pull-off metal or plastic cap which prevents tampering or damage but does not provide sterility (Downie *et al.* 2003, Perry 2007). The vials may be packaged with a specific transfer needle, and the nurse should follow the manufacturer's instructions in these instances.

Syringes

Syringes are commonly plastic and disposable, although some medicines must be administered via glass syringes. They consist of a graduated barrel and a plunger and a tip. It is the tip that classifies the type of syringe as Luer-Lok or

Figure 16.19 Vials.

Figure 16.20 Syringes: Luer-Lok and Luer-Slip.

Luer-Slip (see Figure 16.20). Syringes come in various sizes from 1 to 60 mL. The choice of syringe is made according to the volume of medication to be administered so it is important to choose the smallest syringe possible to ensure accuracy (Downie *et al.* 2003, Perry 2007). Luer-Lok requires the needle to be twisted onto the tip and 'locked' into position. This provides security and these syringes are recommended for use with intravenous medicines, especially cytotoxic medications and any medicines administered via a syringe pump. Luer-Slip syringes tend to be used for intramuscular and subcutaneous injections. Insulin syringes are low-dose syringes and are often calibrated in units and are only used for insulin administration (Downie *et al.* 2003, Perry 2007). There are now a number of pre-prepared syringes that contain 0.9% sodium chloride specifically for flushing or ready to administer medicines often used in emergency situations.

Needles

A needle is composed of three parts (see Figure 16.21):

- the hub which fits onto the tip of a syringe
- the shaft which connects the hub
- the bevel or slanted tip or eye of the needle (different bevels are required depending on use of needle).

Needle sizes are known as gauges, for example 19 G, 21 G (used for IM injections), 23 G (subcutaneous injec-

tions) and 25 G (intradermal injections). This indicates their diameter. The higher the gauge, the finer the needle and selection is made depending on the viscosity of the liquid to be injected (Downie *et al.* 2003, Perry 2007). Needles vary in length from 10 to 16 mm and selection of length will depend on the size and weight of patient, and the type of tissue into which the drug is to be injected, for example longer for IM and shorter for SC. Each needle is enclosed in a removable plastic guard and then sealed in a sterile pack. Filter needles may be used to prevent drawing up glass and rubber particles into the syringe (Downie *et al.* 2003, Perry 2007). There are now a variety of safety needles available to prevent needlestick injury where a plastic guard or sheath slips over the needle after an injection.

Three categories of needle bevel are available.

- *Regular*: for all intramuscular and subcutaneous injections.
- *Intradermal*: for diagnostic injections and other injections into the epidermis.
- *Short*: rarely used.

Medication preparation

Medicines are presented as liquids and can be drawn up directly from the vial or ampoule. If the medicine has been presented in a powder form it will need to be reconstituted. This is usually done using water for injections but some medications will require special diluents which are often supplied with the medication. When adding diluent to a powder, for example 2 mL to a 100 mg vial, the final volume will exceed 2 mL although this is usually not of any consequence if the total dose is to be administered (Downie *et al.* 2003). In order to ensure that the correct volume is withdrawn, it will be necessary to perform a calculation.

Medication calculations

The drug volume required from stock strength:

$$\frac{\text{Strength required}}{\text{Stock strength}} \times \text{Volume of stock solution}$$
$$= \text{Volume required}$$

What you want/What you have got
× Volume of stock solution

It is important to note that the 'use of calculators to determine the volume or quantity of medication should not act as a substitute for arithmetical knowledge and skill' (NMC 2008a).

Single-dose preparations

The volume of the injection in a single-dose container is sufficient to permit the withdrawal and administration of the nominal dose using a normal technique.

| Hub | Shaft | Bevel |

Figure 16.21 Needles.

Multidose preparations

Multidose aqueous injections contain a suitable antimicrobial preservative at an appropriate concentration except when the preparation itself has adequate antimicrobial properties. When it is necessary to present a preparation for parenteral use in a multidose container, the precautions to be taken for its administration and more particularly for its storage between successive withdrawals are given.

Parenteral infusions

Parenteral infusions are sterile, aqueous solutions or emulsions with water; they are free from pyrogens and are usually made isotonic with blood. They are principally intended for administration in large volume. Parenteral infusions do not contain any added antimicrobial preservative (British Pharmacopoeia 2007, Hilary *et al.* 2001).

Specific patient preparations
Reducing pain of injections

Patients are often afraid of receiving injections because they perceive the injection will be painful (Downie *et al.* 2003). Torrence (1989) listed a number of factors that cause pain.

- The needle.
- The chemical composition of the drug/solution.

Box 16.12 Reducing the pain of injections

- Correct length and gauge of needle.
- Correct site.
- Correct angle (90° for IM).
- Correct volume (no more than 3 mL at a site for IM).
- Rotate sites.
- Consider using ice, freezing spray or topical local anaesthetic to numb the skin.
- Listen to views of the experienced patient.
- Explain the benefits of the injection.
- Positioning of the patient so that the muscles are relaxed.
- Use distraction.
- If appropriate, ask the patient to turn their foot inwards (IM).
- Insert and remove the needle quickly.
- Inject medication slowly.

(Dickerson 1992, Downie *et al.* 2003)

- The technique.
- The speed of the injection.
- The volume of drug.

Applying manual pressure to an injection site before performing an injection can be an effective means of reducing pain intensity (Chung *et al.* 2002). Other ways of reducing pain during injections are covered in Box 16.12.

Procedure guideline 16.12 Medication: single-dose ampoule: solution preparation

Essential equipment

- Medication ampoule
- Needle
- Syringe

- Sterile topical swab
- Sharps container
- Ampoule opening aid

Preprocedure

Action	Rationale
1 Wash hands with bactericidal soap and water or bactericidal alcohol handrub.	To prevent contamination of medication and equipment (DH 2007, C).
2 Inspect the solution for cloudiness or particulate matter. If this is present, discard and follow hospital guidelines on what action to take, for example return drug to pharmacy.	To prevent the patient from receiving an unstable or contaminated drug (NPSA 2007d, C).

Procedure

3 Tap the neck of the ampoule gently.	To ensure that all the solution is in the bottom of the ampoule (NPSA 2007d, C).
4 Cover the neck of the ampoule with a sterile topical swab and snap it open. If there is any difficulty, a file or ampoule opening aid may be required.	To minimize the risk of contamination. To prevent aerosol formation or contact with the drug which could lead to a sensitivity reaction. To reduce the risk of injury to the nurse (NPSA 2007d, C).

5	Inspect the solution for glass fragments; if present, discard.	To minimize the risk of injection of foreign matter into the patient (NPSA 2007d, C).
6	Open packaging and attach the needle onto the syringe.	To assemble equipment. E
7	Withdraw the required amount of solution, tilting the ampoule if necessary.	To avoid drawing in any air (NPSA 2007d, C).
8	Replace the sheath on the needle using one-handed scooping method and tap the syringe to dislodge any air bubbles. Expel air (replacing the sheath should not be confused with resheathing used needles). **Or:** An alternative to expelling the air with the needle sheath in place would be to use the ampoule or vial to receive any air and/or drug.	To prevent needlestick injury and aerosol formation (NPSA 2007d, C). To ensure that the correct amount of drug is in the syringe (NPSA 2007d, C).
9	Attach a new needle if required (and discard used needle into appropriate sharps container) or attach a plastic end cap or insert syringe into the syringe packet.	To reduce the risk of contamination of the syringe tip. To avoid tracking medications through superficial tissues and to ensure that the correct size of needle is used for intramuscular or subcutaneous injection. To reduce the risk of injury to the nurse (NPSA 2007d, C).
10	Attach a label to the syringe.	To ensure practitioner can identify medication in syringe (NPSA 2007d, C).

Procedure guideline 16.13 Medication: single-dose ampoule: powder preparation

Essential equipment

- Medication ampoule
- Diluent
- Needle

- Syringe
- Sharps container
- Swab

Preprocedure

Action	**Rationale**
1 Wash hands with bactericidal soap and water or bactericidal alcohol handrub.	To prevent contamination of medication and equipment (DH 2007, C).
2 Open packaging and attach needle to the syringe.	To assemble the equipment. E

Procedure

3 Open the diluent and draw up required volume.	To ensure the correct volume of diluent. E
4 Tap the neck of the ampoule gently.	To ensure that any powder lodged here falls to the bottom of the ampoule (NPSA 2007d, C).
5 Cover the neck of the ampoule with a sterile topical swab and snap it open. If there is any difficulty, an ampoule opening device may be required.	To minimize the risk of contamination. To prevent contact with the drug which could cause a sensitivity reaction. To prevent injury to the nurse (NPSA 2007d, C).
6 Inject the correct diluent slowly into the powder within the ampoule.	To ensure that the powder is thoroughly wet before agitation and is not released into the atmosphere (NPSA 2007d, C).
7 Agitate the ampoule.	To dissolve the drug (NPSA 2007d, C).

(Continued)

Procedure guideline 16.13 *(Continued)*

Action	Rationale
8 Inspect the contents.	To detect any glass fragments or any other particulate matter. If present, continue agitation or discard as appropriate (NPSA 2007d, C).
9 When the solution is clear, withdraw the prescribed amount, tilting the ampoule if necessary.	To ensure the powder is dissolved and has formed a solution with the diluent. To avoid drawing in air (NPSA 2007d C).
10 Replace the sheath on the needle using a one-handed scooping method and tap the syringe to dislodge any air bubbles. Expel air.	To prevent aerosol formation. To ensure that the correct amount of drug is in the syringe (NPSA 2007d, C).
11 Attach a new needle if required (and discard used needle into appropriate sharps container) or attach a plastic end cap or insert syringe into the syringe packet.	To reduce the risk of contamination of the syringe tip. To avoid possible trauma to the patient if the needle has barbed (become bent/hooked), to avoid tracking medications through superficial tissues and to ensure that the correct size of needle is used for intramuscular or subcutaneous injection. To reduce the risk of injury to the nurse. (NPSA 2007d, C).
12 Attach a label to the syringe.	To ensure practitioner can identify medication in syringe (NPSA 2007d, C).

Procedure guideline 16.14 **Medication: multidose vial: powder preparation using a venting needle**

Equipment

- Medication ampoule
- Diluent
- Needle

- Syringe
- Alcohol swab

Preprocedure

Action	Rationale
1 Wash hands with bactericidal soap and water or bactericidal alcohol handrub.	To prevent contamination of medication and equipment (DH 2007, C).
2 Open packaging and attach needle to the syringe	To assemble the equipment. E

Procedure

Action	Rationale
3 Open the diluent and draw up required volume.	To ensure the correct volume of diluent. E
4 Remove the tamper-evident seal and clean the rubber septum with the chosen antiseptic and let it air dry for at least 30 seconds.	To prevent bacterial contamination of the drug, as the plastic lid prevents damage but does not ensure sterility (NPSA 2007d, C).
5 Insert a 21 G needle into the cap to vent the bottle (see Action Figure 5a).	To prevent pressure differentials, which can cause separation of needle and syringe (NPSA 2007d, C).
6 Insert the needle bevel up, at an angle of 45° to 60°. Before completing the insertion of the needle tip, lift the needle to 90° and proceed (see Action Figure 6).	To minimize the risk of coring when inserting the needle into the cap. E

7 Inject the correct diluent slowly into the powder within the ampoule.	To ensure that the powder is thoroughly wet before it is shaken and is not released into the atmosphere (NPSA 2007d, C).
8 Remove the needle and the syringe.	To enable adequate mixing of the solution. E
9 Place a sterile topical swab over the venting needle (see Action Figure 5b) and shake to dissolve the powder.	To prevent contamination of the drug or the atmosphere. To mix the diluent with the powder and dissolve the drug (NPSA 2007d, C).
10 Inspect the solution for cloudiness or particulate matter. If this is present, discard. Follow hospital guidelines on what action to take, for example return drug to pharmacy.	To prevent patient from receiving an unstable or contaminated drug (NPSA 2007d, C).
11 Withdraw the prescribed amount of solution, and inspect for pieces of rubber which may have 'cored out' of the cap (see Action Figure 5c).	To ensure that the correct amount of drug is in the syringe (NPSA 2007d, C). To prevent the injection of foreign matter into the patient (NPSA 2007d, C).
12 Remove air from syringe without spraying into the atmosphere by injecting air back into the vial (see Action Figure 5d) or replace the sheath on the needle using a one-handed scooping method and tap the syringe to dislodge any air bubbles. Expel air.	To reduce risk of contamination of practitioner. To prevent aerosol formation (NPSA 2007d, C).
11 Attach a new needle if required (and discard used needle into appropriate sharps container) or attach a plastic end cap or insert syringe into the syringe packet.	To reduce the risk of contamination of the syringe tip. To avoid possible trauma to the patient if the needle has barbed (become bent/hooked), to avoid tracking medications through superficial tissues and to ensure that the correct size of needle is used for intramuscular or subcutaneous injection. To reduce the risk of injury to the nurse (NPSA 2007d, C).
12 Attach a label to the syringe.	To ensure practitioner can identify medication in syringe (NPSA 2007d, C).

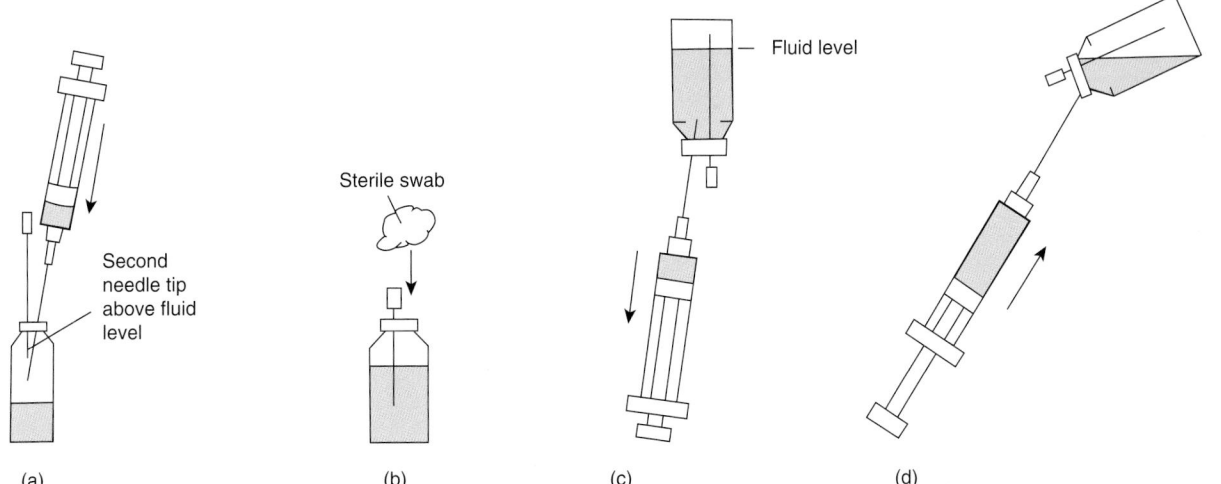

Action Figure 5 Suggested method of vial reconstitution to avoid environmental exposure. (a) When reconstituting vial, insert a second needle to allow air to escape when adding diluent for injection. (b) When shaking the vial to dissolve the powder, push in second needle up to Luer connection and cover with a sterile swab. (c) To remove reconstituted solution, insert syringe needle and then invert vial. Ensuring that tip of second needle is above fluid, withdraw the solution. (d) Remove air from syringe without spraying into the atmosphere by injecting air back into vial.

985

(Continued)

Procedure guideline 16.14 (*Continued*)

45–60°

Action Figure 6   Method to minimize coring.

Procedure guideline 16.15   Medication: multidose vial: powder preparation using equilibrium method

Essential equipment

- Medication vial
- Diluent
- Needle

- Syringe
- Alcohol swab

Preprocedure

Action	Rationale
1 Wash hands with bactericidal soap and water or bactericidal alcohol handrub.	To prevent contamination of medication and equipment (DH 2007, C).
2 Open packaging and attach needle to the syringe	To assemble the equipment. E

Procedure

3 Open the diluent and draw up required volume.	To ensure the correct volume of diluent. E
4 Remove the tamper-evident seal and clean the rubber septum with the chosen antiseptic and let it air dry for at least 30 seconds.	To prevent bacterial contamination of the drug, as the plastic lid prevents damage but does not ensure sterility (NPSA 2007d, C).
5 With the needle sheathed, draw into the syringe a volume of air equivalent to the required volume of solution to be drawn up.	To prevent bacterial contamination of the drug (NPSA 2007d, C).
6 Remove the needle cover and insert the needle bevel up, at an angle of 45–60°, into the rubber septum. Before complete insertion of the needle tip, lift the needle to 90° and proceed (see Action Figure 6 in Procedure guideline 16.14).	To gain access to the vial and reduce the risk of coring. E
7 Invert the vial. Keep the needle in the solution and slowly depress the plunger to push the air into the vial.	To create an equilibrium in the vial (NPSA 2007d, C).
8 Release the plunger so that the solution flows back into the syringe (if a large volume of solution is to be withdrawn, use a push-pull technique).	To create an equilibrium in the vial (NPSA 2007d, C).

9 Inject the diluent into the vial. Keeping the tip of the needle above the level of the solution in the vial, release the plunger. The syringe will fill with the air which has been displaced by the solution.	This 'equilibrium method' helps to minimize the build-up of pressure in the vial (NPSA 2007d, C).
10 With the needle and syringe in place, gently swirl the vial to dissolve all the powder.	To mix the diluent with the powder and dissolve the drug (NPSA 2007d, C).
11 Inspect the solution for cloudiness or particulate matter. If this is present, discard. Follow hospital guidelines on what action to take, for example return drug to pharmacy.	To prevent patient from receiving an unstable or contaminated drug (NPSA 2007d, C).
12 Withdraw the prescribed amount of solution, and inspect for pieces of rubber which may have 'cored out' of the cap (see Action Figure 5c in Procedure guideline 16.14).	To ensure that the correct amount of drug is in the syringe (NPSA 2007d, C). To prevent the injection of foreign matter into the patient (NPSA 2007d, C).
13 Remove air from syringe without spraying into the atmosphere by injecting air back into the vial (see Action Figure 5d in Procedure guideline 16.14) or replace the sheath on the needle using a one-handed scooping method and tap the syringe to dislodge any air bubbles. Expel air.	To reduce risk of contamination of practitioner. To prevent aerosol formation (NPSA 2007d, C).
14 Attach a new needle if required (and discard used needle into appropriate sharps container) or attach a plastic end cap or insert syringe into the syringe packet.	To reduce the risk of contamination of the syringe tip. To avoid possible trauma to the patient if the needle has barbed (become bent/hooked), to avoid tracking medications through superficial tissues and to ensure that the correct size of needle is used for intramuscular or subcutaneous injection. To reduce the risk of injury to the nurse. (NPSA 2007d, C).
15 Attach a label to the syringe.	To ensure practitioner can identify medication in syringe (NPSA 2007d, C).

Procedure guideline 16.16 Medication: injection administration

Essential equipment

- Clean tray or receiver in which to place drug and equipment
- 21 G needle(s) to ease reconstitution and drawing up, 23 G if from a glass ampoule
- 21, 23 or 25 G needle, size dependent on route of administration
- Syringe(s) of appropriate size for amount of drug to be given
- Swabs saturated with isopropyl alcohol 70%
- Sterile topical swab, if drug is presented in ampoule form
- Drug(s) to be administered
- Patient's prescription chart, to check dose, route and so on
- Recording sheet or book as required by law or hospital policy
- Any protective clothing required by hospital policy for specified drugs, such as antibiotics or cytotoxic drugs, such as goggles or gloves (see Chapter 15)

Preprocedure

Action	Rationale
1 Collect and check all equipment.	To prevent delays and enable full concentration on the procedure. E.
2 Check that the packaging of all equipment is intact.	To ensure sterility. If the seal is damaged, discard (NPSA 2007d, C).
3 Wash hands with bactericidal soap and water or bactericidal alcohol handrub.	To prevent contamination of medication and equipment (DH 2007, C).

(Continued)

Procedure guideline 16.16 (*Continued*)

Procedure

4 Prepare needle(s), syringe(s), and so on, on a tray or receiver.	To contain all items in a clean area. E
5 Inspect all equipment.	To check that none is damaged; if so, discard or report to MHRA. C
6 Consult the patient's prescription chart and ascertain the following: (a) Drug (b) Dose (c) Date and time of administration (d) Route and method of administration (e) Diluent as appropriate (f) Validity of prescription (g) Signature of doctor.	To ensure that the patient is given the correct drug in the prescribed dose using the appropriate diluent and by the correct route (NMC 2008a, C; NPSA 2007d, C).
7 Check all details with another nurse if required by hospital policy.	To minimize any risk of error (NMC 2008a, C).
8 Select the drug in the appropriate volume, dilution or dosage and check the expiry date.	To reduce wastage. Treatment with medication that is outside the expiry date is dangerous. Drugs deteriorate with storage. The expiry date indicates when a particular drug is no longer pharmacologically efficacious (NPSA 2007d, C).
9 Proceed with the preparation of the drug, using protective clothing if advisable.	To protect practitioner during preparation (NPSA 2007d, C).
10 Take the prepared dose to the patient and close the door or curtains as appropriate	To ensure patient privacy and dignity. E
11 Check patient's identity	To prevent error and confirm patient's identity (NPSA 2005, C).
12 Evaluate the patient's knowledge of the medication being offered. If this knowledge appears to be faulty or incorrect, offer an explanation of the use, action, dose and potential side-effects of the drug or drugs involved.	A patient has a right to information about treatment (NMC 2008a, C).
13 Administer the drug as prescribed.	To ensure patient receives treatment. E

Postprocedure

14 Record the administration on appropriate charts.	To maintain accurate records, provide a point of reference in the event of any queries and prevent any duplication of treatment (NMC 2008a, C; NMC 2009, C; NPSA 2007d, C).

Intradermal injection

Definition

The intradermal route provides a local rather than systemic effect and is used primarily for administering small amounts of local anaesthetic and skin testing, for example allergy or tuberculin testing (Snyder 2007).

The injection is given into the dermis of the skin just below the epidermis where the blood supply is reduced and drug absorption can occur slowly (Chernecky *et al.* 2002).

Evidence-based approaches

Observation of an inflammatory reaction is a priority, so the best sites are those that are lowly pigmented, thinly keratinized and hairless. Chosen sites are the inner forearms and the scapulae. The injection site most commonly used is the medial forearm area as this allows for easy inspection (Downie *et al*. 2003). Volumes of 0.5 mL or less should be used (Chernecky *et al*. 2002).

Preprocedural considerations
Equipment
The injections are best performed using a 25 or 27 G needle inserted at a 10–15° angle, bevel up, just under the epidermis. Usually a TB (tuberculosis) or 1 mL syringe is used to ensure accuracy of dose.

Procedure guideline 16.17 Medication: intradermal injection

Essential equipment

- Needle 25–27 G
- 1 mL syringe containing medication
- Alcohol swab
- Non-sterile gloves

Preprocedure

Action	Rationale
1 Explain and discuss the procedure with the patient.	To ensure that the patient understands the procedure and gives their valid consent (Griffith and Jordan 2003, E; NMC 2008b, C; NMC 2008c, C).
2 Consult the patient's prescription chart and ascertain the following: (a) Drug (b) Dose (c) Date and time of administration (d) Route and method of administration (e) Diluent as appropriate (f) Validity of prescription (g) Signature of doctor.	To ensure that the patient is given the correct drug in the prescribed dose using the appropriate diluent and by the correct route (NMC 2008a, C; NPSA 2007d, C).

Procedure

3 Close the curtains or door and assist the patient into the required position.	To ensure patient privacy and dignity. E To allow access to the appropriate injection site (Workman 1999, E).
4 Remove appropriate garments to expose the injection site.	To gain access for injection (Workman 1999, E).
5 Assess the injection site for signs of inflammation, oedema, infection and skin lesions.	To promote effectiveness of administration (Workman 1999, E). To reduce the risk of infection (Fraise and Bradley 2009, E; Workman 1999, E). To avoid skin lesions and avoid possible trauma to the patient (Workman 1999, E).
6 Choose the correct needle size and attach the needle.	To minimize the risk of missing the subcutaneous tissue and any ensuing pain (Workman 1999, E).
7 Clean the injection site with a swab saturated with isopropyl alcohol 70% and apply gloves.	To reduce the number of pathogens introduced into the skin by the needle at the time of insertion. (For further information on this action see Skin preparation.)
8 Remove the needle sheath and hold syringe with the dominant hand with the bevel of needle pointing up.	To facilitate needle placement (Perry 2007, E).

(Continued)

Procedure guideline 16.17 *(Continued)*

9 With the non-dominant hand, stretch skin over the site with forefinger and thumb.	To facilitate the needle piercing the skin more easily (Perry 2007, E).
10 With the needle almost against the patient's skin, insert the needle into the skin at an angle of 10–15° and advance through the epidermis so the needle tip can be seen through the skin.	To ensure the needle tip is in the dermis (Perry 2007, E).
11 Inject medication slowly. It is not necessary to aspirate as the dermis is relatively avascular.	To minimize the discomfort at site (Perry 2007, E).
12 While injecting medication, a bleb (resembling a mosquito bite) will form (see Action Figure 12).	To indicate medication is in dermis (Perry 2007, E).
13 Withdraw the needle rapidly and apply pressure gently. Do not massage the site.	To prevent dispersing medication into underlying tissue layers and altering test results (Chernecky *et al.* 2002, E, Perry 2007, E).

Postprocedure

14 Ensure that all sharps and non-sharp waste are disposed of safely and in accordance with locally approved procedures. For example, sharps into sharps bin and syringes into an orange clinical waste bag.	To ensure safe disposal and to avoid laceration or other injury to staff (DH 2005, C; MHRA 2004, C).
15 Record the administration on appropriate sheets.	To maintain accurate records, provide a point of reference in the event of any queries and prevent any duplication of treatment (NMC 2008a, C; NMC 2009, C; NPSA 2007d, C).

Action Figure 12 Intradermal bleb. After Springhouse (2005). Reproduced with permission of Lippincott Williams and Wilkins.

Subcutaneous injection

Definition

These are given beneath the epidermis into the loose fat and connective tissue underlying the dermis and are used for administering small doses of non-irritating water-soluble substances for example insulin, heparin (Downie *et al.* 2003).

Related theory

Subcutaneous tissue is not richly supplied with blood vessels and so medication is absorbed more slowly than when given intramuscularly. The rate of absorption is influenced by factors that affect blood flow to tissues such as physical exercise or local application of hot or cold compresses (Perry 2007). Other conditions can prevent or delay absorption due to an impaired blood flow so in these conditions subcutaeous injections are contraindicated, for example circulatory shock, occlusive vascular disease (Perry 2007).

Evidence-based approaches
Injection sites

Sites recommended are the abdomen in the umbilical region, the lateral or posterior aspect of the lower part of the upper

Figure 16.22 Sites recommended for subcutaneous injection. Reproduced from Elkin *et al.* (2007) with permission.

arm, the thighs (under the greater trochanter rather than mid-thigh) and the buttocks (Downie *et al.* 2003) (Figure 16.22). It has been found that the amount of subcutaneous tissue varies more than was previously thought; this is particularly significant for administration of insulin as inadvertent

intramuscular administration can result in rapid absorption and hypoglycaemic episodes (King 2003). Rotation of sites can decrease the likelihood of irritation and ensure improved absorption. If using the abdominal area then try to inject each subsequent injection 2.5 cm from the previous one (Chernecky *et al.* 2002). Injection sites should be free of infection, skin lesions, scars, birthmarks, bony prominences and large underlying muscles or nerves (Perry 2007).

The skin should be gently pinched into a fold to elevate the subcutaneous tissue which lifts the adipose tissue away from the underlying muscle (Workman 1999). The practice of aspirating to ensure a blood vessel has not been pierced is no longer recommended as it has been shown that this is unlikely to occur (Peragallo-Dittko 1997, Perry 2007). The maximum volume tolerable using this route for injection is 2 mL and drugs should be highly soluble to prevent irritation (Downie *et al.* 2003).

Preprocedural considerations
Equipment

Injections are usually given using a 25 G needle. To ensure medication reaches the subcutaneous tissue, the rule is: if you can grasp 2 inches of tissue, insert the needle at a 90° angle and for 1 inch, insert needle at a 45° angle (Chernecky *et al.* 2002, Perry 2007). With the introduction of shorter needles (13 mm), it is recommended that insulin injections be given at an angle of 90° (King 2003). The length of the needle should be selected by pinching the skin tissue and selecting a needle one-half the width of the skinfold (Chernecky *et al.* 2002). Shorter needles should also be used at a 45° angle in children and underweight adults.

Specific patient preparations

It has been stated that it is not necessary to use an alcohol swab to clean the skin prior to administration of injections providing the skin is socially clean. If unsure or in immunocompromised patients, the skin should be prepared using an antiseptic swab (Dann 1969, Downie *et al.* 2003).

Procedure guideline 16.18 **Medication: subcutaneous injection**

Essential equipment

- Alcohol swab
- Needle
- Syringe containing prepared medication
- Sharps bin
- Non-sterile gloves

Preprocedure

Action	Rationale
1 Explain and discuss the procedure with the patient.	To ensure that the patient understands the procedure and gives their valid consent (Griffith and Jordan 2003, E; NMC 2008b, C; NMC 2008c, C).

(Continued)

Procedure guideline 16.18 (*Continued*)

2 Consult the patient's prescription chart and ascertain the following: (a) Drug (b) Dose (c) Date and time of administration (d) Route and method of administration (e) Diluent as appropriate (f) Validity of prescription (g) Signature of doctor.	To ensure that the patient is given the correct drug in the prescribed dose using the appropriate diluent and by the correct route (NMC 2008a, C; NPSA 2007d, C).
3 Wash hands.	To prevent contamination of medication and equipment (DH 2007, C).

Procedure

4 Close the curtains or door and assist the patient into the required position.	To ensure patient's privacy and dignity. E To allow access to the appropriate injection site (Perry 2007, E).
5 Remove appropriate garments to expose the injection site.	To gain access for injection. E
6 Assess the injection site for signs of inflammation, oedema, infection and skin lesions.	To promote effectiveness of administration (Perry 2007, E). To reduce the risk of infection (Fraise and Bradley 2009, E; Workman 1999, E). To avoid skin lesions and possible trauma to the patient (Perry 2007, E).
7 Pinch the skin of the area and select the correct needle size.	To minimize the risk of missing the subcutaneous tissue and any ensuing pain (Perry 2007, E).
8 Clean the injection site with a swab saturated with isopropyl alcohol 70% and apply gloves.	To reduce the number of pathogens introduced into the skin by the needle at the time of insertion. (For further information on this action see Skin preparation.)
9 Gently pinch the skin up into a fold.	To elevate the subcutaneous tissue, and lift the adipose tissue away from the underlying muscle (Perry 2007, E).
10 Remove the needle sheath and hold syringe between thumb and forefinger of dominant hand as if grasping a dart.	To enable a quick smooth injection (Perry 2007, E).
11 Insert the needle into the skin at an angle of 45° and release the grasped skin (unless administering insulin when an angle of 90° should be used). Inject the drug slowly.	Injecting medication into compressed tissue irritates nerve fibres and causes the patient discomfort (Perry 2007, E). The introduction of shorter insulin needles makes 90° the more appropriate angle (Trounce and Gould 2000, E).
12 Withdraw the needle rapidly. Apply gentle pressure. Do not massage area.	To aid absorption. Massage can injure underlying tissue (Perry 2007, E).

Postprocedure

13 Ensure that all sharps and non-sharp waste are disposed of safely and in accordance with locally approved procedures.	To ensure safe disposal and to avoid laceration or other injury to staff (MHRA, 2004, C; DH, 2005b, C).
14 Record the administration on appropriate sheets.	To maintain accurate records, provide a point of reference in the event of any queries and prevent any duplication of treatment (NMC 2008a, C; NMC 2009, C; NPSA 2007d, C).

Postprocedural considerations

Education of patient and relevant others

Patients often have to administer their own subcutaneous injections, for example insulin for diabetics. The nurse must teach the patient how to prepare and administer self-injection, including aspects such as equipment, storage, handwashing, injection technique and safe disposal of equipment and sharps (Perry 2007).

Complications

Medications collecting within the tissues can cause sterile abscesses, which appear as hardened, painful lumps (Perry 2007). The nurse must monitor and report these.

Subcutaneous infusion

Definition

Continuous infusion of fluids or medication into the subcutaneous tissues (Perry 2007).

Evidence-based approaches

Methods for subcutaneous infusions of fluids (hypodermoclysis)

Hypodermoclysis is a method of infusing fluid into subcutaneous tissue that is easier than administering intravenous fluids (Sasson and Shvartzman 2001). Subcutaneous fluids can be given to maintain adequate hydration in patients with mild or moderate dehydration (Mei and Auerhahn 2009, Sasson and Shvartzman 2001). The use of this route is generally limited to palliative care or elderly patients. It is not recommended for patients needing rapid administration of fluids, and is also contraindicated in patients with clotting disorders or who have problems with fluid overload (such as those with cardiac failure) (Mei and Auerhahn 2009).

A volume of 1000–2000 mL can be given over 24 hours; this can be given as a continuous infusion, over a number of hours (such as overnight) or as intermittent boluses (Moriarty and Hudson 2001). More than one site can be used if greater volumes are required (Moses 2009). It is recommended that electrolyte-containing fluids such as sodium chloride 0.9% or dextrose saline be used although 5% glucose has also been used (Sasson and Shvartzman 2001). More than one site can be used to allow administration of a greater volume of fluid.

Advantages of this route include the following.

- Side-effects are few and not generally significant.
- It is a relatively easy procedure which can be carried out at home, reducing the need for hospitalization.
- May be set up and administered by nurses in almost any setting.

- Low cost.
- Less likely to cause fluid overload.
- Intravenous access can be problematic in elderly or debilitated patients; avoidance of this can reduce anxiety and distress (Mei and Auerhahn 2009, Sasson and Shvartzman 2001).

Side-effects of subcutaneous fluid administration include pain, bruising, local oedema, erythema and local inflammation and can be reduced by changing the site of infusion (Mei and Auerhahn 2009).

Hyaluronidase is an enzyme which temporarily increases the permeability of subcutaneous connective tissue by degrading hyaluronic acid and has been shown to increase the dispersion and absorption of co-administered molecules (Thomas et al. 2009). It can be given as a subcutaneous injection before commencing fluids or added to infusion bags (Sasson and Shvartzman 2001). A randomized study compared absorption and side-effects of administration of subcutaneous fluids with or without hyaluronidase. No significant differences were found although patients not receiving hyaluronidase showed an increase in the size of the limb in which the fluid had been administered, but no differences in pain or local discomfort were found so no clear benefit to the use of hyaluronidase was demonstrated (Constans et al. 1991). Most agree that it is not necessary to use hyaluronidase if the infusion rate is 1 mL/min or less (Mei and Auerhahn 2009, Moses 2009).

Methods for subcutaneous infusions of drugs

This may be the route of choice in patients with problems such as vomiting, diarrhoea or dysphagia and who are unable to tolerate drugs by the oral route; patients with bowel obstruction whose gut absorption may be impaired may also benefit. It is also commonly used for patients who are dying and no longer able to manage medication orally (Dickman et al. 2007, Perry 2007). Continuous subcutaneous infusion of insulin is used in a small number of diabetic patients, particularly when adequate control cannot be achieved with multiple daily insulin doses. Such patients need to be under the care of a multidisciplinary team familiar with the use of such infusions (NICE 2003).

Infusions of a single drug, such as an antiemetic or analgesic, do not generally cause problems with stability. The drug should be diluted with a suitable diluent (sodium chloride is recommended for most drugs) and given over 12–24 hours (Dickman et al. 2007). The use of a combination of drugs can be problematic; there is anecdotal evidence regarding combinations of drugs but not many pharmaceutical studies confirming compatibility. Combinations of up to four drugs have been reported, but if compatibility is uncertain it may be best to use a second syringe pump. It is also important to ensure that the diluent used is compatible with all the drugs in the infusion. It is recommended that infusions are not exposed to direct sunlight or to increased temperatures as drug instability may result (Dickman *et al.* 2007). Hyaluronidase may be used to enhance the pharmacokinetics of drugs such as subcutaneous morphine (Thomas *et al.* 2009).

Preprocedural considerations
Equipment
Access devices

Research has shown that the use of peripheral cannulas rather than steel winged infusion devices results in sites remaining viable for longer (Torre 2002). Incidence of needlestick injuries may also be reduced (Dawkins *et al.* 2000). It is now recommended that subcutaneous infusion be given via a plastic cannula. Administration of infusions of drugs or fluids requires the insertion of a 25 G winged infusion set or a 24 G cannula. These should be inserted at an angle of 45° and secured with a transparent dressing to enable inspection of the site. This may also be appropriate for patients not receiving a continuous infusion but requiring frequent subcutaneous injections; this is common practice in palliative care in order to reduce the number of needles inserted into the patient and the subsequent trauma caused.

Syringe driver

A syringe driver is a portable battery-operated infusion device. It is used to deliver drugs at a predetermined rate via the appropriate parenteral route (e.g. subcutaneous) and is suitable for symptom management and palliative care (Dickman *et al.* 2007, Quinn 2008). The syringe driver should be used for patients who are unable to tolerate oral medication, for example, in nausea and vomiting, dysphagia, intestinal obstruction, local disease or sometimes in intractable pain which is unrelieved by oral medications and where rapid dose titration is required. Drugs administered by subcutaneous infusion include opioid analgesics, antiemetics, anxiolytic sedatives, corticosteroids, non-steroidal anti-inflammatory drugs and anticholinergic drugs (Dickman *et al.* 2007).

The Sims (Graseby) Medical MS16A and MS26 syringe drivers are typical examples of drivers in use; however, other types are available and nurses should follow the manufacturer's instruction manual for details of their use. The MS16A allows drug administration at an hourly rate. This driver is clearly marked with a pink '1 h' in the bottom right-hand corner. The MS26 delivers drugs at a 24-hourly rate. This driver is clearly marked with a yellow '24 h' in the bottom right-hand corner (Figure 16.23). It is important that users are aware that the MS16A syringe driver is calibrated in millimetres per hour, and the MS26 is calibrated in millimetres per day. Confusion between the two drivers in relation to rate settings has resulted in fatal errors (Dickman *et al.* 2007, MHRA 2006a). Most sizes and brands of plastic syringes can be used with these drivers; however, it is recommended to use Luer-Lok syringes to avoid leakage or accidental disconnection.

Figure 16.23 Sims (Graseby) Medical MS26 daily rate syringe driver.

The advantages of the syringe driver are as follows.

- It avoids the necessity of intermittent injections.
- Mixtures of drugs may be administered.
- Infusion timing is accurate, which is particularly advantageous in the community where it is not possible to constantly monitor the rate.
- The device is lightweight and compact, allowing mobility and independence.
- Rate can be increased.
- Simple calculations of dosage are required over a 12- or 24-hour period.
- It allows patients to spend more time at home with their symptoms managed effectively.

The disadvantages are as follows.

- The patient may become psychologically dependent on the device.
- Inflammation or infection may occur at the insertion site of the subcutaneous cannula.
- The rate calculation differs between the Sims (Graseby) Medical MS16A and MS26 syringe drivers and this can be confusing for the nurse.
- The alarm system of some syringe drivers, for example the Sims (Graseby), operates only if the plunger is obstructed. It does not alert the nurse if the flow is too rapid or too slow.

(Dickman *et al.* 2007)

Specific patient preparations
Infusion sites

Choice of site should be based on both thickness of subcutaneous tissue and patient convenience. Sites recommended for subcutaneous infusion of drugs or fluids are the lateral aspects of the upper arms and thighs, the abdomen, the chest and the scapula (Mitten 2001). If the patient is ambulant then the chest or abdomen is the preferred site (Dickman *et al.* 2007). The following areas should not be used.

- Lymphoedematous areas, as absorption may be impaired and infection may be introduced.

- Sites over bony prominences, as there may be insufficient subcutaneous tissue.
- Previously irradiated skin areas, as absorption may be impaired.
- Sites near a joint, as movement may cause the cannula to become dislodged.

- Any areas of inflamed, infected or broken skin (Mitten 2001, Perry 2007).

Rotation of the site every 3 days should be routine in order to minimize site reactions although in some patients this may not be feasible so the infusion site must be monitored regularly and the device resited as necessary (Dickman *et al.* 2007).

Procedure guideline 16.19 Medication: subcutaneous infusion of fluids

Essential equipment

- Clinically clean receiver or tray containing the prepared drug to be administered
- Sharps box
- Isopropyl alcohol 70% swab

- Transparent adhesive dressing
- Infusion fluid
- Administration set
- Winged infusion set or 24 G cannula

Preprocedure

Action	Rationale
1 Explain and discuss the procedure with the patient.	To ensure that the patient understands the procedure and gives their valid consent (Griffith and Jordan 2003, E; NMC 2008b, C; NMC 2008c, C).
2 Before administering any prescribed fluid check that it is due and has not already been given.	To protect the patient from harm (NPSA 2007d, C).
3 Before administering any prescribed fluid, consult the patient's prescription chart and ascertain the following: (a) Type of fluid (b) Volume (c) Date and time of administration (d) Route and method of administration (e) Diluent as appropriate (f) Validity of prescription (g) Signature of doctor (h) The prescription is legible.	To ensure that the patient is given the correct fluid in the prescribed dose using the appropriate diluent and by the correct route. To protect the patient from harm (NMC 2008a, C; NPSA 2007d, C).
4 Wash hands with bactericidal soap and water or bactericidal alcohol handrub, and assemble the necessary equipment.	To minimize the risk of infection (Fraise and Bradley 2009, E; Pratt *et al.* 2007, C).

Procedure

5 Check the name and volume of infusion fluid against the prescription chart.	To ensure that the correct type and quantity of fluid are administered (NMC 2008a, C; NPSA 2007d, C).
6 Check the expiry date of the infusion bag.	To prevent an ineffective or toxic compound being administered to the patient (NPSA 2007d, C).
7 Check that the packaging is intact and inspect the container and contents in a good light for cracks, punctures, air bubbles.	To check that no contamination of the infusion container has occurred (NPSA 2007d, C).
8 Inspect the fluid for discoloration, haziness and crystalline or particulate matter. If this occurs, discard.	To prevent any toxic or foreign matter being infused into the patient (NPSA 2007d, C). To detect any incompatibility or degradation (NPSA 2007d, C).
9 Establish the correct drip rate setting using the correct calculation.	To monitor rate and ensure fluid is infused safely (Pickstone 1999, E).

995

(Continued)

Procedure guideline 16.19 *(Continued)*

10 Place the infusion bag and administration set in a clean receptacle. Wash hands and proceed to the patient.	To minimize the risk of contamination (Pratt *et al.* 2007, C).
11 Check the identity of the patient against the prescription chart, and with the patient.	To minimize the risk of error and ensure the correct fluid is administered to the correct patient (NMC 2006a, C; NMC 2008a, C; NPSA 2007d, C).
12 Place the infusion bag on a flat surface, remove the seal and insert the spike of the administration set fully into the infusion bag port.	To prevent puncturing the side of the infusion and to reduce the risk of contamination (DH 2007, C).
13 Hang the infusion bag from a drip stand.	To allow gravity flow. E
14 Open the roller clamp and allow the fluid through the set to prime it. Close clamp.	To remove air from the set. E
15 Assist the patient into a comfortable position.	To ensure patient comfort during the proedure. E
16 Expose the chosen site for infusion.	To expose the area. E
17 Clean the chosen site with a swab saturated with 70% isopropyl alcohol. Wait until the alcohol evaporates.	To reduce the risk of infection and prevent stinging sensation on insertion of needle (Fraise and Bradley 2009, E; Pratt *et al.* 2007, C).
18 Grasp the skin firmly.	To elevate the subcutaneous tissue. E
19 Insert the infusion needle into the skin at an angle of 45°, bevel up, and release the grasped skin. (If using a cannula, remove the stylet.)	To gain access to the subcutaneous tissue (Moses 2009, E; Sasson and Shvartzman 2001, E).
20 Connect the administration set to the device.	To commence the infusion. E
21 Apply transparent dressing to secure infusion device.	To prevent movement and reduce the risk of mechanical phlebitis and infection (Fraise and Bradley 2009, E; Moses 2009, E; Pratt *et al.* 2007, C; Weinstein and Plumer 2007, E).
22 Open the roller clamp and adjust until the flow rate is achieved. The rate is usually 1 mL/min per site by gravity.	To ensure the correct rate is set (Moses 2009, E).

Postprocedure

23 Complete the patient's prescription chart and other hospital and/or legally required documents. This should include infusion device and site checks.	To comply with local drug administration policies and provide a record in the event of any queries (NMC 2009, C). To prevent any duplication of treatment (NMC 2009, C).
24 Monitor the patient for any infusion- or site-related complications.	To detect complications promptly (Sasson and Shvartzman 2001, E).
25 Ask the patient to report any pain or tenderness at the infusion site.	To ascertain whether there are any problems that may require nursing care and refer to medical staff where appropriate. E.
26 Discard waste, making sure that it is placed in the correct containers, for example sharps into a designated receptacle.	To ensure safe disposal and avoid injury to staff. To prevent reuse of equipment (DH 2005, C; MHRA 2004, C).

Procedure guideline 16.20 Medication: subcutaneous administration using a Graseby syringe driver

Essential equipment

- Clinically clean receiver or tray containing the prepared drug to be administered
- Syringe driver/pump
- Battery (PP3 size, 9 volt alkaline)
- Plastic peripheral cannulas (e.g. 24 G) and microbore driver set (100 cm) with needle-free Y connector injection site (or 100 cm winged infusion set)
- Luer-Lok syringe of suitable size (e.g. 10 mL)
- Isopropyl alcohol 70% swab

- Transparent adhesive dressing
- Drugs and diluent
- Needle (to draw up drug)
- Drug additive label
- Patient's prescription chart
- Recording chart or book as required by law or hospital policy
- Sharps box

Preprocedure

Action	Rationale
1 Explain and discuss the procedure with the patient.	To ensure that the patient understands the procedure and gives their valid consent (Griffith and Jordan 2003, E; NMC 2008b, C; NMC 2008c, C).
2 Before administering any prescribed drug, check that it is due and has not already been given.	To protect the patient from harm (NPSA 2007d, C).
3 Before administering any prescribed drug, consult the patient's prescription chart and ascertain the following: (a) Drug (b) Dose (c) Date and time of administration (d) Route and method of administration (e) Diluent as appropriate (f) Validity of prescription (g) Signature of doctor (h) The prescription is legible.	To ensure that the patient is given the correct drug in the prescribed dose using the appropriate diluent and by the correct route. To protect the patient from harm (NMC 2008a, C; NPSA 2007d, C).
4 Calculate and check dosage of drugs required over a 24-hour period.	To establish correct dosages of drugs (Pickstone 1999, E).
5 Wash hands with bactericidal soap and water or bactericidal alcohol handrub, and assemble the necessary equipment.	To minimize the risk of infection (Fraise and Bradley 2009, E; Pratt *et al.* 2007, C).

Procedure

6 Check the name, strength and volume of subcutaneous drug(s) against the prescription chart.	To ensure that the correct type and quantity of fluid are administered (NMC 2008a, C; NPSA 2007d, C).
7 Check the expiry date of the drug(s).	To prevent an ineffective or toxic compound being administered to the patient (NPSA 2007d, C).
8 Check that the packaging is intact and inspect the container and contents in a good light for cracks, punctures, air bubbles.	To check that no contamination of the infusion container has occurred (NPSA 2007d, C).

(Continued)

Procedure guideline 16.20 (*Continued*)

9 Check the identity and amount of drug to be prepared. Consider: (a) Compatibility of drugs (b) Stability of mixture over the prescription time (c) Any special directions for dilution, for example pH, optimum concentration (d) Sensitivity to external factors such as light (e) Any anticipated allergic reaction. If any doubts exist about the listed points, consult the pharmacist or appropriate reference works.	To minimize any risk of error. To ensure safe and effective administration of the drug. To enable anticipation of toxicities and the nursing implications of these (NPSA 2007d, C).
10 Using a Luer-Lok syringe, draw up drugs required with diluent to measure a total volume (this will depend on type of syringe device used).	To ensure accuracy and avoid any infusion errors. To ensure the drug is prepared correctly (NPSA 2007d, C).
11 Inspect the fluid for discoloration, haziness and crystalline or particulate matter. If this occurs, discard and re-evaluate drug compatability. *Note*: This can occur even if the mixture is theoretically compatible, thus making vigilance essential.	To prevent any toxic or foreign matter being infused into the patient (NPSA 2007d, C). To detect any incompatibility or degradation (NPSA 2007d, C).
12 Establish the correct rate setting of the driver using the correct calculation.	To monitor rate and ensure drug is infused safely (Dickman *et al.* 2007, E; Pickstone 1999, E).
13 Measure stroke length in millimetres. The stroke length is the *length* of fluid to be infused, that is, the distance the plunger has to travel (irrespective of the number of millilitres) (see Action Figure 13).	Example: Stroke length = 48 mm Delivery time = 1 day Rate setting = 48 mm
14 Check the delivery time (previously prescribed) in days. Set rate using screwdriver provided (see Action Figure 14).	To ensure correct rate setting. E
15 Calculate: $$\text{Rate} = \frac{\text{Fluid length}}{\text{Infusion period in days}}$$	See instruction booklets provided with individual syringe driver (manufacturer's instructions, C).
16 Complete the drug additive label and fix it on the syringe.	To identify which drug has been added, when and by whom (NPSA 2007d, C).
17 Wash hands with bactericidal soap and water or bactericidal alcohol handrub.	To minimize the risk of infection (Fraise and Bradley 2009, E; Pratt *et al.* 2007, C).
18 Connect prepared syringe to a 100 cm microbore driver set with needle-free Y connector injection site.	This length of tubing allows patient greater freedom of movement. E.
19 Prime the infusion by gently depressing the plunger of the syringe until the fluid is visible at the end of the infusion set. Priming the infusion set after calculation will reduce the delivery time by approximately half an hour for the first infusion. Do not alter previously calculated rate setting despite volume reduction in barrel of syringe.	This removes extraneous air from the system. E Ensures patient receives drugs immediately and accurately. E
20 Place the syringe and infusion set in a clean receptacle. Wash hands and proceed to the patient.	To minimize the risk of contamination (Pratt *et al.* 2007, C).
21 Check the identity of the patient against the prescription chart, syringe drug additive label and with the patient if possible.	To minimize the risk of error and ensure the correct drug is administered to the correct patient (NMC 2006a, C; NMC 2008a, C; NPSA 2007d, C).

22 Assist the patient into a comfortable position.	To aid patient comfort. E
23 Expose the chosen site for infusion.	To ensure access to site. E
24 Clean the chosen site with a swab saturated with 70% isopropyl alcohol. Wait until the alcohol evaporates.	To reduce the risk of infection and prevent stinging sensation on insertion of needle (Fraise and Bradley 2009, E; Pratt *et al.* 2007, C).
25 Grasp the skin firmly.	To elevate the subcutaneous tissue. E
26 Insert the infusion needle into the skin at an angle of 45° and release the grasped skin. (If using a cannula, remove the stylet and connect the extension set.)	Positioning shallower than 45° may shorten the life of the infusion site. E
27 Apply transparent dressing to secure infusion device.	To prevent movement and reduce the risk of mechanical phlebitis and infection (Fraise and Bradley 2009, E; Pratt *et al.* 2007, C; Weinstein and Plumer 2007, E).
28 Check that the infusion set and syringe are securely connected.	To ensure that there is no disconnection so that the drug(s) are administered correctly. E
29 Connect the syringe to the syringe driver/pump.	To ensure the syringe is connected correctly to the syringe driver/pump. E
30 Place the syringe on the syringe driver along the grooved lines, with barrel clamp firmly in position.	To ensure the syringe is in the correct position. C
31 Secure in place with rubber strap.	To ensure the syringe is securely clamped to the barrel. C
32 Slide the actuator assembly along the lead screw by pressing white release button, as shown in Action Figure 32, until it rests against the end of the plunger.	To enable the pump mechanism to operate correctly. C
33 Secure plunger with additional safety clamp (see Action Figure 33) and clear Perspex container.	To ensure extra security and minimize the risk of errors in infusional rates. C
34 Fit the battery, ensuring contact by flashing light on front of syringe driver.	To ensure device is working. E
35 Press start/test button to commence infusion. The indicator light should flash to indicate functioning syringe pump.	To check the infusion device is operating correctly. C

Postprocedure

36 Complete the patient's prescription chart and other hospital and/or legally required documents. This should include infusion device serial number and infusion device and site checks.	To comply with local drug administration policies and ensure the safe administration and monitoring of the infused drug and accurate records. To provide a record in the event of any queries (NMC 2009, C). To prevent any duplication of treatment (NMC 2009, C).
37 Monitor the patient for any infusion-related complications.	To detect complications promptly (Dickman *et al.* 2007, E; Dougherty 2002, E; MHRA 2010b, C; Pickstone 1999, E; Quinn 2000, E).
38 Ask the patient to report any pain and tenderness at the infusion site and if they experience any change in their symptoms or have new symptoms.	To ascertain whether there are any problems that may require nursing care and refer to medical staff where appropriate. E
39 Discard waste, making sure that it is placed in the correct containers, for example sharps into a designated receptacle.	To ensure safe disposal and avoid injury to staff. To prevent reuse of equipment (DH 2005, C; MHRA 2004, C).

999

(Continued)

Procedure guideline 16.20 (*Continued*)

Action Figure 13   Measuring stroke length.

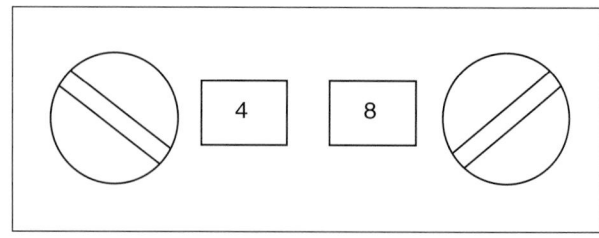

Action Figure 14   Setting the rate.

Action Figure 32   Connecting syringe to syringe driver.

Action Figure 33   Securing the plunger.

Procedure guideline 16.21 Medication: subcutaneous administration using a McKinley T34

Essential equipment

- Clinically clean receiver or tray containing the prepared drug to be administered
- Syringe driver/pump
- Battery (PP3 size, 9 volt alkaline)
- Plastic peripheral cannulas (e.g. 24 G) and microbore driver set (100 cm) with needle-free Y connector injection site (or 100 cm winged infusion set)
- Luer-Lok syringe of suitable size (e.g. 10 mL)
- Swab saturated with isopropyl alcohol 70%

- Transparent adhesive dressing
- Drugs and diluent
- Needle (to draw up drug)
- Drug additive label
- Patient's prescription chart
- Recording chart or book as required by law or hospital policy
- Sharps box

Preprocedure

Action	Rationale
1 Explain and discuss the procedure with the patient.	To ensure that the patient understands the procedure and gives their valid consent (Griffith and Jordan 2003, E; NMC 2008b, C; NMC 2008c, C).
2 Before administering any prescribed drug, check that it is due and has not already been given.	To protect the patient from harm (NPSA 2007d, C).

3 Before administering any prescribed drug, consult the patient's prescription chart and ascertain the following: (a) Drug (b) Dose (c) Date and time of administration (d) Route and method of administration (e) Diluent as appropriate (f) Validity of prescription (g) Signature of doctor (h) The prescription is legible.	To ensure that the patient is given the correct drug in the prescribed dose using the appropriate diluent and by the correct route. To protect the patient from harm (NMC 2008a, C; NPSA 2007d, C). To comply with NMC (2006a, C; 2008a, C).
4 Calculate and check dosage of drugs required over a 24-hour period.	To establish correct dosages of drugs (Pickstone 1999, E).
5 Wash hands with bactericidal soap and water or bactericidal alcohol handrub, and assemble the necessary equipment.	To minimize the risk of infection (Fraise and Bradley 2009, E; Pratt *et al.* 2007, C).

Procedure

6 Check the name, strength and volume of subcutaneous drug(s) against the prescription chart.	To ensure that the correct type and quantity of fluid are administered (NMC 2008a, C; NPSA 2007d, C).
7 Check the expiry date of the drug(s).	To prevent an ineffective or toxic compound being administered to the patient (NPSA 2007d, C).
8 Check that the packaging is intact and inspect the container and contents in a good light for cracks, punctures, air bubbles.	To check that no contamination of the infusion container has occurred (NPSA 2007d, C).
9 Check the identity and amount of drug to be prepared. Consider: (a) Compatibility of drugs (b) Stability of mixture over the prescription time (c) Any special directions for dilution, for example pH, optimum concentration (d) Sensitivity to external factors such as light (e) Any anticipated allergic reaction. If any doubts exist about the listed points, consult the pharmacist or appropriate reference works.	To minimize any risk of error. To ensure safe and effective administration of the drug. To enable anticipation of toxicities and the nursing implications of these (NPSA 2007d, C).
10 Using a Luer-Lok syringe, draw up drugs required with diluent to measure a total volume (this will depend on type of syringe device used). See Box 16.13 for McKinley T34 recommended volumes and Action Figure 10 for a McKinley T34 syringe pump.	To ensure accuracy and avoid any infusion errors. To ensure the drug is prepared correctly (NPSA 2007d, C).
11 Inspect the fluid for discoloration, haziness and crystalline or particulate matter. If this occurs, discard and re-evaluate drug compatability. *Note*: This can occur even if the mixture is theoretically compatible, thus making vigilance essential.	To prevent any toxic or foreign matter being infused into the patient (NPSA 2007d, C). To detect any incompatibility or degradation (NPSA 2007d, C).
12 Establish the correct rate setting of the driver using the correct calculation.	To monitor rate and ensure drug is infused safely (Dickman *et al.* 2007, E; Pickstone1999, E).
13 Complete the drug additive label and fix it onto the syringe without obscuring the markings.	To identify which drug has been added, when and by whom and be able to visually inspect the amount in the syringe (NPSA 2007d, C).

1001

(Continued)

Procedure guideline 16.21 (*Continued*)

14 Wash hands with bactericidal soap and water or bactericidal alcohol handrub.	To minimize the risk of infection (Fraise and Bradley 2009, E; Pratt *et al.* 2007, C).
15 Connect prepared syringe to a 100 cm microbore driver set with needle-free Y connector injection site.	This length of tubing allows patient greater freedom of movement. E
16 Prime the infusion by gently depressing the plunger of the syringe until the fluid is visible at the end of the infusion set. Priming the infusion set after calculation will reduce the delivery time by approximately half an hour for the first infusion. Do not alter previously calculated rate setting despite volume reduction in barrel of syringe.	This removes extraneous air from the system. E Ensures patient receives drugs immediately and accurately. E
17 Place the syringe and infusion set in a clean receptacle. Wash hands and proceed to the patient.	To minimize the risk of contamination (Pratt *et al.* 2007, C).
18 Check the identity of the patient against the prescription chart, syringe drug additive label and with the patient if possible.	To minimize the risk of error and ensure the correct drug is administered to the correct patient (NMC 2006a, C; NMC 2008a, C; NPSA 2007d, C).
19 Assist the patient into a comfortable position.	To aid patient comfort. E
20 Expose the chosen site for infusion.	To gain access to the site. E
21 Clean the chosen site with a swab saturated with 70% isopropyl alcohol. Wait until the alcohol evaporates.	To reduce the risk of infection and prevent stinging sensation on insertion of needle (Fraise and Bradley 2009, E; Pratt *et al.* 2007, C).
22 Grasp the skin firmly.	To elevate the subcutaneous tissue. E
23 Insert the infusion needle into the skin at an angle of 45° and release the grasped skin. (If using a cannula, remove the stylet and connect the extension set.)	Positioning shallower than 45° may shorten the life of the infusion site. E
24 Apply transparent dressing to secure infusion device.	To prevent movement and reduce the risk of mechanical phlebitis and infection (Fraise and Bradley 2009, E; Pratt *et al.* 2007, C; Weinstein and Plumer 2007, E).
25 Check that the infusion set and syringe are securely connected.	To ensure that there is no disconnection so that the drug(s) are administered correctly. E
26 Connect the syringe to the syringe driver/pump.	To ensure the syringe is connected correctly to the syringe driver/pump. E
27 Press the <<FF or >>Back key to adjust the actuator to accommodate the syringe. Lift the barrel arm and ensure the syringe is loaded so as to stop all three sensors (barrel, collar and plunger) flashing.	To ensure the syringe is in the correct position (manufacturer's instructions, C).
28 The pump will detect size and brand of syringe. Check and confirm by pressing YES key.	To enable the pump mechanism to operate correctly (manufacturer's instructions, C).
29 Set a new programme for each syringe.	To clear previous programme and reduce risk of error (manufacturer's instructions, C).
30 Pump measures deliverable volume in syringe. Use down arrow key to select a smaller volume.	May be necessary to allow for KVO volume. E

31 Press Yes to confirm volume to be infused. Press Yes to confirm infusion duration. Pump displays rate calculated on volume and duration set by user. Then press Yes to confirm.	To complete set-up of device (manufacturer's instructions, C).
32 Secure in the clear Perspex lock box.	To ensure extra security and minimize the risk of errors in infusional rates. E

Postprocedure

33 Complete the patient's prescription chart and other hospital and/or legally required documents. This should include infusion device serial number and infusion device and site checks.	To comply with local drug administration policies and ensure the safe administration and monitoring of the infused drug and accurate records. To provide a record in the event of any queries (NMC 2009, C). To prevent any duplication of treatment (NMC 2009, C).
34 Monitor the patient for any infusion-related complications.	To detect complications promptly (Dickman *et al.* 2007, E; Dougherty 2002, E; MHRA 2010b, C; Pickstone 1999, E; Quinn 2000, E).
35 Ask the patient to report any pain and tenderness at the infusion site and if they experience any change in their symptoms or have new symptoms.	To ascertain whether there are any problems that may require nursing care and refer to medical staff where appropriate. E
36 Discard waste, making sure that it is placed in the correct containers, for example sharps into a designated receptacle.	To ensure safe disposal and avoid injury to staff. To prevent reuse of equipment (DH 2005, C; MHRA 2004, C).

Action Figure 10   McKinley T34 syringe pump.

Box 16.13 Volumes for syringe pumps

- 10 mL syringe must be drawn up to 10 mL (approx. rate = 0.42 mL per 24 hours)
- 20 mL syringe must be drawn up to 17 mL (approx. rate = 0.71 mL per 24 hours)
- 30 mL syringe must be drawn up to 22 mL (approx. rate = 0.92 mL per 24 hours)
- 60 mL syringe must be drawn up to 32 mL (approx. rate = 1.33 mL per 24 hours)

Problem-solving table 16.2 Prevention and resolution (Procedure guideline 16.21)

Problem	Cause	Prevention	Action
Precipitation or cloudiness in the syringe	Indicates incompatability	Check compatability prior to mixing. Use www.pallcarematters.co.uk for up-to-date advice	Remove syringe, dispose of contents and prepare a new syringe

Postprocedural considerations
Ongoing care

Accurate documentation of the site, rate, flow, start time and drugs used is imperative in order to avoid confusion and errors amongst staff (Dickman *et al.* 2007, Dougherty 2002, MHRA 2010b, Moses 2009, NMC 2006a, NMC 2008a, NMC 2009, Quinn 2000, Sasson and Shvartzman 2001). Sites and tubing may need to be changed every 1–4 days (Moses 2009).

The frequency of checks should be as follows.

- At start of infusion – record date, time, start volume, infusion rate setting, name of person setting up infusion.
- Based upon the type of infusion and patient's condition; however, at a minimum these should be carried out 15 minutes and 1 hour after the initial set-up and thereafter a minimum of every 4 hours.
- Device must be checked at the start of each shift and/or when setting up an infusion.

Infusion device and infusion checks

- Check and record the date, time, rate and volume remaining and that the battery/syringe driver is working.
- Record any reasons for changing of the drug, dose, rate setting of syringe driver or site.
- Check subcutaneous site for:
  - pain/discomfort
  - swelling/induration
  - erythema
  - leakage of fluid
  - bleeding.

Complications
Skin reactions

Some drugs are particularly likely to cause irritation and may need to be diluted in a greater volume of diluent; cyclizine and levomepromazine are amongst these. This may result in skin sites that break down rapidly or site reactions. The following methods can help to prevent this.

- Check compatibility of drugs and diluents and consider changing the drug combination.
- Dilute the solution as much as possible or change the diluent.
- Rotate the site at least every 72 hours.
- Use of a non-metal cannula.
- Use a different site cleanser.
- Change the dressing used.
- Consider adding dexamethasone 1 mg to the driver; this may be helpful but is not currently recommended for routine use. Care should also be taken as dexamethasone is incompatible with a number of drug combinations (Dickman *et al.* 2007).

Intramuscular injections

Definition

An intramuscular injection deposits medication into deep muscle tissue under the subcutaneous tissue (Chernecky *et al.* 2002). The vascularity of muscle aids the rapid absorption of medication (Perry 2007).

Evidence-based approaches
Site and volume of injection

Selecting the site requires correct identification of the muscle groups by landmarking correct anatomical features (Hunter 2008). Choice will be influenced by the patient's physical condition and age. Intramuscular injections should be given into the densest part of the muscle (Pope 2002). An active patient will probably have a greater muscle mass than older or emaciated patients (Hunter 2008).

The injectable volume will depend on the muscle bed. In children, injectable volumes should be halved because muscle mass is less (Workman 1999). However, it appears that it is the medicine rather than just the volume that affects how a patient tolerates the injection. Malkin (2008) uses Botox injections as an example where a volume of 1–3 mL can be injected into facial muscle groups, supporting the view that tolerance of the drug is more important than the volume.

Current research evidence suggests that there are five sites that can be utilized for the administration of intramuscular injections (Rodger and King 2000, Tortora and Derrickson 2009).

- The *ventrogluteal site* (Figure 16.24a) is relatively free of major nerves and blood vessels and the muscle is large and well defined, making it easy to locate (Greenway 2004). It is located by placing the palm of the hand on the patient's opposite greater trochanter (right hand on left hip). The index finger is then extended to the anterior superior iliac spine to make a V. Injection in the centre of the V will ensure the injection is given into the gluteus medius muscle (Hunter 2008). This is the site of choice for intramuscular injections (Rodger and King 2000) and used for antibiotics, antiemetics, deep intramuscular and Z-track injections in oil, narcotics and sedatives. Up to 2.5 mL can be safely injected into the ventrogluteal site (Rodger and King 2000).
- The *deltoid site* (Figure 16.24b) has the advantage of being easily accessible whether the patient is standing, sitting or lying down. It is found by visualizing a triangle where the horizontal line is located 2.5–5 cm below the acromial process and midpoint of the lateral aspect of the arm, in line with the axilla to form the apex (Hunter 2008). The injection is then given 2.5 cm down from the acromial process, avoiding the radial and brachial nerves. Owing to the small area of this site, the number

(a) The ventrogluteal injection site

(b) The deltoid injection site

(c) The dorsogluteal injection site

(d) The rectus femoris and vastus lateralis injection sites

Figure 16.24   Intramuscular injection sites. Reproduced from Rodger and King (2000) with permission.

and volume of injections which can be given into it are limited. Drugs such as narcotics, sedatives and vaccines, which are usually small in volume, tend to be administered into the deltoid site (Workman 1999). Rodger and King (2000) state that the maximum volume that should be administered at this site is 1 mL.

- The *dorsogluteal site* (Figure 16.24c) or upper outer quadrant is the traditional site of choice and is used for deep intramuscular and Z-track injections. It is located by using imaginary lines to divide the buttocks into four quarters. However, this site carries the danger of the needle hitting the sciatic nerve and the superior gluteal arteries (Workman 1999). The gluteus muscle has the lowest drug absorption rate and this can result in a build-up in the tissues, increasing the risk of overdose (Malkin

2008). The muscle mass is also likely to have atrophied in elderly, non-ambulant and emaciated patients. Finally, it appears that there is a risk that the medication will not reach the muscle due to the amount of subcutaneous tissue in this area (Greenway 2004) and so it is not recommended for routine immunizations due to the poor absorption and risk of nerve injury (DH 2006, WHO 2004). In adults, up to 4 mL can be safely injected into this site (Rodger and King 2000).

- The *rectus femoris site* (Figure 16.24d) is a well-defined muscle found by measuring a hand's breadth from the greater trochanter and the knee joint, which identifies the middle third of the quadriceps muscle (Hunter 2008). It is used for antiemetics, narcotics, sedatives, injections in oil, deep intramuscular and Z-track injections. It is rarely used by nurses, but is easily accessed for self-administration of injections or for infants (Workman 1999). 1–5 mL can be injected (1–3 mL in children).

■ The *vastus lateralis site* (Figure 16.24d) is used for deep intramuscular and Z-track injections. One of the advantages of this site is its ease of access but more importantly, there are no major blood vessels or significant nerve structures associated with this site. It is the better option in the obese patient (Nisbet 2006). Up to 5 mL can be safely injected (Rodger and King 2000).

There is debate over which site to use. The two recommended are the vastus lateralis and the ventrogluteal, but most nurses tend to use the dorsogluteal as it is more familiar (Greenway 2004).

Rate of administration

It is recommended that the plunger is depressed at a rate of 10 seconds per millilitre.

Technique

The Z-track method involves pulling the skin downwards or to one side of the injection site and inserting the needle at a right angle to the skin, which moves the cutaneous and subcutaneous tissues by approximately 1–2 cm (Workman 1999). The injection is given and the needle withdrawn, while releasing the retracted skin at the same time. This manoeuvre seals off the puncture track. An angle of 90° is supported by the DH (2006). The syringe should be held like a pen to insert with a dart-like motion. Aspiration is still an accepted part of an IM injection to ensure that the medication does not enter the capillaries or is inadvertently given intravenously (Hunter 2008), but there is no evidence to support this. Some centres have had to adapt as safety devices do not allow the withdrawal of the plunger as the safety system can then be activated.

Preprocedural considerations

1006

Equipment

The most common size of needle is 21 G (23 G may also be used in a thin patient) but it does depend on the viscosity of the medication. The important aspect of the needle is the length. The correct use of needle length will result in fewer adverse events and reduce complications of abscess, pain and bruising (Malkin 2008). Needles should be long enough to penetrate the muscle and still allow a quarter of the needle to remain external to the skin (Workman 1999). Lenz (1983) states that when choosing the correct needle length for intramuscular injections, it is important to assess the muscle mass of the injection site, the amount of subcutaneous fat and the weight of the patient. It may be necessary to calibrate the BMI to calculate body fat (DH 2006). Without

such an assessment, most injections intended for gluteal muscle are deposited in the gluteal fat. The following are suggested as ways of determining the most suitable size of needle to use.

Deltoid and vastus lateralis muscles

The muscle to be used should be grasped between the thumb and forefinger to determine the depth of the muscle mass or the amount of subcutaneous fat at the injection site.

Gluteal muscles

The layer of fat and skin above the muscle should be gently lifted with the thumb and forefinger for the same reasons as before. Use the patient's weight to calculate the needle length required.

The following are recommended but remembering that women have more subcutaneous tissue than men.

- Children   16 mm needle
- 31.5–40.0 kg   25 mm needle
- 40.5–90.0 kg   25 mm needle
- 90 kg   38 mm needle

(Pope 2002)

Specific patient preparations
Skin preparation

There are many inconsistencies regarding skin cleaning prior to subcutaneous or intramuscular injections. Previous studies have suggested that cleaning with an alcohol swab is not always necessary, as not cleaning the site does not result in infections and may predispose the skin to hardening (Dann 1969, Koivistov and Felig 1978, Workman 1999).

Dann (1969), in a study over a period of 6 years involving more than 5000 injections, found no single case of local and/or systemic infection. Koivistov and Felig (1978) concluded that whilst skin preparations did reduce skin bacterial count, they are not necessary to prevent infections at the injection site. Some hospitals accept that if the patient is physically clean and the nurse maintains a high standard of hand hygiene and asepsis during the procedure, skin disinfection is not necessary (Workman 1999).

In the immunosuppressed patient, the skin should be cleaned as such patients may become infected by inoculation of a relatively small number of pathogens (Downie *et al.* 2003). The practice at the Royal Marsden Hospital is to clean the skin prior to injection in order to reduce the risk of contamination from the patient's skin flora. The skin should be cleaned using an 'alcohol swab' (containing 70% isopropyl alcohol) for 30 seconds and then allowed to dry. If the skin is not dry before proceeding, skin cleaning is ineffective and the antiseptic may cause irritation by being injected into the tissues (Downie *et al.* 2003).

Procedure guideline 16.22 Medication: intramuscular injection

Essential equipment

- Alcohol swab
- Needle
- Syringe containing prepared IM medication

Preprocedure

Action	Rationale
1 Explain and discuss the procedure with the patient.	To ensure that the patient understands the procedure and gives their valid consent (Griffith and Jordan 2003, E; NMC 2008b, C; NMC 2008c, C).
2 Consult the patient's prescription sheet and ascertain the following: (a) Drug (b) Dose (c) Date and time of administration (d) Route and method of administration (e) Diluent as appropriate (f) Validity of prescription (g) Signature of doctor.	To ensure that the patient is given the correct drug in the prescribed dose using the appropriate diluent and by the correct route (NMC 2008a, C; NPSA 2007d, C).

Procedure

3 Close the curtains or door and assist the patient into the required position.	To ensure patient privacy and dignity. E To allow access to the injection site and to ensure the designated muscle group is flexed and therefore relaxed (Workman 1999, E).
4 Remove the appropriate garment to expose the injection site.	To gain access for injection (Workman 1999, E).
5 Assess the injection site for signs of inflammation, oedema, infection and skin lesions.	To promote effectiveness of administration (Workman 1999, E). To reduce the risk of infection (Fraise and Bradley 2009, E; Workman 1999, E). To avoid skin lesions and avoid possible trauma to the patient (Perry 2007, E; Workman 1999, E).
6 Clean the injection site with a swab saturated with isopropyl alcohol 70% for 30 seconds and allow to dry for 30 seconds (Workman 1999).	To reduce the number of pathogens introduced into the skin by the needle at the time of insertion and to prevent stinging sensation if alcohol is taken into the tissues upon needle entry (Hunter 2008, E; Workman 1999, E). (For further information on this action see Skin preparation.)
7 With the non-dominant hand, stretch the skin slightly around the injection site.	To displace the underlying subcutaneous tissues, facilitate the insertion of the needle and reduce the sensitivity of nerve endings (Hunter 2008, E; Workman 1999, E).
8 Holding the syringe in the dominant hand like a dart, inform the patient and quickly plunge the needle at an angle of 90° into the skin until about 1 cm of the needle is left showing.	To ensure that the needle penetrates the muscle (Hunter 2008, E; Workman 1999, E).
9 Pull back the plunger. If no blood is aspirated, depress the plunger at approximately 1 mL every 10 seconds and inject the drug slowly. If blood appears, withdraw the needle completely, replace it and begin again. Explain to the patient what has occurred.	To confirm that the needle is in the correct position and not in a vein (Workman 1999, E). This allows time for the muscle fibres to expand and absorb the solution (Hunter 2008, E; Workman 1999, E). To prevent pain and ensure even distribution of the drug (Perry 2007, E).

1007

(Continued)

Procedure guideline 16.22 *(Continued)*

10 Wait 10 seconds before withdrawing the needle.	To allow the medication to diffuse into the tissue (Perry 2007, E; Workman 1999, E).
11 Withdraw the needle rapidly. Apply gentle pressure to any bleeding point and then apply a small plaster over the puncture site.	To prevent tissue injury and haematoma formation (Perry 2007, E).

Postprocedure

12 Ensure that all sharps and non-sharp waste are disposed of safely and in accordance with locally approved procedures, for example put sharps into sharps bin and syringes into orange clinical waste bag.	To ensure safe disposal and to avoid laceration or other injury to staff (DH 2005, C; MHRA 2004, C).
13 Record the administration on appropriate charts.	To maintain accurate records, provide a point of reference in the event of any queries and prevent any duplication of treatment (NMC 2008a, C; NMC 2009, C; NPSA 2007d, C).

Intravenous injections and infusions

Definition

The introduction of medication or solutions into the circulatory system via a peripheral or central vein (Chernecky *et al.* 2002).

Anatomy and physiology

See Chapter 18 for anatomy and physiology related to the venous system.

Related theory

Intravenous therapy is now an integral part of the majority of nurses' professional practice (RCN 2010). The nurse's role has progressed considerably from being able to add drugs to infusion bags (DHSS 1976) to now assessing patients and inserting the appropriate vascular access device (VAD) prior to drug administration (Gabriel 2005).

Any nurse administering intravenous drugs must be competent in all aspects of intravenous therapy and act in accordance with *The Code* (NMC 2008b), that is, to maintain knowledge and skills (Hyde 2008, RCN 2010). Training and assessment should comprise both theoretical and practical components and include legal and professional issues, fluid balance, pharmacology, drug administration, local and systemic complications, infection control issues, use of equipment and risk management (Hyde 2008, RCN 2010).

The nurse's responsibilities in relation to intravenous drug administration include the following.

- Knowing the therapeutic use of the drug or solution, its normal dosage, side-effects, precautions and contraindications.

- Preparing the drug aseptically and safely, checking the container and drug for faults, using the correct diluent and only preparing it immediately prior to administration.
- Identifying the patient and checking allergy status.
- Checking the prescription chart.
- Checking and maintaining patency of the VAD.
- Inspecting the site of the VAD and managing/reporting complications where appropriate.
- Controlling the flow rate of infusion and/or speed of injection.
- Monitoring the condition of the patient and reporting changes.
- Making clear and immediate records of all drugs administered (Finlay 2008, NMC 2008a, NMC 2008b, RCN 2010).

Evidence-based approaches
Methods of administering intravenous drugs

There are three methods of administering intravenous drugs: continuous infusion, intermittent infusion and direct intermittent injection.

Continuous infusion

Continuous infusion may be defined as the intravenous delivery of a medication or fluid at a constant rate over a prescribed time period, ranging from several hours to several days to achieve a controlled therapeutic response (Turner and Hankins 2010). The greater dilution also helps to reduce venous irritation (Weinstein and Plumer 2007, Whittington 2008).

A continuous infusion may be used when:

- the drugs to be administered must be highly diluted
- a maintenance of steady blood levels of the drug is required (Turner and Hankins 2010).

Pre-prepared infusion fluids with additives such as those containing potassium chloride should be used whenever possible. This reduces the risk of extrinsic contamination, which can occur during the mixing of drugs (Weinstein and Plumer 2007). Only one addition should be made to each bottle or bag of fluid after the compatibility has been ascertained. More additions can increase the risk of incompatibility occurring, for example precipitation (Weinstein and Plumer 2007, Whittington 2008). The additive and fluid must be mixed well to prevent a layering effect which can occur with some drugs (Whittington 2008). The danger is that a bolus injection of the drug may be delivered. To safeguard against this, any additions should be made to the infusion fluid and the container inverted a number of times to ensure mixing of the drug, before the fluid is hung on the infusion stand (NPSA 2007d). The infusion container should be labelled clearly after the addition has been made. Constant monitoring of the infusion fluid mixture (Weinstein and Plumer 2007, Whittington 2008) for cloudiness or presence of particles should occur, as well as checking the patient's condition and intravenous site for patency, extravasation or infiltration (Downie *et al.* 2003).

Intermittent infusion

Intermittent infusion is the administration of a small-volume infusion, that is, 25–250 mL, over a period of between 15 minutes and 2 hours (Turner and Hankins 2010). This may be given as a specific dose at one time or at repeated intervals during 24 hours (Pickstone 1999).

An intermittent infusion may be used when:

- a peak plasma level is required therapeutically
- the pharmacology of the drug dictates this specific dilution
- the drug will not remain stable for the time required to administer a more dilute volume
- the patient is on a restricted intake of fluids (Whittington 2008).

Delivery of the drug by intermittent infusion can be piggybacked (via a needle-free injection port), if the primary infusion is of a compatible fluid, may utilize a system such as a 'Y' set or or a burette set with a chamber capacity of 100 or 150 mL (Turner and Hankins 2010). This is when the drug can be added to the burette and infused while the primary infusion is switched off. A small-volume infusion may also be connected to a cannula specifically to keep the vein open, and maintain patency.

All the points considered when preparing for a continuous infusion should be taken into account here, for example pre-prepared fluids, single additions of drugs, adequate mixing, labelling and monitoring.

Direct intermittent injection

Direct intermittent injection (also known as intravenous push or bolus) involves the injection of a drug from a syringe into the injection port of the administration set or directly into a VAD (Chernecky *et al.* 2002, Turner and Hankins

2010). Most are administered anywhere from 3 to 10 minutes depending upon the drug (Weinstein and Plumer 2007, Whittington 2008).

A direct injection may be used when:

- a maximum concentration of the drug is required to vital organs. This is a 'bolus' injection which is given rapidly over seconds, as in an emergency, for example adrenaline
- the drug cannot be further diluted for pharmacological or therapeutic reasons or does not require dilution. This is given as a controlled 'push' injection over a few minutes
- a peak blood level is required and cannot be achieved by small-volume infusion (Turner and Hankins 2010).

Rapid administration could result in toxic levels and an anaphylactic-type reaction. Manufacturer's recommendations of rates of administration (i.e. millilitres or milligrams per minute) should be adhered to. In the absence of such recommendations, administration should proceed slowly, over 5–10 minutes (Dougherty 2002).

Delivery of the drug by direct injection may be via the cannula through a resealable needle-less injection cap, extension set or via the injection site of an administration set.

- If a peripheral device is *in situ*, the bandage and dressing must be removed to inspect the insertion of the cannula, unless a transparent dressing is in place (Finlay 2008).
- Patency of the vein must be confirmed prior to administration and the vein's ability to accept an extra flow of fluid or irritant chemical must also be checked (Dougherty 2008).

Administration into the injection site of a fast-running drip may be advised if the infusion in progress is compatible in order to dilute the drug further and reduce local chemical irritation (Dougherty 2002). Alternatively, a stop–start procedure may be employed if there is doubt about venous patency. This allows the nurse to constantly check the patency of the vein and detect early signs of extravasation. If the infusion fluid is incompatible with the drug, the administration set may be switched off and a compatible solution may be used as a flush (NPSA 2007d).

If a number of drugs are being administered, 0.9% sodium chloride must be used to flush in between each drug to prevent interactions. In addition, 0.9% sodium chloride should be used at the end of the administration to ensure that all the drug has been delivered. The device should then be flushed to ensure patency is maintained (see Chapter 18) (Dougherty 2008).

The following principles are to be applied throughout preparation and administration.

Asepsis and reducing the risk of infection

Microbes on the hands of healthcare personnel contribute to healthcare-associated infection (Weinstein and Plumer 2007).

Therefore aseptic technique must be adhered to throughout all intravenous procedures (see Chapter 18). The nurse must employ good handwashing and drying techniques using a bactericidal soap or a bactericidal alcohol handrub. If asepsis is not maintained, local infection, septic phlebitis or septicaemia may result (Hart 2008, Pratt *et al.* 2007, RCN 2010).

The insertion site should be inspected at least once a day for complications such as infiltration, phlebitis or any indication of infection, for example redness at the insertion site of the device or pyrexia (RCN 2010). These problems may necessitate the removal of the device and/or further investigation (Finlay 2008).

It is desirable that a closed system of infusion is maintained wherever possible, with as few connections as is necessary for its purpose (Finlay 2008, Hart 2008). This reduces the risk of bacterial contamination. Any extra connections within the administration system increase the risk of infection. Three-way taps have been shown to encourage the growth of micro-organisms. They are difficult to clean due to their design, as micro-organisms can become lodged and are then able to multiply in the warm, moist environment (Finlay 2008, Hart 2008). This reservoir for micro-organisms may then be released into the circulation.

The injection sites on administration sets or injection caps should be cleaned using a 2% chlorhexidine alcohol-based antiseptic, allowing time for it to dry (Pratt *et al.* 2007). Connections should be cleaned before changing administration sets and manipulations kept to a minimum. Administration sets should be changed according to use (intermittent/continuous therapy), type of device and type of solution, and the set must be labelled with the date and time of change (NPSA 2007d, RCN 2010).

To ensure safe delivery of intravenous fluids and medication:

- replace all tubing when the vascular device is replaced (Pratt *et al.* 2007)
- replace solution administration sets and stopcocks used for continuous infusions every 72 hours unless clinically indicated, for example, if drug stability data indicate otherwise (Pratt *et al.* 2007, RCN 2010). Research has indicated that routine changing of administration sets (used for infusing solutions) every 48–72 hours instead of every 24 hours is not associated with an increase in infection and could result in considerable savings for hospitals (Pratt *et al.* 2007, RCN 2010)
- replace solution administration sets used for lipid emulsions and parenteral nutrition at the end of the infusion or within 24 hours of initiating the infusion (Pratt *et al.* 2007, RCN 2010). Certain intravenous fluids including lipid emulsions, blood and blood products are more likely than other parenteral fluids to support microbial growth if contaminated and therefore replacement of the intravenous tubing is required more frequently than 48–72 hours (Pratt *et al.* 2007)

- replace blood administration sets at least every 12 hours and after every second unit of blood (McClelland 2007, Pratt *et al.* 2007, RCN 2010)
- all solution sets used for intermittent infusions, for example antibiotics, should be discarded immediately after use and not allowed to hang for reuse (RCN 2010)
- if administering more than one infusion via a multi lumen extension set or multipl ports, be aware of the risk of back tracking of medication and consider using sets with one way, non return or anti reflux valves (MHRA 2010a).

Inspection of fluids, drugs, equipment and their packaging must be undertaken to detect any points where contamination may have occurred during manufacture and/or transport. This intrinsic contamination may be detected as cloudiness, discoloration or the presence of particles (BNF 2011, RCN 2010, Weinstein and Plumer 2007). Infusion bags should not be left hanging for longer than 24 hours. In the case of blood and blood products, this is reduced to 5 hours (McClelland 2007, RCN 2010).

Safety

All details of the prescription and all calculations must be checked carefully in accordance with hospital policy in order to ensure safe preparation and administration of the drug(s).

The nurse must also check the compatibility of the drug with the diluent or infusion fluid. The nurse should be aware of the types of incompatibilities and the factors which could influence them. These include pH, concentration, time, temperature, light and the brand of the drug. If insufficient information is available, a reference book (e.g. *British National Formulary*) or the product data sheet must be consulted (NPSA 2007d, Whittington 2008). If the nurse is unsure about any aspect of the preparation and/or administration of a drug, they should not proceed and should consult with a senior member of staff (NMC 2008a). Constant monitoring of both the mixture and the patient is important. The preferred method and rate of intravenous administration must be determined.

Drugs should never be added to the following: blood; blood products, that is plasma or platelet concentrate (see Chapter 8); mannitol solutions; sodium bicarbonate solution; and so on. Only specially prepared additives should be used with fat emulsions or amino acid preparations (Downie *et al.* 2003).

Accurate labelling of additives and records of administration are essential (NPSA 2007d, RCN 2010).

Any protective clothing which is advised should be worn, and vinyl gloves should be used to reduce the risk of latex allergy (Hart 2008). Healthcare professionals who use gloves frequently or for long periods face a high risk of allergy from latex products. All healthcare facilities should develop policies and procedures that determine measures to protect staff and patients from latex exposure and outline a treatment plan for latex reactions (Dougherty 2002).

Preventing needlestick injuries should be key in any health and safety programme and organizations should introduce safety devices and needle-free systems wherever possible (NHS Employers 2007). Basic rules of safety include not resheathing needles, disposal of needles immediately after use into a recognized sharps bin and convenient location of sharps bins in all areas where needles and sharps are used (Hart 2008, MHRA 2004, RCN 2010).

Comfort

Both the physical and psychological comfort of the patient must be considered. Comprehensive explanation of the practical aspects of the procedure together with information about the effects of treatment will contribute to reducing anxiety and will need to be tailored to each patient's individual needs.

Legal and professional issues

At least one patient will experience a potentially serious intravenous (IV) drug error every day in an 'average' hospital. IV drug errors have been estimated to be a third of all drug errors. 'Fifteen million infusions are performed in the NHS every year and 700 unsafe incidents are reported each year with 19% attributed to user error' (NPSA 2004, p.1). Between 1990 and 2000, there were 1485 incidents reported to the Medical Devices Agency which involved infusion pumps (MHRA 2010b). In 50% of incidents no cause was established. However, of the remaining incidents, 27% were attributed to user error (e.g. misloading of the administration set or syringe, setting the wrong rate, confusing pump type) and 20% to device-related issues (e.g. poor maintenance, cleaning) (MHRA 2010b, Williams and Lefever 2000). Syringe pumps have given rise to the most significant problems in terms of patient mortality and morbidity (Fox 2000, MHRA 2010b, NPSA 2003).

The high frequency of human error has highlighted the need for more formalized, validated, competency-based training and assessment (MHRA 2010b, NPSA 2003, 2004, Pickstone 2000, Quinn 2000). Nurses must be familiar with the device they are using and not attempt to operate any device that they have not been fully trained to use (Murray and Glenister 2001, NPSA 2003). As a minimum, the training should cover the device, drugs and solutions, and the practical procedures related to setting up the device and problem solving (Medical Devices Agency 2000, MHRA 2010b). Staff should also be made aware of the mechanisms for reporting faults with devices and procedures for adverse incident reporting within their trust and to the MHRA and the NPSA (MHRA 2006b).

A useful checklist (Box 16.14) has been produced by the Medical Devices Agency for staff to follow prior to using a medical device to ensure safe practice (Medical Devices Agency 2000, MHRA 2010b).

Box 16.14 Checklist: how safe is your practice?

- Have I been trained in the use of the infusion device?
- Was the training formalized and recorded or did I just pick it up as I went along?
- How was my competency in relation to the infusion device assessed?
- Have I read the user instructions on how to use the infusion device and am I familiar with any warning labels?
- When was the infusion device last serviced?
- Are there any signs of wear, damage or faults?
- Do I know how to set up and use the infusion device?
- Is the infusion device and any additional equipment in good working order?
- Do I know how the infusion device should perform and the monitoring that needs to be done to check its performance?
- Am I using the correct additional equipment, for example the appropriate disposable administration set for the infusion pump?
- Do I know how to recognize whether the infusion device has failed?
- Do I know what to do if the infusion device fails?
- Do I know how and to whom to report an infusion device-related adverse incident?
- Does checking the infusion device indicate it is functioning correctly and to the manufacturer's specification?
- What action should be taken if the infusion device is not functioning properly?
- Is there up-to-date documentation to record regular checking of the infusion device?
- What are the details (name and serial number) of the infusion device being used?
- What is the cleaning and/or decontamination procedure for the infusion device and what are my responsibilities in this process?
- Do I know how to report an adverse incident?
- Do I have access to MHRA device bulletins of relevance to my area of practice and do I read and take note of hazard and safety notices?

(Adapted from Medical Devices Agency 2000, p.10; 2001, pp.8, 9)

The nurse must have knowledge of the solutions, their effects, rate of administration, factors that affect flow of infusion, as well as the complications which could occur when flow is not controlled (Weinstein and Plumer 2007). The nurse should have an understanding of which groups require accurate flow control in order to prevent complications (Box 16.15) and how to select the most appropriate device for accuracy of delivery to best meet the patient's flow control needs (according to age, condition, setting and prescribed therapy) (Weinstein and Plumer 2007).

The identification of risks is crucial, for example complex calculations, prescription errors (Dougherty 2002, Weinstein and Plumer 2007) and the risks associated with infusions, such as neonatal risk infusions, high-risk infusions, low-risk infusions and ambulatory infusions (MHRA 2010b,

---

Box 16.15 Groups at risk of complications associated with flow control

- Infants and young children.
- The elderly.
- Patients with compromised cardiovascular status.
- Patients with impairment or failure of organs, for example kidneys.
- Patients with major sepsis.
- Patients suffering from shock, whatever the cause.
- Postoperative or post-trauma patients.
- Stressed patients, whose endocrine homoeostatic controls may be affected.
- Patients receiving multiple medications, whose clinical status may change rapidly.

(Adapted from Quinn 2008)

Box 16.17 Criteria for selection of an infusion device

- Rationalization of devices.
- Clinical requirement.
- Education.
- Compatibility with other equipment.
- Disposables.
- Product support.
- Costs.
- Service and maintenance.
- Regulatory issues, for example compliance with European Community Directives.

(Department of Health, Social Services and Public Safety 2006, Health Care Standards Unit, 2007a, 2007b, MHRA 2010b, NHS Litigation Authority 2007, Quinn 2000)

Quinn 2000). The early detection of errors and infusion-related complications, for example over- and underinfusion (Box 16.16), is imperative in order to instigate the appropriate interventions in response to an error or to manage any complications, as serious errors or complications can result in patient death (Dougherty 2002, NPSA 2003, Quinn 2008). Overinfusion accounts for about half of the reported errors involving infusion pumps, with 80% due to user error rather than a fault with the device (Medical Devices Agency 2000). The use of infusion devices, both mechanical and electronic, has increased the level of safety in intravenous therapy. However, it is recommended that a clearly defined structure for management of infusion systems must exist within a hospital (Department of Health, Social Services and Public Safety 2006, MHRA 2010b, NHS Litigation Authority 2007, NPSA 2004) (Box 16.17).

Strategies need to be developed for replacement of old, obsolete or inappropriate devices (Department of Health, Social Services and Public Safety 2006, Health Care Standards Unit 2007a, 2007b, MHRA 2010b, NHS Litigation Authority 2007, Quinn 2000), planned service maintenance programmes and acceptance testing (MHRA 2010b).

Healthcare professionals are personally accountable for their use of infusion devices and they must therefore ensure they have appropriate training before using the pump (MHRA 2008a, Quinn 2008). Records of training should also be maintained.

Improving infusion device safety

A high frequency of human error is reported in the use of infusion device systems, so competence-based training is advocated for users of these systems (MHRA 2010b, NPSA 2004). By rationalizing the range of infusion device types within organizations and the establishment of a centralized equipment library, the number of patient safety incidents will be reduced (MHRA 2010b, NPSA 2004). Smart infusion pumps reduce pump programming errors by the setting of pre-programmed upper and lower dose limits for specific drugs. The pump will alert the nurse when setting the infusion device if the pump has been set outside the preset dose limits (Keohane *et al.* 2005, Weinstein and Plumer 2007, Wilson and Sullivan 2004). Whatever infusion device is used, the need to monitor the patient and the device remains paramount for patient safety (Quinn 2008, RCN 2010).

Box 16.16 Complications of inadequate flow control

Complications associated with overinfusion
- Fluid overload with accompanying electrolyte imbalance.
- Metabolic disturbances during parenteral nutrition, mainly related to serum glucose levels.
- Toxic concentrations of medications, which may result in a shock-like syndrome ('speed shock').
- Air embolism, due to containers running dry before expected.
- An increase in venous complications, for example chemical phlebitis, caused by reduced dilution of irritant substances (Weinstein and Plumer 2007).

Complications associated with underinfusion
- Dehydration.
- Metabolic disturbances.
- A delayed response to medications or below therapeutic dose.
- Occlusion of a cannula/catheter due to slow flow or cessation of flow.

(Quinn 2008, p.195)

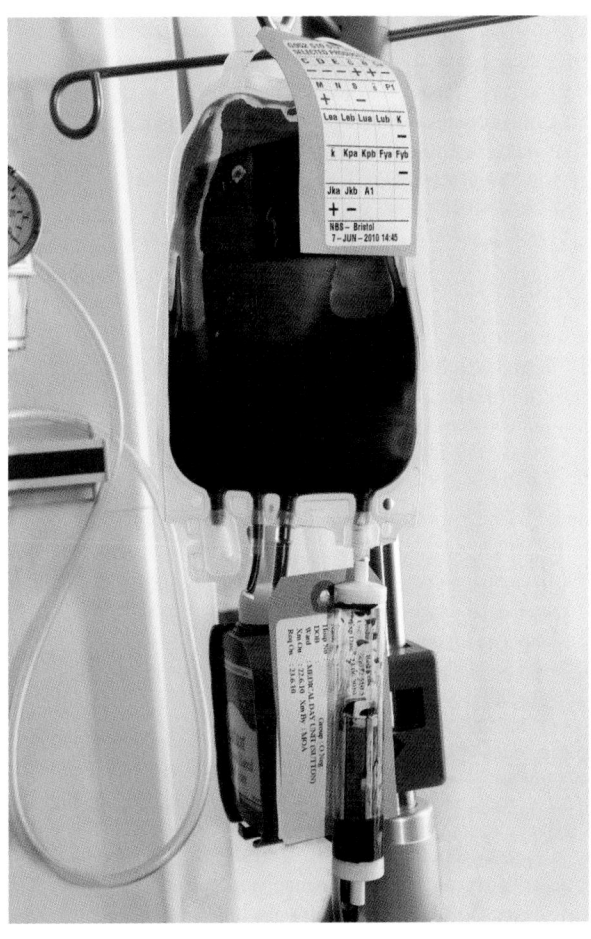

Figure 16.25 Blood administration set.

Figure 16.26 Fluid administration set.

set but should be repositioned along the set at intervals as the tubing can develop a 'memory' and not regain its shape, making it difficult to regulate (Hadaway 2010). It is opened to allow the fluid along the tubing to remove the air and then closed until attached to the patient's VAD. Finally the Luer-Lok end is covered with a plastic cap to maintain sterility until ready to be attached (Downie *et al.* 2003).

There is a variety of sets. A solution set is used to administer crystalloid solutions (it can be used as a primary or secondary set and is also available as a Y-set to allow for dual administration of compatible solutions). Parenteral nutrition is also administered via solution sets. Solution sets may have needle-free injection ports which allow for the administration of bolus injections or connection of secondary infusions. Sets may also have back check valves which

Preprocedural considerations

Equipment

Vascular access devices

For vascular access devices see Chapter 18.

Administration sets

An administration set is used to administer fluids, blood or medications via an infusion bag into a VAD. The set comprises a number of components (see Figures 16.25, 16.26, 16.27). At the top is a spike which is inserted into the infusion container via an entry port. This is covered by a sterile plastic lid which is removed just prior to insertion into the container (Downie *et al.* 2003). The plastic tubing continues from the spike to a drip chamber which may contain a filter. This is filled by squeezing it when attached to the fluid and waiting for the chamber to fill halfway, thus allowing the practitioner to observe the drops. Along the tubing is a roller clamp which allows the tubing to be incrementally occluded by pinching the tubing as the clamp is tightened; this is used to adjust the rate of flow (Hadaway 2010). It is usually positioned on the upper third of the administration

Figure 16.27 Labelled administration set.

Figure 16.28 Extension set with needle-free injection cap.

allow solutions to flow in one direction only and are used especially when a secondary set is used (Hadaway 2010).

Blood and blood products are administered via a blood administration set (Figure 16.25) which has a special filter. Platelets can be administered via blood sets (check with manufacturer) or specialist platelet administration sets. Some medications such as taxanes must be administered via special taxane administration sets as they have a filter.

Extension sets

Extension sets are used to add length (Hadaway 2010). The short extension sets tend to have a needle-free connector (Figure 16.28) and are attached directly to the VAD to provide a closed system and other equipment is then attached via the needle-free connector. The long (50–200 cm) extension sets are used to connect from syringe pumps or drivers to a VAD and usually have a back check or antisyphon valve. They can be single, double or triple and may contain a slide or pinch clamp but do not regulate flow (Hadaway 2010).

Needle-free injection caps

These are caps that are attached to the end of a VAD or extension set (Figure 16.28) to provide a closed system and remove the need for needles when administering medications, thus removing the risk of needlestick injury. There are various types available and differences include the type of septum (split septum or mechanical valve) (Hadaway 2010). Some provide positive or neutral displacement (to reduce risk of blood reflux and occlusion) and others are coated with antimicrobial or antibactericidal solutions on external or internal parts to reduce the risk of infection (Hadaway 2010). These require regular changing in accordance with the manufacturer's instructions as well as cleaning before and after each use (MHRA 2007, 2008).

It has been suggested that needle-free systems can increase the risk of bloodstream infections (Danzig et al. 1995). However, most studies have found no difference in microbial contamination when comparing conventional and needle-free systems (Brown et al. 1997, Luebke et al. 1998, Mendelson et al. 1998). It appears that an increased risk is only likely where there is lack of compliance with cleaning protocols or changing of equipment (Pratt et al. 2007).

Other equipment

Other IV equipment includes stopcocks (used to direct flow) usually three- or four-way devices. These tend to be used in critical care but are discouraged in the general setting due to misuse and contamination issues. If used, they should be capped off (Hadaway 2010).

Infusion devices

An infusion device is designed to accurately deliver measured amounts of fluid or drug via a number of routes (intravenous, subcutaneous or epidural) over a period of time. The infusion device is set at an appropriate rate to achieve the desired therapeutic response and prevent complications (Dougherty 2002, MHRA 2010b, Quinn 2000).

Gravity infusion devices

Gravity infusion devices depend entirely on gravity to deliver the infusion. The system consists of an administration set containing a drip chamber and a roller clamp to control the flow, which is usually measured by counting drops (Pickstone 1999). The indications for use are:

- delivery of fluids without additives
- administration of drugs or fluids where adverse effects are not anticipated and which do not need to be infused with absolute precision
- where the patient's condition does not give cause for concern and no complication is predicted (Quinn 2008).

The flow rate is calculated using a formula that requires the following information: the volume to be infused; the number of hours the infusion is running over; and the drop rate of the administration set (which will differ depending on type of set). The number of drops per millilitre is dependent on the type of administration set used and the viscosity of the infusion fluid. Increased viscosity causes the size of the drop to increase. For example, crystalloid fluid administered via a solution set is delivered at the rate of 20 drops/mL; the rate of packed red cells given via a blood set will be calculated at 15 drops/mL (Quinn 2008).

The rate of administration of a continuous or intermittent infusion may be calculated from the following equation (Pickstone 1999):

$$\frac{\text{Volume to be infused}}{\text{Time in hours}} \times \frac{\text{Drop rate}}{60 \text{ minutes}} = \text{Drops per minute}$$

In this equation, 60 is a factor for the conversion of the number of hours to the number of minutes.

Factors influencing flow rates are as follows.

Type of fluid

The composition, viscosity and concentration of the fluid affect flow (Pickstone 1999, Quinn 2000, Springhouse 2005, Weinstein and Plumer 2007). Irritating solutions may result in venospasm and impede the flow rate, which may be resolved by the use of a warm pack over the cannula site and the limb (Springhouse 2005, Weinstein and Plumer 2007).

Height of the infusion container

Intravenous fluids run by gravity and so any changes in the height of the container will alter the flow rate. The container can be hung up to 1.5 m above the infusion site which will provide a hydrostatic pressure of 110 mmHg (MHRA 2010b, Springhouse 2005). One metre above the infusion site would create 70 mmHg of pressure, which is adequate to overcome venous pressure (normal range in an adult is 25–80 mmHg) (Pickstone 1999). If it is hung too high then it can create too greater pressure within the vein, leading to infiltration of the medication (MHRA 2006a). Therefore any alterations in the patient's position may alter the flow rate and necessitate a change in the speed of the infusion to maintain the appropriate rate of flow (Hadaway 2010, Weinstein and Plumer 2007). Positioning of the patient will affect flow and patients should be instructed to keep the arm lower than the infusion, if the infusion is reliant on gravity (Quinn 2008).

Administration set

The flow rate of the infusion may be affected in several ways.

- Roller clamps (Figure 16.29) or screw clamps, used to adjust and maintain rates of flow on gravity infusions, vary considerably in their efficiency and accuracy which are often dependent on a number of variables such as patient movement and height of infusion container (Hadaway 2010). The roller clamp should be used as the primary means of occluding the tubing even if there is an anti-free flow device (MHRA 2010b).

Figure 16.29 Roller clamp.

- The inner diameter of the lumen and the length of tubing will also affect flow. Microbore sets have a narrow lumen, so flow is restricted to some degree. However, these sets may be used as a safeguard against 'runaway' or bolus infusions by either an integrated antisyphon valve or anti-free flow device (Hadaway 2010, Quinn 2000, Weinstein and Plumer 2007).
- Inclusion of other in-line devices, for example filters, may also affect the flow rate (Hadaway 2010, MHRA 2010b).

Vascular access device

The flow rate may be affected by any of the following.

- The condition and size of the vein; for example, phlebitis can reduce the lumen size and decrease flow (Quinn 2008, Weinstein and Plumer 2007).
- The gauge of the cannula/catheter (MHRA 2010b, Springhouse 2005, Weinstein and Plumer 2007).
- The position of the device within the vein; that is, whether it is up against the vein wall (Quinn 2008).
- The site of the vascular access device, for example, the flow may be affected by the change in position of a limb, such as a decrease in flow when a patient bends their arm if a cannula is sited over the elbow joint (Springhouse 2005).
- Kinking, pinching or compression of the cannula/catheter or tubing of the administration set may cause variation in the set rate (MHRA 2010b, Springhouse 2005).
- Restricted venous circulation; for example, a blood pressure cuff or the patient lying on the limb increases the risk of occlusion of the device and may result in clot formation (Quinn 2008).

The patient

Patients occasionally adjust the control clamp or other parts of the delivery system, for example, change the height of the container, thereby making flow unreliable. Some pumps have tamper-proof features to minimize the risk of accidental manipulation of the infusion device (Hadaway 2010) or unauthorized changing of infusion device controls (Amoore and Adamson 2003).

Advantages and disadvantages of gravity infusion devices

A gravity flow system is simple to set up. It is low cost and the infusion of air is less likely than with electronic devices (Pickstone 1999). However, the system does require frequent observation and adjustment due to:

- the tubing changing shape over time
- creep or distortion of tubing made of polyvinyl chloride (PVC)
- fluctuations of venous pressure which can affect the flow of the solution
- the roller clamp can be unreliable, leading to inconsistent flow rates.

There can also be variability of drop size and if the roller clamp is inadvertently left open, free flow will occur. Infusion rates with viscous fluids can be reduced (particularly if administered via small cannulas) and there is a limitation on the type of infusion as it is not suitable for arterial infusions: this is because viscosity and arterial flow offer a high resistance to flow which cannot be overcome by gravity (Pickstone 1999, Quinn 2008). If more than one infusion is infusing and one is slower than the other or there is no flow in the second set then there is a risk of back tracking which leads to underinfusion or bolus delivery of medicines. The MHRA recommends that in these systems, the sets should include antireflux valves (MHRA 2007).

Gravity drip rate controllers

A controller is a mechanical device that operates by gravity. These devices use standard solution sets and although they look much like a pump, they have no pumping mechanism. The desired flow rate is set in drops per minute and controlled by battery- or mains-powered occlusion valves (MHRA 2010b).

Advantages and disadvantages of gravity drip rate controllers

Although they can maintain a drip rate within 1%, volumetric accuracy is not guaranteed and many of the disadvantages associated with gravity flow still remain. The main advantages are that they are relatively inexpensive and can usually use standard gravity sets. They also incorporate some audible and visual alarm systems (MHRA 2010b).

Infusion pumps

These devices use pressure to overcome resistance from many causes along the fluid pathway, for example length and bore of tubing or particulate matter in the tubing (Hadaway 2010). There are a number of general features required in infusion pumps.

Accuracy of delivery

In order to meet requirements for high-risk and neonatal infusions, pumps must be accurate to within ±5% of the set rate when measured over a 60-minute period although some may be as accurate as ±2% (Hadaway 2010, MHRA 2010b). They also have to satisfy short-term, minute-to-minute accuracy requirements, which demand smoothness and consistency of output (MHRA 2010b).

Occlusion response and pressure

Flow will occur if the pressure at the tip of an intravascular device is just fractionally above the pressure in the vein; the pressure does not need to be excessive. In an adult peripheral vein, pressure is approximately 25 mmHg, while in a neonate it measures 5 mmHg (Quinn 2000). Most pumps have a variable pressure set-ting which allows the user to use their own judgement about the pressure needed to deliver therapy safely. The normal pumping pressure is only slightly lower than the occlusion pressure (Hadaway 2010). Flow is dependent upon pressure divided by resistance. If long extension sets of small internal bore are used, the resistance to flow will increase (Pickstone 1999, Quinn 2000).

If an administration set occludes, the resistance increases and the infusion will not flow into the vein. The longer the occlusion occurs, the greater the pressure and the pump will continue to pump until an occlusion alarm is activated. There are two types of occlusions: upstream, between the pump and the container, and downstream, which is between the pump and the patient. An upstream occlusion alarms when a vacuum is created in the upstream tubing or full reservoir, due to a collapsed or empty plastic fluid container or clamped/kinking tubing. A downstream occlusion is when the pressure required by the pump exceeds a certain pounds per square inch (psi) limit to overcome the pressure created by the occlusion. Downstream occlusion pressures range from 1.5 to 15 psi (Hadaway 2010).

Pumps alarm at 'occlusion alarm pressure' and many pumps allow the user to set the pressure within a range (MHRA 2010b). Therefore, the time it takes to alarm depends on the rate of flow: high rates alarm more quickly. When the alarm is activated, a certain amount of stored medication will be present and it is important that what could be a potentially large bolus is not released into the vein. The release of the stored bolus could lead to rupture of the vein or constitute overinfusion, which may be detrimental to the patient, particularly if it is a critical medication (Amoore and Adamson 2003, MHRA 2010b). With a syringe pump, to prevent a bolus being delivered to the patient, the clamp should not be opened as this will release the bolus: the first action is to remove the pressure by opening the syringe plunger clamp and then deal with the occlusion.

While pressure occlusion may not prevent extravasation, it may minimize the risk of resulting complications (Quinn and Upton 2006). Single-unit variable pressure pump settings which allow an earlier alarm alert are used in neonatal and paediatric units (Quinn 2008).

Air in line

Air-in-line detectors are designed to detect only visible or microscopic 'champagne' bubbles. They should not create anxiety over small particles of air but alert the nurse to the integrity of the system. Most air bubbles detected are too small to have a harmful effect but the nurse should clarify the cause of any alarms (MHRA 2010b).

Antisyphonage

Uncontrolled flow from a syringe is called siphonage; this is a result of gravity or leakage of air into the syringe and administration set. Siphonage can occur whether or not the syringe is fixed into an infusion device (Quinn 2008). It has been reported that 'in practice, a 50 mL syringe attached to a length of administration set with an internal diameter of 3 mm has been shown to empty by siphonage in less than 1 minute' (Pickstone 1999, p.57).

To minimize the risk of siphonage, the following safe practice should be undertaken.

- The syringe (plunger and barrel) should be correctly located and secured.
- Intravenous administration extension sets should always be micro/narrow bore in diameter to increase the resistance to flow; wide-bore extension sets should be avoided.
- Position of the syringe pump should always be the same level as the infusion site (MHRA 2010b).
- Extension sets with an integral antisiphonage/antireflux valve should be used (MHRA 2010b, MHRA 2007, Quinn 2008).

Safety software

Smart pumps contain safety software also known as dose error reduction systems (Hertzel and Sousa 2009). There is an internal drug library, meaning that pumps are programmed to contain information on medications with upper and lower dosing limits (Hadaway 2010). A number of studies have evaluated the effectiveness of using smart pumps to prevent medication errors, showing the success of these systems (Dennison 2007, Fields and Peterson 2005, Larson et al. 2005, Rothschild et al. 2005).

Volumetric pumps

Volumetric pumps (Figure 16.30) pump fluid from an infusion bag or bottle via an administration set and work by calculating the volume delivered (Quinn 2008). This is achieved when the pump measures the volume displaced in a 'reservoir'. The reservoir is an integral component of the administration set (Hadaway 2010). The mechanism of action may be piston or peristaltic (Hadaway 2010). The indications for use are all large-volume infusions, both venous and arterial.

All are mains and battery powered, with the rate selected in millilitres per hour. The accuracy of flow is usually within 5% when measured over a period of time, which is more than adequate for most clinical applications (MHRA 2010b, Pickstone 1999).

Advantages and disadvantages of volumetric pumps

These pumps are able to overcome resistance to flow by increased delivery pressure and do not rely on gravity. This generally makes the performance of pumps predictable and capable of accurate delivery over a wider range of flow rates (MHRA 2010b).

The pumps also incorporate a wide range of features, including air-in-line detectors, variable pressure settings and comprehensive alarms such as end of infusion, keep vein open (KVO, where the pump switches to

Figure 16.30 Volumetric pump.

a low flow rate, for example 5 mL/h, in order to continue flow to prevent occlusion of the device) and low battery. Many have a secondary infusion facility, which allows for intermittent therapy, for example antibiotics. The pump is programmed to switch to a secondary set and, when completed, it reverts back to the primary infusion at the previously set rate. The changing hospital environment has led to an increased demand on volumetric pumps, which in turn has resulted in the development of multichannel and dual-channel infusion pumps. These may consist of two devices with an attached housing or of several infusion channels within a single device (Hadaway 2010).

The disadvantages are that these are usually relatively expensive and often dedicated administration sets are required. The use of the wrong set could result in error even if the pump appears to work. Some are complicated to set up, which can also lead to errors (MHRA 2010b).

Syringe pumps

Syringe pumps (Figure 6.31) are low-volume, high-accuracy devices designed to infuse at low flow rates. The plunger of a syringe containing the substance to be infused is driven forward by the syringe pump at a controlled rate to deliver it to the patient (MHRA 2010b).

Figure 16.31   The Alaris GH syringe pump.

Syringe pumps are useful where small volumes of highly concentrated drugs need to be infused at low flow rates (Quinn 2008). The volume for infusion is limited to the size of the syringe used in the device, which is usually a 60 mL syringe, but most pumps will accept different sizes and brands of syringe.

These devices are calibrated for delivery in millilitres per hour (Weinstein and Plumer 2007).

Advantages and disadvantages of syringe pumps

Syringe pumps are mains and/or battery powered, are usually easy to operate, and tend to cost less than volumetric pumps. The alarm systems are becoming more comprehensive and include low battery, end of infusion and syringe clamp open alarms. Most of the problems associated with the older models, for example free flow, mechanical backlash (slackness which delays the start-up time of the infusion) and incorrect fitting of the syringe, have been eliminated in the newer models (MHRA 2010b, Quinn 2008). The risk of free flow is minimized by the use of an antisiphonage valve which may be integral to the administration set (Pickstone 1999). Despite the use of an antisiphonage valve, the clamp of the administration set must still be used (MHRA 2010b). Where mechanical backlash is an issue and there is a prime or purge option, this should be used at the start of the infusion to take up the mechanical slack (Amoore *et al.* 2001).

Specialist pumps

Patient-controlled analgesia pumps

Patient-controlled analgesia (PCA) devices are typically syringe pumps (although some are based on volumetric designs) (MHRA 2010b) (Figure 16.32). The syringe pump forces down on the syringe piston, collapsing the syringe at a preset rate, but the distinguishing feature is the ability of the pump to deliver doses on demand, which occurs when the patient pushes a button (Hadaway 2010). Whether or not the dose is delivered is determined by preset parameters

in the pump. That is, if the maximum amount of drug over a given period of time has already been delivered, a further dose cannot be delivered.

Patient-controlled analgesia pumps are useful for patients who require pain control. They are used more in the acute setting, but are also useful in ambulatory situations.

Infusion options of a PCA pump are usually categorized into three types.

- *Basal*: a 'baseline' rate can be accompanied by intermittent doses requested by patients. This aims to achieve pain relief with minimal medication, but not necessarily to achieve a pain-free state (Hadaway 2010).
- *Continuous*: designed for the patient who needs maximum pain relief without the option of demand dosing, for example epidural.
- *Demand*: drug delivered by intermittent infusion when button is pushed and can be used alone or supplemented by the basal rate. Doses can be limited by a designated maximum amount (Hadaway 2010).

The PCA pump can dispense a bolus dose, with an initial bolus being called a loading dose. This may benefit patients as the one-time dose is significantly higher than a demand dose in order to achieve immediate pain relief (see Chapter 9).

Advantages and disadvantages of PCA pumps

These devices offer a 'lock-out' feature (when a key or a combination of numbers is necessary to gain access to pump controls), which is designed for patient safety. They have an extensive memory capability which can be accessed through the display via a printer or computer (MHRA 2010b). This facility is critical for the pump's effective use in pain management (Hadaway 2010), as it enables the clinician to determine when and how often demand is made by a patient and what total volume has been infused (Hadaway 2010). It has also been shown that they increase patient satisfaction, patients require less sedation, their

Figure 16.32   The Alaris PCA pump used generally in acute hospital settings. Reproduced by permission of Alaris.

anxiety is reduced and so are their nursing needs and time in hospital (Ripamonti and Bruera 1997).

Anaesthesia pumps

These are syringe pumps designed for delivery of anaesthesia or sedation and must only ever be used for that purpose. They should be restricted to operating theatres or critical care units and should be clearly labelled. They are designed to allow rapid changes in flow rate and bolus to be made while the pump is infusing (Quinn 2008). Total intravenous anaesthesia (TIVA) and target-controlled infusion (TCI) pumps are now available, which have been designed to control the induction, maintenance and reversal phases of anaesthesia (Absalom and Struys 2006).

Epidural pumps

Epidural pumps (Figure 16.33) provide analgesia (most commonly a combination of opioids and anaesthetic agents) via a fine catheter inserted directly into the epidural space. As a form of analgesia delivery, the efficacy of the epidural route has been well highlighted (Block *et al.* 2003, Werawatganon and Charuluxanun 2005, Wheatley *et al.* 2001). See also Chapter 9.

Ambulatory infusion devices

Ambulatory infusion devices were developed to allow patients more freedom and to enable the patient to con-

Figure 16.33 Epidural pump.

tinue with normal activities or to move unencumbered by a large infusion device (Hadaway 2010). Ambulatory devices range in size and weight and are used for small volumes of drugs and are mainly designed for patients to wear and use when ambulant. The solution containers are often more cumbersome than the actual pump itself. Due to their size, the number of alarms may be more limited. Considerations for selection of an ambulatory device include the following.

- Type of therapy.
- Patient's ability to understand how to manage the infusion device.
- Drug stability.
- Frequency of doses.
- Reservoir volumes required.
- Control of flow/flow rates.
- Type of access.
- Cost-effectiveness.
- Portability.
- Convenience.

Ambulatory pumps fall into two categories: mechanical and battery-operated infusion devices.

Mechanical infusion devices

These are simple and compact but may not necessarily be cost-effective as they are usually disposable. The mechanism for delivery is by balloon or simple spring, or they may be gas powered. They are usually very 'user friendly' as they require minimal input from the patient and no battery. They can also be purchased prefilled (Quinn 2008).

Elastomeric balloon devices These are made of a soft rubberized material capable of being inflated to a predetermined volume and the drug is then administered over a very specific infusion time. The balloon is encapsulated inside a rigid transparent container which may be round or cylindrical. The rate of infusion is not controlled by the balloon but by the diameter of the restricting outlet located in the preattached tubing (Quinn 2008). It is designed to supply the patient's need for a single dose infusion of drugs, for example intermittent small-volume parenteral therapies such as delivery of antibiotics. Its small size causes little disruption to the patient's daily activities and it tends to be well tolerated (Hadaway 2010). Figure 16.34 shows an elastomeric device.

Spring mechanism Spring coil piston syringes have a spring which powers the plunger of a syringe in the absence of manual pressure. The volume is restricted by the size of the syringe, which is usually prefilled. The spring coil container tends to be a multidose, small-volume administration device and is a combination of a spring coil in a collapsible flattened disc. Its shape can accommodate many therapies and volumes (Hadaway 2010).

Figure 16.34 Elastomeric device.

Battery-operated infusion devices
Battery-operated pumps are small and light enough to be carried around by the patient without interfering with most everyday activities. They are operated using rechargeable or alkaline batteries but, owing to their size, the available battery capacity tends to be low. The length of time the battery lasts is often dependent on the rate at which the pump is set. Most give an output in the form of a small bolus delivered every few minutes. Most devices have an integral case or pouch which allows the pump and the reservoir/syringe to be worn with discretion by the patient. There are two types: ambulatory volumetric infusion pumps and syringe drivers.

Ambulatory volumetric infusion/syringe pumps An ambulatory volumetric infusion/syringe pump is an infusion device which pumps in the same way as a large volumetric pump, but by nature of its size it is portable and useful in the ambulatory setting (hospital or home care).

This pump is suitable for patients who have been prescribed continuous infusional treatment for a period of time, for example from 4 days to 6 months, and enables the patients, where appropriate, to receive treatment at home, because it is small and portable.

The advantages of the ambulatory pump are as follows.

- Able to deliver drugs continuously or intermittently.
- Infusion routes: central, peripheral venous, epidural, intra-arterial, intrathecal and subcutaneous.
- Delivery of drugs accurately over a set period of time.
- Improving potential outcomes of treatment by delivering treatment continuously.
- Heightening the patient's independence and control by allowing them to be at home and participate in their own care.

- Compact, light and easy to use.
- Has audible alarm systems.

The disadvantages are as follows.

- It may require the insertion of a central venous access device, which has associated complications and problems.
- It could malfunction at home, which could be distressing and dangerous for the patient.
- In spite of its ease of use, some patients may not be able to cope with it at home.
- Patients may have to adapt their lifestyle to cope with living with a pump continuously.

Syringe drivers
See Subcutaneous infusion.

Specific patient preparations
Selecting the appropriate infusion device for the patient

The nurse has a responsibility to determine when and how to use an infusion device to deliver hydration, drugs, transfusions and nutritional support, and how to select the appropriate device in order to manage the needs of the patient. The following factors should be considered when selecting an appropriate infusion delivery system (Quinn 2008).

- Risk to the patient of:
  (a) overinfusion
  (b) underinfusion
  (c) uneven flow
  (d) inadvertent bolus
  (e) high-pressure delivery
  (f) extravascular infusion.
- Delivery parameters:
  (a) infusion rate and volume required
  (b) accuracy required (over a long or short period of time)
  (c) alarms required
  (d) ability to infuse into site chosen (venous, arterial, subcutaneous)
  (e) suitability of device for infusing drug (e.g. ability to infuse viscous drugs).
- Environmental features:
  (a) ease of operation
  (b) frequency of observation and adjustment
  (c) type of patient (neonate, child, critically ill)
  (d) mobility of patient.

Paediatric considerations

The MHRA classifies infusion devices into categories of infusion risk. Neonatal infusions are the highest risk category; high-risk infusions are typically the infusion of fluids in children where accuracy of the flow rate is essential (Medical

Table 16.10 Therapy categories and performance parameters

Therapy category	Therapy description	Patient group	Critical performance parameters
A	Drugs with narrow therapeutic margin	Any	Good long-term accuracy
			Good short-term accuracy
	Drugs with short half-life	Any	Rapid alarm after occlusion
			Small occlusion bolus
	Any infusion given to neonates	Neonates	Able to detect very small air embolus (volumetric pumps only)
			Small flow rate increments
			Good bolus accuracy
			Rapid start-up time (syringe pumps only)
B	Drugs other than those with a short half-life	Any except neonates	Good long-term accuracy
			Alarm after occlusion
	Total parenteral nutrition	Volume sensitive except neonates	Small occlusion bolus
	Fluid maintenance		Able to detect small air embolus (volumetric pumps only)
	Transfusions		
			Small flow rate increments
C	Diamorphine	Any except neonates	Bolus accuracy
	Total parenteral nutrition	Any except volume sensitive or neonates	Long-term accuracy
	Fluid maintenance		Alarm after occlusion
	Transfusions		Small occlusion bolus
			Able to detect air embolus (volumetric pumps only)
			Incremental flow rates

MHRA (2010b). © Crown copyright. Reproduced under the terms of the Click-Use Licence.

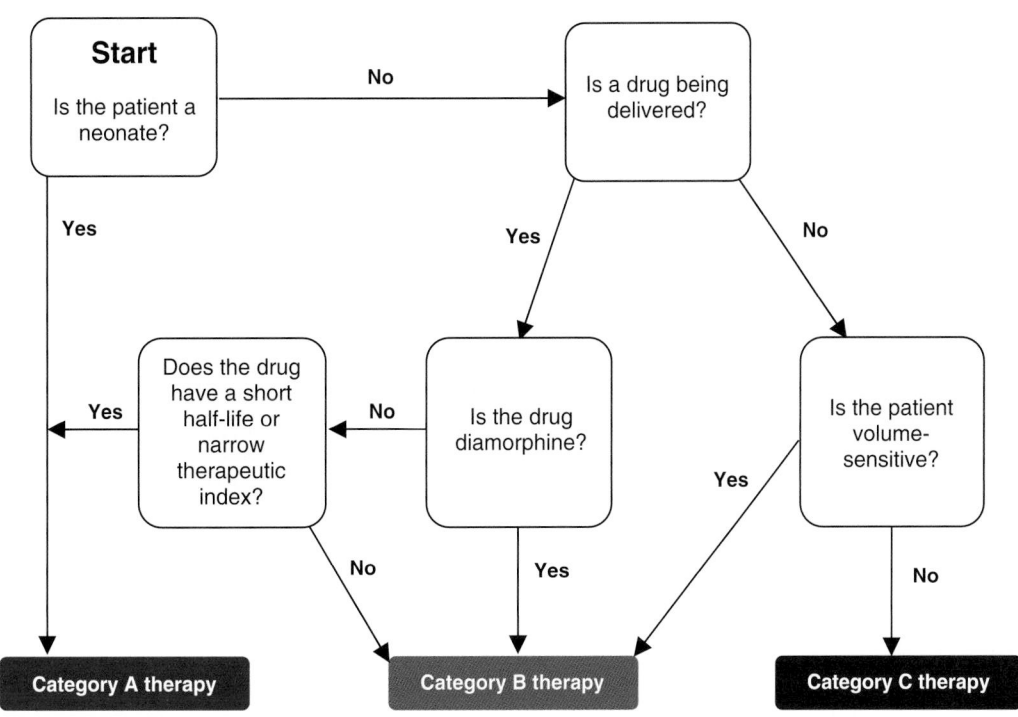

Figure 16.35 Decision tree for selection of infusion device. MHRA (2010b). © Crown copyright. Reproduced under the terms of the Click-Use Licence.

Devices Agency 2003). Infusion therapy within the paediatric setting requires very specific skills (Frey and Pettit 2010). Competency in calculation of paediatric dosages, maintaining a stringent fluid balance, use of paediatric-specific devices and management of complications are paramount.

The MHRA has made recommendations on the safety and performance of infusion devices in order to enable users to make the appropriate choice of equipment to suit most applications (MHRA 2010b). The classification system is divided into three major categories according to the potential risks involved. These are shown in Table 16.10.

A pump suited to the most risky category of therapy (A) can be safely used for the other categories (B and C). A pump suited to category B can be used for B and C, whereas a pump with the lowest specification (C) is suited only to category C therapies (MHRA 2010b) (Figure 16.35). Hospitals are required to label each infusion pump with its category and it is necessary to know the category of the proposed therapy and match it with a pump of the same or better category. A locally produced list of drugs/fluids by their categories will need to be provided to all device users (MHRA 2010b).

Procedure guideline 16.23 Medication: continuous infusion of intravenous drugs

This procedure may be carried out by the infusion of drugs from a bag, bottle or burette.

Essential equipment

- Clinically clean receiver or tray containing the prepared drug to be administered
- Patient's prescription chart
- Recording chart or book as required by law or hospital policy
- Gloves
- Protective clothing as required by hospital policy for specific drugs
- Container of appropriate intravenous infusion fluid
- 2% chlorhexidine swab
- Drug additive label

Preprocedure

Action	Rationale
1 Explain and discuss the procedure with the patient.	To ensure that the patient understands the procedure and gives their valid consent (Griffith and Jordan 2003, E; NMC 2008b, C; NMC 2008c, C).
2 Inspect the infusion in progress.	To check it is the correct infusion being administered at the correct rate and that the contents are due to be delivered on time in order for the next prepared infusion bag to be connected. To check whether the patient is experiencing any discomfort at the site of insertion, which might indicate the peripheral device needs to be resited (NPSA 2007d, C).
3 Before administering any prescribed drug, check that it is due and has not already been given.	To protect the patient from harm (NPSA 2007d, C).
4 Before administering any prescribed drug, consult the patient's prescription chart and ascertain the following: (a) Drug (b) Dose (c) Date and time of administration (d) Route and method of administration (e) Diluent as appropriate (f) Validity of prescription (g) Signature of doctor (h) The prescription is legible.	To ensure that the patient is given the correct drug in the prescribed dose using the appropriate diluent and by the correct route. To protect the patient from harm (NMC 2008a, C; NPSA 2007d, C). To comply with NMC (2008a) *Standards for Medicines Management*.
5 Wash hands with bactericidal soap and water or bactericidal alcohol handrub, and assemble the necessary equipment.	To minimize the risk of infection (DH 2007, C; Fraise and Bradley 2009, E).

6 Prepare the drug for injection as described in Procedure guideline 16.15.	To ensure the drug is prepared (NPSA 2007d, C).
7 Check the name, strength and volume of intravenous fluid against the prescription chart.	To ensure that the correct type and quantity of fluid are administered (NMC 2008a, C; NPSA 2007d, C).
8 Check the expiry date of the fluid.	To prevent an ineffective or toxic compound being administered to the patient (NPSA 2007d, C).
9 Check that the packaging is intact and inspect the container and contents in a good light for cracks, punctures, air bubbles.	To check that no contamination of the infusion container has occurred (NPSA 2007d, C).
10 Inspect the fluid for discoloration, haziness and crystalline or particulate matter.	To prevent any toxic or foreign matter being infused into the patient (NPSA 2007d, C).
11 Check the identity and amount of drug to be added. Consider: **(a)** Compatibility of fluid and additive **(b)** Stability of mixture over the prescription time **(c)** Any special directions for dilution, for example pH, optimum concentration **(d)** Sensitivity to external factors such as light **(e)** Any anticipated allergic reaction. If any doubts exist about the listed points, consult the pharmacist or appropriate reference works.	To minimize any risk of error. To ensure safe and effective administration of the drug. To enable anticipation of toxicities and the nursing implications of these (NPSA 2007d, C).
12 Any additions must be made immediately before use.	To prevent any possible microbial growth or degradation (NPSA 2007d, C).
13 Wash hands thoroughly using bactericidal soap and water or bactericidal alcohol handrub.	To minimize the risk of cross-infection (DH 2007, C; Fraise and Bradley 2009, E).
14 Place infusion bag on flat surface.	To prevent puncturing the side of the infusion bag when making additions (NPSA 2007d, C).
15 Remove any seal present.	To expose the injection site on the container. E
Procedure	
16 Clean the site with the swab and allow it to dry.	To reduce the risk of contamination (NPSA 2007d, C).
17 Inject the drug using a new sterile needle into the bag, bottle or burette. A 23 or 25 G needle should be used. If the addition is made into a burette at the bedside: **(a)** Avoid contamination of the needle and inlet port **(b)** Check that the correct quantity of fluid is in the chamber **(c)** Switch the infusion off briefly **(d)** Add the drug.	To minimize the risk of contamination. To enable resealing of the latex or rubber injection site (NPSA 2007d, C). To minimize the risk of contamination (NPSA 2007d, C). To ensure the correct dilution (NPSA 2007d, C). To ensure a bolus injection is not given (NPSA 2007d, C).
18 Invert the container a number of times, especially if adding to a flexible infusion bag.	To ensure adequate mixing of the drug (NPSA 2007d, C).
19 Check again for haziness, discoloration and particles. This can occur even if the mixture is theoretically compatible, thus making vigilance essential.	To detect any incompatibility or degradation (NPSA 2007d, C).
20 Complete the drug additive label and fix it on the bag, bottle or burette.	To identify which drug has been added, when and by whom (NPSA 2007d, C).

(Continued)

Procedure guideline 16.23 (*Continued*)

21 Place the container in a clean receptacle. Wash hands and proceed to the patient.	To minimize the risk of contamination (DH 2007, C).
22 Check the identity of the patient against the prescription chart and infusion bag.	To minimize the risk of error and ensure the correct infusion is administered to the correct patient (NPSA 2007d, C).
23 Check that the contents of the previous container have been fully delivered.	To ensure that the preceding prescription has been administered (NPSA 2007d, C).
24 Switch off the infusion. Apply gloves. Place the new infusion bag on a flat surface and then disconnect empty infusion bag.	To ensure that the administration set spike will not puncture the side wall of the infusion bag (Finlay 2008, E; NPSA 2007d, C).
25 Push the spike in fully without touching it and hang the new infusion bag on the infusion stand. Insert tubing into an infusion pump where appropriate.	To reduce the risk of contamination (DH 2007, C). To ensure accuracy of delivery (Quinn 2008, E).
26 For gravity infusion, restart the infusion and adjust the rate of flow as prescribed. If via an infusion pump, start the pump and set rate.	To ensure that the infusion will be delivered at the correct rate over the correct period of time (NPSA 2007d, C).
27 If the addition is made into a burette, the infusion can be restarted immediately following mixing and recording and the infusion rate adjusted accordingly.	To ensure that the infusion will be delivered correctly (NPSA 2007d, C).
28 Ask the patient whether any abnormal sensations, and so on, are experienced.	To ascertain whether there are any problems that may require nursing care and refer to medical staff where appropriate. E.

Postprocedure

29 Discard waste, making sure that it is placed in the correct containers, for example sharps into a designated receptacle.	To ensure safe disposal and avoid injury to staff. To prevent reuse of equipment (DH 2005, C; MHRA 2004, C).
30 Complete the patient's recording chart and other hospital and/or legally required documents.	To maintain accurate records. To provide a point of reference in the event of any queries. To prevent any duplication of treatment (NMC 2009, C).

Procedure guideline 16.24 Medication: intermittent infusion of intravenous drugs

Essential equipment

- Patient's prescription chart
- Recording chart or book as required by law or hospital policy
- Protective clothing as required by hospital policy for specific drugs
- Container of appropriate intravenous infusion fluid
- Drug additive label
- Intravenous administration set
- Intravenous infusion stand
- Clean dressing trolley
- Clinically clean receiver or tray containing the prepared drug to be administered
- Sterile needles and syringes
- 10 mL for injection of a compatible flush solution, for example 0.9% sodium chloride or 5% dextrose
- Flushing solution to maintain patency plus sterile injection cap
- 2% chlorhexidine swab
- Gloves
- Alcohol-based hand wash solution or rub
- Sterile dressing pack
- Hypoallergenic tape
- Sharps bin

Preprocedure

Action	Rationale
1 Explain and discuss the procedure with the patient.	To ensure that the patient understands the procedure and gives their valid consent (Griffith and Jordan 2003, E; NMC 2006c, C; NMC 2008b, C).
2 Before administering any prescribed drug, check that it is due and has not been given already. Check that the information contained in the prescription chart is complete, correct and legible.	To protect the patient from harm (NMC 2008a, C; NPSA 2007d, C).
3 Before administering any prescribed drug, consult the patient's prescription chart and ascertain the following: (a) Drug (b) Dose (c) Date and time of administration (d) Route and method of administration (e) Diluent as appropriate (f) Validity of prescription (g) Signature of prescriber.	To ensure that the patient is given the correct drug in the prescribed dose using the appropriate diluent and by the correct route (NMC 2008a, C; NPSA 2007d, C). To protect the patient from harm. To comply with NMC (2008a) *Standards for Medicines Management.*
4 Wash hands with bactericidal soap and water or bactericidal alcohol handrub.	To prevent contamination of medication and equipment (DH 2007, C).
5 Prepare the intravenous infusion and additive as described in Procedure guidelines 16.12, 16.13, 16.14 and 16.15.	To ensure the drug is prepared correctly (NPSA 2007d, C).
6 Prime the intravenous administration set with infusion fluid mixture and hang it on the infusion stand.	To ensure removal of air from set and check that tubing is patent. To prepare for administration (NPSA 2007d, C).
7 Draw up 10 mL of compatible flush solution for injection using an aseptic technique.	To ensure sufficient flushing solution is available. E
8 Draw up solution (as per hospital policy) to be used for maintaining patency, for example 0.9% sodium chloride.	To prepare for administration. E
9 Place the syringes in a clinically clean receiver or tray on the bottom shelf of the dressing trolley.	To ensure top shelf is used for sterile dressing pack in order to minimize the risk of contamination. E
10 Collect the other equipment and place it on the bottom shelf of the dressing trolley.	To ensure all equipment is available to commence procedure. E
11 Place a sterile dressing pack on top of the trolley.	To minimize risk of contamination. E
12 Check that all necessary equipment is present.	To prevent delays and interruption of the procedure. E
13 Wash hands thoroughly using bactericidal soap and water or bactericidal alcohol handrub before leaving the clinical room.	To minimize the risk of cross-infection (DH 2007, C; Fraise and Bradley 2009, E).
14 Proceed to the patient. Check patient's identity against prescription chart and prepared drugs.	To minimize the risk of error and ensure the correct drug is given to the correct patient (NMC 2008a, C; NPSA 2007d, C).

Procedure

15 Open the sterile dressing pack.	To minimize the risk of cross-infection (DH 2007, C; Fraise and Bradley 2009, E).
16 Open the 2% chlorhexidine swab packet and empty it onto the pack.	To ensure the correct cleaning swab is available (DH 2007, E).

(Continued)

Procedure guideline 16.24 *(Continued)*

17 Wash hands with bactericidal soap and water or with a bactericidal alcohol handrub.	To minimize the risk of cross-infection. (DH 2007, C; Fraise and Bradley 2009, E).
18 If peripheral device is *in situ* remove the patient's bandage and dressing.	To observe the insertion site (Dougherty 2008, E).
19 Inspect the insertion site of the device.	To detect any signs of inflammation, infiltration, and so on. If present, take appropriate action (DH 2003c, C).
20 Wash and dry hands.	To minimize the risk of contamination (DH 2007, C).
21 Put on gloves.	To protect against contamination with hazardous substances, for example cytotoxic drugs (NPSA 2007d, C).
22 Place a sterile towel under the patient's arm.	To create a sterile area on which to work. E
23 Clean the needle-free cap with 2% chlorhexidine swab.	To minimize the risk of contamination and maintain a closed system (Pratt *et al.* 2007, C).
24 Inject gently 10 mL of 0.9% sodium chloride for injection.	To confirm the patency of the device. E
25 Check that no resistance is met, no pain or discomfort is felt by the patient, no swelling is evident, no leakage occurs around the device and there is a good backflow of blood on aspiration.	To ensure the device is patent (Dougherty 2008, E).
26 Connect the infusion to the device.	To commence treatment. E
27 Open the roller clamp or insert the tubing into an infusion pump and start pump.	To check the infusion is flowing freely. E
28 Check the insertion site and ask the patient if they are comfortable.	To confirm that the vein can accommodate the extra fluid flow and that the patient experiences no pain. E
29 Adjust the flow rate as prescribed.	To ensure that the correct speed of administration is established (NPSA 2007d, C).
30 Tape the administration set in a way that places no strain on the device, which could in turn damage the vein.	To reduce the risk of mechanical phlebitis or infiltration (Dougherty 2008, E).
31 If a peripheral device is *in situ*, cover it with a sterile topical swab and tape it in place.	To maintain asepsis (Dougherty 2008, E).
32 Remove gloves.	To ensure disposal. E
33 If the infusion is to be completed within 30 minutes, bandaging is unnecessary and the patient may be instructed to keep the arm resting on the sterile towel. Otherwise reapply bandage.	To reduce the risk of dislodging the device. E
34 The equipment must be cleared away and new equipment only prepared when required at the end of the infusion.	To ensure that the equipment used is sterile prior to use. E
35 Monitor flow rate and device site frequently.	To ensure the flow rate is correct and the patient is comfortable, and to check for signs of infiltration (NPSA 2007d, C).
36 When the infusion is complete, wash hands using bactericidal soap and water or bactericidal alcohol handrub, and recheck that all the equipment required is present.	To maintain asepsis and ensure that the procedure runs smoothly (DH 2007 C; Finlay 2008, E).

37 Stop the infusion when all the fluid has been delivered.	To ensure that all the prescribed mixture has been delivered and prevent air infusing into the patient (NPSA 2007d, C).
38 Put on non-sterile gloves.	To protect against contamination with hazardous substances. E
39 Disconnect the infusion set and flush the device with 10 mL of 0.9% sodium chloride or other compatible solution for injection. (A 'minibag' may be used to flush the drug through the tubing but the cost implications of this as well as the risk to patients on restricted intake should be considered before this is adopted routinely.)	To flush any remaining irritating solution away from the cannula. E
40 Attach a new sterile injection cap if necessary.	To maintain a closed system (Hart 2008, E).
41 Flushing must follow.	To maintain the patency of the device (Dougherty 2008, E).
42 Clean the injection site of the cap with 2% chlorhexidine swab.	To minimize the risk of contamination (Hart 2008, E).
43 Administer flushing solution using the push- pause technique and ending with positive pressure.	To maintain the patency of the device and if needle was used, to enable reseal of the injection site (Dougherty 2008, E).
44 If a peripheral device is *in situ*, cover the insertion site and cannula with a new sterile low-linting swab. Tape it in place. Apply a bandage.	To minimize the risk of contamination of the insertion site. To reduce the risk of dislodging the cannula. E
45 Remove gloves.	To ensure disposal. E
46 Assist the patient into a comfortable position.	To ensure the patient is comfortable. E

Postprocedure

47 Record the administration on appropriate charts.	To maintain accurate records, provide a point of reference in the event of any queries and prevent any duplication of treatment (NMC 2009, C).
48 Discard waste, placing it in the correct containers, for example sharps into a designated container.	To ensure safe disposal and avoid injury to staff (DH 2005, C; MHRA 2004, C; NHS Employers 2007, C).

Procedure guideline 16.25 Medication: injection (bolus or push) of intravenous drugs

Essential equipment

- Clinically clean receiver or tray containing the prepared drug(s) to be administered
- Patient's prescription chart
- Protective clothing as required by hospital policy or specific drugs
- Clean dressing trolley
- Sterile needles and syringes
- 0.9% sodium chloride, 20 mL for injection, or compatible solution
- Flushing solution, in accordance with hospital policy
- 2% chlorhexidine swab
- Sterile dressing pack
- Hypoallergenic tape
- Sharps container

Preprocedure

Action
1 Explain and discuss the procedure with the patient.

Rationale
To ensure that the patient understands the procedure and gives their valid consent (Griffith and Jordan 2003, E; NMC 2006c, C; NMC 2008b, C).

Procedure guideline 16.25 *(Continued)*

2 Before administering any prescribed drug, check that it is due and has not been given already. Check that the information contained in the prescription chart is complete, correct and legible.	To protect the patient from harm (NMC 2008b, C).
3 Before administering any prescribed drug, consult the patient's prescription sheet and ascertain the following: **(a)** Drug **(b)** Dose **(c)** Date and time of administration **(d)** Route and method of administration **(e)** Diluent as appropriate **(f)** Validity of prescription **(g)** Signature of prescriber **(h)** The prescription is legible.	To ensure that the patient is given the correct drug in the prescribed dose using the appropriate diluent and by the correct route (NMC 2008a, C; NPSA 2007d, C). To protect the patient from harm. To comply with NMC (2008a) *Standards for Medicines Management.*

Procedure

4 Select the required medication and check the expiry date.	Treatment with medication that is outside the expiry date is dangerous. Drugs deteriorate with storage. The expiry date indicates when a particular drug is no longer pharmacologically efficacious (NPSA 2007d, C).
5 Wash hands with bactericidal soap and water or bactericidal alcohol handrub, and assemble necessary equipment.	To minimize the risk of infection (DH 2007, C; Fraise and Bradley 2009, E).
6 Prepare the drug for injection as Procedure guideline 16.15.	To prepare the drug correctly. E
7 Prepare a 20 mL syringe of 0.9% sodium chloride (or compatible solution) for injection, as described, using aseptic technique.	To use for flushing between each drug (NPSA 2007d, C).
8 Draw up the flushing solution, as indicated by local hospital policy.	To prepare for administration. E
9 Place syringes in a clinically clean receptacle on the bottom shelf of the dressing trolley, along with the receptacle containing any drug(s) to be administered.	To ensure top shelf is used for sterile dressing pack in order to minimize the risk of contamination. E
10 Collect the other equipment and place it on the bottom of the trolley.	To ensure all equipment is available to commence procedure. E
11 Place a sterile dressing pack on top of the trolley.	To minimize the risk of contamination. E
12 Check that all necessary equipment is present.	To prevent delays and interruption of the procedure. E
13 Wash hands thoroughly.	To minimize the risk of infection (DH 2007, C; Fraise and Bradley 2009, E).
14 Proceed to the patient and check identity with prescription chart and prepared drug.	To minimize the risk of error and ensure the correct patient (NPSA 2007d, C).
15 Open the sterile dressing pack and 2% chlorhexidine swab and empty onto pack.	To gain access to equipment and to ensure there is a cleaning swab available (DH 2007, C).
16 Wash hands with bactericidal soap and water or with bactericidal alcohol handrub.	To reduce the risk of infection (DH 2007, C; Fraise and Bradley 2009, E).

17	If a peripheral device is *in situ*, remove the bandage and dressing (if appropriate).	To observe the insertion site. E
18	Inspect the insertion site of the device.	To detect any signs of inflammation, infiltration, and so on. If present, take appropriate action (see Problem-solving table 16.3) (DH 2003c, C).
19	Observe the infusion, if in progress.	To confirm that it is infusing as desired (NPSA 2007d, C).
20	Check whether the infusion fluid and the drugs are compatible. If not, change the infusion fluid to 0.9% sodium chloride to flush between the drugs if necesary.	To prevent drug interaction. Some manufacturers may recommend that the drug is given into the injection site of a rapidly running infusion (NPSA 2007d, C). A compatible fluid must be used to remove the medication and prevent precipitation or drug incompatibility if medications mix in the tubing (Whittington 2008, E).
21	Wash hands or clean them with an alcohol handrub.	To minimize the risk of infection (DH 2007, C; Fraise and Bradley 2009, E).
22	Place a sterile towel under the patient's arm.	To create a sterile field. E
23	Clean the injection site with a 2% chlorhexidine swab and allow to dry.	To reduce the number of pathogens introduced by the needle at the time of the insertion. To ensure complete disinfection has occurred (Pratt *et al.* 2007, C).
24	Switch off the infusion.	To prevent excessive pressure within the vein. To prevent contact with an incompatible infusion fluid. To allow the nurse to concentrate on the site of insertion and injection (NPSA 2007d, C).
25	If a peripheral device is *in situ*, gently inject 0.9% sodium chloride. This may not be necessary if the patient has a 0.9% sodium chloride infusion in progress.	To confirm patency of the vein. To prevent contact with an incompatible infusion solution (NPSA 2007d, C).
26	Open the roller clamp of the administration set fully. Inject the drug at a speed sufficient to slow but not stop the infusion and inject the drug smoothly in the direction of flow at the specified rate.	To prevent backflow of drug up the tubing. To prevent excessive pressure within the vein. To prevent speed shock (NPSA 2007d, C).
27	Ensure used needles and syringes are disposed of immediately into appropriate sharps container (or are returned to tray). Do not leave any sharps on opened sterile pack.	To reduce the risk of needlestick injury and to prevent contamination of pack (RCN 2010, C).
28	Observe the insertion site of the device throughout.	To detect any complications at an early stage, for example extravasation or local allergic reaction (Dougherty 2008, E).
29	Blood return and/or 'flashback' must be checked frequently throughout the injection (that is, every 3–5 mL) but other signs and symptoms must be taken into consideration.	To confirm that the device is correctly placed and that the vein remains patent (Weinstein and Plumer 2007, E). Flashback alone is not an indicator that the vein is patent (Dougherty 2008, E).
30	Consult the patient during the injection about any discomfort, and so on.	To detect any complications at an early stage, and ensure patient comfort (Dougherty 2008, E).
31	If more than one drug is to be administered, flush with 0.9% sodium chloride between administrations by restarting the infusion or changing syringes.	To prevent drug interactions (NPSA 2007d, C).

1029

(Continued)

Procedure guideline 16.25 *(Continued)*

32	At the end of the injection, flush with 0.9% sodium chloride by restarting the infusion or attaching a syringe containing 0.9% sodium chloride.	To flush any remaining irritant solution away from the device site (NPSA 2007d, C).
33	Observe the insertion site of the cannula carefully.	To detect any complications at an early stage. Extra pressure within the vein caused by both fluid flow and injection of the drug may cause rupture of the vessel (Dougherty 2008, E).
34	After the final flush of 0.9% sodium chloride, adjust the infusion rate as prescribed or open the fluid path of the tap/stopcock or administer the flushing solution using pulsatile flush and ending with positive pressure.	To continue delivery of therapy. To maintain the patency of the cannula (Finlay 2008, E).
35	If a peripheral device is *in situ*, cover the insertion site with new sterile low-linting swab and tape it in place.	To minimize the risk of contamination of the insertion site. E
36	Apply a bandage.	To reduce the risk of dislodging the cannula. E
37	Assist the patient into a comfortable position.	To ensure the patient is comfortable. E

Postprocedure

38	Record the administration on appropriate charts.	To maintain accurate records, provide a point of reference in the event of any queries and prevent any duplication of treatment (NMC 2009, C).
39	Dispose of used syringes with needles, unsheathed, directly into a sharps container during procedure or place back on to plastic tray and then dispose of in a sharps container as soon as possible. *Do not* disconnect needle from syringe prior to disposal. Other waste should be placed into the appropriate plastic bags.	To avoid needlestick injury (MHRA 2004, C; NHS Employers 2007, C).

Problem-solving table 16.3 Prevention and resolution (Procedure guidelines 16.23, 16.24 and 16.25)

Problem	Cause	Prevention	Action
Infusion slows or stops (part 1)	Change in position of the following:		
	(a) Patient	Check the height of the fluid container if the patient is active and receiving an infusion using gravity flow	Adjust the height of the container accordingly. The infusion should not hang higher than 1 m above the patient as the increased height will result in increased pressure and possible rupture of the vessel/device (Quinn 2008)
	(b) Limb	Prevent by avoiding inserting peripheral devices at joints of limbs	Move the arm or hand until infusion starts again. Secure the device, then bandage or splint the limb again carefully in the desired position. Take care not to cause damage to the limb

Problem	Cause	Prevention	Action
		Instruct the patient on the amount of movement permitted. Continued movement could result in mechanical phlebitis (Lamb and Dougherty 2008)	
	(c) Administration set	Tape the administration set so that it cannot become kinked or occluded	Check for kinks and/or compression if the patient is active or restless and correct accordingly
	(d) Cannula	Secure the cannula firmly to prevent movement. It may come into contact with the vein wall or a valve. Infusions sited in small veins are prone to this problem	Remove the bandage and dressing and manoeuvre the peripheral device gently, without pulling it out of the vein, until the infusion starts again. Secure adequately
Infusion slows or stops (part 2)	Technical problems:		
	(a) Negative pressure prevents flow of fluid	Ensure that the container is vented using an air inlet	Vent if necessary, using venting needle
	(b) Empty container	Check fluid levels regularly	Replace the fluid container before it runs dry
	(c) Venous spasm due to chemical irritation or cold fluids/drugs	Dilute drugs as recommended. Remove solutions from the refrigerator a short time before use	Apply a warm compress to soothe and dilate the vein, increase the blood flow and dilute the infusion mixture
	(d) Injury to the vein	Detect any injury early as it is likely to progress and cause more serious conditions (see below)	Stop the infusion and resite the cannula
	(e) Occlusion of the device due to fibrin formation	Maintain a continuous, regular fluid flow or ensure that patency is maintained by flushing. Instruct the patient to keep arm below the level of the heart if ambulant and attached to a gravity flow infusion	**If peripheral device**: remove extension set/injection cap and attempt to flush the cannula gently using a 10 mL syringe of 0.9% sodium chloride. If resistance is met, stop and request a resiting of the peripheral device (see Chapter 18)
			If CVAD: remove injection cap and attempt to flush the cannula gently using a 10 mL syringe of 0.9% sodium chloride. If resistance is met, attempt to instil fibrinolytic agent such as urokinase (see Chapter 18)

1031

(Continued)

Problem-solving table 16.3 (*Continued*)

Problem	Cause	Prevention	Action
	(f) The cannula has become displaced either completely or partially, that is, fluid or drug has leaked into the surrounding tissues (infiltration). If the drugs were vesicant in nature this would then be defined as extravasation	Secure the cannula and tape the administration set to prevent pulling and dislodgement. Instruct the patient on the amount of movement permitted with the limb that has the device *in situ* (Fabian 2000)	Confirm that infiltration of drugs has/has not occurred by: (i) inspecting the site for leakage, swelling, and so on (ii) testing the temperature of the skin: it will be cooler if infiltration has occurred (iii) comparing the size of the limb with the opposite limb Once infiltration has been confirmed, stop the infusion and request a resiting of the device. If the infusion is allowed to progress, discomfort and tissue damage will result. Apply cold or warm compresses to provide symptomatic relief, whichever provides the most comfort for the patient. Reassure the patient by explaining what is happening. Document in care plan and monitor site (Lamb and Dougherty 2008) If extravasation, follow hospital policy and procedure (see Chapter 15)
Infusion pump alarming			
(a) Air detected	Air bubbles in administration set	Ensure all air is removed from all equipment prior to use	Remove all air from the administration set and restart the infusion
(b) Tube misload	Administration set has been incorrectly loaded	Ensure set is loaded correctly	Check that the set is loaded correctly and reload if necessary
(c) Upstream occlusion	Closed clamp, obstruction or kink in the administration set is preventing fluid flow	Ensure the container/fluid bag has been adequately pierced by the administration spike	Inspect the administration set and restart the infusion
		Ensure that the tubing is taped to prevent kinking	If tubing is kinked, reposition, tape and restart infusion
		Ensure the regulating (roller) clamp is open	Check the administration set and open the clamp; restart the infusion
(d) Downstream occlusion	Phlebitis/infiltration or extravasation	Observe site regularly for signs of swelling, pain and erythema	Remove peripheral device, provide symptomatic relief where appropriate. Initiate extravasation procedure. Resite as appropriate
	Closed distal clamp	Ensure clamps are open	Locate distal occlusion, restart infusion
(e) KVO alert (keep vein open)	The volume infused is complete and the device is infusing at the KVO rate	Program in a new volume as appropriate	Do not turn the device off. Allow KVO mode to run to maintain patency of device Prepare new infusion or discontinue as appropriate

Problem	Cause	Prevention	Action
Infusion devices malfunctioning (electrical/mechanical)	Not charging at mains	Ensure that the device is kept plugged in where appropriate	Change device and remove device from use until fully charged. Send to works department to check plug
	Low battery	Check lead is pushed in adequately	
	Batteries keep requiring replacement	Do not use small rechargeable batteries in ambulatory devices	
	Technical fault	Ensure all infusion devices are serviced regularly	Remove infusion device from use and contact biomedical engineering department or relevant personnel
	Device soiled inside mechanism	Maintain equipment and keep clean and free from contamination	Remove administration set, wipe pump, reload. Do not use alcohol-based solutions on internal mechanisms
Unstable infusion device	Mounted on old, poorly maintained stands	Ensure that stands are maintained and kept clean. Replace old stands	Remove device from stand. Remove stand and send to works department for repair
	Mounted on incorrect stands	Ensure the correct stands are used	Check the stand and change to appropriate stand
	Equipment not balanced on stand	Ensure that all equipment is balanced around the stand	Remove devices and attach to two stands if necessary. Balance equipment

Postprocedural considerations

Ongoing care

Monitoring of the infusion while in progress includes monitoring of the patient's condition and response to therapy, the VAD site, the rate and volume infused. It may also include the battery life and occlusion pressure. The frequency of monitoring is often based on the type of therapy and patient condition, for example 15 minutes after setting up infusion, at 1 hour and then 4 hourly. This information must be documented on the patient's fluid balance chart or in their notes. The type and make of pump along with the serial number should also be documented (useful if any errors occur) (MHRA 2008a).

Complications

For phlebitis, thrombosis, septicaemia and embolism, see Chapter 18. For infiltration and extravasation, see Chapter 15.

Allergic reaction

This is a complication associated with any medication administration but because it happens more rapidly when IV medication is administered, it is often considered as more of an issue.

An allergic reaction is a response to a medication or solution to which the patient is sensitive and may be immediate or delayed (Lamb and Dougherty 2008, Perucca 2010). Clinical features may start with chills and fever, with or without urticaria, erythema and itching. The patient could then go onto experience shortness of breath with or without wheezing, then angioneurotic oedema and in severe cases anaphylactic shock (Lamb and Dougherty 2008). Prevention is by assessment and recording of patient allergies (drug, food and products) and application of allergy identification wristbands (NPSA 2008, Perucca 2010). In the event of an allergic reaction, the infusion should be stopped immediately, the tubing and container changed and the vein kept patent. The doctor should be notified and any interventions undertaken (Lamb and Dougherty 2008).

1033

Circulatory overload (isotonic fluid expansion)

A critical and common complication of intravenous therapy is circulatory overload, which is *isotonic fluid expansion*. It is caused by infusion of fluids of the same tonicity as plasma into the vascular circulation, for example sodium chloride 0.9%. As isotonic solutions do not affect osmolarity, water does not flow from the extracellular to the intracellular compartment. The result is that the extracellular compartment expands in proportion to the fluid infused (Weinstein and Plumer 2007). Because of the electrolyte concentration,

no extra water is available to enable the kidneys selectively to excrete and restore the balance. It can also occur due to:

- infusing excessive amounts of sodium chloride solutions
- large volume infusions running over multiple days
- rapid fluid infusion into patients with compromised cardiac, liver or renal status (Lamb and Dougherty 2008, Macklin and Chernecky 2004).

Prevention includes thorough assessment of the patient before commencing IV therapy, close monitoring of patient; main-

Table 16.11 Monitoring overinfusion and underinfusion

Type of fluid/electrolyte imbalance	Patients at risk	Signs and symptoms	Treatment
Circulatory overload (isotonic fluid expansion)	Early postoperative or post-trauma patients, older people, those with impaired renal and cardiac function and children	Weight gain A relative increase in fluid intake compared to output A high bounding pulse pressure, indicating a high cardiac output Raised central venous pressure measurements Peripheral hand vein emptying time longer than normal (peripheral veins will usually empty in 3–5 seconds when the hand is elevated and will fill in the same length of time when the hand is lowered to a dependent position) Peripheral oedema Hoarseness Dyspnoea, cyanosis and coughing due to pulmonary oedema and neck vein engorgement	If detected early: withholding all fluids until excess water and electrolytes have been eliminated by the body and/or administration of diuretics to promote rapid diuresis
Dehydration (hypertonic contraction or hypotonic contraction)	*Hypertonic:* elderly, unconscious or incontinent patients *Hypotonic:* infants are at greatest risk, especially if they have diarrhoea. Loss of salt from various sources: excess diuresis, fistula drainage, burns, vomiting or sweating	*Hyper/hypotonic contraction* Weight loss *Hypercontraction* Thirst (although this may be absent in the elderly) Irritability and restlessness and possible confusion Diminished skin turgor Dry mouth and furred tongue *Hypocontraction* Negative fluid balance Weak, thready, rapid pulse rate Increased 'hand filling time' Increased skin turgor	Replacement of fluids and electrolytes

taining infusion rates as prescribed and use of infusion devices where required (Lamb and Dougherty 2008). If circulatory overload is detected early, place the patient in an upright position (Macklin and Chernecky 2004). Treatment consists of withholding all fluids until excess water and electrolytes have been eliminated by the body and/or administration of diuretics to promote rapid diuresis (Weinstein and Plumer 2007). However, careful monitoring should continue to prevent isotonic contraction occurring (where there is loss of fluid and electrolytes isotonic to the extracellular fluid such as blood and large volumes of fluid from diarrhoea and vomiting; Weinstein and Plumer 2007). If fluid administration is allowed to continue unchecked, it can result in left-sided heart failure, circulatory collapse and cardiac arrest (Dougherty 2002).

Dehydration

Dehydration may be categorized as either hypertonic or hypotonic contraction and may be caused by underinfusion. Hypertonic contraction occurs when water is lost without corresponding loss of salts (Weinstein and Plumer 2007) and occurs in patients unable to take sufficient fluids (elderly, unconscious or incontinent patients) or who have excess insensible water loss via skin and lungs or as a result of certain drugs in excess. Hypotonic contraction occurs when fluids containing more salt than water are lost and this results in a decrease in osmolarity of the extracellular compartment (Weinstein and Plumer 2007).

It is important that the nurse recognizes the symptoms of overinfusion or underinfusion and certain factors should be considered when monitoring patients (Weinstein and Plumer 2007) (see Table 16.11).

Speed shock

Speed shock is a systemic reaction that occurs when a substance foreign to the body is rapidly introduced into the circulation (Perucca 2010, Weinstein and Plumer 2007). This complication can manifest following administration of intravenous bolus injections or when large volumes of fluid are given too rapidly (Perucca 2010). This should not be confused with pulmonary oedema, which relates to the volume of fluid infused into the patient. Rapid, uncontrolled administration of drugs will result in toxic concentrations reaching vital organs (Lamb and Dougherty 2008). Toxicity may be manifested by an exaggeration of the usual pharmacological actions of the drug or by signs and symptoms specific for that drug or class of drugs. The most extreme toxic response which can occur if a drug is given at a dose or rate exceeding that recommended is termed the lethal response.

Signs of speed shock may include:

- flushed face
- headache and dizziness
- congestion of the chest
- tachycardia and fall in blood pressure
- syncope
- shock
- cardiovascular collapse (Perucca 2010, Weinstein and Plumer 2007).

Prevention of speed shock involves the nurse having knowledge of the drug and the recommended rate of administration. When commencing an infusion using gravity flow, check that the solution is flowing freely before adjusting the rate and monitored regularly (Perucca 2010). Movement of the patient or the device within the vessel can cause the infusion to flow more or less freely after a few minutes of setting the rate (Weinstein and Plumer 2007). For high-risk medications an electronic flow control device is recommended (RCN 2010). Although most pumps have an anti-free flow mechanism, always close the roller clamp prior to removing the set from the pump (MHRA 2006a, Pickstone 1999). If speed shock occurs, the infusion must be slowed down or discontinued. Medical staff should be notified immediately and the patient's condition treated as clinically indicated (Perucca 2010).

Websites

MHRA. How we regulate medicines section:
www.mhra.gov.uk

WHO. Medicines: safety of medicines – adverse drug reactions. Factsheet No.293:
www.medicines.org.uk/EMC/medicine/21309/SPC/
Kentura+oxybutynin+transdermmal+patch

References

Absalom, A. and Struys, M. (2006) *An Overview of TCI & TIVA*. Academia Press, Ghent, Belgium.

Aldridge, M. (2010) Miscellaneous routes of medication administration, in *Medicines Management* (eds A. Jevon *et al.*). Wiley Blackwell, Oxford, pp. 239–261.

Alexander, M., Fawcett, J. and Runciman P. (2007) *Nursing Practice: Hospital and Home*, 3rd edn. Churchill Livingstone, London.

Amoore, J. and Adamson, L. (2003) Infusion devices: characteristics, limitations and risk management. *Nursing Standard*, **17** (28), 45–52.

Amoore, J., Dewar, D., Ingram, P. and Lowe, D. (2001) Syringe pumps and start up time: ensuring safe practice. *Nursing Standard*, **15** (17), 43–45.

Andrew, S. (2006) Pharmacology, in *Ophthalmic Care* (ed. J. Marsden). Whurr, Chichester, pp. 42–65.

Applebe, G.E. and Wingfield, J. (2005) *Dale and Appelbe's Pharmacy Law and Ethics*, 8th edn Pharmaceutical Press, London.

Armitage, G. (2008) Double checking medicines: defence against error or contributory factor? *Journal of Evaluation in Clinical Practice*, **14** (4), 513–517.

Armitage, G. and Knapman, H. (2003) Adverse events in drug administration: a literature review. *Journal of Nursing Management*, **11**, 130–140.

Arndt, M. (1994) Research and practice: how drug mistakes affect self-esteem. *Nursing Times*, **90** (15), 27–31.

Audit Commission (2001) *A Spoonful of Sugar: Medicines Management in NHS Hospitals*. Audit Commission, London.

Aulton, M.E. (ed.) (1988) *Pharmaceutics. The Science of Dosage Form Design*. Churchill Livingstone, Edinburgh.

Baxter, K. (ed.) (2008) *Stockley's Drug Interactions*, 8th edn. Pharmaceutical Press, London.

Beijnen, J.H. and Schellens, J.H.M. (2004) Drug interactions in oncology. *Lancet Oncology*, 5, 489–496.

Block, B.M., Liu, S., Rowlingson, A. *et al.* (2003) Efficacy of postoperative analgesia: a meta-analysis. *JAMA*, 290, 2455–2463.

BNF (2011) *British National Formulary*. BMJ Group and RPS Publishing, London.

Bridge, J., Hemingway, S. and Murphy, K. (2005) Implications of non medical prescribing of controlled drugs. *Nursing Times*, **101** (44), 32–33.

British Pharmacopoeia (2007) *British Pharmacopoeia*. Stationery Office, London.

Brock, N. and Pohl, J. (1983) The development of mesna for regional detoxification. *Cancer Treat Review*, **10** (suppl A), 33–43.

Brown, J., Moss, H. and Elliot, T. (1997) The potential for catheter microbial contamination from a needleless connector. *Journal of Hospital Infection*, **36** (3), 181–189.

Care Quality Commission (2009) The safer management of controlled drugs. Annual report 2008. Care Quality Commission, London.

Chernecky, C., Butler, S.W., Graham, P. and Infortuna, H. (2002) *Drug Calculations and Drug Administration*. W.B Saunders, Philadelphia.

Chung, J.W.Y., Ng, W.M.Y. and Wong, T.K.S. (2002) An experimental study on the use of manual pressure to reduce pain in intramuscular injection. *Journal of Clinical Nursing*, **11**, 457–461.

Constans, T., Dutertre, J. and Froge, E. (1991) Hypodermoclysis in dehydrated elderly patients – local effects with and without hyaluronidase. *Journal of Palliative Care*, **7** (2), 10–12.

Cookson, S, Ihrig, M., O'Mara, E.M. *et al.* (1998) Increased blood stream infection rates in surgical patients associated with variation from recommended use and care following implementation of a needleless device. *Infection Control and Hospital Epidemiology*, **19** (1), 23–27.

Dann, T.C. (1969) Routine skin preparation before injection: an unnecessary procedure. *Lancet*, ii, 96–97.

Danzig, L.E., Short, L., Collins, K. *et al.* (1995) Bloodstream infections associated with a needleless intravenous infusion system in patients receiving home infusion therapy. *JAMA*, **273** (23), 1862–1864.

Dawkins, L, Britton, D., Johnson, I. *et al.* (2000) A randomised trial of winged Vialon cannulae and metal butterfly needles. *International Journal of Palliative Nursing*, **6** (3), 110–116.

Deeks, P. and Byatt, K. (2000) Are patients who self-administer their medicines in hospital more satisfied with their care? *Journal of Advanced Nursing*, **31** (2), 395–400.

Dennison, R.D. (2007) A medication safety education program to reduce the risk of harm caused by medication errors. *Journal of Continuing Education in Nursing*, **38** (4), 176–184.

Department of Health, Social Services and Public Safety (2006) *Controls Assurance Standards: Medical Devices and Equipment Management*. www.dhsspsni.gov.uk/medical_devices_06_pdf .

DH (1989) *Report of the Advisory Group on Nurse Prescribing (Crown One)*. HMSO, London.

DH (1998) *Review of Prescribing, Supply and Administration of Medicines. A Report on the Supply and Administration of Medicines under Group Protocols (Crown Two)*. HMSO, London.

DH (1999) *Review of Prescribing, Supply and Administration of Medicines. Final Report (Crown Three)*. HMSO, London.

DH (2000) *Patient Group Directions*. HSC 2000/026. Health and Safety Commission, London.

DH (2003a) *Supplementary Prescribing by Nurses and Pharmacists within the NHS in England: a Guide for Implementation*. National Health Service, London.

DH (2003b) *Building a Safer NHS for Patients: Improving Medication Safety*. Department of Health, London.

DH (2003c) *Winning Ways: Working Together to Reduce Healthcare-Associated Infection in England*. Department of Health, London.

DH (2004) *Extending Independent Nurse Prescribing within the NHS in England: a Guide to Implementation*. Department of Health, London.

DH (2005) *Hazardous Waste (England) Regulations*. Department of Health, London.

DH (2007) *Safer Management of Controlled Drugs. A Guide to Good Practice in Secondary Care (England)*. Department of Health, London.

DH (2009) *Changes to Medicines Legislation to Enable Mixing of Medicines Prior to Administration in Clinical Practice*. Department of Health, London. www.dh.gov.uk.

DHSS (1976) *Health Services Development, Addition of Drugs to Intravenous Fluids, HC(76)9 (Breckenridge Report)*. HMSO, London.

Dickerson, R.J. (1992) 10 tips for easing the pain of intramuscular injections. *Nursing*, **92**, 55.

Dickman, A., Schneider, J. and Varga, J. (2007) *The Syringe Driver: Continuous Subcutaneous Infusions in Palliative Care*, 3rd edn. Oxford University Press, Oxford.

Dirckx, J.H. (2001) *Stedman's Concise Medical Dictionary for the Health Professions*, 4th edn. Lippincott Williams and Wilkins, Philadelphia.

Dougherty, L. (2002) Delivery of intravenous therapy. *Nursing Standard*, **16** (16), 45–56.

Dougherty, L. (2008) Obtaining peripheral access, in *Intravenous Therapy in Nursing Practice*, 2nd edn (eds L. Dougherty and J. Lamb). Blackwell Publishing, Oxford.

Downie, G., MacKenzie, J. and Williams, A. (eds) (2003) Medicine management, in *Pharmacology and Medicines Management for Nurses*, 3rd edn. Churchill Livingstone, London, pp. 49–91.

Elkin, M.K., Perry, A.G. and Potter, P.A. (2007) *Nursing Interventions and Clincial Skills*, 4th edn (eds M.K. Elkin, A.G. Perry and P.A. Potter). Mosby Elsevier, St Louis, MO.

Fabian, B. (2000) IV complications: Infiltration. *Journal of Intravenous Nursing*, **23** (4), 229–231.

Fair, R. and Proctor, B. (2007) *Administering Medicines through Enteral Feeding Tubes*, 2nd edn. Royal Hospitals, Belfast.

Fields, M. and Peterson, J. (2005) Intravenous medication safety systems averts high risk medication errors and provides actionable data. *Nursing Administration Quarterly*, **29** (1) 78–87.

Finlay, T. (2008) Safe administration of IV therapy, in *Intravenous Therapy in Nursing Practice*, 2nd edn (eds L. Dougherty and J. Lamb). Blackwell Publishing, Oxford.

Forrester, J., Dick, A.D., McMenamin, P.G. and Lee, W.R. (2002) *The Eye: Basic Science in Practice*, 2nd edn. Saunders, Edinburgh.

Fox, N. (2000) Armed and dangerous. *Nursing Times*, **96** (44), 24–26.

Fraise, A.P. and Bradley, T. (eds) (2009) *Ayliffe's Control of Healthcare-associated Infection: A Practical Handbook*, 5th edn. Hodder Arnold, London.

Frey, A.M. and Pettit, J. (2010) Infusion therapy in children, in *Infusion Nursing: An Evidence-Based Approach*, 3rd edn (eds M. Alexander, A. Corrigan, L. Gorski, J. Hankins and R. Perucca). Saunders Elsevier, St Louis, MO, pp.550–568.

Gladstone, J. (1995) Drug administration errors: a study into the factors underlying the occurrence and reporting of drug errors in a district general hospital. *Journal of Advanced Nursing*, **22** (4), 628–637.

Greenway, K. (2004) Using the ventrogluteal site for intramuscular injection. *Nursing Standard*, 18 (25), 39–42.

Griffith, R. and Jordan, S. (2003) Administration of medicines part 1: the law and nursing. *Nursing Standard*, 18 (2), 47–53.

Hadaway, L.C. (2010) Anatomy and physiology related to infusion therapy, in *Infusion Nursing: An Evidence-Based Approach*, 3rd edn (eds M. Alexander, A. Corrigan, L. Gorski, J. Hankins and R. Perucca). Saunders Elsevier, St Louis, MO, pp.139–177.

Hand, K. and Barber, N. (2000) Nurses' attitudes and beliefs about medication errors in a UK hospital. *International Journal of Pharmacy Practice*, 8, 128–134.

Hardman, J.G.. Limbird, L.E., Molinoff, P.B. *et al.* (eds) (1996) *Goodman and Gilman's The Pharmacological Basis of Therapeutics*, 9th edn. McGraw-Hill, New Jersey.

Harkin, H. (2008) Guidance document in ear care. www.earcarecentre.com/protocols.htm.

Hart, S. (2008) Infection control in IV therapy, in *Intravenous Therapy in Nursing Practice*, 2nd edn (eds L. Dougherty and J. Lamb). Blackwell Publishing, Oxford.

Haw, C., Stubbs, J. and Dickens, G. (2007) An observational study of medication administration: errors in old age psychiatric inpatients. *International Journal of Quality in Health Care*, **19** (4), 210–216.

Healthcare Commission (2007) The Best Medicine. The Management of Medicines in Acute and Specialist Trusts. Healthcare Commission, London.

Health Care Standards Unit (2007a) *First Domain – Safety (Info Bank) C4b*. www.hcsu.org.uk/index.php?option=com_content&task=view&id=197&Itemid=109.

Health Care Standards Unit (2007b) *Updated signpost C4b*. www.hcsu.org.uk/index.php?option=com_content&task=view&id=309&Itemid=111.

Hertzel, C. and Sousa, V.D. (2009) The use of smart pumps for preventing medication errors. *Journal of Infusion Nursing*, **32** (5), 257–267.

Hillery, A., Lloyd, A. and Swarbrick, J. (eds) (2001) *Drug Delivery and Targeting for Pharmacists and Pharmaceutical Scientists*. CRC Press, Boca Raton, FL.

Hilton, S. (1990) An audit of inhaler technique among patients of 34 general practitioners. *British Journal of General Practice*, 40(341), 505–506.

HMSO (1968) *Medicines Act*. HMSO, London.

HMSO (1971) *Misuse of Drugs Act*. HMSO, London.

Ho, C.Y.W., Dean, B.S. and Barber, N. (1997) When do medication administration errors happen to hospital in-patients? *International Journal of Pharmacy Practice*, 5, 91–96.

Howard, R.L, Avery, A., Slavenburg, S. *et al.* (2007) Which drugs cause preventable admissions to hospital? A systematic review. *British Journal of Clinical Pharmacology*, 63 (2), 136–147.

Hutton, M. (1998) Numeracy skills for IV calculations. *Nursing Standard*, 12 (43), 49–56.

Hyde, L. (2008) Legal and professional aspects of IV therapy, in *Intravenous Therapy in Nursing Practice*, 2nd edn (eds L. Dougherty and J. Lamb). Blackwell Publishing, Oxford.

Jarman, H., Jacobs, E. and Zielinski, V. (2002) Medication study supports registered nurses' competence for single checking. *International Journal of Nursing Practice*, 8, 330–335.

Jordan, S., Griffiths, H. and Griffith, R. (2003) Administration of medicines part 2: pharmacology. *Nursing Standard*, 18 (3), 45–54.

Kelly, J. and Wright, D. (2009) Administering medication to adult patients with dysphagia. *Nursing Standard*, **23**, 29, 61–68.

Keohane, C.A., Hayes, J., Saniuk, C. *et al.* (2005) Intravenous medication safety and smart infusion systems. *Journal of Infusion Nursing*, 28 (5), 321–328.

King, L. (2003) Subcutaneous insulin injection technique. *Nursing Standard*, 17 (34), 45–52.

Kirkwood, B. (2006) The cornea, in *Ophthalmic Care* (ed. J. Marsden). Whurr, Chichester, pp. 339–69.

Koda-Kimble, M.A., Young, L.Y., Kradjan, W.A. and Guglielmo, B.J. (eds) (2005) *Applied Therapeutics: The Clinical Use of Drugs*, 8th edn. Lippincott Williams and Wilkins, Philadelphia.

Koivistov, V.A. and Felig, P. (1978) Is skin preparation necessary before insulin injection? *Lancet*, i, 1072–1073.

Lamb, J. and Dougherty, L. (2008) Local and systemic complications of intravenous therapy, in *Intravenous Therapy in Nursing Practice*, 2nd edn (eds L. Dougherty and J. Lamb). Blackwell Publishing, Oxford.

Larson, G.Y., Parker, H., Cash, J. *et al.* (2005) Standard drug concentrations and smart pump technology reduce continuous medication infusion errors in pediatric patients. *Pediatrics*, **116** (1), 21–25.

Latter, S. (2008) Safety and quality in independent prescribing: an evidence review. *Nurse Prescribing*, 6 (2), 59–65.

Latter, S., Maben, J., Myall, M. *et al.* (2005) *An Evaluation of Extended Formulary Independent Nurse Prescribing: Executive Summary of Final Report*. University of Southampton, Southampton.

Laverty, D., Mallett, J. and Mulholland, J. (1997) Protocols and guidelines for managing wounds. *Professional Nurse*, **13** (2), 79–80.

Lenz, C.L. (1983) Make your needle selection right to the point. *Nursing*, 13 (2), 50–51.

Luebke, M.A, Arduino, M., Duda, D. *et al.* (1998) Comparison of the microbial barrier properties of a needleless and conventional needle based intravenous access system. *American Journal of Infection Control*, **26**, 437–441.

Luker, K. and Wolfson, D. (1999) Introduction, in *Medicines Management for Clinical Nurses* (eds K. Luker and D. Wolfson). Blackwell Science, Oxford.

Macklin, D. and Chernecky, C.C. (2004) *IV Therapy*. Saunders, St Louis, MO.

Malkin, B. (2008) Are techniques used for intramuscular injection based on research evidence? *Nursing Times*, 104 (50/51), 48–51.

Mallett, J., Faithfull, S., Guerrero, D. *et al.* (1997) Nurse prescribing by protocol. *Nursing Times*, 93 (8), 50–52.

Marieb, E.N. and Hoehn, K. (2007) *Human Anatomy and Physiology*, 7th edn. Pearson Benjamin Cummings, San Francisco.

Marriott, J.L. and Nation, R.L. (2002) Splitting tablets. *Australian Prescriber*, 25 (6), 133–135.

Martin, P.J. (1994) Professional updating through open learning as a method of reducing errors in the administration of medicines. *Journal of Nursing Management*, 2 (5), 209–212.

Mathijssen, R.H.J., Verweij, J., de Bruijn, P. *et al.* (2002) Effects of St. John's wort on irinotecan metabolism. *Journal of the National Cancer Institute*, 94, 1247–1249.

McClelland, B. (2007) *Handbook of Transfusion Medicine*, 3rd edn. HMSO, London.

McHale, J. (2002) Extended prescribing: the legal implications. *Nursing Times*, 98 (32), 36–38.

Medical Devices Agency (2000) *Equipped to Care*. Medical Devices Agency, London. www.mhra.gov.uk/home/idcplg?IdcService=SS_GET_PAGE&useSecondary=true&ssDocName=CON007425&ssTargetNodeId=575.

Medicines Partnership Programme (2007) *A Competency Framework For Shared Decision-Making With Patients: Achieving*

1037

Concordance For Taking Medicines. NPC plus and Medicines Partnership Programme, Keele.

Mei, A. and Auerhahn, C. (2009) Hyperdermoclysis maintaining hydration in the frail older adult. *Annals of Long Term Care,* **17** (5), 28–30.

Mendelson, M.H., Short, L., Schechter, C. *et al.* (1998) Study of a needleless intermittent intravenous access system for peripheral infusions: analysis of staff, patient and institutional outcomes. *Infection Control and Hospital Epidemiology,* **19** (6), 401–406.

MHRA (2001) *Recommendations on the control and monitoring of storage and transportation of medicinal products.* Medicines and Healthcare Products Regulatory Agency, London.

MHRA (2004) *Reducing Needlestick and Sharps Injuries.* Medicines and Healthcare Products Regulatory Agency, London.

MHRA (2005) *Consultation on Options for the Future of Independent Prescribing by Extended Formulary Nurse Prescribers.* Medicines and Healthcare Products Regulatory Agency, London.

MHRA (2006a) *Free-flow situations.* www.mhra.gov.uk/home/idcplg?IdcService=GET_FILE&dID=20057&noSaveAs=0&Rendition=WEB.

MHRA (2006b) *Reporting adverse incidents and disseminating medical device alerts.* DB2006(01). www.mhra.gov.uk/home/idcplg?IdcService=SS_GET_PAGE&useSecondary=true&ssDocName=CON007304&ssTargetNodeId=572.

MHRA (2007) *Medical Device Alert/2007/089. Intravenous (IV) infusion lines all brands.* Medicines and Healthcare Products Regulatory Agency, London.

MHRA (2008a) *Devices in practice: a guide for professionals in health and social care.* Medicines and Healthcare Products Regulatory Agency, London.

MHRA (2008b) *Medical Device Alert 2008/016. Needle-free intravascular connectors.* All brands. Medicines and Healthcare Products Regulatory Agency, London.

MHRA (2009) *Drug Safety Update: Volume 2, Issue 9.* Medicines and Healthcare Products Regulatory Agency, London.

MHRA (2010a) *Good Pharmacovigilance Practice.* Medicines and Healthcare Products Regulatory Agency, London.

MHRA (2010b) *Device Bulletin Infusion Systems.* DB 2003 (02) v2.0 November. Medicines and Healthcare Products Regulatory Agency, London.

MHRA (2010c) *Patient Group Directions in the Private Sector.* Medicines and Healthcare Products Regulatory Agency, London. www.mhra.gov.uk/Howweregulate/Medicines/Availabilityprescribingsellingandsupplyingofmedicines/ExemptionsfromMedicinesActrestrictions/PatientGroupDirectionsintheprivatesector/index.htm

MHRA (2010d) *Patient Group Directions in the NHS.* Medicines and Healthcare Products Regulatory Agency, London. www.mhra.gov.uk/Howweregulate/Medicines/Availabilityprescribingsellingandsupplyingofmedicines/ExemptionsfromMedicinesActrestrictions/PatientGroupDirectionsintheNHS/index.htm

Mirakian, R., Ewan, P.W., Durham, S.R. *et al.* (2009) BSACI guidelines for the management of drug allergy. *Clinical and Experimental Allergy,* **39,** 43–61.

Mitten, T. (2001) Subcutaneous drug infusions: a review of problems and solutions. *International Journal of Palliative Nursing,* **7** (2), 75–85.

Moriarty, D. and Hudson, E. (2001) Hypodermoclysis for rehydration in the community. *British Journal of Community Nursing,* **6** (9), 437–443.

Moses, S. (2009) Hypodermoclysis technique. www.fpnotebook.com/ER/Procedure/HypdrmclysTchnq.thm.

Murray, W. and Glenister, H. (2001) How to use medical devices safely. *Nursing Times,* **97** (43), 36–38.

NHSCLU (2009) www.corelearningunit.nhs.uk.

NHS Connecting for Health (2009) Electronic prescribing in hospitals: challenges and lessons learned. www2.lse.ac.uk/LSEHealthAndSocialCare/LSEHealth/News/ePrescribing%20Report.pdf

NHS Employers (2007) *The Management of Health, Safety and Welfare Issues for NHS Staff.* NHS Confederation (Employers), London.

NHS Litigation Authority (2007) *NHSLA Risk Management Standards for Acute Trusts.* www.nhsla.com/NR/rdonlyres/F9DA791B-AF6D-4198-AC49-EE9B81A91B17/0/NHSLARiskManagementStandardsforAcuteTrusts200708website.doc.

NICE (2003) *Technology Appraisal Guidance No 57. Guidance on the Use of Continuous Subcutaneous Insulin Infusion for Diabetes.* National Institute for Health and Clinical Excellence, London.

Nisbet, A. (2006) Intramuscular gluteal injections in the increasingly obese population: retrospective study. *BMJ,* **332,** 637–638.

NMC (2001a) Press statement: covert administration of medicines can be justified. Nursing and Midwifery Council, London.

NMC (2001b) *UKCC Position Statement on the Covert Administration of Medicines – Disguising Medicine in Food and Drink.* Nursing and Midwifery Council, London.

NMC (2001c) *Circular 25/2002.* Nursing and Midwifery Council, London.

NMC (2006a) *Medicines Management A–Z Advice Sheet.* Nursing and Midwifery Council. www.nmc-uk.org/aFrameDisplay.aspx?DocumentID=1801.

NMC (2006b) *Standards of Proficiency for Nurse and Midwife Prescribers.* Nursing and Midwifery Council, London.

NMC (2008a) *Standards for Medicines Management.* Nursing and Midwifery Council, London.

NMC (2008b) *The Code: Standards of Conduct, Performance and Ethics for Nurses and Midwives.* Nursing and Midwifery Council, London.

NMC (2008c) *Consent.* Nursing and Midwifery Council, London. www.nmc-uk.org/Nurses-and-midwives/Advice-by-topic/A/Advice/Consent/.

NMC (2009) *Record Keeping: Guidance for Nurses and Midwives.* Nursing and Midwifery Council, London.

NPC (2001) *Maintaining Competency in Prescribing: an Outline Framework to Help Nurse Prescribers.* National Health Service, London.

NPC (2003a) *Supplementary Prescribing. A Resource to Help Healthcare Professionals to Understand the Framework and Opportunities.* National Health Service, London.

NPC (2003b) *Maintaining Competency in Prescribing: an Outline Framework to Help Nurse Supplementary Prescribers.* National Health Service, London.

NPC (2007) *Self Administration of Medicines: 5 Minute Guide Series.* National Prescribing Centre, Keele. www.npci.org.uk/medicines_management/safety/selfadmin/library/library_fivemin_guides.php.

NPC (2009) *Patient Group Directions: A Practical Guide and Framework of Competencies for All Professionals Using Patient Group Directions.* National Prescribing Centre, London. www.npc.co.uk/prescribers/resources/patient_group_directions.pdf

NPSA (2003) *Risk Analysis of Infusion Devices.* National Patient Safety Agency, London.

NPSA (2004) *Safer Practice Notice 01: Infusion Devices.* National Patient Safety Agency, London. www.npsa.nhs.uk/Patientsafety/alerts-and-directives/notices/infusion-device.

NPSA (2005) *Wristbands for Hospital Inpatients Improve Safety (Safer Practice Notice 11).* National Patient Safety Agency, London.

NPSA (2006) *Ensuring Safer Practice with High Dose Ampoules of Morphine and Diamorphine, Alert No. 2006/12*. National Patient Safety Agency, London.

NPSA (2007a) *Safety in Doses: Medication Safety Incidents in the NHS, PSO/4*. National Patient Safety Agency, London.

NPSA (2007b) *Standardising Wristbands Improves Patient Safety*. Safer Practice Notice 0507. NPSA, London,

NPSA (2007c) Patient Safety Alert 19. Promoting Safer Measurement and Administration of Liquid Medicines via Oral and other Enteral Routes. National Patient Safety Agency, London.

NPSA (2007d) Promoting Safer Use of Injectable Medicines. Alert No. 2007/20. National Patient Safety Agency, London. www.npsa.nhs.uk/Patientsafety/alerts-and-directives/alerts/injectable-medicines.

NPSA (2008a) Rapid Response Report 05: Reducing Dosing Errors with Opioid Medicines. National Patient Safety Agency, London.

NPSA (2008b) Rapid Response Report 11: Reducing risk of overdose with midazolam injection in adults. National Patient Safety Agency, London.

NPSA/NICE (2007) Patient Safety Guidance 001. Technical patient safety solutions for medicines reconciliation on admission of adults to hospital. National Patient Safety Agency, London.

NPSA/NRLS (2009) *Safety in Doses. Improving the Use of Medicines in the NHS*. National Patient Safety Agency, London.

Peragallo-Dittko, V. (1997) Rethinking subcutaneous injection technique. *American Journal of Nursing*, 97 (5), 71–72.

Perry, A.G. (2007) Administration of injections, in *Nursing Interventions and Clinical Skills*, 4th edn (eds M.K. Elkin, A.G. Perry and P.A. Potter). Mosby Elsevier, St Louis, MO, pp. 416–446.

Perucca, R. (2010) Peripheral venous access devices, in *Infusion Nursing: An Evidence-Based Approach*, 3rd edn (eds M. Alexander, A. Corrigan, L. Gorski, J. Hankins and R. Perucca). Saunders Elsevier, St Louis, MO, pp.456–479.

Pickstone, M. (1999) *A Pocketbook for Safer IV Therapy*. Medical Technology and Risk Series. Scitech Educational, Kent.

Pickstone, M. (2000) Using the technology triangle to assess the safety of technology-controlled clinical procedures in critical care. *International Journal of Intensive Care*, 7 (2), 90–96.

Pope, B.B. (2002) How to administer subcutaneous and intramuscular injection. *Nursing*, 32 (1), 50–51.

Pratt, R.J., Pellowe, C., Wilson, J. *et al.* (2007) Epic 2: national evidence-based guidelines for preventing healthcare-associated infections in NHS hospitals in England. *Journal of Hospital Infection*, 65 (1) (Suppl), S1–S12.

Quinn, C. (2000) Infusion devices: risks, functions and management. *Nursing Standard*, 14 (26), 35–41.

Quinn, C. (2008) Intravenous flow control and infusion devices, in *Intravenous Therapy in Nursing Practice*, 2nd edn (eds L. Dougherty and J. Lamb). Blackwell Publishing, Oxford, pp. 197–224.

Quinn, C. and Upton, D. (2006) A review of claims against the NHS relating to IV therapy. *Health Care Risk Report*, 12 (14), 15–18.

Rawlins, M.D. and Thompson, J.W. (1977) Pathogenesis of adverse drug reactions, in *Textbook of Adverse Drug Reactions* (ed. D.M. Davies). Oxford University Press, Oxford.

RCN (2010) *Standards for Infusion Therapy*, 3rd edn. Royal College of Nursing, London.

Reckmann, M.H., Westbrook, J.I. and Koh, Y. *et al.* (2009) Does computerised provider order entry reduce prescribing errors for hospital inpatients? A systematic review. *JAMA*, 10, 1197.

Regnard, C. and Hockley, J. (2004) *A Guide to Symptom Relief in Palliative Care*, 5th edn. Radcliffe Medical Press.

Riedl, M.A. and Casillas, A.M. (2003) Adverse drug reactions: types and treatment options. *American Family Physician*, 68, 1781–1790.

Ripamonti, C. and Bruera, E. (1997) Current status of patient controlled analgesia in cancer patients. *Oncology*, 11 (3), 373–380.

Rodger, M.A. and King, L. (2000) Drawing up and administering intra-muscular injection: a review of the literature. *Journal of Advanced Nursing*, 31 (3), 574–582.

Rosenthal, M.M. (2003) Check the wristband. www.webmm.rhq.gov/case.aspx?/caseID=22+searchStr=wristband.

Rothschild, J.M., Keohane, C.A., Cook, E.F. *et al.* (2005) A controlled trial of smart infusion pumps to improve medication safety in critically ill patients. *Critical Care Medicine*, 33, 533–540.

RPSGB (2005) *The Safe and Secure Handling of Medicines. A Team Approach*. Royal Pharmaceutical Society of Great Britain, London.

RPSGB (2007a) *Developing and Implementing Standard Operating Procedures for Dispensing*. Royal Pharmaceutical Society of Great Britain, London.

RPSGB (2007b) *Legal and Advisory Service Fact Sheet Six. Monitored Dosage Systems and Compliance Aids*. Royal Pharmaceutical Society of Great Britain, London.

RPSGB (2009) *Medicines, Ethics and Practice. A Guide for Pharmacists and Pharmacy Technicians*, No. 33. Royal Pharmaceutical Society of Great Britain, London.

Sasson, M. and Shvartzman, P. (2001) Hypodermoclysis: an alternative infusion technique. *American Family Physician*, 64 (9), 1575–1578.

Savage, P. and Tripp, K. (2008) A study of independent double checking processes for chemotherapy administration via an ambulatory infusion pump. 15th International Conference on Cancer Nursing, Singapore 17–21 August 2008. Abstract Q116.

Schulmeister, L. (2008) Patient misidentification. *Clinical Journal of Oncology Nursing*, 12 (3), 495–498.

Sexton, J. (1999) The nurse's role in medicines administration – legal and procedural framework, in *Medicines Management for Clinical Nurses* (eds K. Luker and D. Wolfson). Blackwell Science, Oxford.

Shepherd, M. (2002a) Medicines 2. Administration of medicines. *Nursing Times*, 98 (16), 45–48.

Shepherd, M. (2002b) Medicines 3. Managing medicines. *Nursing Times*, 98 (17), 43–46.

Shuttleworth, A. (2005) Are nurses ready to take on the BNF? *Nursing Times*, 101 (48), 29–30.

Smyth, J. (ed.) (2006) The NEWT guidelines for administration of medication to patients with enteral feeding tubes and swallowing difficulties. North East Wales NHS Trust, Wrexham.

Snyder J. (2007) Administration of nonparenteral medications, in *Nursing Interventions and Clincial Skills*, 4th edn (eds M.K. Elkin, A.G. Perry and P.A. Potter) Mosby Elsevier, St Louis, MO, pp. 379–415.

Springhouse (2005) *Intravenous Therapy Made Incredibly Easy*, 3rd edn (ed. L. Bruck). Lippincott, Williams and Wilkins, Philadelphia.

Stollery, R., Shaw, M. and Lee, A. (2005) *Ophthalmic Nursing*, 3rd edn. Blackwell Publishing, Oxford.

Taxis, K. and Barber, N. (2003) Ethnographic study on the incidence and severity of intravenous drug errors. *BMJ*, 326, 684–687.

Taxis, K., Dean, B. and Barber, N. (1999) Hospital drug distribution systems in the UK and Germany: a study of medication errors. *Pharmacy World and Science*, 21 (1), 25–31.

Taylor, N.J. (2000) Fascination with phlebitis. *Vascular Access Devices*, 5 (3), 24–28.

Thomas, J.R., Wallace, M., Yocum, R. *et al.* (2009) The INFUSE morphine study: use of recombinant human hyaluronidase

1039

(rHuPH20) to enhance the absorption of subcutaneously administered morphine in patients with advanced illness. *Journal of Pain and Symptom Management*, 38, 663–672.

Torrance, C. (1989) Intramuscular injection, part 1 and 2. *Surgical Nurse*, 2 (5), 6–10; 2 (6), 24–7.

Torre, M. (2002) Subcutaneous infusion: non-metal cannulae vs metal butterfly needles. *British Journal of Community Nursing*, 7 (7), 365–369.

Tortora, G.J. and Derrickson, B. (2009) *Principles of Anatomy and Physiology*, 12th edn. John Wiley, Hoboken, New Jersey.

Treloar, A., Beats, B. and Philpot, M. (2000) A pill in the sandwich: covert medication in food and drink. *Journal of the Royal Society of Medicine*, 93, 408–411.

Trounce, J. and Gould, D. (2000) *Clinical Pharmacology for Nurses*, 16th edn. Churchill Livingstone, London.

Turner, M.S. and Hankins, J. (2010) Pharmacology, in *Infusion Nursing: An Evidence-Based Approach*, 3rd edn (eds M. Alexander, A. Corrigan, L. Gorski, J. Hankins and R. Perucca). Saunders Elsevier, St Louis, MO.

Twycross, R., Wilcock, A., Dean, M. and Kennedy, B. (2007) *Palliative Care Formulary*, 3rd edn. www.palliativedrugs.com.

UCL Institute of Child Health (2008) *Information Sheet on G6PD Deficiency*, 2nd edn. UCL Institute of Child Health, London.

Walker, R. and Edwards, C. (2003) *Clinical Pharmacy and Therapeutics*, 3rd edn. Churchill Livingstone, London.

Watt, S. (2003) Safe administration of medines to children: part 2. *Paediatric Nurse*, 15 (5), 40–44.

Weeks, K.W., Lyne, P. and Torrance, C. (2000) Written drug dosage errors made by students: the threat to clinical effectiveness and the need for a new approach. *Clinical Effectiveness in Nursing*, 4, 20–29.

Weeks, K.W., Lyne, P., Mosely, L. and Torrance, C. (2001) The strive for clinical effectiveness in medication dosage calculation problem solving skills: the role of constructivist learning theory in the desing of a computer based 'authentic world' learning environment. *Clinical Effectiveness in Nursing*, 5, 18–25.

Weinstein, S. and Plumer, A. (2007) *Plumer's Principles and Practices of Intravenous Therapy*, 8th edn. Lippincott, Williams and Wilkins, Philadelphia.

Werawatganon, T. and Charuluxanun, S. (2005) Patient controlled intravenous opioid analgesia versus continuous epidural analgesia for pain after intra-abdominal surgery. *Cochrane Database of Systematic Reviews*, 1; CD004088.

Wheatley, R., Schug, S. and Watson, D. (2001) Safety and efficacy of postoperative epidural analgesia. *British Journal of Anaesthesia*, 87 (1), 47–61.

Whittington, Z. (2008) Pharmacological aspects of IV therapy, in *Intravenous Therapy in Nursing Practice*, 2nd edn (eds L. Dougherty and J. Lamb). Blackwell Publishing, Oxford.

WHO (2004) *Immunization in Practice. Module 6: Holding an Immunization Session*. World Health Organization, Geneva.

WHO (2008) Medicines: safety of medicines – adverse drug reactions. Factsheet No.293. www.medicines.org.uk/EMC/medicine/21309/SPC/Kentura+oxybutynin+transdermmal+patch.

Williams, C. and Lefever, J. (2000) Reducing the risk of user error with infusion pumps. *Professional Nurse*, 15 (6), 382–384.

Wilson, K. and Sullivan, M. (2004) Preventing medication errors with smart infusion technology. *American Journal of Health System Pharmacists*, 61 (2), 177–183.

Workman, B. (1999) Safe injection techniques. *Nursing Standard*, 13 (39), 47–52.

Wright, A., Hecker, J. and Lewis, G. (1985) Use of transdermal glyceryl trinitrate to reduce failure of intravenous infusion due to phlebitis and extravasation. *Lancet*, ii, 1148–1150.

Perioperative care

Procedure guidelines

Overview

This chapter relates to the care provided to the patient in the three stages of surgery:

■ preoperative care
■ intraoperative care
■ postoperative care.

Preoperative care

Definition

Preoperative care is the physical and psychological care provided to the patient to help them prepare to undergo surgery.

Related theory

Venous thromboembolism (VTE) is a condition where a blood clot is formed inside a vein. This is normally due to stasis of blood within the vessel, trauma to the vessel or an increase in the ability of the blood to clot. This most frequently happens in the deep veins of the leg which is termed a deep vein thrombosis or DVT. If one of these clots dislodges from the leg and travel to the lung via the bloodstream, it is called a pulmonary embolus or PE. This is a potentially fatal complaint (NICE 2010) (Box 17.1).

Patients should be assessed for the individual risk factors for VTE when hospitalized in order to determine the most appropriate thromboprophylaxis (HoCHC 2005, NICE 2010). Patients at higher risk include those with major illness, for example acute cardiac or respiratory failure, major surgery, older patients, patients who are obese or with a previous history of DVT or PE (NICE 2010, SIGN 2002) (Box 17.2). All patients requiring an inpatient stay for surgery should have prophylactic treatment to reduce the risk of DVT, which may include anticoagulation and mechanical compression methods, for example antiembolic stockings and intermittent pneumatic compression methods (NICE 2010, Roderick et al. 2005, SIGN 2002).

> **Box 17.2** Venous thrombus risk factors
>
> ■ Patient undergoing major surgery or abdominal/pelvic surgery.
> ■ Immobility, for example prolonged bed rest.
> ■ Active cancer.
> ■ Severe cardiac failure or recent myocardial infarction.
> ■ Acute respiratory failure.
> ■ Elderly.
> ■ Previous history of DVT or PE.
> ■ Acute infection/inflammation.
> ■ Diabetes.
> ■ Smoker.
> ■ Obesity.
> ■ Gross varicose veins.
> ■ Paralysis of lower limbs.
> ■ Clotting disorders.
> ■ Hormone replacement therapy.
> ■ Oral contraceptives.
>
> (HoCHC 2005, NICE 2010, Rashid et al. 2005, SIGN 2002)

Patients should be given verbal and written information before surgery about the risks of VTE and the effectiveness of prophylaxis (NICE 2010). It is estimated that 20% of patients undergoing major surgery will develop a DVT with the risk increasing to 40% of patients undergoing major orthopaedic surgery (SIGN 2002). Mechanical compression methods reduce the risk of DVT by about two-thirds when used as monotherapy and by about half when added to pharmacological methods (Roderick et al. 2005). Graduated compression (antiembolic) stockings promote venous flow and reduce venous stasis not only in the legs but also in the pelvic veins and inferior vena cava (Hayes et al. 2002, Rashid et al. 2005, Roderick et al. 2005).

Evidence-based approaches
Rationale

To ensure patient safety at all times and minimize intra/postoperative complications by:

■ delivering the required nursing care for the preoperative patient
■ minimizing potential problems by ensuring patients have carried out certain procedures and are prepared safely for theatre. These include:
  – preoperative fasting
  – skin preparation
  – marking skin for surgery
  – preoperative pregnancy testing
  – preventing toxic shock syndrome from tampons (female only)
  – patient education

> **Box 17.1** Signs of DVT/PE
>
> ■ Complaints of calf or thigh pain.
> ■ Erythema, warmth, tenderness and abnormal swelling of the calf or thigh in the affected limb.
> ■ Numbness or tingling of the feet.
> ■ Dyspnoea, chest pain or signs of shock.
> ■ Pain in the chest, back or ribs which gets worse when the patient breathes in deeply.
> ■ Coughing up blood.

- application of antiembolic stockings (graduated elastic compression stockings)
- assessment for latex allergy
- consent.

Legal and professional issues

Consent

For consent to be valid it must encompass several factors.

- The patient must have capacity – that is, the ability to understand and retain the information provided, especially around the consequences of having or not having the procedure.
- Consent must be given willingly – this is without pressure or undue influence to either undertake or not undertake treatment.
- Has sufficient information been provided? This is so the patient has a understanding of the procedure and the purpose behind it.

(DH 2009)

The person obtaining the patient's consent for surgery should be the surgeon performing the procedure or someone who is sufficiently trained to undertake it (DH 2009).

The gaining of consent, unless it is an emergency, should be treated as a process, rather than a one-off event. For major operations, it should be considered good practice where possible to look for a person's consent to the proposed procedure well in advance, when there is time to respond to the person's questions and provide adequate information. Before the procedure starts, the clinician should check that the person still consents. Gaining a person's signature to confirm their consent immediately before the procedure is due to start, at a time when they may be feeling particularly vulnerable, would shed real doubt as to its validity. Patients should not in any situation be given routine preoperative medication before being asked for their consent to proceed with the treatment (NMC 2008).

Preprocedural considerations

Equipment

Antiembolic stockings (graduated elastic compression stockings thromboembolic deterrent)

For patients with VTE thigh-length graduated compression/antiembolic stockings should be fitted from the time of admission to hospital unless contraindicated, for example if the patient has peripheral arterial disease or diabetic neuropathy (NICE 2007) (Box 17.3). The patient should continue wearing them until they have returned to their usual level of mobility.

Thigh-length stockings are difficult to put on and can roll down, creating a tourniquet just above the knee which restricts blood supply, so patient monitoring and/or assistance should

---

Box 17.3 Contraindications for antiembolus stockings

- Severe peripheral arterial disease.
- Severe peripheral neuropathy.
- Vascular disease resulting from congestive heart conditions.
- Gangrene.
- Pulmonary oedema or massive oedema of the legs.
- Major leg deformity.
- Certain types of skin disease, for example weeping skin lesions/dermatitis. The stockings would hinder healing of local leg conditions, for example dermatitis.
- Recent skin graft.
- Cellulitis.
- Pressure sores to heels. Pressure sores are a complication of antiembolic stockings and stockings should not be applied (NICE 2005).

---

take place to ensure that stockings are fitted smoothly, are not rolled down or the top band not folded down. If thigh-length stockings are inappropriate for a particular patient for reasons of compliance or fit, knee-length stockings may be a suitable alternative. It has been suggested that 15–20% of patients cannot effectively wear thigh-length antiembolic stockings because of unusual limb size or shape (SIGN 2002). In reality, knee-high stockings have the advantage of simplicity, with greater patient compliance and economy (Barker and Hollingsworth 2004, Byrne 2002, Parnaby 2004). When applying the stockings, it is important that correct measurements are taken so that the appropriate stocking size is fitted for optimum effectiveness. The stocking compression profile should be equivalent to the Sigel profile, and approximately 18 mmHg at the ankle, 14 mmHg at the mid-calf and 8 mmHg at the upper thigh (NICE 2007).

During surgery, the use of heel supports which reduce the pressure of the calves on the operating table will also encourage venous return. Intermittent calf compression air boots that promote venous flow during surgery have also been reported to be effective (Davis and O'Neill 2002, NICE 2010). The intermittent calf compression boots can be used in conjunction with antiembolic stockings, providing double protection. The only time this needs to be reviewed is when the patient is placed in the Lloyd Davis position as there is a risk of developing compartment syndrome. In this instance, either the antiembolic stockings or the intermittent calf compression boots should be used: this decision will be made by the surgeon and the anaesthetist.

Namebands

Namebands (otherwise known as identity bands or wristbands) are fundamental in the identification of patients. In the most recent guidance, the information to be included on the namebands is: date of birth, in the format dd.mm.yyyy, name (surname first in capitals followed by the first name with the first letter in capitals) and the patient's 10-digit NHS number (NPSA 2007). The NPSA Alert (2007) 'Standardising wristbands improves patient safety' states that within 2 years all NHS organizations in England and Wales where wristbands are used should generate and print all patient wristbands from the hospital electronic demographic system.

Specific patient preparations
Fasting

General anaesthesia carries the risk of the patient inhaling gastric contents during induction, which could lead to serious complications and can even be fatal although this is relatively rare (Dean and Fawcett 2002). This is due to the potential for airway reflexes (such as coughing or laryngospasm) or gastrointestinal motor responses (such as gagging or recurrent swallowing) occurring during surgery (Asai 2004). Surgery itself can be a factor as manipulation of organs in the chest or abdominal cavities may force gastric contents up the oesophagus (Asai 2004).

Ensuring that the patient understands the rationale for fasting is important in order to reduce anxiety. For elective surgery patients are kept 'nil by mouth' long enough to allow the stomach to empty. This means that patients can have water or clear fluids up to 2 hours before surgery and solid foods up to 6 hours before, provided this is light food (AAGBI 2010, RCN 2005). However, gastric emptying can be delayed by anxiety or the action of some opiates, for example morphine (O'Callaghan 2002), so it is important to be aware of this when deciding when to commence patients 'nil by mouth'. Most patients prefer not to eat but would like to have a drink to keep their mouth moist before surgery and so are happy to comply with only fasting from water and clear fluids for 2 hours prior to surgery. Patients being fed via a nasogastric or gastrostomy tube should have their feed stopped 6 hours prior to surgery but they are able to have water up to 2 hours before surgery. Depriving elderly or unwell patients of fluids for a length of time can be detrimental to their health so in these cases other methods of hydration such as intravenous fluids should be considered (AAGBI 2010).

Skin preparation

Traditionally perioperative preparation has included the removal of body hair from the planned surgical wound site. Hair can interfere with the exposure of the incision, suturing and application of tape or dressings as well as increasing the risk of acquiring a surgical site infection (SSI) due to its associated bacteria (JBI 2008). There is around a 10% incidence of SSIs in UK patients every year, which can increase hospital stay and morbidity by delaying wound healing and causing unnecessary pain (JBI 2008).

Three methods of hair removal are currently used.

- *Shaving*: using a sharp blade held within a razor which is drawn over the patient's skin to cut hair close to the skin's surface.
- *Clipping*: using clippers with fine teeth to cut hair to about 1 mm from patient's skin. Heads of clippers are either disposable or disinfected (JBI 2008).
- *Chemical depilation*: using chemicals to dissolve hair. Cream needs to remain in contact with skin for 5–20 minutes. There is a risk of causing irritation or allergic reaction so a patch test needs to be carried out 24 hours before cream applied.

There have been two systematic reviews examining perioperative shaving (Kjonniksen *et al*. 2002, Tanner *et al*. 2006). Both conclude that shaving is not advisable. Shaving has been found to cause cuts and abrasions whereby microorganisms can enter and colonize these cuts, contaminating the surgical sites, and any exudate produced provides a culture medium which can cause postoperative wound infections (Taylor and Tanner 2005). Clippers do not come into contact with the skin and therefore reduce the risk of cuts and abrasions (Taylor and Tanner 2005).

Research from one systematic review found that the surgical site infection rates amongst patients who had hair removed prior to surgery and those who had not were not significantly different (Tanner *et al*. 2006). However, if hair will interfere with the surgical procedure and removal is essential then the following best practice is advised.

- Hair removal should be done on the day of surgery, in a location outside the operating room such as the anaesthetic room or ward. *Rationale*: prevents infection risk in operating room (Kjonniksen *et al*. 2002, Murkin 2009).
- Only hair interfering with the surgical procedure should be removed (Murkin 2009). *Rationale*: to prevent unnecessary trauma or visible difference for the patient.
- Depilation creams or clipping should be used to remove hair instead of shaving. *Rationale*: causes fewer SSIs than shaving (JBI 2008).
- If clipping is used then the clipper should be single-use electric or battery operated, or a clipper with a reusable head that can be disinfected between patients. *Rationale*: prevents cross-infection (AORN 2008).
- If using clippers it is recommended to do this on the day of surgery. *Rationale*: fewer SSIs (JBI 2008).

Marking skin for surgery

It may be that the surgeon needs to mark an area of the body for surgery. This is normally a limb to be operated on or the position of an organ such as a specific kidney in a patient undergoing a nephrectomy. The marking should be undertaken by the surgeon performing the operation or a deputy who will be present at the surgery, using an indelible pen, to ensure the correct site is marked and this should be checked against the patient's consent form (Haynes *et al.* 2009).

There are some situations in which a specialist nurse may mark the skin. Stoma therapists mark the position on the patient's skin which is the optimum place for the stoma to be placed (see Chapter 6 for further information).

Preoperative pregnancy testing

A review of the literature regarding the concerns that surgery and anaesthesia can cause congenital abnormalities or spontaneous abortion during the early gestation period has shown that there is no increase in the rate of congenital defects (Allaert *et al.* 2007). However, there is an increased risk of spontaneously aborting the foetus when undertaking surgery during the first trimester of pregnancy. It is possible that this is affected by surgical manipulation and the patient's underlying medical condition rather than exposure to anaesthesia (Allaert *et al.* 2007, Kuczkowski 2004).

Recent guidelines suggest that all women who are able to bear children should undergo pregnancy testing preoperatively to rule out this possibility (NPSA 2010). Local procedures and guidelines should be followed to ensure that the possibility of this is excluded, and that all patients have provided informed consent prior to the test being carried out (NPSA 2010).

Prevention of toxic shock syndrome from tampon use

Toxic shock syndrome (TSS) is a rare, life-threatening bacterial infection. It happens when the bacteria *Staphylococcus aureus* and *Streptococcus pyogenes*, which normally live harmlessly on the skin, enter the body's bloodstream and produce poisonous toxins. These toxins cause severe vasodilation which in turn causes a large drop in blood pressure (shock), resulting in dizziness and confusion. They also begin to damage tissue, including skin and organs, and can disturb many vital organ functions. If TSS is left untreated, the combination of shock and organ damage can result in death.

Female patients of menstruating age therefore need to be made aware of the dangers of using tampons which can cause infection leading to toxic shock syndrome.

At the time of admission it is important to ask patients if they are menstruating and to highlight the dangers of using tampons during surgery. If these are left *in situ* for longer than 6 hours, infection may develop. Nurses can offer a sanitary pad as an alternative.

Patient education

Research by several authors has shown that preoperative patient education not only meets patients' information needs but also assists in reducing anxiety levels and promotes the patients' well-being (Bondy *et al.* 1999, Jlala *et al.* 2010, Klopfenstein *et al.* 2000, Walker 2002).

Patient information booklets can also help patients to gain a greater understanding of surgery and what is expected of them.

Preoperative education can address some of the patients' concerns and fears. As pain and anaesthesia are patients' greatest worries, they need to be discussed in the preoperative period so that anxiety can be reduced (Mitchell 2000), which may result in patients requiring less analgesia (Beddows 1997). Preoperative visiting by recovery staff allows patients to ask questions, which could help them to manage their anxiety and provide baseline information about patients, which is important for effective management postoperatively, for example, of pain. It also gives information to the surgical team to allow them to maintain continuity of care in the operating department (Beddows 1997).

The control of pain while the patient is still in the operating theatre and recovering from their surgery is vital to further reduce anxiety and promote general well-being. Use of patient-controlled analgesia (PCA) gives the patient a sense of autonomy, which may decrease anxiety and which will in turn influence the patient's pain perception (Field and Adams 2001). For further information see Chapter 9.

Information about the equipment and intravenous access extension sets that the patient will be attached to postoperatively should also be provided to ensure they know what to expect and are fully informed as this can be disconcerting to both the patient when they return from theatre and the patient's relatives when they see them immediately post surgery. Additional information on when the patient will be expected to mobilize, when they can eat and drink and the length of time they can expect to be in hospital is also important at this time.

Assessment of latex allergy

Latex is a natural rubber composed of proteins and added chemicals. Its durable, flexible properties give it a high degree of protection from many micro-organisms, which make it an ideal fibre to use for many healthcare products. It currently provides the best protection against infection and gives the sensitivity and control needed in the healthcare field. It is found in the following products (AORN 2004, HSE 2004).

- Gloves.
- Airways.
- Intravenous tubing.
- Stethoscopes.
- Catheters.
- Dressings and bandages.

Some of the proteins in the natural rubber latex can cause allergic reactions and sensitivity and the incidence of latex hypersensitivity seems to be increasing (Rose 2005). Sensitivity can be described as the development of an immunological memory to specific latex proteins, which can be asymptomatic. Allergy is the visible reaction of the sensitivity, for example hives, rhinitis, conjunctivitis, anaphylaxis (AORN 2004). Anyone with sensitivity to latex is at risk of an allergic reaction, which can be serious or potentially life-threatening, and therefore sensitivities and allergies should

1045

be treated in the same way (AORN 2004). There are various types of reaction.

- *Irritation*: irritant contact dermatitis, a non-allergenic reaction caused by soaps, gloves, glove powder and hand creams. Symptoms range from dry, crusty, itchy skin to rashes and inflammation, which usually resolves when use is discontinued (AORN 2004, HSE 2004, Rose 2005).
- *Type IV reaction*: delayed hypersensitivity, sometimes known as allergic contact dermatitis caused by exposure to chemicals used in latex manufacturing. Results in red, raised, palpable area with bumps, sores and cracks usually occurring several hours within 6–48 hours of contact (AORN 2004, Rose 2005).
- *Type I reaction*: immediate hypersensitivity, sometimes called immunoglobulin E response. Caused by exposure to proteins in latex on glove surface and/or bound to powder and it can also be caused by proteins in food such as peanuts, watermelons, bananas, avocados, potatoes, tomatoes and some seafood. Symptoms include wheal and flare response, irritant and allergic contact dermatitis, facial swelling, rhinitis, urticaria, respiratory distress and asthma and on rare occasions anaphylactic shock. It occurs within minutes and can fade rapidly after removal of the latex (AORN 2004, Rose 2005).

Once sensitization has taken place, further exposure will cause symptoms to recur and increasing exposure to latex proteins increases the risk of developing allergic symptoms (HSE 2004).

Powdered gloves can create the greatest risk as proteins leak into the powder which can become airborne when gloves are removed and inhaling the powder may lead to respiratory sensitization (AORN 2004, HSE 2004).

Healthcare providers have an ethical responsibility to prevent latex sensitization and because there is no cure, protection must be paramount (AORN 2004).

Employers should have a policy on glove use which will give you information and instruction on risk of latex, safe working methods, recognizing symptoms of sensitization and the action to be taken if a sensitization is suspected (HSE 2004). There is also a voluntary scheme in place for reporting cases of latex sensitization, both of staff and patients, to the Medical Devices Agency (MDA), which is an executive agency of the Department of Health (HSE 2004).

Assessment and monitoring for symptoms of latex allergy in both the conscious and unconscious patient are required at all stages of perioperative care. The assessment should cover the following known risk factors for latex allergy (Box 17.4) (AORN 2004).

If a suspected or confirmed latex sensitivity or allergy is found, this information must be communicated to all members of the healthcare team and departments that the patient may visit, including theatre, recovery, pathology and radiology (AORN 2004, Rose 2005). The anaesthetist will need to be informed so that decisions can be made regarding potential allergy prophylaxis preoperatively (Rose 2005). The patient

1046

Box 17.4 Risk factors for latex allergy

- History of multiple surgeries beginning at an early age (e.g. spina bifida, urinary malformation).
- Known food allergies (avocado, chestnut or banana).
- History of an allergic reaction to latex.
- History of an allergic reaction during an operation.
- Past experience of itchy skin, skin rash or redness when in contact with rubber products.
- Past skin irritation from an examination by a doctor or dentist wearing rubber gloves.
- Past sneezing, wheezing or chest tightness when exposed to rubber.

is normally first on the theatre list or in a theatre that has been allowed to stand clean and empty for at least 2 hours to ensure the removal of any latex dust and products (Rose 2005). They will need to be cared for in a latex-free environment with no latex or latex products used for the patient or in the immediate care environment (AORN 2004). Box 17.5 lists preoperative actions in the event of a latex allergy.

Box 17.5 Preoperative actions in the event of a latex allergy

- Notify operating theatre of potential or confirmed latex allergy 24–48 hours (or as soon as possible) before scheduled procedure.
- Identify the patient's risk factors for latex allergy and communicate them to the healthcare team.
- Schedule the procedure as the first case of the day if the facility is not latex safe.
- Plan for a latex-safe environment of care.
- The theatre must be cleaned with latex-free gloves and equipment.
- All latex products must be removed or covered with plastics so that the rubber elements are not exposed.
- All healthcare staff in direct contact with the patient must wear vinyl gloves during procedures and in the vicinity of the patient.
- Secure latex-free products for all latex-containing items used by surgeons and anaesthetists.
- A latex-free contents box or trolley (this holds stock of all latex-free products that will be required during surgery and anaesthetic) should be ready in every theatre department and recovery room. There should be a list of all latex-free equipment with the manufacturers listed available in the box or trolley.
- Notify surgeon if no alternative product is available.
- Notify anaesthetist if latex-containing product to be used and develop plan of emergency care if necessary.
- Where a type I (immediate hypersensitivity reaction) allergy is suspected, suitable clinical management procedures must be ready for use in the event of the patient having a hypersensitivity reaction.

(AORN 2004)

Further guidance may be sought from the Association of Peri-operative Registered Nurses (AORN) proposed latex guideline at www.aorn.org/proposed/latex.htm.

Preoperative theatre checklist

The preoperative checklist (see Procedure guideline 17.2 and Figure 17.1) is the final check between the ward and the operating theatre and should be completed as fully as possible to reduce the possibility of any complications dur-ing the period that the patient is put under anaesthetic or during surgery itself.

One item on the list is ensuring that blood results and X-rays or imaging accompany the patient. The blood results are important for assessing patient haemoglobin levels which will help in transporting oxygen and also the electrolytes to identify any imbalances such as low sodium or potassium as these can interfere with anaesthetic agents and can cause cardiovascular disturbances such as arrhythmias (see Tables 17.1 and 17.2).

Procedure guideline 17.1 Antiembolic stockings: assessment, fitting and wearing

Essential equipment

- Tape measure
- Antiembolic stockings (calf or thigh length)
- Apron
- Patient records/documentation

Preprocedure

Action	Rationale
1 Assess and record in the patient's documentation the patient's risk factors for VTE, that is, DVT and PE. See Box 17.2.	All patients admitted to hospital should undergo a risk assessment for venous thrombosis to determine the most appropriate preventive measures, that is thromboprophylaxis (HoCHC 2005, C; NICE 2010, C; Roderick *et al.* 2005, C; SIGN 2002, C). The higher the number of risk factors, the greater the risk for VTE (NICE 2010, C; SIGN 2002, C).
2 Assess and record in the patient's documentation the patient's suitability for antiembolic stockings, identifying whether the patient has any contraindications to wearing antiembolic stockings (see Box 17.3).	To comply with national guidelines and hospital policy/guidelines. To ensure that antiembolic stockings are fitted correctly and to reduce the complications associated with antiembolic stockings (All Wales Tissue Viability Nurse Forum 2009, C; HoCHC 2005, C; NICE 2010, C; Rashid *et al.* 2005, E; SIGN 2002, C).
3 Explain and discuss the procedure with the patient and provide written information as follows: (a) reasons for wearing antiembolic stockings (b) how to fit and wear stockings (c) what to report to the nurse, for example any feelings of pain or numbness or skin problems (d) skin care, that is, wash and dry legs daily (e) reasons for early mobilization and adequate hydration (f) reasons for not crossing legs or ankles (g) length of time that the stockings should be worn, for example until the patient returns to their usual level of mobility.	To ensure that the patient understands the procedure and gives their valid consent (NMC 2009, C; NMC 2008, C). To ensure that the patient understands how to fit and wear stockings including self-care measures and what to report to the nurse so as to detect complications early, for example pressure sores, circulation difficulties of wearing antiembolic stockings (NICE 2010, C; SIGN 2002, C).

Procedure

4 Perform hand hygiene and put on apron prior to the procedure.	To prevent cross-infection (Pratt *et al.* 2007, E).
5 Place the tape measure around the calf at the greatest point and measure the calf circumference (and leg measurements) according to the manufacturer's instructions, recording the measurements in the patient's documentation.	To comply with the manufacturer's instructions. C Incorrect sizing causes swelling and bruising to ankles and can constrict blood supply, leading to long-term complications. C

(Continued)

1047

Procedure guideline 17.1 (*Continued*)

6 Check pedal pulses are intact.	To ensure the patient has good circulation to the feet and antiembolic stockings are not contraindicated (NICE 2010, C; SIGN 2002, C).
7 Apply the antiembolic stocking to the legs according to the manufacturer's instructions.	To ensure correct size of stocking is fitted correctly. C

Postprocedure

8 Remove stockings daily, observing for pain, skin damage, circulation difficulties which may arise as a result of wrinkling, and so on, of stocking, but for no more than 30 minutes: confirm size is applicable.	To review calf and/or leg measurements to ensure stockings fit correctly (NICE 2005, C; SIGN 2002, C). Reported complications of wearing antiembolic stockings include pressure sores (NICE 2005, C) and circulation difficulties, for example arterial occlusion, thrombosis, gangrene (SIGN 2002, C). The circulation complications can be linked to the tourniquet effect of bunched-up stockings combined with swelling of the leg (HoCHC 2005 C; SIGN 2002, C).
9 Where worn, ensure that antiembolic stockings are of the correct size and fit smoothly. Check the colour and tips of the toes. *Note:* top band of stockings must not be turned down.	To prevent a tourniquet effect if the stocking rolls down. C To ensure the blood supply is not compromised. C
10 Encourage early mobilization. For patients on bed rest, encourage deep breathing and exercises of the leg hourly, flexion/extension and rotation of the ankles.	To improve venous circulation (NICE 2010, C; SIGN 2002, C).
11 Encourage patient to sit with legs up when resting.	It is recognized that this will reduce limb swelling and promote venous return by its gravitational effect; however, there is little scientific data to clarify that this does reduce the risk of VTE. *Note*: care should be taken with patients with ischaemic legs (NICE 2007, C).
12 Monitor for signs of DVT or PE and report to medical staff immediately (see Box 17.1).	To monitor for signs of DVT and PE (NICE 2007, C; Rashid *et al.* 2005, C).
13 Monitor whether the patient has adequate hydration.	To ensure the patient is adequately hydrated (NICE 2010, C; SIGN 2002, C).
14 Record temperature daily.	To detect infection early and signs of inflammation associated with venous thrombosis. C
15 Launder according to the manufacturer's instructions.	To reduce the risk of cross-infection and promote patient comfort. C
16 On discharge from hospital, check the patient understands the following: (a) signs and symptoms of DVT (b) correct use of prophylaxis at home, for example how to wear antiembolic stocking correctly (c) implications of not using prophylaxis correctly (d) to continue to undertake leg exercises if immobile (e) to avoid long periods of travel for 4 weeks after an operation.	To reduce the risks of developing a DVT or PE after an operation and to ensure that the patient reports any symptoms promptly to enable the early detection and management of DVT and/or PE (NICE 2010, C).

Patient Care Need: Care of the Patient undergoing Surgery (Specify)

....

	◆ Potential anxiety related to a lack of knowledge about forthcoming surgery ◆ Patient safety related to surgery

Anticipated Outcome:
◆ Patient/carer will state they have an understanding of the anaesthetic, operation and the possible complications ◆ Patient will have correct surgical procedure and patient safety will be maintained throughout

Patient Care Interventions:

A	◆ Orientate patient to the ward environment / routine including the nurse call bell system and organisation of care ◆ Explain care of valuables and property
B	**Patient Assessment** ◆ Assess patient's physical and psychological concerns, their understanding of the operation and treatment/post-operative plan ◆ Check allergy status / sensitivities and infection risk e.g. Methicillin-Resistant Staphylococcus Aureus (MRSA) - Is it necessary to contact the Theatre Sister? ◆ Check and confirm pregnancy status on all women of childbearing age ◆ Ensure pre-operative blood tests (Full Blood Count, Urea & Electrolyte's, Group & Save/Cross match and blood ordered, Clotting screen, Glucose, Thyroid tests) & investigations (Chest X ray, ECG, and others – CT Scan) are completed *(see unitguidelines)* Baseline observations undertaken: Date:............... Time:...............

Height cms	Weight kg	Blood Pressure mmHg	Oxygen (O₂) Saturations (on air) %
Temperature °C	Pulse rate/min	Respirations breaths/minute	Peak Flow (if required) Litres/minute

◆ Urinalysis - Abnormalities Yes / No (circle & specify if appropriate)

Post-operative Nausea & Vomiting (PONV) Risk Assessment (Apfel's Model 1999)	**Risk Score*** (*circle)	**Obtain Level of Risk from table below** (based on Apfel's model 1999)	
Previous history of PONV or history of motion sickness	1	**Total Risk Score**	**Level of Risk of PONV**
Female	1	4	High Risk
Non-smoker	1	3	High Risk
Post-operative opioid use	1	2	Moderate Risk
Add Risk Scores & Total	....	1	Low Risk
		0	Minimal Risk

Patient with a moderate to high risk PONV score:
◆ Patients should be offered the choice of acupressure bands pre-operatively (Contact the CNS Pain Management)

Site of Acupressure Band(s)(tick):

☐ Right forearm   ☐ Left forearm   Time sited...............(24 hr clock)

◆ Check for correct placement of the acupressure band(s) site(s) and monitor for any signs of swelling, bruising or discomfort 30 minutes following application and thereafter at 4 hourly intervals
◆ To be transferred from the theatre table to their hospital bed whilst in theatres
NB this does not apply to patients with MRSA or known infections (see PONV guidelines)
Reference: Apfel C., Laara E., Koiuranta M et al (1999) A simplified risk score for predicting postoperative nausea and vomiting. *Anesthesiology* **91** (3) 693-700.

Figure 17.1 Preoperative assessment care plan. (*Continued*)

1049

Patient Care Need: Care of the Patient undergoing Surgery (continued) **Patient Care Interventions continued:**	
C	◆ Patient to Fast from (see pre-operative fasting policy): FOOD .... (24 Hr Clock) FLUIDS .... (24 Hr Clock) ◆ Complete pre-operative checklist and ensure patient has passed urine prior to administration of pre-medication (if prescribed) ◆ Administer pre-medication as prescribed (usually within **two** hours of anaesthetic induction time)
D	**Relevant information to include actual and potential medical, physical, psychological and communication problems e.g. diabetes, sight or hearing problems, pre-operative pain, language differences, phobias, pacemaker, previous surgery and anaesthetic problems** **ALLERGY STATUS** Is the patient allergic or sensitive to: drugs and/or solutions e.g. betadine and/or dressings e.g. elastoplast and/or other products e.g. latex *(NB Inform the theatre sister the day before surgery if patient has pacemaker fitted, has an infection risk or latex allergy if possible)* No Known Allergies or Sensitivities ☐ **OR** Specify allergies/sensitivities (see medical notes/prescription chart)
Patient / Carer Education:	

E	Provide information (verbal and/or written) and check understanding, reinforce as required
	 ◆ The pre-operative assessment process and investigations
	 ◆ The emotional and psychological support available
	 ◆ Inform patient of approximate theatre time for operation and duration of operation
	 ◆ Offer visit to Critical Care Unit if appropriate
	 ◆ Wearing of cotton based underwear and/or consent for the possible removal of underwear. For example if undergoing the insertion of an epidural, urinary catheterisation will be necessary.
	 ◆ Pre-operative fasting
	 ◆ Post-operative care & equipment specific to surgery as appropriate
	     ➔ potential pain/discomfort and teaching on Patient Controlled Analgesia/Epidural Analgesia
	     ➔ potential nausea & vomiting and IV hydration
	     ➔ wounds & drain care, catheters, appliances
	     ➔ anti-embolism stockings
	     ➔ positioning, deep breathing and leg exercises, physiotherapy

Additional Interventions: Tick if appropriate or add more interventions for specific surgery	

	☐ Measure and fit knee length anti-embolism stockings on the morning of the operation
	
	     Calf size ....cms Stocking size: small / medium / large / extra large (circle)
	
	 ☐ Administer bowel preparation if prescribed
	
	     Product.. Time.............................Result.............................
	
	     Enema.. Time.............................Result.............................
	
	     Suppositories................................ Time.............................Result.............................

1050

Figure 17.1 *(Continued)*

Procedure guideline 17.2 Preoperative care: theatre checklist

Essential equipment

- Identification bracelets
- Allergy bands if necessary
- Theatre gown
- Cotton-based underwear or disposable pants can be worn if wearing them does not interfere with surgery
- Antiembolic stockings
- Labelled containers for dentures, glasses and/or hearing aid if necessary

- Hypoallergenic tape
- Patient records/documentation including medical records, consent form, drug chart, X-ray films, blood test results, anaesthetic assessment, record and preoperative checklist

Procedure

Action	Rationale
1 Assess the preoperative education received by the patient and ensure that it is complete and understood.	To ensure that the patient understands the nature and outcome of the surgery to reduce anxiety and possible postoperative complications (Walker 2002, E).
2 Check that the patient has undergone relevant investigative procedures, for example X-ray, electrocardiogram (ECG), blood test and that these are included with the patient's notes.	To ensure all relevant information is available to the nurses, anaesthetists and surgeons (AORN 2000, C).
3 For female patients: (a) check and confirm pregnancy status on all women of childbearing age. If a pregnancy test is required, ensure the result is known to all healthcare professionals involved in the operation (b) if appropriate, ask the patient if she is menstruating and ensure that she has a sanitary towel in place and not a tampon.	To eliminate the possibility of unknown pregnancy prior to the planned surgical procedure. E This is to prevent infection if the tampon is left in place for longer than 2 hours (www.tamponalert.org.uk, C).
4 Check the consent form is correctly completed, signed and dated.	To comply with legal requirements and hospital policy and to ensure that the patient has understood the surgical procedure (NMC 2008, C).
5 Check the operation site is marked correctly.	To ensure the patient undergoes the correct surgery for which they have consented (AORN 2000, C).
6 Check that the patient has undergone preanaesthetic assessment by the anaesthetist.	To ensure that the patient can be given the most suitable anaesthetic and any special requirements for anaesthetic have been highlighted (AORN 2000, C).
7 Record the patient's pulse, blood pressure, respirations, temperature and weight.	To provide baseline data for comparison intra- and postoperatively. The weight is recorded so that the anaesthetist can calculate the correct dose of drugs to be administered (AORN 2000, C).
8 Instruct the patient to shower or bath as close to the planned time of the operation as possible and before a premedication is administered, if appropriate.	To minimize risk of postoperative wound infection and prevent patient accidents (Pratt *et al.* 2007, C).
9 Assist the patient to change into a theatre gown after having a shower/bath.	To reduce the risk of cross-infection, increase ease of access to operation site and avoid soiling of patient's own clothes (Pratt *et al.* 2007: R).
10 Long hair should be held back with a non-metallic tie.	For safety, to prevent hair getting caught in equipment and to reduce the risk of infection. E

(Continued)

Procedure guideline 17.2 *(Continued)*

11 All jewellery, cosmetics, nail varnish and clothing, other than the theatre gown, are to be removed. Wedding rings may be left *in situ*, but must be covered and secured with hypoallergenic tape.	Metal jewellery may be accidentally lost or may cause harm to the patient, for example diathermy burns. Facial cosmetics make the patient's colour difficult to assess. Nail varnish makes the use of the pulse oximeter, used to monitor the patient's pulse and oxygen saturation levels, impossible and masks peripheral cyanosis (Vedovato *et al.* 2004, C).
12 Valuables should be placed in the hospital's custody and recorded according to the hospital policy.	To prevent loss of valuables. E
13 Disposable or cotton underwear could be worn unless the patient is undergoing major urology or gynaecology procedure.	To maintain patient's dignity (NMC 2008, C).
14 Check whether patient passed urine before premedication.	To prevent urinary incontinence when sedated and/or unconscious and possible contamination of sterile area. E
15 Apply antiembolic stockings correctly.	To reduce the risk of postoperative deep vein thrombosis or pulmonary emboli (NICE 2010, C).
16 Ensure the patient is wearing an identification bracelet with the correct information.	To ensure correct identification and prevent possible patient misidentification (AORN 2000, C).
17 Ensure the patient is wearing an allergy alert band if appropriate.	To reduce allergic reactions to known causative agents and to alert all involved in the care of the patient in the operating theatre (AORN 2004, C).
18 Check when patient last had food or drink and ensure that it was at least 6 hours before planned operation time.	To reduce the risk of regurgitation and inhalation of stomach contents on induction of anaesthesia (Asai 2004; Dean and Fawcett 2002, C).
19 Note whether the patient has dental crowns, bridge work or loose teeth.	The anaesthetist needs to be informed to prevent accidental damage. Loose teeth or a dental prosthesis could be inhaled by the patient when an endotracheal tube is inserted. E
20 Ensure prosthesis, dentures and contact lenses are removed. Make a note of irremovable prosthesis (for example pacemaker, knee replacement) on the preoperative checklist.	To promote patient safety during surgery, for example dentures may obstruct airway, contact lenses can cause cornea abrasions. Internal non-removable prosthesis may be affected by the electric current used in diathermy. E
21 Spectacles may be retained until the patient is in the anaesthetic room. Hearing aids may be retained until the patient has been anaesthetized (these may be left in position if a local anaesthetic is being used). Any prosthesis should then be labelled clearly and retained in the recovery room.	To allow the patient to communicate fully, thus reducing anxiety and enabling the patient to understand any procedures carried out. E
22 Complete the preoperative checklist by asking the patient and checking records and notes before giving any premedication.	Questioning premedicated patients is not a reliable source of checking information as the patient may be drowsy and/or disorientated (AORN 2000, C).
23 Give the premedication, if prescribed, in accordance with the anaesthetist's instructions.	Different drugs may be prescribed to complement the anaesthetic to be given, for example temazepam to reduce patient anxiety by inducing sleep and relaxation. E
24 Advise the patient to remain in bed once the premedication has been given and to use the nurse call system if assistance is needed.	To reduce the risk of accidental patient injury as the premedication may make the patient drowsy and disorientated. E

25	Ensure the patient is supported fully on the canvas, especially the head, when transferred from the ward bed to the trolley.	To reduce the risk of injury to the neck, and so on, during transfer from the ward to the operating theatre (AORN 2001, C).
26	Ensure that all relevant information, for example X-rays, notes, blood results, accompany the patient to the operating theatre.	To prevent delays which can increase the patient's anxiety and to ensure that the anaesthetist and surgeon have all the information they require for safe treatment of the patient. E
27	The patient should be accompanied to the theatre by a ward nurse who remains present until the patient has been checked by the anaesthetic assistant/nurse and/or anaesthetized.	To reduce patient anxiety and ensure a safe environment during induction. E
28	The ward nurse should give a full handover to the anaesthetic nurse or operating department practitioner on arrival in the anaesthetic room, using patient records and the preoperative checklist.	To ensure the patient has the correct operation. To ensure continuity of care and to maintain the safety of the patient by exchanging all relevant information (AORN 2000, C).

Table 17.1 Haematology values

Test	Reference range	Functions/additional information
RBC	Men: 4.5–6.5×10^{12}/L Women: 3.9–5.6×10^{12}/L	The main function of the RBC is the transport of oxygen and carbon dioxide
Hb	Men: 13.5–17.5 g/dL Women: 11.5–15.5 g/dL	Haemoglobin (Hb) is a protein pigment found within the RBC which carries the oxygen Anaemia (deficiency in the number of RBC or in the Hb content) may occur for many reasons. Changes to cell production, deficient dietary intake or blood loss may be relevant and need to be investigated further
WBC	Men: 3.7–9.5×10^9/L Women: 3.9–11.1×10^9/L	The function of the white blood cell (WBC) is the defence against infection There are different kinds of WBC: neutrophils, lymphocytes, monocytes, eosinophils and basophils Leucopenia is a WBC count lower than 3.7 and is usually associated with the use of cytotoxic drugs Leucocytosis (high levels of neutrophils and lymphocytes) occurs as the body's normal response to infection and after surgery Leukaemia involves an increased WBC count caused by changes in cell production in the bone marrow. The leukaemic cells enter the blood in increased numbers in an immature state
Platelets	Men: 150–400×10^9/L Women: 150–400×10^9/L	Clot formation occurs when platelets and the blood protein fibrin combine. A patient may be thrombocytopenic (low platelet count) due to drugs/poor production or have a raised count (thrombocytosis) with infection or autoimmune disease
Coagulation/INR	INR range 2–3 (in some cases a range of 3–4.5 is acceptable)	Coagulation occurs to prevent excessive blood loss by the formation of a clot (thrombus). However, a clot that forms in an artery may block the vessel and cause an infarction or ischaemia which can be fatal Aspirin, warfarin and heparin are three drugs used for the prevention and/or treatment of thrombosis It is imperative that patients on warfarin therapy receive regular monitoring to ensure a balance of slowing the clot-forming process and maintaining the ability of the blood to clot

Table 17.2 Biochemistry values

Test	Reference range	Functions/additional information
Sodium	135–145 mmol/L	The main function of sodium is to maintain extracellular volume (water stored outside the cells), acid/base balance and the transmitting of nerve impulses
		Hypernatraemia (serum sodium >145 mmol/L) may be an indication of dehydration due to fluid loss from diarrhoea, excessive sweating, increased urinary output or a poor oral intake of fluid. An increased salt intake may also cause an elevation
		Hyponatraemia (serum sodium <135 mmol/L) may be indicated in fluid retention (oedema)
Potassium	3.5–5.2 mmol/L	Potassium plays a major role in nerve conduction, muscle function, acid/base balance and osmotic pressure. It has a direct effect on cardiac muscle, influencing cardiac output by helping to control the rate and force of each contraction
		The most common cause of *hyperkalaemia* (serum potassium >5.2 mmol/L) is chronic renal failure. The kidneys are unable to excrete potassium. The level may be elevated due to an increased intake of potassium supplements during treatment. Tissue cell destruction caused by trauma/cytotoxic therapy may cause a release of potassium from the cells and an elevation in the potassium plasma level. It may also be observed in untreated diabetic ketoacidosis
		Urgent treatment is required as hyperkalaemia may lead to changes in cardiac muscle contraction and cause subsequent cardiac arrest
		The main cause of *hypokalaemia* (serum potassium <3.5 mmol/L) is the loss of potassium via the kidneys during treatment with thiazide diuretics. Excessive/chronic diarrhoea may also cause a decreased potassium level
Urea	2.5–6.5 mmol/L	Urea is a waste product of metabolism that is transported to the kidneys and excreted as urine. Elevated levels of urea may indicate poor kidney function
Creatinine	55–105 µmol/L	Creatinine is a waste product of metabolism that is transported to the kidneys and excreted as urine. Elevated levels of creatinine may indicate poor kidney function
Calcium	2.20–2.60 mmol/L	Most of the calcium in the body is stored in the bone but ionized calcium, which circulates in the blood plasma, plays an important role in the transmission of nerve impulses and for the functioning of cardiac and skeletal muscle. It is also vital for blood coagulation
		High calcium levels (*hypercalcaemia* >2.6 mmol/L) can be due to hyperthyroidism, hyperparathyroidism or malignancy. Elevation in calcium levels may cause cardiac arrhythmia, potentially leading to cardiac arrest
		Tumour cells can cause excessive production of a protein called parathormone-related polypeptide (PTHrp) which causes a loss of calcium from the bone and an increase in blood calcium levels. This is a major reason for hypercalcaemia in cancer patients (Higgins 2009)
		Hypocalcaemia (<2.20 mmol/L) is often associated with vitamin D deficiency due to inadequate intake or increased loss due to GI disease. Mild hypocalcaemia may be symptomless but severe disease may cause increased neuromuscular excitability and cardiac arrhythmias. It is also a common feature of chronic renal failure (Higgins 2009)
C-reactive protein (CRP)	<10 mg/L	Elevation in the CRP level can be a useful indication of bacterial infection. CRP is monitored after surgery and for patients who have a high risk of infection. The CRP level can help monitor the severity of inflammation and assist in the diagnosis of conditions such as systemic lupus erythematous (SLE), ulcerative colitis and Crohn's disease (Higgins 2009)
Albumin	35–50 g/L	Albumin is a protein found in blood plasma which assists in the transport of water-soluble substances and the maintenance of blood plasma volume
Bilirubin	(total) <17 µmol/L	Bilirubin is produced from the breakdown of haemoglobin; it is transported to the liver for excretion in bile. Elevated levels of bilirubin may cause jaundice

Intraoperative care

Intraoperative care: anaesthesia

Definition

Intraoperative care is the physical and psychological care given to the patient in the anaesthetic room and operating theatre until transfer to the recovery room. In the anaesthetic room the patients are admitted and checked into the operating suite. When they are transferred into theatre they are already anaesthetized and are transferred onto the operating table.

Related theory

Safe administration of anaesthesia has been evolving since the early 1840s. During this time surgery was often seen as a final attempt to save life and very few operations were performed. This was because surgery was very painful and patients were conscious during the procedure and could hear everything that was being said and done. In order to support the patients, surgeons would attempt to administer alcohol, morphine and other sedatives but this would not work and most patients were restrained either with straps or held down. The surgeon had to be speedy and often the patients would either faint from pain or die from the bleeding. Then on 16th October 1846 William Morton publicly administered ether at Massachusetts General Hospital, Boston, followed shortly by James Robinson who administered the first ether anaesthetic in England on 19th December 1846. Thus began the developments in anaesthesia as in 1847, James Simpson, Professor of Obstetrics, introduced chloroform in Edinburgh. Although chloroform had severe side-effects such as sudden death and delayed liver damage, it still became popular because it worked well and was easier to use than ether. This was followed closely by the introduction of local anaesthetic in 1877 which led to infiltration anaesthesia, nerve blocks, spinal and epidural analgesia.

However, it was not until the turn of the 20th century that control of the airway using tubes in the trachea to help breathing and intravenous induction agents was introduced, enabling patients to fall asleep quickly and safely. Muscle relaxants emerged in the 1940s and today anaesthesia is very safe and there are very few deaths. Anaesthetists are highly trained and skilled physicians who provide a range of patient care such as obstetric analgesia and anaesthesia, resuscitation, pain management, major accident plan and emergency medicine in A and E.

Evidence-based approaches

Outcomes

- To ensure that the patient understands what will happen in the operating theatres at all times in order to minimize anxiety.

- To ensure that the patient has the correct surgery for which the consent form was signed.
- To ensure patient safety at all times and minimize postoperative complications by:
  - (a) giving the required care for the unconscious patient
  - (b) ensuring injury is not sustained from hazards associated with the use of swabs, needles, instruments, diathermy and power tools
  - (c) minimizing postoperative problems associated with patient positioning, such as nerve or tissue damage
  - (d) maintaining asepsis during surgical procedures to reduce the risk of postoperative wound infection in accordance with hospital policies on infection control.

Legal and professional issues

The World Health Organization safety checklist is also completed at this point in the operating room which complies with the Safety First Campaign (NPSA 2009). The purpose of this safety checklist is to ensure that the correct procedure is performed on the correct patient, encourage team work and improve communication amongst the surgical teams from all disciplines. The safety checklist comprises three parts: sign in, time out and sign out (Table 17.3, Table 17.4 and Table 17.5). Sign in is completed in the anaesthetic room before the patient is induced. It has to be read out loud with the anaesthetist and the anaesthetic assistant present.

Table 17.3 Pre-theatre safety checklist (part 1)

Action	Rationale
Has the patient confirmed his/her identity, site, procedure and consent? ☐ Yes	This is the final point of confirming the details are correct
Is the surgical site marked? ☐ Yes	To ensure surgery is performed at the correct site
Is the anaesthesia machine and medication check complete? ☐ Yes	To ensure that the equipment and all necessary drugs are at hand and in working order to prevent complications arising during induction
Does the patient have a: Known allergy? ☐ No ☐ Yes	To maintain patient's safety and to be aware of any adverse reactions
Difficult airway/aspiration risk? ☐ No ☐ Yes	To ensure that the relevant equipment and drugs are in the room
Risk of >500 mL blood loss (7 mL/kg in children)? ☐ No ☐ Yes, and adequate IV access/fluids planned?	To ensure that the adequate IV fluids are planned and rapid administration of fluids is possible

1055

Preprocedural considerations

Pharmacological support

Prior to commencing anaesthetic, the following medications may be used to ensure that the patient is comfortable, relaxed and asleep.

- *Analgesia*: this will be administered intravenously with the muscle relaxants and sleep-inducing drugs. Drugs used are very much anaesthetist dependent but could include morphine or fentanyl. This is to ensure that the patient does not feel any pain at the time of skin incision.
- *Antiemetics* are given with analgesia. These medications, such as cyclizine, metoclopramide and chlorpromazine, moderate any side-effects from administering analgesia. Antiemetics are also important to prevent inhalation if the patient vomits on arrival in the anaesthetic room or during the induction of anaesthesia. (Although the patient may have been nil by mouth, some contents may still be in the stomach, which may be vomitted as the muscles relax.)
- *Induction agents* are drugs which help to induce sleep. The mostly commonly used is propofol, a short-acting medication that can be administered twice during a procedure.

- *Inhalation agents*: once the patient has been induced, they can then be kept asleep with inhalation agents although these can cause nausea and vomiting. Examples of inhalation agents are sevoflurane and isoflurane. These are administered through vaporizers which are attached to the anaesthetic machines.
- *Muscle relaxants* are the last drugs to be administered during induction as they relax all muscles and patients are paralysed. This has to be done when the patients are asleep otherwise it can be a very frightening experience for them as they are awake but unable to move. The most commonly used relaxants/paralyzing agents are vecuronium and atracurium.

Specific patient preparation

When the patient arrives in the anaesthetic room, it is important to check the patients and their details to ensure that the correct patient is being received. At this point, consent is verified with the patient and the final phase of the preoperative checklist is completed to ensure that it is the correct patient. This is the final patient check prior to commencing surgery and is crucial to ensuring the patient's safety.

Procedure guideline 17.3 Anaesthesia: caring for patient in anaesthetic room

Equipment

- Suction
- Anaesthetic machine

- Medical gases
- Monitoring equipment

Preprocedure

Action	Rationale
1 Greet the patient by name. Confirm with the ward nurse that it is the correct patient for the scheduled operation.	To reduce patient anxiety. P

Procedure

2 Identify the patient by checking the identification band (name and patient number) against the patient's notes and the operating list.	To safeguard against patient misidentification. Questioning the premedicated patient can be unreliable (AORN 2000, C).
3 Check and confirm the correct completion of the preoperative checklist.	To ensure that all the listed measures have been completed and that any additional information has been recorded. E
4 Check that the results of the investigative procedures, for example blood results, X-rays, and so on, are included with the patient's notes.	To ensure that all the required results are available for the theatre team's use. E
5 Maintain a calm, quiet environment and explain all the procedures to the patient including the monitoring of blood pressure, pulse and oxygen saturation.	To reduce anxiety and enhance the smooth induction of anaesthesia (Mitchell 2009, E).
6 When the patient is anaesthetized, ensure that the eyes are closed and secured with hypoallergenic tape.	To prevent corneal damage due to eyes drying out or accidental abrasion. E

Postprocedure

7 When the patient has been anaesthetized, they are transferred into the operating theatre.

Intraoperative care: theatre

Related theory

Before surgical intervention (skin incision)

The team in theatre includes the anaesthetist, surgeon, registrar, anaesthetic assistant, scrub and circulating assistant. Once the patient has been transferred and positioned on the operating table, before surgical intervention, the theatre team will complete the second section of the safety checklist which is 'time out' (Table 17.4). This ensures that the team is fully aware and readily equipped for any eventuality that may arise during the procedure. WHO checklist (part 2) 'Time out' has to be read out loud for all team members to hear and respond to and has to be completed before the start of the surgical intervention, that is skin incision (Table 17.4).

Control of infection and asepsis in the operating theatre

As part of the intraoperative care, the aim of operating theatres is to provide an area free from infectious agents. Large quantities of bacteria are present in the nose and mouth, on the skin, hair and the attire of personnel; therefore, people entering the operating theatres wear clean scrub suits and lint-free surgical hats to eliminate the possibility of these

Table 17.4 WHO checklist (part 2): time out (before the surgical intervention)

Action	Rationale
Have all team members introduced themselves by name and role? ☐ Yes	For all to understand and accept the roles and responsibilities. Also encourages confidence and team building
Surgeon, anaesthetist and registered practitioner verbally confirmed: ☐ What is the patient's name? ☐ What procedure, site and position are planned?	This is to confirm the identity of the patient and the procedure to be performed and site to prevent wrong site surgery
Anticipated critical events Surgeon: ☐ How much blood loss is anticipated? ☐ Are there any specific equipment requirements or special investigations? ☐ Are there any critical or unexpected steps you want the team to know about?	To ensure that all necessary equipment is ready in theatre and there is no time delay in the procedure and to ensure that every eventuality is covered. Also, the surgeon is aware if there any problems with equipment at the start so that they are prepared
Anaesthetist: ☐ Are there any patient-specific concerns? ☐ What is the patient's ASA grade? ☐ What monitoring equipment and other specific levels of support are required, for example blood?	The ASA grade indicates patient's suitability for anaesthesia
Nurse/ODP: ☐ Has the sterility of the instrumentation been confirmed (including indicator results)? ☐ Are there any equipment issues or concerns? ☐ Levels of support required, for example blood?	
Has the SSI bundle been undertaken? ☐ Yes/Not applicable ☐ Antibiotic prophylaxis within the last 60 minutes ☐ Patient warming ☐ Hair removal ☐ Glycaemic control	This is to minimize the risk of postoperative infection which could lead to increased length of stay in hospital
Has VTE prophylaxis been undertaken? ☐ Yes/Not applicable	To prevent development of DVT on the operating table
Is essential imaging displayed? ☐ Yes/Not applicable	To support the surgeon during the procedure

bacteria, hair or dandruff being shed into the environment (Tammelin *et al.* 2000). Well-fitting shoes with impervious soles should be worn and regularly cleaned to remove splashes of blood and body fluids (Woodhead *et al.* 2002). Facemasks are worn to prevent droplets falling from the mouth into the operating field. The extent to which face masks are capable of preventing droplet spread is disputed (Lipp and Edwards 2002). It is, however, accepted that masks offer protection to the wearer from blood splashes and for safety reasons should be worn by the scrub team. Instruments must be handled carefully and needle holders and forceps used to manipulate sutures to minimize the risk of needlestick or sharps injury.

Minimally invasive surgery (laparoscopic surgery)

Specialties using this technique are:

- general surgery
- gynaecology
- gastrointestinal surgery
- urology.

Laparoscopy involves insufflation of the abdomen with carbon dioxide (CO_2). Prolonged insufflation can cause hypothermia as although the gas temperature in the hose equals room temperature, the temperature in the abdomen can decrease to 27.7°C due to high gas flow and the large amounts of gas used (Jacobs *et al.* 2000). Sharma *et al.* (1997) refer to the increased risk of hypercarbia and surgical emphysema during insufflation with CO_2. Careful monitoring and recording of the patient's vital signs, including oxygen saturation and expiratory gas levels, are therefore essential during laparoscopy. Haemorrhage can occur during the procedure and may be difficult to detect because surgeons have a limited view of the area being operated upon. Electrosurgical injuries to organs may occur as a result of capacitive coupling (the transfer of electrical currents from the active electrode through coupling of stray currents into other conductive surgical equipment) (Wu *et al.* 2000). Theatre staff must be aware of potential complications and ensure that equipment is used safely and according to the manufacturer's instructions.

Evidence-based approaches
Rationale

The position of the patient on the operating table must be such as to facilitate access to the operation site(s) by the surgeon, and the patient's airway for the anaesthetist. It will also be dependent upon the type of surgery being performed, position of monitoring equipment and intravenous devices *in situ*. It should not compromise the patient's circulation, respiratory system or nerves.

Preoperative assessment will identify patients who may need extra precautions during positioning because of their weight, nutritional state, age, skin condition or pre-existing disease. Pre-existing conditions such as backache or sciatica can be exacerbated, particularly if the patient is in the lithotomy position, as the sciatic nerve can be compressed against the poles (AORN 2001). Most postoperative palsies are due to incorrect positioning of the patient on the operating table (Alison and Beckett 2010). Consideration by and the co-operation of all theatre personnel can help prevent many of the postoperative complications related to intraoperative positioning and this remains a team responsibility (AORN 2001, Alison and Beckett 2010).

All movements of the limbs of the unconscious patient should take into account the anatomy and natural planes of movement of that limb to avoid stretching and pressure on the related nerve planes (AORN 2001). Hyperabduction of the arm when placed on a board, for example, could stretch the brachial plexus, causing some postoperative loss of sensation and reduced movement of the forearm, wrist and fingers. To prevent this, the board should be angled at 45° and not 90° with hands facing more towards the feet rather than the head. The ulnar and radial nerves may be affected by direct pressure as a result of insufficient padding on arm supports.

Compartment syndrome is a life-threatening complication of the Lloyd Davies position (Figure 17.2) and occurs when perfusion falls below tissue pressure in a closed anatomical space or compartment such as hand, forearm, buttocks, legs, upper arms and feet. It develops through a combination of prolonged ischaemia and reperfusion of muscle within a tight

Figure 17.2 Patient in Lloyd Davies position.

osseofascial compartment (Malik *et al.* 2009). Untreated, it can lead to necrosis, functional impairment, possible renal failure and death (Callum and Bradbury 2000, Paula 2002). If patients are placed in Lloyd Davies position and Trendelenburg tilt for longer than 4 hours, the legs should be removed from the support every 2 hours, or as close to 2 hours as possible, for a short period of time to prevent reperfusion injury (Raza *et al.* 2004). The use of compression stockings and intermittent compression devices in the Lloyd Davies position needs to be reviewed as this may contribute to compartment syndrome (Malik *et al.* 2009). There is insufficient evidence to suggest that use of one device over another will reduce the risk of compartment syndrome, nor is there enough evidence to recommend use of both devices at the same time because this will place pressure on the calf in the Lloyd Davies position. The use of devices will depend very much on the surgeon and anaesthetist and the patient's co-morbidity.

Methods of infection prevention

It is imperative that during surgical procedure infection prevention is maintained at all times. The area around the patient and the scrub assistant's trolley area are all classified as a sterile field meaning that only those staff who have donned gloves and gowns after washing their hands can access this area. Presurgical handwashing is essential to the maintenance of asepsis in the operating theatre. New research has recommended a 1-minute hand wash with a non-antiseptic soap followed by hand rubbing with liquid aqueous alcoholic solution, prior to each surgeon's first procedure of the day (Tanner *et al.* 2007). Before subsequent procedures the process should be repeated. However, this is applicable to minor cases only. This has been shown to be as effective as traditional hand scrubbing with antiseptic soap in preventing surgical site infections (Parienti *et al.* 2002). However, the traditional 3-minute first scrub of the day is recommended for all intermediate, major and complex cases.

Surgical gloves have a dual role, acting as a barrier for personal protection from the patient's blood and other exudate and preventing bacterial transfer from the surgeon's hand to the operating site. It has been suggested that double gloving significantly reduces the number of perforations to the innermost glove in high-risk surgical patients, thus reducing infection rates during surgical procedures (Tanner and Parkinson 2002).

Legal and professional issues

Transferring and positioning

When a patient is transferred between the trolley or bed and operating table, adequate personnel should be present to ensure patient and staff safety (AORN 2001). It is recommended that an approved rolling or sliding device is used to transfer patients from trolley to operating table, in compliance with legislation on manual handling.

Figure 17.3 Flowtron machine and boots.

Safe manual handling and the safety of the patient depend on the participation of the correct number of staff in the specified handling manoeuvre. There should be a minimum of four staff: one at either end of the patient to support the head and the feet and one on either side. Additional staff may be required if the patient weighs over 90 kg.

Once the patient has been positioned safely, the intermittent compression device is attached. Figure 17.3 shows the Flowtron machine used in prevention of deep vein thrombosis in conjunction with VTE stockings.

Preprocedural considerations
Equipment

In the operating room the staff should ensure that all equipment is ready and checked before the first patient is sent for.

- *Anaesthetic machine and vital signs monitor*: this allows the anaesthetists to administer the correct dosage of oxygen and air whilst the monitor displays what is happening to the cardiovascular system such as heartbeat, blood pressure and also the level of oxygen in the blood.
- *Suction unit* (Figure 17.4): this is attached to the anaesthetic machine and will help in the event of obstruction or aspiration due to vomit.

Figure 17.4 High vacuum suction unit.

- *Vaporizer*: this is also attached to the anaesthetic machine and helps to administer inhaling anaesthetic agents. This allows the patient to remain asleep during the procedure.
- *Scavenging system*: this absorbs and draws away all the anaesthetic gases that the patient exhales so it is important to ensure that this is operational. If it isn't the exhaled gases would be released into the air and can be harmful to the staff (Beths 2006).
- *Operating table*: as part of the equipment check, the operating table is assessed to ensure it is fully operational and performs all the required functions to enable correct positioning of the patient. It is also possible to adjust the height of the operating table in relation to the height of the surgeon and team to prevent any unnecessary strain on the back and neck. The power to the table is provided by a battery. This is charged overnight via the mains.
- *Diathermy machine*: diathermy is used routinely during surgery to control haemorrhage by sealing bleeding vessels or cutting body tissues. It uses heat from electricity and this is achieved by passing normal electrical current through the diathermy machine and converting it into a high-frequency alternating current. There are two types of diathermy.

– *Monopolar*: this works by producing current from an active electrode such as diathermy forceps, which are insulated so that the skin does not come into contact with metal, and then returned back to the machine through another electrode such as a patient diathermy plate/pad. This creates a complete circuit.
– *Bipolar*: this does not require a patient diathermy plate/pad. It works by current coming from the machine down one side of the forceps prong, through the tissue and back to the machine through the other side of the forceps prong.

Diathermy is potentially hazardous to the patient if used incorrectly. The main risk when using diathermy is of thermoelectrical burns. The most common cause is incorrect application of the patient plate or a break in the connecting lead (Vedovato *et al.* 2004) or if the patient is in contact with metal. The machine will automatically switch off or will alarm if the neutral electrodes become loose from the patient, but if the patient is in contact with metal this is a little harder to identify. To prevent these injuries, only equipment fitted with adaptive neutral electrodes should be used. It is important that all theatre nurses know how to test and use all diathermy equipment in their department to prevent patient injury (Molyneux 2001, Wicker 2000). This involves checking that the cables and plugs are not damaged and indicator lights are all in working order. It is also important to check alarms to ensure that these are activated if the circuit is broken in any way during surgery.

Other causes of burns include skin preparation solutions or other liquids pooling around the plate site (Fong *et al.* 2000). With alcohol-based skin preparations especially, the skin should be allowed to dry before diathermy is used, as the alcohol can ignite (Fong *et al.* 2000).

If the patient's position is changed during the operation, the diathermy patient plate should be rechecked to ensure that it is still in contact and that the connecting clamp or lead is not causing pressure in the new position. Use of diathermy and the plate position should be noted on the nursing care plan and the patient's skin condition (plate site, pressure areas, and other areas where exposure to metal could have occurred) should be checked before the patient is transferred to the recovery unit.

The use of an electrosurgical diathermy unit during surgical procedures results in a smoke by-product from the coagulation or cutting of tissue. This smoke plume can be harmful to the perioperative personnel because it can contain:

- toxic gases and vapours such as benzene, hydrogen cyanide and formaldehyde
- bio-aerosols
- dead and live cellular material, including blood fragments
- viruses.

(Allen 2004)

To reduce the risk to staff and patients, an efficient filtered evacuation system should be used, such as a smoke evacuation machine; piped hospital suction must not be used (Scott *et al.* 2004).

Figure 17.5 Laparoscopy equipment.

Figure 17.6 Laparoscopic equipment.

- The *suction unit* is also checked to ensure that it is patent and the suction power is adequate to withdraw excessive bodily fluids from the operating site. This is a mobile unit which has the ability to allow high suction power.
- The *operating lights* need to be bright enough to ensure that the procedure is fully illuminated. These are checked to ensure they are bright and all the lamps are in working order prior to every operation.
- The *Flowtron machine* is the intermittent compression device which is used in prevention of DVT in conjunction with VTE stockings.

Equipment for laparoscopy procedure

- Camera system (consisting of light source, camera, insufflator, DVD recorder and monitors × 2). See Figure 17.5.
- Laparoscope.
- Laparoscopy-specific instruments (scissors, biopsy forceps, grabbers, dissectors, ports, retrieval pouches, insufflating tube, light lead). See Figure 17.6.

The equipment used for laparoscopic surgery is very specialized. The AORN recommends that all equipment is regularly and competently maintained and a maintenance record kept in a log (AORN 2000, Wicker and O'Neill 2006). Policies should be developed for the checking procedure, and all staff thoroughly instructed in the operation of laparoscopic equipment. The staff must be able to 'white balance' the camera to ensure clarity of colour and picture (this is done before use) and set the pressure and flow rate of the insufflator for insufflating the abdomen with carbon dioxide. The surgeon will determine the level to achieve and this will be activated at the beginning of the procedure.

Procedure guideline 17.4 Operating theatre procedure

Procedure

Action	Rationale
1 Prior to transferring the patient from the trolley to the operating table, check with the anaesthetist that the patient's airway is protected, patent and safe.	To prevent complications with breathing. E
2 Ensure that there are adequate staff to transfer the patient onto the operating table. Ensure the brakes on the trolley and operating table have been applied. Ensure the patient's head and limbs are supported when transferring to the operating table.	To prevent patient injury during the transfer between trolley and operating table (AORN 2001, C).
3 When transferring the patient, ensure all limbs are supported and secure on the table. Ensure adequate padding and cushioning of bony prominences. The patient's position will be dictated by the nature of the surgery but must take into account the requirements of the anaesthetist and the physical needs of the patient.	If the patient is unconscious and unable to maintain a safe environment, support is necessary to prevent injury. Nerve damage due to compression or stretching must be prevented.

The patient is especially at risk from damage due to pressure and stretching, so measures to maintain the skin's integrity are vital (AORN 2001, C). |

(Continued)

Procedure guideline 17.4 (*Continued*)

4 Ensure the patient is covered by the gown or blanket. These items should only be removed immediately before surgery.	To maintain the patient's dignity. To help prevent a reduction in body temperature or accidental hypothermia. E
5 Use a warm air mattress on the operating table. Ensure all fluids used are warmed if possible.	To help maintain the patient's body temperature and prevent postoperative complications due to hypothermia. E
6 Ensure the diathermy patient plate is attached securely in accordance with the manufacturer's instructions and hospital policy.	To ensure that no injury is sustained from the use of diathermy during surgery (Molyneux 2001, C).
7 Follow hospital policy for the checking of swabs, needles and instruments.	To ensure that swabs, needles and instruments are accounted for at the end of the operation. C
8 Follow hospital policy for the disposal of sharps and clinical waste that is not needed at this point.	To reduce the risk of injury to the patient and staff (Pratt *et al.* 2007, C).

Intraoperative care: recovery

Definition

Postanaesthetic recovery involves the short-term critical care required by patients during their immediate postoperative period within the recovery room, until they are stable, conscious, orientated and safe to transfer back to the ward. The postanaesthetic recovery room is an area within the operating department specifically designed, equipped and staffed for the support, monitoring and assessment of patients through the reversing stages of anaesthesia.

Evidence-based approaches

Prior to transfer to postanaesthetic recovery unit

Once the procedure in the operating room has been completed and the patient is ready to be transferred to the posta-naesthetic unit, the final part of the WHO checklist (part 3) has to be completed (Table 17.5). This is done before any member of the team can leave the operating theatre.

Postanaesthetic care

Postanaesthetic care can best be described and understood as a series of many nursing procedures performed in sequence and simultaneously on patients who are in an artificially induced and traumatized condition. These patients will display varying degrees of responsiveness and physical and emotional states. It is important to establish a rapport with each individual to gain the patient's confidence and co-operation and to aid assessment. It is also necessary to understand that when emerging from the final stage of anaesthesia, some patients can behave in an emotional and disinhibited fashion, at variance with their normal behaviour (Eckenhoff *et al.* 1961, Radtke *et al.* 2008). These displays are always transient and fortunately patients seldom have any recollection of them. Most patients will have an uneventful recovery following surgery.

Table 17.5 WHO checklist (part 3): sign out (before leaving the operating theatre)

Action	Rationale
Registered practitioner verbally confirms with the team:	
■ Has the name of the procedure been recorded?	This is to ensure that the correct information is recorded as verified by the team and all equipment has been accounted for. Also to ensure that the patient is now safe to be transferred out of theatre
■ Has it been confirmed that instruments, swabs and sharps counts are complete (or not applicable)?	
■ Have the specimens been labelled (including patient's name)?	
■ Have any equipment problems been identified that need to be addressed?	
Surgeon, anaesthetist and registered practitioner	To ensure continuity of care and that the recovery nurse has the information to care for the patient in the PACU
■ What are the key concerns for recovery and management of this patient?	

Hypothermia may be a problem, with the symptoms mimicking those of other postoperative complications, which may result in inappropriate treatment. Hypothermia interferes with the effective reversal of muscle relaxants, so monitor patients who are shivering, restless, confused or with respiratory depression (Feldmann, 1988). Shivering puts an increased demand on cardiopulmonary systems as oxygen consumption is increased (Feldmann, 1988, Frank *et al.* 1993). Other complications such as arrhythmias or myocardial infarct can result and the longer the duration of the postoperative hypothermia, the greater the patient mortality (Crayne and Miner, 1988, Frank *et al.* 1993).

Transfer of patient from operating theatre to peri-anaesthesia care unit

The patient is accompanied from the operating theatre to the peri-anaesthesia care unit (PACU) with the anaesthetist and the scrub assistant. They will refer to the theatre care plan which would have identified care given during the procedure. The anaesthetic assistant will ensure that the patient is monitored for heart rate and oxygen saturations during the transfer and also that portable suction is available.

Preprocedural considerations

The recovery period is potentially hazardous. Therefore, when the patient arrives in the PACU, individual nursing care is required until patients are able to maintain their own airway (AAGBI 2002).

Equipment required in the PACU

Speed, efficiency and economy of movement are essential when time becomes a critical factor in the ultimate safety of the patient in the recovery room.

- *Basic equipment for monitoring airway maintenance*: wall-mounted piped oxygen with tubing and facemask (with both fixed and variable settings), a T-piece and full range of oral and nasopharyngeal airways. Spare oxygen cylinders with flowmeters should also be available in case of piped oxygen failure.
- *Suction*: regulator with tubing and a range of oral and endotracheal suction catheters. An electric-powered portable suction machine should also be available in case of pipeline vacuum failure.
- *Sphygmomanometer and stethoscope*: automatic blood pressure recorders are a valuable means of saving time and minimizing disturbance to patients, especially those in pain or disorientated, leaving the nurse's hands free to attend to other needs. However, such equipment can be non-functioning in certain cases, for example shivering

or profoundly bradycardic patients, or if electrical and mechanical failure occurs. Therefore, manual equipment must always be available.
- *Pulse oximeter.*
- *Miscellaneous items*: receivers, tissues, disposable gloves, sharps container and waste receptacle.

These should be available at the patient's head in each recovery bay and the equipment should be compatible between the operating theatres and the recovery room. This must be arranged for ease of access and always be clean and in full working order.

There should be other equipment centrally available for respiratory and cardiovascular support.

- *Self-inflating resuscitator bag*, for example Ambu-bag and/or Mapleson C circuit with facemask. These allow maintenance of a clear airway by titlting the chin upwards and administering oxygen.
- *Full intubation equipment*: laryngoscopes with spare bulbs and batteries, range of endotracheal tubes, bougies and Magill forceps, syringe and catheter mount. This is to ensure that the patient can be intubated quickly during an emergency.
- *Anaesthetic machine and ventilator*: to ensure that the patient can be reventilated if extubated too early or not fully reversed from the anaesthetic.
- *Wright respirometer*: to measure that the patient is breathing deeply enough to allow adequate gaseous exchange.
- *Cricothyroid puncture set*: to access the thyroid surgical site to release pressure and prevent airway obstruction due to a haematoma. This is an emergency situation.
- *Range of tracheostomy tubes and tracheal dilator*: in case an emergency tracheostomy needs to be performed.
- *Intravenous infusion sets and cannulae, range of intravenous fluids.*
- *Central venous cannulas and manometer*: in case an insertion is required in recovery and to allow manual measurement of the central venous pressure (monitor failure).
- *Emergency drug box/trolley*: contents in accordance with current hospital policy. This is to ensure that all emergency drugs are in one place in the event of a cardiac/respiratory arrest.
- *Defibrillator*: required during a cardiac arrest to restart the heart.

Further support equipment, such as nerve stimulators, should be available centrally, whenever possible being stored on trolleys for ease of transportation (AAGBI 2002).

Procedure guideline 17.5 Transfer to PACU

Procedure

Action	**Rationale**
1 The scrub nurse accompanies the patient with the anaesthetist to the recovery area. A handover is given that includes:	To ensure continuity and effective communication of care for the patient. To ensure that the recovery nurse has all the information required to assess the patient's recovery needs. C
■ the surgical procedure performed	The actual procedure performed may be different from the proposed procedure. E
■ information including allergies or pre-existing medical conditions, for example diabetes mellitus	To highlight specific potential postoperative complications to be assessed and monitored. E
■ the patient's cardiovascular state and pattern of anaesthesia used	To maintain the patient's immediate postoperative safety with cardiovascular system and airway. E
■ the presence, position and nature of any drains, infusions or intravenous or arterial devices	To ensure care and management of these drains are continued and the positioning of the patient is assessed to prevent any occlusion of drains or infusions. E
■ information about any anxieties of the patient expressed before surgery, such as a fear of not waking after anaesthesia or fear about coping with pain	To ensure that appropriate action can be taken as the patient regains consciousness and to enable assessment of the efficacy of nursing interventions used. E
■ specific instructions from the anaesthetist for postoperative care.	To facilitate effective communication of the patient's care and treatment. E

Postprocedure

2 All information is to be recorded in the perioperative nursing care plan.

Procedure guideline 17.6 Patients in PACU

The following recommended actions are not necessarily listed in order of priority. Many will be carried out simultaneously and much will depend on the patient's condition, surgery and level of consciousness. All actions must be accompanied by commentary and explanation regardless of the patient's apparent responsiveness, as the sense of hearing returns before the patient's ability to respond (Levinson 1965, Starritt 1999).

Equipment

- Self-inflating resuscitator bag, for example Ambu-bag and/or Mapleson C circuit with facemask
- Full intubation equipment: laryngoscopes with spare bulbs and batteries, range of endotracheal tubes, bougies and Magill forceps, syringe and catheter mount
- Anaesthetic machine and ventilator
- Wright respirometer
- Cricothyroid puncture set
- Range of tracheostomy tubes and tracheal dilator
- Central venous cannulas and manometer
- Emergency drug box/trolley: contents in accordance with hospital policy
- Defibrillator

Procedure

Action

Action	Rationale
1 Assess the patency of the airway by feeling for movement of expired air.	To determine the presence of any respiratory depression or neuromuscular blockade. Observe chest and abdominal movement, respiratory rate, depth and pattern (Drummond 1991, C).
2 Listen for inspiration and expiration. Apply suction if indicated. Observe any use of accessory muscles of respiration and check for tracheal tug.	To ensure airway is clear and laryngeal spasm is not present. E
3 If indicated, support the chin with the neck extended.	In the unconscious patient the tongue is liable to fall back and obstruct the airway, and protective reflexes are absent. E
4 Suction of the upper airway is indicated if gurgling sounds are present on respiration and if blood secretions or vomitus are evident or suspected, and the patient is unable to swallow or cough either at all or adequately. Suction must be applied with care to avoid damage to mucosal surfaces and further irritation or initiation of a gag reflex or laryngeal spasm.	Foreign matter can obstruct the airway or cause laryngeal spasm in light planes of anaesthesia. It can also be inhaled when protective laryngeal reflexes are absent (Dhara 1997, C).
5 Endotracheal suction is performed following the same procedure as that for suction of tracheostomy tubes (see Chapter 10).	To maintain the patency of the tube and remove secretions (Dhara 1997, C).
6 Apply a facemask and administer oxygen at the rate prescribed by the anaesthetist. If an endotracheal tube or laryngeal mask is in position, check whether the cuff or mask is inflated and administer oxygen by means of a T-piece system.	To maintain adequate oxygenation. Oxygen should be administered to all patients in the recovery room (Nimmo *et al.* 1994, C).
7 Observe skin colour and temperature. Check the colour of lips and conjunctiva, then peripheral colour and perfusion.	Central cyanosis indicates impaired gaseous exchange between the alveoli and pulmonary capillaries. Peripheral cyanosis indicates low cardiac output (Nimmo *et al.* 1994, C).
8 Feel and assess the pulse. The patient's position will probably mean that the head, carotid, facial or temporal arteries will offer the easiest access. Note the rate, rhythm and volume, and record.	To assess cardiovascular function and establish a postoperative baseline for future comparisons (Peskett 1999, C).
9 Obtain full information about:	To ensure effective communication of the patient's care and treatment and to aid the planning of subsequent care. E

- anaesthetic technique, potential problems, and the patient's general medical condition
- surgical procedure performed
- the presence of drains and packs
- amount of blood loss
- specific postoperative instructions, and hand it over verbally to ensure that there is no delay in providing immediate care.

Action	Rationale
10 Record blood pressure, pulse and respiratory rate measurements on reception and at a minimum of 5-minute intervals unless the patient's condition dictates otherwise.	To enable any fluctuations or gross abnormalities in cardiovascular and respiratory functions to be detected immediately (Peskett 1999, C).

(Continued)

Procedure guideline 17.6 *(Continued)*

11 Check the temperature of the patient, especially those who are at high risk of hypothermia (Nunney 2008), for example the elderly, children, those who have undergone long surgery or where large amounts of blood or fluid replacement therapy have been used. Temperature must be measured hourly or half-hourly if hypothermic. Use Bair Hugger blankets (see Action Figure 11) and extra blankets to warm the patient.	More than 70% of patients undergoing surgery experience some degree of postoperative hypothermia (Wagner 2003, C).
12 Check and observe wound site(s),dressings and drains. Note and record leakage/drainage on the postoperative chart and also on the drain bottle/bag.	To assess and monitor for signs of haemorrhage (Eltringham *et al.* 1989, C).
13 Check that intravenous infusions are running at the correct prescribed rate and the site of the venous device is satisfactory.	Care of venous devices/sites prevents complications and ensures that fluid replacement and balance is achieved safely. E
14 Check the prescription chart for medications to be administered during the immediate postoperative period, for example analgesia and antiemetics.	To treat symptoms swiftly and appropriately and to monitor their effectiveness. E
15 Orientate the patient to time and place as frequently as is necessary.	To alleviate anxiety, provide reassurance, and gain the patient's confidence and co-operation. Premedication and anaesthesia can induce a degree of amnesia and disorientation. C
16 Give mouth care (see Chapter 9).	Preoperative fasting, drying gases and manipulation of lips, and so on, leave mucosa vulnerable, sore and foul tasting. E
17 After regional and/or spinal anaesthesia, assess the return of sensation and mobility of limbs. Check that the limbs are anatomically aligned.	To prevent inadvertent injury following sensory loss (AAGBI 2002, C).

Action Figure 11 Bair Hugger.

Problem-solving table 17.1 Prevention and resolution (Procedure guideline 17.6)

Problem	Cause	Prevention	Suggested action
Airway obstruction	Tongue occluding the airway	Do not remove the laryngeal mask or the Guedel airway until the patient starts responding to commands	Support chin forward from the angle of the jaw. If necessary insert a Guedel airway. Use a nasopharyngeal airway if the teeth are clenched or crowned
	Foreign material, blood, secretions, vomitus	Use suction to remove sercretions when removing airway	Apply suction. Always check for the presence of a throat pack
	Laryngeal spasm	Do not remove airway until patient responds to commands and ensure oxygen flow is high (5–10 litres) on arrival in PACU	Increase the rate of oxygen. Assist ventilation with an Ambu-bag and facemask. If there is no improvement, inform anaesthetist and have intubation equipment ready. Offer the patient reassurance by talking to them and telling them what you are doing
Hypoventilation	Respiratory depression from medications, for example opiates, inhalations, barbiturates.	Monitor depth and rate of respiration before administering analgesia	Inform the anaesthetist, keeping oxygen on, and administer antagonist on instruction, for example naloxone (opiate antagonist), doxapram (respiratory stimulant). Note: if naloxone is given it can reverse the analgesic effects of opiates and has a duration of action of only 20–30 minutes. The patient must be observed for signs of returning hyperventilation (Nimmo et al. 1994)
	Decreased respiratory drive from a low partial pressure of carbon dioxide ($PaCO_2$), loss of hypoxic drive in patients with chronic pulmonary disease	Ensure that Venturi masks are available and close to hand in the recovery bay	Administer oxygen using a Venturi mask with graded low concentrations (Atkinson et al. 1982)
	Neuromuscular blockade from continued action of non-depolarizing muscle relaxants, potentiation of relaxants caused by electrolyte imbalance, impaired excretion with renal or liver disease		Inform the anaesthetist, have available neostigmine and glycopyrrolate, or atropine potassium chloride and 10% calcium chloride. Often the blockade is mild and will wear off in minutes without treatment, but it is extremely frightening and patients will need continuous reassurance that their condition is not unnoticed and is resolving and that they will not be left alone
Hypotension	Hypovolaemia	Increase the rate of fluids and ensure more fluids are prescribed	Take manual reading of the blood pressure. Take CVP readings if catheter is in place. Give oxygen. Lower the head of the trolley unless contraindicated, for example hiatus hernia, gross obesity. Check the record of anaesthetic agents used which might cause hypotension, for example enflurane, beta-blockers, nitroprusside, opiates, droperidol, sympathetic blockade following spinal anaesthesia. Check the peripheral perfusion. If the CVP is low, increase intravenous infusion unless contraindicated, for example congestive cardiac failure. Check drains and dressings for visible bleeding and haematoma. Inform the anaesthetist or surgeon

(Continued)

Problem-solving table 17.1 *(Continued)*

Problem	Cause	Prevention	Suggested action
Hypertension	Pain, carbon dioxide retention. This may be due to retention during laparoscopic procedures	Ensure pain is assessed as soon as patient is responding to commands and scores are recorded	Treat pain with prescribed analgesia and provide a quiet environment to enable them to rest/sleep. Pain from certain operation sites can also be alleviated by changing the patient's position
	Fluid overload	Slow the intravenous rate	Check fluid balance sheet and the rate of intravenous infusion
	Distended bladder	Check if cather is patent	Offer a bedpan or urinal and if necessary catheterize the patient
	Some anaesthetic drugs given during reversal of anaesthetic	Ensure the anaesthetist monitors patient when reversing effects of anaesthetic drugs	Check the prescription chart for those patients on regular antihypertensive therapy. If the situation is not resolved, inform the anaesthetist. Also check patient's past medical history
Bradycardia	Very fit patient, opiates, reversal agents, beta-blockers, pain, vagal stimulation, hypoxaemia from respiratory depression	Ensure oxygen is administered and anaesthetist identifies any adverse episodes of bradycardia during surgery	Connect the patient to the ECG monitor to exclude heart block and monitor cardiac activity. Ascertain preoperative cardiac function. Check the prescription chart and anaesthetic sheet for medication administered that may cause bradycardia. Inform and liaise with the anaesthetist
Tachycardia	Pain, hypovolaemia, some anaesthetic drugs, for example ephedrine, septicaemia, fear, fluid overload	Ensure pain is managed and intravenous fluids are adminstered	Assess patient's pain and provide analgesia. Check the anaesthetic chart to ascertain which anaesthetic drugs were used. Connect the patient to the ECG monitor to exclude ventricular tachycardia. Provide reassurance for the patient. Assess fluid balance
Pain	Surgical trauma, worsened by fear, anxiety and restlessness	Adminster analgesia after assessing patient's pain	Provide prescribed analgesia and assess its efficacy. Reassure and orientate the patients, who can be unaware that surgery has been performed, in which case their pain is more frightening. Try positional changes where feasible; for example, experience has shown that after breast surgery some relief can be obtained from raising the back support by 20–40°; patients with abdominal or gynaecological surgery can be more comfortable lying on their side; elevate limbs to reduce swelling where appropriate. Unless significant relief is obtained, inform the anaesthetist and the pain control specialist nurse
Nausea and vomiting	Anaesthetic agents, opiates, hypotension, abdominal surgery, pain; high-risk patients who have a history of postoperative nausea and vomiting	Administer antiemetics with the analgesia and ensure intravenous fluids are administered as prescribed	Administer intravenous antiemetics and monitor effectiveness. Encourage slow, regular breathing. If the patient is unconscious, turn onto the side, tip the head down and suck out pharynx, give oxygen. Note: have wire-cutters available if the jaws are wired

Problem	Cause	Prevention	Suggested action
Hypothermia	Depression of the heat-regulating centre, vasodilation, following abdominal surgery, large infusions of unwarmed blood and fluids	Measure and record the patient's temperature upon arrival in the PACU and maintain temperature using a Bair Hugger	Use extra blankets or a Bair Hugger (Kumar *et al.* 2005). Monitor the patient's temperature. Administer warm intravenous fluids. In the event of bladder irrigation this should also be warmed but care has to be taken that the temperature of the warming cabinet is not too hot as this could burn the patient. The temperature should be the same as normal body temperature
Shivering	Some inhalational anaesthetics, hypothermia	Measure and record the patient's temperature upon arrival in the PACU and maintain temperature using a Bair Hugger Measure temperature every 30–60 mins	Give oxygen, reassure the patient and take their temperature. Provide a Bair Hugger and warm blankets
Hyperthermia	Infection, blood transfusion reaction	Measure and record temperature at least every 30–60 mins	Give oxygen, use a fan or tepid sponging if this is warranted. Medical assessment of antibiotic therapy and obtaining blood cultures. Administer intravenous paracetamol if prescribed
	Malignant hyperpyrexia (above 40°)	This will be identified at the time of induction and all personnel will know the location of the emergency drugs	Malignant hyperpyrexia is a medical emergency and a malignant hyperpyrexia pack with the necessary drugs should be readily available at a central point in theatre. All personnel must know its location
Oliguria	Mechanical obstruction of catheter, for example clots, kinking	Check patency and drainage upon arrival in the PACU and every 30–60 mins	Check the patency of the catheter. Consider bladder irrigation. If clots present, inform surgeon
	Inadequate renal perfusion, for example hypotension, systolic pressures under 60 mmHg, hypovolaemia, dehydration		Take blood pressure and CVP if available. Increase intravenous fluids. Inform the anaesthetist
	Renal damage, for example from blood transfusion, infection, drugs, surgical damage to the ureters		Inform the anaesthetist or surgeon

Postprocedural considerations

Immediate care

Care of patients after local and regional anaesthesia

Patients having surgical procedures performed under local or spinal anaesthesia, whether intra- or extra-(epi)dural, will require a period of postoperative observation. The priorities for their care will be concentrated on considerations such as hypotension, headaches and dizziness (AAGBI 2002) as well as those for general anaesthetic.

Discharge from PACU

Discharge from the recovery room is the responsibility of the anaesthetist but the recovery staff are responsible for keeping the anaesthetist informed about any changes in the patient's condition that may arise during the recovery phase. This could be cardiovascular, respiratory or the level of consciousness. The recovery staff use the discharge criteria as an assessment tool to determine whether the patient has achieved optimum recovery to enable them to return to the ward safely. However, if there are any changes in the patient's condition, this needs to be discussed with the

---

Box 17.6 Discharge criteria from PACU to ward

- The patient is fully conscious, able to maintain own airway, exhibits protective airway reflexes and is orientated.
- Respiratory function and good oxygenation are being maintained.
- The cardiovascular system is stable with no unexplained cardiac irregularity. The specific values of pulse and blood pressure are within normal preoperative limits on consecutive observations.
- There is no persistent or excessive bleeding from wound or drainage sites.
- Patients with urinary catheters have passed adequate amounts of urine (more than 0.5 mL/kg/h) (Eltringham *et al.* 1989).
- Pain and emesis should be controlled and suitable analgesia and antiemetic regimes should be prescribed by the anaesthetist (AAGBI 2002).
- Body temperature is at least 36°C (Kean 2000).

---

anaesthetist who should assess the patient before their return to the ward.

The length of patient stay in the recovery room is dependent on the patient's cardiovascular and respiratory condition and the rate at which that patient recovers physically and emotionally from the anaesthetic. A prior knowledge of the patient's cardiovascular and respiratory parameters as well as past medical history obtained through preoperative contact is of great value when assessing their return to normal state. It also has the advantage of helping the patient to orientate to time and place, as familiarity generates a degree of security and confidence. The patients must meet the criteria in Box 17.6 before they can be discharged from the recovery room to the ward.

Complications

While the majority of patients can be expected to achieve uneventful recovery, 24% of all patients have complications (Hines *et al.* 1992). Although nausea and vomiting are high on the list of complications (Jolley 2001), the most notable are respiratory and circulatory complications. Obstruction of the upper airway is the most common respiratory complication in the immediate postoperative period (Dhara 1997). Close observation and appropriate action can prevent the sequence of respiratory obstruction resulting in hypoxia leading to cardiac arrest (Peskett 1999).

Postoperative care

Definition

Postoperative care is the physical and psychological care given to the patient directly following transfer from the recov-

ery room to the ward. Postoperative care continues until the patient is discharged from hospital, and in some cases continues on as ambulatory care on an outpatient basis.

Related theory
Ineffective breathing pattern

Respiratory function postoperatively can be influenced by a number of factors:

- increased bronchial secretions from inhalation anaesthesia
- decreased respiratory effort from opiate medication
- pain or anticipated pain from surgical wounds
- surgical trauma to the phrenic nerve
- pneumothorax as a result of surgical or anaesthetic procedures
- co-morbidity, for example asthma, chronic obstructive airways disease (COAD).

All factors affecting adequate expansion of the lung and the ejection of bronchial secretions will encourage the development of atelectasis and consolidation of the affected lung tissue (AAGBI 2002).

Haemodynamic instability

Haemodynamic instability is most commonly associated with an abnormal or unstable blood pressure, especially hypotension (Anderson 2003). A reduction in systolic blood pressure following surgery can indicate hypovolaemic shock, a condition in which the blood vessels do not contain sufficient blood (Hatfield and Tronson 2009). Bleeding is the most common cause but other causes can occur when tissue fluid is lost from the circulation, for example bowel obstruction and nausea and vomiting (Hughes 2004). Hatfield and Tronson (2009, p. 348) outline three stages of hypovolaemic shock.

- *Compensated shock*: blood flow to the brain and heart is preserved at the expense of the kidneys, gastrointestinal system, skin and muscles.
- *Decompensated shock*: the body's compensatory mechanisms begin to fail and organ perfusion is severely reduced.
- *Irreversible shock*: tissues become so deprived of oxygen that multiorgan failure occurs.

During compensated shock, some patients can lose up to 30% of their circulatory volume before the effects of hypovolaemia are reflected in the systolic blood pressure measurements or heart rate (Hughes 2004). Therefore, when assessing postoperative patients it is also useful to consider the early signs of reduced tissue perfusion in detecting signs of hypovolaemic shock (Anderson 2003, Hatfield and Tronson 2009, Jevon and Ewens 2007), which include:

- restlessness, anxiety or confusion (as a result of cerebral hypoperfusion or hypoxia)
- increased respiratory rate, becoming shallow (frequently occurring before signs of tachycardia and hypotension)

- rising pulse rate (tachycardia as the heart attempts to compensate for the low circulatory blood volume)
- low urine output of <0.5 mL/kg/h (as the kidneys experience a reduction in perfusion and pressure, which activate the renin-angiotensin system in an attempt to conserve fluid and increase circulatory blood volume)
- pallor (pale, cyanotic skin) and later sweating
- cool peripheries (pale, cyanotic lips and nailbed), resulting in a poor signal on the pulse oximeter
- visible bleeding and haematoma from drains and wounds.

In most cases, if impending hypovolaemic shock is recognized and treated promptly, its progression through the aforementioned stages of shock can be circumvented (Hatfield and Tronson 2009). Irrespective of the cause of hypovolaemic shock, the aim of treatment is to restore adequate tissue perfusion (Hughes 2004). Excessive blood loss might require blood transfusion and occasionally surgical intervention. However, if signs are in the compensatory phase, fluid resuscitation with crystalloid or colloid and increased oxygenation to maintain saturation above 95% are sufficient to promote recovery for many patients.

Evidence-based approaches
Rationale

Although different surgical procedures require specific and specialist nursing care, the principles of postoperative care remain the same, underpinned by the application of evidence-based care. The nursing care given during the postoperative period is directed towards the prevention of those potential complications resulting from surgery and anaesthesia which might be anticipated to develop over a longer period of time. Consideration of the psychological and emotional aspects of recovery will of necessity be altered by the changed state of consciousness, awareness and knowledge of patients and their differing responses to surgery, diagnosis and treatment.

Principles of care
Fluid balance

There are several iatrogenic factors potentially contributing to fluid imbalance (circulating and tissue fluid volumes) in the postoperative patient. Anderson (2003) and Hatfield and Tronson (2009) suggest that these include:

- preoperative bowel preparation
- preoperative fasting times
- potential fluid volume excess
- fluid loss perioperatively
- inappropriate fluid prescription
- reduced intake postoperatively
- ongoing losses from bleeding
- paralytic ileus and/or vomiting.

Postoperatively it is essential that accurate fluid balance charts are maintained, outlining all fluid input (intravenous and oral) and output (e.g. urine, vomiting, wound exudate, drains, nasogastric (NG) drainage, stoma). This will facilitate the early identification of fluid loss or excess, which can be raised with a surgical colleague for appropriate management.

Some patients may require fluid replacement in the postoperative period to ensure an adequate fluid balance, avoiding dehydration and the resulting concentration of the blood that, along with venous stasis, is conducive to thrombus formation (Hughes 2004). Postoperative fluid replacements should be based on the following considerations (Doherty and Way 2006):

- maintenance requirements
- extra needs resulting from systemic factors (pyrexia)
- losses from drains
- requirements resulting from third space losses, for example oedema and ileus.

Daily maintenance fluids for sensible and insensible losses will be dependent upon age, gender, weight and body surface area and will increase with pyrexia, hyperventilation and conditions that increase the catabolic rate. Fluid requirements should be frequently re-evaluated with intravenous orders being rewritten every 12–24 hours or more often if clinically indicated. The most commonly used replacement fluids are crystalloids and colloids, which have different functions. The type and rate of fluid replacement regimen will be dependent upon the type and volume of fluid lost peri- and postoperatively (Hughes 2004).

Surgical drains

Surgical drains are used in many different types of surgery with the aim of decompressing or draining either fluid (blood, pus, gastric fluids and lymph) or air from the area of surgery (Hatfield and Tronson 2009). Drains can be open or closed.

- *Open* drains (including corrugated sheets or rubber or plastic) are 'open' to the air with the fluid 'passively' collecting in gauze or a stoma bag. As these drains are 'open', there is an associated risk of infection.
- *Closed* drains are 'closed' to the air with the fluid collecting into bags or bottles, for example chest drains, nasogastric tubes or abdominal drains. Closed drains are either 'active' (maintained under either low or high suction) or 'passive' (no active suction) (Hatfield and Tronson 2009).

As part of maintaining an accurate fluid balance, it is important that nurses accurately measure and record drainage output postoperatively. In particular, nurses should monitor changes in the character (colour, viscosity, odour) or volume of drainage fluid. Furthermore, as drains can become easily blocked with viscous fluid (e.g. blood clots), drain output alone may be an inaccurate method for determining blood loss. Consequently, it is essential that nurses inspect the skin around the drain site for signs of swelling or haematoma. Depending upon the type of surgery performed, drains are usually removed once the drainage has stopped or become less than approximately 25–50 mL/day. In some instances drains are 'shortened' by withdrawing them gradually (typically 2 cm/day).

Urinary output and catheters

Postoperatively, it is important that patients pass urine within 6–8 hours of surgery or pass more than 0.5 mL/kg/h (i.e. half the patient's bodyweight, for example 60 kg = 30 mL) if a urinary catheter is *in situ* (Doherty and Way 2006). Urinary catheters are used to relieve or prevent urinary retention and bladder distension, or to monitor urine output. Most urinary catheters are inserted urethrally but where this is contraindicated, suprapubic catheters can be used (see Chapter 6).

Bowel function

Gastrointestinal (GI) peristalsis usually returns within 24 hours after most operations that do not involve the abdominal cavity and within 48 hours after laparotomy (Crainic *et al.* 2009). Patients undergoing abdominal surgery experience reduced GI peristalsis due to surgical manipulation of the bowel and postoperative opioid medication (Crainic *et al.* 2009). The motility of the small intestine is affected to a lesser degree, except in patients who have had small bowel resection or who were operated on to relieve small bowel obstruction (Crainic *et al.* 2009). Prolonged inhibition of GI peristalsis (more than 3 days post surgery) is referred to as paralytic ileus (Baig and Wexner 2004). The duration of postoperative ileus correlates with the degree of surgical trauma, occurring less frequently following laparoscopic approaches than open procedures (Baig and Wexner 2004). Traditional interventions to prevent postoperative ileus or stimulate bowel function after surgery include decompression of the stomach until return of bowel function with a nasogastric tube (Nelson *et al.* 2005), reduction in opioid use, early mobilization of the patient to stimulate bowel function and early postoperative feeding (Crainic *et al.* 2009). Normal postoperative ileus leads to slight abdominal distension and absent bowel sounds. Return of peristalsis is often noted by the patient as mild cramps, passage of flatus and return of appetite.

Unless clinically indicated, food or enteral feeds should be withheld until there is evidence of return of normal GI motility. Postoperatively, nurses should monitor and document when patients pass flatus and when bowels have opened and the surgical team should be informed. All postoperative bowel movements should be documented (as per Bristol stool chart). Refer to Chapter 6.

Malnutrition

Surgery may exert a deleterious effect on appetite and the ability to maintain adequate nutritional intake postopera-

tively (Newman *et al.* 1998). Return to adequate nutritional state is necessary for wound healing (see Chapter 19) and it is particularly important that diabetic patients should return to their preoperative insulin/diet to avoid increased risk of metabolic disturbance. Consequently it is essential that nurses continue to undertake ongoing nutritional assessments and highlight to the dietitian/surgeon when there is cause for concern (see Chapter 8).

Unless contraindicated by the surgery performed (e.g. major abdominal or head and neck surgery) or the patient's current clinical status (e.g. risk of pulmonary aspiration, vomiting and/or ileus), the majority of patients will be able to meet their nutritional requirements orally in the postoperative period. In line with *Essence of Care: Food and Nutrition Benchmark* (DH 2001), it is essential that the environment is conducive to enabling patients to eat. This encompasses the implementation of protected mealtimes, assistance to eat and drink (including provision of eating aids), provision of regular snacks and maintenance of oral hygiene. For suggestions on modification of diet for patients experiencing anorexia, sore mouth, dysphagia, nausea and vomiting and/or early satiety in the postoperative period, please refer to Chapter 8.

Any patients unable to meet their nutritional requirements orally may require enteral tube feeding either in the short term or on a more permanent basis. Types of enteral feed tubes include nasogastric, nasoduodenal, nasojejunal, gastrostomy or jejunostomy (see Chapter 8 for information relating to feeding tubes, including potential complications, optimal care and factors to consider prior to terminating feeding).

Whilst enteral feeding is the preferred route of nutritional support (NCCAC 2006), parenteral nutrition may be indicated for some postoperative patients who have undergone major abdominal surgery or those with prolonged ileus, uncontrolled vomiting or diarrhoea, short bowel syndrome or gastrointestinal obstruction (see Chapter 8).

Wounds

Wound closure devices

Wounds are usually closed using one of three devices depending on the type of surgery and determined by surgeon preference: clips, sutures, paper sutures.

All should remain *in situ* and only be removed on surgical advice. For paper sutures, this would usually be 7–10 days and for clips/sutures usually 10–14 days postoperatively.

Dressings for surgical wounds

Turner (1985) wrote that the main functions of a wound dressing are to promote healing by providing a moist environment and to protect the wound from potentially harmful agents or injury. In a closed surgical wound, the main function of the dressing is to absorb blood or haemoserous fluid in the immediate postoperative phase.

When dressings are applied in theatre, it is recommended that they are not removed unless exudate, commonly termed 'strike-through', is evident or clinical signs of local or systemic infection occur (Bale and Jones 2006). However, this is often determined by the type of surgery and surgical advice. Unless contraindicated, dressings changes required within 48 hours of surgery should be undertaken using sterile non-touch technique and sterile normal saline (NICE 2008). NICE (2008) guidelines recommend that patients may shower safely 48 hours postoperatively.

The location of the wound and the method of wound closure usually determine whether the wound is dressed or not. Recent studies have demonstrated that it is unnecessary to dress surgical wounds after 48 hours and that this did not cause an increase in infection rates (Meylan and Tschantz 2001, Sticha et al. 1998). Chrintz et al. (1989) also found that early removal of dressings resulted in cost saving, reduced nursing time spent on dressings and increased ability for patient self-care. However, this is largely dictated by patient choice. Patient education and psychological support will be required prior to exposing a wound as it may cause patient distress.

If a dressing is required, a simple shower-proof, non-adherent dressing should be applied. Care should be taken to avoid applying the dressing under tension as this may blister the skin (Gupta et al. 2002). Gauze-based dressings should not be used to dress surgical wounds, as these can completely adhere to the wound and become part of the healing tissue, causing excessive pain, wound damage and excessive use of nursing time on removal (Hollinworth and Collier 2000, Vermeulen et al. 2005).

When a dressing is applied, it should be changed using aseptic technique, as clinically indicated or as per surgical instructions (see Chapter 19). On discharge, the patient should be referred to a community nurse or educated about how to care for themselves, including observing for signs of infection and swelling/seroma formation, in order to continue wound care at home.

Drain sites should remain uncovered unless there is exudate. If exudate is present, a simple non-adherent dressing should be applied around the drain and reviewed as required or at least every 24 hours.

Surgical wound complications

Dehiscence and infection are the two main complications associated with surgical wounds. Dehiscence can range from splitting open of the skin layers to complete dehiscence of the muscle and fascia, exposing internal organs, and occasionally incisional hernia with outer layers intact (Baxter 2003).

Factors associated with surgical dehiscence include infection, age, malnutrition, being male, long-term steroid use, previous radiotherapy, smoking, diabetes and rheumatoid arthritis, which can impair healing by affecting the microcirculation (Poole 1985). Obesity causes increased subcutaneous dead space, rendering the patient more susceptible to haematoma and seroma formation and increased incidence

of infection (Armstrong 1998). Tight suturing can tear the skin and affect vascularity of the wound edges, and may result in necrosis and wound breakdown (Westaby 1985).

Occasionally wound manager bags are required to drain the excessive exudate from a partially or fully dehisced wound. They are indicated if wound dressings are unable to manage the discharge from a wound and skin integrity is compromised.

Wound infection is characterized by purulent exudates, redness, tenderness, elevated body temperature and wound odour. A swab, pus sample and blood cultures should be taken to identify the causative micro-organism and appropriate treatment commenced to eradicate it. Factors affecting the incidence of wound infection are similar to those affecting dehiscence, although drains and sutures increase the risk of infection and should be removed if infection is indicated (Gilchrist 1999). However, the signs are also seen in the normal postoperative inflammatory response, lasting up to 48 hours. Persistent inflammation beyond this period or the presence of pus or purulent discharge, or pyrexia of the patient may indicate infection.

As with drains, venous access devices, chest drains and indwelling urinary catheters, wound dressings and clips/sutures can also increase the risk of infection. Please refer to Chapter 3. Each should be assessed on a daily basis and/or if infection is apparent to determine if they are still clinically indicated and they should be removed at the earliest opportunity. If infection is apparent, samples from the device and blood cultures should be sent for microbiology and appropriate eradication treatment commenced.

Methods for management of pain

Effective management of pain following surgery requires that information about the patient's goals for pain relief, previous history with analgesics, and type of surgical procedure is used to guide decisions about analgesic regimens (Bell and Duffy 2009, Layzell 2008). Analgesics are selected based on the location of surgery, degree of anticipated pain and patient characteristics, such as co-morbidities, and routes of administration and dosing schedules are determined to maximize the effectiveness and safety of analgesia, while minimizing the potential for adverse events (Layzell 2008). (For further information concerning effective management of pain following surgery, including assessment tools, see Chapter 9.)

Methods for coping with immobility

Postoperatively, patients are at increased risk of developing DVT as a result of muscular inactivity, postoperative respiratory and circulatory depression, abdominal and pelvic surgery, prolonged pressure on calves (e.g. from lithotomy poles), increased production of thromboplastin as a result of surgical trauma and pre-existing coronary artery disease (Rashid et al. 2005, C). To prevent this complication, many patients undergoing surgery will be treated with anticoagulants, for example low molecular weight heparin subcutaneous injections or a continuous heparin infusion if the patient was previously anticoagulated (NICE 2010).

Postoperative instructions should describe any special positioning of the patient. Where a patient's condition allows, early mobilization is encouraged to reduce venous stasis unless otherwise contraindicated. For patients on bed rest, nurses should encourage deep breathing and exercises of the leg (flexion/extension and rotation of the ankles). Where worn, nurses should ensure that antiembolic stockings are of the correct size and fit smoothly and should advise patients against the crossing of legs or ankles to prevent constriction of the blood supply and swelling. Furthermore, patients on bed rest should be encouraged to change position hourly to minimize atelectasis and circumvent the development of pressure sores (Terrence and Serginson 2000).

Anticipated patient outcomes

To ensure patient safety at all times and minimize postoperative complications by:

- delivering the required nursing care for the postoperative patient
- minimizing potential postoperative problems associated with:
  - haemodynamic instability
  - ineffective breathing pattern
  - imbalanced fluid volume
  - malnutrition
  - pain
  - immobility
  - infection
  - self-care deficit
  - patient knowledge deficit
  - psychological and emotional aspects of recovery.

Postprocedural considerations
Ongoing care
Self-care/knowledge deficit

The increase in same-day surgical admissions combined with shorter hospital stays means that more postoperative wound healing and recovery takes place at home. This means that patients need to be self-caring on discharge, having assimilated the knowledge of usual postoperative outcomes and management with the ability to recognize when professional intervention and/or advice are required.

Surgery can be physically and psychologically stressful for patients, resulting in patients forgetting up to 60% of any preoperative information/teaching (Swindale 1989). This demonstrates the need for nurses to reinforce preoperative education postoperatively, ensuring that any information and discussions are tailored to the patient's individual needs, taking into account their level of anxiety and distress (Swindale 1989). Ongoing assessment of the patient's un-

derstanding of the information given should be carried out and documented. Nurses should teach the patient and carers any necessary skills (including how to use equipment), allowing sufficient time to practise before discharge. This will enable the patient to be as independent as possible postoperatively and promote an understanding of any self-care initiatives required on discharge. This should be supported with centralized evidence-based written information concerning postdischarge care at home.

Observations

Postoperative observations include:

- blood pressure: normal range <101–149 mmHg systolic
- pulse (rate, rhythm and amplitude): 51–100 bpm
- respiration rate (rate, depth, effort and pattern): 9–14 rpm
- peripheral oxygen saturation: >95%
- temperature: 36.1–37.9°C
- blood glucose (if clinically indicated): 4–7 mmol/L
- central venous pressure (if clinically indicated): 5–10 cm H_2O
- neurological response (Glasgow Coma Scale) (see Chapter 11).
- accurate fluid balance (to include input and output).
(Bickley *et al.* 2009, DH 2000)

The regularity of these postoperative observations will be determined by the type of surgery performed as well as the method of pain control (e.g. epidural). A clear physiological monitoring plan should be made for each patient, detailing frequency of observations and parameters (NCEPOD 2005). If obtaining blood pressure measurements using electronic sphygomomanometers, the operator should also be aware that errors in measurement (for example, if there is a weak, thready or irregular pulse) may not readily obvious to the operator and that manual blood pressure measurement may be indicated. It is therefore essential that nurses develop the skill and dexterity to monitor patients' vital signs with traditional manual equipment (see Chapter 13). It has also been reported that pulse oximeters can be open to misinterpretation and therefore should not replace a respiratory assessment (NCEPOD 2005). Respiratory assessment is an early and sensitive indicator of deterioration (NCEPOD 2005).

Furthermore, it is imperative that nurses are able to interpret the results of postoperative observations and, if reliant on care assistants to take the observations, that nurses themselves interpret the results, thereby ensuring that patients who require it are given immediate priority. Studies reported by the National Confidential Enquiry into Patient Outcome and Death (NCEPOD) (2005) established that 41% of patients admitted to intensive care units from other parts of the hospital following cardiac arrest had abnormal clinical observations up to 24 hours prior to admission, suggesting that a cardiac arrest could potentially have been avoided if ward staff had responded to the abnormal clinical parameters (Goldhill and McNarry 2004, McQuillan *et al.* 1998, NCEPOD 2005, NPSA 2007). The Modified Early Warning System (MEWS) has been found to be a useful tool for referral of clinically deteriorating postoperative patients (Gardner-Thorpe *et al.* 2006). The MEWS is a simple physiological scoring system, based on the postoperative measurements previously outlined, that identifies patients at risk of deterioration who require increased levels of care (DH 2000, NICE 2007) (see Chapter 13). The primary purpose is to prevent delay in intervention or transfer of critically ill patients. The MEWS enables early identification of patient deterioration and, in conjunction with the SBAR (Situation, Background, Assessment, Recommendation) tool, is intended to improve communication between nursing staff and junior doctors/critical care outreach teams to 'flag up' patients who need to be given immediate priority, as recommended by the NHS Institute for Innovation and Improvement (NHSIIP 2008). The call-out algorithm is intended to ensure that appropriate immediate management is started and that the need for critical care expertise should be considered at an early stage.

Routine postoperative respiratory observations will include:

- listening for audible stridor, wheeze, secretions
- respiratory assessment including rate, depth, pattern (ensure greater than 10 rpm)
- observing for increased effort of breathing
- observing any changes in the patient's colour, that is, peripheral/central cyanosis
- pulse oximetry
- use of oxygen therapy – flow and method of delivery
- any chest drains *in situ*
- airway adjuncts.

Deep breathing exercises (DBE), coughing exercises and early mobilization may be undertaken. DBE helps remove mucus which can form and remain in the lungs due to the effects of general anaesthetic and analgesics (which depress action of cilia of the mucus membranes lining the respiratory tract and the respiratory centre in the brain). DBE prevent pneumonia by increasing lung expansion and preventing the accumulation of secretions. DBE also initiate the coughing reflex; voluntary coughing in conjunction with DBE facilitates the expectoration of respiratory tract secretions. A physiotherapist will often provide pre/postoperative advice and/or assessment for DBE. Note that the patient will require adequate analgesia and support for the wound to enable DBE and mobilization.

Discharge planning

All patients, whether short- or long-stay, those with few needs or those with complex needs, should receive comprehensive discharge planning. Postoperatively, discharge planning needs to be tailored to the individual needs of the patients, particularly in relation to advice and information on recovery and self-management (DH 2004) (see Chapter 2).

Websites

www.nhs.uk/Conditions/Toxic-shock-syndrome/Pages/Introduction.aspx

www.nhs.uk/conditions/toxic-shock-syndrome/pages/prevention.aspx

References

AAGBI (2002) *Immediate Postanaesthetic Recovery.* Association of Anaesthetists of Great Britain and Ireland, London. www.aagbi.org/publications/guidelines/docs/postanaes02.pdf.

AAGBI (2010) *Pre-Operative Assessment and Patient Preparation: The Role of the Anaesthetist: AAGBI Guideline 2.* Association of Anaesthetists of Great Britain and Ireland, London. www.aagbi.org/publications/guidelines/docs/preop2010.pdf.

Allaert, S.E., Carlier, S.P., Weyne, L.P. *et al.* (2007) First trimester anesthesia exposure and fetal outcome: a review. *Acta Anaesthesiologica Belgica,* **58** (2), 119–123.

Allen, G. (2004) Smoke plume evacuation; antibiotic prophylaxis; alcohol's effect on infection; misuse of prophylactic techniques. *AORN Journal,* **79** (4), 866–870.

All Wales Tissue Viability Nurse Forum (2009) Guidelines for best practice: the nursing care of patients wearing antiembolic stockings. *British Journal of Nursing,* special supplement.

Anderson, I.D. (2003) *Care of the Critically Ill Surgical Patient,* 2nd edn. Arnold, London.

AORN (2000) Recommended practices for safety through identification of potential hazards in the perioperative environment. *AORN Journal,* **72** (4), 690–692, 695–698.

AORN (2001) Recommended practices for positioning the patient in the perioperative practice setting. *AORN Journal,* **73** (1), 231–235, 237–238.

AORN (2004) AORN latex guideline. *AORN Journal,* **79** (3), 653–672.

AORN (2008) *Perioperative Standards, Recommended Practices and Guidelines.* AORN, Denver, CO.

Armstrong, M. (1998) Obesity as an intrinsic factor affecting wound healing. *Journal of Wound Care,* **7** (5), 220–221.

Asai, T. (2004) Editorial II: who is at increased risk of pulmonary aspiration? *British Journal of Anaesthesia,* **93** (4), 497–500.

Atkinson, R.S., Rushman, G.B. and Lee, J.A. (1982) *A Synopsis of Anaesthesia,* 9th edn. Wright-PSG, Bristol.

Baig, M.K. and Wexner, S.D. (2004) Postoperative ileus: a review. *Diseases of the Colon and Rectum,* **47** (4), 516–526.

Bale, S. and Jones, V. (2006) *Wound Care Nursing: a Patient-Centred Approach,* 2nd edn. Mosby Elsevier, Edinburgh.

Barker, S.G.E. and Hollingsworth, S.J. (2004) Wearing graduated compression stockings: the reality of everyday deep vein thrombosis prophylaxis. *Phlebology,* **19** (1), 52–53.

Baxter, H. (2003) Management of surgical wounds. *Nursing Times,* **99** (13), 66–68.

Beddows, J. (1997) Alleviating pre-operative anxiety in patients: a study. *Nursing Standard,* **11** (37), 35–38.

Bell, L. and Duffy, A. (2009) Pain assessment and management in surgical nursing: a literature review. *British Journal of Nursing,* **18** (3), 153–156.

Beths, T. (2006) *Setting up the Anesthesia Machine and Scavenging System.* Ross University, Dominica, West Indies. www.rossvet.edu.kn/safetyweb/docs/Setting%20up%20the%20Anesthesia%20Machine%20and%20Scavenging%20System.pdf.

Bickley, L.S., Bates, B. and Szilagyi, P.G. (2009) *Bates' Pocket Guide to Physical Examination and History Taking*, 6th edn. Wolters Kluwer Health/Lippincott Williams and Wilkins, Philadelphia.

Bondy, L.R., Sims, N., Schroeder, D.R. *et al.* (1999) The effect of anesthetic patient education on preoperative patient anxiety. *Regional Anesthesia and Pain Medicine*, **24** (2), 158–164.

Byrne, B. (2002) Deep vein thrombosis prophylaxis: the effectiveness and implications of using below-knee or thigh-length graduated compression stockings. *Journal of Vascular Nursing*, **20** (2), 53–59.

Callum, K. and Bradbury, A. (2000) ABC of arterial and venous disease: acute limb ischaemia. *BMJ (Clinical Research ed.)*, **320** (7237), 764–767.

Chrintz, H., Vibits, H., Cordtz, T.O. *et al.* (1989) Need for surgical wound dressing. *British Journal of Surgery*, **76** (2), 204–205.

Crainic, C., Erickson, K., Gardner, J. *et al.* (2009) Comparison of methods to facilitate postoperative bowel function. *MEDSURG Nursing*, **18** (4), 235–239.

Crayne, H.L. and Miner, D.G. (1988) Thermo-resuscitation for postoperative hypothermia. Using reflective blankets. *AORN Journal*, **47** (1), 222–223, 226–227.

Davis, P. and O'Neill, C. (2002) The potential benefits of intermittent pneumatic compression in the prevention of deep venous thrombosis. *Journal of Orthopaedic Nursing*, **6** (2), 95–101.

Dean, A. and Fawcett, T. (2002) Nurses' use of evidence in preoperative fasting. *Nursing Standard*, **17** (12), 33–37.

DH (2000) *Comprehensive Critical Care: A Review of Adult Critical Care Services*. Department of Health, London. www.dh.gov.uk/prod_consum_dh/groups/dh_digitalassets/@dh/@en/documents/digitalasset/dh_4082872.pdf.

DH (2001) *Essence of Care: Patient Focussed Benchmarking for Health Care Practitioners*. Stationery Office, London.

DH (2004) *Achieving Timely Simple Discharge from Hospital: A Toolkit for the Multi-Disciplinary Team*. Stationery Office, London.

DH (2009) *Reference Guide to Consent for Examination or Treatment*. Department of Health, London. www.dh.gov.uk/prod_consum_dh/groups/dh_digitalassets/documents/digitalasset/dh_103653.pdf.

Dhara, S.S. (1997) Complications in the recovery room. *Singapore Medical Journal*, **38** (5), 190–191.

Doherty, G.M. and Way, L.W. (2006) Current surgical diagnosis and treatment. In: *Lange Medical Book*, 12th edn. Lange Medical Books/McGraw-Hill, New York.

Drummond, G.B. (1991) Keep a clear airway. *British Journal of Anaesthesia*, **66**(2), 153–156.

Eckenhoff, J.E., Kneale, D.H. and Dripps, R.D. (1961) The incidence and etiology of postanesthetic excitment. A clinical survey. *Anesthesiology*, **22**, 667–673.

Eltringham, R., Durkin, M., Andrewes, S. and Casey, W. (1989) *Post-Anaesthetic Recovery: a Practical Approach*, 2nd edn. Springer-Verlag, London.

Feldmann, M.E. (1988) Inadvertent hypothermia: a threat to homeostasis in the postanesthetic patient. *Journal of Post Anesthesia Nursing*, **3** (2), 82–87.

Field, L. and Adams, N. (2001) Pain management 2: the use of pyschological approaches to pain. *British Journal of Nursing*, **10** (15), 971–974.

Fong, E.P., Tan, W.T. and Chye, L.T. (2000) Diathermy and alcohol skin preparations – a potential disastrous mix. *Burns*, **26** (7), 673–675.

Frank, S.M., Beattie, C., Christopherson, R. *et al.* (1993) Unintentional hypothermia is associated with postoperative myocardial ischemia. The Perioperative Ischemia Randomized Anesthesia Trial Study Group. *Anesthesiology*, **78** (3), 468–476.

Gardner-Thorpe, J., Love, N., Wrightson, J. *et al.* (2006) The value of Modified Early Warning Score (MEWS) in surgical in-patients: a prospective observational study. *Annals of the Royal College of Surgeons of England*, **88** (6), 571–575.

Gilchrist, B. (1999) Wound infection. In: Miller, M. and Glover, D. (eds) *Wound Management: Theory and Practice*. Nursing Times Books, London, pp. 96–107.

Goldhill, D.R. and McNarry, A.F. (2004) Physiological abnormalities in early warning scores are related to mortality in adult inpatients. *British Journal of Anaesthesia*, **92** (6), 882–884. 10.

Gupta, S.K., Lee, S. and Moseley, L.G. (2002) Postoperative wound blistering: is there a link with dressing usage? *Journal of Wound Care*, **11** (7), 271–273.

Hatfield, A. and Tronson, M. (2009) *The Complete Recovery Room Book*, 4th edn. Oxford University Press, Oxford.

Hayes, J.M., Lehman, C.A. and Castonguay, P. (2002) Graduated compression stockings: updating practice, improving compliance. *MEDSURG Nursing*, **11** (4), 163–166.

Haynes, A.B., Weiser, T.G., Berry, W.R. *et al.* (2009) A surgical safety checklist to reduce morbidity and mortality in a global population. *New England Journal of Medicine*, **360** (5), 491–499.

Higgins, C. (2009) *Understanding Laboratory Investigations for Nurses and Healthcare Professionals*, 2nd edn. Blackwell Publishing, Oxford.

Hines, R., Barash, P.G., Watrous, G. and O'Connor, T. (1992) Complications occurring in the postanesthesia care unit: a survey. *Anesthesia and Analgesia*, **74** (4), 503–509.

HoCHC (2005) *The Prevention of Venous Thromboembolism in Hospitalised Patients: Second Report of Session 2004–2005*. House of Commons Health Committee. Stationery Office, London. www.publications.parliament.uk/pa/cm200405/cmselect/cmhealth/99/99.pdf.

Hollinworth, H. and Collier, M. (2000) Nurses' views about pain and trauma at dressing changes: results of a national survey. *Journal of Wound Care*, **9** (8), 369–373.

HSE (2004) *Latex and You*. Health and Safety Executive, Sudbury. www.hse.gov.uk/pubns/indg320.pdf.

Hughes, E. (2004) Principles of post-operative patient care. *Nursing Standard*, **19** (5), 43–51.

Jacobs, V.R., Morrison, J.E. Jr, Mundhenke, C. *et al.* (2000) Intraoperative evaluation of laparoscopic insufflation technique for quality control in the OR. *Journal of the Society of Laparoendoscopic Surgeons*, **4** (3), 189–195.

JBI (2008) Pre-operative hair removal to reduce surgical site infection. *Australian Nursing Journal*, **15** (7), 27–30.

Jevon, P. and Ewens, B. (2007) *Monitoring the Critically Ill Patient*, 2nd edn. Blackwell, Oxford.

Jlala, H.A., French, J.L., Foxall, G.L. *et al.* (2010) Effect of preoperative multimedia information on perioperative anxiety in patients undergoing procedures under regional anaesthesia. *British Journal of Anaesthesia*, **104** (3), 369–374.

Jolley, S. (2001) Managing post-operative nausea and vomiting. *Nursing Standard*, **15** (40), 47–52.

Kean, M. (2000) A patient temperature audit within a theatre recovery unit. *British Journal of Nursing*, **9** (3), 150–156.

Kjonniksen, I., Andersen, B.M., Sondenaa, V.G. and Segadal, L. (2002) Preoperative hair removal – a systematic literature review. *AORN Journal*, **75** (5), 928–938, 940.

Klopfenstein, C.E., Forster, A. and van Gessel, E. (2000) Anesthetic assessment in an outpatient consultation clinic reduces preoperative anxiety. *Canadian Journal of Anaesthesia*, **47** (6), 511–515.

Kuczkowski, K.M. (2004) Nonobstetric surgery during pregnancy: what are the risks of anesthesia? *Obstetrical and Gynecological Survey*, **59** (1), 52–56.

Kumar, S., Wong, P.F., Melling, A.C. and Leaper, D.J. (2005) Effects of perioperative hypothermia and warming in surgical practice. *International Wound Journal*, 2 (3), 193–204.

Layzell, M. (2008) Current interventions and approaches to post-operative pain management. *British Journal of Nursing*, **17** (7), 414–419.

Levinson, B.W. (1965) States of awareness during general anaesthesia. Preliminary communication. *British Journal of Anaesthesia*, 37 (7), 544–546.

Lipp, A. and Edwards, P. (2002) Disposable surgical face masks for preventing surgical wound infection in clean surgery. *Cochrane Database of Systematic Reviews (Online)*, (1), CD002929.

Malik, A.A., Khan, W.S., Chaudhry, A. *et al.* (2009) Acute compartment syndrome – a life and limb threatening surgical emergency. *Journal of Perioperative Practice*, 19 (5), 137–142.

McQuillan, P., Pilkington, S., Allan, A. *et al.* (1998) Confidential inquiry into quality of care before admission to intensive care. *BMJ (Clinical Research ed.)*, 316 (7148), 1853–1858.

Meylan, G. and Tschantz, P. (2001) [Surgical wounds with or without dressings. Prospective comparative study]. *Annales de Chirurgie*, **126** (5), 459–462.

Mitchell, M. (2000) Nursing intervention for pre-operative anxiety. *Nursing Standard*, **14** (37), 40–43.

Mitchell, M.J. (2009) Patient anxiety and conscious surgery. *Journal of Perioperative Practice*, **19** (6), 168–173.

Molyneux, C. (2001) Electrosurgery policy. *British Journal of Perioperative Practice*, 11 (10), 424.

Murkin, C. E. (2009) Pre-operative antiseptic skin preparation. *British Journal of Nursing*, 18 (11), 665–669.

NCCAC (2006) *Nutrition Support for Adults: Oral Nutrition, Enteral Support, Enteral Tube Feeding and Parenteral Nutrition: Methods, Evidence and Guidance.* National Collaborating Centre for Acute Care, London. www.nice.org.uk/nicemedia/pdf/cg032fullguideline.pdf.

NCEPOD (2005) *An Acute Problem?* National Confidential Enquiry into Patient Outcome and Death, London. www.ncepod.org.uk/2005report/NCEPOD_Report_2005.pdf.

Nelson, R., Tse, B. and Edwards, S. (2005) Systematic review of prophylactic nasogastric decompression after abdominal operations. *British Journal of Surgery*, **92** (6), 673–680.

Newman, L.A., Vieira, F., Schwiezer, V. *et al.* (1998) **Eating and** weight changes following chemoradiation therapy for advanced head and neck cancer. Archives of Otolaryngology Head and Neck Surgery, 124, 589–592.

NHSIIP (2008) *SBAR Situation-Background-Assessment-Recommendation.* NHS Institute for Innovation and Improvement, Coventry.

NICE (2005) *The Prevention and Treatment of Pressure Ulcers.* National Institute for Health and Clinical Excellence, London. www.nice.org.uk/nicemedia/pdf/CG29QuickRefGuide.pdf.

NICE (2007) *Acutely Ill Patients in Hospital: Recognition of and Response to Acute Illness in Adults in Hospital: NICE Clinical Guideline 50.* National Institute for Health and Clinical Excellence, London. www.nice.org.uk/nicemedia/live/10893/28816/28816.pdf.

NICE (2008) *Surgical Site Infection: Prevention and Treatment of Surgical Site Infection.* National Institute for Health and Clinical Excellence, London. www.nice.org.uk/nicemedia/pdf/CG74NICEGuideline.pdf.

NICE (2010) *Venous Thromboembolism: Reducing the Risk of Venous Thromboembolis Deep Vein Thrombosis and Pulmonary Embolism in Patients Admitted to Hospital.* National Institute for Health and Clinical Excellence, London. http://guidance.nice.org.uk/CG92/Guidance.

Nimmo, W.S., Rowbotham, D.J. and Smith, G. (1994) *Anaesthesia*, 2nd edn. Blackwell Scientific, Oxford.

NMC (2008) *Consent.* Nursing and Midwifery Council, London. www.nmc-uk.org/Nurses-and-midwives/Advice-by-topic/A/Advice/Consent.

NMC (2009) *Record Keeping: Guidance for Nurses and Midwives.* Nursing and Midwifery Council, London.

NPSA (2007) *The Fifth Report from the Patient Safety Observatory, Safer Care for the Acutely Ill Patient: Learning from Serious Incident.* National Patient Safety Agency, London. www.nrls.npsa.nhs.uk/resources/?entryid45=59828.

NPSA (2009) http://www.patientsafetyfirst.nhs.uk/content.aspx?path=/.

NPSA (2010) *Checking Pregnancy Before Surgery: Rapid Response Report: NPSA/2010/RRR011.* National Patient Safety Agency, London. www.nrls.npsa.nhs.uk/resources/?EntryId45=73838.

Nunney, R. (2008) Inadvertent hypothermia: a literature review. *Journal of Perioperative Practice*, 18 (4), 148–154.

O'Callaghan, N. (2002) Pre-operative fasting. *Nursing Standard*, **16** (36), 33–37.

Parienti, J.J., Thibon, P., Heller, R. *et al.* (2002) Hand-rubbing with an aqueous alcoholic solution vs traditional surgical hand-scrubbing and 30-day surgical site infection rates: a randomized equivalence study. *Journal of the American Medical Association*, **288** (6), 722–727.

Parnaby, C. (2004) A new anti-embolism stocking. Use of below-knee products and compliance. *British Journal of Perioperative Practice*, **14** (7), 302–304, 306–307.

Paula, R. (2002) *Compartment Syndrome Extremity.* http://emedicine.medscape.com/article/828456-overview.

Peskett, M. J. (1999) Clinical indicators and other complications in the recovery room or postanaesthetic care unit. *Anaesthesia*, **54** (12), 1143–1149.

Poole, G.V. Jr (1985) Mechanical factors in abdominal wound closure: the prevention of fascial dehiscence. *Surgery*, 97, 631–640.

Pratt, R.J., Pellowe, C.M., Wilson, J.A. *et al.* (2007) epic2: National evidence-based guidelines for preventing healthcare-associated infections in NHS hospitals in England. *Journal of Hospital Infection*, 65 (Suppl 1), S1–64.

Radtke, F.M., Franck, M., Schneider, M. *et al.* (2008) Comparison of three scores to screen for delirium in the recovery room. *British Journal of Anaesthesia*, 101 (3), 338–343.

Rashid, S.T., Thursz, M.R., Razvi, N.A. *et al.* (2005) Venous thromboprophylaxis in UK medical inpatients. *Journal of the Royal Society of Medicine*, **98** (11), 507–512.

Raza, A., Byrne, D. and Townell, N. (2004) Lower limb (well leg) compartment syndrome after urological pelvic surgery. *Journal of Urology*, 171 (1), 5–11.

RCN (2005) *Perioperative Fasting in Adults and Children: An RCN Guideline for the Multidisciplinary Team.* Royal College of Nursing, London. www.rcn.org.uk/__data/assets/pdf_file/0009/78678/002800.pdf.

Roderick, P., Ferris, G., Wilson, K. *et al.* (2005) Towards evidence-based guidelines for the prevention of venous thromboembolism: systematic reviews of mechanical methods, oral anticoagulation, dextran and regional anaesthesia as thromboprophylaxis. *Health Technology Assessment*, 9 (49), iii–iv, ix–x, 1–78.

Rose, D. (2005) Latex sensitivity awareness in preoperative assessment. *British Journal of Perioperative Practice*, 15 (1), 27–33.

Scott, E., Beswick, A. and Wakefield, K. (2004) The hazards of diathermy plume. Part 2. Producing quantified data. *British Journal of Perioperative Practice*, **14** (10), 452, 454–456.

Sharma, K.C., Kabinoff, G., Ducheine, Y. *et al.* (1997) Laparoscopic surgery and its potential for medical complications. *Heart and Lung: Journal of Critical Care*, **26** (1), 52–64.

1077

SIGN (2002) *Prophylaxis of Venous Embolism.* Scottish Intercollegiate Guidelines Network, Edinburgh. www.sign.ac.uk/guidelines/fulltext/62/index.html.

Starritt, T. (1999) Patient assessment in recovery. *British Journal of Theatre Nursing,* **9** (12), 593–595.

Sticha, R.S., Swiriduk, D. and Wertheimer, S.J. (1998) Prospective analysis of postoperative wound infections using an early exposure method of wound care. *Journal of Foot and Ankle Surgery,* **37** (4), 286–291.

Swindale, J.E. (1989) The nurse's role in giving pre-operative information to reduce anxiety in patients admitted to hospital for elective minor surgery. *Journal of Advanced Nursing,* **14** (11), 899–906.

Tammelin, A., Domicel, P., Hambraeus, A. and Stahle, E. (2000) Dispersal of methicillin-resistant *Staphylococcus epidermidis* by staff in an operating suite for thoracic and cardiovascular surgery: relation to skin carriage and clothing. *Journal of Hospital Infection,* **44** (2), 119–126.

Tanner, J. and Parkinson, H. (2002) Double gloving to reduce surgical cross-infection. *Cochrane Database of Systematic Reviews (Online),* (3), CD003087.

Tanner, J., Woodings, D. and Moncaster, K. (2006) Preoperative hair removal to reduce surgical site infection. *Cochrane Database of Systematic Reviews (Online),* (3), CD004122.

Tanner, J., Blunsden, C. and Fakis, A. (2007) National survey of hand antisepsis practices. *Journal of Perioperative Practice,* **17** (1), 27–37.

Taylor, T. and Tanner, J. (2005) Razors versus clippers. A randomised controlled trial. *British Journal of Perioperative Practice,* **15** (12), 518–520, 522–523.

Terrence, C. and Serginson, E. (2000) Surgical Nursing. Baillière Tindall, London.

Turner, T.D. (1985) Wound management product selection. *Journal of Sterile Services Management,* **2** (6), 3–6.

Vedovato, J.W., Polvora, V.P. and Leonardi, D.F. (2004) Burns as a complication of the use of diathermy. *Journal of Burn Care and Rehabilitation,* **25** (1), 120–123; discussion 119.

Vermeulen, H., Ubbink, D.T., Goossens, A. *et al.* (2005) Systematic review of dressings and topical agents for surgical wounds healing by secondary intention. *British Journal of Surgery,* **92** (6), 665–672.

Wagner, V.D. (2003) Impact of perioperative temperature management on patient safety. *SSM,* **9**(4), 38–44.

Walker, J.A. (2002) Emotional and psychological preoperative preparation in adults. *British Journal of Nursing,* **11** (8), 567–575.

Westaby, S. (1985) *Would Closure and Drainage.* Mosby, St Louis, MO.

Wicker, P. (2000) Electrosurgery in perioperative practice. *British Journal of Perioperative Practice,* **10** (4), 221–6.

Wicker, P. and O'Neill, J. (2006) *Caring for the Perioperative Patient.* Blackwell, Oxford.

Woodhead, K., Taylor, E.W., Bannister, G. *et al.* (2002) Behaviours and rituals in the operating theatre. A report from the Hospital Infection Society Working Party on Infection Control in Operating Theatres. *Journal of Hospital Infection,* **51** (4), 241–255.

Wu, M.P., Ou, C.S., Chen, S.L. *et al.* (2000) Complications and recommended practices for electrosurgery in laparoscopy. *American Journal of Surgery,* **179** (1), 67–73.

Chapter 18

Vascular access devices: insertion and management

The Royal Marsden Hospital Manual of Clinical Nursing Procedures, Eighth Edition. Edited by Lisa Dougherty and Sara Lister.
© 2011 The Royal Marsden Hospital. Published 2011 by Blackwell Publishing Ltd.

Overview

This chapter provides an overview of vascular access devices inserted in a vein or an artery. The variety of common devices used for both peripheral and central access will be described along with their insertion, care and removal. The taking of blood samples will be covered in Chapter 11.

Vascular access devices

Definition

A vascular access device (VAD) is a device that is inserted into either a vein or an artery, via the peripheral or central vessels, to provide for either diagnostic (blood sampling, central venous pressure (CVP) reading) or therapeutic (administration of medications, fluids and/or blood products) purposes. There is now a comprehensive range of VADs available which allow for selection based on the device, therapy and the quality-of-life needs of the patient. Table 18.1 lists the main types of VADs.

Anatomy and physiology
Anatomy of veins

Veins consist of three layers.

Tunica intima

The tunica intima is a smooth endothelial lining, which allows the passage of blood cells. If it becomes damaged,

Table 18.1 Vascular access devices

Type of device	Material	Features	Common insertion site (veins)	Recommended indwelling life and common uses
Peripheral cannula	Teflon Vialon	Winged Non-winged Non-ported Ported	Cephalic Basilic Dorsal venous network	48–96 hours for short-term access
Midline catheter	Silicone Polyurethane	Single lumen Dual lumen	Basilic Median cubital Cephalic	Used for 1–6 weeks or longer for short- to intermediate-term access
Peripherally inserted central catheter	Polyurethane Silicone	Dual lumen Single lumen Valved	Antecubital fossa Basilic Cephalic Brachial	Used primarily for patients requiring several weeks or months of intravenous access
Short-term percutaneous central venous catheter (non-tunnelled)	Polyurethane Silicone	Heparin, antibiotic and antiseptic coatings, multiple lumen	Jugular Subclavian Femoral	Intended for days to weeks of intravenous access
Skin-tunnelled catheter	Polyurethane Silicone	Valved Antimicrobial/silver cuff Multiple lumen	Jugular Axillary Subclavian Femoral	Indefinite. Used for long-term intermittent, continuous or daily intravenous access. May be appropriate for short-term use if reliable access needed
Implanted ports	*Catheter* Silicone *Port* Titanium Plastic	Dual ports Peripheral ports Valved Low profile CT compatible	Antecubital fossa Subclavian Femoral	Indefinite. Used for long-term access Intermittent, continuous or daily intravenous access

the lining may become roughened and there is an increased risk of thrombus formation (Weinstein and Plumer 2007). Within this layer are folds of endothelium called valves, which keep blood moving towards the heart by preventing backflow. Valves are present in larger vessels and at points of branching and are present as noticeable bulges in the veins (Weinstein and Plumer 2007).

Tunica media

The middle layer of the vein wall is composed of muscular tissue and nerve fibres, both vasoconstrictors and vasodilators, which can stimulate the vein to contract or relax. This layer is not as strong or stiff as in an artery and therefore veins can distend or collapse as the pressure rises or falls (Waugh et al. 2006, Weinstein and Plumer 2007). Stimulation of this layer by a change in temperature (cold), mechanical or chemical stimulus can produce venous spasm, which can make insertion of a needle more difficult.

Tunica adventitia

The tunica adventitia is the outer layer and consists of connective tissue, which surrounds and supports the vessel.

Anatomy of arteries

By contrast, arteries tend to be placed more deeply than veins and can be distinguished by the thicker walls, which do not collapse, the presence of a pulse and bright red blood. It should be noted that aberrant arteries may be present. These are arteries that are located superficially in an unusual place (Weinstein and Plumer 2007).There are two main types of arteries – muscular and elastic – and they are composed of three layers:

- the tunica intima has elongated endothelial cells
- the tunica media in the elastic artery is thicker with more elastic and fibrous tissue arranged in circular bands while the muscular artery is a large mass of smooth muscle fibres controlling constriction and relaxation
- the tunica adventitia contains both collagen and elastic fibres, nerve bundles and lymphatic vessels (Hadaway 2010).

Veins of the peripheral circulation

The superficial veins of the upper limb are most commonly chosen for cannulation and insertion of midlines and peripherally inserted central catheters (PICCs). These veins are numerous and accessible, ensuring that the procedure can be performed safely and with minimum discomfort (Ernst 2005).

- The cephalic vein.
- The basilic vein.
- The metacarpal veins (used only when the others are not accessible) (Figure 18.1a).

On the lateral aspect of the wrist, the cephalic vein rises from the dorsal veins and flows upwards along the radial border of the forearm as the median cephalic, crossing the antecubital fossa as the median cubital vein. Care must be taken to avoid accidental arterial puncture, as this vein crosses the brachial artery. It is also in close proximity to the radial nerve (Dougherty 2008, Masoorli 2007).

The basilic vein has its origins in the ulnar border of the hand and forearm (Waugh et al. 2006). It may be prominent but is not well supported by subcutaneous tissue, making it roll easily. Owing to its position, a haematoma may occur if the patient flexes the arm on removal of the needle, as this squeezes blood from the vein into the surrounding tissues (McCall and Tankersley 2003, Weinstein and Plumer 2007). Care must also be taken to avoid accidental puncture of the median nerve and brachial artery (Garza and Becan-McBride 2010).

The metacarpal veins are easily visualized and palpated. However, the use of these veins is contraindicated in the elderly where skin turgor and subcutaneous tissue are diminished (Weinstein and Plumer 2007).

Veins of the central venous circulation

A central vein is one near the centre of the circulation, the heart (Chantler 2009). Those more commonly used for central venous catheterization are the internal jugular, subclavian and femoral veins (Figure 18.2). The internal jugular vein emerges from the skull through the jugular foramen and runs down the neck into the carotid sheath (Farrow et al. 2009). The axillary vein is a continuation of the basilic vein. From the lateral edge of the ribs to the sternal edge of the clavicle, the continuation of the axillary becomes the subclavian. It angles upwards as it arches over the first rib and passes under the clavicle, forming a narrow passage for the vein (Galloway and Bodenham 2004, Galloway and Bodenham 2009, Hadaway 2010). Here it joins the internal jugular vein to form the brachiocephalic vein behind the sternoclavicular joint. The left brachiocephalic vein is 6 cm in length, twice as long as the right (Hadaway 2010).

The superior vena cava (SVC) drains venous blood from the upper half of the body and is formed from the confluence of the two brachiocephalic (innominate) veins (2 cm wide) (Farrow et al. 2009). The SVC is 7 cm long in normal adults and descends vertically to the upper part of the right atrium of the heart (Farrow et al. 2009).

The femoral vein drains the majority of blood from the lower limb and enters the thigh as a continuation of the popliteal vein. It ascends through the thigh and becomes the external iliac vein and drains into the inferior vena cava. The inferior vena cava drains the lower half of the body and is formed by the two common iliac veins.

Evidence-based approaches

Rationale
Indications

- To obtain venous and arterial blood samples.
- To administer fluids, nutrition, medication or blood products.
- To monitor central venous pressure and arterial pressure.

(a)

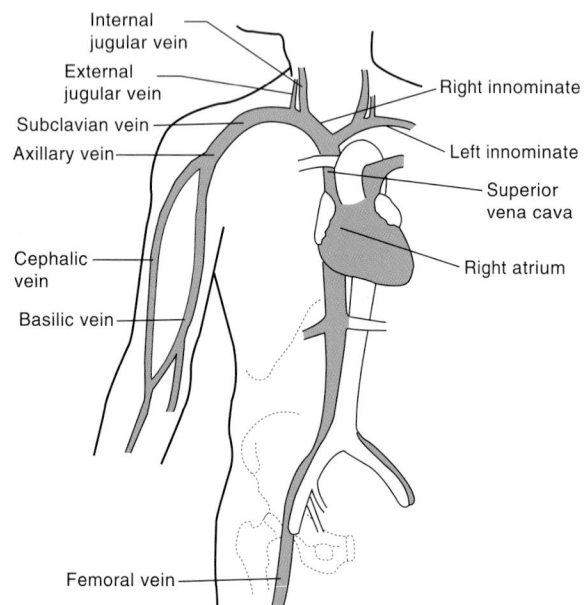

Median nerve

Basilic vein

Brachial artery

Median cubital vein

Basilic vein

Ulnar nerve

Anterior interosseous nerve

Ulnar artery

Median antebrachial vein

Cephalic vein

Radial nerve

Accessory cephalic vein

Radial artery

Cephalic vein

(b)

Cephalic vein

Basilic vein

Dorsal venous arch

Metacarpal veins

Digital veins

(c)

Cephalic

Subclavian

Superior vena cava

Brachiocephalic

Basilic

Figure 18.1 (a) Superficial veins of the forearm. (b) Superficial veins of the dorsal aspect of the hand. (Reproduced with permission from Becton Dickinson and Company.) (c) Veins of the thorax. Redrawn from BD *First PICC Clinical Education Manual* D11 952B 5/98.

Internal jugular vein

External jugular vein

Subclavian vein

Axillary vein

Cephalic vein

Basilic vein

Right innominate

Left innominate

Superior vena cava

Right atrium

Femoral vein

Figure 18.2 The main veins used for central venous access device placement. Reproduced with permission from Dougherty (2006).

Contraindications

There are no specific contraindications for inserting a vascular access device but there may be contraindications for location of the device and the type of medication that can be administered (very few can be administered via an artery).

Principles of care

Regardless of the type of VAD used, the principles of care for the device remain the same.

- To prevent infection.
- To maintain a 'closed' intravenous system with minimal connections to reduce the risk of contamination.
- To prevent damage to the device and associated intravenous equipment.
- To maintain a patent and correctly positioned device.

Each of these principles will be discussed generally and then in more detail under each type of access device.

Methods for prevention of infection at insertion site

Aseptic technique and compliance with recommendations for equipment and dressing changes are essential if microbial contamination is to be prevented (INS 2011, Pratt *et al.* 2007, RCN 2010) (see Chapter 3). Whenever the insertion site is exposed or the intravenous system is broken, aseptic technique should be practised. Where blood or body fluids may be present, gloves should be worn to comply with safe practice (Rowley 2001). It is not necessary to wear sterile gloves when accessing a central venous access devices – clean gloves are adequate (Hemsworth *et al.* 2007).

Cleaning solutions

Most transient flora can be removed from the skin with soap and water using mechanical friction. It is also important to remove dirt as antiseptic solutions are not as effective as they cannot penetrate surface dirt (McGoldrick 2010). Chlorhexidine 2% in 70% alcohol has been shown to be the most effective agent for skin cleaning around the VAD insertion site prior to insertion and between dressing changes (DH 2010, Maki *et al.* 1991, Pratt *et al.* 2007, RCN 2010, Ryder 2001). Seventy percent alcohol acts by denaturing protein and so has excellent properties for destruction of Gram-positive and -negative bacteria, as well as being active against fungi and viral organisms. Alcohol concentration between 70% and 92% provides the most rapid and greatest reduction in microbial counts on skin but does not have any residual activity (Larson 1988). This is where chlorhexidine has an advantage over alcohol used alone, as it has excellent residual activity for 4–6 hours after application (Pratt *et al.* 2007). Solutions should be applied with friction in back and forth strokes for at least 30 seconds and allowed to air dry for 30–60 seconds (INS 2011, McGoldrick 2010). It has been found that 1 minute of application with alcohol is as effective as 12 minutes of scrubbing and reduces bacterial counts by 75%. However, a quick wipe fails to reduce bacterial counts prior to peripheral cannulation (INS 2011, Weinstein and Plumer 2007). Allowing any cleaning solution to dry is vital in order for disinfection to be completed, and in the case of alcohol, which is a plasticizer, it ensures that plastic equipment will not 'glue together' (Dougherty 2006).

Inspection of insertion site and cleaning of equipment

Cleaning solutions should be used not only on insertion sites, but also to clean junctions and connections, and so on. It is recommended that injection caps should be cleaned vigorously with appropriate cleaning agents such as chlorhexidine 2% in alcohol (Brown *et al.* 1997, DH 2010, Pratt *et al.* 2007). The frequency of cleaning the insertion site is debatable; peripheral sites are rarely cleaned once the device is sited because the device is *in situ* for such a short period of time. However, central venous access sites, for example PICCs, may be cleaned weekly (at dressing change) and short-term central venous catheters (CVCs) may be cleaned daily or more frequently (being associated with the highest infection risk). The insertion site should be checked regularly for signs of phlebitis (erythema, pain and/or swelling) or for signs of infection (DH and CMO 2003). Complaints of soreness, unexpected pyrexia and damaged, wet or soiled dressings are reasons for immediate inspection and renewal of the dressing.

Securement and dressings

There are a number of securement devices and dressings available. The aim of a securement device is to secure the device to the skin and prevent movement of the device which in turn will reduce the risk of mechanical phlebitis and infection. They also prevent dislodgement. Types of securement include tape, sutures and self-adhesive anchoring devices applied to the skin, such as Statlocks (Moureau and Iannucci 2003). Suturing can result in inflammation and bacterial colonization of the exit site (Schears 2005) and is no longer recommended (Maki 2002), particularly with PICCs (Nakazawa 2010). Statlocks have been shown to result in significantly longer catheter dwell times and fewer total complications (Gabriel 2001, Maki 2002, Schears 2005, Yamamoto *et al.* 2002).

Types of dressings include sterile gauze and transparent dressings. The recommendation for a central venous access device site is an intact dry adherent transparent semi-occlusive dressing (DH 2010, Pratt *et al.* 2007). These dressings allow observation of the exit site, without the need to remove the dressing. They are also moisture permeable, thereby reducing the collection of moisture under the dressing (Casey and Elliott 2010).

Newer products include a chlorhexidine gluconate antimicrobial transparent dressing which contains a chlorhexidine gel pad which is integral to the dressing and has been shown to allow visualization of the site, facilitating absorption of fluid under the dressing (Moureau *et al.* 2009). It has been shown to prevent the regrowth of microbial skin flora (Maki 2008). This can also be achieved by attaching a hydrophilic polyurethane absorptive foam patch impregnated with CHG under the transparent dressing which has shown to reduce the rate of catheter colonization and demonstrated significant reductions in the associated rate of catheter-related bloodstream infection (Ho and Litton 2006, Ruschulte *et al.* 2009, Timsit *et al.* 2009). However, the foam patch does not enable insertion site visualization.

Methods for maintaining a closed intravenous system

If equipment becomes accidentally disconnected, air embolism or profuse blood loss may occur, depending on the condition and position of the patient (Perucca 2010). Accidental disconnection poses a greater risk in patients with all central venous or arterial access devices than in those with peripheral venous devices. This is because of the amount of air that could be introduced via a CVAD and the speed with which it could enter the pulmonary vessels or the speed of haemorrhage. Luer-Lok provides a more secure connection and all equipment should have these fittings, that is, administration sets, extension sets, injection caps (Dougherty 2006). Needle-free systems provide a closed environment, which further reduces the risk of air entry (Dougherty 2006). Care should be taken to clamp the catheter firmly when changing equipment. Connections must be double checked and precautions taken to prevent the introduction of air into the system when making additions to, or taking blood from, a CVC (Dougherty 2006).

Methods for preventing damage of the VAD and performing a repair

If damage occurs to peripheral devices, they are usually removed and replaced. Catheters are made of non-resealable material so penetration by a needle creates holes and they can rupture if excessive force is exerted (Gorski *et al.* 2010). Pinch-off syndrome can also result in a transected and potentially embolized catheter segment (Gorski *et al.* 2010). Temporary and permanent repairs can be performed depending on where the catheter is damaged and the type of catheter (Dougherty 2006). However, prevention of this occurrence is preferred.

Artery forceps or sharp-edged clamps should not be used to clamp the catheter. A smooth clamp should be placed on the reinforced section of the catheter provided for clamping (Dougherty 2006). If a reinforced section is not present, placing a tape tab over part of the catheter can create one. A second alternative is to move the clamp up or down the catheter at regular intervals to reduce the risk of wear and tear in one place (Dougherty 2006).

Use of the correct syringe size in accordance with manufacturer's guidelines will reduce the risk of catheter rupture (INS 2011). However, syringe size alone will not be sufficient to prevent catheter rupture. If resistance is felt and more pressure is applied to overcome it, catheter fracture could result regardless of syringe size (Hadaway 1998, Macklin 1999). The nurse must be familiar with the action to be taken to minimize any risk to patient safety in this event. Immediate clamping of the catheter proximal to the fracture or split is essential to prevent blood loss or air embolism (Gorski *et al.* 2010). The split area should be covered with an alcohol swab and emergency repair equipment collected, together with sterile gloves to ensure that all manipulations are aseptic. A permanent repair should be performed as soon as possible using the specific equipment provided by the manufacturer or removed if unable to repair. A member of the medical staff or other designated personnel should do this (Dougherty 2006).

Methods for maintaining patency

Patency is defined as the ability to infuse through and aspirate blood from a VAD (Dougherty 2006). It is important

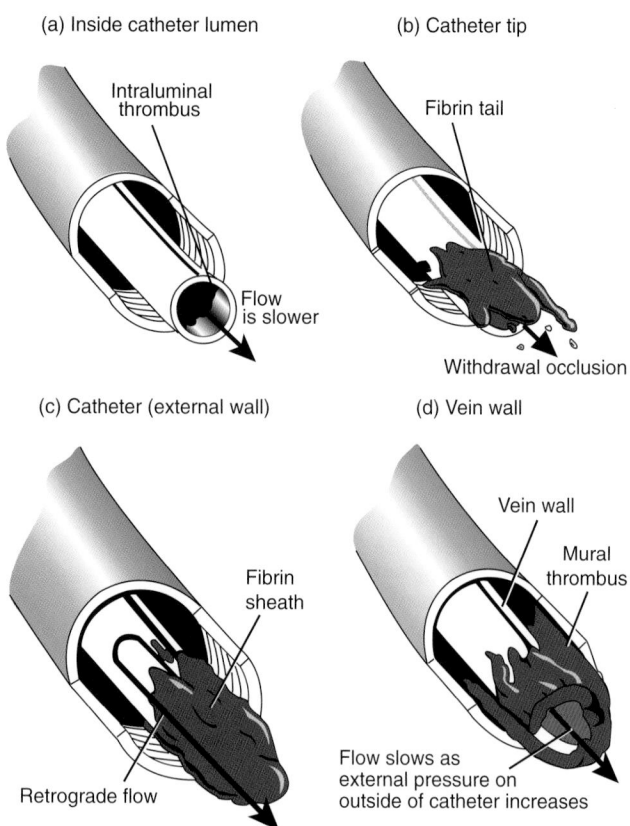

Figure 18.3 Clot formations. Redrawn from Macklin and Chernecky 2004. With permission from Elsevier.

at all times for the patency of the device to be maintained. Blockage predisposes to device damage, infection, inconvenience to patients and disruption to drug delivery. Occlusion of the device is usually the result of:

- clot formation (Figure 18.3) due to: (a) an administration set or electronic infusion device being turned off accidentally and left for a prolonged period; or (b) insufficient or incorrect flushing of the device when not in use. Thrombotic occlusions are responsible for 58% of all occlusions (Hadaway 2010);
- precipitate formation due to inadequate flushing between incompatible medications (Dougherty 2006).

Kinking or pinch-off syndrome may also impair patency of the device. Meticulous intravenous technique will prevent the majority of these problems.

Two main types of solutions are used to maintain patency in VADs: heparin and 0.9% sodium chloride. All devices should be flushed with 10–20 mL 0.9% sodium chloride after blood withdrawal followed by the appropriate flushing solution (Dougherty 2006, Dougherty 2008, INS 2011, RCN 2010).

Maintaining patency can be achieved by:

- a continuous infusion to keep the vein open (KVO), either by the patient being attached to an infusion of 0.9% sodium chloride via a volumetric pump, which reduces

Box 18.1 Advantages and disadvantages of intermittent flushing

The advantages of intermittent flushing compared with a continuous infusion are:

- it reduces the risk of circulatory overload
- it reduces the risk of vascular irritation
- it decreases the risk of bacterial contamination as it eliminates a continuous intravenous pathway
- it increases patient comfort and mobility
- it may reduce the cost of intravenous equipment (Phillips 2005).

One of the disadvantages is the necessity for constant vigilance and regular flushing (Weinstein and Plumer 2007).

comfort and mobility, or by use of an elastomeric device, which is less restrictive and has been able to reduce loss of patency by 50% (Heath and Jones 2001); or

- intermittent flushing (previously known as a 'heparin lock'). See Box 18.1.

When used for intermittent therapy, the device should be flushed after each use with the appropriate flushing solution. (Guidelines for volumes, concentrations and frequency of flushing are commonly established within individual institutions.) It is now well established that flushing with 0.9% sodium chloride can also adequately maintain the patency of the cannula (Goode et al. 1991). This avoids side-effects such as local tissue damage, drug incompatibilities and iatrogenic haemorrhage, which can occur with heparin (Goode et al. 1991). As well as being cost-effective, it appears that daily or twice-daily flushing with a volume of 2–5 mL 0.9% sodium chloride is acceptable (Goode et al. 1991).

There is still no consensus about the solution to use or frequency of flushing (Green et al. 2008) and it also depends on whether the catheter is either open-ended or valved. Heparinized saline is still the accepted solution for maintaining the patency of CVCs for intermittent use or infrequent use (Pratt et al. 2007, RCN 2010), but due to the risk of errors with heparin, its use must be considered carefully (NPSA 2008a). Use of 0.9% sodium chloride alone is not yet widespread, except with certain types of catheters such as the Groshong valve (INS 2011). Flushing regimens, ranging from once daily to once weekly, have been found to be effective. Implanted drug delivery systems such as implanted ports are flushed using a stronger solution of heparin, usually 500 IU heparin in 5 mL 0.9% sodium chloride (Perucca 2010). Recommendations range from monthly (RCN 2010), every 6 weeks (Kefeli et al. 2009) or every 8 weeks (Hoffman 2001) to every 3–4 months when not in use (Hayden and Goodman 2005).

Using the correct techniques to flush the VAD has been highlighted as one of the key issues in maintaining patency (Baranowski 1993, Goodwin and Carlson 1993). There are two stages in flushing.

1 Using a pulsated (push–pause) flush to create turbulent flow when administering the solution, regardless of type and volume. This removes debris from the internal catheter wall (Cummings-Winfield and Mushani Kanji 2008, Goodwin and Carlson 1993, Macklin and Chernecky 2004, Phillips 2005).

2 The procedure is completed using the positive pressure technique. This is accomplished by maintaining pressure on the plunger of the syringe while disconnecting the syringe from the injection cap, which prevents reflux of blood into the tip, reducing the risk of occlusion (Hadaway 2010, INS 2011, Moureau 1999, Phillips 2005).

Manufacturers have now produced needleless injection caps which enable a positive 'displacement' flush and achieve positive pressure without practitioners being required to actively achieve the positive pressure (Weinstein and Plumer 2007). They have been shown to significantly reduce the incidence of catheter occlusions (Berger 2000, Lenhart 2000, Mayo 2001, Rummel et al. 2001) but there has been controversy about these devices and their associated risk of bloodstream infections, resulting in recommendations to carry out a risk assessment prior to routine use (Hadaway 2010). Negative pressure devices require positive pressure on the syringe. Neutral displacement connectors are not dependent upon flushing technique and can be clamped before or after syringe disconnection (Chernecky et al. 2009).

Excessive force should never be used when flushing devices. When a catheter lumen is totally patent, internal pressure will not increase during flushing (Hadaway 1998). However, if resistance is felt (due to partial occlusion) and a force is applied to the plunger, particularly with a small-volume syringe, high pressure could result within the catheter, which may then rupture (Conn 1993, Gorski et al. 2010, Hadaway 1998, Macklin 1999). It is, therefore, recommended that the device is checked first with a 10 mL or larger syringe containing 0.9% sodium chloride (Hadaway 1998, Macklin 2010, RCN 2010). However, smaller syringes should only be used to administer drugs where there is no pressure or occlusion and where it is not possible to further dilute drugs and administer in a large syringe (Hadaway 1998, Macklin 1999). The composition of the individual device determines the maximum pressure that can be exerted.

If a catheter becomes occluded, the nurse should establish the cause of the clot: occlusion or precipitation (INS 2011). If precipitation occurs, then instillation of hydrochloric acid or ethyl chloride may be required (Hadaway 2010, Holcombe et al. 1992, London Standing Committee 2002). There are two types of thrombotic occlusion.

- *Partial withdrawal occlusion* (PWO) (Figure 18.4): this is usually caused by fibrin sheath formation and identified by absent or sluggish blood return whilst fluids can be infused (Nakazawa 2010). Fibrin sheaths can result in seeding of bacteria and drug extravasation (Mayo 2000, 2001) and can be resolved by the instillation of a thrombolytic agent such as urokinase or alteplase (Dougherty

Blood return is absent → Ask patient to cough, deep breathe, change position, stand up or lie with foot of the bed tipped up → Blood return obtained – use central venous catheter as usual

Blood return is still absent

Flush central venous catheter with 0.9% sodium chloride in 10 mL syringe using a brisk 'push pause' technique. Check for flashback of blood → Blood return is still absent → Patient to receive *highly* irritant/vesicant drugs or chemotherapy

Proceed if happy to as long as there are no other complications or pain ← No   Yes

The followings steps should initially be done on admission or prior to drug administration and documented so that all staff are aware that patency has been verified

Step 1
Administer a 250 mL normal saline 'challenge' via an infusion pump over 15 minutes to test for patency – the infusion will probably not resolve the lack of blood return (unless the patient has a high sodium or is on restricted fluid – go to step 2).

If there have been no problems, therapy can be administered as normal. If the patient experiences any discomfort or there are any unexplained problems then stop and seek medical advice. It may be necessary to verify tip location by chest X-ray.

or

Step 2
Instil urokinase 5000 IU in 2 mL and leave for 60 minutes. After this time withdraw the urokinase and assess the catheter again. Repeat as necessary. If blood return is still absent, it may be necessary to verify tip location by chest X-ray.

Figure 18.4 Algorithm for partial withdrawal occlusion, that is, fluids can be infused freely by gravity but blood cannot be withdrawn from the catheter. Adapted from UCL Hospital, Central Venous Catheter Policy.

2006, Fanikos *et al.* 2009, Haire and Herbst 2000, Rinn 2001, Weinstein and Plumer 2007).

- *Total occlusion*: when there is an inability to withdraw blood or infuse fluids or medications. This can be resolved by instillation of a thrombolytic agent (Deitcher *et al.* 2002, Ponec *et al.* 2001, Timoney *et al.* 2002) or by use of an endoluminal brush (Archis *et al.* 2000, Weinstein and Plumer 2007).

If the occlusion is caused by a clot, gentle pressure and aspiration may be sufficient to dislodge it. Silicone catheters expand on pressure and allow fluid to flow around the clot, facilitating its dislodgement. This should only be attempted using a 10 mL or larger syringe. Smaller syringes should never be used as they create a greater pressure (Camp-Sorrell *et al.* 2004, Gorski *et al.* 2010) of mmHg or pounds per square inch (psi). This can result in rupture of the catheter, leading to loss of catheter integrity (Gorski *et al.* 2010). Clearance of a catheter occlusion and instillation of thrombolytic agents should be performed using a three-way tap and negative pressure (Dougherty 2006,

Gabriel 2008, Simcock 2001a). The establishment of negative pressure means creating a vacuum by aspiration of the air or dead space within a catheter (Dougherty 2006, Gabriel 2008, Moureau *et al.* 1999). Another method is use of the percussion technique (Stewart 2001). Unblocking a catheter is not a quick procedure and it can take up to 30 minutes or longer to achieve success.

Methods of maintaining a correctly positioned catheter tip

Tip location is a subject of debate although there are some common recommendations (Chantler 2009).

- The vein should be large with a high blood flow (this dilutes drugs and reduces risk of damage of vein intima).
- The end of the catheter should be in the long axis of the vein and not abutting the vessel wall (to reduce damage to the intima and inaccurate pressure readings).
- The tip should be beyond the last venous valve.

(Chantler 2009)

Figure 18.5 Chest X-ray showing catheter tip correctly positioned (arrow).

The tip location of a CVAD will affect the catheter performance – if the tip is too high, it may be sucked against the adjacent wall when aspiration is applied or if the tip is too far within the right atrium (RA) (Vesely 2002, 2003). A catheter tip positioned against a vascular wall may also become a source of persistent irritation leading to the possible creation of a potential nidus for thrombus formation (Galloway and Bodenham 2004, Mayo 2001). This is reported more frequently in patients who have left-sided placements (Chantler 2009). The arguments for right atrial tip placement are that the tip is in a large chamber, thus preventing contact with the vein wall, and the rapid blood flow also prevents accumulation of thrombin and minimizes irritation of substances. The disadvantages of this tip position are an increase in cardiac arrhythmias (although this may be associated with the insertion of the guidewire as it is reduced by image guidance) and catheter-induced perforation and cardiac tamponade although this has been reduced by using softer materials and imaging guidance (Chantler 2009, Vesely 2002).

The tip position can also change during its time *in situ*. The final position of a PICC is dependent on the insertion site and the position of the patient's arm and the catheter can move at least 2 cm further into the RA on movement (Forauer and Alonzo 2000). If placed in the left arm, it can move more than if in the right arm and when placed in the basilic more than if in the cephalic vein (Vesely 2003). Anatomical changes occur with subclavian and internal jugular insertion when the patient sits upright following insertion and the catheter tip can move upward. In a skin-tunnelled catheter this can be 2–3 cm, particularly in overweight patients of either sex or female patients with substantial breast tissue. Large-diameter catheters can move more than smaller ones and subclavian more than internal jugular placements.

A correctly placed catheter tip will probably be one that undergoes a range of movement between the SVC and upper RA (Dougherty 2006). Tip position is determined by use of a chest X-ray using the posterior anterior (PA) view (Wise *et al.* 2001). See Figure 18.5.

Anticipated patient outcomes

For the patient to have a functioning vascular access device.

Legal and professional issues

Competencies

The nurse inserting devices and/or providing infusion therapy should be competent in all clinical aspects of infusion therapy and have validated competency in clinical judgement and practice, in accordance with the NMC Code to maintain their knowledge and skills (Collins *et al.* 2006, Hyde 2008, NMC 2008a, RCN 2010).

The RCN (2010) recommends that any Registered Nurses undertaking the insertion of VADs or those who manage VADs or administer infusion therapy should have undergone theoretical and practical training in a number of areas (see Box 18.2) (Corrigan 2010, DH 2004, Hyde 2008, MDA 2003, NICE 2003, NPSA 2003, NPSA 2007, Pratt *et al.* 2007). All staff have a professional obligation to maintain their knowledge and skills (NMC 2008a). It is also the responsibility of the organization to support and provide staff with training and education. This may be in the form of study days, practical sessions using a mannequin and a role development workbook (Collins *et al.* 2006, Phillips *et al.* 2011).

Consent

Prior to insertion of a peripheral cannula, it is usual to obtain verbal consent from the patient (Hyde 2008). However, prior to insertion of a CVAD, written consent should be obtained (unless required in an emergency) following an explanation of the procedure, the benefits, the alternatives and the possible complications and the percentage risk of each (these would include pneumothorax, malposition, haemorrhage, thrombosis and infection). This should be provided verbally and in written form (Hamilton 2009).

Preprocedural considerations

Equipment

There are many different types of devices available made of a variety of materials and tip endings and specific equipment associated with VADs includes securement devices and dressings. These will be discussed in more detail in each individual section.

Securement (stabilization) of device and dressings

Devices are secured to prevent movement, which reduces the risk of phlebitis, infiltration, infection and migration

Box 18.2 Required knowledge and skills for:

Vascular access device insertion

- Anatomy and physiology of the circulatory system, in particular, the anatomy of the location in which the device is placed including veins, arteries and nerves and the underlying tissue structures.
- Assessment of patients' vascular access needs, nature and duration of therapy and quality of life.
- Improving venous access, for example the use of pharmacological and non-pharmacological methods.
- Selection of veins and problems associated with venous access due to thrombosed, inflamed or fragile veins, the effects of ageing on veins, disease process, previous treatment, lymphoedema or presence of infection.
- Selection of device and other equipment.
- Infection control issues (handwashing, skin preparation).
- Pharmacological issues (use of local anaesthetics, management of anxious patients, management of haematoma, phlebitis).
- Patient's perspective on living with a vascular access device.
- Risk management in order to reduce the risk of blood spills and needlestick injury.
- Professional and legal aspects (consent, professional guidance, knowledge and skill maintenance, and documentation).
- Performing the procedure.
- Prevention and management of complications during insertion (nerve injury, haematoma).
- Monitoring and care of the site (flushing, dressing, removal).
- Product evaluation.
- Patient information and education.
- Documentation.
- Specific training for insertion of vascular access devices in certain groups, for example neonates, children and oncology patients.

Administration of IV medication and care of VAD *in situ*

- Legal, professional and ethical issues.
- Anatomy and physiology.
- Fluid balance and blood administration.
- Mathematical calculations related to medications.
- Pharmacology and pharmaceutics related to reconstitution and administration.
- Local and systemic complications.
- Infection control issues.
- Use of equipment, including infusion equipment.
- Drug administration.
- Risk management/health and safety.
- Care and management of vascular access devices.
- Infusion therapy in specialist areas covered separately (paediatrics, oncology, parenteral nutrition, transfusion therapy).

(Czaplewski 2010)

(INS 2011, McGoldrick 2010, Moureau and Iannucci 2003, Schears 2005, Yamamoto *et al.* 2002). This can be achieved by suturing, taping or use of stabilizing devices. These all require a dressing over them. The stabilization device should be used in a manner that does not interfere with the assessment and monitoring of the access site (McGoldrick 2010).

The choice of dressing is usually based upon what is most suitable for a particular VAD site or type of skin. An intravenous dressing is applied to minimize the contamination of the insertion site and provide stability of the device (Dougherty 2006). Therefore the ideal intravenous dressing should:

- provide an effective barrier to bacteria
- allow the catheter to be securely fixed
- be sterile
- be easy to apply and remove
- be waterproof
- adhere well
- be comfortable for the patient (Finlay 2004).

There are two main types of dressing: dry, sterile low-linting gauze and transparent dressings. A dry, sterile, low-linting dressing secured with the minimum of hypoallergenic tape is most suitable for patients with skin that is prone to allergy or is thin and tears easily, as transparent dressings can damage the skin if not removed correctly.

The benefits of transparent dressings are that they allow inspection of the insertion site while the dressing is *in situ* and therefore do not require removal; they are waterproof and many are also moisture permeable (McGoldrick 2010). This means that the dressing allows moisture vapour transmission, an important factor related to infection as collection of moisture enhances the proliferation of microorganisms.

When transparent dressings have been compared with sterile gauze, it has been shown that there is no significant difference and that infection rates may have been reduced (DH 2010, Maki and Ringer 1987, RCN 2010). All CVAD dressings must be removed and replaced within 24 hours following insertion of the catheter (Dougherty 2006, RCN 2010, Ryder 2001). This is due to the bacterial colonization, 'biofilm', which occurs 6–18 hours following insertion (Ryder 2002). If gauze is used, it must be replaced when the dressing becomes damp, loosened or soiled or when inspection of the site is necessary (Pratt *et al.* 2007, RCN 2010). Transparent dressings should be changed every 7 days unless manufacturers recommend otherwise or the integrity is compromised, that is, when damp, loose or soiled (INS 2011, Pratt *et al.* 2007, RCN 2010). When the dressing is changed, the insertion site should be inspected for inflammation and/or discharge and the condition of the skin noted (DH 2010).

There are also chlorhexidine-impregnated dressings (for example, protective disc impregnated with chlorhexidine gluconate) which may also be considered for placement at the catheter skin junction. This is done to protect the

1. Patient characteristics		5. Evidence of previous use		• For each risk factor score either 0.1 or 2.
Needle phobia		Evidence of phlebitis		• 0 = risk factor not present.
Confusion		Evidence of infiltration or extravasation		• 1 = risk factor present.
2. Limiting the number of available veins		Visible pin prick or needle marks		• 2 = risk factor present and will complicate a cannulation attempt now.
Hemiplegia, spasticity of upper limb(s), for example post-cerebrovascular accident		Bruising from vasculature use		• Total points to give VAT score.
Radical mastectomy		Dark, stained veins		• Follow action specified below.
Arteriovenous fistula		Cord-like, hard veins		• Re-evaluate patient score at least every three days.
3. Changes in skin integrity		6. Suitability of veins		
Skin graft versus host disease		Flow visible veins		

VAT score	Action
< 3 (easy)	Routine cannulation
4–8 (moderate)	Difficult cannulation Consider alternative IV access device for future therapy
> 9 (difficult)	Expert cannulation. Will require alternative IV access device for therapy to continue

Tattoos, burns, scars, eczema, over veins		Flow palpable veins	
		Few straight veins	
4. Changes in tissue		Veins are mobile	
Oedema		Only short veins identifiable or multiple valves are palpable	
Obesity		7. History	
Cachexia		Previous peripheral chemotherapy	
Radiotherapy to the upper limb(s)		Previous multiple courses of intravenous (IV) antibiotics	
Dark skin		Previous peripheral vesicant chemotherapy	

Figure 18.6   VAT score (Wells 2008).

extraluminal pathway and eliminate or reduce the incidence of infection (McGoldrick 2010).

Assessment and recording tools

Tools have been developed to facilitate venous assessment and venous access device assessment. For example, the venous assessment tool (VAT) consists of a series of risk factors and characteristics that can be assessed to determine if cannulation will be easy, moderate or hard. The VAT score can then be used in the algorithm 'Deciding on Intravenous Access' or DIVA. This guide helps practitioners bring together the proposed therapy and the type of venous access in order to identify the most suitable VAD (Wells 2008). See Figure 18.6.

Pharmacological support
Solutions to maintain patency

Heparin inhibits the conversion of prothrombin to thrombin and fibrinogen to fibrin, thus inhibiting coagulation, and is therefore used to prevent the build-up of fibrin. The standard strength is 10 IU/mL up to a total of 5 mL (50 IU) for all CVADs with the exception of implanted ports where it is usual for the dose to be 100 IU/mL (500 IU total). Sodium chloride 0.9% is used to clean the internal diameter of the device of blood and drugs (Camp-Sorrell et al. 2004). Urokinase is a fibrinolytic agent indicated for the lysis of blood clots in venous catheters that are occluded by fibrin clots. Usually, 5000 IU is dissolved in sterile saline and instilled into the catheter for 20–60 minutes. The drug and any clots are then aspirated and the process can be repeated if necessary (www.emc.medicines).

Specific patient preparations
Education

Patients may be well informed about access devices from the media or via the Internet. They may also have gained knowledge from friends or family experiences. Therefore, involving the patient in the decision-making process is vital (Dougherty 2006). Patient choice about the device or even the site of insertion, for example use of the non-dominant arm, results in better compliance with care of the device and monitoring of problems (Gabriel 2008). It also enables patients to cope better with the changes to their normal activities (Daniels 1995) and the impact on body image can be reduced by involving the individual in the choice and management of the device (Daniels 1995, Dougherty 2006).

Body image and a patient's lifestyle can be issues when living with a CVAD (Dougherty 2006). This is particularly true with an external catheter, which can be distressing and embarrassing for some patients (Hayden and Goodman 2005). It can result in restrictions to normal daily activities, for example bathing, or involvement in sporting activities such as swimming (Gabriel 2000, Molloy et al. 2008, Robbins et al. 2000); some of these can be resolved by the use of an implanted device (Chernecky 2001, Johansson et al. 2009).

The following have been listed as ways in which a CVAD can affect body image.

■   Physical presence and alteration of body appearance and invasion of body integrity.
■   It influences the type of clothes that can be worn.

1089

- It may interfere with physical expressions of closeness and sexuality (Daniels 1995).

The presence of a CVAD could also affect how others view the role function of the individual, particularly if the patient is attached to an infusion pump (Thompson *et al.* 1989). The psychological impact of an indwelling catheter on body image should not be overlooked, especially when patients are sexually active (Gabriel 2000, Oakley *et al.* 2000).

Procedure guideline 18.1 Central venous catheter: insertion site dressing change

This can be adapted to changing a peripheral cannula dressing but this is rarely changed and is usually removed along with the cannula.

Essential equipment

- Sterile dressing pack (containing gallipot, sterile towel and low-linting gauze, sterile gloves)
- Alcohol-based handrub
- Alcohol-based skin cleaning preparation, 2% chlorhexidine in 70% alcohol
- Semi-permeable transparent dressing; sterile low-linting gauze or other appropriate dressing

- Hypoallergenic tape

- Pair of non-sterile gloves
- Apron

Optional equipment

- Securing device
- Bacteriological swab

Preprocedure

Action	Rationale
1 Explain and discuss the procedure with the patient.	To ensure that the patient understands the procedure and gives their valid verbal consent (NMC 2008b, C).

Procedure

2 Perform the dressing using an aseptic technique.	To prevent infection (DH 2010, C). (For further information on asepsis, see Chapter 3.)
3 Screen the bed. Assist the patient into a supine position, if possible.	To allow dust and airborne organisms to settle before the insertion site and the sterile field are exposed. E
4 Wash hands with bactericidal soap and water or bactericidal alcohol handrub.	To reduce the risk of cross-infection (DH 2010, C; Fraise and Bradley 2009, E).
5 Place all equipment required for the dressing on the bottom shelf of a clean dressing trolley.	To reduce the risk of cross-infection (DH 2010, C).
6 Take the trolley to the patient's bedside, disturbing the screens as little as possible.	To minimize airborne contamination (DH 2010, C).
7 Open the sterile dressing pack onto the top of the trolley.	To gain access to equipment. E
8 Attach an orange clinical waste bag to the side of the trolley below the level of the top shelf.	So that contaminated material is below the level of the sterile field (DH 2010, C).
9 Open the other sterile packs, tipping their contents gently onto the centre of the sterile field. Pour lotions into gallipots or into an indented plastic tray where required.	To reduce risk of contamination of contents. E

10 Wash hands with bactericidal alcohol handrub.	Hands may have become contaminated by handling the outer packs, and so on (DH 2010, C).
11 Place the sterile field under the patient's arm or on the chest.	To create a clean working area. E
12 Loosen the old dressing gently.	So that the dressing can be lifted off easily. E
13 Put on clean gloves.	To protect the nurse from any contact with the patient's blood. E
14 Using gloved hands, remove the old dressing and discard it. Remove tapes or securing device if loose or contaminated or due to be changed.	To remove old dressing without contaminating hands (DH 2010, C).
15 If the site is red or discharging, take a swab for bacteriological investigation.	For identification of pathogens. To select appropriate treatment (DH 2010, C).
16 Remove and dispose of gloves and put on sterile gloves from pack.	To minimize the risk of introducing infection (DH 2010, C).
17 Clean the wound with 2% chlorhexidine in 70% alcohol, using back and forth strokes with friction. Allow area to dry prior to applying the dressing.	To enable disinfection process to be completed. To prevent skin reaction in response to the application of a transparent dressing to moist skin (Pratt *et al.* 2007, C).
18 Reapply tapes or securing device if necessary. This may require skin preparation prior to application of securing device.	To secure device and prevent dislodgement and phlebitis (Schears 2005, R5).
19 Apply appropriate dressing, moulding it into place so that there are no folds or creases.	To minimize skin irritation and reduce risk of dressing peeling or becoming damaged. E To ensure security of device and prevent dislodgement. E
20 Document date and time on dressing.	To ensure the dressing is changed as required (DH 2010, C).

Postprocedure

21 Remove gloves and dispose into waste bag.	To dispose of waste. E
22 Fold up the sterile field, place it in the orange clinical waste bag and seal it before moving the trolley. Draw back the curtains. Dispose of waste in appropriate containers.	To prevent environmental contamination (DH 2010, C).
23 Document date and time of dressing and any relevant changes at the insertion site in the patient's records.	To ensure adequate records and to enable continued care of device and patient (NMC 2009, C).

Procedure guideline 18.2 Vascular access devices: maintaining patency

Essential equipment

- Sterile dressing pack (containing gallipot, sterile towel and low-linting gauze)
- Chlorhexidine 2% in 70% alcohol

Medicinal products

- Flushing solution ready prepared in a 10 mL syringe in a clinically clean container

Preprocedure

Action	Rationale
1 Explain and discuss the procedure with the patient.	To ensure that the patient understands the procedure and gives their valid consent (NMC 2008b, C).
2 Wash hands thoroughly or use an alcohol-based handrub.	To reduce the risk of contamination (DH 2010, C; Fraise and Bradley 2009, E).

Procedure

3 Open sterile dressing pack and arrange equipment.	To gain access to equipment. E
4 Clean the needleless injection cap using chlorhexidine 2% in 70% alcohol and apply with friction, rubbing the cap in a clockwise and anticlockwise manner at least five times and allow to air dry.	To minimize the risk of contamination at the connections (DH 2010, C; Pratt et al. 2007, C).
5 Attach the syringe to the needleless injection cap.	To establish connection between cap and syringe. E
6 Using a push–pause method, inject the contents of the syringe (inject 1 mL at a time).	To create turbulence in order to flush the catheter thoroughly (Goodwin and Carlson 1993, E).
7 Maintain pressure on the plunger as the syringe is disconnected from the cap then clamp device tubing if necessary.	To maintain positive pressure and prevent backflow of blood into the catheter, and possible clot formation (Dougherty 2006, E).

Postprocedure

8 Dispose of equipment safely.	To prevent contamination of others (DH 2010, C).
9 Record the procedure.	To maintain accurate records (NMC 2009, C).

Procedure guideline 18.3 Central venous access devices: unblocking an occlusion

Essential equipment

- Sterile dressing pack (containing gallipot, sterile towel and low-linting gauze; sterile gloves)
- Bactericidal handrub
- Alcohol-based skin cleaning preparation, 2% chlorhexidine in 70% alcohol
- 10 mL syringes $\times$ 3
- Needles
- Three-way tap
- Extension set or needleless injection cap
- Apron

Medicinal products

- 0.9% sodium chloride
- Heparin 50 IU in 0.9% sodium chloride
- Fibrinolytic solution if required, for example urokinase

Preprocedure

Action	Rationale
1 Explain and discuss the procedure with the patient.	To ensure that the patient understands the procedure and gives their valid consent (NMC 2008b, C).
2 Perform the procedure using an aseptic technique.	To minimize the risk of infection (DH 2010, C; Fraise and Bradley 2009, E). (For further information on asepsis see Chapter 3.)
3 Wash hands with bactericidal soap and water or bactericidal alcohol handrub. Place all equipment required on bottom shelf.	To minimize the risk of cross-infection (DH 2010, C).
4 Open a sterile pack and empty other equipment onto it.	To create a clean working area (DH 2010, C).
5 Wash hands with bactericidal alcohol handrub.	Hands may have become contaminated by handling the outer packs, and so on (DH 2010, C).

Procedure

6 Clean connections thoroughly with chlorhexidine 2% in 70% alcohol before disconnection.	To minimize infection risk at connection site (DH 2010, C).
7 Remove any extension sets or injection caps.	Occlusion may be in extension set/cap and not in catheter. E
8 Draw up and attempt to flush with 0.9% sodium chloride using a 10 mL syringe.	Smaller syringes create excessive pressure which could result in catheter rupture (Conn 1993, E).
9 If there is pressure within the device lumen, attempt to gently instil the 0.9% sodium chloride using a 'to and fro' motion (push–pull) over a few minutes.	To attempt to clear the catheter (Gabriel 2008, E).
10 If nothing can be aspirated, if a peripheral device then remove the device and resite as necessary. If a central venous access device, attach a three-way tap and to this add an empty 10 mL syringe and a 10 mL syringe containing heparin 50 IU in 5 mL saline.	To commence the negative pressure technique (see Action Figure 10) (Gabriel 2008, E).
11 Attempt to unblock catheter using the negative pressure technique (see Action Figure 11).	This enables the solution to be drawn into the catheter without creating any pressure which could result in catheter rupture (Gabriel 2008, E).
12 If still unable to aspirate, then determine the cause of the occlusion.	
If blood: discuss with doctors who may prescribe a fibrinolytic agent, for example urokinase (5000 IU/mL) or alteplase (see Box 18.3).	To break down fibrin (BNF 2011, C; RCN 2010, C).
Or if precipitation: discuss with pharmacy for best antidote, for example ethyl alcohol or hydrochloric acid.	To break down drug precipitate or fat emulsion (BNF 2011, C).
13 Draw up prescribed solution in a 10 mL syringe.	To prepare appropriate treatment. E
14 Put on clean gloves.	To minimize the risk of introducing infection (DH 2010, C).
15 Instil via a three-way tap using negative pressure technique (see above).	To prevent catheter rupture (Conn 1993, E).
16 Cap off catheter and leave for allotted time, for example 2–4 hours or overnight.	To allow the drug to destroy fibrin (Gabriel 2008, E).

(Continued)

Procedure guideline 18.3 *(Continued)*

17 Clean cap with 2% chlorhexidine in 70% alcohol.	To minimize infection risk at connection site (DH 2010, C).
18 Attach an empty syringe to catheter and attempt to aspirate any clots and solution.	To unblock catheter and ensure no clots are administered into the patient (Gabriel 2008, E).
19 If blood returns, withdraw at least 10 mL and discard.	To ensure no fibrinolytic agent or clots are flushed into the patient (Gabriel 2008, E).
20 Flush catheter with 10 mL 0.9% sodium chloride using a pulsatile flush and then flush with heparinized saline.	To ensure the catheter is flushed and patent (RCN 2010, C).

Postprocedure

21 Remove gloves and dispose of waste.	To prevent contamination of others (DH 2010, C).
22 If still unable to aspirate, discuss the use of a second instillation of fibrinolytic agent. It may be necessary to remove the catheter if a single lumen or if multilumen, to refrain from using the occluded lumen and label not for use.	To maintain some venous access for the patient. If occlusion cannot be removed the catheter is no longer patent. In multilumen catheters there may be another patent lumen for use (Gabriel 2008, E).
23 Document in patient's records.	To ensure adequate records and to enable continued care of device and patient (NMC 2009, C).

Action Figure 10 Turn tap to close off prefilled syringe and open it to empty syringe.

(a)

(b)

Action Figure 11 Unblocking an occluded catheter. (a) Aspirate on an empty syringe, which creates a negative pressure. (b) Turn tap to close off the empty syringe and open to the prefilled syringe. The medication will automatically be aspirated into the catheter. Repeat as necessary. Modified from BD *First PICC Clinical Education Class Manual* D11 952B 5/98.

Box 18.3 Volumes for instillation of urokinase

- Prepare urokinase 5000 IU. (This may require 10,000 IU to be reconstituted in 2 mL water.)
- Volume to be instilled will vary depending on the length of catheter (which will have been dictated by patient's size). These volumes are estimates of the maximum volume required to ensure the urokinase reaches the catheter tip (if blood has tracked back along the length of the catheter then there may be no point in instilling urokinase).
  - *PICC*: remove extension set (if present) and injection cap. Instil 0.5–1 mL into each lumen as required.
  - *Skin-tunnelled catheter:* remove injection cap. Instil 1 mL into each lumen as required.
  - *Implanted port*: remove injection cap. It may be necessary to further dilute the urokinase and instil 2 mL via the needle and integral extension set.

Postprocedural considerations

Immediate care

This will depend on the type of VAD that has been inserted (see each individual VAD).

Ongoing care

Discharging patients home with a VAD in situ

Patients may be discharged home with a VAD *in situ* which will allow them to receive treatment at home (e.g. continuous chemotherapy or intermittent antibiotics) or allow for easier access on each admission (e.g. via implantable ports). An early referral to the community nurses is crucial to ensure adequate support for the patient once at home (Dougherty 2006).

Patients may now receive daily treatment over a 3–5-day period with an indwelling peripheral cannula (Shotkin and Lombardo 1996). The degree of care is minimal compared with a CVC, but patients should receive adequate information about the early signs of phlebitis, such as pain, redness and swelling, and what to do in the case of accidental dislodgement or removal of the cannula.

The dressing of choice for PICC and skin-tunnelled insertion sites is one that is moisture permeable and transparent (NICE 2003, Pratt *et al.* 2007), which usually requires changing once a week, following the initial change within the first 24 hours (RCN 2010, Ryder 2001). This type of dressing may make it difficult for the patient to change the dressing themselves and so a carer or district nurse will need to be involved. At the dressing change, the site should be inspected and any signs of erythema or inflammation should be reported to the hospital at once in order for appropriate treatment to be prescribed (DH 2010). The area should be cleaned using an aseptic technique with a 2% chlorhexidine-based solution (DH 2010, NICE 2003, Pratt *et al.* 2007).

Box 18.4 CVAD flushing kit

A CVAD flushing kit should contain the following when a patient has a skin-tunnelled catheter or PICC *in situ*.

- Needleless injection caps.
- Ampoules of heparinized saline (50 IU heparin in 5 mL 0.9% sodium chloride).
- Chlorhexidine 2% in 70% alcohol wipes.
- Sterile 10 mL Luer-Lok syringes.
- 21 and 23 G needles.
- Instruction leaflet to provide both the community nurse and patient with a point of reference, for example a patient information leaflet on central venous access devices.
- Sharps container.

If a patient wishes to be self-caring, the nurse should observe them carrying out the flushing procedure, either in hospital or in the home setting, until competent to do so without supervision of a nurse (Dougherty 2006, INS 2011). However, some patients prefer the district nurse to take responsibility for maintaining patency. Sufficient equipment (Box 18.4 and Box 18.5) must be supplied to enable the patient or nurse to care for the CVAD from the time of discharge until the patient's next admission.

Education of patient and relevant others

Patients with long-term CVADs *in situ*, such as PICCs or skin-tunnelled catheters, will require instruction and supervision to ensure adequate understanding of the care and maintenance of their devices (Dougherty 2006). This must start early within the discharge planning process along with an assessment of the home environment, the patient's manual dexterity, physical and medical condition (Kayley 2008, Weinstein and Plumer 2007). Patient education is one of the most important aspects of care but to make teaching effective, it is essential to recognize each patient's needs and limitations. It is also vital to acknowledge each patient's past experiences and readiness to learn (Cole 1999, Czaplewski 2010). Education of the patient should encompass care and maintenance of the device as well as signs and symptoms

---

Box 18.5 Contents of pack to take home for patients with PICC

For PICC dressings, a pack containing the following should be sent home with the patient.

- Dressing packs (contains gloves).
- Securing device.
- Gauze.
- Transparent dressings.
- Chlorhexidine 2% in 70% alcohol sponges.
- Bandages.

Figure 18.7 Patient information booklet on central venous access devices.

of complications (Kayley 2008, RCN 2010). Educational packages should be prepared in the form of practical demonstrations and clear, succinct handouts (INS 2011, Kayley 2008, NICE 2003) (Figure 18.7). It is also important to recognize the need to prepare patients carefully to participate in their own self-care and therapy (Czaplewski 2010). The patient, relative and/or carers should understand the following.

- The frequency of changing the dressing and how to care for the site.
- How to maintain patency.
- How to inspect for signs of infection or other complications.
- How to solve problems and where to seek help (RCN 2010).

Patients should be taught what early signs and symptoms to look out for, must know what to do if the catheter becomes occluded or damaged and be told when and who to contact along with a contact name and number in order to be able to seek professional advice. This will help to alleviate any anxiety (Dougherty et al. 1998). Most problems can be managed at home with the involvement of the community nurses and general practitioner.

The most common complications associated with CVADs are infection and thrombosis (Dougherty 2006, Kayley 2008, RCN 2010). The patient should be told to report signs of redness and tracking at the exit site, along the skin tunnel or up the arm, any oozing at the exit site and fevers or rigors. Patients are no longer routinely prescribed prophylactic warfarin as this has been shown to have no

---

Box 18.6 Complications associated with vascular access devices

- Haematoma.
- Arterial puncture.
- Nerve injury.
- Phlebitis.
- Infiltration.
- Extravasation.
- Occlusion.
- Infection.
- Hydrothorax.
- Brachial plexus injury.
- Catheter embolism.
- Arterial puncture and malposition.
- Air embolism.
- Haemorrhage.
- Thoracic duct trauma.
- Thrombosis.
- Pneumothorax.
- Haemothorax.
- Misdirection or kinking.
- Cardiac tamponade.
- Cardiac arrhythmias.

(Dougherty 2006, Dougherty 2008, Weinstein and Plumer 2007)

---

apparent benefit in the prevention of thrombosis (Couban et al. 2005, Young et al. 2005). Therefore it should be stressed to the patient that any of the following signs or symptoms should be reported immediately: breathlessness, pain and/or swelling over the shoulder, across the chest and into the neck and arm. Early reporting may enable effective treatment and avoid removal of the device (Bishop 2009).

Complications

The complications associated with vascular access devices can be found in Box 18.6. Each complication will be discussed in more detail under each device.

Peripheral cannulas

Definition

A cannula is a flexible tube containing a needle (stylet) which may be inserted into a blood vessel (Phillips 2005, RCN 2010, Weller 2005). Cannulas are usually placed in the peripheral veins in the lower arm but may also be placed in the veins of the foot (an area used particularly in paediatric care) (Weinstein and Plumer 2007). However, veins of the lower extremities should not be routinely used in adults due to the risk of embolism and thrombophlebitis (INS 2011, RCN 2010).

Anatomy and physiology

Choice of vein

The main factors to consider prior to inserting a peripheral cannula are the location for siting, condition of the vein, purpose of the infusion (that is, the rate of flow required and the solution to be infused) and the duration of therapy (Dougherty 2008, Phillips 2005).

A suitable vein should always be selected prior to selection of the device. The vein should feel bouncy, refill when depressed, should be straight and free of valves to ensure easy advancement of the cannula. Valves can be felt as small lumps in the vein; some may be visualized at bifurcations, some may be visible to the naked eye in certain vessels. It is best to avoid siting a cannula over a joint as this will lead to an increased risk of mechanical phlebitis and an infusion that will infuse intermittently due to the patient's movement (Dougherty 2008, INS 2011, RCN 2010, Weinstein and Plumer 2007). It can also be very awkward for the patient and may restrict their ability to carry out activities (Macklin and Chernecky 2004, Marsigliese 2001).

The veins of choice are either the cephalic or basilic veins, followed by the dorsal venous network (see Figure 18.1). The practitioner should choose distal veins and then cannulate at proximal points (INS 2011, Perucca 2010). The best vein should always be used (Weinstein and Plumer 2007).

The cephalic vein

The size and position of the cephalic vein make it an excellent vessel for administration of transfusions. It readily accommodates a large-gauge cannula and, by virtue of its position on the forearm, provides a natural splint (Weinstein and Plumer 2007). However, its position at a joint may increase complications such as mechanical phlebitis and even general discomfort. The tendons controlling the thumb obscure the vein during insertion (Hadaway 2010), and care must be taken not to touch the radial nerve (Dougherty 2008).

The basilic vein

The basilic vein is a large vessel, which is often overlooked due to its inconspicuous position on the ulnar border of the hand and forearm. It is found on palpation when the patient's arm is placed across the chest, with the practitioner opposite the patient (Hadaway 2010). Cannulation can be awkward because of its position, mobility and tendency to have many valves (Dougherty 2008, Hadaway 2010).

Dorsal venous network

Using the veins of the dorsal venous network of the hand will allow for cannulation proximally along the veins when resiting the device (Weinstein and Plumer 2007). They can usually be visualized and palpated easily (Hadaway 2010).

- The digital veins are small and may be prominent enough to accommodate a small-gauge needle as a last resort for fluid administration. With adequate taping, the fingers can be immobilized, making it more comfortable as well as preventing the cannula from piercing the posterior wall of the vein (leading to bruising or infiltration) (Springhouse 2002).
- The metacarpal veins are accessible, and easily visualized and palpated. They are well suited for cannulation as the cannula lies flat and the metacarpal veins provide a natural splint (Weinstein and Plumer 2007). The veins tend to be smaller than those in the forearm and therefore may prove difficult to access in infants because they have higher amounts of subcutaneous fat than older children and adults. The use of these veins is contraindicated in the elderly as there is diminished skin turgor and loss of subcutaneous tissue, making the vein difficult to stabilize. They are also more fragile and venous distension is slower (Fabian 2010, Hadaway 2010, Springhouse 2002). Metacarpal veins are a better option for short-term or outpatient intravenous therapy.

Evidence-based approaches

Rationale

The advantages of using a peripheral cannula are that they are usually easy to insert and have few associated complications; however, they are associated with phlebitis (either mechanical or chemical) and require constant resiting (Dougherty 2008, INS 2011, RCN 2010).

Indications

- Short-term therapy of less than a week.
- Bolus injections or short infusions in the outpatient/day unit setting (Hadaway 2010, RCN 2010).

Contraindications

- Long-term intravenous therapy.
- Longer or continous infusions of medications that are vesicant or those that have a pH <5 or >9 (Hadaway 2010).

Methods of improving venous access

Difficult peripheral access is traumatic for the patient. Application of a tourniquet, taping and stroking of veins, vigorous swabbing, clenching the hand to pump up veins, hanging the forearm downwards and application of local warmth are all commonly used aids for cannulation (Dougherty 2008).

The application of the tourniquet promotes venous distension. The tourniquet should be tight enough to impede venous return while not affecting arterial flow (Perucca 2010, RCN 2010). It should be applied around the upper forearm about 6–8 inches above the venepuncture site

(Phillips 2005) to promote dilation of the veins and time should be allowed for the veins to fill. Other methods used to improve venous distension include lowering the extremity below the level of the heart and opening and closing the fist (the action of the muscles forces blood into the veins, causing them to distend) (Phillips 2005). Light tapping of the vein may be useful as this releases histamines beneath the skin and causes dilation (Phillips 2005), but it can be painful and may result in the formation of a haematoma; again, elderly patients and those with fragile veins are most at risk (Witt 2004).

When these methods fail, applying a warm compress in the form of a heat pack, warmed towels or electric heating blanket or immersing the limb in a bowl of warm water for 10–15 minutes helps to increase vasodilation and promote venous filling (Chen 2002, Fink *et al.* 2009, Weinstein and Plumer 2007). Ointments or patches containing small amounts of glycerol trinitrate have been used to improve vasodilation (Gunwardene and Davenport 1990) as well as reducing the incidence of chemical phlebitis and increasing site survival time (Hecker 1988).

Finally new technology can be used, such as transillumination (Venoscope or Accuvein) to illuminate or ultrasound to locate the veins, if the practitioner is unable to palpate them (Phillips 2005, Walker 2009).

Methods of insertion

Skin stabilization is one of the most important elements for successful venepuncture or cannulation (Dougherty 2008, Perucca 2010) (Figure 18.8). Superficial veins tend to roll; to prevent this, the vein must be stabilized by applying traction to the side of the insertion site or below it, using the practitioner's non-dominant hand. This also facilitates a smoother needle entry. Various methods are used (Dougherty 2008).

- The thumb can be used to stretch the skin downwards.
- The hand of the practitioner can be placed under the patient's arm and traction applied with the thumb and forefinger on either side, creating an even traction.
- The vein can be stretched between forefinger and thumb.

Stabilization of the vein must be maintained throughout the procedure until the needle or cannula is successfully sited. If the tension is released halfway through the procedure, the needle may penetrate the opposite wall of the vein, resulting in a haematoma formation (Dougherty 2008).

It is important that the needle enters the skin with the bevel up, as this results in a smooth venepuncture as the sharpest part of the needle will penetrate the skin first, and this also reduces the risk of piercing the posterior wall of the vein (Weinstein and Plumer 2007). The angle at which the needle enters the skin varies with the type of device used and the depth of the vein in the subcuta-

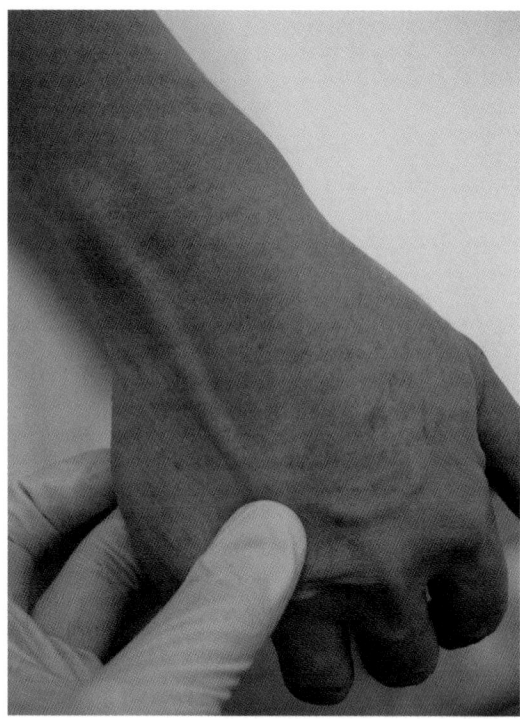

Figure 18.8 Anchoring the vein with the thumb. Reproduced with permission from Dougherty (2008).

neous tissue, from 10° to 45° (Dougherty 2008, Perucca 2010, Weinstein and Plumer 2007). Once the device is in the vein, the angle should always be reduced in order to prevent puncturing the posterior wall of the vein (Perucca 2010).

There are two main methods for approaching the vein.

- The *direct method* is when the device enters through the skin and immediately enters the vein. However, with smaller veins this method may result in puncture of the posterior wall (Dougherty 2008).
- The *indirect method* is when the device is inserted through the skin and then the vein is relocated and the device advanced into the vessel. This method enables a more gentle entry and may be useful in veins which are palpable and visible for only a short section (Dougherty 2008, Perucca 2010, Weinstein and Plumer 2007).

When blood appears in the chamber of a cannula, this is known as 'flashback' and it indicates that the initial entry into the vein has been successful. This may be accompanied by a 'giving way' sensation felt by the practitioner, which occurs because resistance from the vein wall decreases as the device enters the lumen of the vein. This usually occurs with thicker-walled cannulas (Springhouse 2002, Weinstein and Plumer 2007). If the device punctures the posterior wall, the flashback will stop. However, the flashback may be slow with small-gauge cannulas or hypotensive patients.

The cannula should be advanced gently and smoothly into the vein and a number of techniques are used by practitioners. One method which provides the least risk of through puncture but which is more difficult to learn initially, is the one-handed technique (Hadaway 2000, Perucca 2010). The same hand that performs cannulation also withdraws the stylet and advances the cannula into the vein. This allows skin traction to be maintained while the device is advanced and if the patient is unable to co-operate, allows the practitioner to hold onto the patient's arm (Dougherty 2008, Hadaway 2000). If one hand is not used to apply traction then on cannula advancement, there may be unnecessary damage to the endothelium, resulting in phlebitis (Hadaway 2010).

The one-step technique is when the cannula has entered the vein and the practitioner can slide the cannula off the stylet in one movement. The disadvantage with this method is that the stylet must remain completely still in order to prevent damage to the vein. It is best accomplished on a straight vein and when the cannula has a small fingerguard which can be used to 'push' the cannula off (Dougherty 2008).

The two-handed technique is where the practitioner performs the cannulation with one hand but releases the skin traction in order to advance the cannula off the stylet. This method prevents blood spill, but as it necessitates the release of skin traction, it can often lead to the puncturing of the vein wall (Millam 1992).

If the cannulation is unsuccessful, the stylet should not be reintroduced as this could result in catheter fragmentation and embolism (Perucca 2010). A practitioner should not have more than two attempts at cannulation before passing the patient on to a more experienced colleague (Dougherty 2008, INS 2011, Perucca 2010).

Anticipated patient outcomes

The outcome of cannulation is to ensure the patient can receive their intravenous therapy and has a cannula placed that is comfortable and in a convenient position, enabling them to continue daily activities, and finally is secured and dressed to prevent any complications.

Legal and professional issues
Competencies

Pre-registration nurse training does not normally cover cannulation, necessitating the need for postregistration training (Phillips et al. 2011). Postregistration nurses must follow professional guidelines and local policy prior to taking up these skills as it is classified as expanded practice. Nurses must be taught both theory and practical skills in cannulation (RCN 2010). Competencies would include knowledge and skills in anatomy and physiology of the veins, selection of the vein and equipment, ability to improve venous access and prevention and management of complications. One way of achieving these skills is using a structured learning programme (Collins et al. 2006) which provides supervised self-assessment using objective structured clinical examinations (OSCE) (Phillips et al. 2011).

Skilled practitioners who undertake cannulation on a regular basis, for example those in IV teams, can reduce pain and discomfort for patients and reduce local complications such as phlebitis (Dougherty 1994). Patients usually give verbal consent for cannulation (Hyde 2011).

Preprocedural considerations
Equipment
Sizing

A number of different types of peripheral cannula are available. It has been shown that the incidence of vascular complications increases as the ratio of the external diameter of the cannula to vessel lumen increases. Therefore most of the literature recommends the smallest, shortest gauge cannula in any given situation (Macklin and Chernecky 2004, RCN 2010). The measurement used for needles and cannulas is standard wire gauge (swg), which measures the internal diameter; the smaller the gauge size, the larger the diameter. Standard wire gauge measurement is determined by how many cannulas fit into a tube with an inner diameter of 1 inch (25.4 mm) and uses consecutive numbers from 13 to 24. The diameter, for example 1.2 mm, may be expressed as a gauge, for example 18 G (Nauth-Misir 1998). Needles are odd numbers, for example 19 G, 21 G, while cannulas are even numbers, for example 18 G, 20 G (Weinstein and Plumer 2007).

The walls of the device should, therefore, be thin to provide the largest internal diameter without increasing the external diameter. This is to ensure that maximum flow rates may be achieved while reducing complications such as mechanical irritation. Flow rates vary with equipment from different manufacturers. Flow rate through a cannula is related to its internal diameter and is inversely proportional to its length (Table 18.2). However, as the length of the cannula increases, so does the likelihood of vascular complications. For example, a large-gauge device of longer length (1.6–2.0 cm) will fill the vessel, preventing blood flow around it, which could result in mechanical trauma to the vessel and encourage the development of phlebitis (Dougherty 2008, Tagalakis et al. 2002).

1099

Materials

The most suitable material is one that is non-irritant and does not predispose to thrombus formation (Dougherty 2008). The material should also be radiopaque or contain a stripe of radiopaque material for radiographic visualization in the event of catheter embolus (Dougherty 2008, Perucca 2010). Types of material include polyvinylchloride,

Table 18.2 Gauge sizes and average flow rates (using water)

Gauge (G)	Flow rate (mL/min)	General uses
14	350	Used in theatres or emergency for rapid transfusion of blood or viscous fluids
16	215	As 14 G
18	104	Blood transfusions, parenteral nutrition, stem cell harvesting and cell separation, large volumes of fluids
20	62	Blood transfusions, large volumes of fluids
22	35	Blood transfusions, most medications and fluids
24	24	Medications, short-term infusions, fragile veins, children

Teflon, Vialon and various polyurethane and elastomeric hydrogel materials. Studies have compared the different types of material available to ascertain which is most likely to be associated with the lowest potential risk of phlebitis (Karadag and Gorgulu 2000). When considering the results of these studies, however, it must be noted that investigators often use different phlebitis scales and calculations for creating a total score for each device. Other inconsistencies relate to the differences in catheter size, skin preparation, the use of dressings and the type of solution being infused. This makes comparison between catheter materials difficult.

Types of cannula

The 'over the needle' type of cannula is the most commonly used device for peripheral venous access and is available in various gauge sizes, lengths, composition and design features (Dougherty 2008). The cannula is mounted on the needle (known as the stylet) and once the device is pushed off the needle into the vein, the stylet is removed. A sharp-tipped stylet facilitates penetration into the vein and the type of graduation from the cannula to the needle can affect the degree of trauma to the vessel and the cannula tip (Dougherty 2008). A thin smooth-walled cannula tapering to a scalloped end causes less damage than one that is abruptly cut off (Dougherty 2008, Macklin and Chernecky 2004).

Some peripheral cannulas have wings which help with the securing of the device to the skin in order to prevent a piston-like movement within the vein and accidental removal (Dougherty 2008). Some devices may have small ports on the top (these are favoured more in Europe than in the USA) (Figure 18.9). The advantage of a ported device is the ability to administer drugs without interfering with a continuous infusion. However, the caps are often not replaced correctly, which leaves the system exposed to contamination and the possible risk of air entering, so where ported devices are used they should be capped off using a

Figure 18.9 Ported cannula.

needlefree injection connector. It has also been found that the ports cannot be adequately sterilized with a swab, as there is no flat surface. The use of ports may encourage the practitioner not to remove the dressing and inspect the site but merely to administer the drug via the port (Dougherty 2008).

Safety cannulas are now available and have either active or passive mechanisms. In the active devices the practitioner has to push a button in order to activate the safety feature whilst in the passive devices, the stylet has a blunting or shielding facility which is automatically activated on removal from the cannula (Dougherty 2008, RCN 2010) (Figure 18.10).

Assessment and recording tools

The Visual Infusion Phlebitis Scale (VIP) (Figure 18.11) was developed by Jackson (1998) and measures the signs and symptoms of phlebitis, matching them to the appropriate management. Each stage has a numbered score and this is recorded by nursing staff at regular intervals and, where necessary, the corresponding action is taken.

Pharmacological support

The use of local anaesthetic prior to insertion of peripheral cannulas has been advocated to reduce pain and anxiety in children and specific adults (Scales 2005). It is recommended:

- if the cannula is larger than 18 G
- for use of a sensitive site, for example inner aspect of wrist
- at the patient's request (Dougherty 2008, Moureau and Zonderman 2000).

When required, the agent that is the least invasive and/or carries the least risk for allergic reaction should be considered first (RCN 2010).

Local anaesthetic may be applied in a cream/gel, given as an intradermal injection or administered by iontophoresis: a painless dry electrode pushing the local anaesthetic into the skin within 7–10 minutes to a depth of 10 mm (Dougherty

Flashback chamber

Stylet

Figure 18.10 Safety non-ported cannula.

2008, Macklin and Chernecky 2004, Moureau and Zonderman 2000).

The most commonly used local anaesthetic creams are EMLA (eutectic mixture of local anaesthetics: lidocaine and prilocaine) and Ametop (topical amethocaine). These are applied to the skin 30–60 minutes prior to cannulation and covered with an occlusive dressing. A meta-analysis showed that EMLA cream significantly decreased the pain of intravenous cannulation in 85% of adults and children (Fetzer 2002). However, it causes vasoconstriction, making cannulation more difficult. Ametop has been shown to be more effective than EMLA and to cause significantly less vasoconstriction (Browne *et al.* 1999). However, it can result in an erythematous rash if left *in situ* longer than the recommended time (BNF 2011).

Ethyl chloride is a fast-acting vapo-coolant spray that provides rapid, transient, topical local analgesia for minor invasive procedures such as cannulation. It has no anaesthetic properties but the sprayed liquid makes the skin cold and less sensitive as it evaporates, causing instant numbing. The effect lasts about 30–45 seconds (IS Pharma 2009).

Intradermal lidocaine 1% can be slowly injected around the vein to be cannulated after skin sterilization to minimize the discomfort of the procedure. Intradermal injection of lidocaine has been shown to reduce the pain of intravenous cannulation and be less painful than placement of the cannula itself (Brown and Larson 1999). However, it should be used with caution because of the potential to cause an allergic reaction, tissue damage and inadvertent injection of the drug into the vascular system, and it can even obliterate the vein (Dougherty 2011, INS 2011). It is not recommended for routine use (INS 2011, RCN 2010).

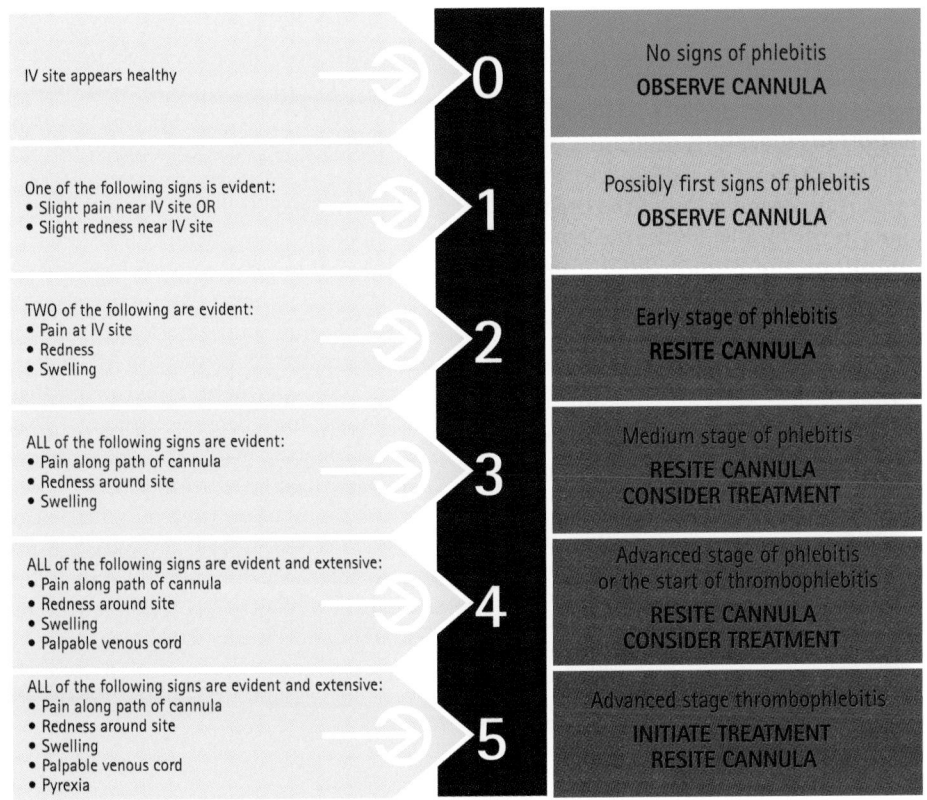

Figure 18.11 Vein Infusion Phlebitis (VIP) Scale. Reproduced from Jackson (1998).

Iontophoresis uses a painless electrical current to facilitate the movement of solute ions across the skin. It has been used to administer lidocaine prior to intravenous cannulation without the need for intradermal injection and has been shown to be as effective as EMLA (Dougherty 2008, Galinkin *et al.* 2002).

Although local anaesthetic reduces the pain of intravenous cannulation, it is not without complications. Irrespective of the method of anaesthesia, there is a risk that the symptoms of extravasation may be obscured or it may even influence the risk of injury occurring (Stanley 2002).

Non-pharmacological support

There are a number of methods for relieving pain using a non-pharmacological approach, including distraction, such as the cough trick (Usichenko *et al.* 2004), massage (Wendler 2003) and transcutaneous electrical nerve stimulation (TENS) (Coyne *et al.* 1995).

Specific patient preparations

Skin preparation

As the most common cause of VAD infection is the patient's own skin flora, it is important to clean the skin adequately prior to cannulation (Figure 18.12). The patient's skin should be washed with soap and water if visibly dirty which will remove most transient flora (Perucca 2010). Then an antiseptic solution such as 2% chlorhexidine solution or 70% alcohol should be applied with repeated back and forth strokes with friction for 30–60 seconds for an area of 4–5 cm (DH 2010, Perucca 2010). A quick wipe fails to reduce bacterial count (Weinstein and Plumer 2007). It should be allowed to air dry for up to 1 minute to ensure coagulation of the organism and to prevent stinging as the needle pierces the skin (INS 2011, RCN 2010, Weinstein and Plumer 2007). Fanning, blowing or blotting the prepared area is contraindicated (Perucca 2010). Once the skin has been cleaned, it must not be touched or repalpated (Dougherty 2008). If it is necessary to repalpate, then the cleaning regimen should be repeated.

Shaving the skin prior to cannulation is not recommended (INS 2011, RCN 2010, Weinstein and Plumer 2007) as the need to remove hair has not been substantiated by scientific evidence (Weinstein and Plumer 2007). Shaving with a razor should not be performed because of the potential for causing micro-abrasions, which increase the risk of infection (INS 2011, Perucca 2010,

Figure 18.12 Cleaning the skin.

RCN 2010). Depilatories should not be used because of the potential for allergic reaction or irritation (Perucca 2010, RCN 2010). If hair removal is necessary then this can be accomplished by clipping with scissors or clippers (Perucca 2010, RCN 2010). These should be cleaned between patients or only used once to prevent cross-infection (RCN 2010).

Psychological preparation

The influence of a bad experience can be overwhelming for a patient and any practitioner performing venepuncture or cannulation must never underestimate either the impact for the patient of undergoing the procedure or how they may view these procedures in the future (Dougherty 2011). Anxiety can be caused by previous bad experience, a degree of needle phobia or dislike of needle procedures (Lavery and Ingram 2005). Many patients will be apprehensive and this anxiety may cause vasoconstriction, making cannulation more difficult for patient and practitioner and more painful for the patient. How nurses approach the patient, their manner and attitude, may have a direct bearing on the patient's response to the procedure (Dougherty 2011). If the patient's history includes complications associated with either procedure, venepuncture or cannulation may be very difficult (Weinstein and Plumer 2007). However, when the procedures are performed by an experienced practitioner and it is a positive experience for the patient, they may feel more comfortable and relaxed. Provision of clear and comprehensive information on the procedure should reduce the patient's anxiety and pain (Dougherty 2011, Lüker and Stahlheber-Dilg 2003, Weinstein and Plumer 2007).

Procedure guideline 18.4 Peripheral cannula insertion

Essential equipment

- Sterile dressing pack
- Various gauge sizes of cannula
- Alcohol-based hand scrub
- Alcohol-based skin preparation, 2% chlorhexidine in 70% alcohol
- Extension set
- Needleless injection cap

- Non-sterile well-fitting gloves
- Hypoallergenic tape
- Bandage, for example light crepe
- 5 mL syringe
- 21 G needle
- Tourniquet
- Sharps container

Optional equipment

- Securing device, for example Statlock
- Topical local anaesthetic

Medicinal products

- 0.9% sodium chloride 5 mL

Preprocedure

Action	Rationale
1 Explain and discuss the procedure with the patient.	To ensure that the patient understands the procedure and gives their valid consent (NMC 2008b, C).
2 If they require topical local anaesthetic, then apply it to chosen venepuncture sites for 30–60 minutes prior to cannulation.	In order to give adequate time for local anaesthetic to be effective (BNF 2011, C).
3 Assemble all the equipment necessary for cannulation.	To ensure that time is not wasted and that the procedure goes smoothly without unnecessary interruptions. E
4 Check all packaging before opening and preparing the equipment to be used.	To ensure all equipment is in date and not contaminated. E

Procedure

5 Carefully wash your hands using bactericidal soap and water or bactericidal alcohol handrub before commencement, and dry.	To minimize the risk of infection (DH 2010, C; Fraise and Bradley 2009, E).
6 Check your hands for any visibly broken skin, and cover with a waterproof dressing.	To minimize the risk of contamination of the nurse by the patient's blood (Pratt et al. 2007, C).
7 In both inpatient and outpatient situations, the correct lighting, ventilation, privacy and position of the patient must be ascertained.	To ensure that the operator and patient are comfortable and that adequate light is available to illuminate the procedure. E
8 Support the chosen limb on a pillow.	To ensure the patient's comfort and ease of access. P, E
9 Apply the tourniquet to the chosen limb.	To dilate the veins by obstructing the venous return. If necessary, use other methods to encourage venous access (Dougherty 2008, E).
10 Assess and select the vein (see Action Figure 10).	To select a vein (Dougherty 2008, E).
11 Release the tourniquet.	To ensure that the patient does not feel discomfort while the device is selected and equipment prepared (Dougherty 2008, E).
12 Select the device based on the vein size.	To reduce damage or trauma to the vein. To reduce the risk of phlebitis (Dougherty 2008, E; RCN 2010, C).

1103

(Continued)

Procedure guideline 18.4 (*Continued*)

13 Wash hands using bactericidal soap and water or bactericidal alcohol handrub.	To minimize risk of infection (DH 2010, C; Fraise and Bradley 2009, E).
14 Open a pack, empty all equipment onto the pack and place a sterile dressing towel under the patient's arm (see Action Figure 14).	To create a clean working area. E
15 Prime the extension set with a syringe of 0.9% sodium chloride (unless taking blood samples immediately after cannulation).	To remove air from the set prior to connection. If taking blood then the sodium chloride will contaminate the sample (Dougherty 2008, E).
16 Reapply the tourniquet.	To promote venous filling (Dougherty 2008, E).
17 Clean the patient's skin and the selected vein for at least 30 seconds using 2% chlorhexidine using back and forth strokes with friction and allow to dry (see Fig.18.12). Do not repalpate the vein or touch the skin.	To maintain asepsis and remove skin flora (DH 2010, C; Dougherty 2008, E; RCN 2010).
18 Put on gloves.	To prevent contamination of the nurse from any blood spill (DH 2010, C).
19 Remove needle guard and inspect the device for any faults (see Action Figure 19).	To detect faulty equipment, for example bent or barbed needles. If these are present, do not use and report to company as faulty equipment (MHRA 2005, C; RCN 2010, C).
20 Anchor the vein with the non-dominant hand by applying manual traction on the skin a few centimetres below the proposed site of insertion.	To immobilize the vein. To provide countertension, which will facilitate a smooth needle entry (Dougherty 2008, E).
21 Holding the cannula in the dominant hand, ensure that it is in the bevel-up position and place the device directly over the vein; insert the cannula through the skin at the selected angle according to the depth of the vein (see Action Figure 21).	To ensure a successful, pain-free cannulation (Dougherty 2008, E).
22 Wait for the first flashback of blood in the flashback chamber of the stylet (see Action Figure 21).	To indicate that the needle has entered the vein (Dougherty 2008, E).
23 Level the device by decreasing the angle between the cannula and the skin. Advance the cannula slightly to ensure entry into the lumen of the vein.	To avoid advancing too far and causing damage to the vein wall. To stabilize the device (Dougherty 2008, E).
24 Withdraw the stylet slightly with the dominant hand and a second flashback of blood will be seen along the shaft of the cannula (see Action Figure 24).	To ensure that the cannula is still in a patent vein. This is called the hooded technique (Dougherty 2008, E).
25 Maintaining skin traction with the non-dominant hand and using the dominant hand, slowly advance the cannula off the stylet and into the vein.	To ensure the vein remains immobilized, thus reducing the risk of a 'through puncture' (Dougherty 2008, E).
26 Release the tourniquet.	To decrease the pressure within the vein. E
27 Apply digital pressure to the vein above the cannula tip and remove the stylet (see Action Figure 27).	To prevent blood spillage. E
28 Immediately dispose of the stylet into an appropriate sharps container (see Action Figure 28).	To reduce the risk of accidental needlestick injury (NHS Employers 2007, C).

29	Attach a primed extension set, needleless injection cap or administration set (see Action Figure 29).	To enable flushing of cannula (Dougherty 2008, E).
30	Tape/secure the cannula using, for example, the method illustrated in Action Figure 30.	To ensure the device will remain stable and secure (Dougherty 2008, E).
31	Aspirate to check for blood flashback then flush the cannula with 0.9% sodium chloride using a pulsatile flush ending with positive pressure.	To ascertain and maintain patency (Goode *et al.* 1991, R1b).
32	Observe the site for signs of swelling or leakage and ask the patient if any discomfort or pain.	To check that the device is positioned correctly and is stable and secure (Dougherty 2008, E)
33	Cover with low-linting swabs or appropriate dressing and bandage firmly.	To ensure patient comfort and security of device (Dougherty 1994, R5).

Postprocedure

34	Discard waste, making sure it is placed in appropriate containers.	To ensure safe disposal in the correct containers and avoid laceration or injury of other staff. To prevent reuse of equipment (NHS Employers 2007, C).
35	Document date and time of insertion, site and size of cannula, number of attempts and sign in patient's notes or care plan.	To ensure adequate records and to enable continued care of device and patient (DH and CMO 2003, C; NMC 2009, C).

Action Figure 10   Palpating the vein.

Action Figure 14   Opening the equipment.

Action Figure 19   Checking the needle tip.

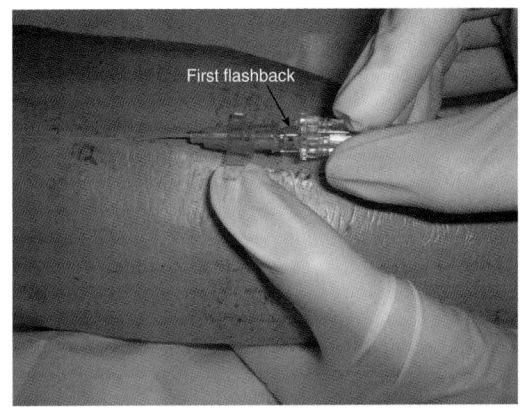

First flashback

Action Figure 21   Inserting the cannula. Waiting for first flashback.

(Continued)

Procedure guideline 18.4 *(Continued)*

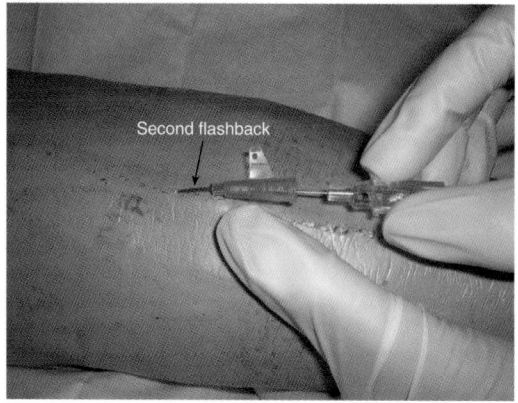

Action Figure 24   Second flashback.

Action Figure 27   Applying digital pressure and removing the stylet.

Action Figure 28   Disposing of the stylet into a sharps bin.

Action Figure 29   Flushing the cannula.

Action Figure 30   Method for taping a peripheral cannula.

Problem-solving table 18.1 Prevention and resolution (Procedure guideline 18.4)

Problem	Cause	Prevention	Action
Anxious patient	Previous traumatic experiences Fear of needles or blood Ignorance about what the procedure involves	Approach the patient in a calm and confident manner Listen to the patient's previous experiences and involve them in site selection Offer a local anaesthetic (by gel or injection) Explain what the procedure involves and show them the equipment if appropriate Offer the patient the opportunity to lie down or recline during the procedure Use all methods of improving venous dilation to ensure success on the first attempt	Refer the patient for psychological support if anxiety and fear are of phobic proportions
Difficulty in locating a suitable vein	Excessive previous use Shock or dehydration Anxiety Fragile, thready veins, for example in the elderly or in patients on anticoagulant therapy Thrombosed veins as a result of treatment, for example cytotoxic therapy	Alternate sites wherever possible to avoid overuse of certain veins Use the methods described above to reduce anxiety	Reassure the patient Use all methods of improving venous access before attempting the procedure, for example use warm water/GTN to encourage venous dilation Assess patient using an assessment tool to ascertain degree of difficulty Do not attempt the procedure unless experienced
Missing the vein on insertion of the cannula	Inadequate anchoring Collapse of the vein Incorrect position of practitioner or patient Inadequate palpation Poor vein choice Lack of concentration Failure to penetrate the vein properly due to incorrect insertion angle	Ensure good position and lighting Better preparation and concentration Use correct technique and accurate vein selection	Withdraw the needle and manoeuvre gently to realign it and correct the angle of insertion Check during manoeuvring that the patient is not feeling any pain If the patient complains of pain, remove the needle If unsuccessful then remove the needle Where necessary, pass to a colleague with more experience

1107

(*Continued*)

Problem-solving table 18.1 (*Continued*)

Problem	Cause	Prevention	Action
Blood flashback seen and then stops	Venospasm Bevel of needle up against a valve Penetration of the posterior vein wall by the device Possible vein collapse	Try to locate valves prior to insertion and insert the device just above the valve Carefully level off once in the vein to prevent penetration of posterior wall Use a good angle of approach to the vein to prevent through puncture	Release and tighten the tourniquet Gently stroke the vein above the needle to relieve venous spasm Withdraw the needle slightly to move the bevel away from the valve If the vein wall is penetrated, remove the device
Difficulty in advancing the cannula	Releasing the tourniquet too soon, causing the vein to collapse Removing the stylet too far and being unable to advance the cannula which is now no longer rigid enough to be advanced Encountering a valve Not releasing the cannula from the needle prior to insertion as per manufacturer's instructions Poor anchoring or stretching of the skin	Ensure the tourniquet remains sufficiently tight until insertion is completed Ensure the cannula is released from the stylet prior to insertion, to allow for smooth advancement Ensure that a sufficient length of the cannula is inserted into the vein before stylet withdrawal Use good technique Assess the vein accurately, observing for valves, and avoid them where possible	In the event of early stylet removal or encountering a valve, connect a syringe of sodium chloride 0.9%, flush the cannula and advance at the same time in an effort to 'float' the device into the vein Tighten the tourniquet and wait for vein to refill
Difficulty in flushing once the cannula is *in situ*	Sometimes, the cannula has been successfully inserted, but on checking patency by flushing, the practitioner has difficulty because: ■ the cannula tip is up against the valve ■ the cannula has pierced the posterior wall of the vein ■ the cannula tip is resting on the wall of the vein ■ there is an occlusion	Avoid areas along the vein where there may be valves Ensure careful insertion to prevent puncturing the posterior wall of the vein	Withdraw the cannula slightly to move it away from the vein wall or valve and attempt to flush If the vein wall is pierced and any swelling is observed, remove the cannula Attempt to withdraw the clot and clear the occlusion

Postprocedural considerations

Immediate care

Once sited, the peripheral cannula should be flushed using a pulsatile flush, ending with positive pressure (Dougherty 2008, RCN 2010, Weinstein and Plumer 2007). The cannula should be secured using clean tape or a securing device (see Figure 18.13). Non-sterile tape should not cover the insertion site and taping should enable the site to remain visible and the cannula stable (Figure 18.14). The procedure shown in Procedure guideline 18.4, Action Figure 30 is recommended (Dougherty 2008, Hadaway 2000, Springhouse 2002). Securement devices are now available and reduce the risk of dislodgement and other complications (Moureau and Iannucci 2003). A dressing should be applied: this can be either a transparent dressing or low-linting gauze (Madeo *et al.* 1997, Perucca 2010). Once the gauze is in place, a bandage may be applied. However, transparent dressings, particularly moisture-permeable dressings, should not be bandaged as the visibility and moisture permeability are obscured.

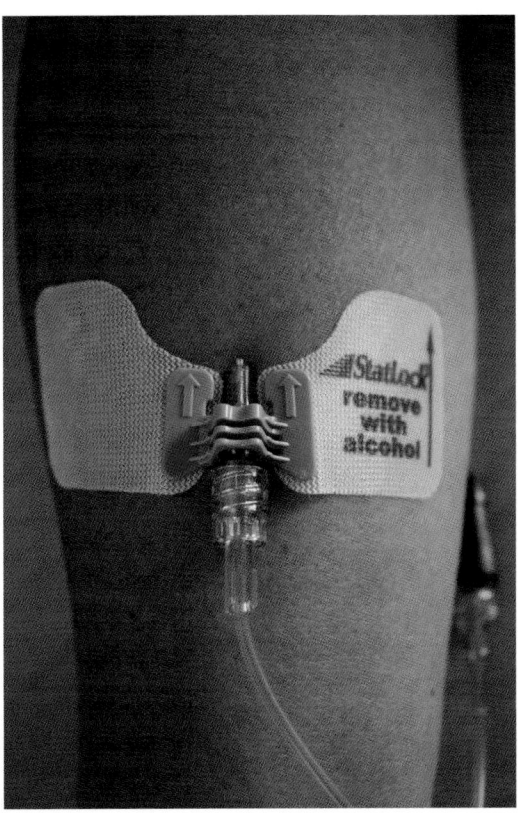

Figure 18.13   Peripheral cannula secured with statlock.

Figure 18.14   Cannula *in situ*.

firm and not involve any rubbing movement. A haematoma will occur if the device is carelessly removed, causing discomfort and a focus for infection (Perucca 2010). The site should be inspected to ensure bleeding has stopped and should then be covered with a sterile dressing (INS 2011). The cannula integrity should be checked to ensure the complete device has been removed (Dougherty 2008, INS 2011, RCN 2010).

Ongoing care

A peripheral cannula should be flushed before and after each use to check for patency prior to administation of a medication, and at least daily if not in use, using 0.9% sodium chloride. The dressing should be changed as required (if transparent) or each time the device is manipulated (gauze). The site should be monitored daily or when the device is used. The site should be inspected for signs of infiltration, extravasation and leakage and using a scale such as the VIP Scale for signs of phlebitis (DH 2010).

Removal

It has been recommended that peripheral devices should be resited every 48–72 hours (Barker *et al.* 2004, DH and CMO 2003, RCN 2010) but some literature supports dwell times (length of time cannula *in situ*) of up to 96 hours with no significant complications providing that non-irritants are administered (Homer and Holmes 1998, McGoldrick 2010). Other studies have found that drug irritation is the most significant predictor of phlebitis and infiltration, rather than dwell time, and that extending the dwell time up to 144 hours could be considered under certain circumstances (Bregenzer *et al.* 1998, Catney *et al.* 2001).

Removal of the intravenous device or cannula should be an aseptic procedure. The device should be removed carefully using a slow, steady movement and pressure should be applied until haemostasis is achieved. This pressure should be

Documentation

On insertion, the practitioner should document the date and time, the site and size of the cannula, the number of attempts and sign their name. This can be as part of a specific cannula care plan or by use of a sticker in the notes (see Figure 18.15) (DH 2010). If a tool is used to monitor the site, for example VIP score, then this should be recorded on a regular basis (e.g. every shift change or at least once a day). The date, time and reason for removal of the cannula must also be documented in the patient's notes (DH and CMO 2003, Dougherty 2008, RCN 2010). This documentation ensures adequate records for the continued care of the device and patient as well as enabling audit and gathering of statistics on rates of phlebitis and infiltration and so on.

Education of patient and relevant others

See Discharging patients home with a VAD *in situ*.

1109

Complications

On insertion

Pain

Pain can be caused by the following:

- tentative stop–start insertion (often associated with hesitant or new practitioners)

Name:	**Hospital No:**	**Need No:**

THE ROYAL MARSDEN

Patient Care Need:

To maintain patient safety related to the management of a **Peripheral Cannula**

♦ Knowledge deficit about the insertion and management of the peripheral cannula
♦ Risk of complications associated with the insertion, the care of a peripheral cannula and its removal

INSERTION OF A PERIPHERAL CANNULA

Anticipated Outcome:

♦ Patient will verbalize an understanding of the insertion of a peripheral cannula and the possible side-effects, complications
♦ Patient will have a peripheral cannula which is correctly positioned and inserted with minimum of discomfort to the patient and trauma to the vein

Nursing Interventions:

A **Patient Assessment**

♦ Assess the patient's anxiety about the insertion of a peripheral cannula and agree any measures that are to be taken e.g. local anaesthetic cream and the type of peripheral cannula
♦ Assess the patient and carer's knowledge and understanding of: the site for the insertion of a peripheral cannula; the potential duration of the peripheral cannula; the care of the peripheral cannula by the nurse and/or the patient, and the need to report any side effects to the nurse
♦ Check that the patient/carer demonstrates an understanding of the intended peripheral cannula
♦ Assess ability to manage a peripheral cannula at home and arrange District Nurse support if required

B **Insertion**

♦ Check with the patient for details of any previous ill effect from vascular access device insertion
♦ Insert a peripheral cannula according to hospital procedure and manage any complications effectively
Possible complications: pain, bruising, haematoma, missed vein, vasovagal reaction

Use for 1st cannulation and then any subsequent resites during the patient's admission (and on subsequent admission) (shaded area to be completed by nurse who cannulates)

*Treatment** * BT – blood transfusion CT – chemotherapy AB – antibiotics FL – fluids Other – please state
*Phlebitis** ** Grade 1 – red OR painful Grade 2 – red and painful OR red and swollen OR swollen and painful *Grade 3 – painful, swollen AND red*

Date	Type and length of Treatment (please specify names of chemo drugs or regimen)	New (N) or Resite (RS)	If resite - Reason for removal (Phlebitis 1, 2 or 3; swelling, occlusion, other state...)	Date and time cannula removed	Site and gauge size of Cannula	No. of attempts	Signature and time of cannulation
Example 20.9.10	Ifos and Doxo 2/7	RS	Phlebitis 1	20.9.10 10.00	L cephalic 22g	2	J.Bloggs 10.30

Instructions For Use:
♦ Date and sign care plan when initiated, enter need number
♦ Individualise as appropriate. Date/time/sign any additional entries/interventions
♦ If need/outcome/interventions are stopped/changed or not applicable – DELETE by drawing a line through the entry, date/time/sign this deletion

Figure 18.15 Care plan related to the insertion of a peripheral cannula. © 2010 The Royal Marsden Hospital NHS Foundation Trust.

Patient Care Need: To maintain patient safety related to the management of a Peripheral Cannula

ONGOING ASSESSMENT & CARE

Anticipated Outcome:
♦ Patient will have a peripheral cannula which is patent, correctly secured and free from signs of phlebitis, infiltration, extravasation and/or infection (and where these complications do occur that they are managed effectively)

Nursing Interventions:
C **Maintaining a patent device**
♦ Flush all devices with 0.9% sodium chloride at start of drug administration, in between drugs and after drug administration
♦ Flush all devices using a turbulent flush and ending with positive pressure
♦ When not in constant use – flush the peripheral cannula once a day with 5 ml 0.9% Sodium Chloride

D **Preventing infection**
♦ Use an aseptic technique whenever the device is manipulated. Use clean non-sterile tape, sterile gauze and a peha crepe bandage – change gauze at each manipulation, and change tape when soiled.

E **Prevent movement or dislodgement of device**
♦ Tape peripheral cannula to secure (as per method in RMH Manual of Clinical Procedures)
♦ Tape administration/extension set to prevent the tubing from pulling on peripheral cannula

F **Monitor site for signs of local complications**
♦ Observe site for erythema, oedema, blanching and ask the patient if any pain or discomfort experienced
♦ If signs or symptoms indicate phlebitis or infiltration, remove cannula
♦ If extravasation indicated – follow extravasation policy
♦ If signs of infection, swab insertion site, remove cannula, send tip to microbiology, inform doctor

G **Inform doctor of any complications during administration of treatment via peripheral cannula**

REMOVAL OF A PERIPHERAL CANNULA

Anticipated Outcome:
♦ Patient will have a peripheral cannula which is removed safely with minimal discomfort and no bruising

Nursing Interventions:
H **Removal of a peripheral cannula**
♦ Remove and apply sterile dressing – check the bleeding has stopped before leaving the patient to ensure no bruising
♦ If further treatment, discuss type of vascular access device required
♦ Record reason for re-siting the cannula *(see page 1)*

Patient/Carer Education:
I Inform and discuss with the patient/carer:
♦ the insertion procedures and the hazards, instructing the patient about the importance of positioning during insertion, and advise the patient to report if during insertion of peripheral cannula the following occurs: pain on insertion, feeling faint, light-headed or dizzy
♦ the function, potential side effects and implication of the peripheral cannula including: potential occlusion, pain/redness at peripheral cannula site and advise the patient how to mobilize and care for the peripheral cannula in situ e.g. during showering
♦ advise the patient of the importance in reporting to the nurse/doctor if they have any symptoms e.g. pain, and that a record is kept for future therapy

J Give the patient the peripheral cannula information leaflet, together with gauze and bandages if required for those patients who have daily outpatient treatment via a peripheral cannula

Additional Interventions:

Date & Time initiated:	Signature: (nurse who initiates care)	Print Name: Job Title:

Figure 18.15(a) (Continued)

SHARING EXPERTISE

THE ROYAL
MARSDEN

Cannula Insertion Record

PATIENT NAME................................... HOSPITAL NO................................

REASON FOR CANNULATION
CHEMOTHERAPY ☐
BLOOD TRANSFUSION ☐
FLUIDS ☐
ANTIBIOTICS ☐
OTHER

| R | L |

Please mark successful
cannulation with an X and
failed cannulations with an F.

FIRST INSERTION ☐   RE-SITE ☐
NUMBER OF ATTEMPTS ☐

INTROCAN SAFETY®
20G ☐   22G ☐   24G ☐

DATE ....

TIME ....

SIGNATURE ....

Cannula Removal Record

DATE AND TIME REMOVED

....

NUMBER OF DAYS IN SITU ☐

CANNULA REMOVED BY

....

Reasons for Removal

PHLEBITIS
I ☐   II ☐   III ☐
INFILTRATION / EXTRAVASATION
☐
OCCLUSION
☐
OTHER (PLEASE STATE)
☐

....

Figure 18.15(b) *(Continued)*

- hitting an artery, nerve or valve
- poor technique – inadequate anchoring causes skin to gather as the needle is inserted
- alcohol is not allowed to dry adequately before insertion, resulting in stinging pain
- using a frequently punctured, recently used or bruised vein
- anxious patient, may have low pain threshold
- use of large-gauge device
- use of veins in sensitive areas (Dougherty 2008).

Pain can be prevented by using methods to relax and relieve anxiety, for example massage, distraction or the use of local anaesthetic creams or injections. The practitioner should avoid the use of bruised, used or sensitive areas. If the patient complains of pain, depending on the cause (e.g. nerve or artery), it may be necessary to remove the device immediately. Reassure the patient and explain, especially in the case of nerve pain, that it may last for a few hours, provide the patient with an information leaflet and document the incident (Dougherty 2008).

Haematoma

This is a swelling of blood under the skin creating a hard painful lump which occurs during the insertion procedure or after removal (Perucca 2010). It can be caused by:

- penetration of the posterior vein wall
- incorrect choice of needle to vein size
- fragile veins
- patients receiving anticoagulant therapy
- spontaneous rupture of the vessel on application of the tourniquet or cleaning of the skin
- inadequate pressure on venepuncture site following removal of the cannula (Dougherty 2008).

Prevention includes good vein and device selection and using a careful technique. The practitioner should always be aware of patients with fragile veins or those on anticoagulant therapy and inexperienced individuals should not attempt cannulation in these individuals (Perucca 2010). A tourniquet should not be applied to a limb where recent venepuncture has occurred and the tourniquet should not be left in place for any longer than necessary.

On removal of the cannula, adequate pressure should be applied to the site. Alcohol pads inhibit clotting and should not be used (Perucca 2010). In the event of a haematoma occurring, the needle should be removed immediately and pressure applied to the site for a few minutes. Elevate the extremity if appropriate and reassure the patient and explain the reason for the bruise. Apply a pressure dressing if required and an ice pack if bruising is extensive. Hirudoid or arnica ointment can help to reduce bruising and discomfort. Arnica is made of dried roots or flower of the arnica plant which stimulates activity of the white blood cells which process congested blood and reduce the bruise (http://emc. medicines.org.uk/medicine/19031/SPC). Hirudoid is a substance similar to heparin which acts by dissolving blood clots and improving blood supply to the skin (http://emc. medicines.org.uk/medicine/5001/SPC/Hirudoid+Cream/). They are both applied directly to the affected arm (BNF 2010). The incident should be documented and the patient given an information sheet with advice about when and who to contact if the haematoma gets worse or they develop any numbness in the limb (Dougherty 2008, Perucca 2010).

Hitting an artery

This is characterized by pain and bright red blood caused by accidental puncture of an artery (Dougherty 2008). It can be prevented by an adequate assessment and recognition of arteries prior to performing the procedure. However, should it occur, the device should be removed immediately and pressure applied to the puncture site for up to 5 minutes. Reassure the patient but do not reapply the tourniquet to the affected limb. The incident must be documented and the patient given a patient information sheet with advice about when and who to contact if they develop numbness or tingling in the limb (Dougherty 2008).

Hitting a nerve

If a nerve is accidentally hit on insertion of the needle into the vein, this will result in severe shooting pain (Masoorli 2003, Yuan and Cohan 1987). Prevention is achieved by ensuring that the location of superficial nerves is known; for example, a common place to hit a nerve is the cephalic vein and this can be avoided by placing three fingers at the wrist and inserting the needle above this (the nerve runs deeper at that point and therefore the practitioner will be less likely to touch it) (Boeson et al. 2000, Masoorli 2007). In the event of touching a nerve, the needle should be removed immediately. Reassure the patient and explain that the pain may last for a few hours and the area may feel numb. Explain that the pain can sometimes last for a few days and that, if it continues or gets worse, medical advice should be sought. Give the patient an information sheet with advice about when and who to contact and document the incident (Dougherty 2008).

Once in situ
Phlebitis

This is inflammation of the intima of the vein (Perucca 2010). It is characterized by pain and tenderness along the cannulated vein, erythema, warmth, streak formation with/without a palpable cord (Mermel et al. 2009).

There are three main types.

- *Mechanical* is related to irritation and damage to a vein by large-gauge cannulas, sited where there is movement, for example antecubital fossa, not secured adequately or increased dwell time.
- *Chemical* is related to chemical irritation from drugs such as antibiotics and chemotherapy.
- *Bacterial* is when the site becomes infected due to poor handwashing or aseptic technique.

(Lamb and Dougherty 2008)

Prevention is key and includes appropriate device and vein selection, dilution of drugs and pharmacological methods, for example application of glyceryl trinitrate (GTN) patches (Dougherty 2008). Treatment includes discontinuing the infusion at the first signs of phlebitis (grade 1). Warm or cold compresses can be applied to the affected site. The patient should be referred to the doctor if the phlebitis rating is over 3. If bacterial phlebitis is suspected then the insertion site should be cultured and the cannula tip sent to microbiology (Dougherty 2008, Macklin and Chernecky 2004, Phillips 2005).

Infiltration and extravasation

See Chapter 15.

Midline catheters

Definition

A midline catheter can be defined as one that is between 7.5 and 20 cm in length (Dougherty 2008, RCN 2010). It provides vascular access in a larger peripheral vein without entering the central venous circulation. It is inserted into an antecubital vein and the tip is extended into the vein of the upper arm for about 20 cm, but it is not extended past the axilla (Hadaway 2010, RCN 2010).

Anatomy and physiology
Choice of vein

The basilic vein is the vein of choice due to its larger size, straighter course for catheter advancement and improved haemodilution capability (Perucca 2010, Weinstein and Plumer 2007). The cephalic and median cubital veins would be the second and third choices (INS 2011).

Evidence-based approaches
Rationale

The midline catheter offers an alternative to peripheral and central venous access. Where patients present with poor peripheral venous access and when the use of a CVC is contraindicated, the midline catheter provides venous accessibility along with easy, less hazardous insertion at the antecubital fossa (Goetz et al. 1998, Weinstein and Plumer 2007). Because the tip of the catheter does not extend beyond the extremities in which it is placed, radiographic confirmation of tip placement is optional and recommended only when there is difficulty in insertion or flushing (Carlson 1999, Weinstein and Plumer 2007). Benefits to the patient include less frequent resiting of the catheter and a subsequent reduction in associated venous trauma (Weinstein and Plumer 2007).

Indications

Midline catheters are indicated in the following circumstances.

- When patients do not have accessible peripheral veins in the lower arm.
- When patients will be undergoing therapy for 1–4 weeks (Carlson 1999), in order to preserve the integrity of the veins and increase patient comfort by removing the need for resites, for example antibiotics.
- Patient preference.

(Dougherty 2008, Hadaway 2010, Perucca 2010)

Contraindications

Should not be used for administration via a midline catheter: vesicant medications, especially by continuous infusion; parenteral nutrition, solutions and/or medications with pH less than 5 or greater than 9 and those with osmolarity greater than 600 mOsm/L (Banton and Leahy-Gross 1998, Hadaway 2010, INS 2011).

Methods of insertion

The insertion is performed via an introducer or using a modified Seldinger technique (i.e. when venous access is established with a needle, a guidewire is threaded through the needle, the

1113

needle is removed and the catheter is threaded over the guide-wire) (Hadaway 2010, Weinstein and Plumer 2007). Adequate assessment of the patient's veins is vital and given the choice, the non-dominant arm should be used. The procedure requires a sterile approach and it is recommended that sterile powder-free gloves are worn (Hayden and Goodman 2005).

Legal and professional issues

The procedure should only be performed by trained and competent nurses who have achieved a high standard of cannulation (Weinstein and Plumer 2007). Competencies would include knowledge of the anatomy and physiology of the veins of the upper arm, ability to select veins and equipment, and prevent and manage complications.

Preprocedural considerations
Equipment

Silicone and polyurethane are the materials most frequently used in the manufacture of midline catheters (Hadaway 2010, Kupensky 1998). Catheters are available as single and double lumen in lengths of up to 20 cm, which can be cut to the desired length following measurement of the arm from the selected vein towards the axilla. They are available in various sizes from 1.9 to 5 French (Dougherty 2008, Hadaway 2010).

Procedure guideline 18.5 **Midline catheter insertion**

Essential equipment

- Sterile minor operation pack (contains sterile drapes and scissors)
- Sterile powder-free gloves
- Alcohol-based hand scrub
- Alcohol-based skin cleaning preparation, such as 2% chlorhexidine in 70% alcohol
- Extension set and needleless injection cap
- Midline catheter

- Introducer
- Transparent dressing
- Securing device and sterile tapes
- 10 mL syringes
- 21 G needle
- Tape measure
- Apron

Medicinal products

- 0.9% sodium chloride
- Topical local anaesthetic

Preprocedure

Action	Rationale
1 Explain and discuss the procedure with the patient.	To ensure that the patient understands the procedure and gives their valid verbal consent (NMC 2008b, C).
2 Apply tourniquet to the arm. Assess venous access in both arms and locate veins by sight and palpation.	To ensure the patient has adequate venous access and to select the vein for catheterization (RCN 2010, C).
3 Apply local anaesthetic cream/gel to chosen venepuncture site and leave for allotted time.	To minimize the pain of insertion (BNF 2011, C).
4 Draw screens and position patient in a comfortable position.	To ensure privacy. To aid insertion and correct placement. E
5 Measure using the tape measure from the selected venepuncture site up the arm, to just below the axilla.	To enable selection of the most suitable catheter length and to know how far to advance the catheter in order for its tip to be located in the correct position. E
6 Take equipment required to patient's bedside. Open outer pack.	To gain access to equipment. E

Procedure

7 Carefully wash hands using bactericidal soap and water.	To minimize the risk of infection (Fraise and Bradley 2009, E; Pratt et al. 2007, C).
8 Put on powder-free sterile gloves; open sterile pack, arranging the contents as required. Draw up the syringe with 0.9% sodium chloride (from assistant).	To prevent contamination. Powder on gloves can increase the risk of mechanical phlebitis. E

9	Remove the cap from the extension set and attach the syringe of 0.9% sodium chloride; gently flush with 2 mL and leave syringe attached.	To check that the catheter is patent and to enable easy removal of guidewire. E
10	If the catheter tip can be trimmed, using the graduated markings along the catheter, select the marking required and pull back guidewire 1 cm from desired new tip, and using sterile scissors trim the catheter. Never trim the guidewire!	To ensure the catheter will be the correct length for placement and to prevent damage to the vein if the guidewire is damaged. E
11	Place sterile towel under patient's arm.	To provide a sterile field to work on. E
12	Clean the skin at the selected site with an appropriate disinfectant, for example 2% chlorhexidine in 70% alcohol, using back and forth strokes with friction, and prepare an area of 15–25 cm.	To ensure skin flora is destroyed and to minimize the risk of infection (Fraise and Bradley 2009, E; RCN 2010, C).
13	Allow the solution to dry thoroughly.	To ensure coagulation of bacteria and completion of disinfection process (Pratt *et al.* 2007, C).
14	Drape the patient with a fenestrated towel.	To provide a sterile field (Pratt *et al.* 2007, C).
15	Inject local anaesthetic intradermally, if required, using a 25 G needle and wait for a few minutes for it to take effect.	To provide adequate anaesthesia (BNF 2011, C).
16	Reapply tourniquet.	To aid venous distension (Dougherty 2008, E).
17	Perform venepuncture with introducer by entering the skin, 1 cm from desired point of entry, at a 15–30° angle. Advance 0.5–1.0 cm once flashback is seen.	To gain venous access (Dougherty 2008, E).
18	Release tourniquet.	To prevent blood loss and 'through puncture' and enable advancement of catheter (Dougherty 2008, E).
19	Position fingers in a V, with index finger on wings and middle finger above sheath tip, and gently remove stylet. Apply pressure.	To contain flashback, prevent contamination of the area with blood and minimize the amount of blood loss from patient (Dougherty 2008, E).
20	Grip catheter 1 cm from the tip and thread through the introducer sheath.	To ensure tip is not contaminated (Dougherty 2008, E).
21	Continue slow advancement of the catheter to the desired length.	To minimize damage to intima of vein (Dougherty 2008, E).
22	Apply pressure above introducer and carefully withdraw the introducer and peel apart.	To ensure there is no movement of the catheter. To remove peel-away introducer (Dougherty 2008, E).
23	Aspirate for blood return and flush catheter with 0.9% sodium chloride.	To check patency of device and ensure continued patency (Dougherty 2008, E).
24	Apply gentle pressure on catheter and slowly withdraw the guidewire.	To ensure there is no withdrawal of catheter (Dougherty 2008, E).
25	Attach needleless injection cap and flush as per local policy.	To ensure patency of the device (Dougherty 2008, E).
26	Secure the catheter with sterile tape or other securing device and a small pressure dressing over the insertion site. Apply a transparent dressing. Apply gauze and a bandage.	To ensure stability of device and protection of the site (Dougherty 2008, E).

1115

(Continued)

Procedure guideline 18.5 *(Continued)*

Postprocedure

27 Remove gloves and dispose of equipment appropriately. Dispose of sharps and clinical waste.	To prevent risk of sharps injurys (NHS Employers 2007, C).
28 Document the procedure in the patient's notes: type, length and gauge of catheter, where it was inserted, any problem, how it was secured.	To ensure adequate records and enable continued care of device and patient (NMC 2009, C).

Problem-solving table 18.2 Prevention and resolution (Procedure guideline 18.5)

Problem	Cause	Prevention	Action
Missed vein (see Cannulation)			
Unable to advance catheter	Valves Choice of vein, for example cephalic narrows above antecubital fossa	Select a vein with fewer valves or one with large lumen	Flush and attempt to advance the catheter Depending on the length advanced, it may be acceptable to leave it and use for short period of time

Postprocedural considerations

Immediate care

It is not usually appropriate to suture these devices *in situ*, as they can be adequately secured with Steristrips or catheter securement devices such as a Statlock (Perucca 2010). The insertion site can then be covered with a moisture-permeable transparent dressing and changed according to the manufacturer's recommendations, for example once a week. The device should be flushed with 0.9% sodium chloride after each use and then with a heparinized solution according to the manufacturer's recommendations, for example weekly.

Ongoing care

Midline catheters can be left *in situ* for extended periods of time; the optimal time interval for removal of a midline catheter is unknown (Hadaway 2010). Therefore it is recommended that maximum dwell times should be limited to 2–4 weeks (INS 2011). Longer dwell times should be decided on site assessment, length of maintaining therapy and patient condition (INS 2011, Kupensky 1998). Once *in situ*, the catheter should be managed exactly as a CVC. If patient goes home with a midline then they should receive information, equipment and support (see Discharging patients home with a VAD *in situ*).

Removal

Removal requires gentle firm traction and the catheter will slide out from the insertion site. Pressure should be applied for at least 3–4 minutes and the site inspected prior to applying a dressing to ensure bleeding has stopped. The catheter integrity should be checked and its length measured to ensure that a complete device has been removed (RCN 2010).

Complications

Mechanical phlebitis is a common side-effect. Close observation and appropriate management such as the application of heat are indicated (see Peripheral cannulas, Complications for more details on management).

Peripherally inserted central catheters (PICC)

Definition

A peripherally inserted central catheter (PICC) is a catheter that is inserted percutaneously via the veins in the arm and is advanced into the central veins, with the tip located in the SVC (usually the lower third) (Hadaway 2010, INS 2011, NAVAN 1998, RCN 2010). It is not to be confused with a midclavicular catheter (often referred to as a 'long line') where the tip is located in a central vein leading to the SVC such as the subclavian or proximal axillary vein (Carlson 1999, Dougherty 2006). Because of the increasing evidence that midclavicular catheters are associated with a high incidence of thrombotic complications (up to 60%), midclavicular placement should only be considered if there are anatomical or pathophysiological reasons, for example SVC syndrome (Carlson 1999, Dougherty 2006).

Anatomy and physiology
Choice of vein

Careful evaluation and adequate assessment of the patient prior to attempting catheter placement go a long way to ensuring success. Examine both arms with a tourniquet in place, palpate for the healthiest, largest vein, and preferably on the non-dominant arm. Problems associated with vein location have been overcome with the use of ultrasound technology. It has been shown that ultrasonography can increase the chance of successful cannulation of the vein on the first attempt (LaRue 2000) compared with using the traditional landmark method (using surface anatomical landmarks and knowing the expected anatomical relationship of the vein to its palpable companion artery) (Dougherty 2006, NICE 2002). However, by using ultrasound, the nurse can position the transducer to obtain a transverse (cross-sectional) or horizontal view of the vein which may aid in the identification of arterial vessels as well as facilitating visualization of solid material, such as a thrombus, in the lumen of the vessel (Hadaway 2010, Weinstein and Plumer 2007). See Figure 18.16.

The basilic and brachial veins

The median basilic vein is the vein of choice for PICC insertions owing to its larger size, straighter course for catheter advancement and improved haemodilution capability (Bullock-Corkhill 2010, NAVAN 1998, RCN 2010) (see Figure 18.17).

Figure 18.16   Ultrasound cross-sectional image of the right internal jugular vein (IJV) without compression through the probe. Image orientation as seen from the head of the patient. CA, carotid artery; T, thyroid; TA, thyroid artery. Depth of field of image is only 2.8 cm, so all structures are very superficial. Reproduced with permission from Hamilton (2009).

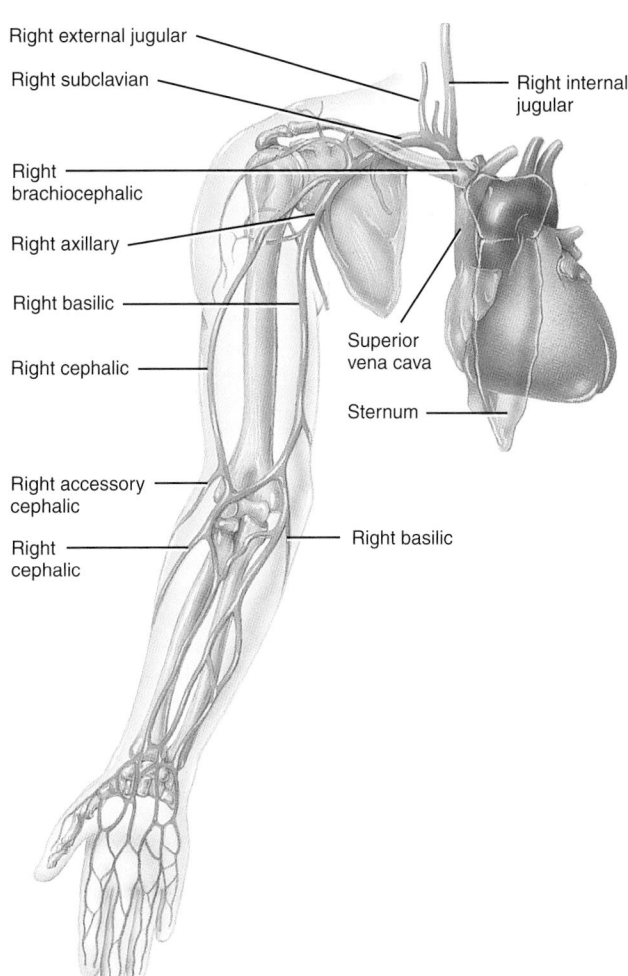

Figure 18.17   Anterior view of superficial veins.

The basilic vein begins in the ulnar (inner aspect) part of the forearm, runs along the posterior, medial surface (back of the arm) and then curves towards the antecubital region, where it is joined by the median cubital vein. It then progresses straight up the upper arm for approximately 5–8 cm and enters the deep tissues. It ascends medially to form the axillary vein (Dougherty 2006, Hadaway 2010). Brachial veins (Figure 18.18) are located deep in the arm alongside the brachial artery and nerve and are slightly smaller than the basilic. They therefore require ultrasound to locate and access them (Hadaway 2010).

The median cubital vein

The median cubital vein (see Figure 18.18) ascends from just below the middle of the antecubital region and commonly divides into two vessels, one of which joins the basilic and the other the cephalic vein. The median cubital vein is commonly used for blood sampling owing to its size and ease of needle entry. If a practitioner is having difficulty locating and/or cannulating the basilic vein, then the median cubital vein may be used as an alternative insertion route (Sansivero 1998). The catheter will then advance into the basilic (or cephalic) vein.

1117

Figure 18.18 Anteromedial view of superficial veins of arm and forearm. Reproduced from Tortora and Derrickson (2009).

The cephalic vein

The cephalic vein begins in the radial side (thumb side) of the hand and ascends laterally (along the outer region of the forearm) into the antecubital region, where it forms a junction with the axillary vein. This vein is usually more accessible than the basilic but its size and the sharp angle where it anastomoses with the subclavian make it more difficult to advance the catheter (Dougherty 2006) and therefore it presents a greater potential for catheter tip malposition (Dougherty 2006, Weinstein and Plumer 2007).

Evidence-based approaches

Rationale

The PICC has many advantages over the other central venous access devices. Firstly, it eliminates the mechanical complications associated with CVC placement, particularly pneumothorax (Dougherty 2006, Gallieni et al. 2009). Secondly, PICCs have been shown to be associated with a reduction in catheter sepsis. This may be related to the temperature of the skin and it has been reported that peripheral sites rarely have more than 50–100 colony-forming units (cfu) of bacteria per 10 cm² of skin compared with 1000–10,000 cfu/cm² on the neck and chest (Carlson 1999, Moureau and Gabriel 2009, Philpot and Griffiths 2003). Thirdly, it is easy to use for both staff and patients (Dougherty 2006) as well as helping to preserve peripheral veins (Gabriel 2000, Oakley et al. 2000, Philpot and Griffiths 2003). It has been shown to reduce patient discomfort and provide a reliable form of access (Costa and Ferguson 2002, Oakley et al. 2000). It has also been shown to be cost-effective when compared with other long-term and short-term catheters and can be inserted at the bedside (Hayden and Goodman 2005, Snelling et al. 2001, Springhouse 2002).

Disadvantages include an increase in self-care, blood withdrawal is not always easy with the smaller gauges and they may occlude (Dougherty 2006, Molloy et al. 2008). Over time, multiple insertions can cause venous scarring and decrease the ability to reuse the site (Hayden and Goodman 2005). It has also been found that compared with skin-tunnelled catheters in patients with gastrointestinal cancers, the advantages of a PICC decrease significantly if treatment lasts more than 120 days (Snelling et al. 2001). PICCs should not be considered as a last resort, but introduced early in treatment (Springhouse 2002).

Indications

- Lack of peripheral access.
- Infusions of vesicant, irritant, parenteral nutrition or hyperosmolar solutions.
- Intermediate to long-term venous access.
- Patient preference.
- Patients with needle phobia, to prevent repeated cannulation.
- Clinician preference if patients are at risk of complications associated with CVAD insertion, for example haemorrhage or pneumothorax, or if other types of devices are contraindicated (Dougherty 2006, Moureau and Gabriel 2009, Philpot and Griffiths 2003).

Contraindications

- Anatomical distortions from surgery, injury or trauma, for example scarring from mastectomy, lymphoedema or burns, which may prevent advancement of the catheter to the desired tip location (Dougherty 2006, Philpot and Griffiths 2003).
- Cardiac pacemaker *in situ*.
- Enlarged axillary/supraclavicular lymph nodes.
- Tumour mass.
- Previous history of thrombosis.
- History of fractured clavicle (may be necessary to avoid that side of patient's body).

Methods of insertion

Venous assessment and selection play key roles in the successful insertion of a PICC, along with the correct positioning of the patient and careful measurement of the patient and the device. To obtain the correct measurement of the length of catheter to be inserted based on anatomical landmarks, using a tape measure, with the arm at 45°, measure diagonally from the selected point for venepuncture to the middle of the clavicle, and then add the length of the clavicle: this gives the measurement for right-sided placement. For left-sided placement, add the width of the manubrium (about 2–4 cm) (Lum 1999). Lum (2004) has since developed a formula-based measurement guide based on a patient's height which provides a more accurate assessment to achieve optimal tip placement (Dougherty 2006) (see Box 18.7).

Box 18.7 Formula to calculate measurement for length of PICC (with PICC located 2.5 cm below the antecubital fossa)

Right PICC	Height in cm $\times$ 3 $\div$ 10
Left PICC	Height in cm $\times$ 3 $\div$ 10 + 4 cm

(Adapted from Lum 2004)

Legal and professional issues

Nurses who wish to undertake this role must be competent in cannulation and receive additional training in theory and practical hands-on instruction at the bedside (Bullock-Corkhill 2010). Competencies would include:

- knowledge and skills in anatomy and physiology of the veins of the upper arm and central veins
- selection of the vein and equipment
- use of ultrasound and local anaesthetic
- prevention and management of complications.

A number of hospitals and companies now provide PICC training days that may also include the use of ultrasound.

Consent

The benefits (the ability to withdraw blood and infuse medications for long-term access) and risks (bleeding, thrombosis, infection, malposition) must be explained to the patient prior to insertion. Written consent should be obtained. An example of the PICC consent form is shown in Figure 18.19.

Preprocedural considerations

Equipment

Peripherally inserted central catheters are available as single- and double-lumen catheters, non-valved or valved, and may be made of silicone or polyurethane (Dougherty 2006, Springhouse 2002). Catheters measure 50–65 cm long, with a diameter of 2–7 Fr. PICCs can be cut to the required length, except for those with valves in the tip (Dougherty 2006) (Figure 18.20). A guidewire within the catheter adds firmness to a silicone catheter, enhancing its advancement. Guidewires are not usually required with a polyurethane catheter (Perucca 2010). The catheter may be inserted through a peel-away introducer or using a modified Seldinger technique with a micro introducer which reduces the trauma to the vein and risk of arterial or nerve damage (Bullock-Corkhill 2010). It can also be used to facilitate placement in a smaller difficult vein, as well as upper arm placement and improving success (Bullock-Corkhill 2010, Sansivero 1998). A cannula is inserted and once the stylet has been removed, a guidewire is advanced, the cannula is removed, and a scalpel is used to enlarge the skin puncture site. Then an introducer is passed over the wire, the wire is removed and the catheter is then advanced via the introducer into the vein (Dougherty 2006, Gabriel 2008, Sansivero 1998).

Pharmacological support

The use of local anaesthetic either topically or by injection should be considered to reduce the pain associated with the initial venepuncture with the introducer or when using the modified Seldinger technique, with or without ultrasound. This ensures that the area where the incision is made or deeper tissues are anaesthetized to reduce pain and discomfort (Hartley Jones 2009). Injectable local anaesthetic such as 1% lidocaine is commonly used and it has been found that intradermal lidocaine is superior to EMLA prior to insertion of PICCs (Fry and Aholt 2001).

Patient identifier/label:

Consent Form 1

(DH) **Department of Health**	Patient's surname/family name
	Patient's first names
	Date of birth
THE ROYAL MARSDEN NHS FOUNDATION TRUST	Responsible health professional
	Job title
	NHS number (or other identifier)
Insertion of a Peripherally Inserted Central Catheter (PICC)	☐ Male ☐ Female
Patient agreement to investigation or treatment	Special requirements (e.g. other language/other communication method)

Name of proposed procedure or course of treatment (including brief explanation if medical term not clear)

Insertion of a peripherally inserted central catheter (PICC)

This catheter is inserted into a vein in your arm and threaded up into the main vein to your heart called the superior vena cava. Before insertion, local anaesthetic will be administered (either as a cream or as an injection) around the vein to minimize the chance of pain during the procedure. The procedure takes about 30 minutes and then you will have a chest X-ray to confirm the correct position of the catheter.

STATEMENT OF HEALTH PROFESSIONAL (to be filled in by health professional with appropriate knowledge of proposed procedure, as specified in Consent Policy)

I have explained the proposed procedure to the patient. In particular, I have explained:

The intended benefits:

☐ This catheter will provide a reliable way to administer your therapy to your vein

☐ _____

_____

_____

_____

_____

To be retained in patient's notes

Figure 18.19   PICC consent form.

Patient identifier/label:

STATEMENT OF HEALTH PROFESSIONAL (Cont.)

Serious or frequently occurring risks:

☐ There are some risks during insertion – firstly that the needle could cause a bruise or swelling.

☐ The catheter may not thread into the correct position and the tip may not be in the correct vein. You would probably be unaware of this. This would be identified on the chest X-ray you have following the procedure. If the tip is not in the correct position it may have to be replaced. This occurs in less than 5% of the procedures.

☐ Once the catheter is in place there is a risk of infection. The risk is usually less than 3% but can be higher depending on many other factors, such as your diagnosis or treatment. Your doctor or nurse will be able to explain the risk to you.

☐ Once the catheter is in place there is a risk of a clot (thrombosis) forming around the catheter. This occurs in less than 3% of patients depending on your diagnosis, treatment or if you have had a clot before. Your doctor or nurse will be able to explain the risk to you.

Any other risks:

_____
_____

Any extra procedures which may become necessary during the procedure:

☐ You may be given a drug called warfarin (a blood thinning agent) to reduce the risk of clot formation while the catheter is in place.

☐ other procedure (please specify) _____

_____
_____

I have also discussed what the procedure is likely to involve, the benefits and risks of any available alternative treatments (including no treatment) and any particular concerns of this patient.

The following leaflet/audiotape has been provided:

☐ **Central Venous Access Devices**

☐ _____

This procedure will involve:

☐ **General and/or regional anaesthesia**   ☐ **Local anaesthesia**

☐ **Sedation**

Signed: **Date:**

Name (Print):   **Job Title:**

To be retained in patient's notes

Figure 18.19   (*Continued*)

Figure 18.20   PICC types.

Procedure guideline 18.6 PICC insertion using a standard introducer

Essential equipment

- Sterile pack containing sterile gown, mask with visor, sterile drapes and scissors
- One pair of sterile powder-free gloves
- Alcohol-based hand scrub
- Alcohol-based skin cleaning preparation, such as 2% chlorhexidine in 70% alcohol
- 10 mL syringes
- Extension set and needleless injection cap
- Introducer
- PICC
- Transparent dressing
- Securing device and sterile tapes
- 23 and 25 G needles
- Tape measure
- Tourniquet
- Sharps container

Medicinal products

- 0.9% sodium chloride
- Heparinized saline

Preprocedure

Action	Rationale
1 Assess patient's medical and intravenous device history.	To ensure the patient has no underlying medical problems and is suitable to undergo the procedure. E
2 Explain and discuss the procedure with the patient. Gain written consent.	To ensure that the patient understands the procedure and gives their valid written consent (NMC 2008b, C).
3 Apply tourniquet and assess venous access, assessing both extremities, and locate veins by sight and palpatation (or by ultrasound).	To ensure the patient has adequate venous access and to select the vein for catheterization (Gabriel 2008, E).

4	Apply local anaesthetic cream/gel to chosen venepuncture site and leave for allotted time.	To minimize the pain of insertion (BNF 2011, C).
5	Draw screens and position patient in a supine position, with patient's arm at a 45° angle from the body.	To ensure privacy. To aid insertion of introducer and then advancement of catheter (Gabriel 2008, E).
6	Measure using the tape measure from the selected venepuncture site diagonally across to the middle of the clavicle, then measure total distance of clavicle. Added together, these will give catheter measurement (see Action Figure 6) or use the formula (see Box 18.7).	To enable selection of the most suitable catheter length and to establish how far to advance the catheter in order for its tip to be located in the correct position, that is, the SVC (Lum 1999, E; Lum 2004, R5).
7	Take equipment required to patient's bedside. Open outer pack. Apply facemask with visor.	To ensure appropriate equipment is available for procedure. E To protect practitioner from blood splash contamination. E

Procedure

8	Carefully wash hands using bactericidal soap and water.	To minimize the risk of infection (Fraise and Bradley 2009, E; Pratt *et al.* 2007, C).
9	Put on sterile gown and powder-free sterile gloves; open sterile tray, arranging the contents as required. Draw up 0.9% sodium chloride into a 10 mL syringe (from an assistant).	To prevent contamination. Powder on gloves can increase the risk of mechanical phlebitis (Elliott 1993, E; Pratt *et al.* 2007, C).
10	Remove the cap from the extension set and attach syringe of 0.9% sodium chloride; gently flush with 2 mL and leave syringe attached.	To check that the catheter is patent and to enable easy removal of guidewire (manufacturer's guidelines, C).
11	If the catheter tip can be trimmed, using the graduated markings along the catheter, select the marking required and pull back guidewire 1 cm from desired new tip, and using sterile scissors trim the catheter. Never trim the guidewire!	To ensure the catheter will be the correct length for SVC tip placement and to prevent damage to the vein if the guidewire is damaged (manufacturer's guidelines, C).
12	Place sterile towel under patient's arm.	To provide a sterile field to work on. E
13	Clean the skin at the selected site with 2% chlorhexidine in 70% alcohol, with friction, and prepare an area of 15–25 cm.	To ensure the removal of skin flora and to minimize the risk of infection (Fraise and Bradley 2009, E; Pratt *et al.* 2007, C).
14	Allow the solution to dry thoroughly.	To ensure coagulation of bacteria and disinfection (Pratt *et al.* 2007, C).
15	Drape the patient with a fenestrated towel.	To provide a sterile field (Pratt *et al.* 2007, C).
16	Inject local anaesthetic intradermally, if required, using a 25 G needle and wait a few minutes for it to take effect.	To enable adequate anaesthesia (BNF 2011, C).
17	Reapply tourniquet.	To aid venous distension (Dougherty 2008, E).
18	Perform venepuncture with introducer by entering the skin, 1 cm from desired point of entry, at a 15–30° angle. Advance 0.5–1.0 cm once flashback is seen.	To gain venous access (Gabriel 2008, E).
19	Release tourniquet.	To prevent blood loss and 'through puncture' and enable advancement of catheter (Gabriel 2008, E).

1123

(Continued)

Procedure guideline 18.6 (*Continued*)

20	Position fingers in a V, with index finger on wings and middle finger above sheath tip, and gently remove stylet. Apply pressure.	To contain flashback, prevent contamination of the area with blood and minimize the amount of blood loss from the patient (Gabriel 2008, E).
21	Continue slow advancement of the catheter and aspirate and flush to check for blood return or resistance.	To minimize damage to intima of vein (Gabriel 2008, E). To check there is no obstruction and that it advances into the correct location.
22	Ask the patient to turn their head towards the arm of insertion and place their chin on the clavicle if possible.	To prevent the catheter entering the jugular vein and to ensure correct advancement of catheter downwards to the SVC (Gabriel 2008, E).
23	Ask patient if they have any aural (behind the ear) sensations on side of catheter insertion.	This could indicate that the catheter has advanced along the internal jugular vein and needs to be withdrawn and readvanced (Dougherty 2006, E).
24	Continue slow advancement of the catheter to the desired length.	To minimize damage to intima of the vein (Gabriel 2008, E).
25	Apply pressure above introducer and carefully withdraw the introducer and peel apart.	To ensure there is no movement of the catheter. To remove peel-away introducer (Gabriel 2008, E).
26	Aspirate for blood return and flush catheter with 0.9% sodium chloride.	To check patency of device and ensure continued patency (Gabriel 2008, E; Pratt *et al.* 2007, C).
27	Apply gentle pressure on catheter and slowly withdraw the guidewire.	To ensure there is no withdrawal of catheter (Gabriel 2008, E).
28	Attach a needleless injection cap and flush as per local policy.	To ensure patency of the device (Gabriel 2008, E; Pratt *et al.* 2007, C).
29	Secure the catheter with a securing device such as a Statlock. Apply a small pad of low-linting gauze directly over the insertion site and secure with sterile tape.	To ensure stability of device and to minimize blood leakage at the site which occurs following insertion (Gabriel 2008, E; Moureau and Iannucci 2003, E; RCN 2010, C).
30	Apply a transparent dressing. Apply low-linting gauze under the extension set and cap, then bandage.	To ensure protection of the site. To prevent the tubing pressing into the patient's skin (Gabriel 2008, E; RCN 2010, C).

Postprocedure

31	Dispose of equipment appropriately. Dispose of sharps and clinical waste.	To prevent sharps injury (NHS Employers 2007, C).
32	Send patient for chest X-ray. Position of catheter to be assessed and documented by the doctor.	To allow position of tip to be assessed. To ensure correct tip location (Wise *et al.* 2001, E).
33	Document the procedure in the patient's notes: type, length and gauge of catheter, where it was inserted, tip confirmation, batch number of catheter and lot number of sterile packs, any problems, how it was secured and patient education.	To ensure adequate records and enable continued care of device and patient (NMC 2009, C). To trace any faulty equipment back to manufacturers (MHRA 2004, C).

Right-sided placement

Measure total distance to end of clavicle and add measurement from intended entry site of PICC to midclavicle

Left-sided placement

Measure total distance of clavicle and manubrium and add to measurement from intended entry site of PICC to midclavicle

Action Figure 6   Preinsertion measurement of a PICC.

Procedure guideline 18.7 PICC insertion using modified Seldinger technique (with or without ultrasound)

Essential equipment

- Sterile pack containing sterile gown, mask with visor, sterile drapes and scissors
- One pair of sterile powder-free gloves
- Alcohol-based hand scrub
- Alcohol-based skin cleaning preparation, such as 2% chlorhexidine in 70% alcohol
- 10 mL syringes
- Extension set and needleless injection cap
- Introducer
- PICC
- Transparent dressing
- Securing device and sterile tapes
- 23 and 25 G needle
- Tape measure
- Tourniquet
- Sharps container

Optional equipment

- Ultrasound machine, gel and sterile probe cover
- MST kit (contains 22 G cannula, wire, 5 mL syringe, introducer/dilator, scalpel, needle)

Medicinal products

- 0.9% sodium chloride
- Heparinized saline
- 1% lidocaine

Preprocedure

Action	Rationale
1 Assess patient's medical and intravenous device history.	To ensure the patient has no underlying medical problems such as taking anticoagulants or previous surgery to arm or chest and so is suitable to undergo the procedure. E
2 Explain and discuss the procedure with the patient. Gain written consent.	To ensure that the patient understands the procedure and gives their valid written consent (NMC 2008b, C).

1125

(Continued)

Procedure guideline 18.7 (*Continued*)

3 Apply tourniquet and assess venous access, assessing both extremities, and locate veins by sight and palpatation (or by ultrasound).	To ensure the patient has adequate venous access and to select the vein for catheterization (Gabriel 2008, E).
4 Apply local anaesthetic cream/gel to chosen venepuncture site and leave for allotted time.	To minimize the pain of insertion (BNF 2011, C).
5 Draw screens and position patient in a supine position, with patient's arm at a 45° angle.	To ensure privacy. To aid insertion of introducer and then advancement of catheter (Gabriel 2008, E).
6 Measure using the tape measure from the selected venepuncture site diagonally across to the middle of the clavicle, then measure total distance of clavicle. Added together, these will give catheter measurement (see Action Figure 6, Procedure guideline 18.6) or use the formula (see Box 18.7).	To enable selection of the most suitable catheter length and to establish how far to advance the catheter in order for its tip to be located in the correct position, that is, the SVC (Lum 1999, E; Lum 2004, R5).
7 Take equipment required to patient's bedside. Open outer pack.	To ensure appropriate equipment is available for procedure. E
8 Apply facemask with visor.	To protect practitioner from blood splash contamination. E

Procedure

9 Carefully wash hands using bactericidal soap and water.	To minimize the risk of infection (Fraise and Bradley 2009, E; Pratt *et al.* 2007, C).
10 Put on sterile gown and powder-free sterile gloves; open sterile tray, arranging the contents as required. Draw up 0.9% sodium chloride into a 10 mL syringe (from an assistant).	To prevent contamination. Powder on gloves can increase the risk of mechanical phlebitis (Elliott 1993, E; Pratt *et al.* 2007, C).
11 Remove the cap from the extension set and attach syringe of 0.9% sodium chloride; gently flush with 2 mL and leave syringe attached.	To check that the catheter is patent and to enable easy removal of guidewire (manufacturer's guidelines, C).
12 If the catheter tip can be trimmed, using the graduated markings along the catheter, select the marking required and pull back guidewire 1 cm from desired new tip, and using sterile scissors trim the catheter. Never trim the guidewire!	To ensure the catheter will be the correct length for SVC tip placement and to prevent damage to the vein if the guidewire is damaged (manufacturer's guidelines, C).
13 Place sterile towel under patient's arm.	To provide a sterile field to work on. E
14 Clean the skin at the selected site with 2% chlorhexidine in 70% alcohol, with friction, and prepare an area of 15–25 cm.	To ensure the removal of skin flora and to minimize the risk of infection (Fraise and Bradley 2009, E; Pratt *et al.* 2007, C).
15 Allow the solution to dry thoroughly.	To ensure coagulation of bacteria and disinfection (Pratt *et al.* 2007, C).
16 Drape the patient with a fenestrated towel. If using ultrasound then apply a sterile ultrasound probe cover.	To provide a sterile field (Pratt *et al.* 2007, C). To ensure all equipment that is in contact with the patient is sterile (Pratt *et al.* 2007, C).
17 Inject local anaesthetic intradermally, if required, using a 25 G needle and wait a few minutes for it to take effect.	To provide adequate anaesthesia (BNF 2011, C).
18 Reapply tourniquet.	To aid venous distension (Dougherty 2008, E).

19 Apply gel to skin and scan for vein.	To identify most suitable vein.
20 Perform venepuncture with cannula. When flashback is seen, advance cannula into vein.	To gain venous access (Gabriel 2008, E). To prevent blood loss and 'through puncture' and enable advancement of catheter (Gabriel 2008, E).
21 Release tourniquet.	To contain flashback, prevent contamination of the area with blood and minimize the amount of blood loss from the patient (Gabriel 2008, E).
22 Remove stylet and advance guidewire through cannula until there is 10–15 cm of wire in vein (see Action Figure 22).	To maintain venous access. E
23 Remove cannula and advance introducer over the wire up to puncture site.	To prepare for insertion. E
24 Infiltrate over the puncture site with 1% lidocaine (intrademally) until a small bleb is observed (see Action Figure 24).	To achieve anaesthesia and minimize patient discomfort. E
25 Check the patient has no sharp sensations at puncture site and then make a small incision (see Action Figure 25).	To ensure area is anaesthetized before proceeding. E
26 Grip the introducer firmly and advance through puncture site (see Action Figure 26).	To enable advancement of dilator. E
27 Remove the wire and then the dilator and grip catheter 1 cm from the tip and thread through introducer sheath.	To enable catheter insertion. E
28 Continue slow advancement of the catheter and aspirate and flush to check for blood return or resistance.	To minimize damage to intima of vein (Gabriel 2008, E). To check there is no obstruction and that it advances into the correct location. E
29 Turn the patient's head towards the arm of insertion and place their chin on the clavicle if possible.	To prevent the catheter entering the jugular vein and to ensure correct advancement of catheter downwards to the SVC (Gabriel 2008, E).
30 Ask patient if they have any aural (behind the ear) sensations on side of catheter insertion.	This could indicate that the catheter has advanced along the internal jugular vein and needs to be withdrawn and readvanced (Dougherty 2006, E).
31 Continue slow advancement of the catheter to the desired length.	To minimize damage to intima of the vein (Gabriel 2008, E).
32 Apply pressure above introducer and carefully withdraw the introducer and peel apart.	To ensure there is no movement of the catheter. To remove peel-away introducer (Gabriel 2008, E).
33 Aspirate for blood return and flush catheter with 0.9% sodium chloride.	To check patency of device and ensure continued patency (Gabriel 2008, E; Pratt *et al.* 2007, C).
34 Apply gentle pressure on catheter and slowly withdraw the guidewire.	To ensure there is no withdrawal of catheter (Gabriel 2008, E).
35 Attach a needleless injection cap and flush as per local policy.	To ensure patency of the device (Gabriel 2008, E; Pratt *et al.* 2007, C).

(Continued)

Procedure guideline 18.7 (*Continued*)

36 Secure the catheter with a securing device such as a Statlock. Apply a small pad of low-linting gauze directly over the insertion site and secure with sterile tape.	To ensure stability of device and to minimize blood leakage at the site which occurs following insertion (Gabriel 2008, E; Moureau and Iannucci 2003, E; RCN 2010, C).
37 Apply a transparent dressing. Apply low-linting gauze under the extension set and cap, then bandage.	To ensure protection of the site. To prevent the tubing pressing into the patient's skin (Gabriel 2008, E; RCN 2010, C).

Postprocedure

38 Remove gloves and dispose of equipment appropriately. Dispose of sharps and clinical waste.	To prevent sharps injury (NHS Employers 2007, C).
39 Send patient for chest X-ray. Position of catheter to be assessed and documented by the doctor (see Figure 18.5).	To allow position of tip to be assessed. To ensure correct tip location (Wise *et al.* 2001, E).
40 Document the procedure in the patient's notes: • type, length and gauge of catheter • where it was inserted • tip confirmation • batch number of catheter and lot number of sterile packs • any problems • how it was secured and • patient education given.	To ensure adequate records and enable continued care of device and patient (NMC 2009, C). To trace any faulty equipment back to manufacturers (MHRA 2004, C).

Action Figure 22   Wire being threaded in cannula.

Action Figure 24   Local anaesthetic injection.

Action Figure 25   Making an incision with a scalpel.

Action Figure 26   Advancing the introducer.

Problem-solving table 18.3 Prevention and resolution (Procedure guidelines 18.6 and 18.7)

Problem	Cause	Prevention	Action
Difficulty when advancing catheter (this may be indicated by resistance when advancing the catheter with or without blood return)	Valves Chosen vein, for example cephalic (size or problems when at junction of axillary vein into subclavian) Muscle spasm in neck	Select a vein with fewer valves or one with large lumen	Flush and attempt to advance the catheter
Aural sensations when flushing	Catheter has advanced into the jugular vein	Get patient to turn their head to side of insertion and tuck chin down on clavicle to help prevent tip malposition	Withdraw catheter until sensation has disappeared, turn patient's head and attempt to readvance, checking for sensations. If it continues, it may be necessary to abandon placement in that vein
Malposition (coiled in vessels, advanced into jugular or accessory veins)	Patient has deviant anatomy Patient not correctly positioned Catheter deflected by valves	Check previous history in case has had previous problems in that vein Position patient correctly Advance catheter slowly	Sit patient upright Withdraw wire a few cm to allow tip to be more flexible and flush vigorously

Postprocedural considerations
Immediate care

Most PICCs are designed with suture wings, so the PICC can be sutured to the patient's skin. However, patients have reported long-term suturing to be uncomfortable; scarring when the device is removed (Gabriel 2000, 2001); and inflammation and bacterial colonization of the exit site (Schears 2005). So suturing is no longer recommended (Maki 2002). PICCs can be adequately secured using Steristrips or securement devices (self-adhesive anchoring devices applied to the skin such as Statlocks (Figure 18.21)). These have been shown to result in significantly longer catheter dwell times and fewer total complications (Gabriel 2001, Maki 2002, Schears 2005, Yamamoto et al. 2002). Bleeding occurs in the first 24 hours so a fold of sterile gauze should be placed over the site under the dressing (Philpot and Griffiths 2003). The insertion site is then covered with a moisture-permeable transparent dressing.

The position of the tip of the PICC should be verified immediately after insertion before any infusion. This is done by a chest X-ray. Ascertaining correct placement is the major reason for ordering a chest X-ray, but a chest X-ray also rules out malposition and pneumothorax and confirms acceptable tip location for the type of medication being administered (Dougherty 2006, INS 2011, RCN 2010, Royer 2001, Wise et al. 2001).

Ongoing care

The initial dressing should be changed at 24 hours and then according to manufacturer's recommendations, for example once a week, to minimize the potential for infection and catheter migration (NICE 2003, Pratt et al. 2007, RCN 2010).

Flushing solution and frequency are usually dependent on the type of catheter and so manufacturer's recommendations

Figure 18.21 Peripheral cannula with securing device.

should be followed. For example, valved catheters are usually flushed once a week with 0.9% sodium chloride, while non-valved catheters are flushed with a heparinized solution (Dougherty 2006, Pratt *et al.* 2007). Care should be taken when using devices such as power injectors for administering intravenous contrast agents via a PICC as the pressure created may lead to catheter rupture. This will depend on the gauge and manufacturer of the catheter (Williamson and McKinney 2001) as most manufacturers now provide computed tomography (CT)-compatible PICCs made specifically to withstand the pressure created during CT scanning. The Medicines and Healthcare Products Regulatory Agency (MHRA 2004) recommends that CT contrast using a pressure injector should not be performed via any CVAD.

Documentation

The following should be documented on insertion.

- Vein used.
- Insertion date and time.
- Length of catheter inserted and external length.
- Size of catheter, manufacturer and batch number.
- Number of cannulation attempts, the veins used and problems encountered.
- Flushing solution used.
- Securement method and dressing.
- Signature of practitioner inserting PICC.
- X-ray confirmation and tip location.
- Type of local anaesthetic used.
- Type of cleaning solutions.

(Moureau and Gabriel 2009)

Education of patients and relevant others

See Discharging patients home with a VAD *in situ*.

Complications

On insertion
Haematoma/arterial puncture/hitting a nerve

See Cannulation.

Once in situ
Mechanical phlebitis

See Cannulation.

Thrombosis

A thrombosis is a clot of blood that can be present at the tip of a catheter or can surround the catheter, for example a thrombosis in the upper arm caused by the presence of a PICC. A SVC thrombus occurs when a catheter chronically rubs against the wall of the SVC, provoking a thrombosis at the site, and is often associated with a fibrin sheath. In order

for a thrombosis to develop, three factors are required, known as Virchow's triad:

1 stasis
2 endothelial damage and
3 hypercoagulable state, caused by the following conditions: diabetes, malnutrition, dehydration, pregnancy, osteomyelitis, smoking, chronic renal failure, cirrhosis, cancer, obesity, sickle cell, surgery, congestive heart failure, oestrogen therapies (Gorski *et al.* 2010).

Symptoms can be very acute or vague. The patient will usually complain of pain in the area such as the arm or the neck, oedema of neck, chest and upper extremity, periorbital oedema, facial tenderness, tachycardia, shortness of breath and sometimes a cough, signs of a co-lateral circulation over the chest area, jugular venous distension and discolouration of the limb (Dougherty 2006).

Thrombosis can be prevented by correct placement of the tip in the SVC, monitoring of catheter function and flushing with pulsatile positive pressure flush (Mayo 2000). The use of prophylactic anticoagulants such as low-dose warfarin has been shown to be of no apparent benefit (Couban *et al.* 2005, Young *et al.* 2005). Full anticoagulation may be necessary if the patient has had previous thromboembolic events (Bishop 2009).

If a thrombosis is suspected then the patient should have a venogram and ultrasound (Dougherty 2006). Treatment can be either catheter removal or anticoagulation as thrombolytic therapy has proved successful in extreme cases and is often dependent on the size of the clot and area of impaired circulation (Gorski *et al.* 2010). If the catheter is to be removed, patients will be prescribed heparin and this may continue for a number of days before they are switched onto an oral anticoagulant such as warfarin. This may then need to continue for up to 3 months following removal (Gorski *et al.* 2010).

Sepsis

Infection is one of the greatest complications associated with a central venous catheter (Dougherty 2006). The catheter provides the ideal opportunity for micro-organisms to either track along the outside of the catheter or be administered via the hub internally into the central venous system. Infections can occur at the insertion site or systemically. Signs of infection at the insertion site include erythema, oedema, tracking along the length of the catheter, tenderness at the site, exudate such as pus, offensive smell. Septicaemia is a systemic infection which is usually characterized by pyrexia, flushing, sweating and rigors (rigors occur particularly when the catheter is flushed). Prevention is good aseptic non-touch technique and use of evidence-based guidelines, for example CVC care bundle (DH 2010). If the patient develops symptoms of an infection then site swabs should be taken along with blood cultures (from the device and peripheral veins). Depending on the clinical condition of the patient, the CVAD may be removed and/or intravenous antibiotics may be commenced (Gorski *et al.* 2010).

Removal of peripherally inserted central catheters

Preprocedural considerations

Removal requires gentle firm traction and the catheter will slide out from the insertion site. A PICC may resist removal because of venous spasm, vasoconstriction, phlebitis, valve inflammation, thrombophlebitis or when a fibrin sheath is present (Gorski *et al.* 2010). Difficulty may occur in 1% of removals (Drewett 2000). Gentle traction and a warm moist compress can be applied to alleviate venous spasm, resulting in easier removal of the catheter (Gorski *et al.* 2010, Marx 1995). If there is difficulty with removal then wait 20–30 minutes and try again or leave for 12–24 hours (Dougherty 2006). Other interventions to aid removal include smooth muscle relaxants, hand and arm exercises or relaxation techniques (Gorski *et al.* 2010, Marx 1995).

Procedure guideline 18.8 PICC removal

Essential equipment

- Dressing pack containing gauze and sterile gloves
- Apron
- Pair of clean gloves
- Cleaning solution
- Occlusive dressing
- Tape
- Bactericidal handrub

Optional equipment

- Sterile scissors
- Specimen container

Preprocedure

Action	Rationale
1 Explain the procedure to the patient.	To ensure that the patient understands the procedure and gives their valid written consent (NMC 2008b, C).
2 Place the patient supine if possible.	To prevent the risk of air embolism (Scales 2008, E).

Procedure

3 Wash hands using a bactericidal handrub and gather equipment required. Apply apron and clean gloves.	To minimize the risk of infection (DH 2010, C; Fraise and Bradley 2009, E).
4 Remove transparent dressing and gently remove securing devices and/or sterile tapes.	To prepare for catheter removal. E
5 Apply sterile gloves and clean the insertion site.	To prevent contamination of the site. E
6 Using a steady and constant motion, gently pull catheter until it is completely removed from exit site.	To remove the catheter and prevent vein damage. E
7 Apply pressure with a finger (digital pressure) over exit site for about 2–3 minutes or until bleeding stops, and apply dressing.	To minimize blood loss and bruising. To provide protection of the entry site. E

1131

(Continued)

Procedure guideline 18.8 *(Continued)*

Postprocedure

8 Check marking of length removed and check it is the same as the length inserted.	To ensure that complete catheter has been removed (RCN 2010, C).
9 If the catheter is removed because of infection, carefully cut off the tip (approximately 5 cm) of the catheter using sterile scissors and place it in a sterile container for microbiological investigation.	To detect any infection related to the catheter and thus provide necessary treatment (DH 2010, C).
10 Remove gloves and dispose of waste.	To ensure safe disposal in the correct containers and avoid laceration or injury of other staff. To prevent reuse of equipment (NHS Employers 2007, C).
11 Document length of catheter removed and reason for removal in care plan.	To ensure adequate records and to enable continued care of device and patient (DH and CMO 2003, C; NMC 2009, C).

Postprocedural considerations

Following removal of the PICC, pressure should be applied for at least 2–3 minutes and the site inspected prior to applying a sterile transparent dressing to ensure bleeding has stopped. The catheter integrity should be checked and its length measured to ensure an intact device has been removed (Dougherty 2006, Springhouse 2002).

Documentation

On removal, the following should be documented: catheter length and integrity, site appearance; dressing applied, reason for removal (Gorski *et al.* 2010).

Short-term percutaneous central venous catheters (non-tunnelled)

Definition

A short-term non-tunnelled percutaneous CVC is a device that enters through the skin directly into a central vein (Dougherty 2006).

Evidence-based approaches

Rationale

Percutaneous non-tunnelled CVCs are commonly used for patients in acute settings and insertion may be in response to an emergency or planned event (Hamilton 2009). Their configuration as a multilumen catheter allows administration of several solutions at once and they are easy to remove (Dougherty 2006, Ives 2009). However, these catheters are associated with an increased risk of complications such as pneumothorax and infection (Chantler 2009) and the catheter material results in irritation of the inner lumen of the vessel and is more thrombogenic than softer silicone catheters (Dougherty 2006, Springhouse 2002).

Indications

- Short-term therapy (a few days up to several weeks).
- CVP readings.
- Emergency use, for example fluid replacement.
- Absence of peripheral veins (Dougherty 2006, Simcock 2001b).

Contraindications

There are few absolute contraindications as these catheters are often placed in an emergency, but where possible they should be avoided in the following situations.

- Patients who have an existing infection.
- Patients with an existing pneumothorax or poor respiratory function.
- Patients with radiation burns to the insertion site, fractured clavicle, and malignant lesion at base of neck or apex of lungs (Dougherty 2006, Scales 2008), SVC syndrome or a history of central placement problems.

Methods of insertion
Choice of vein

These catheters are usually placed in the jugular, subclavian or femoral veins. The shortest catheter and the most direct route are required to create a rapid blood flow around the catheter, which reduces irritation and obstructions, and the risk of complications, and increases the dwell time of the catheter (Springhouse 2002, Weinstein and Plumer 2007). The preferred vein for most CVCs is the subclavian (Weinstein and Plumer 2007). This route has the lowest risk of infection (Chantler 2009, Mermel *et al.* 2001), allows greatest patient mobility after insertion and provides a flatter surface to maintain a dressing (Hadaway 2010). Disadvantages are an increased risk of pneumothorax and difficulty controlling bleeding (Chantler 2009).

The jugular vein approach can be via the internal or external jugular vein. The anatomical location of the internal jugular vein makes it easier to catheterize than the subclavian vein and there is less risk of pneumothorax (Chantler 2009, Hadaway 2010). The external jugular vein is observable and easily entered and insertion complications are rare (Weinstein and Plumer 2007). Disadvantages include catheter occlusion and venous irritation as a result of head movement, difficulty in maintaining an intact dressing, and the position of the catheters being disturbing for patient and family (Chantler 2009, Dougherty 2006, Weinstein and Plumer 2007). The femoral veins are primarily used for short-term access when other sites are not suitable (Springhouse 2002). This route is associated with an increased risk of infection and thrombosis, difficulty in maintaining an intact dressing and inhibiting the patient's mobility (Chantler 2009, Dougherty 2006, Hadaway 2010).

Central venous catheter insertion is a sterile procedure and the insertion requires use of a mask, sterile gloves, a gown and sterile drapes (INS 2011, Pratt *et al.* 2007, RCN 2010). These catheters may be inserted at the patient's bedside, but it is recommended that the procedure is performed in a controlled environment to reduce the risk of contamination (Dougherty 2006). This procedure is usually performed by doctors although more nurses are expanding their roles to include it (Alexandrou *et al.* 2010, Hamilton 2009).

Insertion can be aided by the use of ultrasound (Bodenham 2009). Ultrasound guidance should be used routinely when a CVC is being inserted via the jugular or femoral vein whether in an elective or emergency situation (NICE 2002, Wigmore *et al.* 2007). Ultrasound has been shown to increase success, decreasing failure by 83% and reducing complications by 57% (NICE 2002).

Methods for the Valsalva manoeuvre and Trendelenburg position

Placing the patient in the Trendelenburg position facilitates entry to the vein by distending the vein, increasing CVP and venous blood supply, making veins more visible and accessible (Farrow *et al.* 2009). It also reduces the chance of air embolism because the venous pressure is higher than atmospheric pressure. This is especially important when the catheter is placed using the subclavian approach (Dougherty 2006). A rolled towel may be placed under the back along the spinal cord and between the shoulders to hyperextend the neck and clavicle (Weinstein and Plumer 2007). The Valsalva manoeuvre can be performed by conscious patients to aid insertion of the catheter and also to prevent air embolism (Dougherty 2006, Verghese *et al.* 2002, Weinstein and Plumer 2007). The patient is asked to breathe in and then try to force the air out with the mouth and nose closed (i.e. against a closed glottis). This increases the intrathoracic pressure so that the return of blood to the heart is reduced momentarily and the veins in the neck region become engorged (Dougherty 2006).

Legal and professional issues

Nurses who wish to undertake this role must receive additional training in theory and practical hands-on instruction at the bedside in insertion techniques and ultrasound (Bullock-Corkhill 2010). Competencies would include knowledge of anatomy and physiology of the vasculature of the neck and the chest, selection of the vein and equipment, use of ultrasound and local anaesthetic, and prevention, recognition and management of complications. It is also recommended that nurses have had previous training in critical care or theatre or have advanced life support skills so they can respond appropriately in the event of an emergency during insertion (Hamilton 2009).

Preprocedural considerations
Equipment
Catheters

Most catheters are made of polyurethane and may be single- or multi- (up to five) lumen devices (Figure 18.22). There are a variety of lumen gauges and the catheters vary in length. They are usually open-ended but lumens can exit at staggered points along the catheter (Figure 18.23) (Dougherty 2006, Ives 2009). Multilumen catheters carry a high risk of

Figure 18.22 Non-tunnelled multilumen central venous catheter.

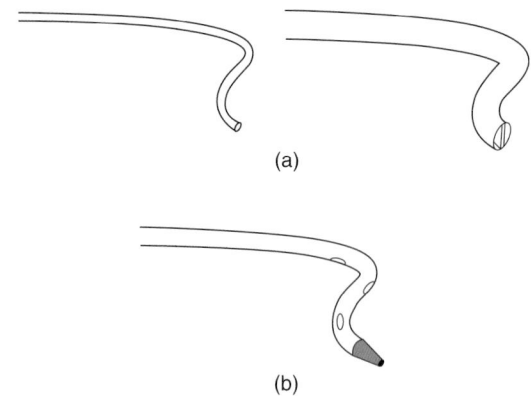

(a)

(b)

Figure 18.23 Types of catheter tips. (a) Open-ended catheter (single and double lumen). (b) Staggered exit open-ended catheter.

Figure 18.24 Ways of achieving the Trendelenburg position.

infection, which has resulted in the manufacture of coated and impregnated catheters, which may have antimicrobial agents such as chlorhexidine or silver sulphadiazine bonded onto the surface. It has been shown that this can reduce the incidence of catheter-related bloodstream infections and their use is strongly recommended by the Department of Health (Bassetti *et al.* 2001, Pratt *et al.* 2007, RCN 2010, Sampath *et al.* 2001).

Pharmacological support

Since these devices are usually in constant use, 0.9% sodium chloride is the flushing solution of choice to reduce the risk of occlusion (Pratt *et al.* 2007). It may be appropriate to use continuous infusions to keep the vein open. 1% Lidocaine is often used to provide anaesthesia prior to cannulation and advancement of the introducer.

Specific patient preparations

When inserting the catheter, the following aspects should be assessed prior to insertion (Hamilton 2009).

- Allergies.
- Physical examination, for example physique, weight (obesity, cachexic), physical features (bull neck, lymphoedema, tracheostomy).
- Vascular assessment.
- Assessment of respiratory, cardiovascular and neurological function.
- Fractures and arthritis, shape of sternum.

- Infection issues.
- Radiological assessment/thrombosis.
- Laboratory assessment, for example biochemistry, coagulation, platelets.

In general, the nurse's responsibilities when assisting another practitioner include the following.

- To ensure, where possible, that the patient understands and has been given a full explanation of the procedure and had the opportunity to discuss any aspects.
- To explain any specific pre- and postprocedure instructions and the appearance and function of the catheter.
- To teach the patient techniques that may be required during insertion, the Valsalva manoeuvre and being placed in the Trendelenburg position (where the patient lies flat with the head lower than the feet; knees may be bent) (Dougherty 2006, Weinstein and Plumer 2007) (Figure 18.24).
- To assemble the equipment requested.
- To prepare local anaesthesia and dressing materials.
- To ensure the correct positioning of the patient during insertion, that is, in the supine or Trendelenburg position.
- To attend to the physical and psychological comfort of the patient during and immediately following the procedure.
- To ensure that no fluid or medication is infused before the correct position of the catheter is confirmed on X-ray by an appropriate clinician and the tip location is documented in the patient's notes.

Procedure guideline 18.9 Short-term central venous catheter (non-cuffed/tunnelled) insertion

Essential equipment

- Sterile pack containing sterile gown and drapes
- One pair of sterile powder-free gloves
- Alcohol-based hand scrub
- Alcohol-based skin cleaning preparation, such as 2% chlorhexidine in 70% alcohol
- 10 mL syringes
- 5 mL syringes
- Needleless injection cap
- Introducer
- Central venous catheter and kit

- Transparent dressing
- Sutures
- 21 G needle
- Cannulas 22 G
- 23 G needle
- 25 G needle
- Labels
- Ultrasound machine
- Ultrasound gel
- Ultrasound probe cover

Optional equipment

- Securing device

Medicinal products

- 0.9% sodium chloride
- 1% plain lidocaine 10 mL

Preprocedure

Action	Rationale
1 Gain consent from doctor to carry out procedure and assess patient's medical and intravenous device history.	To ensure the patient has no underlying medical problems and is suitable to undergo the procedure. E
2 Explain and discuss the procedure with the patient and obtain written consent.	To ensure that the patient understands the procedure and gives their valid written consent (NMC 2008b, C).
3 Draw screens and position patient in a supine position.	To ensure privacy. To aid insertion of introducer and then advancement of catheter (Gabriel 2008, E).
4 Wash hands using a bactericidal handrub.	To minimize the risk of infection (Fraise and Bradley 2009, E; Pratt et al. 2007, C).
5 Take equipment required to patient's bedside. Open outer pack.	To ensure appropriate equipment is available for procedure. E

Procedure

6 Wash hands using a bactericidal handrub.	To minimize the risk of infection (Fraise and Bradley 2009, E; Pratt et al. 2007, C).
7 Put on sterile gown and powder-free sterile gloves; open sterile tray, arranging the contents as required.	To prevent contamination. Powder on gloves can increase the risk of mechanical phlebitis (Elliott 1993, E; Pratt et al. 2007, C).
8 Prefill the syringe with 0.9% sodium chloride and flush each lumen of the catheter and then slide clamp across lumen.	To prevent blood loss and risk of air entry. To ascertain that all lumens are patent. E
9 Place sterile towel under patient's arm.	To provide a sterile field to work on. E
10 Clean the skin at the selected site with 2% chlorhexidine in 70% alcohol, with friction, and prepare an area of 15–25 cm.	To ensure the removal of skin flora and to minimize the risk of infection (Pratt et al. 2007, C).

1135

(Continued)

Procedure guideline 18.9 *(Continued)*

11	Allow the solution to dry thoroughly.	To ensure coagulation of bacteria and disinfection (Pratt *et al.* 2007, C).
12	Drape the patient with a fenestrated towel.	To provide a sterile field (Pratt *et al.* 2007, C).
13	Ask assistant to tip the patient head down into the Trendelenburg position.	To encourage venous filling and reduce risk of air embolism (Farrow *et al.* 2009, E).
14	Ask assistant to apply ultrasound gel to head of probe. Then apply sterile ultrasound probe cover.	To improve conductivity. E To maintain sterility during procedure. E
15	Apply ultrasound gel to neck and scan the side of the neck from below the ear lobe to the clavicle to locate the internal jugular vein and other vessels.	To identify and select suitable vein and vessels to avoid, for example thrombosed vessels or arteries. E
16	Inject local anaesthetic intradermally using a 25 G needle to the area over the selected vessel and wait for it to take effect.	To ensure that the area is anaesthetized and reduce patient discomfort. E
17	Attach an empty 5 mL syringe to the cannula.	To prepare equipment. E
18	Whilst visualizing the vein on the ultrasound machine, insert the cannula directly into the vein at a downward angle of 30–50° (or steeper to get clear visualization on the screen), maintaining gentle suction with the syringe plunger.	To gain venous access (Gabriel 2008, E), reduce risk of arterial puncture and to know when the cannula is in the vein – apposition of the anterior and posterior walls of the vein can occur so blood is often only aspirated on withdrawal rather than insertion (Farrow *et al.* 2009, E).
19	When blood is observed in the syringe, advance cannula off stylet and into the vein. Check that the blood is dark and non-pulsatile.	To ensure the cannula is in the vein and not the artery as it would then be bright red and pulsatile (Farrow *et al.* 2009, E).
20	Remove stylet, apply a digit over the entry and thread the guidewire through cannula until selected depth is reached (this will depend on side used and anatomy of patient). Keep hold of guidewire at all times.	To prevent air entry and to prevent contamination of the area with blood and minimize the amount of blood loss from the patient (Gabriel 2008, E). If placed too deeply, patient will have arrhythmias (Farrow *et al.* 2009, E).
21	Remove cannula and advance dilator over the wire up to puncture site.	To prepare for advancement of dilator. E
22	Make a small incision in the skin at the puncture site.	To aid the advancement of the dilator through the skin. E
23	Advance the dilator using a gentle corkscrew motion to dilate the soft tissues. Advance to about same depth as cannulation and then remove.	To facilitate the passage of the catheter (Farrow *et al.* 2009, E).
24	Remove the catheter from the plastic cover and advance over the wire and into vein via the puncture site.	To maintain sterility until required. To commence insertion of catheter. E
25	As the catheter is advanced along the wire, keep hold of wire from the end of the lumen and ensure it moves freely.	To ensure that the wire is not kinked or stuck within the vessels (Farrow *et al.* 2009, E).
26	Continue slow advancement of the catheter to the desired length (15 cm on right and 17 cm on left) then remove wire.	To minimize damage to intima of vein (Gabriel 2008, E). To check there is no obstruction and that it advances into the correct location (Farrow *et al.* 2009, E).
27	Aspirate and flush all lumens with 0.9% sodium chloride.	To check for blood return or resistance. To check patency of device and ensure continued patency (Gabriel 2008, E; Pratt *et al.* 2007, C).

28	Return the patient to a supine position.	To aid patient comfort. E
29	Attach needlefree caps.	To ensure a closed system. E
30	Clean the insertion site and attach the wings of the catheter to the securing device.	To ensure protection of the site. To prevent the tubing pressing into the patient's skin (Gabriel 2008, E; RCN 2010, C).
31	Suture to the skin or attach to a securing device. Cover with a transparent dressing.	To ensure stability of the device. (Gabriel 2008, E; RCN 2010, C).

Postprocedure

32	Remove gloves and dispose of equipment appropriately. Dispose of sharps and clinical waste.	To prevent sharps injury (NHS Employers 2007, C).
33	Send patient for chest X-ray. Position of catheter to be assessed and documented by the doctor.	To allow position of tip to be assessed. To ensure correct tip location (Wise *et al.* 2001, E).
34	Document the procedure in the patient's notes: ■ type of catheter (number of lumens) ■ number of passes (times needle inserted) ■ length and gauge of cannula ■ vein used ■ any problems ■ ability to aspirate blood ■ how it was secured ■ tip confirmation ■ patient education ■ serial number of catheter and ultrasound machine used.	To ensure adequate records and enable continued care of device and patient (NMC 2009, C).

Problem-solving table 18.4 Prevention and resolution (Procedure guideline 18.9)

Problem	Cause	Prevention	Action
Unable to advance wire, dilator or catheter	Anatomical deviation Valves	Use of ultrasound prior to insertion Good history taking and physical examination prior to commencing procedure	Do not force the wire, dilator or catheter as it may rupture a vessel Remove and reposition patient. If still having problems, remove the wire/catheter and change site or contact a more experienced colleague
Unable to achieve blood flashback	Vein may be transfixed Vein missed	Use of ultrasound to visualize vein	Blood may only be aspirated on withdrawal rather than insertion Withdraw the needle slowly, aspirating gently until flashback seen

1137

Postprocedural considerations
Immediate care

The catheter may be sutured in place but this is no longer recommended due to the risk of infection (Crnich and Maki 2002, Maki 2005). The use of other securement devices is recommended such as a Statlock (Figure 18.25).

Ongoing care

Flushing is recommended after each use of the catheter. The types of dressings used at the insertion site may vary according to the type of patient and unit. Staff in some critical care units do not dress the site but clean it every 4 hours whilst other units may use a moisture-permeable dressing which is changed as necessary, for example weekly (Scales

Figure 18.25 Statlock securement device.

2008). This enables the staff to observe the site regularly for any signs of infection. It is recommended that these types of catheter remain in for 10–14 days. They can then be removed or the site rotated (Timsit 2000) or they can be replaced over a guidewire (Cook *et al.* 1997).

Complications
Pneumothorax

Pneumothorax means presence of air in the pleura (Scales 2008, Weinstein and Plumer 2007). It can occur for a number of reasons but is the most common complication with central venous catheterization. It results from puncture of the pleura during insertion of a central venous catheter. It is is more common with the subclavian approach due to its anatomical proximity to the lung. It is characterized by shortness of breath and sudden onset of chest pain but the patient may be asymptomatic and it may only be discovered on the chest X-ray performed following the procedure. Other symptoms include tachycardia, persistent cough and diaphoresis (Dougherty 2006). Prevention is based on the skill level of the inserting practitioner (Wigmore *et al.* 2007) as well as the use of ultrasound (NICE 2003). If symptoms are noted during insertion, the practitioner may stop the procedure. The patient's colour, respirations and pulse should be monitored and oxygen should be administered. In the case of a small pneumothorax, the patient may feel slightly breathless but no intervention is required and the pneumothorax will heal spontaneously. However, if it is a large pneumothorax then the patient will require the insertion of a chest drain (Scales 2008).

Haemorrhage

This results from damage to the vein and/or artery during or following insertion of a CVAD. It is not usually a serious problem unless the carotid artery is punctured (Bodenham and Simcock 2009, Scales 2008). The use of ultrasound can help to reduce the risk of arterial puncture as the artery can be visualized during insertion. It is important to ensure that the patient is not compromised by having a high international normalized ratio (INR) or a low platelet count, or receiving anticoagulant therapy. These should all be corrected prior to CVAD insertion by administration of platelets, administration of vitamin K, stopping medication a few days prior to insertion, or changing the patient from warfarin to subcutaneous low molecular weight heparin, for example fragmin (Bodenham and Simcock 2009, Dougherty 2006). If symptoms are noted at the time of insertion and the artery can be located then pressure should be applied for at least 5 minutes (longer if the patient has a bleeding disorder). Pressure is not always possible as the ability to apply pressure depends on the location of the artery (Bodenham and Simcock 2009). If symptoms are not recognized immediately then the patient may develop a mediastinal haematoma, which can then lead to tracheal compression and respiratory distress and require surgical intervention (Bodenham and Simcock 2009).

Removal of short-term percutaneous central venous catheters (non-tunnelled)

Procedure guideline 18.10 Short-term central venous catheter (non-cuffed/tunnelled): removal

Essential equipment

- Sterile dressing pack (containing gloves)
- Alcohol-based handrub
- Semi-permeable transparent dressing or other appropriate dressing
- Hypoallergenic tape
- Sterile scissors
- Small sterile specimen container
- Stitch cutter
- Additional sterile low-linting gauze swab and sterile transparent dressing

Medicinal products

■ Alcohol-based skin cleaning preparation, for example 2% chlorhexidine in 70% alcohol

Preprocedure

Action	Rationale
1 Explain and discuss the procedure with the patient.	To ensure that the patient understands the procedure and gives their valid consent (NMC 2008b, C).
2 Screen the bed.	To allow dust and airborne organisms to settle before the insertion site and the sterile field are exposed. E

Procedure

Action	Rationale
3 Wash hands with bactericidal soap and water or bactericidal alcohol handrub. Place all equipment required for the dressing on the bottom shelf of a clean dressing trolley.	To reduce the risk of cross-infection (DH 2010, C; Fraise and Bradley 2009, E).
4 Take the trolley to the patient's bedside, disturbing the screens as little as possible.	To minimize airborne contamination (DH 2010, C).
5 Open the sterile dressing pack.	To gain access to sterile field. E
6 Attach an orange clinical waste bag to the side of the trolley below the level of the top shelf.	So that contaminated material is below the level of the sterile field (DH 2010, C).
7 Open the other sterile packs, tipping their contents gently onto the centre of the sterile field. Pour lotions into gallipots or an indented plastic tray where required.	To reduce risk of contamination of contents. E
8 Discontinue the infusion, if in progress, and disconnect the infusion system from the catheter. Clamp the catheter.	To prevent entry of air or leakage of blood when the catheter is disconnected. E
9 Assist the patient into the Trendelenburg position, that is, head slightly lower than feet.	To prevent air entering vein on catheter removal (Drewitt 2009, E).
10 Wash hands with bactericidal alcohol handwash.	To reduce risk of cross contamination (Fraise and Bradley 2009, E).
11 Loosen the old dressing gently.	So that the dressing can be lifted off easily. E
12 Put on clean gloves.	To protect the nurse from any contact with the patient's blood. E
13 Using gloved hands, remove the old dressing and discard it. Remove tapes or securing device.	To remove old dressing without contaminating hands (DH 2010, C).
14 Remove gloves and put on sterile gloves from pack.	To minimize the risk of introducing infection (DH 2010, C; Fraise and Bradley 2009, E).
15 Clean the wound with 2% chlorhexidine in 70% alcohol using back and forth strokes, with friction.	To prevent contamination of the catheter on removal, and a false-positive culture result (DH 2010, C).
16 Cut and remove any skin suture securing the catheter.	To facilitate removal. E
17 Ask the patient to perform the Valsalva manoeuvre.	To reduce the risk of air embolus (Drewett 2009, E).
18 Cover the insertion site with low-linting gauze.	Swabs are used to discourage the entry of organisms into the insertion site and to absorb any leakage of blood. E

(Continued)

1139

Procedure guideline 18.10 *(Continued)*

19 Hold the catheter with one hand near the point of insertion and pull firmly and gently. As the catheter begins to move, press firmly down on the site with the swabs. Maintain pressure on the swabs for about 5 minutes after the catheter has been removed.	Pressure is applied to prevent haemorrhage and to encourage resealing of the vein wall. It also prevents the entry of air into the vein. E Continued pressure is necessary to allow time for the puncture in the vein to close. E
20 Check the tip is intact.	To ensure that all of the catheter has been removed.
21 If the catheter is removed because of infection, carefully cut off the tip (approximately 5 cm) of the catheter using sterile scissors and place it in a sterile container for microbiological investigation.	To detect any infection related to the catheter, and thus provide necessary treatment (DH 2010, C).

Postprocedure

22 When bleeding has stopped (approximately 5 minutes), cover site with a small gauze pad and a transparent dressing.	To detect any infection at exit site. To prevent air entering the vein via the site (Scales 2008, E).
23 Fold up the sterile field, place it in the orange clinical waste bag and seal it before moving the trolley. Dispose of the equipment in the appropriate containers.	To reduce the risk of environmental contamination (DH 2010, C).
24 Make the patient comfortable.	To ensure patient comfort. E
25 Document date and time and reason for removal in patient's notes or care plan.	To ensure adequate records and to enable continued care of device and patient (NMC 2009, C).

Postprocedural considerations

Immediate care

Major vessels usually heal quickly, but direct pressure must be applied to the site to help this process until cessation of bleeding (Dougherty 2006, INS 2011). A sterile transparent occlusive dressing should be applied (Scales 2008, RCN 2010). Patients should remain flat for a short time after catheter removal to maintain positive intrathoracic pressure and allow the tissue tract time to seal (Drewett 2009).

Ongoing care

The site is assessed daily until it has epithelialized (INS 2011), usually within 72 hours (Springhouse 2002). The integrity of the catheter should be ascertained, and the date, time and reason for removal must be documented (NMC 2009, RCN 2010).

Skin-tunnelled catheters

Definition

A skin-tunnelled catheter is a long-term catheter that lies in a subcutaneous tunnel before entering a central vein (usu-

ally subclavian) (Hadaway 2010). The tunnel commonly exits between the sternum and the nipple. The tip lies at the junction of the SVC and right atrium or within the lower portion of the SVC or the upper right atrium (Dougherty 2006, Galloway and Bodenham 2004) (see Figure 18.26).

Evidence-based approaches

Rationale

Tunnelled silicone catheters were first described by Broviac in Seattle in 1973 and were modified by Hickman and his colleagues, who created a larger lumen of 1.6 mm internal diameter (Bjeletich and Hickman 1980). The special features added included an inert antithrombogenic flexible material and a subcutaneous Dacron cuff attached to the catheter (Ives 2009). The cuff has two functions – to secure the catheter and prevent infection.

Indications

A skin-tunnelled catheter is used when long-term venous access is required or if peripheral vascular access is problematic (Dougherty 2006).

Contraindications

As for other CVADs.

Figure 18.26 Tunnelled catheter. (a) Anatomical positioning of tunnelled catheter. (b) Patient with tunnelled catheter *in situ*.

Methods of insertion

The insertion of a skin-tunnelled catheter is a surgical procedure usually carried out in an operating theatre or designated area, under aseptic conditions, using fluoroscopy and monitoring of the patient by pulse oximetry and electrocardiogram (ECG) to detect arrhythmias (Benton and Marsden 2002, Dougherty 2006, Galloway and Bodenham 2004, Weinstein and Plumer 2007). The procedure is now also performed by nurse specialists at the bedside and within radiology departments (Benton and Marsden 2002, Boland *et al.* 2003, Fitzsimmons *et al.* 1997, Hamilton *et al.* 1995). The procedure is usually performed under sedation along with the use of local anaesthesia (Dougherty 2006). In some patients, for example children, this procedure would be carried out under general anaesthesia.

The aim of the insertion is to place the catheter tip in the right atrium via the subclavian vein and SVC (Galloway and

Bodenham 2004). When there is an SVC obstruction from thrombosis or compression, the femoral vein can be used to access the inferior vena cava. Selection of vessels is as for non-tunnelled CVC. Access may be gained percutaneously using a needle and guidewire or via an open surgical cutdown procedure.

The catheter can be inserted percutaneously when the venepuncture site is made near the subclavian or internal jugular. The tunnelling rod is then passed under the skin and exits at a predetermined point on the chest. The catheter is then attached to the tunnelling rod and drawn through the subcutaneous tunnel. The catheter is then passed into the vein via a peel-away sheath introducer (Davidson and Al Mufti 1997, Galloway and Bodenham 2004, Hadaway 2010). Position is confirmed by the easy aspiration of blood from each lumen and these are then flushed with heparin until correct tip placement has been confirmed. A chest X-ray should be performed after insertion to check for correct placement and pneumothorax (Davidson and Al Mufti 1997, Stacey *et al.* 1991).

Methods for removal

Removal techniques for skin-tunnelled catheters vary. Removal should only be performed by specially trained nurses or doctors. It is recommended that the patient is placed supine and that aseptic technique is used throughout. There are two methods for removal.

Surgical excision

This method involves locating the cuff and performing a minor surgical excision under local anaesthetic. A small incision is made over the site of the cuff and blunt dissection, that is, using forceps, is carried out to prise the tissues apart (Galloway and Bodenham 2004); this causes less damage to the tissues than using a scalpel. The cuff and the catheter are freed from the surrounding fibrous tissue (Dougherty 2006). The proximal section of the catheter is then removed, cut and then the distal end is removed via the exit site. Once the catheter has been removed, the wound is sutured using interrupted sutures, which can be removed after 7 days (Drewett 2009, Galloway and Bodenham 2004).

Traction method

With the traction method, there is a greater risk of the catheter breaking, which could result in a catheter embolism.

The catheter is gripped firmly and constant traction applied until the cuff is loosened in the tunnel (Hayden and Goodman 2005). It may take a few minutes for the catheter and cuff to become loose before sliding free. Constant steady pressure will remove the complete catheter; however, the catheter should be checked on removal to ensure it is complete as breakage and splitting can occur (Hayden and Goodman 2005, INS 2011). The catheter and cuff may be pulled through, but the cuff may remain attached to tissue. This is thought to be of no significance and may be left in place, although some suggest that if the cuff is not removed it could become infected later (Drewett 2000, Galloway and Bodenham 2004). Difficulty with removal or a break in the catheter will require surgical intervention.

Legal and professional issues

Nurses who wish to undertake this role must receive additional training in theory and practical hands-on instruction at the bedside in the removal technique and suturing (Bullock-Corkhill 2010). Competencies would include knowledge in use of local anaesthetic, making an incision/use of scalpel, suturing, and prevention and management of complications.

Preprocedural considerations
Equipment

Polyurethane or silicone skin-tunnelled catheters are available as single-, double- or triple-lumen with a Dacron cuff. The cuff is used to secure the catheter as fibrous tissue grows around it and obliterates part of the subcutaneous tunnel within 1–2 weeks of insertion. It also impedes the migration of micro-organisms, creating a 'barrier' along the subcutaneous tract and therefore reducing the incidence of catheter-related infection (Dougherty 2006, Springhouse 2002, Weinstein and Plumer 2007, Wilson 2006). The cuff is about 1 cm wide (Hadaway 2010) and is usually located about 3–5 cm from the exit site (Stacey *et al.* 1991, Weinstein and Plumer 2007). Knowledge of the distance of the cuff from the bifurcation may assist the practitioner in locating the cuff during removal of the catheter, although it will vary according to the brand of catheter.

The tip of the catheter may be open-ended or closed with a slit valve (Dougherty 2006, Ives 2009). The disadvantage of an open-ended catheter is the problem of blood reflux, resulting in occlusion. Catheters such as the Groshong catheter have a round closed tip which incorporates a two-way valve that remains closed at normal vena caval pressure. Application of a vacuum in order to withdraw blood enables the valve to open inwards; positive pressure into the catheter forces the valve to open outwards (Figure 18.27) (Dougherty 2006). The advantages of valved

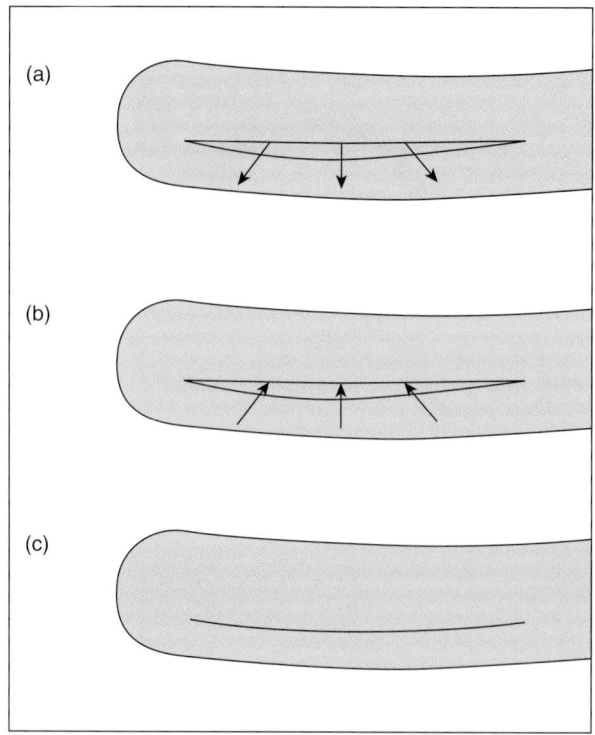

Figure 18.27 Groshong two-way valve catheter. (a) Infusion (positive pressure). (b) Aspiration (negative pressure). (c) Closed (neutral pressure). (Groshong is a registered trademark of CR Bard, Inc. or an affiliate.)

catheters are the reduced risk of bleeding or air emboli on insertion and during subsequent care; the elimination of catheter clamping; and the elimination of the need for heparin along with a reduction in the frequency of flushing (Hoffer *et al.* 1999, Inwood 1999, Weinstein and Plumer 2007). However, if a thrombus forms around the tip, it can result in malfunction and loss of valve competence (Dougherty 2006).

Another type of catheter is the pressure-activated safety valve (PASV). The valve opens with minimal positive pressure for infusion but requires four times as much negative pressure for aspiration (Weinstein and Plumer 2007). This feature reduces the risk of air embolism or bleeding resulting from accidental disconnection (Ives 2009). The valve is incorporated within the hub and not the tip and reduces the risk of reflux even during periods of raised CVP (Weinstein and Plumer 2007).

Procedure guideline 18.11 Central venous catheter (skin-tunnelled): surgical removal

Essential equipment

- Plastic apron
- Sterile gloves
- Minor operations set
- 10 mL Luer-Lok syringe
- 25 G needle
- 21 G needle

- 10 × 10 cm low-linting gauze swabs × 5
- 3/0 Mersilk suture on a curved needle
- Transparent dressing

Optional equipment

- Steristrips (to be used if necessary)
- Specimen container

Medicinal products

- 10 mL plain lidocaine 1%
- Chlorhexidine 2% in 70% alcohol

Preprocedure

Action	Rationale
1 Check the patient's full blood count and clotting profile for that day.	To ensure that the patient is not at risk of bleeding or infection from this invasive procedure. The platelets should be above 100×10^9/L, the white blood count >2 and the INR <1.3 (Dougherty 2006, E). In haematology patients the platelets should be >50 and the INR <1.5.
2 Explain and discuss the procedure with the patient.	To ensure that the patient understands the procedure and gives their valid consent (NMC 2008b, C).
3 Screen the bed and ask patient to remove clothing down to the waist.	To ensure ease of access to the patient's chest. E
4 Ask patient to lie as flat as possible with their arms by their sides.	To minimize the risk of bleeding from gravitational pressure and to dissuade the patient from touching the sterile field (Dougherty 2006, E).

Procedure

5 Palpate and identify the position of the cuff in the patient. This can be done by gently pulling on the catheter and observing for skin pucker.	To locate the area for the incision (Drewett 2009, E; Galloway and Bodenham 2004, E).
6 If the cuff cannot easily be felt, measure up from the bifurcation or hub at the end of the catheter distal to the patient, dependent on the type of catheter *in situ*, then palpate again. If it still cannot be felt, ask for assistance from a more experienced colleague.	The cuff will be positioned differently depending on the type of catheter. To locate the probable site of the cuff. To guard against malplaced incisions (Dougherty 2006, E).
7 Open the outer bag of the minor operation pack.	To gain access to contents. E
8 Put on plastic apron and wash hands, then dry hands on sterile towel provided in the pack.	To reduce risk of infection (DH 2010, C; Fraise and Bradley 2009, E).
9 Put on sterile gloves and assemble all necessary equipment on the sterile pack.	To maintain asepsis and to prepare for the procedure and maximize efficiency (DH 2010, C).
10 Advise the patient that you will explain each step of the procedure as you go along if the patient wishes.	This should take into account the patient's individual wish for information. E

(Continued)

Procedure guideline 18.11 (*Continued*)

11 Clean the area directly over the cuff with 2% chlorhexidine in 70% alcohol, using back and forth strokes, working out from the centre directly over the cuff. Allow the area to dry.	To reduce the risk of infection. To enable disinfection process to be completed. To prevent stinging on insertion of the needle (Dougherty 2006, E).
12 Apply a fenestrated drape.	To create a sterile field to operate within and therefore reduce the risk of infection (Dougherty 2006, E).
13 Inform the patient that you are about to administer the local anaesthetic and that this will cause a stinging sensation.	To prepare the patient. The first injection can be painful and causes a stinging sensation (BNF 2011, C, P).
14 With a 25 G needle, administer the first millilitre of local anaesthetic intradermally directly over the cuff site, causing a raised bleb.	To commence the numbing of the area to be incised. To provide a raised area for the next injection and identification of the site (Macklin and Chernecky 2004, E).
15 Give a further 1–2 mL of local anaesthetic subcutaneously, using the bleb as the area for the insertion of the needle, but directing the needle out and around the area of the cuff site.	To reduce pain for the patient with repeated injections. To ensure all the incision area is numb (Macklin and Chernecky 2004, E).
16 Attach the 21 G needle and with the last remaining 4 mL of local anaesthetic, give two deeper injections to either side of the cuff area.	To ensure anaesthesia at a deeper level during the blunt dissection around the cuff (Macklin and Chernecky 2004, E).
17 Test the area above the cuff for numbness and then make the incision over the cuff site (but slightly to the side of the cuff site in very thin patients). The incision should be longitudinal and about 2 cm in length. Ensure that the incision is through the epidermis and dermis.	To ensure that the patient will not experience any pain. To facilitate identification and removal of the cuff. To allow access to the cuff which is situated below the dermis. To reduce the risk of cutting through the cuff before the cuff has been identified (Dougherty 2006, E; Drewett 2009, E).
18 With one pair of the small artery forceps, commence blunt dissection of tissue from around the cuff. At intervals, place your finger into the site and feel the cuff.	To free the cuff from the surrounding fibrous tissue. To assess the mobility of the cuff. To reduce the risk of bleeding and damage of catheter (Dougherty 2006, E; Drewett 2009, E).
19 Continue with blunt dissection around and under the cuff until it feels mobile.	To facilitate the loosening of the cuff (Dougherty 2006, E).
20 With one pair of artery forceps or the dissecting hook, loop under the cuff and lift it up out of the incision.	To identify the catheter to allow removal (Dougherty 2006, E).
21 Once the cuff is free, still maintaining a grip on the cuff, gently and carefully peel away the thin straw-coloured tissue from the catheter with the blade, ensuring the blade is pulled away from the catheter.	To free the catheter from the anchoring fibrous bands to enable removal. To reduce the risk of accidental incision of the catheter (Dougherty 2006, E).
22 As the last strands of fibre are separated, you should feel the catheter becoming free and you should be able to see the white material of the catheter.	To ensure that you have completely freed the catheter for removal (Dougherty 2006, E).
23 Ask the patient to perform the Valsalva as the proximal portion of the catheter is withdrawn from the vein and apply gentle pressure at the vein exit site.	To remove the catheter and prevent bleeding or air entry (Drewett 2009, E).
24 Remove the distal portion and cut through the catheter using a blade or scissors and remove via the skin exit site.	To remove the distal half of the catheter below the cuff (Dougherty 2006, E).

25	If the catheter is removed because of infection, carefully cut off the tip (approximately 5 cm) of the catheter using sterile scissors and place it in a sterile container for microbiological investigation.	To detect any infection related to the catheter and thus provide necessary treatment (DH 2010, C).
26	Close the incision with three sutures. Commence the first suture in the middle of the incision, with the remaining sutures evenly on either side.	To close the incision efficiently. To ensure that the skin edges and insert are brought together in alignment (Dougherty 2006, E).
27	If there continues to be any bleeding, Steristrips can be applied across the incision over the sutures.	To minimize blood loss (Dougherty 2006, E).
28	It is not usually necessary to suture the exit site.	To leave the exit site to granulate without a suture (Drewett 2009, E).

Postprocedure

29	Apply a small pressure dressing and cover with an airtight dressing.	To absorb any slight bleed and to maintain a clean site (Scales 2008, E).
30	Advise patient that there might be some oozing and to reapply a dry dressing after 24 hours and thereafter once a day until the sutures are removed. Advise the patient that the sutures should be removed in 7 days.	To ensure that the incision has fully closed and healed (Dougherty 2006, E; Drewett 2009, E).
31	Dispose of the equipment in the appropriate containers.	To reduce the risk of environmental contamination (DH 2010, C).
32	Ask the patient to rest on the bed for the next 30–60 minutes, or longer if required, especially patients who are prone to bleeding.	To reduce the risk of bleeding and air embolism as the patient sits or gets up (Dougherty 2006, E).
33	Liaise with the nursing team and document the date, time and reason for removal and any problems in the nursing and medical notes.	To ensure there is good communication between all teams and a written record of the procedure (NMC 2009, C).

Problem-solving table 18.5 Prevention and resolution (Procedure guideline 18.11)

Problem	Cause	Prevention	Action
Unable to locate cuff	Cuff too deep Lack of knowledge of cuff location	Knowledge of all types of catheters and where cuff located as measurement	Contact the catheter manu-facturer for cuff details
Bleeding at site	Low platelets or raised INR Small vessels cut	Not undertaking procedure unless levels are corrected	Apply pressure to site until bleeding stops. May need vessel to be tied off
Cut through catheter/catheter breaks	Removing catheter by traction Incision made too deeply directly over cuff	Only remove catheter by us-ing surgical technique Make incision to side of cuff	Attempt to clamp any remaining catheter with artery forceps Contact surgical team for assistance

Postprocedural considerations

Immediate care

Following insertion

The dressing should be left intact and changed 24 hours after insertion.

Following removal

Since the vein closes following removal of the catheter, there is usually no bleeding. However, there may be slight bleeding at the exit site immediately after removal because of the passage of the cuff.

Following either removal method, pressure should be applied to the site until the bleeding stops, and a dressing may be required for up to 24 hours. The patient should be encouraged to rest flat for 30–60 minutes to allow the tissue tract time to seal (Galloway and Bodenham 2004).

Ongoing care

Following insertion

Healing of the skin tunnel takes approximately 7 days, so at this time the sutures at the entry site may be removed (Dougherty 2006). The exit site sutures should be retained until the fibroblastic response to the Dacron cuff is adequate to secure the catheter, usually in 2–3 weeks (Perucca 2010, Stacey *et al.* 1991, Weinstein and Plumer 2007). A transparent dressing should cover the site and be changed weekly until removal of sutures. Thereafter, a dressing is not usually required unless the patient requests one (Dougherty 2006).

Following removal

Sutures at the incision site should be removed after 7 days (Dougherty 2006).

Education of patient and relevant others

See Discharging patients home with a VAD *in situ*.

Complications

Infection and thrombosis are the main complications – see PICC, Complications.

1146

Implanted ports

Definition

An implanted port is a totally implanted VAD made of two components: a reservoir with a self-sealing septum which is attached to a silicone catheter (Figure 18.28). The port is usually inserted on either the chest or the arm but it can be placed on the lower chest wall/abdomen or thigh, depend-

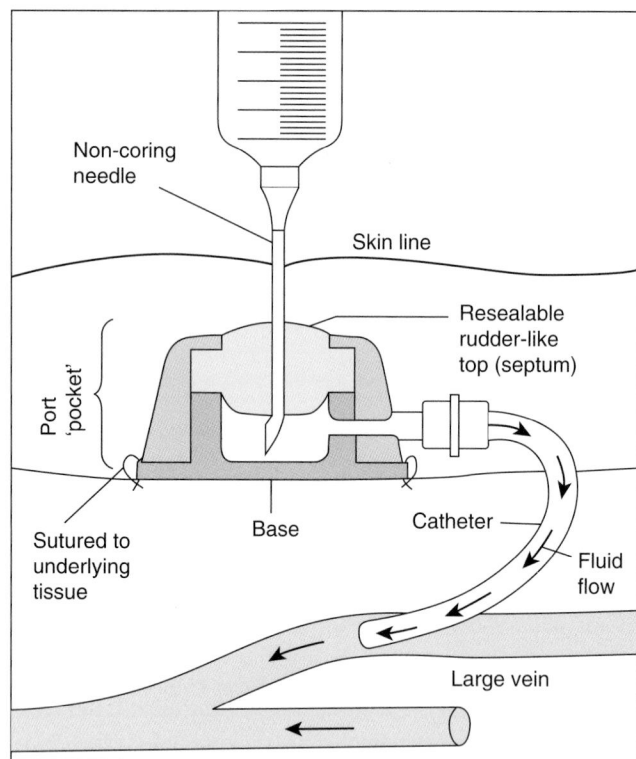

Figure 18.28 Implantable port cross-section, accessed with non-coring needle.

ing on patient needs. It is accessed using a special non-coring needle (Dougherty 2006, Hayden and Goodman 2005, Weinstein and Plumer 2007).

Evidence-based approaches

Rationale

Ports are implanted subcutaneously to provide repeated long-term access (Weinstein and Plumer 2007) to the vascular system (other ports include arterial, epidural and peritoneal ports). Implanted ports require little care of the site because of the intact skin layer over the accessible port, except when accessed. When not in use, the only care required is a monthly flush (Weinstein and Plumer 2007). Other benefits include a reduced risk of infection (Bow *et al.* 1999, Mirro *et al.* 1989, Moureau *et al.* 1999) and less interference with daily activities such as bathing or swimming (Hayden and Goodman 2005), and body image is less threatened than by the presence of an external catheter (Bow *et al.* 1999, Mirro *et al.* 1989). Patients with ports are often very satisfied with their access devices (Chernecky 2001, Johannson *et al.* 2009).

Disadvantages of the port include discomfort when accessing is performed (particularly if placed deeply or in a difficult area to access). This can be overcome with the use of topical local anaesthetic. However, the tissue over the septum becomes calloused or scarred and over time there is loss of sensitivity (Hadaway 2010, Moureau *et al.* 1999). Needle dislodgement with resulting extravasation and needlestick injury are well-documented problems associated with ports (Viale 2003, Nesti and Kovac 2000, Schulmeister and Camp-Sorrell 2000). There are also issues related to occlusion and 'sludge' build-up and newer designs are attempting to reduce this (Stevens *et al.* 2000). Finally there are often problems with obtaining blood return (Moureau *et al.* 1999).

Indications

An implanted port can be used for long-term venous access for all types of therapies, both continuous and intermittent, and if patients have problematic venous access (Dougherty 2006, Springhouse 2002).

Contraindications

Contraindications would be related to location of port, for example not on the chest if there has been bilateral mastectomy or radiation burns, or ability to undergo a general anaesthetic for insertion.

Methods of insertion

Implantation is a surgical procedure usually carried out under general anaesthetic. Some catheters are pre-attached to the reservoir whilst others require attachment on insertion (Dougherty 2006, Hayden and Goodman 2005). The most common veins used are the subclavian, internal jugular and femoral. Ports can also be inserted in the veins of the upper arm (Hadaway 2010, Hayden and Goodman 2005, Weinstein and Plumer 2007).

The catheter is introduced into the SVC via the subclavian or jugular vein and fluoroscopy verifies the placement of the tip. The catheter is then tunnelled to the pocket (Dougherty 2006, Springhouse 2002). The pocket is made just under the skin, usually on a bony prominence for stabilization (Springhouse 2002). The port is then sutured into place to the underlying fascia. The suture line can be lateral, medial, superior or inferior to the port septum to remove it from the area where the port will be accessed because repeated access could cause stress to the suture line (Dougherty 2006, Weinstein and Plumer 2007). The area is tender and oedematous for up to a week following implantation and any manipulation/accessing may be painful. When immediate use is indicated, the port should be accessed and dressed in theatre (Hayden and Goodman 2005).

Legal and professional issues

Although some nurses insert ports (Hadaway 2010), many are responsible for accessing and de-accessing the ports. It is vital that the needle is placed in the port as if it is not then there is a risk of the medications extravasating or infiltrating. Therefore any nurse who wishes to access ports must

Figure 18.29 Implanted ports.

undergo specific training to gain the necessary knowledge and skills to select the correct type and length of needle and access the port successfully with little patient discomfort.

Preprocedural considerations
Equipment

A variety of ports are available and choice is dependent on a number of factors; for example, whether the patient is a child or an adult, the amount of access required and where it is located (Dougherty 2006). Ports are usually single lumen, although double-lumen ports are available (Dougherty 2006). However, double-lumen ports have two septums and therefore require needle access into each septum (Hayden and Goodman 2005). Port reservoirs (Figure 18.29) are about 2.5 cm in height and 0.625 cm in diameter and can weigh from 21 to 28 g; low-profile ports are smaller and often placed in the arm (Ives 2009). Entry can be gained via the side or top but most are accessed by top entry (Hayden and Goodman 2005, Weinstein and Plumer 2007). Catheters are made of silicone and may be open-ended or have a Groshong valve (Biffi *et al.* 2001). The portal body may be made of stainless steel, plastic or titanium, although steel is not often used now as it interferes with electromagnetic imaging procedures and is quite heavy in comparison with other materials (Dougherty 2006). The self-sealing silicone septum can be accessed approximately 2000 times (regular size) (small ports may take only 750), often dependent upon the size of the needle used (Hadaway 2010, Hayden and Goodman 2005).

Non-coring needles have the penetration of a knife so when the needle is removed, the septum closes behind it (Hadaway 2010) (Figure 18.30). The bevel opens on the side of the needle instead of the end (Gabriel 2008, Weinstein and Plumer 2007). They are available in straight or 90° angle configuration with or without extension sets. The needle is available with a metal or plastic hub in gauges 19–24 and lengths from 0.65 to 2.5 cm. Needle gauge is

Figure 18.30 Non-coring needles have the penetration of a knife so when the needle is removed, the septum closes behind it.

selected dependent on type and rate of infusate as well as the location of the port (Dougherty 2006, Weinstein and Plumer 2007). Safety needles are also now available and activate on withdrawal from the port.

Pharmacological support

Prior to accessing a port, topical local anaesthetic may be used over the site (Gorski *et al.* 2010). Whilst the port is accessed, it is usual to flush it with 0.9% sodium chloride and heparinized saline 50 IU in 5 mL but once the needle is due to be removed, a higher strength of heparin is recommended – 100 IU heparin per mL to a total of 5 mL (500 IU).

Procedure guideline 18.12 Implanted ports: insertion and removal of non-coring needles

Essential equipment

- Plastic apron
- Dressing pack (containing sterile gloves)
- 10 mL syringes containing 0.9% sodium chloride × 2
- Non-coring (Huber point) needle with extension set
- Plaster

Optional equipment

- Transparent dressing if needle remaining *in situ*

Medicinal products

- Heparinized saline in 10 mL syringe
- 2% chlorhexidine in 70% alcohol

Preprocedure

Action	Rationale
1 Explain and discuss the procedure with the patient.	To ensure the patient understands the procedure and gives their valid consent (NMC 2008b, C).
2 If required, apply topical local anaesthetic cream for 30–60 minutes.	To reduce the feeling of pain on insertion of the needle. E
3 Place the patient in a comfortable position.	To aid patient comfort and to gain access to port. E
4 Locate the port and identify the septum; assess the depth of the port and thickness of the skin.	In order to select correct length of needle (Dougherty 2006, E).
5 Check length and type of therapy.	In order to select correct gauge and configuration of needle (Camp-Sorrell *et al.* 2004, C; Dougherty 2006, E).

Procedure

6 Wash hands using a bactericidal hand soap.	To minimize the risk of contamination (DH 2010, C).
7 Put on sterile gloves.	To minimize the risk of contamination (DH 2010, C).
8 Flush port needle and extension set with 0.9% sodium chloride.	To check patency of needle and set (Dougherty 2006, E).
9 Clean the skin over the port with 2% chlorhexidine in 70% alcohol using back and forth strokes. Allow to dry.	To minimize the risk of contamination and destroy skin flora (DH 2010, C). To ensure disinfection (DH 2010, C).

10	Holding the needle in the dominant hand, stabilize the port between the forefinger and index finger of the non-dominant hand (see Action Figure 10).	To ensure the port is stabilized and will not move on insertion of the needle (Dougherty 2006, E).
11	Inform the patient you are about to insert the needle.	To prepare the patient for a pushing sensation. P, E
12	Using a perpendicular angle, push the needle through the skin until the needle hits the back plate.	To ensure the needle is well inserted into the portal septum. E
13	Draw back on the syringe and check for blood return.	To check the needle is correctly placed and the port is patent (Camp-Sorrell *et al.* 2004, C; Dougherty 2006, E).
14	Flush with 0.9% sodium chloride and observe the site for any swelling or pain.	To check for patency and correct positioning (Camp-Sorrell *et al.* 2004, C; Dougherty 2006, E).
15	Administer the drug as required.	To carry out instructions as per prescription. E
16	Flush with 10 mL 0.9% sodium chloride.	To ensure all of the drug is administered (RCN 2010, C).
17	If the needle is to remain *in situ*, attach a needlefree injection cap and flush with heparinized saline using a pulsatile flush and ending with positive pressure.	To maintain patency (Camp-Sorrell *et al.* 2004, C; Dougherty 2006, E).
18	Secure the needle by placing gauze under the needle (if necessary) and cover with transparent dressing.	To ensure the needle is well supported and will not become dislodged (Camp-Sorrell *et al.* 2004, C; Dougherty 2006, E).
19	If the needle is to be removed, then heparinize using 500 IU heparin in 5 mL 0.9% sodium chloride.	To maintain patency over a longer period of time, for example 1 month (Camp-Sorrell *et al.* 2004, C; Dougherty 2006, E).
20	Maintain pressure on the plunger as syringe is disconnected from injection cap.	To prevent backflow of blood and possible clot formation (Camp-Sorrell *et al.* 2004, C; Dougherty 2006, E).
21	Press down on either side of the portal of the implanted port with two fingers.	To support the port while removing the needle (P; Camp-Sorrell *et al.* 2004, C; Dougherty 2006, E).
22	Withdraw the needle using steady traction and activate safety device where appropriate. Discard needle in appropriate sharps container.	To prevent trauma to the skin and the risk of needlestick injury (NHS Employers 2007, C).

Postprocedure

23	No dressing is usually required, but a small plaster may be applied.	To prevent oozing at the site. E
24	Document date of access, size and length of needle and number of attempts in patient's notes or care plan.	To ensure adequate records and to enable continued care of device and patient (NMC 2009, C).

(Continued)

Procedure guideline 18.12 (*Continued*)

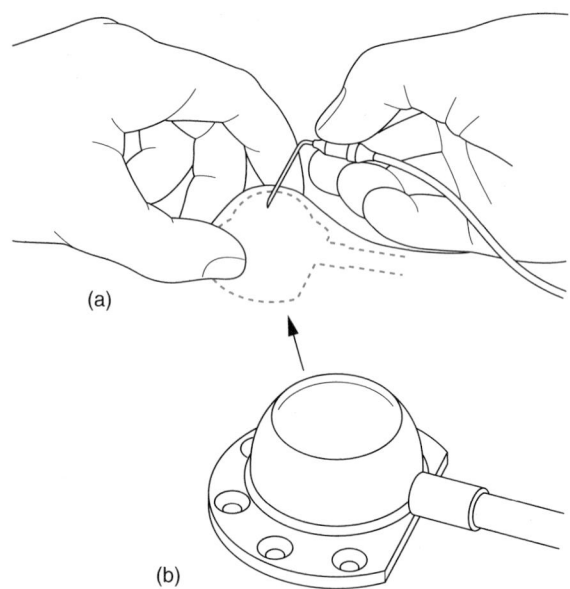

(a)

(b)

Action Figure 10 Flushing a port.

Problem-solving table 18.6 Prevention and resolution (Procedure guideline 18.12)

Problem	Cause	Prevention	Action
Unable to access port	Incorrect selection of length of needle	Choice of correct length needle	Ask for assistance from a colleague to locate port and help to stabilize it
	Port too deep or mobile	Skilled practitioners should access difficult ports	
	Unable to locate port		
Unable to withdraw blood	Needle not in port		Realign needle or remove and ask colleague to access port
	Fibrin sheath		Instil urokinase to remove fibrin

Postprocedural considerations

Immediate care

Once accessed

The needle should be supported with gauze (if necessary) and covered with a transparent dressing to minimize the risk of needle dislodgement.

Ongoing care

Regular assessment of the port when accessed is essential to check for signs of erythema, swelling or discomfort, which could indicate infection, infiltration or extravasation (INS 2011, Springhouse 2002). Most manufacturers recommend that only syringes 10 mL or larger should be used for drug administration or when flushing, to prevent excessive pressure which could result in separation of the catheter from

the reservoir or rupture if the catheter is occluded (Conn 1993). When the port is accessed, the needle can remain *in situ* for 7 days (Dougherty 2006, Gorski *et al.* 2010, Springhouse 2002). When not in use, the port only requires flushing once a month with a concentrated solution of heparin (100 IU in 1 mL), usually a total of 5–6 mL (Gorski *et al.* 2010, Springhouse 2002, Weinstein and Plumer 2007).

Removal

Implanted ports may be surgically removed and after removal the site must be assessed for any signs of inflammation (Galloway and Bodenham 2004).

Education of patient and relevant others

Patients can be taught to access their own ports. See Discharging patients home with a VAD *in situ*.

Complications

As for all other CVADS.

Twiddler's syndrome

This term is used to describe patients who nervously touch and potentially dislodge their ports by turning them over so the septum cannot be accessed (Gorski *et al.* 2010). If this occurs then it may need to be turned back surgically. Explain to patients who 'twiddle' their ports why it can result in problems.

Arterial cannulas

Definition

An arterial cannula is a plastic tube inserted and secured in a peripheral or central artery. When the cannula is electronically transduced, arterial waveforms can be observed in conjunction with continuous blood pressure readings. An arterial cannula is generally inserted into a peripheral artery, most commonly the radial or dorsalis pedis.

Anatomy and physiology

Arteries are elastic and muscular blood vessels which carry oxygenated blood from the left side of the heart. The large pressure generated by the heart and resistance in the arteries ensure that organs and tissues receive highly oxygenated blood (Scales 2008).

The radial artery originates from the brachial artery at the neck of the radius and passes along the lateral aspect of the forearm (Drake *et al.* 2005). The radial artery gives off multiple fasciocutaneous perforators until it reaches the wrist, where it forms the deep palmar arch. The radial artery contributes to the main artery of the thumb and index finger (Wallach 2004). The radial pulse can be felt by gently palpating the radial artery against the underlying muscle and bone (Drake *et al.* 2005).

Related theory

Pulsus paradoxus is a term used when the difference in peak systolic pressure between inspiration and expiration is greater than 10 mmHg. This accentuates the normal pattern and an exaggerated swing in systolic pressure is seen on the monitor. This is caused by:

- pericardial disease, for example cardiac tamponade causing impeded ventricular filling
- exaggerated inspiration by the patient
- changes in intrathoracic pressure, caused by lung pathology, such as asthma
- hypovolaemia, particularly when the patient has concurrent high airway pressures.

If the arterial device is inserted under emergency conditions and asepsis has been compromised, the Communicable Diseases Centre (O'Grady *et al.* 2002) recommends that the cannula should be replaced within 24 hours. Colonization and infection of arterial devices are rare (Minnaganti and Cunha 2000) and are usually related to duration of cannulation.

Data suggest that arterial cannulas may be associated with a substantially lower risk of local cannula-related infection when compared to short-term peripheral venous cannulas which have been left *in situ* for the equivalent length of time (RCN 2010). There is a common risk of catheter colonization but serious soft tissue infection is very rare, which may be related to exposure to high vascular pressures and subsequent local turbulence experienced in arterial cannulas (O'Grady *et al.* 2002). Additionally, if the puncture site is well stabilized and treated with asepsis and all samples are obtained using aseptic technique, this will further minimize the risk of soft tissue infection (Marini and Wheeler 2010). There is also no evidence suggesting any difference in infection rates between femoral or peripheral arterial cannulation (O'Grady *et al.* 2002). However, regular observation of the arterial cannula insertion site is imperative for signs of inflammation which may predispose patients to cannula-related infection. Cannulation for more than 4 days also increases this risk (O'Grady *et al.* 2002).

Evidence-based approaches

Rationale

It is worth noting that morbidity associated with arterial cannulation is less than that associated with five or more arterial punctures (Bersten *et al.* 2009). An arterial puncture describes a one-off insertion of a needle attached to an appropriately heparinized syringe enabling the aspiration of blood from the artery for analysis. Arterial punctures are important and useful in the initial and short-term assessment of acid/base balance and respiratory function. However, multiple puncture attempts will increase the risk of injury, not only due to the direct trauma but also associated with vasospasm (Lipsitz 2004). If the patient requires repetitive blood sampling, it may be more appropriate to admit the patient into a more clinically suitable area where arterial cannulation is possible. This not only minimizes both the distress to the patient and time taken by skilled personnel in obtaining each sample, but reduces the risks associated with multiple punctures.

An arterial cannula provides an invaluable tool in providing continuous monitoring of systemic blood pressure and facilitates frequent arterial blood gas (ABG) and laboratory sampling. Arterial cannulation is most commonly achieved and maintained in the critical care and theatre setting (Mignini *et al.* 2006). Ideally, prior to obtaining any arterial blood gas sample, the patient should be in a respiratory steady state for 15–20 minutes. The oxygen should not be titrated, and if ventilated, suction should not be attempted and ventilation parameters not adjusted (Weinstein and Plumer 2007).

The arterial device is attached to a transducer that enables the mechanical energy of the arterial pressure to be transformed into an electrical signal. This is displayed as a waveform by a haemodynamic monitoring system. An amplifier enhances the signal, which is converted into a digital display and oscilloscope trace (Hazinski 1992). Arterial device tubing should be stiff with low compliance as this prevents the loss of pressure signals through tube expansion, and it must not exceed 120 cm in length because this may alter pressure readings (Daily and Schroeder 1994).

The arterial waveform has three separate components that reflect the cardiac cycle.

1 The upstroke: the positive deflection occurs at the peak of systole.
2 The dicrotic notch occurs with aortic valve closure and reflects the beginning of diastole.
3 The lowest point of the waveform is end-diastole.

Indications

- During and following major anaesthesia.
- Monitoring of acid/base balance and respiratory status in (Adam and Osborne 2005):
  - acute respiratory failure
  - mechanical ventilation, especially in response to alteration of support and oxygenation
  - the period during and after cardiorespiratory arrest
  - severe sepsis
  - shock conditions
  - major trauma
  - acute poisoning
  - acute renal failure
  - severe diabetic ketoacidosis
  - critically ill patients.

Contraindications

- Previous upper extremity surgery (harvested for pedicled/free flaps).
- Previous axillary clearance.
- Peripheral vascular disease.
- Raynaud's disease.
- Diabetes.
- Collagen vascular disease.
- Active upper or lower limb infection.

Principles of care

In critical care, continuous arterial monitoring is invaluable in optimizing and evaluating treatments, particularly in patients receiving intravenous nitrates and inotropes where their effects on mean blood pressure (MBP) can be instantaneous, necessitating appropriate titration (Mignini *et al.*

2006). Arterial devices must be cared for, managed and interpreted by skilled personnel who are able to regularly assess areas distal to the cannula, identify accurate waveforms, distinguish artefact, troubleshoot complications and maintain safe practice. The hazard of disconnection, the necessary monitoring systems, the potential consequence of severe haemorrhage and risks associated with accidental intra-arterial drug administration limit their use outside specialized areas.

Routes of cannulation
Radial arterial cannulation

Cannulation of the radial artery is the most common placement of arterial cannulas (Mignini *et al.* 2006) and is performed in most acute care settings (Box 18.8). The hand has a good collateral blood supply, as the radial artery is near the skin surface, it is readily accessible, easily secured, and the patient is disturbed less (Adam and Osborne 2005, Wallach 2004). However, radial cannulation is not without risk (Wallach 2004); there is an estimated 0.2% risk of serious complications associated with the procedure. In response to these risks, cannulation of the non-dominant hand should be attempted whenever possible (Wallach 2004). Ideally, the cannula should not be positioned close to any intravenous cannula as this may compromise blood flow around the adjoining structures.

Dorsalis pedis cannulation

The dorsalis pedis route for arterial cannulation is, according to Durbin (1995), equally as risky as radial cannulation, and more technically difficult, but provides a safe and easily available alternative when radial arteries are not appropriate.

Blood pressure measured from the dorsalis pedis and radial artery typically have a higher systolic and lower diastolic than centrally measured blood pressure, although the

---

Box 18.8 Complications of arterial cannulation

- Vascular thrombosis.
- Distal embolization (see Box 18.10).
- Proximal embolization: digital ischaemia.
- Local/systemic infection.
- Vascular spasm.
- Skin necrosis of catheter site due to accidental intra-arterial injection.
- Hypovolaemia secondary to accidental disconnection.
- Cannula fracture/breakage.
- Pseudo-aneurysm formation.
- Median nerve palsy (Bersten *et al.* 2009).
- Damage to nearby structures.

mean blood pressure is identical and clinically interchangeable (Mignini *et al.* 2006); this is described as distal pulse amplification (Dorman *et al.* 1998).

Femoral artery cannulation

The femoral artery may be cannulated if it is not possible to cannulate a peripheral artery, particularly if the patient is haemodynamically compromised. The femoral artery is accessible and there is relative ease in palpating even a weak pulse (Adam and Osborne 2005). If a patient has a femoral catheter in place and needs to be positioned at a 45° angle, there is an increased risk of catheter fracture (Ho *et al.* 2003). This is particularly serious as there is no collateral blood supply to the leg and lower limb, and as such fracture may have long-term consequences for the patient.

Brachial cannulation

The brachial artery is the major artery of the arm and divides into the radial and ulnar branches and should be avoided as a site for inserting an arterial cannula. A cannula inserted at the antecubital fossa into the brachial artery may risk cannula fracture in the conscious patient and its placement may inconvenience the patient because they have to minimize arm flexion.

Legal and professional issues

In 2008 the National Patient Safety Agency (NPSA) published a rapid response report which highlighted the many potential errors associated with the use of arterial cannulas. Various recommendations were given and immediate actions had to be in place by January 2009 (www.npsa.nhs.uk/patientsafety/alerts-and-directives/rapidrr/) (Box 18.9).

In order to minimize risks associated with arterial cannulation, sampling should only be done by competent trained staff (NPSA 2008b) (Box 18.9).

Preprocedural considerations
Assessment

It is important prior to any cannulation that the circulation of the hand is assessed: temperature, capillary refill and the colour of the hand (RCN 2010). More than 97% of patients have adequate flow through collateral supply, which prevents ischaemia, should either the radial or ulnar artery be interrupted (Durbin 2001). Although not fully reliable, the Allen test should be completed prior to radial arterial cannulation in order to establish whether there is adequate blood supply to the hand (Figure 18.31). The Allen test consists of simultaneously compressing both the radial and ulnar arteries for approximately 1 minute (Tegtmeyer *et al.* 2006). During this time, the conscious patient rapidly opens and closes the hand to promote local exsanguination. Approxi-

---

Box 18.9 Action required by the National Patient Safety Agency when using arterial catheters

- Sampling from arterial devices is risky and should only be undertaken by competent trained staff. Trusts should raise awareness of the risks and review local guidelines. These should include criteria for requests for blood gas analysis, sampling technique, monitoring and interpretation of results (including unexpected findings).
- Arterial infusion sets must be identified clearly. This means labelling or use of safety solutions such as marked sets adopted by some trusts.
- Any infusion (or additive) attached to the arterial catheter must be prescribed before administration. Further checks should be made at regular intervals and key points (such as shift handover).
- Staff should only use sodium chloride 0.9% to keep catheters open.
- Labels should clearly identify the contents of the infusion bags, even when pressure bags are used. Over time, the manufacturers should develop a universal system to address this problem.

(Reproduced with permission from the NPSA website (www.npsa.nhs.uk))

---

mately 5 seconds after release of one of the arteries (usually the ulnar), the extended hand should blush owing to capillary refilling. If blanching occurs, palmar arch circulation is inadequate and a radial cannula could lead to ischaemia of the hand (Pierce 1995).

Evaluation by a Doppler probe may be carried out as a more reliable alternative (Adam and Osborne 2005). Shiloh *et al.* (2010) suggest that using ultrasound guidance may improve arterial cannulation.

(a)

(b)

Figure 18.31 The Allen test.

1153

Procedure guideline 18.13 Arterial cannula insertion: preparation and setting up of monitoring set

Essential equipment

- 500 mL pressure infuser cuff
- Pressure monitoring system equipment
- Designated arterial cannula
- Sterile intravenous pack
- Non-sterile gloves
- Transparent dressing

- Syringes: various sizes
- A label to identify arterial device
- 2% chlorhexidine in alcohol swab
- Transpore tape
- Bactericidal hand cleanser

Medicinal products

- 500 mL bag of 0.9% sodium chloride
- 1% lidocaine injection

Preprocedure

Action	Rationale
1 Explain the procedure with the patient.	To ensure the patient understands the procedure and gives valid consent wherever appropriate (NMC 2008b, C). *Note*: many patients are anaesthetized when arterial devices are inserted.
2 Wash hands using a bactericidal handrub.	To minimize the risk of infection (Fraise and Bradley 2009, E; Pratt *et al.* 2007, C).
3 Prepare infusion and transducer sets using aseptic technique.	To minimize the risk of infeciton (Fraise and Bradley 2009, E; Pratt *et al.* 2007, C).
4 Check that all Luer-Lok connections are secure.	To prevent disconnection, as equipment is often loose when taken straight from package. E

Procedure

5 Connect transducer to bag of 500 mL 0.9% sodium chloride, which must be prescribed (NPSA 2008b, C).	To prepare infusion, saline is more effective than heparinized flush (O'Grady *et al.* 2002, C; Gamby and Bennett 1995, R3; Kulkarni *et al.* 1994, R3). Only sodium chloride 0.9% must be used as flush (NPSA 2008b, C). To prime the administration set and three-way tap ports. E
6 Open roller clamp fully, squeeze the flush device-actuator (see instructions with set).	To reduce the risk of air embolus, although retrograde air embolus is a rare event after routine radial artery cannula flushing. E
7 Check thoroughly for air bubbles in the circuit.	To reduce the risk of inaccurate pressure readings caused by bubbles in the set (Daily and Schroeder 1994, R4).
8 Insert bag into pressure infuser, inflate the pressure bag to 300 mmHg.	To prevent backpressure of blood into the transducer set by ensuring pressure is higher than arterial blood pressure (Morton and Fontaine 2009, R5). An automatic flush mode is activated within the system which delivers 3 mL per hour, which maintains patency of cannula.
9 Wash hands with bactericidal soap and water or bactericidal handrub.	To reduce the risk of cross-infection (DH 2010, C; Fraise and Bradley 2009, E).

10	Prepare trolley near the patient.	To reduce the risk of cross-infection (DH 2010, C; Fraise and Bradley 2009, E).
11	Complete the Allen test if radial artery is to be used.	To assess whether palmar arch circulation is adequate, although this assessment is not entirely reliable (Wallach 2004, R4).
12	Prepare the insertion site with 2% chlorhexidine swab and place a sterile towel under the appropriate area.	To maintain asepsis. To provide a clean working area (DH 2010, C).
13	Administer adequate local anaesthetic.	To minimize pain during the procedure; this may reduce the sudden movement which could result in through puncture (Lipsitz 2004, R5). Local vasodilation effects of the local anaesthetic may reduce vasospasm, making a successful cannulation more likely (Lipsitz 2004, R5).
14	Apply gloves.	To prevent contamination of hands if blood spillage occurs (Pratt et al. 2007, C).
15	Another nurse may act as an assistant and holds the patient's foot or arm. If the radial artery is cannulated, the wrist must be hyperextended.	To prevent movement and to flex the hand/foot slightly to facilitate insertion. E Prolonged hyperextension may be associated with changes in median nerve conduction, so promptly return the wrist to the neutral position following cannulation (Chowet et al. 2004, R4).
16	Insert the cannula and observe for blood flashback.	To ascertain that the cannula is in the artery. E
17	Attach transducer set and fully open roller clamp.	To commence flush infusion system, and prevent backflow of blood. E
18	Apply transparent dressing over the cannula and tape tubing securely.	To leave the site visible and secure and to allow the observer to recognize immediately any dislodgement, inflammation or disconnection. E
19	Clearly label the device as arterial, on the dressing as well as on the tubing.	To ensure the device is not mistaken for a venous cannula, preventing accidental intra-arterial injection of drugs (E), particularly if the tubing is disconnected and cannula capped off, in the event of a transfer (NPSA 2008b, C), although this practice should be discouraged.
20	Loop the tubing around the thumb, ensuring this is not too tight (see Action Figure 20).	To minimize movement of cannula and damage to the vessel, to prevent ulcer formation. E
21	Connect transducer to monitoring equipment.	Allows checking of arterial waveform and obtaining continuous blood pressure measurements. E
22	Calibrate the arterial device.	The transducer will read an arterial pressure calibrated to atmospheric air which offsets the extraneous atmospheric and hydrostatic pressures. E

Postprocedure

23	Dispose of equipment and clinical waste appropriately.	To prevent sharps injury (NHS Employees 2007, C).
24	Document clearly date and placement of arterial cannula inserted.	To maintain accurate records and provide appropriate reference (NMC 2009, C).

1155

(Continued)

Procedure guideline 18.13 (Continued)

Cannula in position
with criss-cross strapping

Arterial
label

Loop tube loosely
around thumb

Transparent dressing

Action Figure 19 Positioning, securing and labelling of cannula.

Postprocedural considerations

Ongoing care

Arterial cannulas are not replaced routinely so frequent and accurate assessment is essential in order to minimize complications. In the event of a spike in temperature and raised inflammatory markers, removal may be considered.

The arterial cannula site must be assessed at regular intervals to check for appropriate labelling of the device, correct flush fluid, any pain or erythema at the site. There should always be vigilance if the sample taken from the arterial cannula is not within the expected range and staff must be trained in considering and eliminating any risk of contamination which may affect blood results which could in turn determine changes in consequent therapies. The NPSA (2008b) described a number of serious incidents associated with changes in treatment directly associated with arterial blood sampling results. This was because of inappropriate flush agents, predominantly dextrose;

for example, patients had insulin sliding scale infusions titrated in response to contaminated samples where blood glucose was abnormally high and not reflective of the patient's actual serum glucose.

The following volumes of blood should be withdrawn and discarded in order to clear 0.9% sodium chloride, old blood and small emboli from the dead space, the cannula and the three-way tap. Generally, when using a peripheral artery cannula, 3–5 mL must be taken and discarded. A femoral artery cannula is longer and commonly 5 mL should be taken and discarded, but always check manufacturer's instructions.

On each shift it is advisable that the site of the cannulated artery is checked and documented, that an appropriate flush agent is prescribed, that labelling is appropriate and there is absence of pain and colour changes distal to the cannula.

Removal of arterial cannula

Procedure guideline 18.14 Arterial cannula: removal

Essential equipment

- Sterile dressing pack
- Non-sterile gloves
- Hypoallergenic tape
- 2% chlorhexidine in 70% alcohol

Preprocedure

Action	Rationale
1 Explain and discuss the procedure with the patient.	To ensure the patient understands the procedure and gives their valid consent (NMC 2008b, C).
2 Check platelet and coagulation screen.	To prevent delay in removal whilst coagulation is corrected. E
3 Prepare trolley	To reduce the risk of cross-infection (DH 2010, C; Fraise and Bradley 2009, E).
4 Wash hands with bactericidal soap and water or bactericidal alcohol handrub before leaving the clinical room.	To reduce the risk of cross-infection (DH 2010, C; Fraise and Bradley 2009, E).

Procedure

5	Turn three-way tap diagonally or turn off flow switch, depending on arterial product.	To prevent backflow of blood into cannula. E
6	Turn off flush set.	To prevent spillage when removing cannula. E
7	Deflate pressure cuff.	Pressure is no longer required. E
8	Loosen transparent dressing and tape from the cannula site.	To facilitate removal of cannula. E
9	Clean hands with bactericidal skin-cleaning solution.	To minimize the risk of infection (DH 2010, C; Fraise and Bradley 2009, E).
10	Apply gloves.	To prevent contamination of hands with blood (Pratt *et al.* 2007, C).
11	Remove dressing and tape. Clean cannula site area with 2% chlorhexidine swab.	To reduce the risk of infection (DH 2010, C; Fraise and Bradley 2009, E).
12	Place sterile piece of gauze over area and gently remove cannula.	To minimize bleeding and blood spillage (Pratt *et al.* 2007, C).
13	Apply pressure for a minimum of 5 minutes.	To prevent haematoma and blood loss (RCN 2010, C).
14	Apply a clean, sterile, low-linting gauze dressing.	To maintain asepsis and minimize blood loss (E)
15	Secure with tape. Do not create a tourniquet type dressing.	To ensure pressure and prevent haematoma or blood loss. E

Postprocedure

16	Remove gloves and dispose of equipment appropriately.	To prevent sharps injury (NHS Employers 2007, C).
17	Document the date and time of removal in the patient's notes.	To ensure adequate records and enable continued care of device and patient (NMC 2009, C).

Problem-solving table 18.5 Prevention and resolution (Procedure guideline 18.14)

Problem	Cause	Prevention	Action
Backflow of blood into the cannula	The pressure infusor cuff may not be inflated to the optimal	Ensure that the pressure infusor cuff is inflated to 300 mmHg	Check that the pressure infusor cuff is inflated to 300 mmHg and if not, inflate to correct level
Arterial spasm	Forceful flushing or forceful aspiration when withdrawing blood	This pressure is higher than arterial blood pressure and an automatic flush mode is activated in the system which delivers 3 mL per hour. This maintains patency of circuit, cannula and artery (Allan 1984)	Check that the pressure infusor cuff is inflated to 300 mmHg and if not, inflate to correct level
Cerebral embolism	Prolonged, high-pressure flushing can drive a clot or gas bubbles retrograde to produce cerebral embolism	Avoid forceful flushing or aspiration and maintain a slow even pressure when withdrawing blood	Check that the pressure infusor cuff is inflated to 300 mmHg and if not, inflate to correct level

Postprocedural considerations

Immediate care

Following the procedure, check the patient's hand, assessing and documenting the temperature, colour, swelling and any signs of bleeding. Avoid blood pressure measurement being taken manually on the arm where the arterial cannula was removed for 12–24 hours to minimize bleeding or haematoma formation. Medical staff must be informed immediately if the hand or forearm becomes discoloured or swollen, or if the patient complains of pain in the limb. In the event of any complication, careful documentation is essential; consider a request for medical photography to photograph the affected area.

Education

Ask the patient to apply pressure if they notice any oozing from the dressing and immediately inform a member of staff.

Complications

There are a number of complications that can occur as a result of arterial cannulation: see Box 18.8.

Hypovolaemia

Hypovolaemia can occur as a result of severe haemorrhage, which can be caused by (a) accidental disconnection of tubing from the cannula or from one of the connections within the system or (b) dislodgement of the cannula.

The flow from an 18 G cannula can result in blood loss of 250 mL per minute (Bersten *et al.* 2009). Unconscious or delirious patients and children are at particular risk. The risk can be minimized by clear labelling of the arterial cannula (Zideman and Morgan 1981), arterial tubing and sets should be predominantly red in colour, and alarm settings on the monitor must be turned on and audible (Adam and Osborne 2005). The use of Luer-Lok connections, ensuring visibility of the cannula, appropriate nurse/patient ratios and adequate training and competency of nurses caring for patients with arterial cannulas will also help reduce this complication.

The cannula may become dislodged, particularly if the patient is diaphoretic and dressings tend to lift. Securing the cannula using an appropriate cannula-securing device may be useful. Inform the patient about the danger of dislodging the cannula and the amount of movement that is preferred. Staff must also take care when moving the patient, and avoid putting stress on the arm and connections. Ideally, non-invasive blood pressure should not be measured on the same arm which has an arterial cannula. Marini and Wheeler (2010) recommend attempting a minimum of once-daily sphygmomanometry in order to confirm cannula pressure, especially in patients whose vasopressors are titrated to these pressures, and particularly in those patients who are elderly, are hypertensive or those with underlying vascular disease.

Box 18.10 Treatment of distal embolism

- Remove the cannula.
- Arrange for Doppler imaging.
- After consultation with consultant, heparinize (if no contraindications).
- Consider a peripheral vasodilator.

Accidental intra-arterial injection of drugs

Accidental intra-arterial injection of drugs intended for administration through a central or peripheral venous device may cause distal ischaemia and necrosis, sometimes resulting in permanent functional damage (Marieb and Hoehn 2010, Teplitz 1990, Tinker and Zapol 1992). Drugs such as calcium channel blockers and vasopressors are particularly harmful if injected intra-arterially (Marini and Wheeler 2010). Careful and appropriate labelling and appropriate staff training can minimize this risk. In the event of accidental injection of any drug, stop administering the drug and report immediately to medical staff and the senior nurse. The nurse should then attempt to withdraw blood from the three-way tap in order to aspirate any of the drug. Then assess the limb pulse, colour and temperature hourly, or more frequently if required, and complete an accident form and/or other relevant documentation.

Local damage to the artery

Local damage to the artery is the most common complication of arterial cannulation (Marieb and Hoehn 2010). Regular close inspection and assessment of the limb and areas distal to the cannula must be carried out as there is a risk of thrombosis and embolism. Signs and symptoms include pain, a change in temperature in the distal limb, mottling and blanching of the limb when the cannula is flushed. The medical team should be informed if any of the above are discovered (Adam and Osborne 2005). If a distal embolism is suspected, the cannula may have to be removed and limb warming attempted in order to avoid permanent damage (Box 18.10). The risk of ischaemia distal to the cannula is increased when associated with low cardiac output, shock, sepsis and prolonged cannulation (Bersten *et al.* 2009, Gamby and Bennett 1995).

References

Adam, S.K. and Osborne, S. (2005) *Critical Care Nursing: Science and Practice*, 2nd edn. Oxford University Press, Oxford.

Alexandrou, E., Spencer, T.R., Frost, S.A., Parr, M.J., Davidson, P.M. and Hillman, K.M. (2010) A review of the nursing role in central venous cannulation: implications for practice policy and research. *Journal of Clinical Nursing*, **19** (11–12), 1485–1495.

Allan, D. (1984) Care of the patient with an arterial catheter. *Nursing Times*, **80** (46), 40–41.

Archis, C.A., Blacka, J. and Brown, M.A. (2000) Does an endoluminal catheter brush improve flows or unblock haemodialysis catheters? *Nephrology*, **5** (1–2), 55–58.

Banton, J. and Leahy-Gross, K. (1998) Assessing catheter performance: four years of tracking patient outcomes of midline, midclavicular and PICC line program. *Journal of Vascular Access Devices*, **3** (3), 19–26.

Baranowski, L. (1993) Central venous access devices: current technologies, uses, and management strategies. *Journal of Intravenous Nursing*, **16** (3), 167–194.

Barker, P., Anderson, A.D. and MacFie, J. (2004) Randomised clinical trial of elective re-siting of intravenous cannulae. *Annals of the Royal College of Surgeons of England*, **86** (4), 281–283.

Bassetti, S., Hu, J., D'Agostino, R.B. Jr. and Sherertz, R.J. (2001) Prolonged antimicrobial activity of a catheter containing chlorhexidine-silver sulfadiazine extends protection against catheter infections in vivo. *Antimicrobial Agents and Chemotherapy*, **45** (5), 1535–1538.

Benton, S. and Marsden, C. (2002) Training nurses to place tunnelled central venous catheters. *Professional Nurse*, **17** (9), 531–533.

Berger, L. (2000) The effects of positive pressure devices on catheter occlusions. *Journal of Vascular Access Devices*, **5** (4), 31–34.

Bersten, A.D., Soni, N. and Oh, T.E. (2009) *Oh's Intensive Care Manual*, 6th edn. Butterworth-Heinemann, Oxford.

Biffi, R., De Braud, F., Orsi, F. *et al.* (2001) A randomized, prospective trial of central venous ports connected to standard open-ended or Groshong catheters in adult oncology patients. *Cancer*, **92** (5), 1204–1212.

Bishop, L. (2009) Aftercare and management of central access devices, in *Central Venous Catheters* (eds H. Hamilton and A. Bodenham). Wiley-Blackwell, Chichester, pp.221–237.

Bjeletich, J. and Hickman, R.O. (1980) The Hickman indwelling catheter. *American Journal of Nursing*, **80** (1), 62–65.

BNF (2011) *British National Formulary*. BMJ Group and RPS Publishing, London.

Bodenham, A. (2009) Ultrasound-guided venous access, in *Central Venous Catheters* (eds H. Hamilton and A.R. Bodenham). Wiley-Blackwell, Oxford, pp127–141.

Bodenham, A. and Simcock, L. (2009) Complications of central venous access, in *Central Venous Catheters* (eds H. Hamilton and A.R. Bodenham). Wiley-Blackwell, Oxford, pp.175–205.

Boeson, M.B., Hranchook, A. and Stoller, J. (2000) Peripheral nerve injury from intravenous cannulation: a case report, *AANA Journal*, **68** (1), 53–57.

Boland, A., Haycox, A., Bagust, A. and Fitzsimmons, L. (2003) A randomised controlled trial to evaluate the clinical and cost-effectiveness of Hickman line insertions in adult cancer patients by nurses. *Health Technology Assessment*, **7** (36), iii, ix–x, 1–99. www.hta.ac.uk/pdfexecs/summ736.pdf.

Bow, E.J., Kilpatrick, M.G. and Clinch, J.J. (1999) Totally implantable venous access ports systems for patients receiving chemotherapy for solid tissue malignancies: a randomized controlled clinical trial examining the safety, efficacy, costs, and impact on quality of life. *Journal of Clinical Oncology*, **17** (4), 1267.

Bregenzer, T., Conen, D., Sakmann, P. and Widmer, A.F. (1998) Is routine replacement of peripheral intravenous catheters necessary? *Archives of Internal Medicine*, **158** (2), 151–156.

Brown, J. and Larson, M. (1999) Pain during insertion of peripheral intravenous catheters with and without intradermal lidocaine. *Clinical Nurse Specialist*, **13** (6), 283–285.

Brown, J.D., Moss, H.A. and Elliott, T.S. (1997) The potential for catheter microbial contamination from a needleless connector. *Journal of Hospital Infection*, **36** (3), 181–189.

Browne, J., Awad, I., Plant, R. *et al.* (1999) Topical amethocaine (Ametop) is superior to EMLA for intravenous cannulation. Eutectic mixture of local anesthetics. *Canadian Journal of Anaesthesia*, **46** (11), 1014–1018.

Bullock-Corkhill, M. (2010) Central venous access devices: access and insertion, in *Infusion Nursing: An Evidence-Based Approach*, 3rd edn (eds M. Alexander, A. Corrigan, L. Gorski *et al.*). Saunders Elsevier, St Louis, MO, pp.480–494.

Camp-Sorrell, D., Cope, D.G. and Oncology Nursing Society (2004) *Access Device Guidelines: Recommendations for Nursing Practice and Education*, 2nd edn, Oncology Nursing Society, Pittsburgh, PA.

Carlson, K.R. (1999) Correct utilization and management of peripherally inserted central catheters and midline catheters in the alternate care setting. *Journal of Intravenous Nursing*, **22** (6 Suppl), S46–S50.

Casey, A.L. and Elliott, T.S. (2010) Prevention of central venous catheter-related infection: update. *British Journal of Nursing*, **19** (2), 78, 80, 82 passim.

Catney, M.R., Hillis, S., Wakefield, B. *et al.* (2001) Relationship between peripheral intravenous catheter dwell time and the development of phlebitis and infiltration. *Journal of Infusion Nursing*, **24** (5), 332–341.

Chantler, J. (2009) Applied anatomy of the central veins, in *Central Venous Catheters* (eds H. Hamilton and A. Bodenham). Wiley-Blackwell, Chichester, pp.14–33.

Chen, B.H. (2002) Active hand warming eases peripheral intravenous catheter insertion. *BMJ*, **325**, 409–410.

Chernecky, C. (2001) Satisfaction versus dissatisfaction with venous access devices in outpatient oncology: a pilot study. *Oncology Nursing Forum*, **28** (10), 1613–1616.

Chernecky, C., Macklin, D., Casella, L. and Jarvis, E. (2009) Caring for patients with cancer through nursing knowledge of IV connectors. *Clinical Journal of Oncology Nursing*, **13** (6), 630–633.

Chowet, A.L., Lopez, J.R., Brock-Utne, J.G. and Jaffe, R.A. (2004) Wrist hyperextension leads to median nerve conduction block: implications for intra-arterial catheter placement. *Anesthesiology*, **100** (2), 287–291.

Ciano, B.A. (2001) Hemodynamic monitoring, in *Infusion Therapy in Clinical Practice*, 2nd edn (ed. J. Hankins). W.B. Saunders, St Louis, MO, pp.404–417.

Cole, D. (1999) Selection and management of central venous access devices in the home setting. *Journal of Intravenous Nursing*, **22** (6), 315–319.

Collins, M., Phillips, S., Dougherty, L. *et al.* (2006) A structured learning programme for venepuncture and cannulation. *Nursing Standard*, 20 (26), 34–40.

Conn, C. (1993) The importance of syringe size when using an implanted vascular access device. *Journal of Vascular Access Networks*, **3** (1), 11–18.

Cook, D., Randolph, A., Kernerman, P. *et al.* (1997) Central venous catheter replacement strategies: a systematic review of the literature. *Critical Care Medicine*, **25** (8), 1417–1424.

Corrigan, A. (2010) Infusion nursing as a speciality, in *Infusion Nursing: An Evidence Based Approach*, 3rd edn (eds M. Alexander, A. Corrigan, L. Gorski, J. Hankins and R. Perucca). Saunders Elsevier, St Louis, MO, pp1–9.

Costa, N. and Ferguson, E. (2002) Placement of triple lumen peripherally inserted central catheters in critical patients. *Journal of Vascular Access Devices*, **7** (4), 27–30.

Couban, S., Goodyear, M., Burnell, M. *et al.* (2005) Randomized placebo-controlled study of low-dose warfarin for the prevention of central venous catheter-associated thrombosis in patients with cancer. *Journal of Clinical Oncology*, **23** (18), 4063–9.

Coyne, P.J., MacMurren, M., Izzo, T. and Kramer, T. (1995) Transcutaneous electrical nerve stimulator for procedural pain associated with intravenous needlesticks. *Journal of Intravenous Nursing*, **18** (5), 263–267.

1159

Crnich, C.J. and Maki, D.G. (2002) The promise of novel technology for the prevention of intravascular device-related bloodstream infection. II. Long-term devices. *Clinical Infectious Diseases*, 34 (10), 1362–1368.

Cummings-Winfield, C. and Mushani-Kanji, T. (2008) Restoring patency to central venous access devices. *Clinical Journal of Oncology Nursing*, 12 (6), 925–934.

Czaplewski, L. (2010) Clinician and patient education, in *Infusion Nursing: An Evidence-Based Approach*, 3rd edn (eds M. Alexander, A. Corrigan, L. Gorski et al.). Saunders Elsevier, St Louis, MO, pp.71–94.

Daily, E.K. and Schroeder, J.S. (1994) *Techniques in Bedside Hemodynamic Monitoring*, 5th edn. Mosby, St Louis, MO.

Daniels, L.E. (1995) The physical and psychosocial implications of central venous access devices in cancer patients: a review of the literature. *Journal of Cancer Care*, 4 (4), 141–146.

Davidson, T. and Al Mufti, R. (1997) Hickman central venous catheters in cancer patients. *Cancer Topics*, 10 (8), 10–14.

Deitcher, S.R., Fesen, M.R., Kiproff, P.M. et al. (2002) Safety and efficacy of alteplase for restoring function in occluded central venous catheters: results of the cardiovascular thrombolytic to open occluded lines trial. *Journal of Clinical Oncology*, 20 (1), 317–324.

DH (2004) *Building a Safer NHS for Patients – Improving Medication Safety*. Department of Health, London.

DH (2010) *Clean Safe Care. High Impact Intervention: Central Venous Catheter Care Bundle and Peripheral IV Cannula Care Bundle*. Department of Health, London.

DH and Chief Medical Officer (2003) *Winning Ways: Working Together to Reduce Healthcare Associated Infection in England: Report of the Chief Medical Officer*. Department of Health, London.

Dorman, T., Breslow, M.J., Lipsett, P.A. et al. (1998) Radial artery pressure monitoring underestimates central arterial pressure during vasopressor therapy in critically ill surgical patients. *Critical Care Medicine*, 26 (10), 1646–1649.

Dougherty, L. (1994) A Study to Discover How Cancer Patients Perceive the Intravenous Cannulation Experience. Unpublished MSc thesis, University of Guildford.

Dougherty, L. (2006) *Central Venous Access Devices: Care and Management*. Blackwell, Oxford.

Dougherty, L. (2008) Obtaining peripheral vascular access, in *Intravenous Therapy in Nursing Practice*, 2nd edn (eds L. Dougherty and J. Lamb). Blackwell Publishing, Oxford, pp.225–270.

Dougherty, L. (2011) Patients' perspective, in *Venepuncture and Cannulation* (eds S. Phillips, M. Collins and L. Dougherty). Wiley-Blackwell, Chichester.

Dougherty, L., Viner, C. and Young, J. (1998) Establishing ambulatory chemotherapy at home. *Professional Nurse*, 13 (6), 356–358.

Drake, R.L., Vogl, W. and Mitchell, A.W.M. (2005) *Gray's Anatomy for Students*. Elsevier, Philadephia.

Drewett, S.R. (2000) Central venous catheter removal: procedures and rationale. *British Journal of Nursing*, 9 (22), 2304–2315.

Drewett, S.R. (2009) Removal of central venous access devices, in *Central Venous Catheters* (eds. H. Hamilton and A. Bodenham). Wiley-Blackwell, Chichester, pp.238–248.

Durbin, C.G. (1995) Do arterial lines equal unnecessary testing? *Chest*, 108 (1), 7–8.

Durbin, C.G. Jr. (2001) Radial arterial lines and sticks: what are the risks? *Respiratory Care*, 46 (3), 229–231.

Elliott, T.S. (1993) Line-associated bacteraemias. *CDR Review*, 3 (7), R91–96.

Ernst, D.J. (2005) *Applied Phlebotomy*. Lippincott, Williams and Wilkins, Baltimore, MD.

Fabian, B. (2010) Infusion therapy in the older adult, in *Infusion Nursing: An Evidence Based Approach*, 3rd edn (eds M. Alexander, A. Corrigan, L. Gorski, J. Hankins and R. Perucca). Saunders Elsevier, St Louis, MO, pp.571–582.

Fanikos, J., Fudyma, C., Herbst, S. et al. (2009) To aliquot ot not? Optimising use of fibrinolytic agents in the management of catheter occlusions. *Clinical Courier*, 26 (18), 1–4.

Farrow, C., Bodenham, A. and Millo, J. (2009) Cannulation of the jugular veins, in *Central Venous Catheters* (eds H. Hamilton and A. Bodenham). Wiley-Blackwell, Chichester, pp.78–91.

Fetzer, S.J. (2002) Reducing venipuncture and intravenous insertion pain with eutectic mixture of local anesthetic: a meta-analysis. *Nursing Research*, 51 (2), 119–124.

Fink, R.M., Hjort, E., Wenger, B. et al. (2009) The impact of dry versus moist heat on peripheral IV catheter insertion in a hematology-oncology outpatient population. *Oncology Nursing Forum*, 36 (4), E198–E204.

Finlay, T. (2004) *Intravenous Therapy*. Blackwell Science, Oxford.

Fitzsimmons, C.L., Gilleece, M.H., Ranson, M.R. et al. (1997) Central venous catheter placement: extending the role of the nurse. *Journal of the Royal College of Physicians of London*, 31 (5), 533–535.

Forauer, A.R. and Alonzo, M. (2000) Change in peripherally inserted central catheter tip position with abduction and adduction of the upper extremity. *Journal of Vascular and Interventional Radiology*,11, 1315–1318.

Fraise, A.P. and Bradley, T. (eds) (2009) *Ayliffe's Control of Healthcare-associated Infection: A Practical Handbook*, 5th edn. Hodder Arnold, London.

Fry, C. and Aholt, D. (2001) Local anesthesia prior to the insertion of peripherally inserted central catheters. *Journal of Infusion Nursing*, 24 (6), 404–408.

Gabriel, J. (2000) What patients think of a PICC. *Journal of Vascular Access Devices*, 5 (4), 26–30.

Gabriel, J. (2001) PICC securement: minimising potential complications. *Nursing Standard*, 15 (43), 42–44.

Gabriel, J. (2008) Long-term central venous access, in *Intravenous Therapy in Nursing Practice*, 2nd edn (eds L. Dougherty and J. Lamb). Blackwell, Oxford, pp.321–351.

Galinkin, J.L., Rose, J.B., Harris, K. and Watcha, M.F. (2002) Lidocaine iontophoresis versus eutectic mixture of local anesthetics (EMLA) for IV placement in children. *Anesthesia and Analgesia*, 94 (6), 1484–1488.

Gallieni, M., Pittiruti, M, and Biffi, R, (2009) Vascular access in oncology patients. *CA: A Cancer Journal for Clinicians*, 58, 323–346.

Galloway, S. and Bodenham, A. (2004) Long-term central venous access. *British Journal of Anaesthesia*, 92 (5), 722–34.

Galloway, S. and Bodenham, A.R. (2009) Central venous access via the subclavian and axillary veins, in *Central Venous Catheters* (eds H. Hamilton and A.R. Bodenham). Wiley-Blackwell, Oxford, pp101–113.

Gamby, A. and Bennett, J. (1995) A feasibility study of the use of non-heparinised 0.9% sodium chloride for transduced arterial and venous lines. *Intensive and Critical Care Nursing*, 11 (3), 148–150.

Garza, D. and Becan-McBride, K. (2010) *Phlebotomy Handbook*, 8th edn. Pearson Education, New Jersey.

Goetz, A.M., Miller, J., Wagener, M.M. and Muder, R.R. (1998) Complications related to intravenous midline catheter usage. A 2-year study. *Journal of Intravenous Nursing*, 21 (2), 76–80.

Goode, C.J., Titler, M., Rakel, B. et al. (1991) A meta-analysis of effects of heparin flush and saline flush: quality and cost implications. *Nursing Research*, 40 (6), 324–330.

Goodwin, M.L. and Carlson, I. (1993) The peripherally inserted central catheter: a retrospective look at three years of insertions. *Journal of Intravenous Nursing*, 16 (2), 92–103.

Gorski, L., Perucca, R. and Hunter, M. (2010) Central venous access devices: care, maintenance, and potential problems, in *Infusion Nursing: An Evidence-Based Approach*, 3rd edn (eds M. Alexander, A. Corrigan, L. Gorski *et al.*). Saunders Elsevier, St Louis, MO, pp.495–515.

Green, E., Macartney, G., Zwaal, C. *et al.* (2008) Managing central venous access devices in cancer patients: a clinical practice guideline. www.cancercare.on.ca/common/pages/UserFile.aspx?serverId=6&path=/File%20Database/CCO%20Files/PEBC/pebc16-1s.pdf,

Gunwardene, R.D. and Davenport, H.T. (1990) Local application of EMLA and glycerol trinitrate ointment before venepuncture. *Anesthesia*, 45, 52–54.

Hadaway, L. (1998) Catheter connection... are large syringes necessary? *Journal of Vascular Access Devices*, 3 (3), 40–41.

Hadaway, L. (2000) Peripheral IV therapy in adults, in *Self Study Workbook*. Hadaway Associates, Georgia.

Hadaway, L.C. (2010) Anatomy and physiology related to infusion therapy, in *Infusion Nursing: An Evidence-Based Approach*, 3rd edn (eds M. Alexander, A. Corrigan, L. Gorski *et al.*). Saunders Elsevier, St Louis, MO, pp.139–177.

Haire, W.D. and Herbst, S.F. (2000) Consensus statement on the use of t-PA to restore immediate function in the treatment of thrombotic catheter dysfunction. *Journal of Vascular Access Devices*, 5 (2), 28–36.

Hamilton, H. (2009) Patient examination and assessment: choice of devices, in *Central Venous Catheters* (eds H. Hamilton and A. Bodenham). Wiley-Blackwell, Chichester, pp.34–56.

Hamilton, H., O'Byrne, M. and Nicholai, L. (1995) Central lines inserted by clinical nurse specialists. *Nursing Times*, 91 (17), 38–39.

Hartley Jones, C. (2009) Problems and practical solutions during insertion of catheters, in *Central Venous Catheters* (eds H. Hamilton and A.R. Bodenham). Wiley-Blackwell, Oxford, pp157–174.

Hayden, M.K. and Goodman, M. (2005) Chemotherapy: principles of adminstration, in *Cancer Nursing: Principles and Practice*, 6th edn (eds C.H. Yarbro, M. Goodman and M.H. Frogge). Jones and Bartlett, Sudbury, MA, pp.351–411.

Hazinski, M.F. (1992) *Nursing Care of the Critically Ill Child*, 2nd edn. Mosby Year Book, St Louis, MO.

Heath, J. and Jones, S. (2001) Utilization of an elastomeric continuous infusion device to maintain catheter patency. *Journal of Intravenous Nursing*, 24 (2), 102–106.

Hecker, J. (1988) Improved technique in i.v. therapy. *Nursing Times*, 84 (34), 28–33.

Hemsworth, S., Selwood, K., van Saene, R. and Pizer, B. (2007) Does the number of exogenous infections increase in paediatric oncology patients when sterile surgical gloves are not worn for accessing central venous access devices? *European Journal of Oncology Nursing*, 11, 442–447.

Ho, K.M. and Litton, E. (2006) Use of chlorhexidine-impregnated dressing to prevent vascular and epidural catheter colonization and infection: a meta-analysis. *Journal of Antimicrobial Chemotherapy*, 58 (2), 281–287.

Hoffer, E.K., Borsa, J., Santulli, P. *et al.* (1999) Prospective randomized comparison of valved versus nonvalved peripherally inserted central vein catheters. *American Journal of Roentgenology*, 173 (5), 1393–1398.

Hoffman, K.R. (2001) Subcutaneous ports used for vascular access need only be flushed every eight weeks to maintain patency. *Proceedings of the American Society of Clinical Oncology*, 20, 1634.

Holcombe, B.J., Forloines-Lynn, S. and Garmhausen, L.W. (1992) Restoring patency of long-term central venous access devices. *Journal of Intravenous Nursing*, 15 (1), 36–41.

Homer, L.D. and Holmes, K.R. (1998) Risks associated with 72- and 96-hour peripheral intravenous catheter dwell times. *Journal of Intravenous Nursing*, 21 (5), 301–305.

Hyde, L. (2008) Legal and professional aspects of IV therapy, in *IV Therapy in Practice* (eds L. Dougherty and J. Lamb). Churchill Livingstone, Edinburgh.

Hyde, L. (2011) Legal and professional aspects, in *Venepuncture and Cannulation* (eds S. Phillips, M. Collins and L. Dougherty). Wiley-Blackwell, Chichester.

INS (2011) Infusion Nursing Standards of Practice 2011. *Journal of Infusion Nursing*, 34 (1), Supplement.

Inwood, S. (1999) A preliminary assessment of an innovative valved catheter. *Journal of Vascular Access Devices*, 4 (2), 30–33.

IS Pharma (2009) Cryogesic taking the pain out of needle procedures. www.ispharma.plc.uk.

Ives, F. (2009) Catheter design and materials, in *Central Venous Catheters* (eds H. Hamilton and A. Bodenham). Wiley-Blackwell, Chichester, pp.57–77.

Jackson, A. (1998) Infection control – a battle in vein: infusion phlebitis. *Nursing Times*, 94 (4), 68, 71.

Johansson, E., Engervall, P., Bjorvell, H. *et al.* (2009) Patients' perceptions of having a central venous catheter or a totally implantable subcutaneous port system – results from a randomised study in acute leukemia. *Supportive Care Cancer*, 17, 137–143.

Karadag, A. and Gorgulu, S. (2000) Effect of two different short peripheral catheter materials on phlebitis development. *Journal of Intravenous Nursing*, 23 (3), 158–166.

Kayley, J. (2008) Intravenous therapy in the community, in *Intravenous Therapy in Nursing Practice*, 2nd edn (eds. L. Dougherty and J. Lamb). Blackwell, Oxford, pp. 352–374.

Kefeli,U., Dane, F., Yumuk, P.F. *et al.* (2009) Prolonged interval in prophylactic heparin flushing for maintenance of subcutaneous implanted port care in patients with cancer. *European Journal of Cancer Care*, 18, 191–194.

Kulkarni, M., Elsner, C., Ouellet, D. and Zeldin, R. (1994) Heparinized saline versus normal saline in maintaining patency of the radial artery catheter. *Canadian Journal of Surgery*, 37 (1), 37–42.

Kupensky, D.T. (1998) Applying current research to influence clinical practice. *Journal of Intravenous Nursing*, 21 (5), 271–274.

Lamb, J. and Dougherty, L. (2008) Local and systemic complications of intravenous therapy, in *Intravenous Therapy in Nursing Practice*, 2nd edn (eds L. Doughterty and J. Lamb). Blackwell Publishing, Oxford, 167–196.

Larson, E. (1988) Guideline for use of topical antimicrobial agents. *American Journal of Infection Control*, 16 (6), 253–266.

LaRue, G.D. (2000) Efficacy of ultrasonography in peripheral venous cannulation. *Journal of Intravenous Nursing*, 23 (1), 29–34.

Lavery, I. and Ingram, P. (2005) Venepuncture: best practice. *Nursing Standard*, 19 (49), 55–65.

Lenhart, C. (2000) Prevention versus treatment of venous access device occlusions. *Journal of Vascular Access Devices*, 5 (4), 34–35.

Lipsitz, E.C. (2004) Cannulation injuries of the radial artery. *American Journal of Critical Care*, 13 (4), 314, 319.

London Standing Committee (2002) *Standards of Care of External Central Venous Catheters in Adult Cancer Patients*. London Standing Committee, London.

Lüker, P. and Stahlheber-Dilg, B.A. (2003) Pain related to Optiva 2, biovalve and Venflon 2 intravenous catheters. *British Journal of Nursing*, 12 (22), 1345–1351.

Lum, P. (1999) Techniques for optimising catheter tip position. NAVAN 13th Annual Conference, Orlando.

Lum, P. (2004) A new formula-based measurement guide for optimal positioning of central venous catheters. *Journal of the Association for Vascular Access*, 9 (2), 80–86.

Macklin, D. (1999) What's physics got to do with it? A review of the physical principles of fluid administration. *Journal of Vascular Access Devices*, **4** (2), 7–11.

Macklin, D. (2010) Catheter management. *Seminars in Oncology Nursing*, **26** (2), 113–120.

Macklin, D. and Chernecky, C.C. (2004) *IV Therapy*. Saunders, St Louis, MO.

Madeo, M., Martin, C. and Nobbs, A. (1997) A randomized study comparing IV 3000 (transparent polyurethane dressing) to a dry gauze dressing for peripheral intravenous catheter sites. *Journal of Intravenous Nursing*, **20** (5), 253–256.

Maki, D.G. (2002) The promise of novel technology for the prevention of intravascular device related blood stream infections. NAVAN, San Diego, CA.

Maki, D.G. (2005) *Renowned Expert Dennis Maki Addresses Catheter Related Infections*. Infection Control Today. www.infectioncontroltoday.com/articles/402/402_511feat3.html.

Maki, D.G. (2008) *A Novel Integrated Chlorhexidine Impregnated Transparent Dressing for Prevention of Catheter Related Blood Stream Infection: A Prospective Comparative Study in Healthy Volunteers*. 18th Annual Scientific Meeting of the Society of Healthcare Epidemiology of America. Orlando, Florida.

Maki, D.G. and Ringer, M. (1987) Evaluation of dressing regimens for prevention of infection with peripheral intravenous catheters. Gauze, a transparent polyurethane dressing, and an iodophor-transparent dressing. *JAMA*, **258** (17), 2396–2403.

Maki, D.G., Ringer, M. and Alvarado, C.J. (1991) Prospective randomised trial of povidone-iodine, alcohol, and chlorhexidine for prevention of infection associated with central venous and arterial catheters. *Lancet*, **338** (8763), 339–343.

Marieb, E.N. and Hoehn, K. (2010) *Human Anatomy and Physiology*, 8th edn. Benjamin Cummings, San Francisco.

Marini, J.L. and Wheeler, N.P. (2010) *Critical Care: The Essentials*, 3rd edn. Lippincott, Williams and Wilkins, Philadelphia.

Marsigliese, A.M. (2001) Evaluation of comfort level and complication rates as determined by peripheral intravenous catheter sites. *Canadian Intravenous Nurses Association*, **17**, 26–39.

Marx, M. (1995) The management of the difficult peripherally inserted central venous catheter line removal. *Journal of Intravenous Nursing*, **18** (5), 246–249.

Masoorli, S. (2003) Extravasation injuries associated with the use of central vascular access devices. *Journal of Vascular Access Devices*, **8** (1), 21–23.

Masoorli, S. (2007) Nerve injuries related to vascular access insertion and assessment. *Journal of Infusion Nursing*, **30** (6), 346–350.

Mayo, D.J. (2000) Catheter-related thrombosis. *Journal of Vascular Access Devices*, **5** (2), 10–20.

Mayo, D.J. (2001) Catheter-related thrombosis. *Journal of Intravenous Nursing*, **24** (3 Suppl.), S13–S22.

McCall, R.E. and Tankersley, C.M. (2003) *Phlebotomy Essentials*, 3rd edn. Lippincott, Williams and Wilkins, Philadelphia.

McGoldrick, M. (2010) Infection prevention and control, in *Infusion Nursing: an Evidence-Based Approach*, 3rd edn (eds M. Alexander, A. Corrigan, L. Gorski *et al.*). Saunders Elsevier, St Louis, MO, pp.204–228.

MDA (2003) *Infusion Devices Bulletin DB 2003(02)*. Medical Devices Agency, London. www.mhra.gov.uk/publications/safetyguidance/devicebulletins/CON007321.

Mermel, L.A., Farr, B.M., Sherertz, R.J. *et al.* (2001) Guidelines for the management of intravascular catheter-related infections. *Journal of Intravenous Nursing*, **24** (3), 180–205.

Mermel, L.A., Allon, M., Bouza, E. *et al.* (2009) Clinical practice guidelines for the diagnosis and management of intravascular catheter-related infection: 2009 Update by the Infectious Dis-

eases Society of America. *Clinical Infectious Diseases*, **49** (1), 1–45.

MHRA (2004) *Medical Device Alert MDA/2004/010 Central Venous Catheters (All Manufacturers) (25/2/04)*, 1–3. Medicines and Healthcare Products Regulatory Agency, London.

MHRA (2005) *Alert MDA 2005/01 and Device Bulletin DB 2005 (01): Reporting Adverse Incidents and Disseminating Medical Device Alerts*. Medicines and Healthcare Products Regulatory Agency, London.

Mignini, M.A., Piacentini, E. and Dubin, A. (2006) Peripheral arterial blood pressure monitoring adequately tracks central arterial blood pressure in critically ill patients: an observational study. *Critical Care*, **10** (2), R43.

Millam, D.A. (1992) Starting i.v.s: how to develop your venipuncture expertise. *Nursing*, **22** (9), 33–46.

Minnaganti, V.R. and Cunha, B.A. (2000) *Acinetobacter baumanii*-associated arterial line infection. *American Journal of Infection Control*, **28** (5), 376–377.

Mirro, J. Jr., Rao, B.N., Stokes, D.C. *et al.* (1989) A prospective study of Hickman/Broviac catheters and implantable ports in pediatric oncology patients. *Journal of Clinical Oncology*, **7** (2), 214–222.

Molloy, D., Smith, L.S. and Aitchison, T. (2008) Cytotoxic chemotherapy for incurable colorectal cancer: living with a PICC line. *Journal of Clinical Nursing*, **17**, 2398–2407.

Morton, P.G. and Fontaine, D.K. (eds) (2009) *Critical Care Nursing: A Holistic Approach*, 11th edn. Lippincott Williams and Wilkins, Philadelphia.

Moureau, N. and Gabriel, J. (2009) Peripherally inserted central catheters, in *Central Venous Catheters* (eds. H. Hamilton and A. Bodenham). Wiley-Blackwell, Chichester, pp.114–126.

Moureau, N. and Iannucci, A.L. (2003) Catheter securement: trends in performance and complications associated with the use of either traditional methods or adhesive anchor devices. *Journal of Vascular Access Devices*, **8** (1), 29–33.

Moureau, N. and Zonderman, A. (2000) Does it always have to hurt? Premedications for adults and children for use with intravenous therapy. *Journal of Intravenous Nursing*, **23** (4), 213–219.

Moureau, N., Thompson McKinnon, B. and Douglas, C.M. (1999) Multi disciplinary management of thrombotic catheter occlusions in vascular access devices. *Journal of Vascular Access Devices*, **4** (2), 22–29.

Moureau, N., Deschneau, M. and Pyrek, J. (2009) Evaluation of the clinical performance of a chlorhexidine gluconate antimicrobial transparent dressing. *Journal of Infection Prevention*, **10** (Supplement), S13–S17.

Nakazawa, N. (2010) Infectious and thrombotic complications of central venous catheters. *Seminars in Oncology Nursing*, **26** (2), 121–131.

Nauth-Misir, N. (1998) Intravascular catheters. *Professional Nurse*, **13** (7), 463–471.

NAVAN (1998) Tip location of peripherally inserted central catheters. *Journal of Vascular Access Devices*, **3** (2), 8–10.

Nesti, S.P. and Kovac, R. (2000) 5-Fluorouracil extravasation following port failure. *Journal of Intravenous Nursing*, **23** (3), 176–180.

NHS Employers (2007) Needlestick injury, in *The Healthy Workplaces Handbook*. NHSE, London.

NICE (2002) *Guidance on the Use of Ultrasound Locating Devices for Placing Central Venous Catheters*. National Institute for Clinical Excellence, London. www.nice.org.uk/nicemedia/live/11474/32461/32461.pdf.

NICE (2003) *Infection Control: Prevention of Healthcare-Associated Infection in Primary and Community Care: NICE Clinical Guide-*

line 2. National Institute for Clinical Excellence, London. www.nice.org.uk/nicemedia/live/10922/29117/29117.pdf.

NMC (2008a) *The Code: Standards of Conduct, Performance and Ethics for Nurses and Midwives*. Nursing and Midwifery Council, London.

NMC (2008b) *Consent*. Nursing and Midwifery Council, London. www.nmc-uk.org/Nurses-and-midwives/Advice-by-topic/A/Advice/Consent/.

NMC (2009) *Record Keeping: Guidance for Nurses and Midwives*. Nursing and Midwifery Council, London.

NPSA (2003) *Risk Analysis of Infusion Devices*. National Patient Safety Agency, London.

NPSA (2007) *Alert 20. Promoting the Safer Use of Injectable Medicines*. National Patient Safety Agency, London.

NPSA (2008a) *Risks with Intravenous Heparin Flush Solutions*. National Patient Safety Agency, London.

NPSA (2008b) *Infusions and Sampling from Arterial Lines*. National Patient Safety Agency, London.

Oakley, C., Wright, E. and Ream, E. (2000) The experiences of patients and nurses with a nurse-led peripherally inserted central venous catheter line service. *European Journal of Oncology Nursing*, 4 (4), 207–18.

O'Grady, N.P., Alexander, M., Dellinger, E.P. *et al.* (2002) Guidelines for the prevention of intravascular catheter-related infections. *Morbidity and Mortality Weekly Report*, 51 (RR-10), 1–30.

Perucca, R. (2010) Peripheral venous access devices, in *Infusion Nursing: An Evidence-Based Approach*, 3rd edn (eds M. Alexander, A. Corrigan, L. Gorski *et al.*). Saunders Elsevier, St Louis, MO, pp.456–479.

Phillips, L.D. (2005) *Manual of I.V. Therapeutics*, 4th edn. F.A. Davis, Philadelphia.

Phillips, S., Collins, M. and Dougherty, L. (eds) (2011) *Venepuncture and Cannulation*. Wiley-Blackwell, Chichester.

Philpot, P. and Griffiths, V. (2003) The peripherally inserted central catheter. *Nursing Standard*, 17 (44), 39–46.

Pierce, L.N.B. (1995) Non-invasive respiratory monitoring and invasive monitoring of direct and derived tissue oxgenation variables, in *Guide to Mechanical Ventilation and Intensive Respiratory Care*. W.B. Saunders, Philadelphia, London. pp.29

Ponec, D., Irwin, D., Haire, W.D. *et al.* (2001) Recombinant tissue plasminogen activator (alteplase) for restoration of flow in occluded central venous access devices: a double-blind placebo-controlled trial. The cardiovascular thrombolytic to open occluded lines (COOL) efficacy trial. *Journal of Vascular and Interventional Radiology*, 12 (8), 951–955.

Pratt, R.J., Pellowe, C.M., Wilson, J.A. *et al.* (2007) epic2: National evidence-based guidelines for preventing healthcare-associated infections in NHS hospitals in England. *Journal of Hospital Infection*, 65 (Suppl 1), S1–64.

RCN (2010) *Standards for Infusion Therapy*, 3rd edn. Royal College of Nursing, London.

Rinn, T.L. (2001) Fibrinolytic therapy in CVC occlusion. *Journal of Intravenous Nursing*, 24 (Suppl 3), S9–S12.

Robbins, T.L., Cromwell, P. and Korones, D.N. (2000) Swimming and central venous catheter related infections in children with cancer, in *Measuring Patient Outcomes* (eds M.T. Nolan and V. Mock). Sage Publications, Thousand Oaks, CA, pp.169–184.

Rowley, S. (2001) Theory to practice. Aseptic non-touch technique. *Nursing Times*, 97 (7), VI–VIII.

Royer, T. (2001) A case for posterior, anterior, and lateral chest x-rays being performed following each PICC placement. *Journal of Vascular Access Devices*, 6 (4), 9–12.

Rummel, M.A., Donnelly, P.J. and Fortenbaugh, C.C. (2001) Clinical evaluation of a positive pressure device to prevent central venous catheter occlusion: results of a pilot study. *Clinical Journal of Oncology Nursing*, 5 (6), 261–265.

Ruschulte, H., Franke, M., Gastmeier, P. *et al.* (2009) Prevention of central venous catheter related infections with chlorhexidine gluconate impregnated wound dressings: a randomized controlled trial. *Annals of Hematology*, 88 (3), 267–272.

Ryder, M. (2001) The role of biofilm in vascular catheter related infections. *New Developments in Vascular Disease*, 2 (2), 15–25.

Ryder, M. (2002) Biofilm – unlocking the mystery of catheter-related infections. NAVAN 15th Annual Conference, Virginia.

Sampath, L.A., Saborio, D.V., Yaron, I. and Modak, S. (2001) Safety and efficacy of an improved antiseptic catheter impregnated intraluminally with chlorhexidine. *Journal of Infusion Nursing*, 24 (6), 395–403.

Sansivero, G.E. (1998) Venous anatomy and physiology. Considerations for vascular access device placement and function. *Journal of Intravenous Nursing*, 21 (5 Suppl), S107–S114.

Scales, K. (2005) Vascular access: a guide to peripheral venous cannulation. *Nursing Standard*, 19 (49), 48–52.

Scales, K. (2008) Anatomy and physiology related to intravenous therapy, in *Intravenous Therapy in Nursing Practice*, 2nd edn (eds L. Dougherty and J. Lamb), Blackwell Publishing, Oxford, pp. 23–48.

Schears, G.J. (2005) The benefits of a catheter securement device on reducing patient complications. *Managing Infection Control*, 5 (2), 14–25.

Schulmeister, L. and Camp-Sorrell, D. (2000) Chemotherapy extravasation from implanted ports. *Oncology Nursing Forum*, 27 (3), 531–538.

Shiloh, A.L., Sural, R.H., Paiulin, L.M. and Eisen, L.A. (2010) Ultrasound guided catheterisation of the radial artery: a systematic review and meta analysis of randomized controlled trials. *Chest*, 10, 919.

Shotkin, J.D. and Lombardo, F. (1996) Use of an indwelling peripheral catheter for 3–5 day chemotherapy administration in the outpatient setting. *Journal of Intravenous Nursing*, 19 (6), 315–320.

Simcock, L. (2001a) Managing occlusion in central venous catheters. *Nursing Times*, 97 (21), 36–38.

Simcock, L. (2001b) The use of central venous catheters for IV therapy. *Nursing Times*, 97 (18), 34–35.

Snelling, R., Jones, G., Figueredo, A. and Major, P. (2001) Central venous catheters for infusion therapy in gastrointestinal cancer. A comparative study of tunnelled centrally placed catheters and peripherally inserted central catheters. *Journal of Intravenous Nursing*, 24 (1), 38–47.

Springhouse (2002) *Intravenous Therapy Made Incredibly Easy*. Lippincott, Williams and Wilkins, Philadelphia.

Stacey, R.G., Filshie, J. and Skewes, D. (1991) Percutaneous insertion of Hickman-type catheters. *British Journal of Hospital Medicine*, 46 (6), 396–398.

Stanley, A. (2002) Managing complications of chemotherapy administration, in *The Cytotoxics Handbook*, 4th edn (eds M. Allwood, A. Stanley and P. Wright). Radcliffe Medical Press, Oxford, pp.119–192.

Stevens, B., Barton, S.E., Brechbill, M., Moenter, S., Piel, A.L. and Shankle, D. (2000) A randomized, prospective trial of conventional vascular ports vs the Vortex "Clear-Flow" reservoir port in adult oncology patients. *Journal of Vascular Access Devices*, 5 (2), 37–40.

Stewart, D. (2001) The percussion technique for restoring patency to central venous catheters. *Care of the Critically Ill*, 17 (3), 106–107.

Tagalakis, V., Kahn, S.R., Libman, M. and Blostein, M. (2002) The epidemiology of peripheral vein infusion thrombophlebitis: a critical review. *American Journal of Medicine*, 113 (2), 146–151.

1163

Tegtmeyer, K., Brady, G., Lai, S. *et al.* (2006) Videos in Clinical Medicine. Placement of an arterial line. *New England Journal of Medicine*, **354** (15), e13.

Teplitz, L. (1990) Arterial line disconnection. *Nursing*, **20** (5), 33.

Thompson, A.M., Kidd, E., McKenzie, M. *et al.* (1989) Long term central venous access: the patient's view. *Intensive Therapy and Clinical Monitoring*, **10** (5), 142–145.

Timoney, J.P., Malkin, M.G., Leone, D.M. *et al.* (2002) Safe and cost effective use of alteplase for the clearance of occluded central venous access devices. *Journal of Clinical Oncology*, **20** (7), 1918–1922.

Timsit, J.F. (2000) Scheduled replacement of central venous catheters is not necessary. *Infection Control and Hospital Epidemiology*, **21** (6), 371–374.

Timsit, J.F., Schwebel, C., Bouadma, L. *et al.* (2009) Chlorhexidine-impregnated sponges and less frequent dressing changes for prevention of catheter-related infections in critically ill adults: a randomized controlled trial. *JAMA*, **301** (12), 1231–1241.

Tinker, J. and Zapol, W.M. (1992) *Care of the Critically Ill Patient*, 2nd edn. Springer-Verlag, New York.

Usichenko, T.I., Pavlovic, D., Foellner, S. and Wendt, M. (2004) Reducing venipuncture pain by a cough trick: a randomized crossover volunteer study. *Anesthesia and Analgesia*, **98** (2), 343–345.

Verghese, S.T., Nath, A., Zenger, D. *et al.* (2002) The effects of the simulated Valsalva maneuver, liver compression, and/or Trendelenburg position on the cross-sectional area of the internal jugular vein in infants and young children. *Anesthesia and Analgesia*, **94** (2), 250–254.

Vesely, T.M. (2002) Optimal positioning of CVC's. *Journal of Vascular Access Devices*, **7** (3), 9–12.

Vesely, T.M. (2003) Central venous catheter tip position: a continuing controversy. *Journal of Cardiovascular and Interventional Radiology*, **14** (5), 527–534.

Viale, P.H. (2003) Complications associated with implantable vascular access devices in the patient with cancer. *Journal of Infusion Nursing*, **26** (2), 97–102.

Walker, E. (2009) Piloting a nurse-led ultrasound cannulation scheme. *British Journal of Nursing*, **18** (14), 854–859.

Wallach, S.G. (2004) Cannulation injury of the radial artery: diagnosis and treatment algorithm. *American Journal of Critical Care*, **13** (4), 315–319.

Waugh, A., Grant, A., Chambers, G. and Ross, J.S. (2006) *Ross and Wilson Anatomy and Physiology in Health and Illness*, 10th edn. Churchill Livingstone/Elsevier, Edinburgh.

Weinstein, S. and Plumer, A.L. (2007) *Plumer's Principles and Practice of Intravenous Therapy*, 8th edn. Lippincott Williams and Wilkins, Philadelphia.

Weller, B.F. and Royal College of Nursing (2005) *Baillière's Nurses' Dictionary*, 24th edn. Elsevier, Edinburgh.

Wells, S. (2008) Venous access in oncology and haematology patients: part two. *Nursing Standard*, **23** (1), 35–42.

Wendler, M.C. (2003) Effects of Tellington touch in healthy adults awaiting venipuncture. *Research in Nursing and Health*, **26** (1), 40–52.

Wigmore, T., Smythe, J.F., Hacking, M.B. *et al.* (2007) Effect of the implementation of NICE guidelines for ultrasound guidance on the complication rates associated with central venous catheter placement in patients presenting for routine surgery in a tertiary referral centre. *British Journal of Anaesthesia*, **99** (5), 662–665.

Williamson, E.E. and McKinney, J.M. (2001) Assessing the adequacy of peripherally inserted central catheters for power injection of intravenous contrast agents for CT. *Journal of Computer Assisted Tomography*, **25** (6), 932–937.

Wilson, J. (2006) *Infection Control in Clinical Practice*, 3rd edn. Baillière Tindall Elsevier, Edinburgh.

Wise, M., Richardson, D. and Lum, P. (2001) Catheter tip position: a sign of things to come! *Journal of Vascular Access Devices*, **6** (2), 18–27.

Yamamoto, A.J., Solomon, J.A., Soulen, M.C. *et al.* (2002) Sutureless securement device reduces complications of peripherally inserted central venous catheters. *Journal of Vascular and Interventional Radiology*, **13** (1), 77–81.

Young, A.M., Begum, G., Billingham, L.J. *et al.* (2005) WARP: a multi-centre prospective randomised controlled trial (RCT) of thrombosis prophylaxis with warfarin in cancer patients with central venous catheters (CVCs). Abstract 8804. *Journal of Clinical Oncology*, **23** (16S).

Yuan, T.R.W. and Cohan, M.D. (1987) Lateral antebrachial cutaneous nerve injury as a complication of phlebotomy. *Journal of the Canadian Intravenous Nurses Association*, **3** (3), 16–17.

Zideman, D.A. and Morgan, M. (1981) Inadvertent intra-arterial injection of flucloxacillin. *Anaesthesia*, **36** (3), 296–298.

Wound management

The Royal Marsden Hospital Manual of Clinical Nursing Procedures, Eighth Edition. Edited by Lisa Dougherty and Sara Lister.
© 2011 The Royal Marsden Hospital. Published 2011 by Blackwell Publishing Ltd.

Overview

The aim of this chapter is to provide an overview of wound care principles and current practice in managing acute surgical wounds, plastic surgical approaches and wounds related to oncology and cancer treatment.

Wounds

Definition

A wound can be defined as an injury to living tissue, breaking its continuity (Martin 2010). Wounds can be divided into six basic categories:

1 contusion (bruise)
2 abrasion (graze)
3 laceration (tear)
4 incision (cut)
5 puncture (stab)
6 burn.

Both external and internal factors can contribute to the formation of a wound.

- *External*: mechanical (friction, surgery), chemical, electrical, temperature extremes, radiation, micro-organisms.
- *Internal*: circulatory system failure (venous, arterial, lymphatic), endocrine (diabetes), neuropathy, haematological (porphyria cutanea tarda, mycosis fungoides), malignancy (fungating wound, Marjolin's ulcer (Naylor *et al.* 2001)).

Anatomy and physiology

The skin is the largest organ in the body and makes up about 10% of the adult total bodyweight (Hess 2005). The skin is important as it functions as an outer boundary for the body and helps preserve the balance within (Solomon *et al.* 1990). The skin needs to remain intact to perform vital functions (Timmons 2006) and without it humans would not survive insults from bacterial invasion or heat and water loss (Marieb and Hoehn 2010).

The skin varies in thickness from 1.5 to 4 mm depending upon which part of the body it is covering (Marieb and Hoehn 2010). The skin is made up of two main layers, the dermis and epidermis, which have six main functions: protection, sensation, thermoregulation, metabolism, excretion and non-verbal communication (Hess 2005, Timmons 2006).

The *epidermis* is the outermost layer and is avascular and thin. It regenerates every 4–6 weeks and functions as a protective barrier, preventing environmental damage and micro-organism invasion (Hess 2005). The thickness of the epidermis varies and it is thicker over the palms of the hands and soles of the feet (Marieb and Hoehn 2010).

The *dermis* provides support and transports nutrients to the epidermis. It contains blood and lymphatic vessels, sweat and oil glands and hair follicles. The dermis is made up of collagen and fibroblasts, elastins and other extracellular proteins which bind it together and keep it strong (Hess 2005). Its extracellular matrix (ECM) contains fibroblasts, macrophages and some mast cells and white blood cells (Marieb and Hoehn 2010). The connective tissue within the dermis is highly elastic and provides strength to maintain the skin's integrity and combat everyday stretching and wear and tear (Timmons 2006).

The subcutaneous layer just below the dermis is the deepest extension and binds the skin to underlying tissues (Solomon *et al.* 1990). This layer is known as the *hypodermis* or superficial fascia and stores fat. It also assists the body as a protective layer and allows movement (Marieb and Hoehn 2010).

Related theory
Classification of wounds

There are many different wound classification systems available and choice depends on the type of information required. A wound may be classified simply according to the method of healing, for example primary, secondary or tertiary intention (Miller and Dyson 1996), but this does not provide any information about the wound's characteristics. Further simple classification systems include whether the wound is acute (of short duration), chronic (of long duration) or according to the amount of tissue loss (Dealey 2005). A classification system that contains an appraisal of tissue loss is considered most useful (Flanagan 1996). Superficial, partial-thickness wounds are usually traumatic and painful, but retain the hair follicles or sweat glands and part of the dermis and are usually considered *acute wounds*, whilst full-thickness wounds destroy the dermis and some deeper layers may also be involved (Dealey 2005). Full-thickness wounds take longer to heal and can be life threatening if necrosis or infection complicates healing (Hampton and Collins 2004), and are therefore *chronic wounds*.

Evidence-based approaches
Methods of wound healing

Wound healing is the process by which damaged tissue is restored to normal function. Healing may occur by primary, second or tertiary intention. Healing by *primary intention* involves the union of the edges of a wound under aseptic conditions, for example, a laceration or incision that is closed with sutures or skin adhesive (Dealey 2005, Miller and Dyson 1996).

Healing by *secondary intention* occurs when the wound's edges cannot be brought together. The wound is left open and allowed to heal by contraction and epithelialization. Epithelialization encourages restoration of the skin's integrity (Giele and Cassell 2008). Wounds that heal by secondary intention include surgical or traumatic wounds where a large amount of tissue has been lost, heavily infected wounds, chronic wounds or, in some cases, where a better cosmetic or functional result will be achieved (Calvin 1998, Miller and Dyson 1996).

Healing by *tertiary intention*, or delayed primary closure, occurs when a wound has been left open and is then closed primarily after a few days' delay, usually once swelling, infection or bleeding has decreased (Giele and Cassell 2008).

Phases of wound healing

Wound healing is a cellular and biochemical process which relies essentially on an inflammatory process (Hampton and Collins 2004). These processes are dynamic, depend upon each other and overlap (Dealey 2005, Timmons 2006). It is important to support a wound-healing environment that encourages progression from one phase to the next without bacterial contamination, as this increases slough and necrosis (Hampton and Collins 2004).

The generally accepted stages of healing are:

1 haemostasis
2 inflammatory phase
3 proliferation or reconstructive phase
4 maturation or remodelling phase.

(Dealey 2005)

There are a number of internal and external factors that may influence normal wound healing and cause a delay in progress through these stages (Table 19.1). Growth factors involved throughout these phases act on individual cells to promote cell growth.

Haemostasis (minutes)

Vasoconstriction occurs within a few seconds of tissue injury and damaged blood vessels constrict to stem the blood flow. When platelets come into contact with exposed collagen from damaged blood vessels, they release chemical messengers that stimulate a 'clotting cascade' (Flanagan 2000, Hampton and Collins 2004, Timmons 2006). Platelets adhere to vessel walls and are stabilized by fibrin networks to

Table 19.1 Factors that delay wound healing

Extrinsic factor	Action	Intrinsic factor	Action
Cold	Any drop in temperature delays healing by up to 4 hours	Age	The elderly have a thinning of the dermis and underlying structural support for the wound (i.e. less moisture and subcutaneous fat). The metabolic process and circulation also slow with age
Excessive heat	Temperature over 30°C reduces tensile strength and causes vasoconstriction	Medical and general health conditions	Diabetes, cardiopulmonary disease, hypovolaemic shock, rheumatoid arthritis, anaemia, obesity
Chronic excessive exudate	Wounds should not be too wet or too dry (see moisture balance section in Table 19.2)	Malnutrition or protein–energy malnutrition	Poor healing, decreased tensile strength and higher risk of wound dehiscence and infection. Low serum albumin causes oedema
Poor dressing application and techniques	Gaping of dressing material or multiple layers Tape/adhesive not fastened securely and allowing slipping of wound exudates/dressing materials and/or bandaging too tight/loose	Psychosocial factors	Alcohol and smoking (carbon monoxide affects the blood vessels and circulation of oxygen), poor mobility, stress, isolation, anxiety and altered body image
Poor surgical technique	Prolonged operating time, inappropriate use of diathermy and drains can lead to haematomas and infection	Drugs	Steroids and non-steroidal anti-inflammatories, anti-inflammatories, immunosuppressives, cytotoxic chemotherapy

From Bale and Jones (2006), ConvaTec (2004), Hampton and Collins (2004).

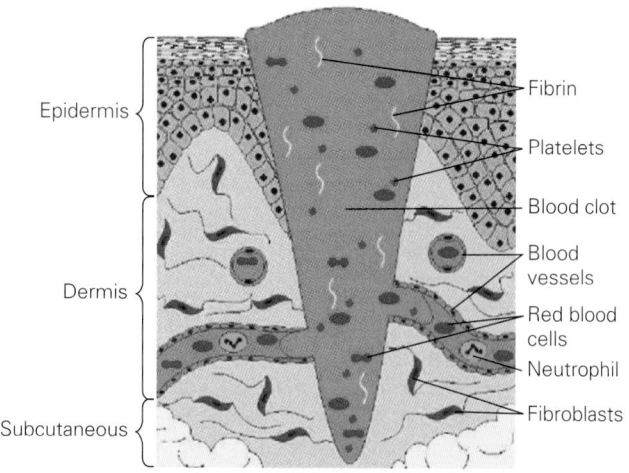

Figure 19.1 Haemostasis in a wound. Reproduced by kind permission of Wayne Naylor.

form a clot. Bleeding ceases when the blood vessels thrombose, usually within 5–10 minutes of injury (Hampton and Collins 2004). See Figure 19.1.

Inflammatory phase (1–5 days)

With the activation of clotting factors comes the release of histamine and vasodilation begins (Dowsett 2002, Flanagan 1996). The liberation of histamine also increases the permeability of the capillary walls and plasma proteins, leucocytes, antibodies and electrolytes exude into the surrounding tissues. The wound becomes red, swollen and hot. These signs are accompanied by pain and tenderness at the wound site, last for 1–3 days and can be mistaken for wound infection (Hampton 2008). See Figure 19.2.

Polymorphonuclear leucocytes and macrophages migrate to the wound within hours and these phagocytose debris

and bacteria and begin the process of repair (Hart 2002). If the number and function of macrophages are reduced, as may occur in disease, for example diabetes (Springett 2002), or due to treatment, for example chemotherapy in cancer patients (Tobias and Hochhauser 2010), healing processes are affected. Nutrients and oxygen are required to produce the cellular activity and therefore malnourished patients and hypoxic wounds are more susceptible to infection (Dealey 2005, Timmons 2006). The breakdown of debris causes an increased osmolarity within the area, resulting in further swelling. A chronic wound can get stuck in this phase of wound healing (Collier 2002, Dealey 2005, Hampton and Collins 2004) with prolonged healing, tendency to infection and high levels of exudate (Timmons 2006).

Proliferative phase (3–24 days)

Acute wounds will start to granulate within 3 days, but the inflammatory and proliferative phases can overlap, with both granulation and sloughy tissue present (Timmons 2006). See Figure 19.3.

The fibroblasts are activated to divide and produce collagen by processes initiated by the macrophages (Timmons 2006). Newly synthesized collagen creates a 'healing ridge' below an intact suture line, thus giving an indication of how primary wound healing is progressing. Wound healing by secondary intention will also have a healing rim around it as the wound contracts. This mechanism is dependent on the presence of iron, vitamin C and oxygen. Vitamin C (ascorbic acid) and lactate are stimulants for fibroblast activity (Hampton and Collins 2004). Fibroblasts are also dependent on the local oxygen supply (Dealey 2005). The wound surface and the oxygen tension within encourage the macrophages to instigate the process of angiogenesis, forming new blood cell vessels (Dealey 2005, Hampton and Collins 2004). These vessels branch and join other vessels, forming loops. The fragile capillary loops are held within a framework

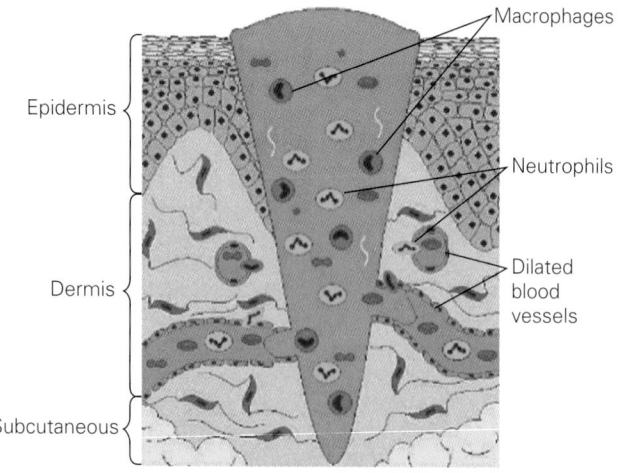

Figure 19.2 The inflammatory phase of wound healing. Reproduced by kind permission of Wayne Naylor.

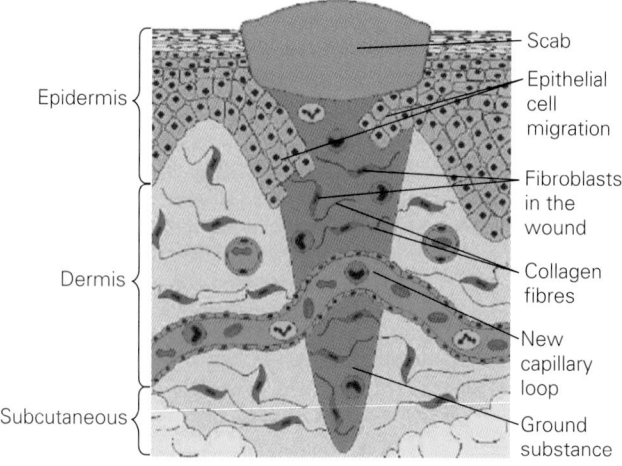

Figure 19.3 The proliferative phase of wound healing. Reproduced by kind permission of Wayne Naylor.

of collagen. This complex is known as granulation tissue. At this stage, the wound will appear pink and moist with raised red bumps (Hampton and Collins 2004).

The process of wound contraction can significantly reduce the size of the wound and the area that new tissue must cover. It is extremely important and only observable in open wounds healing by secondary intention. There is debate about the exact method by which wound contraction occurs (Tejero-Trujeque 2001).

Re-epithelialization of the wound usually begins within 24 hours of injury (Calvin 1998, Garrett 1997). Macrophages produce a number of growth factors including keratinocyte growth factor (KGF) which stimulates a proliferation of cells within the wound bed (Timmons 2006). Epithelial cells (keratinocytes) may migrate from hair follicles and sweat glands within the wound or from the perimeter of the wound (Moore and Foster 1998). Endothelial buds grow and the fibroblasts continue the process of repair by laying down fibrous tissue (Hampton and Collins 2004). Epithelial cells will burrow under contaminated debris and unwanted material (Waldorf and Fewkes 1995) while also secreting an enzyme that separates the scab from underlying tissue. Dissolving dry eschar requires nearly 50% of the cell's metabolic energy (Dealey 2005). Through a mechanism called contact inhibition, epithelial cells will cease migrating when they come into contact with other epithelial cells (Garrett 1997).

Epithelialization (migration, mitosis and differentiation) occurs at an increased rate in a moist wound environment, as do the synthesis of collagen and formation of new capillaries (Flanagan 1999). Wound contraction is a function of myofibroblasts, which are prominent in granulating tissue. The extent of wound contraction is dependent on the number of myofibroblasts present and it is maintained by collagen deposition and cross-linking (Giele and Cassell 2008). The rate of epithelialization is influenced by growth factors (Timmons 2006) but little is known about the reality of growth factor activity in chronic wounds (Hampton and Collins 2004).

Maturation phase (21 days onward)

This stage begins at around 21 days following the initial injury (Figure 19.4). Maturation or remodelling of the healed wound may last for more than a year. Collagen is reorganized, the fibres becoming enlarged and orientated along the lines of tension in the wound (at right angles to the wound margin) (Silver 1994). This occurs via a process of lysis and resynthesis. Intermolecular cross-linking aids the tensile strength of the wound. During this reorganization fibroblasts may constrict the neighbouring collagen fibres surrounding them, causing contraction of the tissue and reduction of blood vessels within the scar (Cho and Hunt 2001). Maximum strength is reached in approximately 3 months, although the scar will only achieve about 70–80% of normal skin strength (Calvin 1998, Ehrlich 1998). At the end of the maturation phase, the delicate granulation tissue of the wound will have been replaced by stronger avascular scar tissue. Rationalization of the blood vessels also results

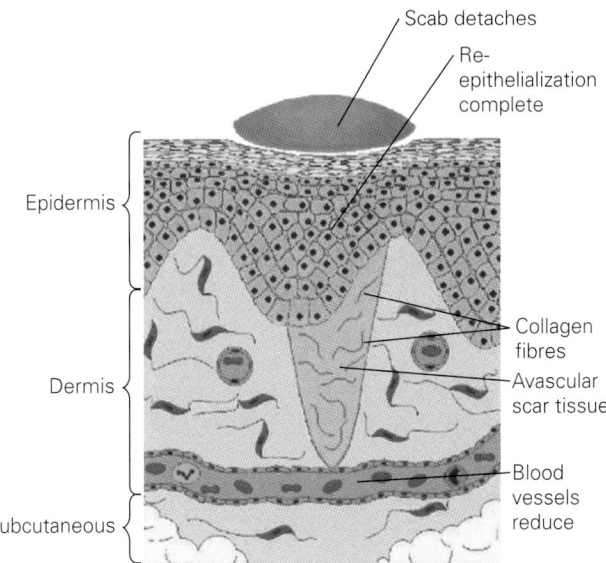

Figure 19.4 The maturation phase of wound healing. Reproduced by kind permission of Wayne Naylor.

in thinning and fading of the scar, although it is not fully known why this varies amongst people (Dealey 2005).

Methods of wound assessment

In order to provide a method of wound assessment and a simple way of selecting appropriate dressings, an international group of wound care experts developed a concept using 'TIME' (tissue, infection/inflammation, moisture balance and edge advancement) as an acronym to identify the key barriers to healing (Dowsett and Ayello 2004, Werdin et al. 2008) (see Table 19.2).

Wound bed preparation

Wound bed preparation (WBP) focuses on controlling and optimizing the wound environment for healing (Falanga 2000). It provides a means of bringing together a cohesive plan of both patient and wound care (Ayello et al. 2004, Vowden and Vowden 2002).

Tissue factors affecting wound healing

The rate of wound healing varies depending on the general health of the individual, the location of the wound, the degree of damage and the treatment applied. It is necessary when treating a wound to appraise all potential detrimental factors and minimize them, where possible, in order to provide the optimum systemic, local and external conditions for healing.

Factors that may delay healing include disease (including malignancy), poor nutritional state and infection. Other influences involve the local microenvironment of the wound, including temperature, pH, humidity, air gas composition, oxygen tension, blood supply and inflammation (Storch and Rice 2005). Whether this influence is positive or negative

Table 19.2 TIME principles for wound bed preparation

TIME	Status	Problem	Solution
Tissue	Tissue not viable	Defective matrix cell debris impairing healing	Debridement
Inflammation and infection	Colonized → infection continuum	Wound healing delayed	Topical antimicrobials dependent on bacterial load
Moisture balance	Dry → excessive moisture	Maceration potential	Restore moisture balance
			Prevent maceration to peri-wound margins
Edge of wound	Non-migrating keratinocytes	Wound not closing	Reassess cause or consider corrective therapies

Adapted from Schultz *et al.* (2003); permission granted by Smith & Nephew.

may depend on the stage of wound healing that has been reached. Other important considerations are external variables such as continuing trauma, possibly caused by treatment or the presence of foreign bodies. Factors known to affect wound healing are listed in Table 19.1.

Achieving a well-vascularized wound bed

Improving the blood flow to the wound bed will increase the availability of nutrients, oxygen, active cells and growth factors within the wound environment (Collier 2002). This may be achieved through the use of compression therapy, topical negative pressure therapy or wound management products that exert an osmotic pull on the wound bed, increasing capillary growth, for example Vacutex (Collier 2002).

Debridement of devitalized tissue

Surgical debridement is the most effective method of removing necrotic tissue (Wolcott *et al.* 2009). It is performed by a surgeon and usually involves excision of extensive or deep areas of necrosis, usually to the point of bleeding viable tissue to 'kickstart' healing (Hampton and Collins 2004). While this option is very effective, it carries the risks associated with general anaesthesia. An alternative method of rapid debridement is 'sharp' debridement, which may be utilized for the removal of loose, devitalized, superficial tissue only (Vowden and Vowden 1999). Sharp debridement can be performed at the patient's bedside by an experienced healthcare professional with relevant training (Poston 1996). However, this can be a dangerous practice in inexperienced hands and is controversial (Fairbairn *et al.* 2002). Potentially, ligaments may be severed as they can have the appearance of sloughy tissue or vascular damage could occur (Hampton and Collins 2004). It is also acknowledged that informed patient consent is required as this is an invasive procedure with potential risks and complications (Fairbairn *et al.* 2002).

Autolytic debridement is recommended as a less invasive technique which utilizes the body's natural debriding mechanism. This effect is enhanced in a moist wound environment, which can be achieved through the use of hydrogel dressings or semi-occlusive dressings that maintain moisture at the wound surface. Many dressings are designed for this purpose and break down necrotic tissue naturally (Hampton and Collins 2004, Hess 2005) (Table 19.3).

Inflammation and infection (or bacterial burden)

It is generally agreed that all chronic wounds harbour a variety of bacteria to some degree and this can range from contamination through colonization to infection. There is also a stage between colonization and infection called 'critical colonization' where the bacterial load has reached a level just below clinical infection (Collier 2002). When a wound becomes infected, it will display the characteristic signs of heat, redness, swelling, pain, heavy exudate and malodour. The patient may also develop generalized pyrexia. However, immunosuppressed patients, diabetic patients or those on systemic steroid therapy may not present with the classic signs of infection. Instead, they may experience delayed healing, breakdown of the wound, presence of friable granulation tissue that bleeds easily, formation of an epithelial tissue bridge over the wound, increased production of exudate and malodour and increased pain (Cutting 1998, Gilchrist 1999). Careful wound assessment is essential to identify potential sites for infection, although routine swabbing of the area is not considered to be beneficial (Donovan 1998).

Methods available for the management of wound infection or to decrease the bacterial burden in the wound include debridement, antimicrobial dressings, for example those containing iodine or silver, topical negative pressure therapy and antibiotic therapy. Honey and essential oils have also been used and there is a growing body of literature to this effect (see Fungating wounds). Appropriate antibiotic treatment of the infection should be determined from a positive wound swab(s).

Moisture balance

Wound exudate usually performs a useful function of cleaning the wound and providing nutrients to the healing wound bed. However, in the presence of excess exudate, the process of wound healing can be adversely affected. This is especially so in chronic wounds where wound fluid may actually prevent the proliferation of cells vital to wound healing, such as fibroblasts, keratinocytes and endothelial cells (Vowden and Vowden 2002).

Table 19.3 Dressing groups. Please refer to manufacturer's recommendations with regard to individual products

Dressings	Description	Advantages	Disadvantages
Activated charcoal	Contains a layer of activated charcoal that traps and reduces odour-causing molecules *Example*: Carbonet, Clinisorb	Easy to apply as either primary or secondary dressing; can be combined with another dressing with absorbency *Example*: Kaltocarb	Need to obtain a good seal to prevent leakage of odour; some dressings lose effectiveness when wet[a]
Adhesive island	Consists of a low adherent absorbent pad located centrally on an adhesive backing *Example*: Mepore and Pad, Opsite Post-Op	Quick and easy to apply; protects the suture line from contamination and absorbs exudate/blood	Only suitable for light exudate; some can cause skin damage (excoriation, blistering) if applied incorrectly
Alginates	A textile fibre dressing made from seaweed; the soft woven fibres gel as they absorb exudate and promote autolytic debridement. Available as a sheet, ribbon or packing *Example*: Kaltostat, Sorbsan, Algisorb	Are suitable for moderate to heavy exudate; can be used on infected wounds; useful for sinus and fistula drainage; have haemostatic properties; can be irrigated out of wound with warm saline	Cannot be used on dry wounds or wound with hard necrotic tissue (eschar); sometimes a mild burning or 'drawing' sensation is reported on application[a]
Antimicrobials	These topical dressings can be used as primary or secondary dressings and are available as a primary layer (*example*: Acticoat) and impregnated in other dressings (*examples*: Aquacel Ag, Mepilex Ag, Allevyn Ag) or as a cream (*example*: Flamazine)	Suitable for chronic wounds with heavy exudate that need protection from bacterial contamination by providing a broad range of antimicrobial activity; can reduce or prevent infection	Cannot be used during radiotherapy; sometimes sensitivity occurs with the use of silver and some skin staining can occur; instructions vary with products and dressings are expensive Evidence base for use is controversial and needs monitoring[a]
Capillary wound dressings	Composed of 100% polyester filament outer layers and a 65% polyester and 35% cotton woven inner layer; outer layer draws exudate, interstitial fluid and necrotic tissue into the inner layer via a capillary action *Example*: Vacutex	Suitable for light to heavy exudate; debride necrotic tissue; protect and insulate the wound; maintain a moist environment and prevent maceration; encourage development of granulation tissue; can be cut to any shape and are available in large rolls; can be used as a wick to drain sinus and cavity wounds	Can be hard to cut and are quite stiff to fit into wounds; cannot be used on malignant wounds or where there is the risk of bleeding due to the 'drawing' action and resultant increase in blood flow to the wound bed Expensive and should be used on a named patient basis
Collagen	This protein is fibrous and insoluble and produced by fibroblasts. Collagen encourages collagen fibres into the granulation tissue. It is available in sheets/gels *Example*: Promogran	Conforms well to wound surface, maintains a moist environment, suitable for most wounds to accelerate healing. Supports ECM	Not recommended for necrotic wounds[a]
Foams	Produced in a variety of forms, most being constructed of polyurethane foam and may have one or more layers; foam cavity dressings are also available *Examples*: Allevyn, Mepilex, Biatain, PolyMem	Suitable for use with open, exuding wounds; highly absorbent, non-adherent and maintain a moist wound bed Available for low-high exudates and/or bordered to simplify dressing choice	May be difficult to use in wounds with deep tracts and need a combined approach with an alginate or in fungating wounds
Honey – most widely used is Manuka honey	Available as tubes of liquid honey (*example*: Actibalm) or impregnated dressings (*example*: Activon Tulle; Mesitran (with hydrogel sheet))	Suitable for acute and chronic infected, necrotic or sloughy wounds; provides a moist wound environment; non-adherent; antibacterial; assists with wound debridement; eliminates wound malodour; has an anti-inflammatory effect	Can be messy to use and causes leakage if excess exudate is present[a] May have a burning/drawing effect when first applied

(Continued)

Table 19.3 (*Continued*)

Dressings	Description	Advantages	Disadvantages
Hydrocolloid	Usually consists of a base material containing gelatin, pectin and carboxymethylcellulose combined with adhesives and polymers; base material may be bonded to either a semi-permeable film or a film plus polyurethane foam; some have a border	Suitable for acute and chronic wounds with low to no exudate; provides a moist wound environment; promotes wound debridement; provides thermal insulation; waterproof and barrier to micro-organisms; easy to use	May release degradation products into the wound; strong odour produced as dressing interacts with exudate; some hydrocolloids cannot be used on infected wounds
Hydrofibre	Same consistency as hydrocolloid but in a soft woven sheet (also available with silver or combined with Duoderm in Combiderm) *Example*: Aquacel	Forms a soft, hydrophilic, gas-permeable gel on contact with the wound and manages exudate whilst preventing maceration of wound edge Easy to remove without trauma to wound bed	Does not have haemostatic property of alginates[a]
Hydrogels	Contain 17.5–90% water depending on the product, plus various other components to form a gel or solid sheet *Examples*: AquaForm Gel, Granugel, Geliperm (Sheet)	Suitable for light exudate wounds; absorb small amounts of exudate; donate fluid to dry necrotic tissue; reduce pain and are cooling; low trauma at dressing changes; can be used as carrier for drugs	Cool the wound surface; use with caution in infected wounds; can cause skin maceration due to leakage if too much gel is applied or the wound has moderate to heavy exudate[a] Moderate care of sheets so they do not dry out
Semi-permeable films	Polyurethane film with a hypoallergenic acrylic adhesive; have a variety of application methods often consisting of a plastic or cardboard carrier *Examples*: Tegaderm, Opsite	Only suitable for shallow superficial wounds; prophylactic use against friction damage; useful as retention dressing; allow passage of water vapour; allow monitoring of the wound	Possibility of adhesive trauma if removed incorrectly; do not contain exudate and can macerate, slip or leak Should not be used to cover an Allevyn dressing
Skin barrier film	Alcohol-free liquid polymer that forms a protective film on the skin *Example*: Cavilon (also comes as a barrier cream)	Non-cytotoxic; does not sting if applied to raw areas of skin; high wash-off resistance; protects the skin from body fluids, friction and shear and the effects of adhesive products	Requires good manual dexterity to apply; may cause skin warming on application

Dealey (2005); Hess (2005).
[a]Requires a secondary dressing.
Dressing Data Cards are also available from World Wide Wounds (2004).

The control of oedema or lymphoedema and lessening the bacterial burden on the wound will undoubtedly help in the reduction of wound exudate. However, if the methods for achieving these goals are unsuccessful or contraindicated then exudate must be managed through the use of wound management products. These include such products as absorbent wound dressings (e.g. alginates, hydrofibre, foams), non-adherent wound contact layers with a secondary absorbent pad, wound manager bags and topical negative pressure therapy (White 2001). It is also vital to protect the skin surrounding the wound from maceration by excess exudate and excoriation from corrosive exudate. Useful products for skin protection include ointments/pastes (e.g. zinc oxide BP), alcohol-free skin barrier films and thin hydrocolloid sheets used to 'frame' the wound.

Edge non-advancement

The clearest sign that the wound is failing to heal is when the epidermal edge is not advancing over time (Dowsett and Ayello 2004). In this case a thorough assessment should commence using the TIME principles and interventions.

Principles of wound cleaning

The aim of wound cleaning is to help create the optimum local conditions for wound healing by removal of excess debris, exudate, foreign and necrotic material, toxic components, bacteria and other micro-organisms.

If the wound is clean and little exudate is present, repeated cleaning is contraindicated since it may damage new tissue, decrease the temperature of the wound unnecessarily and remove exudate (Morison 1989). A fall in the temperature of the wound of 12°C is possible if the procedure is prolonged or the lotions are cold. It can take 3 hours or longer for the wound to return to normal temperature, during which time the cellular activity is reduced and therefore the healing process slowed (Collier 1996).

Sodium chloride (0.9%) is a physiologically balanced solution that has a similar osmotic pressure to that already present in living cells and is therefore compatible with human tissue (Lawrence 1997). Used at body temperature, it is the safest and best cleaning solution for non-contaminated wounds (Fletcher 1997, Miller and Dyson 1996). Although sodium chloride has no antiseptic properties, it dilutes bacteria and is non-toxic to tissue (Thomas 2009). Tap water is also advocated for cleaning chronic wounds (Riyat and Quinton 1997). A study demonstrated that, in comparison with sterile 0.9% sodium chloride, lower rates of infection were found in the group where tap water was used (Angeras *et al.* 1992).

Principles of dressing a wound

With the exception of wounds where the main aim is to ameliorate symptoms such as malignant wounds, an ideal wound dressing must be capable of fulfilling the following functions.

- Removes excess exudate and toxic components.
- Maintains a high humidity at the wound–dressing interface.
- Allows gaseous exchange.
- Provides thermal insulation.
- Is impermeable to bacteria.
- Is free from particulate or toxic components.
- Allows change without trauma.
- Is acceptable to the patient.
- Is highly absorbent (for heavily exuding wounds).
- Is cost-effective.
- Provides mechanical protection.
- Is conformable and mouldable.
- Is able to be sterilized.
  (Field and Kerstein 1994, Hampton 1999, Morgan 2000)

In addition, the dressing should minimize pain, odour and bleeding and be comfortable when in place.

A moist wound environment has been shown to affect a wound in the following ways. It:

- increases rate of epithelial migration
- reduces the lag phase between epithelial cell proliferation and differentiation
- encourages synthesis of collagen and ground substance
- promotes formation of capillary loops
- decreases length of inflammatory phase
- reduces pain and trauma due to dressing adherence
- promotes breakdown of necrotic tissue
- speeds wound contraction.
  (Flanagan 1999, Garrett 1997, Miller and Dyson 1996, Williams and Young 1998)

Preprocedural considerations

Equipment

Dressings are named and categorized to make choices more clear (see Table 19.3 for details of groups of dressings). The dressing that is applied directly over the wound bed is the **primary** dressing. Dry dressings (such as gauze) do not provide most of the criteria for an ideal dressing and should not be used as a primary contact layer as they are likely to adhere and disturb healing (Dealey 2005). This depends on the definition of 'dry' dressing as some dressings appear dry but 'gel' on contact with the wound, which maintains a moist environment, and are non-adhesive, thus becoming 'wet' (examples include Aquacel, alginates and hydrocolloids). The wound itself has the ability to produce moisture.

Wet dressings, such as hydrogels, can make a wound too wet and be responsible for maceration if used inappropriately (Hampton and Collins 2004).

Occlusive dressings achieve many of the criteria for an ideal dressing. They affect the wound and healing in several ways. They have the ability to maintain hydration and prevent the formation of an eschar. As they are designed for moderate exudates, chronic wounds (or fungating wounds) and pressure sores are often dressed with occlusive dressings that are bordered with adhesive. They have a combined primary and secondary layer (examples include Mepilex, Lyofoam, Allevyn and Granuflex). If patients have sensitive skin (or are undergoing radiotherapy) and adhesive borders are traumatic, dressings should be held in place with netting (Netelast) or bandages. A simple secondary dressing is a gauze layer or dressing pad and tape or bandage to secure (see Table 19.3).

Care should be taken with wounds that are difficult shapes to treat. These include long, narrow cavities which require a dressing that can be comfortably inserted into the space but removed easily without leaving any fibres behind and without trauma (Bale 1991).

Dressings should be changed when leakage occurs or the dressing no longer absorbs exudates, around every 2–7 days or as instructed (Hess 2005).

Assessment and recording tools

The wound should be evaluated each time a dressing is applied or if it gives cause for concern. The aim of evaluating the wound is to assess healing and to establish which treatment will best provide the ideal environment for healing. The surface area or volume of the wound should be measured and recorded. Photography also provides a useful record of wound progression (Vowden 1995).

A list of variables that require regular assessment is shown in Table 19.1. Figure 19.5 is an example of a wound assessment chart. Teare and Barrett (2002) recommend that the underlying cause of the wound should also be assessed, with the primary focus on details such as size and depth as well as the stage of healing. Links can then be made between the wound dressing and the optimal healing environment. The

THE ROYAL MARSDEN WOUND ASSESSMENT CHART
Complete one chart for each wound

Patient name:						
Hospital number:						
Date of assessment (weekly)						

Wound dimensions

Max length (cm)						
Max width (cm)						
Max depth (cm)						

Wound bed – approximate % cover (enter %)

Necrotic (BLACK)						
Slough (YELLOW)						
Granulating (RED)						
Epithelializing (PINK)						

Skin around wound

Intact						
Healthy						
Fragile						
Dry						
Scaly						
Erythema						
Maceration						
Oedema						
Eczema						
Skin nodules						
Skin stripping						
Dressing allergy						
Tape allergy						
Other (please state)						

Exudate level

None						
Low						
Moderate						
High						
Amount increasing						
Amount decreasing						

Odour (see over for rating scale)

None						
Slight						
Moderate						
Strong						

Bleeding

None						
Slight						
Moderate						
Heavy						
At dressing change						

Pain from wound (see over for rating scale)

Level (0–10)						
Continuous						
At specific times (specify)						

Wound infection suspected

Swab taken (Y/N)						
Swab result						
Treatment						
Assessment review date						
Initials of Assessor						

Figure 19.5 Wound assessment chart. Reproduced courtesy of the Royal Marsden Hospital NHS Foundation Trust.

Location (mark diagram):	Visual Analogue Scale (VAS) for Patient's Rating of Pain.

Right   Left   Left   Right

VAS scale: 0 1 2 3 4 5 6 7 8 9 10
No pain ... Worst pain imaginable

Rating Scale for Odour	
Score	Assessment
None	No odour evident, even when at the patient's bedside with the dressing removed.
Slight	Wound odour is evident at close proximity to the patient when the dressing is removed.
Moderate	Wound odour is evident upon entering the room (1.5 to 3 metres from patient) with the dressing removed.
Strong	Wound odour is evident upon entering the room (1.5 to 3 metres from patient) with the dressing intact.

Diagram of wound if appropriate (or attach tracing/photograph):

Date: _____	Date: _____
Date: _____	Date: _____
Date: _____	Date: _____

Notes on use
Use one chart per wound.
Complete a wound assessment at least once a week.
Measure the wound at its widest points using a clean ruler, use a sterile wound swab or blunt probe to measure wound depth.
For the 'skin around wound' assessment more than one box may be ticked.
Odour and pain should be assessed using the scales at the top of page 2.
Following the assessment a wound management care plan should be written and updated if necessary after each reassessment.

Figure 19.5 (*Continued*)

use of this type of documentation to assist in the assessment process is recommended to:

- facilitate continuity of care by providing a central reference point for wound progression
- facilitate appropriate evaluation of all relevant parameters
- fulfil legal and professional requirements (Teare and Barrett 2002).

Procedure guideline 19.1 Dressing a wound

Essential equipment

- Sterile dressing pack containing gallipots or an indented plastic tray, low-linting swabs and/or medical foam, disposable forceps, gloves, sterile field, disposable bag
- Fluids for cleaning and/or irrigation
- Hypoallergenic tape
- Appropriate dressing

- Appropriate hand hygiene preparation
- Any other material will be determined by the nature of the dressing; special features of a dressing should be referred to in the patient's nursing care plan
- Detergent wipe
- Total traceability system for surgical instruments and patient record form

Optional equipment

- Sterile scissors

Preprocedure

Action	Rationale
1 Explain and discuss the procedure with the patient.	To ensure that the patient understands the procedure and gives his or her valid consent (NMC 2008a, C; Wilson 2005, E).
2 Clean hands with bactericidal alcohol rub.	Hands must be cleaned before and after every patient contact and before commencing the preparations for aseptic technique, to prevent cross-infection (Fraise and Bradley 2009, E).
3 Clean trolley with detergent wipe.	To provide a clean working surface (Fraise and Bradley 2009, E).
4 Place all the equipment required for the procedure on the bottom shelf of the clean dressing trolley.	To maintain the top shelf as a clean working surface. E
5 Screen the bed area and provide privacy. Position the patient comfortably so that the area to be dealt with is easily accessible without exposing the patient unduly.	To allow any airborne organisms to settle before the sterile field (and in the case of a dressing, the wound) is exposed (Fraise and Bradley 2009, E). Maintain the patient's dignity and comfort. E
6 If the procedure is a dressing and the wound is infected or producing copious amounts of exudate, put on a disposable plastic apron.	To reduce the risk of cross-infection (Fraise and Bradley 2009, E).
7 Take the trolley to the treatment room or patient's bedside, disturbing the screens as little as possible.	To minimize airborne contamination (Fraise and Bradley 2009, E).

Procedure

8 Loosen the dressing tape.	To make it easier to remove the dressing. E
9 Clean hands with a bactericidal alcohol handrub.	To reduce the risk of wound infection (Fraise and Bradley 2009, E).
10 Check the pack is sterile (i.e. the pack is undamaged, intact and dry), open the outer cover of the sterile pack and slide the contents onto the top shelf of the trolley.	To ensure that only sterile products are used (Fraise and Bradley 2009, E).
11 Open the sterile field using only the corners of the paper.	So that areas of potential contamination are kept to a minimum. E

12	Where appropriate, loosen the old dressing.	The dressing can then be lifted off without causing trauma. E
13	Clean hands with a bactericidal alcohol handrub.	Hands may become contaminated by handling outer packets, dressing, and so on. (Fraise and Bradley 2009, E).
14	Using the plastic bag in the pack, arrange the sterile field. Pour cleaning solution into gallipots or an indented plastic tray.	The time the wound is exposed should be kept to a minimum to reduce the risk of contamination. To prevent contamination of the environment. To minimize risk of contamination of cleaning solution. E
15	Remove dressing by placing a hand in the plastic bag, lifting the dressing off and inverting the plastic bag so that the dressing is now inside the bag. Thereafter use this as the 'dirty' bag.	To reduce the risk of cross-infection. To prevent contamination of the environment. E
16	Attach the bag with the dressing to the side of the trolley below the top shelf.	Contaminated material should be below the level of the sterile field. E
17	Assess wound healing with reference to Table 19.2.	To evaluate wound care (Dealey 2005, E; Hampton and Collins 2004, E; Hess 2005, E).
18	Put on gloves.	To reduce the risk of infection to the wound and contamination of the nurse. Gloves provide greater sensitivity than forceps and are less likely to traumatize the wound or the patient's skin. E
19	If necessary, gently clean the wound with a gloved hand using 0.9% sodium chloride, unless another solution is indicated. If appropriate, irrigate by flushing with water or 0.9% sodium chloride.	To reduce the possibility of physical and chemical trauma to granulation and epithelial tissue (Hess 2005, E).
20	Apply the dressing that is most suitable for the wound using the criteria for dressings (see Table 19.3).	To promote healing and/or reduce symptoms. E
21	Remove gloves; fasten dressing as appropriate with hypoallergenic tape/Netelast/bandage/tapeless retention dressing.	To prevent irritation of skin and to avoid trauma to wound. E
22	Make sure the patient is comfortable and the dressing is secure.	A dressing may slip or feel uncomfortable as the patient changes position. E

Postprocedure

23	Dispose of waste in orange plastic clinical waste bags. Remove gloves.	To prevent environmental contamination. Orange is the recognized colour for clinical waste (DH 2005, C).
24	Draw back curtains and ensure the patient is comfortable.	
25	Check that the trolley remains dry and physically clean. If necessary, wipe with detergent wipe.	To reduce the risk of spreading infection (Fraise and Bradley 2009, E).
26	Record assessment in relevant documentation at the end of the procedure.	To maintain an accurate record of wound-healing progress (NMC 2009, C).

Problem-solving table 19.1 Prevention and resolution (Procedure guideline 19.1)

Problem	Cause	Prevention	Management
Bleeding	The wound is invading small blood vessels Because of their fragile vascular condition and capillary ooze, fungating wounds frequently bleed (Wilson 2005) Dry dressings are not soaked off and traumatize the friable tissues common to fungating wounds	Tranexamic acid can be taken regularly (10 day oral course; Alexander 2009) by patients known to have bleeding wounds or applied topically to specific points to minimize blood loss. It works by increasing clot formation	Ensuring that the surface of the wound has enough moisture to prevent trauma and adherence of dressings Using Kaltostat or similar calcium alginate and gentle compression is effective for small bleeds (Wilson 2005) Palliative radiotherapy (either a single fraction or short course; Tobias and Hochhauser 2010) Administer blood transfusion if indicated and patient is symptomatic
Malodour	Fatty acids are the by-product of the necrotic tissue within the wound and these produce malodour (Hampton 2008) Malodour can also be due to bacterial infection and a wound swab ought to be taken Lund-Neilsen et al. (2005) found that the 12 patients with malignant wounds in their study categorized odour into ordinary wound liquid and decay	Patient education Essential oils infusers (at least 2 in combination) Keeping room air circulating or windows open Allowing the patient to shower gently to remove old dressings and clean their wounds naturally Metrotop gel or oral antibiotics if infection present	Using dressings that absorb odour, and ensuring they are in contact with the wound bacteria (i.e. charcoal, silver as this is antimicrobial) Changing dressings when strike-through occurs Clearing of necrotic tissue by autolytic debridement (honey or Aquacel kept moist enough to gel either with saline or exudates) Honey has antibacterial properties and should be applied directly to the wound (impregnated versions are available to incorporate a suitable secondary dressing for absorption)
Pain	Combined causes, including general cancer burden in advanced disease The wound could be in an uncomfortable position	Soak off any dressings and use a skin barrier (i.e. Cavilon) to prevent tapes sticking Promoting a comfortable position for the patient Maintaining skin integrity	Provide analgesia on a continuous basis with a break-through dose as needed prior to changing dressing Minimize checking the dressing and changing it as appropriate Psychosocial support can relieve the emotions that increase pain and distress
Heavy exudates	Large tumours and advanced disease stages produce excessive volumes of exudates in fungating wounds and additional factors can be due to inappropriate dressings or infection (Selby 2009)	Absorption via appropriate dressings which allow vapour transfer at the wound surface into an absorbent backing layer	Whilst fungating wounds are often in challenging shapes, foam dressings are designed to hold excess moisture and are sponge-like, with some having a gentle wound contact layer that prevents maceration A drainage bag (stoma) system is suitable for those that need changing 2–3 times a day (Wilson 2005)

Postprocedural considerations

Ongoing care

Dressings need to be changed when 'strike-through' occurs, that is, the dressing becomes soiled and damp at the surface or edge or leakage of wound exudates occurs (see individual dressing packs for instructions to guide practice). The medical team may take the dressing down to view the wound and the nurse should be present to monitor this and reapply an appropriate dressing. Record any changes and/or instructions in the patient's notes or wound care plan (NMC 2009). Included in the notes should be the amount of exudate, any signs of inflammation or odour and appearance of the tissue (Lippincott Williams and Wilkins, 2008). Measuring or photographing the wound can also benefit ongoing assessment as long as this is appropriate and acceptable to the patient.

Fungating wounds

Definitions

A fungating wound is the result of a cancerous mass that infiltrates the epithelium and surrounding lymph and blood vessels (Pearson and Mortimer 2004). It can present as an ulcerating crater with a distinct margin or a raised fungating nodule (Bennett and Moody 1995). Fungating wounds are diagnosed based on histological assessment and disease may be recurrence, advanced local disease or metastasis (Grocott 2007, Hampton and Collins 2004).

Related theory

It has been estimated that around 5–10% of people with metastatic cancer will develop such a wound (Haisfield-Wolfe and Rund 1997). Fungating wounds tend to occur in older patients (60–70 years old) with advanced cancer and usually develop during the last 6 months of life (Haisfield-Wolfe and Rund 1997, Ivetic and Lyne 1990). Fungating wounds can occur almost anywhere on the body. They arise most commonly from cancer of the breast (62%) or head and neck (24%), melanoma, soft tissue sarcoma and some cancers of the genitourinary system (Naylor 2001, Thomas 1992, Wilkes et al. 2001).

Evidence-based approaches

Principles of care

The goals of care are palliative and focused on controlling symptoms and improving the patient's quality of life, rather than curing (Grocott 2007, Laverty et al. 1997). They signify progressive and life-threatening disease which affects the patient's well-being and quality of life (Naylor 2002).

The nurse needs to be aware of these psychosocial issues and allow the patient to express their fears and concerns.

Excellent communication skills coupled with empathy and sensitivity can be of great benefit to the patient when having to readjust to their changing situation (Naylor et al. 2001). It is impossible to completely understand the impact that a fungating wound has on patients and their family, but it is possible to offer a realistic and holistic approach to their care that affords them the opportunity to live as full a life as possible within the limitations of their wound and their disease.

The chronic nature of malignant wounds means that patients are involved in an ongoing process of adjustment. Wounds are also a constant reminder to patients of advanced disease and possible impending death (Laverty et al. 1997, Naylor et al. 2001). They may also feel embarrassment, especially with regard to their relationship with their partner (Bird 2000). Leakage of exudate and strong odour may lead them to live separate lives and may make the continuation of a sexual relationship extremely difficult, if not impossible (Hallett 1995).

Preprocedural considerations

Assessment

Assessment and evaluation of a wound are discussed earlier in the chapter, but it is important to emphasize that an accurate history of a malignant lesion should be taken and that the management of the wound should be documented clearly from the beginning. The aim of management is to control symptoms rather than encouraging the wound to heal (Laverty et al. 1997). A wound assessment tool to record the amount and type of odour/exudate/pain, and the dressings used, is a helpful means of evaluating care strategies (see Problem-solving table 19.1 and Figure 19.5).

Applying the wound bed preparation principles (Vowden and Vowden 2002) and TIME (Table 19.2) is advocated in palliative wound care (Grocott 2007, Lo et al. 2007) as autolytic debridement and moisture management can enhance quality of life. Approaches for managing the side-effects of fungating wounds are listed in Problem-solving table 19.1 (NB: the table is designed to guide the nurse whilst following Procedure guideline 19.1). Effectively controlling symptoms can increase independence and help patients regain a measure of control over their lives (Grocott 2007).

Specific patient preparations

Each patient responds individually to having such a wound, the consequences of which impinge on physical, psychological, social, sexual as well as spiritual well-being. The highest level of nursing expertise is required. Informing patients can lead them to understand their signs and symptoms and enable them to report accurately and live more positively with their wound (Lo et al. 2008).

Whilst their appearance and presenting symptoms are unique (Young 2005), the four most common symptoms associated with fungating wounds are bleeding, malodour, pain and heavy exudates (Grocott 2007, Hampton 2008, Lund-Nielsen et al. 2005).

Postprocedural considerations

Immediate care

Tapes should only be applied to healthy skin in order to avoid further tissue damage. Care should be taken to leave a large margin around the wound, including any existing cutaneous nodules. Plain bandaging or the use of Netelast/Tubifast is helpful where a wound is positioned in a difficult area (Naylor 2002).

Ongoing care

Along with dressings, the patient can benefit from a course of palliative radiotherapy to reduce exudate and bleeding or palliative chemotherapy which can reduce tumour bulk and the aforementioned side-effects for a period of time (Alexander 2009). Silver creams or dressings should be avoided during radiotherapy treatment. For hormone-receptive tumours (i.e. breast), hormone therapy can reduce the rate at which a fungating wound progresses and deteriorates (Fairbairn 1993). Chemotherapy is occasionally used for this purpose, but hormone therapy has fewer side-effects and can enhance the patient's sense of well-being.

Complementary therapies

The use of complementary therapies in wound management is based very much on anecdotal evidence. However, there have been trials using essential oils in wound care, in particular for the relief of pain and wound odour (Baker 1998, Price and Price 2007). Complementary therapies such as relaxation, massage, visualization, imagery and distraction may be very useful in the reduction of wound pain, especially that which is associated with procedures such as dressing changes (Naylor 2001). Other complementary therapies for pain management include acupuncture, acupressure, autogenic therapy and hypnosis (Rankin-Box 2001).

Radiotherapy skin reactions

Definition

Radiotherapy skin reactions may present as skin irritation, erythema and/or flaking or peeling of skin within a field of radiotherapy treatment. These reactions develop over a period of weeks as repeated ionizing radiation causes an inflammatory response (Simonen et al. 1998) and reduces the opportunity for tissue healing due to neutrophilic infiltration of the epidermis and apoptosis (Bernier et al. 2008). The skin tries to compensate by increasing mitotic activity, but this results in scaly, thickened skin (dry desquamation) as the cells are immature and vulnerable. As the damage continues, the basal layer breaks down and the epidermis sloughs off (moist desquamation), patchily at first but with general oedema (NHSQIS 2010). Chronic radiation dam-

Table 19.4 Categories of acute radiotherapy skin reactions

Category	Description
Erythema	Reddened skin, which may be oedematous and feel hot and irritable
Dry desquamation	Dry, flaky or peeling skin that may be itchy
Moist desquamation	Peeling skin with exposure of the dermis and exudate production, often painful and may become infected
Necrosis	Death of tissue; skin may darken and turn black

age due to the loss of collagen and supporting structures within the dermis causes fibrotic changes and reduced or complete hair loss and a fragile epidermal skin covering, and will leave the skin prone to poor healing and sun damage (Bernier et al. 2008, NHSQIS 2010). These changes are summarized in Table 19.4 and Table 19.5.

Anatomy and physiology

Radiation impairs stem cell division within the basal layer of the epidermis, disrupting or sometimes halting the normal process of skin regeneration (Archambeau et al. 1995). There are four main types of radiation skin reaction, which are classified according to the appearance of the skin (see Table 19.8). Table 19.6 lists the factors that increase the risk of skin reactions in radiotherapy.

Related theory

The degree of skin reaction depends on the prescribed radiotherapy treatment and a number of patient and environmental factors (Naylor et al. 2001, NHSQIS 2010, Wells and MacBride 2003).

Radio-sensitizing chemotherapy drugs used concomitantly will increase the side-effects, including the skin reaction to radiotherapy. Monoclonal antibody treatment that targets the epidermal growth factor is known to produce an acne-like rash which varies in severity (Saltz et al. 2004) but particularly affects treatment fields in head and neck areas (Ang 2008).

Patients treated with combination therapy are at a greater risk of developing skin reactions which may begin with the skin feeling tight or tender and progress to an open wound with exposed nerve endings which requires dressing (Goldberg and Mcgynn-Byer 2000, Myers 2004).

Evidence-based approaches

Methods of skin care during radiotherapy

Preventive measures to help maintain skin integrity during radiotherapy are institutional and given to patients prior to treatment (Bernier et al. 2008, Kedge 2009, Laverty et al. 2000, NHSQIS 2010). However, there is a consensus that

Table 19.5 Skin care advice during radiotherapy

Do	Avoid	Rationale
Gently wash skin using warm water with a mild soap and pat the skin dry especially in skinfolds (e.g. under breast)	Perfumes or solutions containing alcohol or metals, including make-up and deodorants (within the field)	Daily washing improves skin condition and general well-being for patients
Apply a hydrophilic moisturizer to the treatment area (before treatment and allow it to soak in)	Applying moisturizer shortly before treatment Using creams other than those recommended by team	Application of cream promotes comfort, but a layer of cream and/or Vaseline on the lips will create a bolus effect (increasing the dose and damage to the area) and need time to soak in
Apply cream more frequently as needed 2–3 times daily once skin becomes itchy/dry	Corticosteroids for pruritus (unless a low dose – 1% cream is prescribed for a short period in severe pruritus)	Steroids can thin the skin and use should be limited or avoided if possible
Use an electric razor (for male head and neck patients)	Friction from wet shaving and after-shave	Protect epidermis and reduce irritation/ friction
Wear comfortable cotton clothes and silk scarves around the neck	Tight clothes and woolly or synthetic fibres	These can increase friction and discomfort in the treatment area
Protect the skin from sunlight, wind or extremes of temperature	Exposure to the sun and ensure that this continues life-long within the treatment field	Skin is vulnerable to sunburn and alters during treatment
Attend weekly skin and symptom review clinics	Using any sticky plaster or tape in the treatment field	Reviewing skin and reinforcing advice is vital

patients should avoid heat and environmental factors and be gentle with skin care (Kedge 2009, Myers 2004). It is important to follow recognized guidelines to assess the skin (NHSQIS 2010; see Table 19.8).

Legal and professional issues

Competencies

Oncology nurses caring for patients with radiotherapy skin reactions should have read the radiotherapy department skin care policy or the related section within the hospital wound care guidelines. Advice should be sought from the appropriate nurse or radiographer responsible for day-to-day review of patients whilst undergoing radiotherapy. Before making recommendations for patients, the evidence or lack of evidence supporting nursing practice should be understood or sought (Kedge 2009, McQuestion 2006).

Therapy radiographers treating patients daily with radiotherapy are responsible for daily assessment and information, referring to allied health professionals as necessary and assisting patients with making informed choices about treatment.

Preprocedural considerations

Recent recommendations use the available literature and expert opinion to draw up national guidelines in Scotland (NHSQIS 2010) and the Cancer Care Ontario Supportive Care Guidance Group (SCGG) (Bolderston et al. 2006). There has been an emphasis on using the principles of wound healing to address moist desquamation and it is

Table 19.6 Factors that increase the risk of skin reactions to radiotherapy

Treatment factors	Patient factors	Environmental factors
Concomitant chemotherapy or epidermal growth factor receptor (EGFR)	Age (older age has thinning and drying effect on the skin, which extends healing time)	Use of 'bolus' materials (e.g. a wax blanket) to increase the dose of radiotherapy to the skin
Total dose and fractionation of radiotherapy	Steroid or immunosuppressant therapy	Chemical irritants (see Table 19.5)
Large volume of normal tissue included in the area of treatment	Co-morbidities: diabetes, obesity or malnutrition	Treatment to the skin in vulnerable places prone to moisture and friction (i.e. the breast, perineum, head and neck or skinfolds)
Entry and exit sites of radiation	Smoking	Chronic sun exposure

Table 19.7 Recommended treatments for acute radiotherapy skin reactions

Radiation skin reaction	Suggested treatment
Erythema and dry desquamation (may be managed in the same way)	<ul><li>Hydrophilic and moisturizing creams, for example aqueous cream: provide symptomatic relief (number of applications per day increase as treatment progresses)</li><li>1% hydrocortisone: for itchy, irritable or burning feelings of the skin within the treatment field; should be applied sparingly, twice a day, but *not to areas of broken or infected skin* (*use of moisturizing creams should continue and be applied before the steroid*)</li></ul>
Moist desquamation	<ul><li>Hydrogel sheets: reduce discomfort and promote healing (soothing and cooling) in early stages where area is weeping and sore (rather than sloughy); can be used alone with instructions for patients to rehydrate and refrigerate or with suitable secondary dressing, e.g. dressing pad with bandage or Tubifast</li></ul>Examples from practice:<ul><li>amorphous hydrogels: useful in head and neck (especially behind ears), skinfolds or the perineum, and can be reapplied as comfortable/patient preference</li><li>use with Mepitel (or suitable meshed non-stick primary dressing) and secondary dressing</li><li>Mepitel and secondary dressing may be sufficient alone (Macmillan *et al.* 2007)</li><li>Activon Tulle (impregnated with honey) followed by secondary dressing (best left intact post treatment for 2–3 days)</li><li>modern absorbent dressings (especially if sloughy), for example alginate (Kaltostat/Sorbsan), hydrofibre (Aquacel), with a secondary dressing, foam (Mepilex/Allevyn) or PolyMem which comes in a useful roll for head and neck and contains an antiseptic: http://www.PolyMem.eu</li><li>hydrocolloid sheets: may be applied to areas of moist desquamation *once radiotherapy treatment has finished (as during treatment it can become warm and sticky)*</li></ul>
Necrosis	Debride eschar/slough; manage according to TIME/WBP

Bolderston *et al.* (2006), Heggie *et al.* (2002), McQuestion (2006), Naylor *et al.* (2001), Patwardhan *et al.* (2002), Wells and MacBride (2003), Wickline (2004).

important that nurses have an understanding of this and radiation effects on the skin. Limited evidence supports the use of hydrogels and hydrocolloid but patients have reported improved comfort (Kedge 2009, Macmillan *et al.* 2007, Myers 2004). See Table 19.7.

Assessment

Assessment of the treatment area is imperative and should be ongoing. A baseline assessment should note the current

Table 19.8 Radiation Therapy Oncology Group (RTOG)

Score	Description
RTOG 0	No visible change
RTOG 1	Faint or dull *erythema*
RTOG 2 (a)	Tender or bright *erythema* with or without *dry desquamation*
RTOG 2 (b)	Patchy *moist desquamation;* moderate oedema
RTOG 3	Confluent *moist desquamation; pitting oedema*

Reproduced with permission from the Society of Radiographers.

condition of the skin, the risk factors listed below and the educational needs of the patient and their family or carers (Maher 2005). Measures to minimize and delay skin breakdown and promote comfort should be initiated early on in the treatment plan. Special note should be made of concurrent illness (i.e. diabetes) or skin changes (i.e. scars, eczema) which may affect healing (Noble-Adams 1999). Table 19.7 has drawn an example of managing radiation skin reactions from sources and experience.

Weekly review encompassing holistic skin assessment and records throughout the course of treatment and identification of high-risk patients prior to treatment (i.e. elderly, malnourished and/or fair complexions) are essential. Each patient should be treated on a case-by-case basis if they progress to confluent moist desquamation as it requires specialist wound care (Bernier *et al.* 2008).

Postprocedural considerations

Patients should be given contact numbers for a named professional once their treatment has finished as radiation damage continues and peak skin reaction can occur up to 14 days after radiation treatment. If skin breakdown occurs, they should seek advice and return to the department for assessment and treatment if possible. Referrals to district nurses can be made but ideally the radiation centre will monitor closely until the acute side-effects of treatment subside.

Pressure ulcers

Definition

A pressure ulcer usually results from compromised circulation secondary to pressure over time and is a local site of cell death (Hess 2005).

Measures for preventing and detecting pressure ulcers have been discussed in Chapter 4 and are briefly described here to facilitate dressing choices.

Anatomy and physiology

The European Pressure Ulcer Advisor Panel (EPUAP) and National Pressure Ulcer Advisory Panel (2009) classify ulcers according to depth in four stages. The first is superficial damage which is characterized by local inflammation and may present as a persistent area of redness with no breach of the epidermis. The second stage is partial loss of the epidermis or dermis, often with a blistering or abrasion. The third stage involves damage to the dermis and subcutaneous layers of tissue and clinically appears as an ulcer but does not involve the underlying fascia. The fourth stage involves tissue necrosis and full-thickness skin loss, often with tunnelling sinus tracts (Hess 2005).

Evidence-based approaches

Bryant (2000) lists four principles of wound care for pressure sore assessment.

- Eliminate the source (i.e. cause of pressure damage).
- Ensure the microenvironment is optimal (to promote wound healing).
- Support the host (using appropriate pressure-relieving aids and ensuring adequate nutritional balance and skin care regimen).
- Provide education (explaining to the patient and caregivers the principles of caring for their skin and pressure areas).

Wound dressings that maintain a moist environment facilitate healing and after a thorough assessment, selections can be made according to the depth of the ulcer and degree of damage from the dressings (see Table 19.3).

Preprocedural considerations

Nurses must consistently question whether they are employing measures for preventing pressure ulcers and whether the patient and caregivers are following the care plan

(recording tools are listed in Chapter 4). Documentation should be made if the patient refuses care and/or evaluation of whether the patient improves or deteriorates should be recorded to keep the care plan up to date (Bryant 2000). Nutritional status and the patient's ability to self-care and mobilize should also be evaluated and documented (EPUAP 2009).

Assessment using the TIME principles (Dowsett and Ayello 2004) and following the procedure for changing a dressing should be practised.

Administration of analgesia as prescribed and the seting of a time frame with the patient's agreement are recommended to improve the experience for the patient (EPUAP 2009). Nurses should consult additional guidance if unfamiliar with the patient or regimen (http://www.epuap.org/guidelines/Final_Quick_Treatment.pdf) (NMC 2009).

Assessment

The EPUAP (2009) recommends the use of a pressure ulcer classification system to estimate tissue loss, and that the skin is assessed by colour, temperature and consistency (i.e. firm/turgid or soft/boggy).

Stages 1–2 with light exudates: for reddened areas, barrier cream and relief of pressure are recommended, whilst superficial ulcers require dressing with transparent films (e.g. Opsite, Tegaderm) as they effectively retain moisture and prevent friction (Bluestein and Javaheri 2008). For fragile skin, a skin barrier (e.g. Cavilon) may be used under the film or a light hydrocolloid (e.g. Duoderm Thin). Appropriate measures such as removal of pressure, positioning the patient and protective dressings will prevent the condition from worsening (Falanga 2000).

Stage 3 ulcers should be dressed with synthetic dressings rather than gauze as these cause less pain and require less frequent changes (Bluestein and Javaheri 2008, EPUAP 2009). These dressings include alginates, hydrocolloids and foams and are often available in site-specific shapes to ease application and removal and minimize leakage.

Surgical wounds

Evidence-based approaches

Methods of wound closure

There are four main methods of wound closure:

- sutures
- adhesive skin closure strips
- tissue adhesive
- staples.

See Table 19.9 for advantages and disadvantages of each method.

Table 19.9 Advantages and disadvantages of methods of wound closure

Method	Advantages	Disadvantages
Sutures: interrupted sutures are separate sutures each with its own knot and are used on the majority of wounds because they are the most versatile A *continuous* suture is one long thread that spirals along the entire suture line at evenly spaced intervals	*Non-absorbable* sutures are more widely used for skin closure where the material causes little reaction or rejection. A monofilament nylon is a strong single-stranded nylon providing continued strength; silk is a braided strand and fairly easy to handle *Absorbable* sutures degrade rapidly and thus allow the deep tissues within a wound to be closed successfully. They are also useful for patients who may not remember they have had sutures or will not attend for follow-up Sutures can be removed once healing has occurred, normally 5–10 days after injury	Suturing must be performed by an experienced practitioner Requires local anaesthetic Suture material is a foreign body in the wound and thus increases the risk of infection Interrupted sutures are not recommended for fragile skin Sutures tied too tightly can damage tissues and when too loose they may delay healing If skin layers are not aligned then patients can be left with a scar Forceps used to lift skin may crush the tissue
Adhesive skin closure strips	Available in a variety of widths Useful for superficial wounds that are not subject to tension Strips are cheap and easy to use and remove No local anaesthetic required and tissue damage is minimal	Strips do not adhere to sweaty or hairy skin If there is tissue oedema it makes it difficult to achieve good apposition of the wound edges May be suitable over some joints but where skin is taut or subject to movement, they do not provide optimum closure
Tissue adhesive	Surgical 'superglues' are now popular for emergency settings Good cosmetic results Less painful than suturing Wound complication rates are low	It is expensive Not suitable over joints and areas of high tension Needs second person to assist in getting skin edges aligned
Staples	Staples are made of stainless steel wire Provide greatest tensile strength Quick method and offers low level of tissue reactivity and better resistance to infection than sutures Can be performed without local anaesthetic	Staples are more expensive than sutures and may be confined to wounds where needlestick injury is a high risk Must be inserted by an experienced practitioner Failure to align tissue edges may cause scar deformity Only useful for superficial skin layers

From Elkin *et al.* (2004), Jay (1999), Richardson (2007).

Wounds may vary and therefore careful assessment is required before the method of closure is selected and attempted (Richardson 2007). Richardson (2007) lists the following guiding principles to assist with decision making.

- What is the aim of the wound closure? For example, eliminating dead space where a haematoma can develop, realigning tissue correctly or holding aligned tissues until healing has occurred.
- What is the history of the wound? This informs the practitioner about the depth of the wound and likelihood of infection.
- What is the wound site pattern? This and biomechanical properties may rule out some methods of closure.

Suturing

Evidence-based approaches

Rationale

Suturing as a method for wound closure is appropriate for managing deep, large wounds and ideally wounds that are less than 6 hours old.

Indications

This method is used to promote healing, realign tissue layers and hold the skin edges until they have healed by first

Table 19.10 Common suturing errors

Error	Resulting problems
Sutures too loose	Fails to bring wound edges together, leading to gaps
	Sutures may fall out
Sutures too tight	Does not allow for normal wound swelling
	May induce vascular compromise of the wound edges leading to necrosis, delayed healing, poor cosmetic results
Wound edge overlapping	Interferes with wound healing and may cause a ridge, leading to a more obvious scar
Sutures too near the wound edge	These are likely to pull out

Adapted from Castille (1998) with permission.

intention and no longer require artificial support (Castille 1998). There are a number of common suturing errors as listed in Table 19.10.

Contraindications

Experts are usually required to manage wounds of a certain depth or in complex areas such as the face or hand. This is to minimize scarring and not restrict movement by poor technique. Therefore local policy will probably prevent nurses from suturing these wounds (Castille 1998, Reynolds and Cole 2006).

Legal and professional issues

Competencies

Nurses should decline to carry out procedures that they have not been prepared for (NMC 2008b). Suturing wounds requires skill and should be performed by practitioners who have undergone appropriate training. This includes the principles of wound assessment and healing (Castille 1998, Reynolds and Cole 2006).

Preprocedural considerations

The environment should be comfortable, quiet, relaxed and private prior to suturing (Castille 1998). It is advisable to lie the patient down to relieve anxiety and prevent further injury that could occur if the patient faints (Reynolds and Cole 2006).

Before closing the wound by any method, the wound must be thoroughly cleansed to minimize the risk of wound infection and ensure that any dirt or foreign bodies are removed (Reynolds and Cole 2006). Dirty wounds should be cleansed with running water or sterile solution of 0.9% sodium chloride under pressure (Castille 1998, Reynolds and Cole 2006).

The wound area needs to be prepared by administering local anaesthetic and as a result suturing is more painful and takes longer than other methods of wound closure (Reynolds and Cole 2006). Contaminated wounds may need to be treated with a broad-spectrum antibiotic to prevent possible infection (Castille 1998).

Procedure guideline 19.2 Suturing a simple wound

Essential equipment

- Plastic apron
- Sterile gloves
- Suture pack (containing needle holder, tissue forceps, dressing forceps, scissors, low-linting swabs, solution pot)
- Sutures in varying gauges and materials
- Local anaesthetic (1% lidocaine hydrochloride)
- Sterile 0.9% sodium chloride solution
- 10 mL syringe and needles (21 and 25 G)
- Dressing

Preprocedure

Action	Rationale
1 Explain and discuss the procedure with the patient.	To ensure that the patient understands the procedure and gives their valid consent (NMC 2008a, C).
2 Follow the procedure for aseptic technique.	To reduce the risk of contamination (Fraise and Bradley 2009, E).

1185

(Continued)

Procedure guideline 19.2 *(Continued)*

Procedure

3 Using a bright light, assess the wound and decide the type of material and gauge of needle to use.	To ensure that the wound is closed using most appropriate material to promote healing (Reynolds and Cole 2006, E).
4 The area surrounding the wound may require shaving.	To prevent hairs from becoming trapped in the closed wound (Castille 1998, E).
5 Draw up and administer the local anaesthetic slowly along the wound edge, drawing back first to ensure that the needle is not inserted far enough into a vessel to raise a small blister (Reynolds and Cole 2006).	To prevent any pain during the procedure, but explain that a slight tugging sensation will still be felt (Castille 1998, E). Accidental injection of local anaesthetic into a blood vessel can result in convulsions or cardiovascular shock (Reynolds and Cole 2006, E).
6 After a couple of minutes check that the areas are anaesthetized by testing with a small needle.	This will ensure full anaesthesia in 2 minutes, with peak time around 10–25 minutes (BNF 2011, C) and procedure is pain free (Reynolds and Cole 2006, E).
7 Inspect the site.	To ascertain how to match the wound edges (Castille 1998, E).
8 With linear wounds, suturing should begin at the centre.	To create good apposition of the edges (Castille 1998, E).
9 Select the tissue forceps, needle and needle holder.	To prepare the equipment for the procedure. E
10 The needle should be grasped in the needle holder on its flattened area about a third of the way along from the suture material (see Action Figure 10).	To prepare the suture material for use (Jay 1999, E).
11 The needle holder should be held in the dominant hand and support the wound edge with the tissue forceps.	To allow adequate control by the practitioner of the equipment and to support the tissue during the procedure (Castille 1998, E).
12 The needle should be inserted at a 90° angle to the skin, taking a full-thickness 'bite' about 5 mm from the edge of the wound (see Action Figure 12).	To create good apposition of the edges without excessive tension (Castille 1998, E). (NB: see Postprocedural considerations for rationale.)
13 Bring the needle up in between the wound edges and pull the suture through the tissue until a short tail remains at the initial skin entry site (see Action Figure 13).	To ensure there is enough suture to use for knotting. E
14 Reinsert the needle at a 90° angle from the base of the wound on the other side and pull the suture through the tissue (see Action Figure 14).	To bring wound edges together (Jay 1999, E).
15 Hold the needle parallel to the skin and, grasping the needle end of the suture, make two clockwise loops around the needle holder (see Action Figure 15).	To begin to create a knot (Castille 1998, E).
16 Grasp the tail of the suture with the needle holder and pull it through the loop with the needle holder pulled towards you (see Action Figure 16).	To 'set a throw' (Castille 1998, E).
17 Follow this by a single anti-clockwise loop around the needle holder and move the needle to the opposite side of the wound (see Action Figures 17a, 17b).	To square the knot (Castille 1998, E).
18 Then create a third throw of one loop.	To ensure that the knot is tied securely but not too tightly (Castille 1998, E).
19 The suture can then be cut free from the knot, leaving tails of about 5 mm (see Action Figure 19).	To enable easy removal of the suture (Castille 1998, E).

20 Insert each suture in the same way until completed.	To close the wound effectively. E
21 Once completed, discard needle in sharps bin.	To prevent potential sharps injury to practitioner (NHSE 2005, C).

Postprocedure

22 Clean any blood from the surrounding area using aseptic technique and sterile saline solution of 0.9% sodium chloride.	To prevent any possible wound infection (Fraise and Bradley 2009, E).
23 Apply a suitable dressing.	To protect the wound from further trauma or contamination and ensure optimum healing (Castille 1998, E; Reynolds and Cole 2006, E).
24 Record the date, time and name of the practitioner, amount of local anaesthetic used and size and type of suture material and number of sutures on the appropriate charts.	To maintain accurate records and provide a point of reference in the event of any queries (NMC 2009, C; Reynolds and Cole 2006, E).
25 The need for analgesia after the local anaesthetic has worn off should be explained (Castille 1998).	Pain assessment is ongoing following the procedure to maintain patient comfort. E
26 Provide the patient with written and verbal advice regarding wound care and when the sutures should be removed.	To ensure optimum care for the wound and correct removal (Castille, 1998, E).

Action Figure 10 Grasp the needle.

Action Figure 12 Insert the needle at a 90° angle.

Action Figure 13 Bring the needle up between the wound edges.

Action Figure 14 Reinsert the needle on the other side.

(Continued)

Procedure guideline 19.2 *(Continued)*

Action Figure 15 Make two clockwise loops.

Action Figure 16 Grasp the tail of the suture with the needle holder.

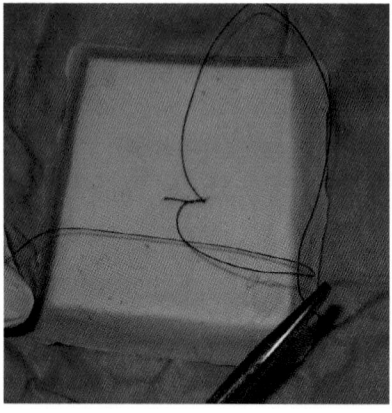

Action Figure 17a Loop the suture around the needle holder.

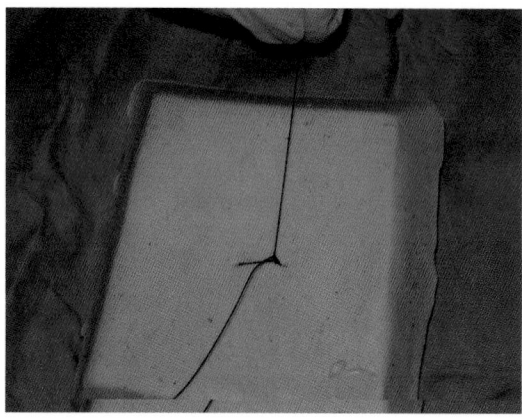

Action Figure 17b Move the needle to the opposite side of the wound.

Action Figure 19 The suture can be freed from the knot.

Postprocedural considerations

The tension of the sutures can affect healing and cosmetic appearance (Hampton and Collins 2004), with inflammation occurring when they are too tight which can lead to devitalized tissue (Reynolds and Cole 2006). If too loose, the scar will not align and hold the wound edges in apposition (Clark 2004, Reynolds and Cole 2006). See Table 19.10 for common suturing errors.

Evidence-based approaches

Rationale

Removal of sutures is usually performed between 7 and 10 days post insertion, but this is dependent on where the wound is and whether it has healed. Routinely, every other suture or staple is removed first, with the rest removed if the incision remains securely closed. If any sign of suture line separation is evident during the removal process, the remaining sutures are left in place and reported to the medical team (Elkin *et al.* 2004). Note that staples have replaced clips (Pudner 2005).

Preprocedural considerations

Assess the wound, as the time period for removal of sutures depends upon the patient's underlying pathology, condition of their skin and the wound position (Pudner 2005). Surgical notes and instructions should also be taken into account along with the skills of the practitioner (NMC 2009). Analgesia may be offered depending on the patient and wound site.

Procedure guideline 19.3 Suture removal

Essential equipment

- Sterile dressing pack containing gallipots or an indented plastic tray, low-linting swabs and/or medical foam, disposable forceps, gloves, sterile field, disposable bag
- Fluids for cleaning and/or irrigation
- Hypoallergenic tape
- Appropriate dressing
- Appropriate hand hygiene preparation
- Any other material will be determined by the nature of the dressing; special features of a dressing should be referred to in the patient's nursing care plan

- Detergent wipe for cleaning trolley
- Total traceability system for surgical instruments and patient record form

Optional equipment

- Any extra equipment that may be needed during procedure, for example sterile scissors, stitch cutter, staple remover, sterile adhesive sutures

Preprocedure

Action	Rationale
1 Explain and discuss the procedure with the patient.	To ensure that the patient understands the procedure and gives their valid consent (NMC 2008a, C).
2 Perform procedure using aseptic technique.	To prevent infection (see Chapter 3, Procedure guideline 3.9) (Fraise and Bradley 2009, E).

Procedure

3 Clean the wound with an appropriate sterile solution such as 0.9% sodium chloride.	To prevent infection (Fraise and Bradley 2009, E).
4 Lift knot of suture with metal forceps. Snip stitch close to the skin. Pull suture out gently towards the side that has been cut. For intermittent sutures, alternate sutures may be removed first before remaining sutures are removed (Pudner 2005).	Plastic forceps tend to slip against nylon sutures. E To prevent infection by drawing exposed suture through the tissue (Pudner 2005, E). To ensure wound closure and predict dehiscence (Pudner 2005, E).
5 Use tips of scissors slightly open or the side of the stitch cutter to gently press the skin when the suture is being drawn out.	To minimize pain by counteracting the adhesion between the suture and surrounding tissue. E

1189

(Continued)

Procedure guideline 19.3 (*Continued*)

Postprocedure

6 Record condition of suture line and surrounding skin (amount of exudate, pus, inflammation, pain, and so on).	To document care and enable evaluation of the wound (Bale and Jones 2006, E; Dealey 2005, E; NMC 2009, C).
7 Use of adhesive skin tapes should be monitored and they are usually left in place until they fall off by themselves.	To improve cosmetic effect and support tensile strength of the wound post suture removal, when indicated (Pudner 2005, E).

Procedure guideline 19.4 Staple removal

Essential equipment

- Sterile dressing pack containing gallipots or an indented plastic tray, low-linting swabs and/or medical foam, disposable forceps, gloves, sterile field, disposable bag
- Fluids for cleaning and/or irrigation
- Hypoallergenic tape
- Appropriate dressing
- Appropriate hand hygiene preparation
- Any other material will be determined by the nature of the dressing; special features of a dressing should be referred to in the patient's nursing care plan
- Detergent wipe for cleaning trolley
- Total traceability system for surgical instruments and patient record form

Optional equipment

- Any extra equipment that may be needed during procedure, for example sterile scissors, stitch cutter, staple remover, sterile adhesive sutures

Preprocedure

Action	Rationale
1 Explain and discuss the procedure with the patient.	To ensure that the patient understands the procedure and gives their valid consent (NMC 2008a, C).
2 Perform procedure using aseptic technique.	To prevent infection (see Chapter 3, Procedure guideline 3.9) (Fraise and Bradley 2009, E).

Procedure

3 Clean the wound with an appropriate sterile solution such as 0.9% sodium chloride.	To prevent infection (Fraise and Bradley 2009, E).
4 Slide the lower bar of the staple remover with the V-shaped groove under the staple at an angle of 90°. Squeeze the handles of the staple removers together to open the staple.	To release the staple atraumatically from the wound. If the angle of the staple remover is not correct, the staple will not come out freely (Pudner 2005, E).
5 If the suture line is under tension, use free hand to gently squeeze the skin either side of the suture line.	To reduce tension of skin around suture line and lessen pain on removal of staple. E
6 If the wound gapes use adhesive sutures to oppose the wound edges.	To improve the cosmetic effect. E

Postprocedure

7 Record condition of suture line and surrounding skin (amount of exudate, pus, inflammation, pain, etc.).	To document care and enable evaluation of the wound (Bale and Jones 2006, E; Dealey 2005, E; NMC 2009, C).
8 Use of adhesive skin tapes should be monitored and they are usually left in place until they fall off by themselves.	To improve cosmetic effect and support tensile strength of the wound post suture removal, when indicated (Pudner 2005, E).

Wound drains

Evidence-based approaches

The purpose of a drain within the wound is to prevent haematoma formation or excess fluid build-up within the wound bed as these can lead to infection and irritation of the tissues (Walker 2007). Suboptimal conditions put surgical wounds at risk of dehiscence, which can be indicated by a sudden discharge of fluid or cellulites along the suture line (Hampton and Collins 2004), particularly in abdominal wounds where an abscess may develop, or the patient may report a 'popping' sensation (Beitz et al. 2008).

Nurses are ideally placed to observe the postoperative patient and often are involved in managing drainage systems (Walker 2007). Surgical wounds will heal rapidly if blood perfusion is maximized (Hampton and Collins 2004).

Preprocedural considerations

Check the patient's operation notes to establish the number and site(s) of internal and external sutures. Explain the procedure to the patient and gain their consent (NMC 2008a).

Giving information about the proposed procedure helps to relieve anxiety and relax the patient. The easiest way to control pain is via the patient-controlled analgesia (PCA), if *in situ* (Hampton and Collins 2004). Offer the patient analgesia as per chart or encourage self-administration via the PCA pump to promote comfort (NMC 2008b). Another member of staff may be needed to reassure the patient during the procedure.

An aseptic technique should always be used and the drainage system should be handled as little as possible to minimize infection risk (Pudner 2005).

Equipment

- *Open drains*, for example Yates, Penrose, corrugated, are usually sutured in place and covered with a dressing (exudates passively ooze into the dressing from the surgical wound bed).
- *Closed drains*, for example Redivac and concertina-type, have perforated tubing along the incision and have a suction mechanism that exerts pressure (active drainage from the wound bed).

Procedure guideline 19.5 Wound drainage systems: changing the dressing around the drain site and observation/management

Essential equipment

- Sterile dressing pack containing gallipots or an indented plastic tray, low-linting swabs and/or medical foam, disposable forceps, gloves, sterile field, disposable bag
- Fluids for cleaning and/or irrigation
- Hypoallergenic tape
- Appropriate absorbent dressing
- Appropriate hand hygiene preparation
- Any other material will be determined by the nature of the dressing; special features of a dressing should be referred to in the patient's nursing care plan
- Detergent wipe
- Total traceability system for surgical instruments and patient record form

Optional equipment

- Any extra equipment that may be needed during procedure, for example sterile scissors, metal forceps, stitch cutter

Preprocedure

Action	Rationale
1 Explain and discuss the procedure with the patient.	To ensure that the patient understands the procedure and gives their valid consent and participates in care (NMC 2008a,C; Walker 2007, C).
2 Perform procedure using aseptic technique.	To prevent infection (Fraise and Bradley 2009, E).

Procedure

3 Clean the surrounding skin with an appropriate sterile solution such as 0.9% sodium chloride.	To prevent infection and remove excess debris. E
4 Check condition of surrounding skin.	To assess for any excoriation of the skin. E

(Continued)

1191

Procedure guideline 19.5 (*Continued*)

5 Ensure that the skin suture holding the drain site in position is intact.	To prevent the drain from leaving the wound. E
6 Cover the drain site with a non-adherent, absorbent dressing.	To protect the drain site, prevent infection entering the wound and absorb exudate. E

Postprocedure

7 Tape securely.	To prevent drain coming loose. E
8 Ensure that the drain is primed or that the suction pump is in working order.	To ensure continuity of drainage. Ineffective drainage can result in oedema/haematoma (Hess 2005, E).

Procedure guideline 19.6 Wound drainage systems: changing the vacuum bottle of a closed drainage system

Essential equipment:

- Sterile dressing pack containing gallipots or an indented plastic tray, low-linting swabs and/or medical foam, disposable forceps, gloves, sterile field, disposable bag
- Clamp (usually part of the system in place)
- Redivac drainage bottle
- Marker pen and chart

Procedure

Action	Rationale
1 Use aseptic technique and sterile equipment (as listed above).	To prevent infection (Fraise and Bradley 2009, E; Walker 2007).
2 Ensure sterile drainage system is readily available.	To ensure sterility during change of system. E
3 Measure the contents of the bottle to be changed and record this in the appropriate documents.	To maintain an accurate record of drainage from the wound and enable evaluation of state of wound (NMC 2009, E).
4 Clamp the tube with the tubing clamps on the drainage tube and bottle connector and remove the bottle.	To prevent air and contamination entering the wound via the drain. E
5 Clean the end of the tube and attach it to the sterile bottle.	To maintain sterility. E
6 Unclamp the tubing clamps.	To re-establish the drainage system. E
7 Place used vacuum drainage system into the clinical waste bag.	To safely dispose of used system. E

Postprocedure

8 Document in patient's notes that the drainage bottle has been changed.	To record the change (NMC 2009, C).

Procedure guideline 19.7 Wound drain removal (closed drainage system, for example, Redivac or concertina)

Essential equipment

- Sterile dressing pack containing gallipots or an indented plastic tray, low-linting swabs and/or medical foam, disposable forceps, gloves, sterile field, disposable bag
- Scissors or stitch cutter (refer to patient notes for directions if dressing in place)
- Sterile absorbent dressing to place over drainage site
- Wound swab/sterile pot (to be used if infection suspected)

Procedure

Action	Rationale
1 Use aseptic technique and sterile equipment (as listed above).	To prevent infection (Fraise and Bradley 2009, E; Pudner 2005, E; Walker 2007, E).
2 Release the vacuum (active drainage system) by clamping the tubing with the clamp provided (Walker 2007).	This releases the vacuum and prevents suction and traumatic removal during the procedure which may damage the tissue. E
3 Only clean the wound if necessary, using an appropriate sterile solution, such as 0.9% sodium chloride.	To reduce risk of infection. E
4 If the drain is sutured in place, hold the knot of the suture with metal forceps and gently lift upwards.	Plastic forceps tend to slip against nylon sutures. To allow space for the scissors or stitch cutter to be placed underneath. E
5 Cut the shortest end of the suture as close to the skin as possible.	To prevent infection by allowing the suture to be liberated from the drain without drawing the exposed part through tissue (Pudner 2005, E).
6 Warn the patient of the pulling sensation they will experience and reassure throughout (Walker 2007).	To promote comfort and co-operation. E
7 Grasp the drain close to the skin and remove gently. If there is resistance, place free gloved hand against the tissue to oppose the removal from the wound.	To minimize pain and reduce trauma (E). Drains that have been left in for an extended period will sometimes be more difficult due to tissue growing around the tubing (Walker 2007, E).
8 The edge of the drain should be clean cut and not jagged.	This clean appearance ensures that the whole drain has been removed. E
9 Cover the drain site with a sterile dressing and tape securely.	To prevent infection entering the drain site. E
10 If the site is inflamed or there is a request for the tip to be sent to microbiology, cut it cleanly and send it in a sterile pot.	Recognize and treat suspected infection (Fraise and Bradley 2009, E; Walker 2007, E).

Postprocedure

Action	Rationale
11 Measure and record the contents of the drainage bottle in the appropriate documents.	To maintain an accurate record of drainage from the wound and enable evaluation of state of wound (NMC 2009, C).
12 Dispose of used drainage system in clinical waste bag.	To ensure safe disposal. E

Procedure guideline 19.8 Wound drain shortening (open drainage systems, for example, Penrose, Yates or corrugated)

Essential equipment

- Sterile dressing pack containing gallipots or an indented plastic tray, low-linting swabs and/or medical foam, disposable forceps, gloves, sterile field, disposable bag
- Scissors or stitch cutter (refer to patient notes for directions if dressing in place)
- Sterile absorbent dressing to place over drainage site
- Wound swab/sterile pot (to be used if infection suspected)

Procedure

Action	Rationale
1 Use aseptic technique and sterile equipment (as listed above).	To prevent infection (Fraise and Bradley 2009, E; Pudner 2005, E; Walker 2007, E).
2 If the drain is sutured in place, hold the knot of the suture with metal forceps and gently lift upwards.	Plastic forceps tend to slip against nylon sutures. To allow space for the scissors or stitch cutter to be placed underneath. E
3 Cut the shortest end of the suture as close to the skin as possible.	To prevent infection by allowing the suture to be liberated from the drain without drawing the exposed part through tissue (Pudner 2005, E).
4 Using gloved hand, gently ease the drain out of wound to the length requested by surgeons.	To allow healing to take place from base of wound. E
5 Using gloved hand, place a sterile safety pin through the drain as close to the skin as possible, taking great care not to stab either yourself or the patient.	To prevent retraction of drain into the wound and minimize the risk of cross-infection and sharps injury. E
6 Cut same amount of tubing from distal end of drain as withdrawn from wound.	So there is a convenient length of tubing to drain into the bag. To ensure patient comfort. E
7 Place a sterile, suitably sized dressing or drainage bag over the drain site (depending upon the expected amount of exudates).	To allow effluent to drain, prevent excoriation of the skin and contain any odour. E
8 Check dressing/bag is secure and comfortable for the patient.	For patient comfort. E

Postprocedure

9 Record by how much the drainage tube was shortened, or example 1–2 cm every 24–28 hours (Pudner 2005, E).	To ensure the length remaining in the wound is known (NMC 2009, C).

Postprocedural considerations

Check wound and drain site for signs of infection and obtain a wound swab if appropriate. Report any unusual signs or complications and record (Fraise and Bradley 2009, NMC 2009).

Plastic surgery

Definition

Plastic surgery is the collective term that refers to surgical procedures that are performed to restore function and assist in the healing of exposed or non-union fractures, soft tissue defects or to improve natural contours (McCarthy 1990).

This is achieved by using flaps and skin grafts for reconstruction purposes, in addition to using the natural elasticity and mobility of the skin. Surgical reconstruction is often required following extensive surgery for cancers of the breast, head and neck, skin, soft tissue and genitourinary system. The aim is to perform a simple procedure that will provide the best aesthetic and functional outcome (Achauer and Eriksson 2000).

Anatomy and physiology

A surgical flap is a strip of tissue, usually consisting of skin, underlying fat, fascia, muscle and/or bone, which is transferred from one part of the body (known as the donor site) to another (known as the recipient site) (Storch and Rice 2005).

A skin graft is living but devascularized (separated from its blood supply) tissue consisting of all or some of the layers of the skin which is removed from one area of the body and applied to a wound on another area of the body. The common methods of skin grafting are full-thickness skin grafts (FTSG), in which the entire epidermis and dermis is removed, split-thickness or split skin graft (SSG), which consists of the epidermis and the upper part of the dermis only (Giele and Cassell 2008).

Evidence-based approaches

Principles of care

Each patient will require individually planned, and therefore unique, surgery. Reconstructive surgery of this type often results in altered anatomy, in both appearance and function, which may affect the psychological and physical well-being of the patient. Preoperative patient assessment must be as detailed as possible; this should include information on past and present medical conditions that may delay wound healing. For certain patient groups, for example those with recurrence of head and neck cancer, anatomy may already have been altered, through previous surgery, thereby narrowing down the possible options for reconstruction.

The complexity of the surgery will often require intensive nursing care. Postoperative observation of the wound sites, dressings and drains is crucial as deterioration of a wound can occur suddenly, for example fluid-filled seromas, necessitating the need for prompt nursing action. The main aim following flap reconstruction is to allow easy access for observation and to ensure that circulation and overall care are monitored efficiently during the crucial first 72 hours. Figure 19.6 shows a flap observation chart. These should adhere to medical notes and instructions as per patient. The principles are clarified in the procedure guidelines (e.g. change of wound dressing, removal of drains).

Seroma

Following surgery, it is normal for haemoserous fluid to collect postoperatively at the site of excision. Fluid

---

Name: .... Hospital No: .... Ward:..

THE ROYAL MARSDEN

Flap Observation Chart

Instructions	Criteria for Assessment	Normal	Arterial Insufficiency	Venous Congestion
1. **Confirm with the surgeon the frequency of flap observations (see medical notes / nursing care plan)** Suggested immediate post-op assessment frequency: • every 15 minutes for first 4 hours, • every 30 minutes for the next 4 hours, • hourly for 24–36 hours, • then 2–4 hourly thereafter 2. **If signs of venous or arterial occlusion seek immediate help** 3. **At each handover, confirm flap status/observations at the bedside**	**Colour** • If it is an external flap then check with the donor site for original colour • If it is an internal flap then monitor for extremes of colour	Usual skin tone	Paler than usual skin tone	Blue / Purple / Mottled
	Temperature • An external or internal flap should always feel warm to touch • If the flap feels cool or has increased warmth, **seek medical assessment immediately** • A warmer flap may be due to an abnormal inflammatory response, e.g. infection	Warm	Cold	Increased warmth
	Turgidity (Texture) • The flap should usually feel soft (spongy), not hard or flaccid • Hard or swollen flap indicates possible oedema or haematoma	Soft	Flaccid	Turgid (hard)
	Capillary Refill (Blanching) • If possible this should be timed (in seconds) • If timing not possible and an alteration in perfusion is suspected, **seek medical assessment immediately**	2–3 seconds	Absent / Sluggish > 6 seconds	Brisk < 3 seconds
	Specific Monitoring Instructions (e.g. Monitor the tension on the flap and check for kinking)			

Type & Location of Flap: .... Donor Area (if appropriate): ....

....

Timing		Colour (tick one)			Temperature (tick one)			Turgidity (Texture) (tick one)			Capillary Refill (Blanching) (tick one)			Specific Instructions (specify):	Signature and Print Name
Date	Time	Usual skin tone	Paler than usual skin tone	Blue / purple / mottled	Warm	Cold	Increased warmth	Soft	Flaccid	Turgid (hard)	2–3 seconds	Absent / sluggish > 6 seconds	Brisk < 3 seconds		

Title: Flap Observation Chart	Version No: 2 Issue Date: March 2005 Unique Identification Number: NR027	Document Type: Clinical Record - Chart
Department: Nursing & Rehabilitation – Nursing	Page 1 of 2	© 2005 The Royal Marsden Hospital

Figure 19.6 Flap observation chart.

collects where there is a space created by tissue removal and it will continue to do so until the underlying tissues adhere (Harmer 2003).

A seroma is defined as a clinically identifiable collection of serous fluid within any *surgical* cavity (Woodworth *et al.* 2000). There appears to be no relationship between seroma formation and the patient's age, tumour size, grade or Body Mass Index (Woodworth *et al.* 2000). Seroma formation is a common sequel rather than a complication following breast surgery, particularly when axillary dissection has been undertaken (Agrawal *et al.* 2006) and the extent of dissection, mastectomy versus breast-conserving surgery and the number of lymph nodes removed have all been shown to influence seroma formation (Cregan 2006). The sentinel lymph node biopsy technique introduced in recent years seems to confer a lower risk of seroma formation (Vitug and Newman 2007).

It is common for serous fluid to collect after removal of the drain. Patients who develop seromas will commonly report a bulging wound and experience pain or discomfort, which may in turn prevent them from performing postoperative exercises, such as arm exercises, which are recommended to restore mobility and minimize the risk of lymphoedema. Seroma formation can also impair the healing process and hinder the patient's recovery phase due to the risk of wound infection, wound dehiscence, flap necrosis, a delay in commencing further treatment and an increase in the number of postoperative clinic visits required for seroma surveillance (Agrawal *et al.* 2006). Depending on the amount that has collected, a surgeon or specialist nurse may aspirate this as required. Symptomatic seromas can be drained by simple percutaneous fine needle aspiration according to individual hospital protocol (Warren 2008).

Negative pressure wound therapy

Definition

Negative pressure wound therapy (NPWT) is the application of a uniform negative pressure across the wound bed to promote healing (Ubbink *et al.* 2008). The benefits of NPWT are improving exudates management, reduction of odour and infection rates and increasing local blood flow to the wound (KCI 2007, NICE 2009, Ubbink *et al.* 2008).

Evidence-based approaches

Rationale

The advantage of using NPWT is that it stimulates granulation in an enhanced well-vascularized wound bed and promotes wound healing. It creates a moist wound environment and removes exudates and bacteria from the wound (KCI 2007). The interstitial fluid that mechanically compromises

healing is gently removed whilst the capillary circulation is increased (Ubbink *et al.* 2008). Pressures are set at the level best suited to the wound type and can be set on continuous or intermittent according to the therapy required (Benbow 2006). Maintaining the vacuum seal is essential in providing this therapy. It has proven to be cost efficient, safe and effective as a treatment modality for wound care (KCI 2007). The benefits to chronic wound healing of using NPWT versus other treatments have been shown in a number of clinical trials, but further research is needed with fewer methodological flaws and clearer reporting of infection rates and length of hospital stay (NICE 2009, Ubbink *et al.* 2008).

Indications

NPWT is indicated for:

- chronic wounds
- pressure ulcers
- dehisced wounds and incisions
- partial-thickness burns
- flaps and grafts.

(KCI 2007)

See Figure 19.7 for an example of a patient with a wound being treated with the NPWT device.

Contraindications

Negative pressure wound therapy is contraindicated in grossly contaminated wounds, malignant wounds, untreated osteomyelitis, non-enteric and unexplored fistulae or necrotic tissue with eschar present and areas with exposed tendons (KCI 2007).

Precautions should be exercised when there is active bleeding in the wound, difficult haemostasis or when the patient is taking anticoagulants (Benbow 2006). The wound site must be carefully assessed to ensure that NPWT is indeed the appropriate treatment modality. If signs of infection or

Figure 19.7 Negative pressure wound therapy: right inguinal wound.

Figure 19.8 Negative pressure wound therapy: VAC dressing.

Figure 19.9 Negative pressure wound therapy: VAC pump.

complications develop, the therapy should be discontinued (KCI 2007). There is currently not enough evidence to recommend NPWT for open abdominal wounds (NICE 2009).

Preprocedural considerations

Consulting the appropriate company representative for training is essential as application and approach are individually determined and KCI, for example, have their own comprehensive clinical guidelines (KCI 2007). If the wound is bigger than the largest foam dressing, more than one piece of foam may be used as long as the edges of the foam are in contact with each other. KCI also has recommendations for changing the type of foam once the exudates decrease (KCI 2007). Using several smaller pieces of film to cover the

area is recommended for larger wounds as they are easier to apply and maintaining an air-tight seal is more successful (KCI 2007).

Equipment

Figures 19.7, 19.8 and 19.9 show the vacuum-assisted closure or VAC therapy system (KCI International). See the Websites and useful addresses at the end of the chapter for contact details for VAC and KCI, amongst others. Other methods for NPWT are available and use similar principles (Hampton and Collins 2004). All equipment used should be the manufacturer's recommended materials for the relevant system (KCI 2007).

Procedure guideline 19.9 Negative pressure wound therapy

Essential equipment

- NPWT unit
- NPWT dressing pack
- NPWT canister and tubing
- Sterile scissors
- Sterile gloves
- Apron
- Dressing procedure pack
- Sterile 0.9% sodium chloride for irrigation (warmed to approx. 37°C in a jug of warm water)
- Clamp (Spencer Wells forceps)

Optional equipment

- Extra semi-permeable film dressings to seal any leaks
- Non-adherent wound contact layer to prevent foam adhering to wound bed
- Alcohol-free skin barrier film to protect any fragile or macerated skin around the wound

1197

(Continued)

Procedure guideline 19.9 (*Continued*)

Preprocedure

Action	Rationale
1 Explain and discuss the procedure with the patient.	To ensure the patient understands the procedure and other options available and gives their valid consent (NMC 2008a C).
2 Provide routine analgesia prior to dressing procedure.	To prevent unnecessary procedural pain. E
3 Ensure there is adequate lighting and the patient is comfortable and in a position where the wound can be accessed and viewed easily. Assemble all necessary equipment.	To allow access to area for dressing change. Dressing application can be complicated and take a long time so the patient should be in a comfortable position for the procedure (Beldon 2006, E)

Procedure

4 Use aseptic technique and sterile equipment (as listed above).	To prevent infection (Fraise and Bradley 2009, E; Pudner 2005, E; Walker 2007, E).
5 To remove the NPWT dressing, put on a pair of non-sterile gloves.	To reduce the risk of cross-infection (Fraise and Bradley, E).
6 Clamp the dressing tubing and disconnect it from the canister tubing. Allow any fluid in the canister tubing to be sucked into the canister. Switch off the pump and clamp the canister tubing.	To prevent spillage of body fluid waste from the tubing or canister. E
7 Remove and discard the canister (if full or at least weekly).	To prevent pump alarming and for infection control. E
8 Carefully remove the occlusive film drape by gently lifting one edge and then stretching the drape horizontally and slowly pulling up from the skin.	To prevent damage to the peri-wound skin. E
9 Carefully remove the foam dressing from the wound bed. Irrigate with sterile 0.9% sodium chloride if required.	To prevent damage to newly formed tissue within the wound bed and prevent pain. E
10 Clean the wound with sterile 0.9% sodium chloride.	To prevent infection and remove surface debris/necrotic tissue (Dealey 2005, E).
11 Debride the wound if applicable.	To remove loose necrotic tissue that may be a focus for infection (Vowden and Vowden 2002, C).
12 To apply the dressing, cut the NPWT foam to fit the size and shape of the wound, including tunnelling and undermined areas.	The foam should fit the wound exactly to ensure full benefit of the negative pressure therapy (Beldon 2006, E).
13 Avoid cutting the foam over the wound bed.	To prevent loose particles of foam falling into the wound. E
14 Place the foam into the wound cavity.	The whole wound bed must be covered with foam. If the foam is touching, it will transfer the negative pressure to the next piece. E
15 If the wound bed is friable/granulating and likely to bleed, Mepitel may be used under the foam to protect the extracellular matrix (ECM).	The ECM requires a trauma-free dressing removal and once exudates subside, the wound bed may become less moist (alternatively, white foam, slightly damp, is recommended by KCI; (KCI 2007, C).
16 Cut the occlusive film drape to size and apply over the top of the foam, ensuring a 3–5 cm border onto intact skin, NPWT gel strip or hydrocolloid. (NB: do not compress the foam into the wound.)	To obtain a good seal around the wound edges. E

17 Choose a location on the sealed occlusive film drape to apply the tubing where the tubing will not rub or cause pressure. Cut a hole through the film, approximately 2 cm in diameter, leaving the foam intact.	To reduce the risk of pressure injury to skin. E
18 Place the TRAC pad on the film with the hole in the centre of the elbow joint directly over the hole in the film drape. Gently press around the TRAC pad (KCI 2007).	To ensure correct position and seal of the pad. (NB: TRAC is used for the vacuum-assisted closure (VAC) system; follow manufacturer's individual instructions) (KCI 2007, C).
19 To commence the NPWT, insert the canister into the pump until it clicks into place.	Indicates the canister is positioned correctly and is secure (Beldon 2006, E).
20 Connect the dressing tubing to the canister tubing and open clamps.	The pump will alarm if the tubing is clamped or not connected. E
21 Press POWER button and follow the on-screen instructions to set the level and type of pressure required according to instructions from the patient's medical/surgical team.	To ensure the therapy is set to the individual requirements of the patient. E
22 Start the pump by pressing THERAPY ON/OFF: the foam should contract into the wound.	Any small air leak will prevent the foam dressing from contracting and reassessment is required. E

Postprocedure

23 Document the dressing and setting in the patient's notes.	To provide a record (NMC 2009, C).

Postprocedural considerations

Ongoing care

Careful monitoring of the peri-wound area for signs of infection or oedema and checking the equipment whilst *in situ* are imperative to ensure patient safety. The dressings should be changed every 48–72 hours to observe and monitor the wound for signs of infection. The NPWT unit should not be switched off for more than 2 hours and regular assessments should be made (KCI 2007).

Websites and useful addresses

Aspen Medical (Sorbsan, Aquaform, Polymem, Mesitran): www.aspenmedicaleurope.com/Pages/Specialist WoundCare.asp
Coloplast (biatain): www.coloplast.co.uk/ECompany/GBMED/ Homepage. nsf/(VIEWDOCSBYID)/CC89E227B1FD573-B41256A06002A0DE5
Convatec (aquacel. combiderm, duoderm, granuflex): www.convatec.co.uk
www.hydrofiber.co.uk/engb/cvthy-products/hy-internapag/0/accessser/0/3377/7947/hydrofiber-technology.html
World Wide Wounds: Dressings Datacards: www.worldwidewounds.com/Common/ProductDatacards.html#top
World Wide Wounds: Product Reviews: www.wounds-uk.com/woundessentials/03_product_review.pdf
Insight Medical for tracheostomy dressings and Actibalm Honey: www.insightmedical.net/product.asp?ID=47
KCI for VAC therapy: topical negative pressure: www.kci-medical.com
Molnlycke Health Care (Mepitel, Mepilex) www.molnlycke.com/item.asp?id=3273&lang= 2&si=14

Smith and Nephew (Allevyn): www.wound.smith-nephew.com/uk/Home.asp
For 'TIME' wound bed preparation (assessment principles): www.wound.smith-nephew.com/uk/node.asp?NodeId= 3104

Society of Radiographers
Telephone: 020 7740 7200
Website: www.sor.org/public/patient_info.htm
RTOG Skin Assessment Tool with pictures available from: www.sor.org/public/contact/contact_us.htm

NHS Quality Improvement Scotland
Telephone: 0131 623 4300
Website: www.nhshealthquality.org
Best Practice Statement – April 2004 Skincare of Patients Receiving Radiotherapy

Wound Care Society
Telephone: 01480 434401
Website: www.woundcaresociety.com
Wound Care Alliance UK
Telephone: 0121 331 7083
Website: www.wcauk.org/about/php

References

Achauer, B.M. and Eriksson, E. (2000) *Plastic Surgery: Indications, Operations, and Outcomes*. Mosby, St Louis, MO.

Agrawal, A., Ayantunde, A.A. and Cheung, K.L. (2006) Concepts of seroma formation and prevention in breast cancer surgery. *ANZ Journal of Surgery*, **76** (12), 1088–1095.

Alexander, S. (2009) Malignant fungating wounds: managing pain, bleeding and psychosocial issues. *Journal of Wound Care*, **18** (10), 418–425.

Ang, K.K. (2008) Multidisciplinary management of locally advanced SCCHN: optimizing treatment outcomes. *Oncologist*, **13** (8), 899–910. theoncologist.2007–2015

Angeras, M.H., Brandberg, A., Falk, A. and Seeman, T. (1992) Comparison between sterile saline and tap water for the cleaning of acute traumatic soft tissue wounds. *European Journal of Surgery*, **158** (6–7), 347–350.

Archambeau, J.O., Pezner, R. and Wasserman, T. (1995) Pathophysiology of irradiated skin and breast. *International Journal of Radiation Oncology, Biology, Physics*, **31** (5), 1171–1185.

Ayello, E.A., Dowsett, C., Schultz, G.S. *et al.* (2004) TIME heals all wounds. *Nursing*, **34** (4), 36–41.

Baker, J. (1998) Essential oils: a complementary therapy in wound management. *Journal of Wound Care*, **7** (7), 355–357.

Bale, S. (1991) A holistic approach and the ideal dressing. Cavity wound management in the 1990s. *Professional Nurse*, **6** (6), 316, 318, 320–323.

Bale, S. and Jones, V. (2006) *Wound Care Nursing: A Patient-Centred Approach*, 2nd edn. Mosby Elsevier, Edinburgh.

Beitz, J.M., Bonner, M. and Calianno, C. (2008) *Wound Care Made Incredibly Visual*, Lippincott Williams and Wilkins, Philadelphia.

Beldon, P. (2006) Topical negative pressure dressings and vacuum-assisted closure. *Wound Essentials*, **1**, 110–114.

Benbow, M. (2006) An update on VAC therapy... vacuum assisted closure. *Journal of Community Nursing*, **20** (4), 28–32.

Bennett, G. and Moody, M. (1995) *Wound Care for Health Professionals* Chapman and Hall, London.

Bernier, J., Bonner, J., Vermorken, J.B. *et al.* (2008) Consensus guidelines for the management of radiation dermatitis and co-existing acne-like rash in patients receiving radiotherapy plus EGFR inhibitors for the treatment of squamous cell carcinoma of the head and neck. *Annals of Oncology*, **19** (1), 142–149.

Bird, C. (2000) Supporting patients with fungating breast wounds. *Professional Nurse*, **15** (10), 649–652.

Bluestein, D. and Javaheri, A. (2008) Pressure ulcers: prevention, evaluation, and management. *American Family Physician*, **78** (10), 1186–1194.

BNF (2010) *British National Formulary 59*. BMA/RPSGB, London.

Bolderston, A., Lloyd, N.S., Wong, R.K. *et al.* (2006) The prevention and management of acute skin reactions related to radiation therapy: a systematic review and practice guideline. *Supportive Care in Cancer*, **14** (8), 802–817.

Bryant, R.A. (ed) (2000) *Acute and Chronic Wounds: Nursing Management*, 2nd edn Mosby, St Louis, MO.

Calvin, M. (1998) Cutaneous wound repair. *Wounds: A Compendium of Clinical Research & Practice*, **10** (1), 12–33.

Castille, K. (1998) Suturing. *Nursing Standard*, **12** (41), 41–46.

Cho, M. and Hunt, T.K. (2001) The overall approach to wounds. In: Falanga, V. (ed) *Cutaneous Wound Healing*. Martin Dunitz, London. pp. xii.

Clark, A. (2004) Understanding the principles of suturing minor skin lesions. *Nursing Times*, **100** (29), 32–34.

Collier, M. (1996) The principles of optimum wound management. *Nursing Standard*, **10** (43), 47–52; quiz 53–54.

Collier, M. (2002) Wound-bed preparation. *Nursing Times*, **98** (2), 55–57.

ConvaTec (2004) *ConvaTec Wound Care Reference Guide*, ConvaTec, Uxbridge.

Cregan, P. (2006) Review of concepts of seroma formation and prevention in breast cancer surgery. *ANZ Journal of Surgery*, **76** (12), 1046.

Cutting, K.F. (1998) *Wounds and Infection*. Wound Care Society, Huntingdon.

Dealey, C. (2005) *The Care of Wounds: A Guide for Nurses*, 3rd edn. Blackwell Science, Oxford.

DH (2005) *Hazardous Waste (England) Regulations*. Department of Health, London.

Donovan, S. (1998) Wound infection and wound swabbing. *Professional Nurse*, **13** (11), 757–759.

Dowsett, C. (2002) The role of the nurse in wound bed preparation. *Nursing Standard*, **16** (44), 69–72, 74, 76.

Dowsett, C. and Ayello, E. (2004) TIME principles of chronic wound bed preparation and treatment. *British Journal of Nursing*, **13** (15), S16–S23.

Ehrlich, H.P. (1998) The physiology of wound healing. A summary of normal and abnormal wound healing processes. *Advances in Wound Care: The Journal for Prevention and Healing*, **11** (7), 326–328.

Elkin, M.K., Perry, A.G. and Potter, P.A. (2004) Skill 22.3 removing staples and sutures. In: *Nursing Interventions and Clinical Skills*, 3rd edn. Mosby, St Louis.

EPUAP (2009) *International Guideline: Treatment of Pressure Ulcers: Quick Reference Guide*. European Pressure Ulcer Advisory Panel and National Pressure Ulcer Advisory Panel, Washington D.C. http://www.epuap.org/guidelines/Final_Quick_Treatment.pdf.

Fairbairn, K. (1993) Towards better care for women. Understanding fungating breast lesions. *Professional Nurse*, **9** (3), 204, 206, 208 passim.

Fairbairn, K., Grier, J., Hunter, C. and Preece, J. (2002) A sharp debridement procedure devised by specialist nurses. *Journal of Wound Care*, **11** (10), 371–375.

Falanga, V. (2000) Classifications for wound bed preparation and stimulation of chronic wounds. *Wound Repair and Regeneration*, **8** (5), 347–352.

Field, F.K. and Kerstein, M.D. (1994) Overview of wound healing in a moist environment. *American Journal of Surgery*, **167** (1A), 2S–6S.

Flanagan, M. (1996) A practical framework for wound assessment. 1: Physiology. *British Journal of Nursing*, **5** (22), 1391–1397.

Flanagan, M. (1999) The physiology of wound healing. In: Miller, M. and Glover, D. (eds) *Wound Management: Theory and Practice*. Nursing Times Books, London: pp. 14–22.

Flanagan, M. (2000) The physiology of wound healing. *Journal of Wound Care*, **9** (6), 299–300.

Fletcher, J. (1997) Wound cleansing. *Professional Nurse*, **12** (11), 793–796.

Fraise, A.P. and Bradley, T. (eds) (2009) *Ayliffe's Control of Healthcare-associated Infection: A Practical Handbook*, 5th edition. Hodder Arnold, London.

Garrett, B. (1997) The proliferation and movement of cells during re-epithelialisation. *Journal of Wound Care*, **6** (4), 174–177.

Giele, H. and Cassell, O. (2008) *Plastic and Reconstructive Surgery*. Oxford University Press, Oxford.

Gilchrist, B. (1999) Wound infection. In: Miller, M. and Glover, D. (eds) *Wound Management: Theory and Practice*. Nursing Times Books, London: pp. 96–107.

Goldberg, M.T. and Mcgynn-Byer, P. (2000) Oncology-related skin damage. In: Bryant, R.A. (ed) *Acute and Chronic Wounds: Nursing Management*, 2nd edn. Mosby, St Louis, MO: pp. 367–386.

Grocott, P. (2007) Care of patients with fungating malignant wounds. *Nursing Standard*, **21** (24), 57–58, 60, 62 passim.

Haisfield-Wolfe, M.E. and Rund, C. (1997) Malignant cutaneous wounds: a management protocol. *Ostomy/Wound Management*, **43** (1), 56–60, 62, 64–66.

Hallett, A. (1995) Fungating wounds. *Nursing Times*, **91** (39), 81–82, 85.

Hampton, S. (1999) Choosing the right dressing. In: Miller, M. and Glover, D. (eds) *Wound Management: Theory and Practice*. Nursing Times Books, London: pp. 116–128.

Hampton, S. (2008) Malodorous fungating wounds: how dressings alleviate symptoms. *British Journal of Community Nursing*, **13** (6), S31–S32, S34, S36 passim.

Hampton, S. and Collins, F. (2004) *Tissue Viability: The Prevention, Treatment, and Management of Wounds*, Whurr Publishers, London.

Harmer, V. (2003) Surgery as a treatment for breast cancer. In: Harmer, V. (ed) *Breast Cancer: Nursing Care and Management*. Whurr Publishers, London: pp. 82–101.

Hart, J. (2002) Inflammation. 1: Its role in the healing of acute wounds. *Journal of Wound Care*, **11** (6), 205–209.

Heggie, S., Bryant, G.P., Tripcony, L. *et al.* (2002) A Phase III study on the efficacy of topical aloe vera gel on irradiated breast tissue. *Cancer Nursing*, **25** (6), 442–451.

Hess, C.T. (2005) *Wound Care*, 5th edn. Lippincott Williams and Wilkins, Philadelphia.

Ivetic, O. and Lyne, P.A. (1990) Fungating and ulcerating malignant lesions: a review of the literature. *Journal of Advanced Nursing*, **15** (1), 83–88.

Jay, R. (1999) Suturing in A + E. *Professional Nurse*, **14** (6), 412–415.

KCI (2007) *VAC Therapy Clinical Guidelines: A Reference Source for Clinicians*. KCI Licensing, Kidlington. http://www.kci1.com.

Kedge, E.M. (2009) A systematic review to investigate the effectiveness and acceptability of interventions for moist desquamation in radiotherapy patients. *Radiography*, **15** (3), 247–257.

Laverty, D., Mallett, J. and Mulholland, J. (1997) Protocols and guidelines for managing wounds. *Professional Nurse*, **13** (2), 79–781.

Laverty, D., Naylor, W., Mallett, J. and Mulholland, J. (2000) *Wound Management Guidelines*. Royal Marsden NHS Foundation Trust, London.

Lawrence, J.C. (1997) Wound irrigation. *Journal of Wound Care*, **6** (1), 23–26.

Lippincott Williams and Wilkins (2008) *Wound Care Made Incredibly Visual!* Wolters Kluwer Health/Lippincott Williams and Wilkins, Philadelphia.

Lo, S.F., Hsu, M.Y. and Hu, W.Y. (2007) Using wound bed preparation to heal a malignant fungating wound: a single case study. *Journal of Wound Care*, **16** (9), 373–376.

Lo, S.F., Hu, W.Y., Hayter, M. *et al.* (2008) Experiences of living with a malignant fungating wound: a qualitative study. *Journal of Clinical Nursing*, **17** (20), 2699–2708.

Lund-Nielsen, B., Muller, K. and Adamsen, L. (2005) Malignant wounds in women with breast cancer: feminine and sexual perspectives. *Journal of Clinical Nursing*, **14** (1), 56–64.

Macmillan, M.S., Wells, M., MacBride, S. *et al.* (2007) Randomized comparison of dry dressings versus hydrogel management of radiation-induced moist desquamation. *International Journal of Radiation, Oncology, Biology, Physics*, **68** (3), 864–872.

Maher, K.E. (2005) Radiation therapy: toxicities and management. In: Yarbro, C.H., Frogge, M.H. and Goodman, M. (eds) *Cancer Nursing: Principles and Practice*, 6th edn. Jones and Bartlett, Sudbury, MA: pp. 283–314.

Marieb, E.N. and Hoehn, K. (2010) *Human Anatomy and Physiology*, 8th edn. Benjamin Cummings, San Francisco.

Martin, E.A. (2010) *Concise Colour Medical Dictionary*, 5th edn. Oxford University Press, Oxford.

McCarthy, J.G. (ed) (1990) *Plastic Surgery: Volumes 1–8*. W.B. Saunders, Harcourt and Brace, Philadelphia.

McQuestion, M. (2006) Evidence-based skin care management in radiation therapy. *Seminars in Oncology Nursing*, **22** (3), 163–73.

Miller, M. and Dyson, M. (1996) *Principles of Wound Care*. Macmillan Magazines, London.

Moore, P. and Foster, L. (1998) Acute surgical wound care. 2: The wound healing process. *British Journal of Nursing*, **7** (19), 1183–1187.

Morgan, D.A. (2000) *Formulary of Wound Management Products: A Guide for Healthcare Staff*, 8th edn. Euromed Communications, Haslemere.

Morison, M.J. (1989) Wound cleansing – which solution? *Professional Nurse*, **4** (5), 220–225.

Myers, B.A. (2004) *Wound Management: Principles and Practice*. Prentice Hall, Upper Saddle River, NJ.

Naylor, W. (2001) Assessment and management of pain in fungating wounds. *British Journal of Nursing*, **10** (22 Suppl), S33–6, S38, S40, passim.

Naylor, W. (2002) Malignant wounds: aetiology and principles of management. *Nursing Standard*, **16** (52), 45–53.

Naylor, W., Laverty, D. and Mallett, J. (2001) *The Royal Marsden Hospital Handbook of Wound Management in Cancer Care*. Blackwell Science, Oxford.

NHSE (2005) *The Management of Health, Safety and Welfare Issues for NHS Staff*. NHS Employers, London.

NHSQIS (2010) *Best Practice Statement: Skincare of Patients Receiving Radiotherapy*. NHS Quality Improvement Scotland. http://www.nhshealthquality.org/nhsqis/files/SKINRADIO_BPS_MAR10.pdf.

NMC (2008a) *Consent*. Nursing and Midwifery Council, London www.nmc-uk.org/Nurses-and-midwives/Advice-by-topic/A/Advice/Consent.

NMC (2008b) *The Code: Standards of Conduct, Performance and Ethics for Nurses and Midwives*. Nursing and Midwifery Council, London.

NMC (2009) *Record Keeping: Guidance for Nurses and Midwives*. Nursing and Midwifery Council, London.

Noble-Adams, R. (1999) Radiation-induced skin reactions. 2: Development of a measurement tool. *British Journal of Nursing*, **8** (18), 1208–1211.

Patawardhan, A., Sharma, V. and Dinshaw, K.A. (2002) Duoderm CGF vs Gentian violet 1 % dressing in the treatment of radiation induced ulcers. *World Council of Enterostomal Therapists Journal*, **22** (2), 32–38.

Pearson, I. and Mortimer, P.S. (2004) Skin problems in palliative medicine. In: Doyle, D., Hanks, G., Cherny, N. and Calman, K.(eds) *Oxford Textbook of Palliative Medicine*. Oxford University Press, Oxford: pp.618–627.

Poston, J. (1996) Sharp debridement of devitalized tissue: the nurse's role. *British Journal of Nursing*, **5** (11), 655–656, 658–662.

Price, S. and Price, L. (2007) *Aromatherapy for Health Professionals*, 3rd edn. Churchill Livingstone Elsevier, Edinburgh.

Pudner, R (2005) Wound healing in the surgical patient. In: *Nursing the Surgical Patient*, 2nd edn. Elsevier, Edinburgh: pp. 45–69.

Rankin-Box, D.F. (2001) *The Nurse's Handbook of Complementary Therapies*, 2nd edn. Baillière Tindall, in association with the Royal College of Nursing, Edinburgh.

Reynolds, T. and Cole, E. (2006) Techniques for acute wound closure. *Nursing Standard*, **20** (21), 55–64.

Richardson, M. (2007) Exploring various methods for closing traumatic wounds. *Nursing Times*, **103** (5), 30–31.

Riyat, M.S. and Quinton, D.N. (1997) Tap water as a wound cleansing agent in accident and emergency. *Journal of Accident and Emergency Medicine*, **14** (3), 165–166.

1201

Saltz, L.B., Meropol, N.J., Loehrer, P.J. Sr. et al. (2004) Phase II trial of cetuximab in patients with refractory colorectal cancer that expresses the epidermal growth factor receptor. *Journal of Clinical Oncology*, **22** (7), 1201–1208.

Schultz, G.S., Sibbald, R.G., Falanga, V. *et al.* (2003) Wound bed preparation: a systematic approach to wound management. *Wound Repair and Regeneration*, **11** (s1), S1–S28.

Selby, T. (2009) Managing exudate in malignant fungating wounds and solving problems for patients. *Nursing Times*, **105** (18), 14–17.

Silver, I. (1994) The physiology of wound healing. *Journal of Wound Care*, **3** (2), 106–109.

Simonen, P., Hamilton, C., Ferguson, S. *et al.* (1998) Do inflammatory processes contribute to radiation induced erythema observed in the skin of humans? *Radiotherapy and Oncology*, **46** (1), 73–82.

Solomon, E.P., Adragna, P.J. and Schmidt, R.R. (1990) *Human Anatomy and Physiology*. W.B. Saunders, Philadelphia.

Springett, K. (2002) The impact of diabetes on wound management. *Nursing Standard*, **16** (30), 72–74, 76, 78–80.

Storch, J.E. and Rice, J. (2005) *Reconstructive Plastic Surgical Nursing: Clinical Management and Wound Care*. Blackwell, Oxford.

Teare, J. and Barrett, C. (2002) Using quality of life assessment in wound care. *Nursing Standard*, **17** (6), 59–60, 64, 67–68.

Tejero-Trujeque, R. (2001) How do fibroblasts interact with the extracellular matrix in wound contraction? *Journal of Wound Care*, **10** (6), 237–242.

Thomas, S. (1992) *Current Practices in the Management of Fungating Lesions and Damaged Skin*. Surgical Materials Testing Laboratory, Bridgend.

Thomas, S. (2009) *Formulary of Wound Management Products*, 10th edn. Euromed Communications, Liphook.

Timmons, J. (2006) Skin function and wound healing physiology. *Wound Essentials*, (1), 8–17. Wound-UK. www.wounds-uk.com/woundessentials/01_physiology.pdf.

Tobias, J.S. and Hochhauser, D. (2010) *Cancer and Its Management*, 6th edn. Wiley-Blackwell, Chichester.

Ubbink, D.T., Westerbos, S.J., Evans, D., Land, L. and Vermeulen, H. (2008) Topical negative pressure for treating chronic wounds. *Cochrane Database of Systematic Reviews*, 3, CD001898.

Vitug, A.F. and Newman, L.A. (2007) Complications in breast surgery. *Surgical Clinics of North America*, **87** (2), 431–451.

Vowden, K. (1995) Common problems in wound care: wound and ulcer measurement. *British Journal of Nursing*, **4** (13), 775–776, 778–779.

Vowden, K.R. and Vowden, P. (1999) Wound debridement, Part 2: Sharp techniques. *Journal of Wound Care*, **8** (6), 291–294.

Vowden, K. and Vowden, P. (2002) *Wound Bed Preparation*. World Wide Wounds. www.worldwidewounds.com/2002/april/Vowden/Wound-Bed-Preparation.html.

Waldorf, H. and Fewkes, J. (1995) Wound healing. *Advances in Dermatology*, **10**, 77–96.

Walker, J. (2007) Patient preparation for safe removal of surgical drains. *Nursing Standard*, **21** (49), 39–41.

Warren, M. (2008) Collaboration in developing a protocol for nurse-led seroma aspiration. *British Journal of Nursing*, **17** (15), 956–960.

Wells, M. and MacBride, S. (2003) Radiation skin reactions. In: Faithfull, S. and Wells, M. (eds) *Supportive Care in Radiotherapy*. Churchill Livingstone, Edinburgh: pp. 135–159.

Werdin, F., Tenenhaus, M. and Rennekampff, H.O. (2008) Chronic wound care. *Lancet*, **372** (9653), 1860–1862.

White, R. (2001) Managing exudate. *Nursing Times*, **97** (14), 59–60.

Wickline, M.M. (2004) Prevention and treatment of acute radiation dermatitis: a literature review. *Oncology Nursing Forum*, **31** (2), 234–247.

Wilkes, L., White, K., Smeal, T. and Beale, B. (2001) Malignant wound management: what dressings do nurses use? *Journal of Wound Care*, **10** (3), 65–69.

Williams, C. and Young, T. (1998) *Myth and Reality in Wound Care*. Quay Books, Salisbury.

Wilson, V. (2005) Assessment and management of fungating wounds: a review. *British Journal of Community Nursing (Supplement)*, **10** (3), S28–34.

Wolcott, R.D., Kennedy, J.P. and Dowd, S.E. (2009) Regular debridement is the main tool for maintaining a healthy wound bed in most chronic wounds. *Journal of Wound Care*, **18** (2), 54–56.

Woodworth, P.A., McBoyle, M.F., Helmer, S.D. and Beamer, R.L. (2000) Seroma formation after breast cancer surgery: incidence and predicting factors. *American Surgeon*, **66** (5), 444–451.

Young, C.V. (2005) The effects of malodorous fungating malignant wounds on body image and quality of life. *Journal of Wound Care*, **14** (8), 359–362.

The Code

The Code
Standards of conduct, performance and ethics for nurses and midwives

The people in your care must be able to trust you with their health and well-being. To justify that trust, you must:

- make the care of people your first concern, treating them as individuals and respecting their dignity
- work with others to protect and promote the health and well-being of those in your care, their families and carers, and the wider community
- provide a high standard of practice and care at all times
- be open and honest, act with integrity and uphold the reputation of your profession.

As a professional, you are personally accountable for actions and omissions in your practice and must always be able to justify your decisions.

You must always act lawfully, whether those laws relate to your professional practice or personal life.

Failure to comply with this Code may bring your fitness to practise into question and endanger your registration.

This Code should be considered together with the Nursing and Midwifery Council's rules, standards, guidance and advice available from www.nmc-uk.org.

Make the care of people your first concern, treating them as individuals and respecting their dignity

Treat people as individuals

- You must treat people as individuals and respect their dignity
- You must not discriminate in any way against those in your care
- You must treat people kindly and considerately
- You must act as an advocate for those in your care, helping them to access relevant health and social care, information and support

Respect people's confidentiality

- You must respect people's right to confidentiality
- You must ensure people are informed about how and why information is shared by those who will be providing their care
- You must disclose information if you believe someone may be at risk of harm, in line with the law of the country in which you are practising

Collaborate with those in your care

- You must listen to the people in your care and respond to their concerns and preferences
- You must support people in caring for themselves to improve and maintain their health
- You must recognize and respect the contribution that people make to their own care and well-being
- You must make arrangements to meet people's language and communication needs
- You must share with people, in a way they can understand, the information they want or need to know about their health

Ensure you gain consent

- You must ensure that you gain consent before you begin any treatment or care
- You must respect and support people's rights to accept or decline treatment and care
- You must uphold people's rights to be fully involved in decisions about their care
- You must be aware of the legislation regarding mental capacity, ensuring that people who lack capacity remain at the centre of decision making and are fully safeguarded
- You must be able to demonstrate that you have acted in someone's best interests if you have provided care in an emergency

Maintain clear professional boundaries

- You must refuse any gifts, favours or hospitality that might be interpreted as an attempt to gain preferential treatment
- You must not ask for or accept loans from anyone in your care or anyone close to them
- You must establish and actively maintain clear sexual boundaries at all times with people in your care, their families and carers

Work with others to protect and promote the health and well-being of those in your care, their families and carers, and the wider community

Share information with your colleagues

- You must keep your colleagues informed when you are sharing the care of others
- You must work with colleagues to monitor the quality of your work and maintain the safety of those in your care
- You must facilitate students and others to develop their competence

Work effectively as part of a team

- You must work co-operatively within teams and respect the skills, expertise and contributions of your colleagues
- You must be willing to share your skills and experience for the benefit of your colleagues
- You must consult and take advice from colleagues when appropriate
- You must treat your colleagues fairly and without discrimination
- You must make a referral to another practitioner when it is in the best interests of someone in your care

Delegate effectively

- You must establish that anyone you delegate to is able to carry out your instructions
- You must confirm that the outcome of any delegated task meets required standards
- You must make sure that everyone you are responsible for is supervised and supported

Manage risk

- You must act without delay if you believe that you, a colleague or anyone else may be putting someone at risk
- You must inform someone in authority if you experience problems that prevent you working within this Code or other nationally agreed standards
- You must report your concerns in writing if problems in the environment of care are putting people at risk

Provide a high standard of practice and care at all times

Use the best available evidence

- You must deliver care based on the best available evidence or best practice
- You must ensure any advice you give is evidence based if you are suggesting health-care products or services
- You must ensure that the use of complementary or alternative therapies is safe and in the best interests of those in your care

Keep your skills and knowledge up to date

- You must have the knowledge and skills for safe and effective practice when working without direct supervision
- You must recognize and work within the limits of your competence
- You must keep your knowledge and skills up to date throughout your working life
- You must take part in appropriate learning and practice activities that maintain and develop your competence and performance

Keep clear and accurate records

- You must keep clear and accurate records of the discussions you have, the assessments you make, the treatment and medicines you give and how effective these have been
- You must complete records as soon as possible after an event has occurred
- You must not tamper with original records in any way
- You must ensure any entries you make in someone's paper records are clearly and legibly signed, dated and timed
- You must ensure any entries you make in someone's electronic records are clearly attributable to you
- You must ensure all records are kept confidentially and securely

Be open and honest, act with integrity and uphold the reputation of your profession

Act with integrity

- You must demonstrate a personal and professional commitment to equality and diversity
- You must adhere to the laws of the country in which you are practising
- You must inform the NMC if you have been cautioned, charged or found guilty of a criminal offence
- You must inform any employers you work for if your fitness to practise is impaired or is called into question

Deal with problems

- You must give a constructive and honest response to anyone who complains about the care they have received
- You must not allow someone's complaint to prejudice the care you provide for them
- You must act immediately to put matters right if someone in your care has suffered harm for any reason
- You must explain fully and promptly to the person affected what has happened and the likely effects
- You must co-operate with internal and external investigations

Be impartial

- You must not abuse your privileged position for your own ends
- You must ensure that your professional judgement is not influenced by any commercial considerations

Uphold the reputation of your profession

- You must not use your professional status to promote causes that are not related to health
- You must co-operate with the media only when you can confidently protect the confidential information and dignity of those in your care
- You must uphold the reputation of your profession at all times

Information about indemnity insurance

The NMC recommends that a registered nurse, midwife or specialist community public health nurse, in advising, treating and caring for patients/clients, has professional indemnity insurance. This is in the interests of clients, patients and registrants in the event of claims of professional negligence.

Whilst employers have vicarious liability for the negligent acts and/or omissions of their employees, such cover does not normally extend to activities undertaken outside the registrant's employment. Independent practice would not be covered by vicarious liability. It is the individual registrant's responsibility to establish their insurance status and take appropriate action.

In situations where an employer does not have vicarious liability, the NMC recommends that registrants obtain adequate professional indemnity insurance. If unable to secure professional indemnity insurance, a registrant will need to demonstrate that all their clients/patients are fully informed of this fact and the implications this might have in the event of a claim for professional negligence.

Contributors to previous editions

First edition edited by

A. Phylip Pritchard
Research Assistant, Department of Nursing Research
Valerie-Anne Walker
Research Assistant, Department of Nursing Research

Second edition edited by

A. Phylip Pritchard
Assistant to the Director of In-Patient Services/Chief
 Nursing Officer
Jill A. David
Director of Nursing Research

Third edition edited by

A. Phylip Pritchard
Formerly Co-ordinator of European Educational
 Initiatives, The Royal Marsden Hospital, and
 Executive Secretary, European Oncology Nursing Society
Jane Mallett
Research and Practice Development Co-ordinator

Fourth edition edited by

Jane Mallett
Research and Practice Development Manager
Christopher Bailey
Macmillan Research Practitioner, Macmillan Practice
 Development Unit, Centre for Cancer and Palliative
 Care Studies, Institute of Cancer Research

Fifth edition edited by

Jane Mallett
Research and Practice Development Manager,
 The Royal Marsden Hospital
Lisa Dougherty
Clinical Nurse Specialist Intravenous Services,
 The Royal Marsden Hospital

Sixth and seventh editions edited by

Lisa Dougherty
Nurse Consultant Intravenous Therapy, The Royal
 Marsden Hospital
Sara Lister
Assistant Chief Nurse/Head of School, The Royal Marsden
 Hospital School of Cancer Nursing and Rehabilitation

Contributors

Karen Allan, Senior Staff Nurse (Smithers Ward)
Emma Allum, Senior Staff Nurse (Wiltshaw Ward)
Sarah Aylott, formerly Practice Development Facilitator
Caroline Badger, formerly Senior Nurse (Lymphoedema)

Christopher Bailey, Macmillan Research Practitioner,
 Institute of Cancer Research
Michael Bailey, Senior Staff Nurse (Wilson Ward)
Sophie Baty, Sister (Recovery Theatre)
Rachel Bennett, formerly Ward Sister (Wilson Ward)
Chris Berry, formerly Back Care Advisor
Judith Bibbings, formerly Sister (Gastrointestinal/
 Genitourinary)
Peter Blake, Consultant Clinical Oncologist
Yannette Booth, formerly Lecturer in Cancer Nursing
Derryn Borley, formerly Assistant Director of Nursing
 Services
David Brighton, Professional Development Facilitator (IT)
Jo Bull, Senior Staff Nurse (Burdet Coutts Ward)
Monica Burchall, formerly Sister (High Dependency)
Nancy Burnett, Senior Nurse Manager
Susannah Button, formerly Ward Sister (Ellis Ward)
Antoinette Byrne, formerly Dietitian
Jill Carter, formerly Clinical Nurse Specialist (Palliative Care)
Neve Carter, Senior Staff Nurse (Horder Ward) and
 Practice Development Facilitator
Patrick Casey, formerly Clinical Nurse Specialist/Unit
 Manager (Gastrointestinal/Genitourinary)
Anne Chandler, Clinical Nurse Specialist in Pain
 Management
Belinda Crawford, Matron (Neurointensive Care),
 Atkinson Morley Hospital
Sharyn Crossen, Nursing Sister (Wilson Ward)
Gay Curling, Clinical Nurse Specialist (Breast Diagnostic)
Lisa Curtis, formerly Macmillan Lecturer, Institute of
 Cancer Research
Tonia Dawson, Clinical Nurse Specialist (Pelvic Cancer)
Barbara Dicks, Director of Patient Services/Chief
 Nursing Officer
Emma Dilnutt, formerly Clinical Nurse Specialist
 (Palliative Care)
Nigel Dodds, Lead Nurse, Hospital and Home Programme
Anne Doherty, formerly Staff Nurse (Operating Theatres)
Ann Duncan, Ward Sister (Smithers Ward)
Nuala Durkin, formerly Clinical Nurse Specialist/Unit
 Manager (High Dependency)
Jean Edwards, Senior Nurse Manager/Private Patient
 Co-ordinator
Stephen Evans, Radiation Protection Adviser
 (Physics Department)
Sarah Faithfull, CRC Nursing Fellow, Institute of Cancer
 Research
Deborah Fenlon, formerly Group Clinical Nurse Specialist
 (Breast Care Services)
Emma Foulds, Lecturer Practitioner, The Royal Marsden
 Hospital School of Cancer Nursing and Rehabilitation

Tracey Gibson, Senior Staff Nurse (Critical Care)

Aileen Grant, Staff Nurse (Children's)

Jacqueline Green, Senior Dietitian

Douglas Guerrero, Clinical Nurse Specialist (Neuro-oncology)

Rachel Hair, formerly Senior Nurse (Neuro-oncology)

James Neale Hanvey, Divisional Nurse Director, Rare Cancers Division

Shujina Haq, Specialist Registrar (Occupational Health)

Sarah Hart, Clinical Nurse Specialist, Infection Control, Radiation Protection

Cathryn Havard, formerly Senior Nurse (Gastrointestinal/ Genitourinary)

Pauline Hill, Clinical Nurse Specialist (Community Liaison)

Hilary Hollis, formerly Programme Leader

Lynne Hopwood, Assistant Chief Nurse (Operations)

Sian Horn, formerly Sister (High Dependency)

Elizabeth Houlton, formerly Senior Nurse (Community Liaison/Self-Care)

Nest Howells, formerly Information Officer, CancerLink

Jennifer Hunt, Director, Nursing Research Initiative for Scotland

Patricia Hunt, Lecturer Practitioner

Maureen Hunter, Rehabilitation Services Manager

Elizabeth Janes, formerly Dietitian

Margareta Johnstone, formerly Clinical Nurse Specialist (High Dependency)

Penelope A. Jones, formerly Clinical Nurse Specialist (Community Liaison/Palliative Care)

Audrey Kelly, Specialist Sister (Breast Care)

Danny Kelly, formerly Lecturer in Cancer Nursing, Institute of Cancer Research

Jennifer Kelynack, Nursing Sister (Critical Care)

Betti Kirkman, formerly Clinical Nurse Specialist (Breast Diagnostic)

Glynis Knowles, Senior Staff, Breast Care (Outpatients Department, Sutton)

Diane Laverty, Clinical Nurse Specialist (Palliative Care)

Maria Law, Ward Sister (Kennaway Ward)

Susan J. Lee, formerly Occupational Health Manager

Sally Legge, Clinical Nurse Specialist (Gastrointestinal)

Annie Leggett, formerly Clinical Nurse Specialist (Intravenous Therapy)

Anne Lister, formerly Clinical Nurse Specialist/Unit Manager (Palliative Care)

Philippa A. Lloyd, Senior Staff Nurse (Wiltshaw Ward)

Nicholas Lodge, Clinical Group Research Nurse (Gynaecology)

E. Lopez-Verdugo, Senior Technician/Theatre Manager

Jane Machin, Specialist Speech and Language Therapist

Hazel Mack, formerly Acting Ward Sister (Horder Ward)

Elizabeth MacKenzie, Sister (Critical Care)

Jean Maguire, Ward Sister/Specialist Sister for Lung Cancer

Jane Mallett, Research and Practice Development Manager

Neve Mann, formerly Practice Development Facilitator

Glynis Markham, formerly Director of Nursing Services

David Mathers, Deputy Charge Nurse, University Hospitals of Leicester NHS Trust

Anne McLoughlin, Nursing Specialist Sister (Breast Care)

Lisa Mercer, Senior Dietitian

Catherine Miller, formerly Senior Nurse (Continuing Care)

Jennifer Miller, Senior Occupational Therapist, Occupational Therapy Department

Marion Morgan, formerly Research Sister (Gynaecology)

Wayne Naylor, Clinical Nurse Specialist, Wellington Cancer Centre, New Zealand, formerly Wound Management Research Nurse, The Royal Marsden Hospital

Katrina Neal, formerly Clinical Nurse Specialist/Unit Manager (Palliative Care)

Liz O'Brien, Clinical Team Leader, District Nursing, Croydon Primary Care Trust

Emma Osenton, Ward Sister (Wiltshaw Ward)

Evelyn Otunbade, Backcare Adviser

Buddy Joe Paris, Staff Nurse (Critical Care)

Sinéad Parry, Project Lead, End of Life Care, Learning Disabilities, Trinity Hospice, formerly Complex Discharge Co-ordinator, Royal Marsden Hospital

Rachelle Pearce, formerly Sister (Medical Day Unit)

Emma Pennery, formerly Senior Clinical Nurse Specialist/ Honorary Clinical Research Fellow

Helen Jayne Porter, formerly Clinical Nurse Specialist (High Dose Chemotherapy)

Joanne Preece, formerly Head of Risk Management

Judith Pretty, formerly Clinical Nurse Specialist (Head and Neck)

Barry Quinn, Lecturer Practitioner (Haemato-oncology)

Ffion M. Read, Senior Staff Nurse (Medical Day Unit)

Elizabeth Rees, formerly Research Nurse Palliative Care

Francis Regan, formerly Senior Staff Nurse (Burdett Coutts Ward)

Frances Rhys-Evans, formerly Clinical Nurse Specialist/ Ward Manager (Head and Neck and Thyroid Cancer)

Louise-Ann Ritchie, Nurse Practitioner (Haematology)

Jean Maurice Robert, Staff Nurse (Critical Care)

Helen Roberts, formerly Senior Nurse (Head and Neck)

Tim Root, Chief Pharmacist

Corinne Rowbotham, Senior Staff Nurse (IV Services)

Ray Rowden, formerly Director of Nursing Services

Miriam Rushton, formerly Senior Nurse (Gynaecology)

Kevin Russell, Charge Nurse (Critical Care)

1213

Patricia Ryan, Senior Sister (Haemato-oncology)

Lena Salter, formerly Patient Services Manager

Mave Salter, Complex Discharge Co-ordinator

Catherine Sandsund, Senior Physiotherapist, Physiotherapy Department

Neelam Sarpal, Teaching Sister

Kate Scott, Clinical Nurse Specialist (Psychological Care)

James Smith, formerly Chaplain

Caroline Soady, Clinical Nurse Specialist (Head and Neck)

Catherine South, Specialist Sister (Head and Neck)

Val Speechley, Patient Information Officer

Moira Stephens, Clinical Nurse Specialist (Haemato-oncology)

Mavis Stork, formerly Theatre Services Manager

Mary Anne Tanay, Research Nurse (Head and Neck)

June Toovey, formerly Sister (Intravenous Therapy Team)

Anne Topping, formerly Senior Nurse (Gastrointestinal/ Genitourinary)

Jennie Treleaven, Consultant Haematologist

Robert Tunmore, formerly Clinical Nurse Specialist (Psychological Support)

Beverley van der Molen, formerly Clinical Nurse Specialist/ Unit Manager (General Oncology)

Rebecca Verity, formerly Senior Staff Nurse (Bud Flanagan Ward)

Chris Viner, Clinical Nurse Specialist (Ambulatory Chemotherapy)

Caro Watts, Nurse Consultant (Transitional Care (Cancer))

Clare Webb, Specialist Sister in Psychological Care

Richard Wells, formerly Rehabilitation Services Manager

Alexandra Westbrook, Programme Leader

Isabel White, Head of Undergraduate Cancer Care Studies

Jane Wilson, formerly Group Theatre Manager

Miriam Wood, Senior Practice Development Facilitator (supporting role)

Karen Wright, formerly Research Assistant Nursing Research Unit

Karen Young, formerly Physiological Measurement Technician

Index

The Royal Marsden Hospital Manual of Clinical Nursing Procedures, Eighth Edition. Edited by Lisa Dougherty and Sara Lister.
© 2011 The Royal Marsden Hospital. Published 2011 by Blackwell Publishing Ltd.